Hardikar's

Orthopaedic Operations

Text and Atlas

Hardikar's
Orthopaedic Operations
Text and Atlas

Editor-in-Chief

Sharad M Hardikar MB FRCS (Edn)
Professor Emeritus Orthopaedics
Chief Orthopaedic Surgeon
Chairman
Hardikar Hospital
Pune, Maharashtra, India

Co-Editors

Shrinivas S Shintre MS (Ortho)
Professor and Head
Department of Orthopaedics
BJ Government Medical College and Sassoon General Hospital
Pune, Maharashtra, India
Fellowship, Joint Replacement Surgery (New York, US)

Vijay M Panchanadikar D Ortho DNB (Ortho)
Consultant Orthopaedic Surgeon
Deenanath Mangeshkar Hospital
Pune, Maharashtra, India

Forewords

SM Tuli
S Rajasekaran

JAYPEE BROTHERS MEDICAL PUBLISHERS
The Health Sciences Publisher
New Delhi | London | Panama

Jaypee Brothers Medical Publishers (P) Ltd

Headquarters
Jaypee Brothers Medical Publishers (P) Ltd
4838/24, Ansari Road, Daryaganj
New Delhi 110 002, India
Phone: +91-11-43574357
Fax: +91-11-43574314
E-mail: jaypee@jaypeebrothers.com

Overseas Offices
JP Medical Ltd
83 Victoria Street, London
SW1H 0HW (UK)
Phone: +44 20 3170 8910
Fax: +44 (0)20 3008 6180
E-mail: info@jpmedpub.com

Jaypee-Highlights Medical Publishers Inc
City of Knowledge, Bld. 235, 2nd Floor
Clayton, Panama City, Panama
Phone: +1 507-301-0496
Fax: +1 507-301-0499
E-mail: cservice@jphmedical.com

Jaypee Brothers Medical Publishers (P) Ltd
Bhotahity, Kathmandu, Nepal
Phone: +977-9741283608
E-mail: kathmandu@jaypeebrothers.com

Website: www.jaypeebrothers.com
Website: www.jaypeedigital.com

Hardikar's Orthopaedic Operations: Text and Atlas

First Edition: **2019**

ISBN: 978-93-5270-697-6

Printed at Replika Press Pvt. Ltd.

Dedicated to

My teachers, patients and wife Leela

—Sharad M Hardikar

My father Mr SG Shintre, Late Mother Usha, wife Pradnya, teachers, colleagues

—Shrinivas S Shintre

My mother Ranjana and wife Anjali, teachers and students

—Vijay M Panchanadikar

Contributors

Abhijeet L Wahegaonkar MBBS D Ortho DNB MCh (Ortho) FACS MBA
Adjunct Professor of Hand Surgery
Distinguished Clinical Tutor in Orthopaedic Surgery
Head and Fellowship Director
Department of Upper Limb, Hand and Microvascular Reconstructive Surgery
Sancheti Institute for Orthopaedics and Rehabilitation
Jehangir Hospital
Pune, Maharashtra, India

Abhishek Ranjan MBBS DNB (Ortho)
Chief Resident
Department of Orthopaedics
Rajarshee Chhatrapati Shahu Maharaj Government Medical College and CPR Hospital
Kolhapur, Maharashtra, India

Aditya Upase MBBS D Ortho Fellow Arthroscopy and Sports Medicine (Pune and South Korea)
Consultant Orthopaedic and Arthroscopy Surgeon
Upase Orthopaedic Clinic
Amravati, Maharashtra, India

Ajay Chandanwale MS (Ortho)
Dean JJ Hospital
Mumbai, Maharashtra, India

Ajinkya Nitin Deshpande MBBS DNB (Ortho) (Pune)
Senior Resident
Rajarshee Chhatrapati Shahu Maharaj Government Medical College and CPR Hospital
Kolhapur, Maharashtra, India

Ajit N Damle MS(Gen Sug) MS (Ortho) D Ortho
Consultant Orthopaedic Surgeon
Joshi and Ratna Hospitals
Pune, Maharashtra, India

Alaric Aroojis MS (Ortho) D'Ortho DNB (Ortho)
Consultant Pediatric Orthopaedic Surgeon and Medical Director
Miraclefeet India and Global Operations
Bai Jerbai Wadia Hospital for Children
Mumbai, Maharashtra, India

Ambrish Mathesule MS DNB MNAMS (Ortho)
Associate Professor and Head of Unit
Department of Orthopaedic
BJ Government Medical College and Sassoon General Hospital
Pune, Maharashtra, India

Ameya Bindu MBBS MS (Gen Surgery) MCh DNB Plastic Surgery (Gold medal)
Consultant Plastic, Hand and Reconstructive Microvascular Surgeon
BJ Government Medical College and Sassoon General Hospital
Pune, Maharashtra, India

Amit R Kale MS (Otho) DNB MNAMS MCh (UK)
Professor and Unit Head
Dr DY Patil Medical College Hospital and Research Center
Pune, Maharashtra, India

Amit Swamy MS DNB MNAMS MRCS FICS FIGOF
Professor in Orthopaedics
Swamy Hospital
Aditya Birla Memorial Hospital
Moraya Hospitals
PGI YCM Hospital
Pune, Maharashtra, India

Amol J Rege MBBS MS (ortho) DNB FRCS (Glasg) Mch(L'pool) AO
International Spine—Fellow (Autralia)
Consultant Spine Surgeon
Deenanath Mangeshkar Hospital
Pune, Maharashtra, India

Anshu Shekhar MBBS MS (Ortho)
Associate Consultant
The Orthopaedic Speciality Clinic
Pune, Maharashtra, India

Anup S Bansode MBBS MS (Ortho) Fellow in Hand and Microvascular Surgery
Consultant Hand Surgeon
Hand Surgery Clinics
Giridarshan Society
Pune, Maharashtra, India

Anurag Daxini MBBS D'ortho (DNB Ortho)
Deenanath Mangeshkar Hospital
Pune, Maharashtra, India

Arun Salunkhe MS (Ortho)
Consulting Orthopaedic Surgeon and Ex-Hon Professor
BJ Government Medical College and Sassoon General Hospital
Hardikar Hospital
Pune, Maharashtra, India

Arvind Bhave MS (Ortho) IPTM (Israel) Fellow Spinal Injuries center (Japan)
Fellow Minimally Invasive Spine Surgery (S. Korea)
Spine Surgeon (Spine Endoscopy and MISS)
Deenanath Mangeshkar Hospital
Pune, Maharashtra, India

Ashish Ratnani MBBS D Ortho
Hardikar Hospital
Pune, Maharashtra, India

Ashish S Ranade MS (Ortho)
Consultant Orthopaedic Surgeon
Deenanath Mangeshkar Hospital
Visiting Pediatric Orthopaedic Surgeon
BJ Government Medical College and Sassoon General Hospital
Pune, Maharashtra, India

Ashutosh Sabnis
Consultant Spine Surgeon
Deenanath Mangeshkar Hospital
Pune, Maharashtra, India

Avi Pranay Shah MBBS MS (Ortho) FPO (India USA UK)
Clinical Young Adult Hip and Limb Reconstruction Fellow
Sheffield Children's Hospital
Sheffield, South Yorkshire, UK

Bansi Vasudev Naik Khaunte MS Orthopaedic Surgery
Fellowship in Pediatric Orthopaedics
Orthopaedic Surgeon
Hospicio Hospital
Directorate of Health
Margao, Goa, India

Chaitanya Karande Patil MBBS MS (Ortho) Fellow in Hand and Microvascular Surgery
Consultant Hand Surgeon
Hand Surgery Clinics
Giridarshan Society
Pune, Maharashtra, India

Chandan V Bhole MBBS D Ortho DNB (Ortho)
Assistant Professor
BJ Government Medical College and
Sassoon General Hospital
Pune, Maharashtra, India

Chandrashekhar Dixit D Ortho DNB (Ortho)
Consultant Orthopaedic Surgeon
Jupitor Hospital
Pune, Maharashtra, India

Chandrashekhar Sathaye MS (Ortho)
Consultant Orthopaedic Surgeon
Alibag, Maharashtra, India

Chittanand Mendhe
Senior Resident
BJ Government Medical College and
Sassoon General Hospital
Pune, Maharashtra, India

Devashish Raval MBBS MD D Ortho
Consultant Orthopaedic Surgeon
BKL Walawalkar Rural Medical College
Sawarde, Maharashtra, India

Dudani Baldev MS (Ortho)
Professor Orthopaedics
Ruby Hall Clinic and Inlaks and
Budhrani Hospital
Pune, Maharashtra, India

Gautam Salunkhe MS (Ortho)
Orthopaedic Surgeon
Nirmala Memorial Hospital
Pune, Maharashtra, India

Girish Bartakke MS (Ortho)
Professor and Head
Department of Orthopaedic
Government Medical College
Miraj, Maharashtra, India

Hardik Shah
Senior Resident
Deenanath Mangeshkar Hospital
Pune, Maharashtra, India

Harshal Saogi MBBS D Ortho
Hardikar Hospital
Pune, Maharashtra, India

Hitesh J Mangukiya MS (Ortho)
Consultant Orthopaedic Surgeon
Ashutosh Hospital
Surat, Gujarat, India

J Clement Joseph MS (Ortho)
Head
Orthopaedics and Sports Medicine
Gleneagles Global Health City
Chennai, Tamil Nadu, India

Jignesh Yeshwant Tandel MBBS
Junior Resident 2nd Year
BJ Government Medical College and
Sassoon General Hospital
Pune, Maharashtra, India

Kapil Gangwal MS DNB (Ortho)
Honorary Consultant Orthopaedics
Santokba Durlabhji Memorial Hospital
Jaipur, Rajasthan, India

Kartikeya Promod Joshi MBBS DNB
Panel Consultant
Deenanath Mangeshkar Hospital
Jupiter Hospital
Jehangir Specialty Hospital
Faculty
Bharti Hospital and Research Center
Pune, Maharashtra, India

Kaustubh Kale MS (Ortho)
Senior Resident
Department of Orthopaedics
BJ Government Medical College and
Sassoon General Hospital
Pune, Maharashtra, India

Keshav Shenoy S MBBS MS (Ortho)
Associate Professor
SDM College of Medical Sciences and
Hospital
Dharwad, Karnataka, India

Kiran Kharat MS MSc (Ortho) (London)
Consultant
Joint Replacement Surgeon
Founder Director of Joint Replacement Unit at
Ruby Hall Clinic and Birla Hospitals
Pune, Maharashtra, India

Kumar Kanishk
Senior Resident
Hardikar Hospital
Pune, Maharashtra, India

Madan Hardikar MS (Ortho) D Ortho
Consultant Orthopaedics Surgeon
Associate Professor
Hardikar Hospital
Pune, Maharashtra, India

Madhav Khadilkar MS (Ortho)
Professor of Orthopaedics
Bharati Hospital
Pune, Maharashtra, India

Mahaveer S Dugad DNB (Ortho)
Fellowship in Arthroplasty
Joint Replacement Surgeon
Hardikar Hospital
Pune, Maharashtra, India

Mahesh Kulkarni MS FRCS MCh FRCS(Ortho)
Consultant Joint Replacement Surgeon
Deenanath Mangeshkar Hospital
Columbia Asia Hospital and
Jehangir Hospital
Pune, Maharashtra, India

Mahesh Mone MBBS MS (Ortho)
Consultant Orthopeadic Surgeon
Deenanath Mangeshkar Hospital
Pune, Maharashtra, India

Mandar Agashe MBBS MS (Ortho)
Consultant Pediatric Orthopaedic Surgeon
Agashe Pediatric Superspeciality Clinic
Kurla
Assistant Honorary
BJ Wadia Hospital for Children
Mumbai, Maharashtra, India

Manish R Dastane MBBS DNB MCh Arthroplasty Fellow (USA) AO Fellow (Australia)
Consultant Arthroplasty and
Orthopaedic Surgeon
Deenanath Mangeshkar Hospital
Pune, Maharashtra, India

Manoj Todkar MS DNB MRCS (Glasg) MCh (Ortho) (UK) FICS (USA)
Honorary Associate Professor in
Orthopaedic Surgery
BJ Government Medical College and
Sassoon General Hospital
Hardikar Hospital
Pune, Maharashtra, India

Mayur Purandare DNB (Ortho) MNAMS
Consultant Orthopaedic Surgeon
Orion Hospital and
Jogalekar Hospital and
Sanjeevan Hospital
Pune, Maharashtra, India

Milind Modak MS DNB (Ortho) AO Fellow
Consultant Orthopaedics Surgeon
Yogesh Hospital and
Deenanath Mangeshkar Hospital
Pune, Maharashtra, India

Mohan V Belthur MS DNB MD FRCSC FRCS (Tr and Ortho)
Attending Pediatric Orthopaedic Surgeon
Phoenix Children's Hospital
Clinical Associate Professor
University of Arizona College of Medicine
Phoenix Children's Hospital
Department of Orthopaedics
Phoenix, Arizona, USA

Nagesh Naik MS (Ortho) DNB DNBPMR
Head
Department of Orthopaedic
Prakash Institute of Medical
Sciences and Research
Sangli, Maharashtra, India

Nakul Shah MS DNB (Ortho) MNAMS FICS
Consultant Joint Replacement and
Reconstruction Surgeon
Ex-Associate Professor
Orthopaedic Surgery
Head of Joint Replacement and
Reconstruction at Sanjeevan
MJM Poonawalla Memorial Hospital
Pune, Maharashtra, India

Namdeo Gorgile

Neelkamal Sourav
Senior Resident
Deenanath Mangeshkar Hospital
Pune, Maharashtra, India

Nikhil Mamoria MBBS
BJ Government Medical College and
Sassoon General Hospital
Pune, Maharashtra, India

Nikhil Shah FRCS FRCS MCh (Ortho) (Liv) MS (Ortho) DNB (Ortho) MBBS
Consultant Trauma and
Orthopaedic Surgeon
Wrightington Hospital, UK
Salford Royal Hospital, UK

Nilesh Dattatray Darawade MS(Ortho) D Ortho FNB (Hand and Microsurgery)
Shubhamkar Hand Clinic and
Associate Professor
Smt Kashibai Navale Medical College and
General Hospital
Pune, Maharashtra, India

Niranjan Chavan MBBS Dip (Ortho) DNB
Consultant and Director
GEM Hospital
Jalgaon, Maharashtra, India

Nishant Goyal D Ortho DNB Ortho
DNB Resident
Deenanath Mangeshkar Hospital
Pune, Maharashtra, India

Nitish Agrawal D Ortho
Hardikar Hospital
Pune, Maharashtra, India

Onkar Lande D Ortho
Orthopaedic Surgeon
Hardikar Hospital
Pune, Maharashtra, India

Onkar Sudame
Resident
Deenanath Mangeshkar Hospital
Pune, Maharashtra, India

Pankaj Jindal MBBS MS (Ortho)
Clinical Fellowship in Hand Surgery Grand
Rapids Michigan, USA
Clinical Fellowship in
Hand Surgery Nancy, France
Clinical Fellowship in Hand Surgery
Louisville, USA

Parag Sahasrabudhe MS MCh Plastic Surgery
Professor and Head
Department of Plastic Surgery
BJ Government Medical College and
Sassoon General Hospital
Deenanath Mangeshkar Hospital
Pune, Maharashtra, India

Pavan K Kohli MS DNB(Ortho) MNAMS Fellow Arthroplasty Sports Medicine (Singapore, Germany)
Professor
BKL Walawalkar Medical College
Ratnagiri, Maharashtra, India
Oyster and Pearl Hospitals
Pune, Maharashtra, India

Prahalad Kumar Singhi D'Ortho DNB Ortho FISM Germany Adelaide AOTIF USA
Consultant Arthroscopy and
Trauma Surgeon
Preethi Hospitals (P) Ltd
Madurai, Tamil Nadu, India

Prasad Joshi DNB MS (Ortho)
Joint Replacement Consultant
Joshi Hospital Pvt Ltd
Satara, Maharashtra, India

Prasanna Baindoor MBBS D.Ortho
Associate Professor
SDM College of Medical
Sciences and Hospital
Dharwad, Karnataka, India

Prashant Mall
Senior Resident
Hardikar Hospital
Pune, Maharashtra, India

Prateek Charuchandra Joshi MBBS
Chief Resident
Department of Orthopaedics
BJ Government Medical College and
Sassoon General Hospital
Pune, Maharashtra, India

Pushkar Deshpande MBBS MS Mch (Plastic Surgery)
Consultant Plastic Surgeon
Hardikar Hospital
Perfection Plastic Surgery Clinic
Pune, Maharashtra, India

Rachit Vipul Shah MBBS
Resident
Department of Orthopaedics
BJ Government Medical College and
Sassoon General Hospital
Pune, Maharashtra, India

Raghav Barve MS DNB (Orth)
Fellow Oxford UK
Consultant Arthroscopy and Joint
Replacement Surgeon
Ruby Hall and Deenanath
Mangeshkar Hospital
Joshi and Ratna Hospital
Pune, Maharashtra, India

Raghvendra Singh Raghuvanshi MBBS MS (Ortho)
Spine Fellow
Department of Spine Surgery
Deenanath Mangeshkar Hospital
Pune, Maharashtra, India

Rahul Chaudhari MS (Ortho) ECFMG (USA) Spine/Scoliosis Surgery (USA)
Consultant Spine Surgeon
Hardikar Hospital
Jehangir Hospital
KEM Hospital
Columbia Asia Hospital
7 Orange Hospital
Pune, Maharashtra, India

Rahul Puranik MS MBBS
Associate Professor
Department of Orthopaedic
BJ Government Medical College and
Sassoon General Hospital
Pune, Maharashtra, India

Rajeev Nene MS (Ortho)
Consultant Orthopaedic Surgeon
Nene Hospital
Panel Consultant
Ruby Hall Clinic-Inlaks and
Budhrani Hospital
Pune, Maharashtra, India

Rajkumar Ekambaram MBBS
Cheif Resident
Department of Orthopaedics
BJ Government Medical College and
Sassoon General Hospital
Pune, Maharashtra, India

Rajkumar Mahato
Senior Resident
Hardikar Hospital
Pune, Maharashtra, India

Rajendra Latkar DNB (Ortho)
Consultant Orthopaedic Surgeon
Pune, Maharashtra, India

Ranjit Deshmukh MS DNB(Ortho)
Consultant Orthopaedic Surgeon
Deenanath Mangeshkar Hospital
Pune, Maharashtra, India

Ranjit Mohan Modak DNB(Ortho) MRCS
Fellow
Department of Joint Replacement
Deenanath Mangeshkar Hospital
Pune, Maharashtra, India

Ranjit Rajure
Resident
Department of Orthopaedics
Deenanath Mangeshkar Hospital
Pune, Maharashtra, India

Rishikesh Ghalke DNB (Ortho)
Lecturer
Department of Orthopaedics
Deenanath Mangeshkar Hospital
Pune, Maharashtra, India

Rohit K Jain DNB (Ortho) D.Ortho Fellow in Pediatric orthopaedics (MUHS)
Clinical Fellow in Pediatric Orthopaedics
National University Hospital
Singapore

Rujuta Mehta MS DNB (Ortho)
Head
Department of Pediatric Orthopaedics
Bai Jerbai Wadia Hospital for Children
Consultant Pediatric Orthopaedic Surgeon
Nanavati Superspeciality Hospital
Jaslok Hospital and Shushrusha Hospital
Mumbai, Maharashtra, India

Rupesh Kadam
Senior Resident
BJ Government Medical College and
Sassoon General Hospital
Pune, Maharashtra, India

S Prakash MS (Ortho)
Senior Orthopaedic Surgeon
Hardikar Hospital
Pune, Maharashtra, India

Sachin Nagapurkar MBBS D.Ortho
Fellow Joint Replacement Surgery
(Zimmer USA)
Consultant Orthopaedic and Joint
Replacement Surgeon
Hardikar Hospital
ONE Hospital
Sahyadri Hospital
Mulshi Multispeciality Hospital
Pune, Maharashtra, India

Sachin Ramchandra Tapasvi MBBS MS (Ortho) DNB FRCS (Glasgow)
Chief Consultant
The Orthopaedic Speciality Clinic
Pune, Maharashtra, India

Sagar Gengaje MBBS
BJ Government Medical College and
Sassoon General Hospital
Pune, Maharashtra, India

Sameer Desai MS (Ortho) DNB MRCS
Pediatric Orthopaedic Surgeon
Jehangir Hospital
KEM Hospital
Sahyadri Hospital
Pune, Maharashtra, Pune

Samrat K Taori MBBS DNB(Ortho) MNAMS(Ortho) FHS-Fellowship in Hand and Reconstructive Microsurgery
Hand Surgeon
Specialist in Hand, Wrist Upper Limb and
Peripheral Nerves including Brachial Plexus
Narmada Ratan Taori Hospital and
Taori Hand and Upper Limb Surgery Center
Nagpur, Maharashtra, India

Sandeep Patwardhan MS (Orthopaedic Surgery) D Orthopaedic Surgery
Professor
Pediatric Orthopaedic Specialist
Sancheti Institute for Orthopaedics and
Rehabilitation
Visiting Specialist
Bharati Vidyapeeth Medical Hospital
Pune, Maharashtra, India

Sandeep Vaidya MBBS MS (Ortho) DNB
Consultant Pediatric Orthopaedic Surgeon
Pinnacle Hospital
Jupiter Hospital
Thane, Maharashtra, India
Assistant Honorary
BJ Wadia Hospital for Children
Mumbai, Maharashtra, India

Santosh Jeevannavar MBBS DNB (Ortho)
Consultant Orthopaedic Surgeon
Professor and Head Unit 2
SDM College of Medical
Sciences and Hospital
Dharwad, Karnataka, India

Sarang Kasture D Ortho DNB, FRCS Ed (T&O)
Wales Fellow European Board of Trauma and
Orthopaedics, Dip. SICOT
Speciality Doctor Trauma
Orthopaedics Gwynedd Hospital
Bengaluru, Karnataka, India

Satish A Mane MBBS D Ortho Fellow in Hand and Microvascular Surgery
Consultant Hand Surgeon
Hand Surgery Clinics
Giridarshan Society
Pune, Maharashtra, India

Shaishav Shah MBBS MS (Ortho)
Spine Fellow
Department of Spine Surgery
Deenanath Mangeshkar Hospital
Pune, Maharashtra, India

Shantanu Sudhakar Patil MBBS MS (Ortho)
Head
Department of Translational
Medicine and Research
SRM Medical College and Hospitals
SRM Institute of Science and Technology
Kattankulathur, Tamil Nadu, India

Shrikant Sagane MS (Ortho)
Assistant Professor
Department of Orthopaedic
BJ Government Medical College and
Sassoon General Hospital
Pune, Maharashtra, India

Shrinivas S Shintre MS (Ortho)
Professor and Head
Department of Orthopaedics
BJ Government Medical College and
Sassoon General Hospital
Pune, Maharashtra, India
Fellowship, Joint Replacement Surgery
(New York, US)

Siddharth Hardikar
Senior Resident
Hardikar Hospital
Pune, Maharashtra, India

Siddharth Jaiswal
Senior Resident
Hardikar Hospital
Pune, Maharashtra, India

Sharad M Hardikar MB FRCS (Edn)
Professor Emeritus Orthopaedic
Chief Orthopaedic Surgeon
Chairman
Hardikar Hospital
Pune, Maharashtra, India

Snehal Dantkale
Senior Resident in Orthopaedic
Deenanath Mangeshkar Hospital
Pune, Maharashtra, India

Sunil Nadkarni MS (Orth) FRCS (Ed) MCh (Liverpool)
Consultant Spine Surgeon
Hardikar Hospital
Deenanath Mangeshkar Hospital
Tulip ONP Hospital
Ratna and Joshi Hospitals
Pune, Maharashtra, India
Walawalkar Hospital
Dervan, Maharashtra, India

Sushrut Pulgaonkar MS DNB (Ortho)
BJ Government Medical College and
Sassoon General Hospital
Pune, Maharashtra, India

Swapnil Keny MS (Ortho) FCPS
Consultant Pediatric Orthopaedic Surgeon
Saifee Hospital
Apollo Hospital
Associate Professor
Department of Orthopaedics
Grant Medical College
Mumbai, Maharashtra, India

Trimbak Dapkekar MS (Ortho)
Consultant Orthopaedic Surgeon
Associate Professor
Hardikar Hospital
Pune, Maharashtra, India
Sunrise Global Superspeciality Hospital
Nanded, Maharashtra, India

Uday Pote MBBS D.Ortho DNB Orthopaedics Spine Fellow
Consultant Orthopaedic Spine Surgeon
Hardikar Hospital
Chellaram Multispeciality Hospital
Oyster and Pearl Hospital
Ratna Memorial Hospital
Jupiter Hospital
Pune, Maharashtra, India

Umesh Birole MBBS DNB (Ortho) MRCS (England)
Specialist Registrar
Trauma and Orthopaedic
Ealing Hospital (LNWH NHS Trust)
London, UK

Umesh Jadhav MBBS D.Ortho FCPS (Ortho) Fellow Arthroscopy and Sports Medicine (ISAKOS Spain and USA)
Arthroscopy and Sports Injury Specialist
PanOrtho Hospital
Pune, Maharashtra, India

Varun Rao MBBS DNB (Ortho)
Assistant Professor
(Orthopaedic and Spine Surgeon)
Parul Institute of Medical Sciences and Research
Vadodara, Gujarat, India

Vijay M Panchanadikar D Ortho DNB (Ortho)
Consultant Orthopaedic Surgeon
Deenanath Mangeshkar Hospital
Pune, Maharashtra, India

Vijay Kakatkar MS (Ortho) D' ortho
Director and Consultant Orthopaedic Surgeon
Jay Hospital
Nashik, Maharashtra, India

Vinay Gautam
Senior Resident in Orthopaedics
Deenanath Mangeshkar Hospital
Pune, Maharashtra, India

Viraj U Shingade MS DNB(Ortho) Fellow Paed Orth (UK, South Korea)
Director
Children Orthopaedic Care Institute
Pravira Hospital
President
Nagai Narayanji Memorial Foundation
Nagpur, Maharashtra, India

Vishal Patil
Associate Professor
BJ Government Medical College and Sassoon General Hospital
Pune, Maharashtra, India

Vivek Mukund Badhe MBBS D Ortho
Senior Resident
Department of Orthopaedics
BJ Government Medical College and Sassoon General Hospital
Pune, Maharashtra, India

Wasudeo M Gadegone MS (Ortho) MS (Gen Surgery) MNAMS (Ortho) SICOT Fellow
Professor of Orthopaedics
Government Medical College
Chandrapur, Maharashtra, India

Yash K Shah MBBS MS (Ortho) DNB MNAMS Diploma in Sports Medicine
Consultant Orthopaedic Surgeon Matruseva Hospital
Assistant Professor
MIMER Medical College
Pune, Maharashtra, India

YJ Mahale MS (Ortho) FRCS (England) FICS (USA) Dip Med Rehab (London)
Professor and Head
Department of Orthopaedics
ACPM Medical College
Consultant Orthopaedic Surgeon
Mahale Accident Hospital
Director
OM Multispeciality Hospital
Nirnay Diagnostic Centre
Nirnay Janseva Blood Bank
Dhule, Maharashtra, India

Foreword

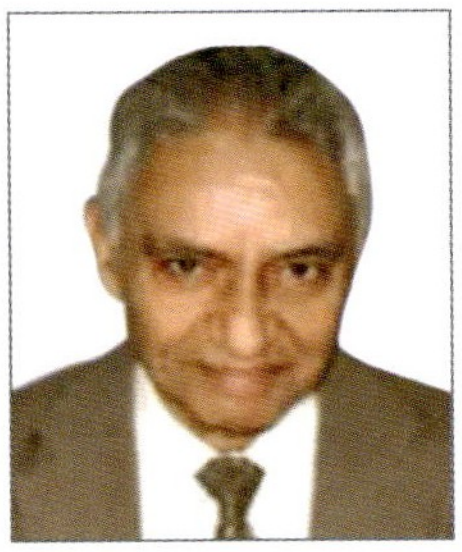

At the time of ever-increasing flow and use of electronic information, it is pleasant to see an effort by the orthopaedic professionals to take time, reflect back on the methodologies of performing orthopaedic operations. The basic concept of this book is to offer to the readers the stepwise pictures of the operative steps with relevant descriptions and discussion. The whole text has been arranged into various sections such as Pediatric Orthopaedics, Arthroscopy, Spine, Wrist and Hand Surgery, Arthroplasty, Ankle and Foot, General Orthopaedics, Traumatology, Bone Tumors and Plastic Surgery. There are many methods to perform the same operative procedure, the illustrations here help you to choose the safest under the circumstances one is working.

Many new orthopaedic procedures have been added in clinical practice in the last 30 years. Previously considered untreatable conditions (e.g. congenital pseudarthrosis, shortening of lower limbs, ankylosed hip or knee, gross deformities of spine) can now be successfully treated by appropriate operative procedures at a suitable time. This book would meet the academic expectations of an orthopaedic neophyte and an experienced surgeon. I am confident that this will help raise the proficiency and safety of orthopaedic operations in general.

The book has been edited by three experienced orthopaedic surgeons to bring in the uniformity in the style and to minimize unnecessary repetitions. This book is recommended to be placed in all medical libraries and in the operating room of all practicing orthopaedic surgeons.

SM Tuli
Senior Consultant
Department of Orthopaedics
VIMHANS-NAYATI Hospital
New Delhi, India
Former Professor
Department of Orthopaedics
Banaras Hindu University and University of Delhi

Foreword

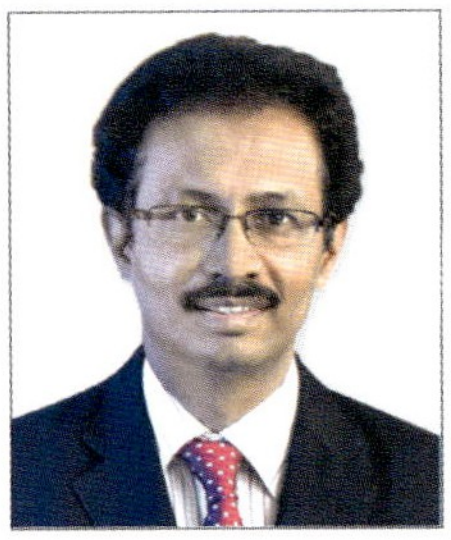

It is an honor for me to write a foreword for '*Hardikar's Orthopaedic Operations: Text and Atlas*' which fills in an important need for not only surgeons in training but also surgeons in practice.

Many pathological conditions, especially in orthopaedics, require surgery for improvement and the recent advances have the capacity to remove pain, restore mobility and give a second life to patients. Although there are many factors affecting the outcome of surgical procedures, one of the determining factors is the surgeon himself and the execution of a perfect surgical procedure. Any surgery has numerous steps and the final outcome depends on the perfect execution of every step. However, the rapid advances in every subspecialty brings in new surgical procedures and the practicing surgeon would have great benefit from a surgical atlas that illustrates the entire procedure with clarity. This book will form a valuable addition to every library in the field of orthopaedic surgery as it has practical tips drawn from experience that will help every surgeon from the junior trainee to the well experienced.

The Editor-in-Chief of the book is Dr Sharad M Hardikar, who is one of the most respected postgraduate teachers and a professional leader in the field of orthopaedics and spine surgery for many decades. His numerous scientific lectures, orations and publications stand testimony for his mastery and experience in this field. I would like to congratulate him and his Co-Editors, Dr Shrinivas S Shintre and Dr Vijay M Panchanadikar, for this effort of bringing to print the pearls of success in a wide variety of surgical procedures.

Professor S Rajasekaran
Chairman
Department of Orthopaedics
Trauma and Spine Surgery
Ganga Hospital
Coimbatore, Tamil Nadu, India
Chair, AO Spine International Board
Past President, SICOT
Past President, Indian Orthopaedic Association

Preface

The very concept of this book is to enable orthopaedic surgeons to perform an operation looking at the serial photographs from instrument trolley to closure of the operation wound. The book covers common operations of all orthopaedic subspecialties. It is expected of practicing orthopaedic surgeons to brush up surgical anatomy and important operative steps before performing the operation. While the book is meant for all orthopaedic surgeons, it will be particularly useful to upcoming surgeons and senior residents who can perform the operation with confidence after reading the chapters. Senior orthopaedic surgeons will also benefit when they have to perform an operation after a gap.

The emphasis being on serial photographs for an operation, text is brief but adequate and only important list of further reading is provided at the end of the procedure. We have included 122 chapters in the book.

The book also will be a good companion for all orthopaedic surgeons, especially for those who have just started their practice in cities and peripheral small towns and wish to do an operation on their own. The book will also be a unique surgical manual for operation theater nursing staff while setting instrument trolley and for operation theater assistants to position the patients.

We are confident that this book will be a proud possession of all orthopaedic surgeons including orthopaedic residents. We propose to include more operative procedures to the book in the course of time.

Sharad M Hardikar
Shrinivas S Shintre
Vijay M Panchanadikar

Acknowledgments

Writing this book was much harder than we expected and more gratifying than we had imagined. This book is the realization of the efforts of so many people. This would be a suitable opportunity to thank all the people who have been a part of this journey.

First and foremost, we would like to thank Shri Jitendar P Vij (Group Chairman), Mr Ankit Vij (Managing Director) and Ms Chetna Malhotra Vohra (Associate Director—Content Strategy) of M/s Jaypee Brothers Medical Publishers (P) Ltd, New Delhi, India, for trusting us to undertake the responsibility to write such a unique book. The support extended by Jaypee team, particularly Mr Sabarish Menon, Mrs Nedup Denka Bhutia (Development Editor) was commendable for completion of the book.

Our sincerest thanks to Orthopaedic Departments, Administrations and Staff of Hardikar Hospital, BJ Government Medical College and Sassoon General Hospital and Deenanath Mangeshkar Hospital, Pune, Maharashtra, India, for their co-operation and contribution.

Our special thanks to Dr Ajay Chandanwale, Dean, BJ Government Medical College and Sassoon General Hospital, Pune for his encouragement and guidance to the book.

We would also like to mention Mrs Rupali Rajesh Sonawane (Jawale) for her relentless efforts in making this book come alive.

We express our special thanks to Dr Umesh Vaidya for providing valuable help. We would like to appreciate the hard work by Drs Rajkumar Ekambaram, Prateek Charuchandra Joshi and Nitish Agrawal.

This work could not have been completed without the support and patience of family and friends, who have been with us throughout this journey.

Finally, we take this opportunity to express our gratitude for our colleagues and their hospital administrators who have supported directly or indirectly to complete the book.

Contents

SECTION 1 Pediatric Orthopaedics

Section Editor: *Ashish S Ranade*

PART 1: CONGENITAL CONDITIONS

PART 2: INFECTIONS

PART 3: PEDIATRIC TRAUMA

SECTION 2 Arthroscopy

Section Editor: *Umesh Jadhav*

SECTION 3 Spine

Section Editor: *Amol J Rege*

SECTION 4 Wrist and Hand Surgery

Section Editor: *Nilesh Dattatray Darawade*

SECTION 6 Ankle and Foot

Section Editors: *Amit Swamy, Amit R Kale*

SECTION 7 General Orthopaedics

Section Editor: *Santosh Jeevannavar*

SECTION 8 Traumatology

Section Editors: *Shrinivas S Shintre, Vijay M Panchanadikar*

PART 1: INJURIES AROUND SHOULDER

PART 2: INJURIES OF ELBOW AND FOREARM

PART 6: FRACTURES AROUND KNEE AND LEG

SECTION 9 Bone Tumors

Section Editor: *Arun Salunkhe*

SECTION 10 Plastic Surgery

Section Editor: *Pushkar Deshpande*

SECTION 1

PEDIATRIC ORTHOPAEDICS

Section Editor: *Ashish S Ranade*

CHAPTER 1

Osteotomies for Clubfoot Correction

Viraj U Shingade

INTRODUCTION

Ponseti's technique has revolutionized the treatment of clubfoot deformity across the world. It has given a mini-invasive approach for treating a clubfoot, when baby presents in early infancy. But in developing countries, we still face the major burden of neglected and relapsed clubfoot deformities; where children present to us at 3–18 years of age, either not treated in the past, or deformities have recurred after open surgeries (Figs. 1A to C). These deformities (Dimeglio III/IV) usually require some kind of bony correction which will be discussed in this chapter.

PATHOLOGICAL ANATOMY

The bones are severely deformed. The normal anatomical relationship of tarsal bones is usually lost. The midtarsal bones act like heel due to abnormal weight bearing. The tendo Achillis is short keeping heel in equinus and varus.

CLINICAL FEATURES

These children tend to walk on dorsum or dorsolateral aspect of foot. It is not possble for them to use normal footwear. They are prone to injuries while playing games and walking long distances. They suffer from repeated wounds at callosities, formed over dorsum of foot. Squatting is difficult for them, which is the most common position, used for day-to-day activities like toileting.

RADIOLOGICAL IMAGING

Standard anteroposterior and lateral view of foot and ankle can be taken before surgery. For evaluating the results of surgery, standing anteroposterior and lateral views of foot and ankle are required during postsurgery follow-up period.

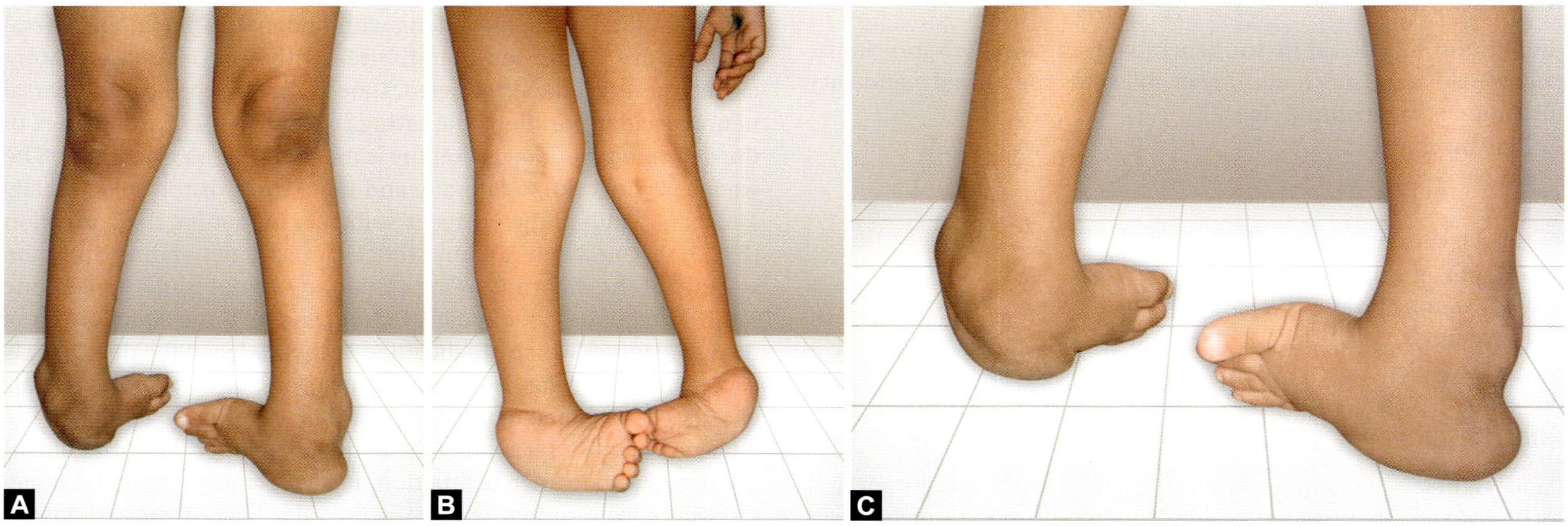

Figs. 1A to C: A 6-year-old girl with bilateral neglected clubfeet. These feet are prone for injuries at callosities formed at dorsum of feet.

TREATMENT OPTIONS

Various types of osteotomies are available depending upon age of the child, severity of deformity, flexibility of the foot, and failure of previous procedures.

For the flexible deformity, Ponseti's-extended indications can still be tried, which means serial corrective plasters at weekly interval followed by tendo Achilles tenotomy.

For Dimeglio grade II deformity and a 4–8 years child, calcaneo-cuboid fusion described by Dilwyn Evans or by Lichtblau (anterior part of calcaneum removed as wedge) can be done.

For a 3–4 years child with persistent heel varus and equinus, open medial wedge calcaneal osteotomy by Dwyer can be performed. In this procedure, the graft can be taken from tibia.

For a 5–8 years child with persistent severe cavus and grossly deformed metatarsals, metatarsal osteotomy described by Heyman (basal osteotomy of lateral four metatarsals) can be done.

For a 4–8 years child, recurrent deformity open wedge osteotomy of medial cuneiform as described by Hofmann can be performed.

Triple arthrodesis (child more than 10 years age) is usually reserved as a last-resort salvage procedure for a very painful, stiff foot, with poor function, and where multiple surgeries have failed.

Many times, we come across situations where patients present with *Dimeglio grades III /IV deformities, with severe deformation of bones (age above 5 years) and they demand one-time procedure.* Many times, they are either neglected due to poverty and other factors or they present with recurrence with previously failed two to three surgeries. These patients are difficult to treat, surgical procedures like Ilizarov are expensive and frequent visits to hospital are required, technique of dorsolateral corrective wedge osteotomy is an affordable and one time procedure that results in a plantigrade foot on which shoes can be fitted.

A study conducted by our institute to measure the outcome of this procedure in neglected as well as relapsed clubfoot deformities has shown favourable results. It was published in the year 2012 with good follow-up. In fact, subsequently, we included patients of neglected and relapsed cases of clubfoot associated with myelomeningocele and found good results and this work was published in the year 2014.

OPERATIVE TECHNIQUE

Instruments

In addition to general instruments like retractors, scissors, knife, needle holder, and mosquito forceps, following specialized mandatory instruments are required (Fig. 2):

- Drill machine
- K-wires
- Plier
- Bone levers (spikes)
- Straight and curved osteotomes
- Periosteum elevator
- Hammer
- Bone nibbler

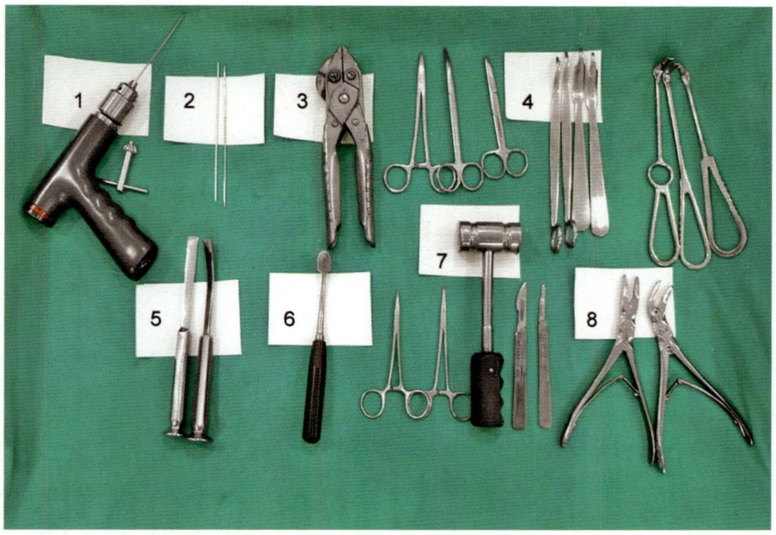

Fig. 2: Mandatory instruments on trolly: (1) Drill machine, (2) K-wires, (3) Plier, (4) Bone levers (spikes), (5) Straight and curved osteotomes, (6) Periosteum elevator, (7) Hammer, and (8) Bone nibbler.

Anesthesia

Patient is placed in a supine position. Epidural anesthesia is preferred for better pain relief postoperatively. Painting and draping of the lower limb is done and the tourniquet is inflated.

Surgical Steps

Step 1: Correction of cavus: Cavus is corrected by releasing the plantar fascia. The knife is passed from the medial aspect of the sole through a small nick (Fig. 3A). The foot needs to be stretched manually for confirmation of completeness of release of plantar fascia.

Step 2: Correction of equinus and heel varus: A small nick is given on posteromedial aspect, a centimeter above the heel. The knife is inserted. A complete Achilles tenotomy is done transversely (Fig. 3B). The foot usually needs to be dorsiflexed manually for getting the correction. The tenotomy unlocks the heel and gives correction for equinus as well as varus of the heel. In rare cases if deformity is severe and is associated with scarring of previous surgery, then we can do the posterior ankle capsular release from the same small incision.

Step 3: Dorso-lateral closing wedge osteotomy: On the dorso-lateral aspect, at the apex of the deformed foot, an elliptical skin incision is made (Fig. 3C). The extension of the incision should be from the lateral border of the foot to just short of the medial border. This skin is usually extra and gets folded after closure of the osteotomy, and hence should be removed along with underlying bursa. The dorsal muscles are gently separated, lifted with a periosteal elevator/chisel, preserved, and retracted. Care is taken to protect the dorsal neurovascular bundle while lifting the soft tissues. At the apex of the deformed foot the osteotomy is marked with an osteotome. The wedge is wider dorso-laterally and taper towards the sole. Usually 1 to 2 cm width of the wedge is sufficient for getting the correction (Fig. 3D). The width of bony wedge can vary depending upon the severity of the deformity. One can always remove additional bone if the correction is inadequate. Cuboid and all three cuneiforms are the usual bones which are included in the wedge. If the deformity is severe, the navicular or distal calcaneus or base of the metatarsals can also be included in the wedge. In rare case, impingement of the navicular against the head of the talus can hamper the correction of the deformity. In such a situation naviculectomy should be done. Occasionally, terminal portion of the talar head is excised, taking care of subtalar joint. The cartilage should be removed from the

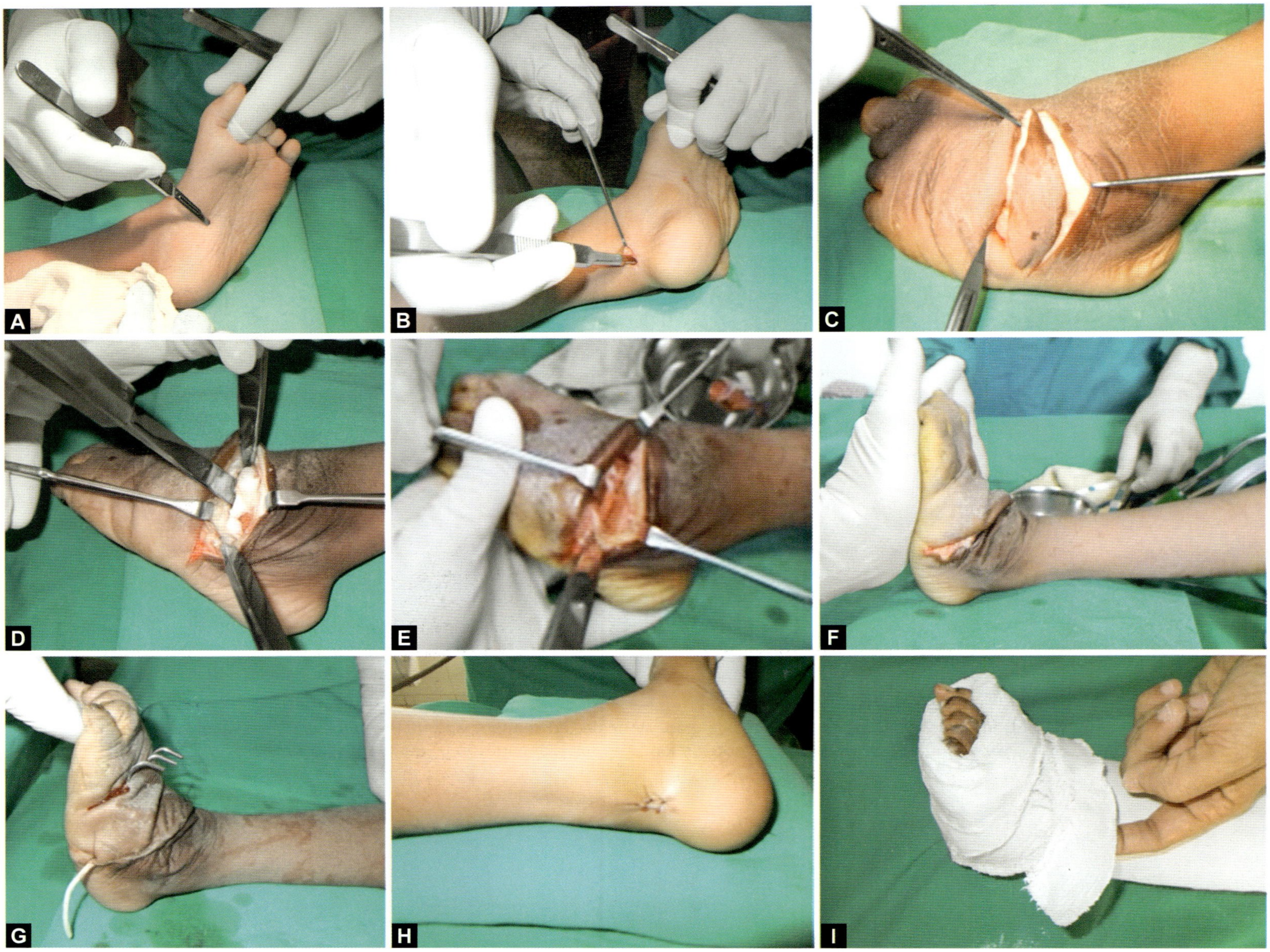

Figs. 3A to I: (A) Correction of cavus is done by percutaneous plantar fasciotomy; (B) Correction of equinus is done by percutaneous tendo Achilles tenotomy. In rare cases of relapsed deformity, if equinus is not corrected completely, the posterior ankle capsular release can be done through same incision; (C) An elliptical skin incision placed dorsolaterally at the apex of deformity; (D) After preserving dorsal structures, osteotomy is marked with osteotome at apex of the deformed foot. The wedge is wider dorsolaterally (1–2 cm) and tapers toward sole; (E) After removal of wedge, deformity is corrected by closing space manually by everting and dorsiflexing the foot; (F) Bony surfaces are approximated and the deformity is completely corrected; (G) Stabilization of forefoot to hindfoot with three K-wires. A rubber drain is kept in situ for drainage of hematoma; (H) View from back—complete correction of equinus as well as heel—varus; and (I) Plaster window made for wound check.

osteotomy bed and approximating edges to prevent nonunion and pseudarthrosis. Usually the subtalar joint is kept untouched.

Step 4: Closure of the osteotomy and fixation: The deformity is finally corrected by following maneuver. The forefoot is manually everted and dorsiflexed. By this maneuver the bony surfaces are approximated, like a closure of an open book (Figs. 3E and F). The stabilization of forefoot to the hindfoot is done with three Kirschner-wires passed from the metatarsals to the calcaneus (Fig. 3G).

The resected wedge consists of the cancellous bone which is used as a graft at the osteotomy closure site. This leaves no chance for the non union. A simple rubber drain is kept (Fig. 3G), wounds are closed (Fig. 3H), the tourniquet is deflated. An above-knee cast is given. A window is made in the cast for wound-check (Fig. 3I), and the limb is elevated on pillows.

POSTOPERATIVE PROTOCOL

Three days of intravenous antibiotics are given to prevent infection along with epidural top-ups for pain relief. On the 3rd postoperative day, the wound is inspected through the window in the cast. Hematoma, if present is drained and the drain is removed. Patients are discharged on the 4th postoperative day. They are advised nonweight for 6 weeks. After 6 weeks, the Kirschner wires and cast are removed. A plastic molded ankle-foot orthosis is applied to be worn for a period of 6 months. Squatting is encouraged at home as per tolerence. Patients are likely to have foot discomfort and plantar pain for few months after cast removal. This is caused by sensitivity of the sole and disuse osteoporosis of the calcaneus and metatarsals.

A few clinical examples are shown in Figures 4 and 5.

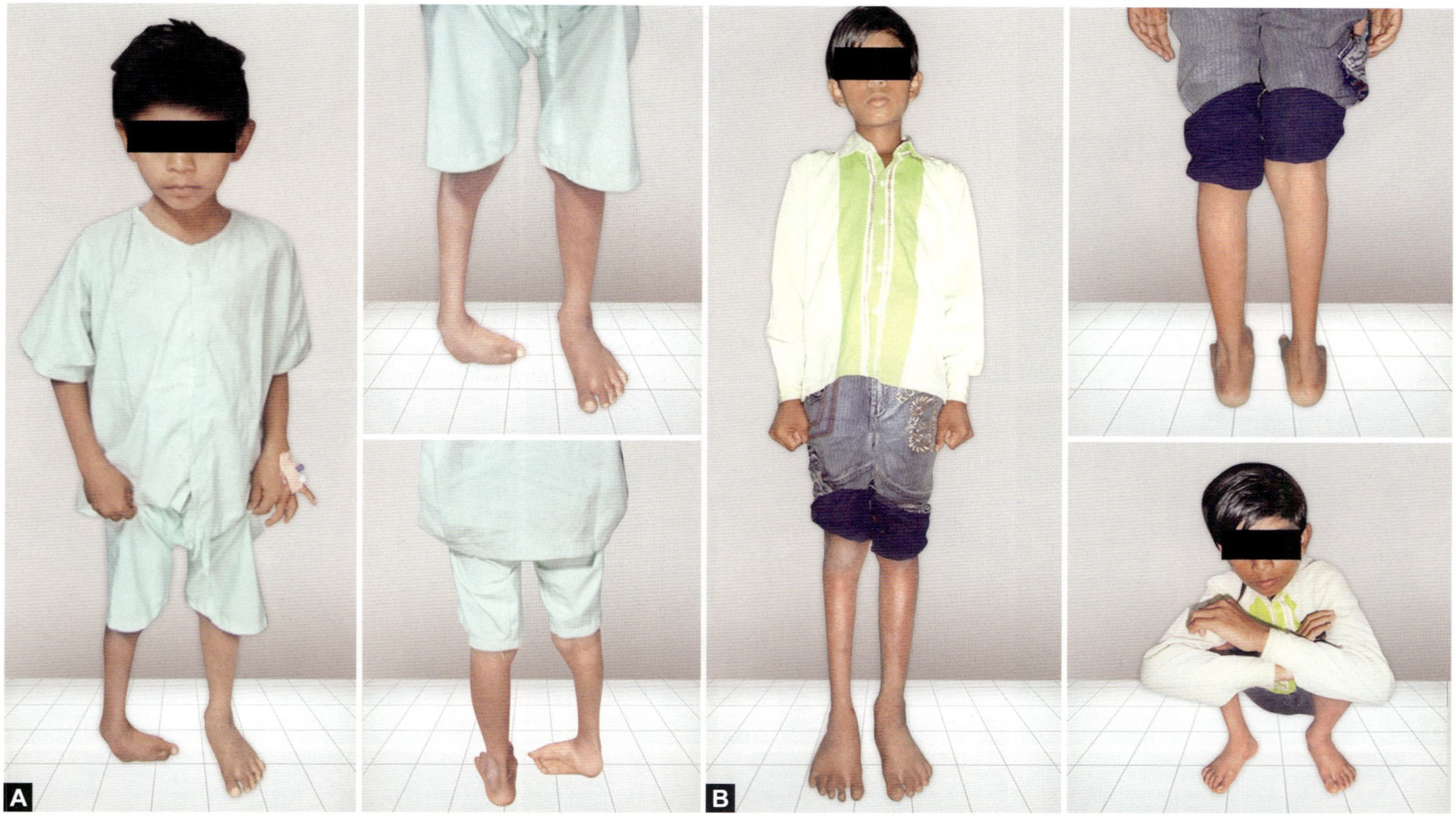

Figs. 4A and B: A 7-year-old male with right side grade IV neglected clubfoot; and (B) Postsurgery 5 years follow-up with good maintenance of hindfoot, forefoot, and midfoot correction. Squatting is possible.

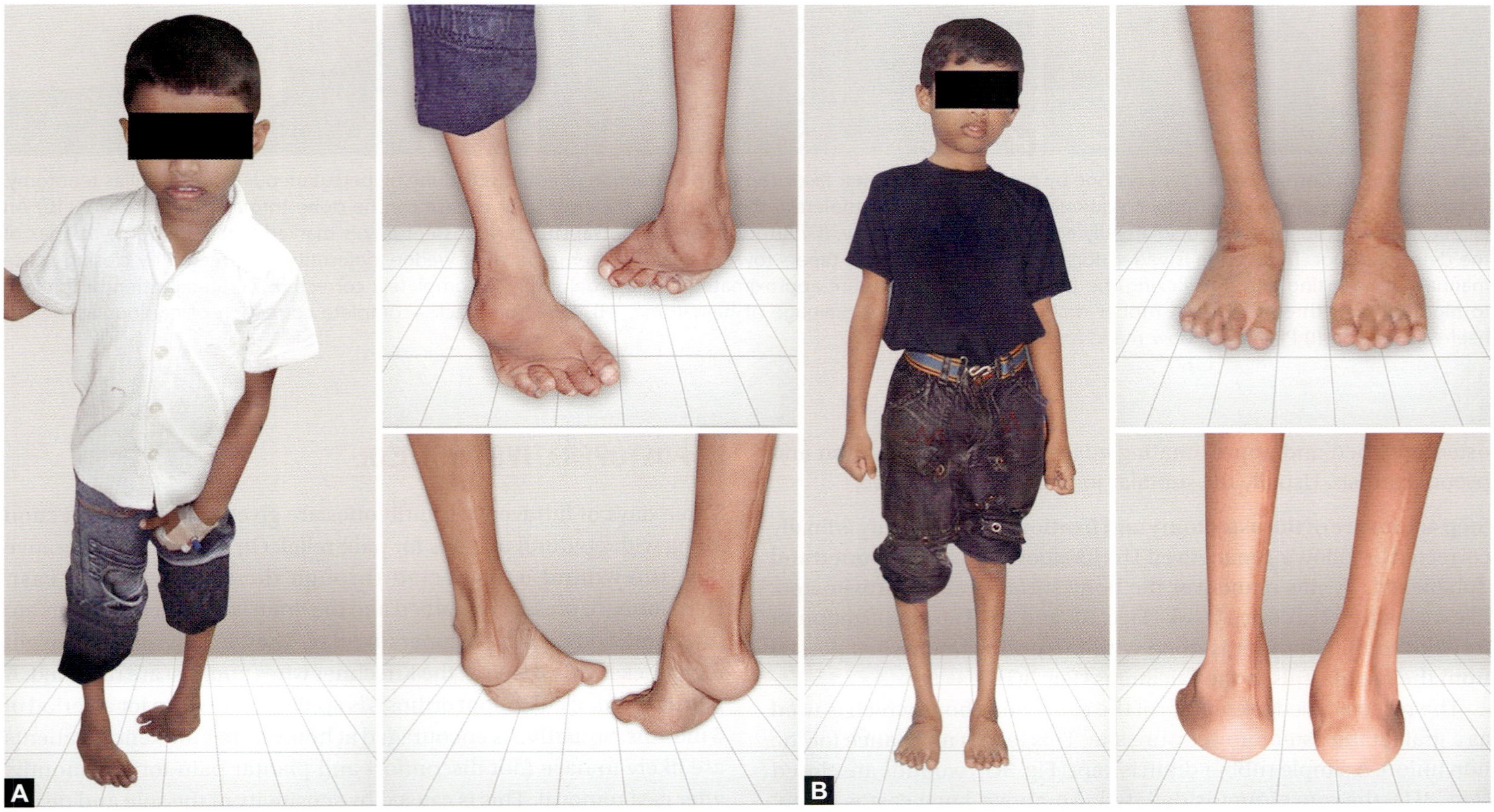

Figs. 5A and B: (A) An 8-year-old male with bilateral grade IV relapsed clubfeet. Extensive scars of previous two attempts of surgical correction are seen clearly; and (B) Postsurgery 3 years follow-up with good maintenance of correction. The technique is equally effective in relapsed cases.

KEYPOINTS

- The technique is equally effective for neglected as well as relapsed clubfoot deformities
- We advice it to be done after 4 years of age
- The tissue handling should be delicate to prevent problem of skin necrosis at edges
- In cases of bilateral deformity, both feet can be operated at same sitting
- In long-term follow-up of more than 10 years, none of the patient developed arthritis.

SUGGESTED READING

1. Bensahela H, Kuo K, Duhaime M, et al. Outcome evaluation of the treatment of clubfoot: the international language of clubfoot. J Pediatr Orthop B. 2003;12(4):269-71.
2. Diméglio A, Bensahel H, Souchet P, et al. Classification of clubfoot. J Pediatr Orthop B. 1995;4(2):129-36.
3. Lourenço AF, Morcuende JA. Correction of neglected idiopathic club foot by the Ponseti method. J Bone Joint Surg Br. 2007;89(3):378-81.
4. Shingade V, Shingade R, Ughade S. Correction of neglected or relapsed clubfoot deformity in an older child by single staged procedure: early results. Curr Orthop Pract. 2012;23(2):122-9.
5. Shingade V, Shingade R, Ughade S. Single-stage correction for clubfoot associated with myelomeningocele in older children: early results. Curr Orthop Pract. 2014;25(1):64-70.

CHAPTER 2

Congenital Muscular Torticollis: Unipolar, Bipolar Sternocleidomastoid Muscle Release

Sandeep Patwardhan, Bansi Vasudev Naik Khaunte

INDICATIONS

Congenital muscular torticollis after ruling out other causes of torticollis, which persists beyond 1 year of age.

If 6 months of controlled manual stretching fails to produce results and evidence of tumor or tight band in the SCM, with restricted range of motion to the tune of 15° or more in rotation, surgical intervention is preferred.

There is no evidence to support contraindication for delayed release, thence no upper age limit in neglected cases, however remodeling of craniofacial abnormality is best if surgery is done before 4 years of age. Head tilt and range of motion improves if the release is done at a later stage, however facial asymmetry cannot be addressed.

CONTRAINDICATIONS

Below 1 year of age, the tissue is very small to handle and there are reports of tethering of scar with deeper tissues resulting in relapse of deformity.

Non-muscular Torticollis. Exclusive muscle release will not correct the head tilt.

POSITIONING

The patient is placed in supine position under general anesthesia, with a bolster placed underneath the ipsilateral shoulder the neck is turned to the opposite side. This position will minimally extend the neck and tense the SCM muscle (Fig. 1).

TECHNIQUE

Regional anatomy is depicted in Figure 2.

Distally make a 4–5-cm long incision in the cervical skin crease after stretching the skin downward so that when relaxed, the incision ends up a fingerbreadth above the medial end of clavicle and sternal notch (Fig. 3A).

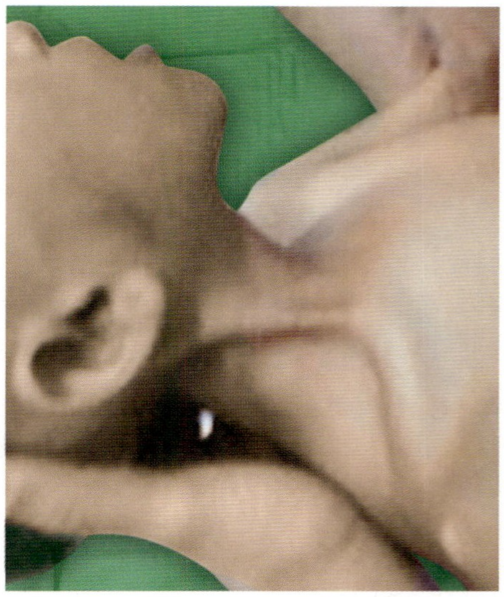

Fig. 1: Prominent right sternocleidomastoid muscle.

In order to expose clavicular and sternal attachments, subcutaneous tissue and platysma muscle are split along the incision. Carefully avoid vital structures underneath, the anterior and external jugular veins and the carotid vessels in the sheath while isolating the muscle.

The clavicular head is a muscular insertion and is completely separated from the bone.

Neck is gently maneuvered to stretch the muscle after Z-lengthening of the sternocleidomastoid sternal attachment up to the middle of the tendon before suturing the ends (Fig. 3B).

Technique described above is unipolar release, which if fails to relieve the tight muscle proceed with releasing the proximal attachment.

Over the mastoid process, a short transverse incision of about 2–3 cm to be made behind the ear so that half of its scar will be camouflaged by the hair line (Fig. 3A).

Skin, subcutaneous tissue, and superficial fascia incised. Wound retracted with blunt retractors.

Once the incision is made, look for the proximal end of the muscle which appears to be stout and gleaming insertion on the mastoid process.

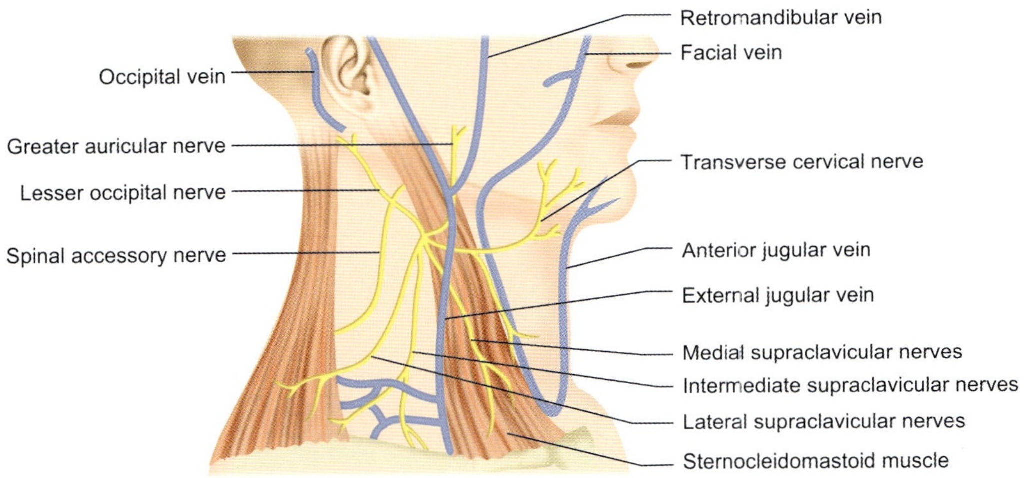

Fig. 2: Regional anatomy.

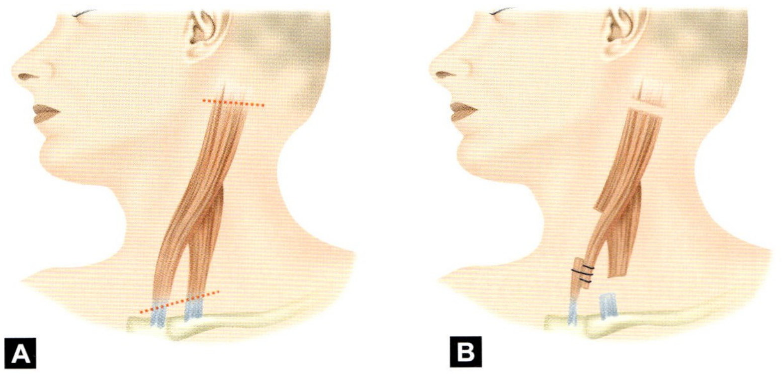

Figs. 3A and B: (A) Incisions; (B) Z-lengthening of sternal attachment.

As the muscle is released and allowed to slide distally, suture holding the lower end is given a gentle tug to palpate and confirm adequacy of the release.

Advantage of this limited incision is that the spinal accessory nerve remains away from the surgical field.

Infrequently, release of contracted bands of fascia or muscle in addition to the above procedure is necessary before closure to gain the desired results.

In order to preserve cosmetic V-appearance of the neck; the tendon ends are sutured or can also be done by releasing the sternal head 2 cm proximal to the attachment and suturing the released clavicular head to distally attached sternal head of sternocleidomastoid with 3-0 monofilament absorbable material in stretched position.

Skin is closed in layers for both wounds to reduce intensity of the scar.

3-0 absorbable monofilament/braided material for subcutaneous tissue, and 3-0 absorbable/nonabsorbable monofilament suture for subcuticular closure.

DANGERS

Carotid vessels within the sheath lie just underneath the sternocleidomastoid muscle. Thus, intraoperatively bradycardia has to be watched for whilst stretching the neck.

In children less than 2 years of age, mastoid is not well developed thus facial nerve exiting from stylomastoid foramen lies just medial and posterior to the proximal attachment of sternocleidomastoid.

Subclavian vessels run just posterior to clavicular head of sternocleidomastoid.

Spinal accessory nerve may take an anomalous route, and may traverse the usual incision site.

Greater auricular nerve is at risk for traction injury causing sensory disturbances over the pinna which recover over period of time.

Ugly scar in front of the neck if incision not planned and taken on the bone.

POSTOPERATIVE CARE

A soft cervical collar is prescribed in the immediate postoperative period and continued until 3 months postoperative.

Preoperatively patients are known to keep their heads turned on the same side of the SCM contracture thence 2 weeks post-release patients are encouraged to sleep prone on the released side with face turned on the opposite side to stretch the sternocleidomastoid.

Postoperatively, passive range of motion exercises is started at 3 weeks. After 6 weeks, active range of motion and physiotherapy is continued until at least 3 months, in order to prevent contracture of the scar and gain neck muscle balance.

SUGGESTED READING

1. Cheng JC, Tang SP, Chen TM, et al. The clinical presentation and outcome of treatment of congenital muscular torticollis in infants—a study of 1,086 cases. J Pediatr Surg. 2000;35(7):1091-6.
2. Cheng JC, Wong MW, Tang SP, et al. Clinical determinants of the outcome of manual stretching in the treatment of congenital muscular torticollis in infants. A prospective study of eight hundred and twenty-one cases. J Bone Joint Surg Am. 2001;83-A(5):679-87.
3. Ferkel RD, Westin GW, Dawson EG, et al. Muscular torticollis. A modified surgical approach. J Bone Joint Surg Am. 1983;65(7):894-900.
4. Gupta A, Kothari SY. Lower pole release in congenital muscular torticollis—retrospective analysis of outcomes in 15 cases. Indian J Phys Med Rehabil. 2016;27(3):46-8.
5. Ho BC, Lee EH, Singh K. Epidemiology, presentation and management of congenital muscular torticollis. Singapore Med J. 1999;40(11):675-9.
6. Patwardhan S, Shyam AK, Sancheti P, et al. Adult presentation of congenital muscular torticollis. J Bone Joint Surg Br. 2011;93(6):828-32.
7. Shim JS, Noh KC, Park SJ. Treatment of congenital muscular torticollis in patients older than 8 years. J Pediatr Orthop. 2004;24(6):683-8.

CHAPTER 3

External Stabilization System for Clubfoot

Rujuta Mehta, Alaric Aroojis, Rohit K Jain

INTRODUCTION

Clubfoot is one of the most common congenital anomalies, its incidence being 5–6 per 1000 live births. The goal of treating clubfoot is to obtain a painless, plantigrade, functionally supple foot. Ponseti is now the gold standard treatment for the clubfoot that present very early. But in developing countries where patients present late and are neglected and in relapsed clubfoot patients, surgeries like posteromedial releases and bony osteotomies are treatment options. But these lead to increase tissue fibrosis and stiffer foot with decreased foot size. In such cases, Joshi's external stabilization system (JESS) and Ilizarov fixators based upon the principle of distraction histogenesis have reported good outcomes.

External fixators have been in use since the last century. Codivilla has been credited as the first physician to perform limb lengthening in 1904. In the early 20th century, various external fixators were used wherein the patients were confined to the bed for bone regeneration. In 1950s, Dr Gavril Ilizarov developed circular external fixator with transosseous tensioned wires using the principle of distraction histogenesis. His technique was unknown to North America until Paley introduced it after studying for 6 months in Italy and Soviet Union. It has now being used extensively for limb lengthening and deformity corrections. JESS developed by Dr BB Joshi is another cheap, less technically demanding external fixator as compared with Ilizarov ring fixators. Both of these techniques have some advantages over soft tissue releases and bony osteotomies such as having supple foot with maintained foot size.

JESS is abbreviation of Joshi's external stabilization system. It was devised by Dr BB Joshi in 1990. The fixator is cheap, versatile, simple, and based upon the principle of tissue histogenesis similar to Ilizarov fixators wherein the tissues are subjected to measured and sustained stretch.

INDICATIONS

- Rigid nonidiopathic syndromic clubfeet
- Neglected clubfeet in older child
- Postsurgical relapse clubfoot
- Neurogenic clubfoot.

PRINCIPLES OF JOSHI'S EXTERNAL STABILIZATION SYSTEM

The principle of JESS is same as that of Ilizarov system—distraction histogenesis. But it differs from Ilizarov in following ways: (a) Wires are not tensioned, (b) the construct is unconstrained, and (c) differential distraction is used to correct the deformity. Physiological stress and tension applied to the tissue promotes tissue histogenesis stimulates. Controlled differential distraction gradually corrects the deformities. Since the deformities in clubfoot are present in the forefoot, the hindfoot and the leg, the JESS frame for clubfoot consists of 3 blocks –, the forefoot block, the hindfoot block and the leg block for correction of these deformities (Figs. 1A to C). As differential distraction can

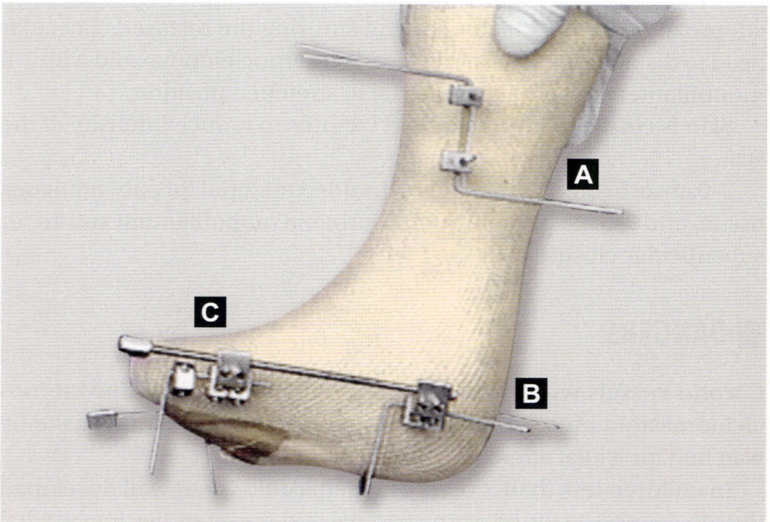

Figs. 1A to C: (A) Leg block; (B) Hindfoot block; and (C) Forefoot block.

correct deformities in two planes, uncoupling of the distractors from the frame is required for correcting the deformities in all the three planes which is followed by manipulation and reconnecting the distractors with the K-wires and completing the frame.

TECHNIQUE OF JOSHI'S EXTERNAL STABILIZATION SYSTEM FIXATOR APPLICATION

The patient is placed in supine position under general anesthesia.

Following are the steps of JESS frame construction (a) insertion of pins, (b) creation of blocks and (c) connecting the blocks via distractors.

Insertion of Pins

Technique of Hindfoot Pins

In the hind foot the first pin is the co-axial K-wire. It is inserted along the long axis of the calcaneum starting on its posterior aspect distal to the insertion of tendo-Achilles in the midline. Then 2 parallel K-wires are passed through the calcaneal tuberosity from medial aspect to lateral aspect, perpendicular to the first co-axial K wire. These 2 wires are in the plane of the deformity. Precautions should be taken while passing these wires, as there are neurovascular structures on the medial side. At the end of it the pins should mirror the deformity.

Technique of Forefoot Pins

3 K wires are passed in the forefoot. A transfixing K-wire is inserted lateral to medial through the necks of 1st and 5th metatarsal engaging only these two metatarsals. 2 parallel K wires are inserted 10 to 12 mm apart, one from medial side through the 1st and 2nd metatarsals and second one through the 3rd, 4th and 5th metatarsals. The 3rd metatarsal should not be engaged from both the sides.

Technique of Leg Pins

The patient is in supine position with the hip and knee extended. Two K-wires parallel to each other are inserted from lateral to medial side in the proximal tibial diaphysis keeping a distance of 3 to 4 cm from each other. The Z rod is used as guide to pass these wires distal to the tibial tuberosity and parallel to the knee joint. One more additional K wire may be used in older children to augment the stability. One additional pin in the antero-posterior direction is inserted to prevent rocking and loosening of the construct.

Attachment of Connecting Rods

Connecting rods are then attached to the three blocks of the frame. For the leg block, two 'Z' rods are attached to the tibial K wires one on the medial side and the other on the lateral side with the distal arm facing posteriorly. Two straight rods are attached to the 'Z' rods anteriorly and posteriorly in the frontal plane. Two L rods are attached to the metatarsal K wires one on the medial side and other on the lateral side to complete the forefoot block. Similarly, for the hindfoot block two L rods are attached to the calcaneal wires one on the medial side and other on the lateral side of the foot. The arms of the L rods should be pointing inferiorly and posteriorly. One straight rod is connected to these posterior arms of the L rods engaging the calcaneal half pin with it and completing the hindfoot block. Care should be taken to prestress all the wires before tightening the joints of the connecting rods.

Attachment of Distractors

Finally, the distractors are attached to complete the construct. The forefoot block is connected to the hindfoot block with calcaneo-metatarsal distractors that are attached to the metatarsal and calcaneal K wires on both sides of the foot. The leg block is connected to the hindfoot block with tibio-calcaneal distractors that are attached to the transverse rods on both sides of the hindfoot and leg. Distraction is carried out on all the four distractors until some kind of resistance is felt. The K wires are cut beyond two finger breadths. A static tibio-metatarsal rod is connected to the anterior straight connecting rod of the tibia and the metatarsals to maintain tension and prevent crushing of the articular cartilage.

Pin sites are cleaned and ends are protected.

DISTRACTION SCHEDULE (FIG. 2)

Differential distraction is started after the 2nd post-operative day at the rate of 0.25 mm every 6 hours (1 mm/day) over the medial tibio-calcaneal and calcaneo-metatarsal distractors and at the rate of 0.25 mm every 12 hourly (0.5 mm/day) over the lateral tibio-calcaneal and calcaneo-metatarsal distractors.

Manual Repositioning

Distraction is carried out for 1 week after which patient is called into the OPD for manual repositioning of the frame. All the four distractors are disconnected keeping the three blocks intact and the foot is manipulated and derotated into a lesser deformed position. The distractors are then reconnected to the blocks and distraction protocol is continued for another one week. This process is continued every week until the foot is over corrected.

Maintenance Phase

Once the over correction is achieved with the foot in plantigrade functional position, distraction is stopped and this over corrected position is maintained in the frame for 6 to 8 weeks (Figs. 3A to F).

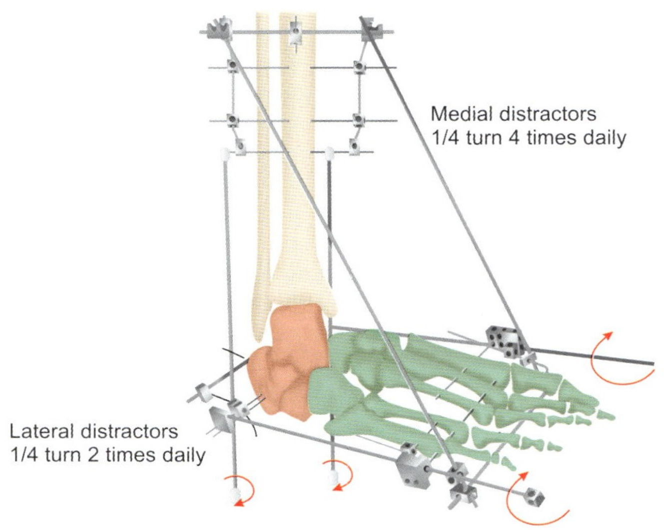

Fig. 2: Distraction schedule.

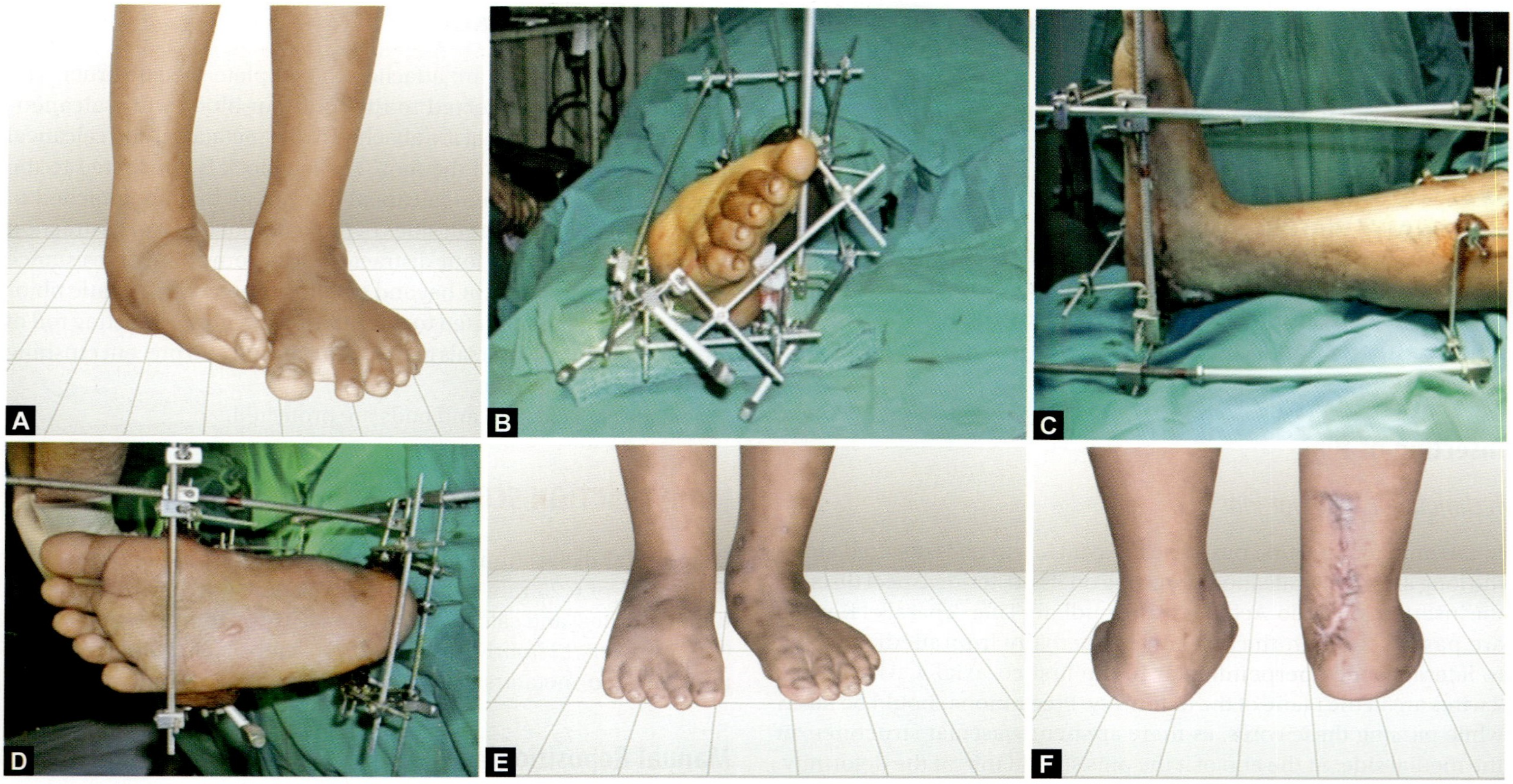

Figs. 3A to F: A 14-year-old boy with right neglected rigid clubfoot gradually corrected to plantigrade foot by Joshi's external stabilization system (JESS) and posterior soft tissue release. (A) Preoperative clinical photograph; (B to D) Gradual correction by JESS; and (E and F) Clinical photograph after complete correction.

Joshi's External Stabilization System Removal

After the completion of the maintenance phase, the frame is removed completely under general anesthesia and well-molded cast is applied in the corrected position. The child is encouraged to walk full weight bearing in the cast. The cast is continued for another 6–8 weeks.

Bracing Phase

At the end of 6–8 weeks of cast application, the cast is removed and is put on a brace and continued to maintain a corrected position.

Advantages

- All the deformities are corrected in the 3 planes by gradual differential distraction.
- Due to tissue histogenesis by distraction, it adds to the tissues and does not decrease the foot size which happens after surgical correction by bony and soft tissue procedures.
- Forceful manipulation causes chondrolysis with compression of the articular cartilage which is avoided with JESS.

Disadvantages

- Pin track infections
- Clawing of toes due to shortening and stretching of toe flexors—managed by giving toe straps.
- Skin necrosis due to acute distraction
- Loosening of components.

CORRECTION OF RELAPSED RESISTANT CLUBFOOT BY ILIZAROV RING FIXATOR

Ilizarov technique is another technique to correct complex foot deformities in relapsed and neglected clubfoot. Ilizarov is an ideal surgical technique to correct the complex three-dimensional deformities in relapsed resistant clubfoot.

Advantages of Ilizarov Technique

- Minimally invasive technique with minimal risk of neurovascular injuries.
- Correction can be both acute and gradual. Also, correction can be adjusted in the postoperative period.
- Along the foot deformities, tibial deformities and limb length discrepancies can be addressed.

Disadvantages

- Pin tract infections
- Prolonged period of treatment
- Clawing of toes.

Technique

- *K-wire insertion*:
  - *Proximal tibial wires*: Two K wires of 1.8 mm diameter are inserted at the junction of proximal 1/3rd and middle 1/3rd . First wire is inserted from lateral to medial one finger breadth

lateral and posterior to shin of tibia and exiting medially anterior to the medial border of the tibia. Second wire is passed through the fibula one finger breadth anterior to its anterior border and exiting through the shin of the tibia one finger breadth postero-medially about 5 mm distal to first wire.

- *Distal tibial wires*: Two K wires of 1.8 mm diameter are similarly inserted at the junction of middle 1/3rd and distal 1/3rd of tibia. The first wire is inserted through fibula and exiting through the shin of the tibia one finger breadth postero-medially. The second wire is passed through the safe middle zone into the tibia exiting just anterior to the medial border of tibia.
- *Calcaneal wires*: One K-wire inserted from anteromedial to posterolateral direction and second wire inserted from posteromedial to anterolateral direction.
- *Forefoot wires*: Two olive wires are used for the forefoot. The first olive wire is passed from the lateral side through the 5th metacarpal neck and is advanced to engage the fourth and third metacarpal neck exiting on the dorsal surface of the foot. The second olive wire is passed from the medial side through the first metacarpal neck and advanced obliquely through second metacarpal neck after lifting it up and exiting through the dorsum of the foot.

• *Rings*: The rings for the tibia are full rings which should allow two fingerbreadth clearance from the maximum girth of the tibia (Figs. 4A to F).

- *Proximal tibial ring*: A full ring is placed at the junction of proximal 1/3rd and the middle 1/3rd of the tibia.
- *Distal tibial ring*: A full ring is placed at the junction of the middle 1/3rd and distal 1/3rd about 10–12 cm proximal to the ankle joint at the junction of middle one-third and distal one-third. Proximal tibial and distal tibial rings are connected with four threaded rods. The calcaneum half ring is connected to the distal tibial ring by hinges placed posteriorly. Medially, and laterally while the forefoot ring is connected to the calcaneum ring by medial and lateral hinges. The proximal tibial ring is connected to the forefoot ring by two threaded rods on either side for correcting the equinus and supination deformities. The hinge allows the rods to move without bending and also prevent the subluxation of joint during distraction. Half ring over the calcaneum is used as a distractor, and compression is achieved through the half ring over dorsum of the forefoot.

Distraction Schedule

Distraction is started from 2nd postoperative day. The sequence of the deformity correction is gradual differential distraction over medial side 1 mm/day and lateral side 0.5 mm/day to correct cavus and forefoot adduction through distractors connected between the forefoot and hindfoot rings. After correction of forefoot adduction and pronation, hindfoot varus is corrected through differential

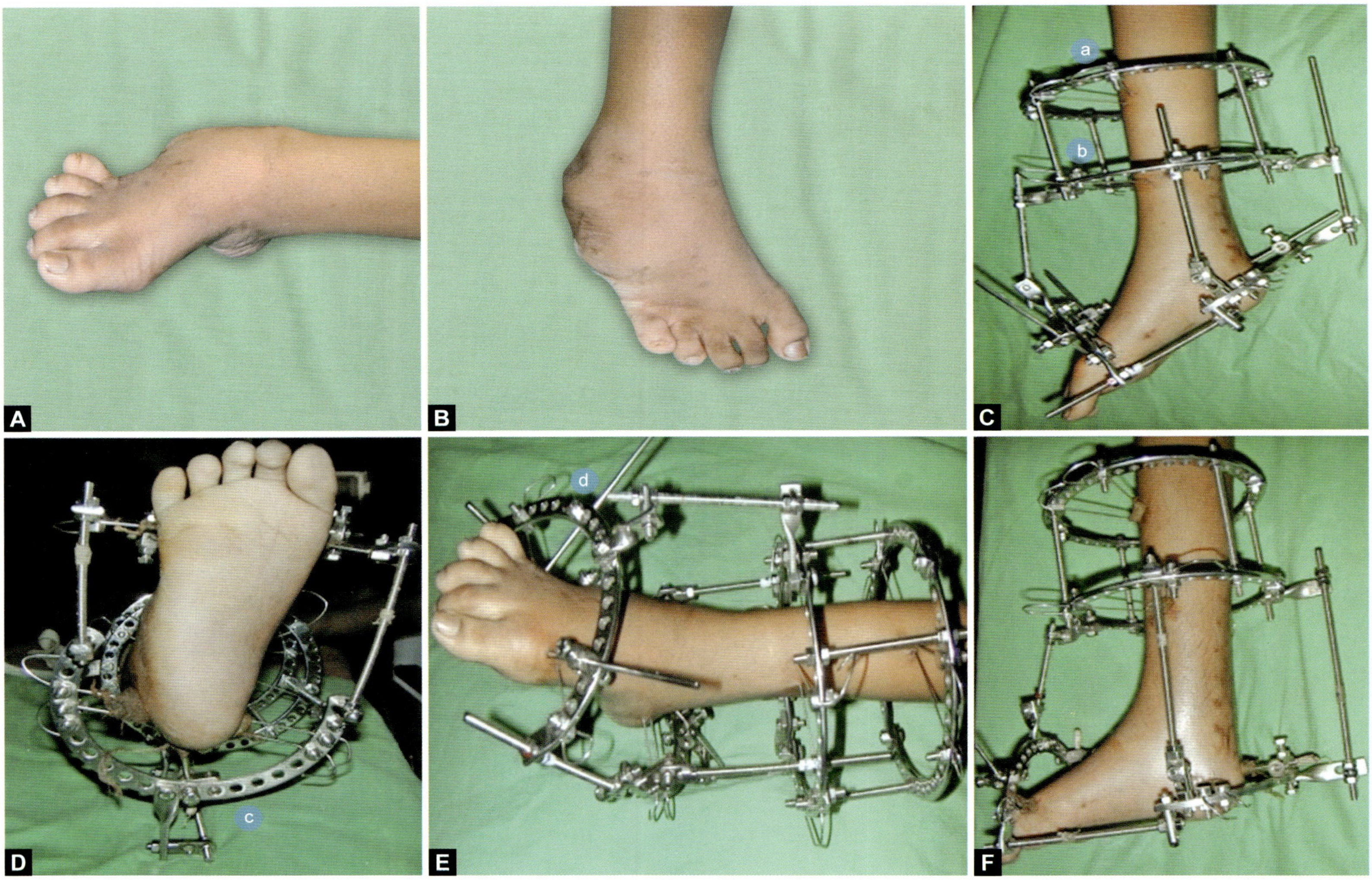

Figs. 4A to F: Relapsed clubfoot treated with Ilizarov ring fixator. (A and B) Preoperative clinical photographs; (C to E) Ilizarov ring frame [(a) proximal tibial ring, (b) distal tibial ring, (c) calcaneal half ring, (d) forefoot metatarsal half ring]; and (F) Complete correction.

distraction of the distractors connecting the tibial rings and calcaneal ring and finally equinus is corrected through distractors connecting the proximal tibial rings and forefoot ring anteriorly.

- Over the course of distraction, soft tissue tension and neurovascular status of the foot clinically and dislocation or subluxation of tarsal and ankle joint radiologically should be closely observed. Deformities are overcorrected up to 10° leading to overlengthening of soft tissue avoiding the recoil that can occur after frame removal.
- Pin tracts are cleaned and dressed with normal saline, betadine and dry gauzes. Once over correction is achieved, distraction is stopped and the Ilizarov frame is locked and maintained in the over corrected position for a further period of 4–6 weeks. After 4–6 weeks of maintenance phase the fixator is removed and the pin tracts are thoroughly cleaned, washed and dressed. A short below knee walking cast is applied for 2 weeks. After 2 weeks, the cast is removed to check the pin tract wounds and again a short below knee walking cast is applied for 4 weeks. After 6 weeks of cast application, foot is braced in an ankle foot orthosis (AFO) for 3 months

Clinical photographs of the patient are obtained preoperatively, postoperatively, at the time of removal of fixator, at orthosis prescription, and at follow-up.

SUGGESTED READING

1. Anwar MH, Arun B. Short term results of correction of CTEV with JESS distractor. J Orthop. 2004;1:e3.
2. Bradish CF, Noor S. The Ilizarov method in the management of relapsed club feet. J Bone Joint Surg Br. 2000;82(3):387-91.
3. Codivilla A. On the means of lengthening, in the lower limbs, the muscles and tissues which are shortened through deformity. 1904. Clin Orthop Relat Res. 1994;301:4-9.
4. Galante VN, Molfetta L, Simone C. The treatment of club foot with external fixation—A review of results. Curr Orthop. 1995;9(3):185-8.
5. Grill F, Franke J. The Ilizarov distractor for the correction of relapsed or neglected clubfoot. J Bone Joint Surg Br. 1987;69(4):593-7.
6. Ikeda. K. Conservative treatment of idiopathic clubfoot. J Pediatr Orthop. 1992;12(2):217-23.
7. Joshi BB, Laud NS, Warrier S, et al. Treatment of CTEV by Joshi's external stabilization system (JESS). In: Kulkarni GS (Ed). Textbook of Orthopedics and Trauma, 1st edition. New Delhi: Jaypee Brothers Medical Publishers (P) Ltd; 1999.
8. Kocaoğlu M, Eralp L, Atalar AC, et al. Correction of complex foot deformities using the Ilizarov external fixator. J Foot Ankle Surg. 2002;41(1):30-9.
9. Paley D. Current techniques of limb lengthening. J Pediatr Orthop. 1988;8(1):73-92.
10. Paley D. The correction of complex foot deformities using Ilizarov's distraction osteotomies. Clin Orthop Relat Res. 1993;293:97-111.
11. Ponseti IV, Smoley EN. The classic: congenital club foot: the results of treatment. 1963. Clin Orthop Relat Res. 2009;467(5):1133-45.
12. Suresh S, Ahmed A, Sharma VK. Role of Joshi's external stabilisation system fixator in the management of idiopathic clubfoot. J Orthop Surg (Hong Kong). 2003;11(2):194-201.

CHAPTER 4

Septic Hip Drainage

Sameer Desai

INTRODUCTION

Septic arthritis of the hip is very common in children. The epiphysis is intracapsular in children and hence, it is one of the most common joint involved. Neonates, preterm babies, children with neonatal intensive care unit (NICU) admission, and children with associated comorbidities are more prone for septic hip. The child will present with history of fever and not bearing weight on limb. On examination, the hip will have an attitude of flexion. Abduction and internal rotation will be painful and restricted. Blood examination will show raised white blood cell (WBC) count and C-reactive protein (CRP). However, these parameters may be only slightly raised in neonates and hence, a high index of suspicion is required. A radiograph will show in increase in joint space, associated subluxation, metaphyseal involvement, and periosteal elevation. However, one should not wait till appearance of signs on radiographs, as it may be too late by then. An ultrasound of the hip will give you additional information regarding status of ossific nucleus (which is important for prognosis and preoperative counseling), presence of pus, septae, and periosteal elevation. In very early cases, a bone scan can be used to diagnose early acute osteomyelitis when the pus is not visible on USG. An MRI is advised if one is in doubt and if one wants to see the amount of metaphyseal involvement.

STEPS OF SURGERY (FIGS. 1 TO 10)

- Patient is in supine position under general anesthesia.
- Mark the iliac crest and anterior superior iliac spine (ASIS).
- Take a bikini incision of about 3 cm just below the ASIS, one-third lateral to the ASIS and two-thirds medial to it (Fig. 1).
- Dissect the fat and fascia and look for the interval between the sartorius which originates from the ASIS and tensor fascia latae (TFL) which lies lateral to it (Fig. 2).
- Look for the lateral cutaneous nerve of thigh which lies between the interval of the two muscles and retract it laterally. Sometimes, its position may vary.

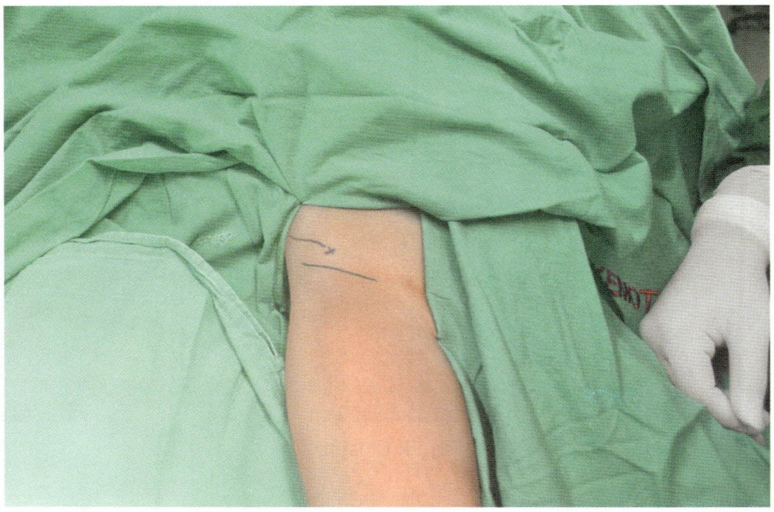

Fig. 1: Skin incision [iliac crest, anterior superior iliac spine (ASIS), and incision].

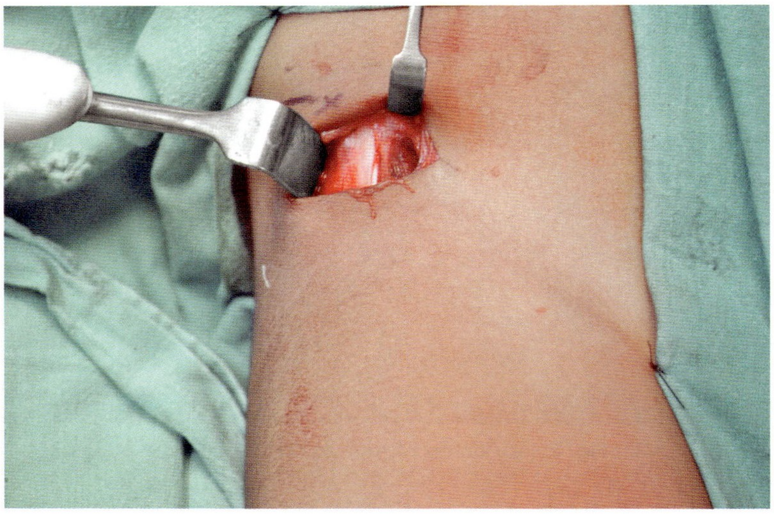

Fig. 2: Tensor fascia latae (TFL) laterally, sartorius medially, and nerve in between

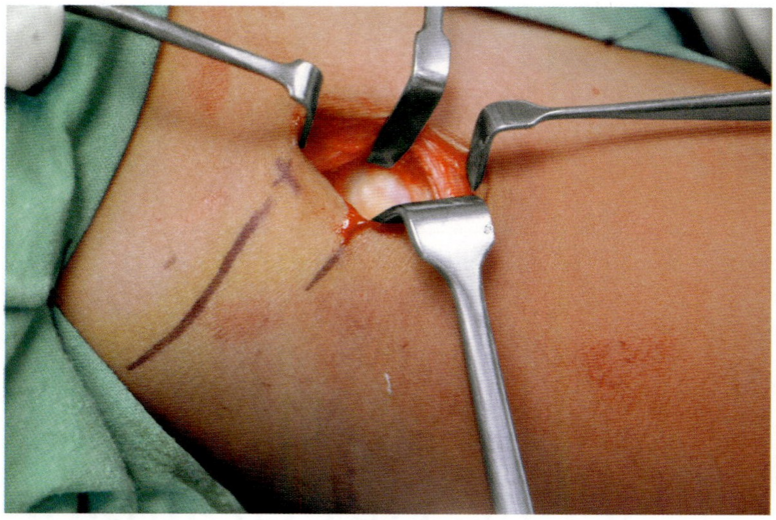

Fig. 3: Retracting the muscles to identify the rectus which originates from the anterior inferior iliac spine (AIIS).

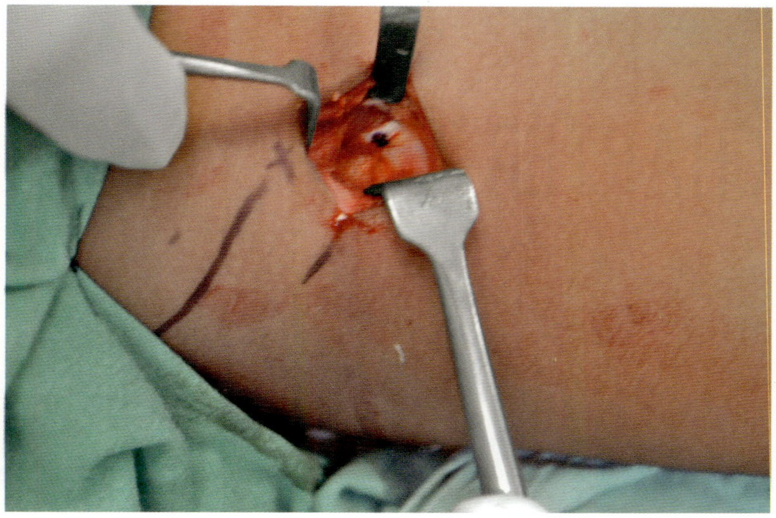

Fig. 4: Blue dot showing rectus.

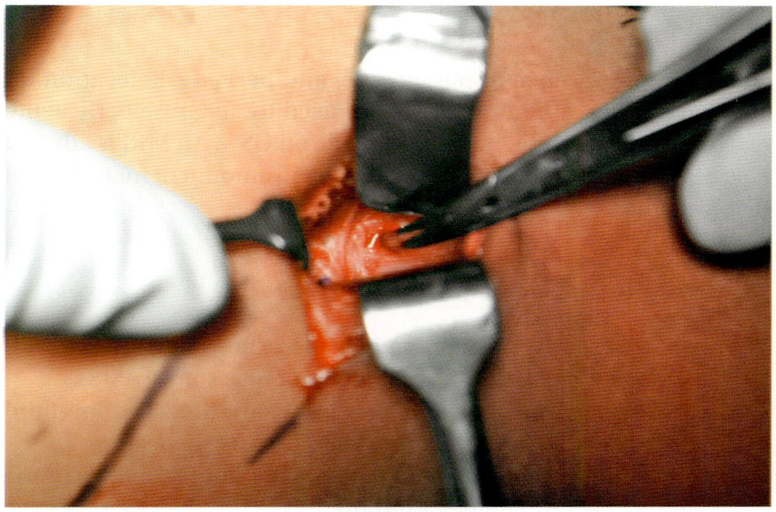

Fig. 5: Dissecting the rectus.

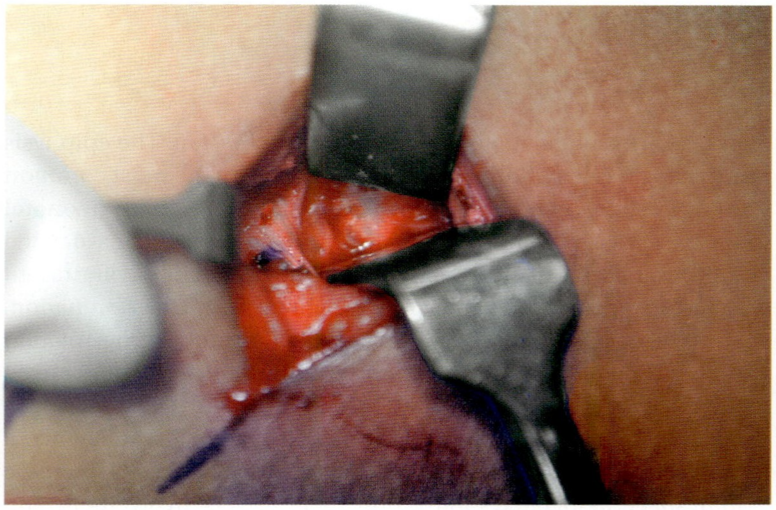

Fig. 6: Retracting the rectus laterally to show the capsule.

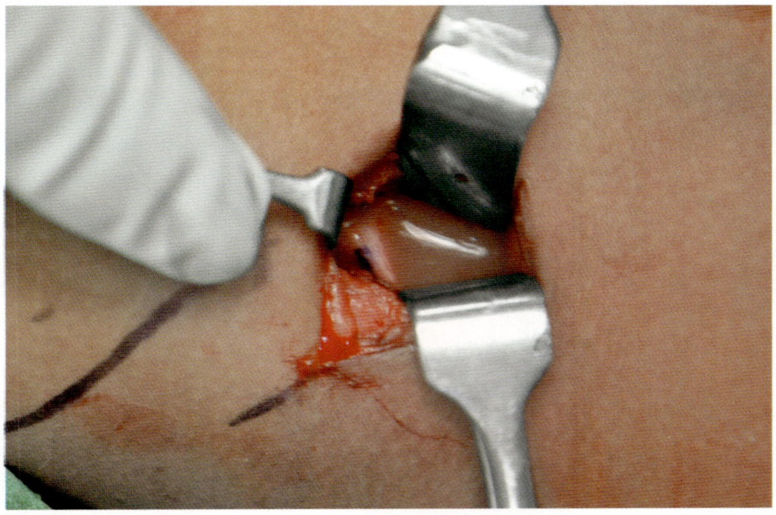

Fig. 7: Incision on capsule to drain the pus.

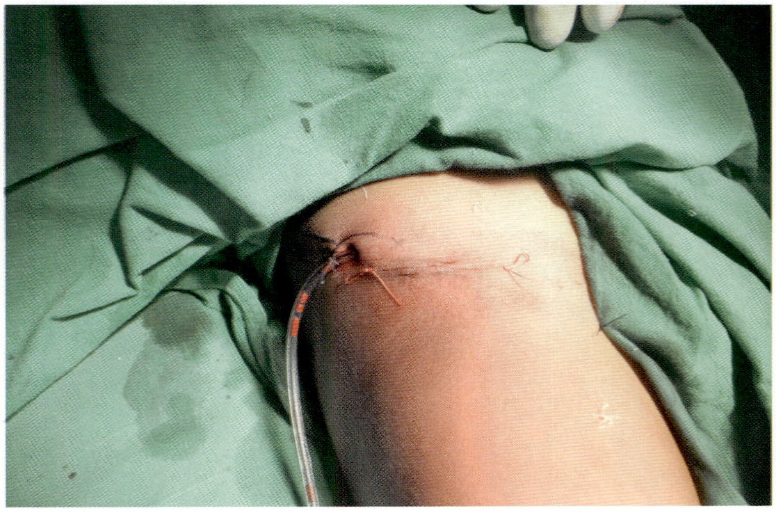

Fig. 8: Closure.

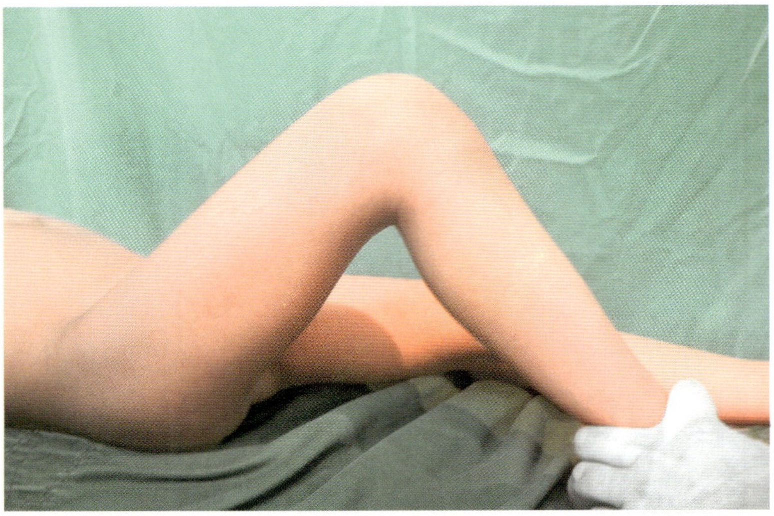

Fig. 9: Preoperative.

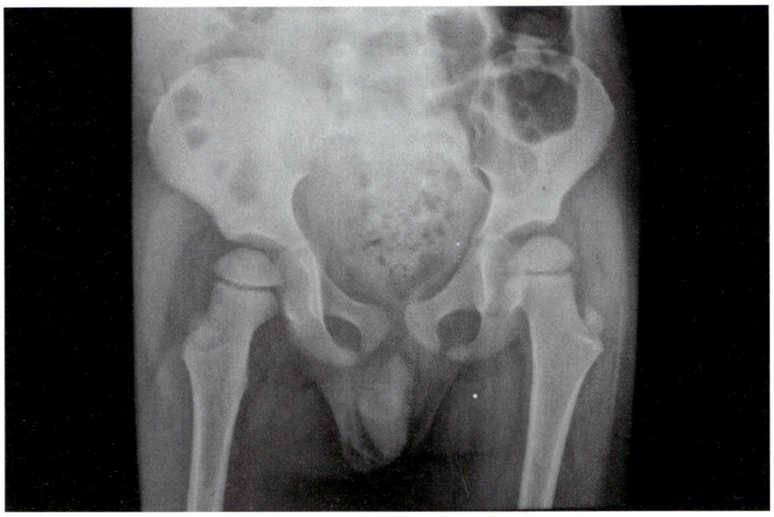

Fig. 10: Preoperative X-ray.

- Retract the sartorius medially and TFL laterally (Fig. 3).
- Just below and medially, one will find the rectus femoris which originates from the anterior inferior iliac spine (Figs. 4 and 5).
- Dissect the muscle and retract it laterally (Fig. 6).
- Below it, you will find the capsule which appears glistening white.
- Make an incision over it to drain the pus (Fig. 7).
- Give adequate wash.
- Put a suction drain and close the wound (Fig. 8).
- Hip spica/traction may be advised in children if it was found to be unstable or subluxated preoperatively (Fig. 9).
- Intravenous antibiotics are to be administered for 1–6 weeks depending on the culture report, clinical response of the child, and blood parameters.
- X-ray image (Fig. 10).

CHAPTER 5

Supracondylar Humerus Fractures Pinning

Ashish S Ranade

INTRODUCTION

Displaced supracondylar humerus fracture is one of the most common pediatric fracture that needs surgical treatment. Over the years, closed reduction and percutaneous K-wire fixation have become standard of care for these fractures. Timely fracture fixation has helped to reduce complications such as compartment syndrome leading to Volkmann ischemic contracture and cubitus varus due to malunion.

INDICATIONS

Preferred method for displaced supracondylar humerus fracture.

CONTRAINDICATIONS

Failed closed reduction, dysvascular limb after closed reduction.

It is usually done within 24 hours. Emergency treatment is done for fractures with poor hand perfusion, fractures with associated median nerve injury.

The steps of operative treatment for closed reduction and K-wire fixation of displaced supracondylar humerus fracture are as follows.

IMPLANTS AND INSTRUMENTS

K-wires of various sizes 1.6 mm, 1.8 mm, and 2 mm are kept ready. A battery-operated drill with wire driver/collate attachment is useful (Figs. 1 and 2).

PATIENT POSITION

Patient is positioned supine on operating table and the affected extremity is placed on radiolucent hand table. C-arm is brought in

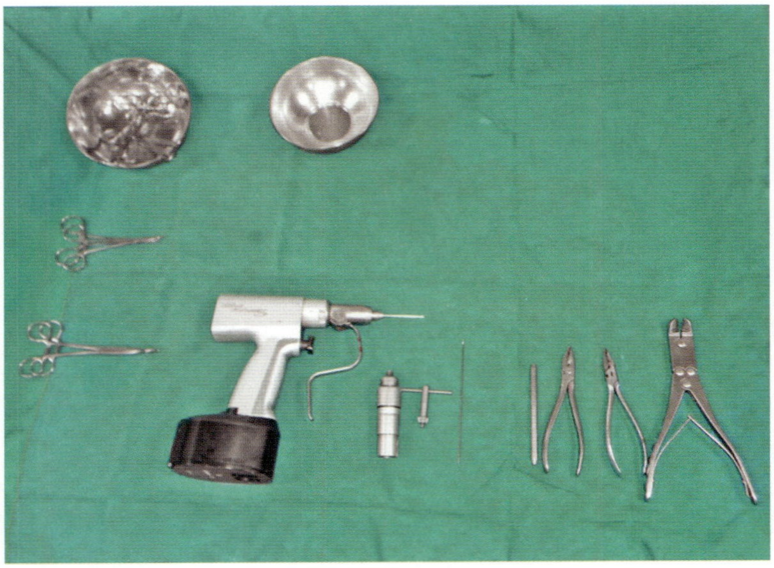

Fig. 1: Instruments for the surgery.

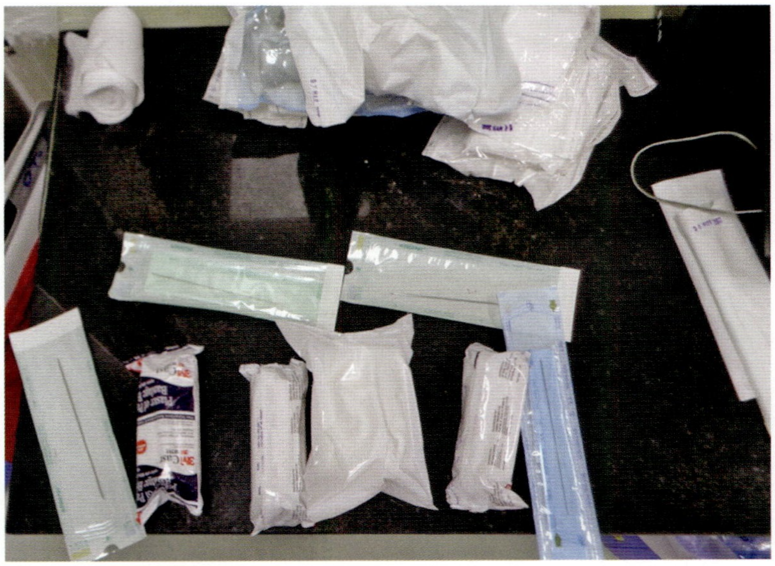

Fig. 2: Necessary implants and plaster materials.

from foot end parallel to table and C-arm screen is placed on opposite side of the surgeon. The whole upper extremity is prepared and draped from shoulder to hand. Hand is prepped so as to palpate radial pulse during/after surgery (Figs. 3 to 5).

REDUCTION OF THE FRACTURE

Under general anesthesia, longitudinal traction is applied while keeping elbow in flexion. A folded sheet or towel is kept underneath the arm to lift the elbow off the ground.

No pressure is exerted in cubital fossa. Medial or lateral translation is corrected, C-arm image is checked. Varus or valgus malalignment is corrected.

Maintaining the traction and by placing pressure over olecranon process elbow is flexed to correct the extension deformity of the distal fragment (Fig. 6).

Rule of thumb is used for determining the position of the forearm to lock the fragments and hold the reduction. For posterolaterally displaced fractures, forearm is kept in supination and for posteromedially displaced fractures, forearm is kept in pronation.

Elbow is flexed till fingers touch shoulder.

At this point, C-arm is checked for shoot through anteroposterior (AP) view (Jones view), oblique views to look for medial and lateral columns and lateral view (Figs. 7 to 10).

Adequacy of reduction is assessed by anterior humeral line passing through anterior one-third of the capitellum, correct restoration of rotation, and look for comminution of medial column if any (Fig. 11).

At the end, radial pulse is checked, and nail bed circulation is checked.

K-WIRE FIXATION

Starting point and trajectory are checked by holding the K-wire. Divergent K-wires are passed from lateral side—1.6-mm or 1.8-mm wires are used. Usually, two K-wires are used, however, sometimes if reduction is not stable, then three lateral entry K-wires may be used.

Elbow is maintained in hyperflexion while passing the K-wires. Pins should engage medial and lateral columns and should be in divergent or parallel fashion. It is acceptable to cross olecranon fossa (Figs. 12 to 15).

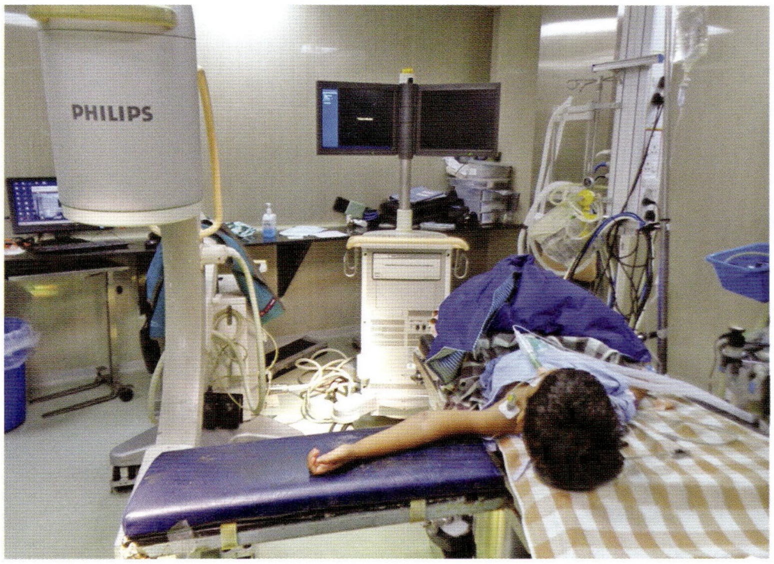

Fig. 3: Patient position.

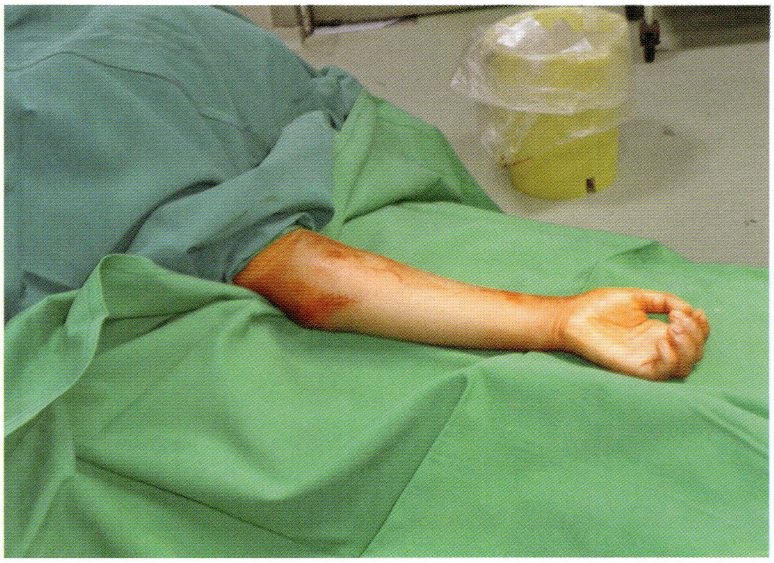

Fig. 4: Preparation and draping of the whole extremity.

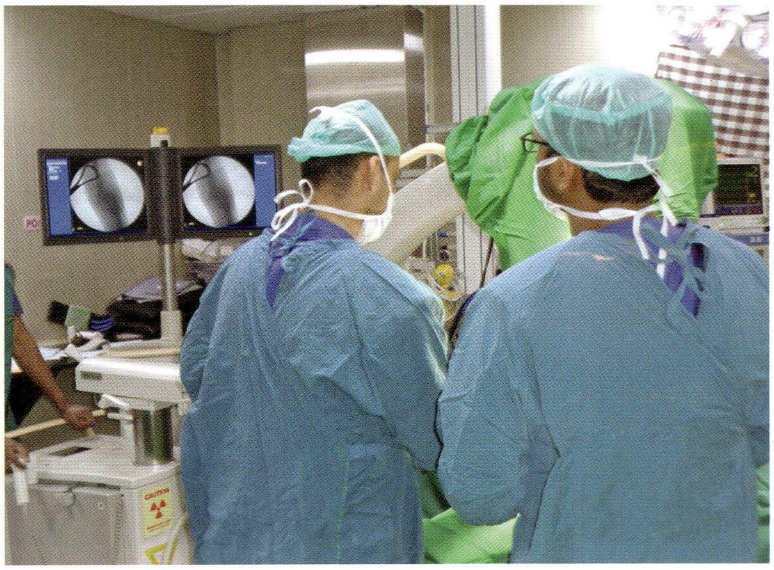

Fig. 5: Position of the C-arm monitor and surgeon.

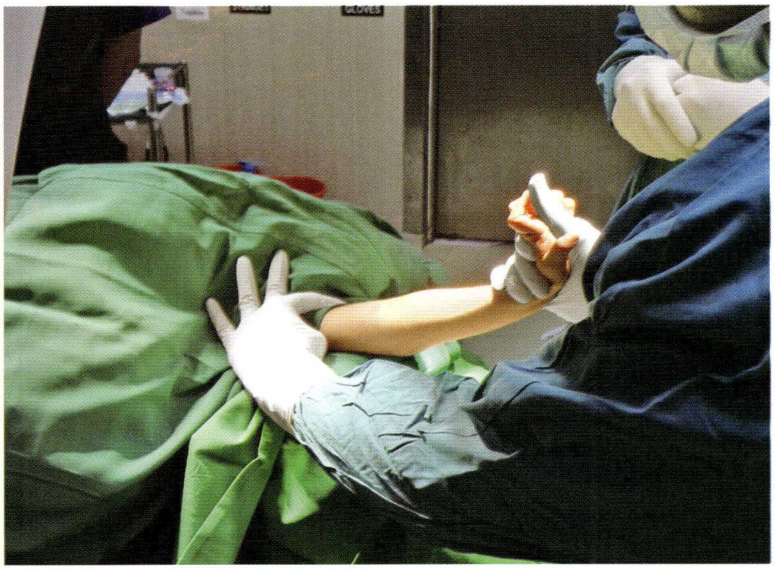

Fig. 6: Reduction maneuver.

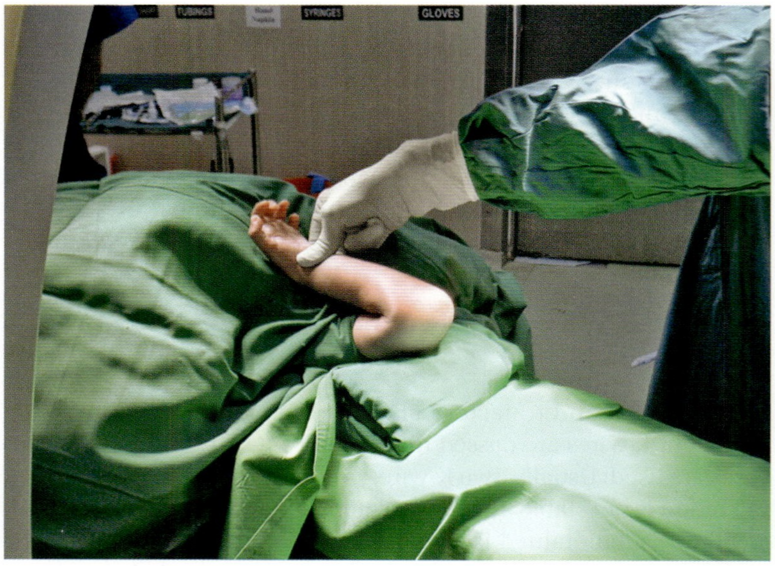

Fig. 7: Hyperflexion at the elbow and positioning for obtaining shoot through anteroposterior (AP) view on C-arm.

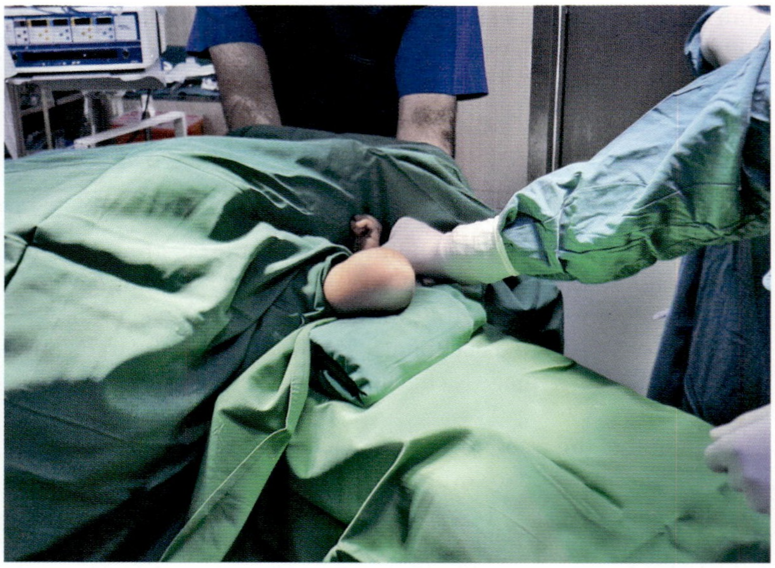

Fig. 8: Lateral position of rotating the arm through the shoulder to obtain lateral view on C-arm.

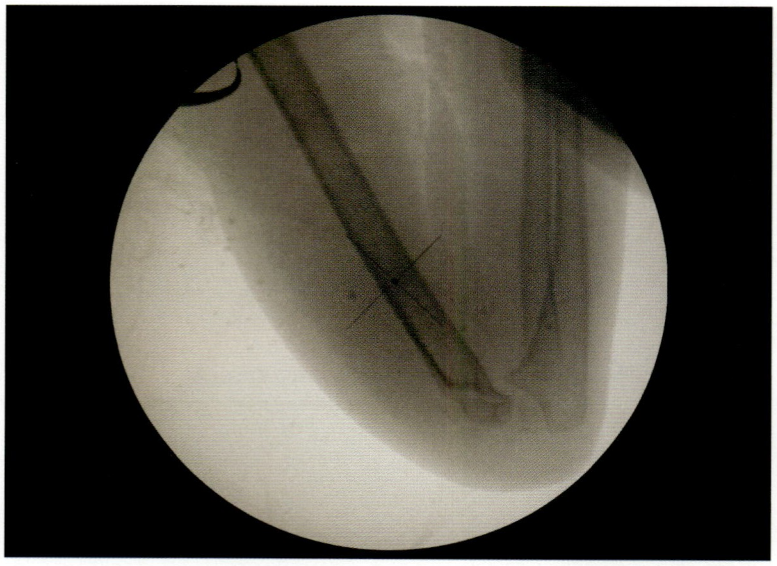

Fig. 9: Lateral view of the elbow.

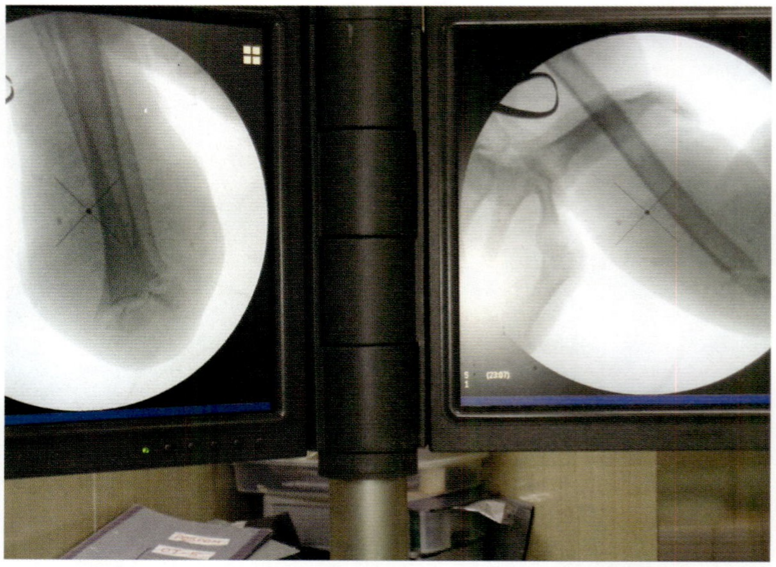

Fig. 10: Shoot through anteroposterior view of the distal humerus.

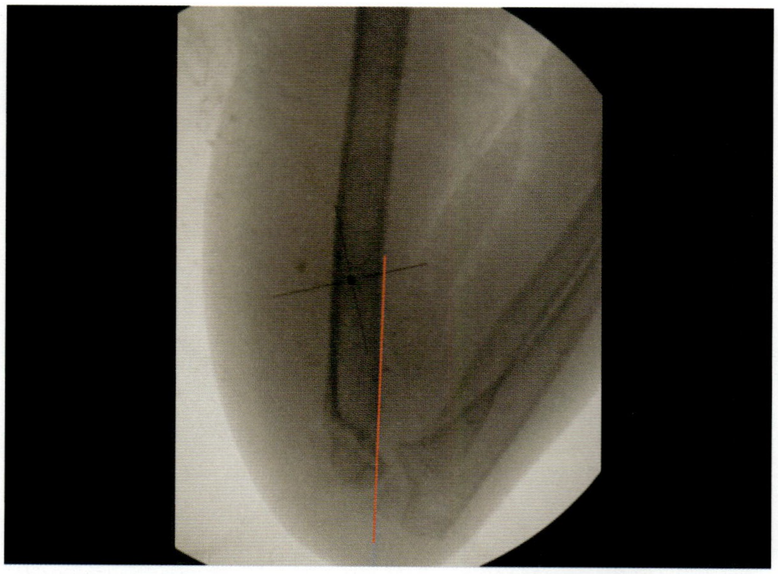

Fig. 11: Lateral view showing anterior humeral line passing through the center of the capitellum.

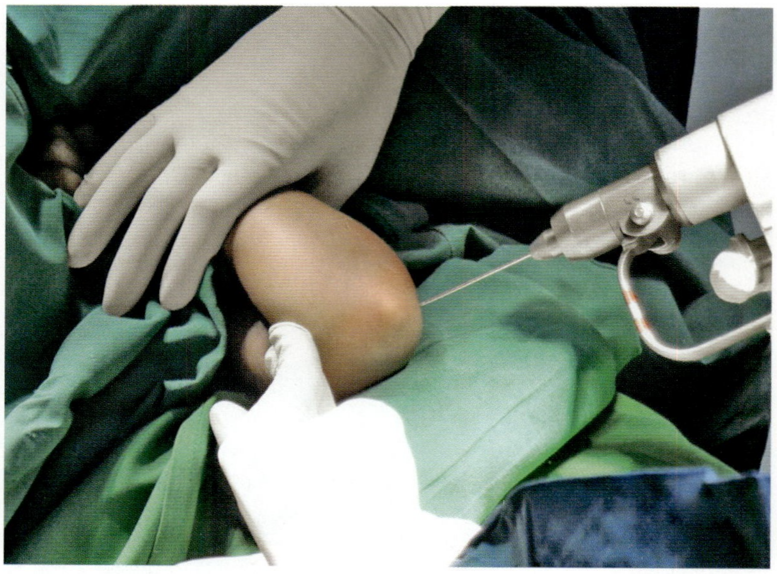

Fig. 12: Placement of first lateral entry of K-wire.

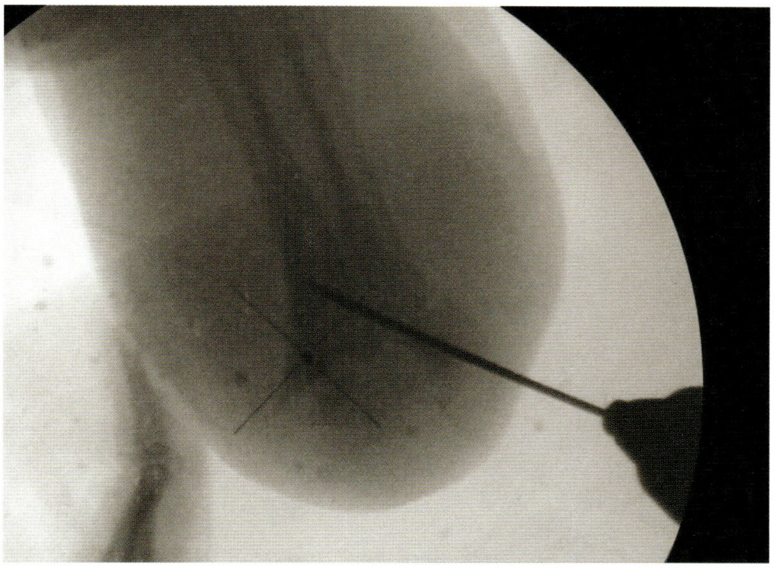

Fig. 13: Shoot through anteroposterior (AP) view showing K-wire trajectory and position.

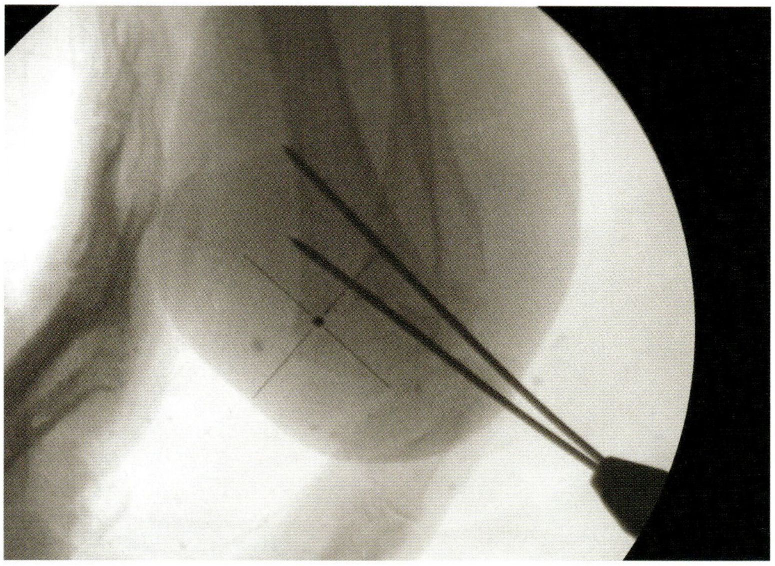

Fig. 14: Divergent K-wires.

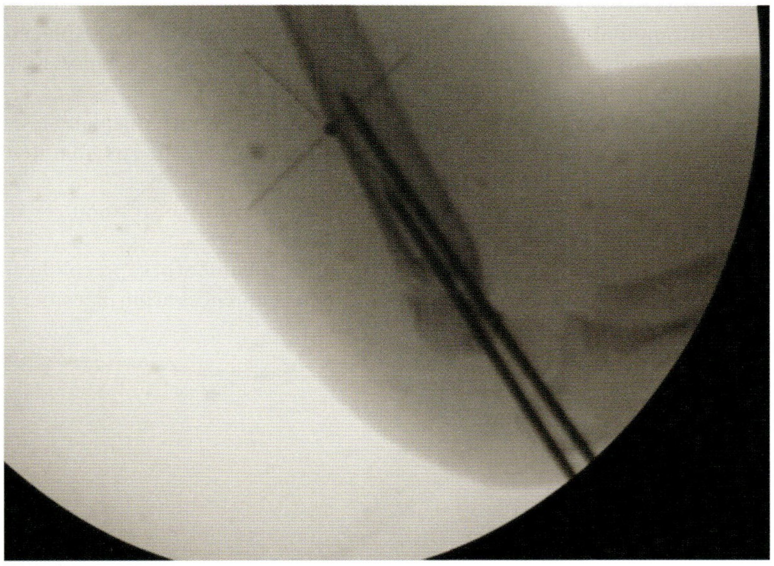

Fig. 15: Lateral view of elbow.

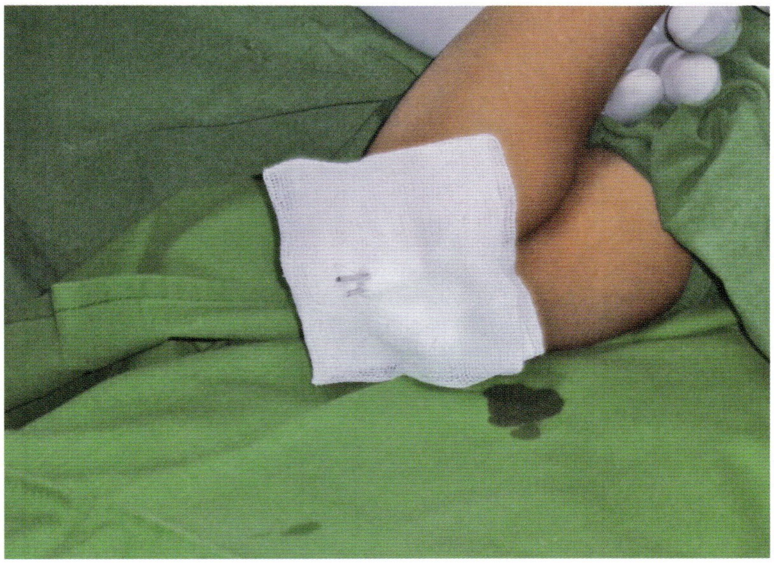

Fig. 16: Cut wire ends outside skin.

STABILITY ASSESSMENT

Under live fluoroscopy, elbow is carried out through range of motion—varus valgus stress and in lateral view. Watch for opening at the fracture site.

When to use medial pin?

Over preference is to use lateral entry K-wires for most the times and to use medial entry K-wire for following indications:

- Medial communition—to avoid varus collapse
- Oblique fractures
- Unstable fractures.

How to minimize ulnar nerve injury?

- Keep elbow in extension
- Start anteriorly on medial epicondyle
- Make a small incision over medial epicondyle and use drill guide to protect soft tissues.

K-wires are cut leaving approximately 2 cm outside skin and the tip is bent and sterile gauze is applied. Well-padded cast is applied while maintaining elbow at 70° of flexion (Figs. 16 to 18).

POSTOPERATIVE PROTOCOL

Elbow elevation on a pillow for 24 hours. Thereafter, upper extremity is supported in arm sling pouch.

At 3–4 weeks, check X-ray is obtained and if signs of union are seen, then K-wires are removed in outpatient clinic. Patient is instructed to use arm sling pouch for 1 week and to do elbow range of motion (ROM) exercises. Formal physiotherapy is usually not recommended unless significant elbow ROM has not been gained by 6 weeks after surgery. At 6–8 weeks after surgery, patient is advised to return to sports and other activities without any restrictions.

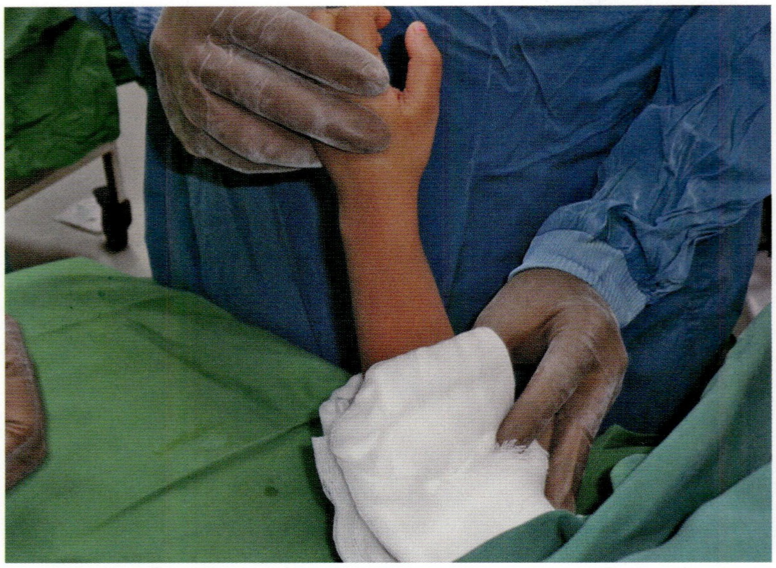

Fig. 17: Placement of sterile dressing over cut and bent K-wire ends.

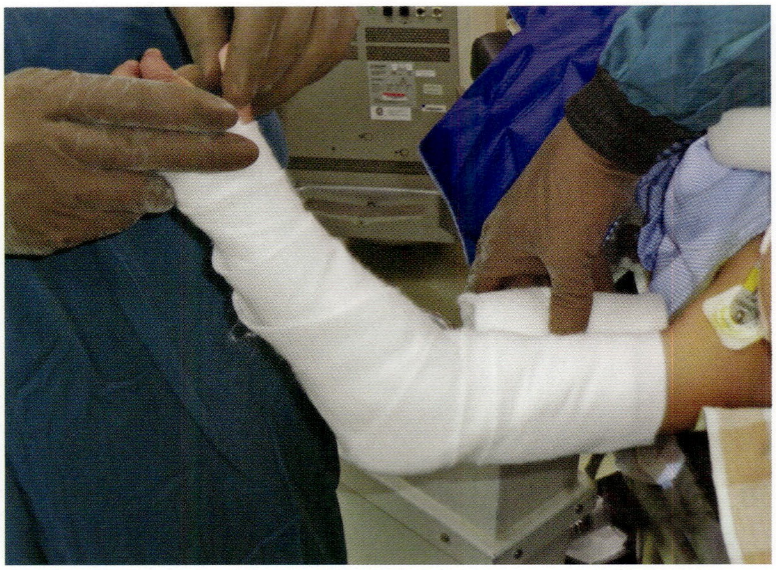

Fig. 18: Well-padded upper extremity with elbow in 70° of flexion before cast application.

COMPLICATIONS

Complications are uncommon. There might be loss of reduction in postoperative period. If it is noticed, then revision of K-wire may be necessary. Pin site infection is a rare complication.

SUGGESTED READING

1. Brauer CA, Lee BM, Bae DS, et al. A systematic review of medial and lateral entry pinning versus lateral entry pinning for supracondylar fractures of the humerus. J Pediatr Orthop. 2007;27(2):181-6.
2. Kocher MS, Kasser JR, Waters PM, et al. Lateral entry compared with medial and lateral entry pin fixation for completely displaced supracondylar humeral fractures in children. A randomized clinical trial. J Bone Joint Surg Am. 2007;89(4):706-12.
3. Larson L, Firoozbakhsh K, Passarelli R, et al. Biomechanical analysis of pinning techniques for pediatric supracondylar humerus fractures. J Pediatr Orthop. 2006;26(5):573-8.
4. Omid R, Choi PD, Skaggs DL. Supracondylar humeral fractures in children. J Bone Joint Surg Am. 2008;90(5):1121-32.
5. Skaggs DL, Hale JM, Bassett J, et al. Operative treatment of supracondylar fractures of the humerus in children. The consequences of pin placement. J Bone Joint Surg Am. 2001;83(5):735-40.

CHAPTER 6

Lateral Condylar Humerus Fracture Pinning

Mohan V Belthur

INTRODUCTION

Lateral humeral condyle fractures are intra-articular physeal injuries in skeletally immature patients. These are the second most common elbow fractures in children and represent about 15–20% of all pediatric elbow fractures. The average age of occurrence of a lateral condylar fractures is 6 (3–9) years old. Historically, these fractures have had worse outcome than other distal humerus fractures. Recently, controversy has developed regarding the optimal treatment options for these fractures which include nonoperative cast immobilization, closed reduction and internal fixation with percutaneous pins/screws, and finally open reduction and percutaneous pinning/screw fixation.

PATHOLOGICAL ANATOMY AND CLASSIFICATION

Anatomy

- The distal humerus is largely cartilaginous in children. The ossification centers appear in a fairly predictable pattern as shown in Figure 1.
- The lateral humeral condyle gets its blood supply from the profunda brachii artery. The artery is located on the posterior aspect of the distal humerus and can be disrupted if the surgical dissection is continued posteriorly on the distal humerus (Fig. 2).
- The soft tissue attachments include the common extensor—supinator muscle origin from the metaphysis of the lateral condyle and the lateral collateral ligament complex (radial collateral ligament, lateral ulnar collateral ligament, and the annular ligament).

Mechanism of injury: Two mechanisms of injury are thought to produce lateral humeral condylar humerus fractures.

- *Push off theory*: Fall onto an outstretched hand with a flexed elbow causes the radial head to impact the lateral condyle resulting in a lateral humeral condylar fracture.
- *Pull off theory*: Fall onto an outstretched hand with elbow extended and forearm supinated causes an avulsion fracture from the adduction force on the forearm and pull from the common extensor muscles.

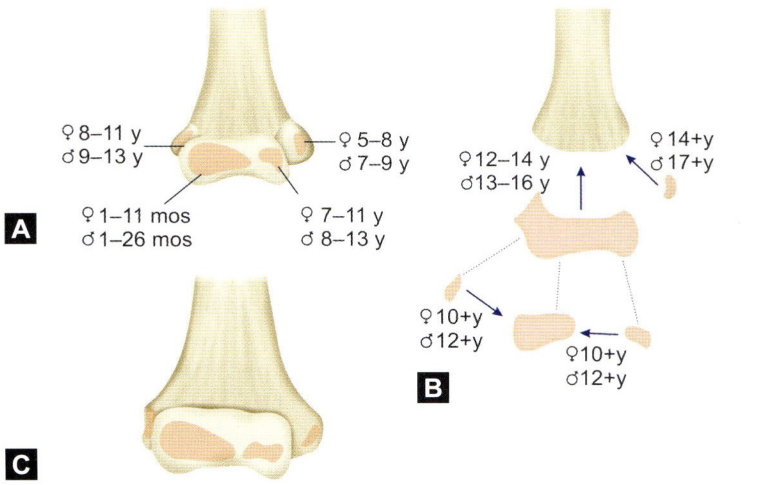

Figs. 1A to C: Appearance of ossification centers in the distal humerus.

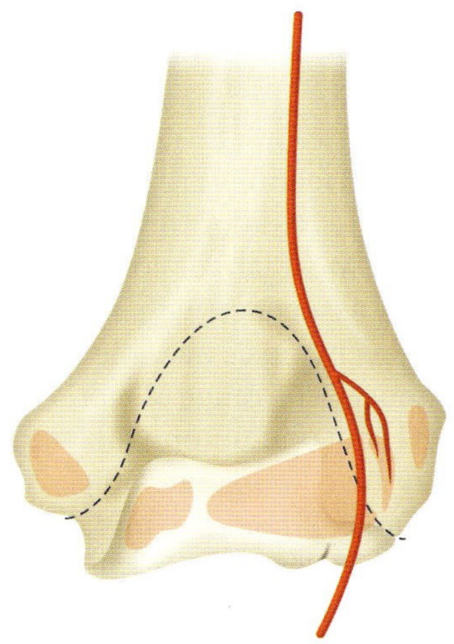

Fig. 2: Posterior view of the distal humerus showing the arterial supply to the lateral condyle.

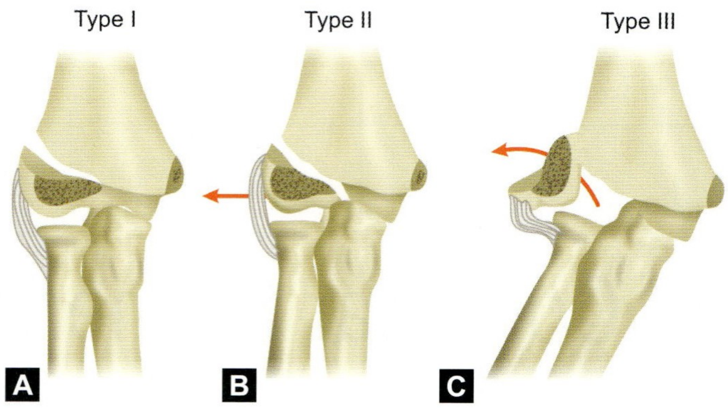

Fig. 3: Jakob classification of the distal humerus.

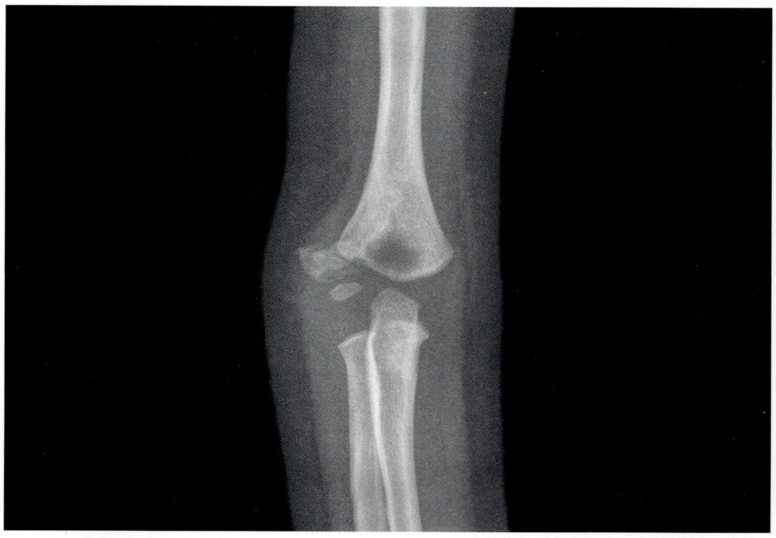

Fig. 4: An anteroposterior radiograph of the right elbow showing a displaced lateral condyle fracture of the distal humerus.

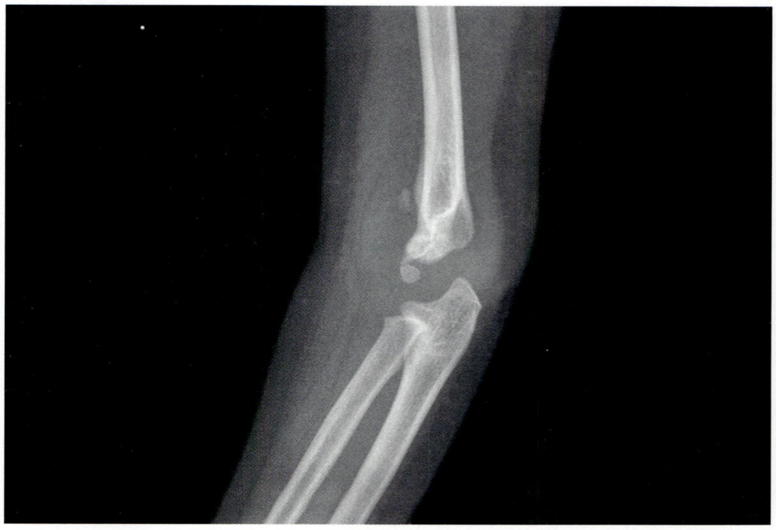

Fig. 5: A lateral radiograph of the right elbow showing a displaced lateral condyle fracture of the distal humerus.

Classification

Milch Classification

It is a radiographic classification based on the path of the fracture through the distal humerus. This is less frequently used as it does not help selecting treatment options.

Type 1: Fracture line is lateral to trochlear groove and is considered stable. This is the less common type.

Type 2: Fracture line extends into trochlear groove and is considered unstable. This is the most common fracture type.

Jakob Classification

This is based on the degree of displacement and therefore helps understand fracture stability and implies articular alignment. This is more useful for making treatment decisions (Fig. 3).

Type 1: Less than 2 mm displacement, intact cartilage hinge

Type 2: 2–4 mm displacement, disrupted cartilage hinge but no malrotation

Type 3: More than 2–4 mm displacement with disrupted articular surface and malrotation.

CLINICAL FEATURES

The most common clinical features are pain, swelling over the lateral aspect of the elbow. The joint deformity is less than what is seen in supracondylar fractures. Most lateral condyle fractures are isolated fractures and not usually associated with injuries in other areas of the body. Tenderness and ecchymosis over the lateral elbow are helpful in proper clinical diagnosis. The range of motion of the affected elbow is restricted by pain. It is not uncommon for lateral humeral condylar fractures to present to the orthopaedic office 2–3 weeks after initial injury due to families mistaking the elbow injury to be just a minor injury or even due to missed diagnoses of minimally displaced fracture by other healthcare providers. These fractures should still be treated to prevent long-term complications. The diagnosis is really confirmed with radiographs of the elbow. Radiographs are also important for treatment decision making.

RADIOLOGICAL IMAGING

- Anteroposterior and lateral radiographs are mandatory for diagnosis of lateral humeral condyle fractures (Figs. 4 and 5). Internal rotation radiograph of the distal humerus is the best view to judge displacement of the fracture fragment.
- An elbow arthrogram can also help classify the fracture displacement.
- Advanced imaging with an MRI can also be obtained to assess fracture displacement.
- *Fat pad sign*: Elevation of the posterior fat pad noted on the lateral X-ray represents joint distension from an intracapsular injury. This can indicate an intra-articular fracture, supracondylar fracture, elbow dislocation with spontaneous reduction or infection.

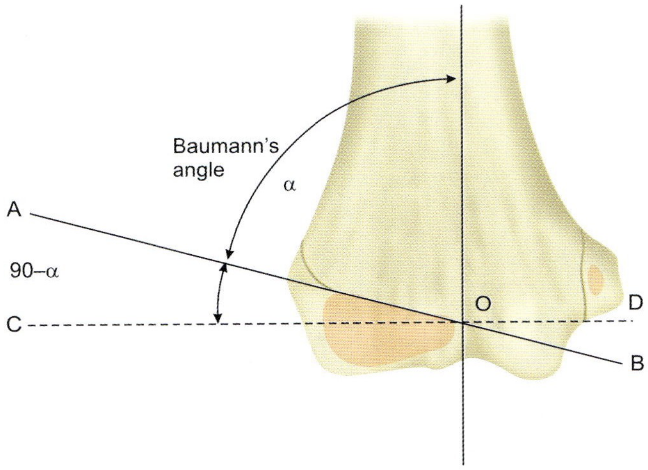

Fig. 6: Baumann's angle. The angle formed by the physeal line and the long axis of the humerus.

- *Baumann's angle*: The angle formed by the capitellar physeal line and the long axis of the humerus can be used to monitor alignment of the distal humerus. Normal angle is between 70–75° (Fig. 6).
- Comparison X-rays of the contralateral elbow can sometimes help differentiate between normal and abnormal anatomy in a pediatric elbow.
- Associated injuries although rare may need to be identified. These include radial neck, olecranon, Monteggia fractures, elbow dislocations and floating elbow injuries.

TREATMENT OPTIONS

- Jakob type I fractures can be treated nonoperatively with a long arm cast but need careful follow-up with anteroposterior, lateral, and internal oblique radiographs.
- Jakob type II fractures can be treated with closed or open reduction and stabilization with percutaneous Kirschner wires or screws.
- Jakob type III fractures usually require open reduction and stabilization with Kirschner wires or screws.

Nonoperative Treatment with Immobilization

Indications

Fractures with less than 2 mm of displacement and no joint incongruity noted on the internal rotation X-rays or noted on advanced imaging such as an MRI. About 40% of fractures can be treated with immobilization alone. The period of immobilization is usually from 4–6 weeks and can be discontinued once radiographic signs of bone healing are visible.

Procedure

- Immobilize in a long arm cast with elbow flexed between 70° and 90° and forearm in neutral position.
- X-rays are obtained out of the cast for the first 2 weeks. Continue cast treatment if no displacement is noted.
- Immobilization is continued for 4–6 weeks until fracture is fully healed.

Closed Reduction and Percutaneous Stabilization

Indications

Fractures with 2–4 mm of displacement at the articular surface and joint incongruity but no malrotation noted on the internal rotation X-rays or noted on advanced imaging such as an arthrogram.

Structures at Risk

The median nerve is at risk with K-wires that are placed too far through the medial distal humerus cortex.

Procedure

- Closed reduction is performed with direct pressure over the fracture fragment with the elbow flexed, the forearm supinated and wrist dorsiflexion.
- Two diverging pins are placed through the lateral distal humerus across the fracture site and into the intact medial column engaging the far cortex.
- Alternatively, if the metaphyseal part of the fracture is large enough a single 4.0 mm lateral cannulated lag screw can be placed for fracture stabilization.
- Joint congruity is confirmed with an arthrogram.
- Open reduction is preformed if closed reduction fails
- Immobilize in a well-padded long arm bivalve cast.

Open Reduction and Stabilization

Indications

- Fractures with greater than 2–4 mm of displacement, joint incongruity and malrotation noted on the internal rotation X-rays or noted on advanced imaging such as an arthrogram, MRI or CT scan.
- Failed closed reduction in Jakob type two fractures.
- Nonunion.

The procedure is preformed through a lateral or posterolateral approach to the elbow.

Structures at Risk

- The median nerve is at risk with K-wires that are placed too far through the medial distal humerus cortex. It is also at risk if any retractors such as Homan's are placed over the anterior and medial humerus.
- The blood supply to the fracture fragment is located on the posterior aspect of the distal humerus. The surgical dissection should stay on the anterior aspect of the humerus.

Procedure

(For Procedure *see* Figures 7 to 28)

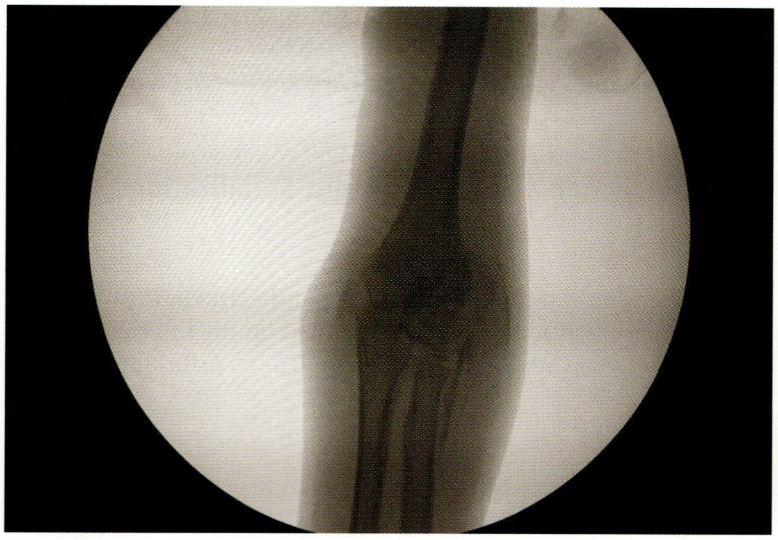

Fig. 7: X ray—intraoperative C-arm anteroposterior image of the left distal humerus with arthrogram showing a displaced lateral condyle fracture of the humerus.

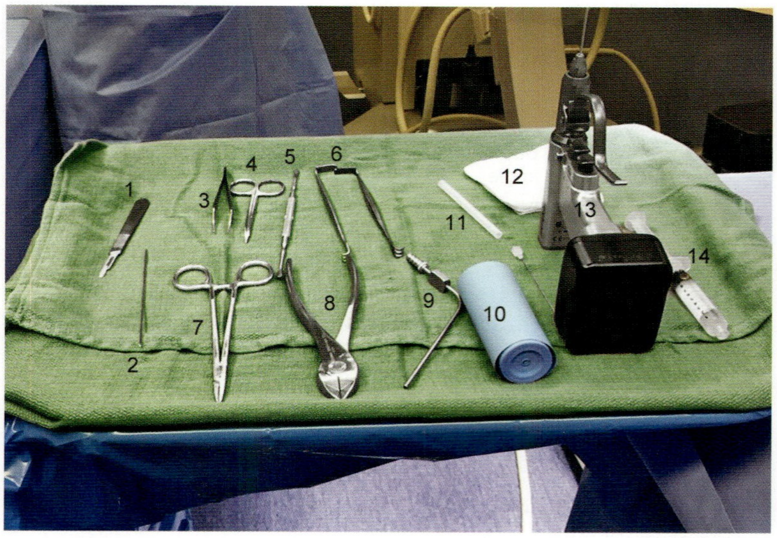

Fig. 8: Instruments—(1) 15 blade on a scalpel, (2) 0.062 or 2 mm K-wires, (3) Forceps, (4) Tenotomy scissors, (5) Freer elevator, (6) Senn retractor, (7) Heavy needle driver, (8) Wire cutter, (9) Frazier tip suction, (10) Esmarch tourniquet bandage, (11) Spinal needle, (12) Sponges, (13) K-wire power driver, (14) Arthrogram solution in syringe. Optional equipment not shown: sterile tourniquet, reduction forceps, arm navy retractor, Weitlaner retractor, Hohmann retractors, Headlamp for visualization.

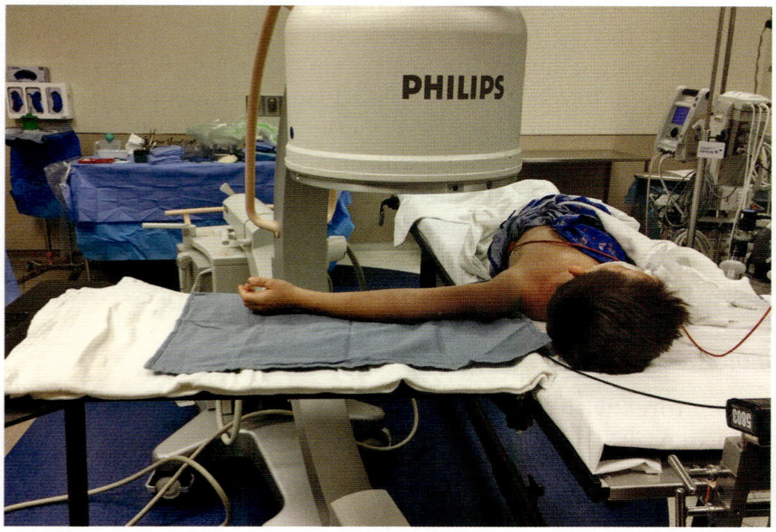

Fig. 9: Position—under general anesthesia patient is positioned supine on operating table with affected upper extremity positioned on a hand table. The surgeon is positioned near the head of the patient and C-arm is positioned at the end of the hand table or at the axilla of the patient.

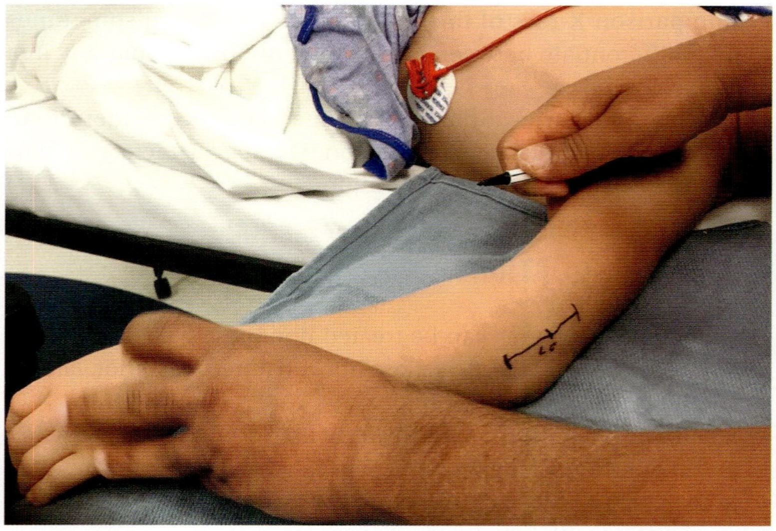

Fig. 10: Incision marking—lateral approach: curved incision 5–6 cm, centered over the lateral epicondyle, two-thirds of the incision should be proximal to the joint line. The incision should be slightly more anterior than standard Kocher approach to allow for pins to be placed through the skin posteriorly.

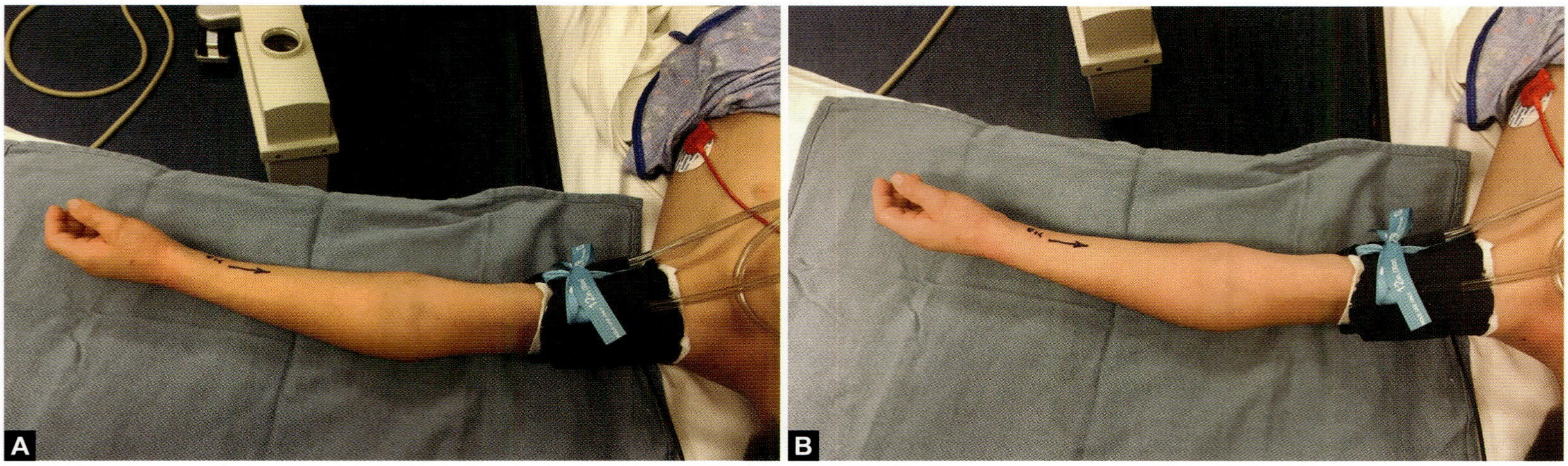

Figs. 11A and B

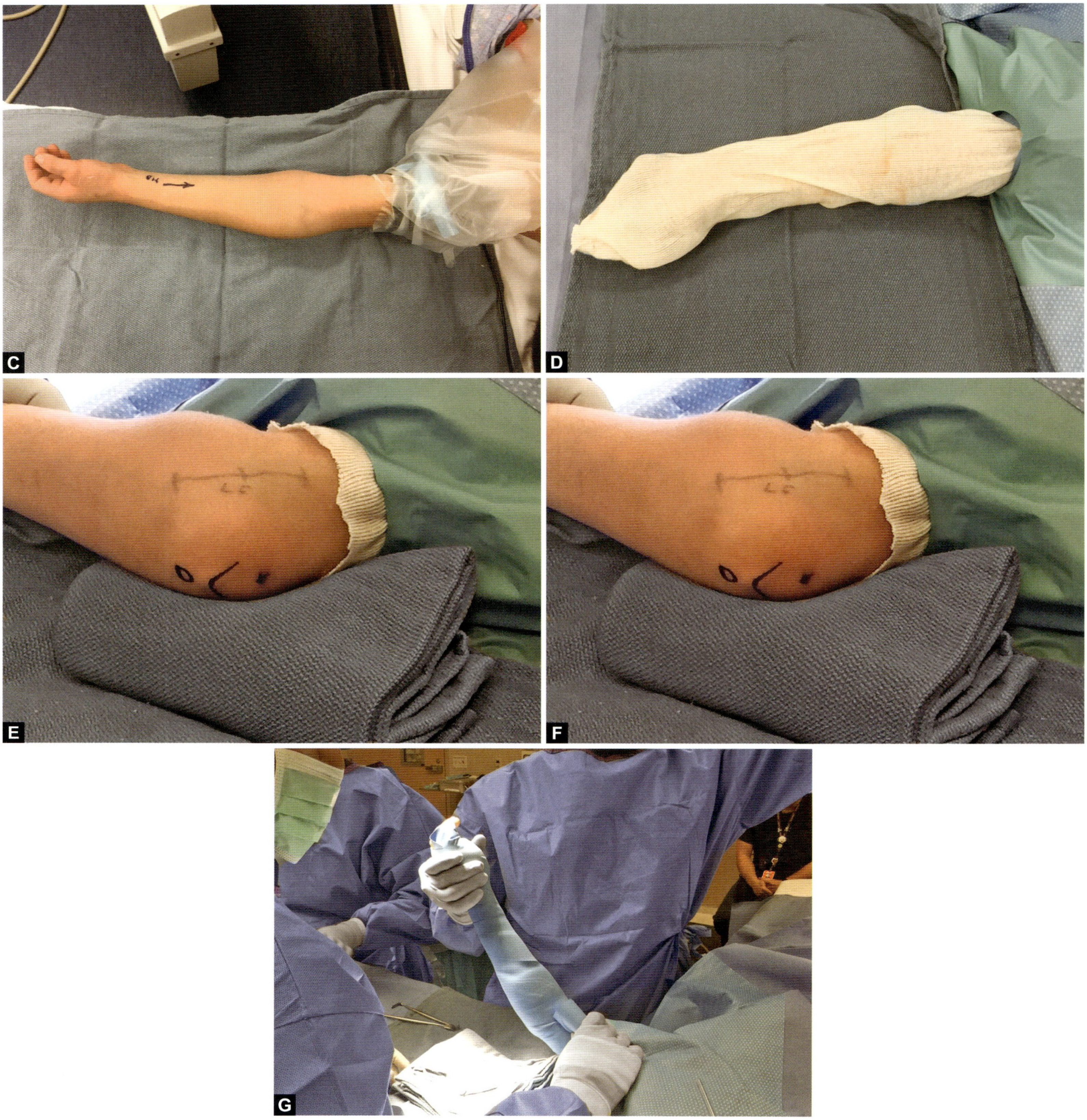

Figs. 11C to G

Figs. 11A to G: Draping—upper limb draped separately for ease of manipulation. Arm is exsanguinated with an Esmarch bandage and tourniquet is inflated.

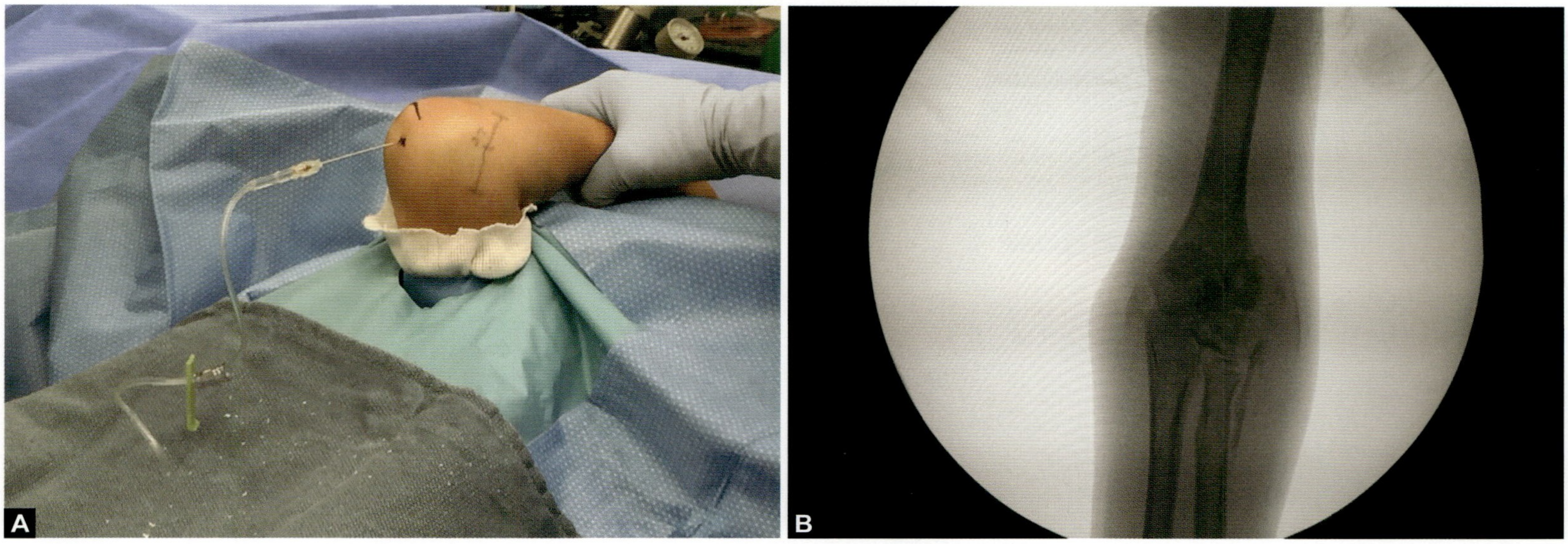

Figs. 12A and B: Imaging—an elbow arthrogram is obtained by placing a spinal needle about 1 cm proximal to the top of the olecranon into the olecranon fossa and elbow joint. The anteroposterior C-arm image confirms the displaced lateral humeral condyle fracture.

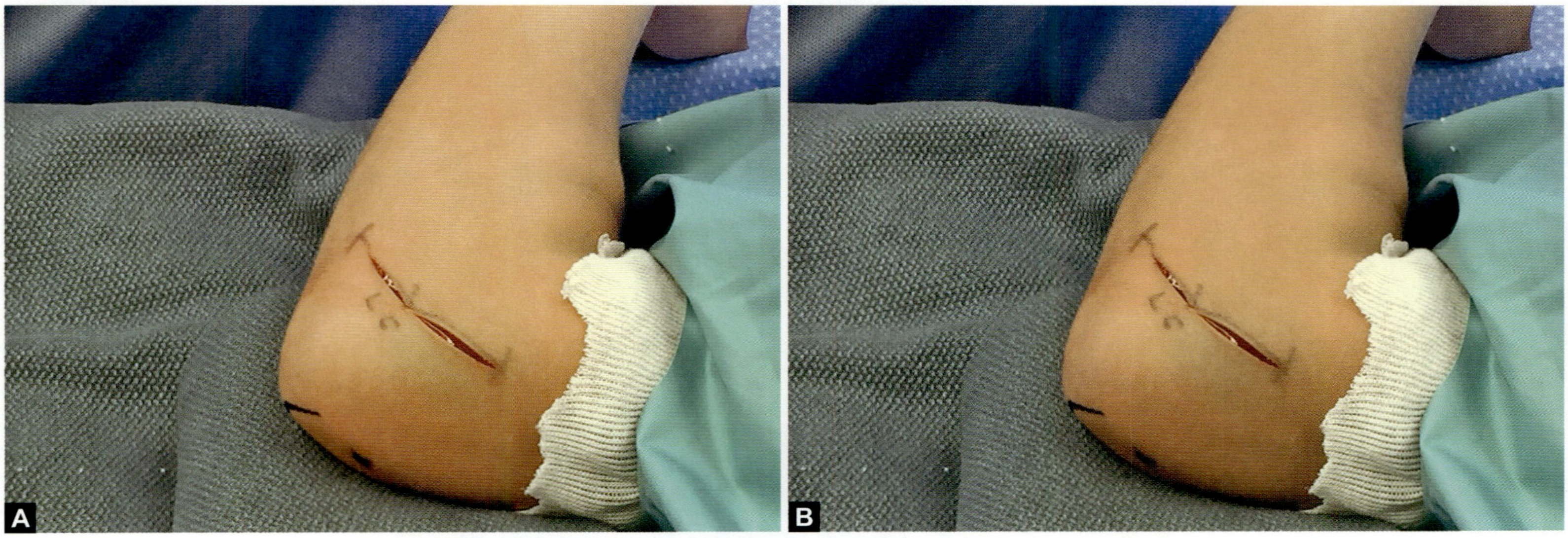

Figs. 13A and B: Skin incision is made with a number 15 blade.

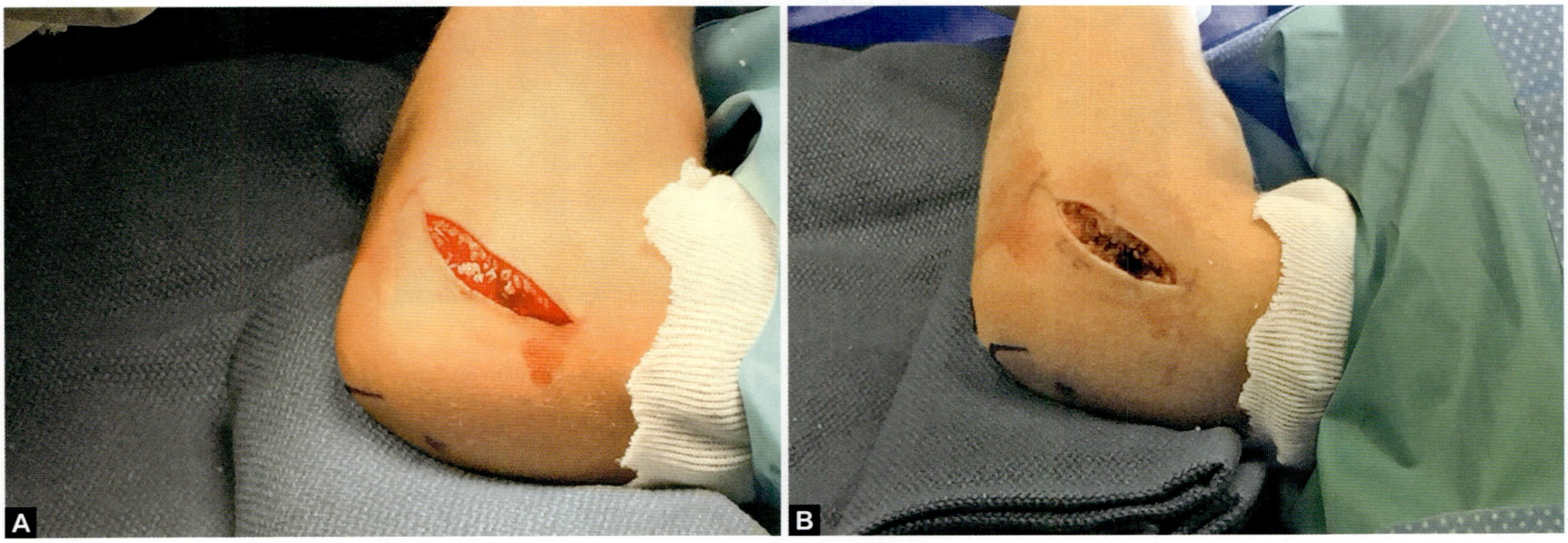

Figs. 14A and B

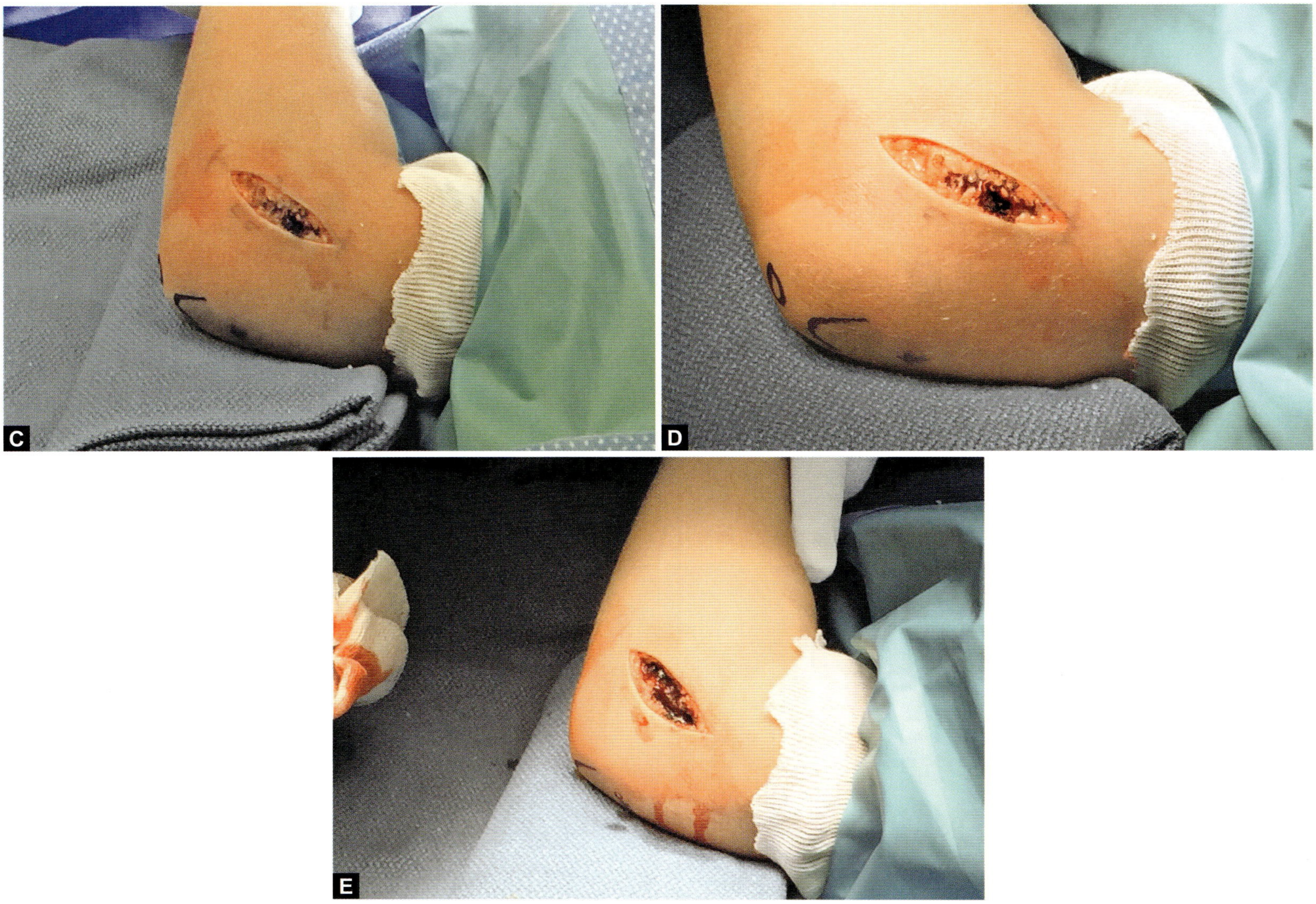

Figs. 14C to E

Figs. 14A to E: Blunt subcutaneous dissection and cauterization of bleeders.

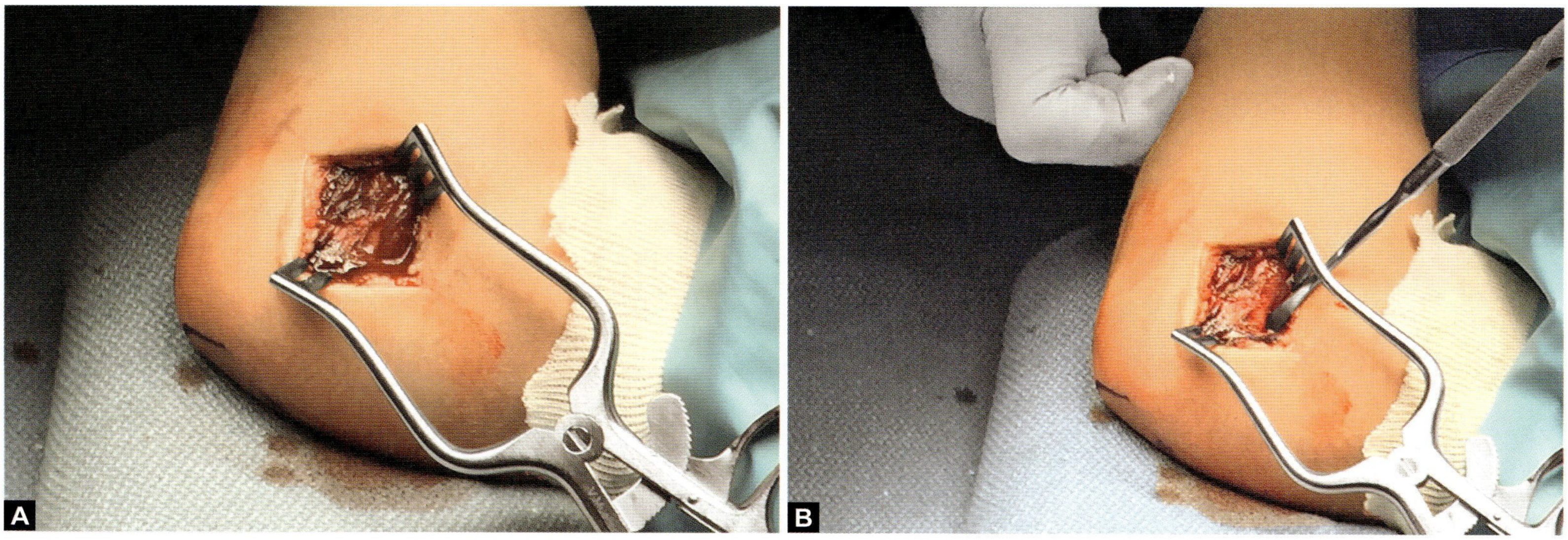

Figs. 15A and B: The interval is between the brachioradialis anteriorly and the triceps posteriorly. Many times the fracture hematoma dissects the brachioradialis and leads to the fracture site.

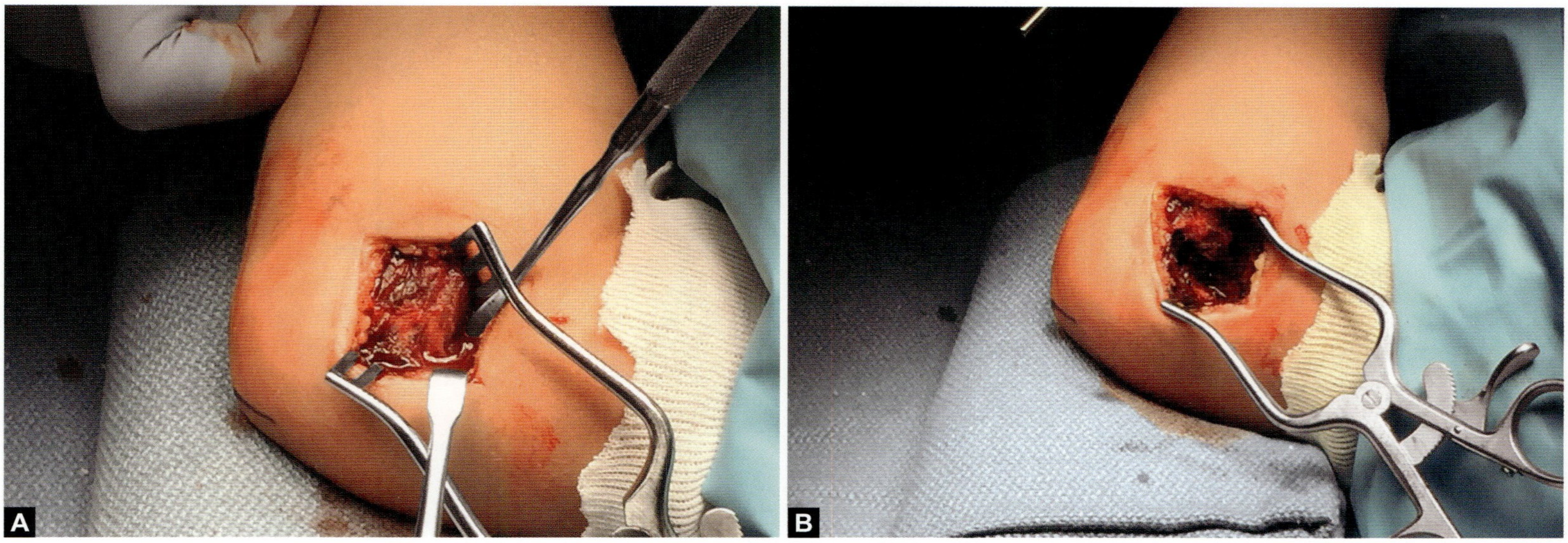

Figs. 16A and B: The anterior humerus is exposed dissecting common extensor mass. Do *not* dissect posteriorly.

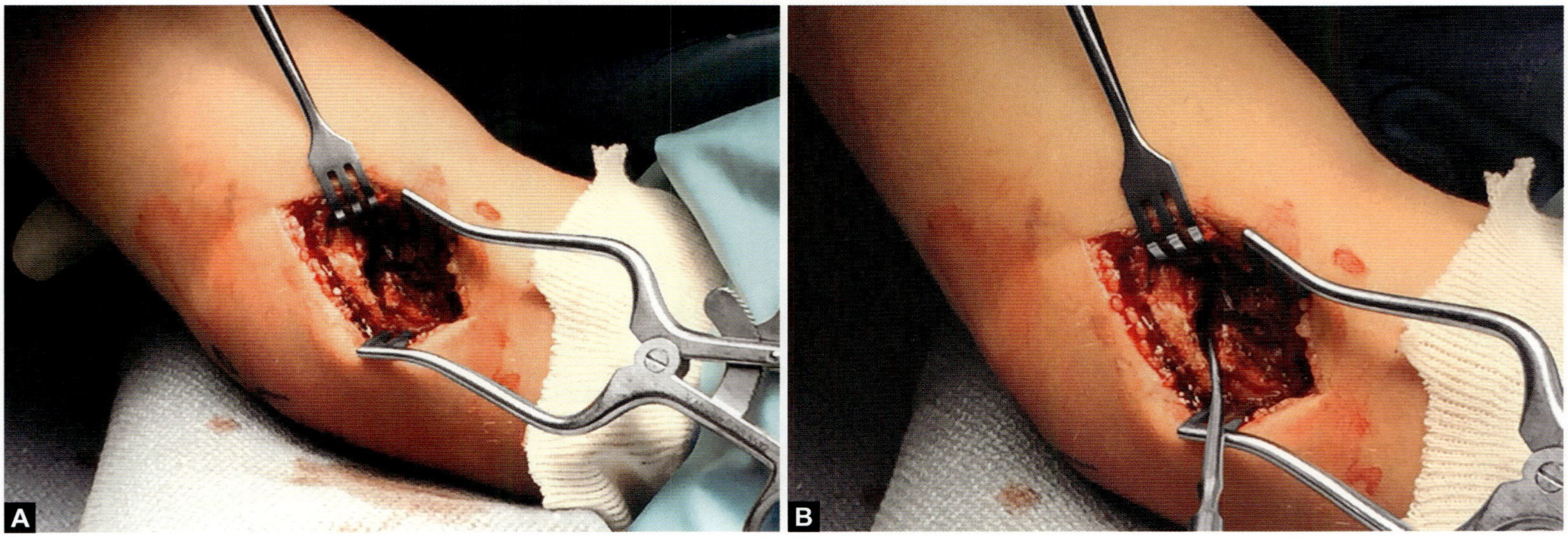

Figs. 17A and B: Identify the displaced and rotated lateral codylar fragment.

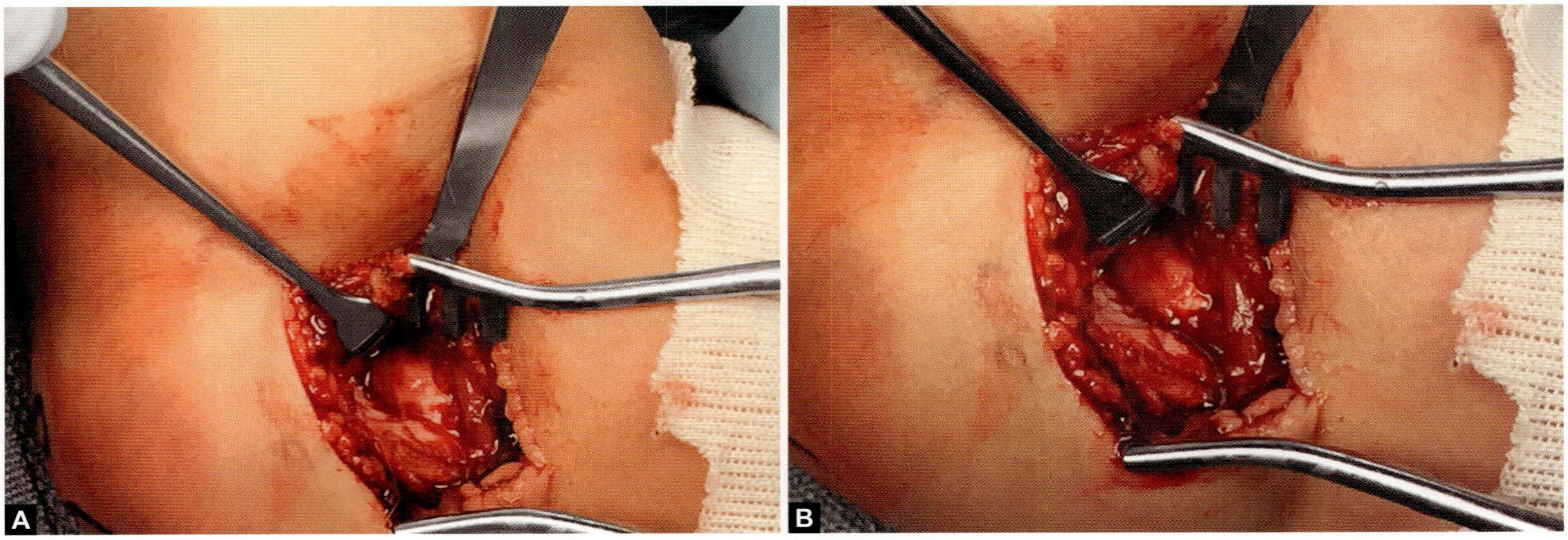

Figs. 18A and B

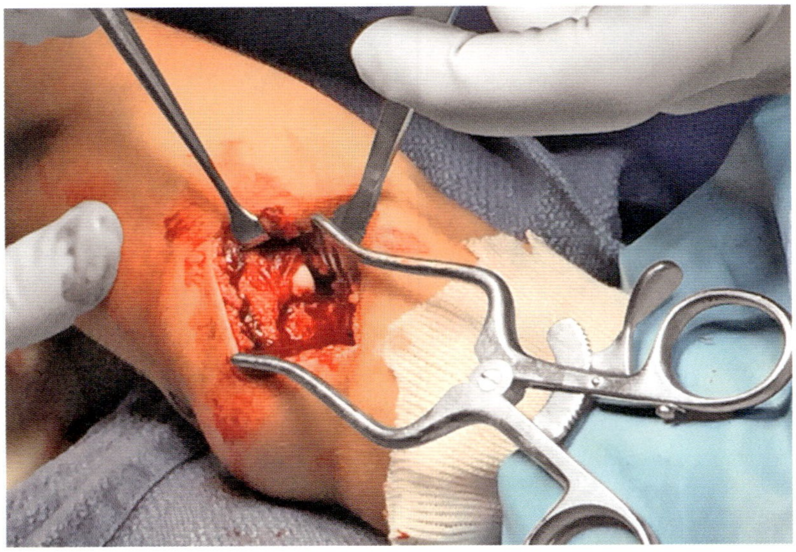

Fig. 18C

Figs. 18A to C: Retraction of the anterior cubital structures with Hohmann or Army-Navy retractor to better visualize fracture site. Headlamp can illuminate fracture site better.

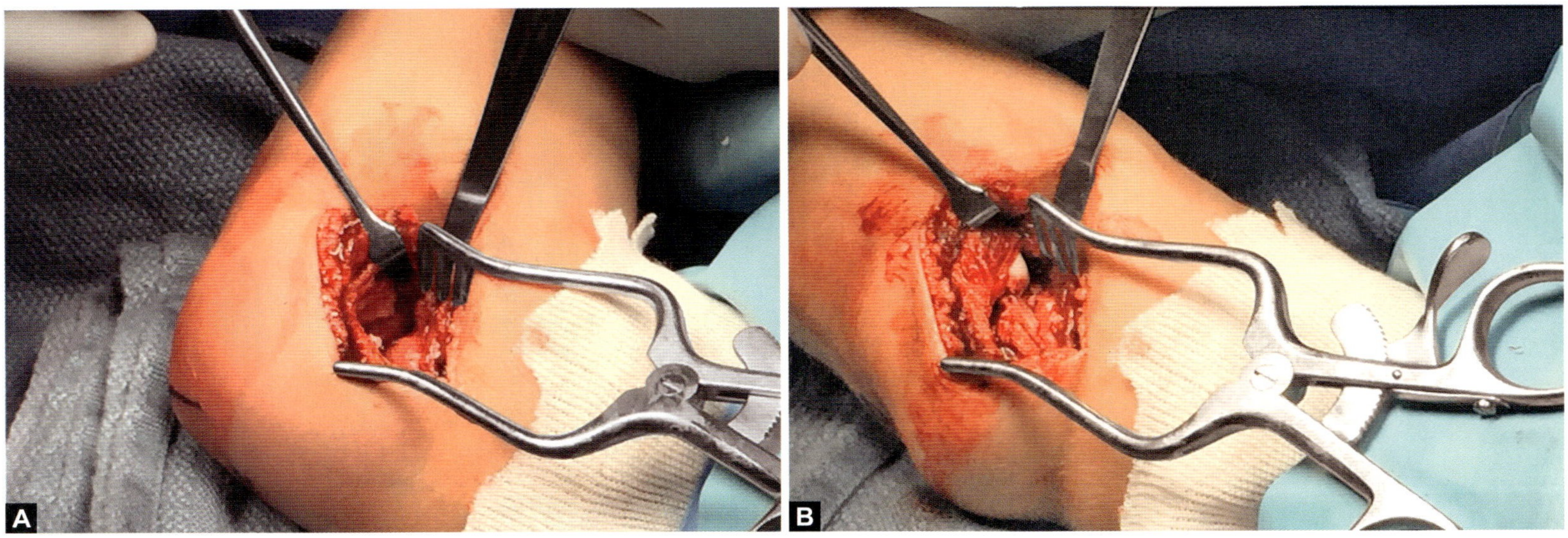

Figs. 19A and B: Fracture site after irrigation and debridement of fracture hematoma.

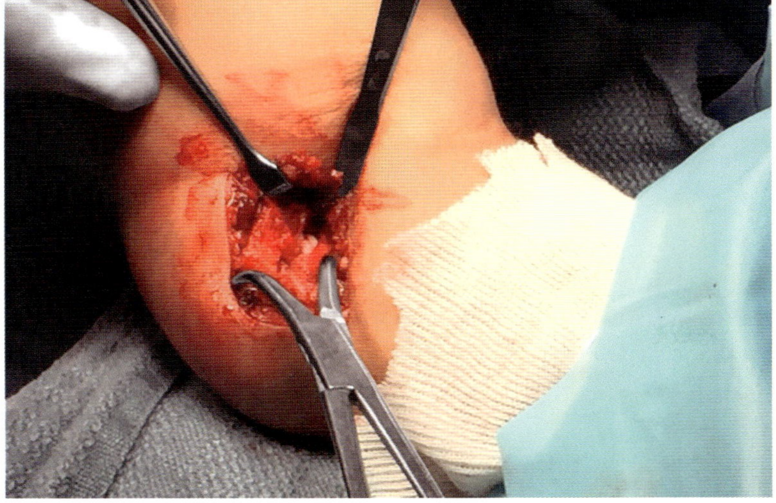

Fig. 20: Fracture reduction using small pointed reduction forceps, the reduction can be held making a small hole in the proximal metaphysis. One prong of the reduction forceps is placed into the hole and the other prong is placed over the lateral condylar fragment to hold the reduction and to allow compression of the fracture. The fracture can also be reduced with digital reduction if a reduction forceps could not be placed.

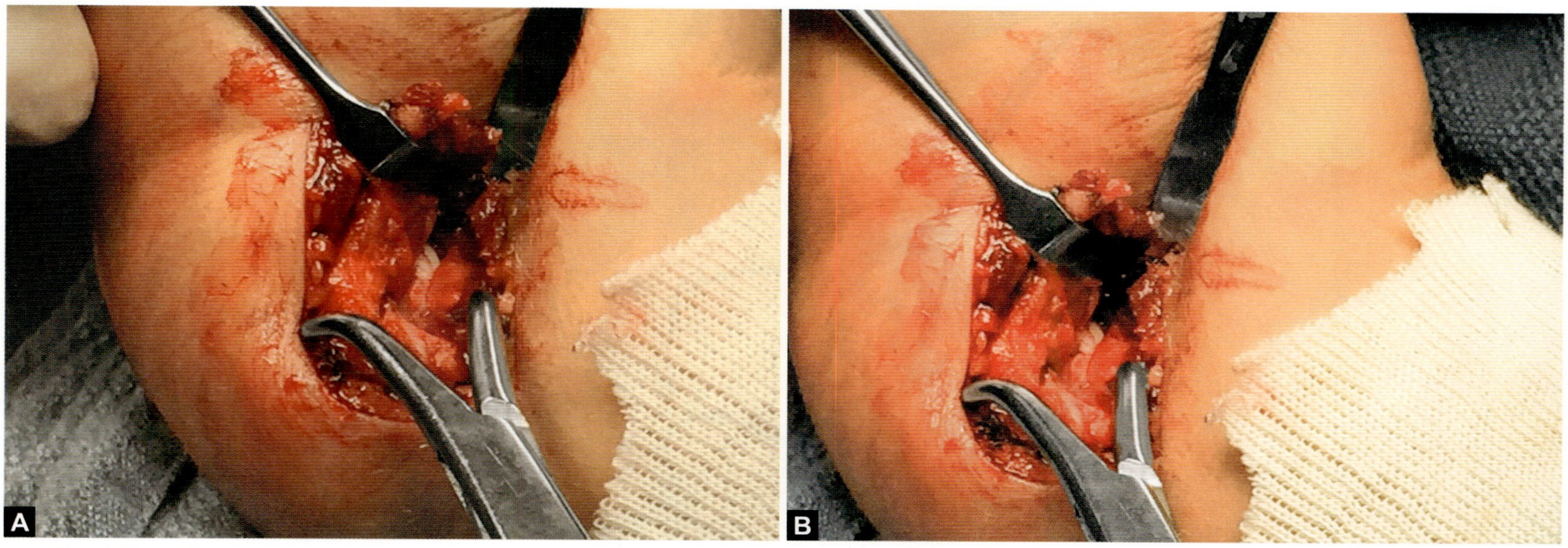

Figs. 21A and B: The reduction should be confirmed under direct visualization. Use the joint line to assess the fracture reduction. Do not use the metaphysis as metaphyseal comminution is common and can cause fracture malreduction if used to evaluate the reduction.

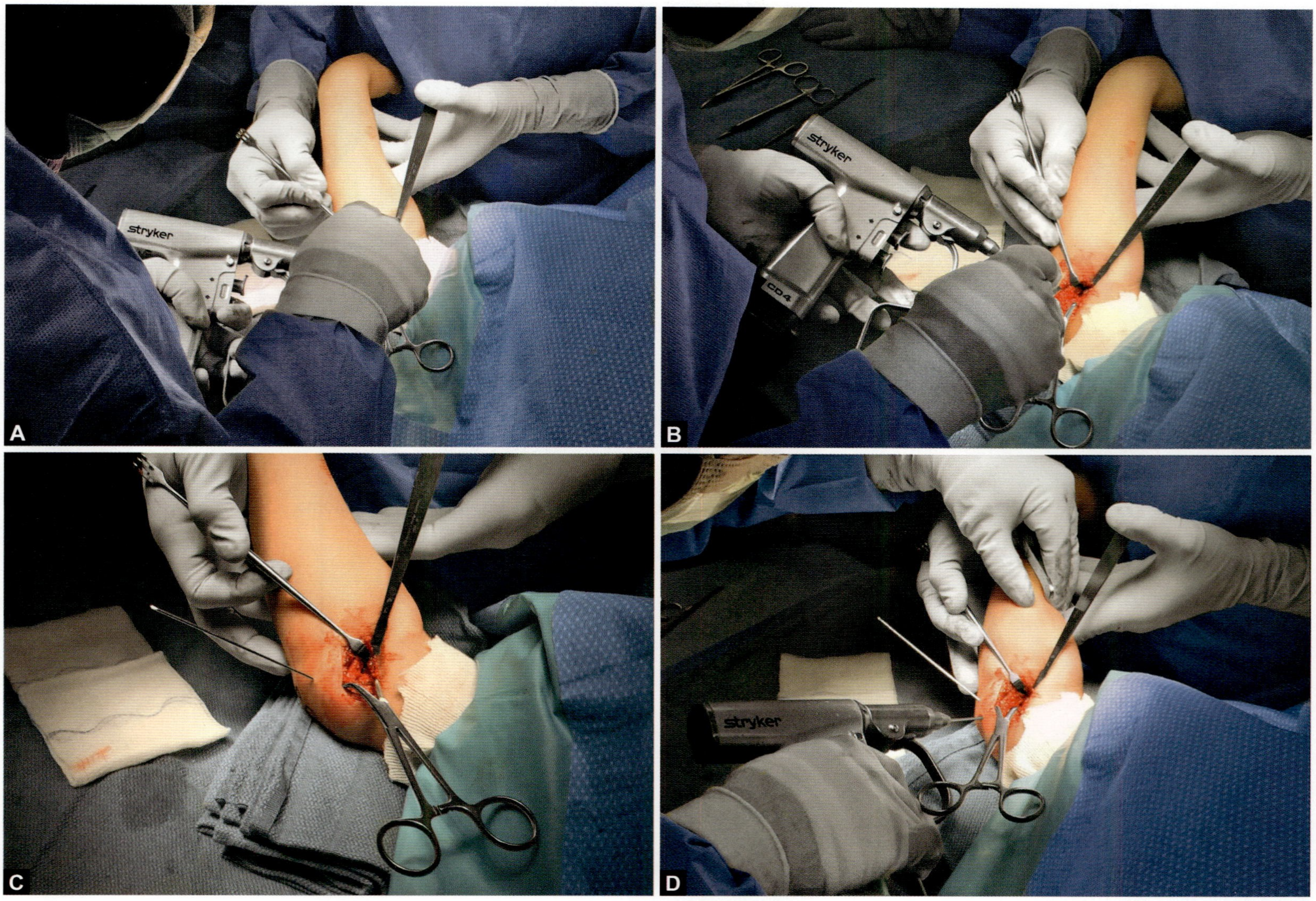

Figs. 22A to D

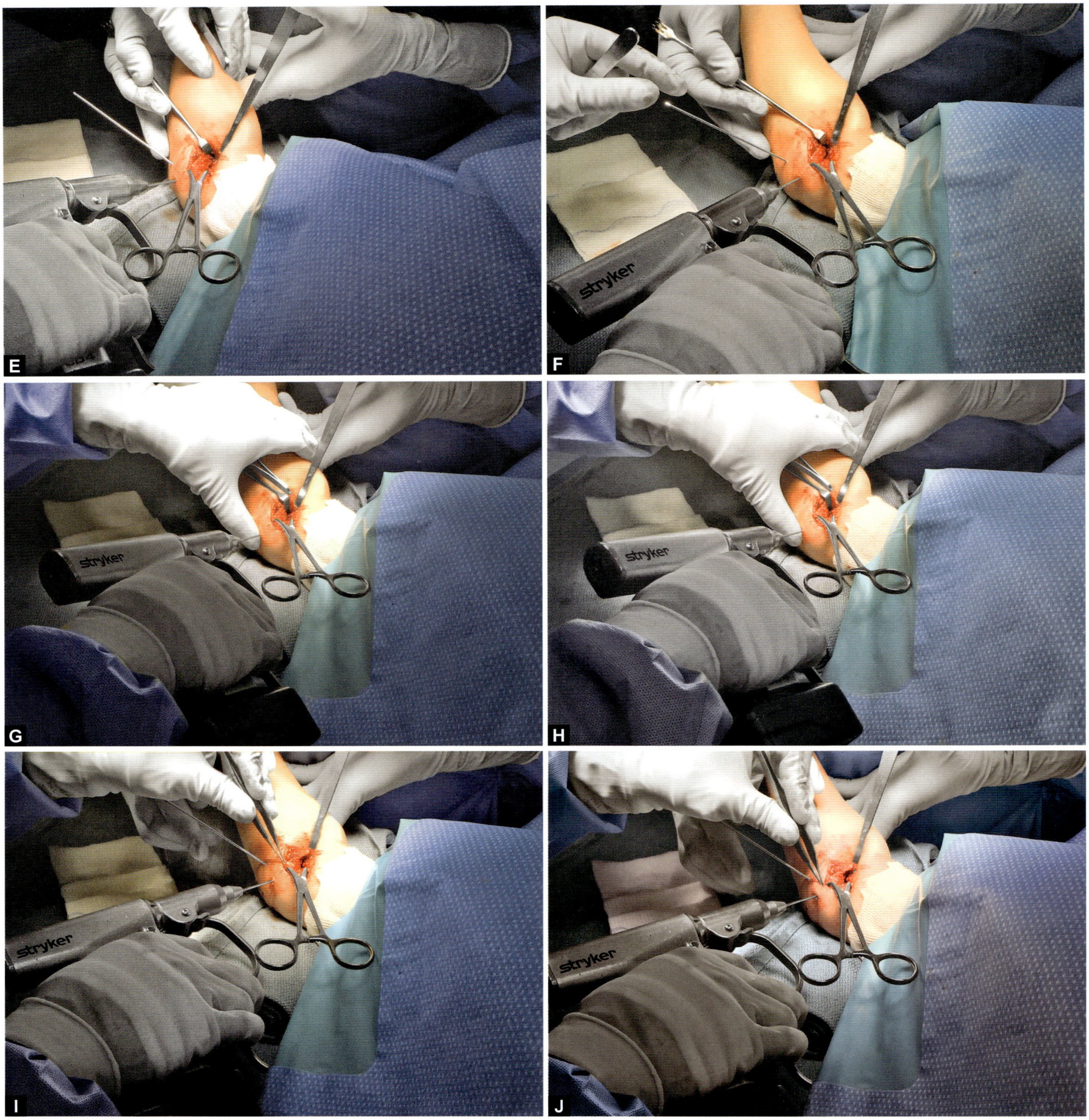

Figs. 22E to J

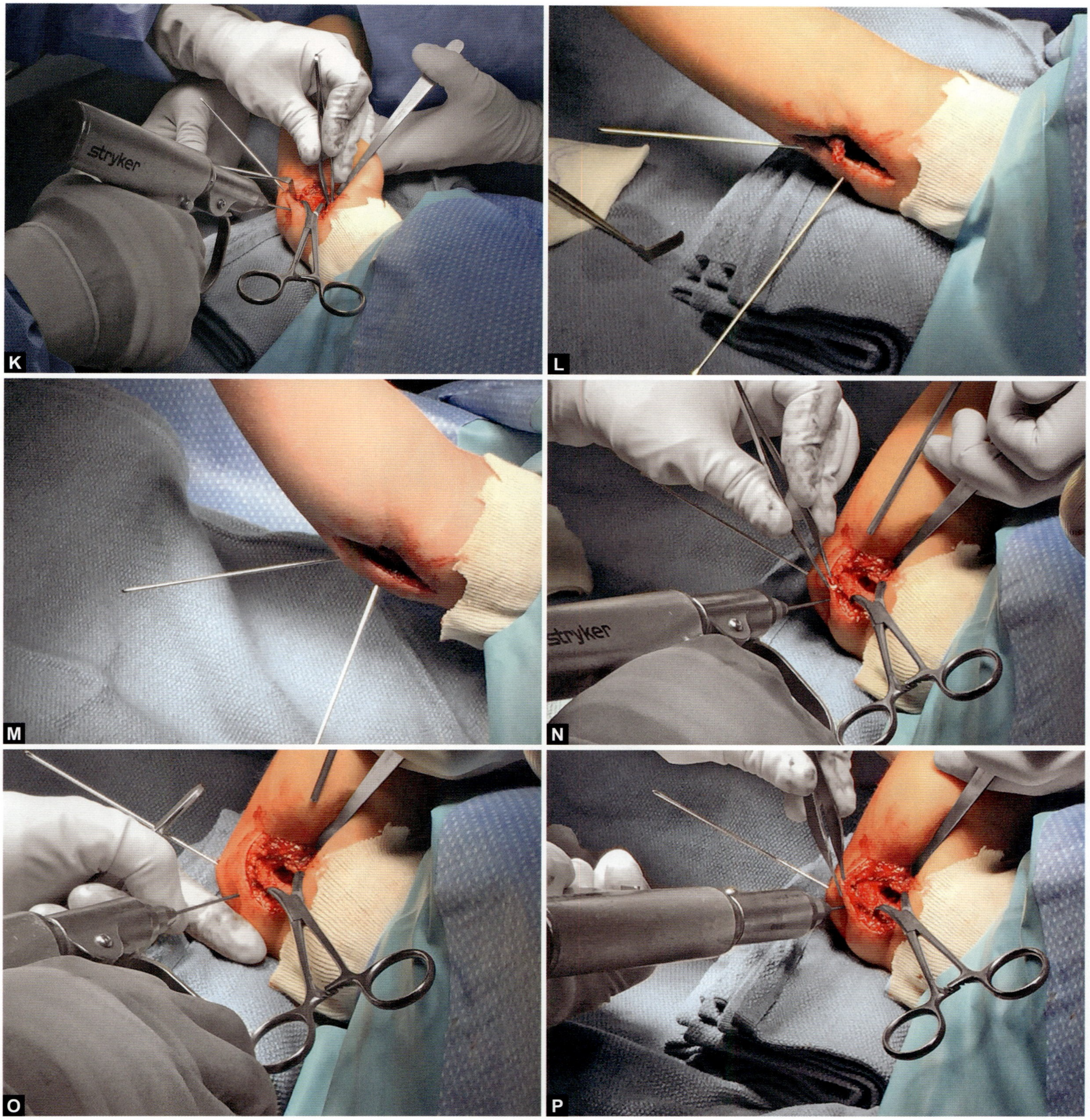

Figs. 22K to P

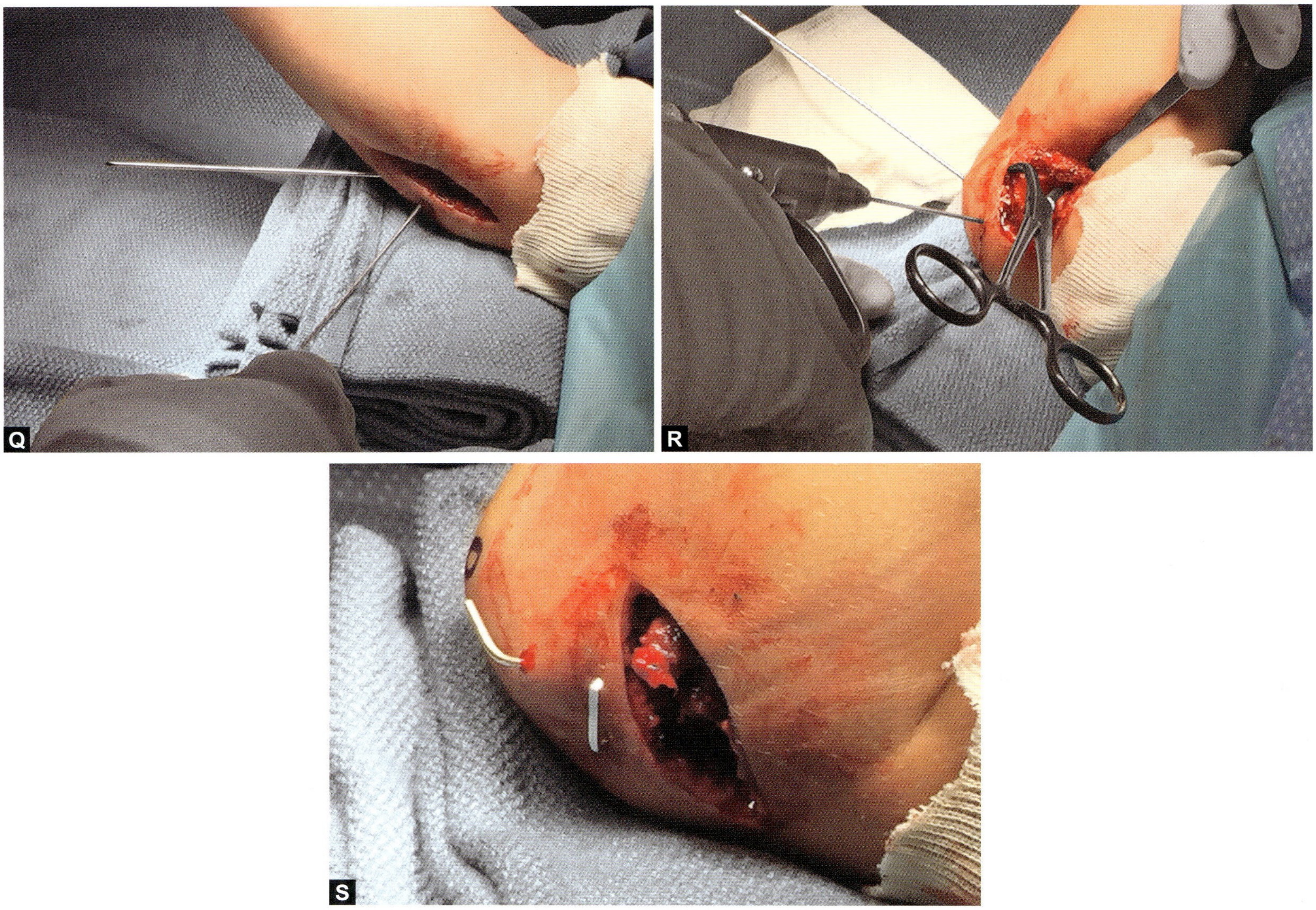

Figs. 22Q to S

Figs. 22A to S: Two K-wires are placed through the skin posterior to the incision from the lateral distal humerus then proximally and medially across the fracture site. The pins should be divergent as much as possible.

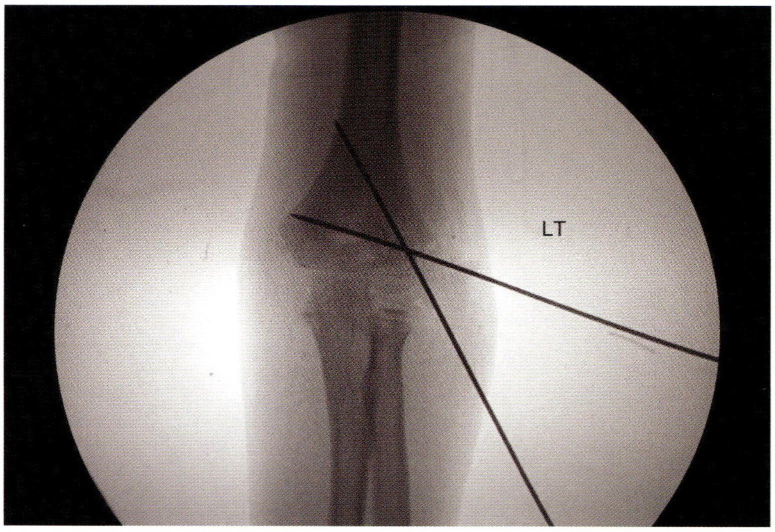

Fig. 23: C-arm imaging with an arthrogram is shown confirming proper reduction of the fracture.

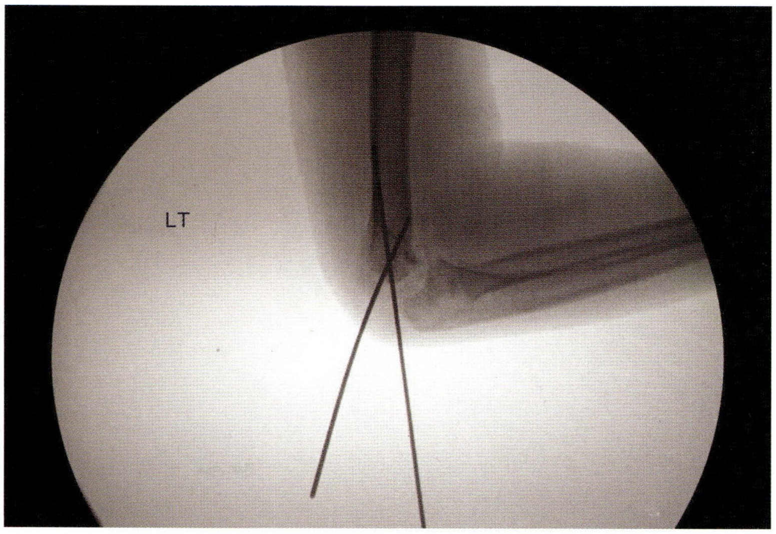

Fig. 24: Lateral view with C-arm imaging of the distal humerus confirms fracture reduction.

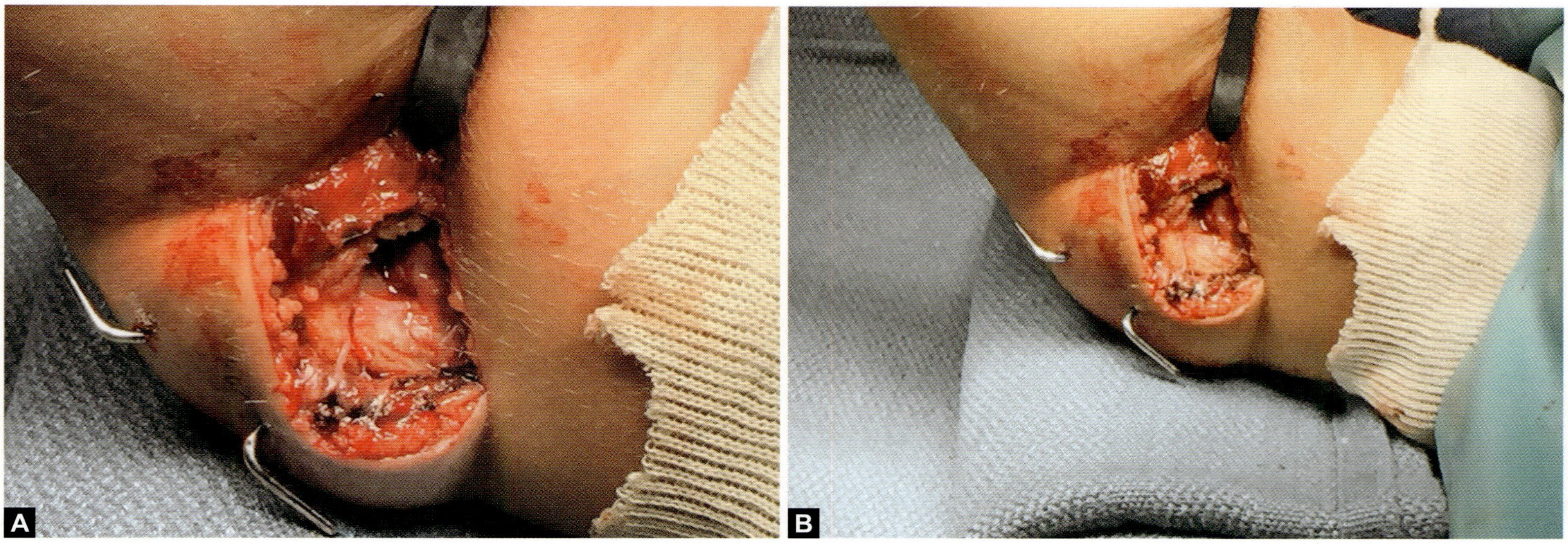

Figs. 25A and B: The K-wires are bent and cut once a proper reduction is noted on X-ray and under direct visualization.

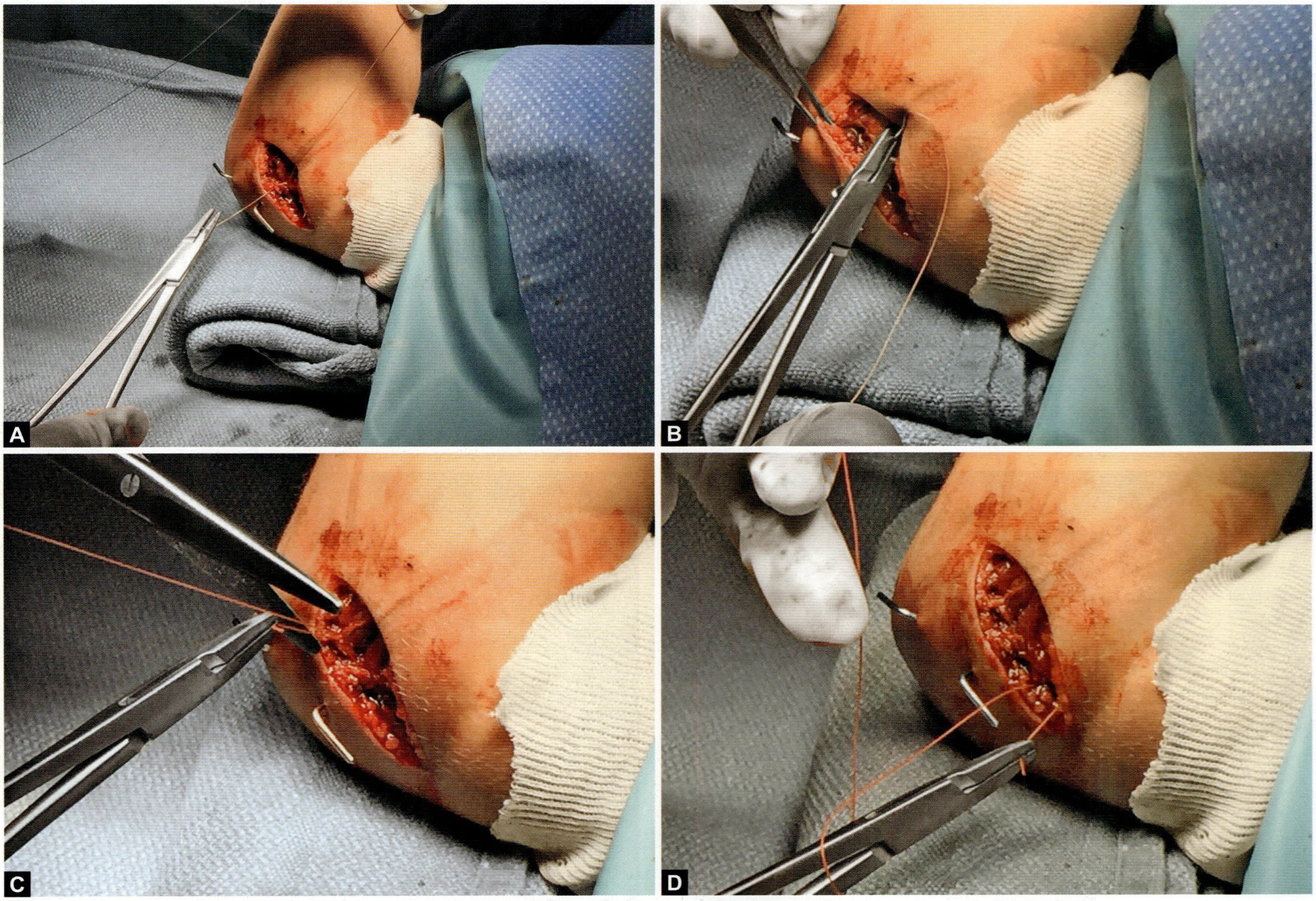

Figs. 26A to D: Hemostasis, irrigation, and subcutaneous closure sutured with 2-0 absorbable inverted interrupted sutures.

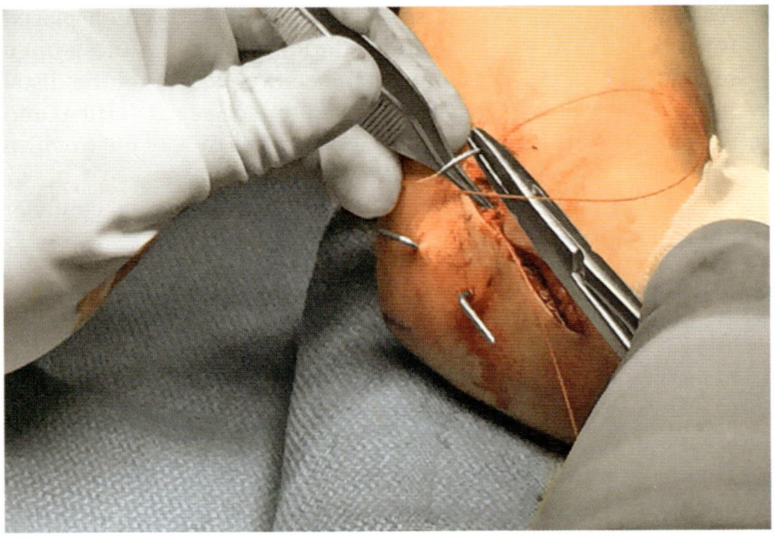

Fig. 27: Closure is obtained with skin closure using a running 3-0 absorbable subcuticular stitch. Soft dressing and felt are placed around K-wires. 4 × 4 gauze dressing is placed over the incision and sterile cast padding is placed to hold the dressing.

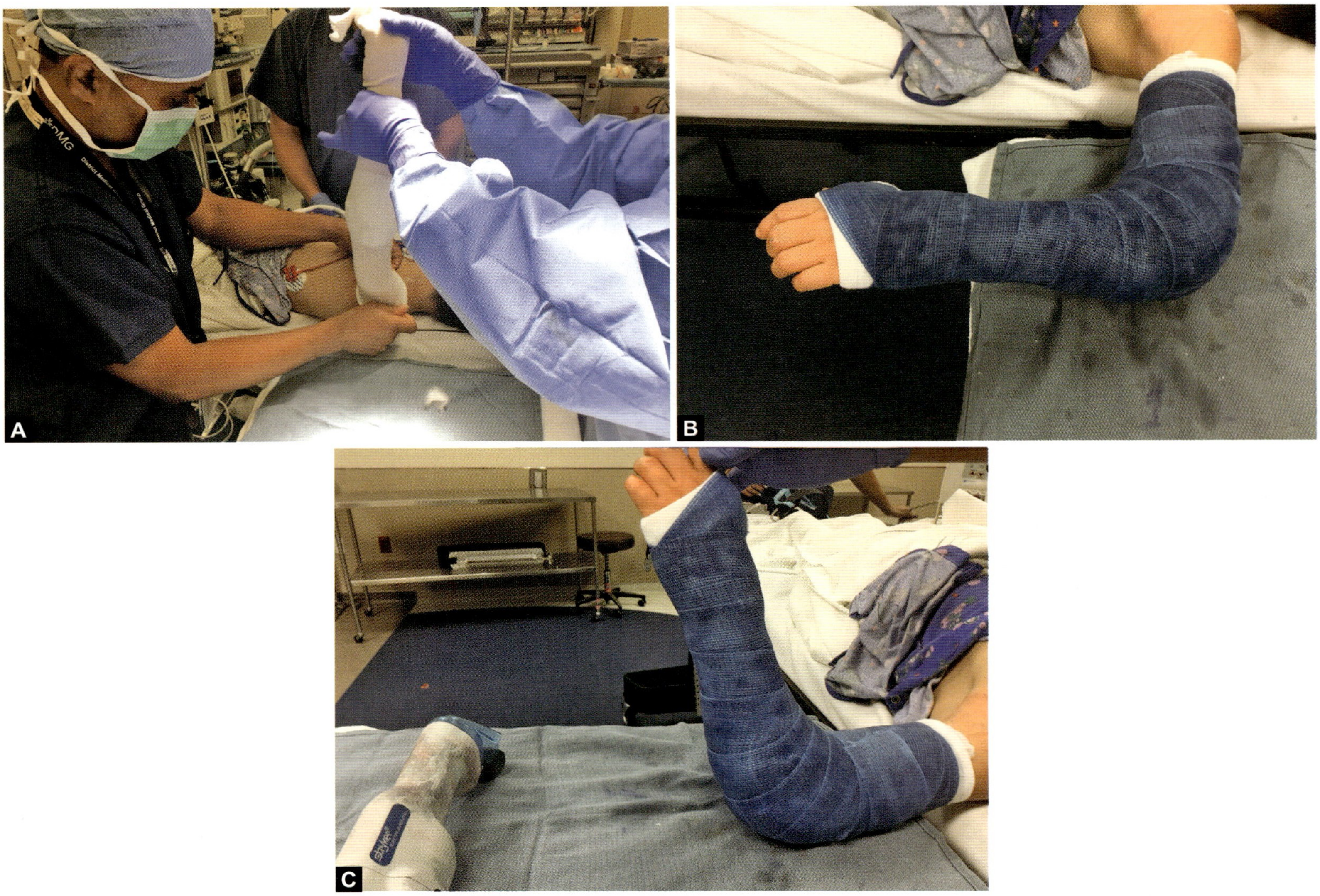

Figs. 28A to C: A long arm bivalve cast is placed with the elbow flex to 90°.

POSTOPERATIVE PROTOCOL

- Patient is placed into a well-padded bivalve long arm cast after surgery with forearm in supination and wrist extended.
- Follow-up in 2 weeks for repeat X-rays and cast overwrap.
- Follow-up in 5 weeks for repeat X-rays. Cast removal and possible pin removal if fracture has good signs of healing. It may need to leave pins in up to 6–8 weeks.
- Allow patient to use arm as tolerated once pins are removed. Patient should refrain from any activity that can cause the patient to fall and reinjure his elbow.
- Follow-up at 3 months for a range of motion check. If the patient still has restricted ROM a referral to physical therapy is warranted. The patient may go back to full activity once full range of motion is achieved.

POTENTIAL COMPLICATIONS

- Elbow stiffness is the most common complication due to increased immobilization time needed for fracture healing. It may need referral to physical therapy.
- Lateral overgrowth and spurring is seen in up to 50–75% of patients. This is most likely due to periosteal disruption at the fracture site and is of no functional significance.
- Superficial pin track infections and/or pin migration is more common than supracondylar fractures. Pins left out of the skin have fewer infection complications than buried pins. These may need pin removal and oral antibiotics.
- Deep infections including septic arthritis and osteomyelitis may need incision and drainage and IV antibiotics.
- Nonunions are more common in this fracture pattern than with supracondylar humerus fractures. It may require reoperation with internal fixation and bone grafting.
- Malunions are also more common in lateral humeral condyle fractures. These may require an intra-articular osteotomy and reconstruction.
- Tardy ulnar nerve palsy may develop from a nonunion or lateral humeral growth arrest leading to cubital valgus and stretch of the ulnar nerve.
- Cubitus valgus and varus (>5° from normal alignment) may develop in lateral condyle fractures. Cubitus varus is more common but rarely requires an osteotomy.
- Avascular necrosis may be associated with displaced or undisplaced fractures and sometimes with posterior dissection during open reductions. The blood supply to the central portion of the distal humerus physis, epiphysis and articular surface is vertical and with minimal cross anastomosis. This makes AVN of the trochlea a potential risk with all distal humerus fractures.
- Fishtail deformity may develop with lateral and medial condylar physeal injuries.

KEY POINTS

- Keep dissection only on the anterior aspect of the distal humerus to prevent disruption of the blood supply to the lateral condylar fragment.
- The distal humerus internal rotation X-ray is used to evaluate fracture displacement on plain radiographs.
- Utilize an arthrogram to evaluate the fracture reduction with both the open and closed techniques.
- The fracture is often rotated, displaced and difficult to reduce during open reduction. Flexing the elbow to 90° can facilitate finding and reducing the fragment.
- Leave enough skin posterior to the incision for percutaneous pinning.

SUGGESTED READING

1. Jakob R, Fowles JV, Rang M, et al. Observations concerning fractures of the lateral humeral condyle in children. J Bone Joint Surg Br. 1975;57:430-6.
2. Mintzer CM, Waters PM, Brown DJ, et al. Percutaneous pinning in the treatment of displaced lateral condyles fractures. J Pediatric Orthop. 1994;14:462-5.
3. Pennock A, Salgueiro L, Upasani V, et al. Closed Reduction and Percutaneous Pinning Versus Open Reduction and Internal Fixation for Type II Lateral Condyle Humerus Fractures in Children Displaced >2 mm. J Pediatr Orthop. 2016;36(8):780-6.
4. Song KS, Kang CH, Min BW, et al. Closed reduction and internal fixation of displaced unstable lateral condylar fractures of the humerus in children. J Bone Joint Surg Am. 2008;90:2673-81.
5. Stein BE, Ramji A, Hassanzadeh H, et al. Cannulated Lag Screw Fixation of Displaced Lateral Humeral Condyle Fractures Is Associated With Lower Rates of Open Reduction and Infection Than Pin Fixation. J Pediatr Orthop. 2017;37(1):7-13.

CHAPTER 7

Dome Osteotomy for Cubitus Varus

Kapil Gangwal

INTRODUCTION

Cubitus varus is a common complication following a supracondylar fracture of humerus in children. Occasionally, it can be encountered following lateral condylar fractures and other pathologies causing growth disturbances at the distal humerus.

The natural history of cubitus varus is one of persistence. The deformity produces a cosmetically unacceptable appearance of the elbow and also interferes with function causing instability, ulnar nerve dysfunction, and predisposition to lateral condylar fractures in some instances.

The management of the deformity is by a supracondylar corrective osteotomy. Numerus techniques of achieving the correction have been described. Commonly performed procedures include a lateral closing wedge osteotomy, fixator-assisted correction with a percutaneous or open osteotomy, and the dome osteotomy.

Dome osteotomy was described by Tien et al.[1] The technique has several advantages compared to the lateral closing wedge procedure, particularly pertaining to circumventing the lateral condylar prominence which is a known and common postoperative complication of the latter procedure. There is further advantage of tailoring the correction to the desired amount intraoperatively without adjusting bone cuts. Also, the osteotomy is inherently stable, which adds to the ease of intraoperative adjustments. The procedure is technically more demanding compared to the commonly performed lateral closing wedge osteotomy.

TIMING OF PROCEDURE

Any age between 4 years and 10 years is good for performing the corrective procedure. It is generally recommended to wait till the child regains full range of movement of the elbow following a fracture before a corrective surgery is undertaken. The author usually gives a gap of 6–18 months following the injury before attempting a corrective procedure. K-wire fixation suffices for the younger children while a more rigid fixation with a plate is needed for older children, adolescents, and adults.

CLINICAL ASSESSMENT (FIGS. 1A TO C)

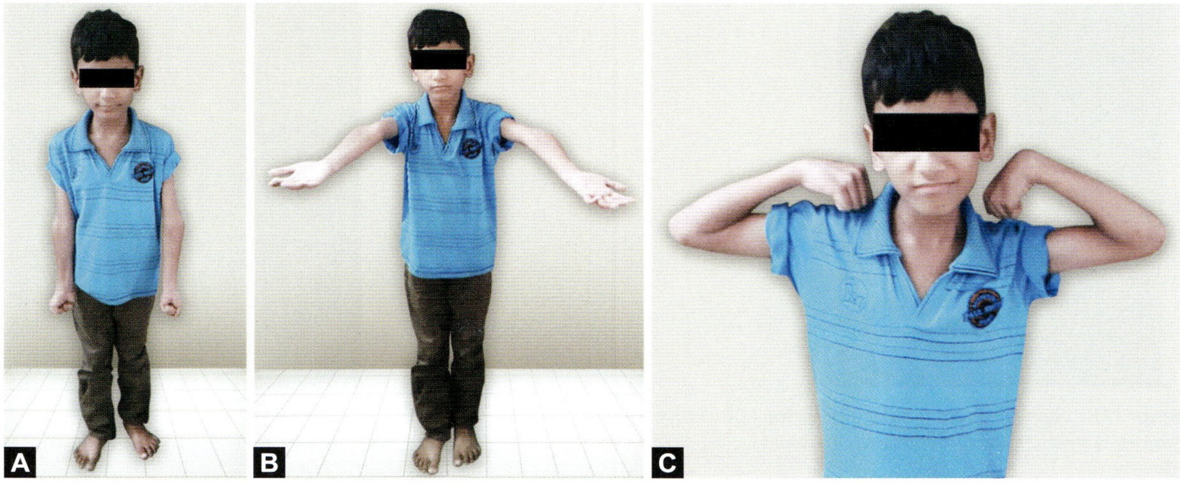

Figs. 1A to C: Preoperative evaluation and documenting the deformity and range of motion.

Clinical Examination (Figs. 1A to C)

Proper documentation of the deformity in the coronal and sagittal plane is required. A photographic documentation of the deformity should be done for comparison with postoperative outcomes. Range of motion must be checked to document any loss of flexion and extension. A neurologic evaluation is done to document radial ulnar and median nerve function. A note needs to be made of the skin condition and of any scars from previous surgery which may interfere with the surgical approach.

Imaging (Figs. 2 and 3)

An anteroposterior X-ray of the upper limb from mid-arm to wrist with the forearm in supination and elbow in extension should be obtained. This will show the extent of the deformity. Usually, X-rays of the contralateral normal limb are obtained to allow for comparison and to calculate the deformity on the X-ray. A lateral view of the elbow is also obtained to check for any angular deformation of the distal humerus in the coronal plane. Special imaging like CT and MRI scans are usually not required.

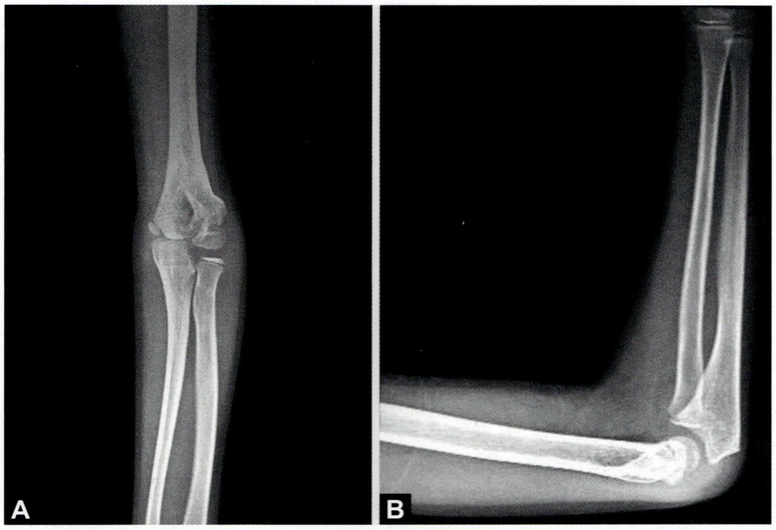

Figs. 2A and B: Anteroposterior (AP) view elbow extended and forearm supinated humerus to wrist and lateral view of elbow.

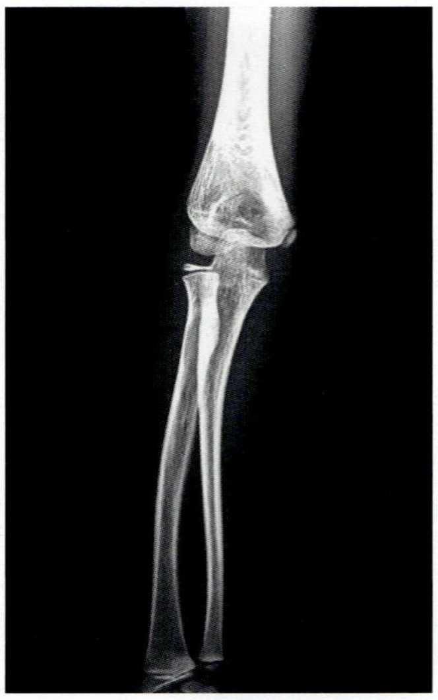

Fig. 3: Anteroposterior (AP) view of normal side elbow for comparison limb extended and supinated humerus to wrist.

PREOPERATIVE COUNSELING

A discussion regarding the potential risks and complications of the procedure should be done prior to undertaking the procedure. There is a possibility of residual deformity, delayed union, nonunion, hardware failure, infection, nerve injury, stiffness, and lateral condylar prominence.

OPERATIVE PROCEDURE

Decision Making

Several types of osteotomies are described for correcting the deformity. The commonly performed procedures are lateral closing wedge osteotomy, dome osteotomy, step cut osteotomy, and the more complex multiplanar osteotomy.

This chapter describes the technique of the dome osteotomy.

PREOPERATIVE PLANNING (FIGS. 4 TO 6)

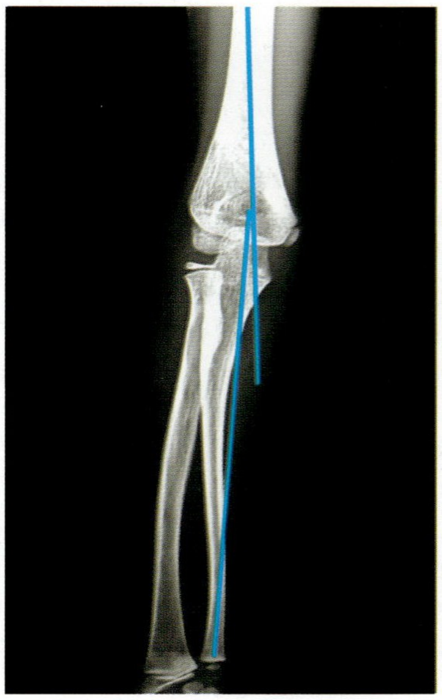

Fig. 4: Humeroulnar alignment of normal limb.

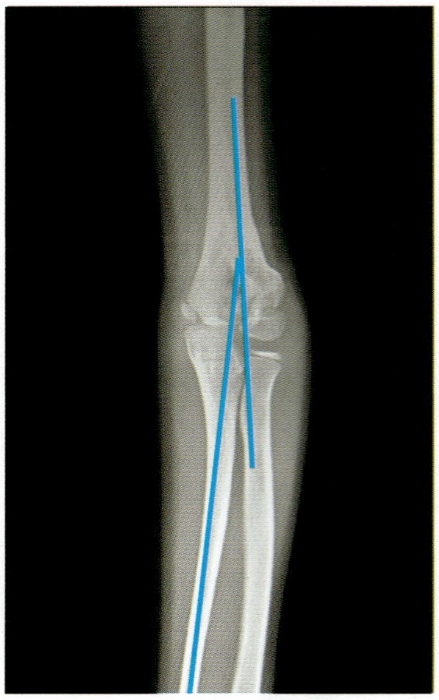

Fig. 5: Humeroulnar alignment of deformed limb.

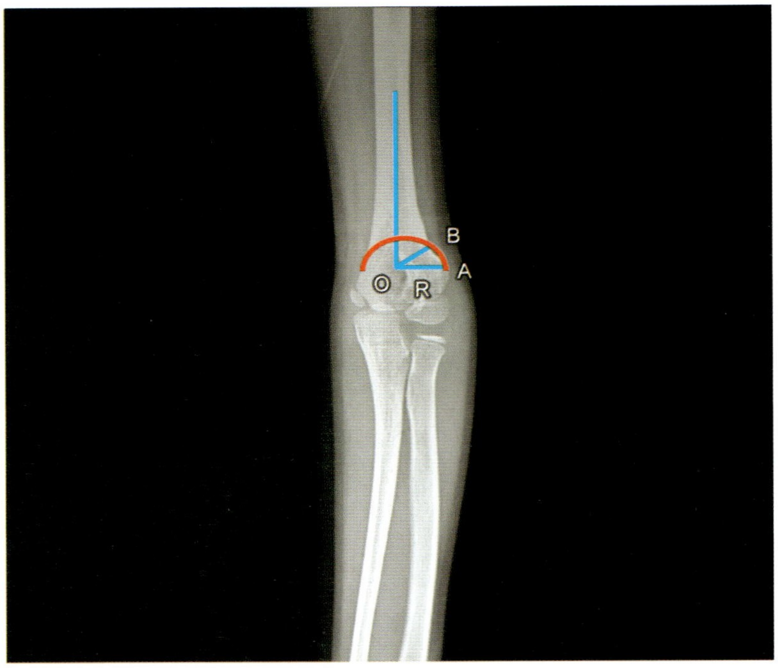

Fig. 6: Preoperative planning of the osteotomy. (1) Draw long axis of humerus. Intersect at tip of olecranon fossa "O", (2) Draw perpendicular from O to lateral cortex humerus "R", (3) Point where R intersects the lateral cortex is point "A", (4) Draw arc of osteotomy from point A to medial cortex using R as the radius of curvature and O as the center point, and (5) Amount of translation marked on lateral cortex as point "B" after calculating the angle of correction AOB to match the humeroulnar angle of the normal side.

ANESTHESIA

General anesthesia.

POSITIONING (FIGS. 7A AND B)

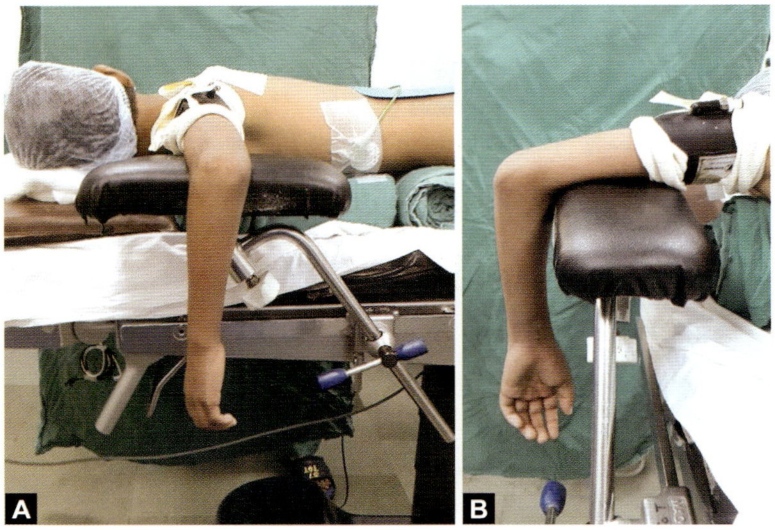

Figs. 7A and B: Child is placed prone on the operating table and arm is rested on a side arm rest with forearm and hand dangling by the edge of the arm rest. A pneumatic tourniquet is applied to the upper arm.

OPERATING TABLE SETUP (FIG. 8)

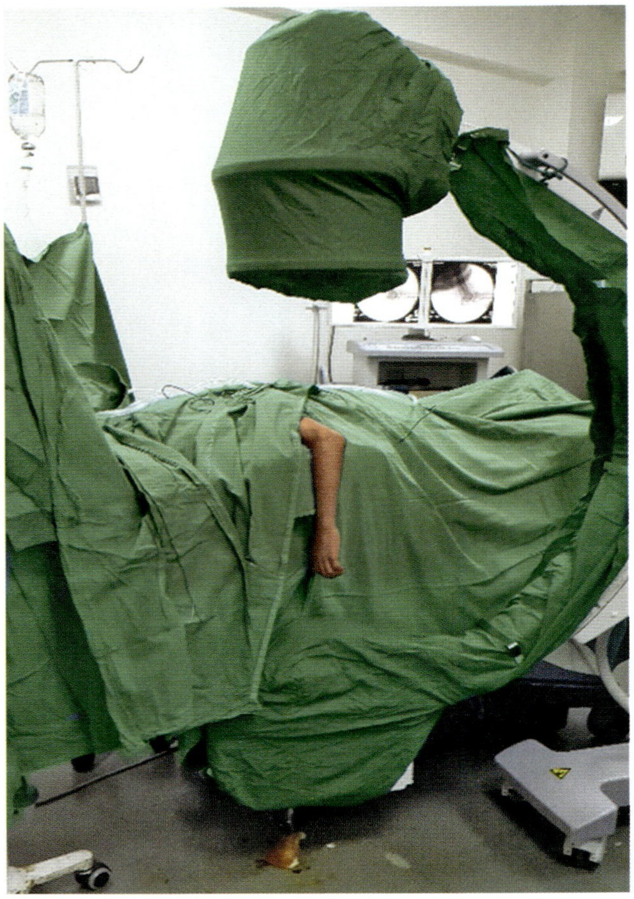

Fig. 8: Image intensifier is brought in to visualize the distal humerus without obstructing the operative field.

INSTRUMENTS (FIG. 9)

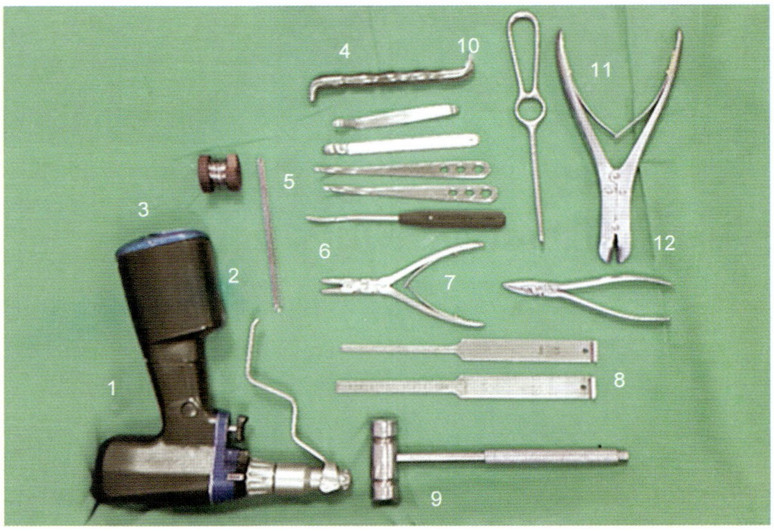

Fig. 9: Instruments: (1) Drill with wire attachment, (2) K-wire 1.6 mm, (3) SS wire, (4) Wire bender, (5) Bone levers blunt and sharp pointed, (6) Periosteum elevator, (7) Bone nibbler, (8) 1/4" and 1/2" osteotomes, (9) Mallet, (10) Bone hook, (11) Pliers, and (12) Wire cutter.

INCISION (FIGS. 10A AND B)

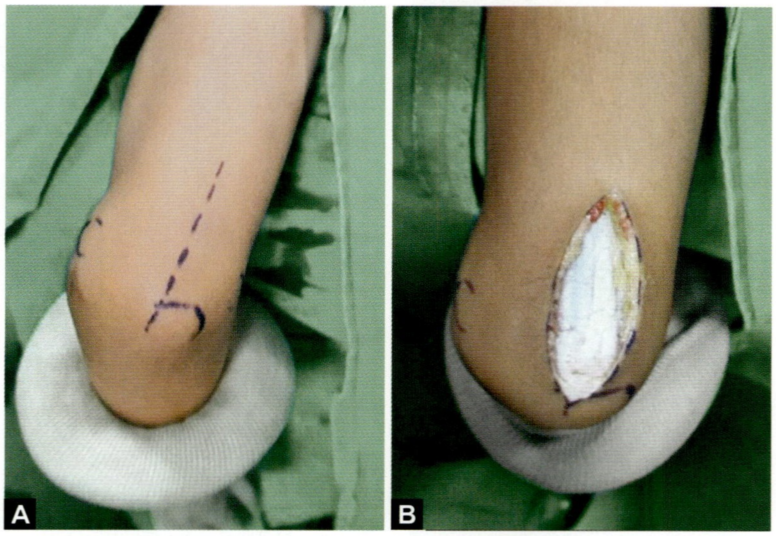

Figs. 10A and B: (A) Mark lateral epicondyle, medial epicondyle and tip of olecranon. Mark longitudinal incision in lower arm till olecranon; (B) Expose triceps aponeurosis.

DEEP DISSECTION (FIGS. 11A AND B)

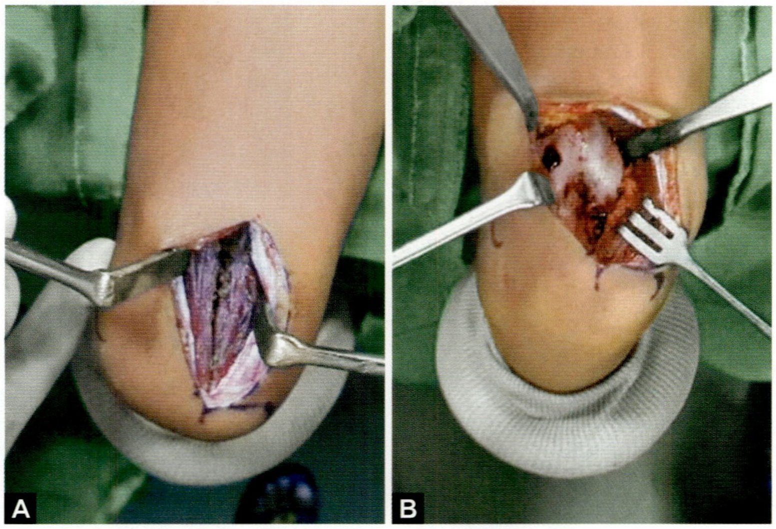

Figs. 11A and B: (A) Incise triceps in the midline; (B) Expose bone subperiosteally, place bone levers medially and laterally.

MARKING THE OSTEOTOMY (FIGS. 12A TO C)

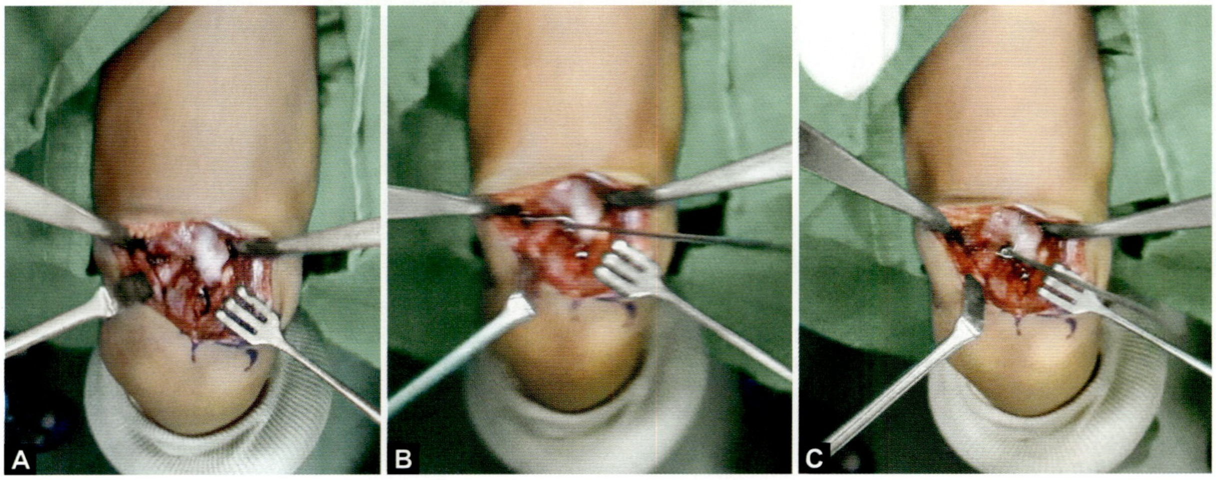

Figs. 12A to C: (A) Make a hole at tip of olecranon fossa; (B) Insert a K-wire in the hole and loop a SS wire with arm equal to the distance from tip of olecranon fossa to lateral condylar column of humerus; (C) Mark the osteotomy by moving the tip of the SS wire from lateral column to medial column keeping the tip of olecranon fossa as the center point.

MAKING THE CUTS (FIGS. 13 AND 14)

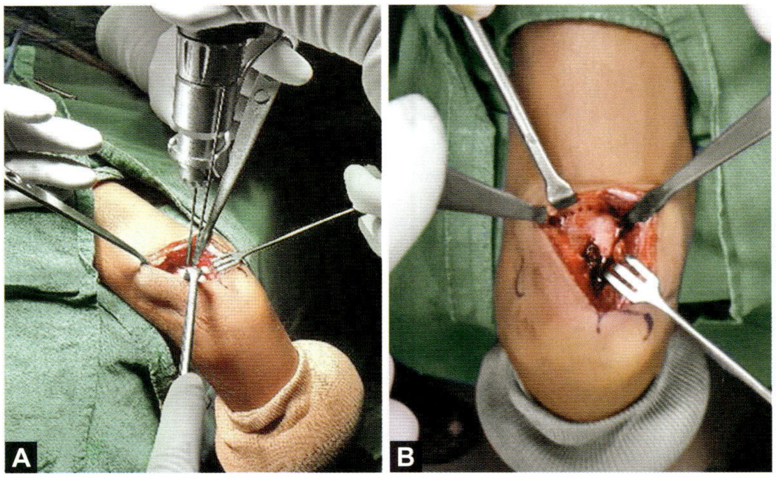

Figs. 13A and B: Use a 1.8 to 2 mm K-wire to mark bi-cortical holes along the planned osteotomy site.

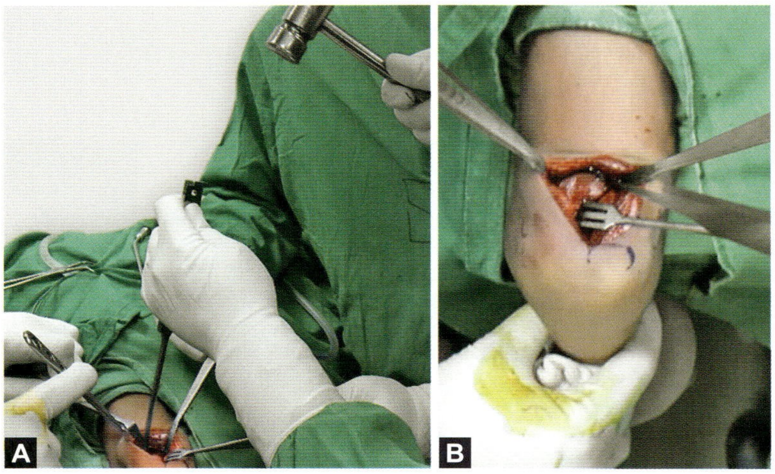

Figs. 14A and B: Use a 1/4″ osteotome to osteotomize the bone by connecting the holes. First cut the near cortex and then cut the far cortex for better control.

DISPLACING THE OSTEOTOMY (FIGS. 15A TO C)

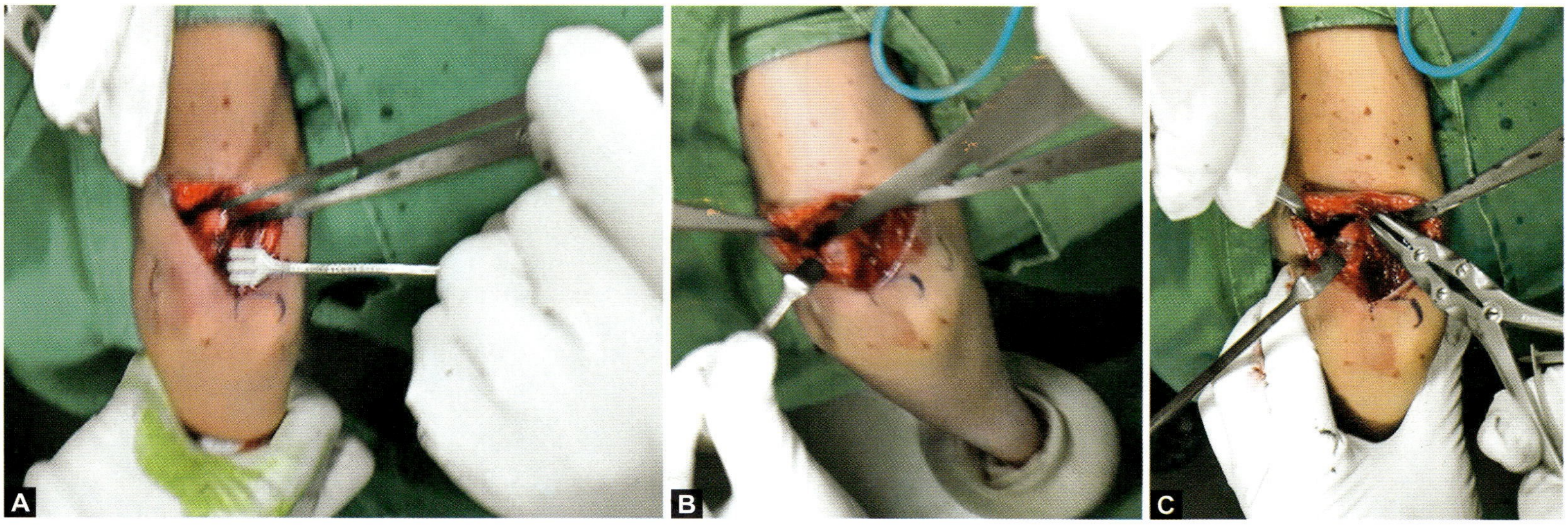

Figs. 15A to C: (A and B) Insert the 1/2″ osteotome in the osteotomy and turn it 90° to translate the osteotomy. This moves the bone fragments over each other like a cogwheel; (C) The sharp edge on the lateral side of proximal fragment needs to be trimmed with a nibbler to shape it to fit the contour of the distal fragment.

FIXATION OF THE OSTEOTOMY (FIGS. 16 TO 19)

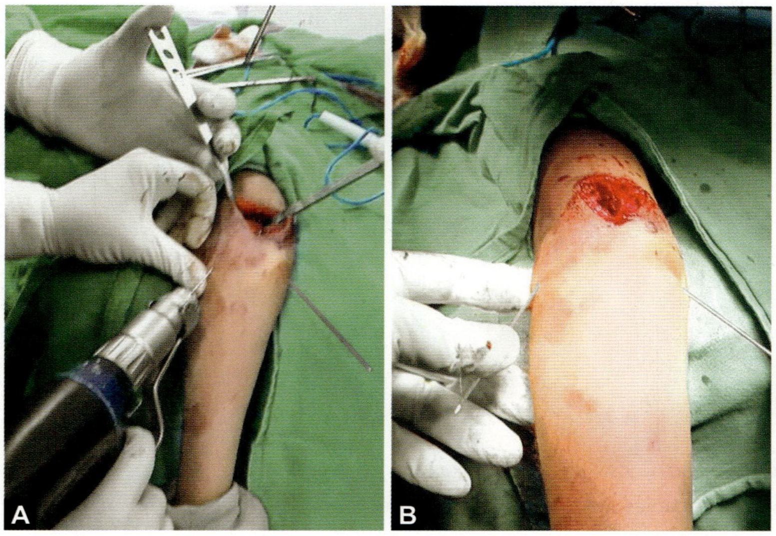

Figs. 16A and B: After confirming correction to match the opposite side, the osteotomy is fixed with 1.6 mm K-wires. The position is confirmed on IITV. Two lateral diverging and one medial wire are placed in the standard manner as pinning a supracondylar humerus fracture.

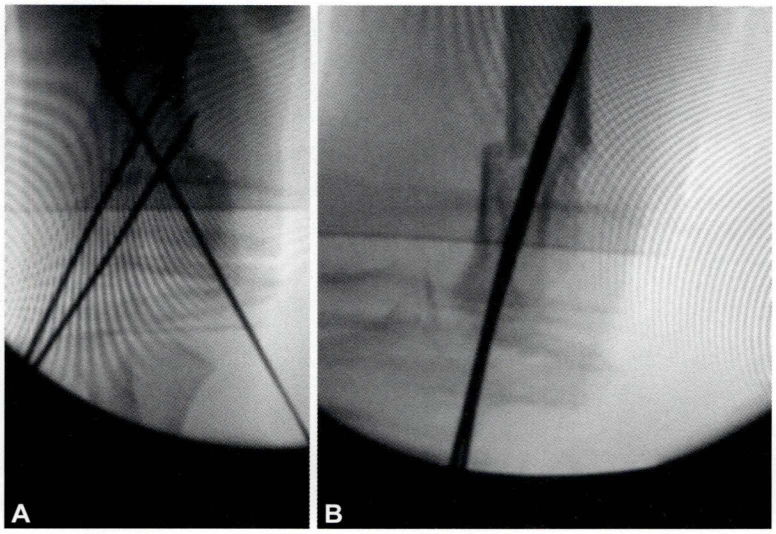

Figs. 17A and B: The position of the osteotomy and the wires is confirmed on IITV.

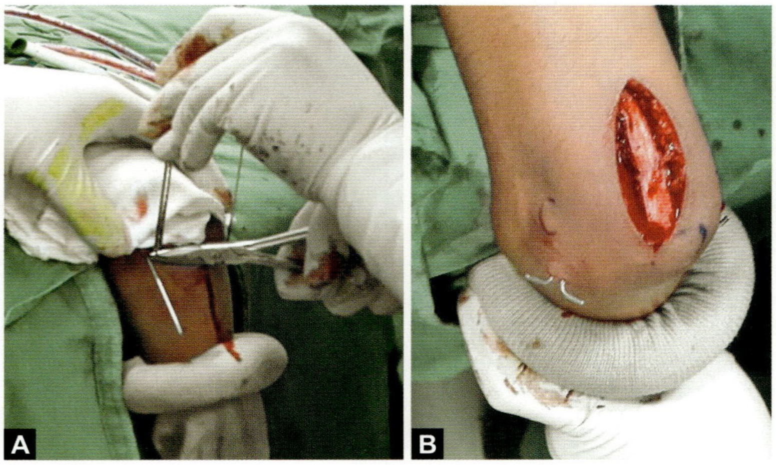

Figs. 18A and B: Wires are bent and cut.

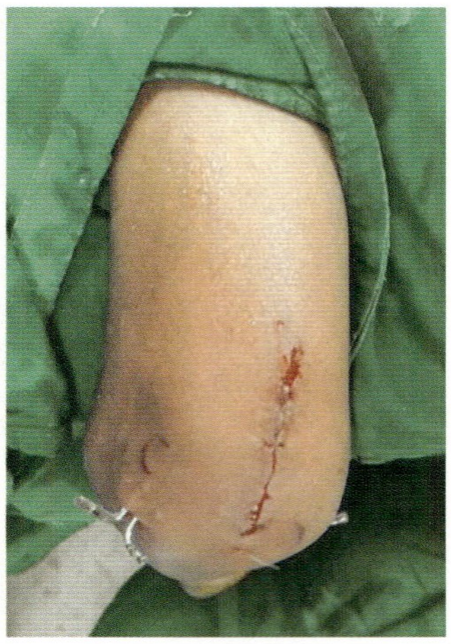

Fig. 19: Wound is closed in the standard fashion.

SPLINTAGE (FIG. 20)

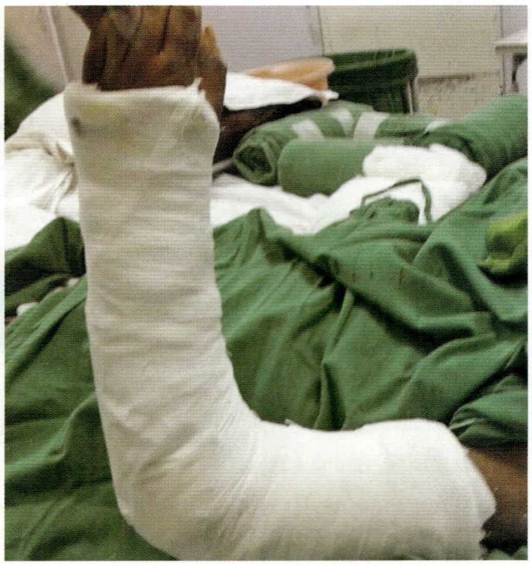

Fig. 20: Above elbow plaster splint is applied for postoperative immobilization.

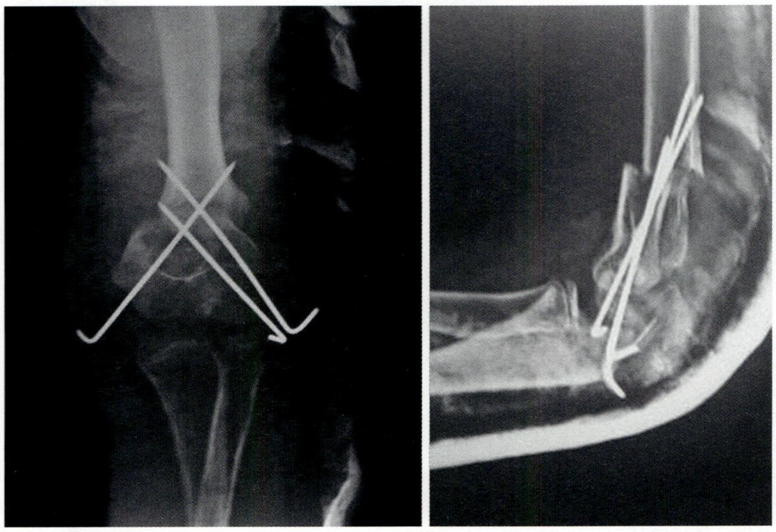

Fig. 21: Postoperative X-ray.

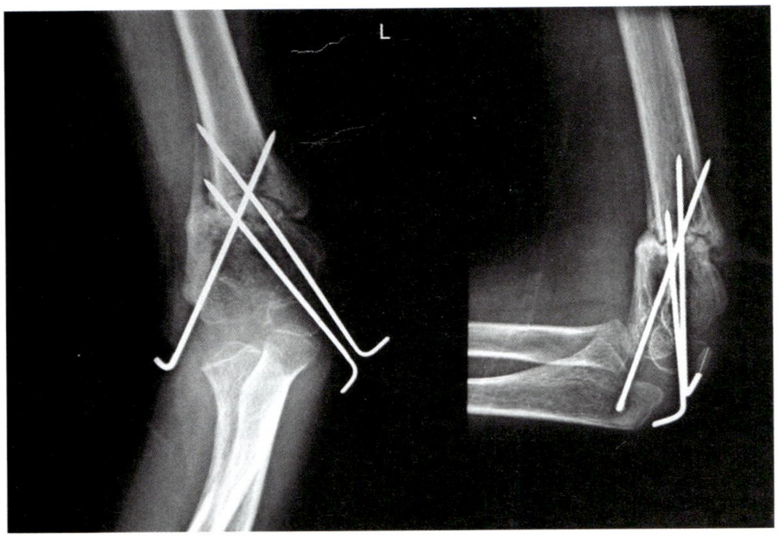

Fig. 22: X-ray at 4 weeks showing healing of osteotomy.

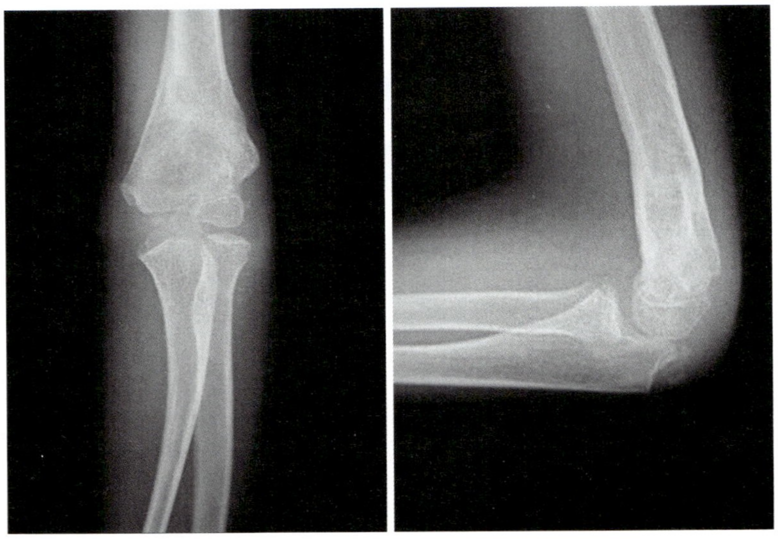

Fig. 23: X-ray at 6 months postoperative.

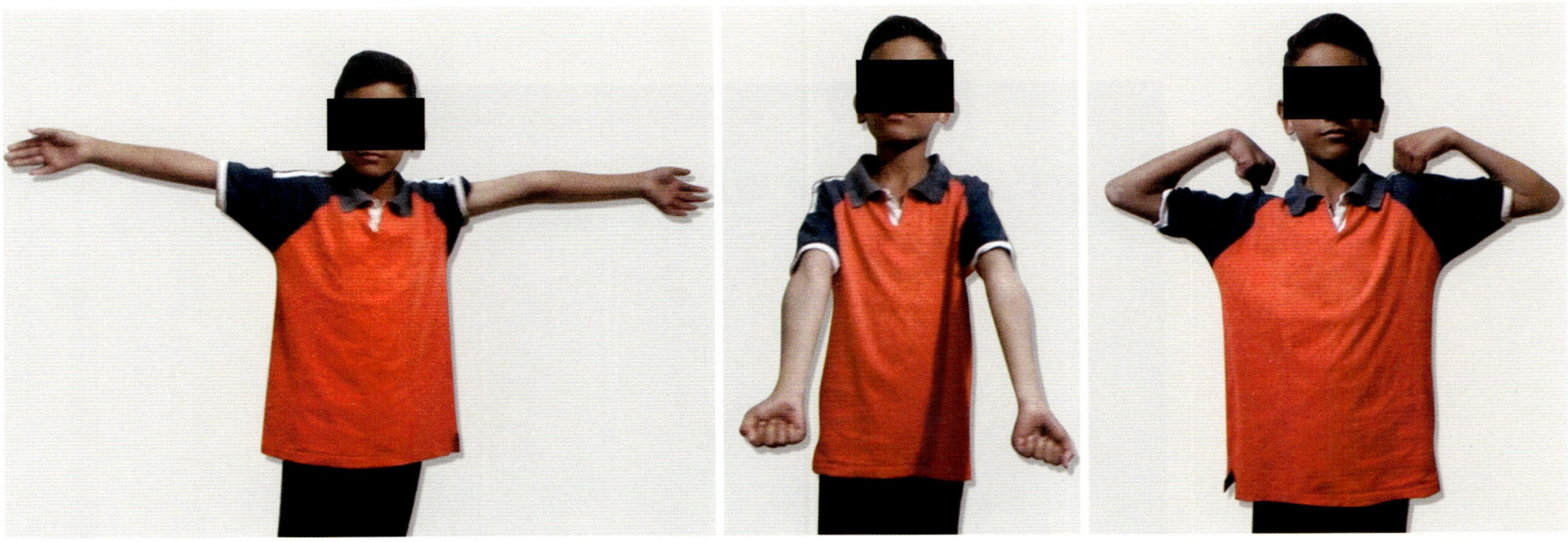

Fig. 24: Clinical picture 6 months following surgery showing range of motion and correction of deformity.

POSTOPERATIVE PLAN

1st follow-up visit is at 1 week from surgery. A X-ray is obtained to check for any interval displacement. After confirming correct position of osteotomy an above elbow cast is applied. 2nd follow up visit is at 4 weeks from surgery. A X-ray out of cast is obtained. K-wires are removed after confirming union of osteotomy and active range of motion exercises of elbow are started.

COMPLICATIONS

Common complication is prominence of lateral condyle if closing wedge osteotomy is done. This is less of a problem with dome osteotomy. Elbow stiffness and mismatch of carrying angles are other possible complications.

REFERENCE

1. Tien YC1, Chih HW, Lin GT, Lin SY. Dome corrective osteotomy for cubitus varus deformity. Clin Orthop Relat Res. 2000;(380):158-66.

SUGGESTED READING

1. Ali AM, Abouelnas BA, Elgohary HS. Dome osteotomy using the paratricipital (triceps-sparing) approach for cubitus varus deformity in children: a surgical technique to avoid lateral condylar prominence. J Pediatr Orthop B. 2016;25(1):62-8.
2. Bauer AS, Pham B, Lattanza LL. Surgical Correction of Cubitus Varus. J Hand Surg Am. 2016;41(3):447-52.
3. Ho CA. Cubitus Varus-It's More Than Just a Crooked Arm! J Pediatr Orthop. 2017;37 Suppl 2:S37-41.
4. Pankaj A, Dua A, Malhotra R, et al. Dome osteotomy for posttraumatic cubitus varus: a surgical technique to avoid lateral condylar prominence. J Pediatr Orthop. 2006;26(1):61-6.

CHAPTER 8

Corrective Osteotomy for Cubitus Varus

Kaustubh Kale, Shrinivas S Shintre, Rajkumar Ekambaram

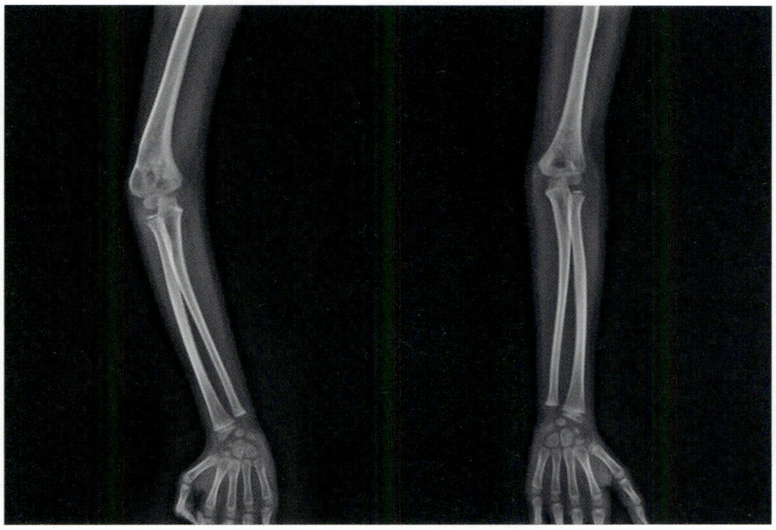

Fig. 1: Preoperative X-ray of a case of cubitus varus due to malunited supracondylar fracture of humerus.

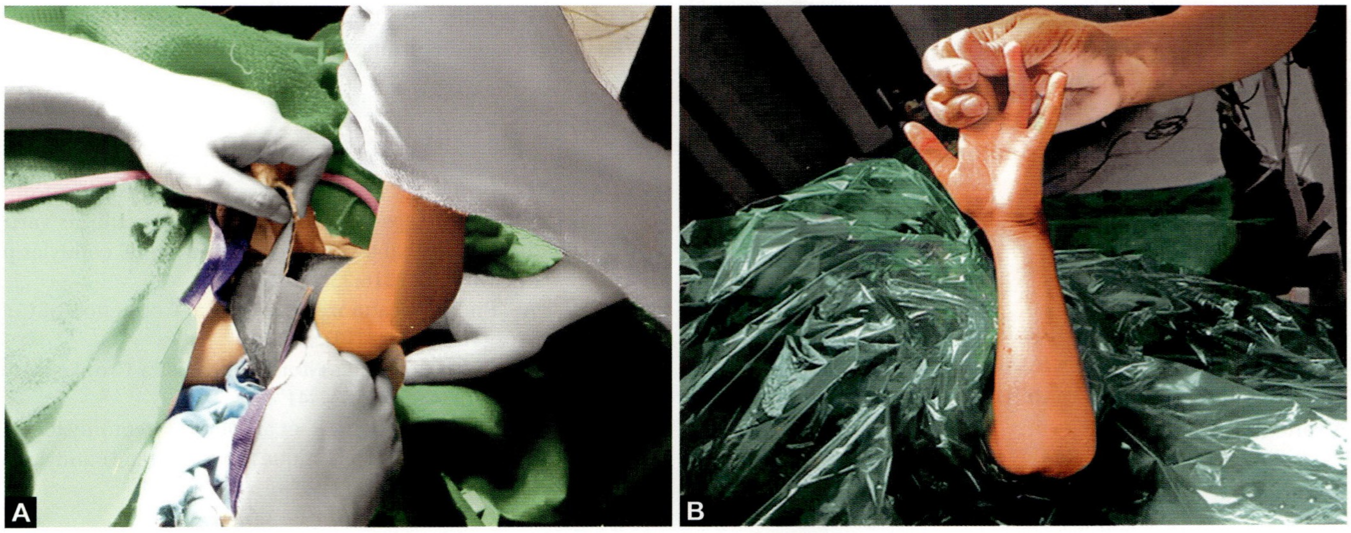

Figs. 2A and B: Preoperative preparation: (A) Supine position is given to the patient with a radiolucent board as an arm rest. A pediatric tourniquet is applied to the arm, proximal to the incision site; (B) The operative limb is scrubbed thoroughly, followed by painting and draping.

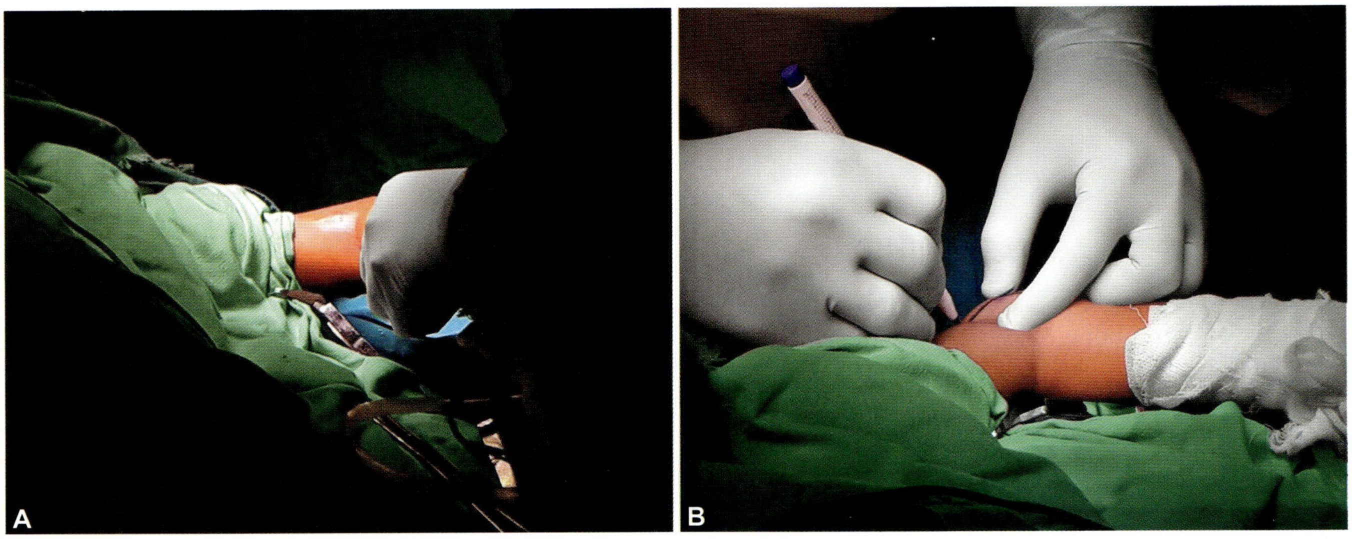

Figs. 3A and B: Painting and draping, skin marking: (A) Standard preparation of the operative limb, draping and tourniquet inflation; (B) Palpating the landmarks, a posterolateral incision line of adequate length is marked with a skin marker.

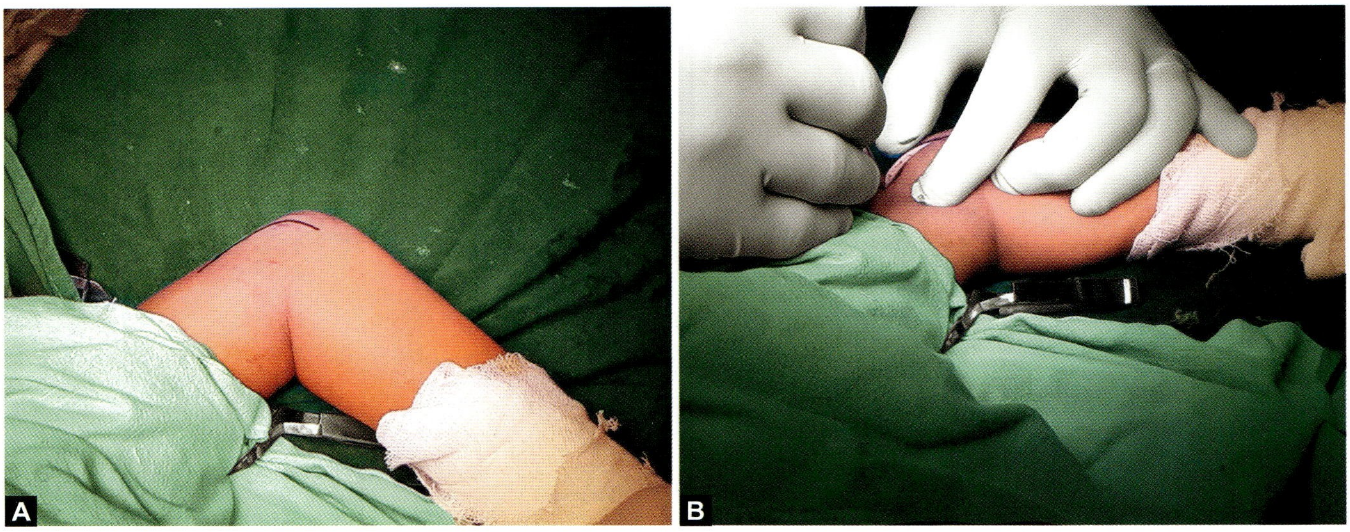

Figs. 4A and B: (A) A posterolateral incision line marked with a marker; (B) Make a gently curved incision along the line, around 5 cm in length.

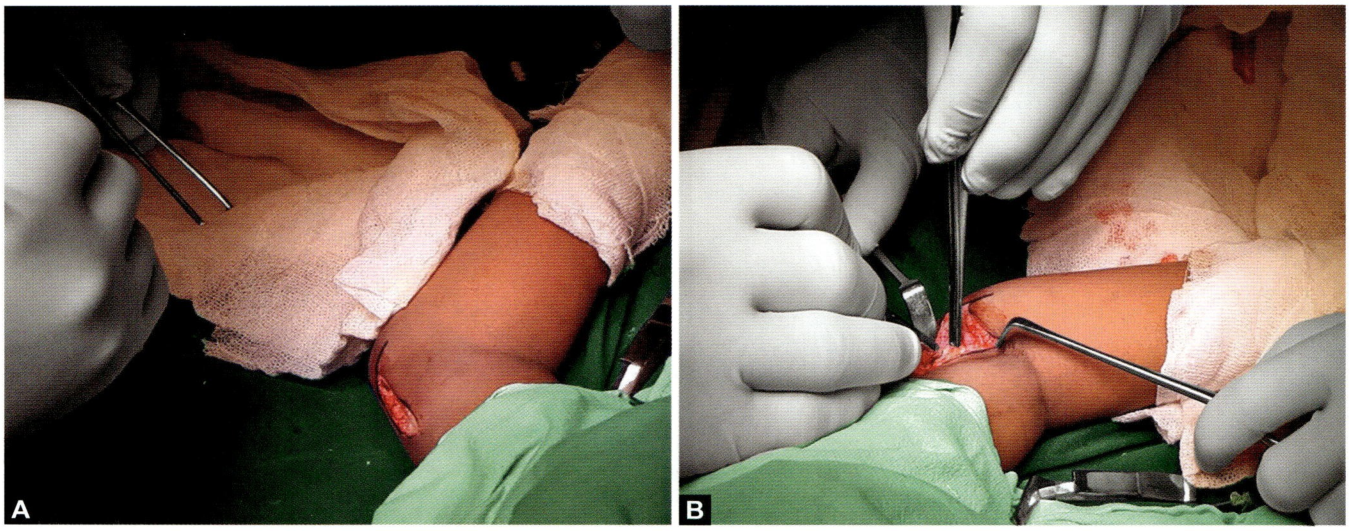

Figs. 5A and B: (A) Extending the incision as required; (B) Incise the deep fascia in line with the skin incision and dissection of the subcutaneous tissue and fat.

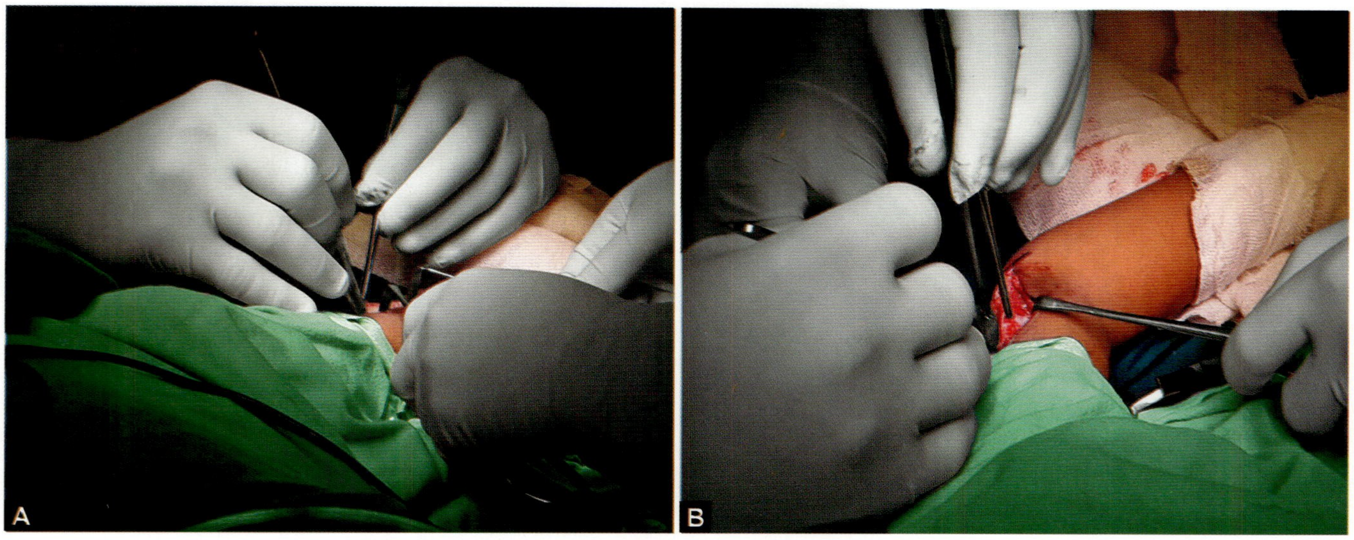

Figs. 6A and B: Retracting the dissected facia and soft tissues.

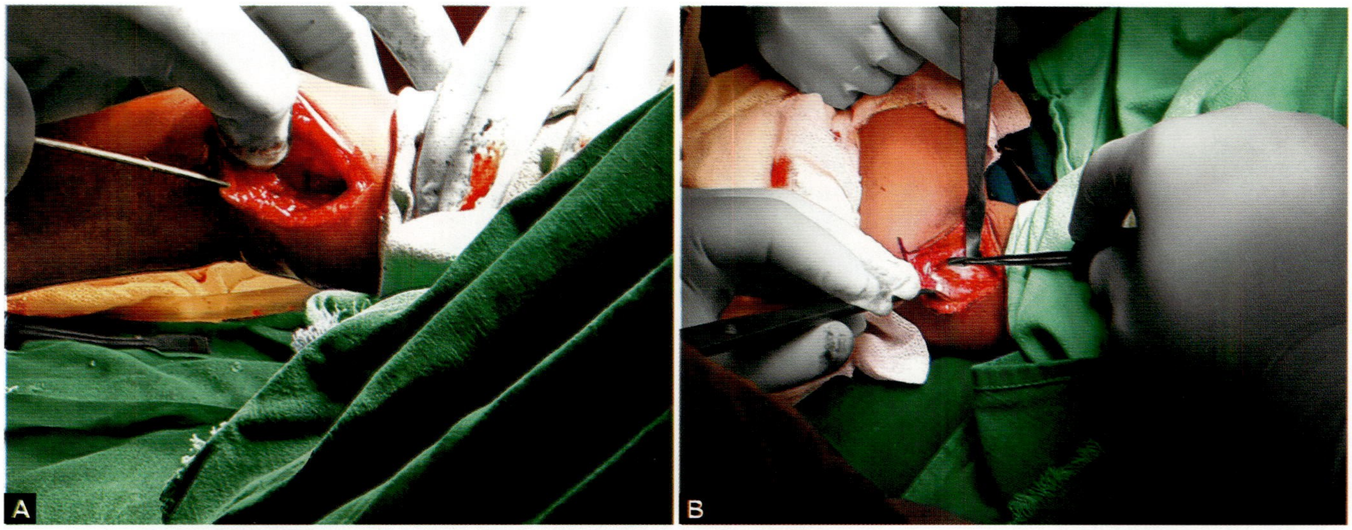

Figs. 7A and B: (A) Deeper dissection through an internervous plane, till the lateral border of distal humerus is reached; (B) Elevating the periosteum along the bone with a periosteum elevator, detaching the lateral half of triceps muscle.

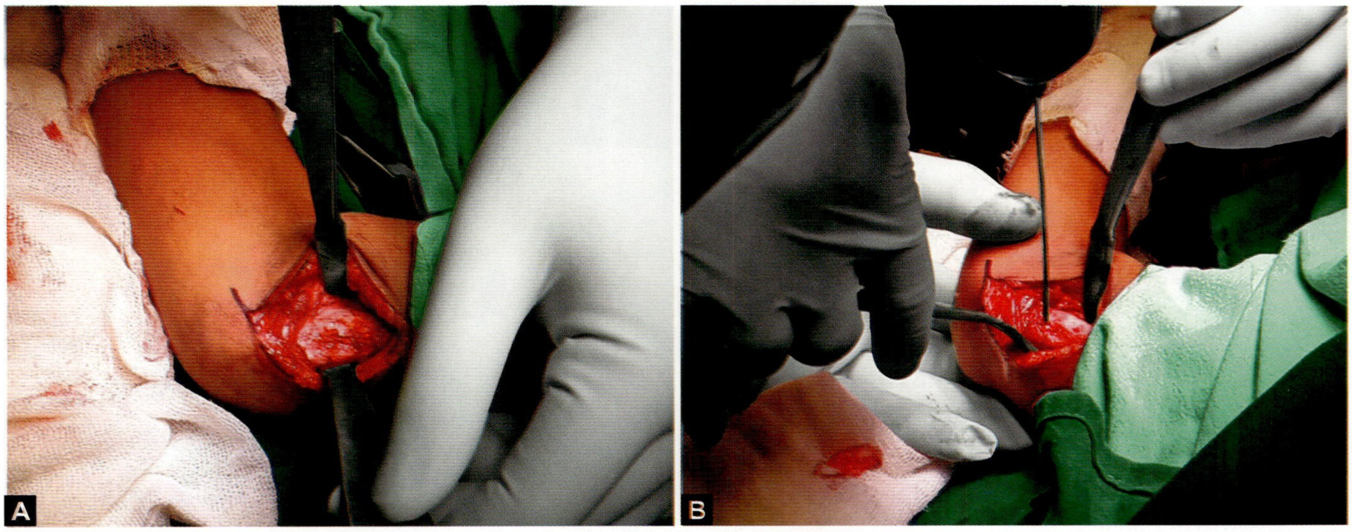

Figs. 8A and B: (A) Visible lateral surface of the distal humerus through the plane between triceps and brachialis; (B) The first of the two K-wires that are to be inserted under fluoroscopic guidance.

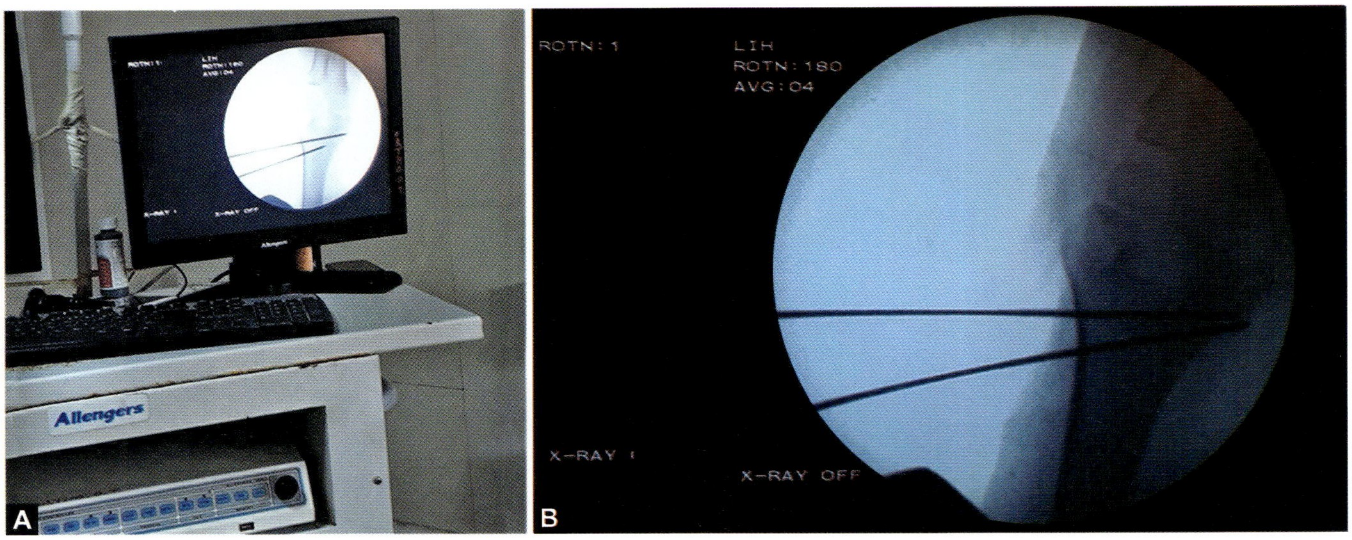

Figs. 9A and B: Two K-wires inserted under fluoroscopic guidance at a preoperatively decided site and angle, corresponding to the planned cuts.

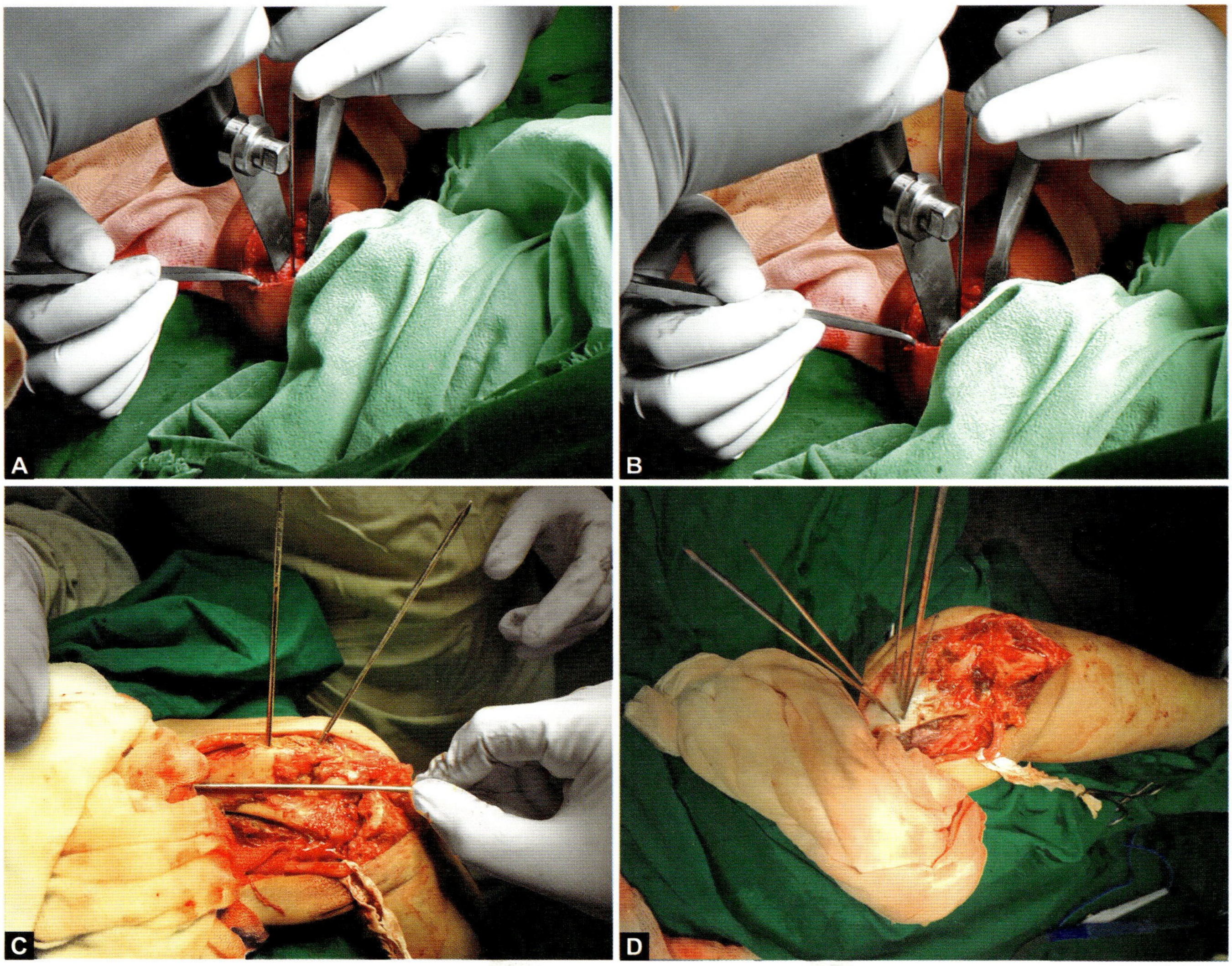

Figs. 10A to D: (A and B) Osteotomy for pure Varus - using 2 K-wires as guide in Medio-Lateral planes using Power saw, keeping the medial cortex intact; Osteotomy for Varus and posterior tilt-marking osteotomy using multiple K-wires, checking them with C-arm and joining the holes (created by K-wires) with power saw or chisel and mallet to perform the osteotomy; (C) K-wire is placed over posterior surface of shaft of humerus corresponding to its long axis. Another K-wire is passed to denote superior cut of osteotomy which is perpendicular to this axis. Inferior cut of osteotomy is denoted by another K-wire passed parallel to inter epicondylar line; (D) Multiple K-wires passed marking a wedge with posterolateral base and anteromedial apex. All the K-wires should meet each other before apex is reached so that anteromedial cortex will be kept intact which can be greensticked in order to maintain the stability of osteotomy.

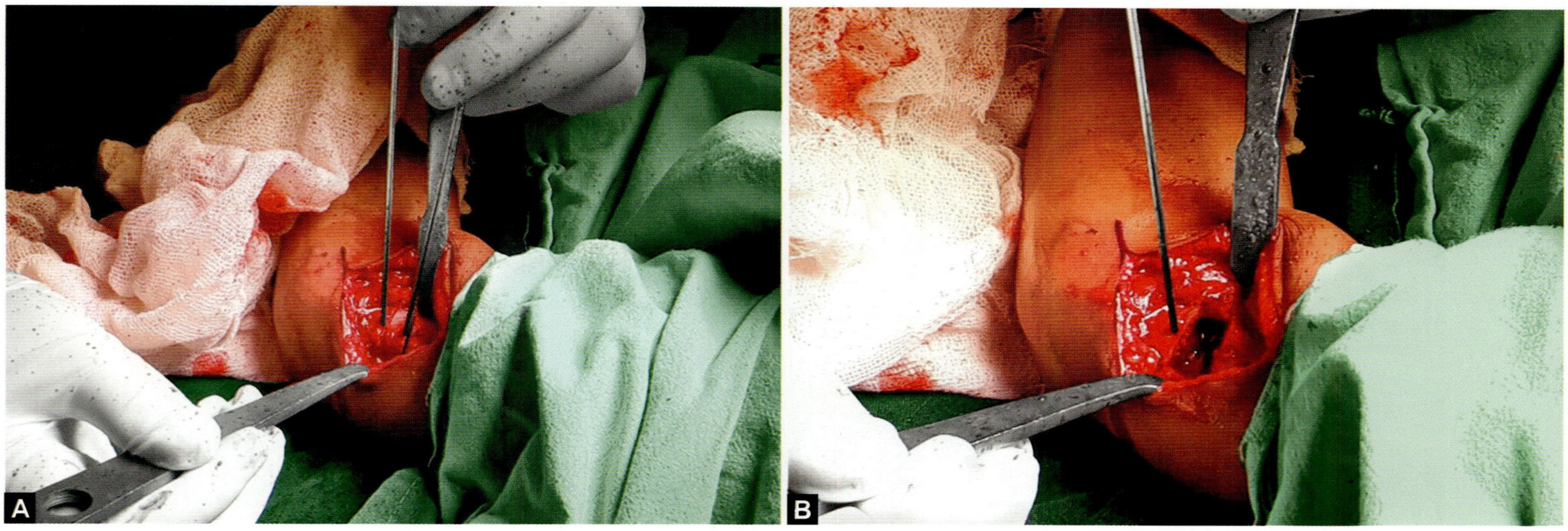

Figs. 11A and B: Bone cuts are seen and the wedge of the bone removed.

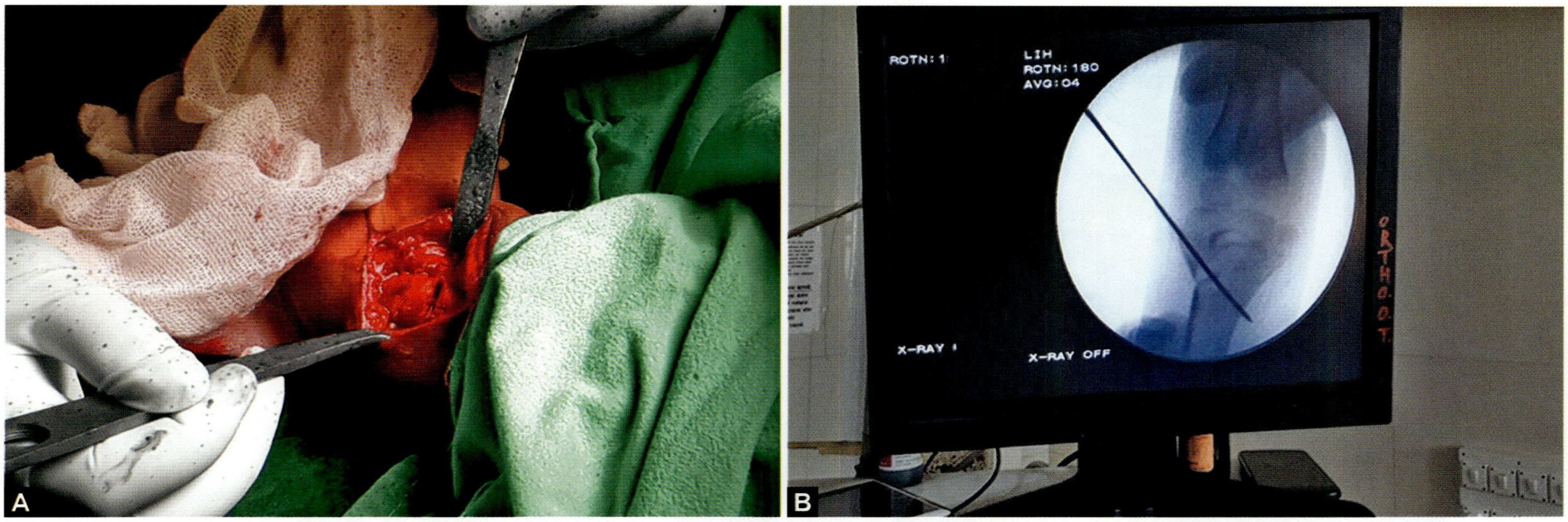

Figs. 12A and B: The proximal and distal fragments of humerus are reduced and fixed with K-wires.

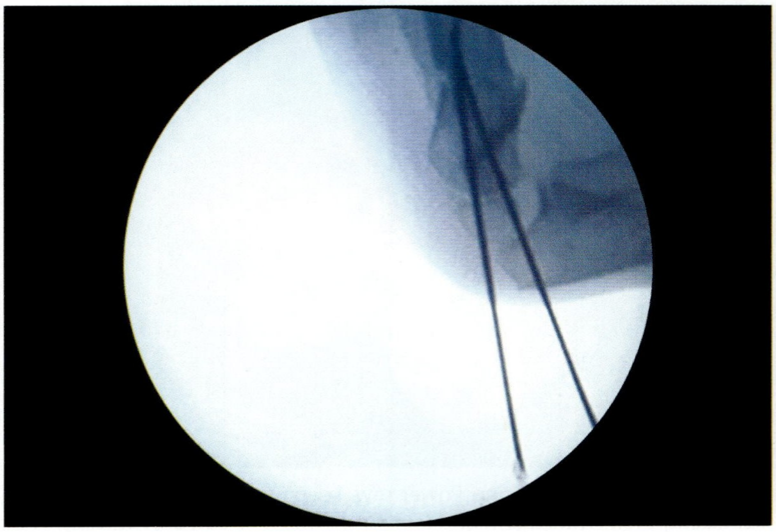

Fig. 13: Correction of the anterior humeral line (AHL) on a lateral view, fixation achieved with 2 K-wires.

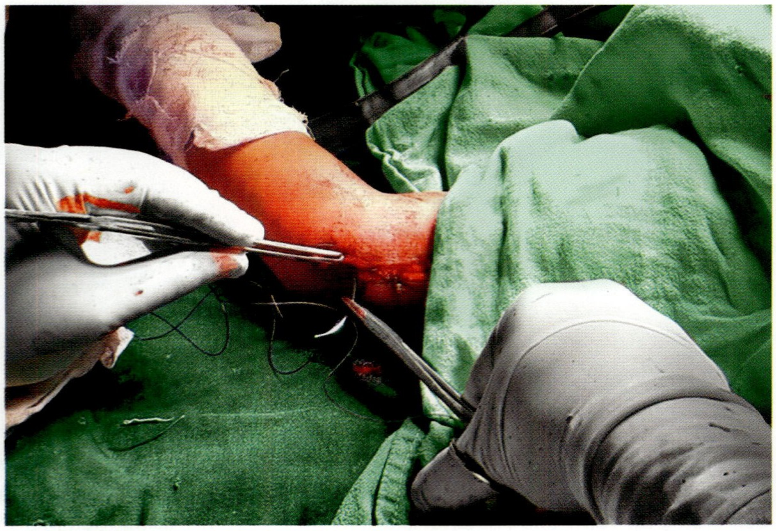

Fig. 14: Wound is washed thoroughly with normal saline, and closed in layers with absorbable suture material 2-0 and nonabsorbable suture material 2-0. Wound dressed properly and tourniquet deflated. Capillary refill assessed at finger tips and nail beds.

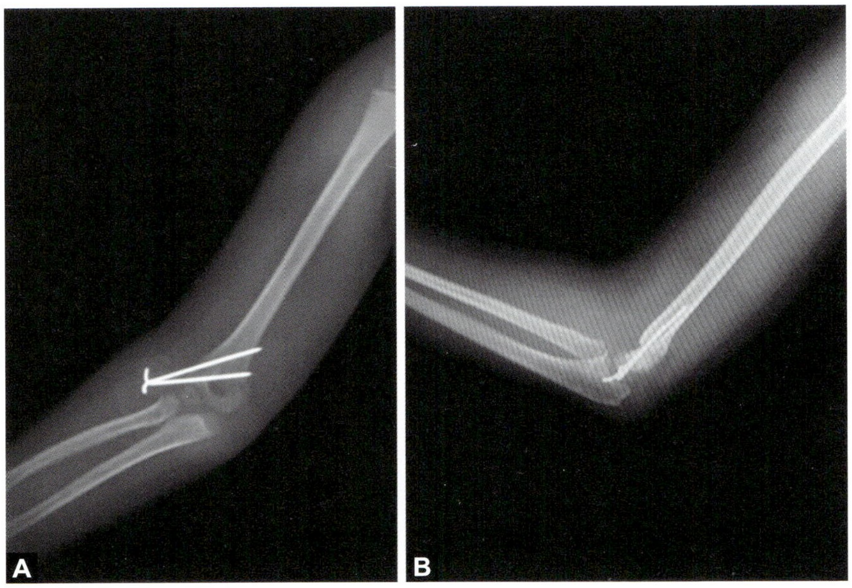

Figs. 15A and B: Postoperative X-ray AP and lateral view respectively.

CHAPTER 9

Forearm Nailing

Swapnil Keny

IMPLANTS AND INSTRUMENTATION (FIG. 1)

A set of elastic stable intramedullary nails typically consists of nails of diameters varying from 2 mm to 4 mm which are color coded as per their diameter for easy identification. Each nail is 440 mm in length and can be cut to size to fit the length of long bones in children.

The set also consists of instruments to insert the nail, help facilitate the reduction, hold the nail while inserting it, cutting the nail to a desired size, and instruments to help seat the nail in its final position.

POSITIONING OF THE PATIENT (FIGS. 2A TO C)

The patient is positioned supine with the arm supported on a radiolucent arm support. Considering that it is a closed procedure, it is always prudent to confirm easy maneuverability of the image intensifier to get the desired images prior to the surgical preparation. An axillary support at times can assist in countertraction when traction is applied. Preparation of the arm and forearm is then done under sterile conditions.

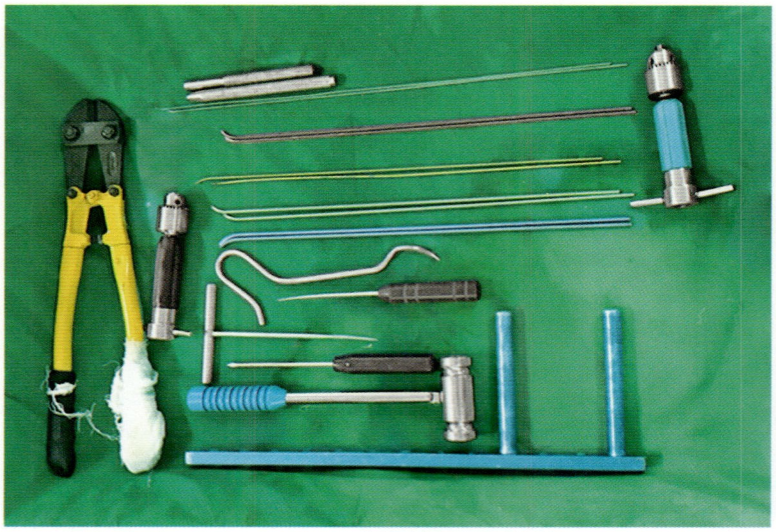

Fig. 1: Elastic nail—implant and instrumentation set.

PREOPERATIVE SIZING OF THE NAIL DIAMETER (FIGS. 3A AND B)

Nails of varying diameters are juxtaposed against the forearm bones while imaging them to determine the ideal nail size which will be a perfect fit for the medullary canal.

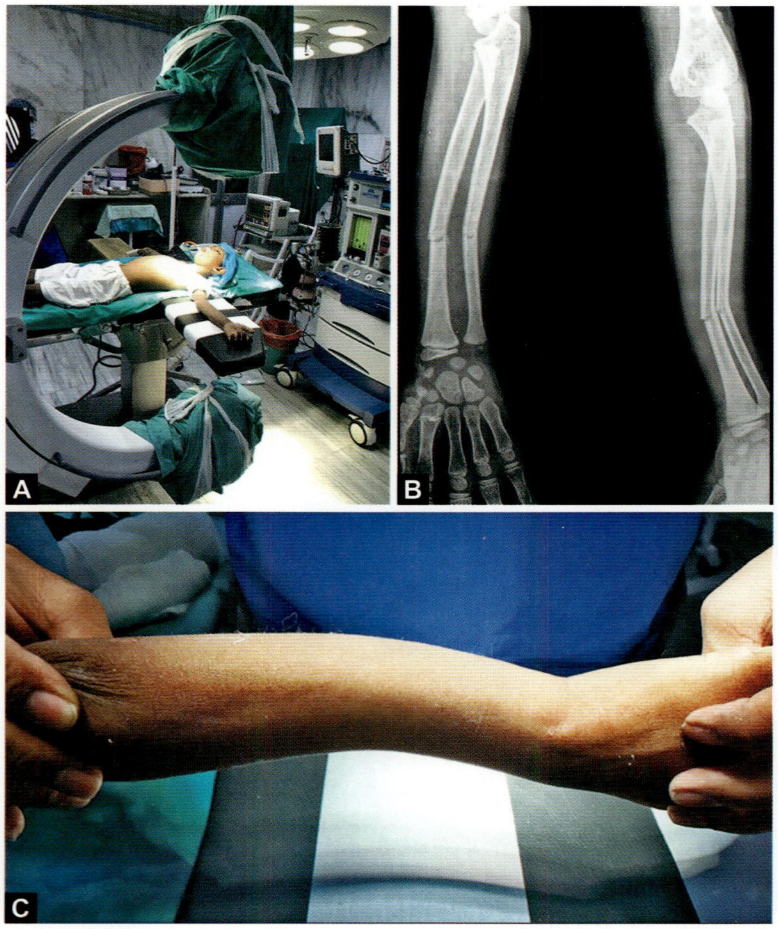

Figs. 2A to C: Preoperative radiographs and patient positioning.

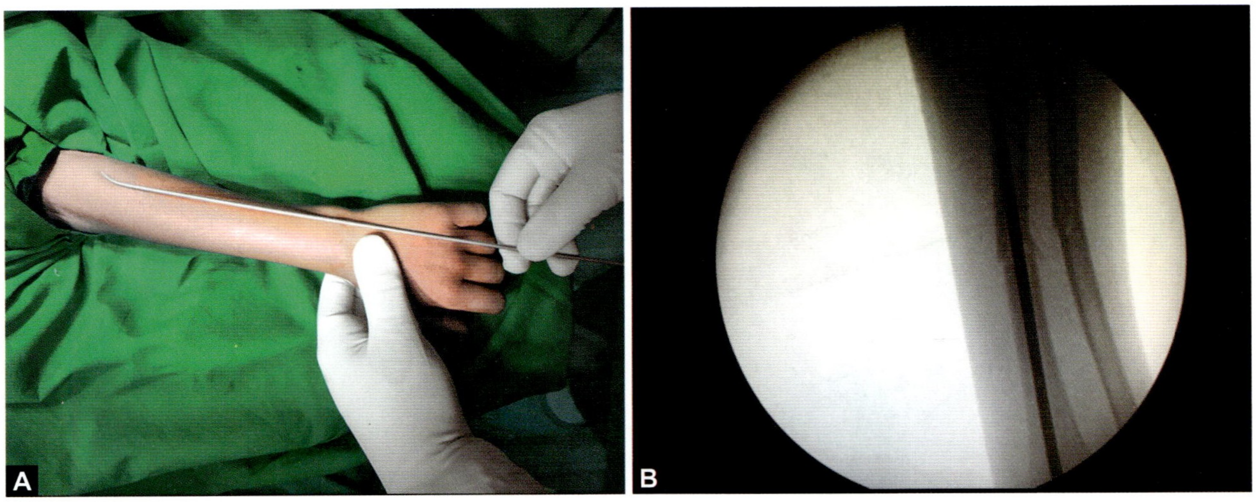

Figs. 3A and B: Preoperative determination of nail diameter.

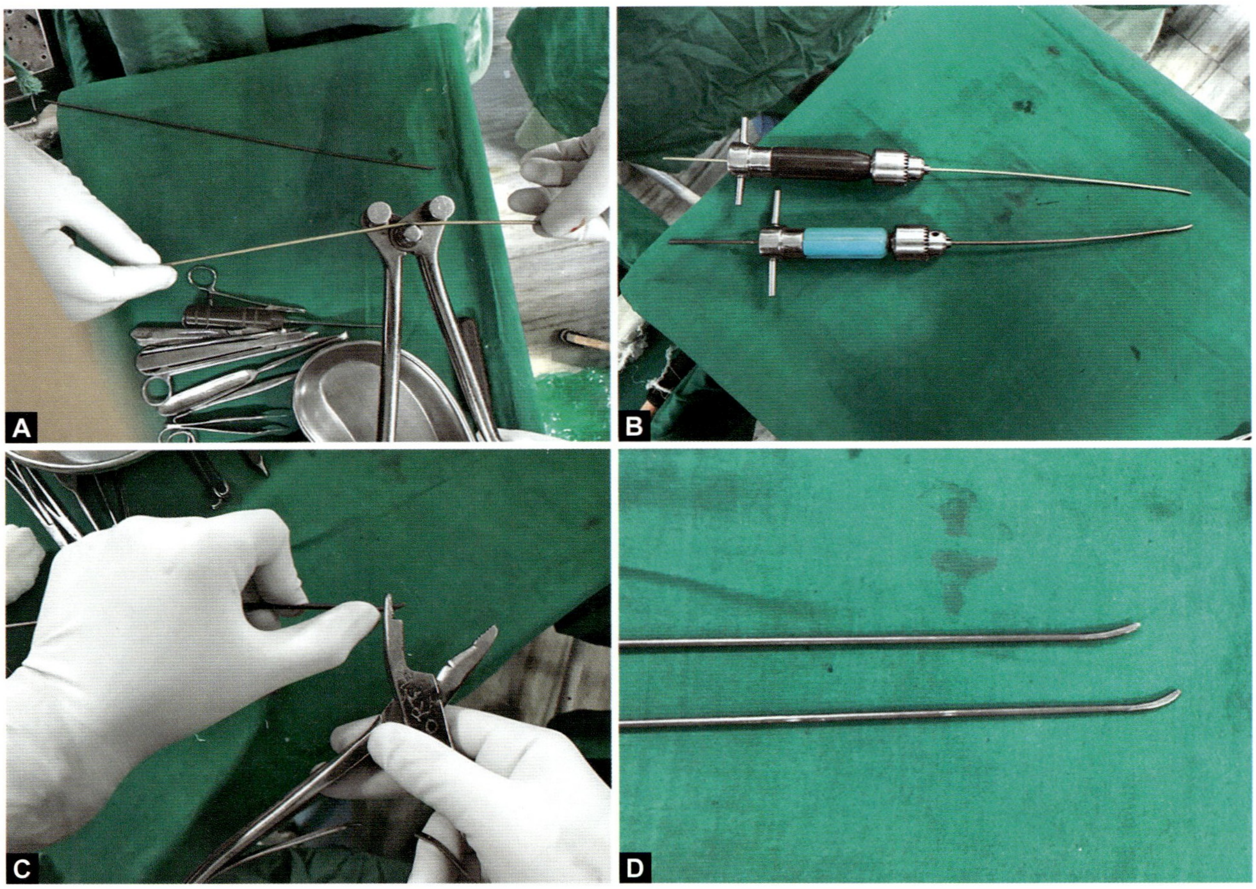

Figs. 4A to D: Contouring the nail and bending of the nail tip.

CONTOURING OF NAIL AND BENDING OF NAIL TIPS (FIGS. 4A TO D)

Unlike a long bone fracture, contouring of elastic nails for forearm fractures is done to maintain the interosseous space between the two forearm bones. Nail tips are bent to facilitate entry and nail passing with minimum amount of endosteal irritation.

MAKING A RADIAL ENTRY POINT (FIGS. 5A TO D)

The radial entry point is made in the center of the distal radial metaphysis after confirming it on an image intensifier. A 2-cm incision is made and the extensor tendons are dissected by blunt dissection. The periosteum of the distal radius is reached and incised. The entry point is reconfirmed by imaging and a small bone awl is used to make a unicortical hole in the distal radius.

FACILITATING INSERTION OF THE RADIAL NAIL (FIGS. 6A AND B)

Once the radial entry point is made with an awl, the awl is angulated to make a track for the nail slide into the radial medullary canal. This track is serially widened with instruments till for smooth entry of the radial nail. Once the nail is advanced to the fracture site, the fracture is reduced with traction and F tool and the nail is guided into the proximal fragment.

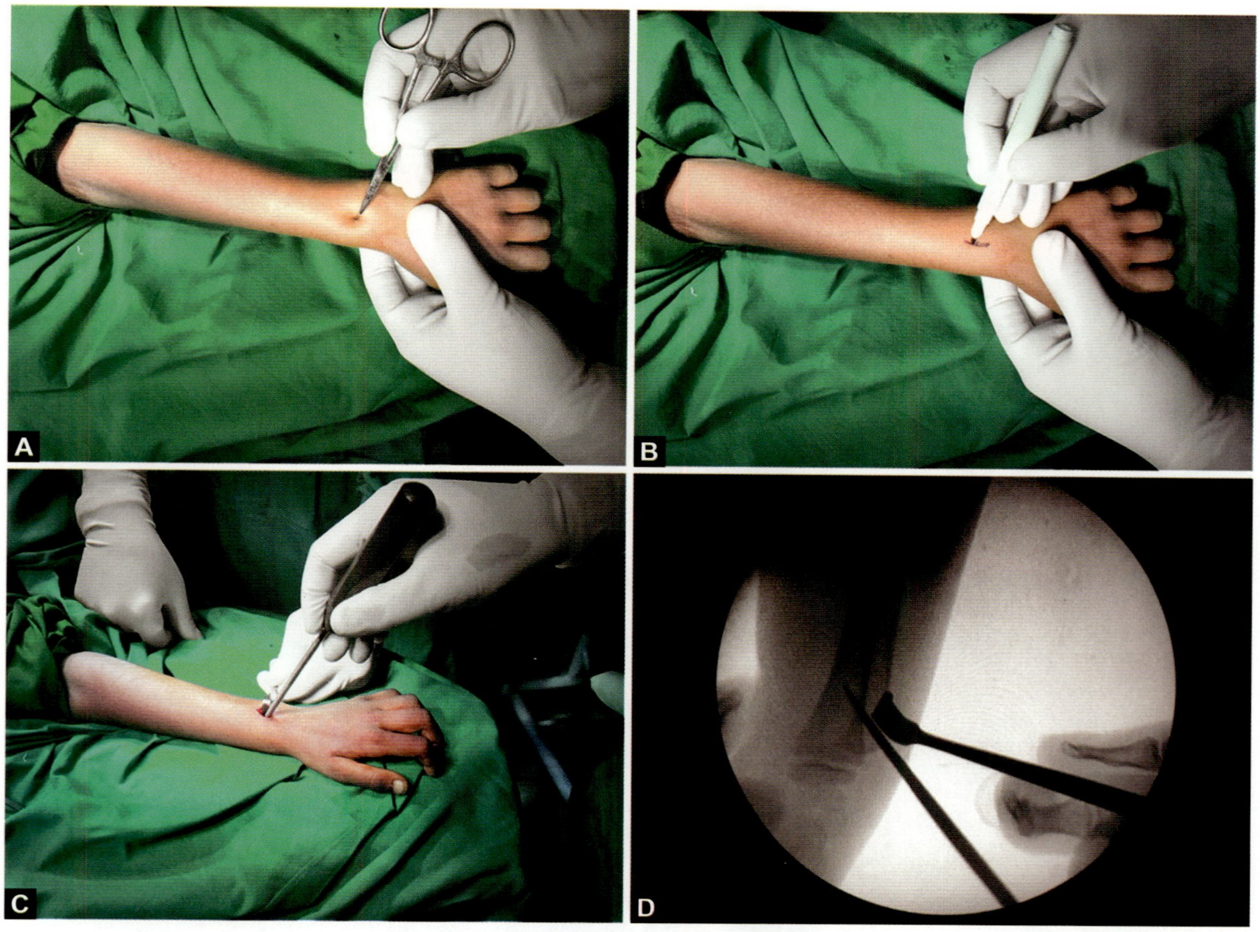

Figs. 5A to D: Making a radial entry point.

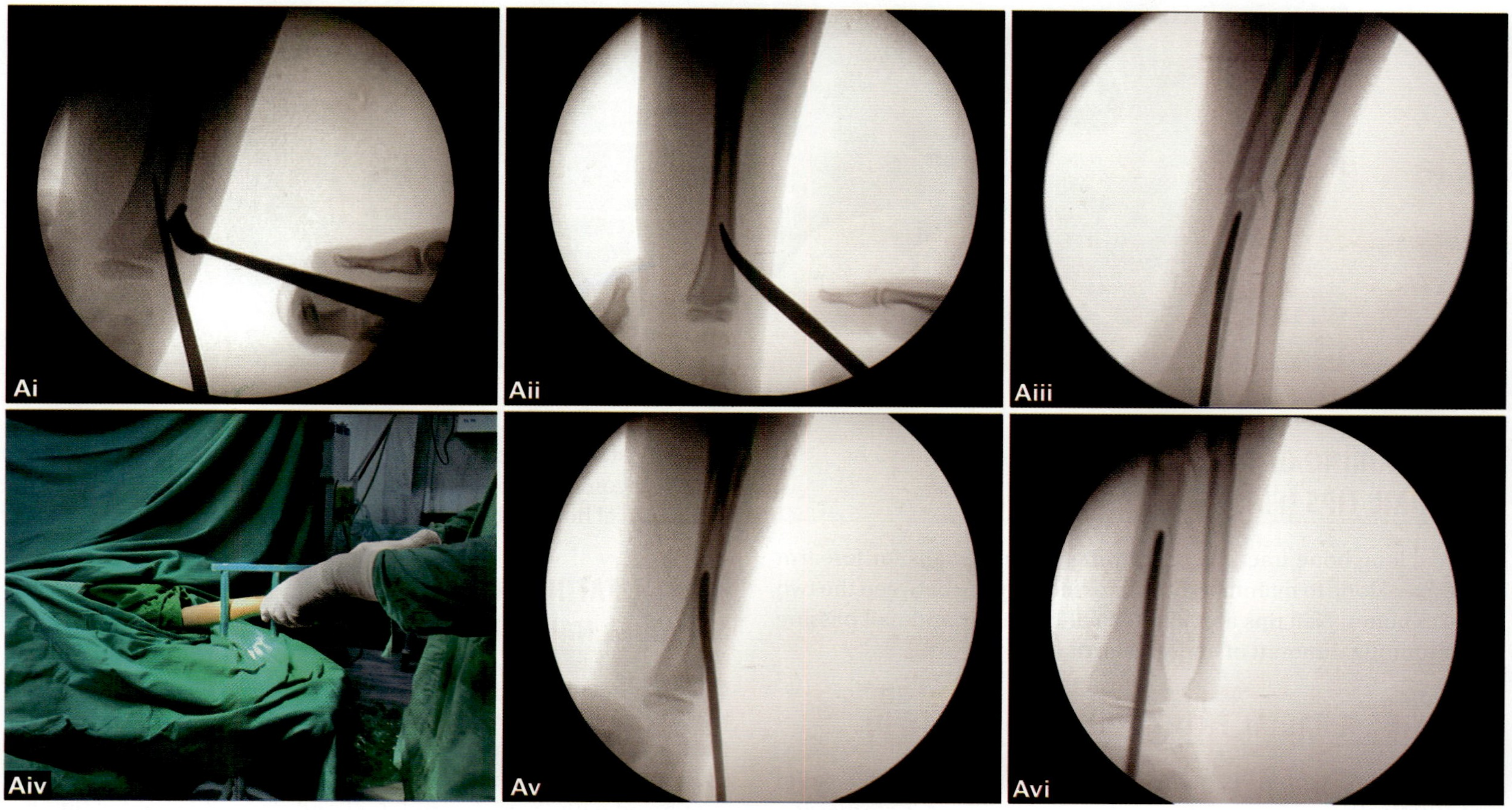

Figs. 6A(Ai to Avi): Facilitating radial nail entry.

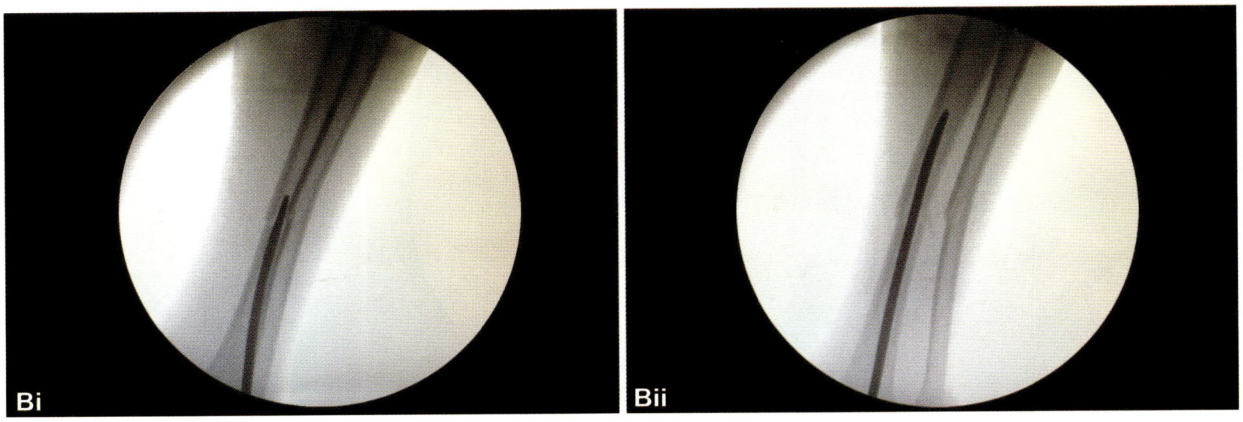

Figs. 6B(Bi and Bii): Radial fracture reduction and nail insertion.

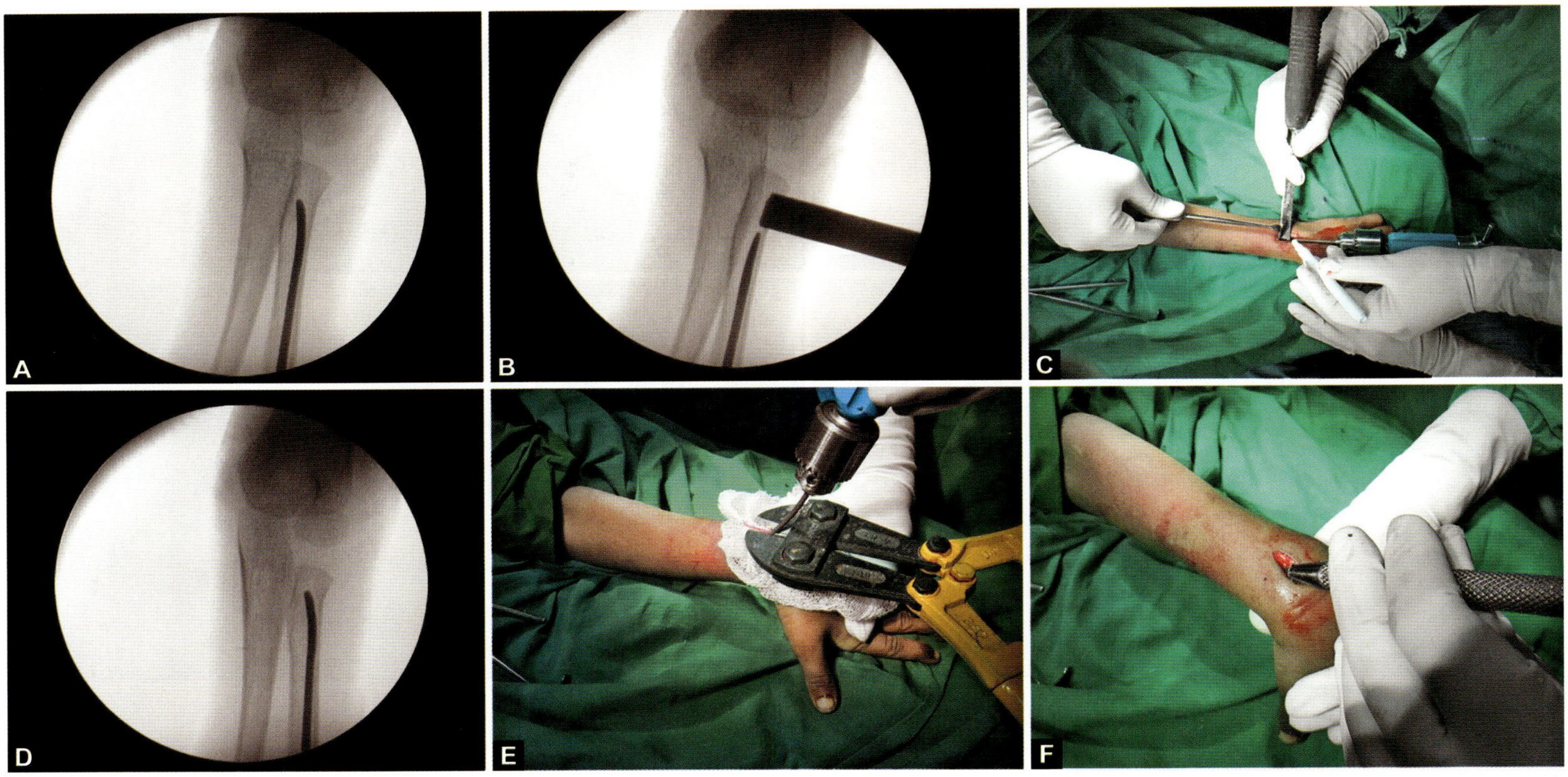

Figs. 7A to F: Final seating of the nail.

FINAL SEATING OF THE RADIAL NAIL (FIGS. 7A TO F)

Once the nail is propagated at considerable distance across the fracture site into the medullary cavity, the final seating point of the tip of the nail in the bone is determined and its distance from the tip is measured. This distance is then marked at the distal end of the nail by measuring it from the point of entry. The nail is cut at this mark and slowly pushed with a specially designed hollow tipped punch and a mallet to its final seating point.

ULNA NAILING (FIGS. 8A TO J)

The entry point for the ulna nail is the proximal metaphysis of the ulna, at least 2 cm away from the olecranon apophysis. The metaphyseo-diaphyseal entry of the nail is facilitated similarly to that of the radial nail and the maneuvers for reduction and nail insertion are the same as that for the radius.

The wounds are closed in layers and the patient's limb is immobilized in a soft bandage.

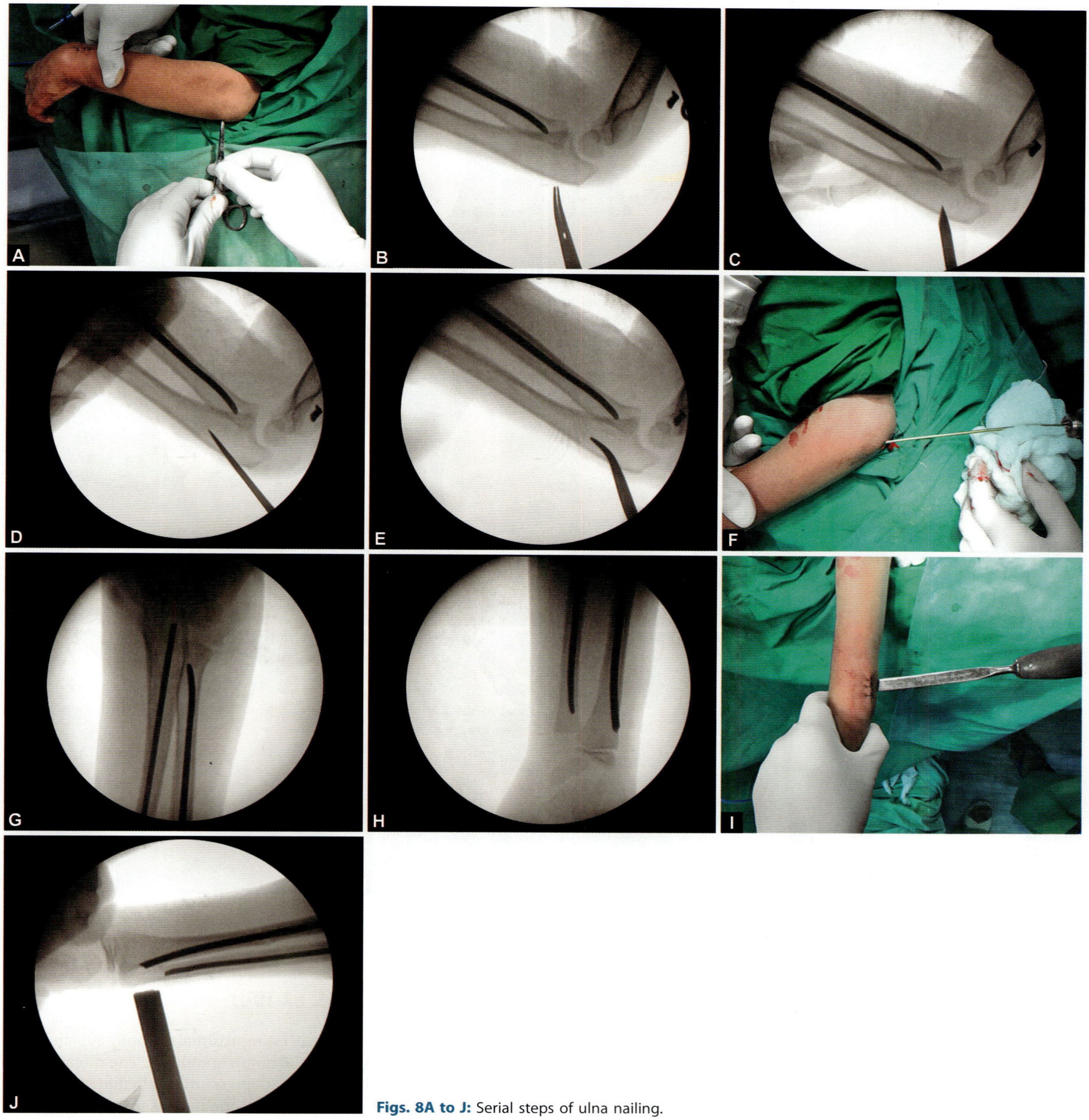

Figs. 8A to J: Serial steps of ulna nailing.

CHAPTER 10

Pediatric Fracture Neck Femur

Avi Pranay Shah, Sandeep Vaidya, Mandar Agashe

INTRODUCTION

Fractures of the neck of the femur in pediatric and adolescent age group are quite rare injuries. In fact, these injuries constitute less than 1% of all fractures in the pediatric population. This low incidence is attributed to the thick and strong periosteum cover and to the tough strong bone of children. Hence, as a result, most of these fractures (80–90%) are due to high-energy trauma and associated with other injuries. Despite their rare occurrence, these fractures are associated with a high complication rate, which make it an important clinical entity to understand.

Fractures of the hip in children are orthopaedic emergencies, requiring prompt and aggressive management within the first few hours after presentation. The anatomy of the pediatric hip differs from the anatomy of adult hips and this accounts for differences in treatment and complications. A thorough understanding of anatomy is important to ensure proper treatment and to understand associated complications to prevent high morbidity rates.

PATHOPHYSIOLOGY

The proximal femoral physis contributes greatly to the metaphyseal growth of the femoral neck with a minimal growth of the femoral head. The trochanteric apophysis also contributes to an extent toward the metaphyseal growth. The most important anatomy to understand is the blood supply of the proximal femur which is derived from two main arterial supplies: the medial circumflex artery and its branches being the main supply and the lateral circumflex artery and its branches. Extracapsular arterial ring is formed at the base of the femoral neck, the ascending cervical branches of the arterial ring at the surface of the femoral neck, and the arteries of the ligamentum teres. There is significant anastomosis among the various arteries in the proximal femur in approximately two-thirds of the cases (Fig. 1).

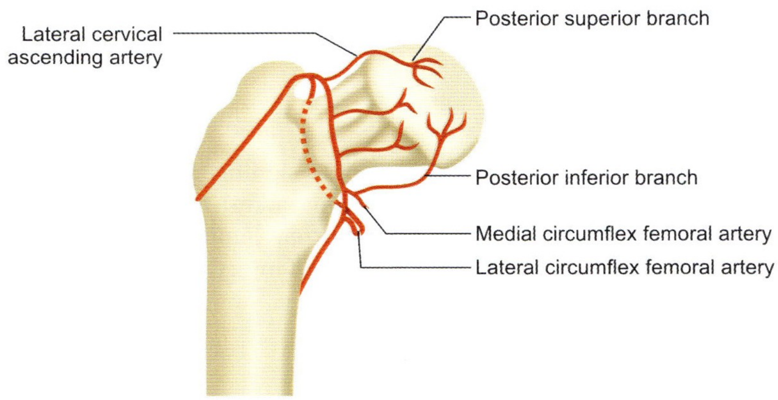

Fig. 1: Schematic diagram showing the blood supply of the proximal femur.

CLASSIFICATION

Delbet was the first person to classify pediatric neck of femur fractures and is the most widely used and acceptable classification. Colonna modified this classification and this is still being used extensively to describe the anatomical location of the fracture. This classification backed by literature gives excellent correlation with the rates of complications, especially AVN with type I having an AVN rate of as much as 80–100% while type IV has an AVN rate of as less as 1–2% (Fig. 2 and Table 1).

CLINICAL FINDINGS

Children are unable to bear weight on the injured extremity. The extremity may be shortened and externally rotated. These fractures may be associated with other polytrauma injuries (head injuries, abdominal injuries, etc.) due to the high velocity required for such injuries.

IMAGING STUDIES

Plain radiographs are the primary standard imaging modality to diagnose and classify a pediatric femoral neck fracture. When attempting a cross-table lateral radiograph, care should be taken

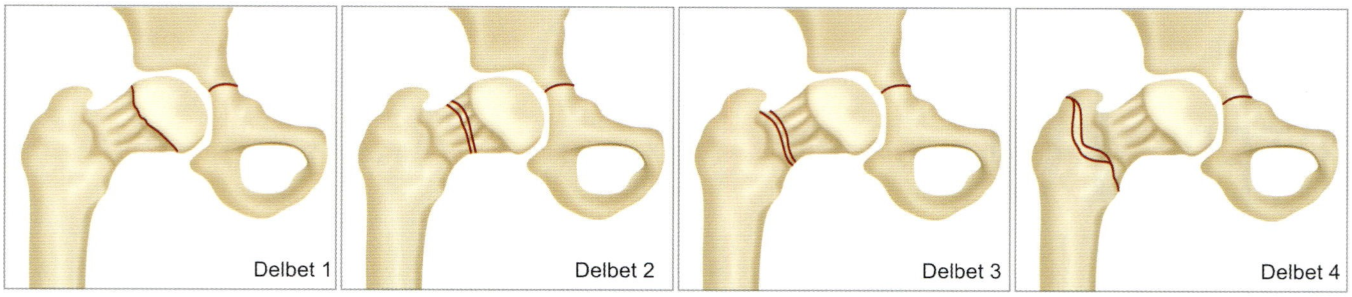

Fig. 2: Schematic representation of the Delbet classification.

TABLE 1: Delbet classification.

Type	*Description*	*Incidence*	*AVN*	*Nonunion*
Type I	Transphyseal IA—without dislocation of epiphysis from acetabulum IB—with dislocation of epiphysis	<10%	38% (AVN 100% in type IB)	
Type II	Transcervical	40–50%	28%	15%
Type III	Cervicotrochanteric (or basicervical)	30–35%	18%	15–20%
Type IV	Intertrochanteric	10–20%	5%	5%

(AVN: avascular necrosis)

to move the uninjured limb so as not to significantly displace the fracture on the injured side. CT or MRI may play a role in diagnosing undisplaced or stress fractures or concurrent femoral neck fracture-dislocations to better define the pattern of injury. They also have a role in diagnosing pathologic fractures.

TECHNIQUES

Nonoperative treatment can be used in children less than 1 year may be by using either a Pavlik harness or abduction brace. Spica cast in abduction can also be used with radiographs at weekly interval.

In older children treated nonoperatively by a spica cast the plaster should be applied past the knee. There are no outcome studies on spica or brace treatment but a spica cast should only be considered in younger children up to 5 years with nondisplaced fractures.

Nonoperative and spica cast treatment alone is not optimal in older children as the potential for nonunion is too great as well as high incidence of coxa vara after conservative methods. A supplemental spica cast is recommended for children that are not near skeletal maturity.

CAPSULOTOMY

Emergent reduction and capsulotomy (<24 h) may diminish risk of AVN by restoring blood flow through kinked vessels. Aspiration with large bore needle through sub-adductor approach or anterior hip approach can be done to reduce the tamponade effect and reduce the risk of AVN.

Open capsulotomy also can be done by performing a hip arthrotomy through the anterior approach using the smith Peterson interval.

Surgical Steps (Capsulotomy)

- *OR table*: Radiolucent
- *Position/positioning aids*: Supine with a "bump" under the thoracolumbar spine to the posterior-superior iliac spine to access the greater trochanter for screw insertion.
- *Fluoroscopy location*: Opposite surgeon
- Mark the anterior incision with hip in 90° flexion to develop. Draw a line that is in line with the skin crease of the anterior hip. The incision should be 2 cm medial and 2 cm lateral to the anterior superior iliac spine (ASIS).
- Perform sharp dissection through the skin and subcutaneous tissue.
- Externally rotate the leg and identify the sartorius.
- Identify the interval between the sartorius and tensor fascia lata (Smith–Petersen interval)
- Open the interval using use Metzenbaum scissors, small blunt retractors, or a hemostat
- Expose the joint capsule with a Cobb elevator for blunt dissection to expose this deeper layer
- Retract the head of the rectus femoris muscle medially this exposes the capsular iliacus and deep capsule of the hip joint
- Create arthrotomy window
- Drain the hip effusion.

CLOSED REDUCTION AND PERCUTANEOUS PINNING/ INTERNAL FIXATION

The child is placed on a radiolucent table with a small radiolucent bump under the ipsilateral buttock. Before draping, it is essential to check whether good-quality AP and frog-lateral C-arm pictures are easily obtained. The entire leg is draped free. The prominent bony markings such as ASIS, greater trochanter, and the lateral femoral condyle are marked with a sterile marking pen. Gentle closed reduction is attempted either by the assistant or the fracture table apparatus to give traction and internal rotation. Once the reduction is checked under fluoroscopy pinning can be done. Depending on the age of the child and type of fracture the choice of implant can be chosen. In younger children aged 2 years, 2-mm smooth pins should be used crossing the physis. The children older than 3 years, 4.5-mm cannulated cancellous (CC) screws can be applied in standard configuration keeping in mind not to cross the physis. Older children and adolescents 6.5-mm or 7.3-mm CC screws can be used in standard configuration.

If reduction cannot be achieved open reduction can be done. The choice of approach depends on the fracture displacement. The standard Watson Jones approach is the most commonly used approach but if posterior displaced femoral head is present which is more commonly seen with type 1b then a posterior approach can be used.

Surgical Steps (Closed Reduction and Percutaneous Pinning)

- *OR table*: Radiolucent
- *Position/positioning aids*: Supine with a "bump" under the thoracolumbar spine to the posterior-superior iliac spine to access the greater trochanter for screw insertion or placing the patient on a fracture table.
- *Fluoroscopy location*: Opposite surgeon
- Closed reduction of fracture by adduction and internal rotation.
- Mark position of guidewire using fluoroscopy on AP and lateral views
- Stab incision and place guidewire in standard position using fluoroscopy
- Insert smooth pins and cross physis (do not penetrate articular surface of femoral head). In older children or adolescents use appropriate screw length. Avoid crossing the physis in children younger than 10 years.

OPEN REDUCTION AND INTERNAL FIXATION

The child is placed on a radiolucent table with a small radiolucent bump under the ipsilateral buttock. Before draping, it is essential to check whether good-quality AP and frog-lateral C-arm pictures are easily obtained. The entire leg is draped free. The prominent bony markings such as ASIS, greater trochanter, and the lateral femoral condyle are marked with a sterile marking pen. After failure of gentle closed reduction open reduction is attempted using the Watson–Jones (anterolateral approach. A lateral incision is made over the proximal femur, slightly anterior to the greater trochanter. The fascia lata is incised longitudinally. The innervation of the tensor muscle by the superior gluteal nerve is 2–5 cm above the greater trochanter, and care should be taken not to damage this structure. The tensor muscle is reflected anteriorly. The interval between the gluteus medius and the tensor muscles will be used. The plane is developed between the muscles and the underlying hip capsule. If necessary, the anterior-most fibers of the gluteus medius tendon can be detached from the trochanter for wider exposure. After clearing the anterior hip capsule, longitudinal capsulotomy is made along the anterosuperior femoral neck. A transverse incision can be added superiorly for wider exposure. Once the hip fracture is reduced, guidewires for cannulated screws can be passed perpendicular to fracture line. 4.5-mm screws are used for children under 8 years and 6.5-mm or 7.3-mm screws used for older children and adolescents.

Displaced type IV fractures in all children more than 3 years should be treated with internal fixation with a pediatric or juvenile compression hip screw or pediatric locking hip plate placed into femoral neck short of the physis. It is important to place an antirotation wire before drilling and tapping the neck for the dynamic hip screw.

Surgical Steps (Open Reduction and Fixation)

- *OR table*: Radiolucent
- *Position/positioning aids*: Supine with a "bump" under the thoracolumbar spine to the posterior-superior iliac spine to access the greater trochanter for screw insertion or placing the patient on a fracture table.
- *Fluoroscopy location*: Opposite surgeon
- Attempt gentle closed reduction of fracture by adduction and internal rotation.
- A lateral incision is made over the proximal femur, slightly anterior to the greater trochanter.
- *Watson–Jones approach*: The interval between gluteus medius and the tensor muscles made.
- Under direct visualization reduction of fracture done.
- Once the hip fracture is reduced, guidewires for cannulated screws can be passed perpendicular to fracture line. Screws inserted in standard fashion.
- In older children and adolescents pediatric dynamic hip screw (DHS) system used with three hole plate or proximal femoral locking plates can be used.

Fixation with Dynamic Hip Screw and Cannulated Cancellous Screws/130 degrees Proximal Femur Locking Plate (Technical Steps) (Figs. 3 to 7)

- *OR table*: Radiolucent
- *Position/positioning aids*: Supine with a "bump" under the thoracolumbar spine to the posterior-superior iliac spine to access the greater trochanter for screw insertion or placing the patient on a fracture table
- *Fluoroscopy location*: Opposite surgeon
- Applicable in older children and adolescents
- Gentle closed fracture reduction is carried. If unable to correct open reduction can to done.
- If is reduced, it is provisionally fixed using two thick K-wires.
- Lateral approach to hip used and dissection done in layers.
- Once reduction is obtained, the guidewire for the proximal screw is placed in the inferior quadrant on the AP view and central on the lateral view. This will allow either one more screw above the first screw.
- The screw is predrilled and kept slightly loose and not completely seated in the bone.
- Cannulated cancellous screw just superior and parallel to the central screw for added stability and compression.
- Standard pediatric DHS is applied in standard fashion.
- Similarly after reduction, guidewire for 130° proximal femur locking plate inserted.
- 130-degrees proximal femur locking plate inserted in standard manner.

Fixation with Dynamic Hip Screw/Proximal Femoral Locking Plate with Valgus Osteotomy (Technical Steps)

- *OR table*: Radiolucent
- *Position/positioning aids*: Supine with a "bump" under the thoracolumbar spine to the posterior-superior iliac spine to access the greater trochanter for screw insertion or placing the patient on a fracture table.
- *Fluoroscopy location*: Opposite surgeon
- Applicable in older children and adolescents with delayed presentation and high Pauwel's angle.

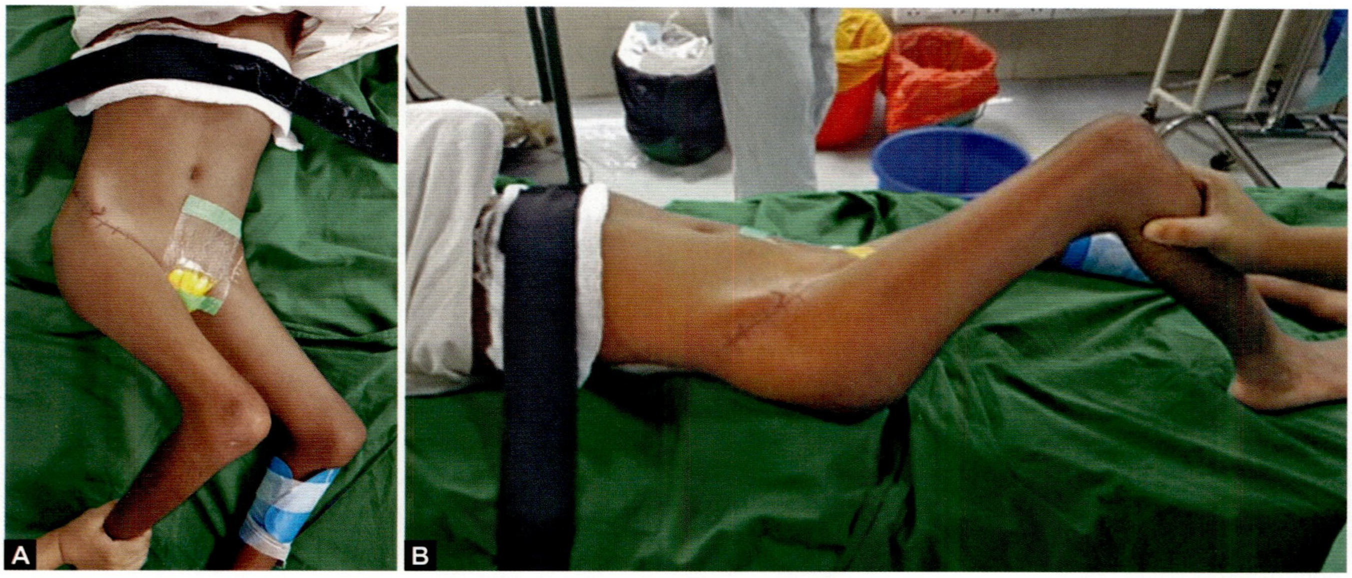

Figs. 3A and B: Position of the child. The authors preferred method is a simple radiolucent table with a small "bump" under the ipsilateral buttock. The C-arm would be from the opposite side. The limb can be gently taken to the frog-leg position for a lateral view. A fracture table can be used for bigger adolescent kids.

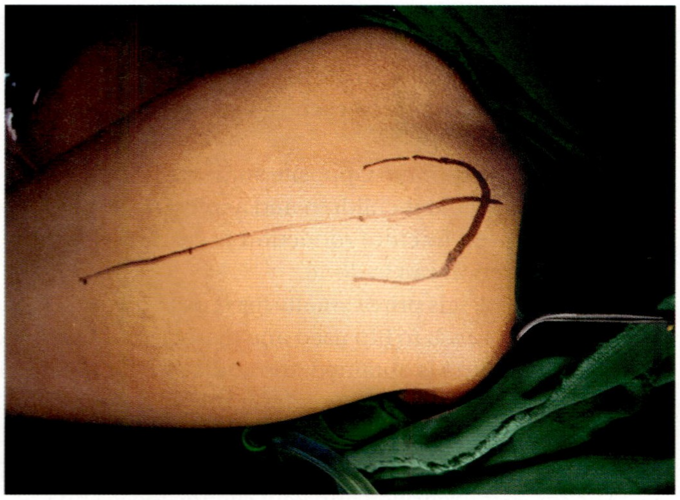

Fig. 4: The reduction is obtained by flexion, abduction and external rotation and once the reduction is obtained, it becomes stable by keeping in extension. The incision is a straight incision from the greater trochanter going distally for about 10–15 cm.

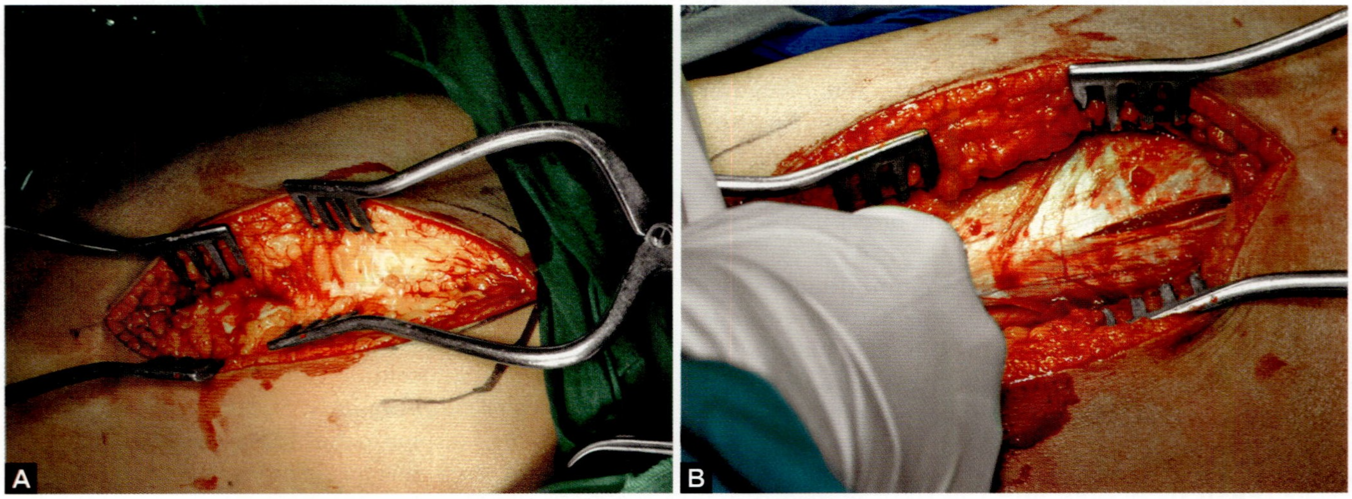

Figs. 5A and B: After the skin, subcutaneous tissue and the fascia lata are incised in the direction of the skin incision, the vastus lateralis muscle is exposed. At the level of the lesser trochanter but on the posterior aspect, the insertion of the gluteus maximus on the linea aspera is identified (also known as the gluteal sling). The entire vastus lateralis can be lifted off the femur safely by inserting a Homann spike at this level under the vastus lateralis and cutting the vastus lateralis distally just anterior to the lateral intermuscular septum, taking care to identify and coagulate the perforators which arise from the posterior compartment and come anteriorly. The proximal end of the vastus is lifted off the vastus ridge over the GT by an L-shaped incision.

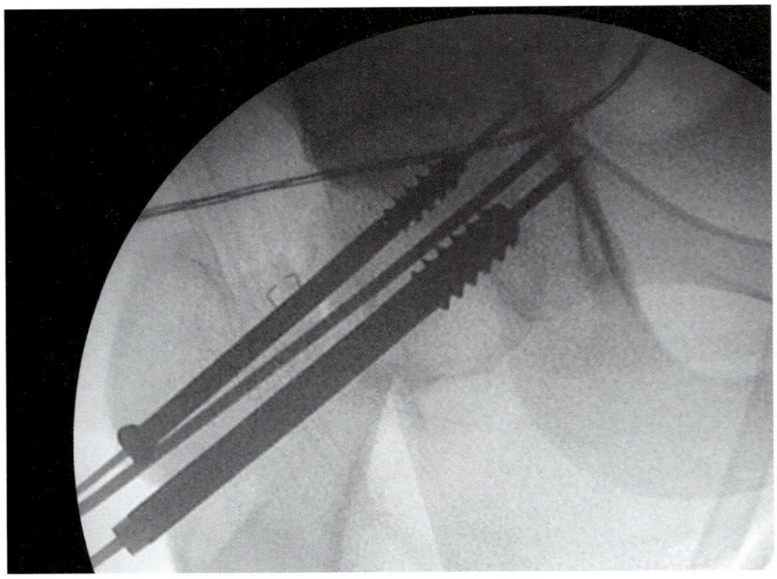

Fig. 6: The guidewire for the dynamic hip screw (DHS) is placed parallel to the neck but slightly inferior to the center deep into the femoral head. It may sometime be advisable to transfix the wire especially in subcapital fractures.

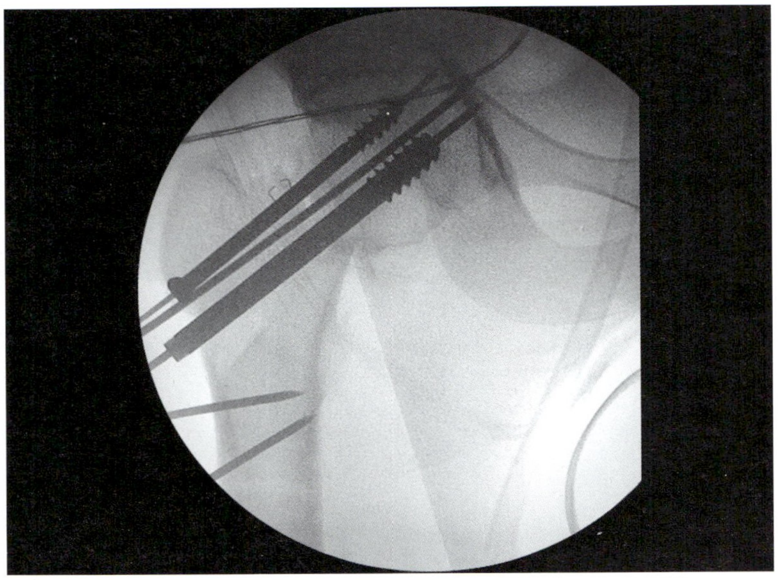

Fig. 7: One or two more wires are placed parallel to the dynamic hip screw (DHS) wire—one for the cannulated cancellous (CC) screw and one if required for the fibula. The DHS is triple reamed and DHS placed according to size, along with the CC screw.

- Gentle closed fracture reduction is carried. If unable to correct open reduction can to done.
- If reduced it is provisionally fixed using two thick K-wires.
- Standard lateral approach to hip used and dissection done in layers.
- Once reduction is obtained, the guidewire for the proximal screw is placed in the central quadrant on the AP view and central on the lateral view if using the DHS system or centrally 5 mm below superior border of the neck. When using the locking plates.
- 140°–150° degrees locking plates are used for valgus osteotomy.
- A subtrochanteric osteotomy is done below lesser trochanter. A lateral closing wedge can be removed with an angle to recreate the required the neck shaft angle when using a DHS system or a transverse osteotomy when using the locking plates.
- Standard pediatric DHS or proximal femoral locking plate is applied.
- It is important to lateralize the distal segment to keep the mechanical axis aligned.

Fixation with Dynamic Hip Screw/Proximal Femoral Locking Plate with Valgus Osteotomy and Nonvascularized Fibula Graft (Technical Steps) (Figs. 8 to 12)

- *OR table*: Radiolucent
- *Position/positioning aids*: Supine with a "bump" under the thoracolumbar spine to the posterior-superior iliac spine to access the greater trochanter for screw.
- *Fluoroscopy location*: Opposite surgeon
- Applicable in children and adolescents with delayed presentation/nonunions and high Pauwel's angle.
- Gentle closed fracture reduction is carried out. If unable to correct open reduction can to done.
- If is reduced, it is provisionally fixed using two thick K-wires.
- The femur is exposed using the standard lateral approach incision
- Once reduction is obtained, the guidewire for the proximal screw is placed in the inferior quadrant on the AP view and central on the lateral view. This will allow either one more screw or fibula just above the first screw.

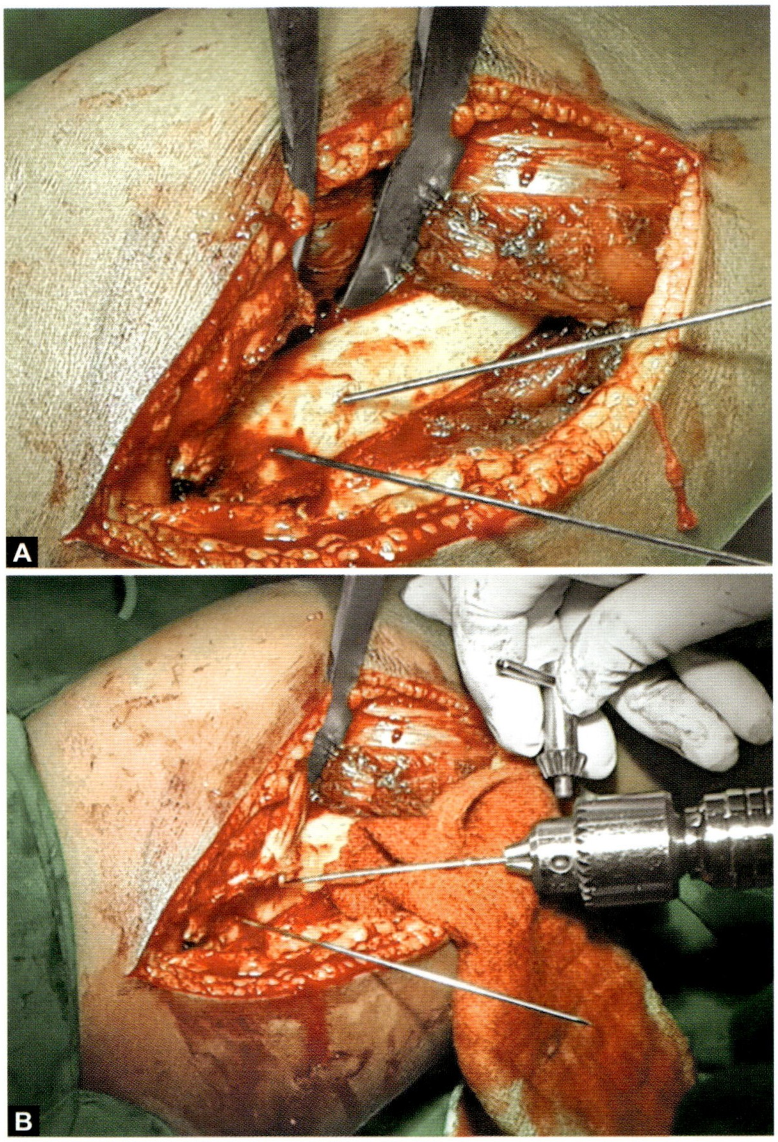

Figs. 8A and B: If required, a valgus osteotomy is performed. The first marking wire is just subtrochanteric and parallel to the dynamic hip screw (DHS) wire and the second wire at an angle which is the angle for correction.

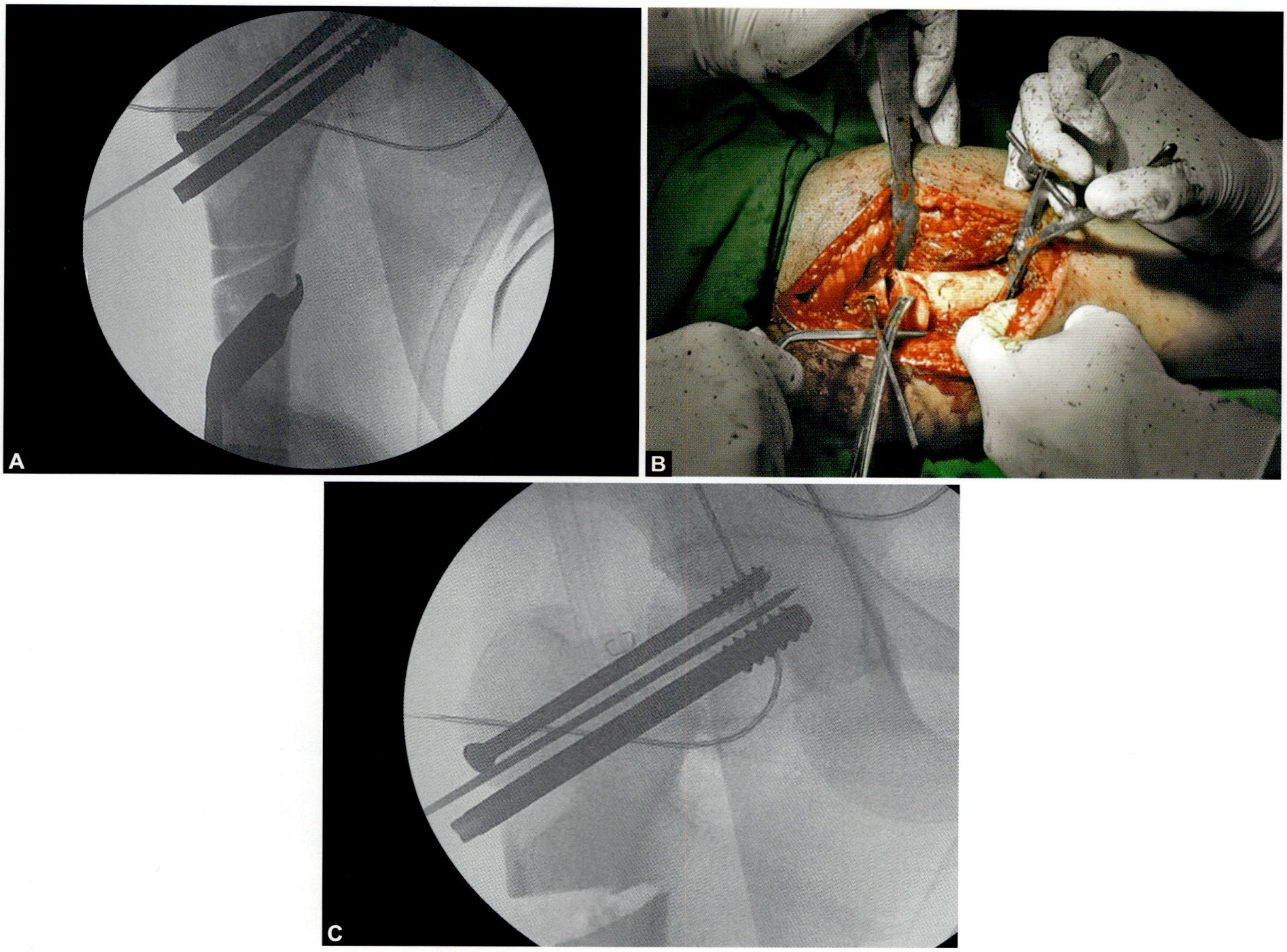

Figs. 9A to C: Once the angle is confirmed, osteotomy is performed using oscillating saw.

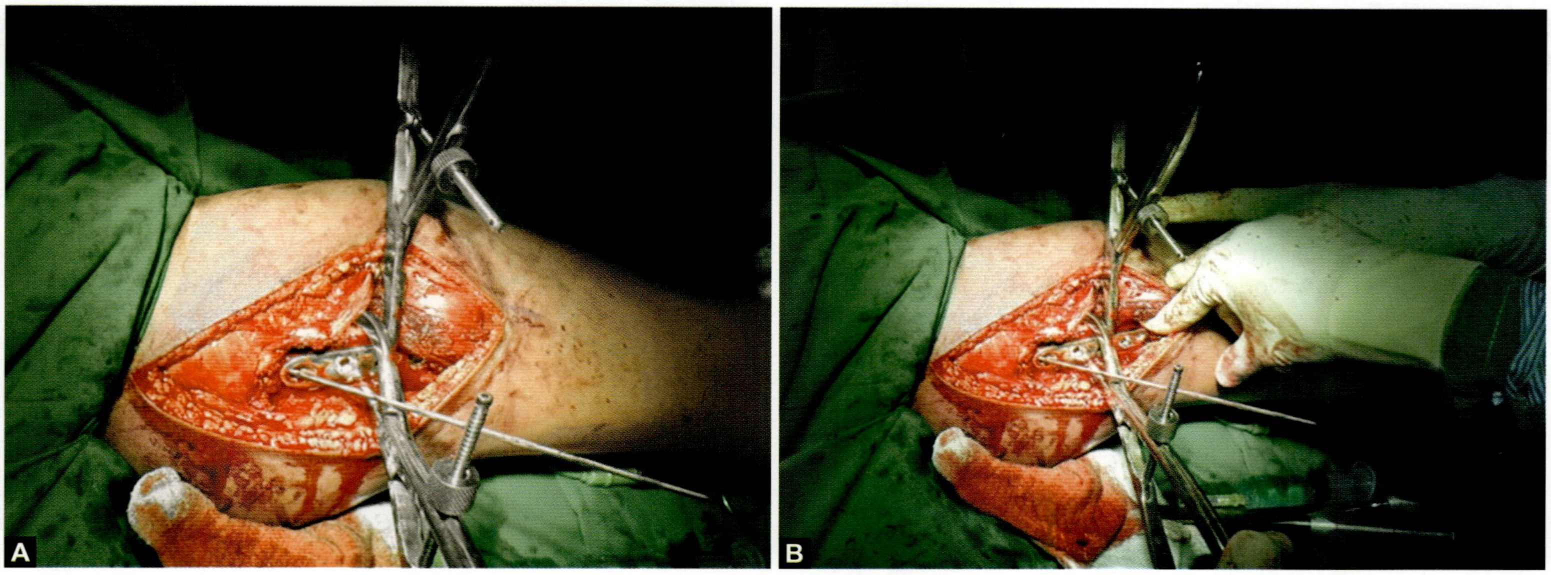

Figs. 10A and B

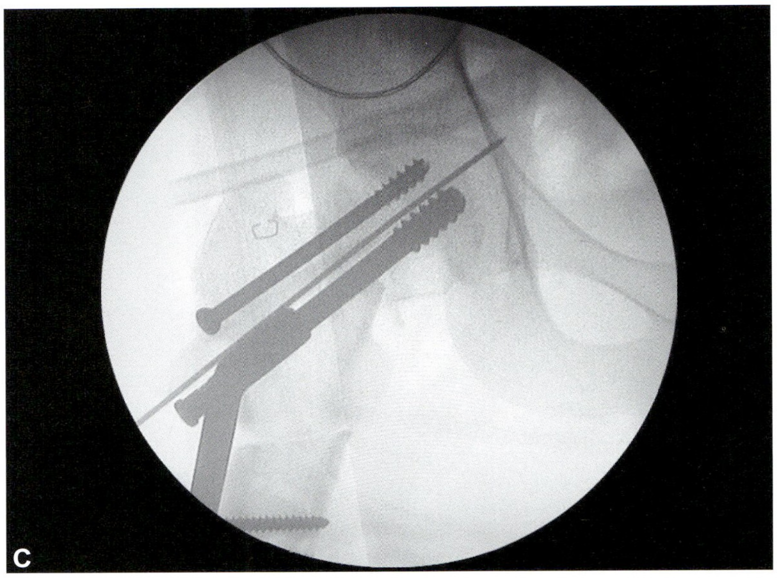

Figs. 10A to C: The proximal fragment is then abducted and the shaft is lateralized in order to align it with the plate which is of an angle of around 140–145°. The plate is then fixed using cortical screws.

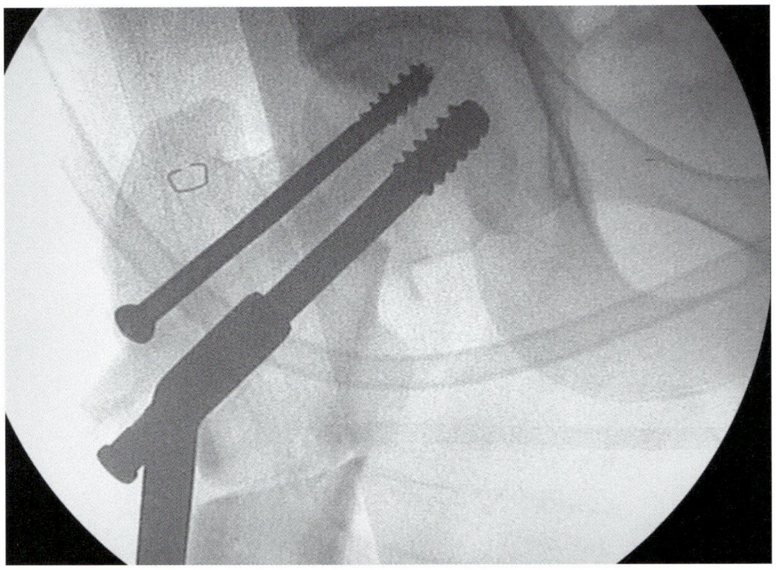

Fig. 11: A segment of nonvascularized fibula is then hammered in the proximal wire which has been reamed with a triple reamer. This fibula should reach the subchondral bone.

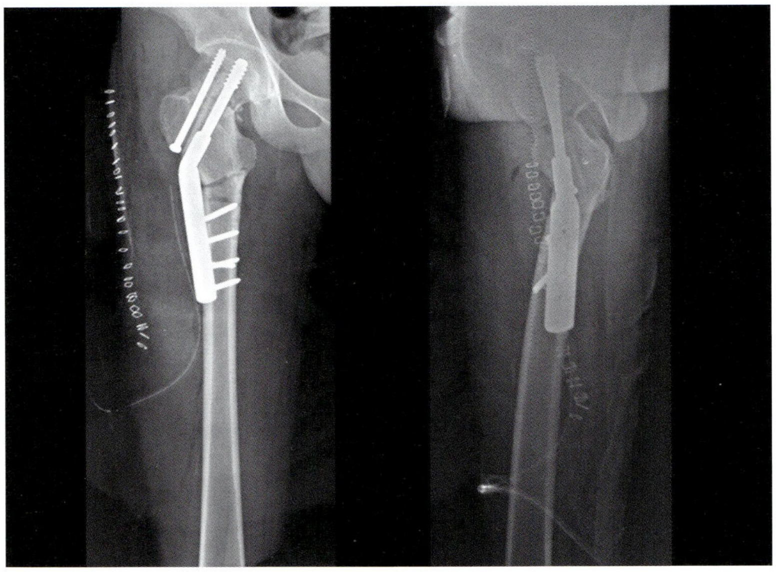

Fig. 12: Final postoperative X-ray after dynamic hip screw (DHS) fixation, valgus subtrochanteric osteotomy and fibula grafting.

- Subtrochanteric osteotomy is then planned just below the lesser trochanter. A wedge equal to the angle of correction is osteotomized and lateral-based wedge is closed.
- The distal fragment is then lateralized and the side plate or locking plate is placed.
- About 6–8 cm of fibular graft is harvested from the middle third. The graft width and length is measured. The size of the expected fibular graft is exactly measured and it is cut to that size. The width (diameter) of the graft is usually 6–7 mm, and if thicker than that, the graft is shingled to that size.
- To prepare the tract at the superior border of the femoral neck, sequential reaming is performed using cannulated drill bits and finally by a triple reamer so as to make the canal of adequate size.
- It is very important to see to it that the canal is dilated adequately
- The fibula is passed over the guidewire and gently tapped using a bone punch.
- The seating of the graft is ensured till approximately 5 mm of the subchondral surface.
- The extra portion of the fibular graft is cut
- If gap between the fracture fragments is too large, it is sometimes necessary to fill the graft using iliac crest cancellous bone grafts.
- DHS or pediatric hip locking plate placed in standard manner.

POSTOPERATIVE CARE

Supplementary casting should be considered for the majority of patients with proximal femoral fractures. Casting is indicated in all type I fractures in younger children. Type II and III fractures, it is recommend to use a hip spica cast for at least 6 weeks, especially in patients whose implants do not cross the femoral physis.

Children older than 12 years can be treated with transphyseal fixation that is stable enough to avoid cast fixation. But, the use of a postoperative cast depends on the stability of fracture fixation and the patient's compliance.

Fractures treated with a hip screw and side plate do not require cast immobilization. Formal physiotherapy usually is not required unless persistent limp, stiffness is seen which is rare.

SECTION 2

ARTHROSCOPY

Section Editor: *Umesh Jadhav*

CHAPTER 11

Anterior Cruciate Reconstruction

Umesh Jadhav, Aditya Upase

INTRODUCTION

The Anterior Cruciate Ligament (ACL) is most commonly injured ligament of the knee. It is commonly injured ligament in two wheeler accidents and sports like basketball, soccer, skiing and gymnastics, etc.

PATHOANATOMY

ACL is composed of the anteromedial and posterolateral bundles. These bundles originates from the medial and anterior aspect of the tibial plateau and runs superiorly, posteriorly and laterally toward its insertion on the lateral femoral condyle. It provides restraining force of anterior translation, prevent excessive rotation and prevents varus and valgus stress. Together with the posterior cruciate ligament (PCL), ACL controls joint kinematics.

GRADES OF INJURY

Injured ligaments are classified as:

- *Grade 1 sprain:* Ligament is partially damaged and slightly stretched with stable knee joint.
- *Grade 2 sprain:* Partial tear of the ligament with minimal instability of the joint.
- *Grade 3 sprain:* Complete tear of the ligament resulting in gross instability of the knee joint.

CLINICAL FEATURES

- *Symptoms*: Patient usually presents with history of injury to knee, pain, swelling, restriction of movement, and difficulty in weight bearing.
- *Signs*: Physical examination reveals effusion and joint line tenderness although clinical objective signs of ligament instability are difficult to demonstrate in acute inflammatory phase. Once acute inflammatory phase subsides, following clinical tests may indicate instability:
  - Lachman's test
  - Anterior drawer test
  - Pivot shift test.

IMAGING

- *X-rays*: Helpful to rule out bony injury.
- *Magnetic resonance imaging (MRI) scans:* MRI is diagnostic and will show torn ACL and other associated injuries of knee joint.

TREATMENT OPTIONS

Treatment will have to be individualized depending upon the patient's age and lifestyle.

Young sportsman will invariably need surgery whereas sedentary and older individual can be managed nonoperatively.

Arthroscopic Anterior Cruciate Ligament Reconstruction using Hamstring Tendon Graft—Surgical Technique

Available graft options:

- Hamstring tendon
- Quadriceps tendon
- Bone patellar tendon bone graft
- Peroneus longus tendon
- Achilles tendon.

SURGICAL STEPS (FIGS. 1 TO 28)

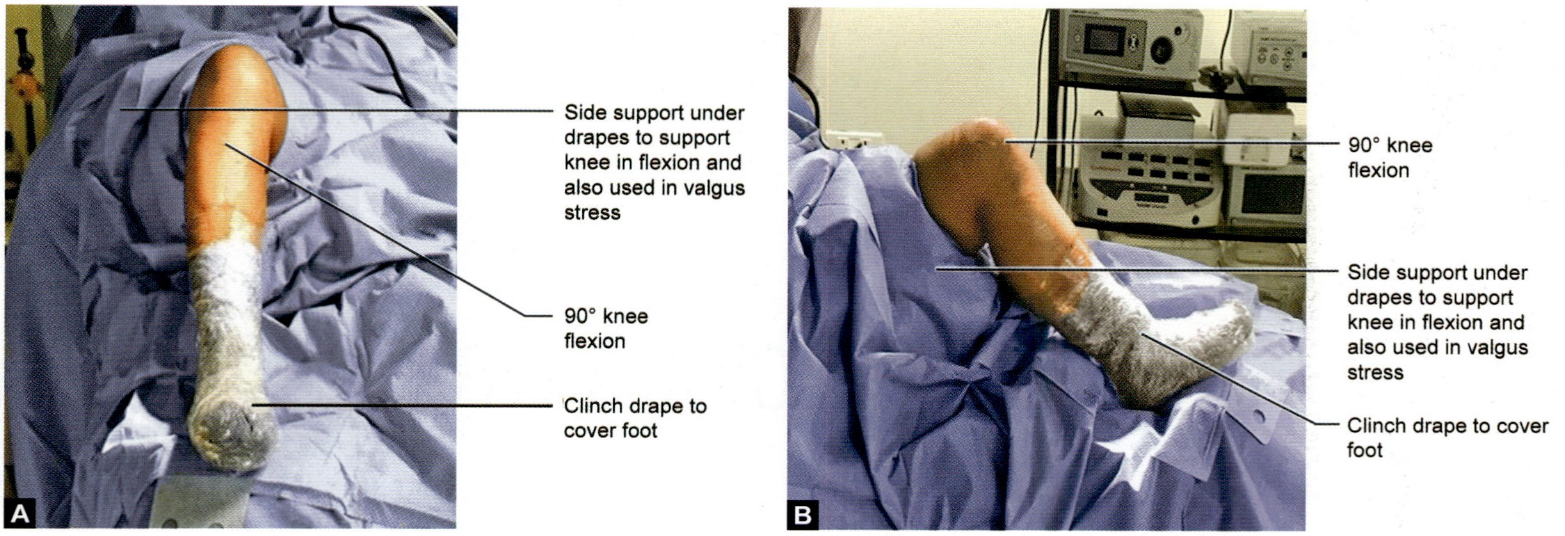

Figs. 1A and B: Patient is positioned supine after spinal anesthesia with side support for valgus stress and knee with 90° flexion. All aseptic precaution should be followed and lower limb is primarily scrubbed, painted, and draped in standard fashion.

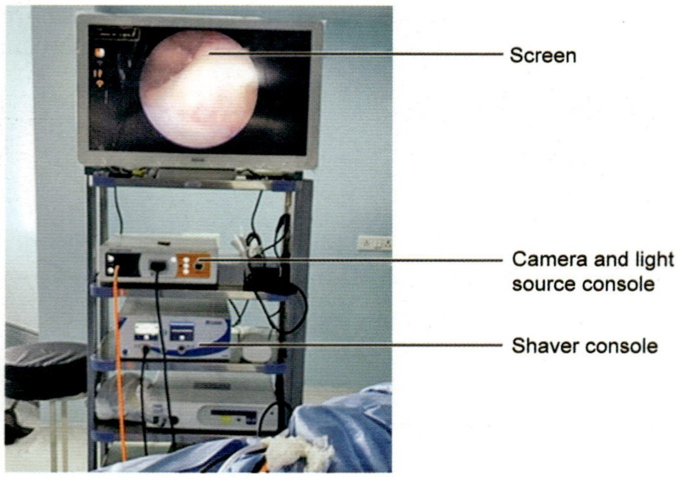

Fig. 2: Arthroscopy setup includes TV screen, camera and light source console, and shaver console. It should be arranged on the contralateral side and surgeon standing on ipsilateral side.

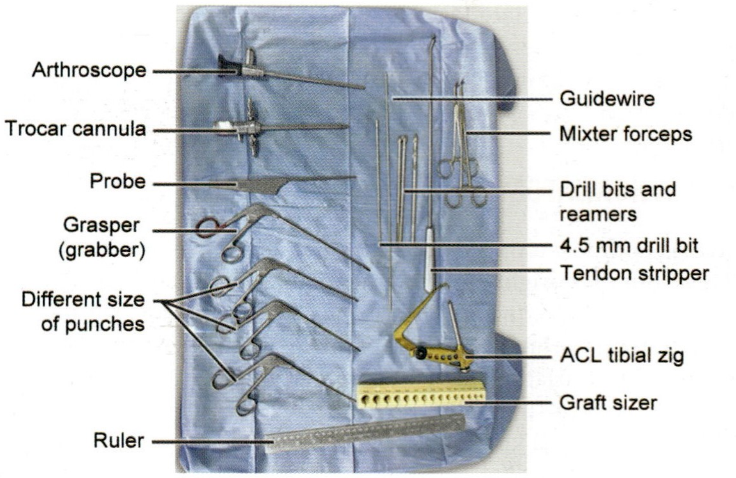

Fig. 3: Check for instrument trolley for all the necessary instruments during the surgical procedure and arranged them properly on the trolley.

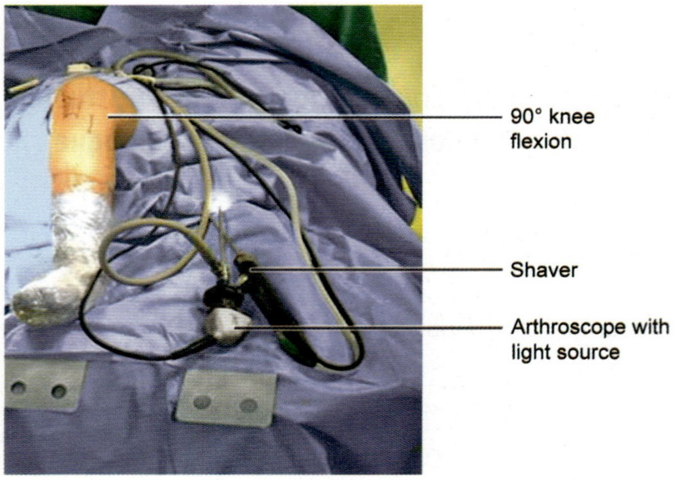

Fig. 4: All required set of instruments must be ready as per standard protocol and can be placed as per surgeon comfort.

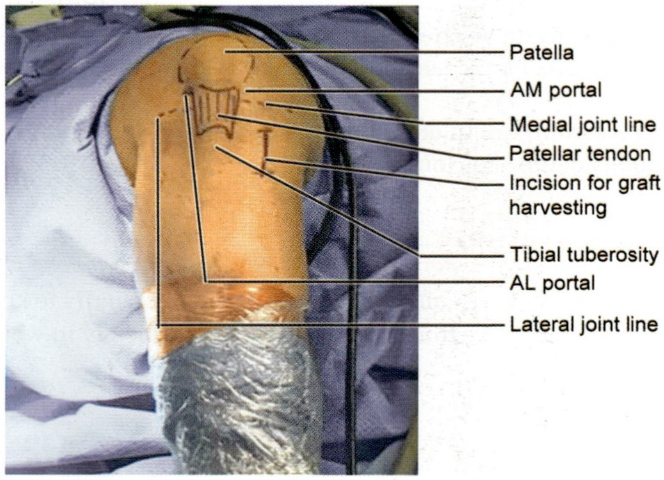

Fig. 5: Identification and marking of landmarks during every surgical procedure is important.

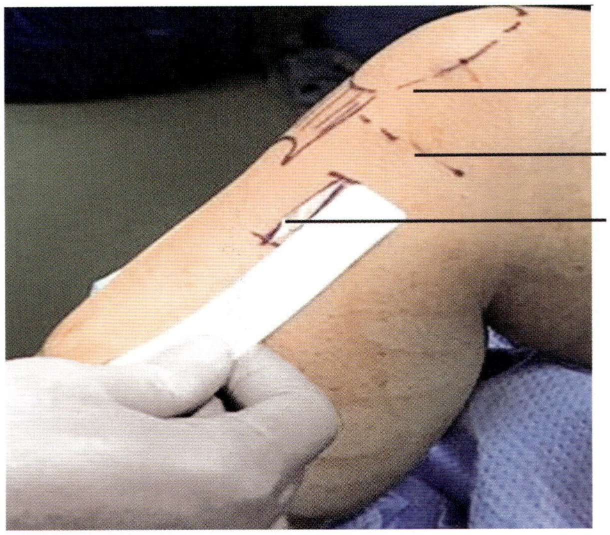

Fig. 6: With knee in 90° flexion, make straight incision two fingerbreadths below the inferior pole of patella and one thumb breadth medial to tibial tuberosity.

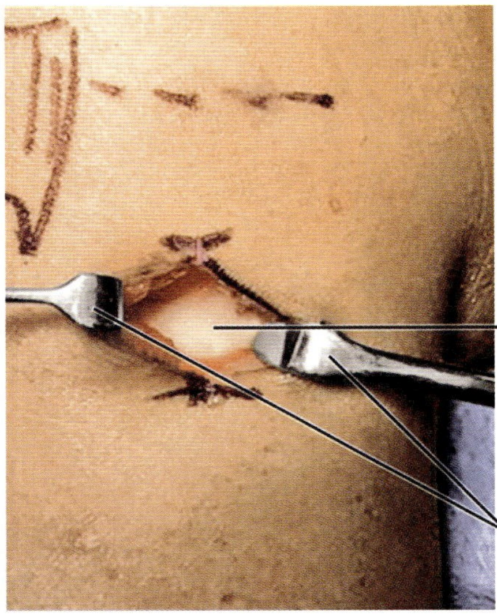

Fig. 7: Expose the sartorius fascia properly, run a finger to palpate the tendons, and incise fascia along the direction of tendons to visualize it.

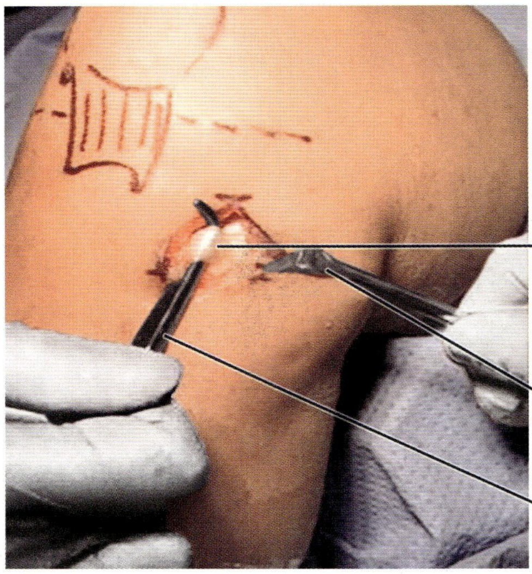

Fig. 8: Run a Mixter forceps from inferior border of hamstring tendons to pull it out. Identification and differentiation of semitendinosus-gracilis tendons is important step here.

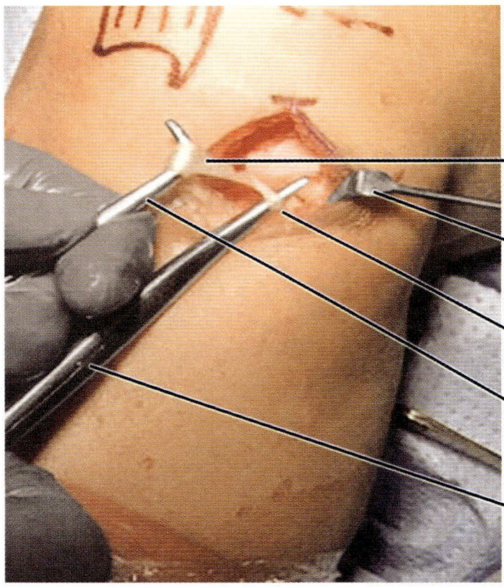

Fig. 9: Palpate all sides of tendon to ensure that there are no fibrous extensions. Vinculi has to be identified and released before harvesting tendon. Feel free excursion of tendons before harvesting.

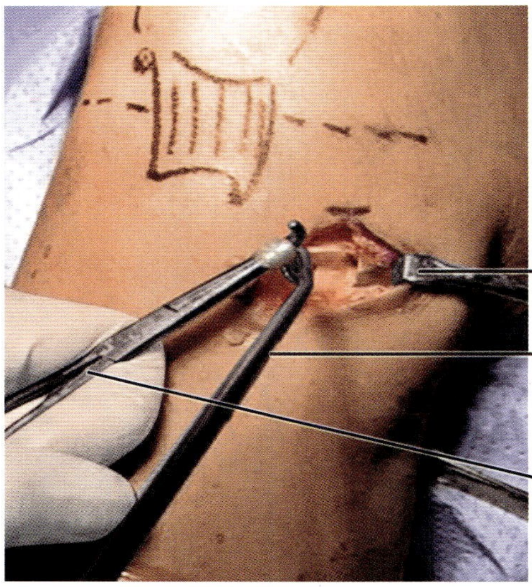

Fig. 10: After careful dissection of adhesions, introduce the tendon stripper to harvest the graft. We recommend to harvest semitendinosus first and then if needed we harvest gracilis.

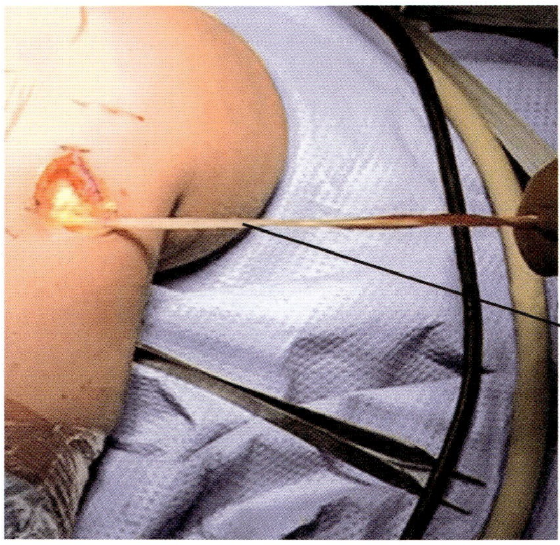

Fig. 11: Check out for muscle tendon junction to see if graft is amputated. Calculate the length of tendon.

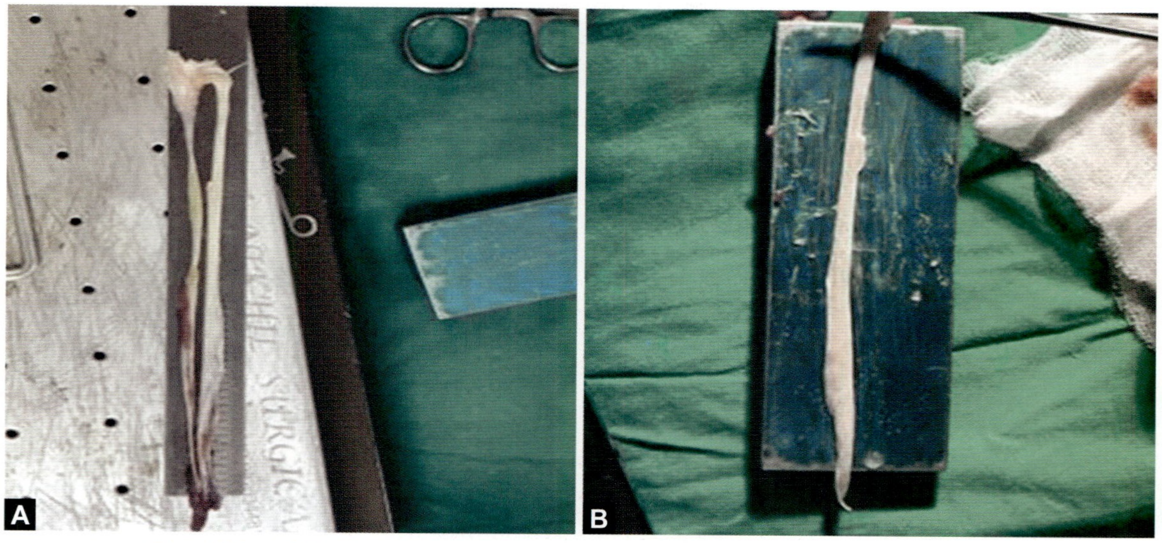

Figs. 12A and B: Measure the graft length to achieve desired length and thickness. Graft preparation has to proceed with removal of muscle portion from the tendon.

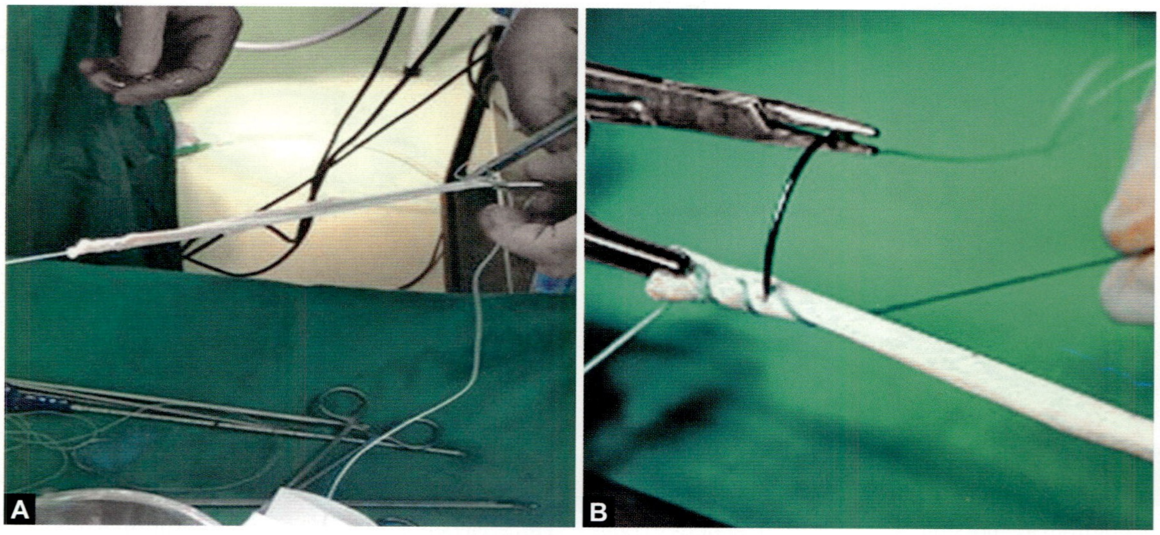

Figs. 13A and B: Graft preparation part includes whip stitching at both the ends of graft. We recommend using number 2 Nonabsobable suture for whip stitching.

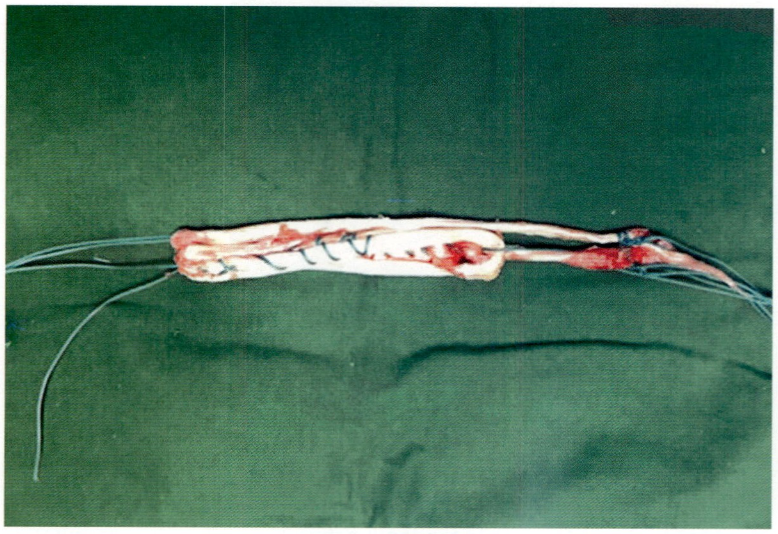

Fig. 14: We recommend five strands hamstring graft preparation (semitendinosus and gracilis).

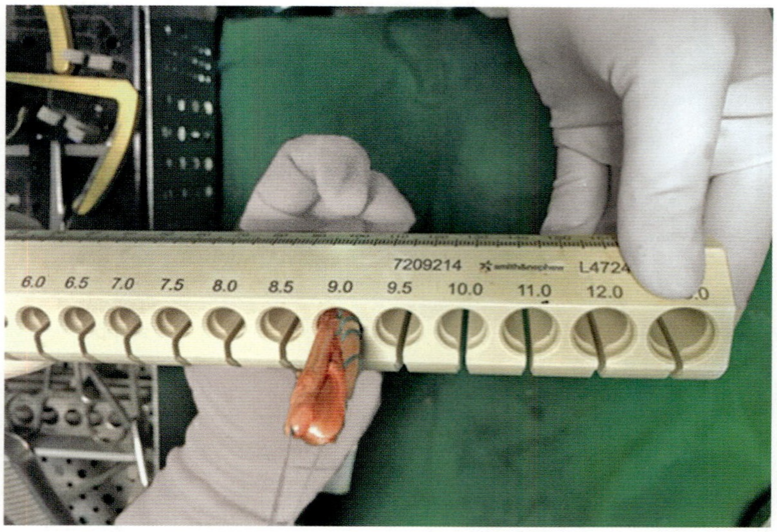

Fig. 15: Measure graft size and length to proceed for tunnel drilling and preparation.

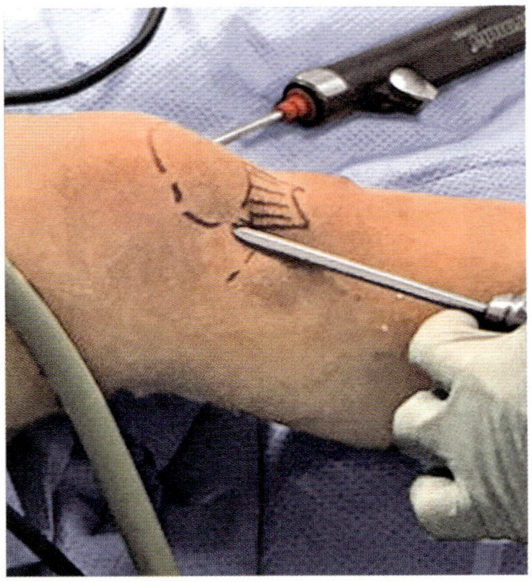

Fig. 16: Diagnostic arthroscopy performed taking AL and AM portals. Check for ACL tear, PCL, lateral meniscus, medial meniscus, any chondral lesion, and popliteus tendon. (AL: anterolateral; AM: anteromedial; ACL: anterior cruciate ligament; PCL: posterior cruciate ligament)

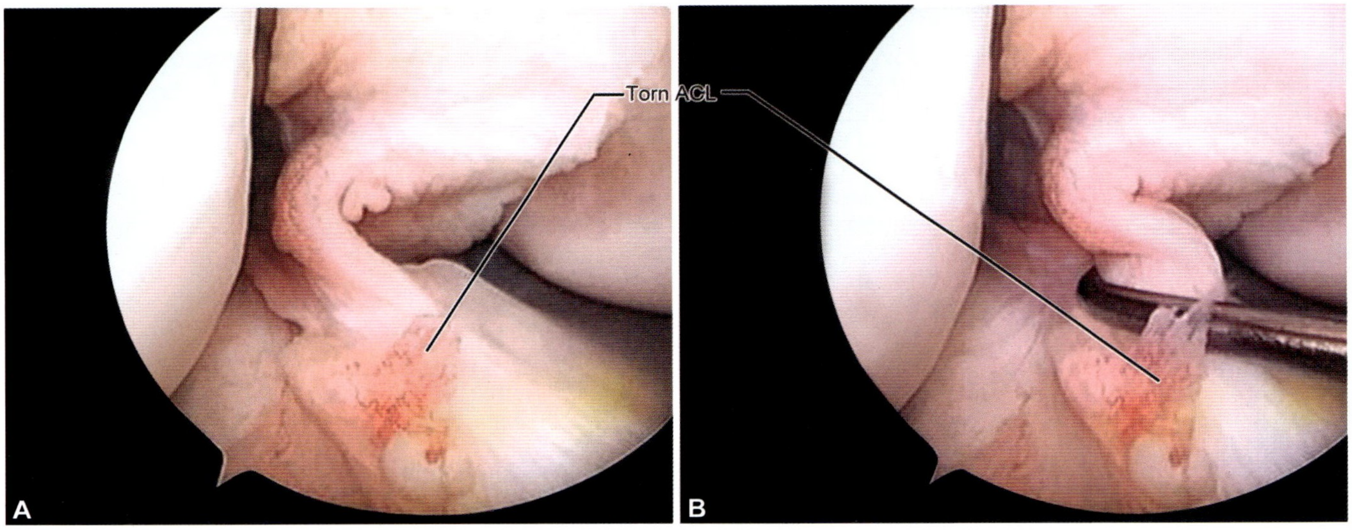

Figs. 17A and B: Evaluate anterior cruciate ligament (ACL) tear, debridement, and shaving inflamed ACL part though we recommend ACL remnant preservation in noninflamed torn ACL.

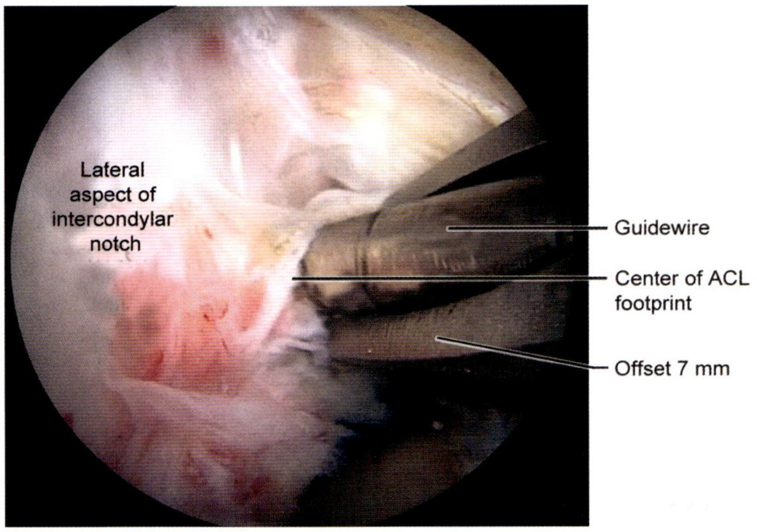

Fig. 18: Put the guidewire at anatomic anterior cruciate ligament (ACL) footprint at femoral attachment. A offset of 7 mm (in case of 9-mm graft thickness) can be used while putting guidewire or 9-mm drill bit also can be used to direct the guidewire position at footprint. Knee should be in 120° flexion at this stage.

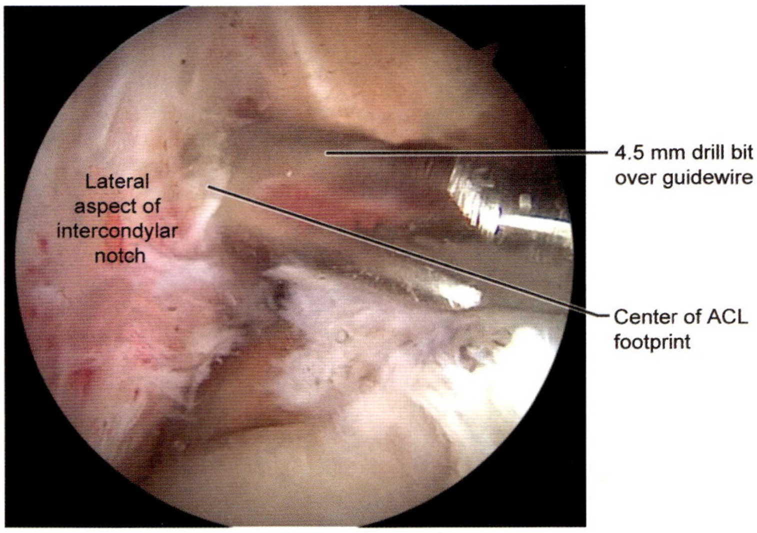

Fig. 19: 4.5 mm drilling should be done across the length of femoral tunnel over guidewire.

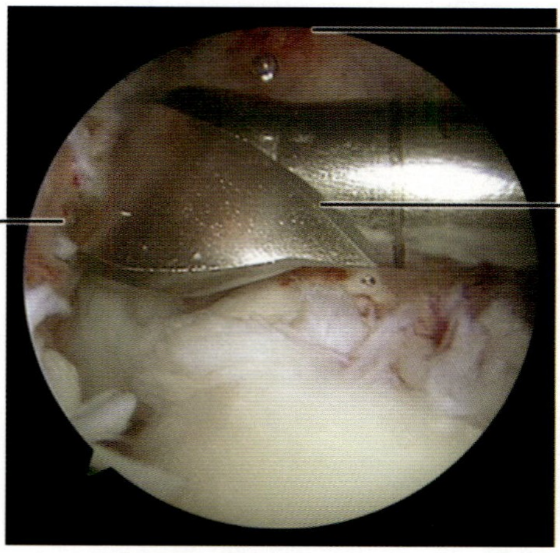

Fig. 20: Measure the tunnel length and proceed for 9-mm femoral tunnel drilling keeping in mind to put 20 mm graft inside the tunnel. A 2-mm posterior wall has to be intact.

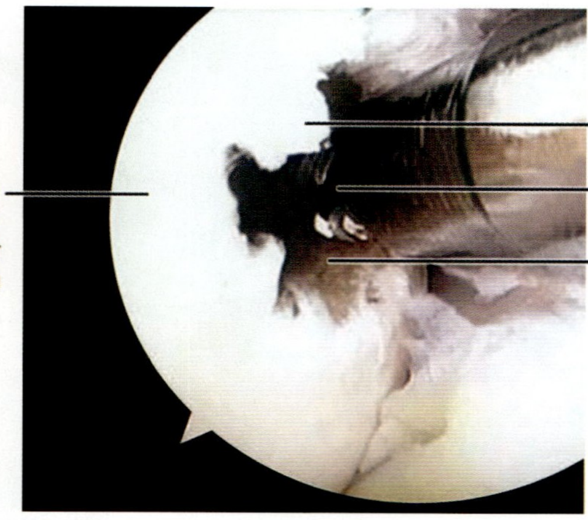

Fig. 21: Remove additional bone debris at femoral tunnel with shaver in provide smooth passage for prepared graft.

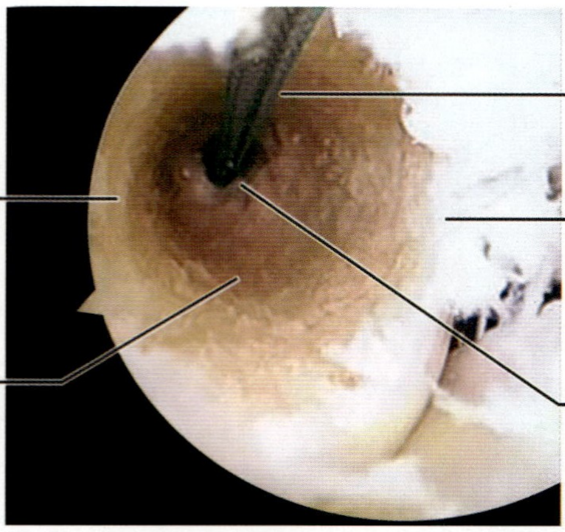

Fig. 22: Pass Nonabsobable suture loop into femoral tunnel, extract two loose ends from lateral aspect through skin, and loop should be secured from anteromedial (AM) portal in order to complete femoral tunnel preparation.

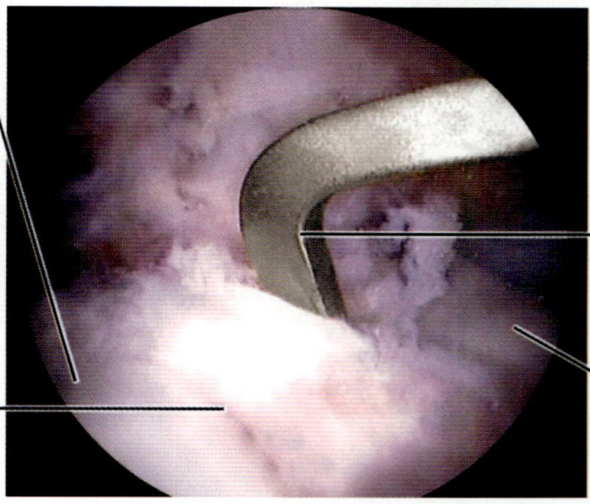

Fig. 23: Anterior cruciate ligament (ACL) tibial zig (tip aimer or elbow aimer) has to be used to secure expected guidewire position of tibial tunnel to be placed. We recommend the guidewire should be placed in line of posterior border of anterior horn of lateral meniscus and as medial as possible.

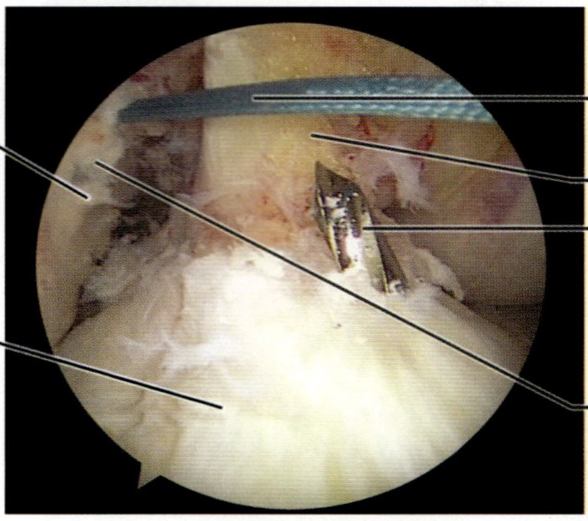

Fig. 24: Check for guidewire position and continue drilling with 9 mm. Remove excess bone debris at both ends of tibial tunnel in order to provide smooth passage for graft. Take out the Nonabsobable suture loop from tibial tunnel.

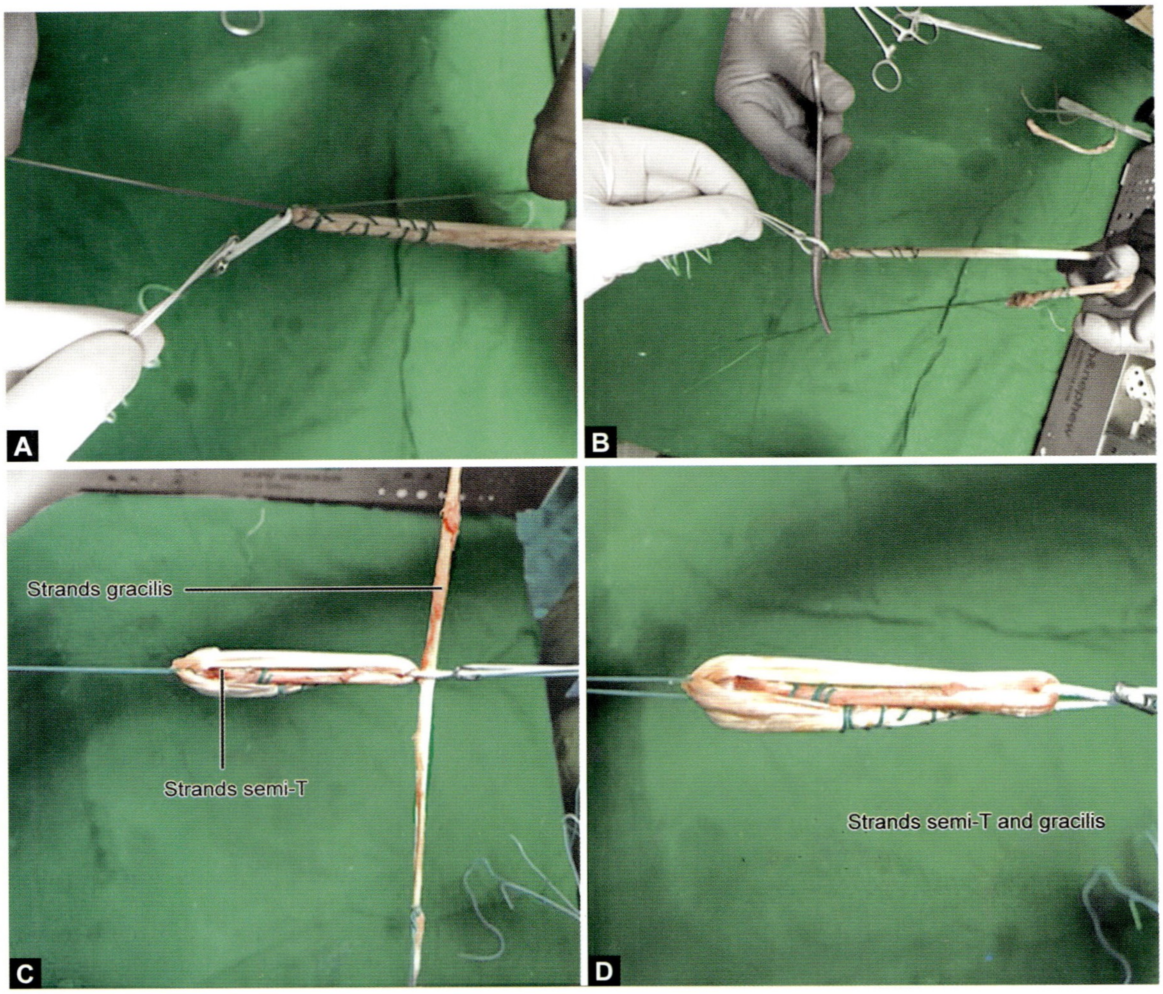

Figs. 25A to D: While preparing three strands of semitendinosus, one end (muscle-tendon end) is sutured to button loop and is tightened and relooped again to make it three strands. To convert it to five strands, gracilis graft has to pass through button loop as shown in figures.

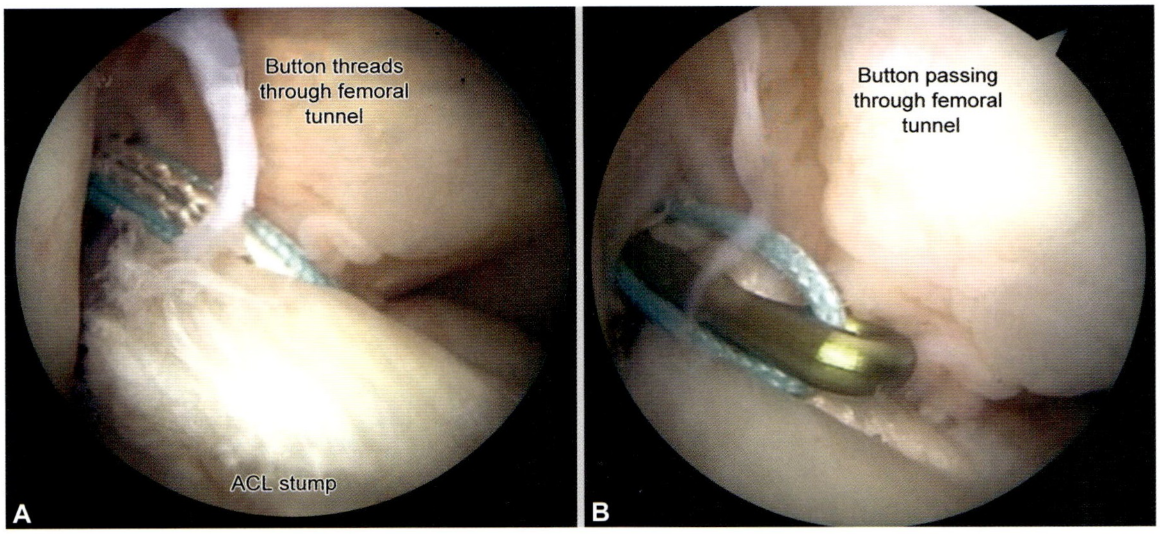

Figs. 26A and B: Put button threads into Nonabsobable suture loop and pull it out from femoral end. After passage of threads, graft should be pulled into the tunnel and button should be flipped (check for dancing movement of button). Pull the graft tightly from tibial tunnel and put bioscrew (one size higher than graft thickness) in 30° of knee flexion, apply posterior drawer to knee.

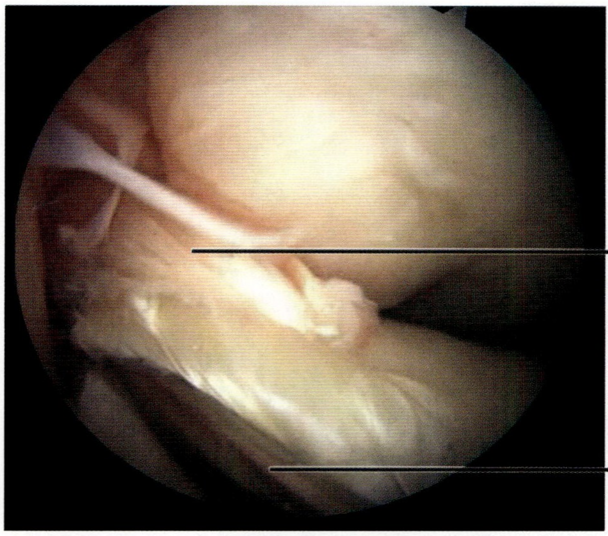

Fig. 27: Tension should be checked after final fixation with probe. Clinically, anterior drawer test at the end of surgical procedure gives firm endpoint.

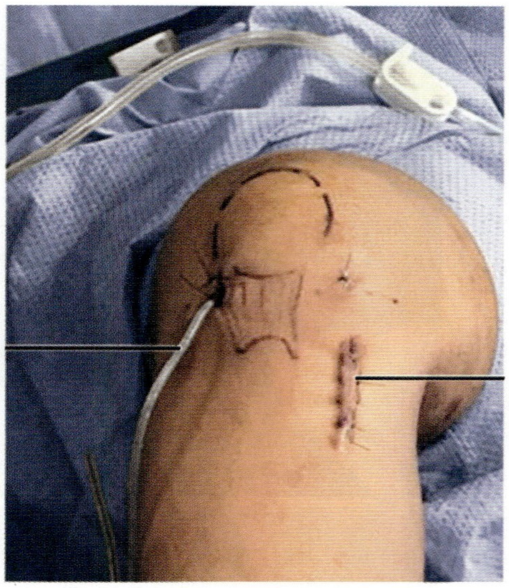

Fig. 28: Graft site subcutaneous closure with Absorbable suture number 2-0 and skin closure with 3-0 nonabsorbable suture after putting suction drain number 12 tubing inside suprapatellar pouch. Compression dressing should be applied for 48 hours. We recommend drain removal after 48 hours.

REHABILITATION

We recommend to start with ankle pumps, static knee exercises, and range of motion (ROM) till 90° with full weight-bearing ambulation wearing long knee brace for 3 weeks. After 3 weeks, we recommend to shift the patient to hinge knee brace, full ROM exercises along with knee strengthening exercises.

SUGGESTED READING

1. Andersson D, Samuelsson K, Karlsson J. Treatment of anterior cruciate ligament injuries with special reference to surgical technique and rehabilitation: an assessment of randomized controlled trials. Arthroscopy. 2009;25(6):653-85.
2. Barber FA, Elrod BF, McGuire DA, et al. Is an anterior cruciate ligament reconstruction outcome age dependent? Arthroscopy. 1996;12(6): 720-5.
3. Benjaminse A, Gokeler A, van der Schans CP. Clinical diagnosis of an anterior cruciate ligament rupture: a meta-analysis. J Orthop Sports Phys Ther. 2006;36(5):267-88.
4. Brand J, Weiler A, Caborn DN, et al. Graft fixation in cruciate ligament reconstruction. Am J Sports Med. 2000;28(5):761-74.
5. Briggs KK, Lysholm J, Tegner Y, et al. The reliability, validity, and responsiveness of the Lysholm score and Tegner activity scale for anterior cruciate ligament injuries of the knee: 25 years later. Am J Sports Med. 2009;37(5):890-7.
6. Carey JL, Dunn WR, Dahm DL, et al. A systematic review of anterior cruciate ligament reconstruction with autograft compared with allograft. J Bone Joint Surg Am. 2009;91(9):2242-50.

CHAPTER 12

Arthroscopic Fixation for Anterior Cruciate Ligament Avulsion Fracture

Umesh Jadhav, Aditya Upase

INTRODUCTION

Tibial attachment of anterior cruciate ligament (ACL) avulsion fracture is a common injury in children and adolescents.

ANATOMY

Anterior cruciate ligament insertion extends to medial and lateral tibial eminence. It inserts 10–14 mm behind anterior border of tibia.

MECHANISM OF INJURY

Anterior cruciate ligament avulsion fracture injury is usually traumatic. Hyperextension injury to the knee or by a direct force over the distal femur with the knee in flexion can cause these injuries.

CLASSIFICATION

Meyers and McKeever have classified these injuries depending on the amount of displacement of the ACL tibial fragment:

- *Type 1*—Minimal or undisplaced fracture fragment
- *Type 2*—Elevation of only the anterior half of the fragment
- *Type 3*—Complete displacement of the fragment
- *Type 4 (modified by Zaricznyj)*—Comminution of the displaced fragment.

CLINICAL FEATURES

- *Symptoms*: Pain in knee, swelling, and difficulty in movements at knee
- *Signs*: Knee effusion, limited range of motion (ROM) secondary to pain, and anterior drawer test is positive.

IMAGING

- *Radiographs*: Knee radiographs anteroposterior and lateral views reveal fracture at tibial spine.
- *CT scan*: Helpful for preoperative planning of fracture fixation
- *MRI scans*: To determine associated ligamentous/meniscal injuries.

TREATMENT OPTIONS

- *Nonoperative:* Aspiration of hemarthrosis from knee joint, closed reduction, and immobilization in full extension is indicated in undisplaced type I and reducible type II fractures.
- *Operative*: Open reduction and internal fixation (ORIF) versus arthroscopic fixation.
  - *Indications*:
    - Type III or type II fractures that cannot be reduced
    - Block to extension.

Open reduction and internal fixation involves arthrotomy, soft tissue dissection, and prolong immobilization resulting in high chance of knee stiffness.

The arthroscopic technique is the preferred treatment modality as it allows magnified vision, accurate reduction, minimal soft tissue dissection, stable fixation, and management of associated intra-articular pathologies.

The fixation options include wires, staples, screw, and sutures.

The advantage of using sutures is that they provide very stable and rigid fixation and do not need removal.

Arthroscopic Anterior Cruciate Ligament Avulsion Fracture Fixation-Surgical Approach

Numerous techniques for treatment of *ACL avulsion fractures* have been described in literature. We are focusing here on arthroscopic fixation of ACL avulsion fracture with two tunnel suture bridge technique.

SURGICAL STEPS (FIGS. 1 TO 17)

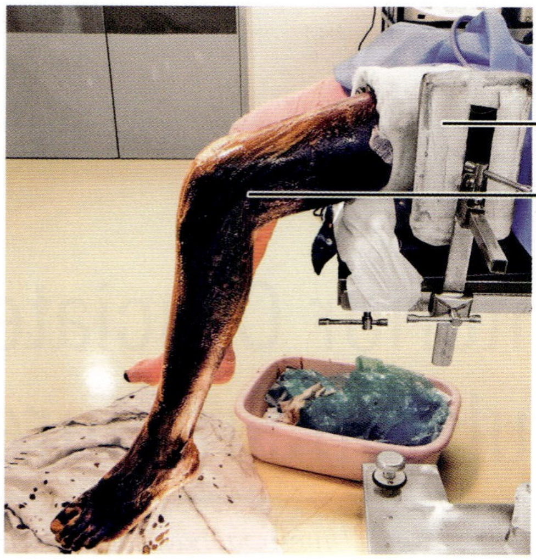

Fig. 1: Patient position is supine under suitable anesthesia with leg hanging down the table with lateral side support as shown. Other lower limb should be wrapped with elastic crape bandage.

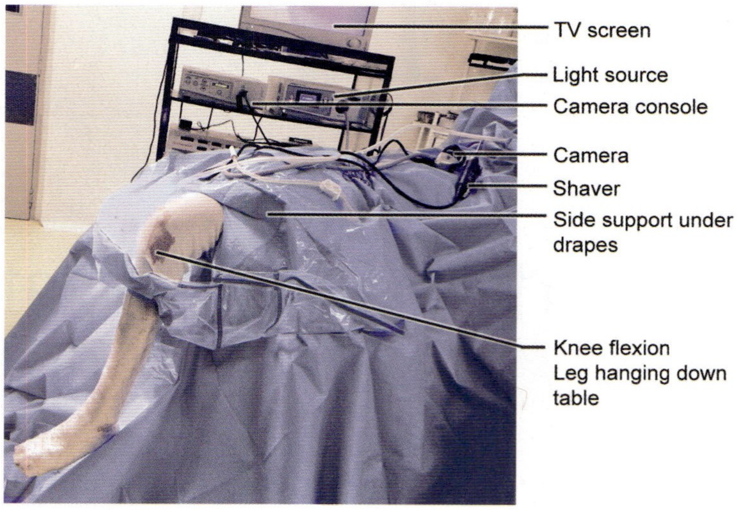

Fig. 2: Painting and draping should be done in standard fashion after primary scrubbing the parts. Arthroscopy setup should be arranged on contralateral side with TV screen, light source, camera console, and shaver console. Operating surgeon should stand on ipsilateral side.

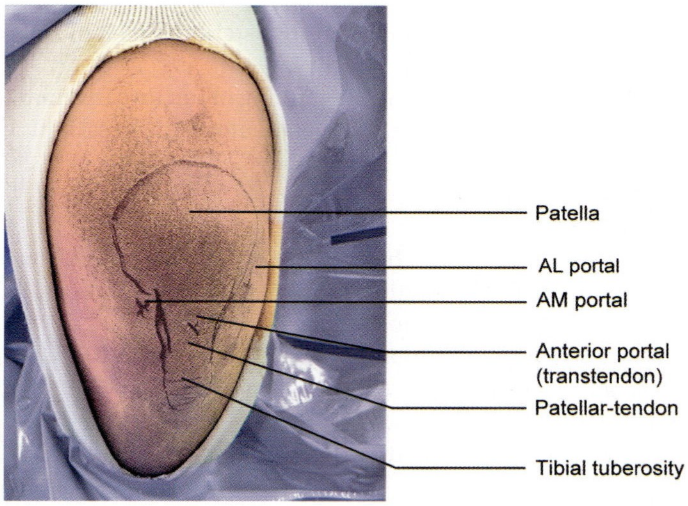

Fig. 3: Surface makings are important in every surgical procedure. Anterolateral (AL) portal should be placed 1 cm lateral to patellar tendon and 1 cm inferior to patella. Anteromedial (AM) portal should be placed 1 cm medial to patellar tendon and 1 cm inferior to patella.

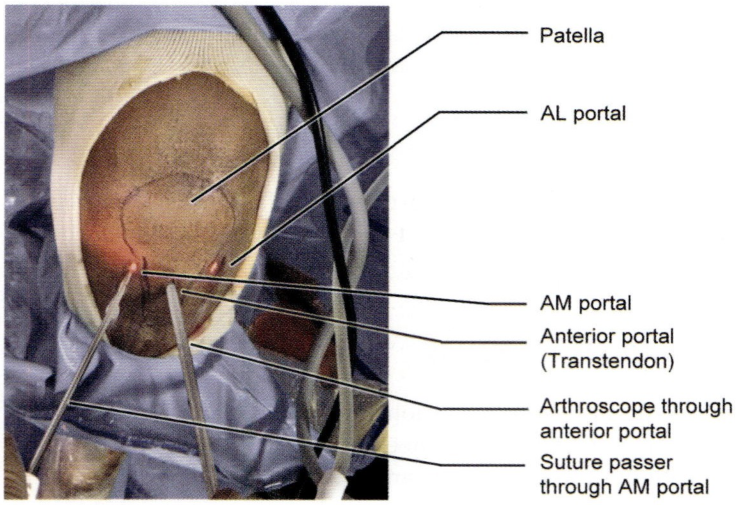

Fig. 4: We require additional portal here in the form of anterior portal, i.e. viewing portal that should be place 1 cm below the lower pole of patella in the center of tendon. AM and AL portals are working portals. (AL: anterolateral; AM: anteromedial)

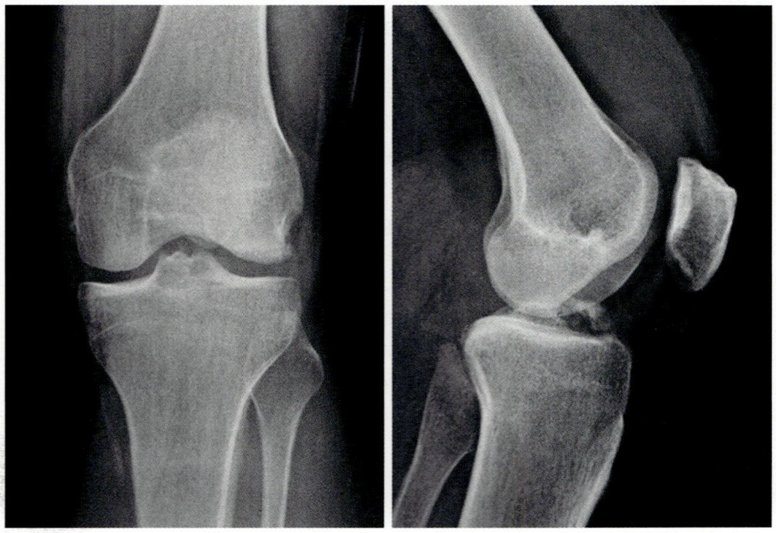

Fig. 5: We are showing here a case of young male having post-traumatic anterior cruciate ligament (ACL) avulsion fracture.

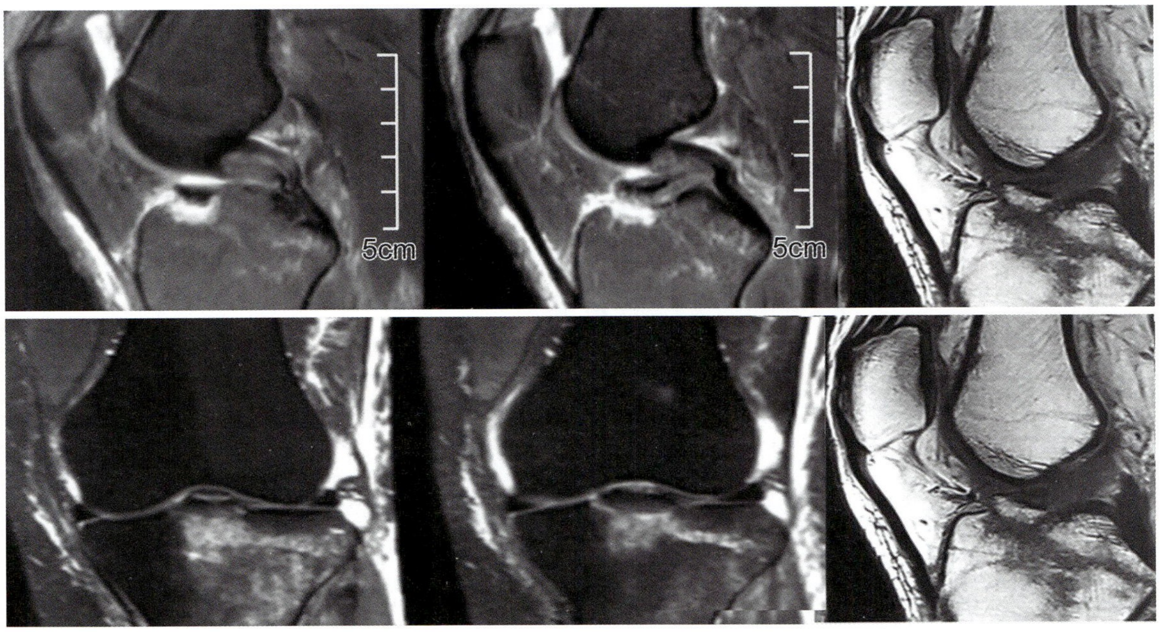

Fig. 6: MRI of the knee joint should be performed in order to rule out any other soft tissue injury. MRI confirmed anterior cruciate ligament (ACL) avulsion injury with intact ACL.

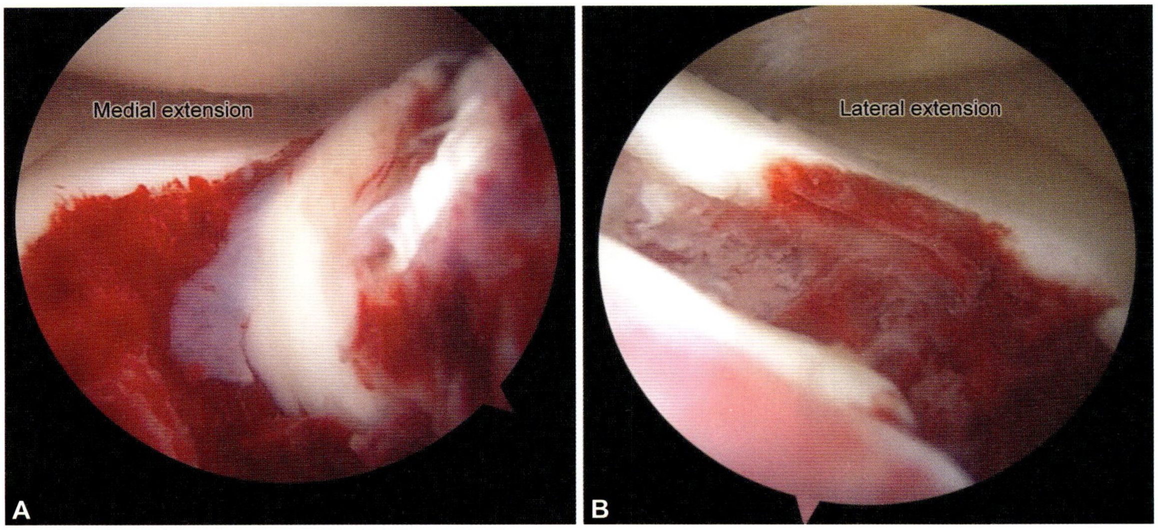

Figs. 7A and B: Arthroscopic evaluation of knee joint should be done in standard fashion. Define the extent of fracture medially, laterally, and also see fracture comminution.

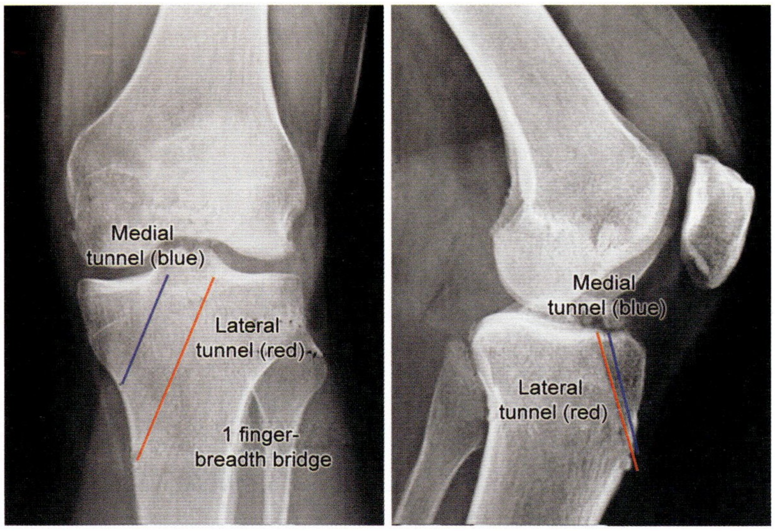

Fig. 8: Fracture crater should be free from soft tissue. Use shaver to clean crater and prepare it. See the fracture reduction with probe and maintain it.

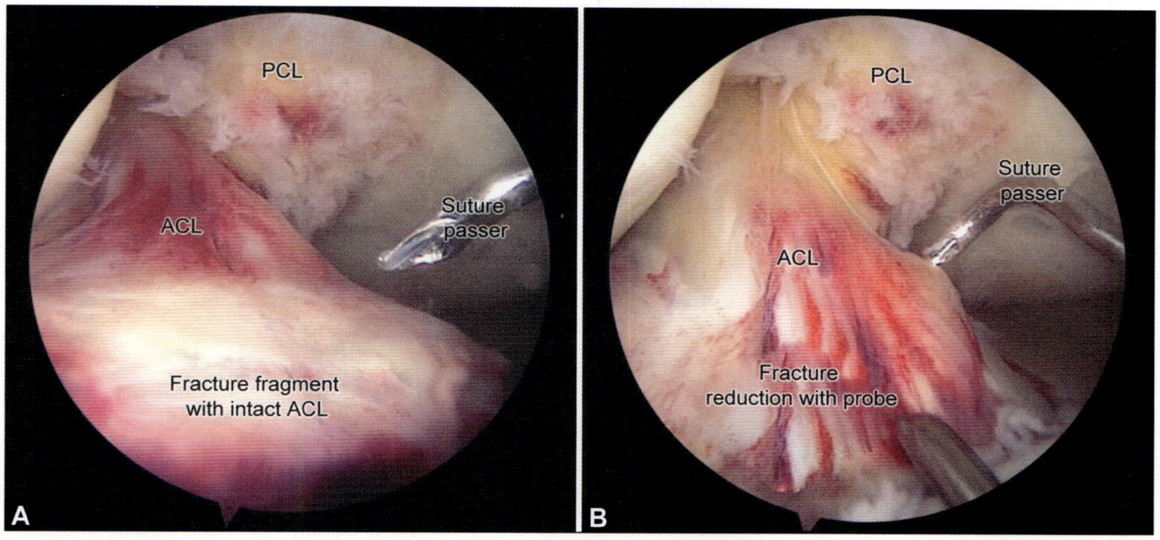

Figs. 9A and B: We use two tunnel drilling technique with 4.5 mm over guidewire, one tunnel medial, and another tunnel lateral to crater. Minimum one fingerbreadth distance should be there between two tunnels as bridge as shown in figure 8.

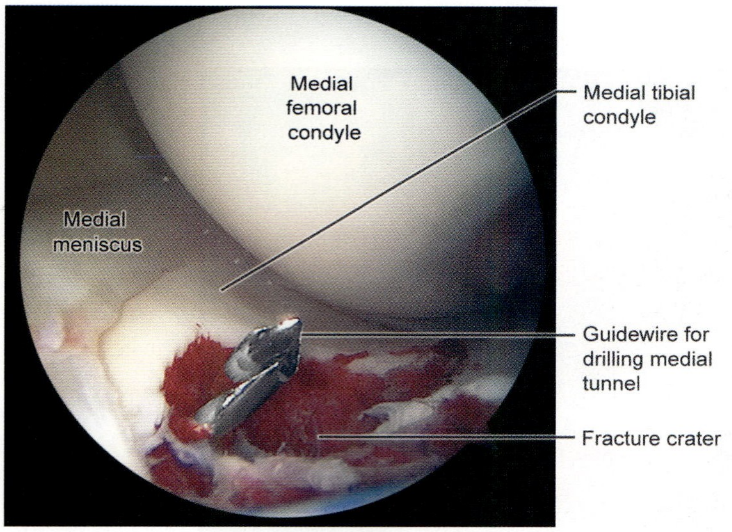

Fig. 10: Before final drilling of tunnel, guidewire should be put just medial and lateral to crater and then 4.5 mm tunnel drilling should be done over guidewire.

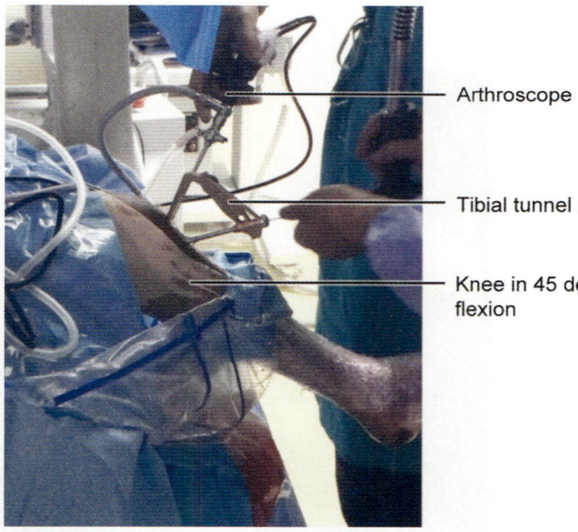

Fig. 11: We use tibial zig for medial and lateral tibial tunnels drilling in 45–50° knee flexion. One can use C-arm guidance while drilling tunnels for confirmation.

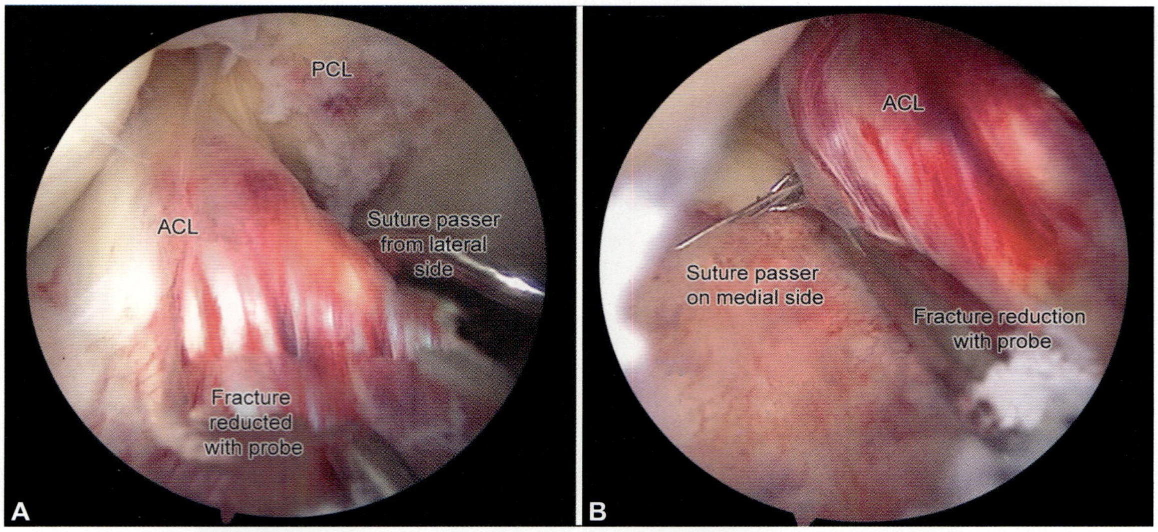

Figs. 12A and B: Pass the suture passer (curved) in midsubstance of anterior cruciate ligament (ACL) from lateral to medial maintaining reduction of fracture fragment pressing it down with probe.

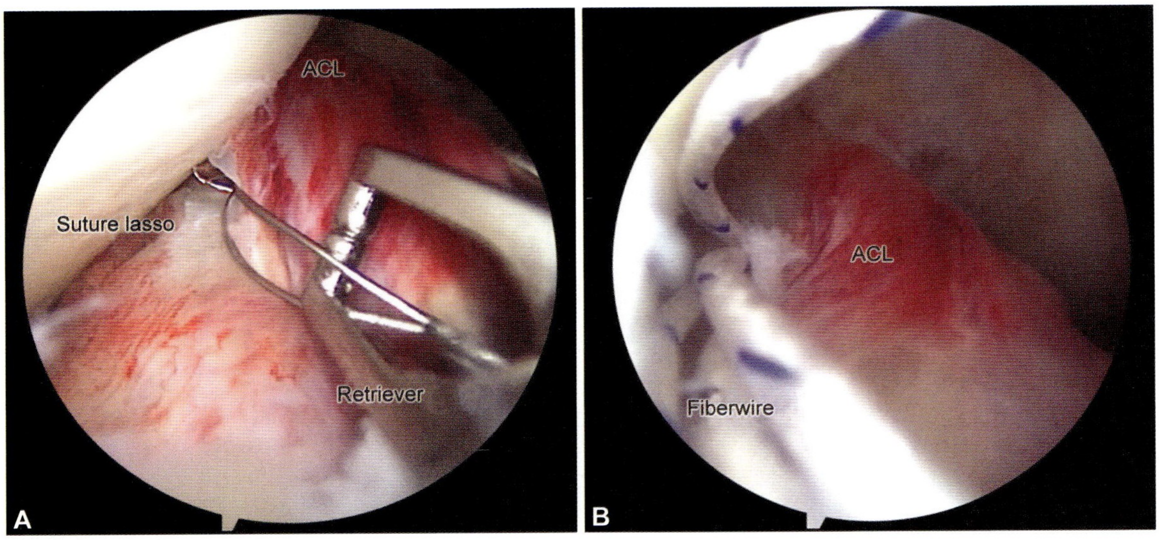

Figs. 13A and B: Bring suture lasso in vision and retrieve it from AM portal, put fiberwire/suturetape/fibertape in lasso, pull it across the substance of ACL laterally, and retrieve it from AL portal. (AL: anterolateral; AM: anteromedial; ACL: anterior cruciate ligament)

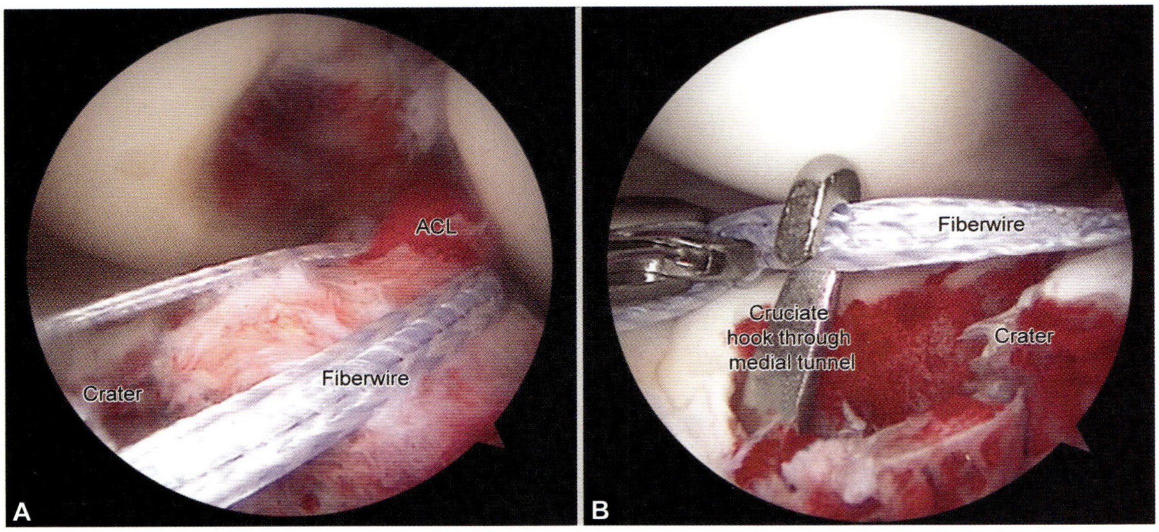

Figs. 14A and B: Bring cruciate hook in action from tibial tunnels and retrieve both the ends out. Check for fracture reduction by pulling threads down and tie it to one another over suture bridge or over suture disc by maintaining fracture reduction with probe.

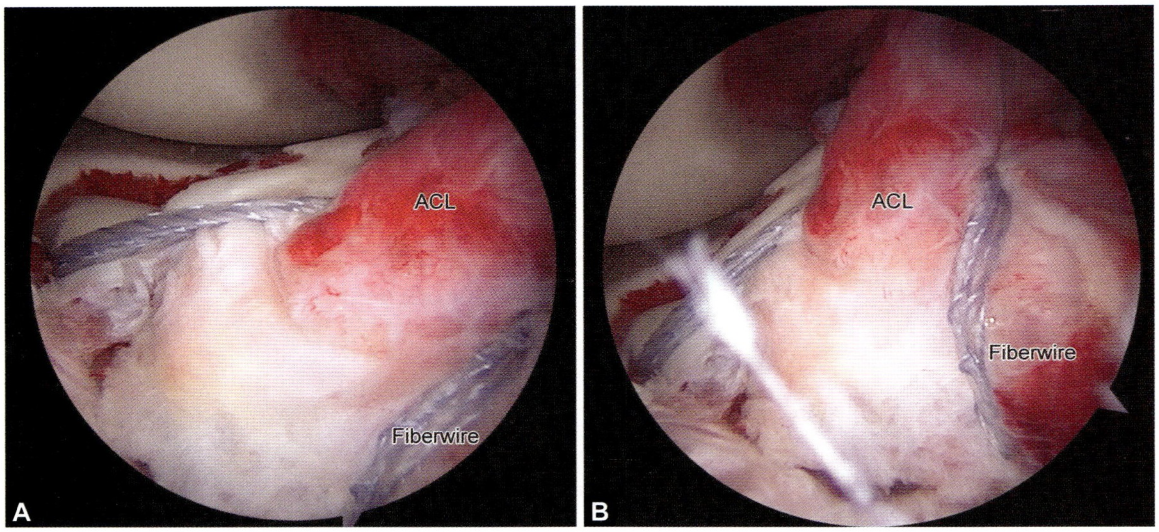

Figs. 15A and B: Final arthroscopic images showing reduction of avulsed fragment after suturing fiberwire over bridge.

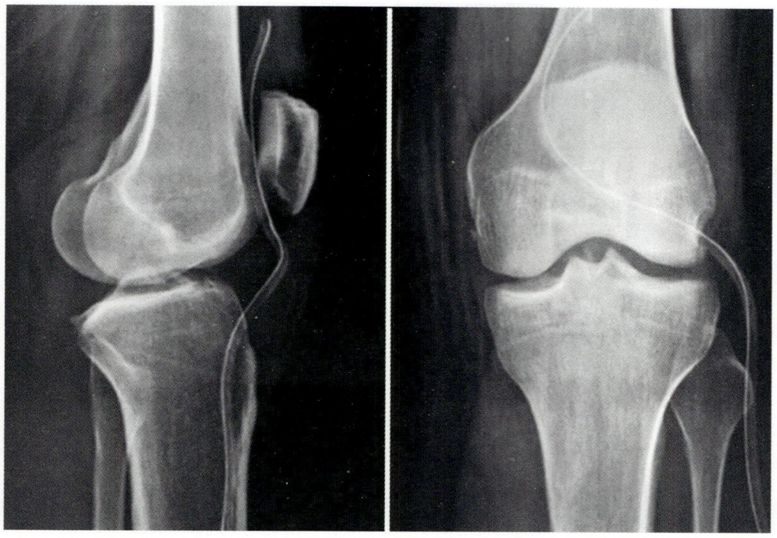

Fig. 16: We prefer to keep drain for 48 hours. Immediate postoperative X-ray shows good fracture reduction.

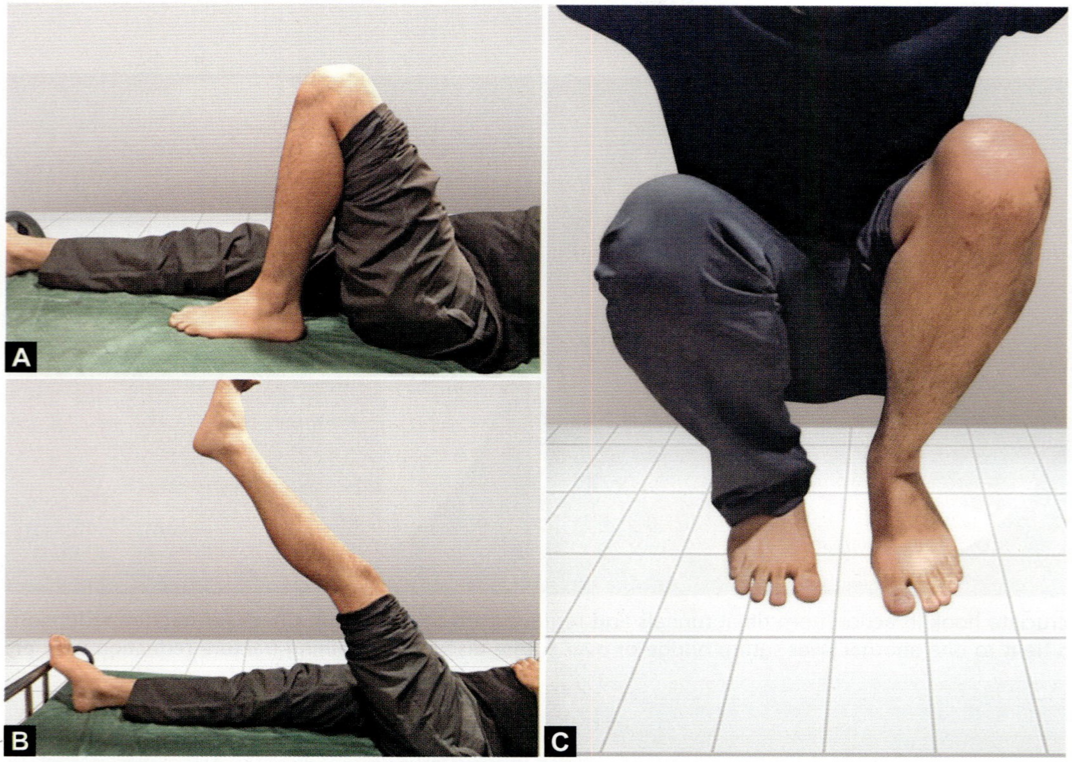

Figs. 17A to C: At the end of 2 months, patient is mobilized full weight bearing with full knee range of motion (ROM).

REHABILITATION

We prefer to keep patient in long knee brace with nonweight-bearing ambulation with walker for 3 weeks. We start ankle pump and static knee exercises immediately.

After 3 weeks partial weight-bearing ambulation wearing long knee brace with walker and range of motion exercises should be initiated.

At the end of 6 weeks, we start full weight-bearing ambulation without walker without brace.

SUGGESTED READING

1. Gans I, Baldwin KD, Ganley TJ. Treatment and management outcomes of tibial eminence fractures in pediatric patients: A systematic review. Am J Sports Med. 2014;42(7):1743-50.
2. Horibe S, Shi K, Mitsuoka T. Nonunited avulsion fractures of the intercondylar eminence of the tibia. Arthroscopy. 2000;16(7):757-62.
3. Huang TW, Hsu KY, Cheng CY. Arthroscopic suture fixation of tibial eminence avulsion fractures. Arthroscopy. 2008;24(11):1232-8.
4. In Y, Kim JM, Woo YK. Arthroscopic fixation of anterior cruciate tibial avulsion fractures using bioabsorbable suture anchors. Knee Surg Sports Traumatol Arthrosc. 2008;16(3):286-9.
5. Sundararajan SR, Rajasekaran S, Bernard SL. Displaced anterior cruciate ligament avulsion fracture: Arthroscopic staple fixation. Indian J Orthop. 2011;45(4):324-9.
6. Zhao J, Huangfu X. Arthroscopic treatment of nonunited anterior cruciate ligament tibial avulsion fracture with figure-of-8 suture fixation technique. Arthroscopy. 2007;23(4):405-10.

CHAPTER 13

Arthroscopic Meniscectomy

Umesh Jadhav, Aditya Upase

INTRODUCTION

Injury to meniscus causes pain and functional impairment to knee joint. Menisci are important structures inside the knee joint for normal biomechanics. During arthroscopic meniscal surgeries aim should be towards preserving maximum portion of meniscus in order to delay or prevent degenerative arthritis.

ANATOMY

The menisci are wedge-shaped fibro-cartilaginous structures located between the femur and the tibia condyles medially and laterally. Meniscus is divided into roots, horns and body. Transverse ligament connects anterior horns of medial and lateral mensci.

FUNCTION

Meniscus is a vital structure for chondroprotection, proprioception, joint stabilization, joint lubrication and articular cartilage nutrition.

MECHANISM OF INJURY

Injury to meniscus usually occurs as a result of rotational force to a flexed knee (usually with twisting sports activities). Valgus force to foot fixed to ground with flexed knee with external rotation force results in lateral meniscus tears.

CLASSIFICATION

Classification is based on the tear patterns observed during arthroscopy.

- Vertical longitudinal tears [most often associated with acute anterior cruciate ligament (ACL) injury]
- Oblique tears
- Circumferential tears
- Complex tears
- Transverse or radial tears (radial tears of the posteromedial compartment are the most frequently seen tears)
- Horizontal cleavage tears.

Degenerative complex tears that generally start from the posterior horn are common in older patients.

CLINICAL FEATURES

- *Symptoms*: Knee pain, knee swelling, locking, catching or cracking sensation. Pop-like feeling when suddenly changing directions or suddenly stopping while running (common in athletes).
- *Signs*: Tenderness on palpation over joint line, McMurray test, and Apley test results positive.

IMAGING

- *X-rays*: Although they will not show any injury to your ligaments or menisci, X-rays can show whether the injury is associated with a broken bone.
- *Magnetic resonance imaging (MRI) scans*: MRI scan is important for diagnosis and also shows tear pattern with high sensitivity.

TREATMENT OPTIONS

For decision making—location, tear pattern and vascularity are important factors. Most of the meniscal tears do not heal spontaneously. According to blood supply and healing prognosis, meniscus is divided into red-red, red-white, or white-white zones. The red-red zone has excellent healing prognosis. The red-white zone has good healing prognosis. The white-white zone has a poor prognosis.

Conservative

Not all meniscal injuries require surgical intervention. Older patients with degenerative meniscus tears without mechanical symptoms can be treated non-operatively with properly guided physical therapy.

Operative

- *Meniscus repair*: Vascular zone tears, young individual with repairable tears.
- *Meniscectomy (partial/total)*: Avascular zone tears, degenerative meniscal tears, and irreparable tears.

Arthroscopic Partial Medial Meniscectomy—Surgical Technique

Following technique is important in dealing with complex tear involving medial meniscus, a step-by-step approach to arthroscopy setup and surgical procedure in the form of arthroscopic partial medial meniscectomy.

SURGICAL STEPS (FIGS. 1 TO 24)

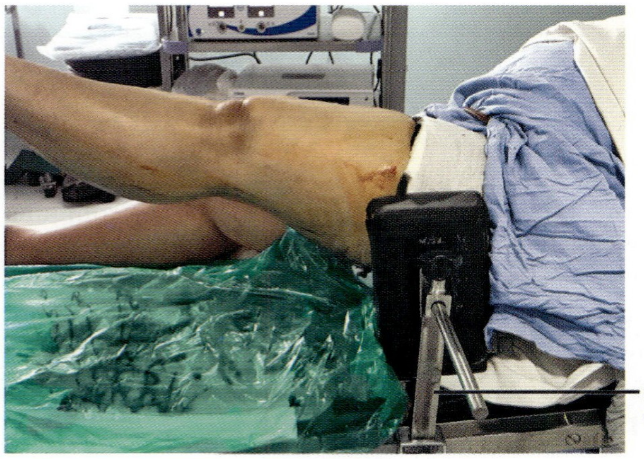

Fig. 1: Patient position is supine under spinal anesthesia with side support for valgus stress during procedure.

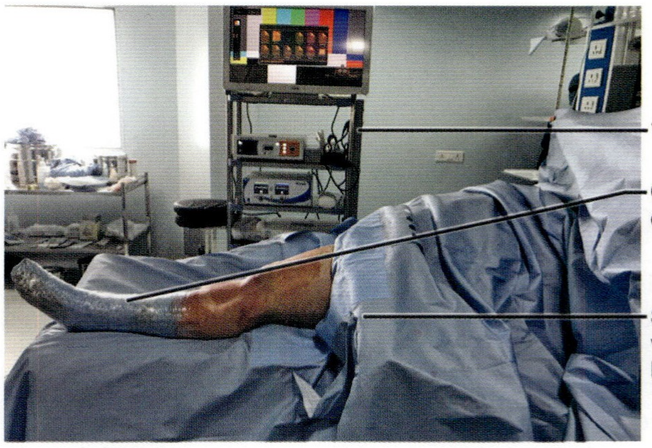

Fig. 2: All aseptic precautions must be followed in order to be ready for surgical procedure. Surgeon is standing on ipsilateral side with video trolley on contralateral side.

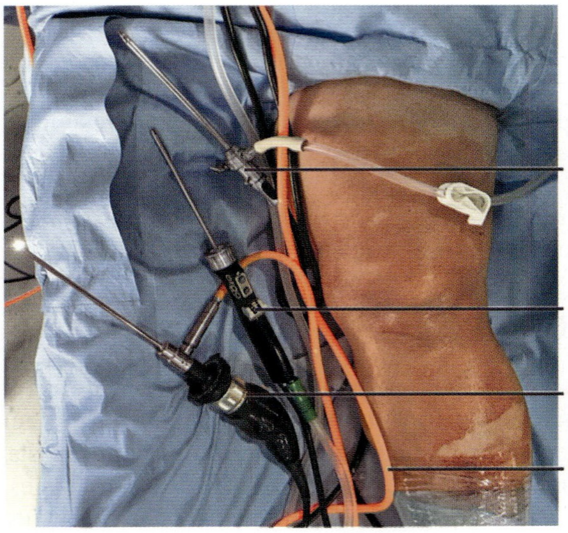

Fig. 3: All required set of instruments must be arranged as per standard protocol.

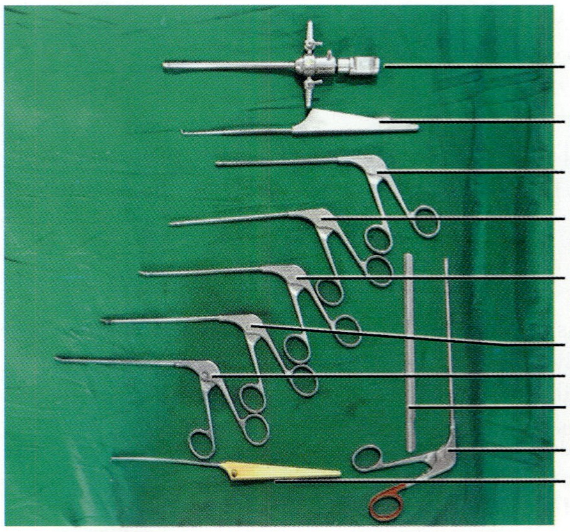

Fig. 4: All instruments have to be ready on the instrument trolley before start of the procedure.

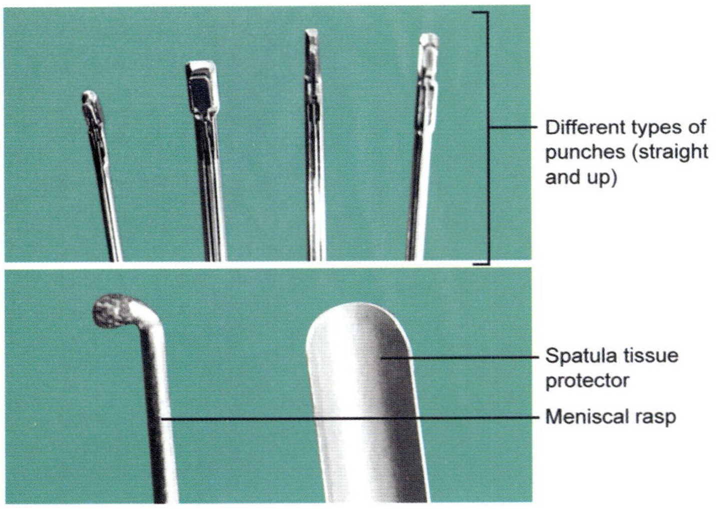

Fig. 5: There are few instruments in every surgery which makes the procedure easy. Meniscal rasp and spatula tissue protector is important while doing meniscus repair.

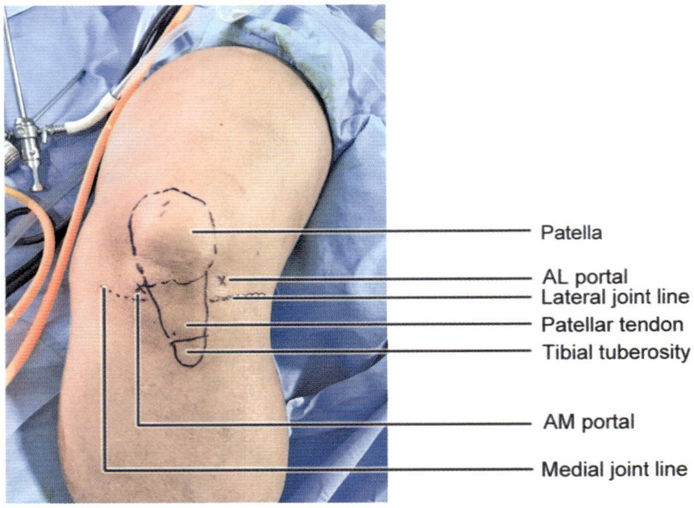

Fig. 6: Identification and marking of landmarks during every surgical procedure is important.

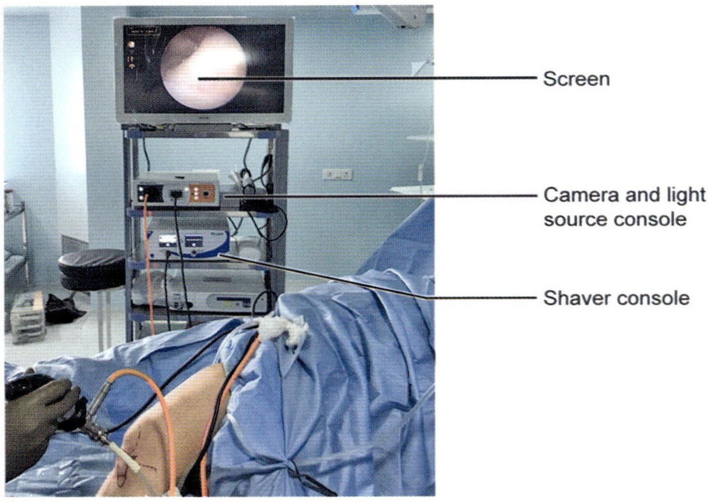

Fig. 7: Arthroscopy setup includes TV screen, camera and light source console, and shaver console. It should be arranged on the contralateral side and surgeon standing on ipsilateral side.

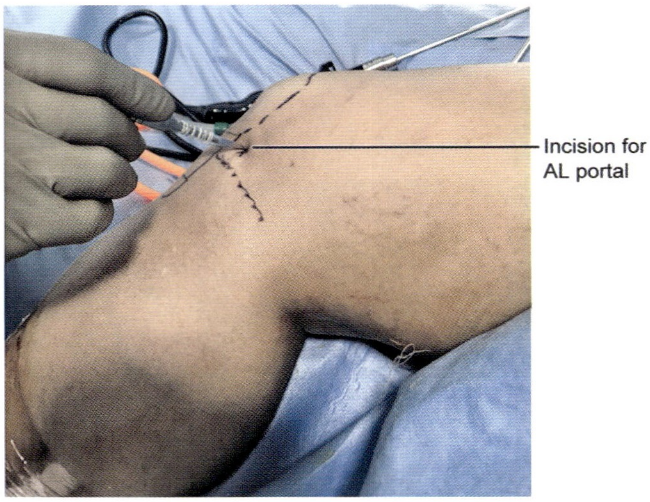

Fig. 8: Take anterolateral (AL) portal incision with 11 number blade. AL portal should be placed 1 cm lateral to patellar tendon and 1 cm inferior to patella.

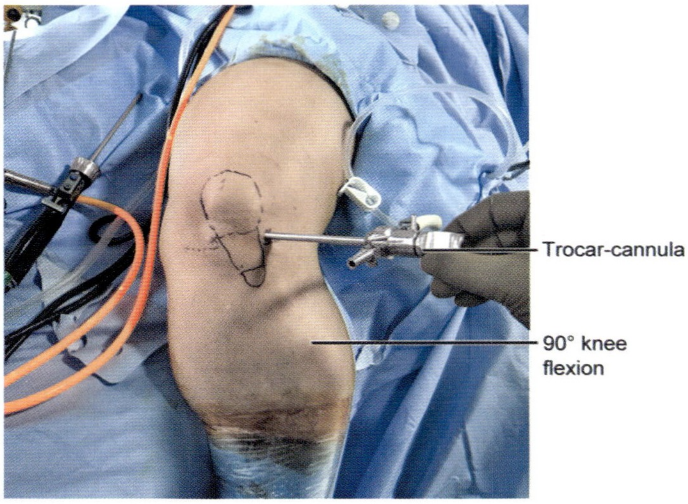

Fig. 9: Trocar cannula should be introduced with direction toward medial aspect of intercondylar notch in knee 90° of flexion. Care should be taken to avoid damage to cartilage.

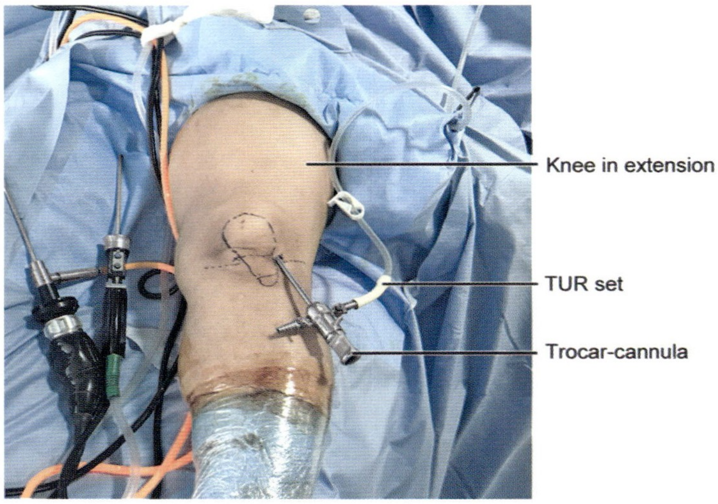

Fig. 10: Then withdraw the trocar cannula little bit, extend the knee and direct it and slide it between the medial femoral condyle and patella to advance it to suprapatellar pouch. Start diagnostic arthroscopy in standard fashion.

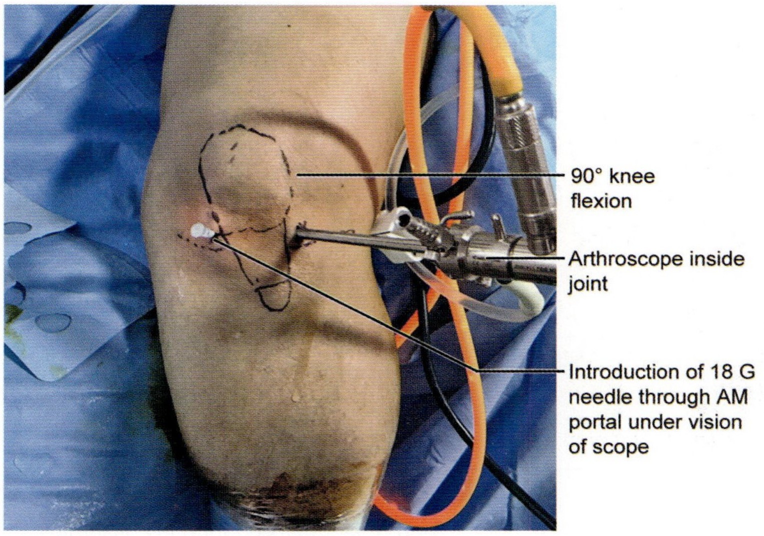

Fig. 11: Direct arthroscope into medial compartment and put 18G needle from marked anteromedial (AM) portal in 90° knee flexion, visualize needle with scope. AM portal should be placed 1 cm medial to patellar tendon and 1 cm inferior to patella.

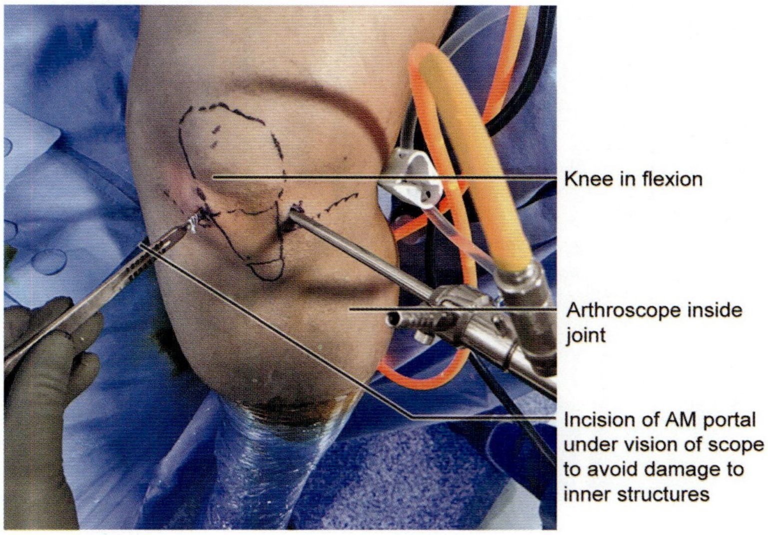

Fig. 12: Withdraw the needle and take incision for AM portal with 11 number blade under arthroscope vision to avoid injury to cartilage, ACL, and menisci. (AM: anteromedial; ACL: anterior cruciate ligament)

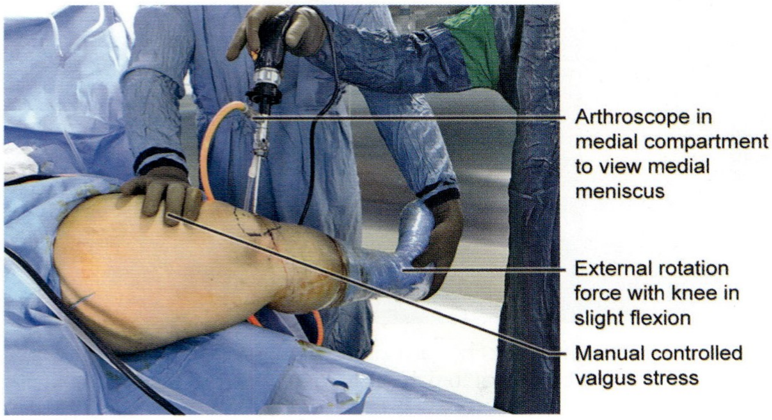

Fig. 13: Combined valgus stress and external rotation of tibia to look for posterior horn of medial meniscus. Side post is important for valgus stress.

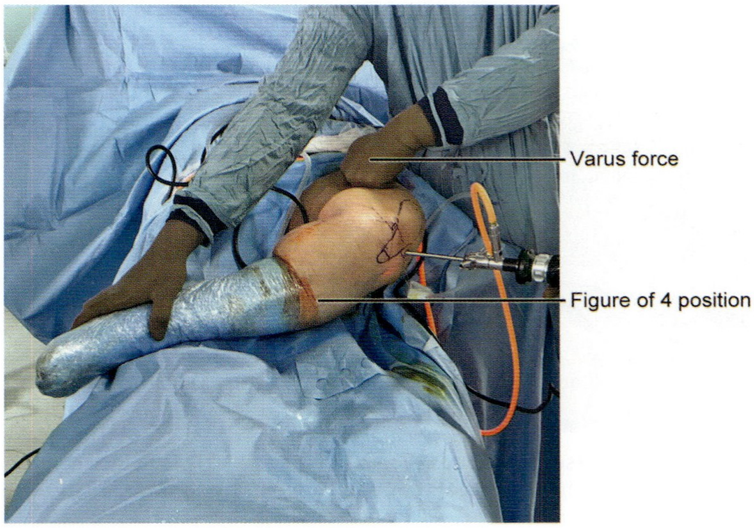

Fig. 14: Figure of four positions with pressing knee joint downward (varus stress) help to open lateral compartment to check for lateral meniscus.

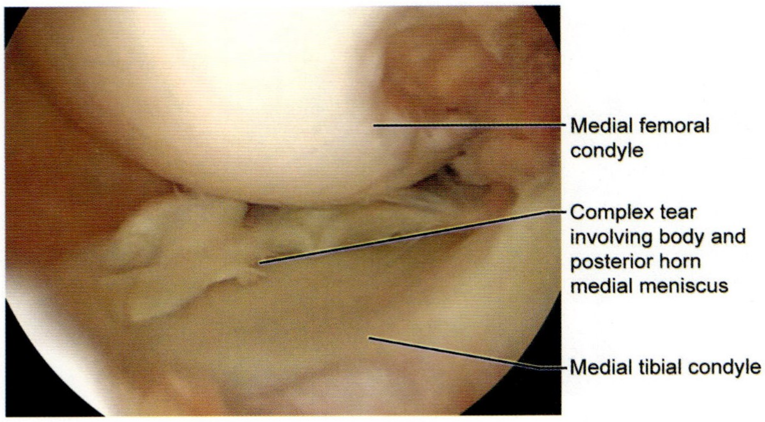

Fig. 15: Complex meniscus tear is irreparable so needs meniscectomy and balancing.

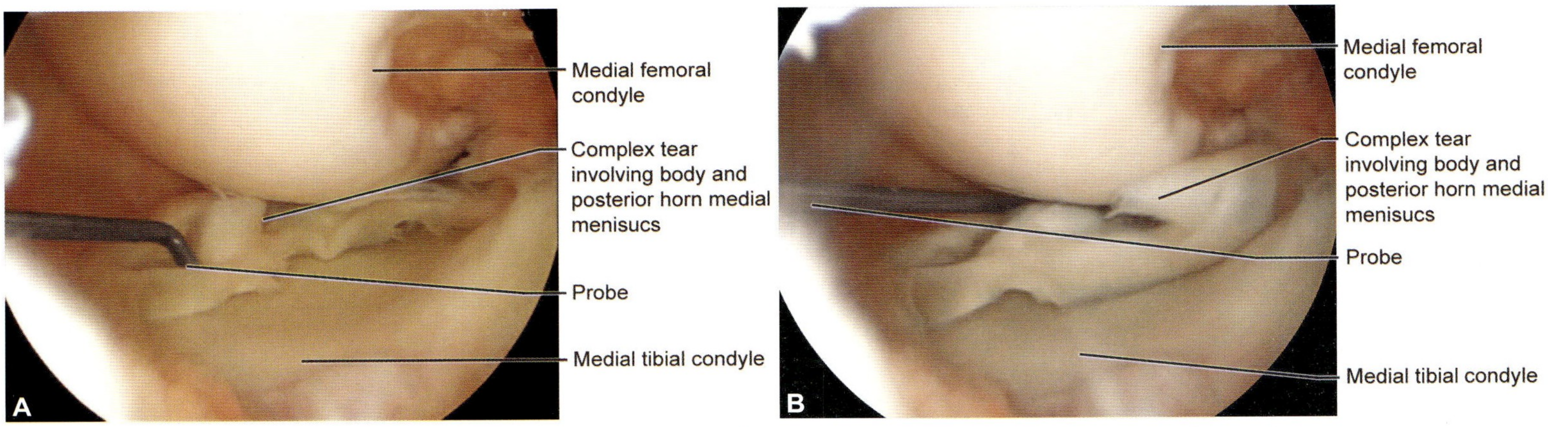

Figs. 16A and B: Meniscus should be probed to identify margins and tear extent in order to plan the meniscectomy.

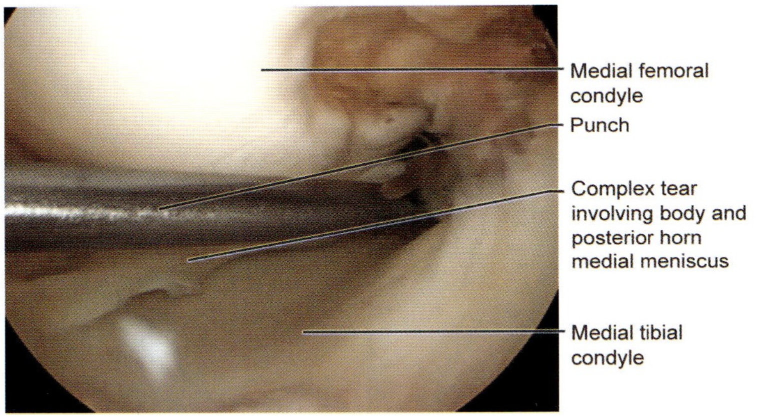

Fig. 17: Begin the technique with partial division of the posterior attachment of meniscal fragment with basket punch.

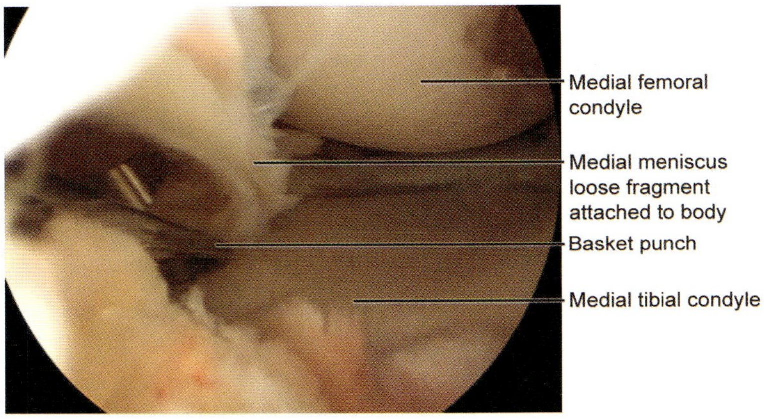

Fig. 18: Divide the anterior most attachment of torn meniscal loose fragment with basket punch in order to remove it.

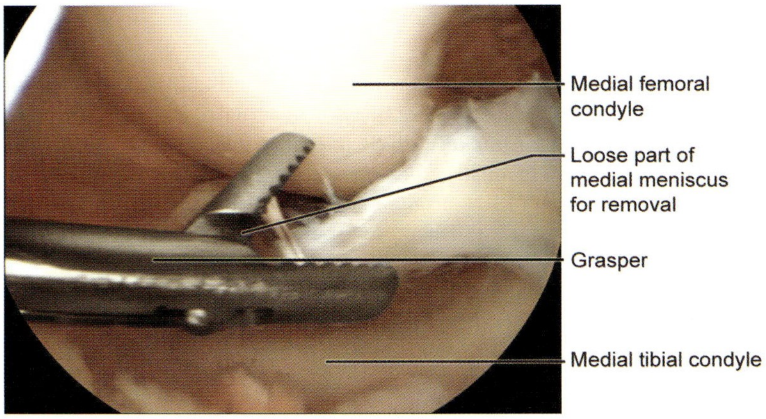

Fig. 19: Insert a grasper through same portal, grasp the loose fragment from one end, twist and rotate the grasper, and take out grasper to remove meniscal loose fragment.

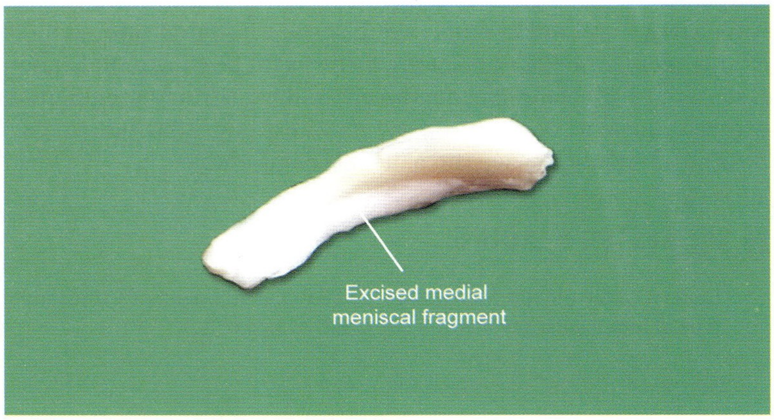

Fig. 20: Large loose medial meniscus fragment removed with the help of grasper.

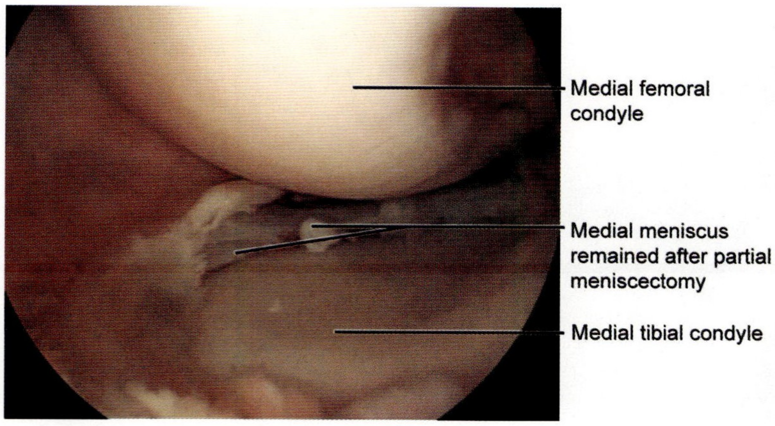

Fig. 21: Observe the joint if there are any other torn fragments.

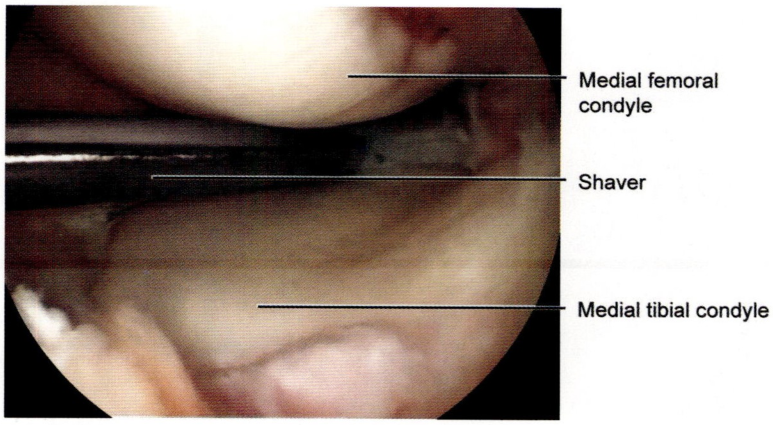

Fig. 22: If there are no further tears, use motorized meniscal shaver to smooth the remaining rim.

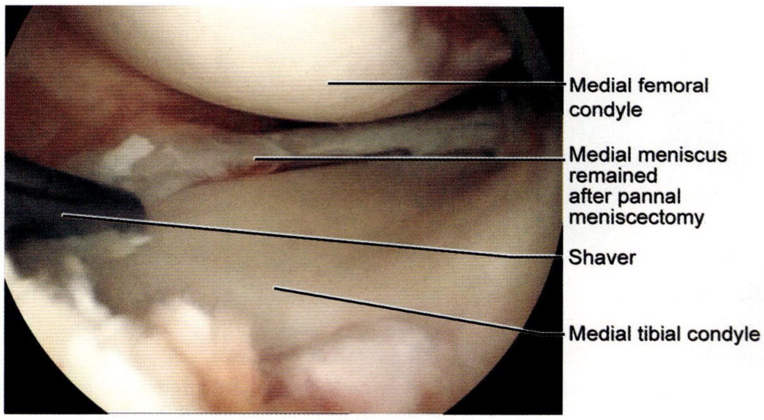

Fig. 23: Smoothening of meniscal rim with shaver completes the partial meniscectomy.

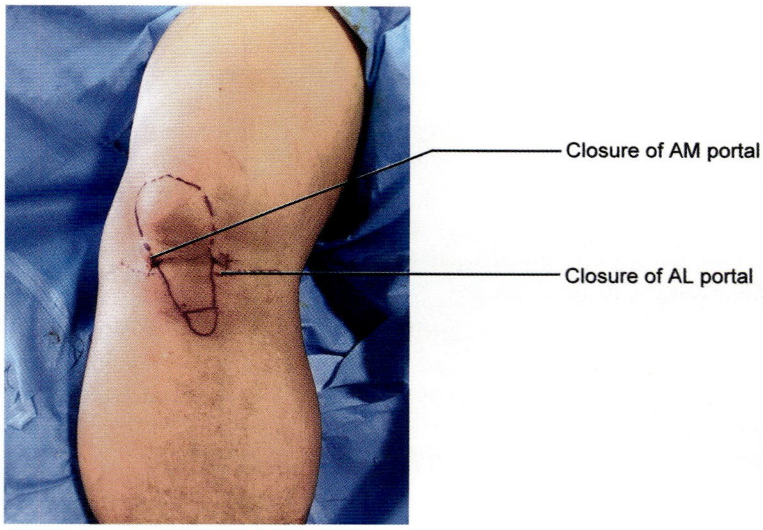

Fig. 24: Closure of two portals in one stitch for each portal. Compression dressing should be done for 48 hours.

REHABILITATION

Knee statics and ankle pump exercises are initiated immediately after surgery. After 24 hours, toe touch weight bearing mobilization is started. Range of motion, quadriceps and hamstring strengthening exercises have to be started from very next day. Start full weight-bearing ambulation when the patient is comfortable.

SUGGESTED READING

1. Burks RT, Metcalf MH, Metcalf RW. Fifteen-year follow-up of arthroscopic partial meniscectomy. Arthroscopy. 1997;13(6):673-9.
2. McNicholas MJ, Rowley DI, McGurty D, et al. Total meniscectomy in adolescence. A thirty-year follow-up. J Bone Joint Surg Br. 2000;82(2):217-21.
3. Mordecai SC, Al-Hadithy N, Ware HE, et al. Treatment of meniscal tears: An evidence based approach. World J Orthop. 2014;5(3):233-41.
4. Shelbourne KD, Dersam MD. Comparison of partial meniscectomy versus meniscus repair for bucket-handle lateral meniscus tears in anterior cruciate ligament reconstructed knees. Arthroscopy. 2004;20(6):581-5.
5. Williams RJ, Warner KK, Petrigliano FA, et al. MRI evaluation of isolated arthroscopic partial meniscectomy patients at a minimum five-year follow-up. HSS J. 2007;3(1):35-43.
6. Zarins B, Boyle J, Harris BA. Knee rehabilitation following arthroscopic meniscectomy. Clin Orthop Relat Res. 1985;198:36-42.

CHAPTER 14

Open Fixation for Posterior Cruciate Ligament Avulsion

Shrinivas S Shintre, Rahul Puranik, Vivek Mukund Badhe

INTRODUCTION

It is an uncommon injury. Isolated posterior cruciate ligament (PCL) disruption is due to avulsion of large piece of posterior part of tibial spine due posteriorly directed force in a flexed knee.

Posterior cruciate ligament injuries are less common than anterior cruciate ligament (ACL) injuries because PCL is stronger than ACL. For the same reason PCL avulsion fracture is more commonly seen than PCL ligament tear.

MECHANISM

Such patients present with history of direct blow on flexed knee, forceful hyperextension. Common is two-wheeler and four-wheeler vehicle accidents (dashboard injury):

CLINICAL FEATURES

Patients usually present with complaints of severe pain over and behind knee joint following history of trauma. Mild swelling may present. Posterior joint tenderness can be elicited. Range of motion is terminally restricted.

Posterior drawer test, posterior sag signs are demonstrated. Lachman test (false positive) may be elicited on clinical examination.

RADIOLOGICAL IMAGING

Plain radiographs in anteroposterior and lateral views are obtained. CT images are useful to know the orientation of fragments and plain fixation.

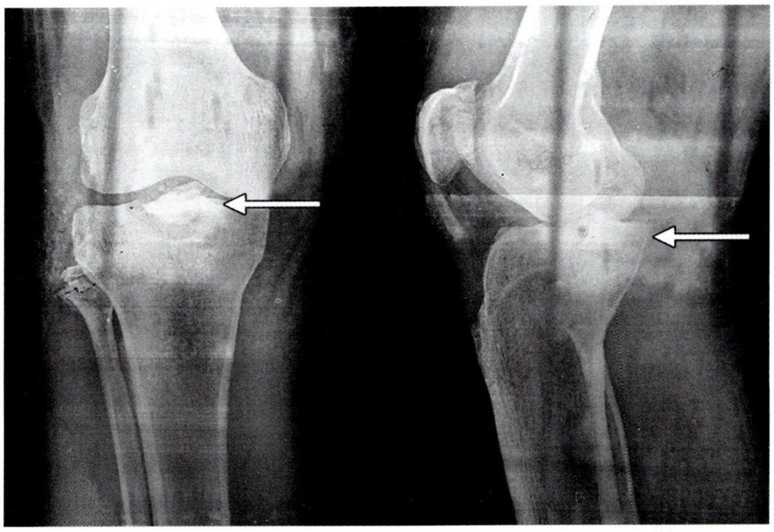

Fig. 1: Anteroposterior and lateral roentgenograph views showing avulsed fragment.

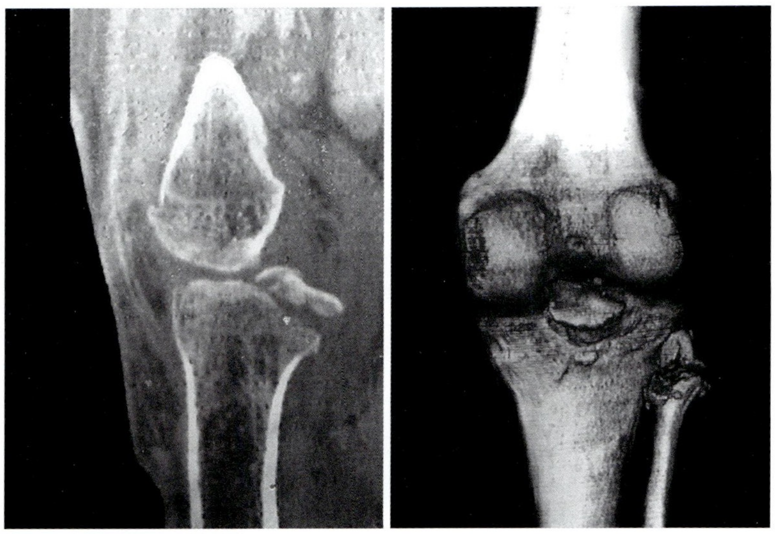

Fig. 2: CT images

TREATMENT

In acute PCL avulsion case, if fragment is small and posterior tibial translation is less than 10 mm, then quadriceps rehabilitation is done. For posterior tibial translation, more than 10 mm PCL reconstruction is choice. In case of large fragment, open reduction and internal fixation is the method of choice.

OPEN REDUCTION AND INTERNAL FIXATION

Burks and Schaffer's posteromedial approach is commonly used for ORIF of PCL avulsion fracture as described here.

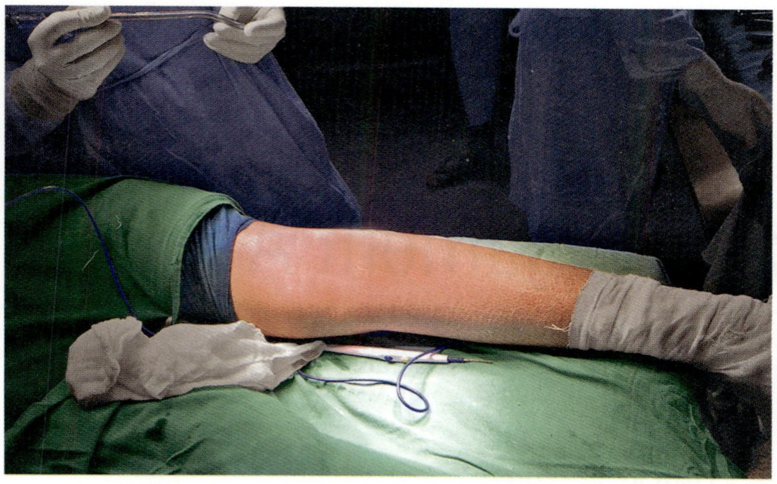

Fig. 3: Tourniquet at level of thigh is applied. Patient is positioned in prone position on operation table and scrubbing, painting, and draping is done under all aseptic precautions.

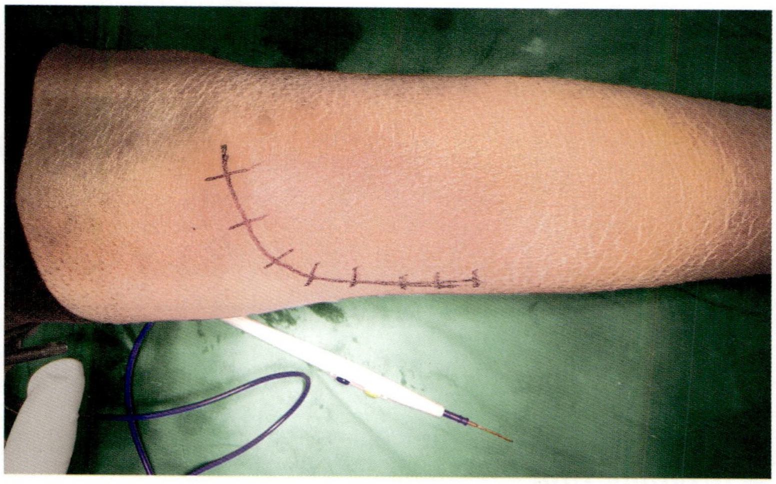

Fig. 4: A curved incision line is marked starting horizontal parallel to posterior flexure crease of knee from lateral to medial which then curved inferiorly as shown in figure.

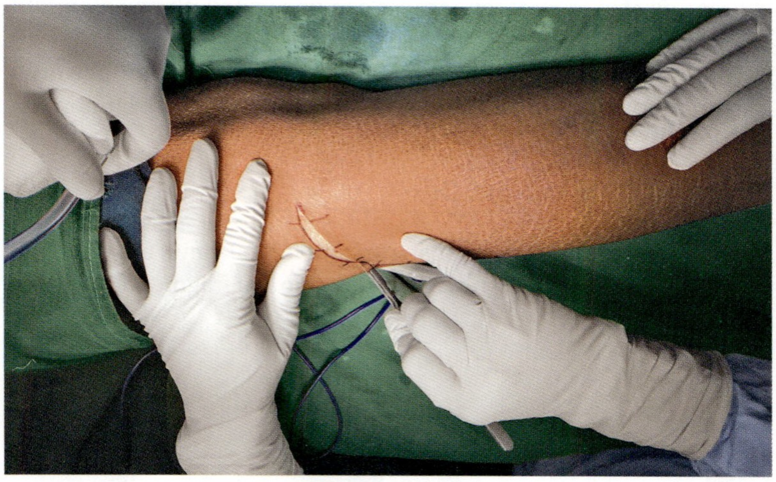

Fig. 5: Skin incision.

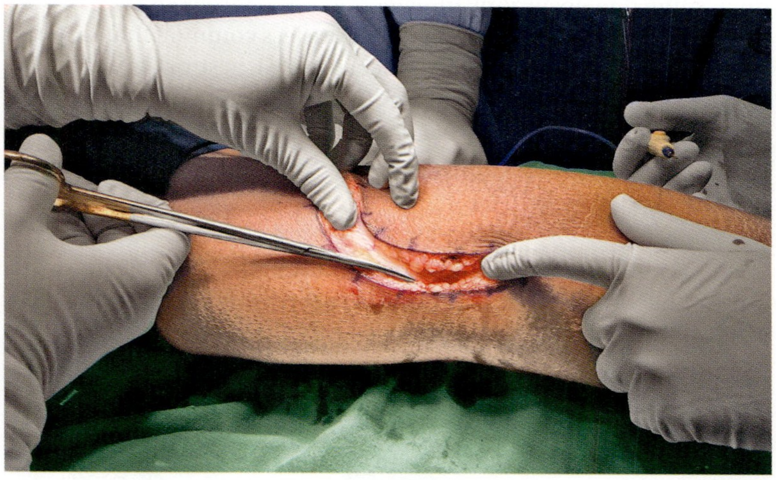

Fig. 6: Subcutaneous tissue and superficial fascia are dissected.

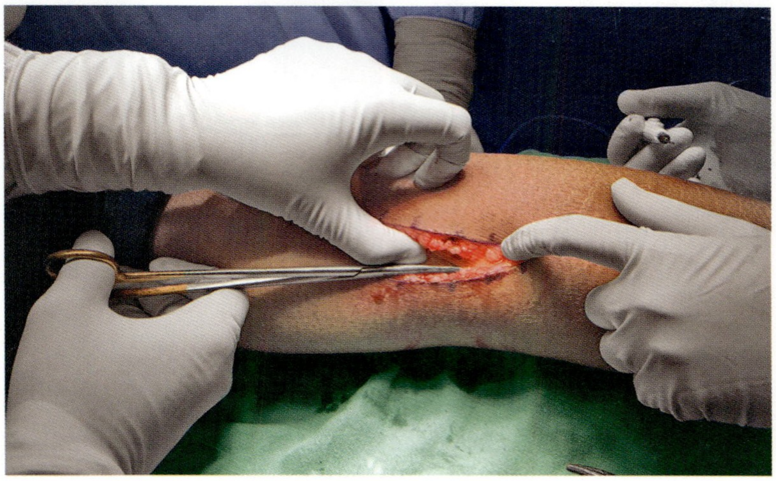

Fig. 7: Deep fascia is dissected.

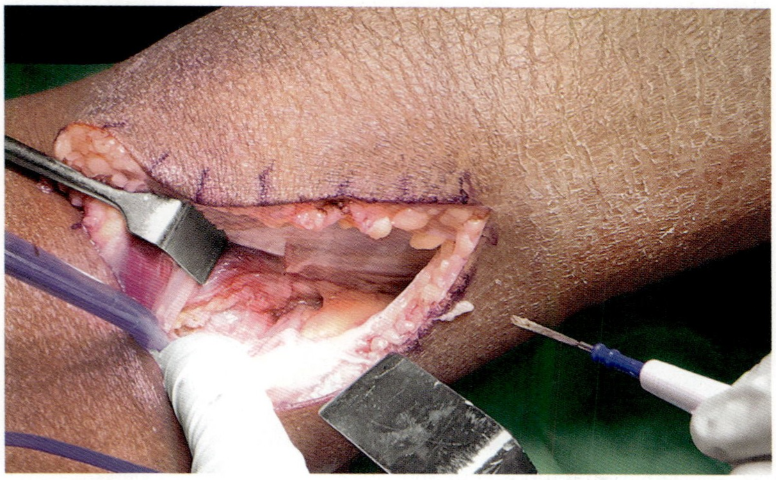

Fig. 8: Medial head of gastrocnemius is separated from semimembranosus using blunt dissection. Medial head of gastrocnemius is retracted laterally.

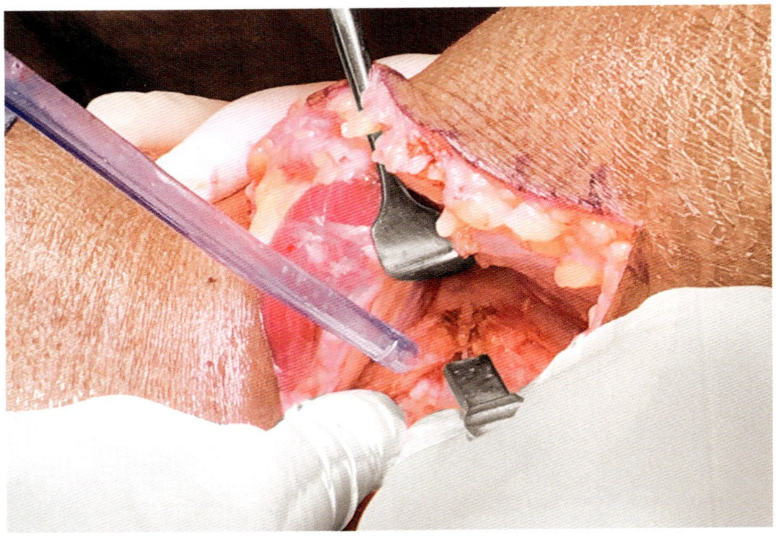

Fig. 9: Avulsed fragment is located. Edges are cleared with periosteum elevator.

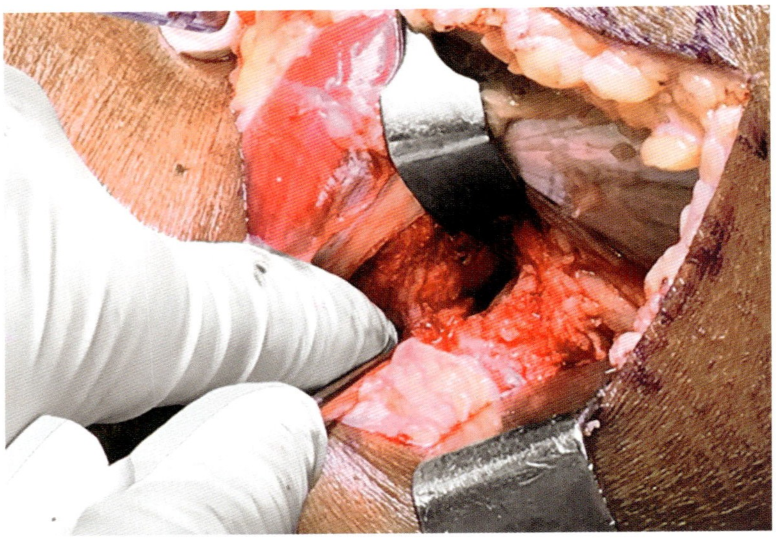

Fig. 10: Fracture surfaces are freshened using scoop.

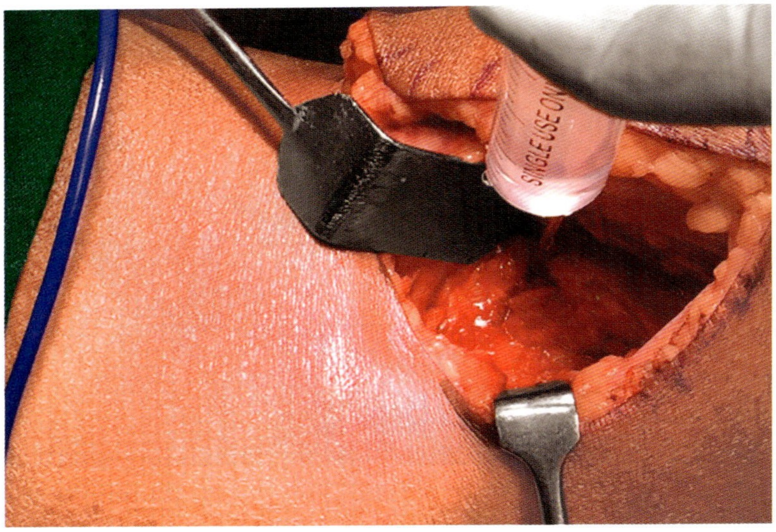

Fig. 11: Adequate wash is given with normal saline.

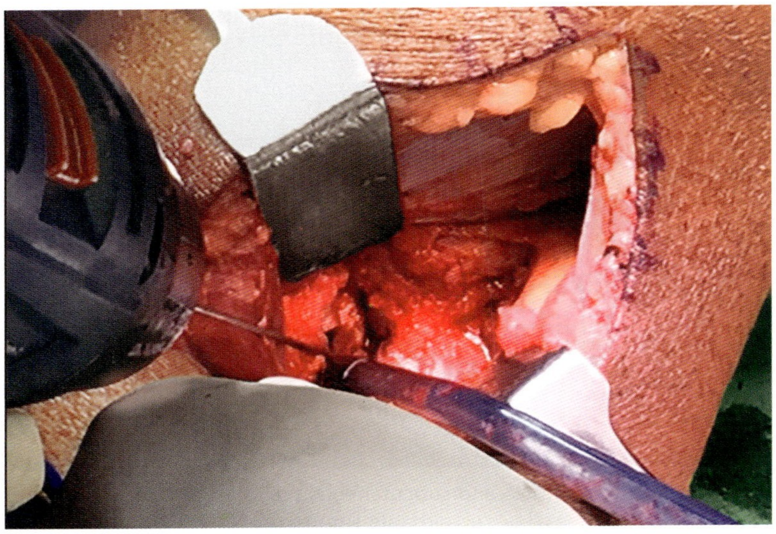

Fig. 12: Temporary fixation is obtained using a K-wire.

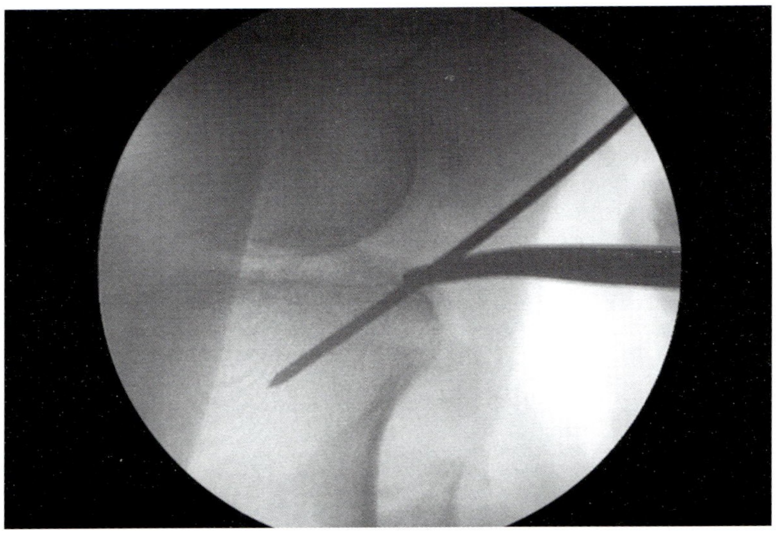

Fig. 13: Temporary fixation is confirmed over fluoroscopy.

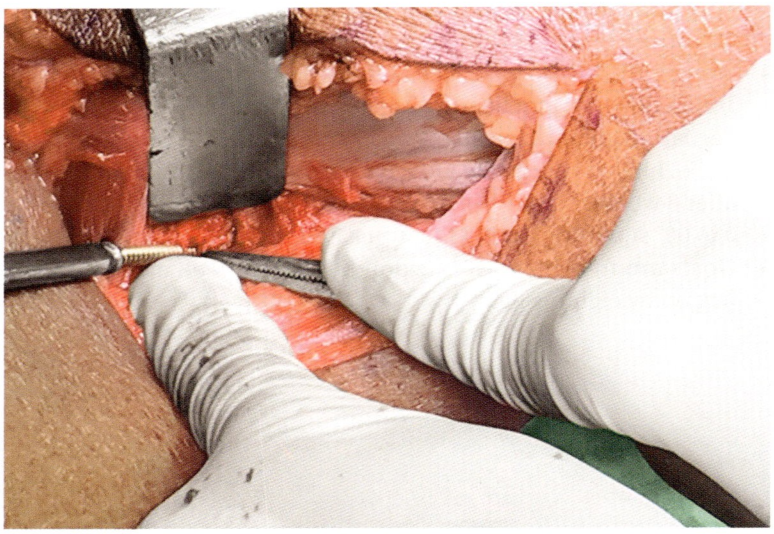

Fig. 14: Final fixation—a 4 mm cancellous screw is achieved.

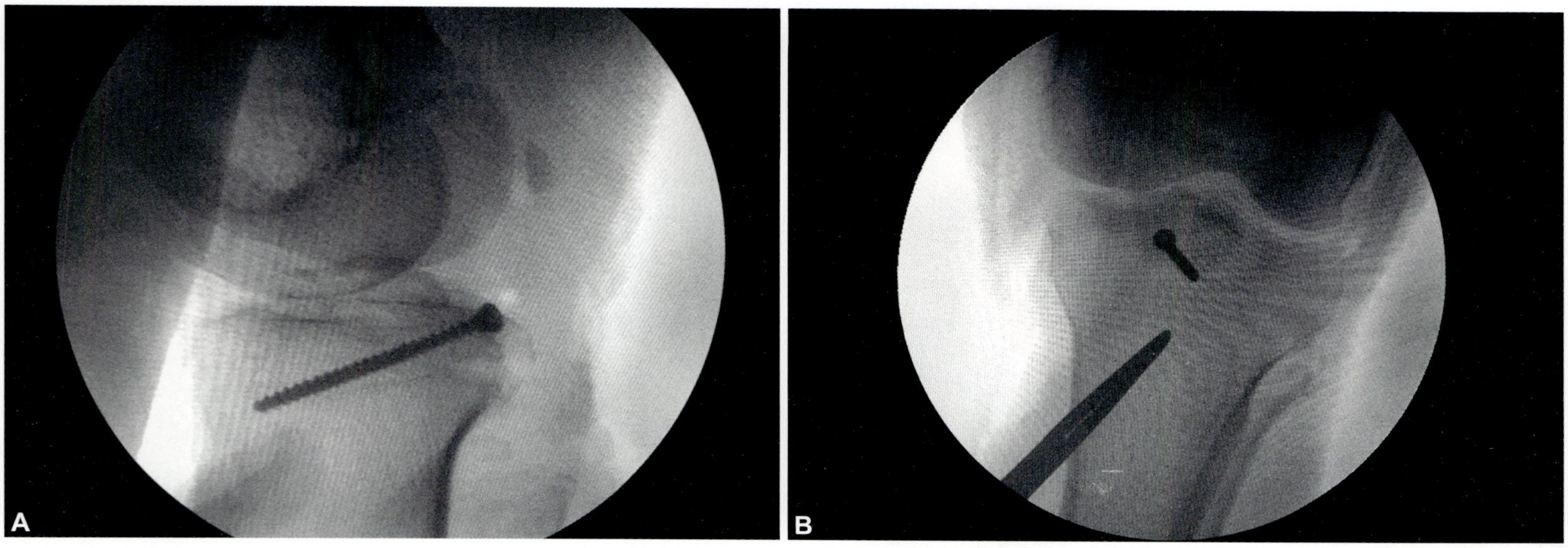

Figs. 15A and B: Final reduction confirmed on fluoroscopy imaging.

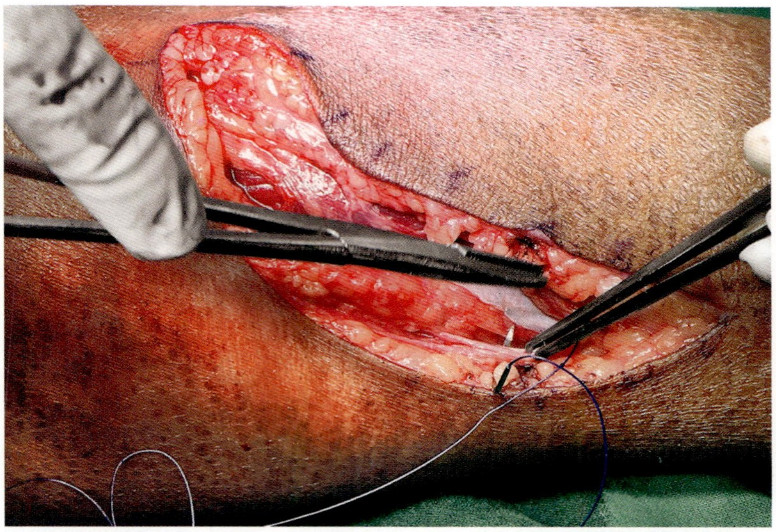

Fig. 16: Deep fascia and subcutaneous tissue are sutured with absorbable suture.

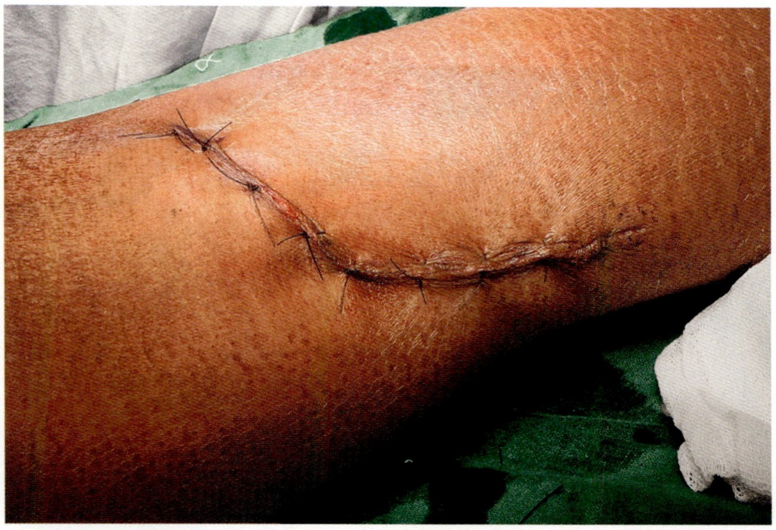

Fig. 17: Skin closure obtained with nonabsorbable intermittent sutures. Sterile dressing is applied.

POSTOPERATIVE CARE

- A long posterior knee brace is applied to immobilize knee in extension.
- Straight leg raises, quadricep and calf pump exercises are advised.
- Touch down weight bearing is given in first week.
- Partial weight bearing after 2 weeks.
- Use of hinged knee brace after 4–6 weeks and discontinued usually after 8 weeks.
- 0 to 60° squatting during first week and up to 90° by third week.
- Goals are to achieve 90° flexion by fourth week and 120° knee flexion by eighth week.

SUGGESTED READING

1. Nicandri GT, Klineberg EO, Wahl CJ, et al. Treatment of posterior cruciate ligament tibial avulsion fractures through a modified open posterior approach: operative technique and 12-to 48-month outcomes. J Orthop Trauma. 2008;22(5):317-24.
2. Veselko M, Saciri V. Posterior approach for arthroscopic reduction and antegrade fixation of avulsion fracture of the posterior cruciate ligament from the tibia with cannulated screw and washer. Arthroscopy. 2003;19(8):916-21.
3. Yang CK, Wu CD, Chih CJ, et al. Surgical treatment of avulsion fracture of the posterior cruciate ligament and postoperative management. Journal of Trauma and Acute Care Surgery. 2003;54(3):516-9.

CHAPTER 15

Management of Chondral Defects of the Knee

Anshu Shekhar, Shantanu Sudhakar Patil, Sachin Ramchandra Tapasvi

INTRODUCTION

The articular lining of synovial joints is made up of hyaline cartilage, which is a composite gel with about 5% cellular material (chondrocytes) in an extracellular matrix of proteoglycans, constrained by a collagen network of mainly type II and type IX collagen fibers. This cartilage is an elastic and resilient structure mainly due to the presence of proteoglycans in the matrix. Histologically, the articular cartilage is divided into four layers depending upon the arrangement and orientation of cells and collagen fibers: (1) superficial tangential layer, (2) transitional layer, (3) radial layer, and (4) the calcified zone.

Damage to the cartilage cover can occur from multiple etiologies, trauma being the most common. Management of a cartilage defect depends on multiple factors as illustrated in Table 1. It is important to consider all the factors prior to choosing the method to be employed.

There are several methods to classify the depth of the cartilage lesion including those described by Outerbridge, Insall, and Noyes. The International Cartilage Repair Society (ICRS) has proposed a classification system to avoid confusion in documentation of these lesions (Table 2).

Treatment algorithms are based on the earlier enumerated factors and a particular method of managing the lesion is chosen. The various options available are basically divided into the following:

1. *Marrow stimulation techniques*—Chondroplasty, subchondral drilling, or microfracture
2. *Osteochondral transfer*—Autograft or allograft
3. Autologous chondrocyte implantation (ACI).

The technical aspect specific to each technique is described. Most of the cartilage restoration procedures can be performed arthroscopically but there are some indications where an open surgery may be required, either due to issues related to accessibility or extent.

MARROW STIMULATION

These methods of management are restricted to ICRS grade 3 and 4 lesions in any location. The common steps in these techniques include:

- *Identification and classification*: During the diagnostic round of arthroscopy, the lesion is identified and meticulous probing with a hook probe is performed to assess the extent of the lesion, stability of margins, and presence of loose flaps (Figs. 1 and 2).
- *Debridement*: This is done for ICRS grade 3 and 4 defects after adequate exposure of the lesion has been obtained. The aim of this exercise is to achieve stable, vertical walls all around the defect and removal of any internal osteophytes in the subchondral bone (Figs. 3 and 4).
- *Assessment of depth and size of defect*: The final analysis of the depth and size of the lesion is performed only after the debridement is complete (Figs. 5A and B).

TABLE 1: Factors to consider in the management of cartilage defects.

Sl. No	*Etiology*	*Traumatic or osteonecrosis or endocrinal or any other*
1.	Size of defect	Measured at least in two planes perpendicular to each other
2.	Depth of defect	Based on thickness of cartilage loss and subchondral bone status
3.	Location	Whether weight-bearing area involved and which bone
4.	Containment	Regarding the condition of surrounding cartilage
5.	Stability	Ligamentous stability in all planes is important
6.	Meniscus status	Loss of meniscus tissue directly impacts stress on the cartilage
7.	Alignment	Can be judged from weight-bearing scanograms
8.	Previous management	Whether some form of restorative procedure has been performed

TABLE 2: International Cartilage Repair Society classification.

Grade 1	Superficial lesions
A	Soft indentation
B	Superficial fissures or cracks
Grade 2	Lesion extending to <50% thickness of the cartilage
Grade 3	Lesion extending to >50% thickness of the cartilage
A	Up to calcified layer
B	Through the calcified layer
C	Up to subchondral bone plate
D	Blisters
Grade 4	Osteochondral defects
A	Extending through subchondral bone plate
B	Extending into trabecular bone

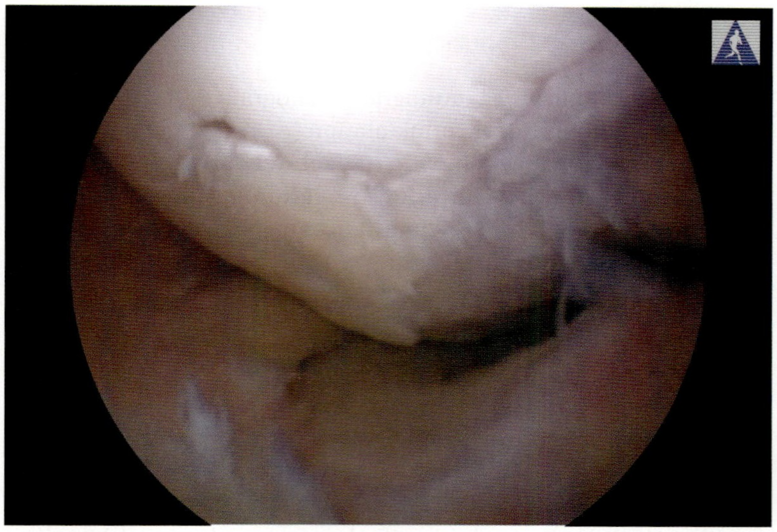

Fig. 1: A fissure seen over the weight-bearing surface of medial femoral condyle would be classified as grade 2 International Cartilage Repair Society (ICRS) lesion.

a. *Chondroplasty*: Chondroplasty is a technique of cartilage restoration where the uneven cartilage surface is treated to obtain a smooth surface. This is typically applied for partial thickness defects like ICRS grade 2 or 3. The loss of superficial layer leads to release of proteoglycans which incites synovitis by release of cytokines and further chondral damage by various chemical pathways. The aim of chondroplasty is to stop this process and stimulate a healing response. There are two methods of performing chondroplasty: (1) mechanical—by using a shaver (also called abrasion chondroplasty), or (2) thermal—by using a radiofrequency probe. Detailed discussion on these technologies and comparison is beyond the scope of this chapter, but there is some evidence that using a radiofrequency device is the better alternative. An illustrative example of chondroplasty for extensive chondromalacia of the patella is shown here (Figs. 6 to 8).
b. *Subchondral drilling*: The technique of subchondral drilling was first described by Pridie in 1959. It is based on the premise that penetration of the subchondral bone causes opening up of vascular channels for migration and proliferation of mesenchymal cells into the area of cartilage defect and their differentiation to form fibrocartilage. This is different from the articular hyaline cartilage and lacks its mechanical qualities leading to its breakdown over a period of time but does offer a reasonable substitute and relief of symptoms. The preparation of the defect is as described in the section earlier (Figs. 9 and 10).
c. *Microfracture*: The creation of multiple holes to allow egress of marrow element and form a "superclot" was first described by Steadman in 1997. This is achieved by using specially designed awls and the integrity of the subchondral bone is preserved. However, there has been some criticism of this technique recently as well (Figs. 11 and 12).

OSTEOCHONDRAL TRANSFER

Marrow stimulating techniques lead to formation of fibrocartilage, which is mechanically much inferior to hyaline cartilage. Also, these techniques can be used for smaller defects only and are contraindicated in the presence of "kissing" lesions. Transfer of

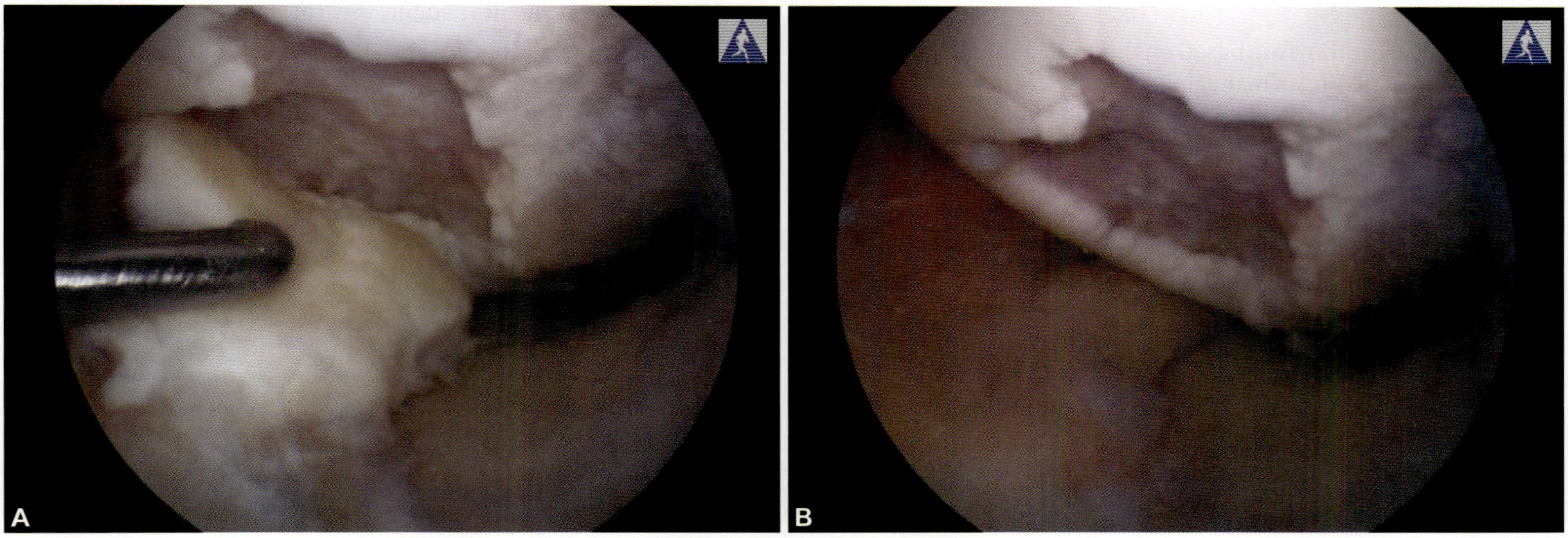

Figs. 2A and B: (A) Probing of the same lesion as in Figure 1 reveals a loose chondral flap with presence of internal osteophytes; and (B) Excision of the loose flap reveals the extent of the lesion which now becomes a grade 4 defect.

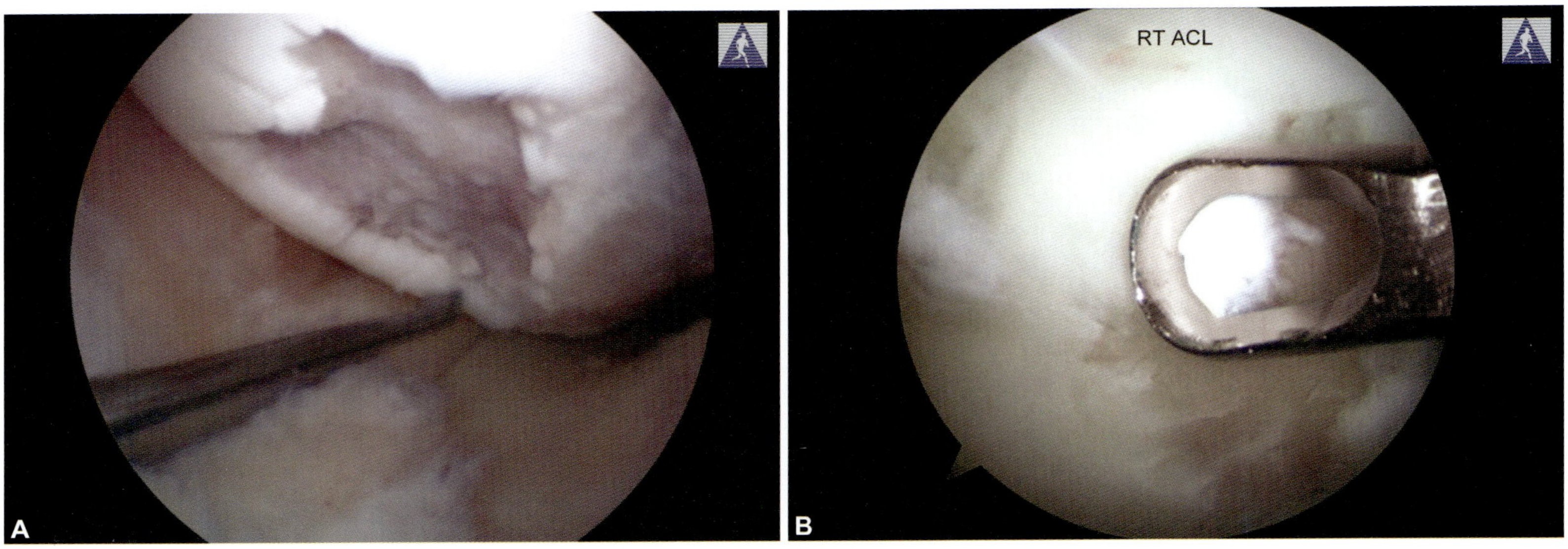

Figs. 3A and B: (A) An arthroscopic curette is used to create stable, vertical walls at the periphery of the lesion; and (B) A ring curette is especially suitable for this procedure. (ACL: anterior cruciate liagment)

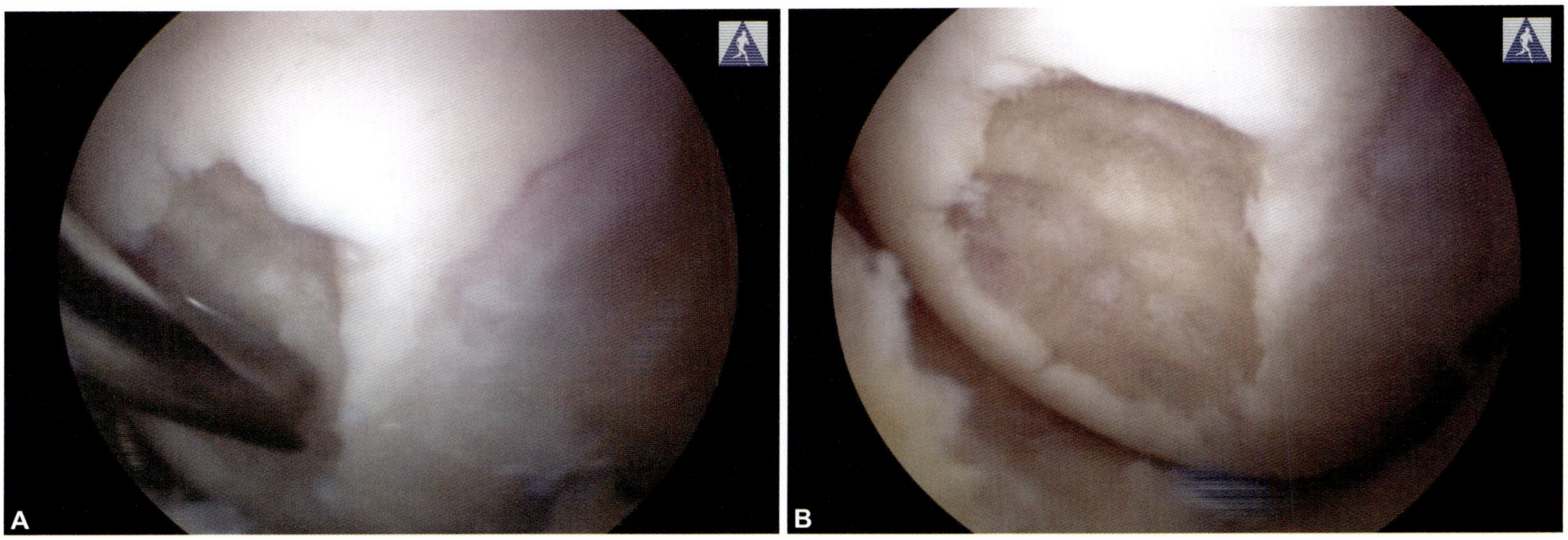

Figs. 4A and B: (A) An arthroscopic full radius shaver is then used for completing the mechanical debridement of the floor of the lesion. This is started at the center of the defect and progressed peripherally in sweeping movement; and (B) A radiofrequency device can also be used for this purpose and causes thermal debridement with similar efficacy. The defect after debridement appears larger and deeper.

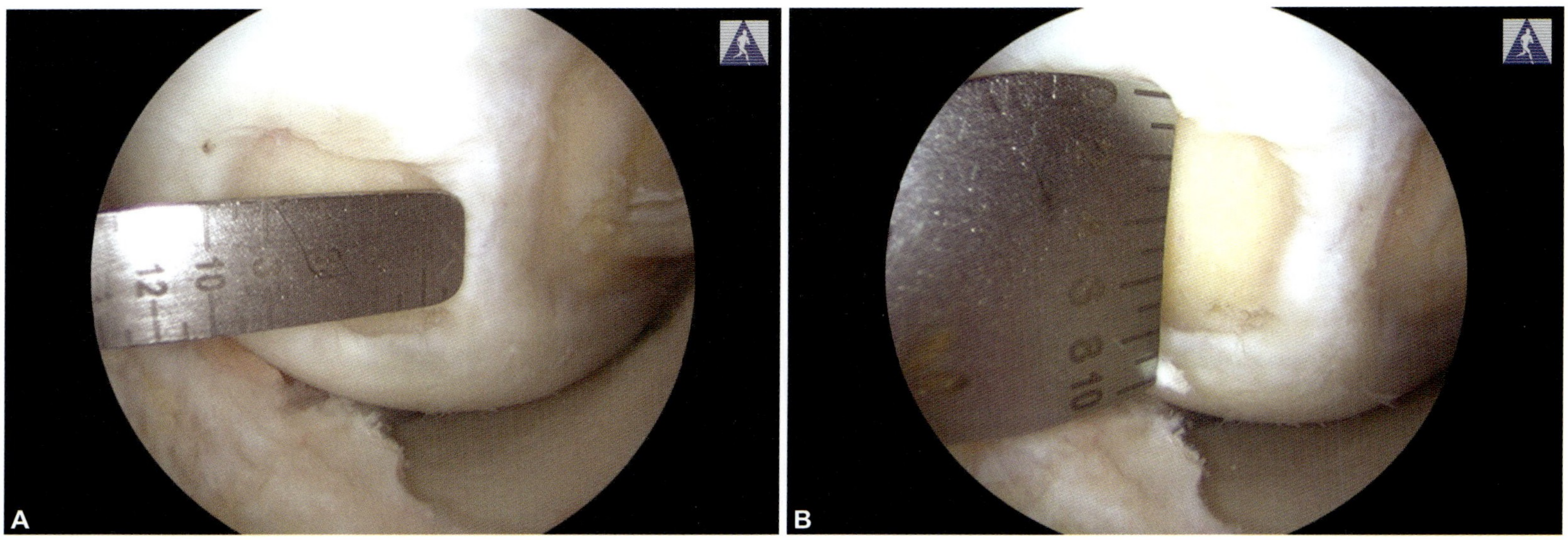

Figs. 5A and B: (A and B) An arthroscopic ruler is used to measure the size of the defect. The measurement must be performed at least in two planes perpendicular to each other and at the widest possible dimensions.

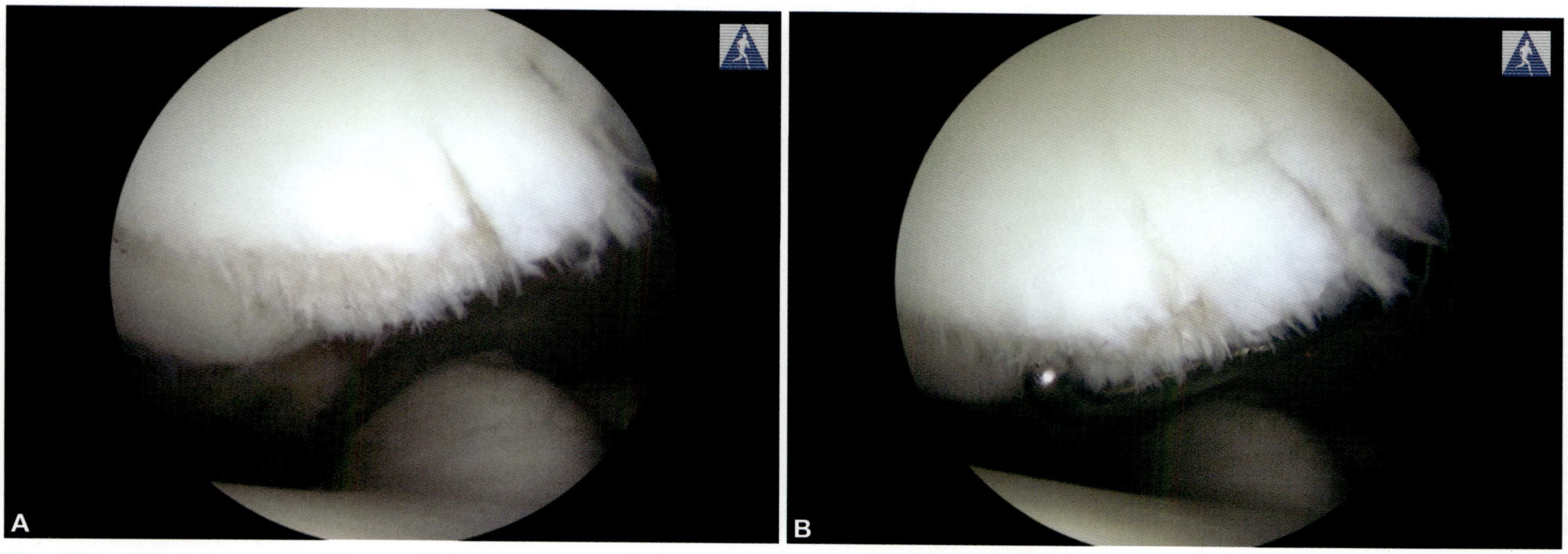

Figs. 6A and B: Arthroscopy of the patellofemoral joint is performed with the knee in full extension. Chondromalacia of the patella is seen best when viewed from the superolateral portal. (A) The typical "crabmeat" appearance is seen; and (B) Probing is done to evaluate the surface and presence of any loose chondral flap.

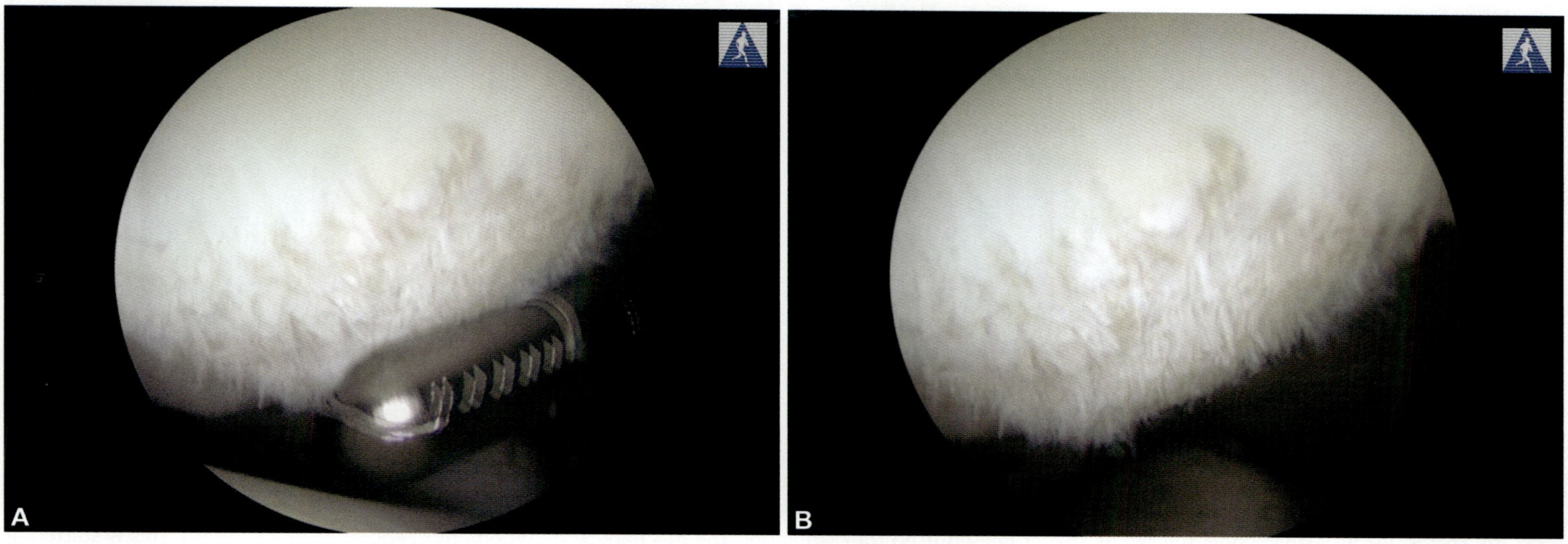

Figs. 7A and B: The superolateral portal is used as the viewing portal and a superomedial portal is created for instrumentation. (A) A shaver is introduced and the frayed cartilage is debrided by moving the shaver in sweeping motion; and (B) Abrasion chondroplasty significantly reduces the fraying but does not produce a completely smooth surface.

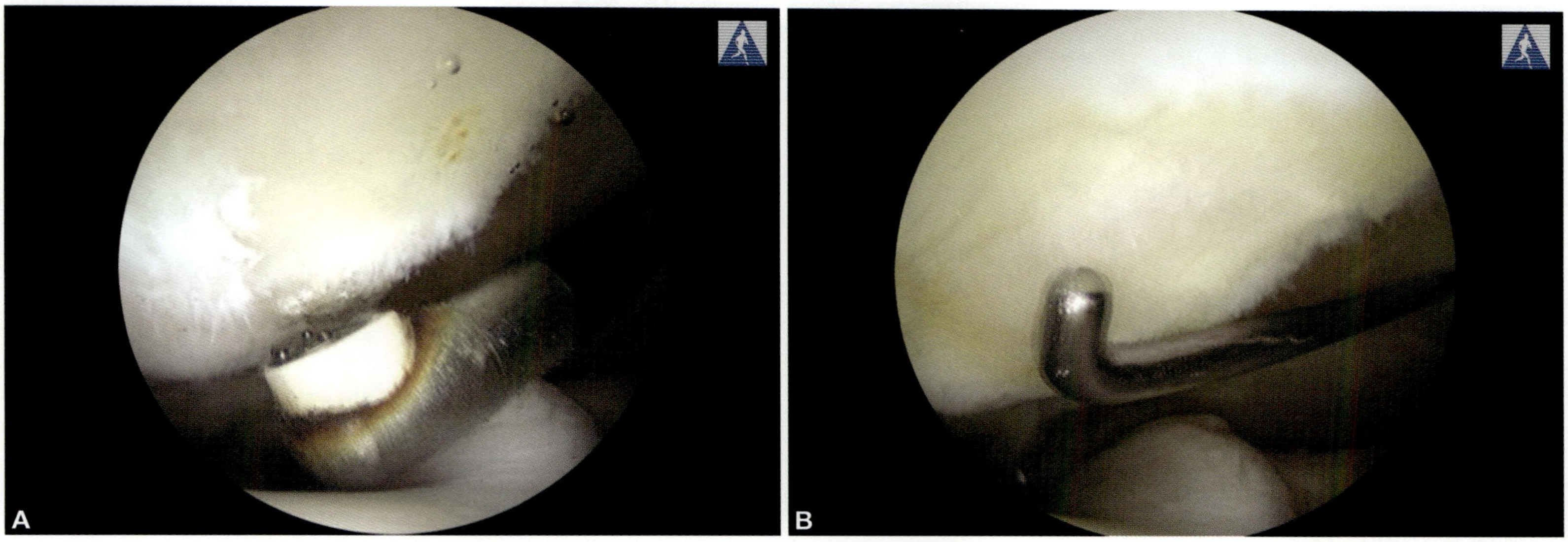

Figs. 8A and B: (A) Thermal chondroplasty is performed by introduction of a radiofrequency probe from the superomedial portal; and (B) The result obtained at the end of the procedure is probed again.

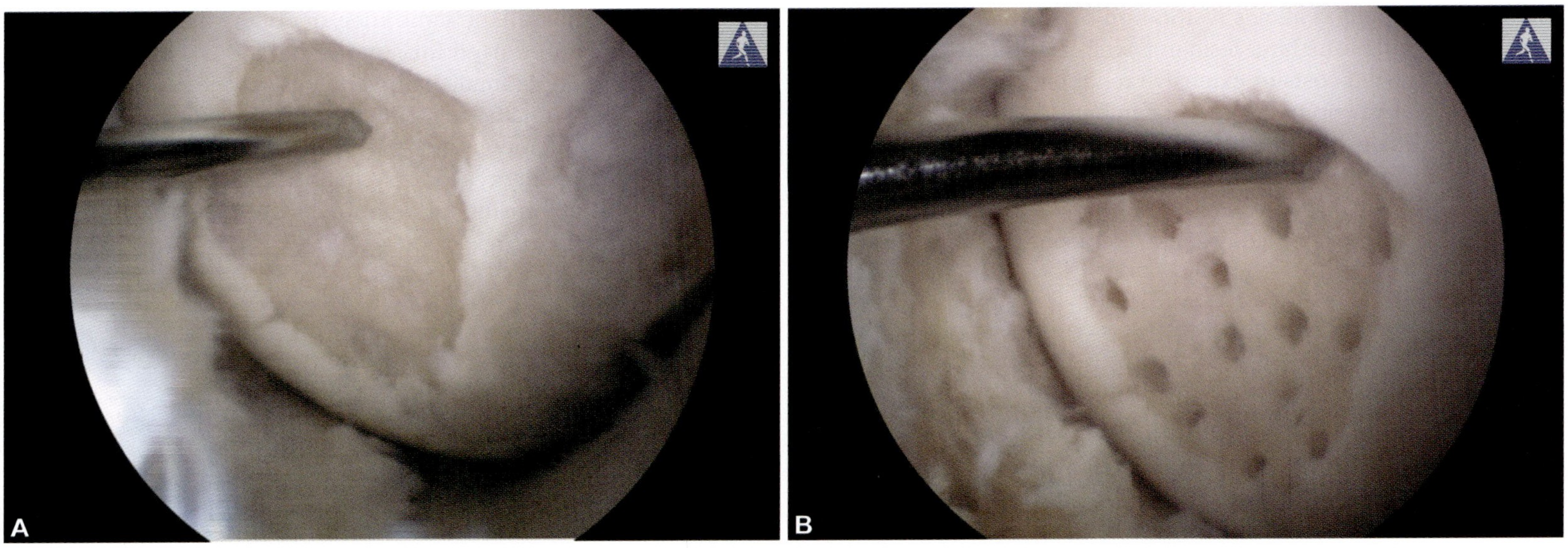

Figs. 9A and B: Drilling can be performed with a 1.6 mm Kirschner wire. The trajectory of the wire at the defect must be perpendicular to its surface. This may be achieved by inserting the wire into the joint through any of the standard portals or percutaneously if needed. (A) Drilling is initiated near the central area of the defect till penetration of the subchondral bone is achieved and advanced peripherally; and (B) Multiple drill holes are created 3–4 mm apart to achieve a honeycomb pattern and coalescence is avoided.

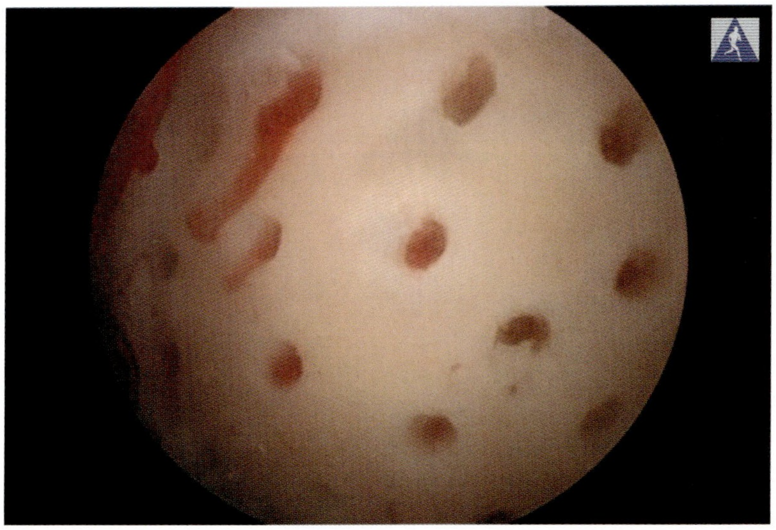

Fig. 10: Adequacy of the procedure is confirmed by the presence of bleeding from the holes. The tourniquet may be deflated and saline infusion stopped to better appreciate this. The holes which do not bleed or emit fat globules may need to be drilled deeper.

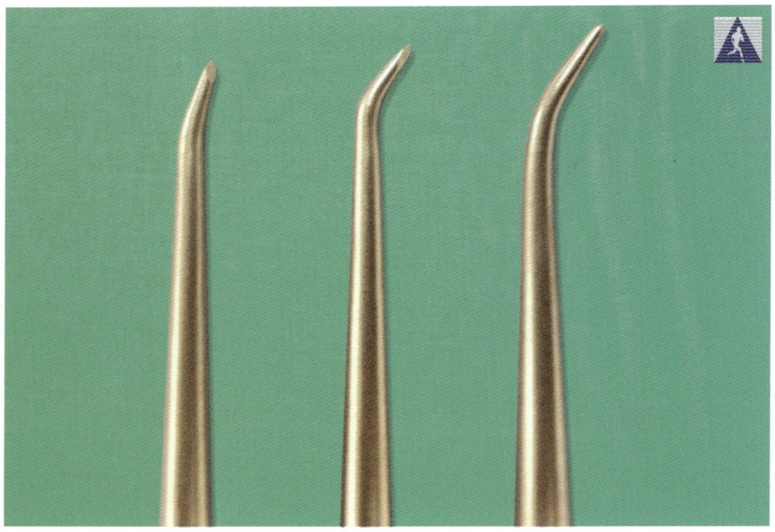

Fig. 11: Microfracture awls are available in various angles and have a trocar tip. This prevents slippage while tapping the awl and helps achieve a perpendicular trajectory to the bone surface.

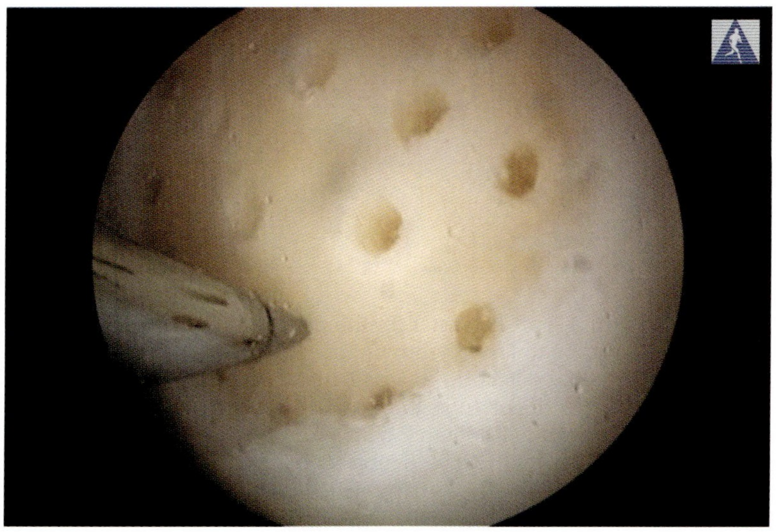

Fig. 12: The awl is inserted from any suitable standard arthroscopy portal after preparation of the defect. The process of creation of the holes is started at the periphery and advanced centrally, maintaining a bridge of 3–4 mm and avoiding coalescence.

osteochondral plug(s) allows restoration of hyaline cartilage at the defect and is suitable for large lesions as well. It is done in a single stage without aggravated costs or extensive rehabilitation later. Although suitable for defects up to 2.5 cm^2, it can be used to cover defects as large as 4 cm^2. The disadvantage of this technique is related to donor site morbidity (for autografts) and contour mismatch.

This surgery can be done using grafts harvested from a nonweight-bearing area like the lateral margin of lateral femoral condyle, above the sulcus terminalis in the same knee, or obtained from an allograft. A single plug can be used for smaller defect of 8 mm or 10 mm diameter but multiple small diameter plugs may be needed for larger defects. All issues related to stability, alignment, and menisci must be managed simultaneously or prior to cartilage surgery. There are multiple commercially available systems in various sizes, to perform an osteochondral transfer and one such system is shown in Figures 13A to E (OATS™, Arthrex, Naples, FL).

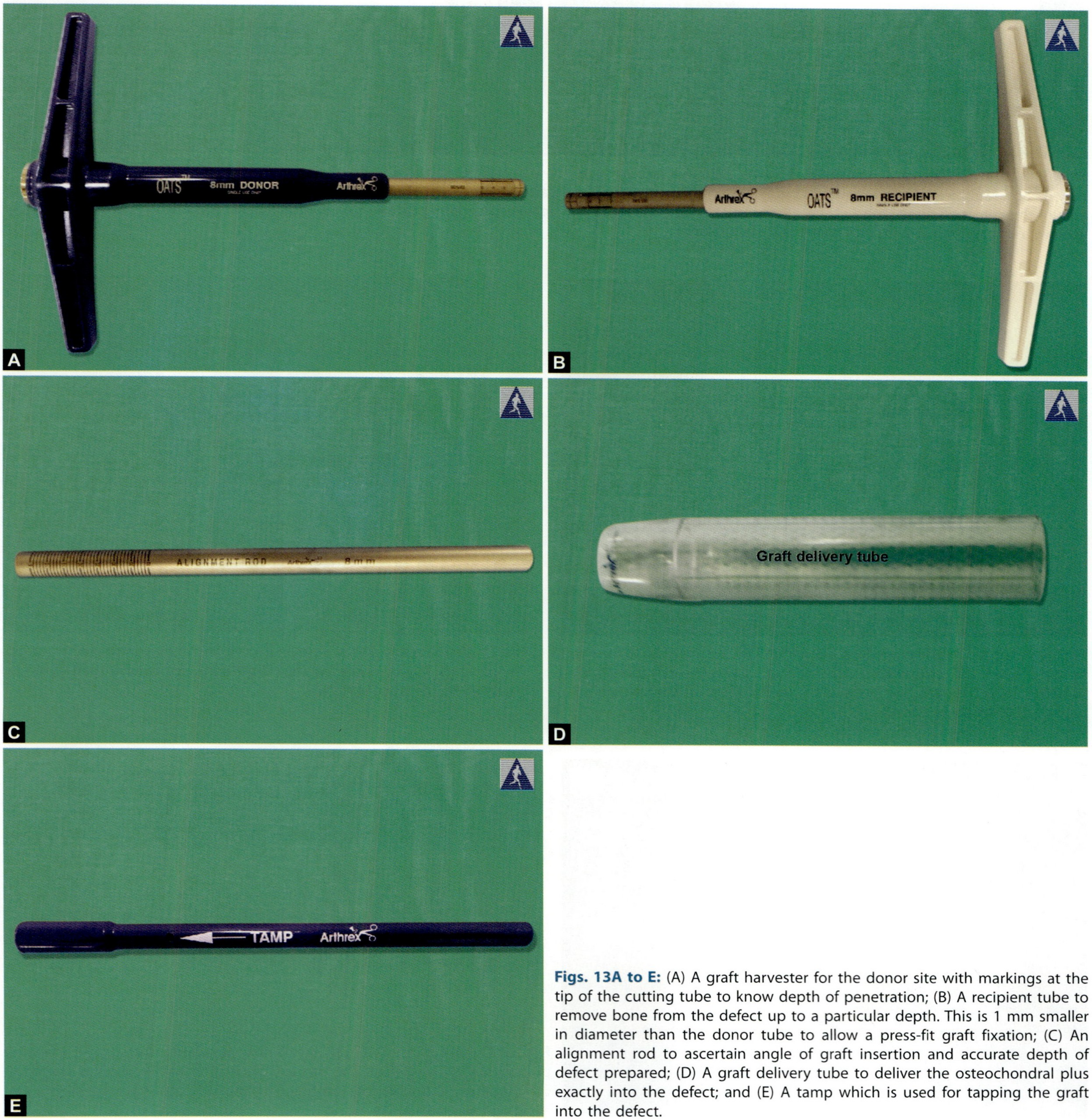

Figs. 13A to E: (A) A graft harvester for the donor site with markings at the tip of the cutting tube to know depth of penetration; (B) A recipient tube to remove bone from the defect up to a particular depth. This is 1 mm smaller in diameter than the donor tube to allow a press-fit graft fixation; (C) An alignment rod to ascertain angle of graft insertion and accurate depth of defect prepared; (D) A graft delivery tube to deliver the osteochondral plus exactly into the defect; and (E) A tamp which is used for tapping the graft into the defect.

The essential steps and principles in osteochondral transfer surgery are enumerated here:

- *Step 1—Approach*: Most lesions in the femoral condyles can be managed arthroscopically but tibial or patellar defects necessitate open surgery. When arthroscopy is planned, a needle inserted up to the defect must be able to be placed perpendicular to bone surface. This requires the knee to be placed in a suitable flexion angle (hyperflexion for femoral condyle weight-bearing areas) and allow good arthroscopic visualization. If neither is possible, a mini-arthrotomy must be performed. Illustrated here is arthroscopic osteochondral autograft transfer for a right knee lateral femoral condyle ICRS grade 4 defect (Figs. 14A and B).
- *Step 2—Preparation of defect*: The defect is prepared in the standard fashion as previously described (Fig. 15).
- *Step 3—Graft harvest*: The autograft can be harvested arthroscopically from a nonweight-bearing area of the knee with confirming geometry. For the convex femoral condyle, grafts harvested from margin of lateral or medial condyle, proximal to sulcus terminalis are suitable (Figs. 16 and 17).
- *Step 4—Donor site preparation*: A cylindrical socket has to be created at the site of chondral defect which will allow insertion of the osteochondral plug. This is done by using the recipient tube which is undersized by 1 mm to enable press-fit implantation later (Figs. 18A and B).
- *Step 5—Conformation of alignment*: The direction and orientation of the recipient site socket is determined by using an alignment rod. This instrument also helps confirm the exact depth of the socket to avoid the plug from being proud after insertion. This must never be lesser than the length of the plug obtained. If this is the case, either the plug length must be shortened accordingly or the alignment rod impacted by a millimeter or two (Figs. 19A and B).
- *Step 6—Graft insertion*: The graft plug is delivered into the joint through the graft delivery tube and placed at the recipient site through the same portal. The portal may be enlarged as needed to avoid struggle and soft tissue entrapment. Arthroscopic visualization is maintained continuously. The osteochondral plug is inserted into the delivery tube maintaining proper orientation for sphericity and tamp placed over it to prevent extrusion due to the saline. The saline infusion may be stopped for a while when this is being done. Insertion of the graft must be done very gently by tapping with a small mallet and under vision to avoid sinking of the graft in the socket (Figs. 20A to D).
- *Step 7—Confirmation of congruity and stability*: The placement and insertion of the osteochondral plug must be done meticulously to obtain desired contour and to avoid graft from sinking or staying proud. The stability is also tested by gentle probing and taking the knee through a full range of motion (Figs. 21A and B).

CHONDROCYTE IMPLANTATION

Large or multifocal defects of the cartilage are not optimally managed with either marrow stimulation or osteochondral plug transfer. The option for cartilage restoration in these patients is chondrocyte implantation at the site of defect. This can either be autologous cultured and concentrated cartilage cells or stem cells from allogenic tissue. As the understanding of cartilage regeneration improved, the technique of chondrocyte implantation has also evolved and is generally described as "generations".

- *First generation*: Involved a two-stage procedure, where autologous cartilage was harvested in the first stage and expanded. These cells were then implanted at the defect site and covered with a periosteal or collagen patch to seal the defect with either sutures or fibrin glue.
- *Second generation*: This also involves a two-stage procedure with the first stage being similar to first generation. However, the implantation of cultured cells was greatly simplified by using a scaffold for cell placement. These scaffolds are either hydrogels or membranes based on structure and either may be natural or synthetic or composite based on origin. A large number of such products are commercially available.
- *Third generation*: The implantation is done in one stage only using allogenic or autologous stem cells which are embedded in a scaffold of hydrogel or membrane. This is based on the premise that pluripotent stem cells would differentiate into chondrocytes induced by appropriate environment.

We describe briefly the surgical principles and technique of a second-generation ACI system which is gel-based (Chondron®) and approved for use in India. This procedure is performed in two

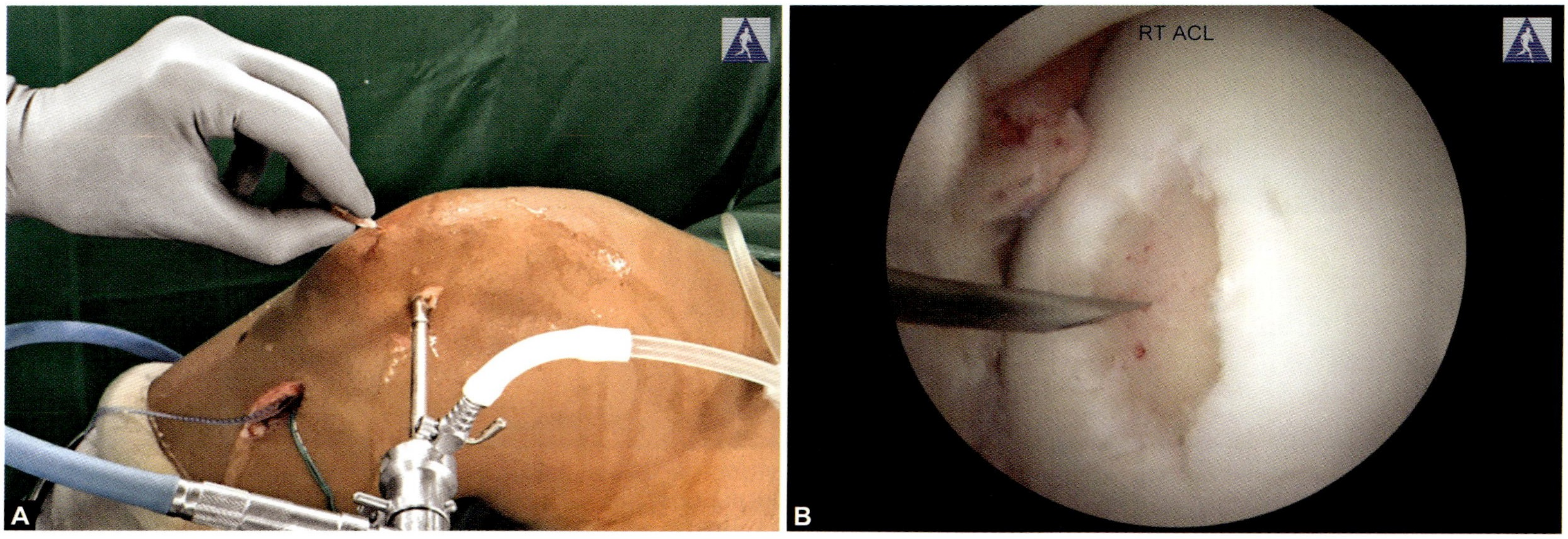

Figs. 14A and B: An International Cartilage Repair Society (ICRS) grade 4 defect is seen arthroscopically on the lateral femoral condyle of the right knee. (A) The arthroscope is inserted from the standard anteromedial portal with the knee in 90° flexion while an 18-gauge needle is inserted from the anterolateral portal pointing toward the defect; and (B) The trajectory of the needle is confirmed to be perpendicular to the bone and decision to proceed with arthroscopic surgery is made.

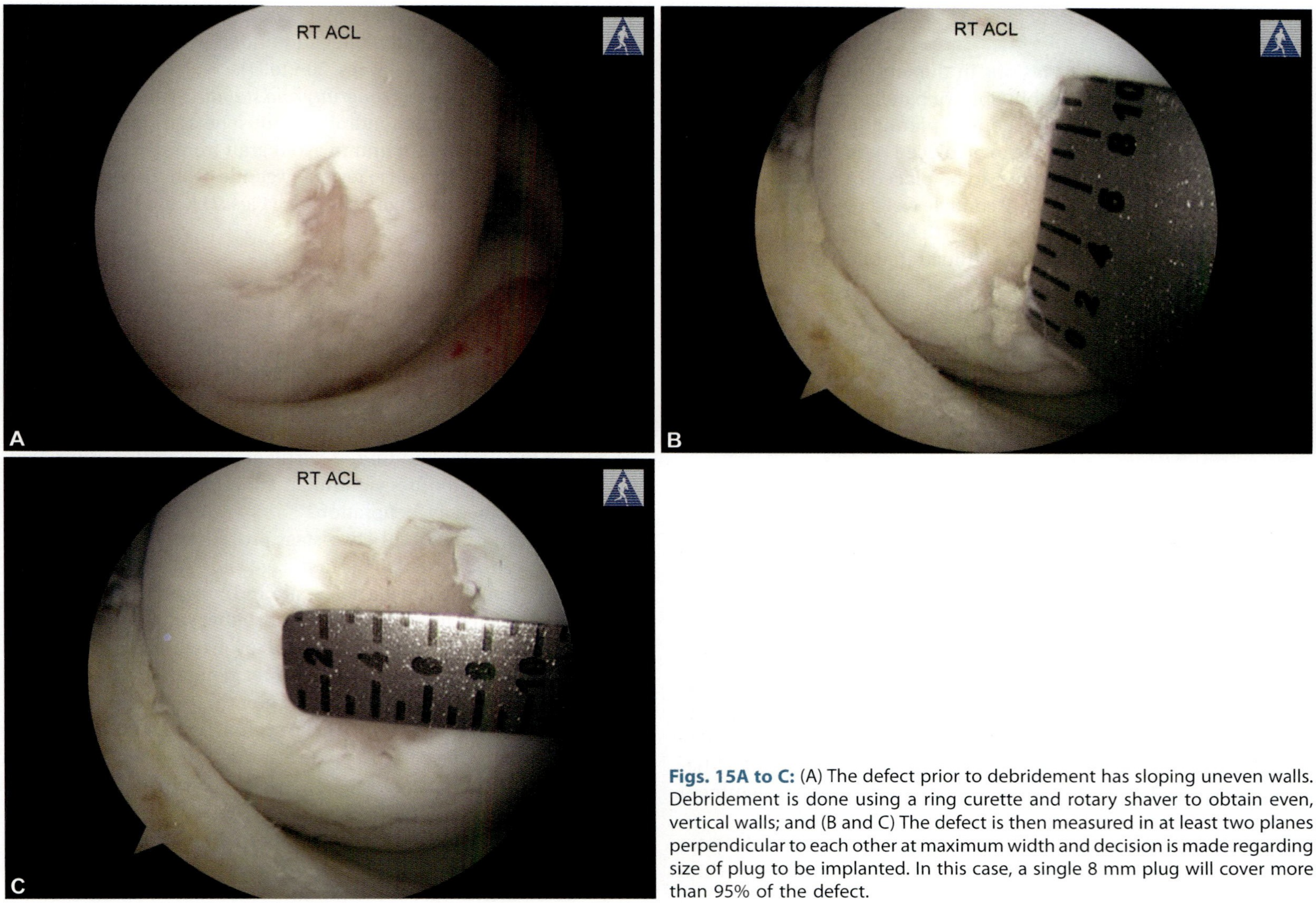

Figs. 15A to C: (A) The defect prior to debridement has sloping uneven walls. Debridement is done using a ring curette and rotary shaver to obtain even, vertical walls; and (B and C) The defect is then measured in at least two planes perpendicular to each other at maximum width and decision is made regarding size of plug to be implanted. In this case, a single 8 mm plug will cover more than 95% of the defect.

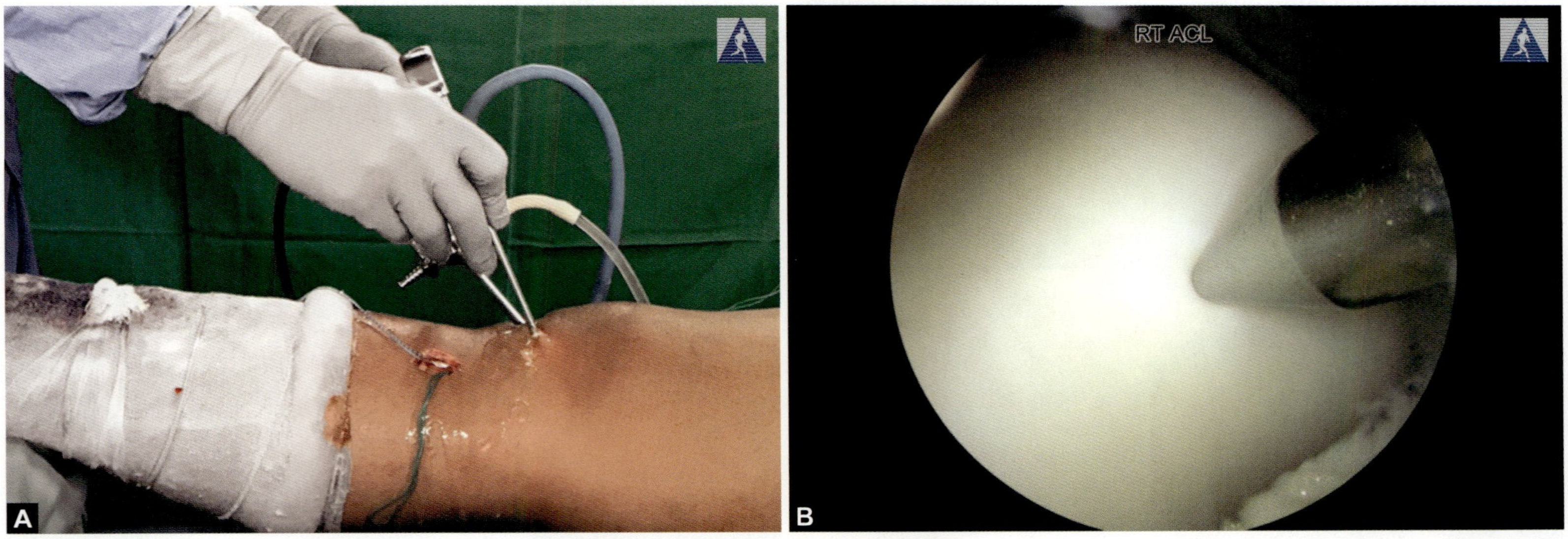

Figs. 16A and B: Graft harvest is planned from medial femoral condyle margin. (A) The knee is brought into full extension and arthroscope is shifted to the anterolateral portal for viewing; and (B) A blunt trocar is inserted up to site of planned donor area to check for perpendicular trajectory. If this is not possible through a standard anteromedial portal, an additional portal must be created to achieve this trajectory.

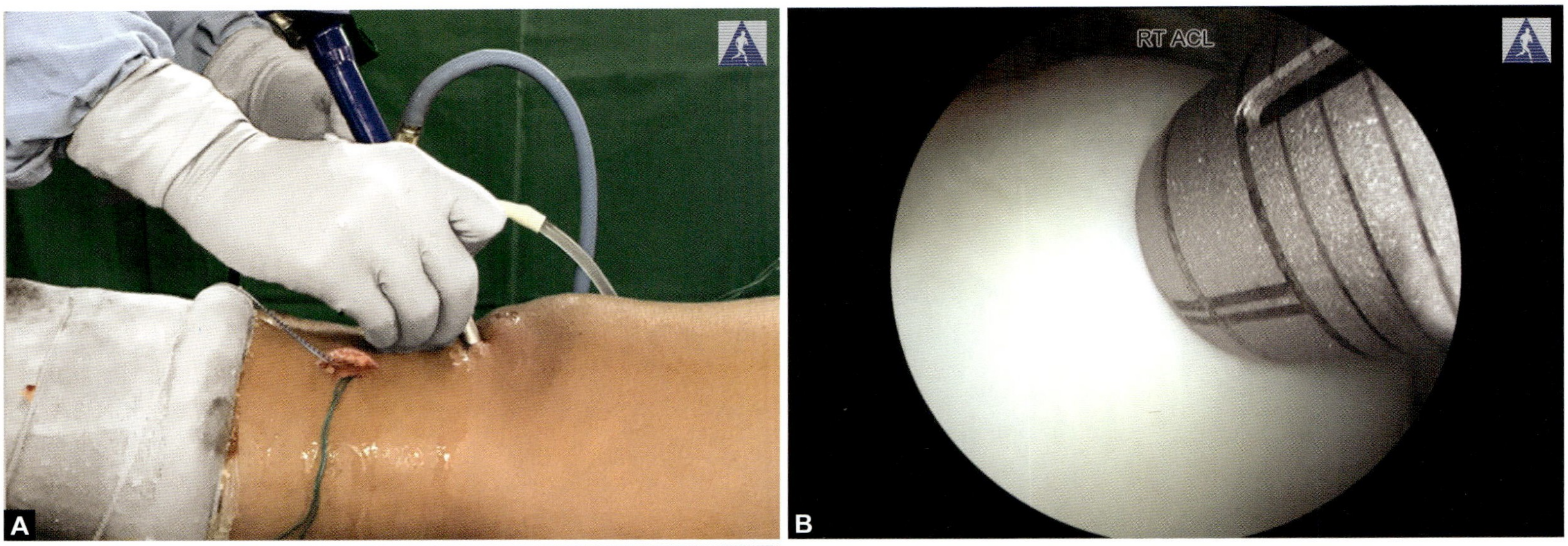

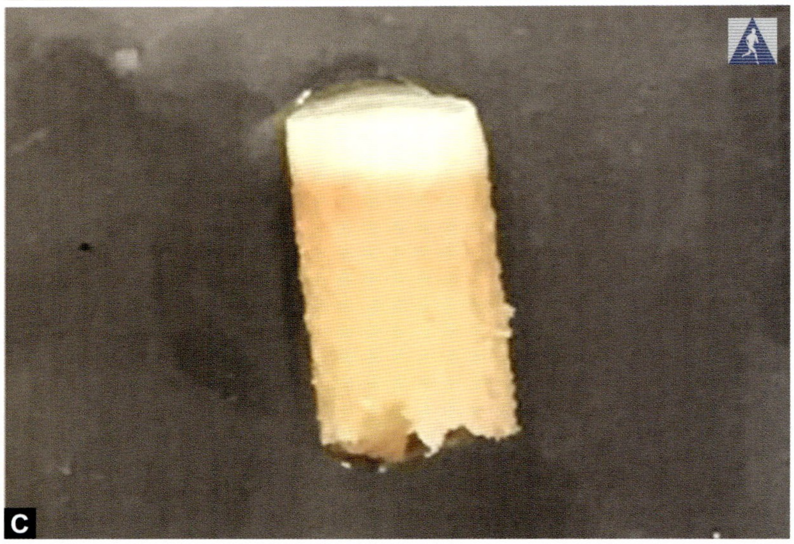

Figs. 17A to C: (A and B) With the knee kept in full extension and viewing from the anterolateral portal, the donor harvest tube of 8 mm is inserted from a separate stab incision and placed at the site as determined. The tube is tapped gently and advanced till about 15–18 mm depth mark under vision. This must be done carefully and a small mallet is used for tapping; and (C) The graft is then delivered out of the donor tube and its length is measured.

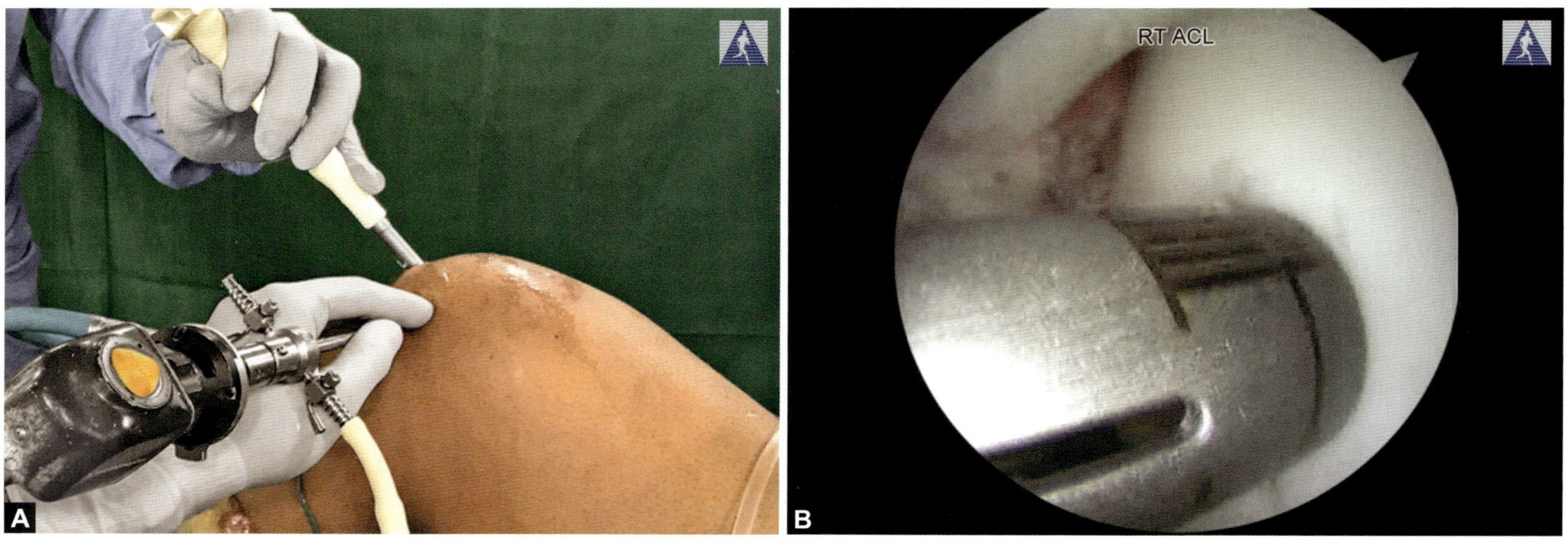

Figs. 18A and B: The arthroscope is shifted to the anteromedial portal for viewing and knee is kept in 90° flexion. (A and B) The recipient tube is placed at the defect and gently tapped in up to the depth required, based on the length of the donor plug, which is 18 mm in this case. Removal of the tube creates an even socket.

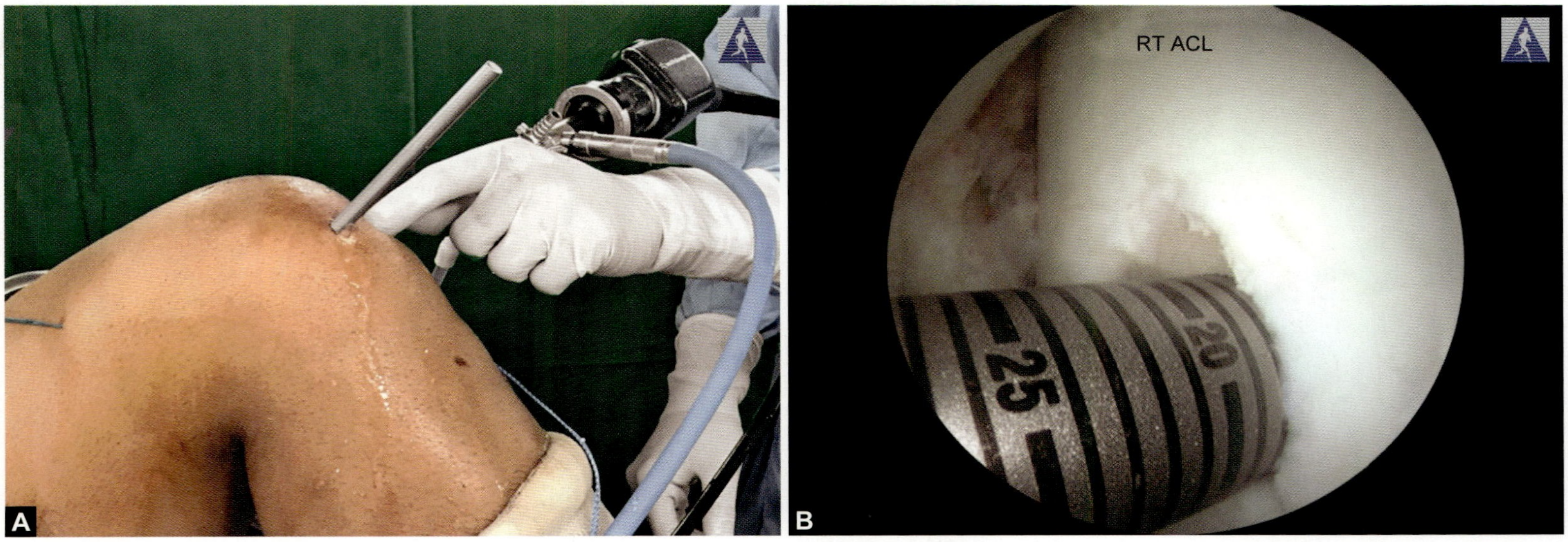

Figs. 19A and B: (A and B) The alignment rod is inserted from the same portal which was used for recipient tube insertion. The direction of socket is seen and depth of the socket read off the markings on the rod.

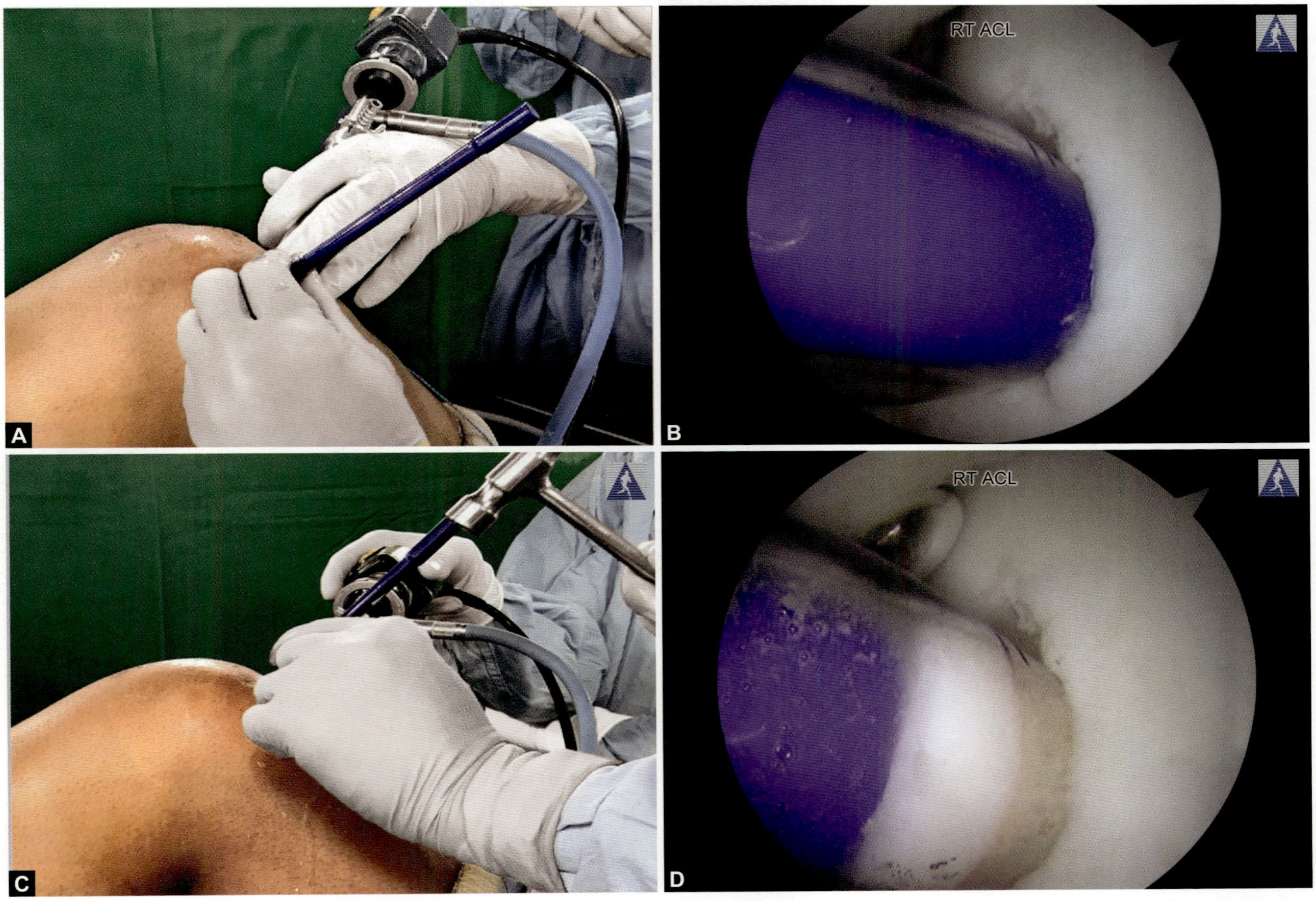

Figs. 20A to D: (A and B) The tamp is inserted into the graft delivery tube and placed at the recipient site through the same portal. The tamp is then withdrawn, saline infusion stopped, and osteochondral plug inserted into the delivery tube; and (C and D) Gentle tapping is done under continuous vision to insert the graft till it completely seated in press fit fashion.

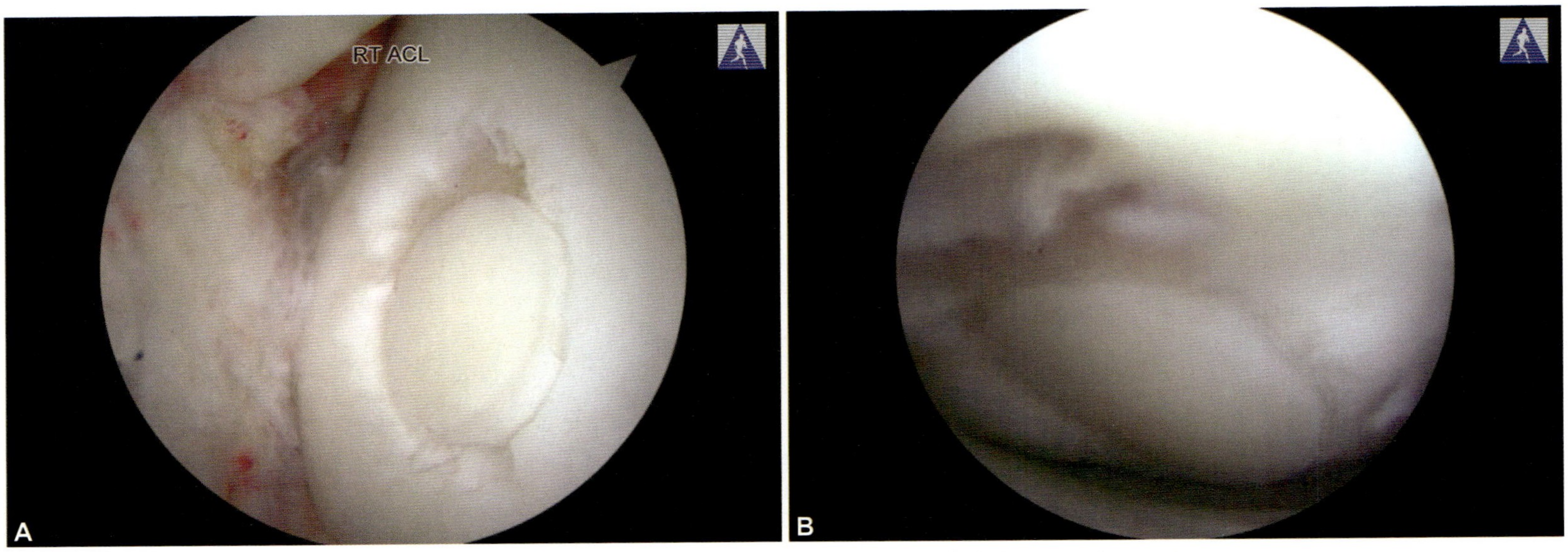

Figs. 21A and B: (A) Final appearance after osteochondral plug insertion; and (B) The knee is taken through a full range of motion to assess stability and congruity.

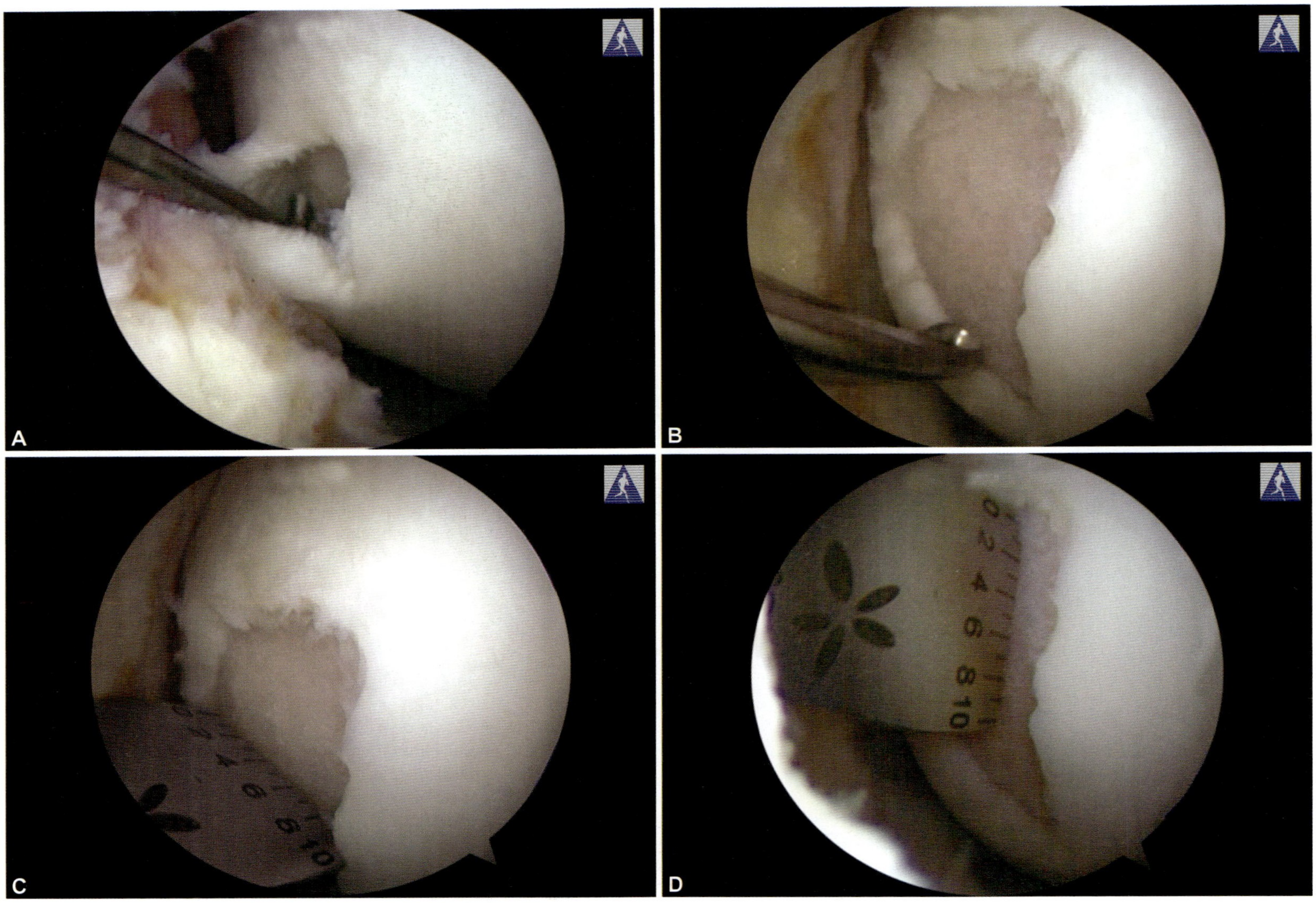

Figs. 22A to D: (A) A chondral flap is detected over the medial femoral condyle on probing; (B to D) Debridement of this lesion is done in the standard fashion as described previously and the defect is sized after final preparation.
Courtesy: Dr Sachin Tapasvi.

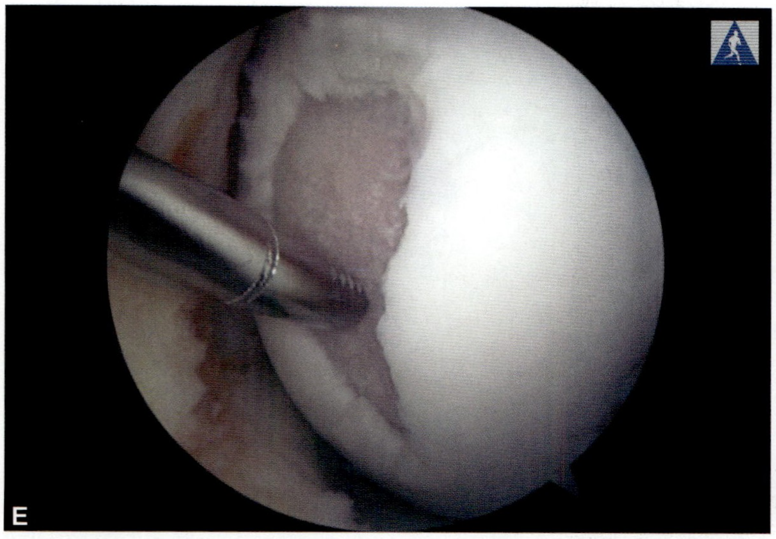

Fig. 22E: Abrasion chondroplasty is performed for the lesion using a rotary shaver to achieve punctate bleeding.
Courtesy: Dr Sachin Tapasvi.

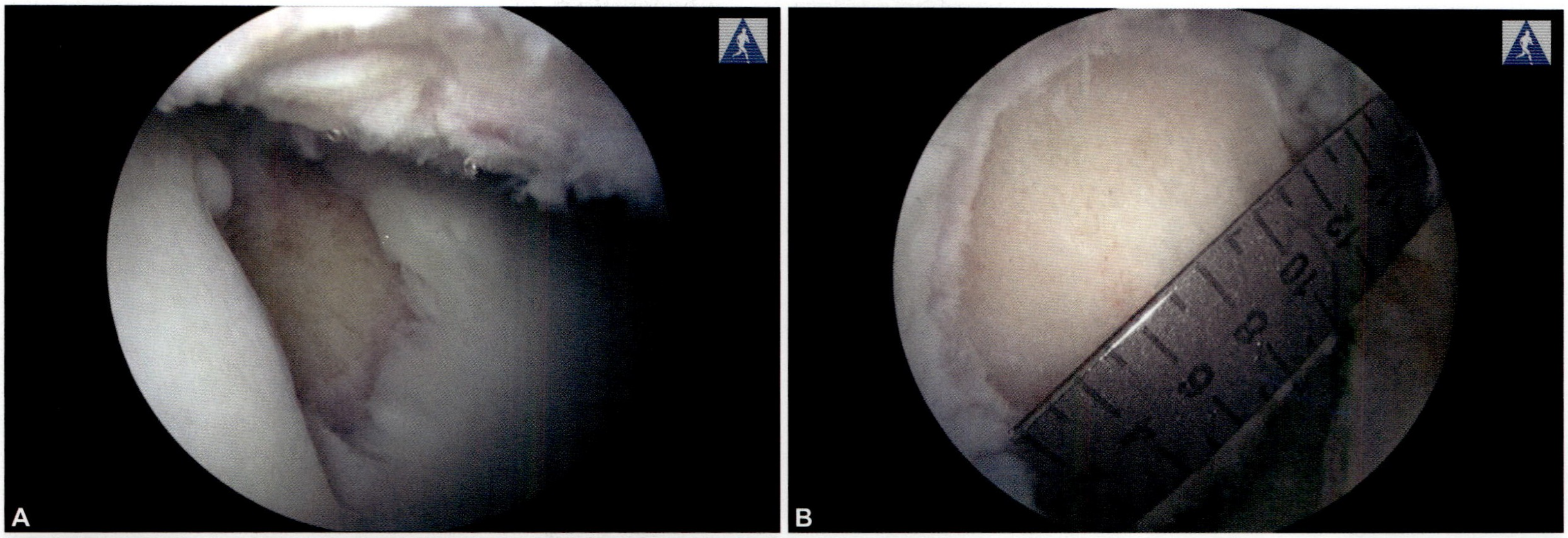

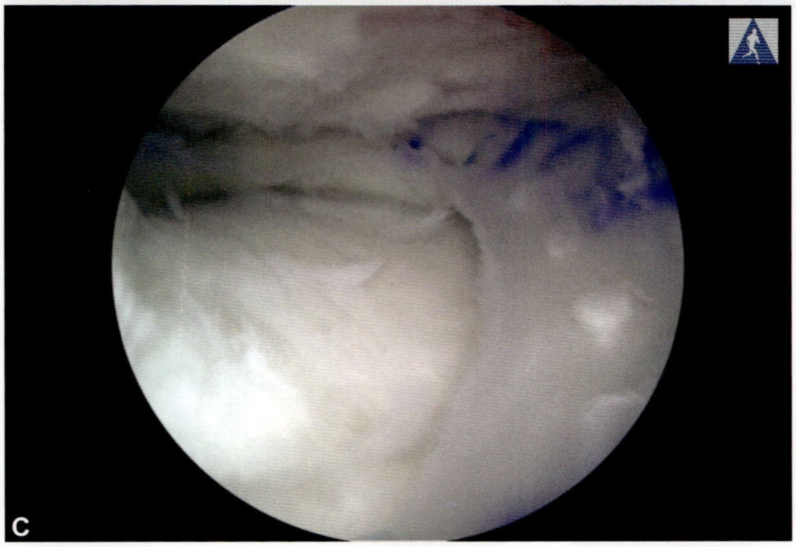

Figs. 23A to C: (A and B) Grade 4 ICRS chondral defects were also present over the trochlea and lateral femoral condyle; and (C) Lateral meniscus allograft transplantation was performed at this stage. The ACL and PCL were confirmed to be stable. (ACL: anterior cruciate ligament; ICRS: International Cartilage Repair Society; PCL: posterior cruciate ligament)
Courtesy: Dr Sachin Tapasvi.

stages and an illustrative example is provided. This patient had large chondral defects over both the femoral condyles and trochlea. These were detected when an arthroscopy was performed for lateral meniscus allograft transplantation as he had undergone a subtotal lateral meniscectomy about 1 year prior. Considering the presence of large multifocal defects, decision was taken to perform ACI for this patient. His alignment and stability were acceptable (Figs. 22 and 23).

Stage 1 Surgery

- *Step 1—Cartilage biopsy*: Cartilage is harvested for culture and cell expansion from a nonweight-bearing area. Either strips of cartilage or osteochondral bone plugs can be harvested from the edge of lateral or medial femoral condyle, superior to sulcus terminalis or adjacent to the notch. About 200–300 mg of cartilage is needed to grow adequate chondrocytes. The harvested cartilage is transported to the laboratory in appropriate medium like Dulbecco's Modified Eagle Medium (DMEM) (Figs. 24A to E).
- *Step 2—Cell culture and expansion in the laboratory*: The cartilage sample is processed in the laboratory as per proprietary technology under strict aseptic precautions. The cartilage is digested and chondrocytes grown till at least 48 million viable cells are produced. These cells are supplied in four vials with each 0.4 mL vial containing 12 million cells (cellular density of 3×10^7 cells/cc). For gel-based ACI, 3–4 million cells/cm^2 of defect are required. It takes about 4–6 weeks for this process to be completed.

Stage 2 Surgery

- *Step 3—Exposure and preparation of the defect*: The second stage is performed as open surgery. A mini-arthrotomy—medial or lateral parapatellar is necessary for adequate exposure and Hoffa's fad is excised to improve visualization. The edges of the defect(s) are freshened and any fibrous tissue removed from the floor with a curette. Drill holes are created with a 1.8 mm drill bit up to 5 mm depth and about 5–7 mm apart from each other. If tourniquet was used till now, this is deflated and hemostasis is achieved. Ooze from the drill holes is stopped by applying firm pressure or using epinephrine-soaked gauze (Fig. 25).
- *Step 4—Implantation of cultured chondrocytes*: The cultured cells are supplied in vials with 1.2×10^7 cells/vial. The final preparation is done after the lesion is ready for implantation. This requires a specially designed delivery system with two 1 mL syringes and a Y-shaped mixing adaptor. One syringe is filled with 1 mL fibrinogen and the second syringe is filled with 0.9 mL of cell suspension

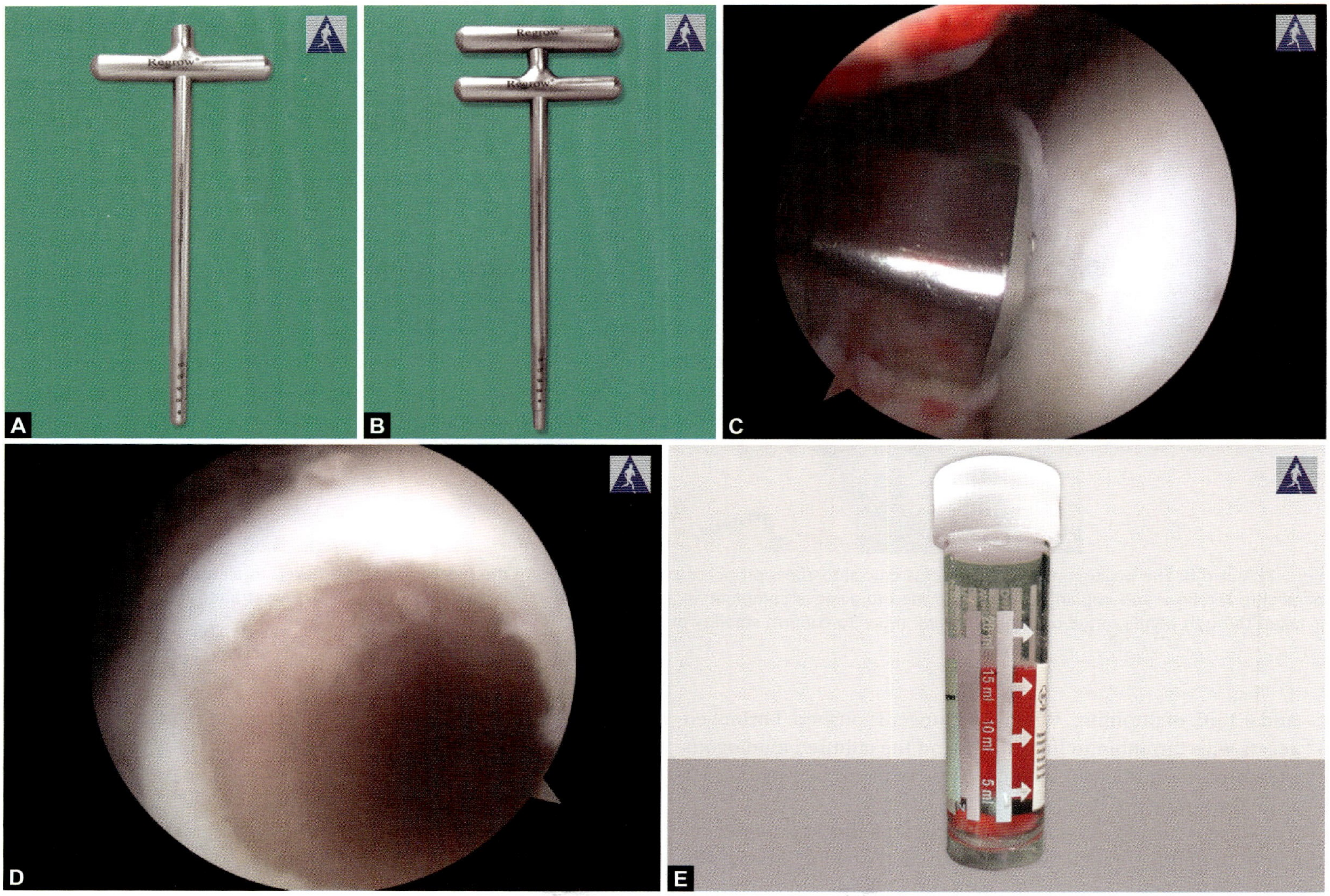

Figs. 24A to E: (A and B) Cartilage harvest for culture can be performed using specially designed instrument, which allows harvesting of a 7-mm osteochondral plug. This consists of a hollow outer tube and an inner obturator; (C) The harvest is performed arthroscopically from the superomedial margin of the medial femoral condyle or superolateral margin of the lateral femoral condyle in the non-articular areas. The donor tube is inserted from the anteromedial portal and viewing from the anterolateral portal with the knee in full extension is done; (D) A socket-like defect is left after the harvest; and (E) The harvested plug is placed in a vial containing the transport medium.
Courtesy: Dr Sachin Tapasvi (Figs. C and D).

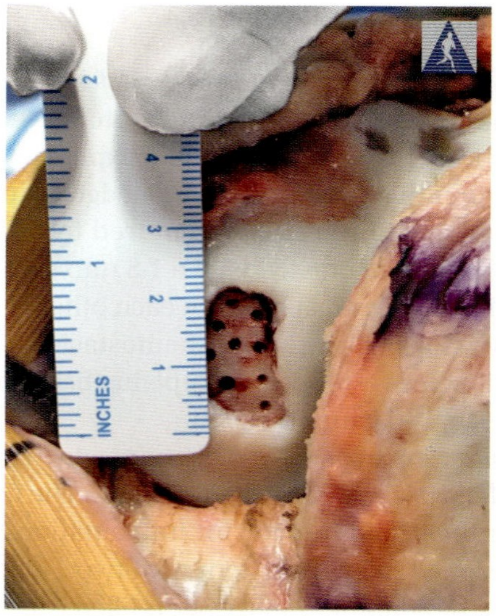

Fig. 25: The defect over medial femoral condyle is prepared by freshening the edges and floor. 1.8 mm drill holes and made about 5–7 mm apart and lesion is sized again. The tourniquet is deflated and hemostasis is achieved prior to implantation.

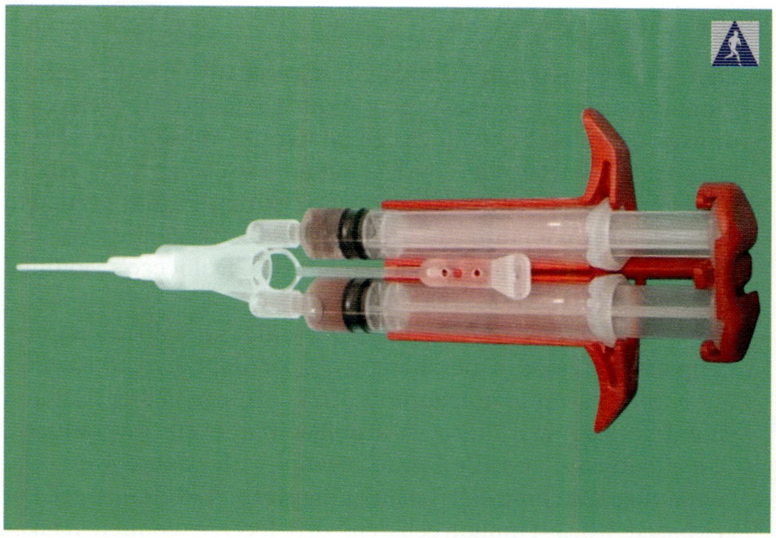

Fig. 26: The delivery devices used for gel-based autologous chondrocyte implantation (ACI) are two 1 mL syringes and a Y-shaped mixing adaptor.

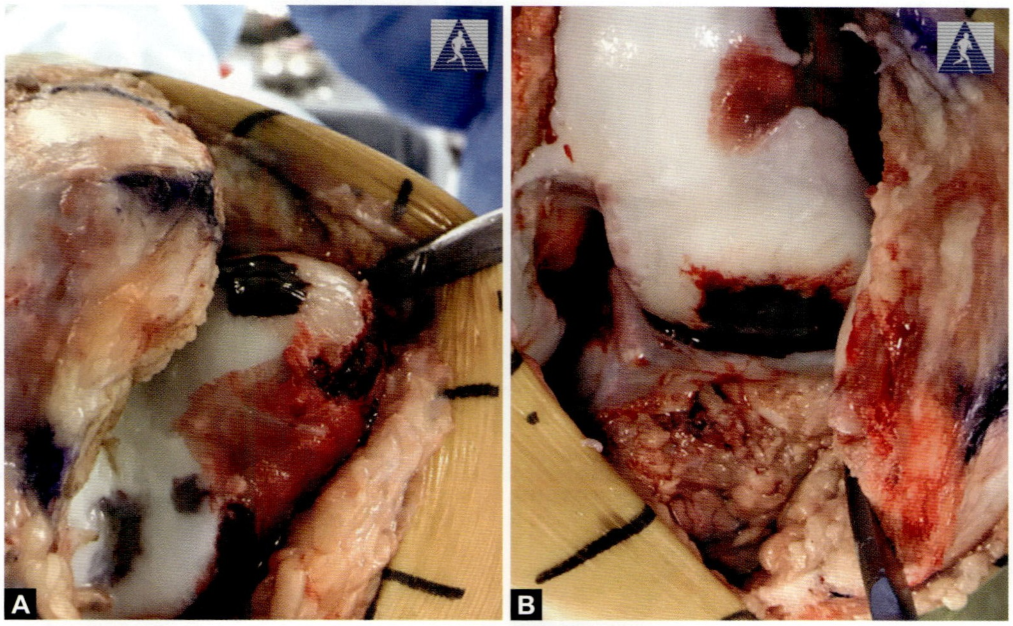

Figs. 27A and B: The positioning of the defect is crucial to allow proper implantation. (A) Here the hip and knee are flexed to almost 90° to get the defect parallel to the floor and implantation is performed to achieve complete fill and adequate contour; and (B) Once the gel is set after about 7 minutes, knee is taken through gentle range of motion several times to confirm stability of the implant.

and 0.1 mL of thrombin. When the plunger is pushed, fibrinogen reacts with thrombin to form fibrin and the cultured autologous chondrocytes and fibrin are mixed and released in a ratio of 1:1 from the nozzle tip (Fig. 26).

The knee is positioned is such a way that the defect is parallel to the floor to eliminate the effect of gravity and flowing away of the suspension while it is setting to a gel form. Adequate retraction to expose the defect is crucial. The plunger of the delivery device is pushed gently so that the suspension is released slowly into the defect and spreads over. Adequate suspension is release to completely cover the defect and achieve a proper contour. The fibrin glue sets in about 7 minutes and has self-adhesive properties. Once the implant in dry and stuck, the knee is taken through range of motion several times to confirm its stability. Wound closure is then done in the standard fashion (Figs. 27A and B).

CONCLUSION

Cartilage lesions may present as isolated pathology or in association with other ligament or meniscal issues. They can be managed successfully by any strategy employing regeneration (marrow stimulation techniques), restoration (osteochondral transfer), or replacement (chondrocyte implantation) of cartilage tissue. Each technique has its advantages and pitfalls but when applied prudently in the presence of suitable indication, they are known to give good results. Cartilage surgery is challenging and strict adherence to surgical principles is imperative for successful outcome.

SUGGESTED READING

1. Bert JM. Abandoning microfracture of the knee: Has the time come? Arthroscopy. 2015;31(3):501-5.
2. Choi NY, Kim BW, Yeo WJ, et al. Gel-type autologous chondrocyte (Chondron) implantation for treatment of articular cartilage defects of the knee. BMC Musculoskelet Disord. 2010;11(1):103.
3. Dewan AK, Gibson MA, Elisseeff JH, et al. Evolution of autologous chondrocyte repair and comparison to other cartilage repair techniques. BioMed Res Int. 2014;2014:1-11.
4. Insall J. Current Concepts Review: patellar pain. J Bone Joint Surg Am. 1982;64(1):147-52.
5. Kosy JD, Schranz PJ, Toms AD, et al. The use of radiofrequency energy for arthroscopic chondroplasty in the knee. Arthroscopy. 2011;27(5): 695-703.
6. Lotto ML, Wright EJ, Appleby D, et al. Ex vivo comparison of mechanical versus thermal chondroplasty: assessment of tissue effect at the surgical endpoint. Arthroscopy. 2008;24(4):410-5.
7. Noyes FR, Bassett RW, Grood ES, et al. Arthroscopy in acute traumatic hemarthrosis of the knee. Incidence of anterior cruciate tears and other injuries. J Bone Joint Surg Am. 1980;62(5):687-95.
8. Outerbridge RE. The etiology of chondromalacia patellae. J Bone Joint Surg Br. 1961;43-B:752-7.
9. Pridie KH. A method of resurfacing osteoarthritic knee joints. J Bone Joint Surg Br. 1959;41(3):618-9.
10. Steadman JR, Rodkey WG, Singleton SB, et al. Microfracture technique for full-thickness chondral defects: Technique and clinical results. Oper Tech Orthop. 1997;7(4):300-4.

CHAPTER 16

Surgery for Medial Knee Instability: Repair to Reconstruction

Sachin Ramchandra Tapasvi, Anshu Shekhar, Shantanu Sudhakar Patil

INTRODUCTION

The medial side of the knee is the most commonly injured site which can result from either contact or noncontact trauma. This region consists of ligaments, tendons, and fascial structures which provide stability to the knee joint. The most important ligamentous structures are:

- Superficial medial collateral ligament (sMCL)
- Medial patellofemoral ligament (MPFL)
- Deep medial collateral ligament (dMCL)
- Posterior oblique ligament (POL).

The anatomy of the medial side and presence of these structures in a layered arrangement were described by Warren and Marshall. They described three layers with layer I comprising of the crural or sartorius fascia, layer II consisting of the sMCL, MPFL, and ligaments in the posteromedial corner, and layer III consisting of the capsule and dMCL with its meniscofemoral and meniscotibial components. The tendons of sartorius, gracilis (GR), and semitendinosus (ST) are present between layers II and III. These layers are best appreciated in the middle third, with layer I fusing with layer II in anterior third and layer III fusing with layer II in the posterior third to form a composite structure along with the tendon sheath of semimembranosus. The posterior oblique ligament is another important constituent of the "posteromedial corner" and consists of three parts: (1) a superior or capsular arm, (2) the largest central or tibial arm, and (3) a superficial arm. LaPrade et al. published their seminal work quantifying the anatomy of the medial side of the knee which has revolutionized surgical management of this injury. They described the attachments of the sMCL, POL, and dMCL with respect to three osseous landmarks—(1) medial epicondyle, (2) adductor tubercle, and (3) gastrocnemius tubercle on the femur and on the tibia (Fig. 1).

Biomechanically, the medial structures provide stability to the knee in the coronal and axial planes. The sMCL is the primary restrain against valgus forces at all higher flexion angles, while the POL and posteromedial capsule performs this function at or near full extension. The sMCL is also a stabilizer of both internal and external rotation at all flexion angles whereas the POL is an important stabilizer against internal rotation and posterior drawer in extension. The dMCL is an important restrain to external rotation but not so much to valgus stability.

A number of clinical and MRI-based classification systems have been devised to classify medial instability but the Fetto and Marshall classification system is the one which provides some rationale for treatment (Table 1).

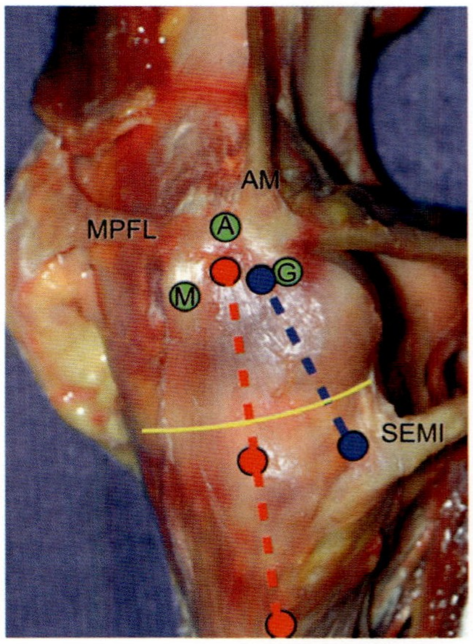

Fig. 1: The anatomy of medial side of knee based on descriptions by LaPrade. The three important bony landmarks are: (1) the medial epicondyle (M), (2) adductor tubercle (A), and (3) gastrocnemius tubercle (G) and easily recognizable. No ligament or tendon attaches to any of these points. The sMCL (red dash) attaches on the femur at a point about 3.2 mm proximal and 4.8 mm posterior to the medial epicondyle. It has two tibial attachments—(1) the major distal insertion is about 6.1 cm distal to the joint line (yellow line), posterior to the hamstring tendons insertion and (2) a proximal insertion about 1.2 cm distal to the joint line. The total length of the sMCL is, thus, about 94.8 mm. The POL (blue dash) inserts on the femur at a point which is about 1.4 mm distal and 2.9 mm anterior to the gastrocnemius tubercle. The tibial attachment is just anterior to the insertion of the direct head of semimembranosus (SEMI) at posteromedial tibia. (AM: adductor magnus tendon, MPFL: medial patellofemoral ligament; POL: posterior oblique ligament; sMCL: superficial medial collateral ligament)

TABLE 1: Fetto and Marshall classification.

Grades	*Feature*	*Interpretation*
I	No valgus laxity	Full anatomic integrity
II	Valgus laxity at 30° flexion only, hard endpoint	Partial disruption of sMCL only
III	Valgus laxity at 0° and 30° flexion, no endpoint	Complete anatomic disruption of sMCL, POL, and posteromedial capsule

(POL: posterior oblique ligament; sMCL: superficial medial collateral ligament)

TABLE 2: Fanelli and Harris classification.

Grades	*Feature*	*Interpretation*
A	Axial plane rotational instability	Posteromedial capsular laxity
B	Combined axial rotational and valgus laxity with firm endpoint	Posteromedial capsular + superficial medial collateral ligament (sMCL) laxity
C	Combined axial rotational and valgus laxity with no endpoint	Disruption or avulsion of posteromedial capsule + sMCL

Another classification described by Fanelli and Harris also takes into account the importance of assessing rotational or axial stability as the medial structures control this movement as well (Table 2). This is, however, applicable in case of chronic medial instability.

SURGICAL OPTIONS: REPAIR AND RECONSTRUCTION

There is no consensus on the management of medial knee injuries but the vast majority of these can be managed nonsurgically with good outcomes. There, however, are situations which necessitate surgical management in both acute and chronic settings. The chronicity of the injury, limb alignment, presence of bony avulsions, and associated ligament injuries were considered in an algorithm provided by Bonasia et al. Grade 3 tears are more complicated often coexist with other ligament(s) and meniscal tears making surgical management a preferred approach. The literature comparing contemporary repair and reconstruction is sparse but there is some evidence that even a nonanatomic reconstruction provides better rotational stability than repair for acute grade 3 tears. A thorough understanding of the anatomy of medial structures is absolutely essential whether one performs a repair or reconstruction.

Repair

A repair of the medial and posteromedial structures is done by open surgery in the acute setting. This can be done for femoral or tibial-sided avulsions or midsubstance tears. The principles of performing the repair are as follows:

- Arthroscopy may be performed with gravity-assisted infusion only, prior to the open surgery to check the status of intra-articular structures.
- A tourniquet aids in better identification of anatomy but this must be deflated and hemostasis achieved prior to closure to avoid hematoma formation.
- The skin incision extends from 2 cm proximal to medial epicondyle up to 6 cm distal to the joint line on the tibia. The straight incision is taken with the knee in extension and flexion causes the incision to appear like a J.
- A limited fasciocutaneous flap is raised, avoiding any dissection in the subcutaneous tissue to preserve the vascularity. Superficial structures like the infrapatellar branch of saphenous nerve and vein must be preserved.
- The sartorius fascia (layer I) is incised in line with the skin incision and the pes tendons, sMCL, and MPFL are identified and their integrity assessed. The torn sMCL can then be retracted to assess the status of the dMCL, its meniscal attachments, POL, and posteromedial capsule (layer III) (Figs. 2A and B).
- Repair is performed in a layered fashion, proceeding from deep to superficial (Layer III–I). Nonabsorbable or absorbable sutures can be used for end-to-end or end-to-side repairs. Where tissue is deficient, suture anchors provide a better repair platform.
- Layer III is repaired first. The meniscofemoral and/or meniscotibial components of the dMCL are best repaired using single-loaded suture anchors. The POL and posteromedial capsule can be sutured end-to-end or to the semimembranosus tendon or fixed with 2.8-mm suture anchors directly keeping the knee in full extension (Figs. 3A and B). It must be possible to bring the knee to full extension after POL repair and prevent overconstraint.
- Layer II is repaired next. Bony avulsions of the sMCL from the femur or tibia can be fixed using partially threaded cannulated cancellous screws with washer (4.5 mm or 6.5 mm depending on size of the bony fragment). Midsubstance tears can be repaired end-to-end with nonabsorbable sutures like No. 2 FiberWire® (Arthrex) or No. 2 Ultrabraid® (Smith and Nephew) using a Bunnell type suture configuration. Soft tissue peels offs from the femur or tibia are more commonly seen and are best repaired using 5.0-mm suture anchors placed at its anatomic attachment sites as described earlier. The knee is kept in 30° flexion, neutral rotation, and varus reduction when the sutures are being tightened (Figs. 4A and B).
- Augmentation of repair can be performed when the tissue is of poor quality or in case of midsubstance sMCL tear. This is discussed in greater detail below.
- The MPFL and medial retinaculum must be sutured if torn, keeping the knee in 20° flexion and avoiding medial constraint of patellar glide.
- Layer I or sartorius fascia is then identified and sutured using continuous or intermittent sutures in its entirety (Figs. 5A to C).
- The tourniquet is now deflated and hemostasis is achieved. A closed suction drain may be kept but is not always necessary. The fat, subcutaneous tissue and skin are sutured and a Jones compression dressing is applied.

Augmentation of Repairs

There exists the concern that the repaired tissue will fail or stretch out over a period of time, especially in the presence of midsubstance tear repairs. This also causes the surgeon to go slow with rehabilitation and range of motion initiation which in turn risks stiffness and

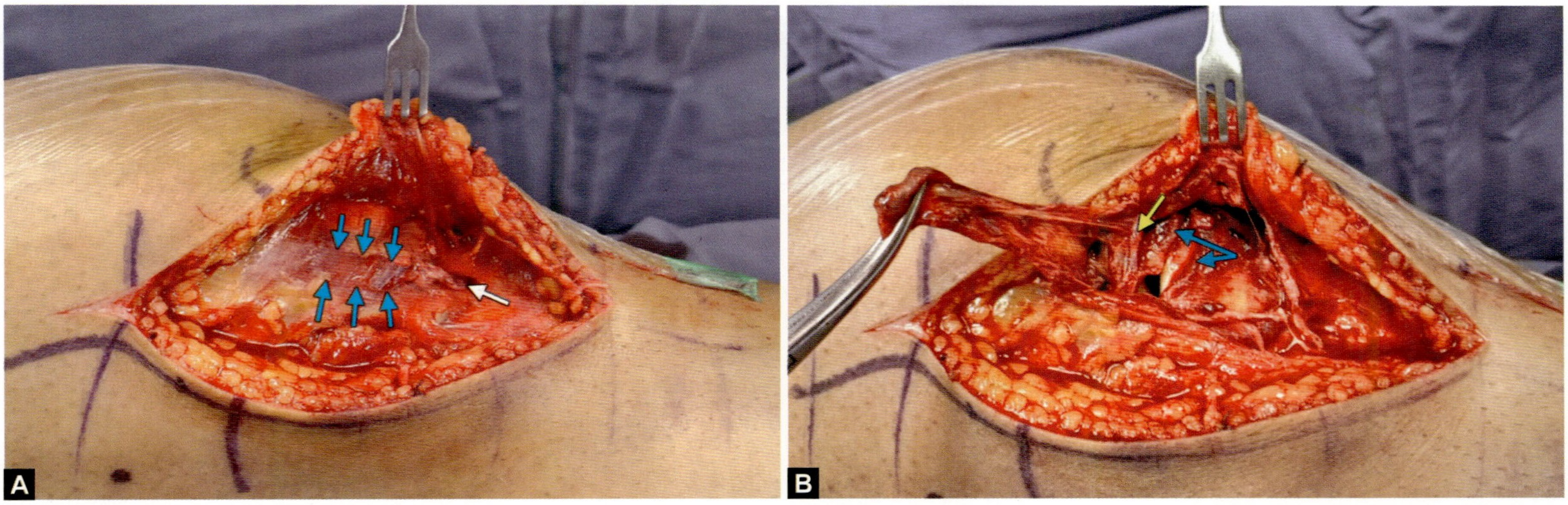

Figs. 2A and B: Medial dissection of the left knee with full-thickness fasciocutaneous flaps raised. (A) The sartorius fascia (layer I) has been incised along the skin incision (blue arrows) and the torn end of sMCL on the tibial side is seen (white arrow); and (B) Proximal retraction of the torn sMCL reveals disruption of layer III in the meniscotibial fibers of dMCL (blue arrows) and extending to the posteromedial capsule. (dMCL: deep medial collateral ligament; sMCL: superficial medial collateral ligament)

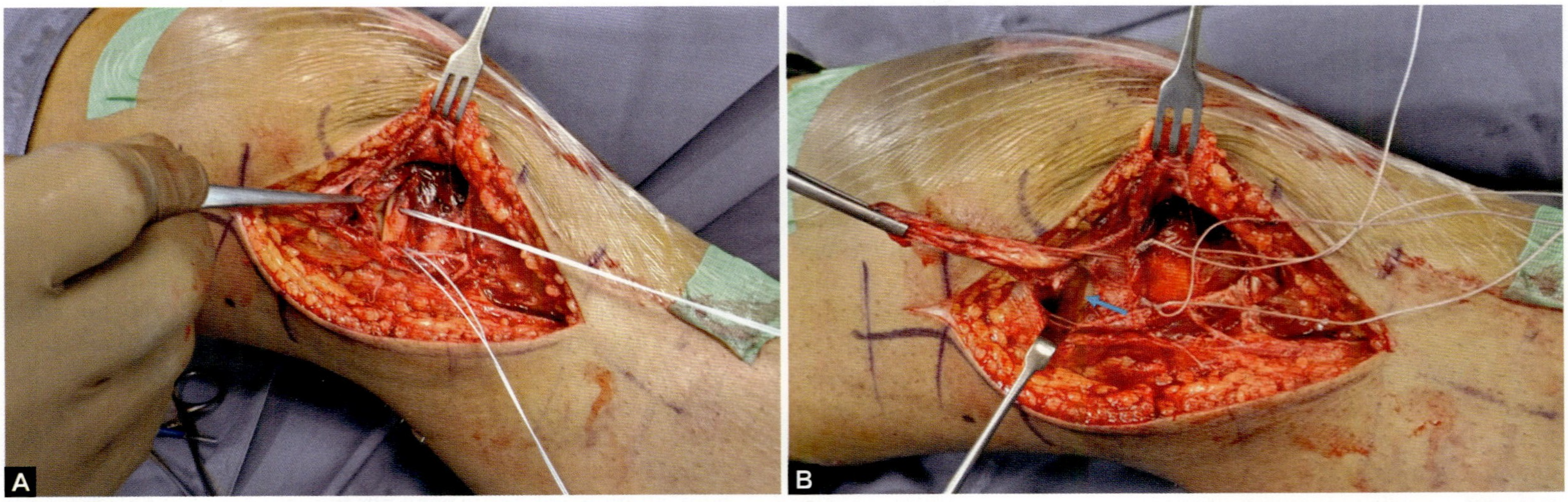

Figs. 3A and B: Two single-loaded 2.8 mm titanium suture anchors have been inserted in the tibia. (A) The anterior anchor will be used for repair of the meniscotibial fibers of the dMCL while the posteriorly placed anchor will be used to repair the POL and posteromedial capsule back to its tibial insertion; and (B) Repair of the dMCL and posteromedial capsule reveals a tear in the meniscofemoral portion of the dMCL as well (blue arrow). This can be repaired using another single-loaded 2.8 mm titanium suture anchor. (dMCL: deep medial collateral ligament; POL: posterior oblique ligament)

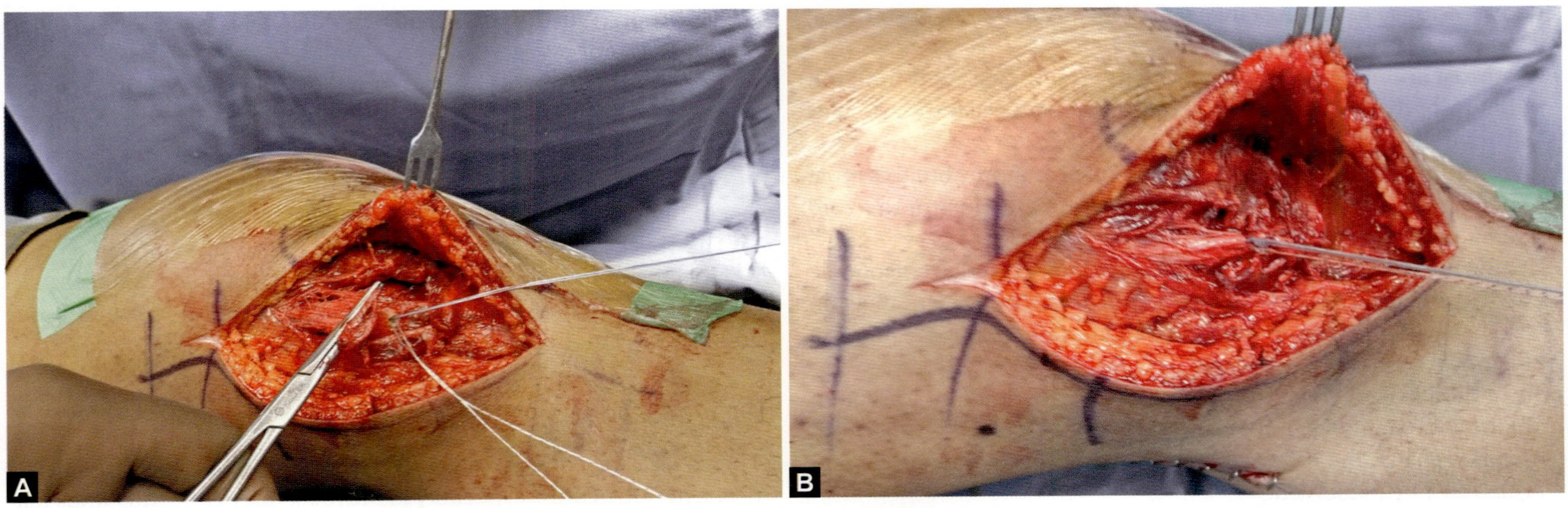

Figs. 4A and B: (A) The tibial avulsion of superficial medial collateral ligament (sMCL) is held and reduced to its attachment site about 6 cm distal to the joint line of the tibia; and (B) A 5.0-mm double-loaded suture anchor is inserted at this point and the sMCL is sutured back.

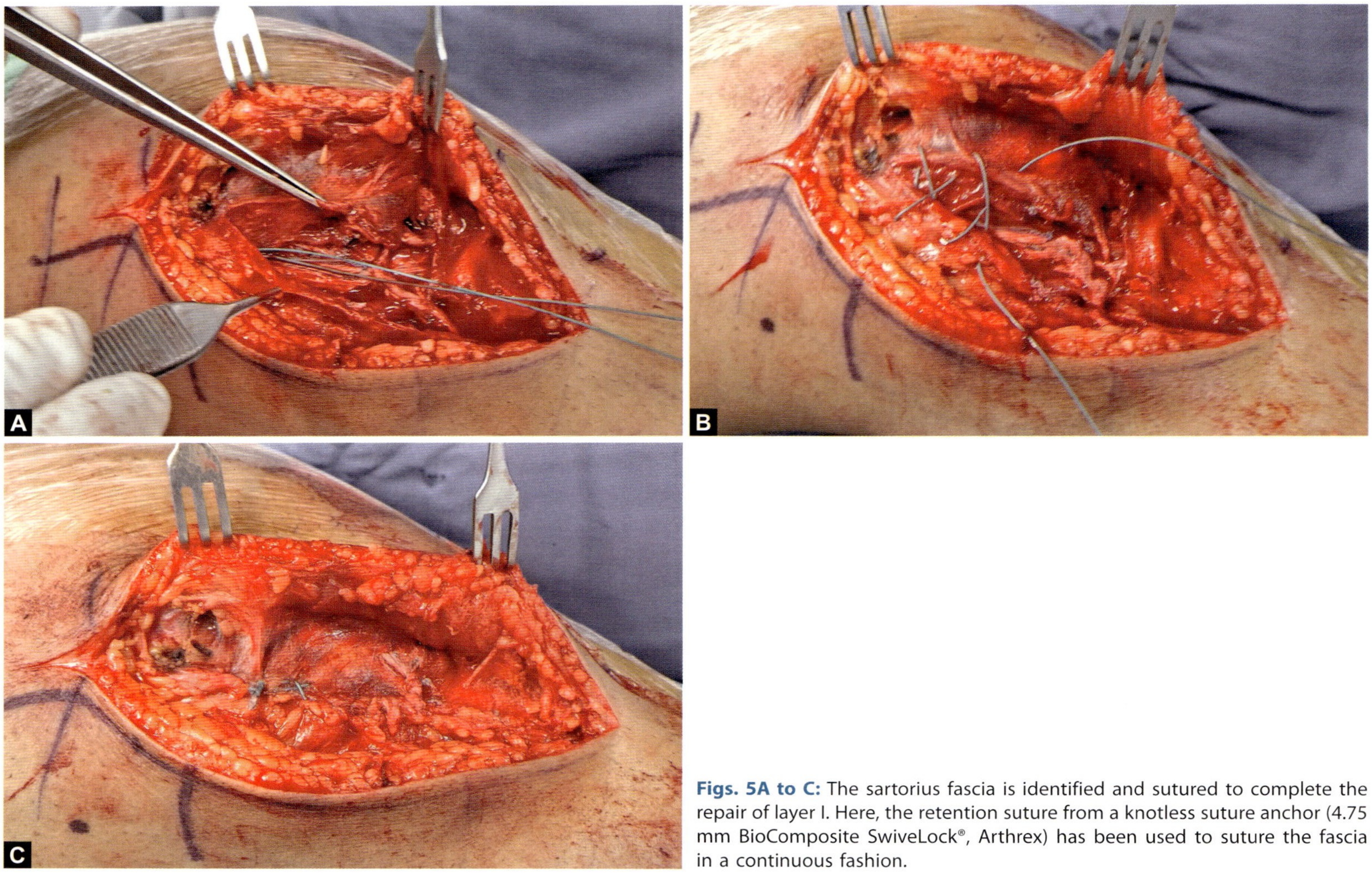

Figs. 5A to C: The sartorius fascia is identified and sutured to complete the repair of layer I. Here, the retention suture from a knotless suture anchor (4.75 mm BioComposite SwiveLock®, Arthrex) has been used to suture the fascia in a continuous fashion.

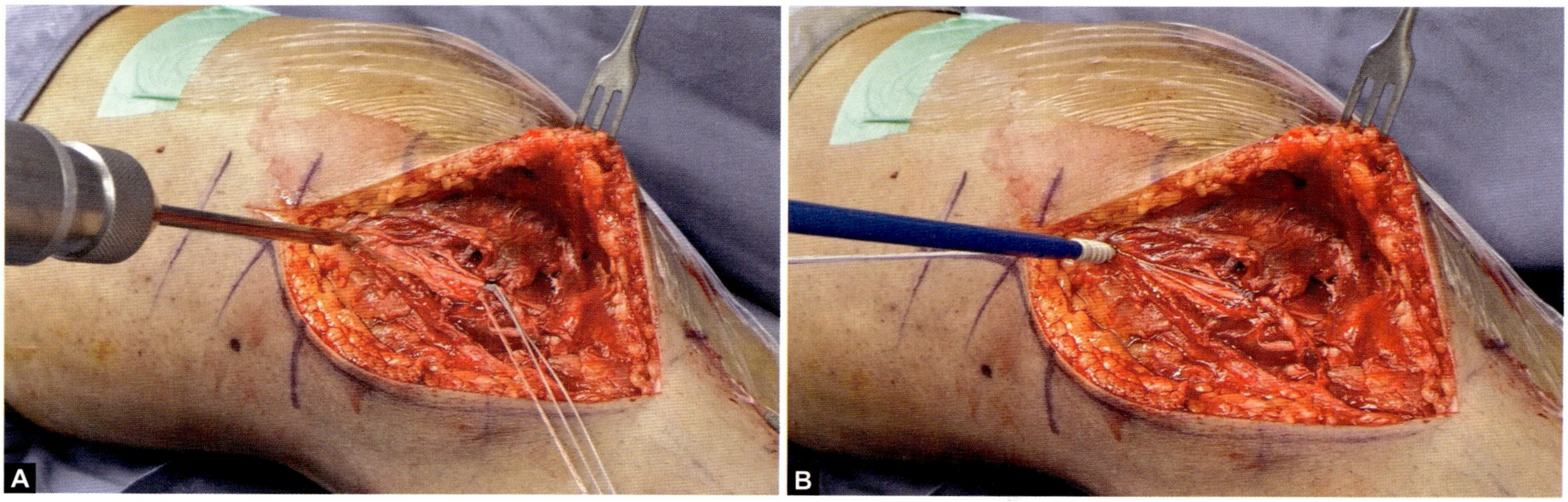

Figs. 6A and B: A method of augmenting the superficial medial collateral ligament (sMCL) repair in the illustrative case as earlier. (A) The high strength sutures from the double-loaded anchor used for sMCL tibial repair are loaded onto a 4.75 mm PEEK SwiveLock® (Arthrex) anchor. The anatomic insertion site on the femur is located and a drill hole made using a 4.5-mm drill bit; and (B) The anchor is then inserted at this point. The sutures, thus, bridge the repair and acts like a synthetic augment.

arthrofibrosis. The concept of augmentation of the repairs has, thus, recently gained traction with the purported advantages of protecting the repair and allowing early range of motion and weight bearing (Figs. 6A and B). Lubowitz et al. first described augmentation of the repair with ultrahigh molecular-weight polyethylene/polyester suture tape (FiberTape®, Arthrex) and knotless bone anchors (4.75 mm PEEK SwiveLock®, Arthrex) in what was called as "internal bracing" (Figs. 7A to D). A minimally invasive augmentation technique has also been described by van der List and DeFelice using the same material. Gilmer et al. have shown in cadaveric specimens that this type of "internal brace" is biomechanically superior to repair alone and equivalent to allograft reconstruction.

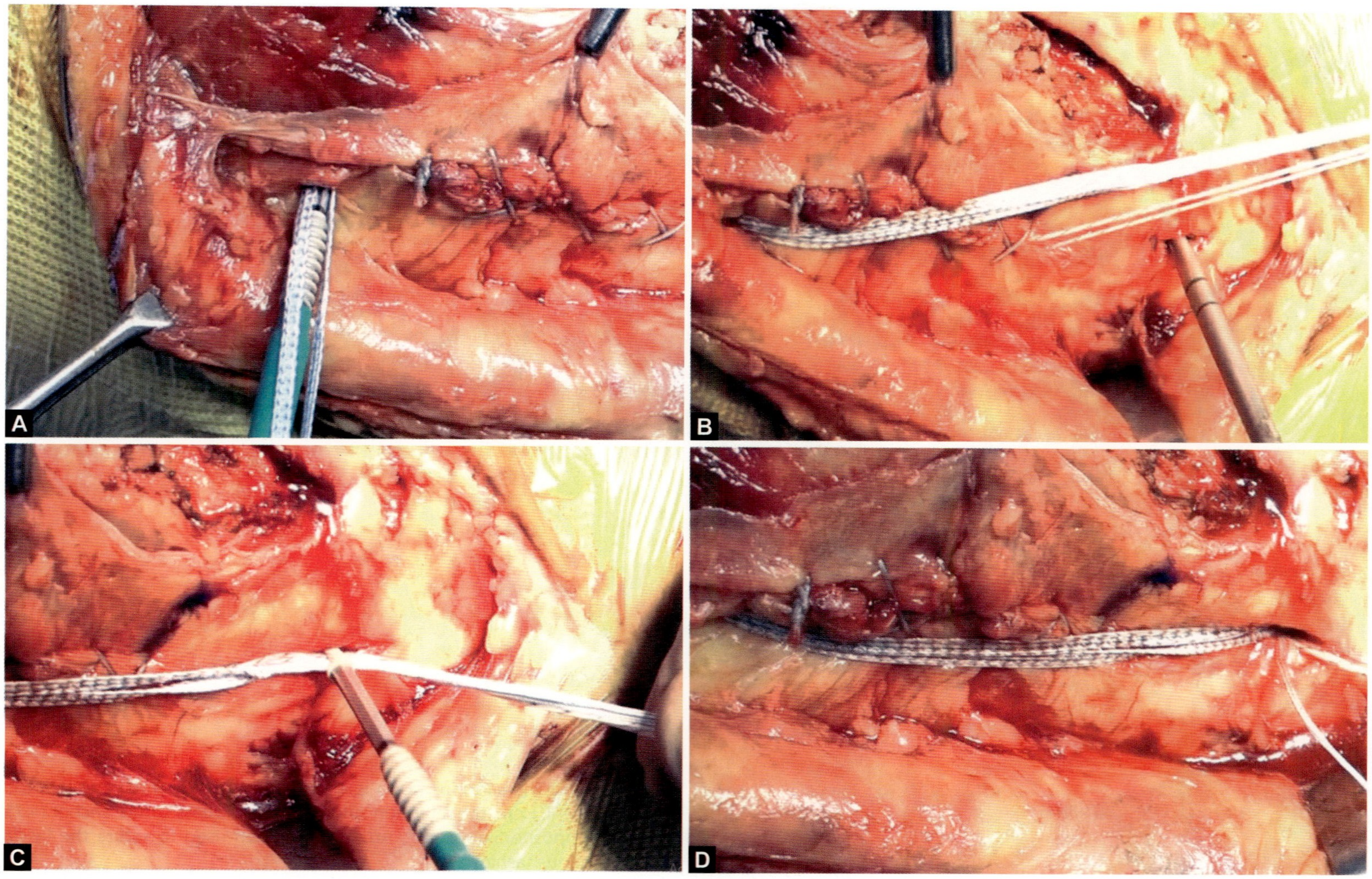

Figs. 7A to D: (A) The InternalBrace™ technique of augmentation of superficial medial collateral ligament (sMCL) repair using tape (FiberTape®, Arthrex) and knotless bone anchors (4.75 mm SwiveLock®, Arthrex). The anchor is loaded with the tape and tapped and inserted at sMCL insertion on femur; (B) The tibial sMCL insertion is located 6 cm distal to joint line and a 4.5-mm drill hole is made followed by a tap insertion since this is hard cortical bone; (C) The other end of the tape and repair sutures are loaded onto the eyelet of another anchor and this is inserted similarly; and (D) The final result is a doubled tape spanning the sMCL and bracing it internally.

Reconstruction

The reconstruction for medial knee instability can be performed with autograft or allograft tissue. Based on which kind of technique is being used, the reconstruction can either be anatomic or nonanatomic.

- *Anatomic*: The anatomic medial knee reconstruction is based on the principle of reconstructing both the sMCL and POL at their anatomic insertions using separate femoral and tibial tunnels and tensioning the grafts at different flexion angles with an aim of replicating both the anatomy and biomechanics of the medial side. This technique has been described by Coobs, Wijdicks, and LaPrade et al. Reconstruction is usually performed in the chronic setting and hence, issues related to incision placement, graft choice and availability, concomitant other ligament reconstruction, and tunnel placement must be planned prior to surgery. The principles of anatomic medial knee reconstruction are as follows:
  - *Graft selection*: The reconstruction can be performed using either autograft or allografts. The ipsilateral semitendinosus (ST) and/or gracilis (GR) tendons can be harvested free and used for reconstruction. LaPrade et al. have reported that usually a 16-cm long sMCL and 12-cm long POL graft are needed to allow 25 mm graft tissue in both the sockets. Thus, if the ST tendon is about 28 cm long, then this alone must be harvested for the reconstruction, sparing the GR tendon. Suitable allografts include tibialis anterior or peroneal tendons.
  - *Graft preparation*: Both ends of the chosen grafts are stitched using baseball stitches. Close placement of sutures and using a high strength suture material reduces chances of graft laceration during fixation with interference screws later. The grafts are marked and sutured for a distance of 25 mm. The ends of the sutures are used to create loops at both ends which will allow graft insertion (Figs. 8A and B).
  - *Surgical dissection*: The knee is kept in extension and a straight incision is taken extending from 2 cm proximal to medial epicondyle on femur to 6 cm distal to the joint line on tibia (Fig. 9). When the knee is in flexion, this becomes like a J. Full-thickness fasciocutaneous flaps are raised and the infrapatellar branch of saphenous nerve is identified and protected if possible. The sartorius fascia is incised in line with the skin incision. The reconstruction is done over layer II with minimal dissection to isolate adductor magnus tendon, medial tendon of gastrocnemius and posteromedial capsule, and direct head of semimembranosus. The femoral osseous landmarks of medial epicondyle, adductor tubercle, and gastrocnemius tubercle are

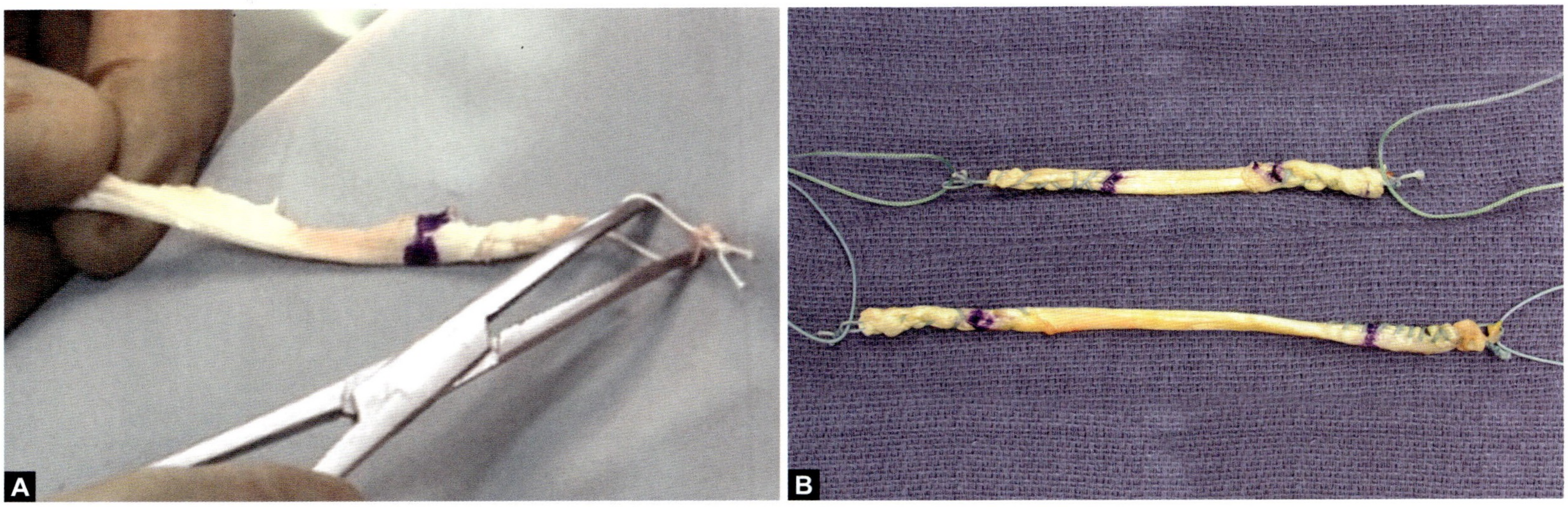

Figs. 8A and B: (A) The graft end is marked at 25 mm and sutured using closely placed baseball stiches. A loop is then created at the end; and (B) Both grafts are prepared in a similar fashion and sutures passed through the loops at both ends.

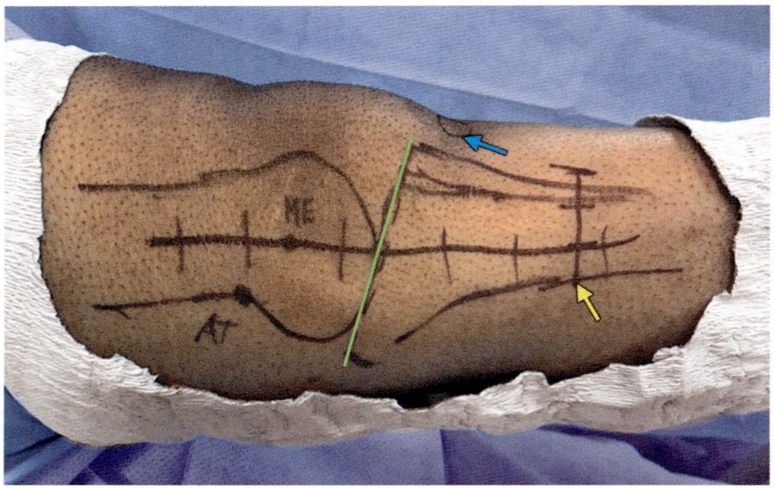

Fig. 9: The incision for reconstruction extends from about 2 cm proximal to medial epicondyle (ME) to about 7 cm distal to the joint line (green line). This provides easy access to the distal sMCL attachment on the tibia which is 6 cm distal to the joint line (yellow arrow). (AT: adductor tubercle; sMCL: superficial medial collateral ligament; blue arrow: tibial tuberosity)

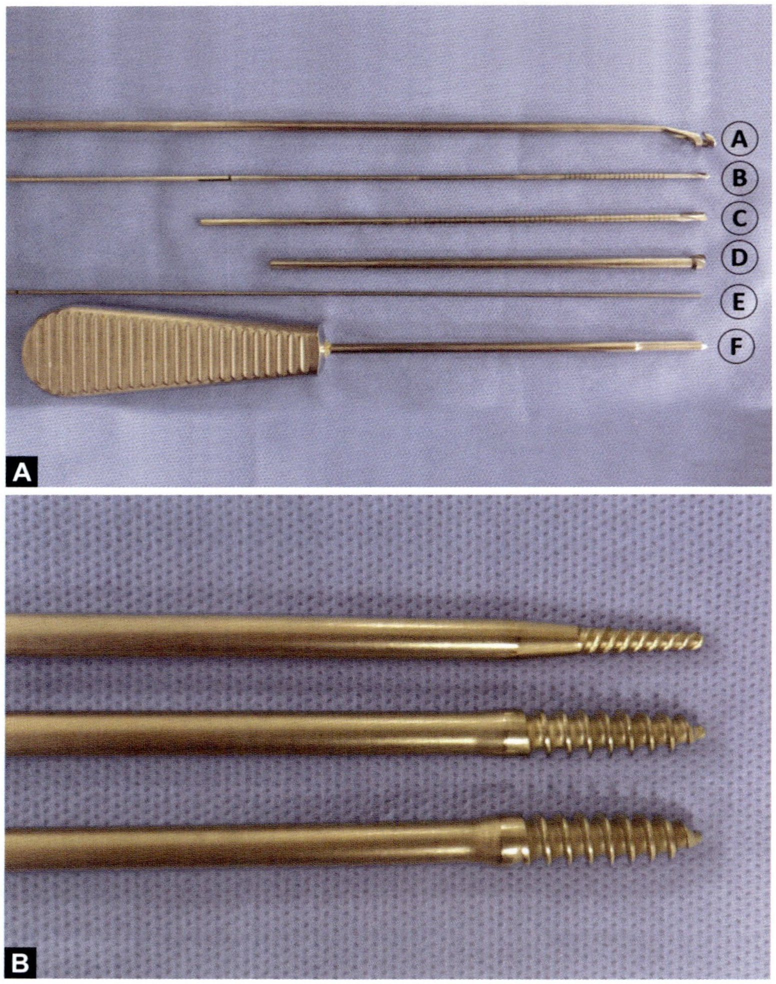

Figs. 10A and B: (A) The specific instruments needed for a reconstruction include: (1) an open tendon stripper, (2) a 2.4-mm drill tip passing pin, (3) a 4.5-mm cannulated drill bit, (4) a 7-mm flower-tip reamer, (5) guidewire, and (6) screw driver for biodegradable interference screw; and (2) Where the bone is hard, especially in the tibia, specially designed taps for biodegradable interference screw must be used to prevent graft laceration during screw insertion.

identified. The femoral sMCL attachment at a point about 3.2 mm proximal and 4.8 mm posterior to the medial epicondyle is marked. Its two tibial attachments one about 6.1 cm distal to the joint line and proximal insertion about 1.2 cm distal to the joint line are also marked. The POL femoral insertion at a point 1.4 mm distal and 2.9 mm anterior to the gastrocnemius tubercle and tibial attachment just anterior to the insertion of the direct head of semimembranosus at posteromedial tibia are similarly marked. The specific instruments needed for a reconstruction are described in Figure 10A and B.

- *Socket placement*: Once all the four points have been located on the femur and tibia for socket placement, these are sequentially created as explained in Figure 11A to E. It is advised to create the femoral sockets followed by tibial ones. When the landmarks are not easily appreciable, an image intensifier can be used for guiding the socket placement. The sockets in the femur for both sMCL and POL are directed slightly proximally. The tibial sMCL socket is drilled transverse and POL socket is drilled pointing towards the Gerdy's tubercle. At the end, we will have four sockets with suture loops placed in each of them (Fig. 12).

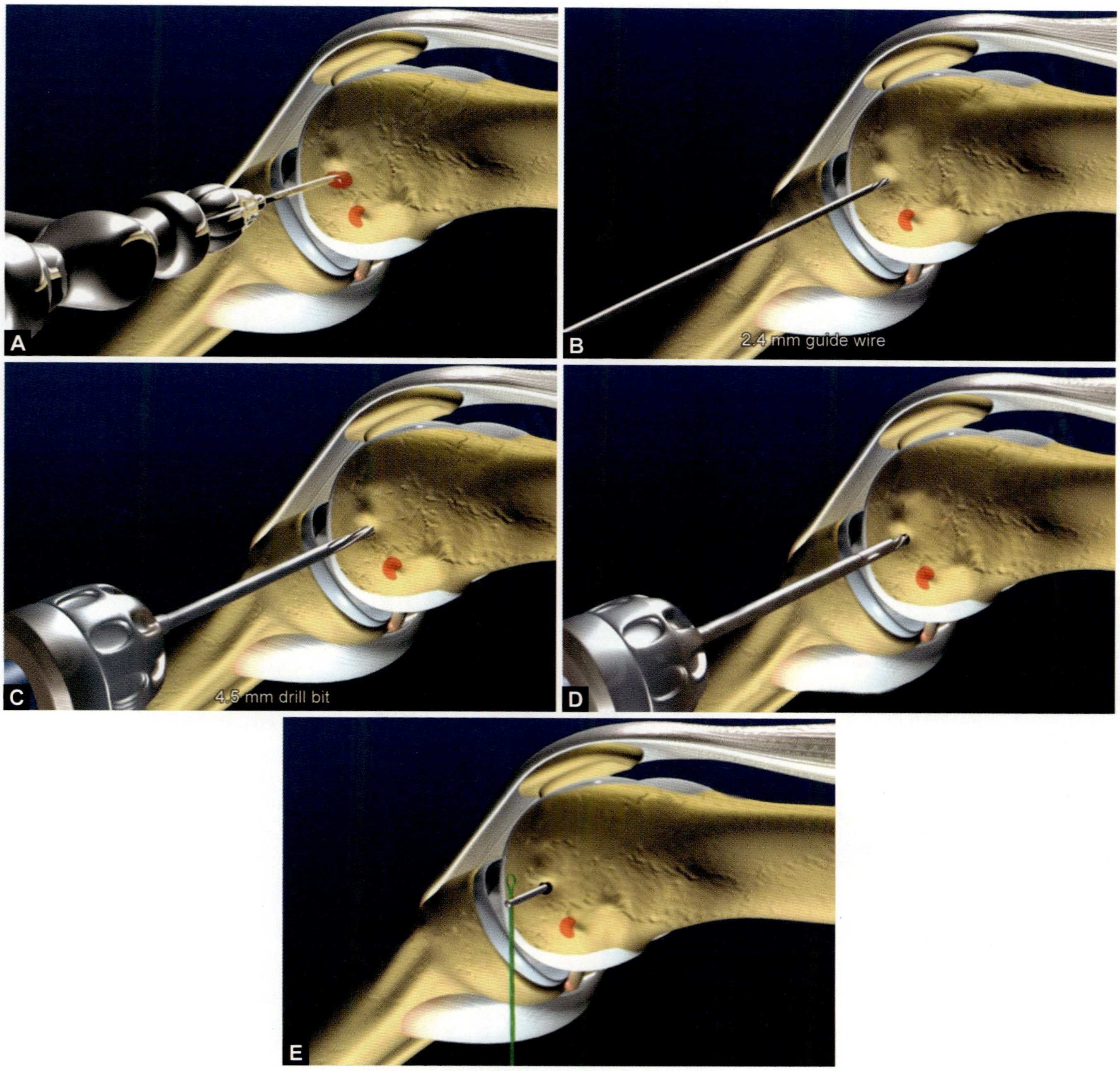

Figs. 11A to E: Steps in socket placement. (A and B) The point is marked with a microfracture awl and a 2.4-mm drill tip passing pin with eyelet is drilled across: in the recommended direction (C) A 4.0-mm cannulated drill bit is drilled over the guide pin through both cortices; (D) A femoral reamer is then drilled for a depth of 25 mm over the guide pin to create a socket; and (E) A suture loop is inserted in the eyelet of the drill pin and this is pulled out from the other side so that the loop side is at the socket opening.

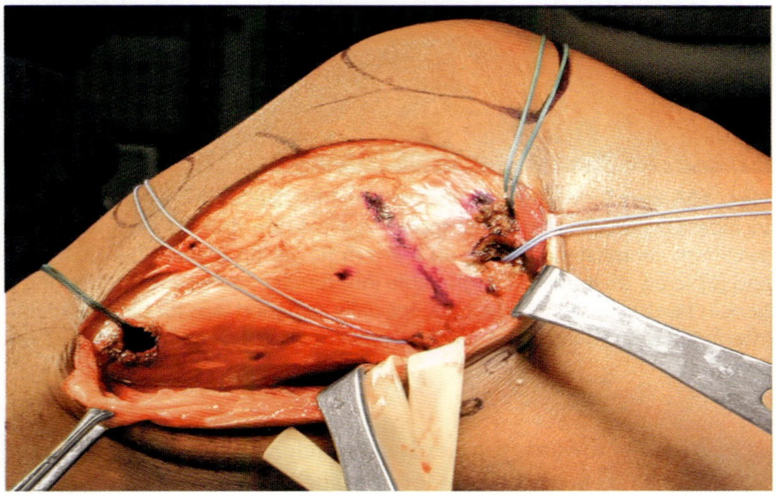

Fig. 12: The four sockets are seen each with a suture loop which will be used for graft insertion.

- *Graft insertion, tensioning, and fixation*: The POL graft is passed and fixed first followed by the sMCL graft. The femoral side of the POL graft is inserted into the socket and fixed with a 23 mm or 25 mm long, 7 mm diameter bioabsorbable or PEEK interference screw. The knee is brought to full extension, graft inserted into the tibial socket, and fixed with a similar screw. The sMCL graft is then inserted and fixed on the femoral side, knee kept in 30° flexion, neutral rotation, varus reduction force applied, and graft passed and fixed in the tibial socket with an interference screw. A 3.5-mm single-loaded titanium suture anchor is then inserted 12 mm distal to the joint line on the tibia and the sMCL graft is tied to it. This recreates the proximal tibial insertion of sMCL which is more important for valgus stability (Figs. 13A to C).
- *Closure*: If a tourniquet was used, this is deflated and hemostasis is achieved. Sartorius fascia is closed with absorbable intermittent sutures. A closed suction drain is inserted and wound closed in layers. A Jones type compression dressing is applied.

- *Nonanatomic*: This method of reconstruction is called so because it does not strictly adhere to the anatomic landmarks for graft placement and fixation. A number of techniques have been described including those by Kim, Lind, and Stannard. These techniques vary in their method of graft fixation but all employ only a single femoral point of fixation guided more by isometricity than by anatomy. They, thus, create a triangular configuration with separate sMCL and POL components and fixations on the tibia from a common femoral anchor point (Fig. 14).

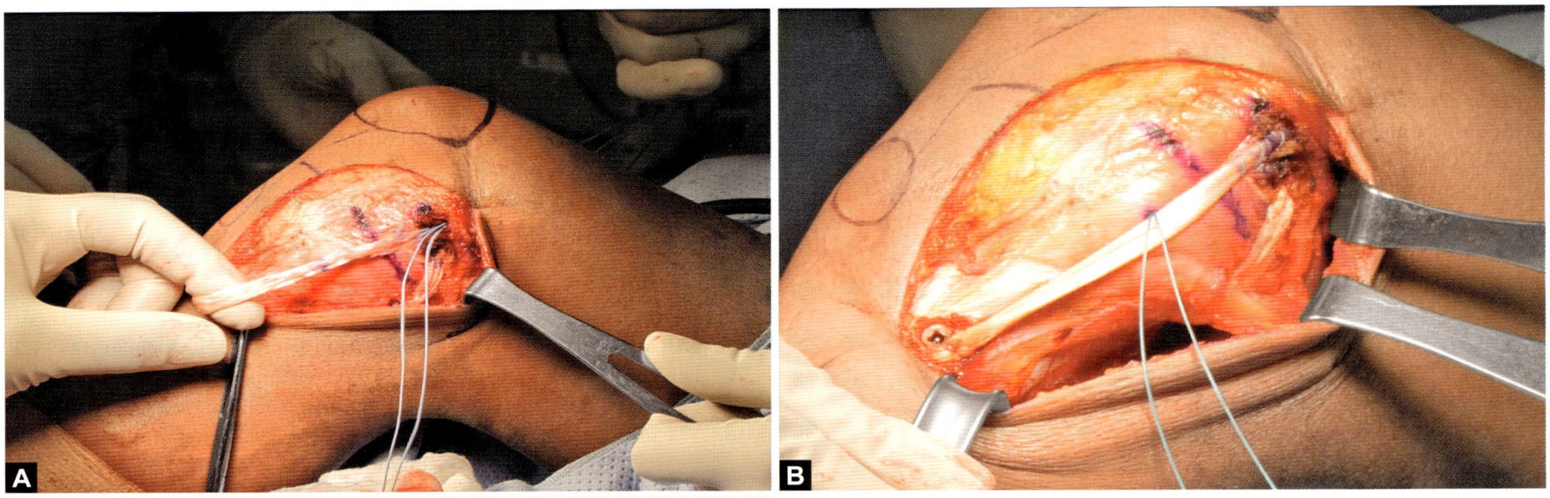

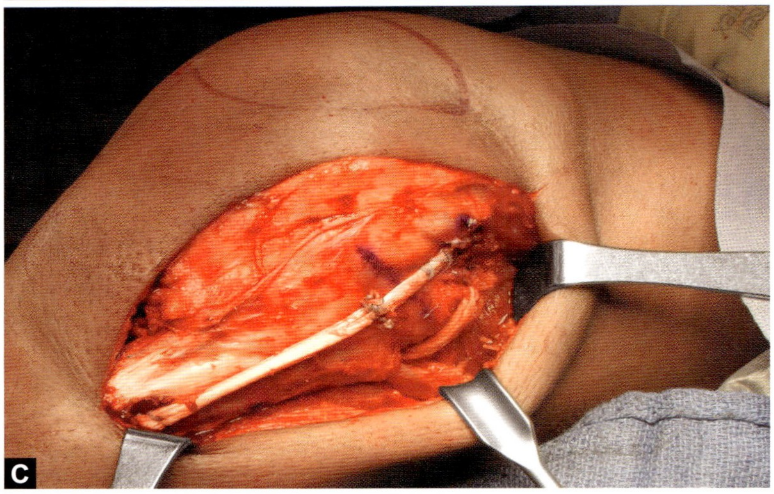

Figs. 13A to C: (A) A suture is passed through the suture loop at the end of the graft and then through the suture loop at the socket opening. The grafts are subsequently pulled into the sockets and fixed with interference screws; POL in full extension and sMCL in 30° flexion; (B) A single-loaded suture anchor is inserted 12 mm distal to joint line on the tibia to reconstruct the proximal insertion of sMCL; and (C) Appearance after completed anatomic reconstruction. (POL: posterior oblique ligament; sMCL: superficial medial collateral ligament)

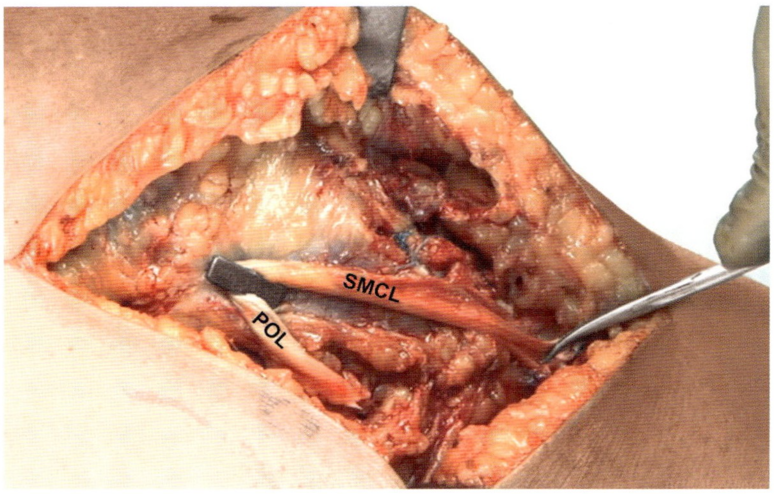

Fig. 14: A nonanatomic reconstruction with semitendinosus graft. The sMCL part of the graft is fixed on the tibia with an interference screw. A common femoral fixation using a ligament staple is performed just proximal and posterior to the medial epicondyle. The POL portion of the graft is fixed on the tibia again with an interference screw to achieve a triangular configuration. (POL: posterior oblique ligament; sMCL: superficial medial collateral ligament)

CONCLUSION

The understanding of anatomy of medial knee structures has evolved recently leading to a concurrent evolution of surgical techniques for management of injuries of medial knee structures. Although majorly managed conservatively, surgical treatment by a repair or reconstruction is sometimes necessary. While repair is performed in the acute setting, anatomic reconstruction is reserved for chronic and residual cases with anteromedial instability. The surgical principles detailed earlier are based on validated studies from current literature.

SUGGESTED READING

1. Andrews K, Lu A, McKean L, et al. Review: Medial collateral ligament injuries. J Orthop. 2017;14(4):550-4.
2. Black B, Azbell C, Volgas D, et al. Posteromedial corner injury in knee dislocations. J Knee Surg. 2012;25(5):429-34.
3. Bollen S. Epidemiology of knee injuries: diagnosis and triage. Br J Sports Med. 2000;34(3):227-8.
4. Bonasia DE, Bruzzone M, Dettoni F, et al. Treatment of medial and posteromedial knee instability: indications, techniques, and review of the results. Iowa Orthop J. 2012;32:173-83.
5. Coobs BR, Wijdicks CA, Armitage BM, et al. An in vitro analysis of an anatomical medial knee reconstruction. Am J Sports Med. 2010;38(2):339-47.
6. Dong J, Wang XF, Men X, et al. Surgical treatment of acute grade III medial collateral ligament injury combined with anterior cruciate ligament injury: anatomic ligament repair versus triangular ligament reconstruction. Arthroscopy. 2015;31(6):1108-16.
7. Fanelli GC, Harris JD. Late medial collateral ligament reconstruction. Tech Knee Surg. 2007;6(2):99-105.
8. Fetto JF, Marshall JL. Medial collateral ligament injuries of the knee. Clin Orthop Relat Res. 1978;132:206-18.
9. Gilmer BB, Crall T, DeLong J, et al. Biomechanical analysis of internal bracing for treatment of medial knee injuries. Orthopedics. 2016;39(3):e532-7.
10. Grood ES, Noyes FR, Butler DL, et al. Ligamentous and capsular restraints preventing straight medial and lateral laxity in intact human cadaver knees. J Bone Joint Surg. 1981;63(8):1257-69.
11. Kim SJ, Lee DH, Kim TE, et al. Concomitant reconstruction of the medial collateral and posterior oblique ligaments for medial instability of the knee. J Bone Joint Surg Br. 2008;90-B(10):1323-7.
12. LaPrade RF, Engebretsen AH, Ly TV, et al. The anatomy of the medial part of the knee. J Bone Joint Surg Am. 2007;89(9):2000-10.
13. LaPrade RF, Wijdicks CA. Surgical technique: development of an anatomic medial knee reconstruction. Clin Orthop Relat Res. 2011;470(3):806-14.
14. Lind M, Jakobsen BW, Lund B, et al. Anatomical reconstruction of the medial collateral ligament and posteromedial corner of the knee in patients with chronic medial collateral ligament instability. Am J Sports Med. 2009;37(6):1116-22.
15. Lubowitz JH, MacKay G, Gilmer B. Knee medial collateral ligament and posteromedial corner anatomic repair with internal bracing. Arthrosc Tech. 2014;3(4):e505-8.
16. Petersen W, Loerch S, Schanz S, et al. The role of the posterior oblique ligament in controlling posterior tibial translation in the posterior cruciate ligament-deficient knee. Am J Sports Med. 2008;36(3):495-501.
17. van der List JP, DiFelice GS. Primary repair of the medial collateral ligament with internal bracing. Arthrosc Tech. 2017;6(4):e933-7.
18. Warren LF, Marshall JL. The supporting structures and layers on the medial side of the knee. J Bone Joint Surg. 1979;61(1):56-62.

CHAPTER 17

Posterolateral Corner Reconstruction of Knee Joint

Vishal Patil, Shrinivas S Shintre, Nagesh Naik, Jignesh Yeshwant Tandel, Rupesh Kadam

INTRODUCTION

Posterolateral corner (PLC) injuries are comparatively rare and are commonly associated with anterior cruciate ligament (ACL) or posterior cruciate ligament (PCL) tears. Isolated PLC injuries amount to around 28%. A number of studies and literature of this topic have led to a better understanding of the PLC, and its reconstruction techniques. Failure to detect PLC injuries is shown to be an important cause of recurrent instability and is a common cause of ACL reconstruction failure. It could result in altered knee biomechanics that may lead to early degenerative changes of the joint.

ANATOMY

The structures comprising the PLC are classified as static and dynamic structures.

Following are the three important static stabilizers of the PLC: (1) the lateral collateral ligament (LCL), (2) the popliteus tendon (PLT), and (3) the popliteofibular ligament (PFL).

- *Lateral collateral ligament:* The lateral collateral ligament (LCL) extends obliquely backward and downward from the lateral epicondyle of the femur proximally, to the head of the fibula distally. The LCL is less prone to injury and more flexible than medial collateral ligament.
- *Popliteus tendon:* It arises at the lateral condyle of the femur and the posterior horn of the lateral meniscus. From there, it runs medially and caudally toward the tibia and inserts proximal and near the origin of the soleus muscle.
- *Popliteofibular ligament:* The PFL arises at the musculotendinous junction of the popliteus. The PFL has two divisions anterior and posterior.
- Lateral capsule
- Arcuate ligament.

The *dynamic* structures which help to stabilize the knee are:

- *Biceps femoris:* Inserts on the posterior aspect of the fibula and posterior to LCL
- Popliteus muscle
- *Iliotibial (IT) tract:* It is the most superficial, broad layer on the lateral aspect of the knee. It inserts on to Gerdy's tubercle in the anterolateral part of the tibia.
- Lateral head of the gastrocnemius.

FUNCTION

The PLC structures act as the primary restrictors to varus forces of the knee and also of posterolateral rotation of the tibia relative to the femur. These structures are important secondary stabilizers to anterior and posterior tibial translation when cruciate ligaments are injured. The primary restraint to varus stress across the knee is provided by LCL and the rest of the posterolateral structures act as secondary varus stabilizers. The LCL and the popliteus complex are the primary restrictors for tibial external rotation, especially between 30° and 40° of flexion and the PCL acts as only as a secondary restraint. Thus, combined PCL and PLC injuries are more vulnerable to external rotation forces. For preventing internal rotation the ACL is the main stabilizer in lower flexion angles and anterolateral ligament (ALL) in higher flexion angles and the PLT is a minor primary stabilizer. The remaining PLC structures are secondary restraints to internal rotation. In full extension and with ACL-or PCL-deficient knees minimal contribution of the PLC has been quoted for anteroposterior tibial translation.

CLASSIFICATION

- Grade I (0–5 mm of lateral opening and minimal ligament disruption)
- Grade II (5–10 mm of lateral opening and moderate ligament disruption)

- Grade III (>10 mm of lateral opening and severe ligament disruption and no endpoint).

MECHANISM OF TRAUMA

- Direct blow over anteromedial knee
- Varus blow to flexed knee
- Dislocation of knee joint
- Hyperextension injuries.

SYMPTOMS

- Pain
- Side-to-side instability near extension
- Patients complain of increased difficulty in walking on uneven ground or stair climbing
- Swelling
- Paresthesia or foot drop due to common peroneal nerve injury. Rare.

EXAMINATION

- *Varus stress test*:
  - Varus laxity at 0° indicates both LCL and cruciate (ACL or PCL) injury
  - Varus laxity at 30° indicates LCL injury.

  Special tests like dial test, reverse pivot shift and external rotation recurvatum test will aid in diagnosis.

IMAGING

- *Radiographs*: Avulsion fracture of the fibula (arcuate fracture) or femoral condyle may be seen.
  MRI is diagnostic study of choice.
- *MRI*: May show injury to the LCL, popliteus, and biceps tendon.
  Bone bruising of medial femoral condyle and medial tibial plateau.

TREATMENT

Nonoperative

In isolated PLC grade I or II injuries: Immobilization of knee in full extension with partial weight bearing for 2 weeks followed by progressive functional rehabilitation focusing on quadriceps strengthening.

Operative

Posterolateral corner repair: Only in isolated PLC injuries with bony or soft tissue avulsion, should be performed within 2–3 weeks of injury.

TECHNIQUES

Lateral-sided repairs are approached laterally irrespective of site of injury.

- Incision starts at the fibular head/neck junction continuing till about 2 cm proximal to lateral epicondyle.
- IT band is the first structure to be identified and three windows are created.
  1. *Window 1*: Just proximal to lateral epicondyle and extending to Gerdy's tubercle.
  2. *Window 2*: Between posterior band of IT band and posterior border of rectus femoris.
  3. *Window 3*: Posterior to biceps femoris near common peroneal nerve.
- Identification of LCL, biceps femoris tendon, popliteal fibular ligament, PLT, PL capsule, and lateral head of gastrocnemius is done.
- Locking sutures passed in the LCL and the biceps tendon and passed through drill holes in the fibular head and LCL and biceps tendon attached to bone.
- In case of fibular head fractures, head is fixed with a titanium screw.

POSTEROLATERAL CORNER RECONSTRUCTION

It is advised for grade III injuries and when repair is not possible because of weakened structures.

Techniques

Aim is to reconstruct LCL and the PFL using a free tendon graft (semitendinosus or Achilles).

SURGICAL STEPS

- Incision is taken on the lateral aspect as described earlier and dissection is carried out till the IT band, the three windows are created, common peroneal nerve is identified and protected.
- Drill a tunnel at lateral epicondyle of femur from lateral to medial side using a guidewire and drill (Fig. 1).
- The harvested semitendinosus graft is folded on itself and secured in this drill hole using an interference screw for fixation in femur such a way that fold is inside tunnel and two tails are outside (Fig. 2).
- A track is created between the popliteal hiatus and posterior aspect of fibula and graft tails are passed through it.
- Another tunnel is created in tibia 2 cm below joint line starting from where popliteus tendon crosses the tibia exiting anteriorly near the tibial tuberosity (Fig. 3A). Second tail of graft is passed in this tunnel from posterior to anterior and fixed with interference screw (Fig. 3B).
- A fibular head tunnel is created by drilling from anterolateral head of fibula to posteromedial tubercle. One tail of graft is then passed through this tunnel posteroanteriorly and sutured on itself (Fig. 4).
- Final reconstruction (Fig. 5)
  - Sutures are passed through the capsule and tied to approximate the capsule.
  - The lateral gastrocnemius is tightened to the back of biceps.
  - Wound is closed in layers.

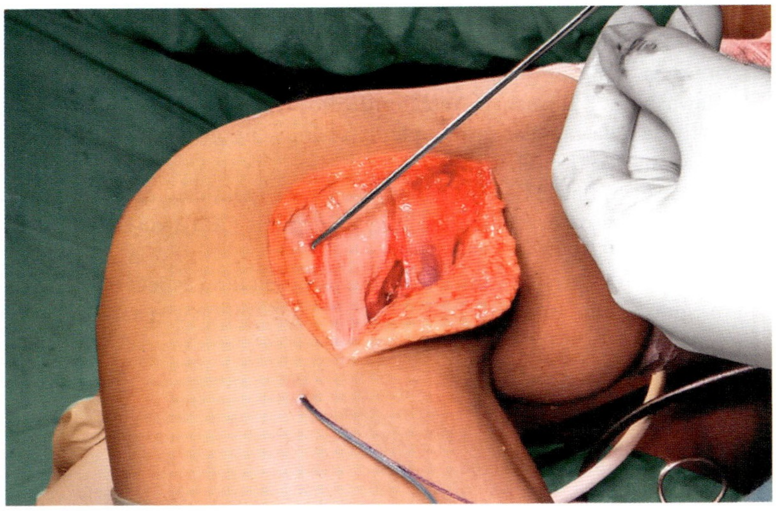

Fig. 1: Drilling of tunnel in femur.

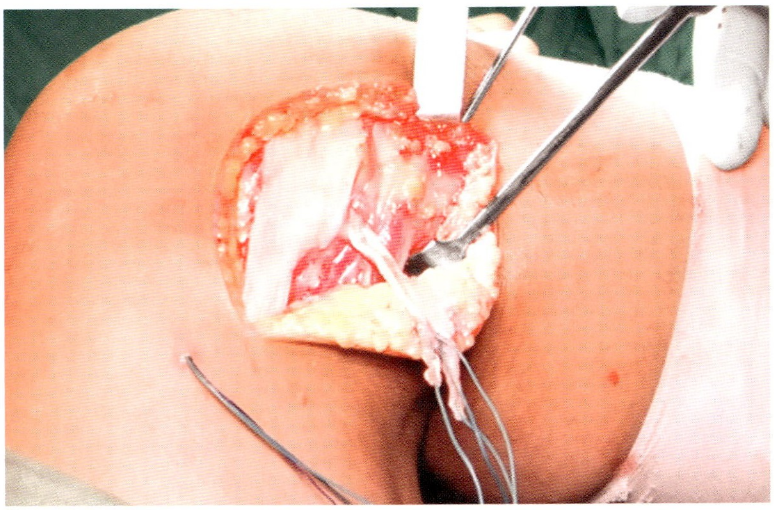

Fig. 2: Semitendinosus graft fixed in femoral tunnel.

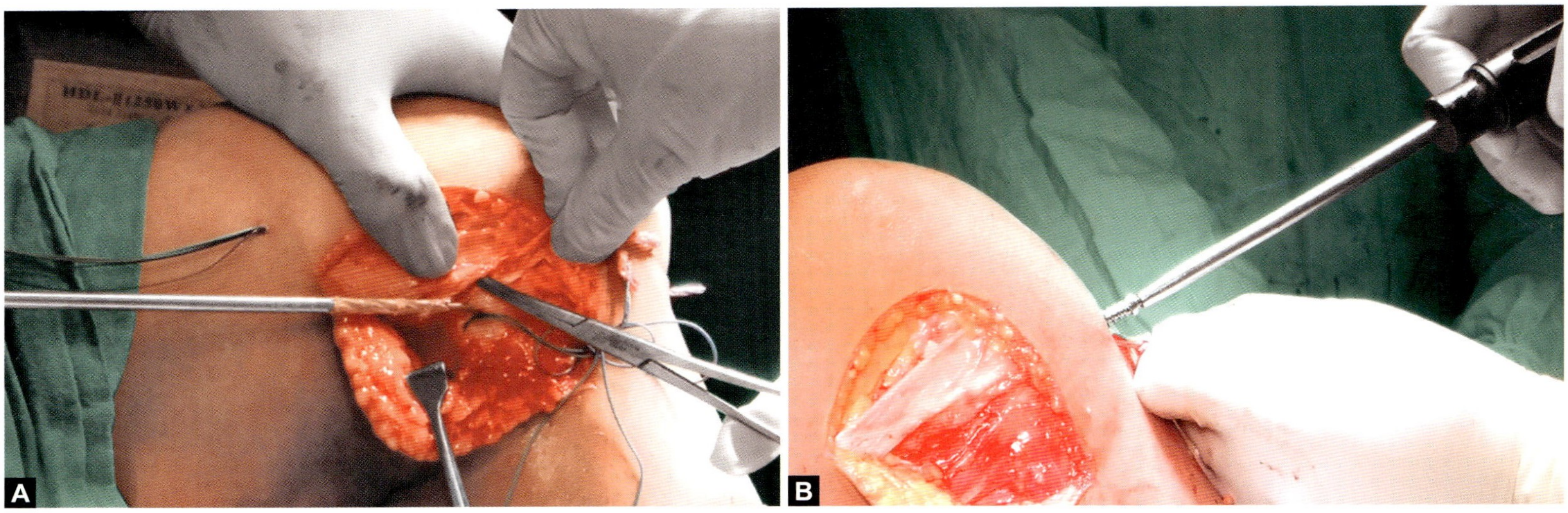

Figs. 3A and B: (A) Tunnel is created in tibia; (B) Graft one tail fixed in tibial tunnel with interference screw.

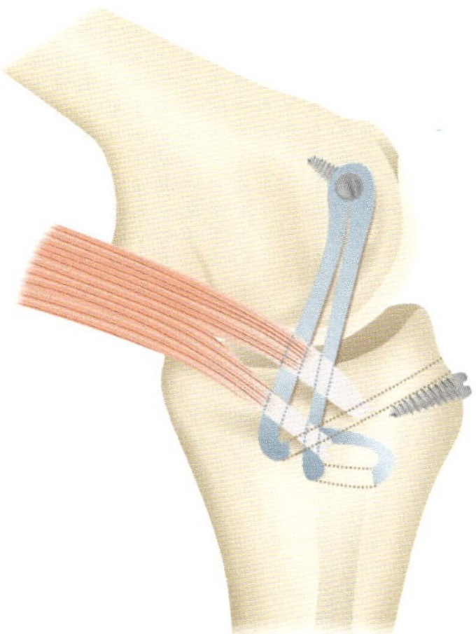

Fig. 4: Graft second tail passed in tunnel in fibula head and sutured on itself.

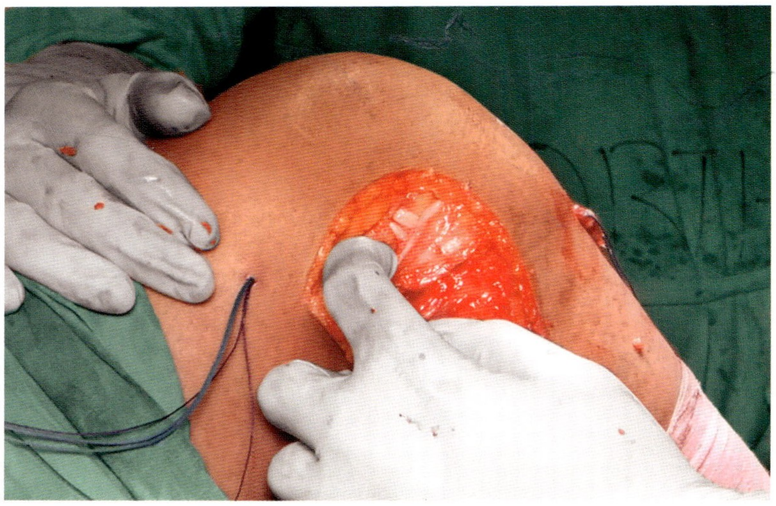

Fig. 5: Final reconstruction.

REHABILITATION

Postoperatively immobilization and protected weight bearing for 4 weeks (long leg casts are preferred as these control leg external rotation better than brace).

- Start passive range of motion (ROM) at 4 weeks for avoiding arthrofibrosis.
- Active hamstring exercises to be avoided for they will stress the PLC.
- Full active extension is encouraged

BIBLIOGRAPHY

1. Cooper DE. Tests for posterolateral instability of the knee in normal subjects. Results of examination under anesthesia. J Bone Joint Surg Am. 1991;73(1):30-6.
2. Geeslin AG, Moulton SG, LaPrade RF. A systematic review of the outcomes of posterolateral corner knee injuries, part 1: surgical treatment of acute injuries. Am J Sports Med. 2015;44(2):1-7.
3. Kawashima T, Takeishi H, Yoshitomi S, Ito M, Sasaki H. Anatomical study of the fabella, fabellar complex and its clinical implications. Surg Radiol Anat. 2007;29(8):611-6.
4. Ranawat A, Baker CL, 3rd, Henry S, Harner CD. Posterolateral corner injury of the knee: evaluation and management. J Am Acad Orthop Surg. 2008;16(9):506-18
5. LaPrade RF, Terry GC. Injuries to the posterolateral aspect of the knee. Association of anatomic injury patterns with clinical instability. Am J Sports Med. 1997;25(4):433-8.

CHAPTER 18

Arthroscopic Bankart Repair

Namdeo Gorgile, Shrinivas S Shintre, Chittanand Mendhe

SURGICAL PROCEDURE

Anesthesia

We prefer interscalene nerve block with hypotensive general anesthesia (mean BP 65 mm Hg).

Position

Even though Bankart repair to be done in lateral decubitus and beach chair position, we prefer lateral decubitus with 30° posterior tilt with arm abduction of 30–45° and a forward flexion of 15° with weight of approximately 5 kg.

Portals

We use three portals, i.e. posterior portal for visualization, lateral coracoid portal for anchor placement and knot tying, and antero-superior portal for suture shuttle.

Surgical Procedure

After giving the general anesthesia, it is very important to confirm the clinical and radiological diagnosis by special tests like apprehension test, anterior/posterior drawer test and relocation tests. It is also very important to note the degree of external rotation in abduction at which the humeral head is dislocating out of joint to know the severity of glenoid bone loss and size of Hill-Sachs defect. Once the clinical diagnosis is made, start the arthroscopic Bankart repair by posterior portal which is typically 2 cm medial and inferior to the posterolateral angle of acromion. Pass the high-flow trocar or sheath by targeting the coracoid anteriorly. Start the diagnostic round of arthroscopy and look for the rotator interval, whole glenoid labrum or biceps-labrum complex, inferior glenohumeral ligament (IGHL), subscapularis, supraspinatus and infraspinatus, and glenoid bone loss (distance from bare spot) Hill-Sachs defect. If there is no or minimal glenoid bone loss with small or shallow Hill-Sachs defect, proceed with arthroscopic Bankart repair by thoroughly releasing the capsulolabral tissue from the glenoid neck by using the glenoid liberator and rasp. After releasing the capsulolabral tissue adequately and preparing the glenoid neck thoroughly from 6 o'clock to 2 o'clock position. Start placing the anchors usually required three one by one (single/double loaded) from inferior to superior with a gap of 5–7 mm, i.e. 5 o'clock to 2 o'clock respectively. During this procedure, posterior portal is used as a visualization portal, lateral coracoid portal (8 mm cannula) for suture anchor placement and knot tying and anterosuperior portal (5.5 mm cannula) as a suture shuttle portal. Usually our preference for knot tying is first sliding knot followed by three half hitches, alternatively. It is very important to shift the capsule from inferior to superior direction and try to recreate a glenoid labrum bumper effect. Usually the inferior two anchors fix the anterior band of Inferior Glenohumeral Ligament (IGHL) that is the key step in arthroscopic Bankart repair. It is very important to avoid taking middle glenohumeral ligament into the repair which will limit the patient's external rotation grossly. If there is a Hill-Sachs defect, Hill-Sachs remplissage should be done before anterior labral repair by a bigger anchor. After the final repair, you will see the centralized humeral head.

Rehabilitation

Continue shoulder immobilizer for a period of 3–4 weeks. Continue simple arm sling for further 3–4 weeks. Start elbow and finger movements immediately after the surgery. Shoulder rehabilitation started with pendulum exercises at 3–4 weeks, supine passive forward flexion followed by active assisted/active exercises gradually. Usually the patient regains full range of motion at 6–8 weeks. Also, it is important to avoid the extreme degree of abduction and external rotation for at least 3–4 months postoperatively.

DISCUSSION

Arthroscopic anterior Bankart repair is a minimally invasive well documented procedure with good functional outcome for the anteroinferior labral tear. The best indication for this procedure will be a case of anteroinferior instability with an anteroinferior labral tear with a very minimum glenoid bone loss and small-shallow Hill-Sachs defect. Usually, the repair is carried out with 2.8 mm suture anchors or with the recently available 1.8 mm all suture anchors which will reduce the size of hole in the glenoid. Care should be taken to place the anchors over the glenoid face with proper trajectory instead of glenoid margin which minimizes the anchor pull-out. The anchor knots must be away from the glenoid cartilage and humeral head to prevent chondral erosion. Now, with the availability of advanced diagnostic techniques, its becoming easy to diagnose bipolar bone loss and other associated shoulder pathologies. The failure of arthroscopic Bankart repair which is common within 2 years of repair is usually correlated with the uni-bi polar bone loss, poor quality of capsulolabral tissue, faulty repair technique and inability to identify humeral avulsion of glenohumeral ligament lesion. There are different varieties of Bankart lesions that exist, i.e. Perthes, anterior labroligamentous periosteal sleeve avulsion (ALPSA), glenolabral articular disruption (GLAD). Usually, the preferred modality to measure the glenoid bone loss and Hill–Sachs defect accurately is the 3D CT scan. The stability of repaired Bankart reduces gradually with the increasing size of bipolar bone loss. Also, it is very important to rule out the multidirectional shoulder instability (bilateral) from anteroinferior instability (unilateral). The choice of procedure for anteroinferior shoulder instability is to be selected on case-to-case basis according to the knowledge and skill of the surgeon. Arthroscopic Bankart procedure is associated with certain complications like anchor pull-out, glenoid rim fractures, synovitis, chondrolysis, loss of external rotation and stiffness. Other known procedures for anteroinferior instability are open Bankart repair, arthroscopic latarjet, open latarjet, iliac crest grafting and other old capsular plication procedures.

SURGICAL STEPS (FIGS. 1 TO 7)

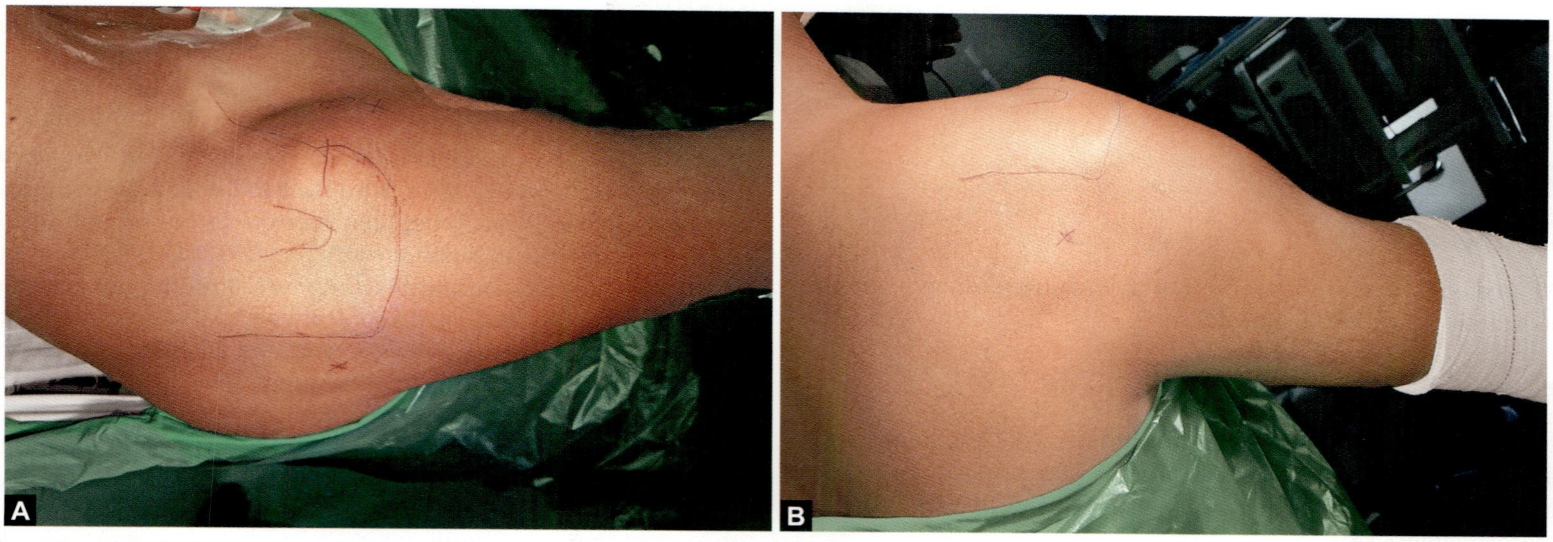

Figs. 1A and B: Bankart repair to be done in lateral decubitus with 30° posterior tilt with arm abduction of 30–45° and a forward flexion of 15°. It can be done in beach chair position. Bony landmarks and portal entry sites marks. Three portals, i.e. posterior portal for visualisation, lateral coracoid portal for anchor placement and knot tying, and anterosuperior portal for suture shuttle.

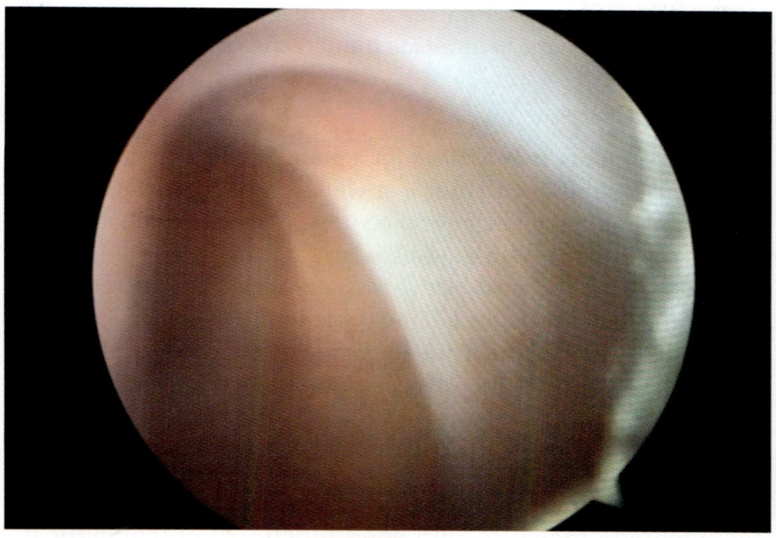

Fig. 2: Start the arthroscopic Bankart repair by posterior portal which is typically 2 cm medial and inferior to the posterolateral angle of acromion. Pass the high-flow trocar or sheath by targeting the coracoid anteriorly. Start the diagnostic round of arthroscopy and look for the rotator interval, whole glenoid labrum or biceps-labrum complex, inferior glenohumeral ligament, subscapularis, supraspinatus and infraspinatus.

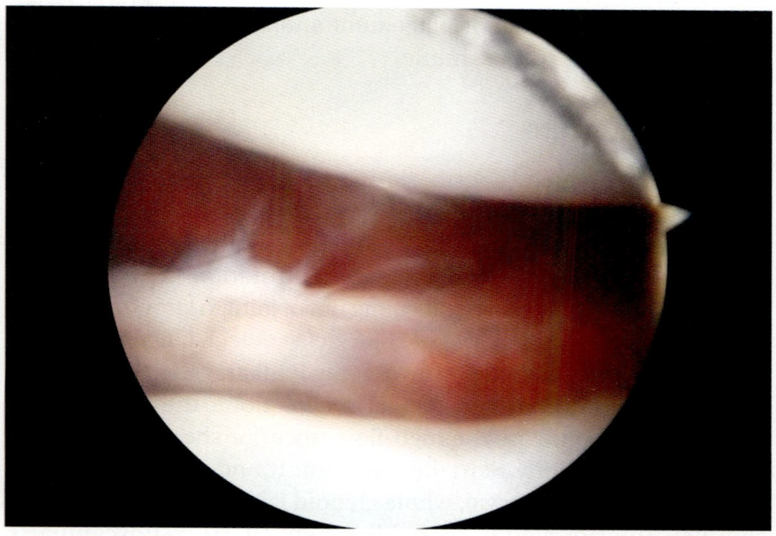

Fig. 3: Glenoid bone loss (distance from bare spot) Hill–Sachs defect. If there is no or minimal glenoid bone loss with small or shallow Hill–Sachs defect.

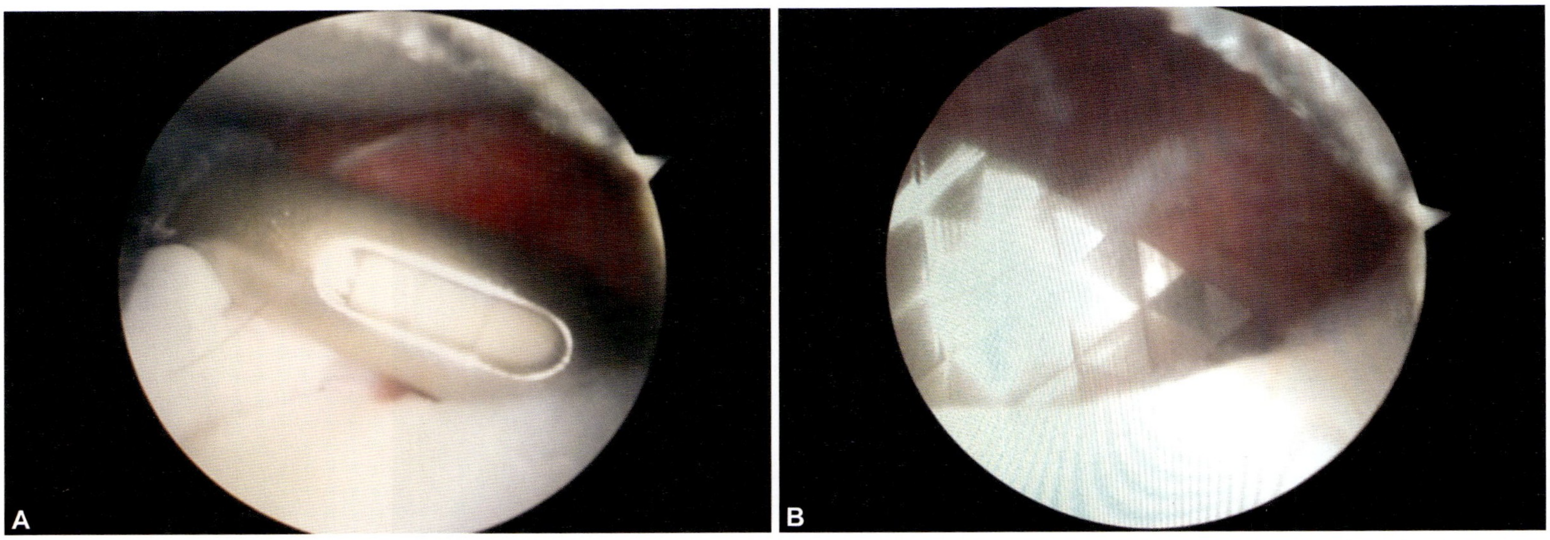

Figs. 4A and B: Thoroughly releasing the capsulolabral tissue from the glenoid neck by using the glenoid liberator and rasp. After releasing the capsulolabral tissue adequately and preparing the glenoid neck thoroughly from 6 o'clock to 2 o'clock position.

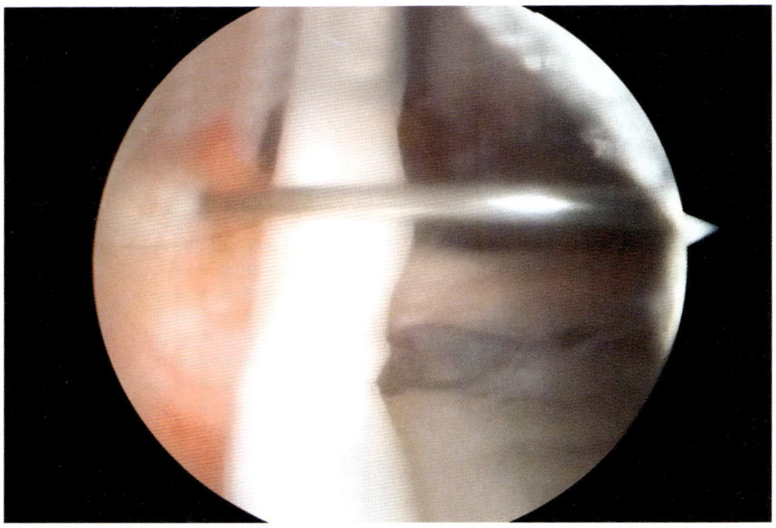

Fig. 5: Start placing the anchors usually required three one by one (single/double loaded) from inferior to superior with a gap of 5–7 mm, i.e. 5 o'clock to 2 o'clock subsequently. During this procedure, posterior portal is used as a visualisation portal, lateral coracoid portal (8 mm cannula) for suture anchor placement and knot tying, and anterosuperior portal (5.5 mm cannula) as a suture shuttle portal.

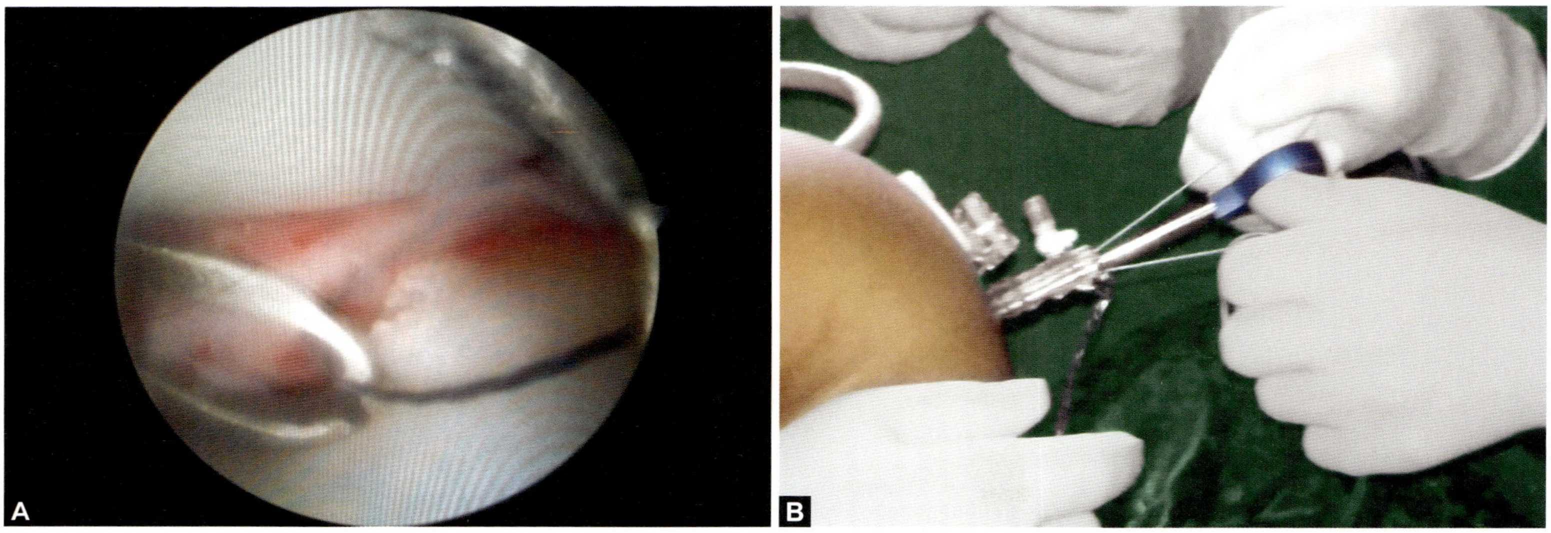

Figs. 6A and B: Knot tying is first sliding knot followed by three half hitches alternatively. It is very important to shift the capsule from inferior to superior direction and try to recreate a glenoid labrum bumper effect. Usually, the inferior two anchors fix the anterior band of inferior glenohumeral ligament that is the key step in arthroscopic Bankart repair. It is very important to avoid taking middle glenohumeral ligament into the repair which will limit the patient's external rotation grossly.

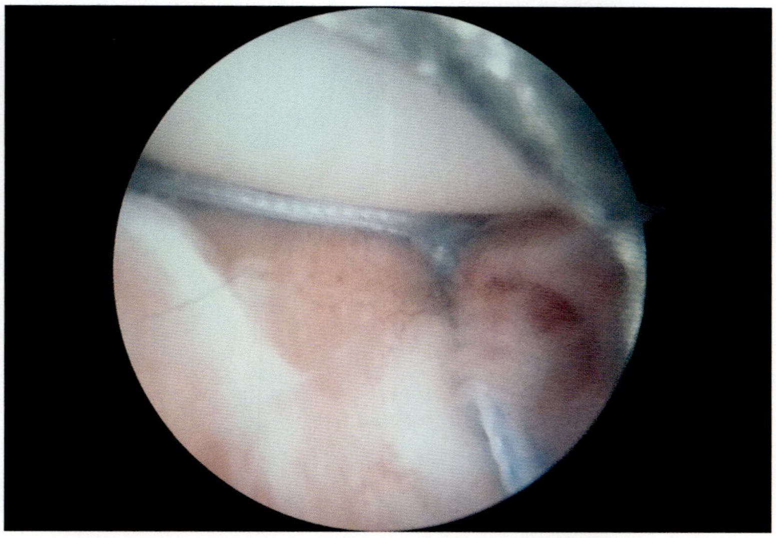

Fig. 7: After the final repair, you will see the centralized humeral head.

CHAPTER 19

Open Latarjet Procedure

J Clement Joseph

INTRODUCTION

The shoulder is the most commonly dislocated joint in the body with 90–95% being anterior dislocations. Operative treatments have become the standard, given the redislocation rates of up to 100% in skeletally immature and as high as 96% for adolescents and young adults less than 30 years of age.

While arthroscopic Bankart repairs have become more successful, still recurrence rates of 11–25% are reported especially in patients with glenoid bone loss and large Hill-Sachs lesions. The Latarjet procedure was introduced by Latarjet in 1954. It involved osteotomizing 2 cm of coracoid along with conjoint tendon and transferring to the anterior inferior glenoid neck. This procedure has evolved with modifications (Box 1) to remain a very useful and successful procedure. The technique that will be described here is open technique, which can be easily reproduced with minimum need for sophisticated equipment. Adding a capsular repair eliminates the end-range apprehension and also lessens the chances of osteoarthritis (OA) by making the coracoid extra-articular (Table 1).

Box 1: Technical modifications of Latarjet procedure.

1. Two bicortical screws instead of one
2. CA ligament 1 cm cuff left attached to coracoid for suturing the capsule
3. Using suture anchors for capsulolabral repair
4. Congruent arc—placing the medial surface of the coracoid on the anterior glenoid
5. Coracoid and glenoid drill guides
6. Cannulated screws with miniplates
7. Arthroscopic Latarjet procedures

TABLE 1: Complications of Latarjet procedure.

Complications	*Tips to avoid*
Neurological up to 20%	• Avoid forceful retraction and large retractors to avoid injury to axillary nerve • Do not dissect and expose medial border of conjoint tendon (musculocutaneous nerve)
Stiffness	• Early mobilization • Capsular repair with arm in full external rotation
Nonunion	• Proper decortication and flat surfaces • Use inferior surface of coracoid on glenoid • Bicortical fixation
Bone block fracture	• Avoid overtightening • Screw holes in coracoid—adequately spaced • Old age—to be careful
Bone block resorption	Avoid Latarjet in patients without glenoid bone loss. Avoid bioabsorbable screws
End-range apprehension	Can be improved by adding a capsular repair either with suture anchors or suturing to CA ligament cuff left attached to coracoid

INDICATIONS FOR LATARJET PROCEDURE

- Glenoid bone loss more than 20%
- Significant Hill-Sachs lesion
- Hyperlaxity
- Recurrence after a soft tissue repair
- Contact sports (relative indication).

KEY INSTRUMENTS

- Fukuda retractor
- Gelpi pointed retractors two numbers
- 3 mm Steinmann pin
- Darrach's retractor
- Hohman's retractors of various sizes
- 2.7 mm drills for 4.0 mm cannulated screws
- 3.2 drill bits for 4.5 mm malleolar screws
- Curved osteotome 20 mm
- Powered saw 10 mm short blades.

ANESTHESIA

Brachial plexus block + General anesthesia + Hypotension.

SURGICAL TECHNIQUE (FIGS. 1 TO 26)

While the traditional arthrotomy is done lateral to the labrum and the labrum is excised to expose the glenoid, we prefer to incise the medial scapular periosteum 5-10 mm medial to joint line and elevating along with labrum and capsule as a layer medially. This helps in preserving the labrum and allows a tension free Bankart repair at the end. It is important to place one or two absorbable sutures to the capsular tissue at this stage, which will help in identification later.

Once the arthrotomy is done, a Fukuda retractor is placed inside the joint, head is retracted, and a good view of glenoid is obtained.

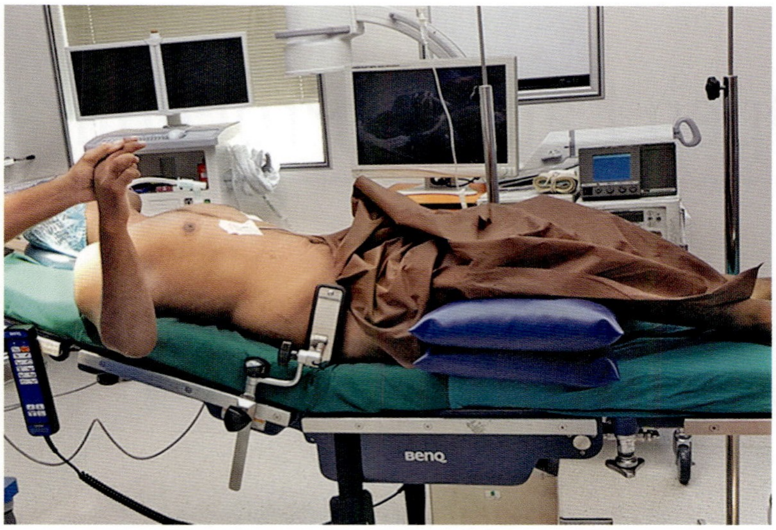

Fig. 1: Positioning: Semi-beach chair (30° up). Pillows under the knees and pelvic and trunk side supports and arm free by the side of table.

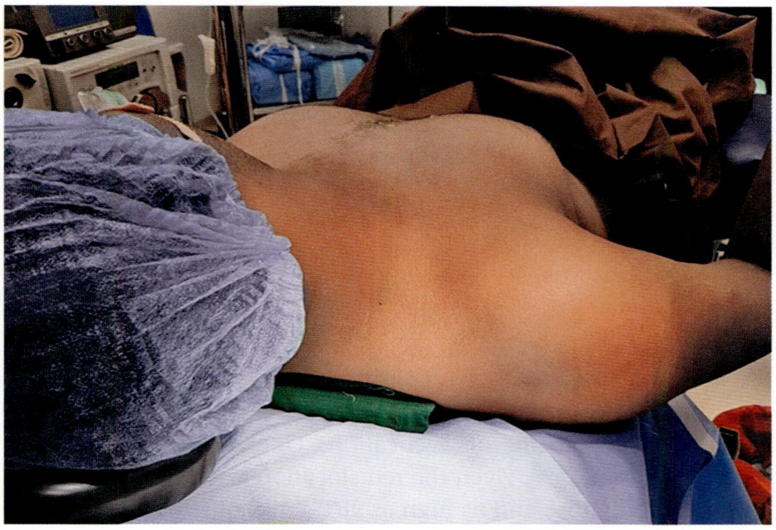

Fig. 2: A folded sheet or towel is placed in the interscapular area, which will make the coracoid more horizontal and easily approachable from the medial aspect for osteotomizing with an osteotome. Further improvements to coracoid access can be obtained by tilting the table laterally during surgery.

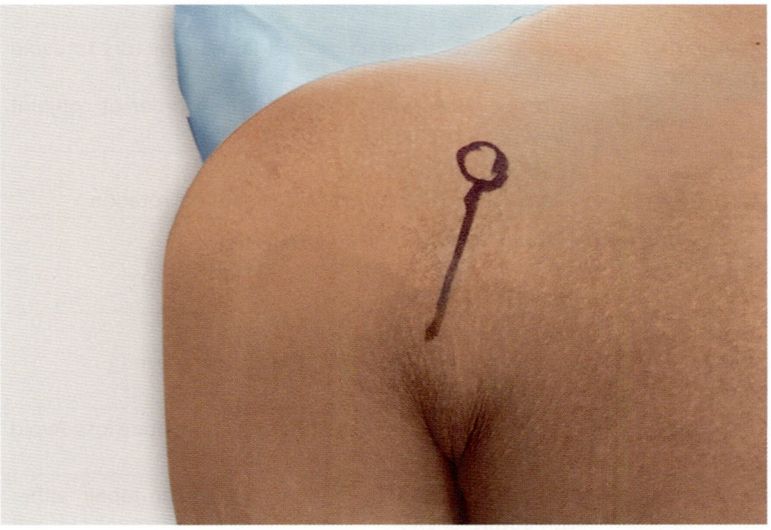

Fig. 3: Incision: A 5–6 cm deltopectoral incision is made from the tip of coracoid toward the axillary fold.

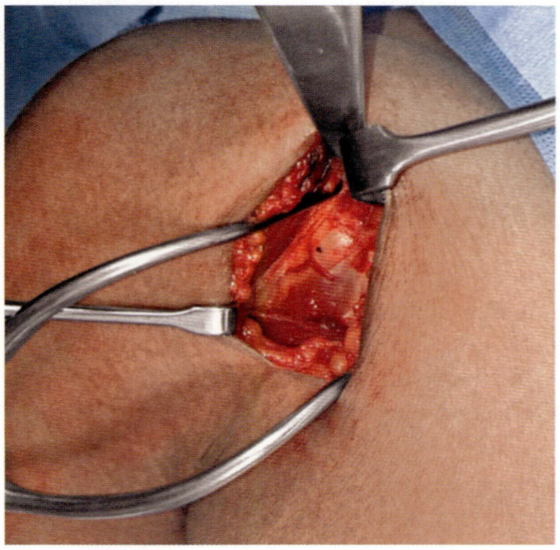

Fig. 4: The cephalic vein is identified in the deltopectoral interval and since most of its tributaries are lateral, it is retracted laterally to avoid bleeding. A Gelpi retractor is used to retract the deltopectoral interval.

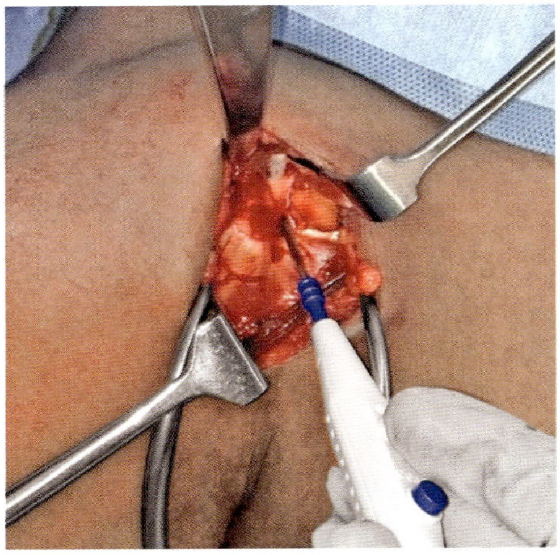

Fig. 5: The clavipectoral fascia is cleared to expose the conjoint tendon and the coracoid. The pectoralis minor is erased from the medial surface of the coracoid. The cautery should be always on the bone and dissection or exposure around the medial border of conjoint tendon is not necessary and is avoided to protect musculocutaneous nerve.

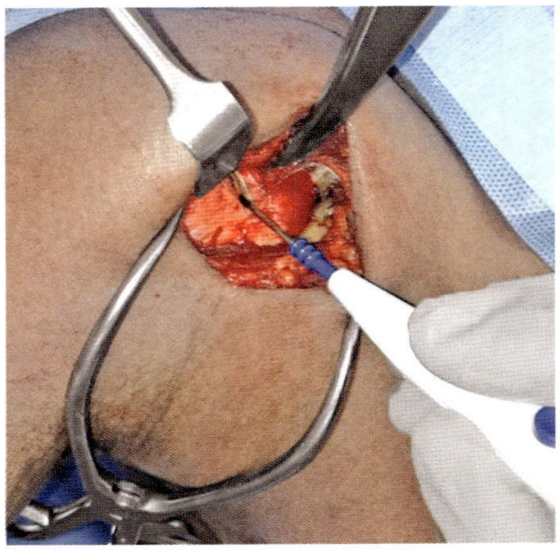

Fig. 6: The arm is now abducted to relax the deltoid and a Darrach's retractor or a large Hohmann retractor is inserted under the deltoid into the subacromial space. The coracohumeral ligament, lateral to the conjoint tendon is released and continuing upward, the coracoacromial ligament is identified and is released close to coracoid. Alternatively, a 1 cm cuff of CA ligament can be left attached to the coracoid, (as shown in figure) which can then be used to suture the capsule at the end of the procedure.

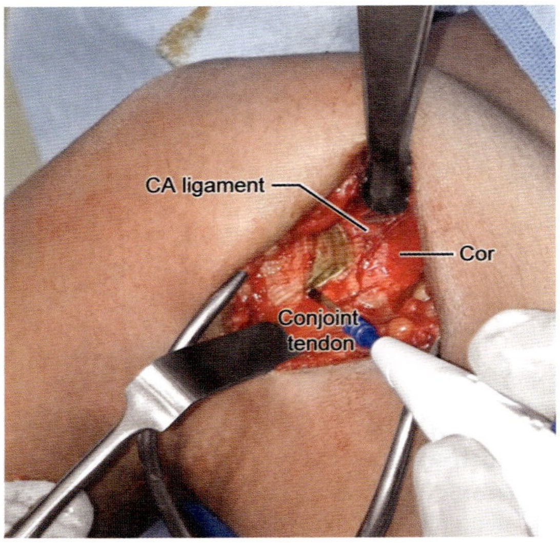

Fig. 7: The lateral margin of the conjoint tendon is exposed and the coracohumeral ligament is divided.

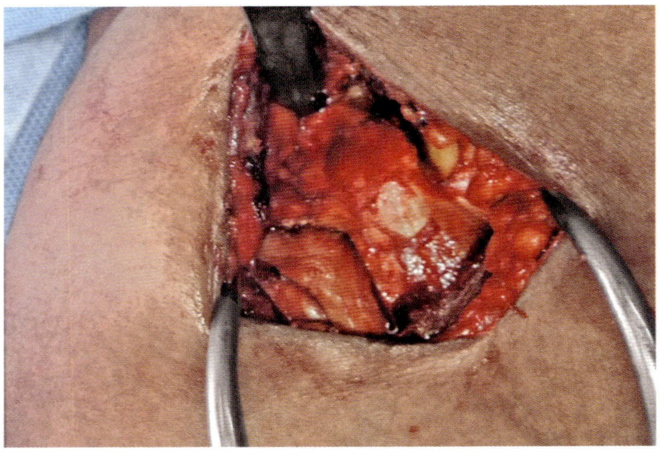

Fig. 8: Another Hohmann is inserted on the superior aspect of coracoid to expose the full profile of coracoid. A mark is made at 2 cm from the tip of coracoid with cautery. Now one should be able to place the curved osteotome comfortably on the mark on the medial aspect of the coracoid just near its elbow. To improve approach, the OT table can be tilted laterally at this stage.

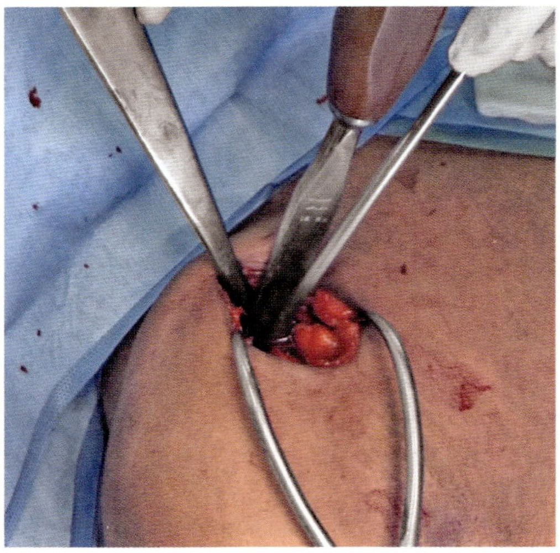

Fig. 9: The osteotome is advanced laterally with gentle firm taps to complete the osteotomy. The potential complications at this stage are splintering of the coracoid or propagation of fracture into the scapula.

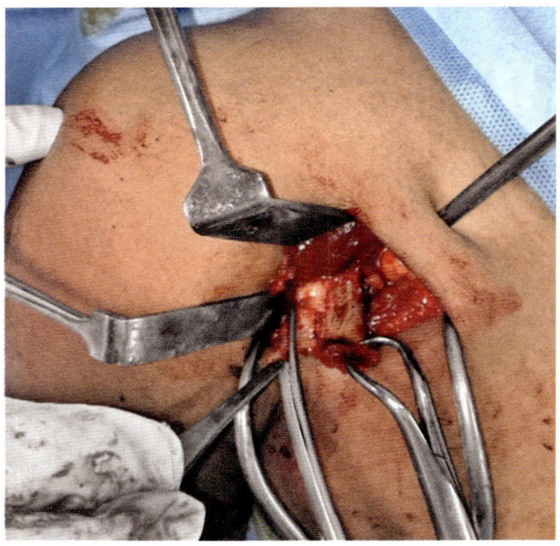

Fig. 10: The osteotomized coracoid is cleared from its bed, edges are trimmed with a nibbler, and gently mobilized (avoid dissecting and exposing around the medial border of conjoint tendon) so that the coracoid can just be delivered out of the skin incision.

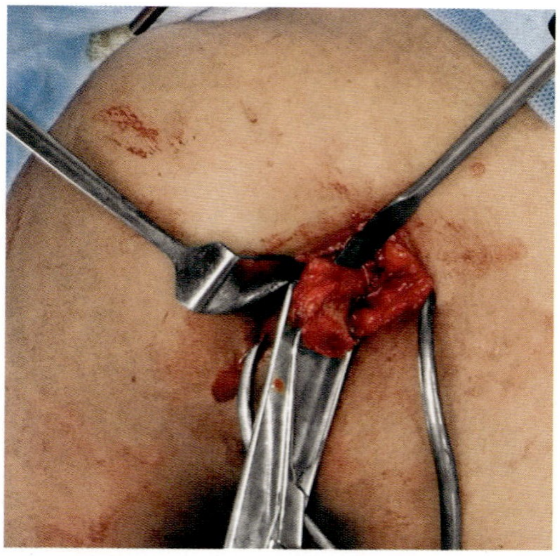

Fig. 11: The flipped coracoid, with its inferior surface facing anteriorly is held with a Kocher and placed on a flat osteotome.

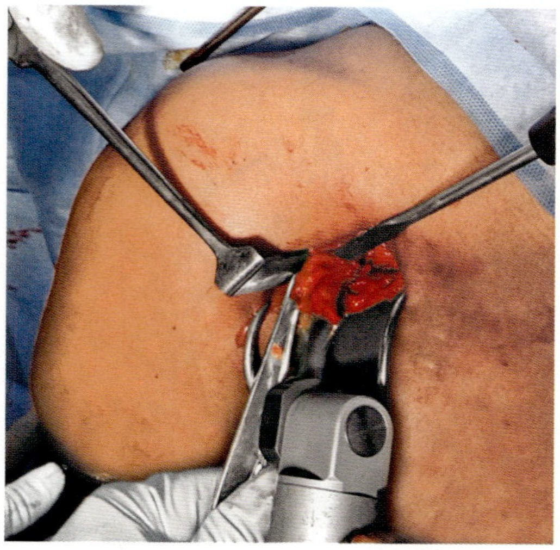

Fig. 12: An oscillating saw is used to decorticate the undersurface of the coracoid.

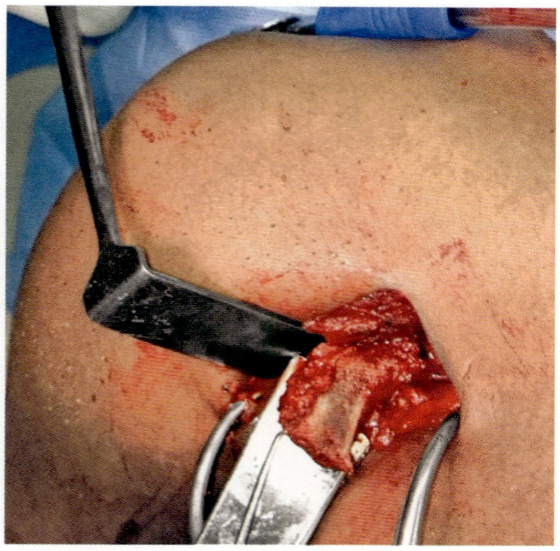

Fig. 13: The decorticated undersurface of coracoid.

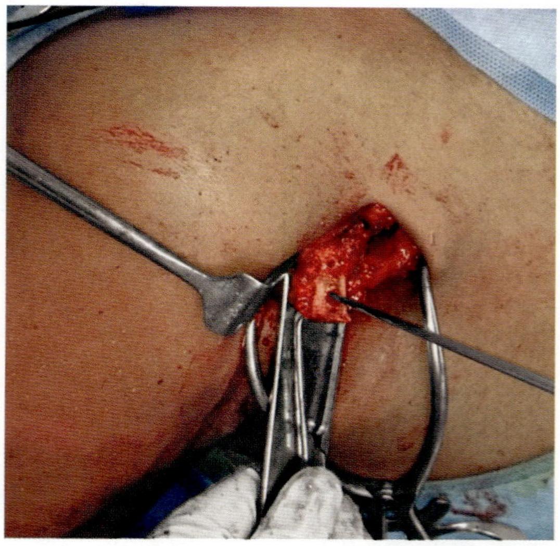

Fig. 14: After decorticating, two drill holes are made in the coracoid with 2.7 mm cannulated drill bits (if malleolar screws are used, 3.2 mm drill bits are used). The coracoid is pushed inferiorly out of the field.

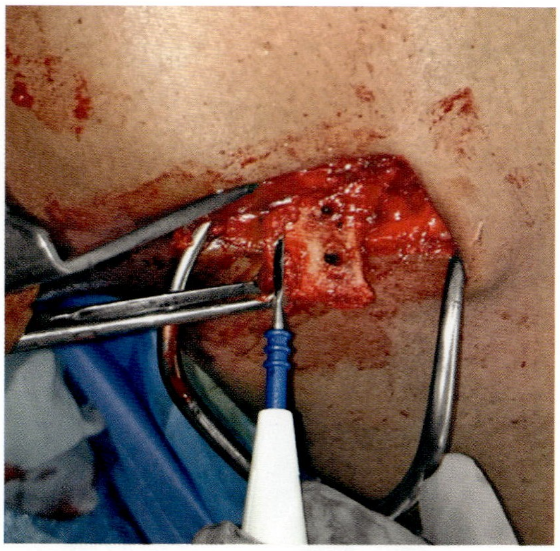

Fig. 15: The drill holes should be evenly spaced out (7–8 mm between the holes). The cuff of CA ligament still attached to the lateral border of coracoid can be seen here. The depth of the drill holes as well the distance of the lower hole from the lateral border and tip of coracoid is measured.

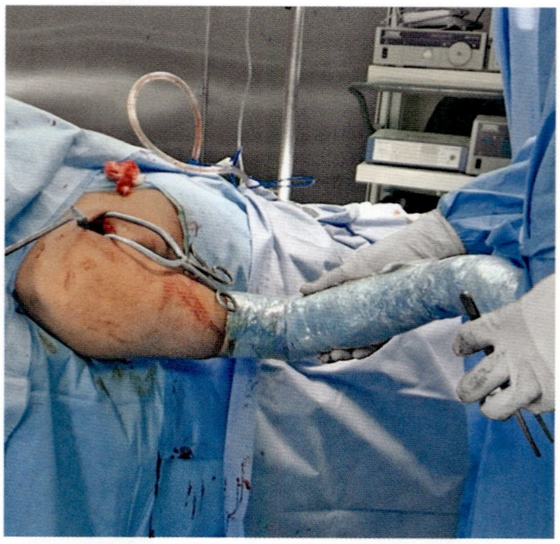

Fig. 16: Now, the arm is adducted and externally rotated. This maneuver brings the muscular portion of the subscapularis to the field, which is easier to split and expose the joint.

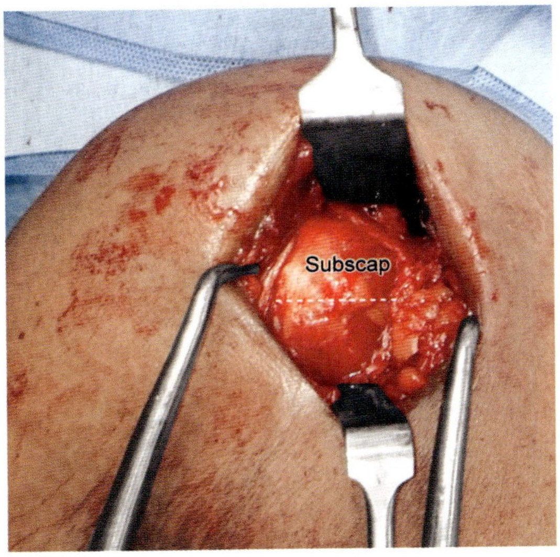

Fig. 17: The anterior aspect of subscapularis is cleared to expose the three veins ("three sisters"). The horizontal muscle split is done approximately between the upper two-thirds and lower one-third of the muscle.

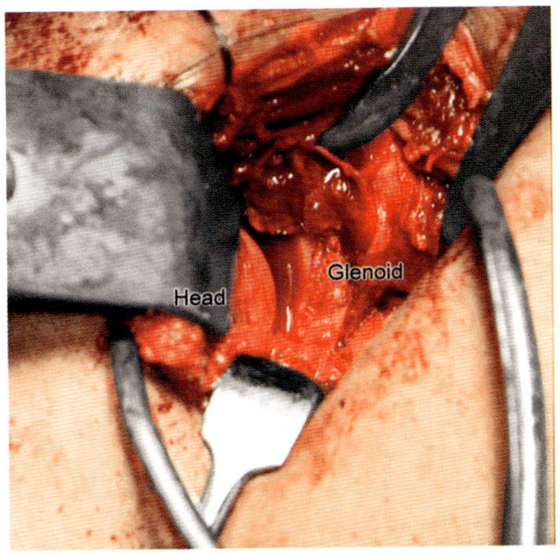

Fig. 18: Another Gelpi retractor is used to open up the subscapularis split and a Hohmann's retractor is placed in the subscapularis fossa (over the medial scapula) and another narrow Hohmann retractor under the lower subscapularis and over the inferior glenoid. The superior subscapularis can be retracted by a retractor and held with 3 mm Steinmann pin.

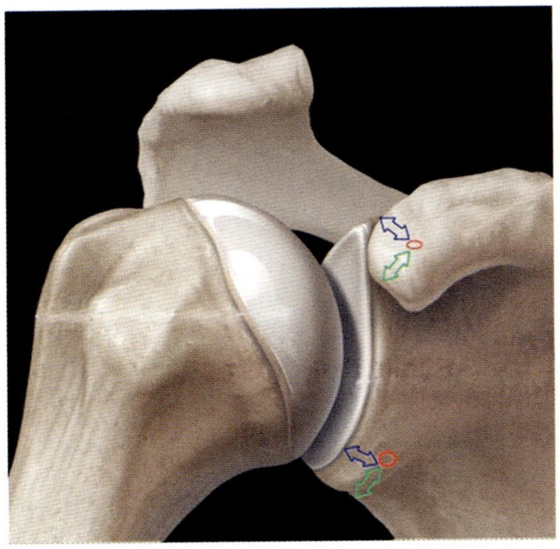

Fig. 19: The starting point for the lower hole on the glenoid is chosen corresponding to the distance of the lower hole in the coracoid from its lateral border and from the tip.

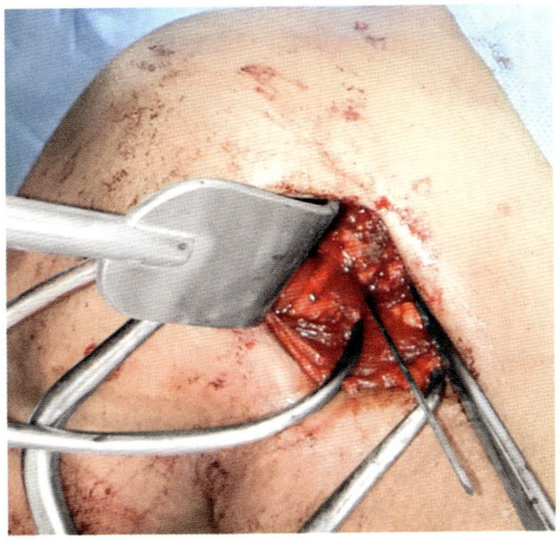

Fig. 20: Guidewire for a cannulated drill.

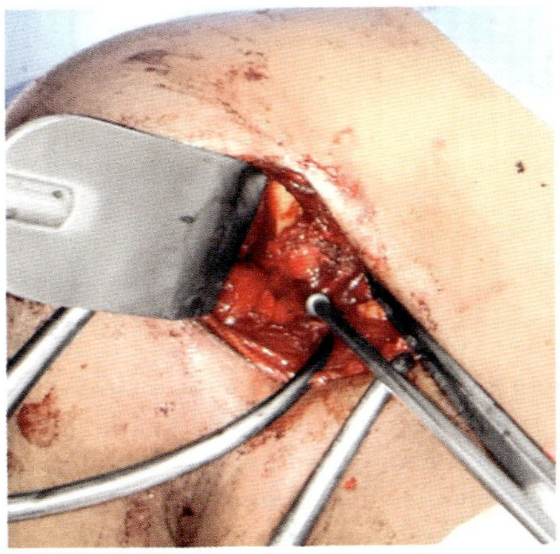

Fig. 21: The coracoid is positioned on the inferior glenoid neck and the guidewire is passed across the holes and a titanium 3.75 mm (Arthrex) screw is being inserted. Alternatively, a 4.5-mm malleolar screw can also be used with a 3.2 mm drilling. In that case, the coracoid is tapped, the screw is fully inserted in the coracoid and the tip is engaged in the hole, and the coracoid is slowly pushed against the glenoid as the screw is being tightened. Before tightening, the glenoid is positioned in such a way that its lateral border is in line with the articular margin or 2–3 mm medially. Overhang should be avoided.

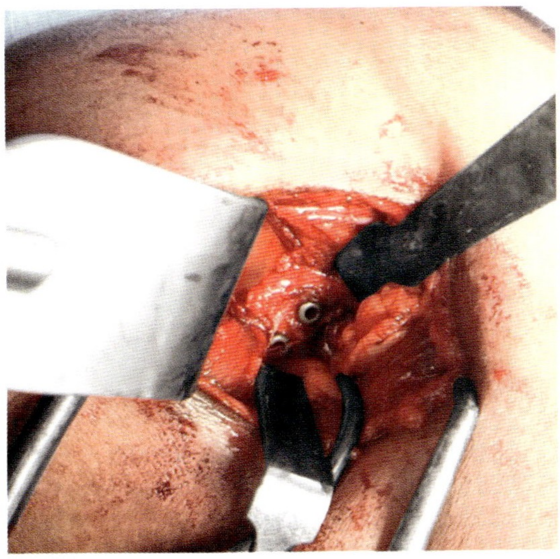

Fig. 22: After positioning the coracoid, the superior drill hole is made in the glenoid through the superior hole in the coracoid and appropriate sized screw is inserted. Overtightening should be avoided and a two-finger technique should be used to tighten. Any overhanging of graft at this stage can be smoothened with an oscillating saw.

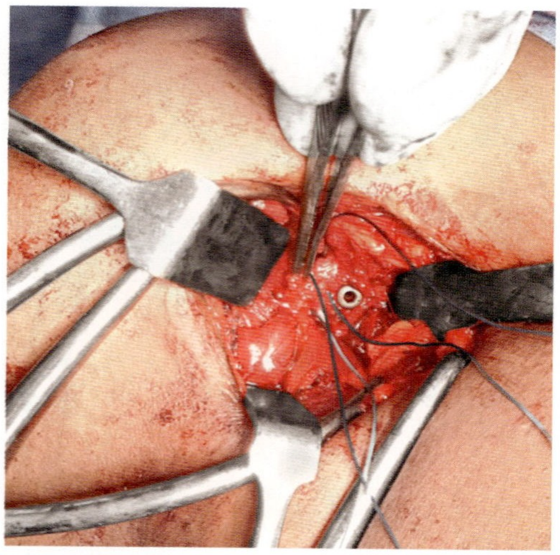

Fig. 23: A Bankart repair can be done at this stage. The capsulolabral tissue can be either sutured to the CA ligament cuff (as in this case) or repaired to the glenoid rim with suture anchors.

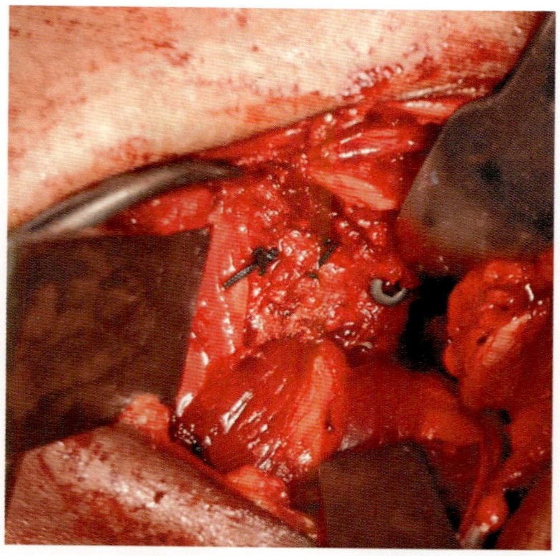

Fig. 24: The repair is done with the shoulder in maximum external rotation with arm by the side of the body to avoid loss of external rotation. The subscapularis is closed with few interrupted absorbable sutures and subcutaneous and skin layers are closed over a drain.

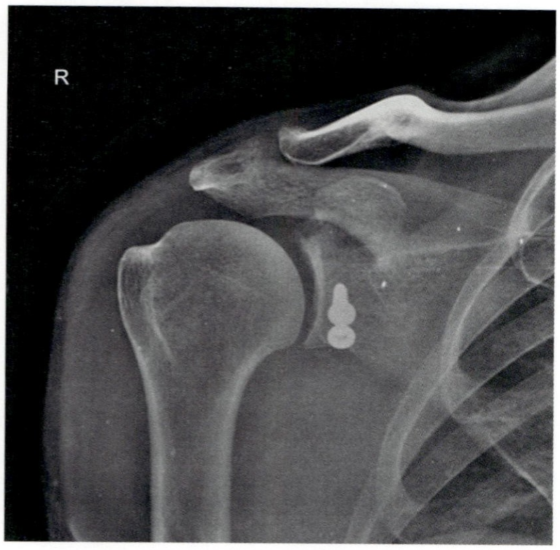

Fig. 25: Postoperative X-ray—anteroposterior (AP) view.

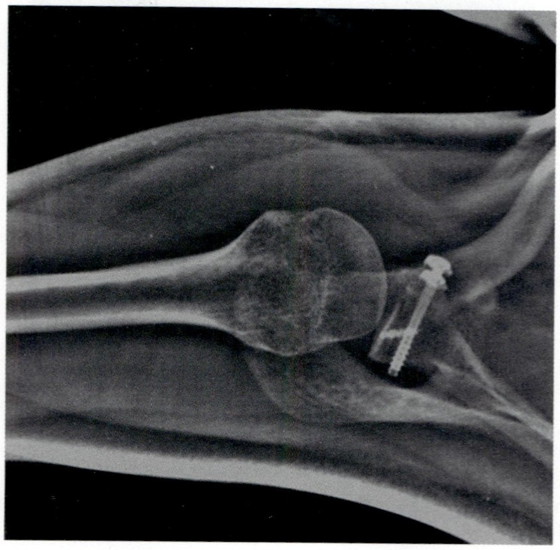

Fig. 26: Postoperative X-ray: Axillary view.

POSTOPERATIVE PROTOCOL

- Sling for a week
- Allow shoulder level activities as tolerated by pain
- Gradual overhead movements after 6 weeks.

SUGGESTED READING

1. Allain J, Goutallier D, Glorion C. Long-term results of the Latarjet procedure for the treatment of anterior instability of the shoulder. J Bone Joint Surg Am. 1998;80(6):841-52.
2. Burkhart SS, De Beer JF, Barth JR, et al. Results of modified Latarjet reconstruction in patients with anteroinferior instability and significant bone loss. Arthroscopy. 2007;23(10):1033-41.
3. Burkhart SS, De Beer JF. Traumatic glenohumeral bone defects and their relationship to failure of arthroscopic Bankart repairs: Significance of the inverted-pear glenoid and the humeral engaging Hill-Sachs lesion. Arthroscopy. 2000;16(7):677-94.
4. Gupta A, Delaney R, Petkin K, et al. Complications of the Latarjet procedure. Curr Rev Musculoskelet Med. 2015;8(1):59-66.
5. Latarjet M. Treatment of recurrent dislocation of the shoulder. Lyon Chir. 1954;49(8):994-7.
6. Shah AA, Butler RB, Romanowski J, et al. Short-term complications of the Latarjet procedure. J Bone Joint Surg Am. 2012;94(6):495-501.
7. Walch G, Boileau P. Latarjet-Bristow procedure for recurrent anterior instability. Tech Shoulder Elbow Surg. 2000;1(4):256-61.
8. Yang JS, Mazzocca AD, Cote MP, et al. Recurrent anterior shoulder instability with combined bone loss: treatment and results with the modified latarjet procedure. Am J Sports Med. 2016;44(4):922-32.

SECTION 3

SPINE

Section Editor: *Amol J Rege*

CHAPTER 20

Anterior Cervical Discectomy and Fusion

Rahul Chaudhari, Varun Rao, Nitish Agrawal

INTRODUCTION

Cervical radiculopathy results from compression and inflammation of a cervical nerve root at or near the neuroforamen through which it exits. The neural compression most commonly occurs due to cervical spondylosis and disc herniation. Cervical nerve roots 1–7 exit above the correspondingly numbered vertebrae and 8th nerve exits between C7 and T1.

PATHOANATOMY

Cervical disc herniation is the most common cause of acute radiculopathy. It has been classified as intraforaminal, posterolateral, and central. Intraforaminal is the most common variety which usually results into sensory symptoms, posterolateral causes motor weakness and central herniation causes myelopathy.

Classification of cervical disc:
- Foraminal
- Peracentral
- Central (Figs. 1A to C)

CLINICAL SYNDROME

Cervical nerve root pain usually starts from neck with radiation along the scapular, shoulder, and upper extremity region. It may be associated with sensory disturbances and motor weakness depending upon the nerve root compression (Table 1).

Other tests which elicit the nerve root compression are Spurling maneuver, Valsalva maneuver, compression test, and shoulder abduction relief sign.

INVESTIGATIONS

Radiographs X-rays

Radiographs usually consists of AP, lateral and right and left oblique X-rays to evaluate reduction in disc height, vertebral osteophytes. Foraminal stenosis can be judged on oblique X-rays. Also sometimes flexion extension lateral views are taken to evaluate instability.

Computed Tomography Scan

CT scan is required to understand the foraminal stenosis, disc calcification and posterior longitudinal ligament ossification. Computed tomography (CT) myelogram sometimes is indicated if magnetic resonance imaging (MRI) is contraindicated.

Magnetic Resonance Imaging

It is gold standard investigation to evaluate disc degeneration, nerve compression, and also to detect abnormal cord signals such as myelomalacia.

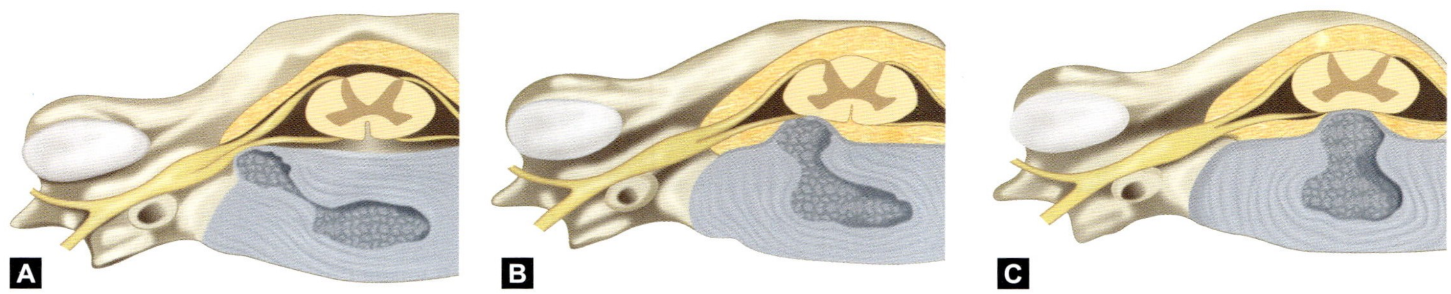

Figs. 1A to C: Types of soft cervical disc herniation. Type A: Infraforaminal herniation; Type B: Posterolateral herniation; Type C: Midline herniation

TABLE 1: Nerve roots and corresponding neurology.

Disc level	*Root*	*Pain*	*Sensory loss*	*Muscles affected*	*Reflex affected*
C3-C4	C4	Lower neck , Trapezius	Lower neck, upper part of shoulder	-	-
C4-C5	C5	Neck, shoulder, outer arm	Lateral arm	Deltoid, biceps	Biceps
C5-C6	C6	Neck, dorsal lateral arm, thumb	Lateral forearm, thumb	Biceps, wrist extension	Brachioradialis
C6-C7	C7	Neck, dorsal lateral forearm, middle finger	Dorsal forearm, middle finger	Triceps, wrist flexion	Triceps
C7-C8	C8	Neck, inner forearm, ulnar digits	Medial forearm, ulnar digits	Finger flexion	
C8-T1	T1	Inner forearm	Medial forearm	Finger intrinsics	

Electromyography

It helps in differentiating nerve entrapment syndrome from cervical radiculopathy.

TREATMENT OPTIONS

4 to 6 weeks of conservative management should be considered for patients of cervical radiculopathy without any neurodeficit or signs of myelopathy. Conservative treatment consists of rest analgesics anti-inflammatory and physical therapy such as interferential therapy (IFT), traction and sometimes cervical pain blocks can be considered. Most patients report significant improvement in few months time. Recent studies have shown that a longer duration of symptoms preoperatively corresponds to worse outcomes after surgery and it is therefore recommended 6 months as the cutoff for nonoperative management.

Here we describe anterior cervical decompression and fusion surgery:

- Position
- Level identification and incision marking with respect to anatomical landmarks
- Incision and exposure
- Anterior cervical retractor placement
- Neuro drill use and Caspar disc distractor placement
- Bone grafting or cage placement
- Plating
- Closure.

SURGICAL STEPS (FIGS. 2 TO 26)

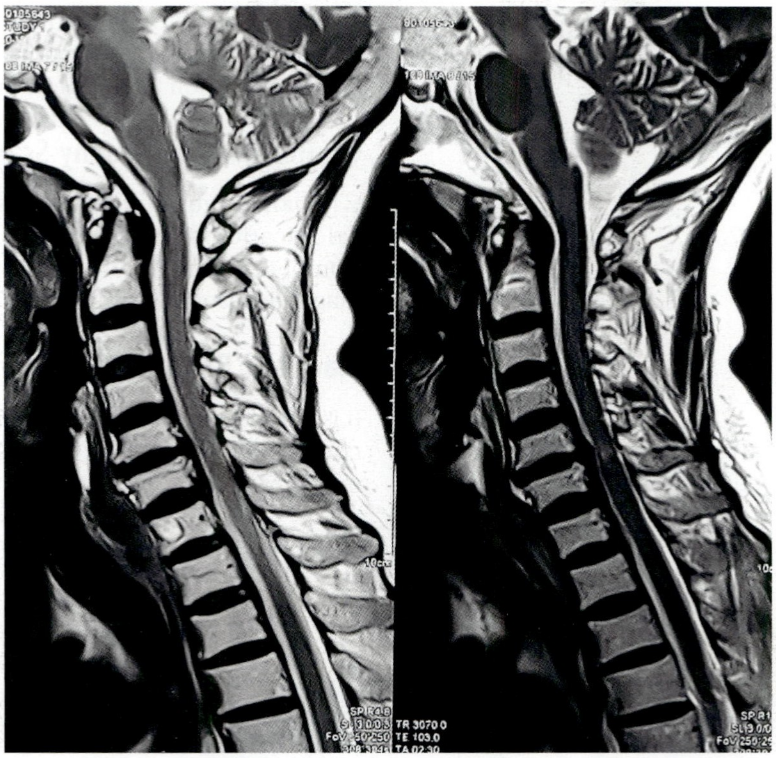

Fig. 2: A 60-year-old female present with 2 months history of right-sided upper limb radiculopathy with walking imbalance with hyper-reflexia in lower extremities. Patient has tried 2 months of conservative trial elsewhere with no relief. So patient has undergone anterior cervical discectomy with interbody spacer with bone graft with plating. Magnetic resonance imaging (MRI) cervical spine T2 sagittal view—C5-C6 and C6-C7 level with disc prolapsed compressing central and lateral recess and foraminal stenosis at C5-C6 and C6-C7 level.

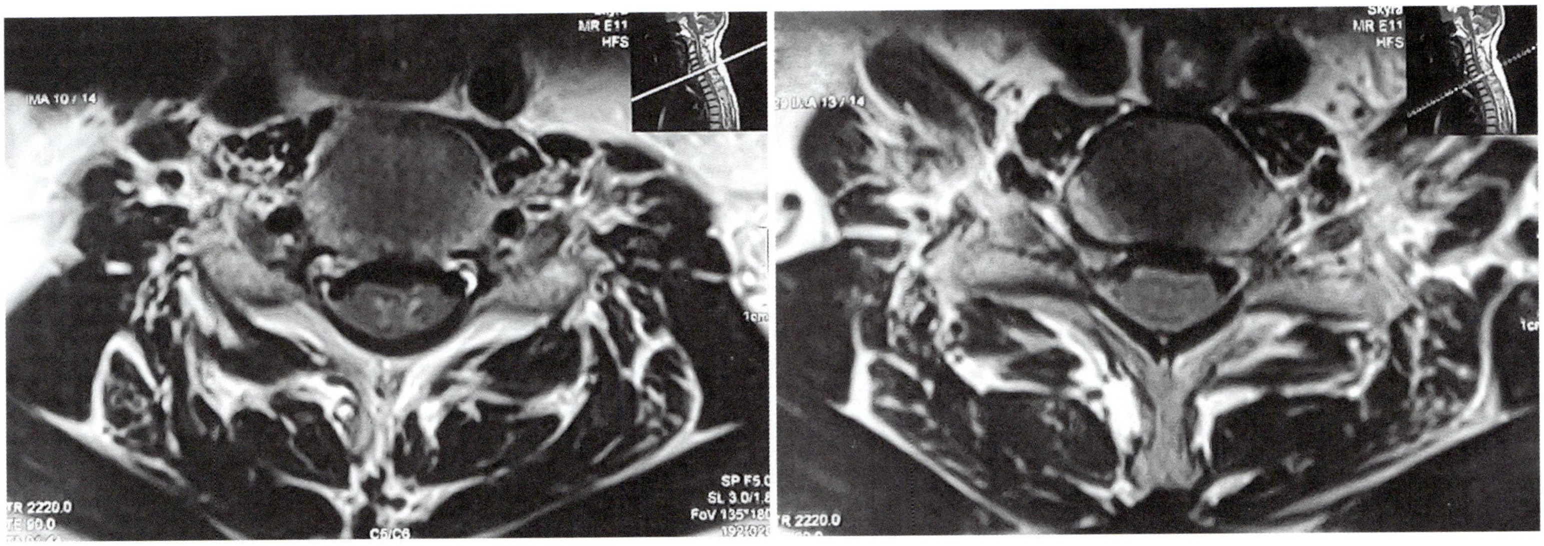

Fig. 3: Magnetic resonance imaging (MRI) cervical spine axial view.

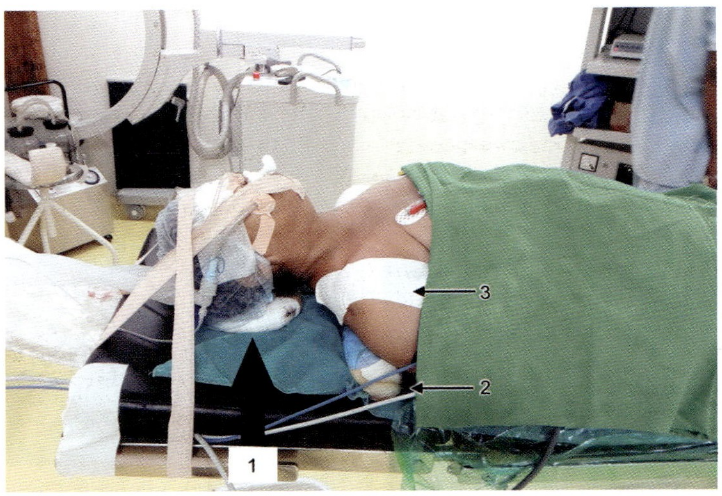

Fig. 4: Supine position (general anesthesia): (1) Head supported on head ring and fixed to the table, (2) Shoulder support given to keep the neck in extension, (3) Arms were pulled down and fixed to the table. Ryle's tube was inserted. Eyes were well padded.

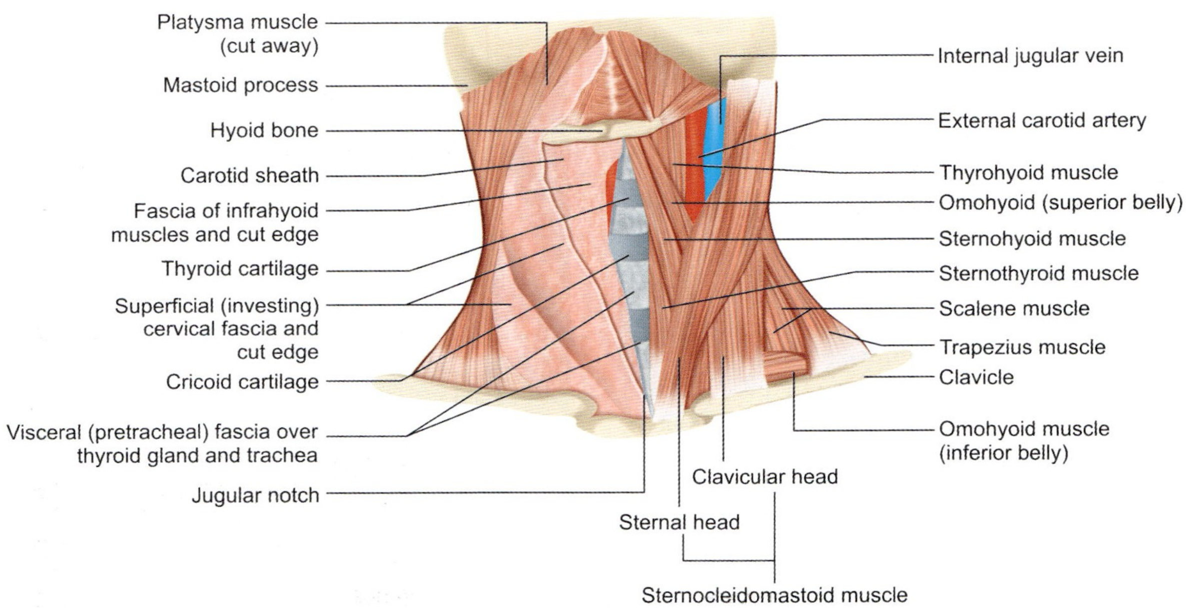

Fig. 5: Different anatomical landmarks for cervical vertebrae levels and anterior neck muscles along with fascia, carotid sheath, and carotid vessels:

- Angle of mandible—C2 level
- Hyoid bone—C3 level
- Thyroid cartilage—C5 level
- Cricoids cartilage—C6 level
- Manubrium—T3-4 level.

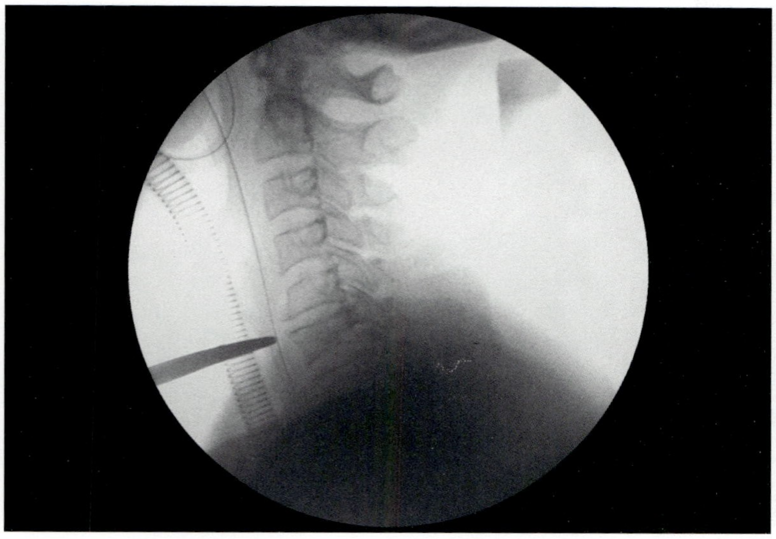

Fig. 6: C5-C6 level was identified under C-arm.

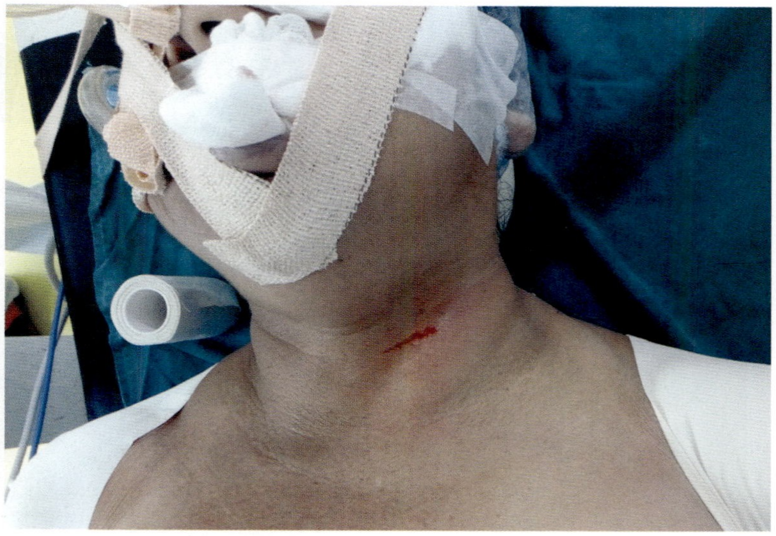

Fig. 7: Level was marked over on left side neck.

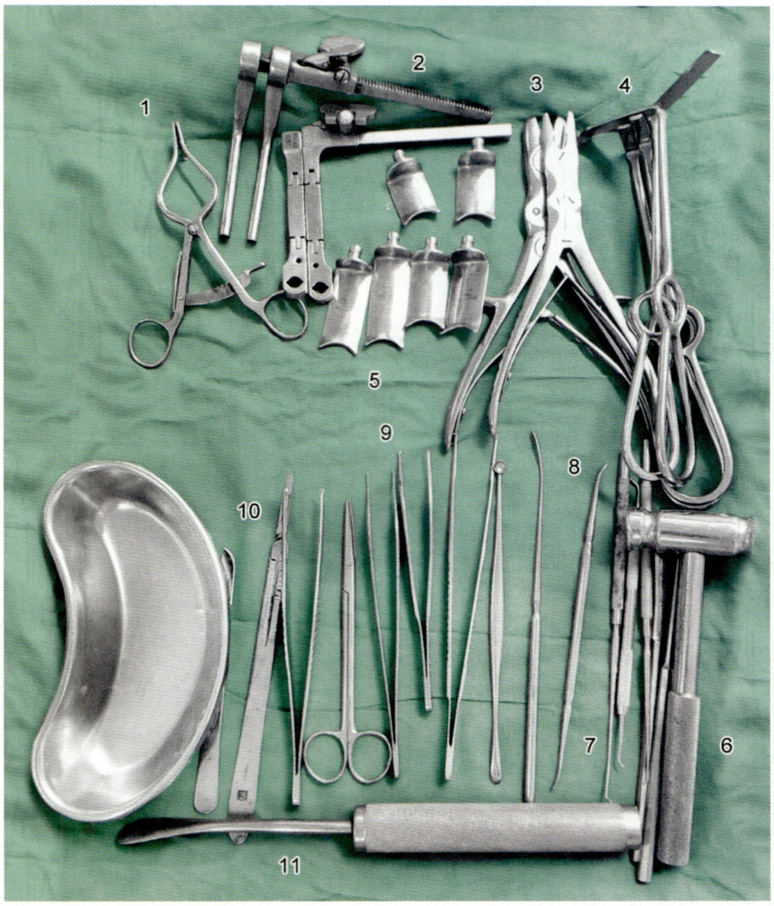

Fig. 8: (1) Self-retaining retractor, (2) Caspar distractor, (3) Bone Nibbler/ Rongeur, (4) right angle retractor, (5) anterior cervical retractor, (6) hammer, (7) ball tip nerve probe, (8) dural dissector, (9) tooth forceps, (10) Bard-Parker handle with blade, and (11) Cobb elevators.

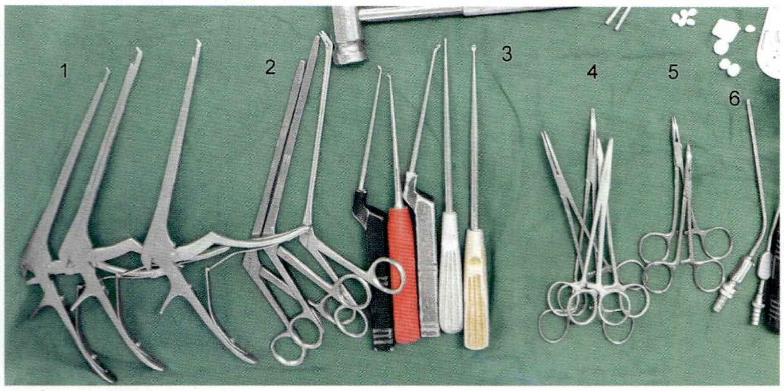

Fig. 9: (1) Kerrison punch, (2) disc forceps/tissue graspers with shark teeth, (3) curettes, (4) artery forceps, (5) mosquito forceps, and (6) suction tube.

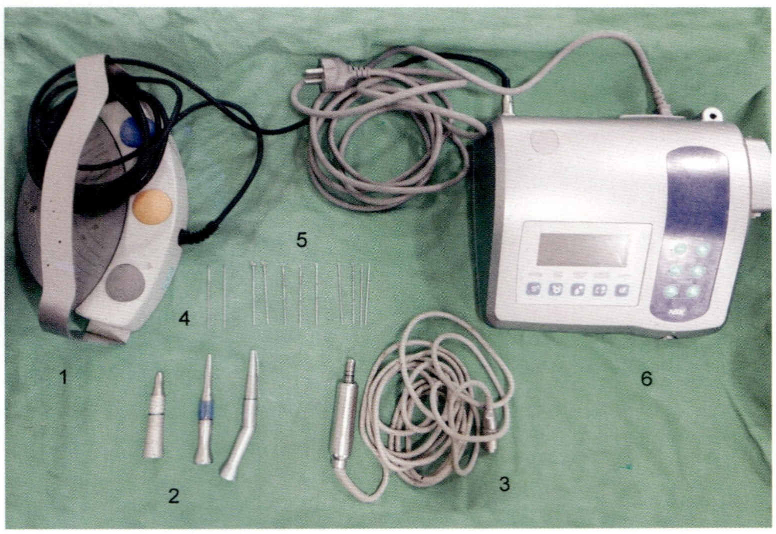

Fig. 10: (1) Foot switch, (2) hand piece, (3) shaft with cable, (4) diamond burr, (5) burr, and (6) advance torque control surgical system.

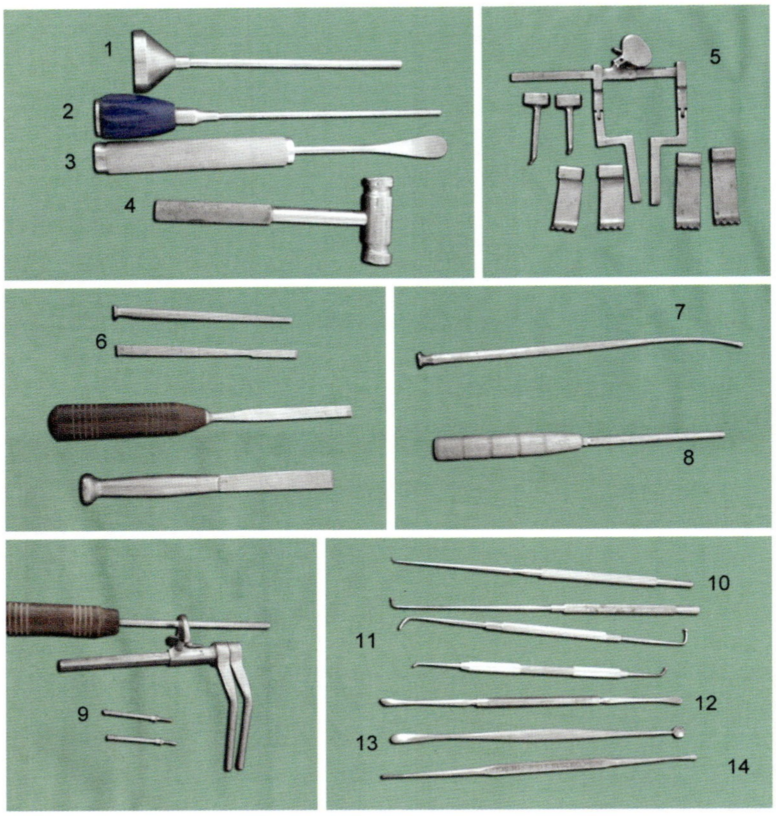

Fig. 11: Additional instruments required. (1) Bone graft funnel, (2) bone graft pusher, (3) Cobb elevators, (4) hammer, (5) anterior cervical retractor, (6) osteotome, (7) angled bone graft punch, (8) straight bone graft punch, (9) Caspar distractor, (10) bone hook, (11) ball tip nerve probe, (12) dural dissector, (13) curette with dural dissector, and (14) dural dissector.

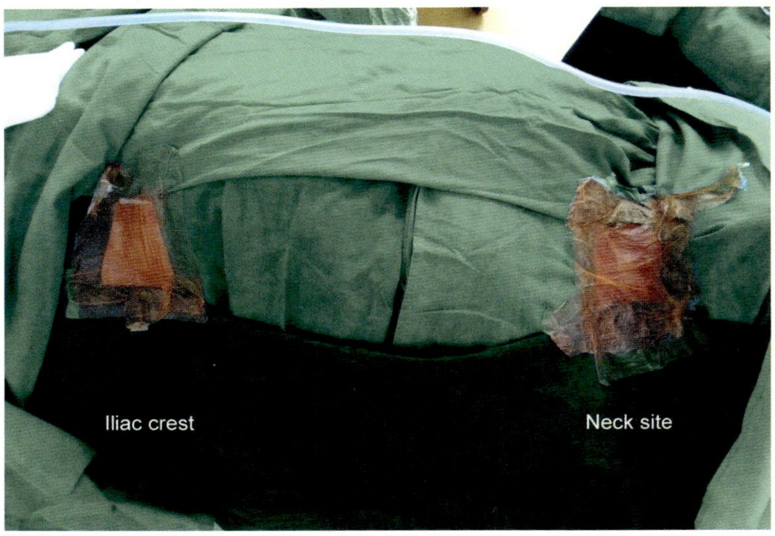

Fig. 12: Iliac crest graft site and neck site was prepped and draped.

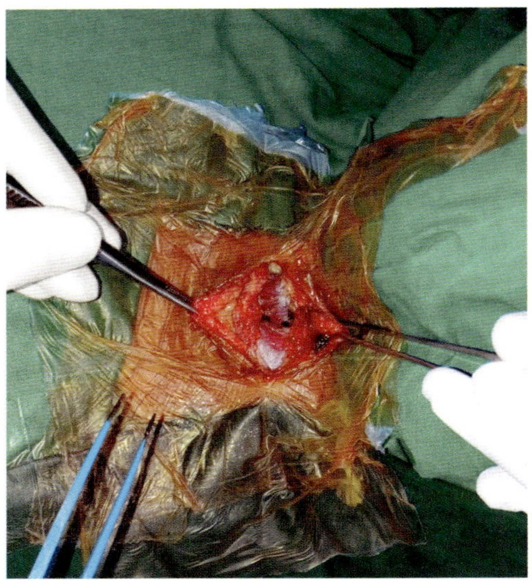

Fig. 13: Horizontal incision taken at cricoid level on left side of neck. Vertical incision can also be taken for multiple levels. Subcutaneous fat and fascia dissected with cautery. The platysma muscle is carefully cut in line with the incision to avoid cutting the large superficial veins just beneath it. Beneath the platysma muscle, the deep cervical fascia is identified and divided laterally to the anterior border of the sternocleidomastoid muscle, where it is dissected inferiorly and superiorly off of the muscle belly. Further dissection is done medial to the sternocleidomastoid. Feel for carotid pulse and always go medial to carotid pulse by finger blunt dissection done to reach prevertebral fascia. So eventually you have esophagus and trachea medially and carotid fascia covered with sternocleidomastoid muscle laterally.

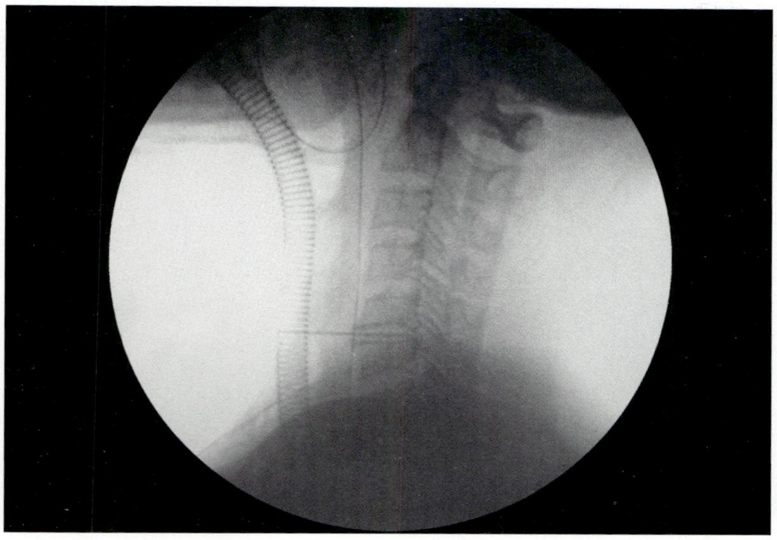

Fig. 14: C5-C6 and C6-C7 level was identified under C-arm on lateral view.

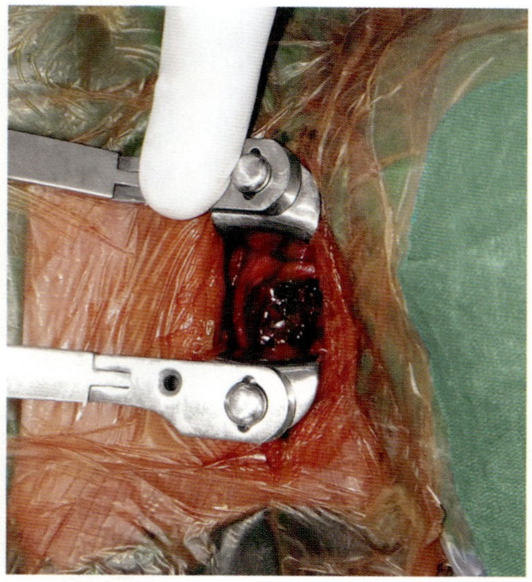

Fig. 15: Prevertebral fascia and longus colli muscle identified and longus colli muscle dissected from bone laterally and anterior cervical retractor protecting trachea and esophagus medially and protecting carotid fascia laterally.

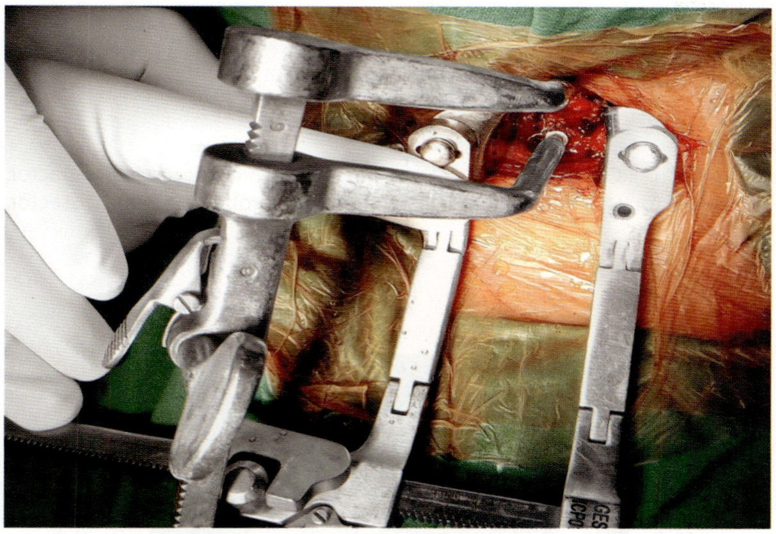

Fig. 16: Casper distractor was placed and the disc space distracted. Burr disc space between C5-C6 and C6-C7 level. Disc removed with curette and pituitary forceps and drilled to reach posterior border of upper and lower vertebral body.

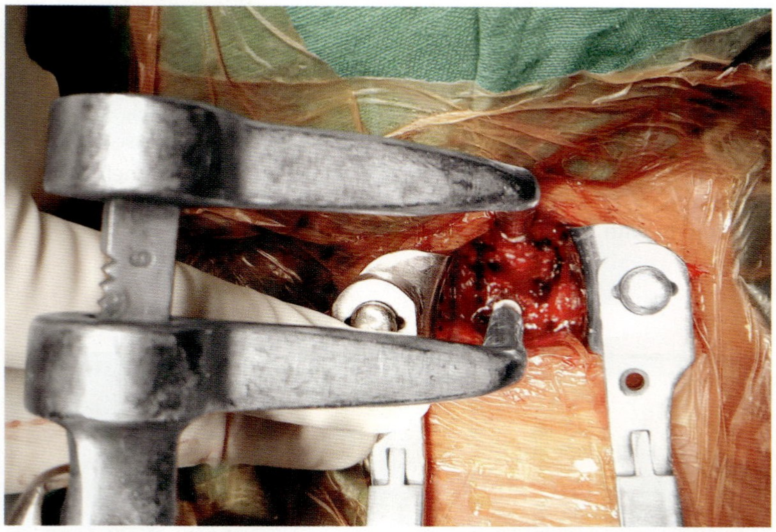

Fig. 17: Caspar distractor was further distracted so it helps to remove the posterior lips and osteophytes of upper and lower vertebral body with Kerrison punch. Thorough central and lateral recess decompression done and foraminal and nerve root area checked with 90° angled nerve root probe or hook to confirm adequate decompression or any remaining loose disc fragments.

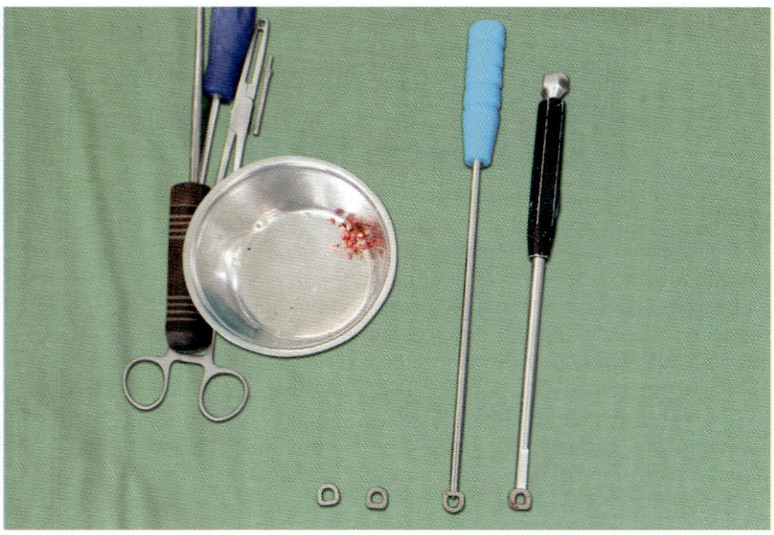

Fig. 18: Interbody spacer and autologous bone graft harvested from iliac crest.

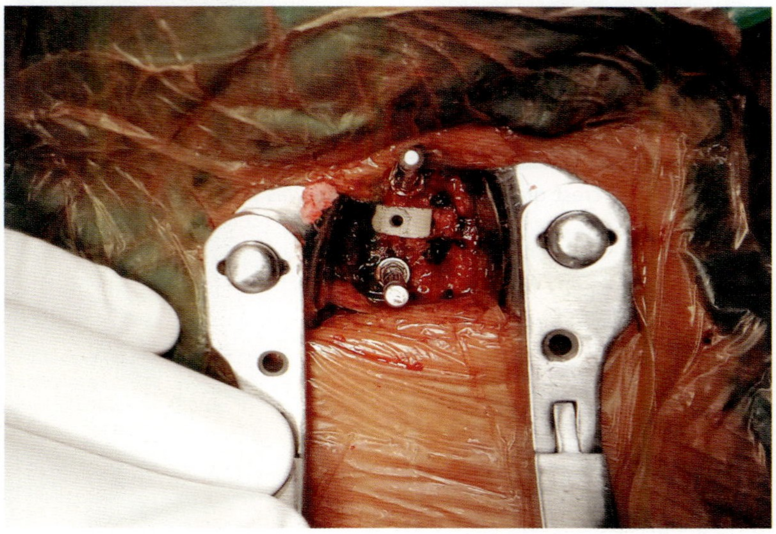

Fig. 19: The disc space is measured and an appropriately sized interbody spacer filled with autologous bone graft is placed in C5-C6 disc space.

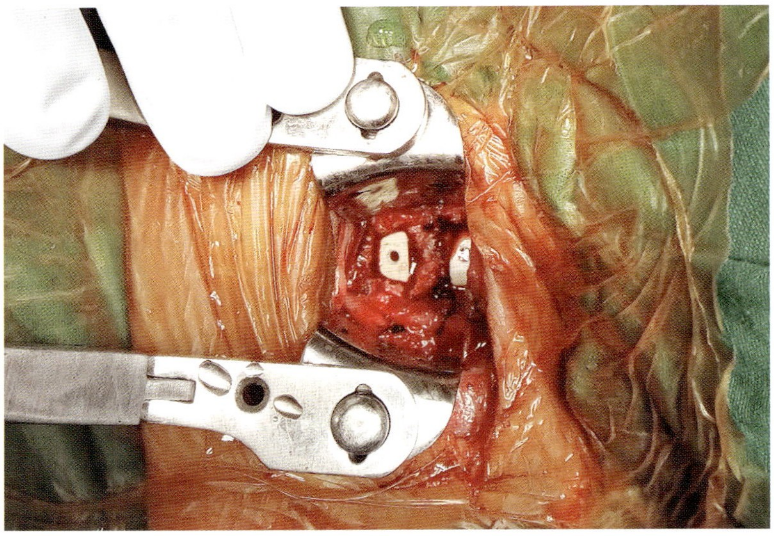

Fig. 20: Similarly disc space between C6-C7 is measured and an appropriately sized interbody spacer filled with autologous bone graft is placed in C6-C7 disc space.

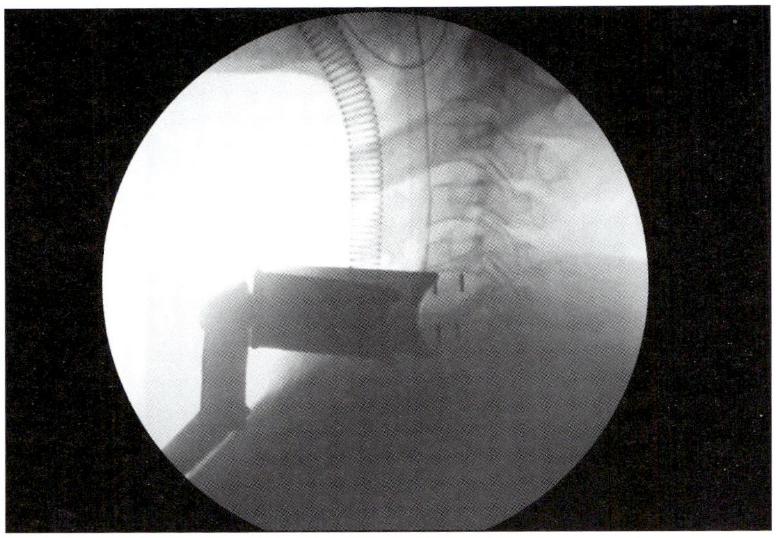

Fig. 21: Position of interbody spacer confirmed in C-arm by judging the radio-opaque markers.

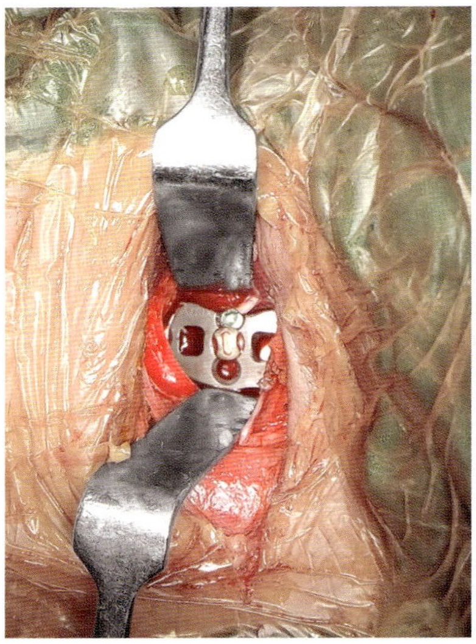

Fig. 22: An appropriate-sized plate is then chosen for fixation.

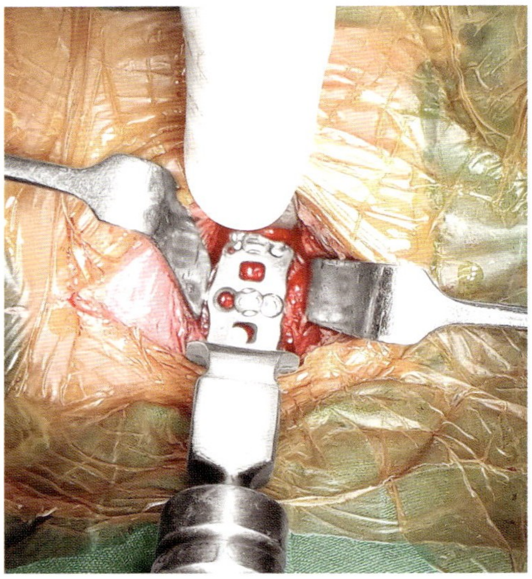

Fig. 23: Anterior cervical locking plate and screws (2 in C5, 1 in C6, and 2 in C7) fixation was done from C5 to C7. Care is taken when drilling screw holes to choose a length that will be contained in the vertebral body and be parallel with the endplate of the disc space.

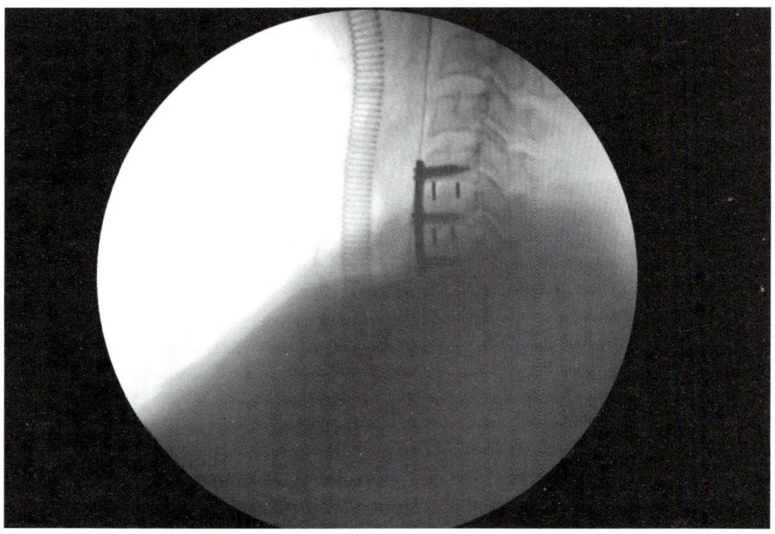

Fig. 24: Plate position and screw sizes confirmed in C-arm on lateral view.

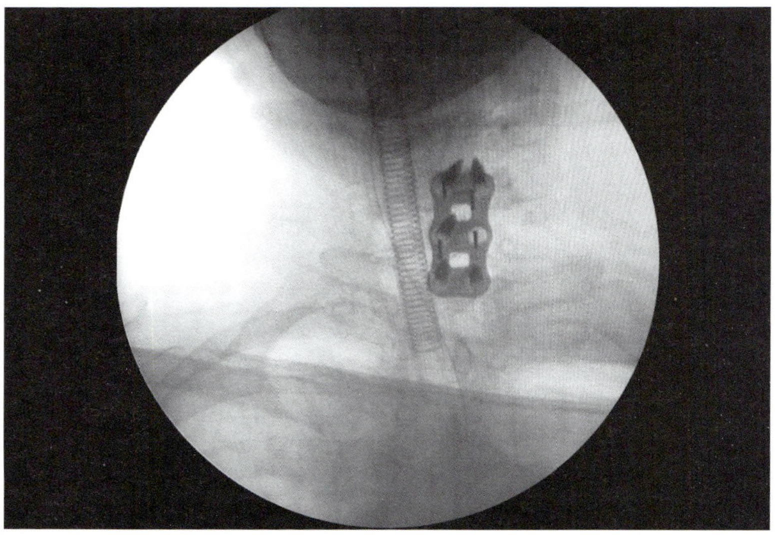

Fig. 25: Fixation confirmed over C-arm anteroposterior (AP) view.

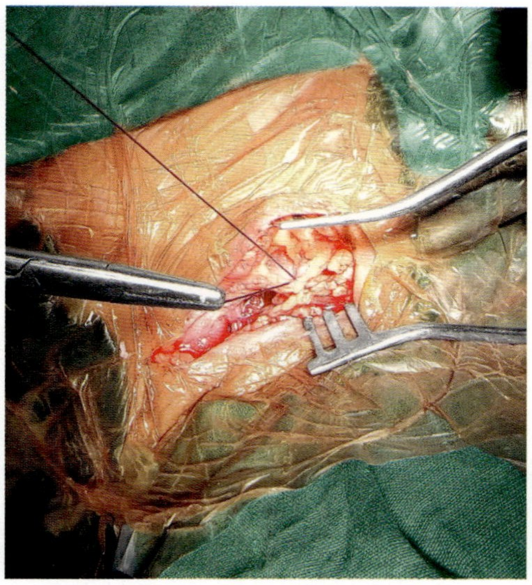

Fig. 26: Platysma and subcutaneous tissue are then closed with interrupted absorbable sutures. Skin suturing done (suction drain can be kept if required). Sterile dressing applied.

POSTOPERATIVE MANAGEMENT

- Neurological evaluation and limb movements checked immediately after extubation and Philadelphia collar was given.
- Patient was kept in intensive care unit (ICU) for observation. 30° propped-up position is given (to decrease swelling in the neck).
- Patient was kept NBM till coming morning.
- Routine IV antibiotics and analgesics were given.

Checklist

- Vitals, neurological status, urine output, and wound soakage if any.
- *Postoperative day 1*:
  - Patient was allowed to sit and oral fluids started on day 1.
  - Patient was given all four limb exercises.
- Oral food started on day 2 and patient was allowed to walk with support if comfortable.
- Urine catheter was removed on postoperative day 3 and patient was allowed to go to bathroom.
- Patient was shifted on oral medicines on day 3.
- Patient was counseled about dysphagia for next few days.

SUGGESTED READING

1. McAnany SJ, kim JS, Overly SC, et al. A meta-analysis of cervical foraminotomy: open versus minimally-invasive technically. Spine. 2015;15(5):849-56.
2. Miller LE, Block JE. Safety and effectiveness of bone allografts in anterior cervical discectomy and fusion surgery. Spine (Phila Pa 1976). 2011;36(24):2045-50.
3. Setton LA, Chen J. Mechanobiology of the intervertebral disc and relevance to disc degeneration. J Bone Joint Surg AM. 2006;88(Suppl 2):52-7.

CHAPTER 21

Cervical Laminectomy

Rahul Chaudhari, Sharad M Hardikar, Nitish Agrawal, Siddharth Hardikar

INTRODUCTION

Cervical spondylotic myelopathy is the most common cause of nontraumatic spastic paraparesis and quadriperesis. About 23.6% of patients presenting with nontraumatic myelopathic symptoms had cervical spondylotic myelopathy.

PATHOGENESIS

- Ligamentum flavum hypertrophy—static as well as dynamic compression of cord
- Encroaching of cervical spinal canal due to bulging disc, osteophytes formation from the vertebral body or uncovertebral joint and ligamentum flavum infolding
- Disc degeneration with disc bulge in spinal canal ossification of posterior longitudinal ligament
- Dynamic factors include abnormal forces on the spinal cord during loading and movement.

CLINICAL MANIFESTATION

- Loss of fine motor skills—fastening buttons or changes in handwriting
- Gait dysfunction or stiffness of the legs
- Neck stiffness and axial pain may be present.
- Loss of sphincter control or urinary symptoms—rare.

PHYSICAL EXAMINATION

Myelopathy is defined by the presence of long-tract findings.

- Deep tendon reflexes—hyperreflexia.
- Increased muscle tone
- Clonus
- Presence of Babinski sign—a slow tonic dorsiflexion of the great toe with fanning of the lesser toes
- Hoffmann sign—positive
- Inverted radial reflex
- Finger escape sign.

IMAGING STUDIES

- Plain radiography gives information related to sagittal balance, deformity, fractures, congenital abnormalities, and instability. Flexion/extension X-rays are used to diagnose instability in segments that may be a cause of motion-induced pain.
- CT myelography is currently the best overall single investigation for cervical spine disorders
- Magnetic resonance imaging (MRI) is a noninvasive and radiation-free procedure
- MRI is excellent imaging to see neural elements and intrinsic cord disease
- Deformation of the dura can be seen on T2 weighted images using movement artifact suppression techniques (MAST)
- Electromyography (EMG) can help diagnose cervical radiculopathy, cervical spondylotic myelopathy.

TREATMENT

Medical Care

- Neck immobilization
- Neck immobilization with a cervical collar
- Nonsteroidal anti-inflammatory drugs (NSAIDs)—reducing inflammation and pain
- Muscle relaxants
- Steroids for severe radiculopathy
- Gabapentin controlling neuropathic pain
- Lifestyle modification and workplace modifications.

Physiotherapy

Heat, ultrasound, and intermittent cervical traction.

Operative Treatment

Primary indications of operative treatment are as follows:

- Failure to pain management conservatively
- Increasing neurological deficit

- Cervical myelopathy that is likely to progress
  - Determined by the position and type of lesion
  - For soft central or hard disc anterior cervical discectomy and fusion is done and for soft lateral disc posteriorly foraminotomy is done.
  - Anterior, posterior, and lateral approach.

Anterior Approach

Anterior approach, cervical discectomy, and interbody fusion.
- The Robinson interbody fusion—tricortical iliac crest wedge
- Simmons technique keystone-shaped graft
- Bailey and Badgley.
- Anterior cervical corpectomy and fusion
- Microsurgical anterior foraminotomy
- Anterior plate fixation in degenerative conditions
- Lateral cervical fusion (Hodgson).

Posterior Approach

Advantages of posterior approach are as follows:
- Multiple levels easily addressed usually reserved for three or more levels
- No risk to vital anterior structures
- Less risk of neurological injury
- Can avoid fusion.

Disadvantages of posterior approach are as follows:
- Less effective in kyphosis as it relies on posterior cord "drift"
- Can result in kyphosis (10–50%)
- Increased pain from approach
- Dura exposed with possible peridural scar.

Laminectomy

Removal of the bony arches of the spinal canal (lamina) to decrease pressure on the spinal cord.
- Neck must be lordotic, or neutral
- Must avoid facet joint removal
- En bloc resection safest
- Beware postoperative palsy specially C5 due to posterior cord drift and resultant nerve root traction.

Complications of laminectomy are:
- Bleeding
- Infection
- Blood clots
- Never injury
- Spinal fluid leak
- Spinal cord injury
- Persistent pain.

Laminoplasty

- Bone not removed. Bones are spread open to widen the space.
- Provides effective canal decompression and neurological improvement.
- Avoids problems of postoperative kyphosis, stiffness from fusion and instrumentation and maintains cervical mobility.
- Not suitable for kyphotic neck because cord cannot fall away.
- For best results the procedure should be performed before cord changes develop.

SURGICAL STEPS (FIGS. 1 TO 18)

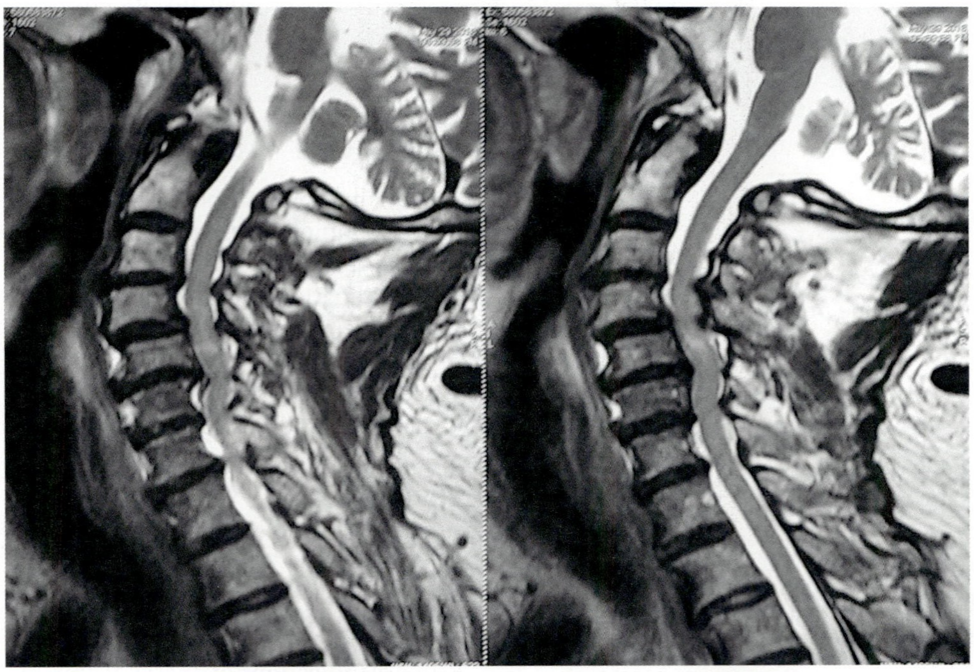

Fig. 1: T2 sagittal image of cervical magnetic resonance imaging (MRI) showing degenerative cervical spine with multilevel spinal stenosis with hypertrophy of ligamentum flavum at C4 and C5 level.

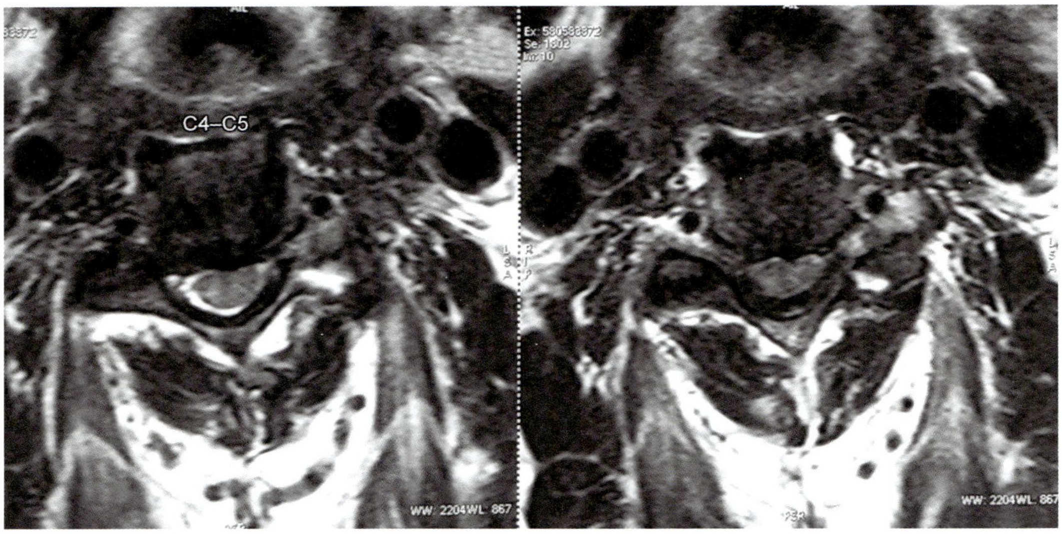

Fig. 2: T2 axial image of C4-C5 level.

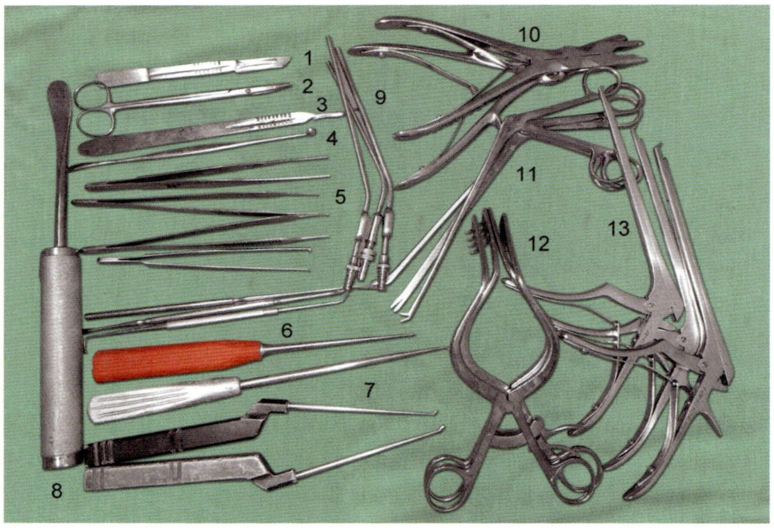

Fig. 3: (1) Knife blade no. 21, (2) dissecting scissors, (3) knife blade no. 15, (4) penfield dura retractor, (5) tissue forceps, (6) ball tip nerve probe, (7) curette, (8) Cobb elevators, (9) suction catheter, (10) Bone Nibbler/Rongeur, (11) disc forceps/tissue graspers with shark teeth, (12) self-retaining retractors, and (13) Kerrison punch.

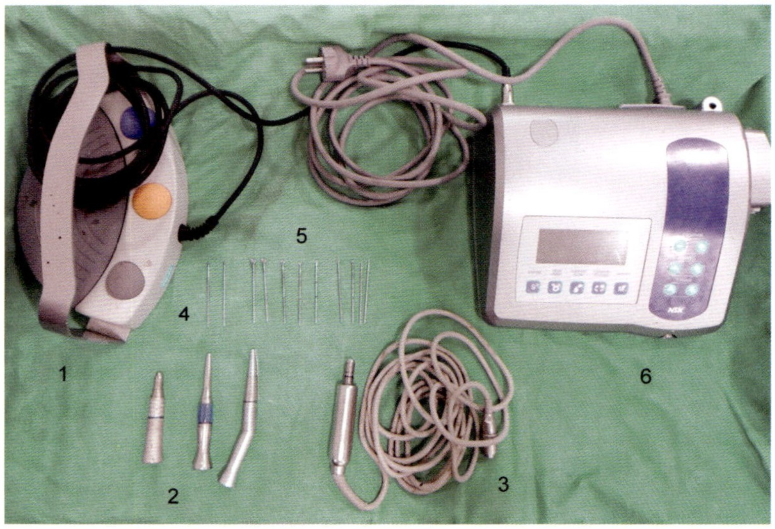

Fig. 4: (1) Foot switch, (2) hand piece, (3) shaft with cable, (4) diamond burr, (5) burr, and (6) advance torque control surgical system.

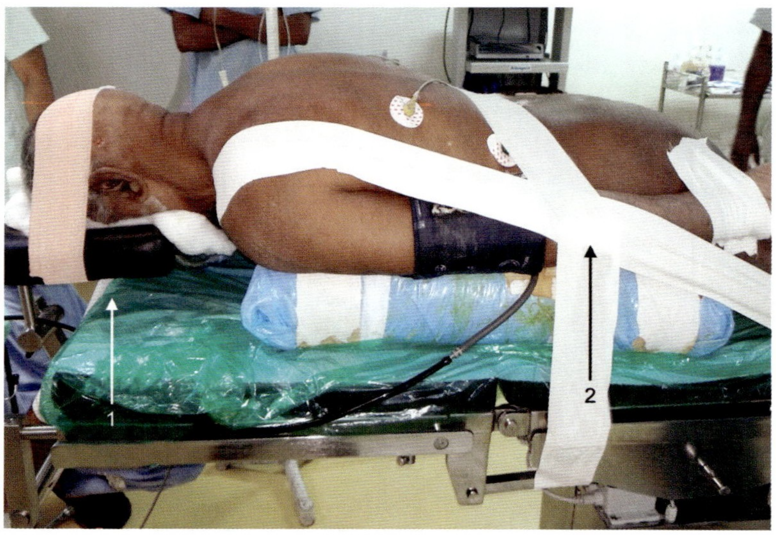

Fig. 5: Prone position. (1) Head rested on horseshoe shaped support and fixed with elastic adhesive strap. (2) Arms pull down and strapped to table. Eyes well padded.

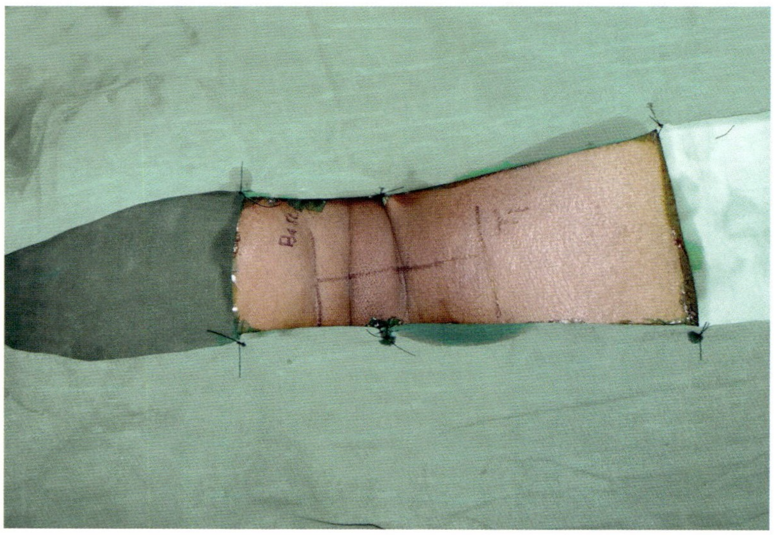

Fig. 6: Occipital protuberance and T1 spinous process marked.

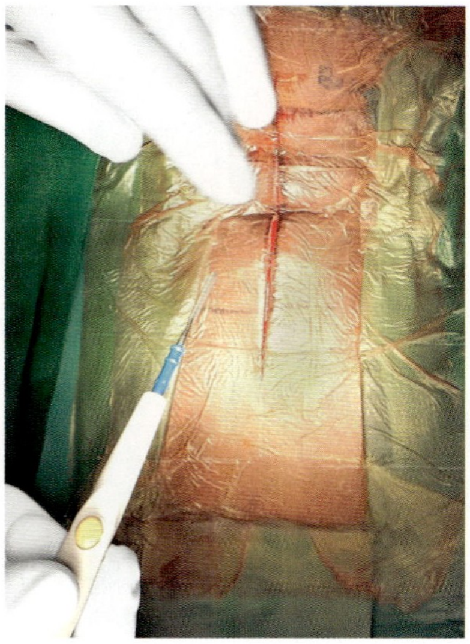

Fig. 7: After standard painting and draping, midline incision taken from C2-C7 level.

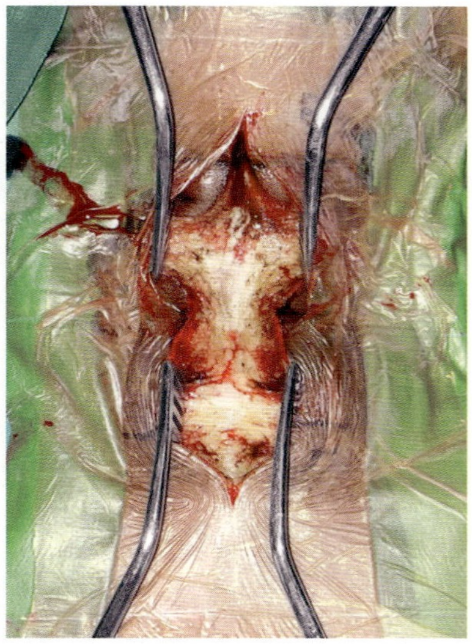

Fig. 8: Subcutaneous fat and fascia dissected with cautery and self-retaining retractor applied for proper exposure.

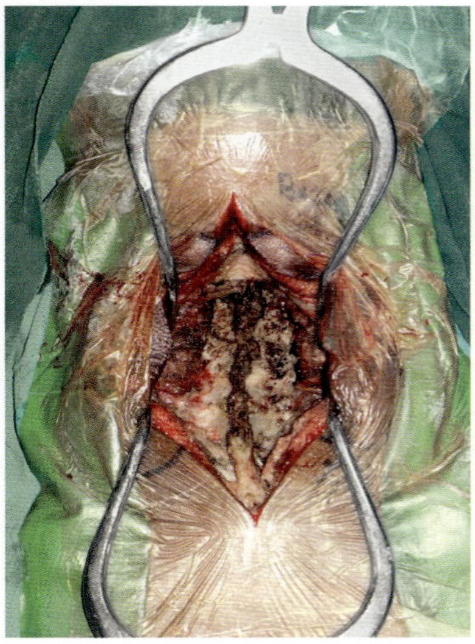

Fig. 9: Muscles detached subperiosteally with the help of cautery. One should not run the cautery in the muscle mass and all the dissection should strictly involve detachment of muscles from spinous process and lamina to avoid excessive bleeding. Spinous process and lamina from C2-C7 exposed with cautery.

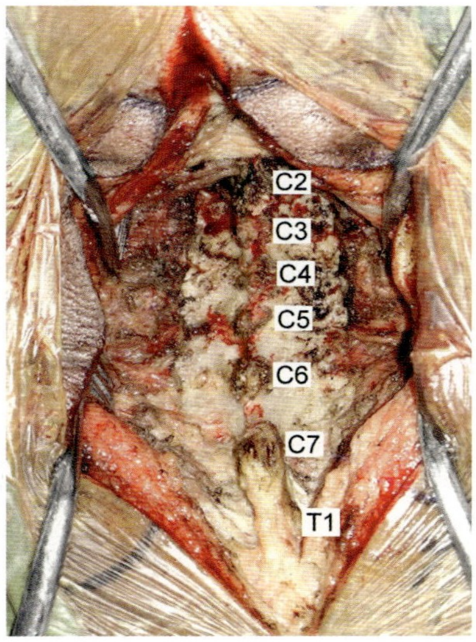

Fig. 10: Interspinous ligament removed from C2 to C7 level by Bone Nibbler.

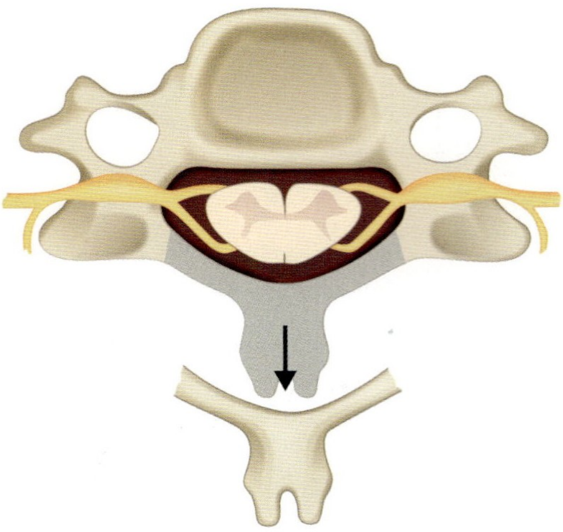

Fig. 11: Single vertebrae axial view showing removal of lamina, spinous process, and hypertrophied ligamentum flavum.

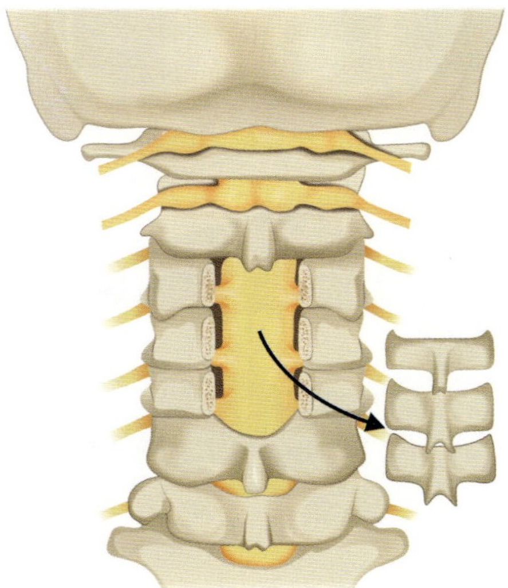

Fig. 12: Diagrammatic representation of cervical spine coronal view showing removal of lamina, spinous process, and hypertrophied ligamentum flavum. Care should be taken not to remove facet joints to preserve movements.

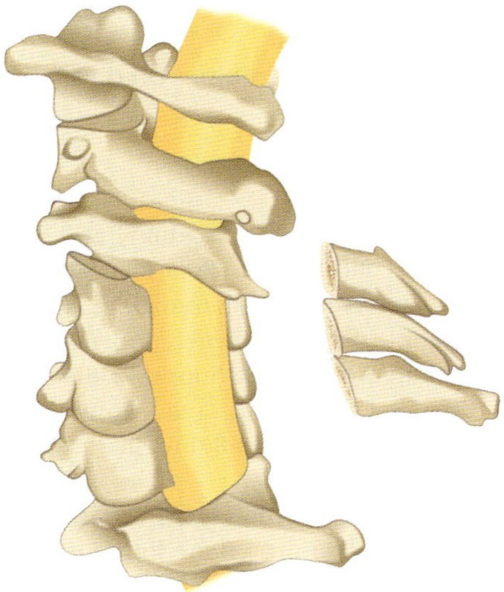

Fig. 13: Diagrammatic representation of cervical spine sagittal view showing removal of lamina, spinous process and hypertrophied ligamentum flavum. Care should be taken not to remove facet joints to preserve movements.

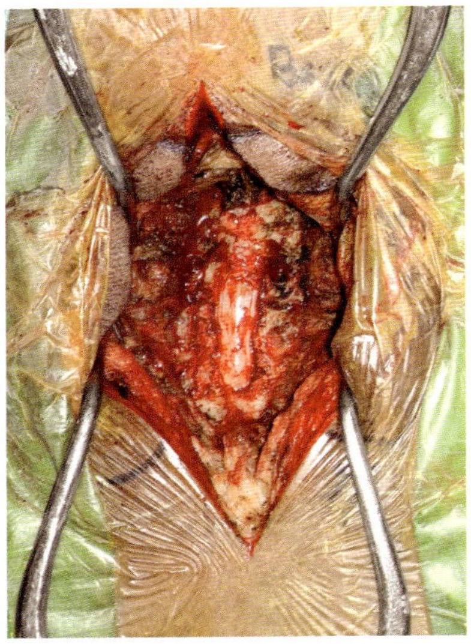

Fig. 14: Spinous process of C3, C4, C5, C6, and C7 removed with Bone Nibbler. Lamina and hypertrophied ligamentum flavum of C4, C5, C6, and C7 removed with burr drill and Kerrison punch.

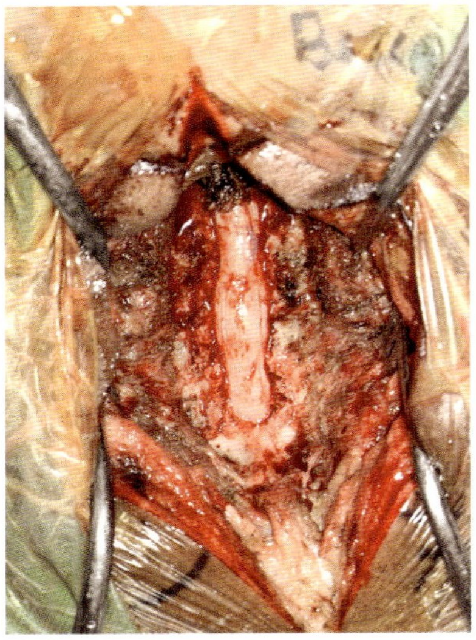

Fig. 15: Lamina of C3 also removed with burr and Kerrison punch. Wide decompression done till medial border of facet joint from C3 to C7 levels.

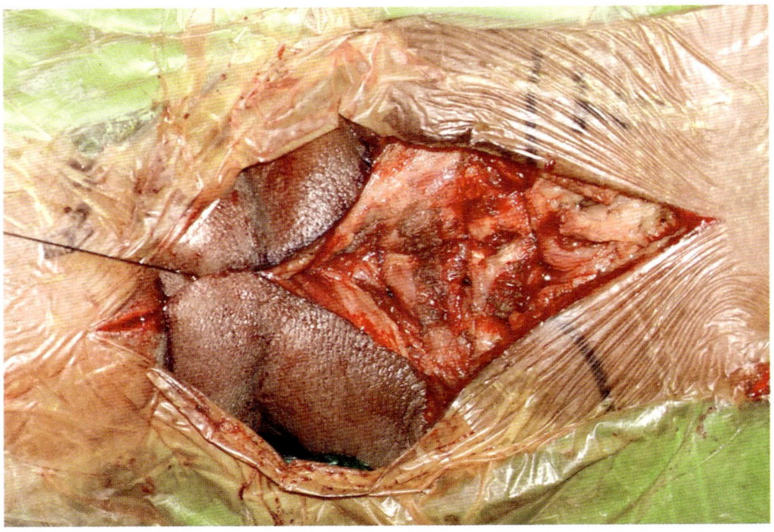

Fig. 16: Wash given with normal saline. Muscle layer loosely sutured and fascia layer tightly sutured with absorbable material over the suction drain.

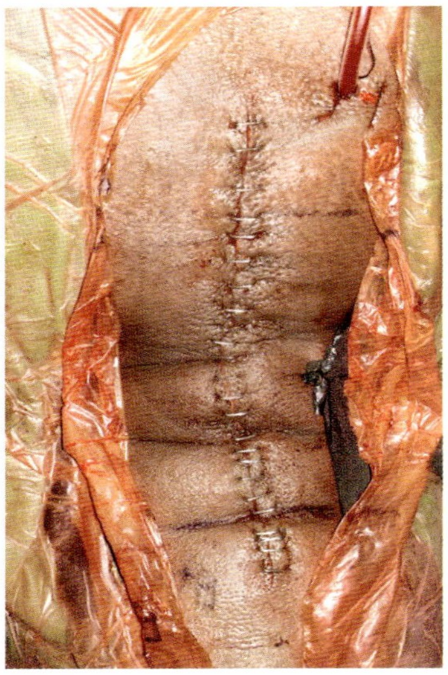

Fig. 17: Subcutaneous suturing done with absorbable material. Skin is sutured with staple sutures and suction drain fixed with absorbable suture material.

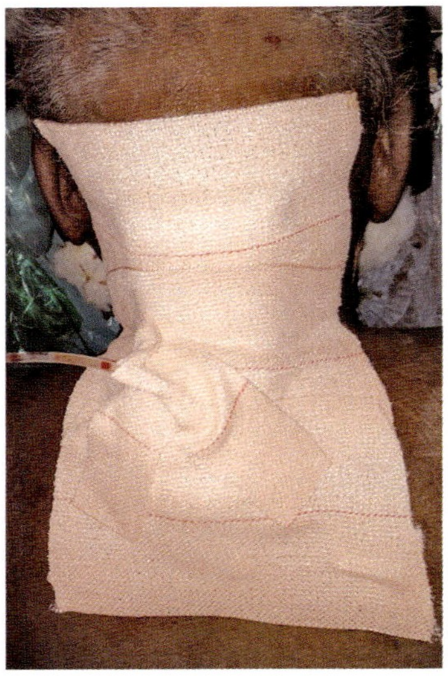

Fig. 18: Compression dressing given with elastic adhesive bandage.

POSTOPERATIVE MANAGEMENT

- Neurological evaluation and limb movements checked immediately after extubation and soft cervical collar was given.
- Patient was kept in intensive care unit (ICU) for observation in propped-up position.
- Oral food started after 6 hours.
- Routine intravenous (IV) antibiotics and analgesics were given.

Checklist

- Vitals, neurological status, drain output, urine output, and wound soakage if any.
  - *Postoperative day 1:*
  - Patient is allowed to sit and walk with support if comfortable
  - Patient was given all four limb exercises and chest physiotherapy with spirometer
- Drain was removed on day 3 (when drain output is less than 50 mL in last 24 hours)
- Urine catheter was removed on postoperative day 3 and patient was allowed to go to bathroom
- Patient was shifted on oral medicines on day 3.

SUGGESTED READING

1. Hadjipavlou AG, Tzermiadinos MN, Bogduk N, et al. The pathophysiology of disc degeneration: a critical review. J Bone Joint Surg. 2008;90(10):1261-70.
2. Lotz JC, Ulrich JA. Innervation, inflammation, and hypermobility may characteristics pathologist disc degeneration: review of animals modal data. J Bone Joint Surg Am. 2006;88 Supple 2:76-82.
3. McAnany SJ, Kim JS, Overley SC, et al. A meta-analysis of cervical foraminotomy: open versus minimally invasive technically. Spine J. 2015; 15:849-56.
4. Setton LA, Chen J. Mechanobiology of the intervertebral disc and relevance to disc degeneration. J Bone Joint Surg Am. 2006;88(Suppl 2):52-7.
5. Vernon-Robert B, Moore RJ, Fraser RD. The natural history histology of age-related disc degeneration: the influence of age and pathology on cell population in the L4-L5 disc. Spine (Phila Pa 1976). 2008;33(25):2767-73.

CHAPTER 22

Anterior Cervical Fixation and Fusion with Plate and Cage

Girish Bartakke, Shrinivas S Shintre, Chittanand Mendhe

SURGICAL STEPS (FIGS. 1 TO 21)

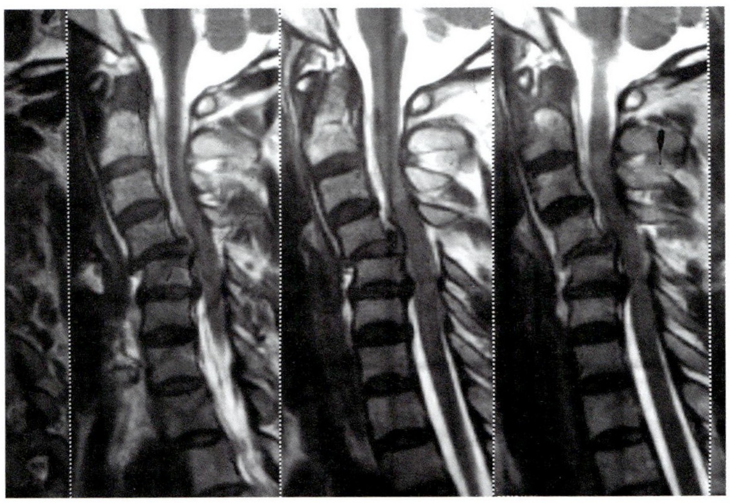

Fig. 1: MRI sagittal view showing C4-C5 anterolisthesis causing the compression over the spinal cord.

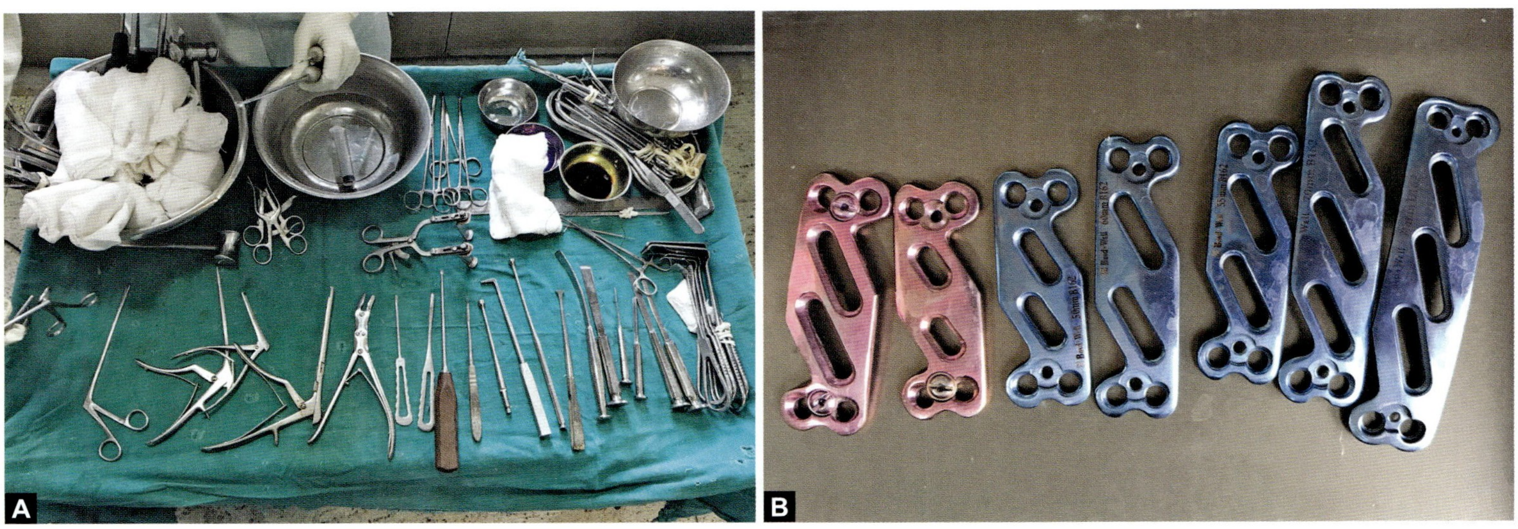

Figs. 2A and B: Trolly contains different sizes of Kerrison rongeurs, nibblers, osteotomes, self-retaining retractor general instruments and different sized anterior cervical plates.

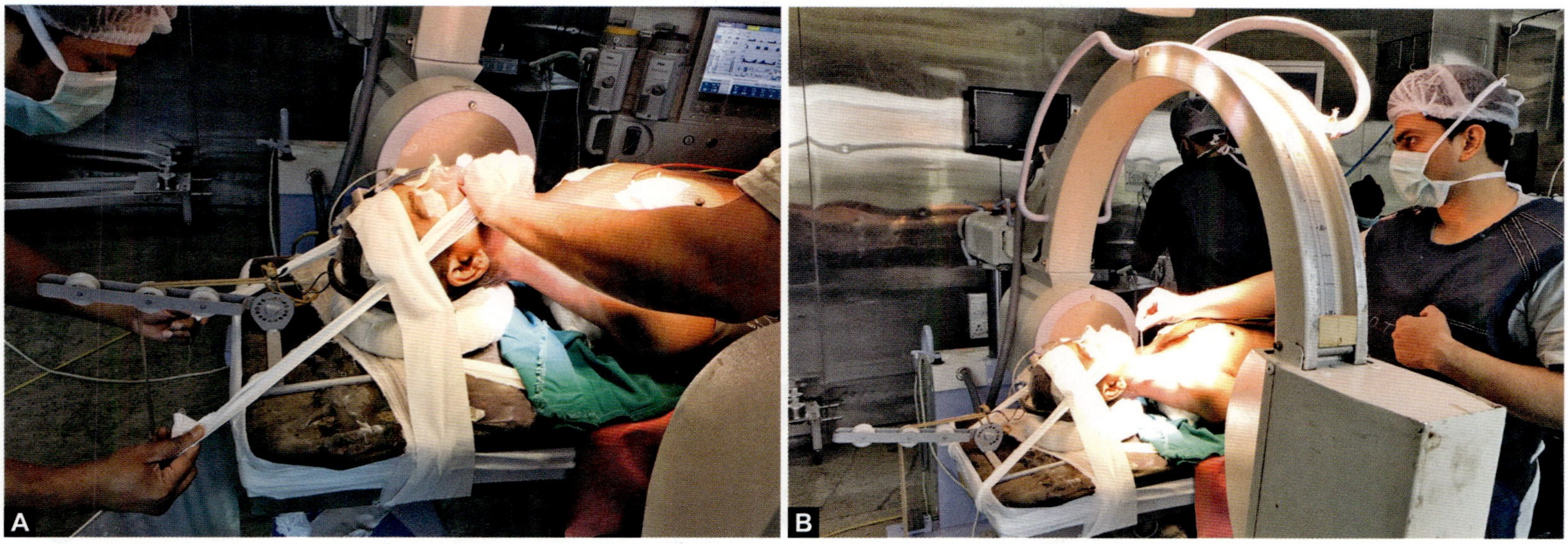

Figs. 3A and B: Position of patient supine with neck in extension and traction given through tongs. Position of C-arm lateral view to identify the vertebral position with the help of metallic rod.

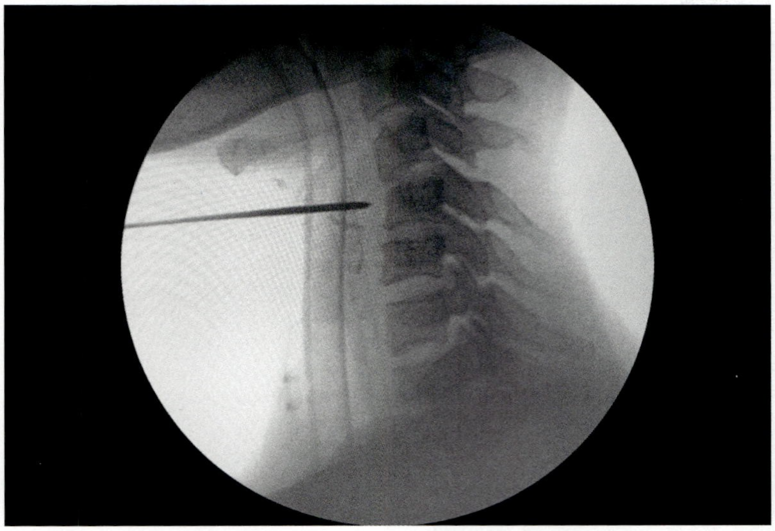

Fig. 4: Confirm the vertebral level under C-arm.

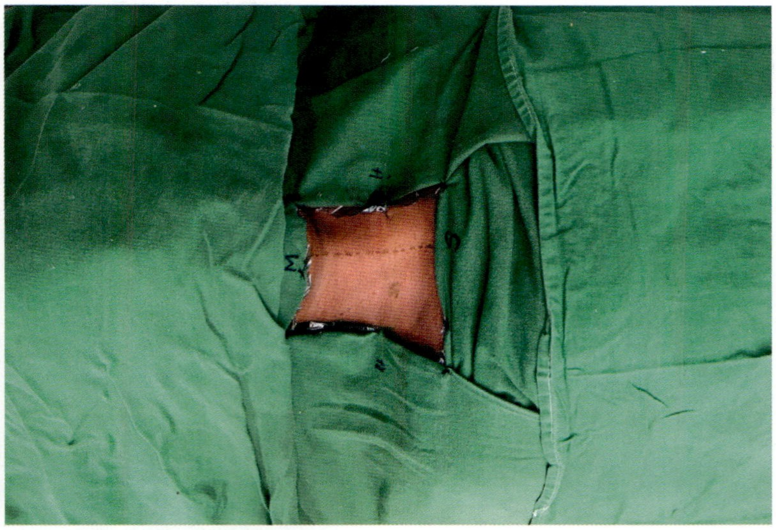

Fig. 5: Painting and draping done from mandible to sternal notch.

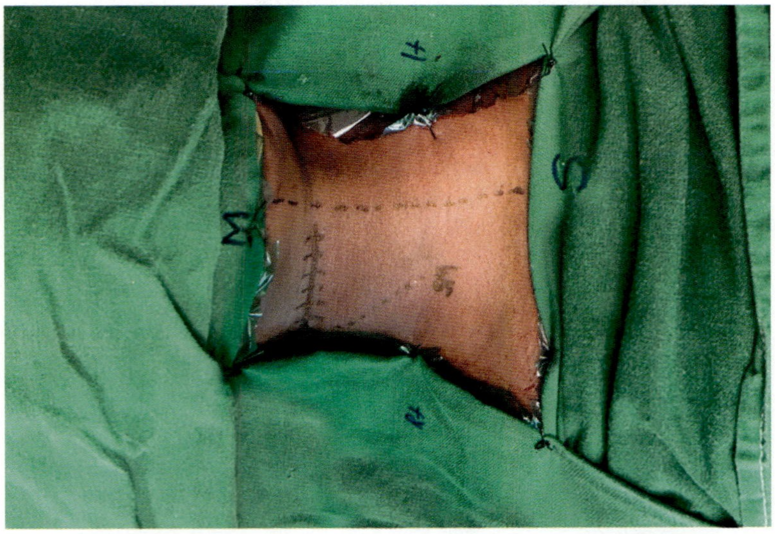

Fig. 6: Mark transverse incision from medial border of sternocleidomastoid muscle to midline of neck.

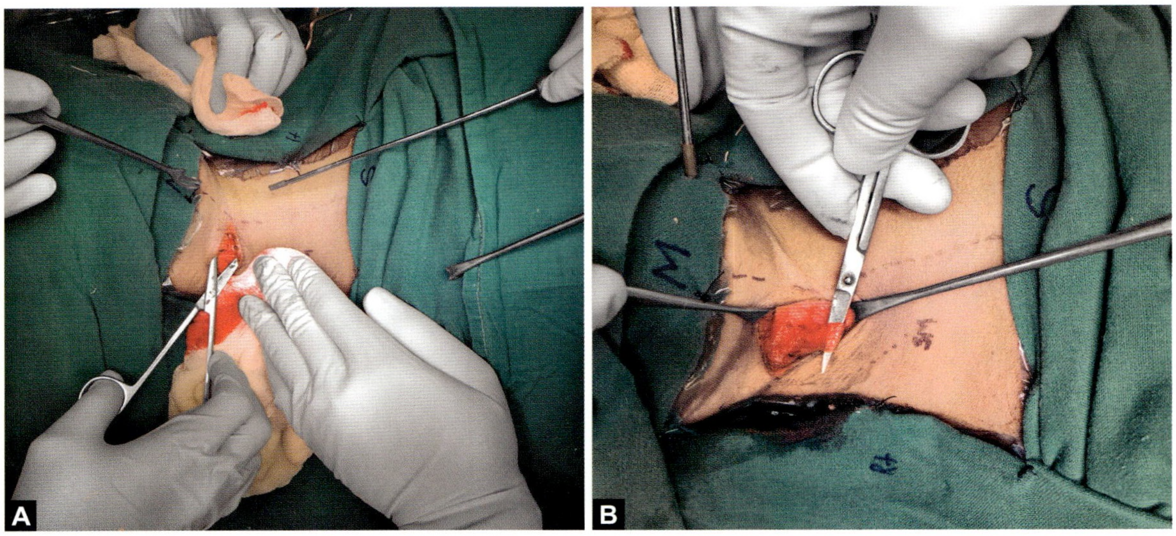

Figs. 7A and B: Take transverse incision over skin, identify platysma muscle and cut platysma muscle in line of skin incision or perpendicular.

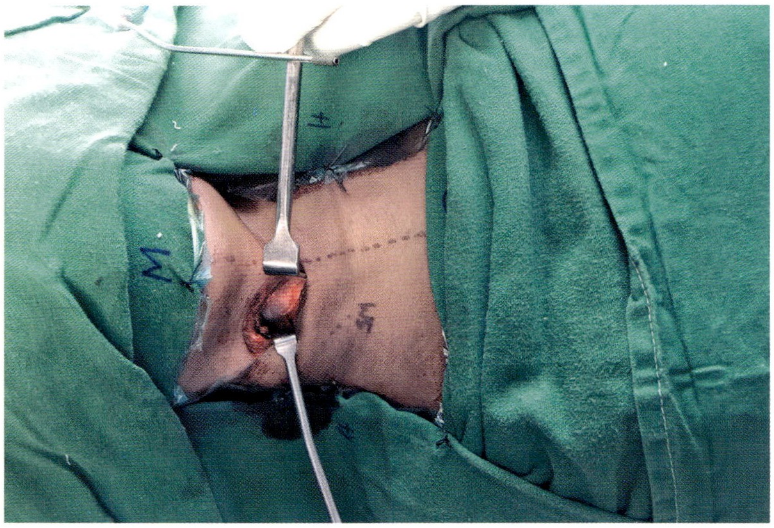

Fig. 8: Identify medial border of sternocleidomastoid and look for carotid pulse in incised deep cervical fascia.

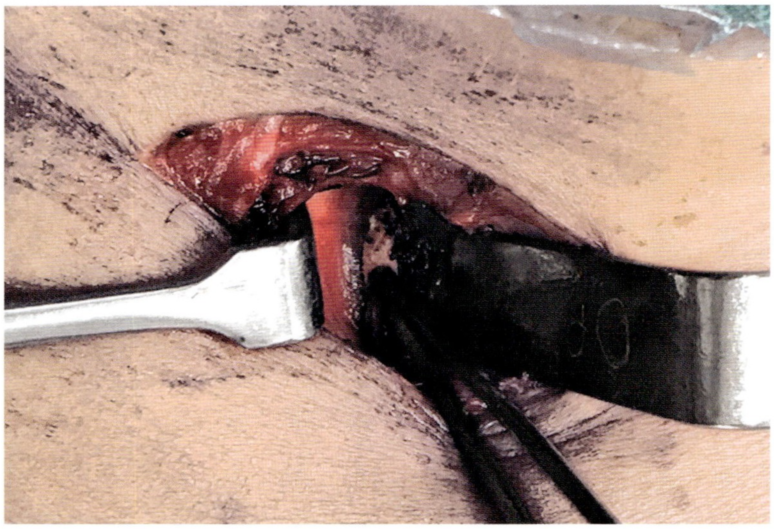

Fig. 9: Retract sternocleidomastoid and carotid vessels laterally and esophagus trachea and thyroid medially.

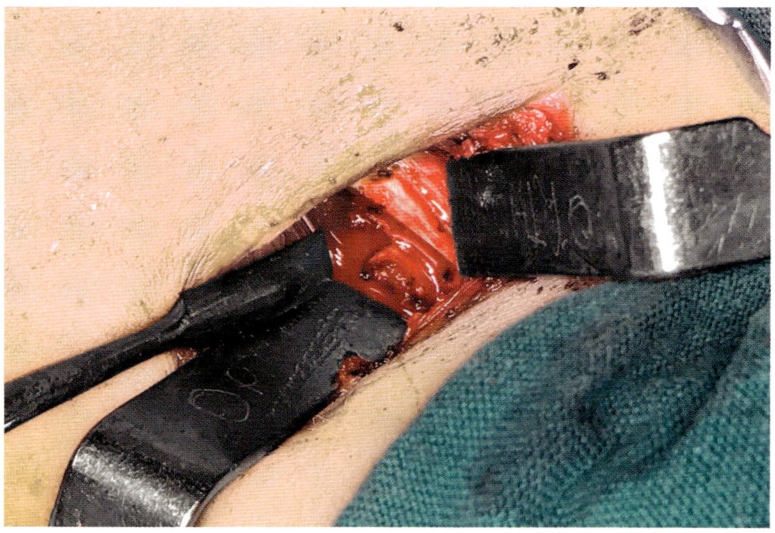

Fig. 10: Perform blunt dissection and divide prevertebral fascia to reach vertebrae. Identify intervertebral disc in between C4-C5.

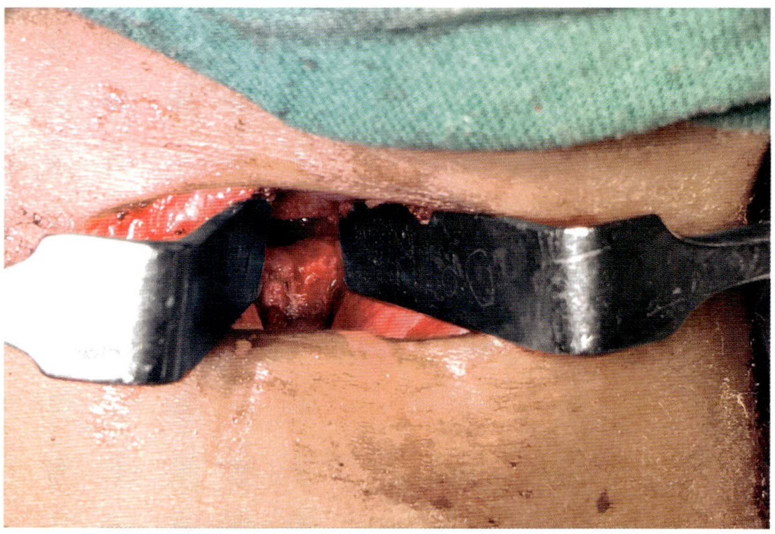

Fig. 11: Discectomy done with help of disc removal forceps.

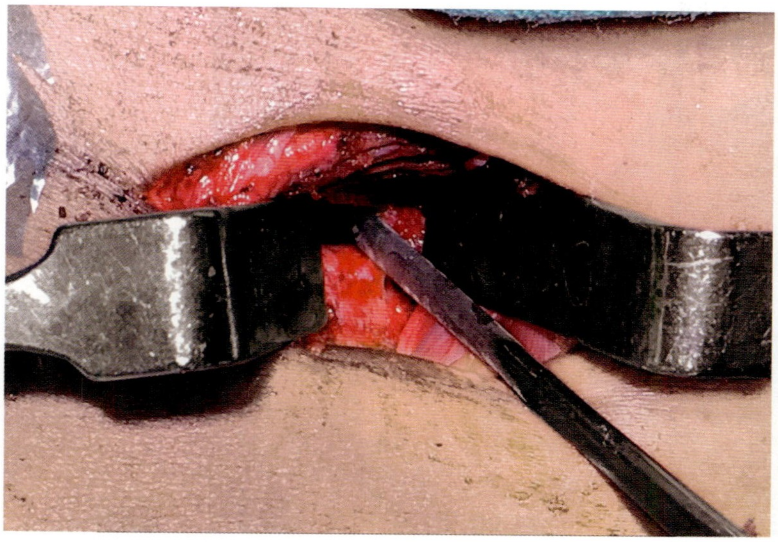

Fig. 12: Measure the width of discs for replacement with cage.

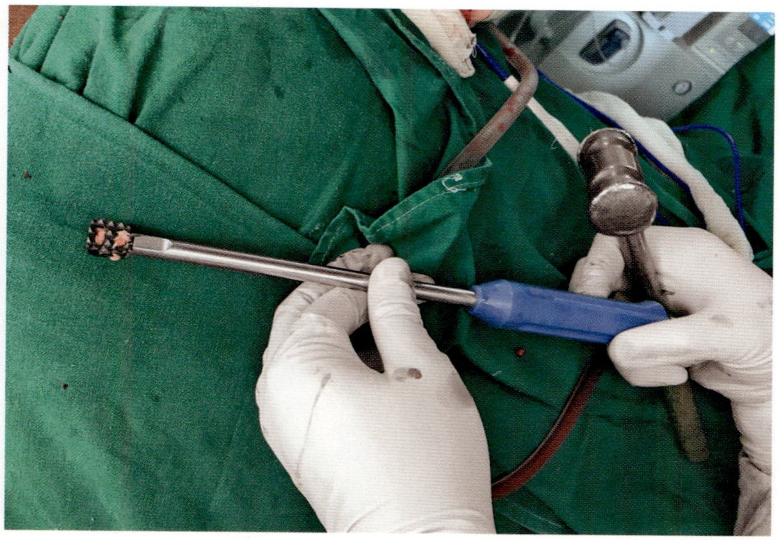

Fig. 13: Appropriate size cage with bone graft. Bone graft harvested from iliac crest.

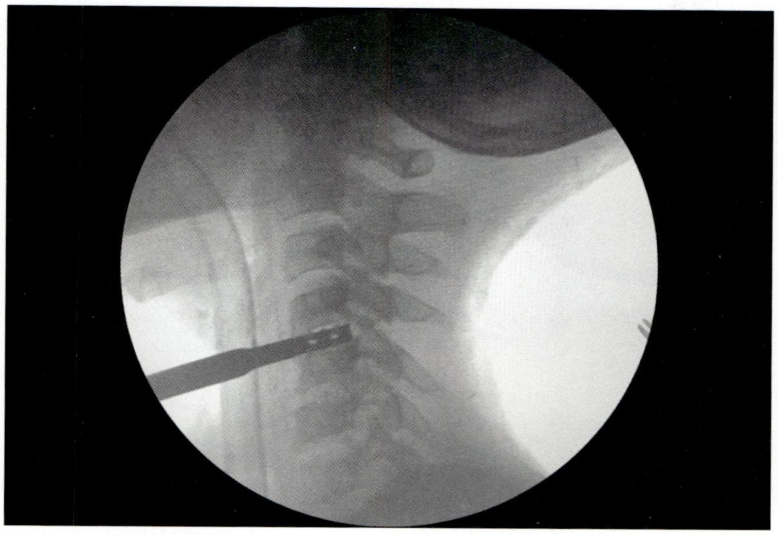

Fig. 14: Place the cage in between C4-C5; confirm with C-arm image.

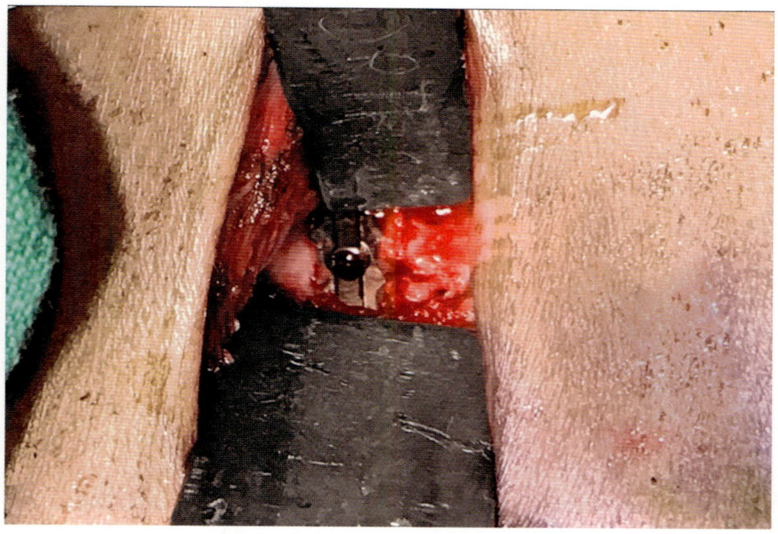

Fig. 15: Intraoperative image of cage placement in disc space C4-C5. Avoid sustained traction over esophagus, trachea and carotid vessels as it may cause pressure effects.

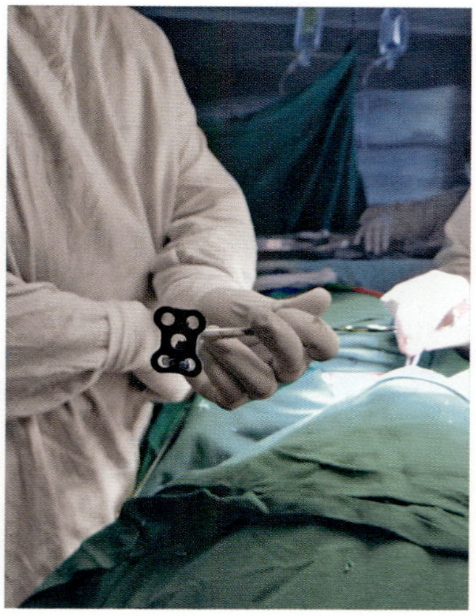

Fig. 16: Anterior cervical plate with four holes.

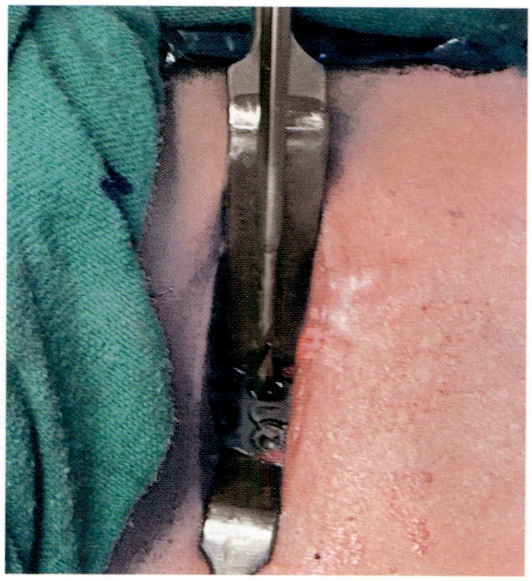

Fig. 17: Place plate over C4 and C5 covering the disc space. Perform drilling.

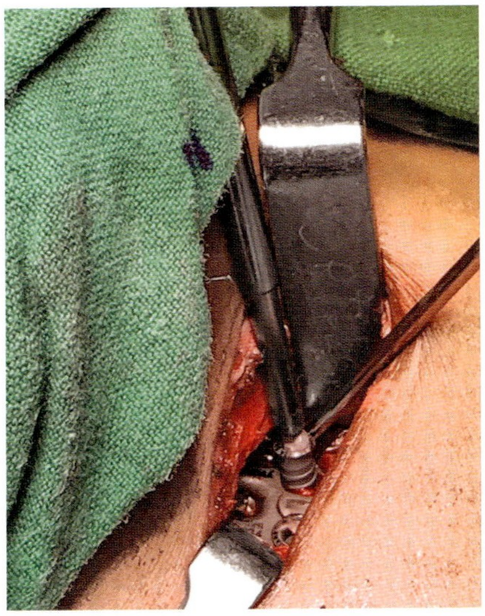

Fig. 18: Insert the screw in predrilled hole.

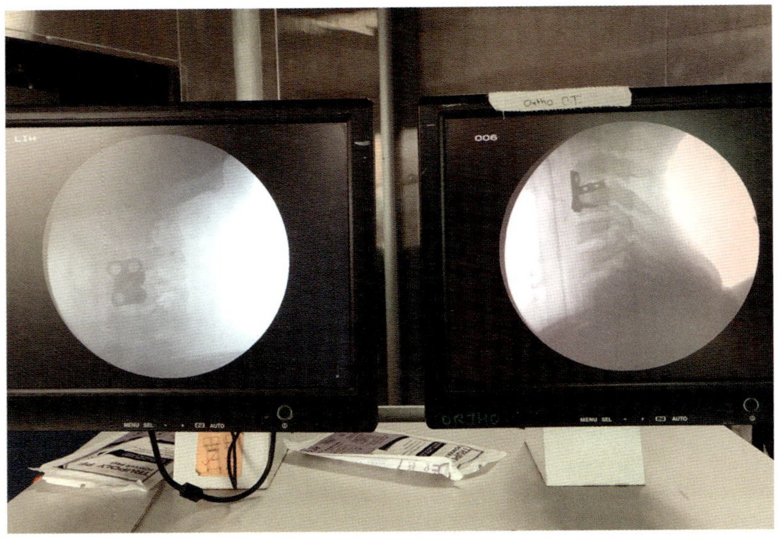

Fig. 19: Confirm placement of screw and plate by C-arm image.

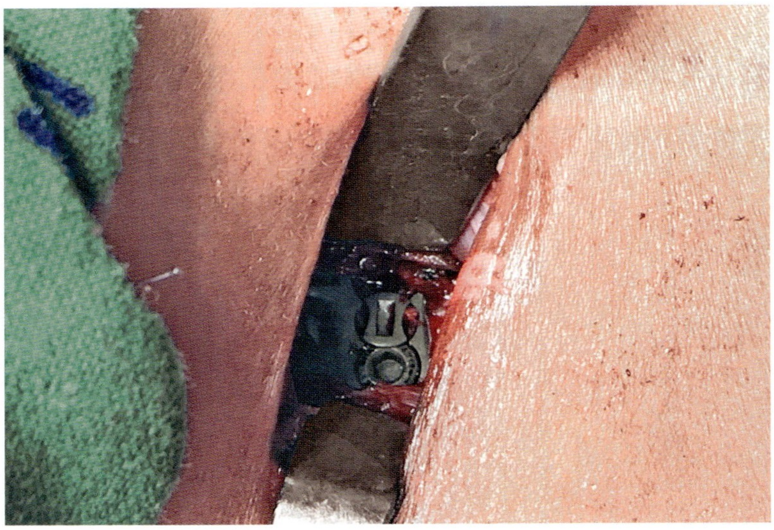

Fig. 20: Drill remaining holes, insert screws and confirm with C-arm.

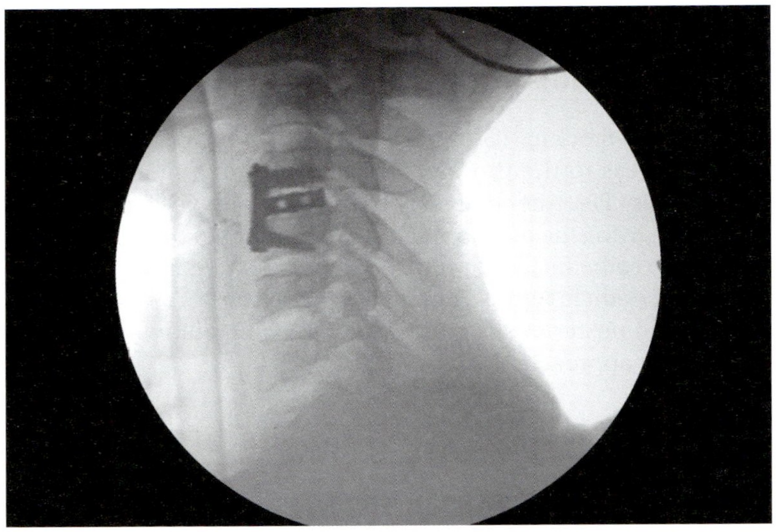

Fig. 21: Final image after placing all four screws in lateral view of C-arm.

After normal saline irrigation, wound is inspected for any bleed and then closed in layers over suction drain.

CHAPTER 23

Transthoracic Approach for Thoracic Spinal Tuberculosis

Shaishav Shah, Raghvendra Singh Raghuvanshi, Amol J Rege

INTRODUCTION

Hodgson and Stock in 1956 reported series of transthoracic approach for the access to the thoracic spine for the treatment of spinal tuberculosis (TB). After that there have been multiple changes in the approach, giving the best approach to the various anterior structures of thoracic spine including vertebral body (VB), intervertebral disc, ipsilateral pedicle and epidural abscess, apart from contralateral pedicle and posterior structures which are difficult to access from the anterior approach.

INDICATIONS FOR SURGERY IN TUBERCULAR SPINE

- The patients with no improvement in the neurology after a conservative and medical trial of at least 6–12 weeks.
- The patients who were neurologically normal when antitubercular treatment started, but developed neurological complications during the conservative treatment.
- The patients who worsened in spite of the medical treatment.
- The patients who have had a recurrence of neurological complication.
- The patients in whom the neurological complications are advanced for instance flaccid paraplegia and in elderly patients in whom recumbency risks are more harmful than surgical risks.

CONTRAINDICATIONS

- Absolute contraindication includes severe lung disease that precludes intraoperative one lung ventilation.
- Relative contraindications include severe adhesions, previous chest injury or surgery.

PREOPERATIVE PLANNING

A clinical evaluation and further pulmonary function tests along with physiological assessment of pulmonary functions and cardiac ailments.

EQUIPMENT AND INSTRUMENTS (FIG. 1)

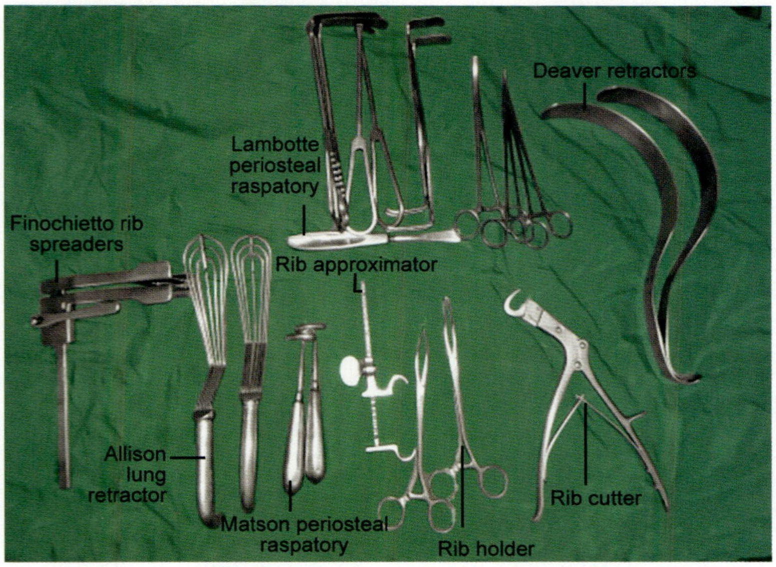

Fig. 1: Equipment for thoracotomy.

POSITIONING

The patient is positioned in the right lateral decubitus position, with shoulders and hips perpendicular to the floor. This helps in proper imaging of the spine intraoperatively and allows for spinal instrumentation to be anatomically correct. All pressure points are well padded.

ANTERIOR THORACIC EXPOSURE OF THORACIC SPINE

Incision

After proper painting and draping the skin incision is to be initiated approximately four centimeters lateral to the spinous process, continuing along the selected rib, and goes anteriorly up to the costochondral junction. The selection of the rib to be removed

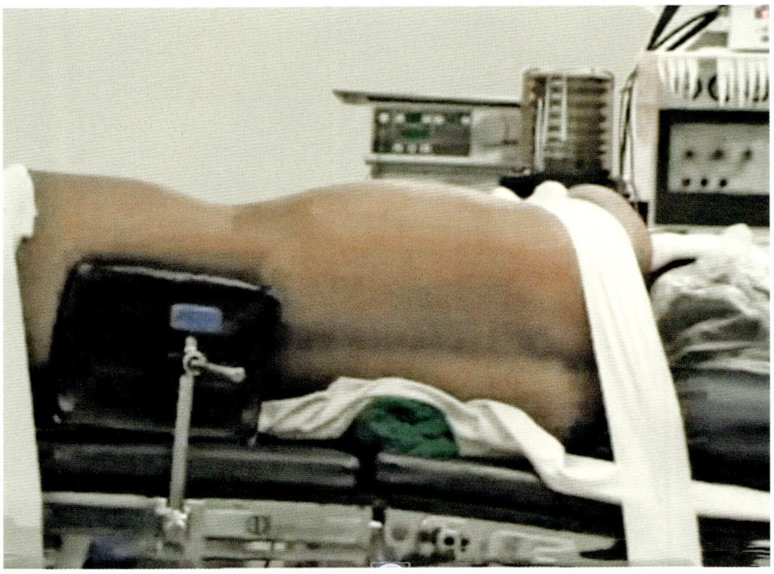

Fig. 2: Position right lateral decubitus with left-side up.

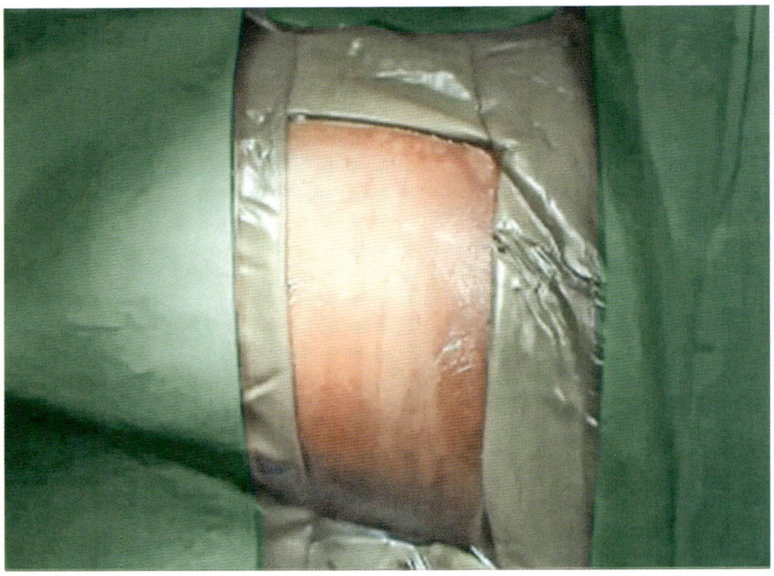

Fig. 3: Painting and draping for left sided approach.

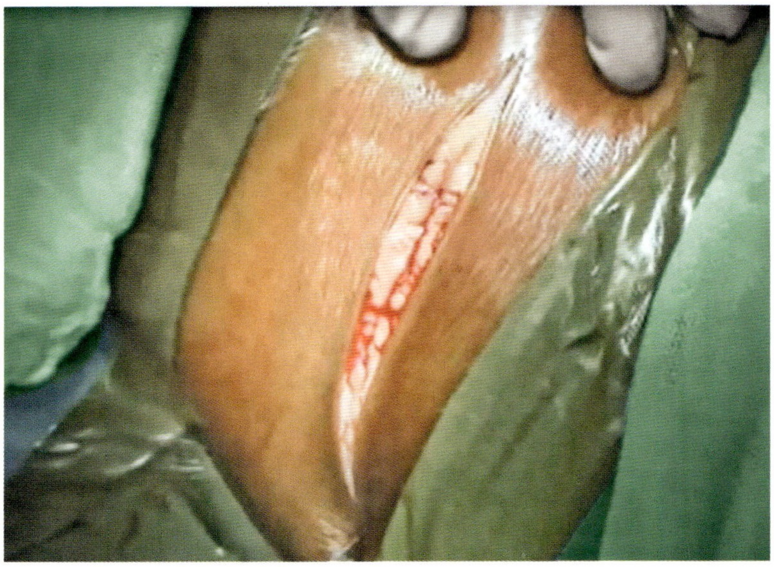

Fig. 4: Skin incision from around four centimetres lateral from spinous process to costochondral junction.

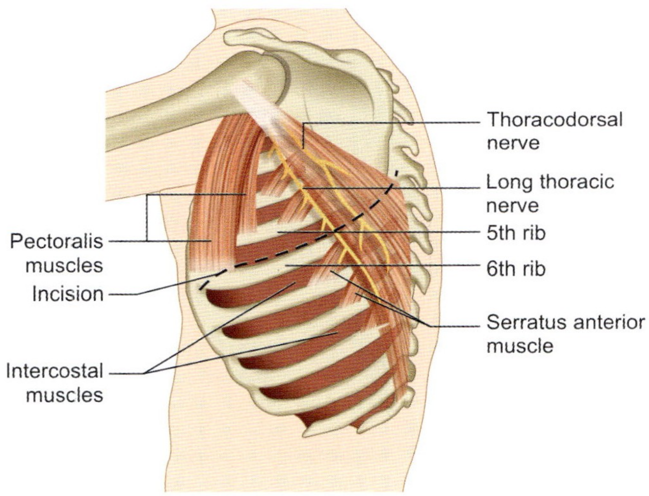

Fig. 5: The interspace that lies two levels above the involved VB is entered (here between 5th and 6th ribs to reach D8) and the rib below it (i.e. 6th) is resected.

depends on the site of the lesion. On the lateral X-rays, the rib that overlies the pathological VB can be visualized. Usually, the interspace that lies two levels above the involved vertebra should be entered, and the rib below this is resected. Hence, the incision is made over this selected rib to be resected.

After the skin is incised, the subcutaneous tissue and fat are incised in line with the skin incision.

Superficial Dissection

The latissimus dorsi muscle is the incised perpendicular to its fibers. After this anteriorly lies serratus anterior muscle and posterior lies trapezius muscle. While severing this muscle the dissection should be as far distal as possible to avoid injuring the long thoracic nerve. The outer periosteum of the selected rib is incised sharply and stripped with a periosteal elevator to visualize its edges properly. Care is taken to perform the dissection of the rib on its superior border to avoid damage to the intercostal bundle that includes a nerve, artery, and a vein, which run along the inferior border. The intercostal muscles (external intercostal, internal intercostal, and innermost intercostal) are stripped off the rib starting from the superior edge. When preparing to resect the rib it should be freed from all its sides,

for this a small dissector is used to free the inner periosteum from the underlying pleura. A rib raspatory or a gauze is introduced, elevating the inner periosteum posteriorly from the rib angle to anteriorly up to costal junction.

Rib Resection

A rib cutter is used to remove the rib. Depending on the level/s of surgery, a single or double level rib resection is performed. The rib is preserved for further strut bone grafting.

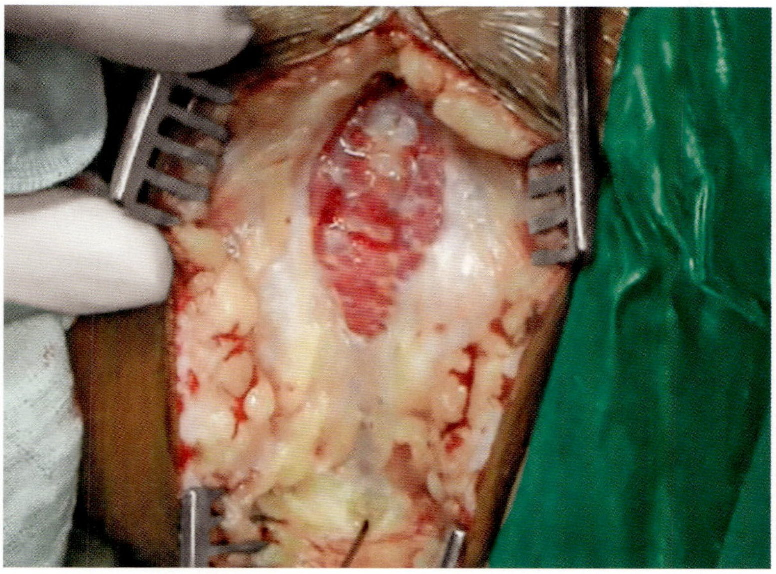

Fig. 6: This photograph depicts the superficial dissection.

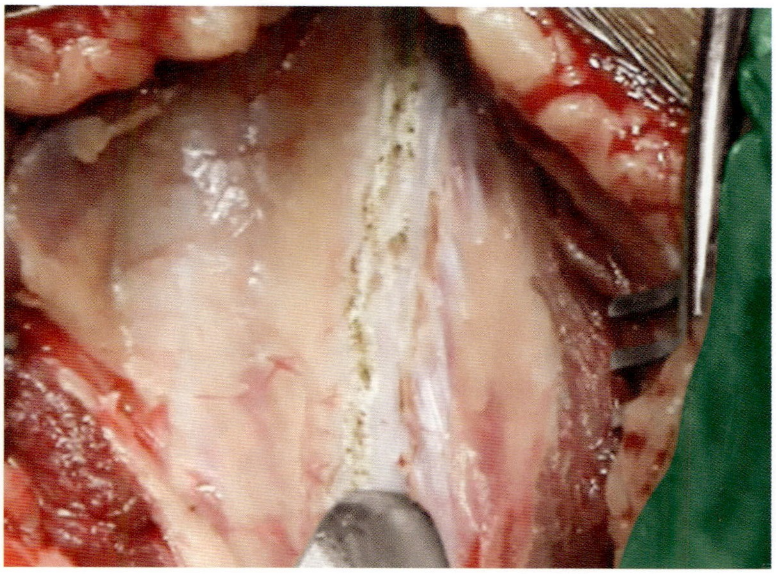

Fig. 7: Periosteal dissection over the rib.

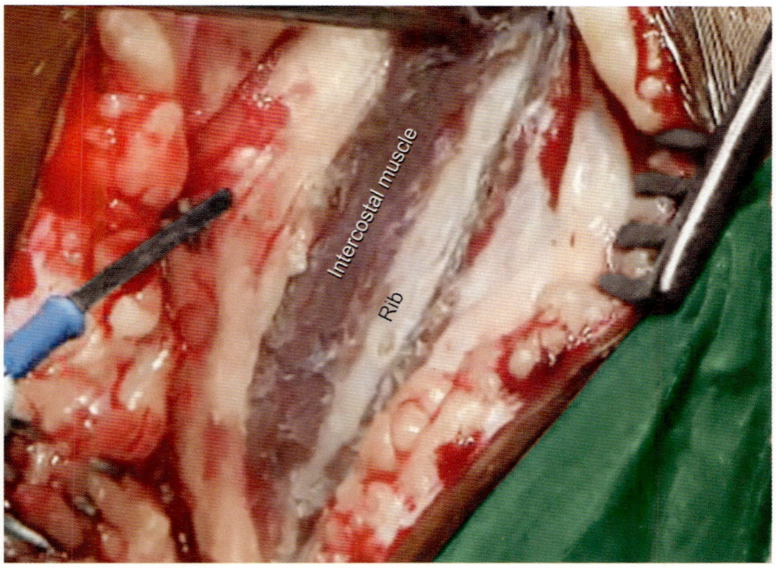

Fig. 8: Dissection till the intercostal muscles.

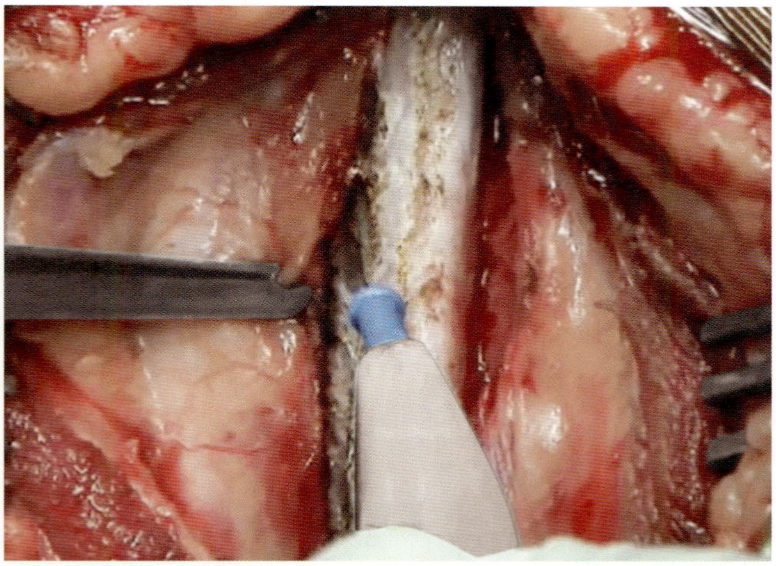

Fig. 9: Subperiosteal dissection from upper aspect of rib to avoid injury to neurovascular bundle that lies in the inferior aspect to the respective rib.

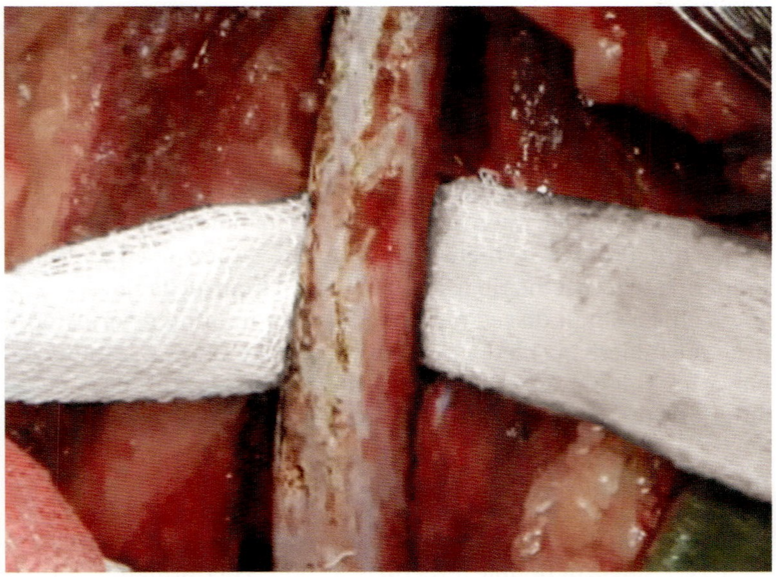

Fig. 10: Inner periosteum is released.

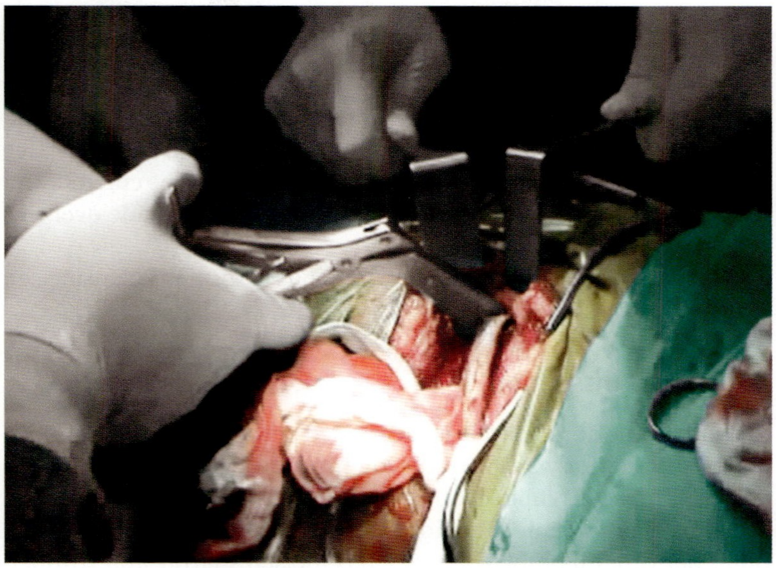

Fig. 11: Rib resection that can be used as bone graft.

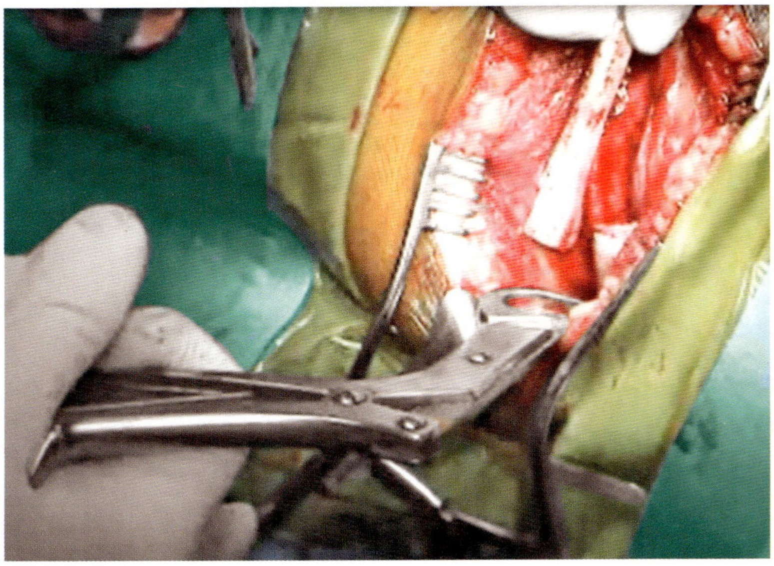

Fig. 12: Rib resection with rib cutter.

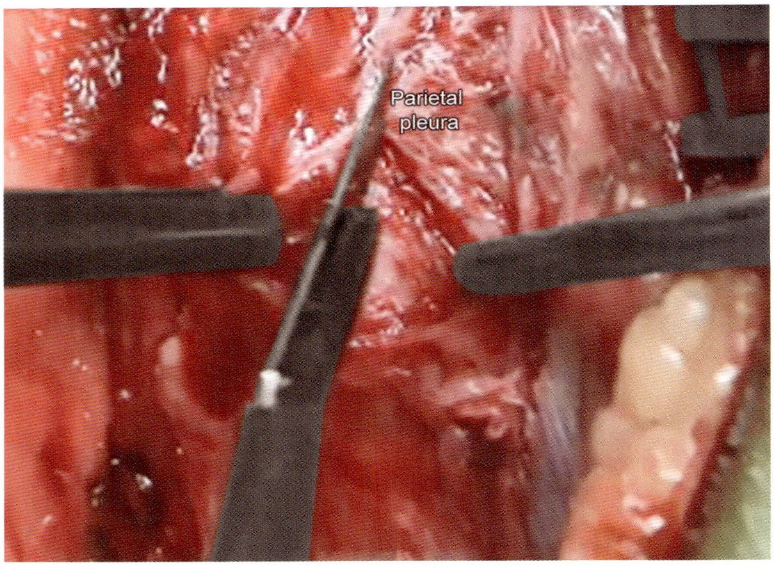

Fig. 13: The parietal pleura is identified and an opening is made with 15 no. knife carefully.

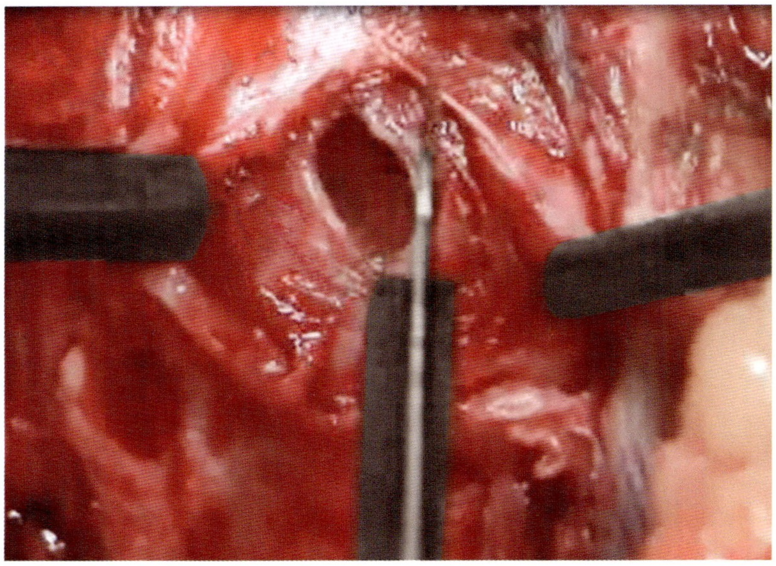

Fig. 14: Incise the parietal pleura with Metzenbaum scissors.

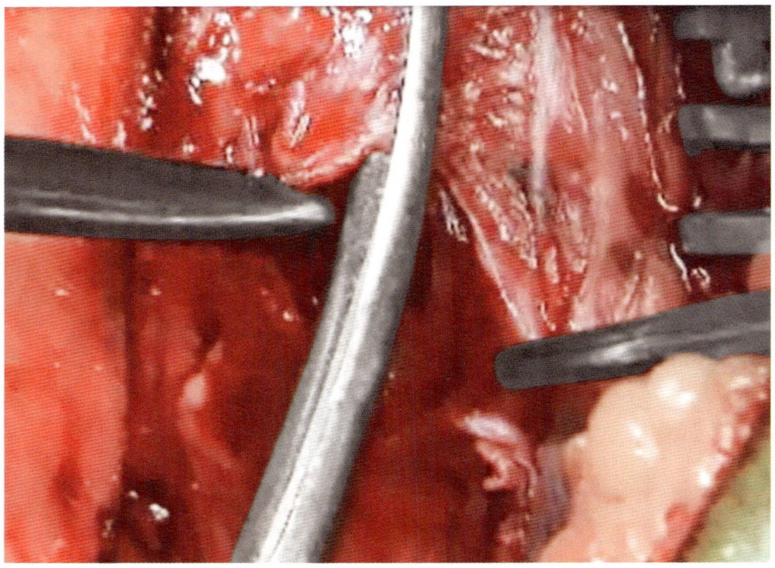

Fig. 15: Complete incising parietal pleura.

Exposure of the Thoracic Cavity

The thoracic cavity is opened in the bed of the resected rib.

The lung is retracted anteriorly with blunt Allis retractor and the vertebral body (VB) is exposed with the parietal pleura covering it. Below the parietal pleura, the rib head is seento be in contact with the intervertebral disc. On digital palpation, the intervertebral disc spaces are palpable, and the segmental vessels usually traverse the middle portion of the VB.

A horizontal incision of parietal pleura is made along the rib head and disc space which are palpable so as to expose segmental vessels. Usually, the dissection goes from the adjacent vertebra adjacent to the diseased vertebra, for instance, exposure of D8 should begin from D7 or D9. The parietal pleurae overlying the segmental vessels are coagulated with a monopolar coagulator or may ligate them.

DEBRIDEMENT AND CORPECTOMY (VERTEBRAL BODY RESECTION)

Once the parietal pleura is dissected and the segmental vessels are managed, the corpectomy starts. The posterior cortical part of the

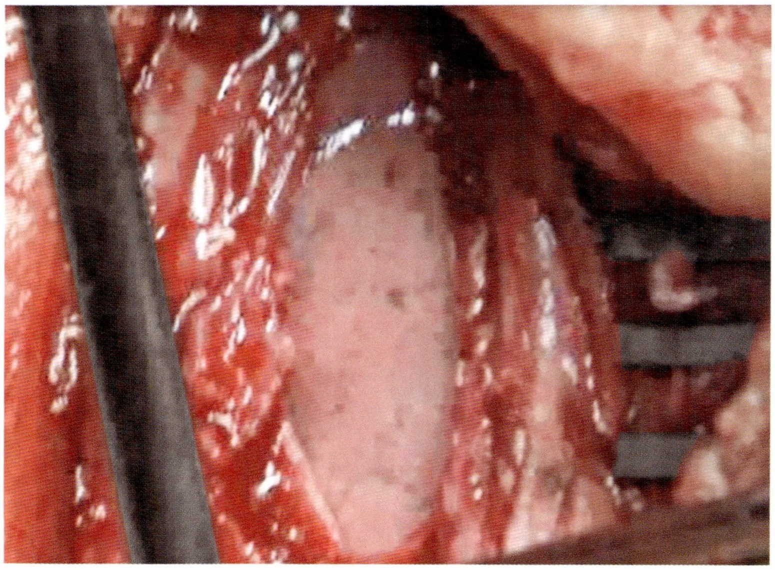

Fig. 16: Lung is exposed.

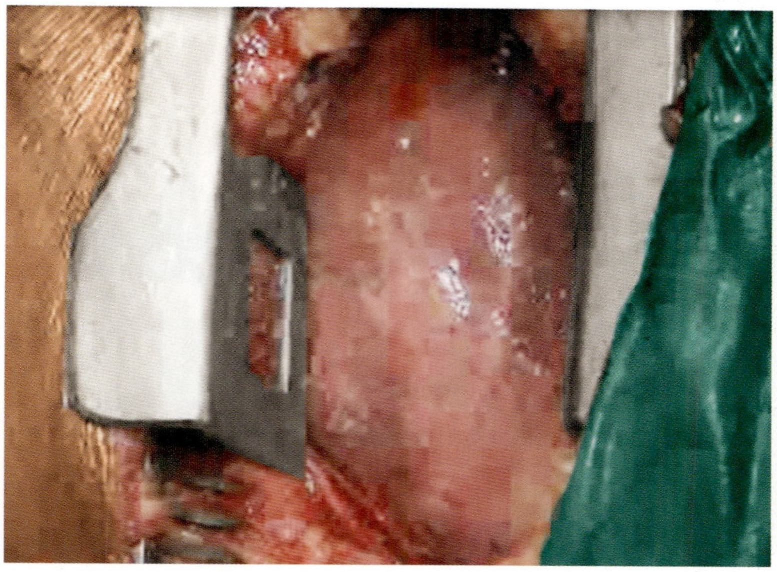

Fig. 17: Ribs retracted with Finochietto retractors.

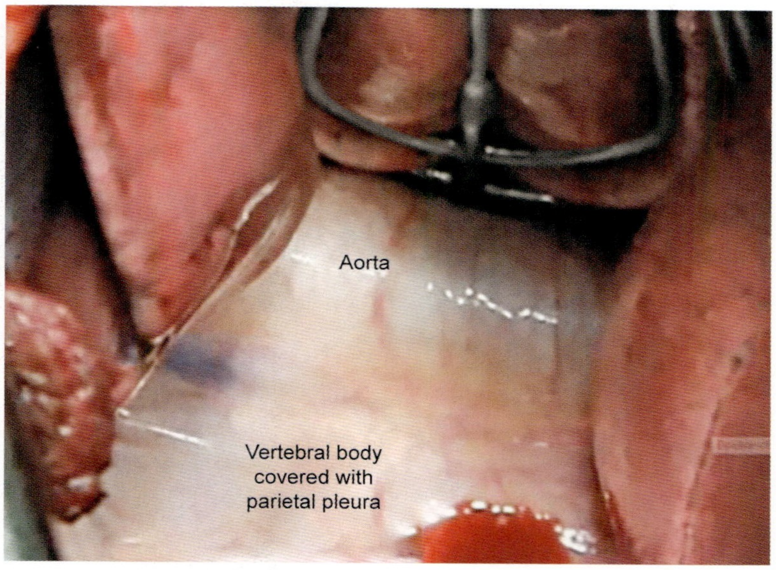

Fig. 18: Lungs are retracted with blunt Allis retractors.

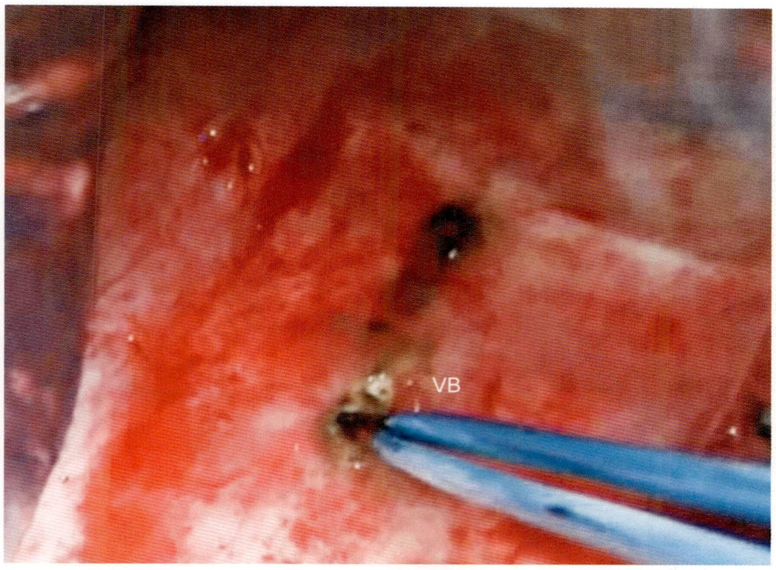

Fig. 19: Parietal pleura over the VB is dissected and segmental vessels cauterized.

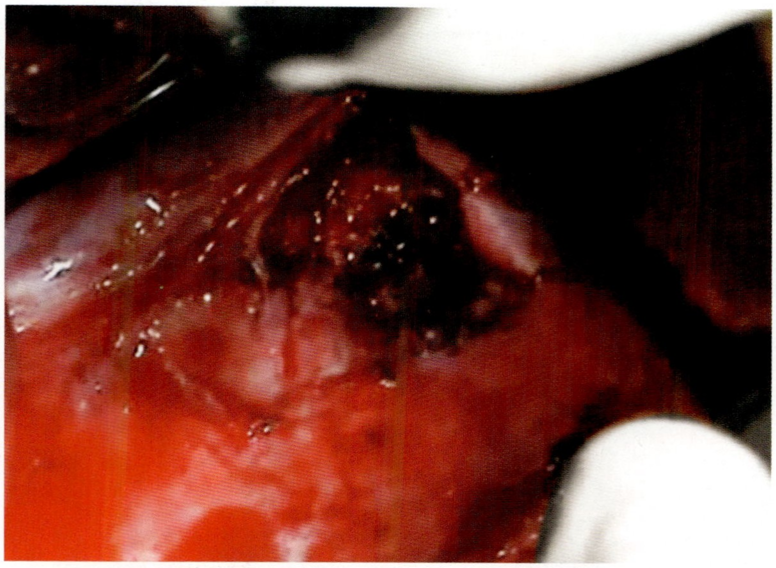

Fig. 20: Adjacent disc removal adjacent to the diseased body is completed with an osteotome and pituitary forceps. The infected body is slightly soft and friable.

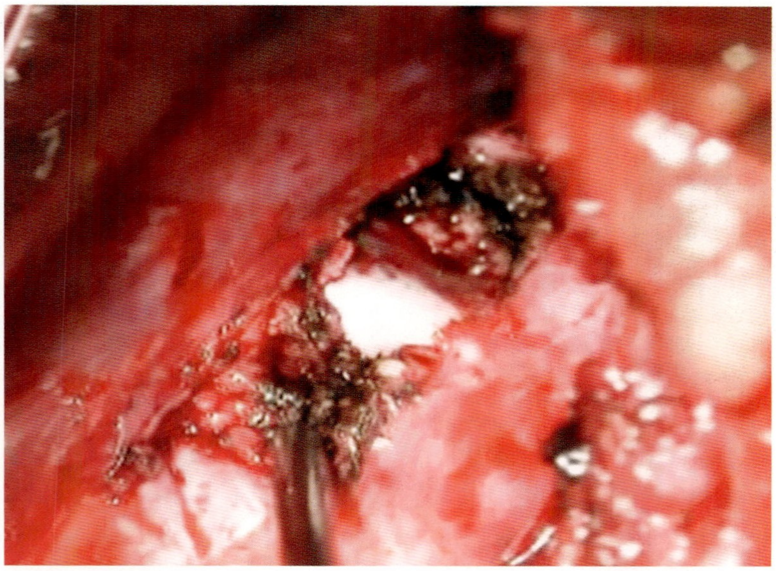

Fig. 21: Discectomy completed first before starting removing the body.

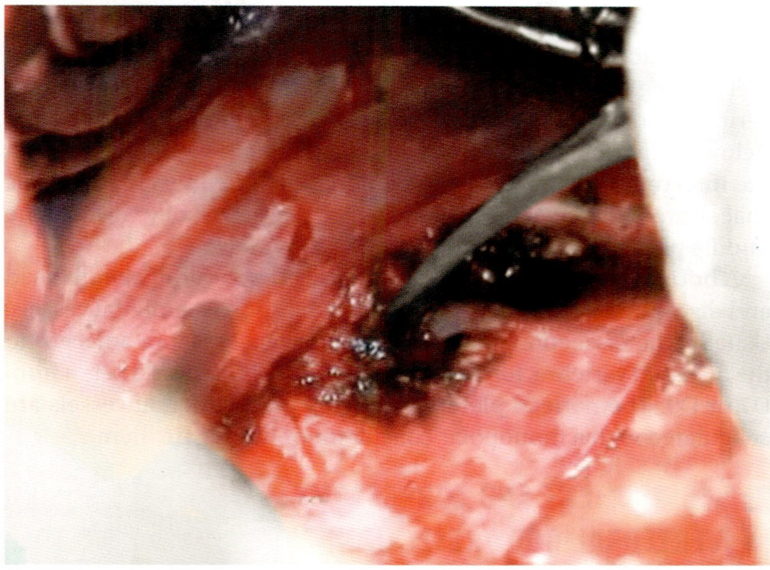

Fig. 22: The resection boundary is marked and controlled with an osteotome, and internal debulking is performed with pituitary forceps, curettes, Kerrison rongeurs, and burr.

CHAPTER 24

Thoracolumbar Fractures: Posterior Surgical Technique

Shaishav Shah, Raghvendra Singh Raghuvanshi, Amol J Rege

INTRODUCTION

- Most common site for vertebral fractures is thoracolumbar spine (60–70%).
- The commonest vertebral fracture occurs at L1 (34.40%). Commonest nonjunctional vertebral fracture occurs at T7 (3.9%)
- In the thoracic spine compression fractures (52%) is the most common injury. In the lumbar spine transverse process fractures (48%) is the commonest injury.
- Spinal cord injury was present in one in four patients of thoracolumbar fractures.

ADVANTAGES

- The posterior structures are easily accessible through posterior midline approach.
- There are very few vital structures at risk while approaching bony lamina and posterior structures routinely.
- The morbidity is also less compared to other approaches.

DISADVANTAGES

- Anterior structures are difficult to access through midline approach.
- Biomechanically posterior only fixation is considered a weak construct as in spine main load bearing is anterior.

PREOPERATIVE PLANNING

The preoperative planning depends on the type of fracture that the patient suffers.

Preoperative X-rays, magnetic resonance imaging (MRI), and computed tomography (CT) scans help guide the approach to the fracture over and above the clinical findings.

Thoracolumbar Injury Classification and Injury Severity Score (TLICS)

Parameters

- Morphology
  - Compression fracture—1 point
  - Burst fracture—2 points
  - Translational rotational injury—3 points
  - Distraction injury—4 points
- Posterior ligamentous complex
  - Intact—0 points
  - Suspected injury or indeterminate—2 points
  - Injured—3 points
- Neurologic involvement
  - Intact—0 points
  - Nerve root—2 points
  - Cord/conus medullaris (incomplete)—3 points
  - Cord/conus medullaris (complete)—2 points
  - Cauda equina—3 points.

TREATMENT AND PROGNOSIS

The total number of points help determine a management plan along with presence of other injuries and comorbidities. Patient with a score of:

- Less than 4: Usually treated nonoperatively.
- Equal to 4: May be treated operatively or nonoperatively.
- More than 4: Usually considered for operative management.

EQUIPMENT AND INSTRUMENTS

General orthopaedic and spine surgery instruments are must. In addition specialized instrumentation as shown in Figure 1 is required.

POSITIONING

- The position of the patient is prone with two horizontally placed well-padded bolsters (one at the level of sternum and another one at the level of anterior-superior iliac spine) or a frame over a radiolucent operating table.
- The abdomen should be free in order to avoid increased intraabdominal pressure due to compression to prevent excessive bleeding.
- Adequate padding needs to be provided to elbows and knees to avoid pressure sores and other neurological complications.
- The head is rested over a soft cushioned horseshoe ring or a jelly to avoid pressure on the eyes.

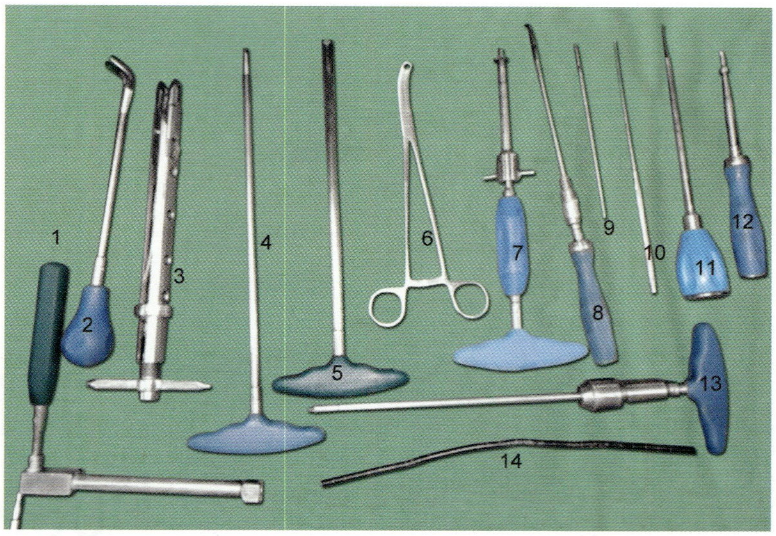

Fig. 1: (1) Final tightener, (2) rod rocker, (3) rod reducer, (4 and 13) set screw driver, (5) rod pusher, (6) rod holder, (7) pedicle screw driver, (8 and 9) bone tap, (10) pedicle sound, (11) pedicle probe, (12) starter with stopper, and (14) rod sizer.

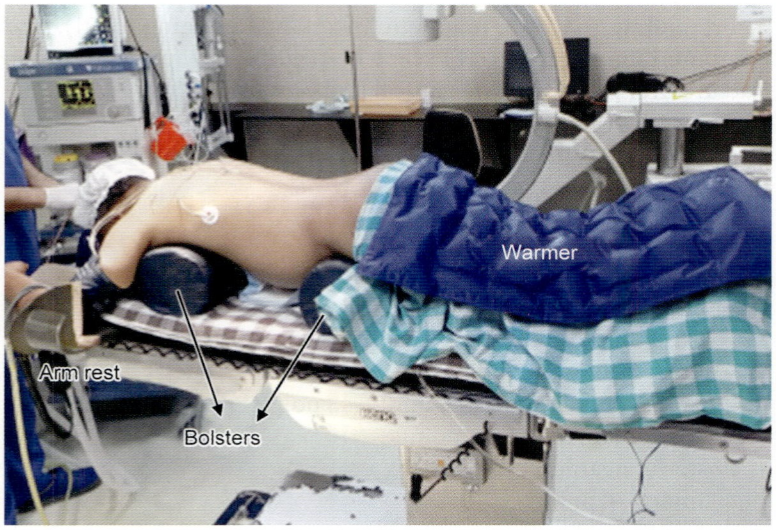

Fig. 2: Proper positioning of the patient with proper cushioning of bony prominencies.

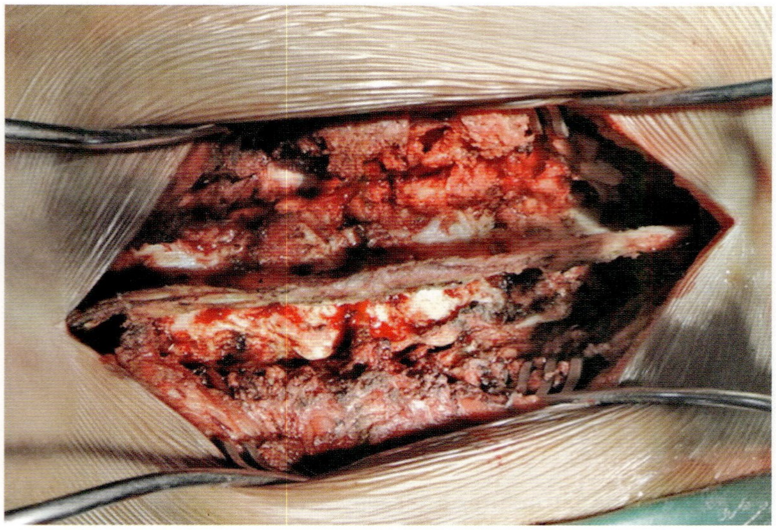

Fig. 3: Adequate posterior exposure for pedicle screw insertion.

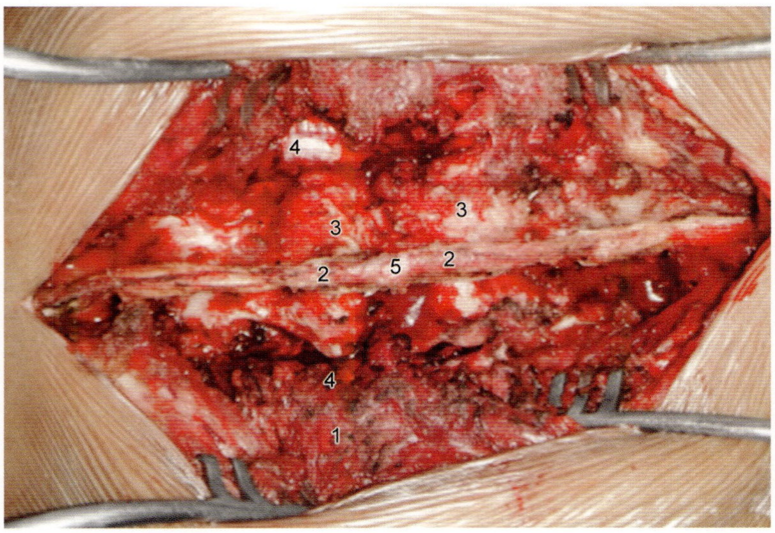

Fig. 4: (1) Paraspinal musculature, (2) spinous process, (3) lamina, (4) facet capsule, and (5) interspinous ligament.

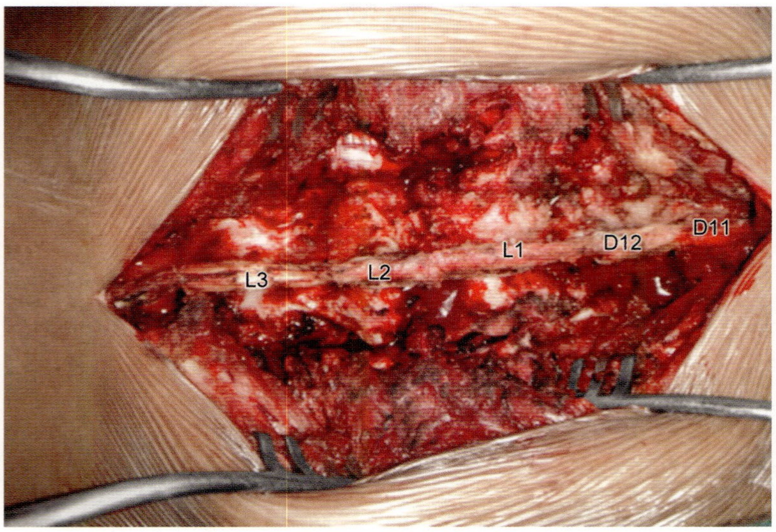

Fig. 5: L1 fracture with exposure of D11 to L3.

EXPOSURE

- The level to be exposed is marked with the needle under C-arm guidance.
- A skin incision is made over the palpable and marked level with the skin knife up to the level of the subcutaneous fat.
- Continuing the sharp dissection the fascia over the paraspinous musculature is reached. Fascia is then dissected and the paraspinous muscles are then stripped off the spinous process and lamina till the facet capsule with the use of diathermy.
- Care has to be taken for exposure of certain fractures for instance, fractures with posterolateral corner (PLC) injured one-sided exposure followed by fixation of that side should follow exposure of the opposite side as both sided exposure at once can make the fracture more mobile and the neurological injury can increase.
- One has to be cautious enough to avoid unnecessary stripping off the capsule of the facets of the terminal vertebrae to be fixed to avoid destabilization of the joints and residual instability.

PEDICLE SCREW PLACEMENT

There are three techniques for pedicle screw placement:
1. Intersection technique
2. Pars interarticularis technique
3. Mammillary process technique.

Entry Point for Lumbar Spine

The entry point of the pedicle screw is determined as the confluence of any of the four lines:
1. Pars interarticularis
2. Mammillary process
3. Lateral border of the superior articular facet
4. Mid transverse process.

Entry Point for Thoracic Spine

In the lower thoracic segments pedicle screw entry point is defined after determining the intersection of the mid portion of the facet joint and the superior edge of the transverse process. The specific entry point is to be just lateral and caudal to this intersection.
- Both the pedicles of L2 are entered and checked under C-arm.
- After the entry, pedicle probe helps track down through the isthmus of the pedicle into the vertebral body.
- For controlled and appropriate pedicle probe navigation anatomically it should direct towards the opposite transverse process, this will take care of the craniocaudal trajectory.
- Likewise, the mediolateral angulation is also important with difference at different levels for instance 45° at L5 and 0° at D5.

Every step in pedicle screw insertion should be checked with pedicle sound to confirm correct placement of the screw as margin for error is minimal.

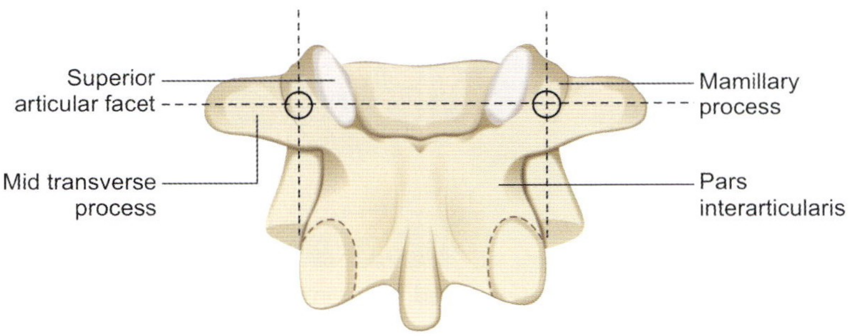

Fig. 6: Entry point for lumbar spine.

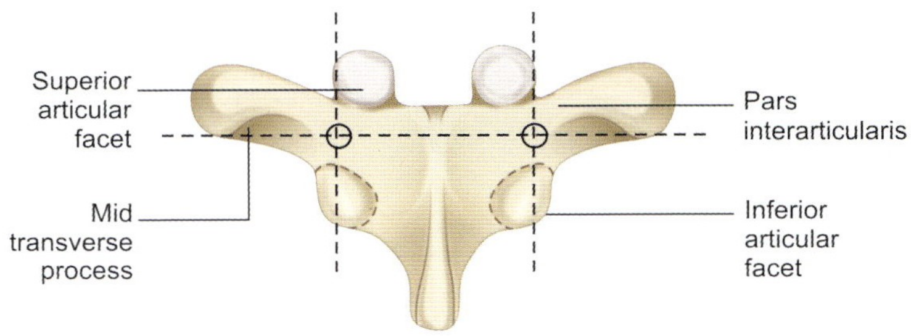

Fig. 7: Entry point for thoracic spine.

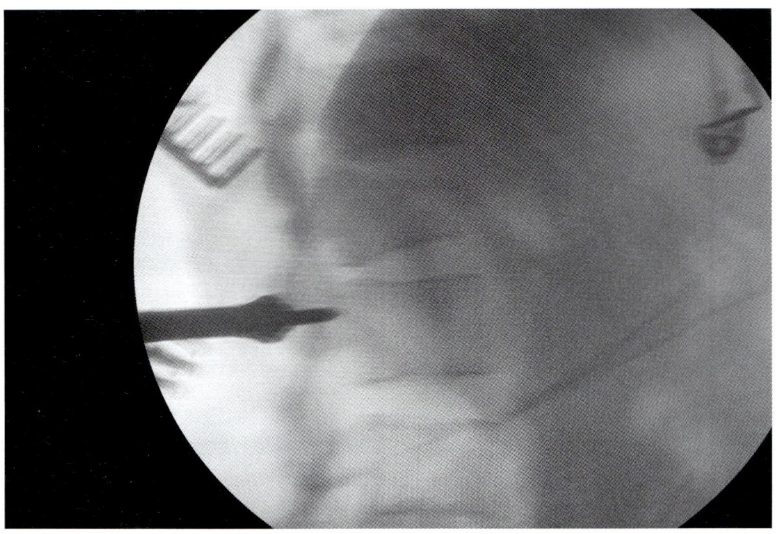

Fig. 8: L2 pedicle entry by starter with stopper. Open the superficial cortex of the entry point by a burr/rongeur or by hammering the starter.

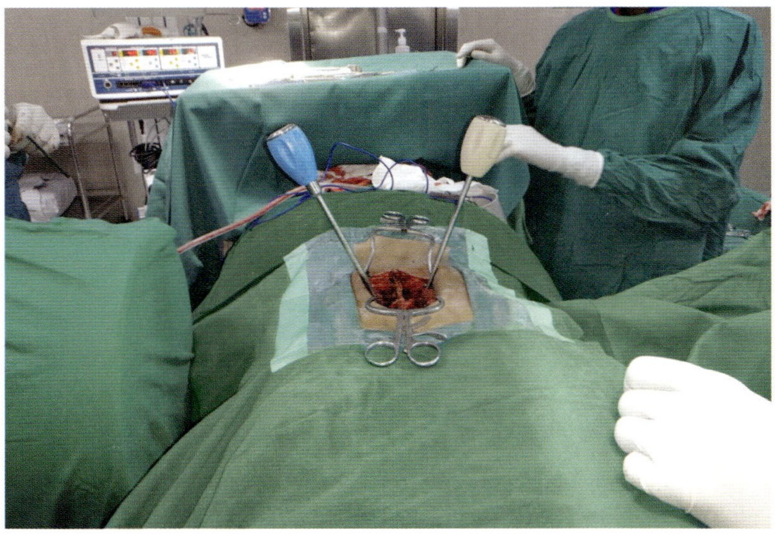

Fig. 9: Both the pedicles entered and their positions checked with C-arm.

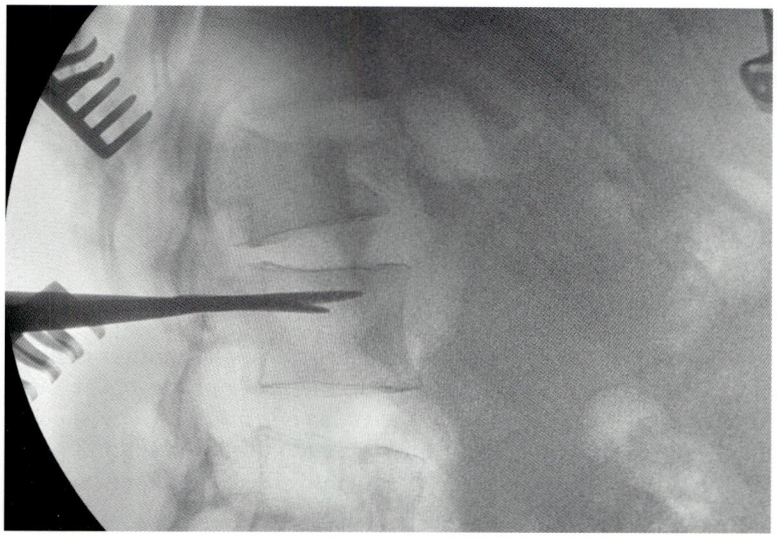

Fig. 10: C-arm guided pedicle probe insertion.

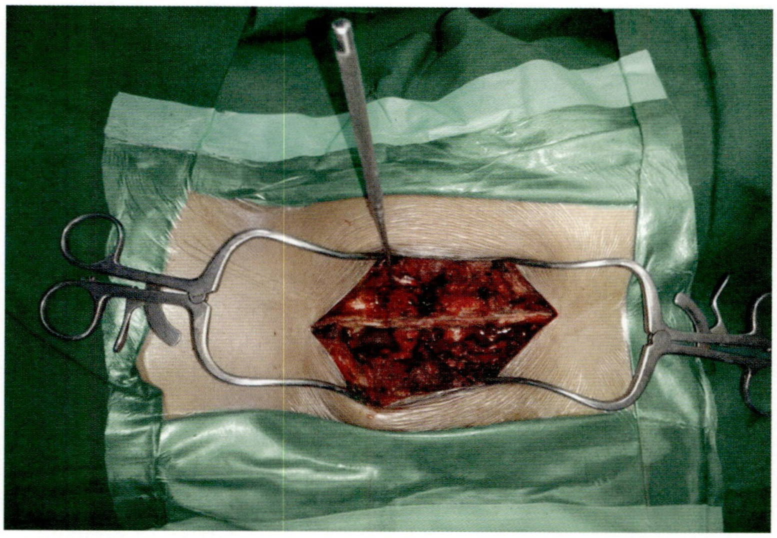

Fig. 11: Checking all walls at every step with pedicle sound.

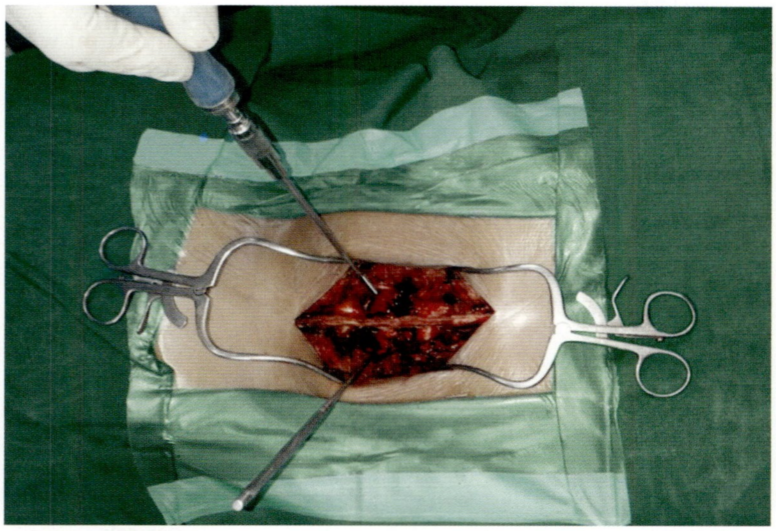

Fig. 12: Tap the tract and again check it for the walls with pedicle sound.

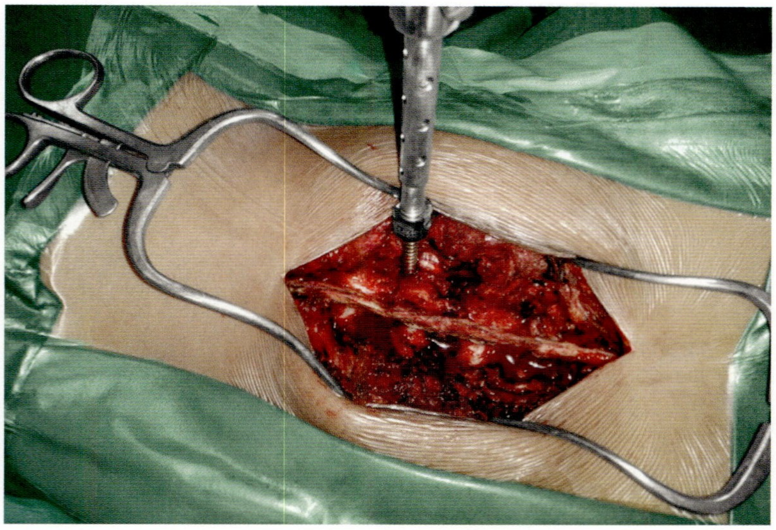

Fig. 13: Controlled screw insertion.

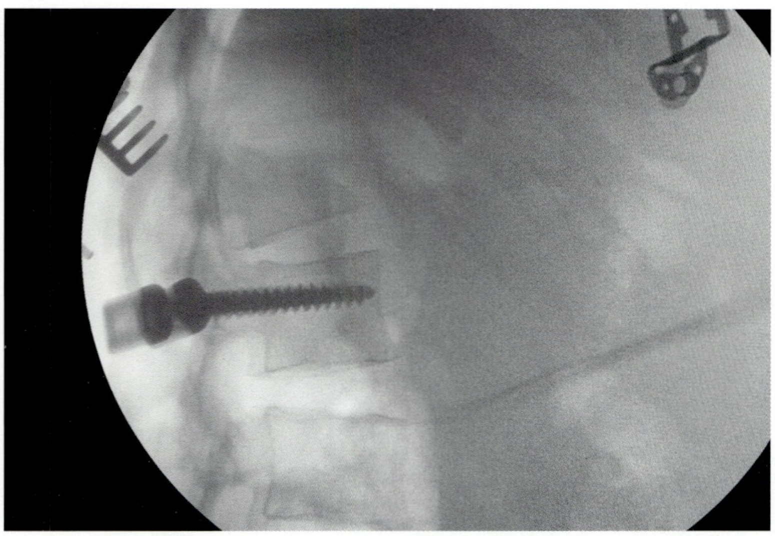

Fig. 14: Intraoperative X-ray always whenever needed to confirm the progress and proper placement as well as proper length of the screw.

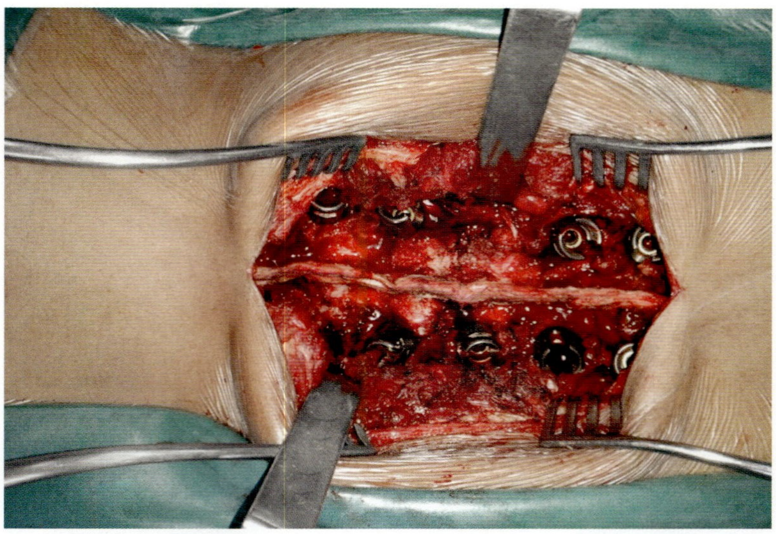

Fig. 15: Depending on the fracture pattern, the screws are inserted into the levels above and below. Usually short segment (one level above and one level below) can suffice, but at thoracolumbar junction being the transitional area long segment (two levels above and two levels below) fixation is necessary for stability of the construct.

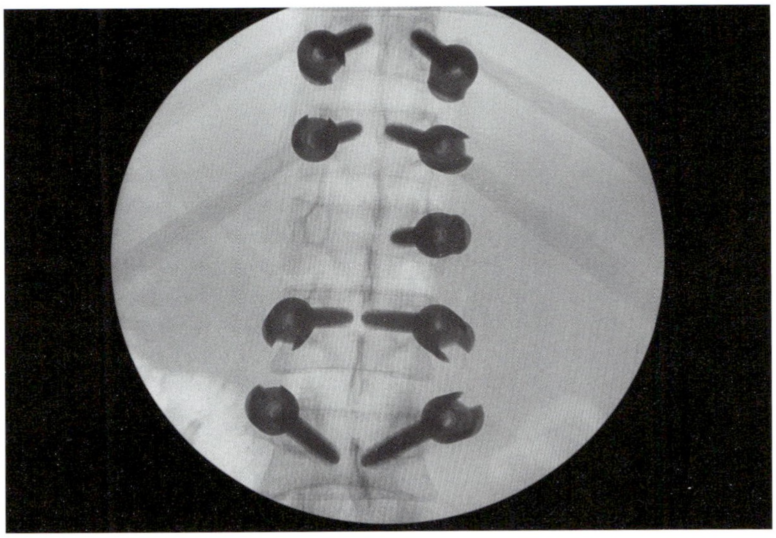

Fig. 16: Final X-ray to confirm correct placement of screws AP view.

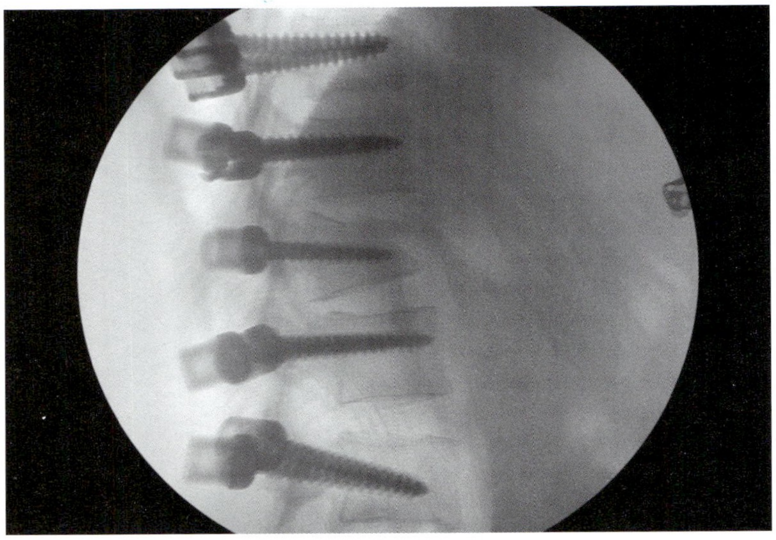

Fig. 17: Final C-arm X-ray to confirm correct placement of screws lateral view.

- There should be bony feel on all four sides of the pedicle, if there is deficit of any, then the tract is improper and the screw should be redirected accordingly.
- Among these four, inferior (exiting nerve root) and medial (spinal cord and traversing root) walls are important, and if breached can injure their respective structures.

There should be proper preoperative planning regarding the fracture pattern and the involvement of the pedicles of the involved vertebra. If possible, always try and insert the screw into the fractured vertebra, as it is mechanically more stable a construct.

In this case, it was possible to insert the pedicle screw only in one pedicle of the fractured vertebra.

ROD PLACEMENT

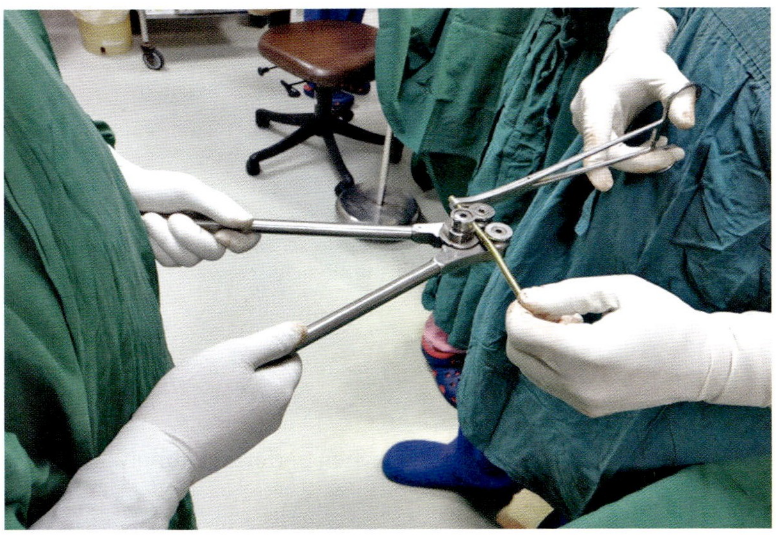

Fig. 18: Rods are given apt bend for the respective levels. Here being the junctional area, double curve is given, i.e. kyphotic curve for thoracic levels and lordotic for lumbar levels to normalize the curvature of spine.

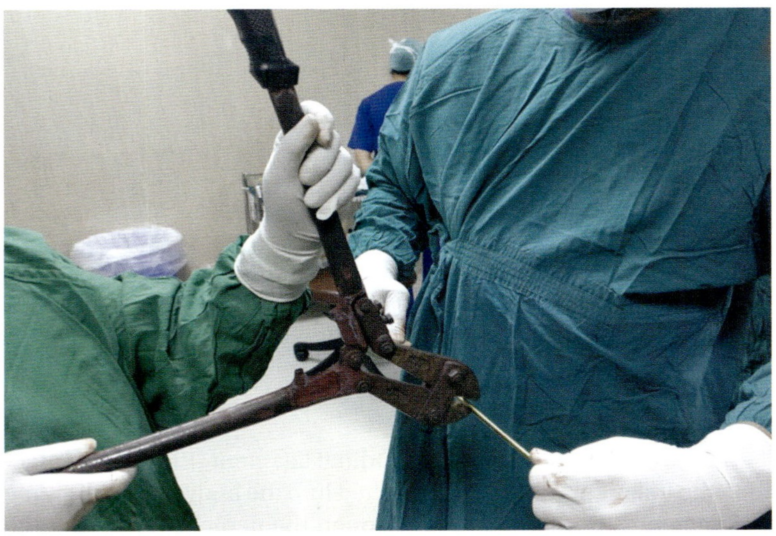

Fig. 19: Rods are cut appropriately to fit in the screws, they should not be too long to impinge adjacent vertebrae neither too short for the construct.

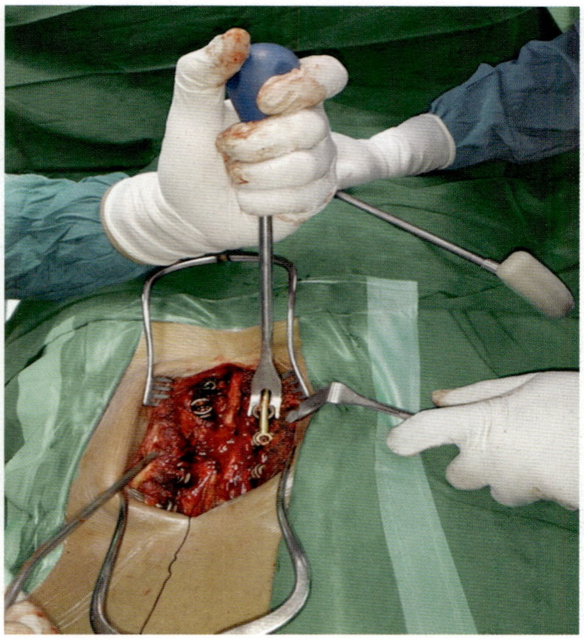

Fig. 20: Many times the rods do not fit in easily, here comes the role of rod reducers and rockers that help in reduce the rods to the screw heads.

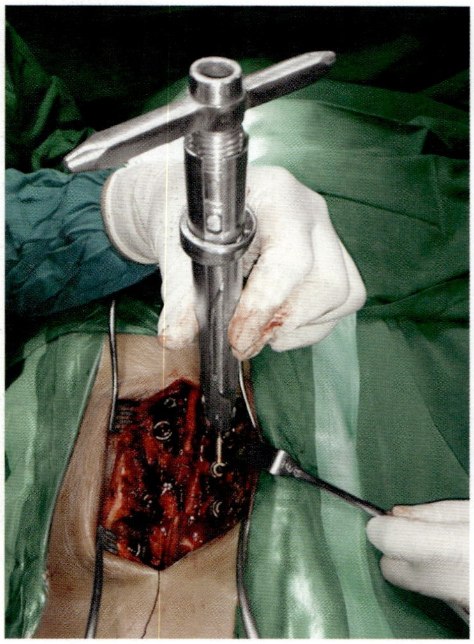

Fig. 21: Rod reducer used to reduce fracture and proper rod insertion

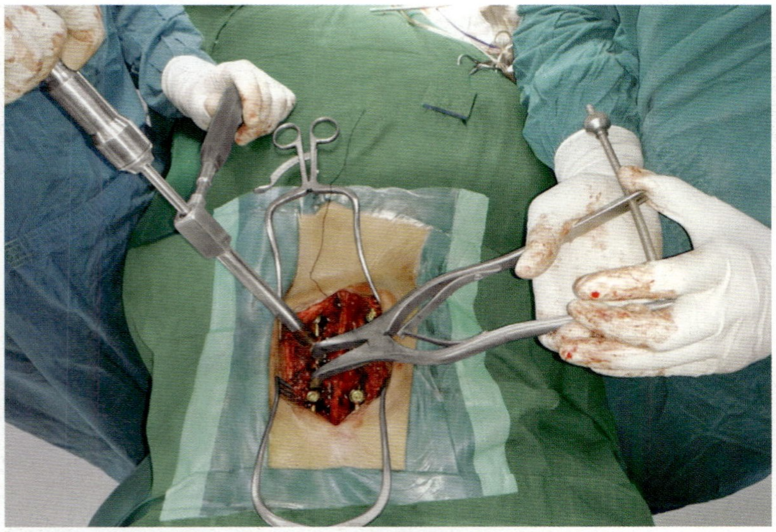

Fig. 22: Distraction of the fractured segment helps reduce the retropulsed fragments into the spinal cord due to ligamentotaxis (if posterior longitudinal ligament is intact). For Chance fractures, the scenario is different where the fracture site is to be compressed for proper healing.

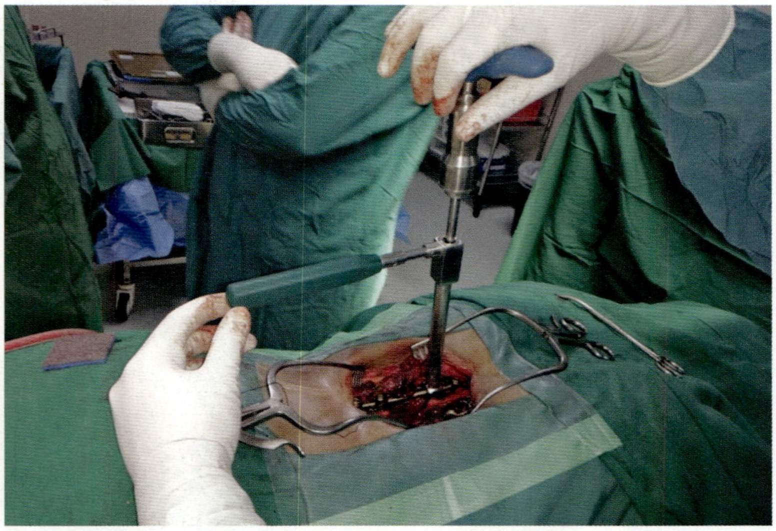

Fig. 23: Final tightening of the screws once the rods are affixed to the pedicle screws.

But sometimes posterior longitudinal ligament (PLL) is not intact then the fragments have to be punched into the body by approaching the fragments posterolaterally (through the pedicle or through the facet). This maneuver is useful only when performed timely i.e. within 3 days.

DECOMPRESSION (FIG. 24)

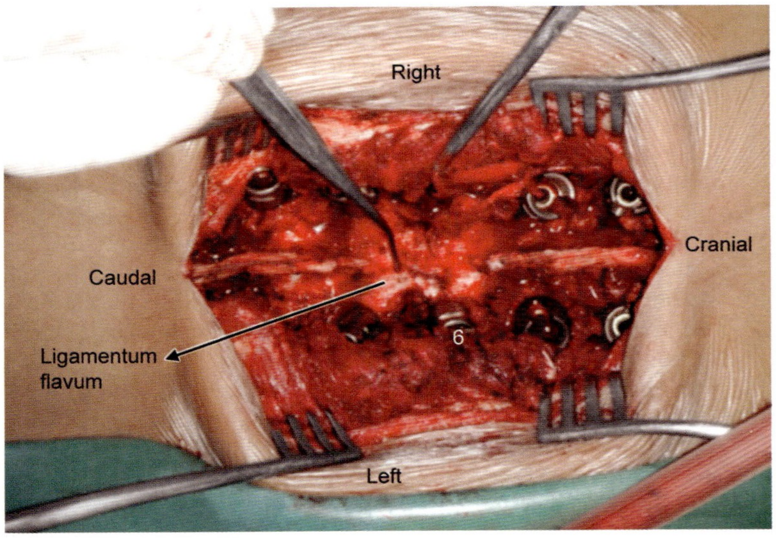

Fig. 24: Decompression of the spinal cord at the fractured level. Spinous process cut lamina of L1 removed and ligamentum flavum excised. But care has to be taken in certain fracture types as one may encounter dural tears and trapped nerve roots. Fractures with vertical lamina fractures have high probabilities of entrapped spinal cord. If so, one must be ready to suture dura mater back, or if too small can use a fascial graft or fibrin glue.

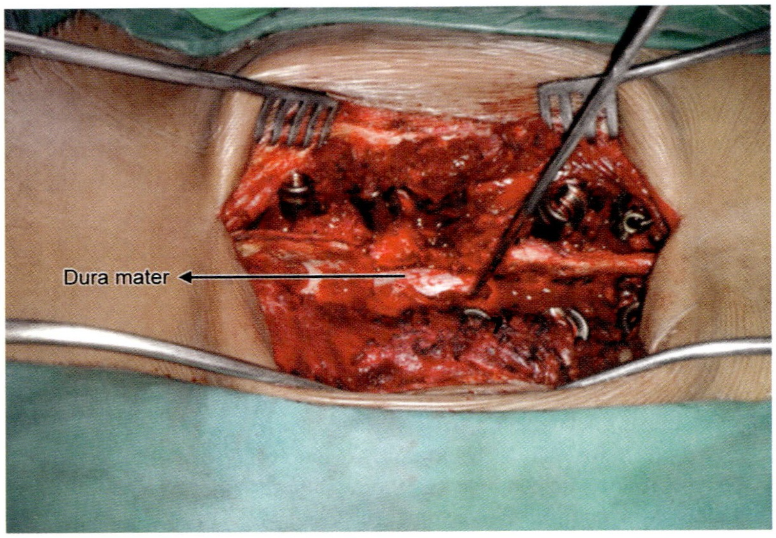

Fig. 25: Adequate decompression.

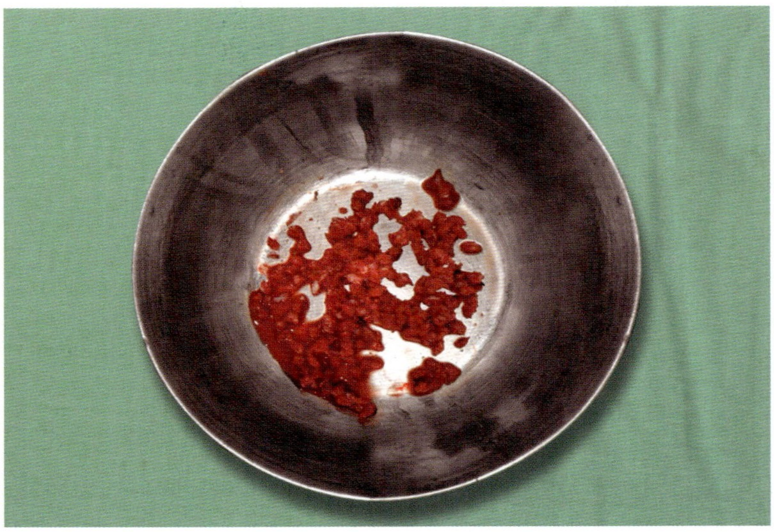

Fig. 26: Bone graft from the local site after decompression separated from soft tissue.

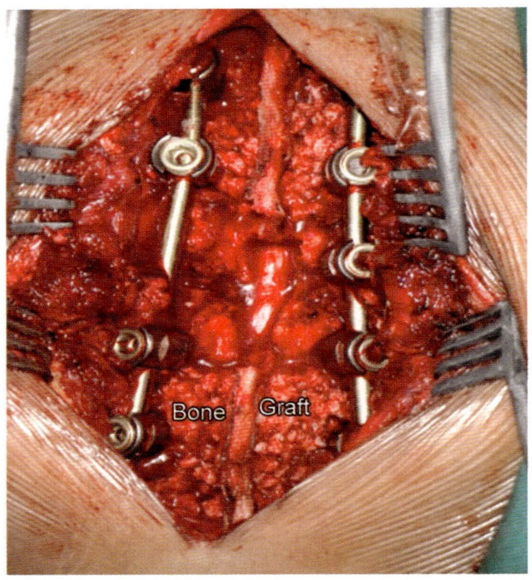

Fig. 27: Bone graft inserted for posterolateral fusion.

CLOSURE

Once the surgical fixation and decompression has been achieved, tight closure of the muscle and fascial layer is performed with continuous or interrupted sutures with absorbable suture material.

POSTOPERATIVE CARE AND REHABILITATION

The patient is mobilized on the first postoperative day with an orthosis unless other injuries that prevent from doing so. The orthosis is continued for 8–12 weeks, depending on resolution of pain and radiographic follow-up for evidence of healing and functional output.

COMPLICATIONS

- *Vascular complications*: Major vessel injuries when going too anterior while placement of pedicle screws may injure aorta or vena cava.
- *Neurological complications*: Nerve root injury to the nerve root inferior to the respective pedicle, if the inferior wall of the pedicle is breached. Cord/cauda injury, if too medial a screw placement.
- Dural tear.

SUGGESTED READING

1. Baaj AA, Reyes PM, Yaqoobi AS, et al. Biomechanical advantage of the index-level pedicle screw in unstable thoracolumbar junction fractures. J Neurosurg Spine. 2011;14:192-7.
2. Carbone JJ, Tortolani PJ, Quartararo LG. Fluoroscopically assisted pedicle screw fixation for thoracic and thoracolumbar injuries: technique and short-term complications. Spine. 2003;28:91-7.
3. Carl AL, Tromanhauser SG, Roger DJ. Pedicle screw instrumentation for thoracolumbar burst fractures and fracture-dislocations. Spine (Phila Pa 1976). 1992;17:S317-24.
4. Chance GQ. Note on a type of flexion fracture of the spine. Br J Radiol. 1948;21(249):452-3.
5. Delamarter RB, Sherman J, Carr JB. Pathophysiology of spinal cord injury: recovery after immediate and delayed decompression. J Bone Joint Surg Am. 1995;77:1042-9.
6. Esses SI, Sachs BL, Dreyzin V. Complications associated with the technique of pedicle screw fixation: a selected survey of ABS members. Spine (Phila Pa 1976). 1993;18(15):2231-8.
7. Gertzbein SD, Crowe PJ, Fazl M, et al. Canal clearance in burst fractures using the AO internal fixator. Spine. 1992;17:558-60.
8. Guven O, Kocaoglu B, Bezer M, et al. The use of screw at the fracture level in the treatment of thoracolumbar burst fractures. J Spinal Disord Tech. 2009;22:417-21.
9. Holmes JF, Miller PQ, Panacek EA. Epidemiology of thoracolumbar spine injury in blunt trauma. Acad Emerg Med. 2001;8(9):866-72.
10. Katsuura Y, Osborn JM, Cason GW. The epidemiology of thoracolumbar trauma: A meta-analysis. J Orthop. 2016;13(4):383-8.
11. Krag MH, Weaver DL, Beynonn BD, et al. Morphometry of the thoracic and lumbar spine related to transpedicular screw placement for surgical spinal fixation. Spine. 1988;13:27-32.
12. Leucht P, Fischer K, Muhr G, et al. Epidemiology of traumatic spine fractures. Injury. 2009;40:166-72.
13. McLain RF, Sparling E, Benson DR. Early failure of short-segment pedicle instrumentation for thoracolumbar fractures: a preliminary report. J Bone Joint Surg Am. 1993;75:162-7.
14. R Vaccaro, Alexander & Oner, Cumhur & K Kepler et al. AOSpine & Knowledge Forum, Trauma. (2013). AOSpine Thoracolumbar Spine Injury Classification System: Fracture Description, Neurological Status, and Key Modifiers. Spine. 38. 2028- 27.10.1097/BRS.0b013e3182a8a381.
15. Scholl BM, Theiss SM, Kirkpatrick JS. Short segment fixation of thoracolumbar burst fractures. Orthopedics. 2006;29:703-8.
16. Stambough JL. Posterior instrumentation for thoracolumbar trauma. Clin Orthop Relat Res. 1997;335:73-88.
17. Vaccaro AR, Lehman RA, Hulbert RJ, et al. A new classification of thoracolumbar injuries: the importance of injury morphology, the integrity of the posterior ligamentous complex, and neurologic status. Spine. 2005;30:2325-33.
18. Vaccaro AR, Zeiller SC, Hulbert RJ, et al. The thoracolumbar injury severity score: a proposed treatment algorithm. J Spinal Disord Tech. 2005;18:209-15.
19. Wood KB, Bohn D, Mehbod A. Anterior versus posterior treatment of stable thoracolumbar burst fractures without neurologic deficit: a prospective, randomized study. J Spinal Disord Tech. 2005;18 (Supp l): S15-23.

CHAPTER 25

Vertebroplasty for Osteoporotic Fractures

Arvind Bhave

INTRODUCTION

Vertebral compression fractures are commonest complications of osteoporosis. It causes progressive pain, deformity, disability, and finally affecting the quality of life and morbidity.

Standard conservative treatment consists of analgesics, bed rest, and use of braces. It temporarily reduces pains, but dependence of drugs, and narcotics progressively increases. Also lying in bed causes further bone loss, and kyphotic deformity leading to substantial limitation of activities of life.

Vertebroplasty is currently accepted minimally invasive treatment of stabilizing the fractured vertebra with cementing material usually PMMA [polymethyl methacrylate cement]. It was initially done in France and published in 1987 for hemangioma. Later on it was widely popularized in United States.

PATIENT EVALUATION AND PREPROCEDURAL WORK-UP

Vertebroplasty is good MISS procedure which eliminates the risk of major spine surgery, reducing pains considerably, mobilizing early in already compromised old, geriatric patients and through prompt pain relief, may provide early mobilization and rehabilitation for elderly multimorbid patients.

Duration of Pain Prior to Vertebroplasty

The indications from the consensus guidelines for vertebroplasty developed by the Standards of Practice Committee of the Society of Interventional Radiology are:

- Painful primary and secondary osteoporotic vertebral compression fractures refractory to medical therapy
- Painful vertebrae with extensive osteolysis or invasion secondary to benign or malignant tumors
- Painful vertebral fracture associated with osteonecrosis.

Contraindications to Vertebroplasty

Contraindications to vertebroplasty are:

- Uncontrolled bleeding disorder
- Vertebral body fracture without symptoms
- Infection
- Bone cement allergy
- Tumor mass extending to spinal canal.

TECHNICAL CONSIDERATIONS

Image-guided Approach

Visualization of needle insertion and bone cement injection is crucial in achieving a low incidence of complications. Vertebroplasty is carried out under single-plane or biplanar fluoroscopy control. It is very important to detect leakage of cement under direct fluoroscopic control. In case of cement leakage, the procedure should be immediately aborted. Computed tomography (CT) is suggested by some clinicians to reduce the operative time and facilitate accurate visualization of the needle position and bone cement distribution.

Technique

Venogram

Effectiveness of venography as a tool to identify potential routes of cement extravasation into vein is debated.

Uni/bipedicular approach: Percutaneous vertebroplasty can be done successfully via a single pedicle approach is possible in cases of vertebral osteonecrosis with intraosseous vacuum clefts, such as Kummel's disease.

Anesthesia: General Anesthesia versus Local Anesthesia

Vertebroplasty can be performed under local anesthesia.

Material

The high-viscosity PMMA system is safe and effective for clinical use. It reduces extravasation rate and thus related complications.

A biomechanical study revealed that about 3.5 cm of PMMA largely restored normal stress distributions to fractured and adjacent vertebral bodies.

Many devices for doing vertebroplasty are available. The author has devised a device termed "AB-needle". Advantages of this needle assembly are as follows:

- The design of the vertebroplasty needle in such a way that gives better spreadability of the cementing materials through multiple portals.
- It possesses a unique locking system at the neck of the vertebroplasty needle, which prohibits or restricts the movement of the vertebroplasty needle while hammering it, at the time of operation. The luer locking knob of the stylet and groove in it aligns the direction of the flanged tip of the needle; deep inside the body at the time of surgery.
- The vertebroplasty needle that possesses a unique system at the proximal end, which can accept any syringe or cement delivery system available for the delivery of the cementing material.

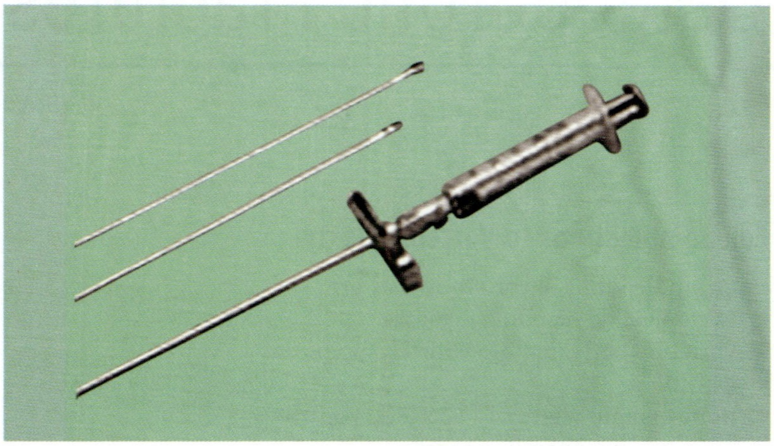

Fig. 1: Assembly of AB-needle for vertebroplasty.

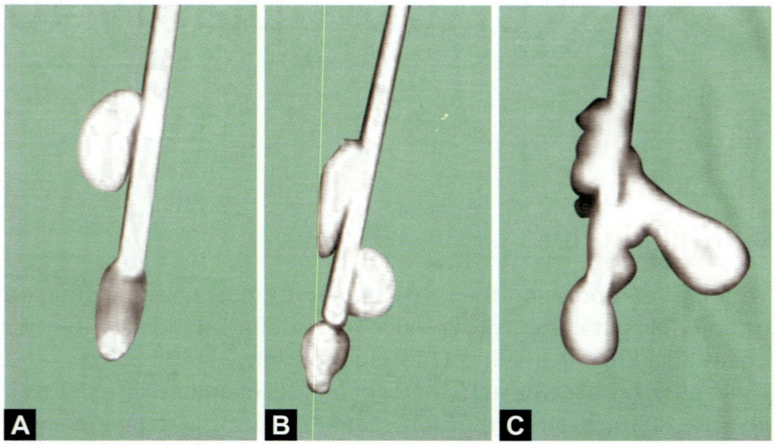

Figs. 2A to C: Peculiarity of side holes making it possible to have 360° filling of the fractured cavity.

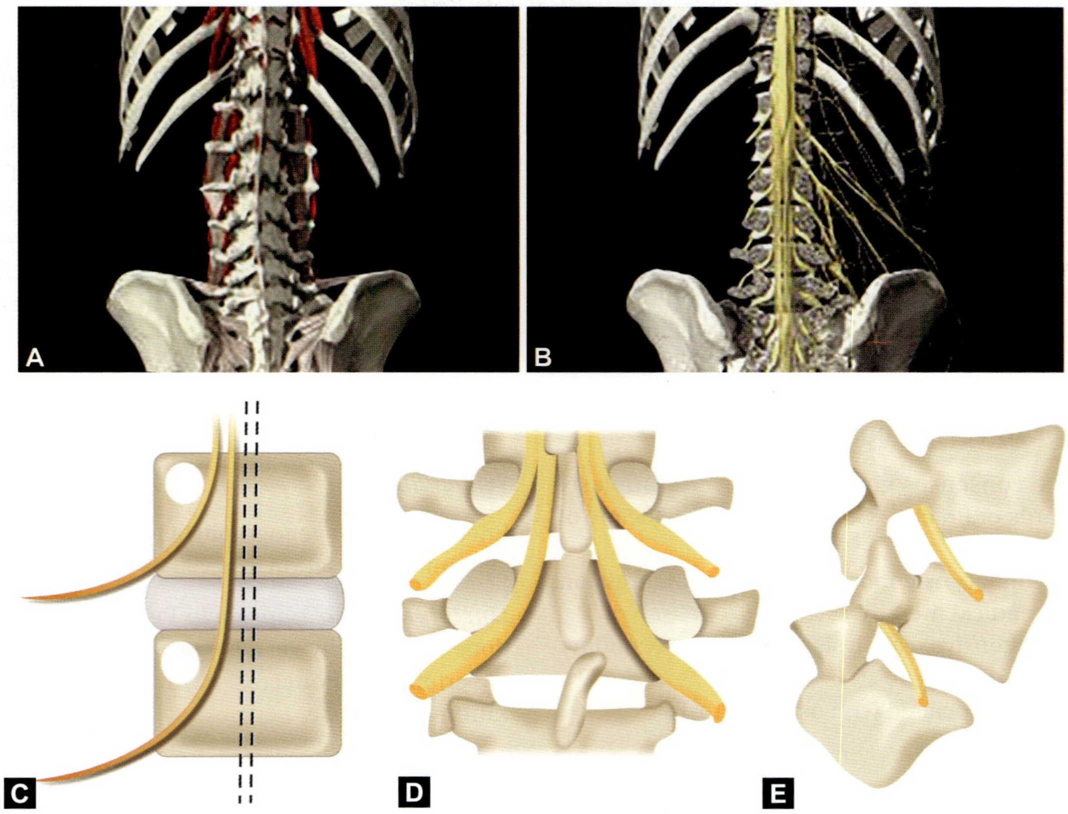

Figs. 3A to E: Anatomical structures involved relation to spinal cord and nerves and pedicles of the vertebral bodies.

POSITION OF THE PATIENT

With the patient in prone position, where the area to be operated, spine can be visualized under C-arm image intensifier. The anatomical landmarks of the vertebral body must be clearly visible.

MONITORING

C-arm should be able to give anteroposterior (AP), lateral, and oblique pictures if required continuously during the procedure. All steps right from the positioning, needle placement, and cement injections should be carefully monitored continuously, at least in biplanar positions of the C-arm. It is essential to have true AP and lateral views. The anatomical landmarks seen on AP view are superior and inferior endplates, the lateral borders of the vertebral body, the spinous process in the center, and medial and lateral pedicle margins. The landmarks as seen on the lateral view are: the anterior and the posterior vertebral borders, superior and inferior endplates, posterior aspect of the spinal canal and superior and inferior contours, and borders of the pedicles. Identifying these landmarks one should be able to remove the parallax have true views of the vertebra to be operated.

OPERATING TABLE

Should be radiolucent, and can allow extension of the spine to achieve dynamic reduction wherever possible to restore the height of the vertebra.

POSITIONING

The patient is rolled gently in prone position. Extreme caution is during the positioning is essential to protect skin and the fragile osteoporotic bones. The extremities and the bony prominences should be well padded. Once the positioned the imaging for the affected vertebrae should be seen very carefully. Use of skin marking pen can be made to mark entry points corresponding to the bony landmarks under C-arm/fluoroscopic visualization.

- Patient's comfort in prone position is the key.
- Arm rests near head of table.

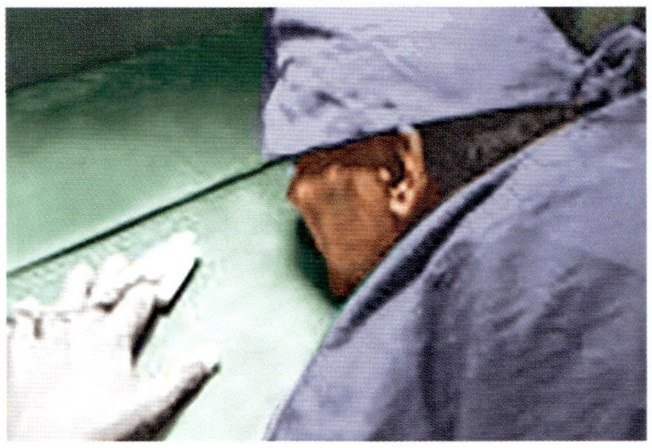

Fig. 4: Positioning of the patient in prone comfortable position.

ANESTHESIA

Identification of the pedicle margins under C-arm control is done. The entry points in the pedicle are at about 10 o'clock position on the left pedicle and about 2 o'clock position in right pedicle. Local anesthesia is infiltrated over the skin till the periosteum of the vertebral body to be operated after identifying the vertebral level. Levels to be injected are marked and 2% lignocaine is infiltrated. Additionally intravenous sedation may be administered as per the requirement of the individual patient.

At some centers general anesthesia, monitored anesthesia [midazolam, fentanyl, and dexmedetomidine] is also used depending upon the surgeon, anesthesiologist's, experience, patient's condition and so on.

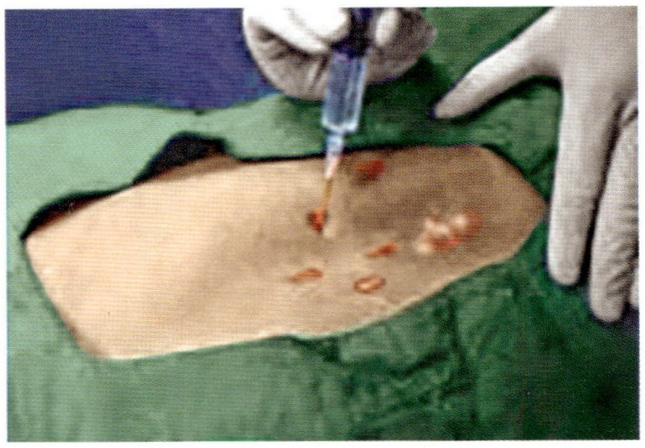

Fig. 5: Infiltration till pedicle with local anesthesia.

After draping and preparation one can skin mark the site as per C-arm image intensifier guidance.

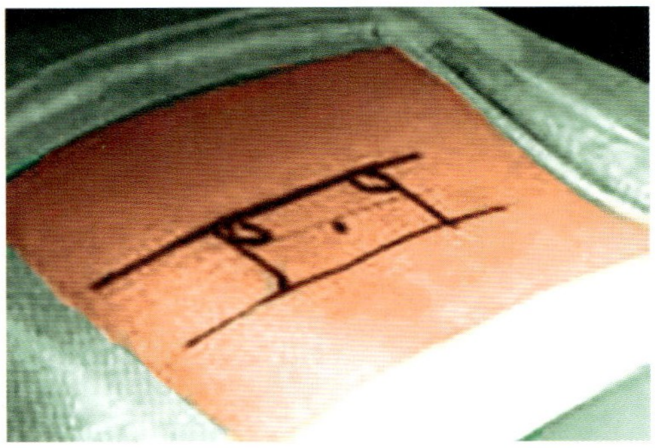

Fig. 6: Skin marking for pedicle and extrapedicular approach.

INCISION

Skin stab incision is taken suitable for insertion of the needle.

Insertion of the AB Needle

The entry point is taken from the superolateral cortex of the pedicle. The insertion of the needle with trocar is done manually under fluoroscopy. Gentle tapping with mallet is done whenever necessary under fluoroscopy control. This takes the needle tip to preplanned trajectory, depending upon the transpedicular or extrapedicular approach is planned. Major resistance is felt to the tapping hand is at the insertion at the pedicle, then at the posterior vertebral cortex.

In osteoporotic bone usually the needle can be gently passed with hand rotational movements without resistance.

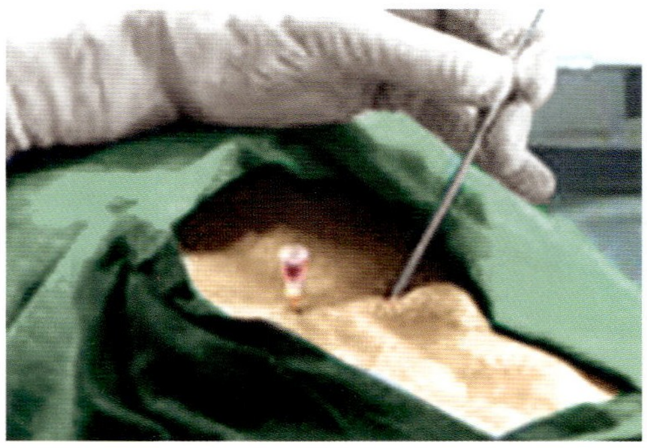

Fig. 7: Insertion of AB needle through the anesthetized skin through stab incision.

One should be extremely cautious to avoid the penetration of the anterior cortex. The medial and the inferior cortices of the pedicles are to be strictly avoided until the needle is totally inside the vertebral bodies. In lateral view monitoring of the needle placement is necessary depending upon the fracture anatomy and to avoid ventral penetration of the needle.

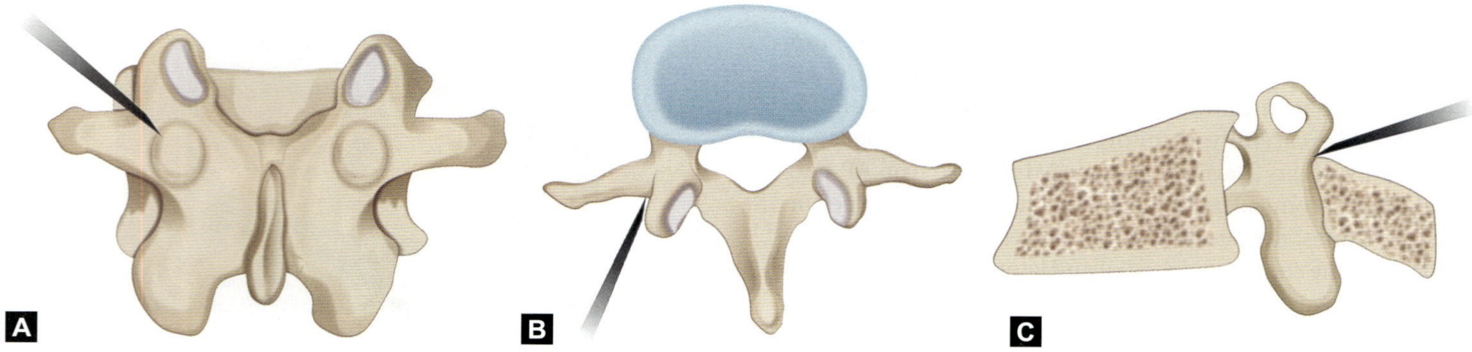

Figs. 8A to C: Anatomical drawing and C-arm picture for proper needle insertion technique [transpedicular technique].

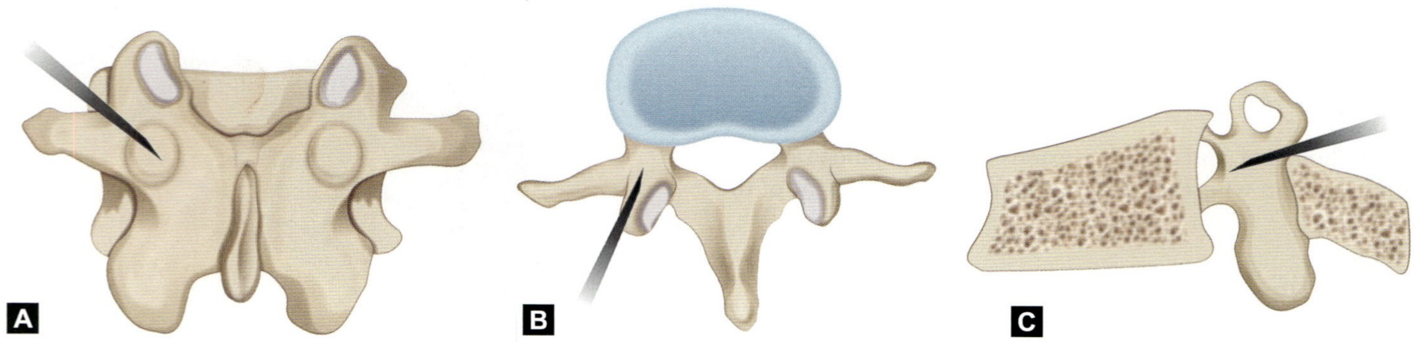

Figs. 9A to C: Midpedicular proper placement of the needle.

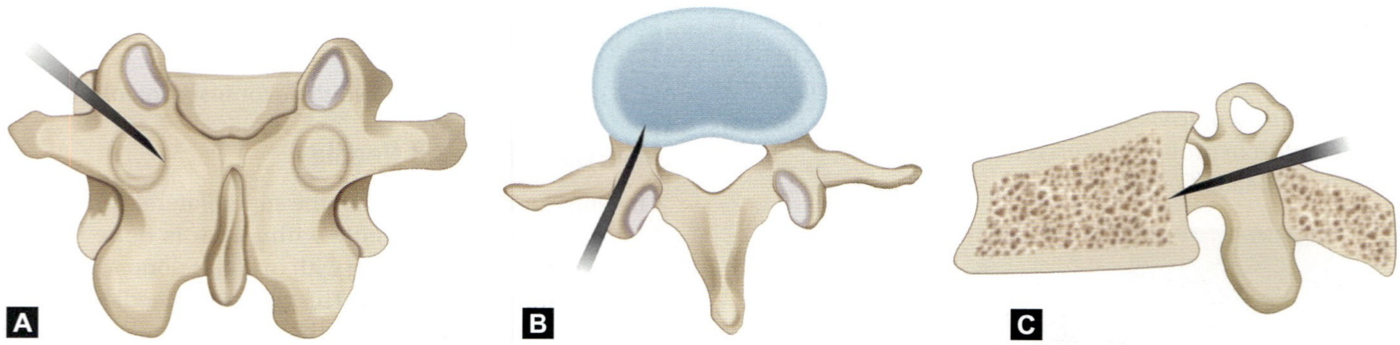

Figs. 10A to C: Suggested proper placement at the entrance at the posterior vertebral wall.

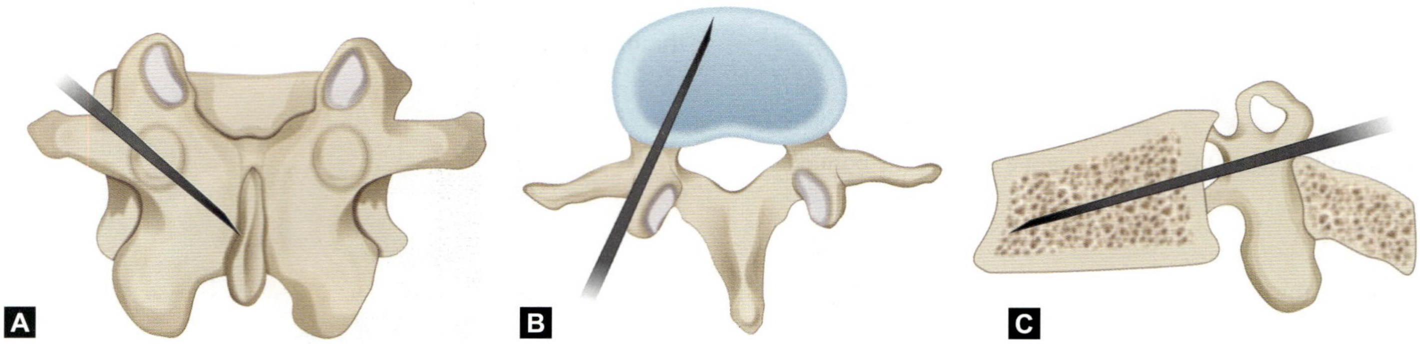

Figs. 11A to C: Safe placement of the needle in the vertebral body.

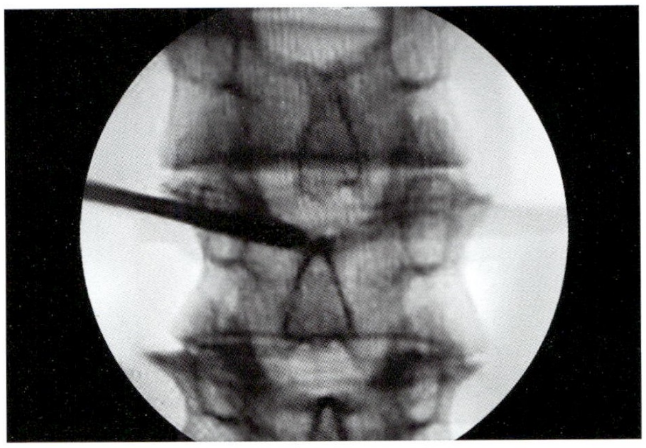

Fig. 12: Final C-arm view.

STEPS OF PREPARATION OF CEMENT (FIGS. 13 TO 20)

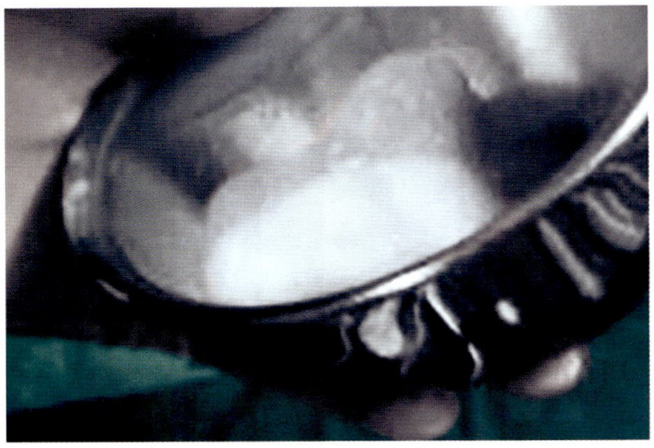

Fig. 13: Collect the powder in a bowl.

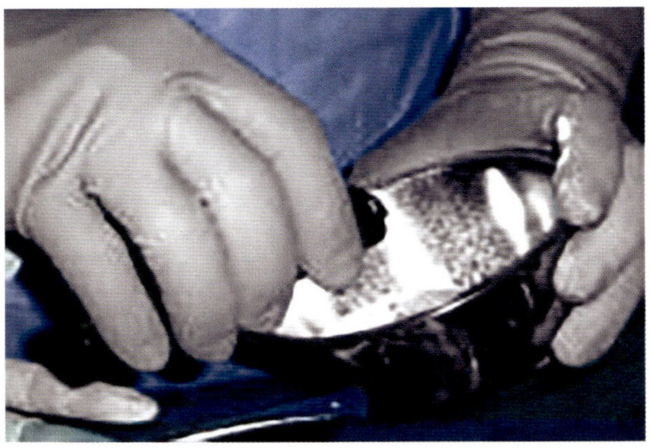

Fig. 14: Open the bottle containing the monomer.

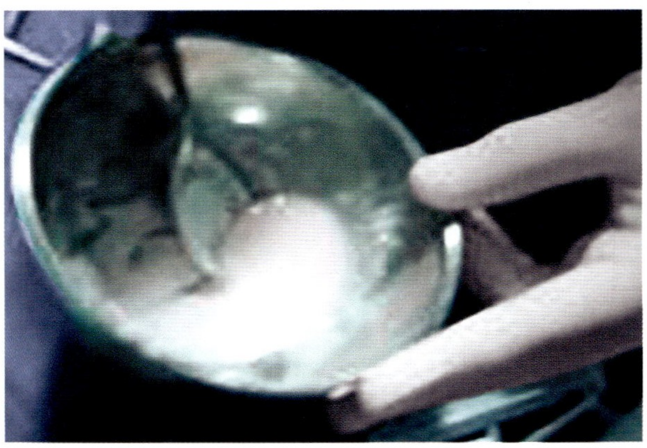

Fig. 15: Thorough mixing of the powder [polymer] and the monomer. This can be done in a bowl or in a mixing chamber of some vertebroplasty system.

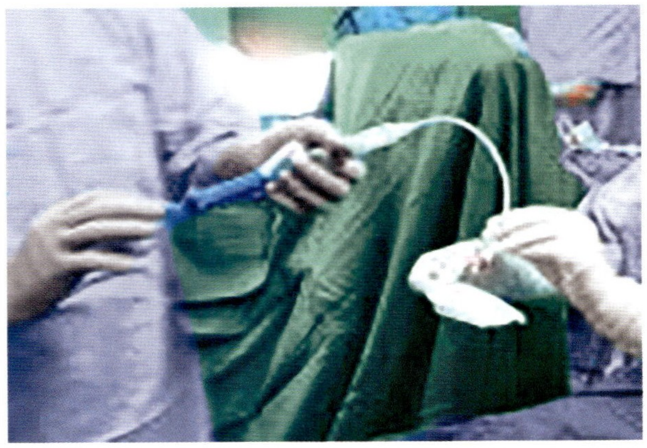

Fig. 16: Fill-up the syringe or syringes.

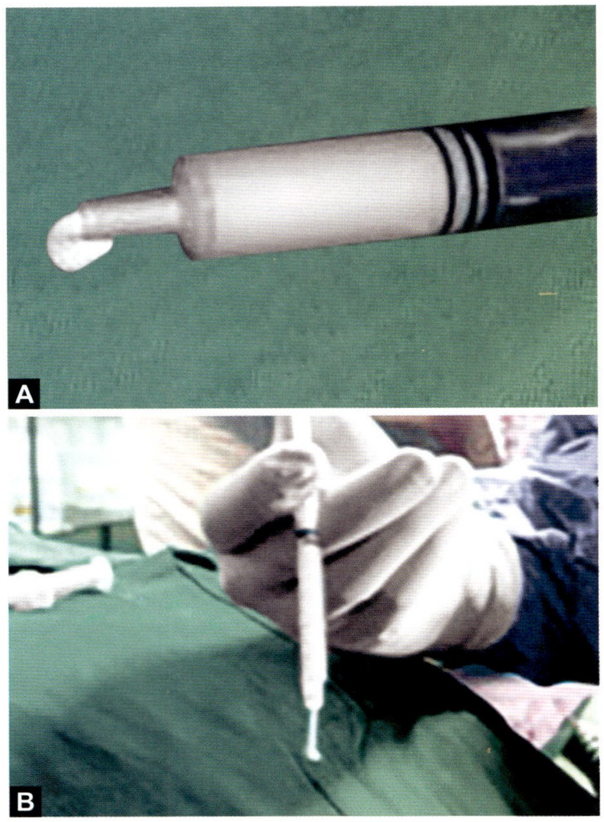

Figs. 17A and B: Wait till the cement has consistency like toothpaste.

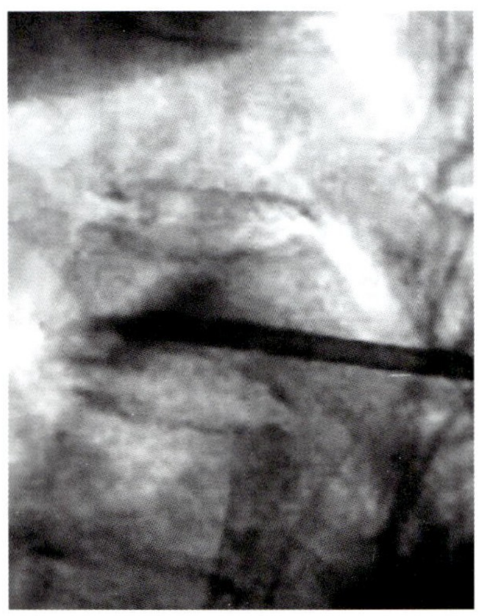

Fig. 18: Under C-arm/fluoroscopy, control monitor the filling of the cement in at least two axes, usually anteroposterior and lateral views. Sometimes take help of oblique views when in doubt.

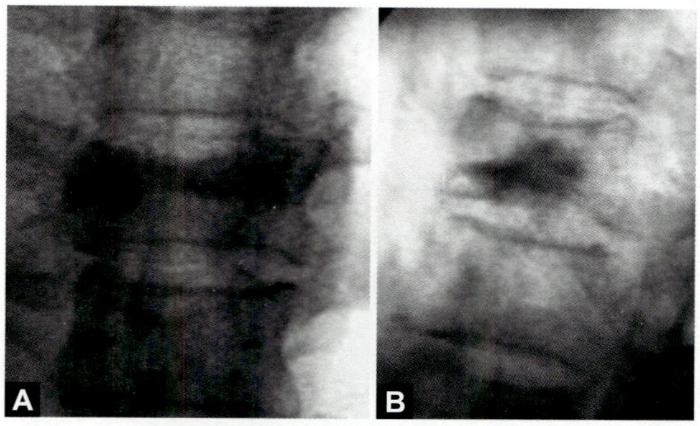

Figs. 19A and B: The C-arm pictures at the end of the procedure (anteroposterior and lateral views).

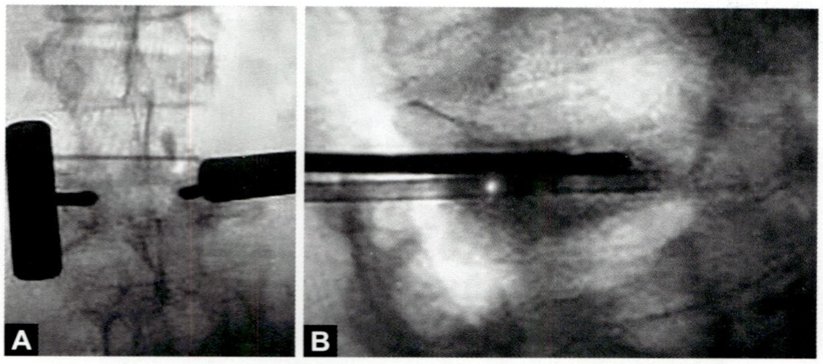

Figs. 20A and B: Treated by bipedicular approach.

MULTILEVEL VERTEBROPLASTY (FIGS. 21 TO 24)

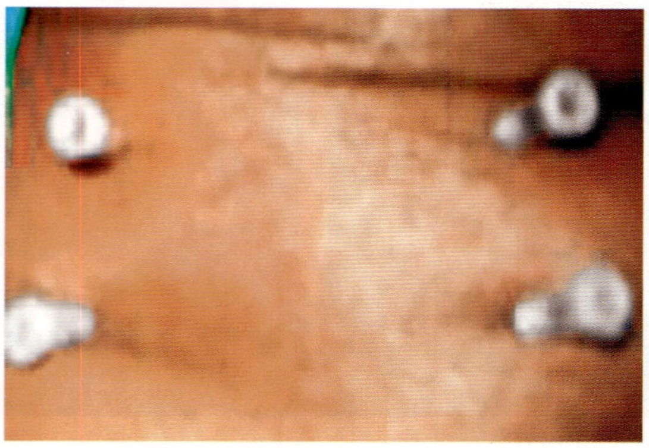

Fig. 21: Local anesthesia till periosteum of the vertebral body.

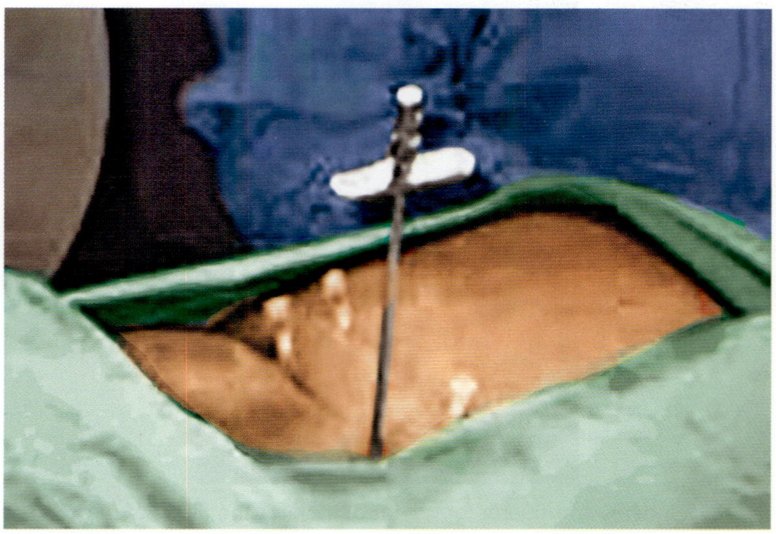

Fig. 22: Insertion of the needle.

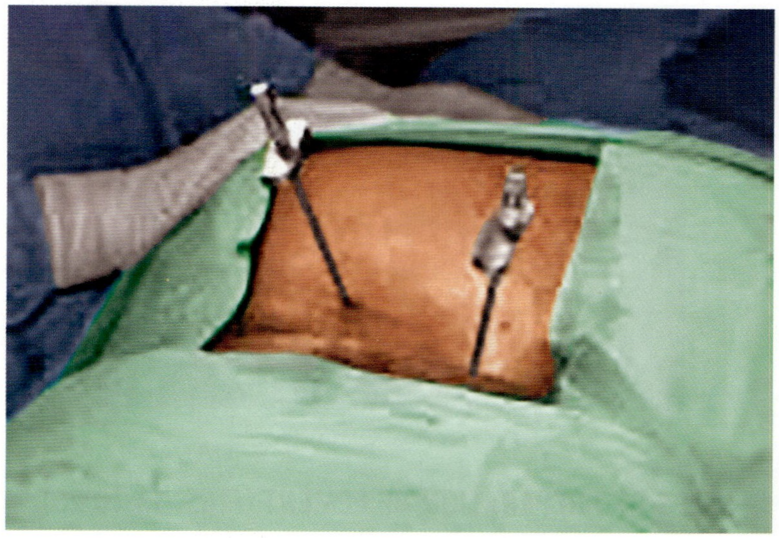

Fig. 23: Insertion of needles at required levels.

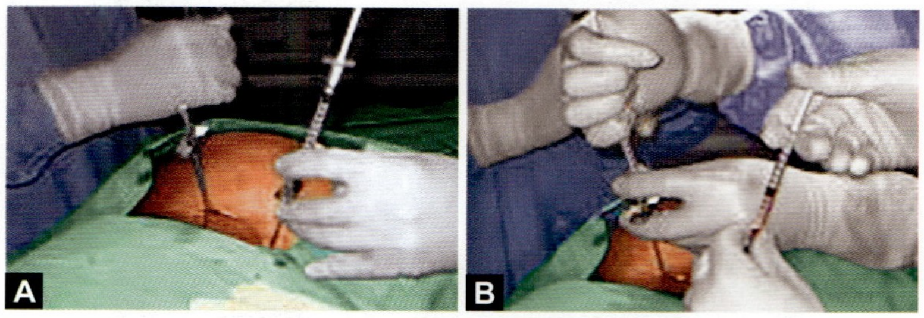

Figs. 24A and B: Injection of the cement.

ILLUSTRATIVE CASE (FIGS. 25 TO 27)

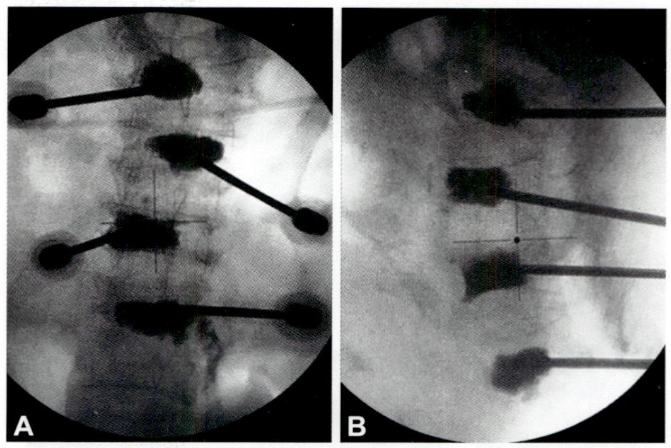

Figs. 25A and B: C-arm pictures of multilevel vertebroplasties in single sitting.

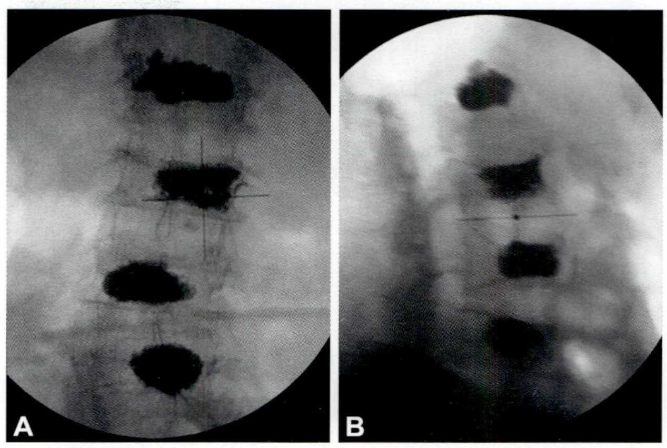

Figs. 26A and B: At completion of the procedure.

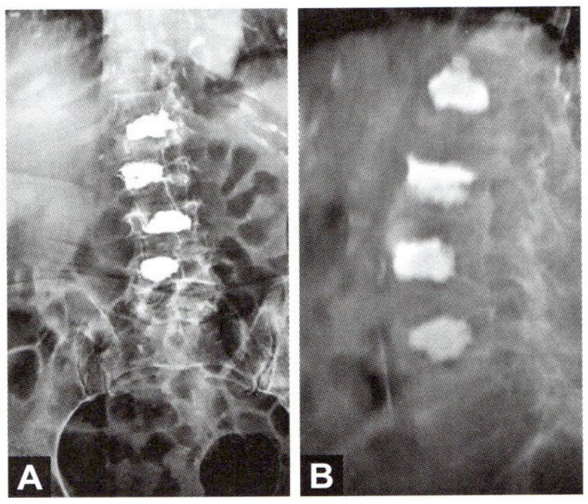

Figs. 27A and B: Long-term 4 years follow-up.

SUGGESTED READING

1. Anselmetti GC, Zoarski G, Manca A, et al. Percutaneous vertebroplasty and bone cement leakage: clinical experience with a new high-viscosity bone cement and delivery system for vertebral augmentation in benign and malignant compression fractures. Cardiovasc Interv Radiol. 2008;31:937-47.
2. Bhave A. Emerging techniques in Spine surgery. 1st edition. New Delhi, India: Jaypee Brothers Medical Publishers (P) Ltd.; 2009. pp. 57-74.
3. Bhave A. Vertebroplasty Made Easy. 1st edition. New Delhi, India: Jaypee Brothers Medical Publishers (P) Ltd.; 2008. pp. 37-79.
4. Chen JF, Lee ST, Lui TN, et al. Percutaneous vertebroplasty for the treatment of osteoporotic vertebral compression fractures: a preliminary report. Chang Gung Med J. 2002;25:306-14.
5. Chen JF. Percutaneous vertebroplasty for treatment of thoracolumbar spine bursting fracture. Surg Neurol. 2004;62:494-500.
6. Chen LH, Lai PL, Chen WJ. Unipedicle percutaneous vertebroplasty for spinal intraosseous vacuum cleft. Clin Orthop Relat Res. 2005;435:148-53.
7. Chen LH, Niu CC, Yu SW, et al. Minimally invasive treatment of osteoporotic vertebral compression fracture. Chang Gung Med J. 2004;27:261-7.
8. Denaro L, Longo UG, Denaro V. Vertebroplasty and kyphoplasty: reasons for concern? Orthop Clin North Am. 2009;40:465-71.
9. Deramond H, Depriester C, Galibert P, et al. Percutaneous vertebroplasty with polymethylmethacrylate. Technique, indications, and results. Radiol Clin North Am. 1998;36:533-46
10. Galibert P, Deramond H, Rosat P. Preliminary note on the treatment of vertebral angioma by percutaneous acrylic vertebroplasty. Neurochirurgie. 1987;33:166-8.
11. Gangi A, Guth S, Imbert JP, et al. Percutaneous vertebroplasty: indications, technique, and results. Radiographics. 2003;23(2):e10.
12. Laredo JD, Hamze B. Complications of percutaneous vertebroplasty and their prevention. Skelet Radiol. 2004;33:493-505.
13. Luo J, Daines L, Charalambous A, et al. Vertebroplasty: only small cement volumes are required to normalize stress distributions on the vertebral bodies. Spine J. 2009;34:2865-73.
14. Mathis JM. Percutaneous vertebroplasty: complication avoidance and technique optimization. AJNR Am J Neuroradiol. 2003;24:1697-706.
15. McGraw JK, Cardella J, Barr JD, et al. Quality improvement guidelines for percutaneous vertebroplasty. J Vasc Interv Radiol. 2003;14:827-31.
16. Silverman SL. The clinical consequences of vertebral compression fracture. Bone. 1992;13:S27-31.
17. Tam AL, Mohamed A, Pfister M, et al. C-arm cone beam computed tomography needle path overlay for fluoroscopic guided vertebroplasty. Spine (Phila Pa 1976). 2010;35:1095-9.
18. Vasconcelos C, Gailloud P, Beauchamp NJ, et al. Is percutaneous vertebroplasty without pretreatment venography safe? Evaluation of 205 consecutives procedures. AJNR Am J Neuroradiol. 2002;23:913-7.
19. Yu SW, Yang SC, Kao YH, et al. Clinical evaluation of vertebroplasty for multiple-level osteoporotic spinal compression fracture in the elderly. Arch Orthop Trauma Surg. 2008;128:97-101.
20. Zampini JM, White AP, McGuire KJ. Comparison of 5766 vertebral compression fractures treated with or without kyphoplasty. Clin Orthop Relat Res. 2010;468:1773-80.
21. Zoarski GH, Snow P, Olan WJ, et al. Percutaneous vertebroplasty for osteoporotic compression fractures: quantitative prospective evaluation of long-term outcomes. J VascInterv Radiol. 2002;13:139-48.

Some material in this chapter is sourced from the book-Vertebroplasty–made easy, Author Dr Arvind Bhave [Jaypee Brothers Medical Publishers (P) Ltd. New Delhi.]

CHAPTER 26

Endoscopic Lumbar Discectomy

Amit R Kale, Ashutosh Sabnis, Rajkumar Mahato

INTRODUCTION

Outpouching of disc nucleus pulposus through an annulus tear is referred to as ruptured/herniated/prolapsed/slipped disc. Lumbar disc herniation 15 times more common than cervical. Lumbar discs are responsible for over 90% of all organic symptoms attributable to low backache.

STAGES OF DISC HERNIATION

- Disc degeneration
- Protrusion
- Extrusion
- Sequestration or sequestered disc.

VARIATIONS

- Interforaminal protrusion
- Dorsal/central protrusion
- Lateral type

CLINICAL FEATURES

- Pain in low back
- Referred pain in sacroiliac region, buttocks, and posterior thigh
- Radicular pain extends below knee and follows dermatome of involved nerve root with motor and sensory symptoms (sciatica)
- *Muscle spasm*: Erector spinae muscle
- Abnormalities of posture
- *Joint derangement*: Flattening of lordosis
- *Motor changes*: Muscle weakness and wasting due to prolonged and severe root irritation
- Diminution/complete loss of the reflex tendon jerks of affected root—early and reliable sign of root involvement
- *Sensory charges*: Tingling/pins and needles or blunting or loss of sensitivity.

PHYSICAL EXAMINATION

- *Inspection*: Antalgic gait
- *Palpation*: Tenderness on palpation and with paraspinal muscle spasm
- *Straight leg test*: Passive-positive in 90% cases
- Bowstring test
- Figure of "4" [Flexion ABduction External Rotation (FABER) test]
- Contralateral straight leg raising test (Fajersztajn test)
- Lasegue test
- Femoral nerve stretch test.

INVESTIGATION

- X-ray
  - Anterior-posterior L-S spine X-ray
  - Lateral L-S spine, oblique L-S spine
  - Flexion and extension views
- Myelography: Not recommended nowadays as noninvasive and accurate tests are available
- Computed tomography (CT) scan
- Magnetic resonance imaging (MRI) scan—superior in detection of disc degeneration.
  - T1 (spine-lattice): Good anatomic display of cord, nerve roots and highlight fat and marrow space
  - T2 (spine-spin): Highlight fluid in lumbar dural sac and differentiate nucleus from annulus fibrosus.

TREATMENT

- Strict bed rest
- Nonsteroidal anti-inflammatory drugs (NSAIDs), muscle relaxants, and night sedation
- *Physiotherapy*: Passive extension of spine, proper body posture, and body mechanics education. Transcutaneous electrical nerve stimulation, ultrasound, and diatherapy
- Epidural steroid
- *Chemonucleolysis*: Chymopapain.

Surgical Treatment

Indications

- Paraplegia or acute bladder paralysis due to cauda equina compression.
- Peripheral neurological deficit and neurological claudication failure of conservative treatment of 4–6 weeks.

Approaches:

- Posterior approach:
  - Laminectomy and discectomy—standard
  - Fenestrated operation—limited laminectomy
  - Microsurgical laminectomy with disc fragment excision
- Anterior approach with or without interbody fusion
- Percutaneous approach—suction, laser or arthroscopic discectomy or endoscopic discectomy.

SURGICAL STEPS (FIGS. 1 TO 23)

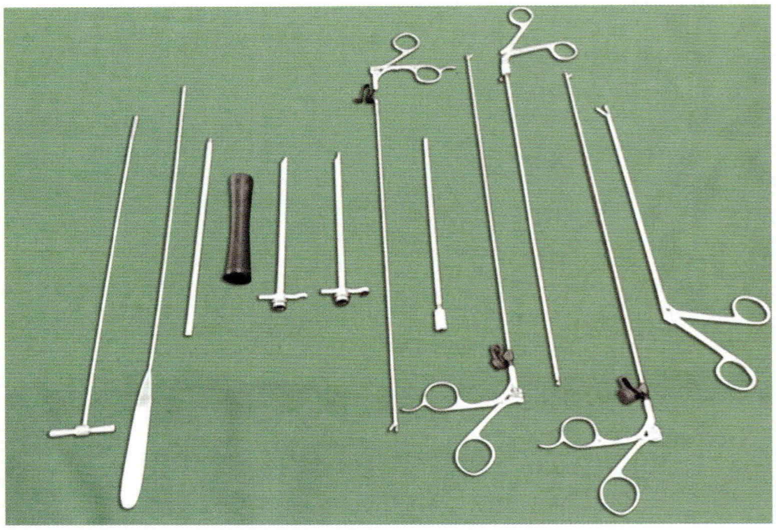

Fig. 1: Instrument trolley.

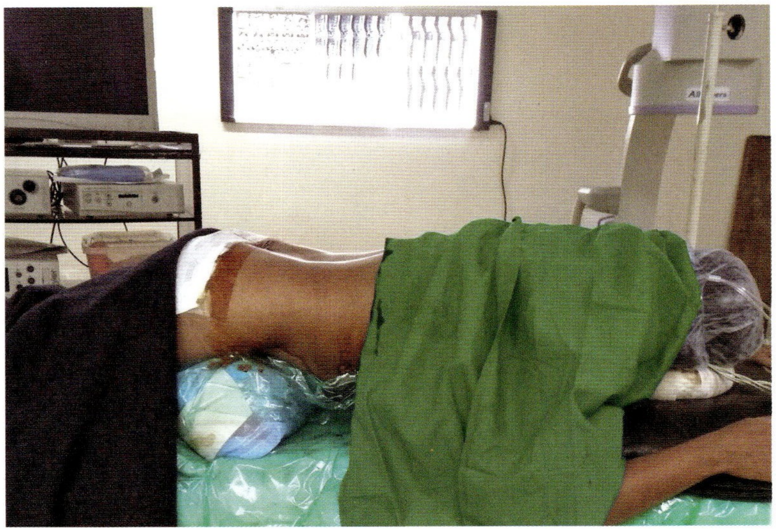

Fig. 2: Patient is lying prone on the table, head on the right side.

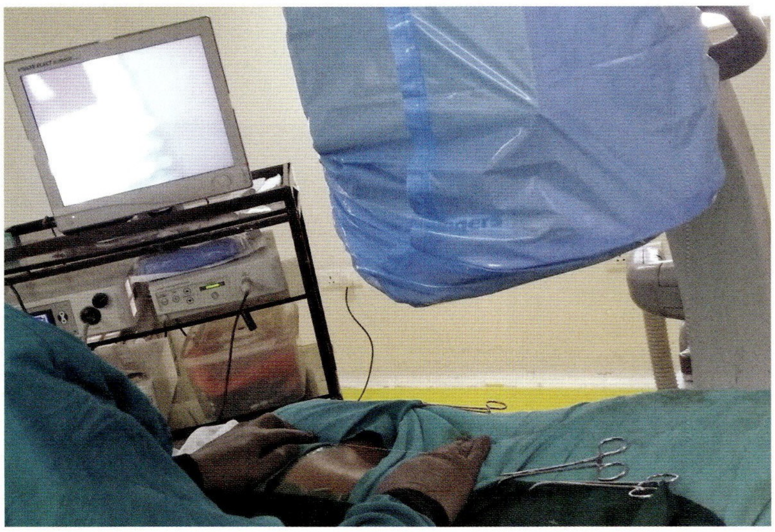

Fig. 3: C-arm is lined up to exactly center over the affected area, exact anteroposterior (AP) image is assured by confirming that both the pedicles at L5-S1 are equidistance from midline spinous process. Pedicles are seen end on. All areas of body likely to have pressure are properly padded, patient is awake and aware throughout the procedure. A metallic marker is used to mark a midline under C-arm, skin is marked with a permanent marker, midline marking is essential for proper orientation.

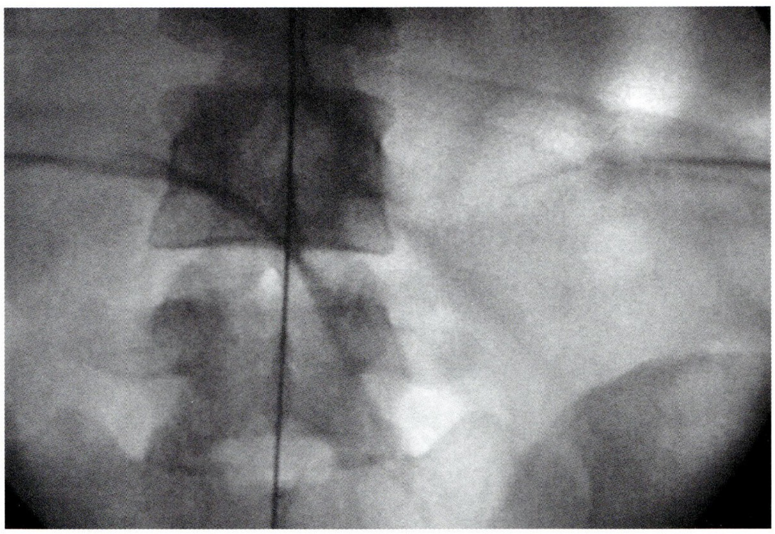

Fig. 4: C-arm image shows metallic marker is on the center of the vertebral bodies corresponding to the spinous processes.

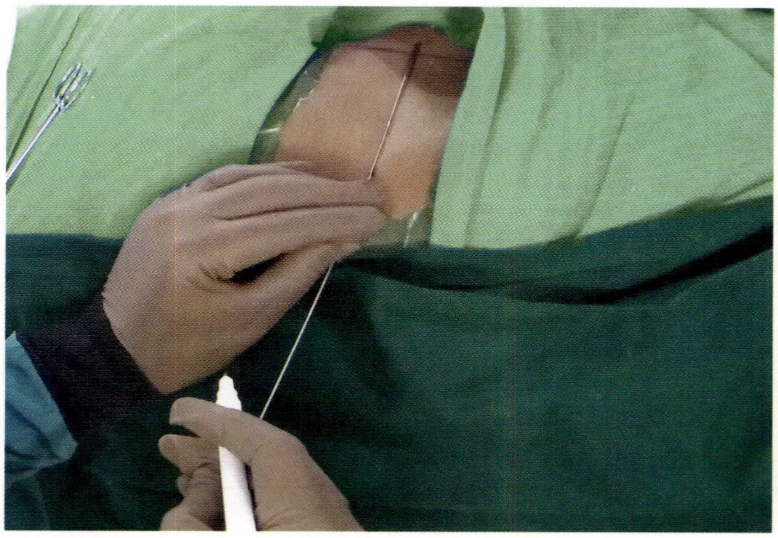

Fig. 5: The disc space is being marked as is seen in the anteroposterior image.

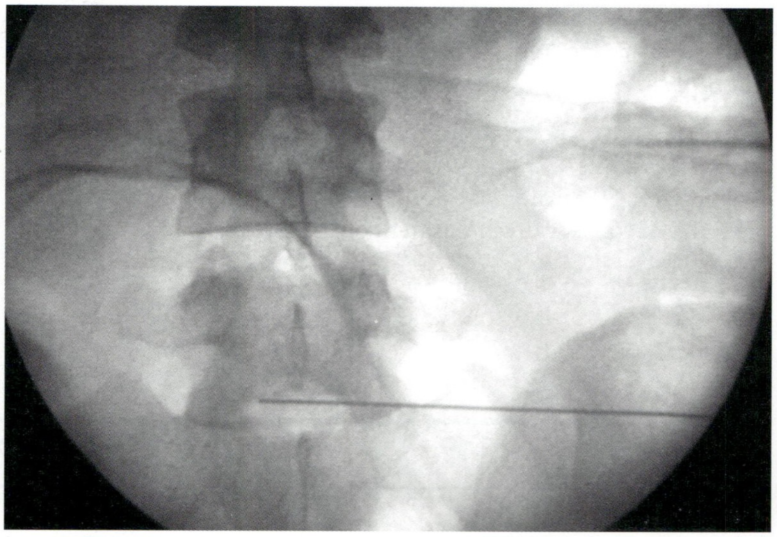

Fig. 6: C-arm image shows metallic marker in L5-S1 disc space, which is to be operated.

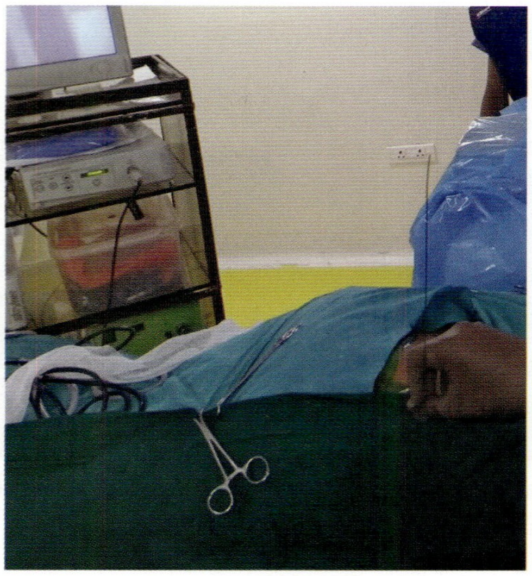

Fig. 7: First step is to line it up exactly in lateral view, that we remove any parallax between the C-arm and the disc end plates, ensure that both the end plates are parallel to each other. The marking is done for disc inclination and depth of the disc space.

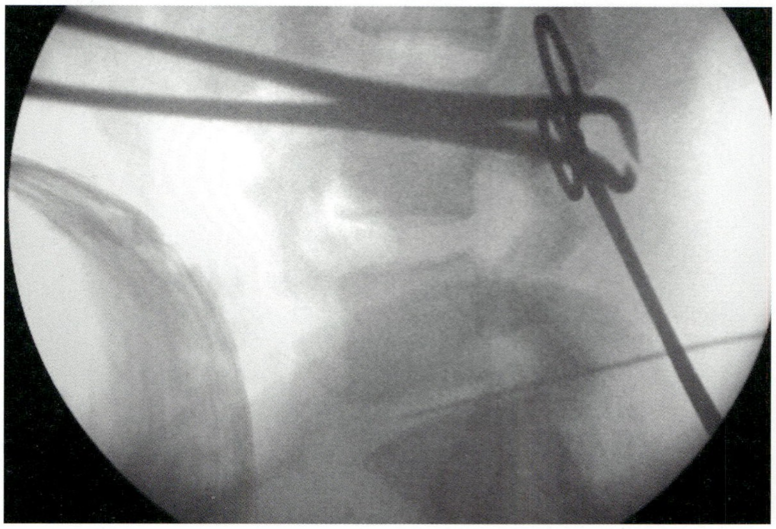

Fig. 8: Disc marking is done with a marker line in line with the disc seen in C-arm.

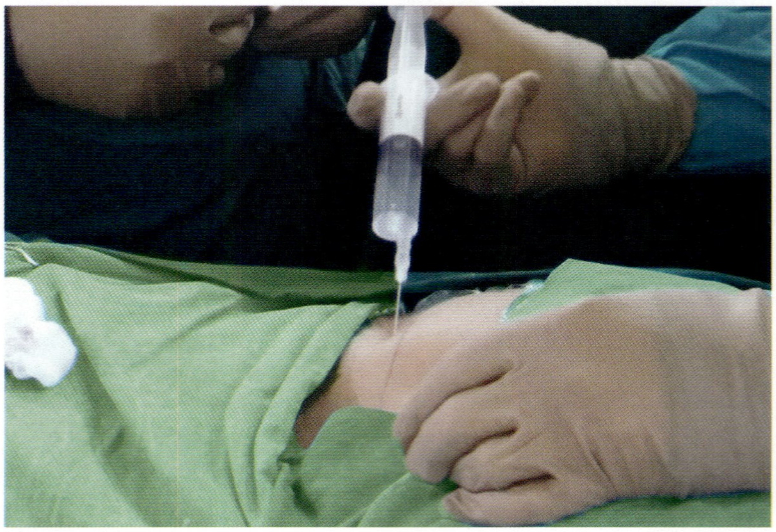

Fig. 9: Local anesthetic agent 2% plain lignocaine without adrenaline is injected to numb skin and subcutaneous tissue, a wheel is raised by injection.

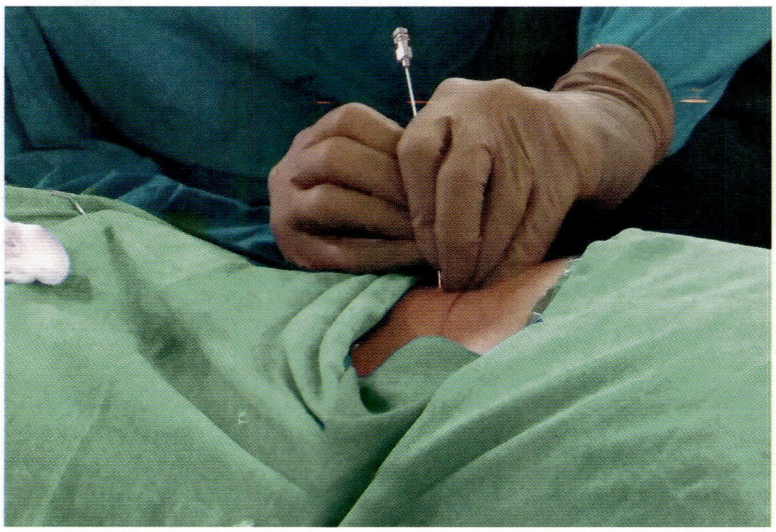

Fig. 10: The needle is inserted with an angle of 25° to the horizontal. The tip is advanced to the intervertebral foramen and is visualized all along before proceeding.

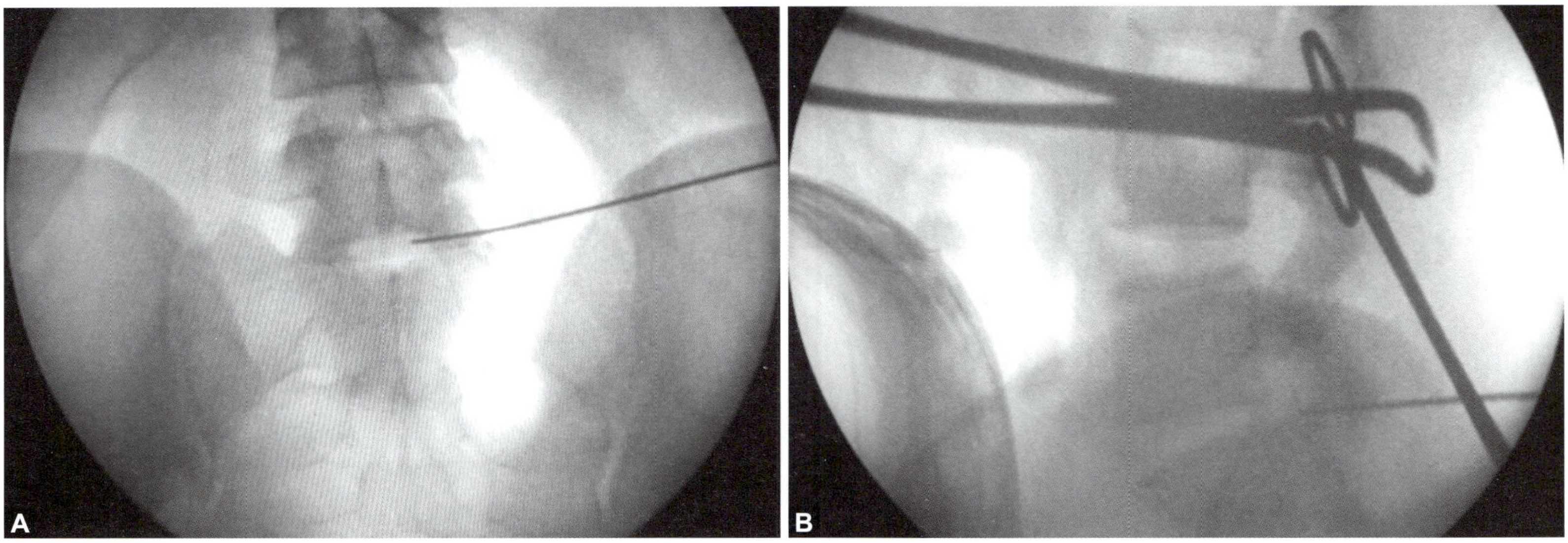

Figs. 11A and B: The anteroposterior view (A) of C-arm image shows its tip in the medial pedicle line which it is not supposed to cross. The medial pedicle line is the lateral edge of the dural sac, the tip of the needle is lateral to the medial pedicle line and on lateral view (B) it is on the posterior annulus, this is an ideal placement.

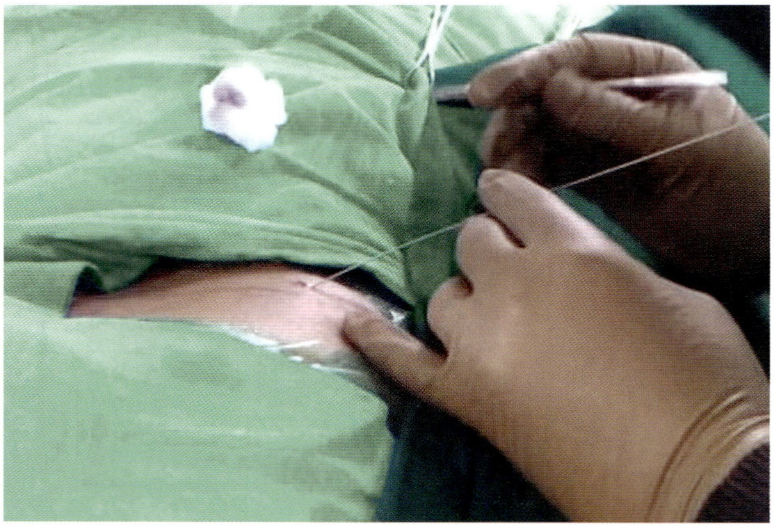

Fig. 12: The stylet of the needle is replaced by the guidewire.

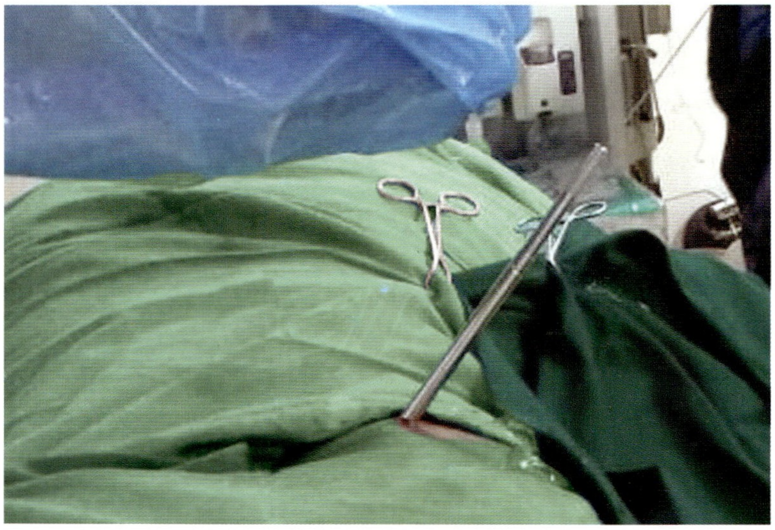

Fig. 13: Skin incision is now taken with No. 11 blade and a dilator which will gently dilate the muscle and is introduced over the guidewire. The tip of the dilator is blunt and very safe. The dilator is introduced up to the annulus, on reaching it, the patient experiences pain.

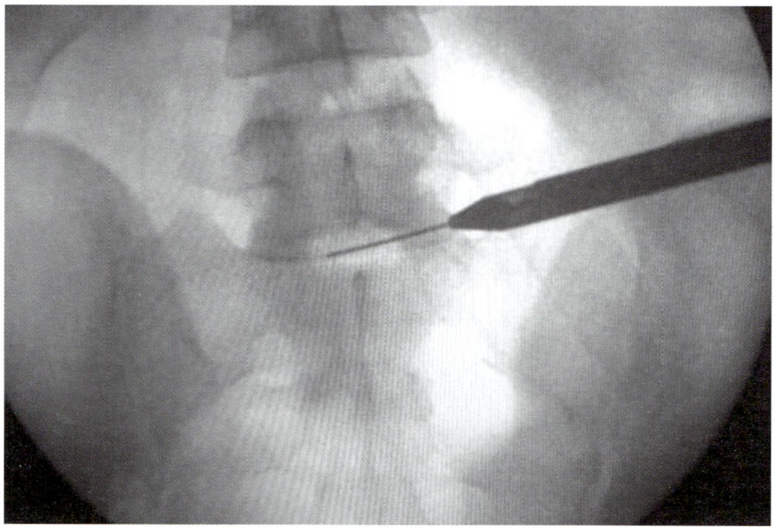

Fig. 14: The tip is checked over anteroposterior view and a cannula is inserted over this dilator. The cannula is pushed with the hand with small rotating movements over the dilator, until we reach the annulus.

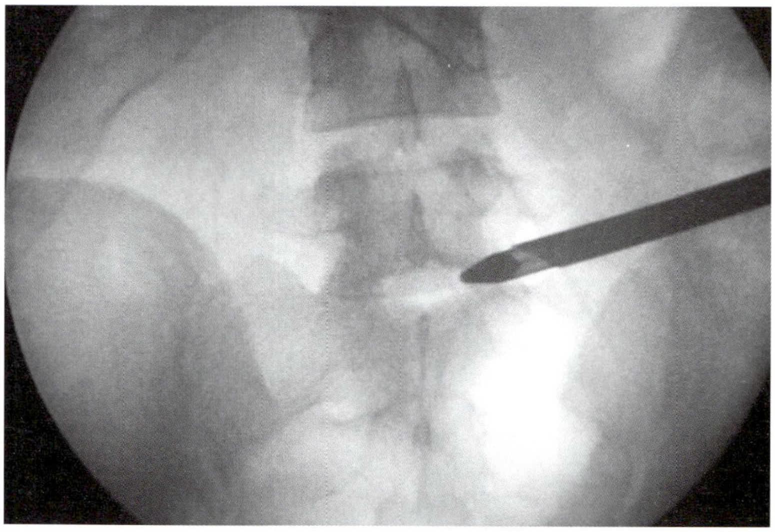

Fig. 15: C-arm image shows dilator along with cannula within the disc space after removing the guidewire.

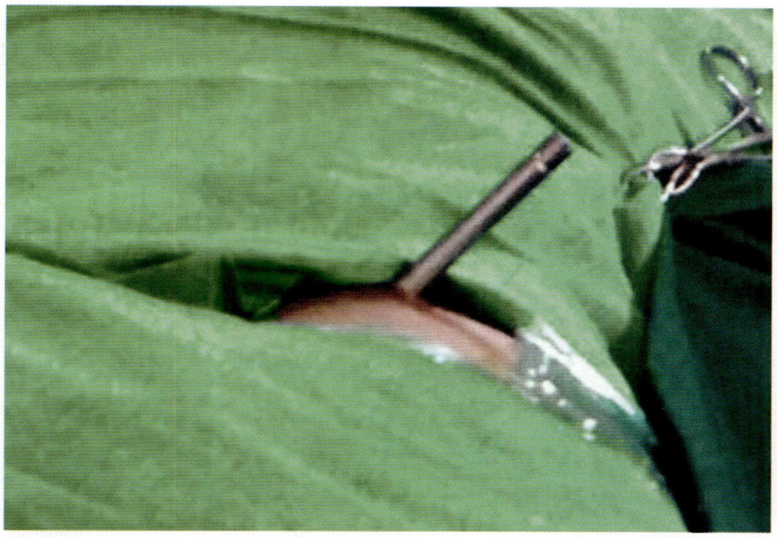

Fig. 16: Cannula in situ and the dilator has been removed.

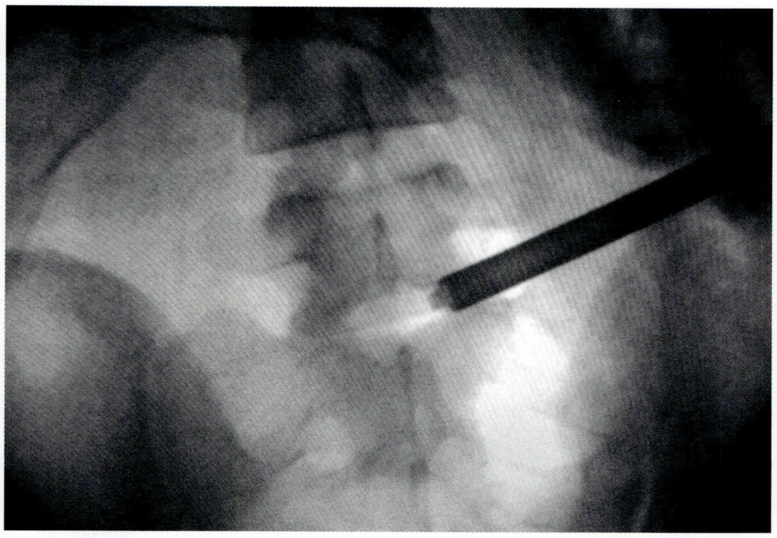

Fig. 17: The tip of the cannula can be seen inside the disc in the anteroposterior view of C-arm image.

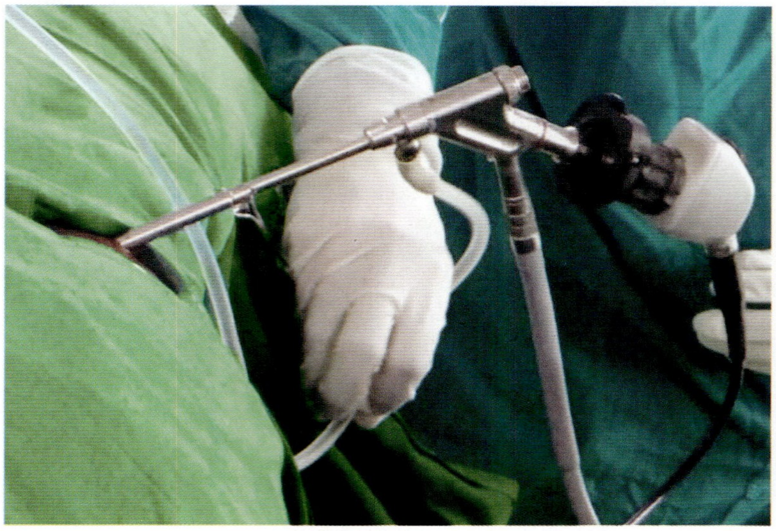

Fig. 18: The cannula guides the scope inside.

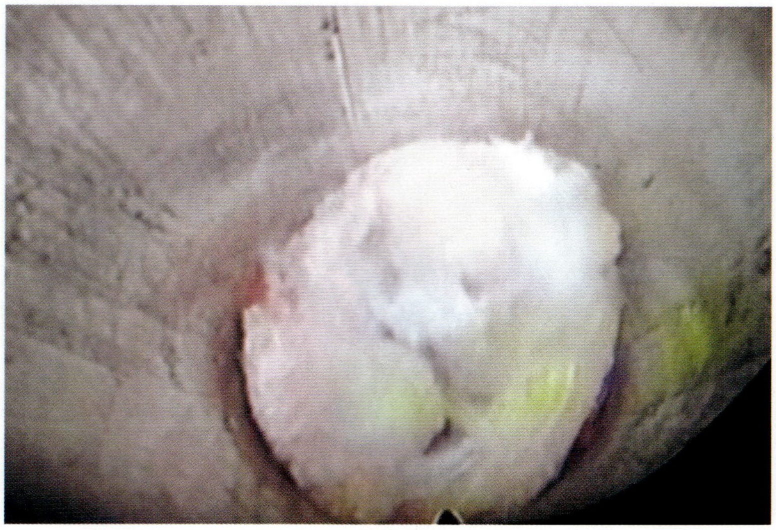

Fig. 19: Targeted fragment is seen after inserting the scope.

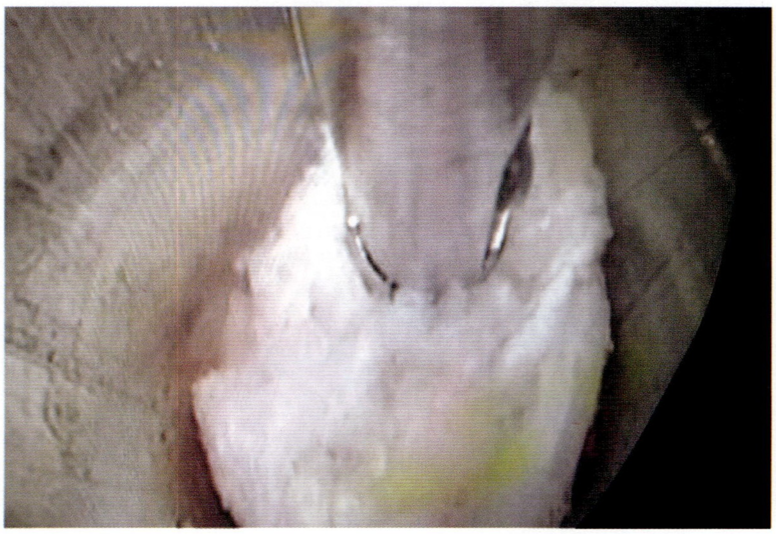

Fig. 20: Targeted fragmentectomy is done with the grasper under the endoscopic guidance.

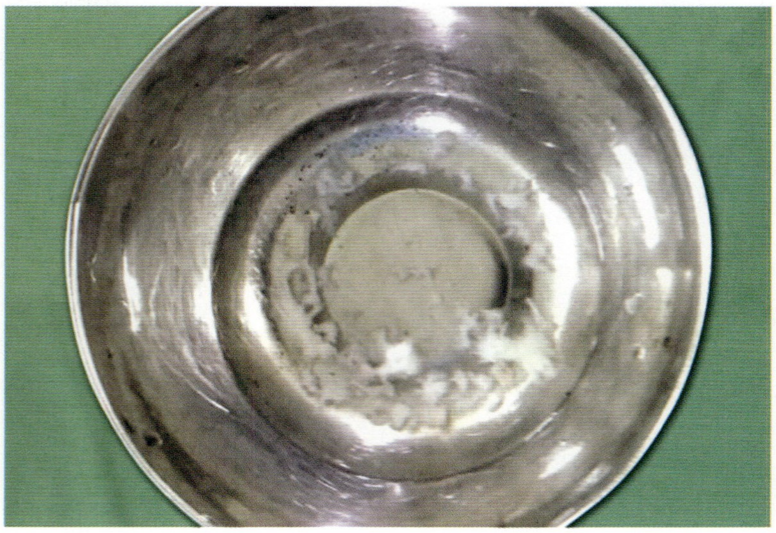

Fig. 21: Removed disc fragments.

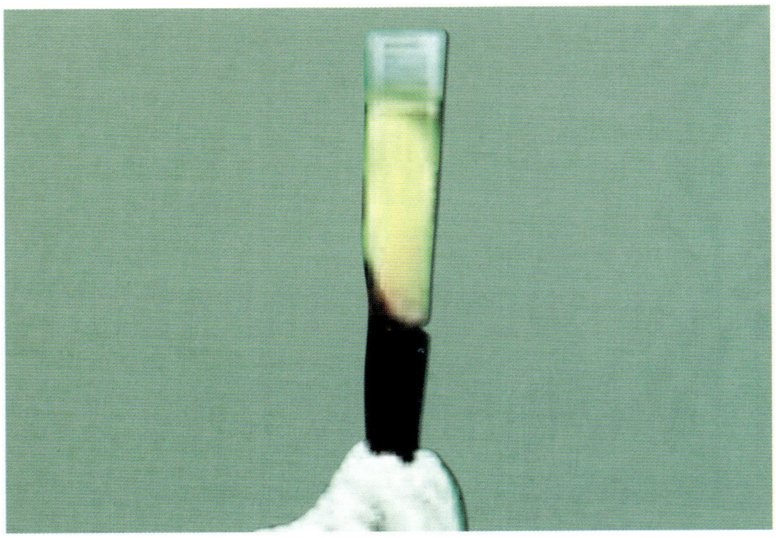

Fig. 22: Test tube containing separated platelet rich fibrin above, which has been separated from the whole blood of patient by centrifugation.

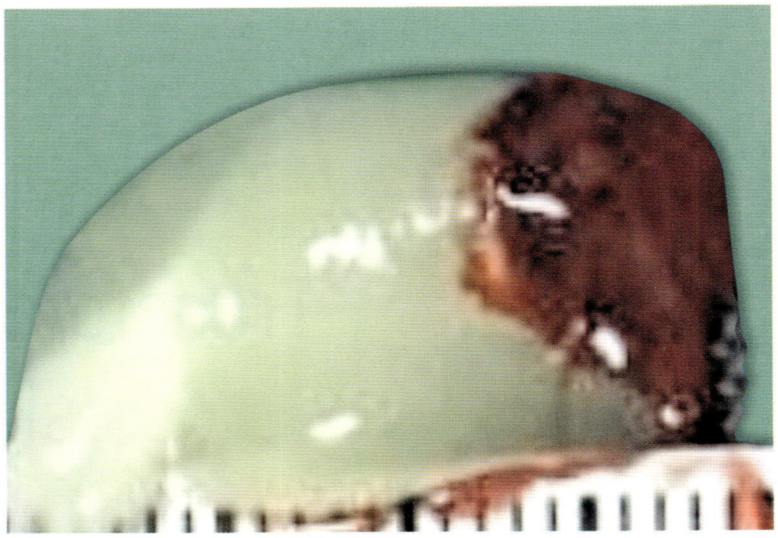

Fig. 23: Platelet rich fibrin, which is to be inserted after the completion of the procedure through the cannula. Procedure was completed, cannula was removed and dressing is done.

COMPLICATIONS

- *Infection*:
  - Superficial wound infection
  - Deep disc space infection
- Thrombophlebitis/deep vein thrombosis
- Pulmonary embolism
- *Dural tears*: Pseudomeningocele, cerebrospinal fluid (CSF) leak, and meningitis
- Postoperative cauda equina lesions
- Neurological damage or nerve root injury
- Urinary retention or urinary tract infection.

SUGGESTED READING

1. Wilson DH, Harbaugh RE. Lumbar discectomy: a comparative study of microsurgical and standard techniques. In: Hardy RW (Ed). Lumbar Disc Disease. New York: Raven Press; 1982. pp. 147-56.
2. Wilson DH, Kenning J. Microsurgical lumbar discectomy: preliminary report of 83 consecutive cases. Neurosurgery. 1979;4:137-40.
3. Yasargil MG. Microsurgical operation of herniated lumbar disc. Adv Neurosurg. 1977;4:81-2.

CHAPTER 27

Transforaminal Lumbar Interbody Fusion by Minimally Invasive Surgery Technique

Raghvendra Singh Raghuvanshi, Shaishav Shah, Amol J Rege

INTRODUCTION

Lumbar interbody fusion technique with unilateral access to the interbody space, Transforaminal lumbar interbody fusion (TLIF) can be performed through an open procedure or minimally invasive surgery (MIS) technique with smaller incisions.

INDICATIONS

- Spondylolisthesis
- Recurrent disc herniation.

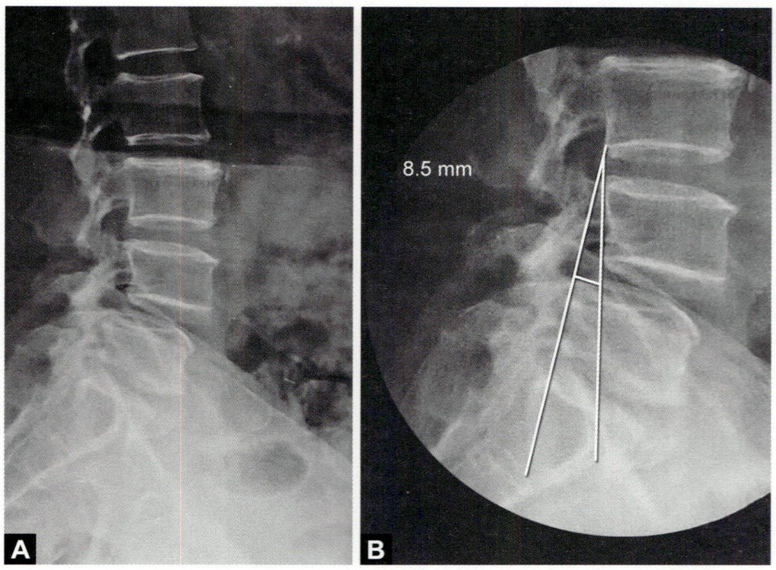

Figs. 1A and B: Listhesis at L4-5 level.

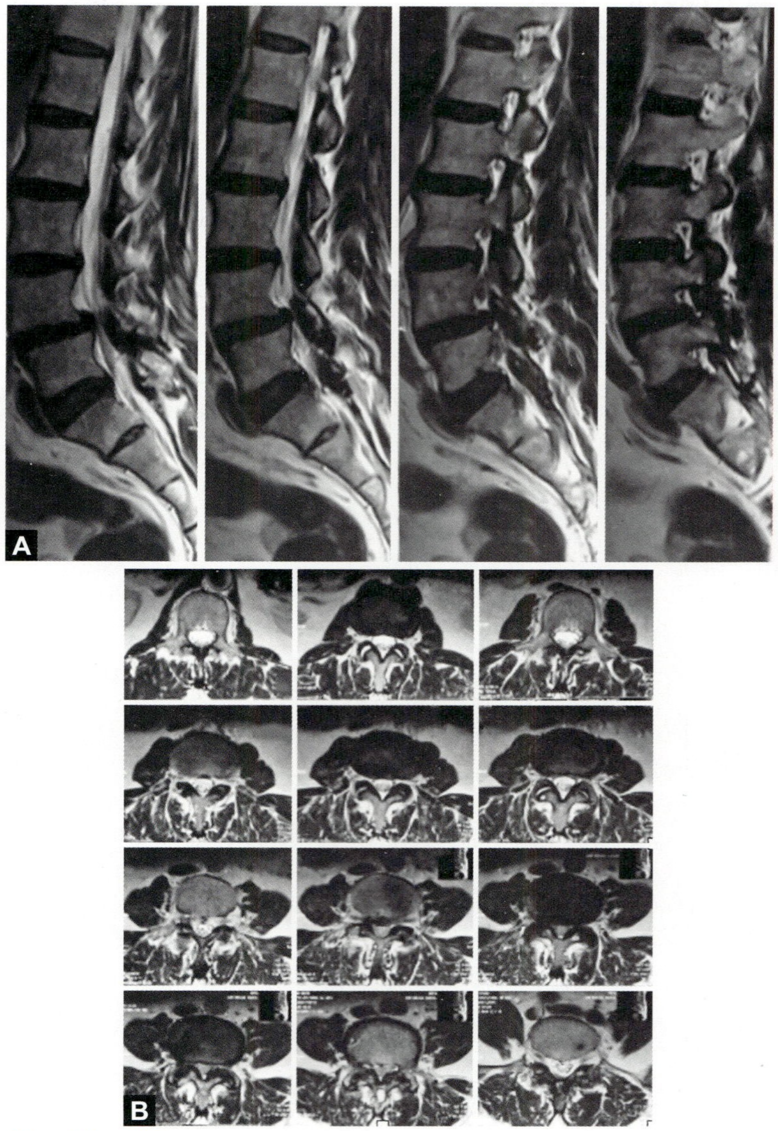

Figs. 2A and B: Listhesis at L4-5 level with canal narrowing at same level.

ADVANTAGES VIA MINIMALLY INVASIVE SURGERY

- By opening the neural foramen on one side only, damage to important anatomical structures such as nerve roots, dura, and ligamentum flavum is reduced.
- Using a MIS mini-open incision reduces access-associated muscle injury, minimize bleeding and improve postoperative recovery.
- Lesser chances of infection.

LIMITATIONS

- Difficult to correct more than grade 3 listhesis
- Learning curve
- Radiation exposure.

CONTRAINDICATIONS

- Epidural scaring
- Arachnoiditis.

PREOPERATIVE PLANNING

- X-ray L-S spine four views—anteroposterior (AP), lateral, lateral dynamic-flexion, and extension.
- Magnetic resonance imaging (MRI)
- How many levels require fusion
- Symptomatic site right or left.

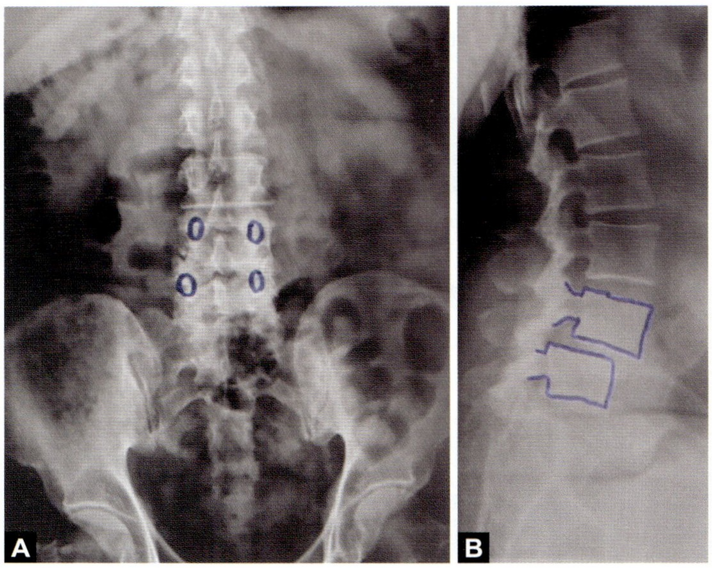

Figs. 3A and B: Preoperative planning with level of fusion and number of screws required.

POSITION

- After the patient is put under general anesthesia, patient is catheterized, shifted to prone position over radiolucent table with bolsters keeping abdomen free.
- Antibiotic prophylaxis given.
- *Part preparation*: Under all aseptic precautions, scrubbing, painting, and draping done.

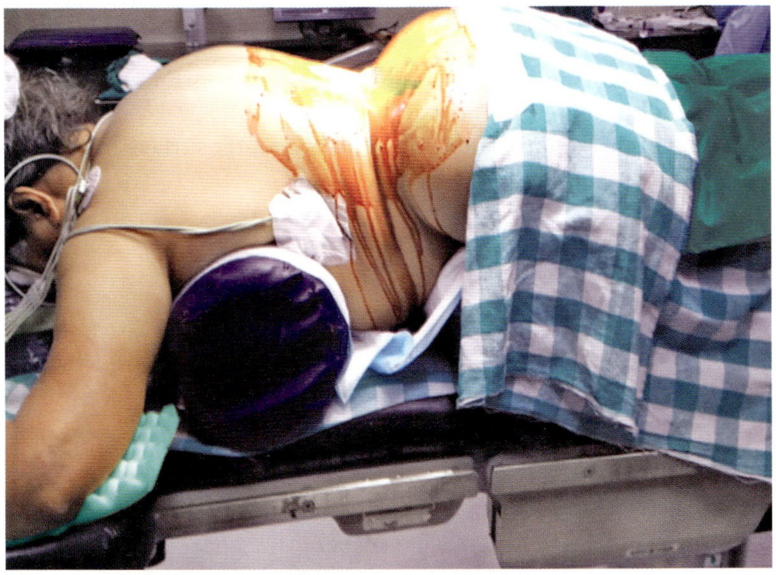

Fig. 4: Positioning and part preparation.

INSTRUMENTS

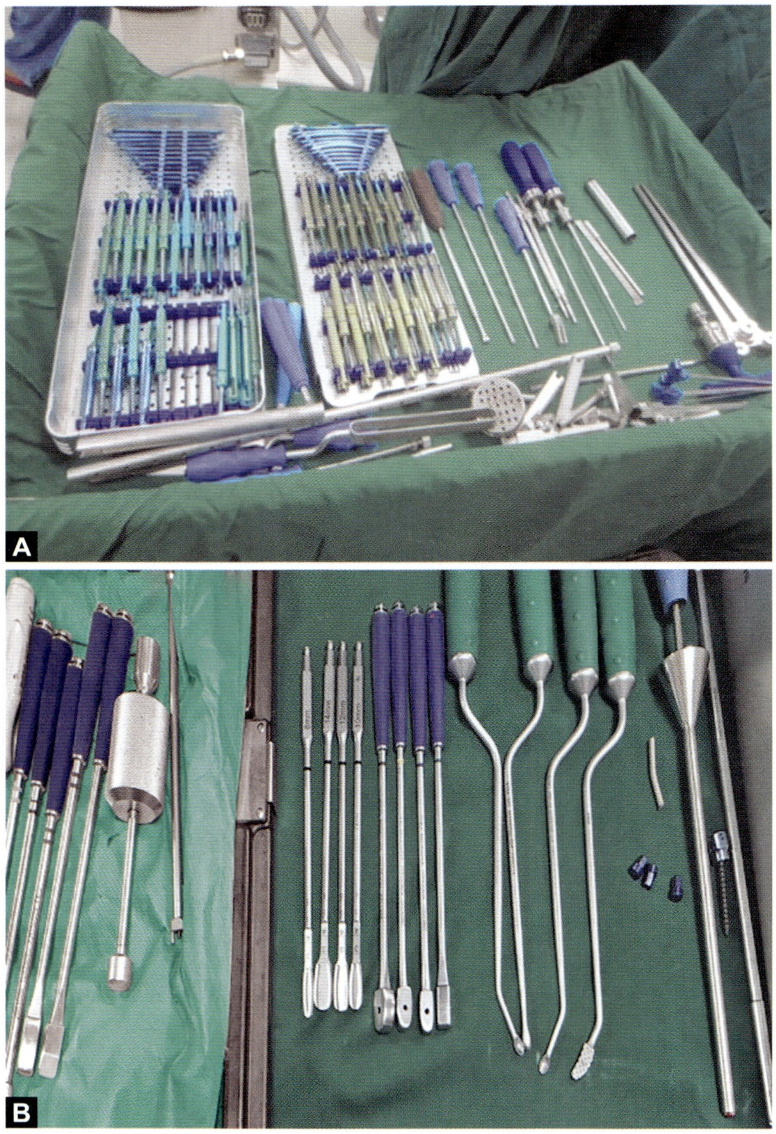

Figs. 5A and B: Instruments required for minimally invasive system.

INCISION PLANNING

- Level is confirmed under C-arm guidance in both anteroposterior and lateral view.
- Extent and location of incision is planned after surface marking.

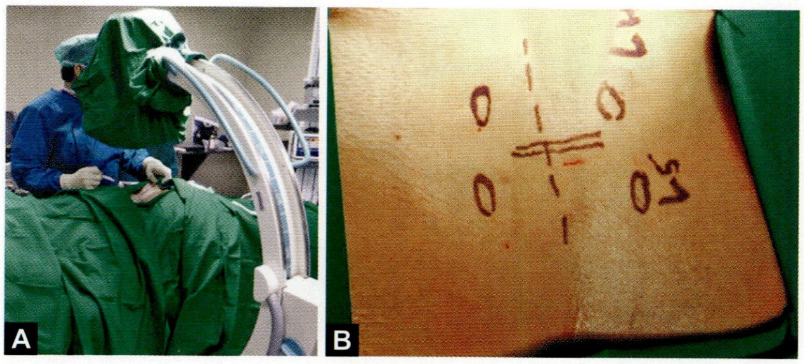

Figs. 6A and B: (A) Confirmation of level under C-arm; (B) Surface marking.

Percutaneous Pedicle Screw Fixation

Needle with trocar is inserted through a small stab incision and advanced till it reaches tip of transverse process on its posterior aspect, then it is advanced medially till its base, at this junction under C-arm guidance it is advanced through the pedicle taking precaution not to breach the medial and inferior border of the pedicle under C-arm guidance.

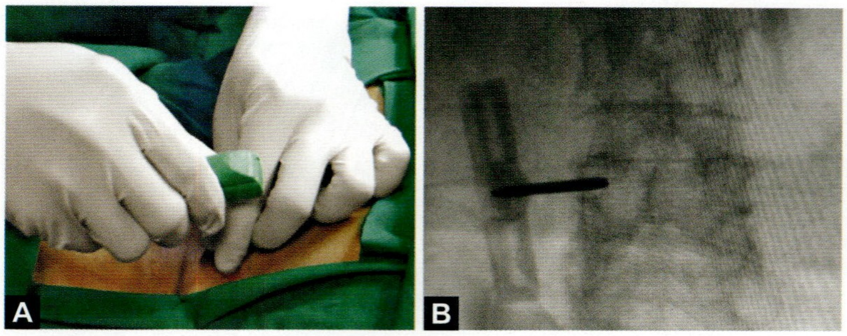

Figs. 7A and B: Percutaneous pedicle screw fixation.

Trocar Removed and Exchanged with Guidewire

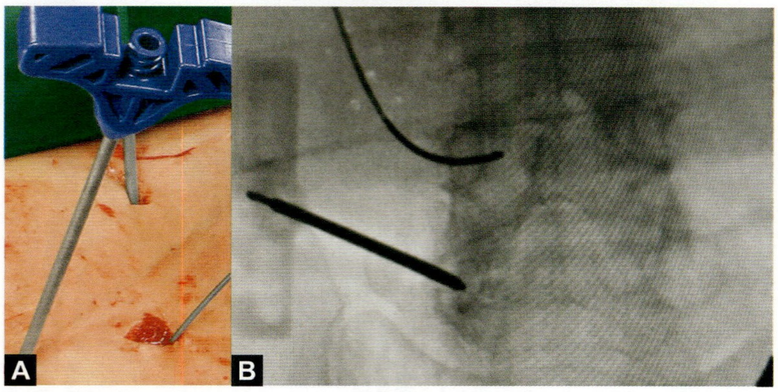

Figs. 8A and B: Trocar removed and exchanged with guidewire.

Pedicle Screw Insertion

After sequential tubular dilatation, tapping done with 1 mm smaller sized tap comparing with desired screw size, tap removed, cannulated pedicle screw inserted through the guidewire and position confirmed on C-arm, similarly pedicle screw inserted into inferior pedicle on same side.

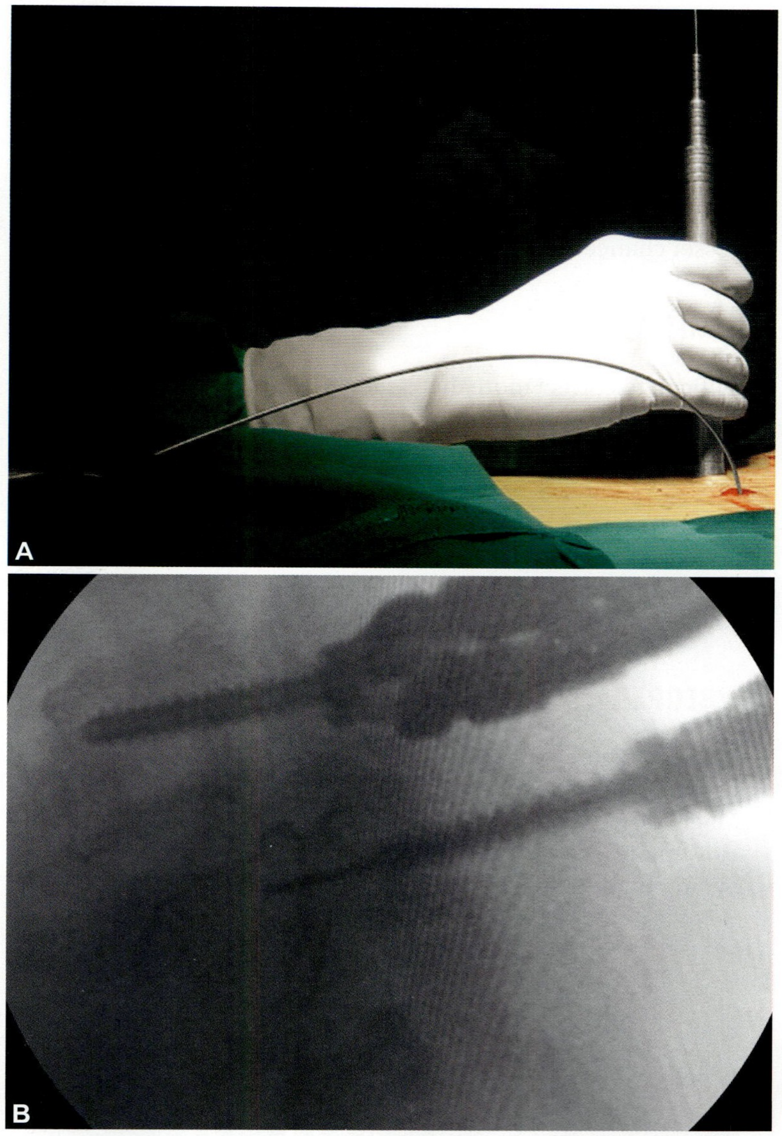

Figs. 9A and B: Serial dilators and pedicle screw fixation.

Tubular System is Aligned and Jig is Placed

After inserting all screws on one side the tubular system is aligned and jig is placed.

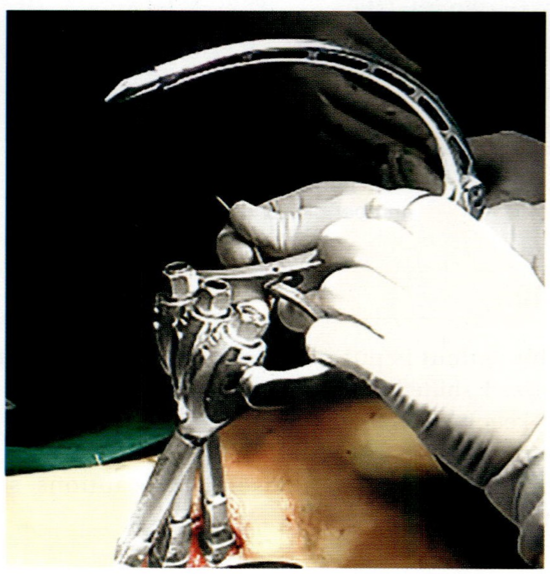

Fig. 10: Tubular system is aligned and jig is placed.

Rod Insertion

After jig placement, rod length to be used is determined, based upon calibration on jig scale.

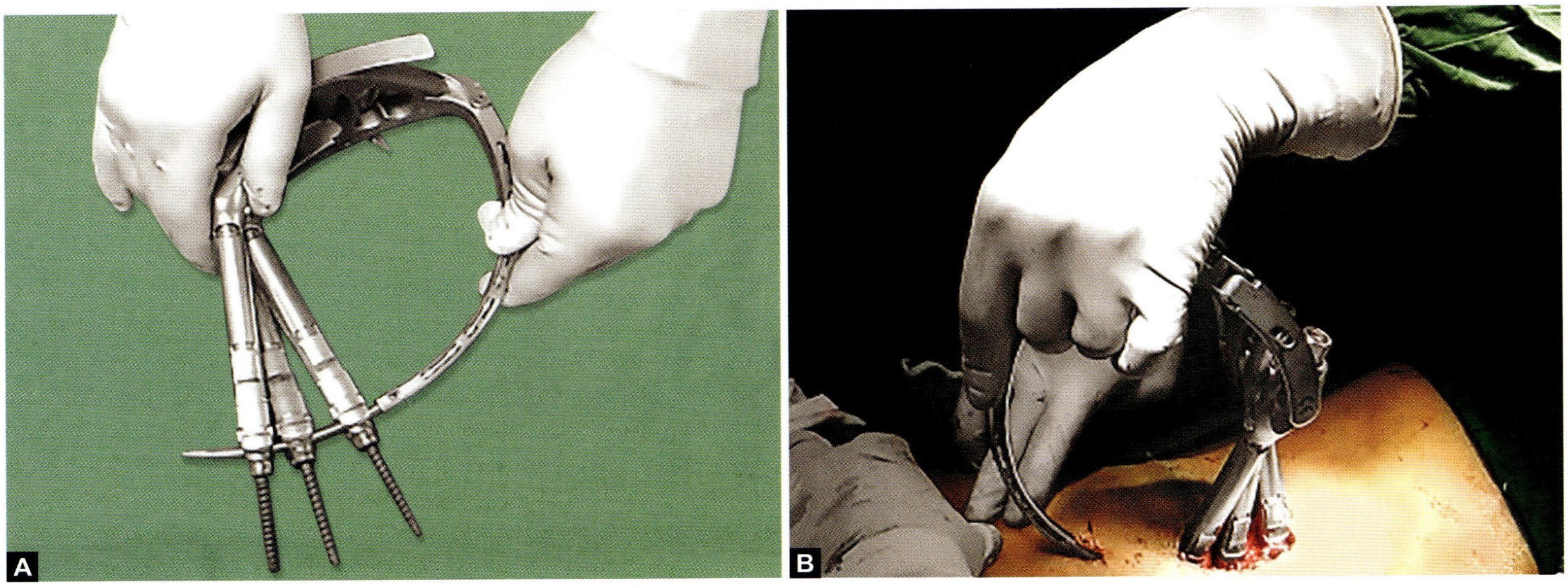

Figs. 11A and B: Rod insertion through jig.

Reduction of Listhesis

Tightening over the rod reduces the listhesis, and is confirmed under C-arm guidance.

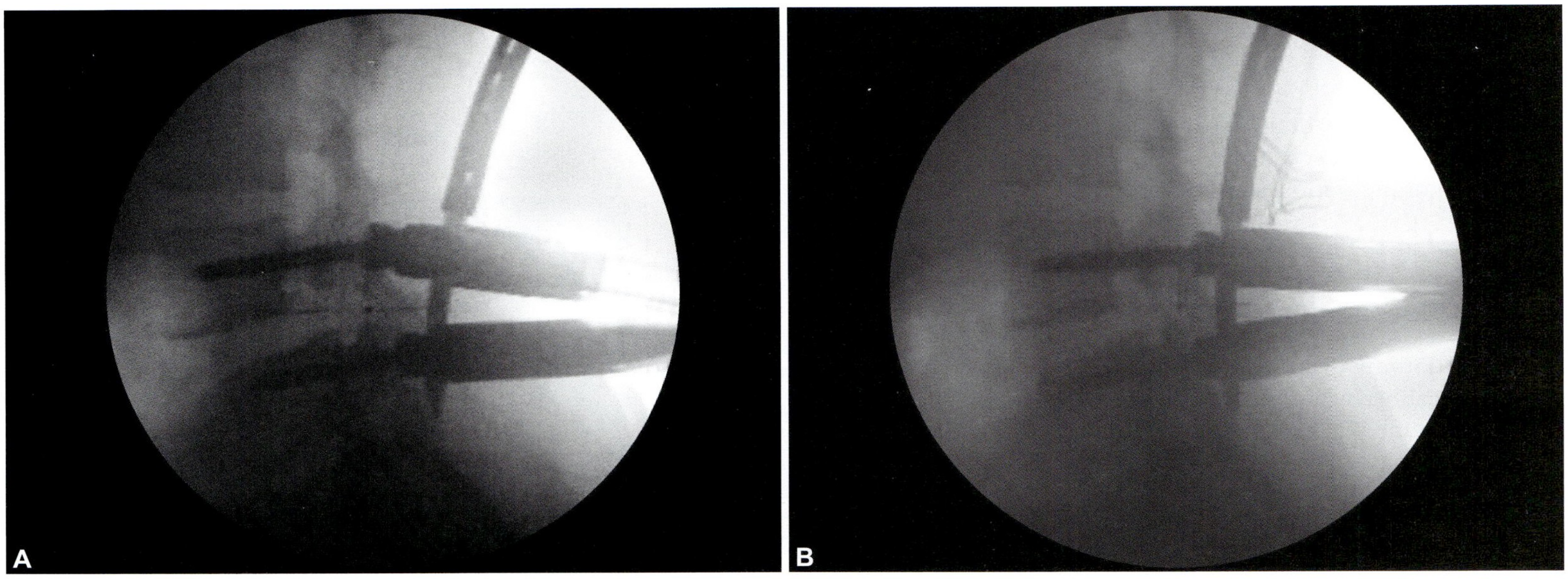

Figs. 12A and B: Sequential tightening over the rod reducing the listhesis as shown.

After rod placement distraction is achieved to open up the disc space for operative convenience and cage insertion.

Exposure on the Other Side

A small straight paramedian insertion given on other side, guidewires are placed over both pedicles and exposure done till facet joint are visible at targeted disc level to be fuse.

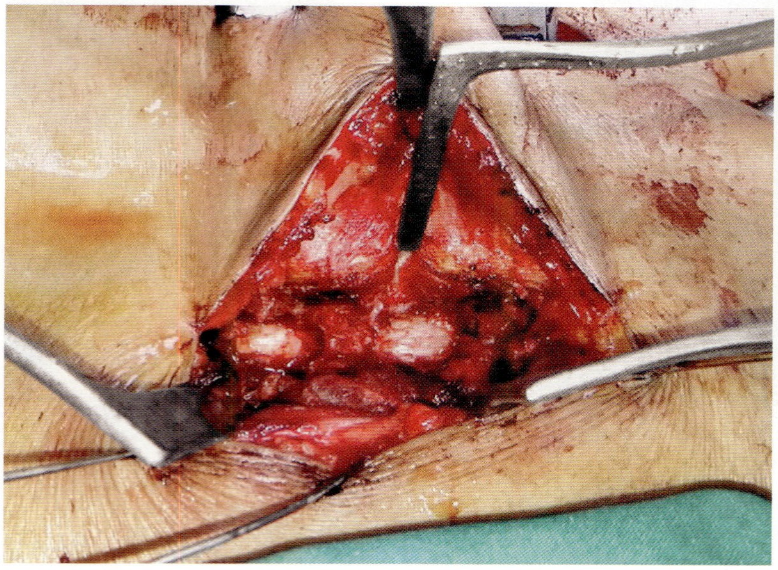

Fig. 13: Exposure done till facet joint are visible at disc level to be fused.

Decompression

Lamina exposed and hemilaminectomy performed and inferior articular facetectomy done to expose transforaminal space, part of superior articular facet can also be osteotomized to further increase the space, all the bone fragments are collected and kept as graft material.

End Plate Preparation

After annulotomy disc is removed, shavers inserted in gradually increasing caliber, with rotatory movements all the disc is shaved off till grating sound is achieved, angled curette and rounguers are used to further increase the raw area over the vertebral surfaces, the loose disc pieces are removed, appropriate cage size is measured.

Cage Insertion

Graft is filled into the disc space, graft also incorporated into the cage and with slow hammers inserted into the targeted intervertebral space prefilled with graft, after cage insertion position is confirmed under C-arm guidance and pedicle screws are inserted, rod is inserted after jig placement, and compression achieved from both sides.

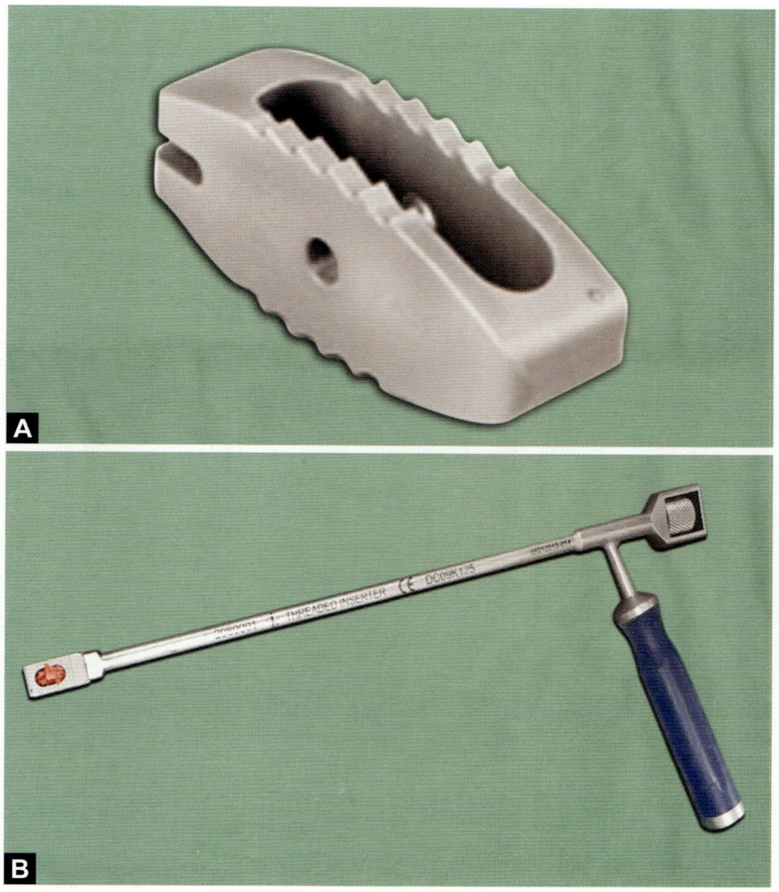

Figs. 14A and B: Polyetheretherketone (PEEK) cage with space for graft placement.

Compression

Rod inserted through the jig and compression achieved from both sides.

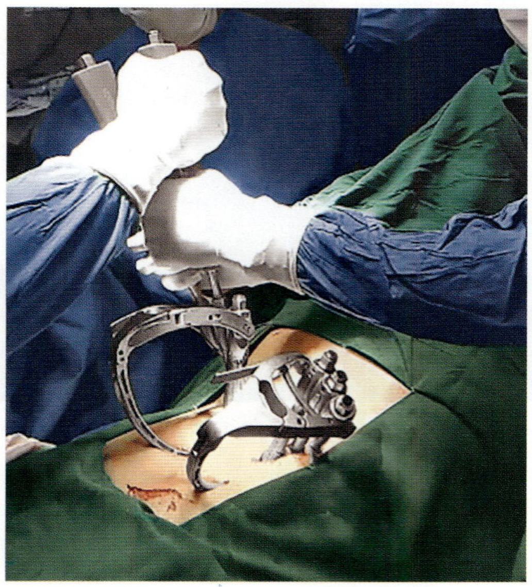

Fig. 15: Compression at targeted fusion level.

After final compression, rod and cage position is confirmed under C-arm, pedicle screws are fully tightened and jig assemble is disengaged.

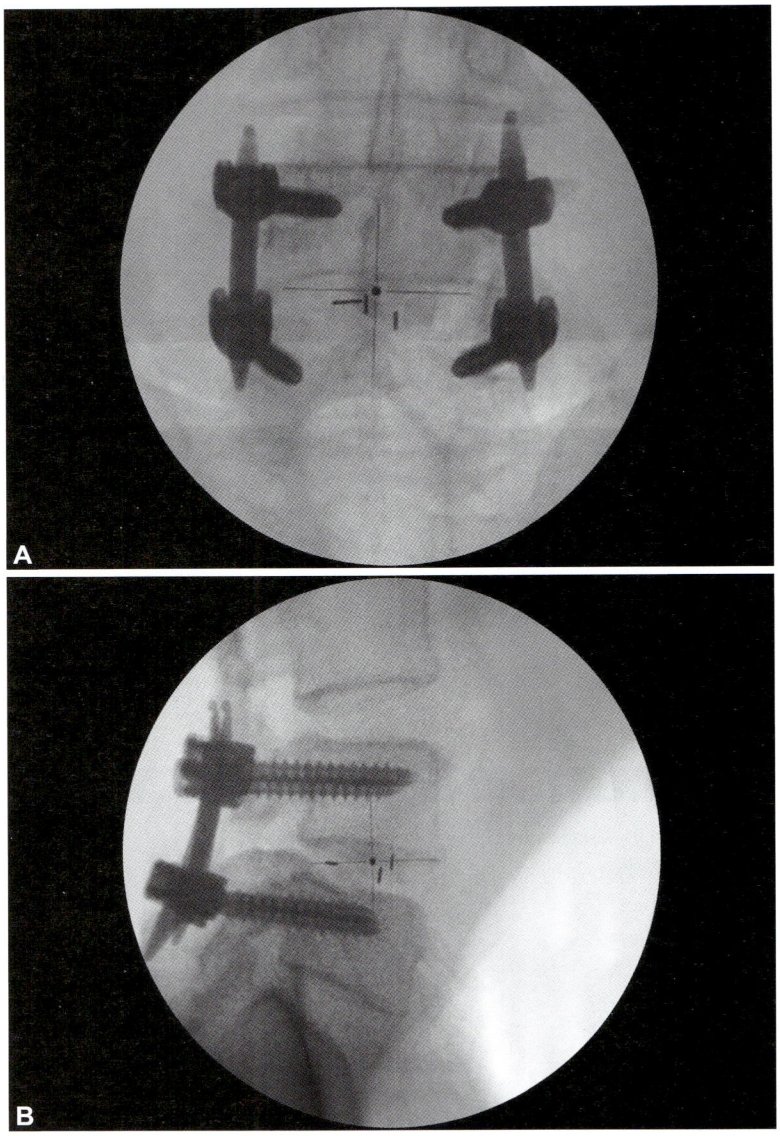

Figs. 16A and B: Final satisfactory listhesis reduction.

CLOSURE

- After copious saline irrigation, wound closure performed in layers over drain.
- Skin closure done with absorbable suture.

SURGICAL SCAR

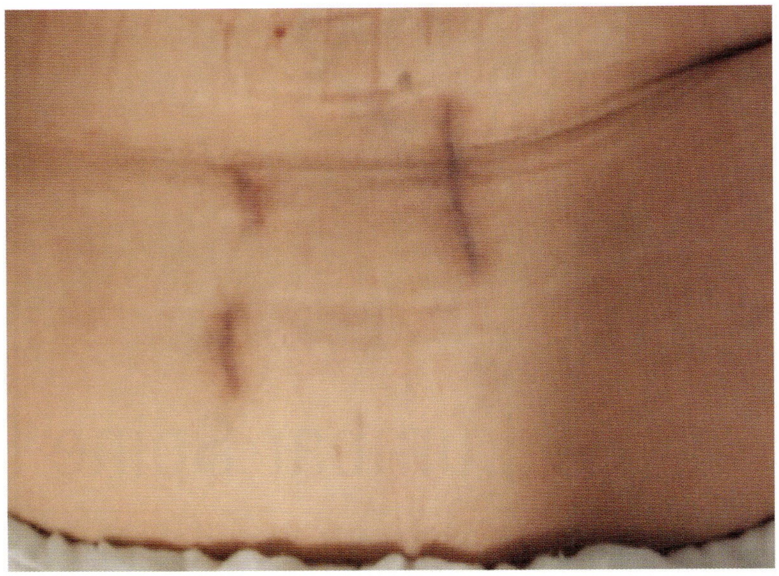

Fig. 17: Minimal surgical scar 2 weeks after surgery.

COMPLICATIONS

- Adjacent segment degeneration.
- Persistent dermatomal pain or numbness.
- Infection.

SUGGESTED READING

1. German JW, Foley KT. Minimal access surgical techniques in the management of the painful lumbar motion segment. Spine (Phila Pa 1976). 2005;30:S52-9.
2. Khoo LT, Palmer S, Laich DT, et al. Minimally invasive percutaneous posterior lumbar interbody fusion. Neurosurgery. 2002;51:S166-81.
3. Park P, Foley KT. Minimally invasive transforaminal lumbar interbody fusion with reduction of spondylolisthesis: technique and outcomes after a minimum of 2 years' follow-up. Neurosurg Focus. 2008;25(2):E16.
4. Peng CW, Yue WM, Poh SY, et al. Clinical and radiological outcomes of minimally invasive versus open transforaminal lumbar interbody fusion. Spine (Phila Pa 1976). 2009;34:1385-9.
5. Schwender JD, Holly LT, Rouben DP, et al. Minimally invasive transforaminal lumbar interbody fusion TLIF: technical feasibility and initial results. J Spinal Disord Tech. 2005;18 (Suppl):S1-S6.

CHAPTER 28

Lumbar Spine Fixation by Open Method

Rahul Chaudhari, Sharad M Hardikar, Nitish Agrawal

INTRODUCTION

Degenerative lumbar stenosis is common cause of disabling back and claudicating leg pain in older population. It usually results due to narrowing of the spinal canal due to bulging intervertebral disc, hypertrophy of ligamentum flavum and degeneration of facet joints. The general incidence of stenosis ranges from 1.7% to 8%. Symptoms usually develop in fifth or sixth decade of life.

PATHOANATOMY

Anatomically spinal canal shapes have been described in three shapes: round, oval, and trefoil (Fig. 1). Trefoil canal have smallest cross sectional area and are more prone for symptomatic stenosis.

Areas of stenosis in spinal canal (Figs. 2A and B) need to be understood before considering decompression surgery:

- Central
- Lateral recess
- Foraminal.

Arnoldi et al. classified lumbar stenosis as congenital, acquired or combined (Box 1).

Box 1: Classification of lumbar spinal stenosis.

Congenital (developmental) stenosis
- Chondrodystrophy
- Idiopathic

Acquired stenosis
- Degenerative
- Spondylolytic
- Iatrogenic
- Post-traumatic
- Miscellaneous

Combined (degenerative changes superimposed on a congenitally narrow spinal canal)

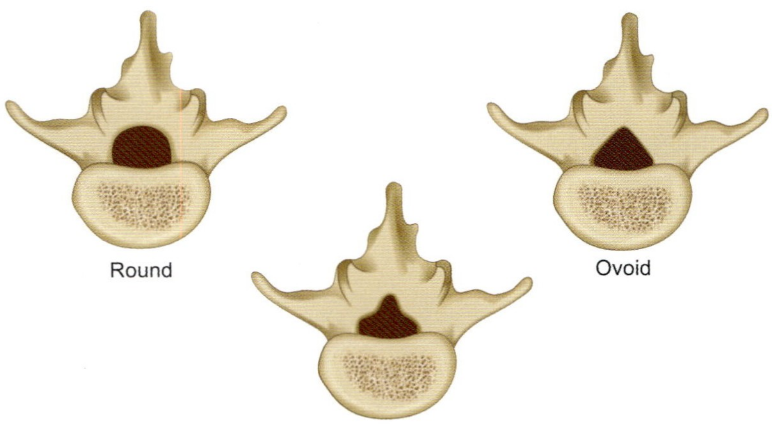

Fig. 1: The three typical shapes of the spinal canal. Trefoil canals have the smallest cross-sectional area.

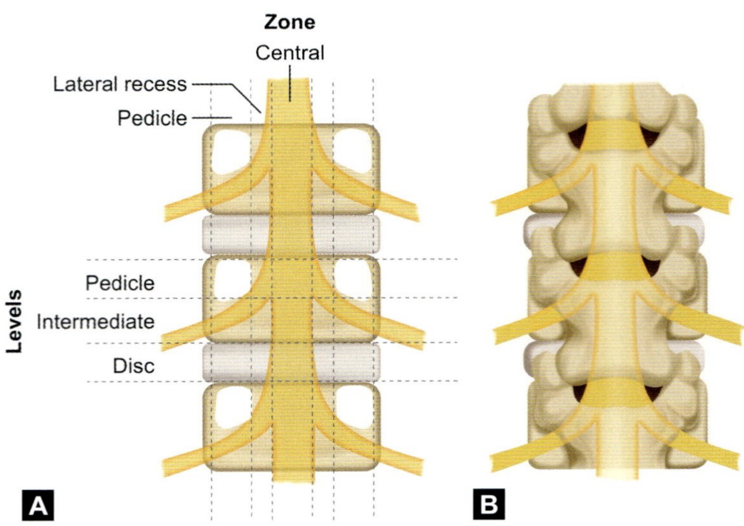

Figs. 2A and B: Areas of stenosis in spinal canal.

CLINICAL SYNDROME

Neurogenic claudication means sensation of pain, heaviness, tightness, and subjective weakness in lower extremities, worse with standing activity or lumbar extension and relieved by sitting down or leaning forward. Incidence of symptoms is back pain (95%) claudication (91%) leg pain (71%) weakness (33%), and voiding disturbances (33%).

DIFFERENTIAL DIAGNOSIS

Peripheral vascular claudication should be differentiated from neurogenic claudication.

INVESTIGATIONS

- *X-rays*: Spondylosis with or without hypertrophic facets and narrowing of interlaminar spaces. Dynamic X-rays are helpful for evaluating instability. Degenerative spondylolisthesis or scoliosis is suggestive of stenosis.
- *Magnetic resonance imaging (MRI)*: Gold standard investigation to confirm the clinical diagnosis. It allows to study the disc, facet joint, and ligamentum flavum components and their contribution towards stenosis.
- *Computed tomography (CT) scan*: Usually required to study bony element of the stenosis such as facetal osteophytes or calcified disc or ligamentum flavum.
- *Myelogram*: These are helpful if MRI is contraindicated to study nerve root compressions and to assess dynamic component of stenosis. CT myelography especially helpful in iatrogenic stenosis if planning for revision lumbar decompression.
- *Electrophysiological studies*: Electromyography, nerve-conduction velocity, and somatosensory evoked potentials are not part of the routine assessment. About 80% of patients with symptomatic stenosis will demonstrate electromyogram (EMG) changes. EMG and somatosensory evoked potential (SSEP) may be helpful in patients with diabetes and lumbar stenosis. SSEPs pre- and postexercise may help to identify specific nerve roots involved.

SURGICAL INTERVENTION

Initially all patients without significant neurological deficit are subjected to conservative line of treatment by rest, physiotherapy and medication and if needed epidural steroids. If conservative treatment fails or if there is significant neurological deficit then surgery will have to be undertaken and in most patients it will involve decompression and instrumented spinal fusion.

LUMBAR SPINE FIXATION

Introduction

Earlier uninstrumented spinal surgeries were performed but currently fusion surgeries are only instrumented. Pedicle screw fixation is common type of fixation to perform spinal fusion procedures.

Indication of Lumbar Spine Fixation

- Degenerative lumbar spine with instability
- Disc induced back pain
- Lumbar spine infection
- Fracture spine
- Spinal deformities
- Vertebral tumors

Types of Spinal Fixation

(A) Vertebral
  (1) Posterior pedicle screw with rod fixation – Open or percutaneous
  (2) Lateral vertebral screw with rod fixation
(B) Interbody fixation
  (1) Posterior lumbar interbody fusion (PLIF) – Posterior approach
  (2) Transforaminal lumbar interbody fusion (TLIF) – Posterior approach
  (3) Lateral lumbar interbody fusion (LLIF) – Lateral retroperitoneal approach
  (4) Oblique lumbar interbody fusion (OLIF) – Lateral retroperitoneal approach
(C) Sacropelvic screw fixation
  (1) Sacral screw
  (2) Sacrum Ala screw
  (3) Iliac screw

Entry point for pedicle screw insertion in lumbar spine:
The entry point of the pedicle screw is defined as the confluence of any of the four lines:
1. Pars interarticularis
2. Mamillary process
3. Lateral border of the superior articular facet
4. Mid-transverse process

Intersection of vertical line tangential to lateral border of superior articular process and horizontal line bisecting the transverse process and lateral to pars interarticularis with mediolateral inclination is 5–10° in upper lumbar spine and and 10–15° in lower lumbar spine.

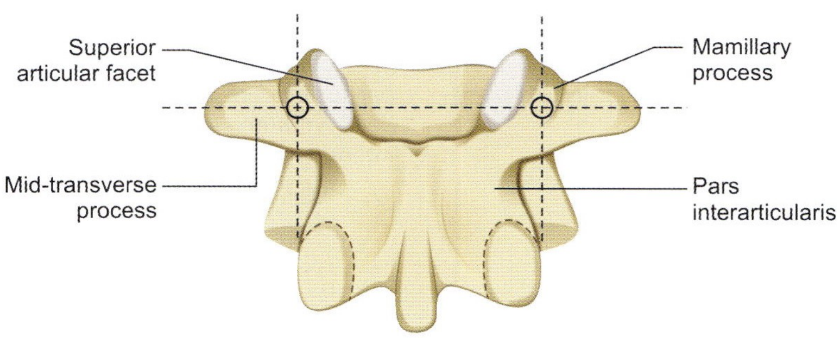

Fig. 3: The entry point.

SURGICAL STEPS (FIGS. 4 TO 27)

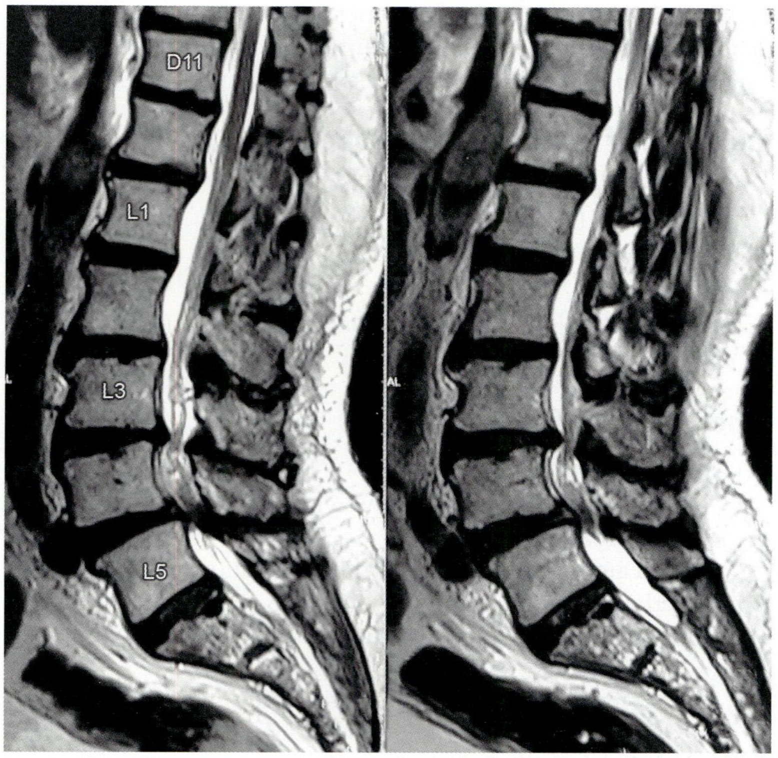

Fig. 4: Magnetic resonance imaging (MRI) L-S spine T2 sagittal view showing lumbar canal stenosis at L3-L4 and L4-L5 level with listhesis between L4 and L5.

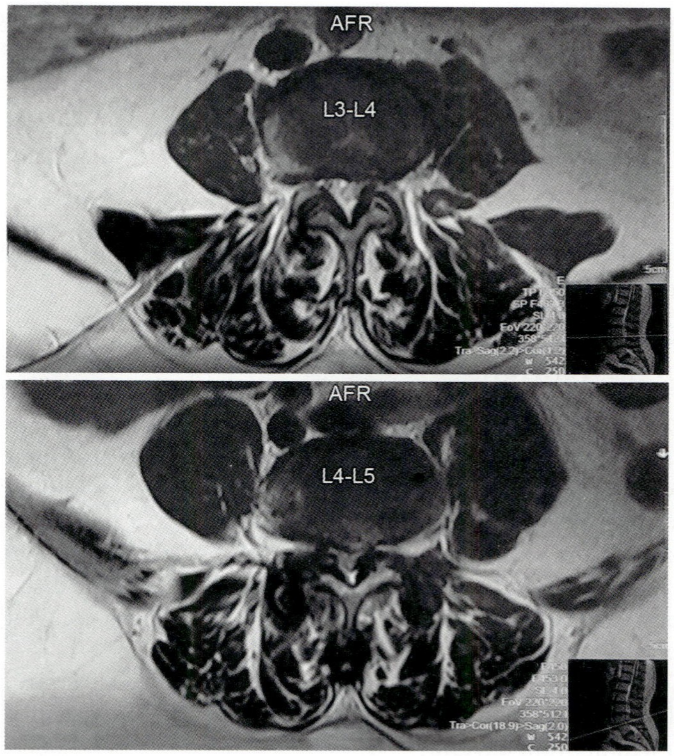

Fig. 5: Magnetic resonance imaging L-S spine T2 axial view.

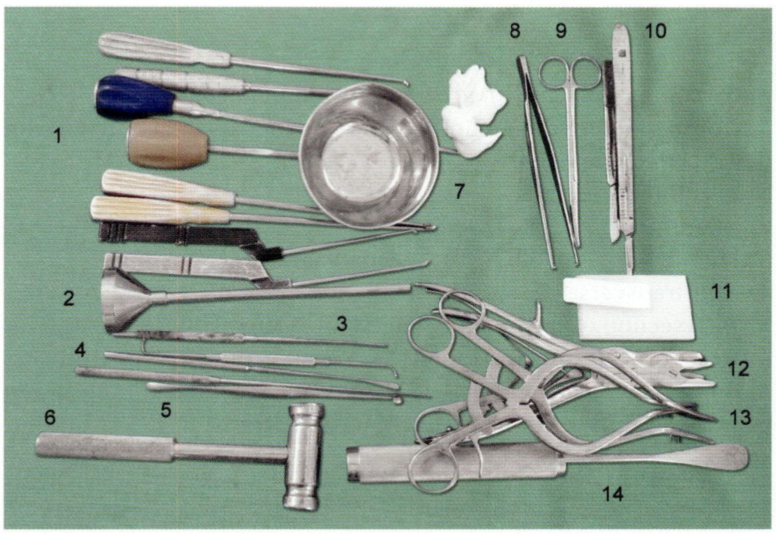

Fig. 6: (1) Curette, (2) Bone graft funnel, (3) Bone hook, (4) Dural dissector, (5) Curette with dural dissector, (6) Hammer, (7) Sterile container, (8) Tooth forceps, (9) Scissor, (10) Knife, (11) Gel foam, (12) Bone nibbler, (13) Self-retaining retractors, (14) Cobb elevator.

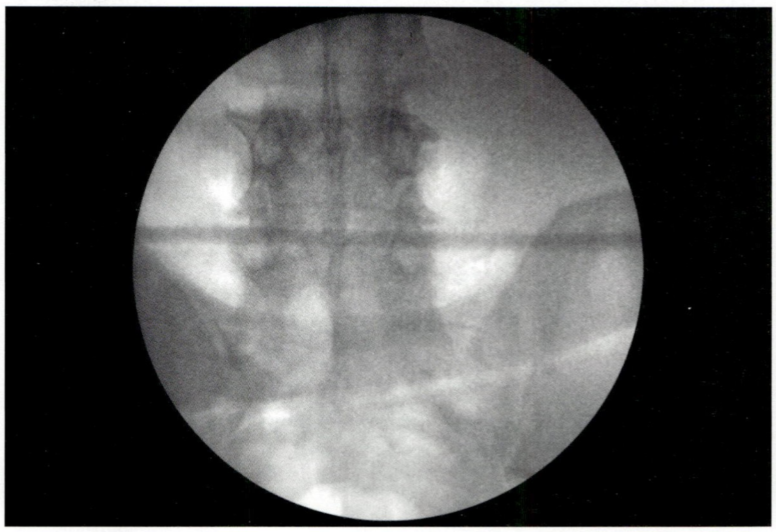

Fig. 7: Prone position given on operating table. The patient should be positioned in spinal lordosis. This is particularly important when long lumbar fusions are planned. It diminishes the possibility of postoperative flat back syndrome and spinal dysfunction. L5 level identified over C-arm image intensifier on anteroposterior view and marked.

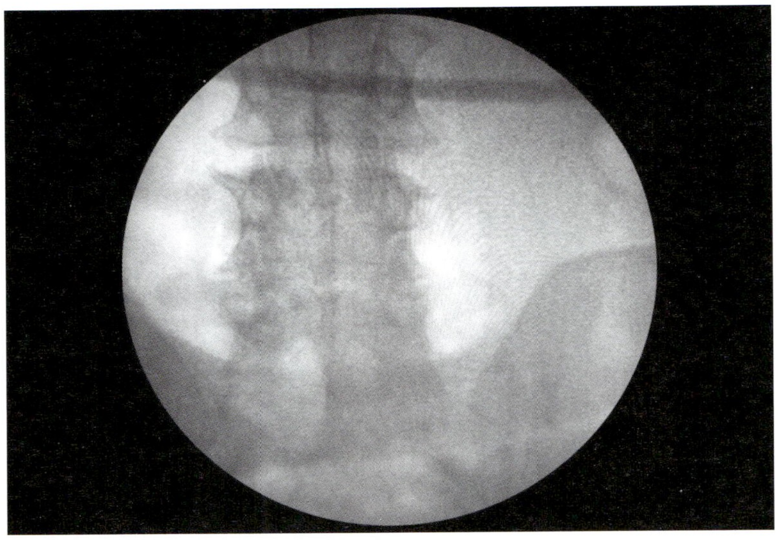

Fig. 8: L3 level identified over C-arm image intensifier on anteroposterior (AP) view and marked.

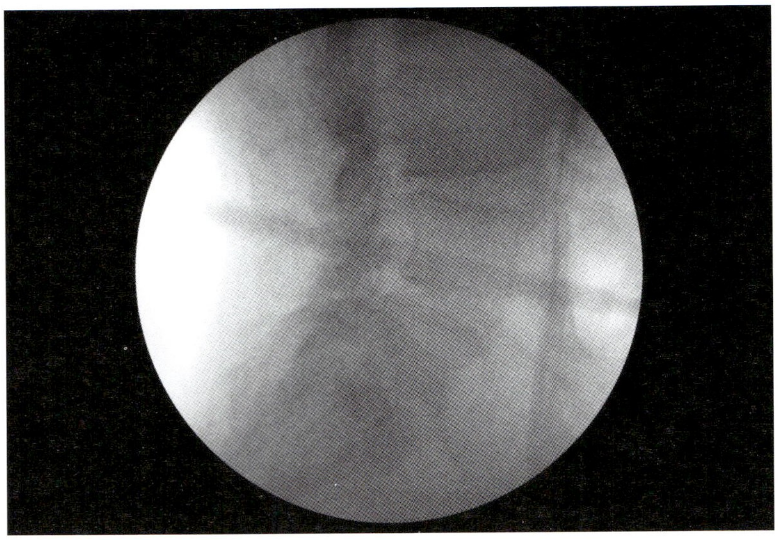

Fig. 9: L4 level identified over C-arm II on lateral view and marked.

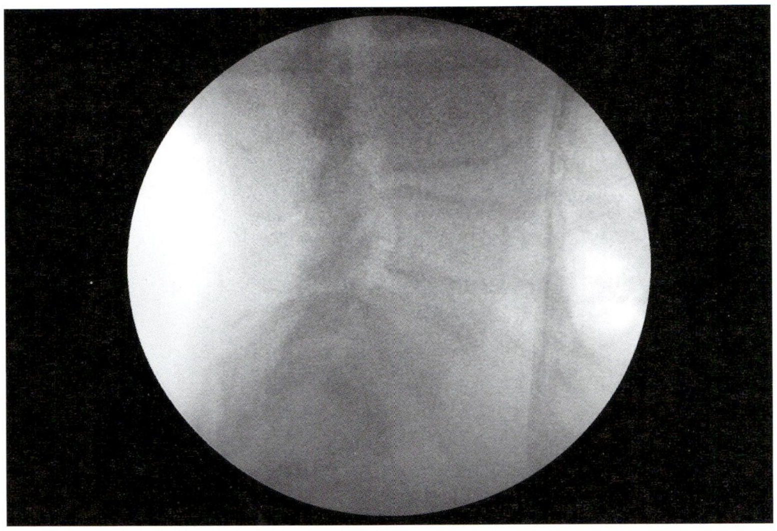

Fig. 10: L3 level identified over C-arm II on lateral view and marked.

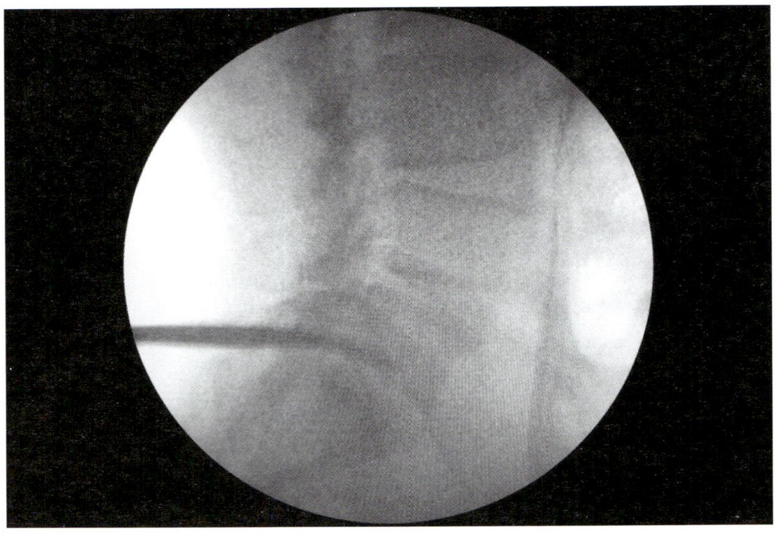

Fig. 11: L5 level identified over C-arm II on lateral view and marked.

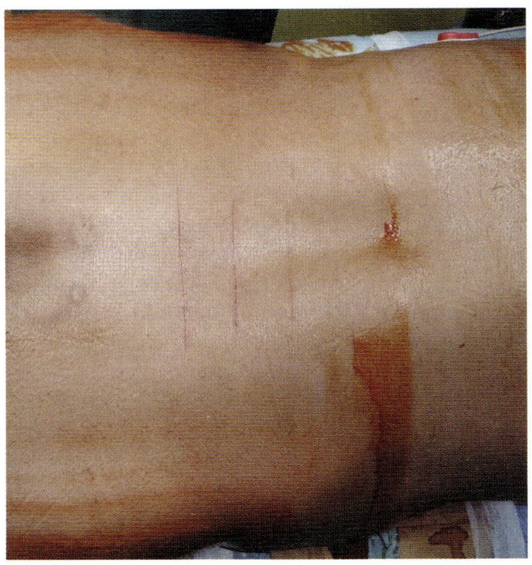

Fig. 12: L3, L4, and L5 levels are marked on skin with needle No. 18.

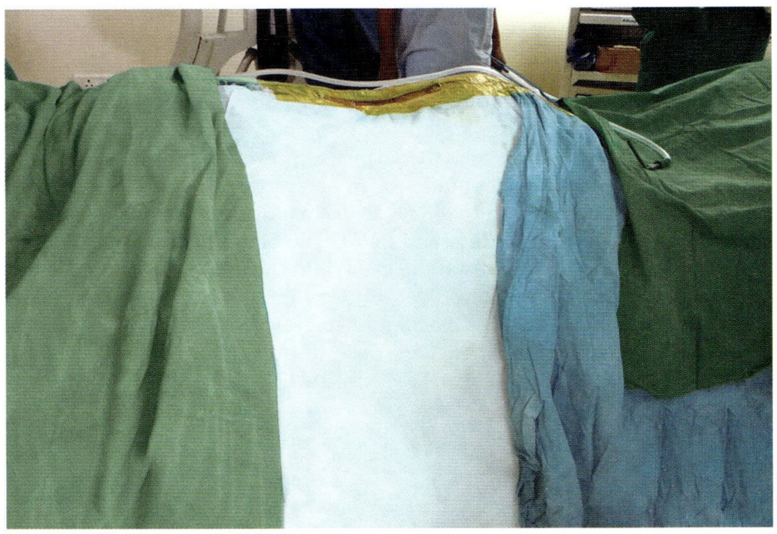

Fig. 13: Painting and draping done in standard manner.

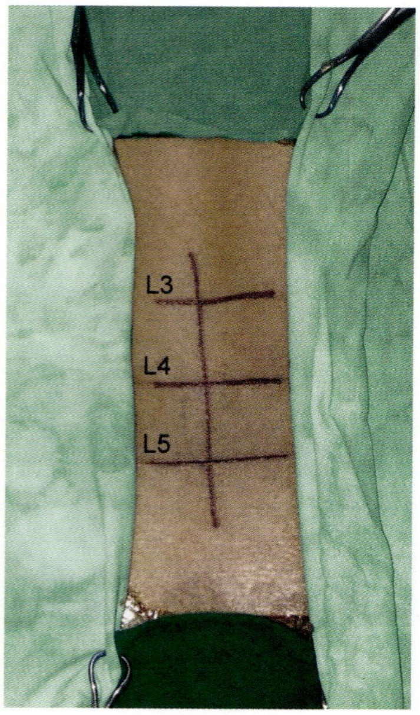

Fig. 14: L1-S1 spinal area exposed. Midline incision site and L3, L4 and L5 level marked with marker pen.

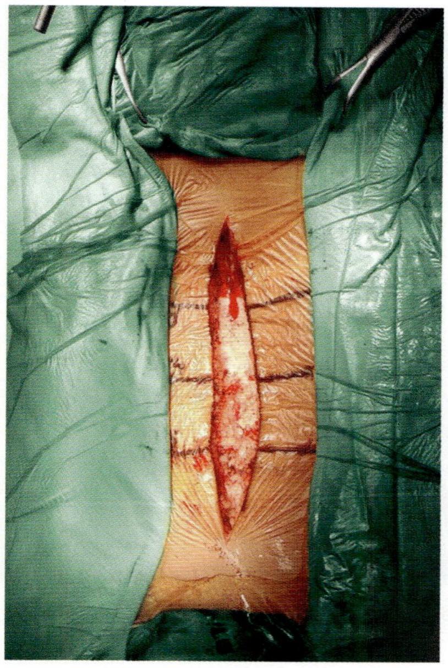

Fig. 15: Incision taken with knife (incision extended proximally till L2-L3 level and distally till L5-S1 level).

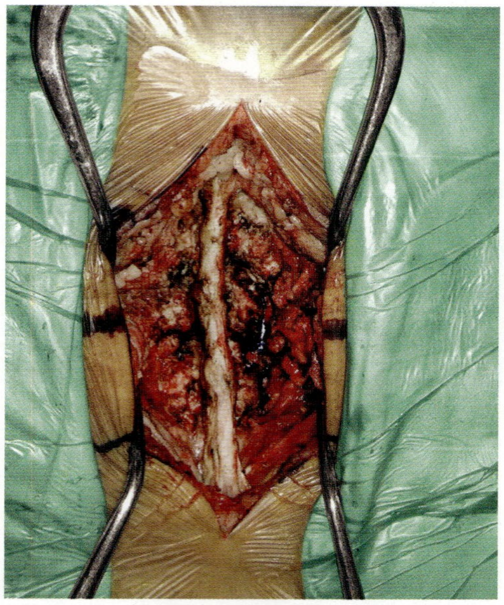

Fig. 16: Superficial fat, subcutaneous tissue, fascia, and muscle layers are dissected from midline with unipolar cautery, bipolar cautery, and cobb elevator. Posterior spinal muscles separated from spinous process subperiosteally. Paravertebral soft tissue dissection should proceed in a caudal-cephalad direction due to the caudal-cephalad orientation of the paravertebral muscle attachments. Self-retaining retractors are applied for proper exposure of operating field. L3, L4, L5 lamina, transverse process, and superior and inferior facets are exposed with cautery. One should not run the cautery in the muscle mass and all the dissection should strictly involved detachment muscles from spinous process and lamina to avoid excessive bleeding. Avoid blood pooling, which occurs if the lordotic cephalad segments are decorticated first.

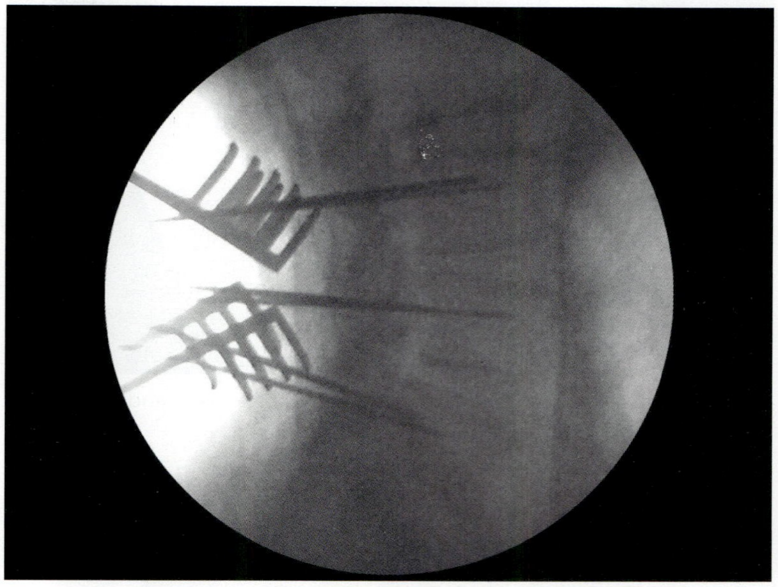

Fig. 17: Entry point in lumbar spine intersection of vertical line tangential to lateral border of superior articular process and horizontal line bisecting the transverse process trajectory converse by 10–15 towards from midline. Remove bone by nibbler. Bleeding of bones controlled by bone wax. Use pedicle owl for initial entry then further by pedicle probe till anterior cortex. K wires are inserted after that. This process is done first for L3, L4, L5 on left side and then L3, L4, L5 on right side. Total 6 K wires are inserted in 6 screw hole. K wire positions confirmed on C-arm II on lateral view. The facet immediately cephalad to the fusion must be preserved to avoid iatrogenic instability. The majority of the decortication is carried out using sharp instruments such as osteotomes, curettes, and roungers.

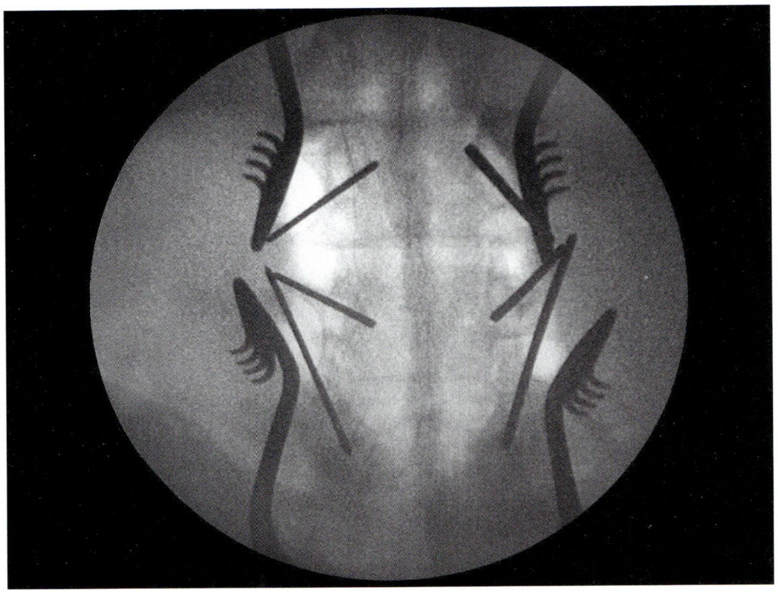

Fig. 18: K-wire positions confirmed on C-arm II on lateral view.

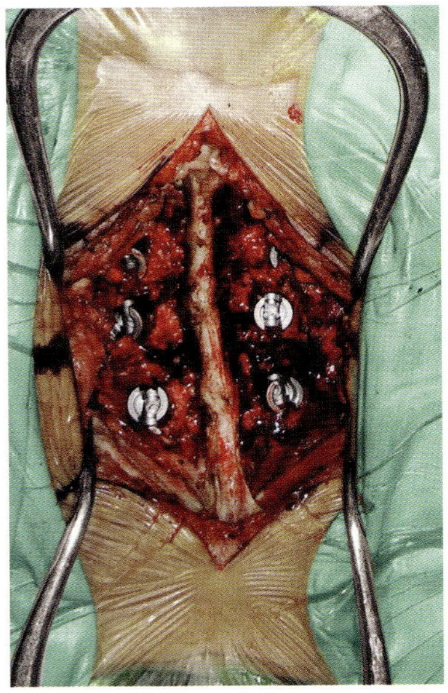

Fig. 19: Now screws are inserted on L3, L4, and L5 vertebrae on left side then inserted on L3, L4, and L5 vertebrae on right side. First take measurement then use tap for entry into cortex and appropriate length pedicle screw fixed on each vertebrae. Avoid prolonged muscle refraction. Self-retaining retractors should be relaxed every hour and the wound reirrigated. This allows reperfusion of the paravertebral muscles and diminishes the possibility of infection. If there is excessive tension on the muscles, the incision can be lengthened. Facet joints should be thoroughly cleared of all soft tissues and the intra-articular portion of the joint denuded of cartilage.

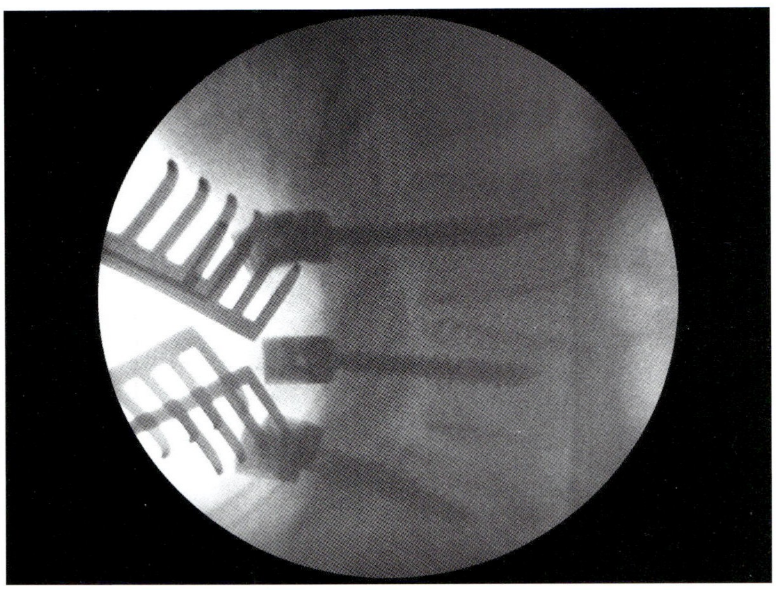

Fig. 20: Screw positions confirmed on C-arm II.

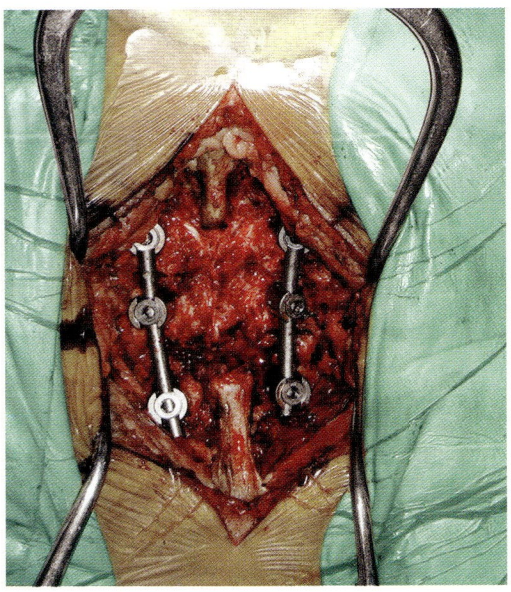

Fig. 21: Interspinous ligament of L3-4, L4-5 level, and L4 spinous process removed with bone nibbler. Bone is preserved for further bone grafting. Now rod size taken and both side fixation done with appropriate size rods. Distraction done by McBride refractor/spreader and tightened with screwdriver. Decompression done by this technique at L3-L4 level and L4-5 level on both right and left side.

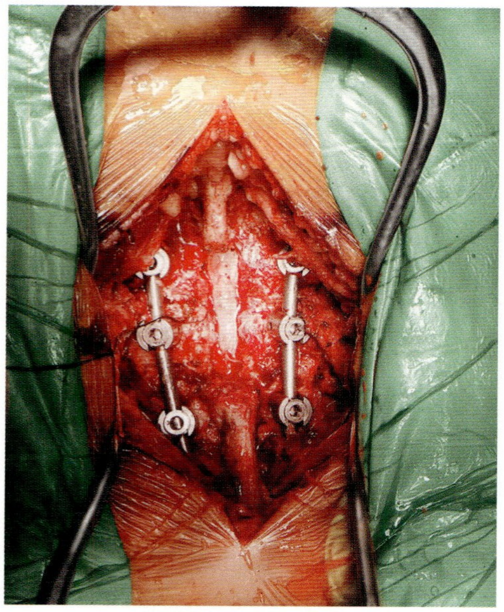

Fig. 22: Lamina of L4 removed with Kerrison punch and bone nibbler. Ligamentum flavum between L3-4, L4-5 removed with dural dissector and Kerrison punch. Stenosis checked with ball tip. Decompression done with disc forceps and dura retractor on central, paracentral, lateral recess, foraminal, and extra foraminal sites. Fibrosis around dura removed.

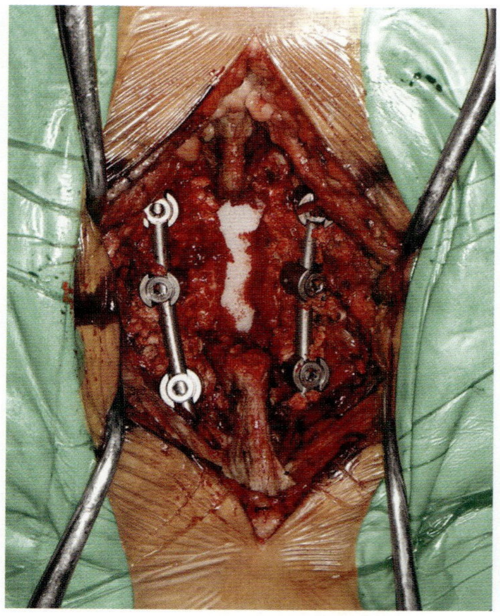

Fig. 23: Decompression confirmed with ball tip and nerve root probe. Bleeding site cauterized with bipolar cautery. Wash given with normal saline. Gel foam placed for hemostasis. Final tightening of screws done and bone graft placed between screws and rods. Avoid using an inadequate amount of bone graft; occasionally harvesting of both iliac crests may be necessary and/or augmentation with allograft bone may be needed. Avoid bony fragment extrusion into the spinal canal. Dissection should extend to the tips of the spinous processes bilaterally and to the lateral aspect of the facet joints. All soft tissues should be denuded to allow maximal surface area of bony fusion. If a lumbar decompression has been performed prior to the fusion, the exposed dura should be protected with cottonoids to diminish the likelihood of an iatrogenic dural laceration.

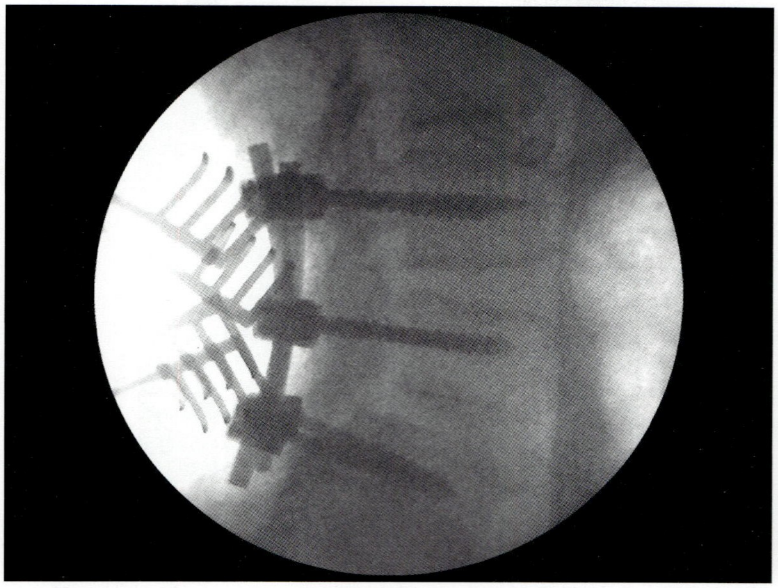

Fig. 24: Final fixation confirmed over C-arm II on lateral view.

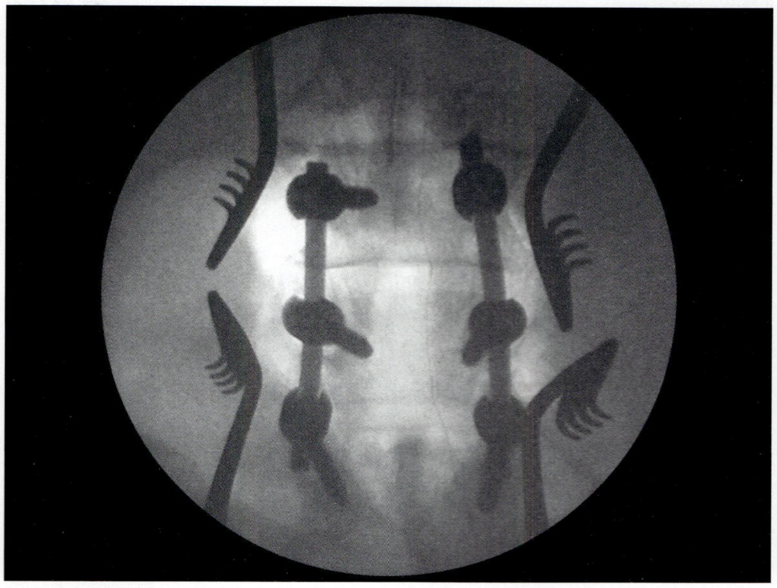

Fig. 25: Final fixation confirmed on C-arm II on anteroposterior (AP) view.

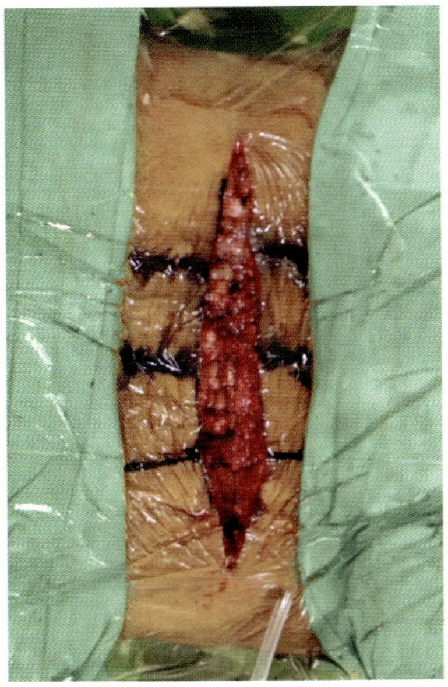

Fig. 26: Drain No. 12 placed. Fascia layer closed lightly with absorbable mateial continuous locking sutures.

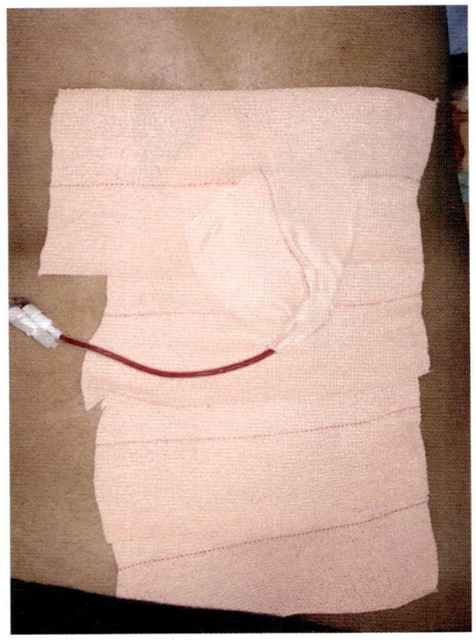

Fig. 27: Subcutaneous suturing done with absorbable material and skin suturing done with nonabsorbable suture material and drain fixed with non-absorbable suture material. Compression dressing done with elastic adhesive bandage at operative site and drain.

POSTOPERATIVE MANAGEMENT

- Neurological evaluation and limb movements checked immediately after extubation.
- Patient was kept in intensive care unit (ICU) for observation in supine position.
- Oral food started after 6 hours.
- Routine intravenous (IV) antibiotics and analgesics were given.

Checklist

- Vitals, neurological status, drain output, urine output and wound soakage if any.
- Postoperative day 1:
  - Patient is allowed to log roll and patient was given all four limb exercises and chest physiotherapy with spirometer.
  - Lumbosacral (LS) belt was given and patient is allowed to sit and walk with support if comfortable.
- Drain was removed on day 3 (when drain output is less than 50 mL in last 24 hours).
- Urine catheter was removed on postoperative day 3 and patient was allowed to go to bathroom.

BIBLIOGRAPHY

1. Genevay S, Atlas SJ. Lumbar spinal stenosis, Best Pract Res Clin Rheumatol. 2010;24:253.
2. Kaptan H, Kasimcan O, Cakiroglu K. Lumbar spinal stenosis in elderly patients. Ann NY Acad Sci. 2014;1100:173.
3. Lee JY, Whang PG. Lumbar spinal stenosis. Instr Course Lect. 2013; 62:383.

CHAPTER 29

Spinal Extradural Tumor

Sunil Nadkarni, Onkar Sudame, Siddharth Hardikar

INTRODUCTION

Epidural tumors can be broadly classified into soft tissue tumors and bony tumors. These again can be classified as benign and malignant tumors (Flowchart 1).

Clinical presentation of soft tissue and bony tumors is different. Epidural tumors present with localized pain, radicular pain, gait disturbances, weakness, dysesthesia (common in soft tissue tumors) and sphincter abnormality (more common with bony tumors). Benign tumors have a long duration as compared to malignant tumors. Bony destruction and instability is more common with bony and malignant tumors.

Tumor excision techniques can be classified as:

- Curettage
- Intralesional/debulking
- En bloc resection.

Surgical approaches change according to grading, staging, survival, and type of tumor. For example, vascular tumors require embolization prior to definitive surgery, high-grade tumors may not be amenable to en bloc excision and may have to do away with debulking.

Detailed surgical approaches required for different types of tumors are beyond the scope of this book. We present a case of a thoracic spine dorsal epidural angiolipoma.

CLINICAL PRESENTATION

A 47-year-old female housewife came to us with complaints of weakness and heaviness of both legs associated with tingling and numbness of both feet which increased since 2 months. She also had a couple of falls while walking during this period. She said she had insidious onset of back pain, heaviness in both legs with tingling in both feet with gradual progression since last 7–8 months, which she attributed to her recent weight gain and overall sedentary lifestyle. Back pain was continuous dull aching not relieved with rest. She did not have any girdle pain or sphincter abnormalities.

Flowchart 1: Classification of spinal epidural tumors.

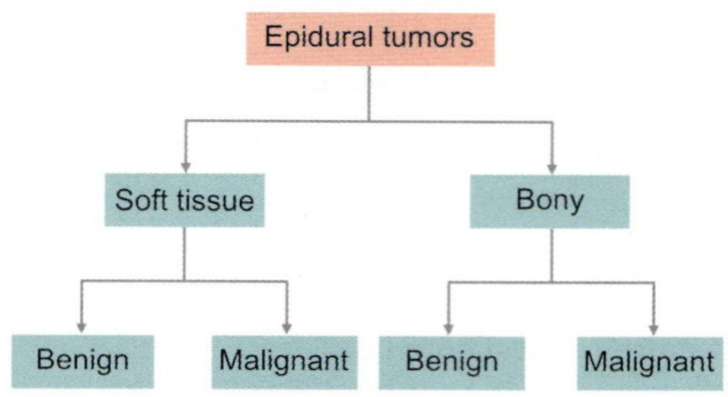

On examination, she was walking with support. Crude touch sensation was partially reduced in bilateral L4, L5, and S1 dermatomes. Position sense of both great toes was absent. Rest lower limb position sense was present. Temperature perception of both lower limbs was present. Her lower limbs had grade 3 power. Bilateral knee jerk and ankle jerk were brisk. Bilateral Babinki's sign was positive.

Magnetic resonance imaging (MRI) revealed and epidural dorsal angiolipoma extending from D7 to D10 vertebra levels with maximum compression and cord changes at D8–D9 levels (Figs. 1 to 4).

Her lab reports were normal with erythrocyte sedimentation rate (ESR) 12 and C-reactive protein (CRP) 20.

INSTRUMENTS (FIG. 5)

Other than the routine general surgical and orthopaedic instruments following instruments are needed for this surgery:

- Spinous process cutter
- Nerve hook
- McDonald retractor
- Penfield's dura retractor
- Kerrison's rongeur
- Bone curettes (straight and angled of all sizes)
- Burr handle
- Burr tips (cutting and diamond tips of various sizes).

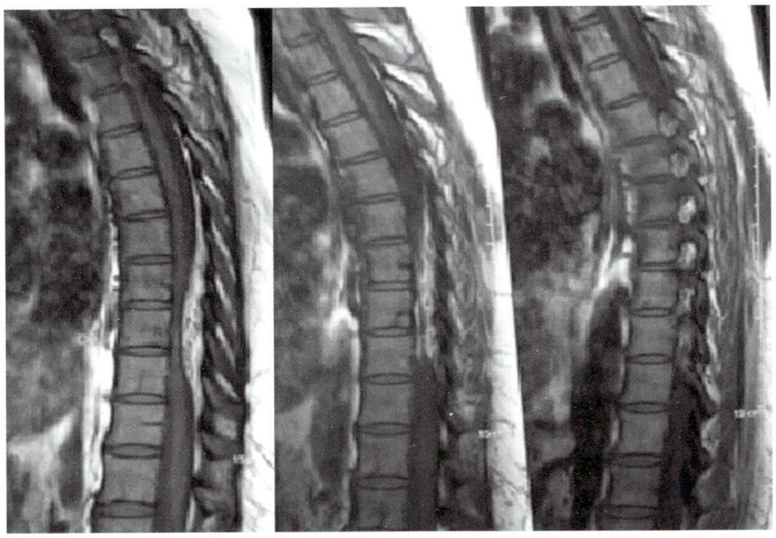

Fig. 1: T1 weighted sagittal magnetic resonance imaging (MRI) images showing epidural lesion extending from D7 to D10 with hyperintensity (following subcutaneous fat intensity) extending into the left intervertebral foramens. A few intermixed hypointense dots (representing intervening vessels) are seen within the lesion.

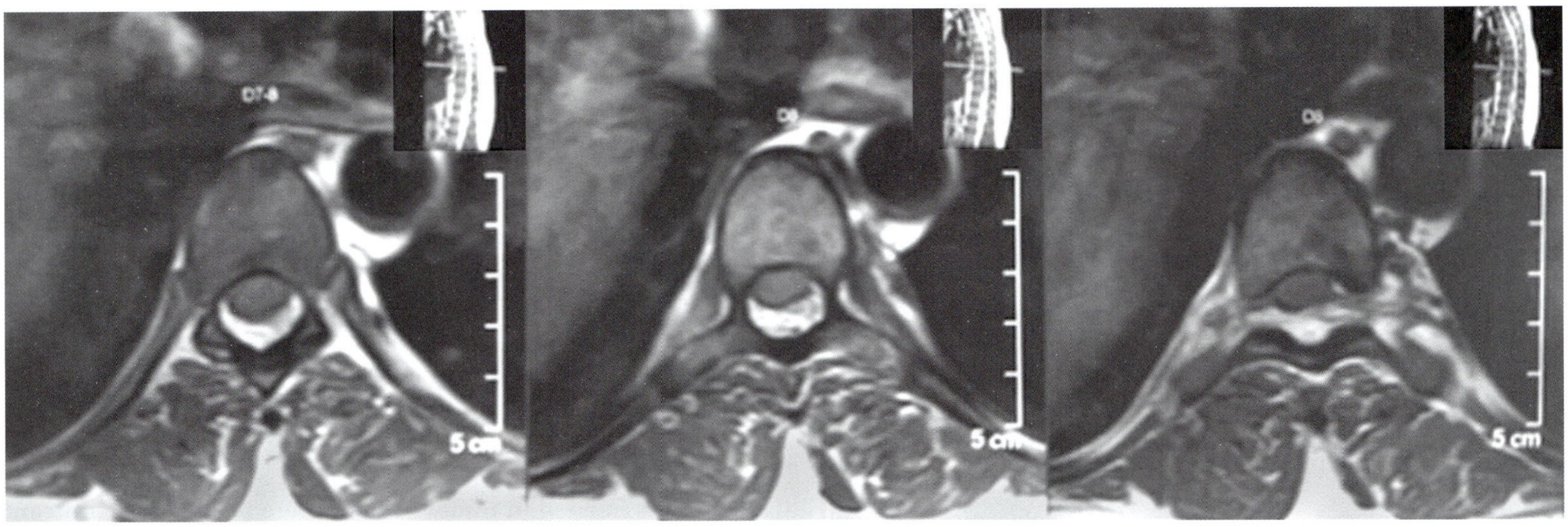

Fig. 2: T1 weighted axial magnetic resonance imaging (MRI) images showing the tumor dorsally at D7 and D8 level.

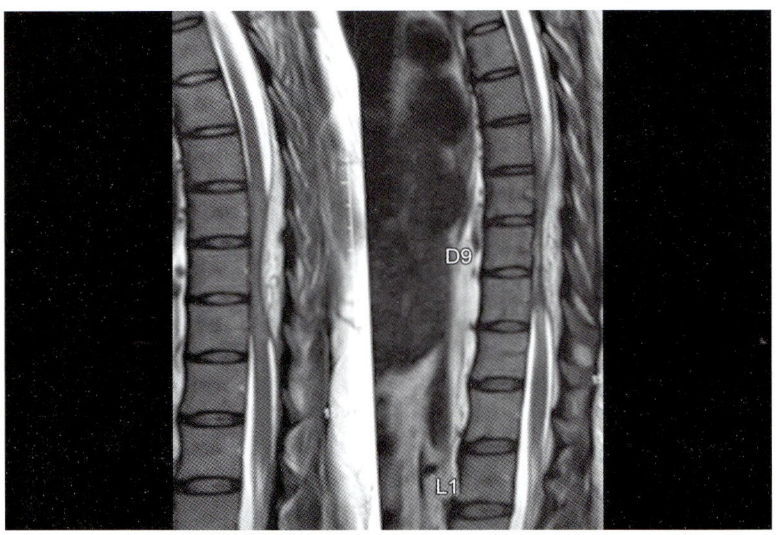

Fig. 3: T2 weighted sagittal magnetic resonance imaging (MRI) scan.

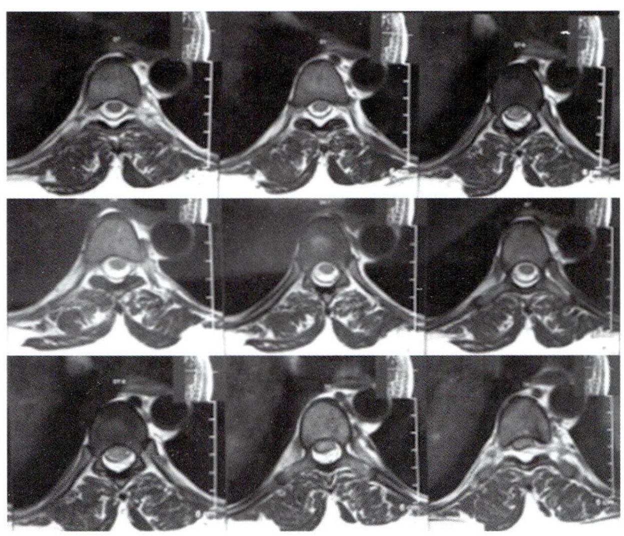

Fig. 4: T2 weighted axial magnetic resonance imaging (MRI) scan.

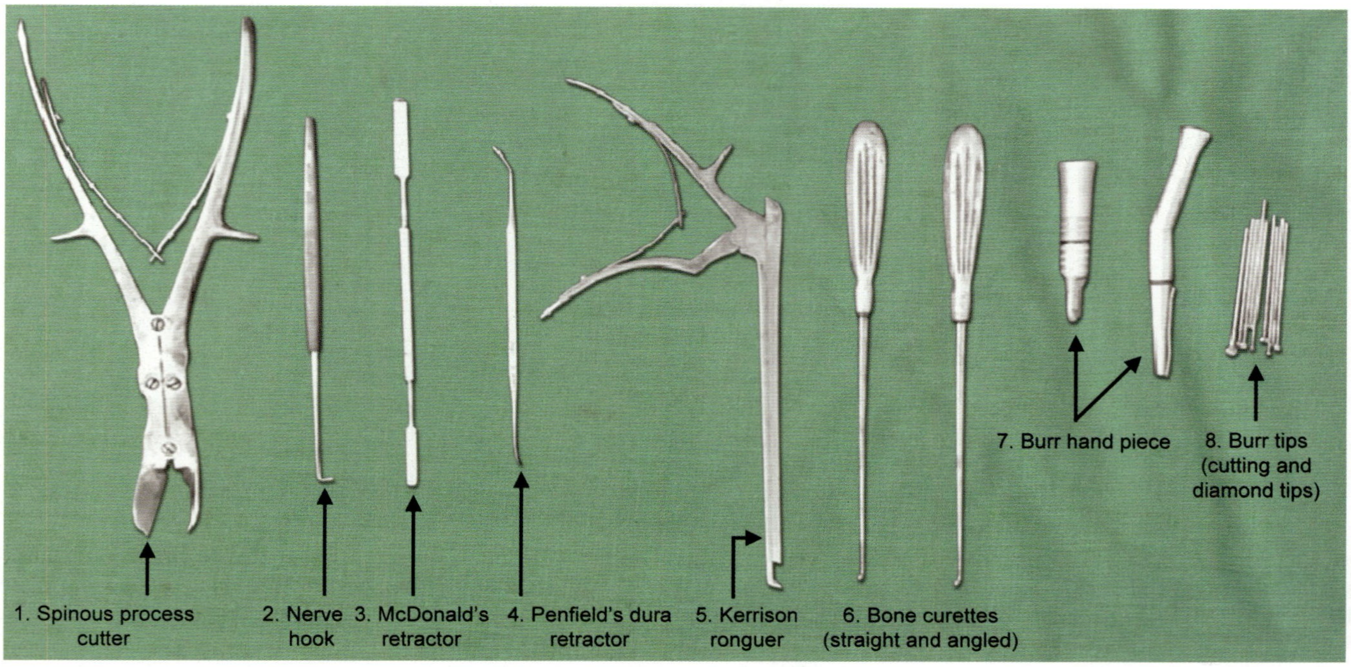

Fig. 5: Instruments commonly used for performing surgery on spinal epidural tumors.

SURGICAL PROCEDURE (FIGS. 8 TO 23 THE HEAD END IS ON THE LEFT SIDE)

Position (Fig. 6)

After general anesthesia patient was given prone position taking care of the head while turning. Her head, chest, pelvis, knees, legs, and elbows were well padded. Abdomen must be free off any pressure. Both arms must not be abducted too much.

Trolley and C-arm Position (Fig. 7)

C-arm is to be placed opposite to the trolley placement. Principal surgeon stands at the side of the trolleys. Trolleys are usually placed at the side where screw placement, facetectomy or cage placement is contemplated so that the C-arm can easily come from front and the surgeon can easily see the screen (placed at patients foot end) without being disturbed by C-arm positioning.

Scrubbing, Painting, and Draping (Fig. 8)

An assistant scrubs up and scrubs the part to be operated and also a generous part of the skin beyond the operative field with betadine scrub and solution. The part is painted with betadine solution (preferably 10%). The part to be operated is kept exposed and the drapes are put over carefully so as to include at least 3 inches of painted part from all sides each. The operative field can then be sealed off with a sterile transparent drape (e.g. ioban).

Incision (Fig. 9)

After marking the level of vertebra to be exposed under C-arm guidance, take skin incision with No. 22 blade followed by subcutaneous incision through same line. Further dissection can be made with Bowie's cautery. It is important to coagulate oozers as we go deeper because then tend to ooze in the operative field.

Deep Dissection (Figs. 10 and 11)

After reaching the fascia, dissect the fascia, and the multifidus muscle of the spinous process bilaterally to expose the required levels of lamina (in this case we exposed from D7 pedicle level to D11 pedicle because we were contemplating fixation from D7 to D11). Clear the lamina off any soft tissue till laterally exposing the respective transverse process.

Fixation

Fixation is needed in tumors where there is already significant destruction causing instability or in order to dissect out the tumor you are likely to destabilize the spine with facetectomy. Putting pedicle screws prior to decompression laminectomy is preferred because the anatomical landmarks are still intact.

Laminectomy (Figs. 12 to 16)

With the use of spinous process cutter and bone nibbler spinous processes are cut. Lamina is thinned out as much as possible with a bone nibbler. With the use of a bone burr remaining lamina is thinned out till the bone appears bluish, which is the end point of burring. Burr is preferable in thoracic and cervical spine because it restricts the use of Kerrison's rounger. Kerrison's ronguer's use is to be restricted in these regions because:

- In the thoracic region the canal diameter is small as compared to lumbar region
- The foot plate placement between the cord and lamina can cause cord injury how much ever small ronguer you use.

After thinning out the lamina, an angled curette is used. Edge of the curette is hooked at the edge of bone and pulled up gently away from dura taking care not to have pinched the dura while doing so. Curette must not be introduced between lamina and dura.

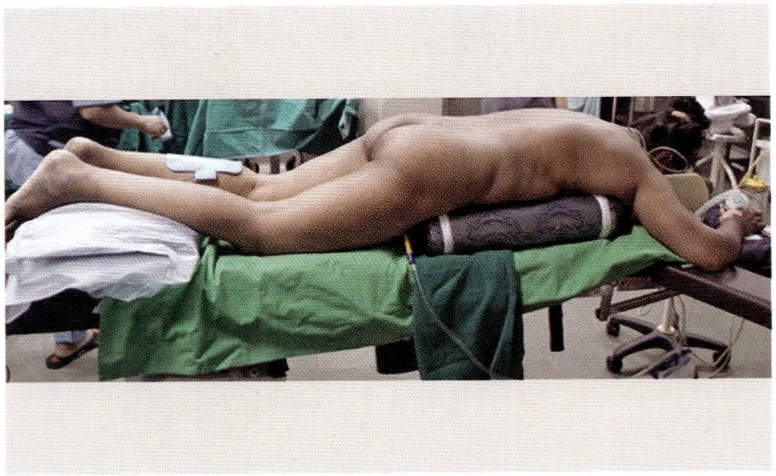

Fig. 6: Position.

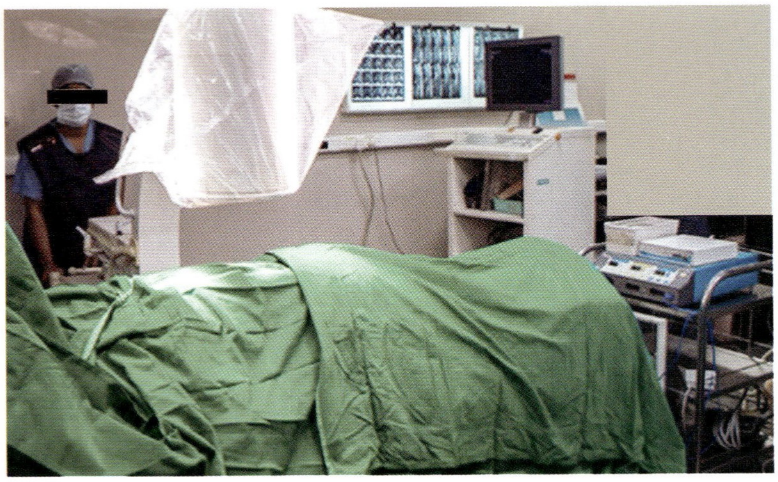

Fig. 7: Head end to the left with draping, C-arm positioning, and C-arm screen positioning.

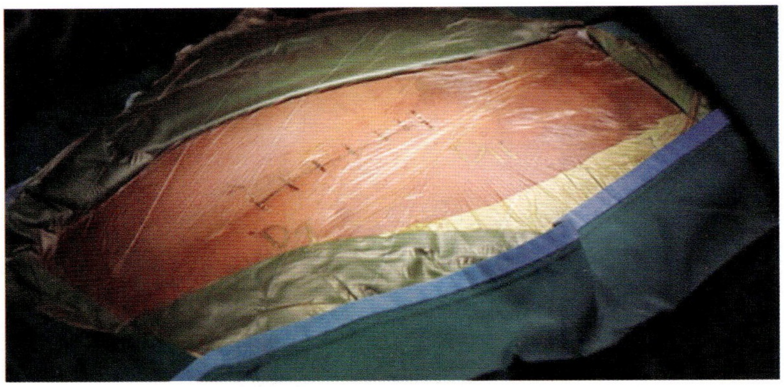

Fig. 8: Draping and marking of the levels to be exposed.

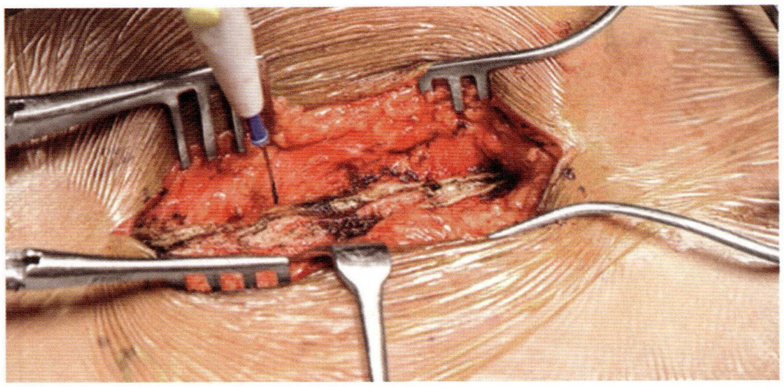

Fig. 9: After taking the skin incision, with the Bowie's cautery we dissect through the subcutaneous tissue till the fascia is exposed.

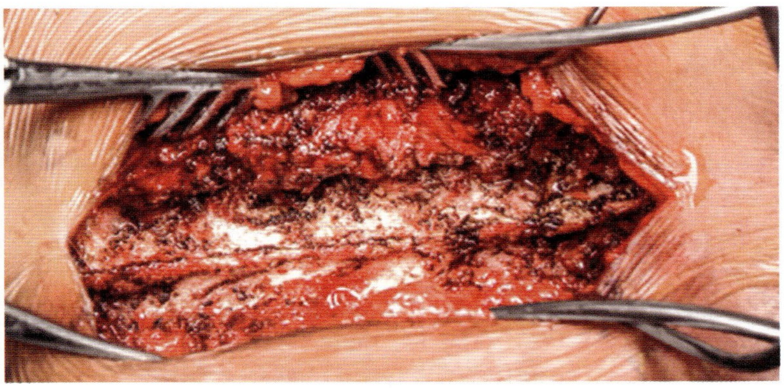

Fig. 10: Fascia and multifidus muscle is dissected off the lamina exposing D7 to D11 lamina and laterally till the respective transverse process.

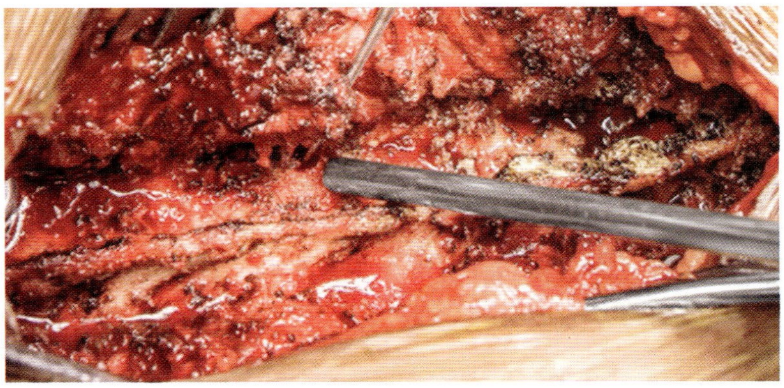

Fig. 11: Suction tip pointing at the exposed transverse process.

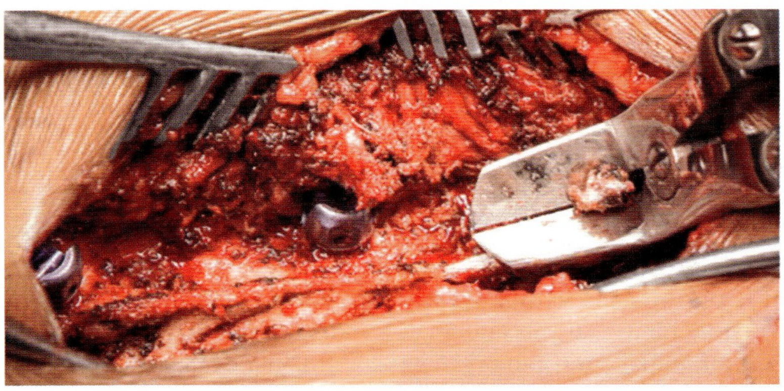

Fig. 12: With the use of a spinous process cutter the spinous processes of the respective vertebra.

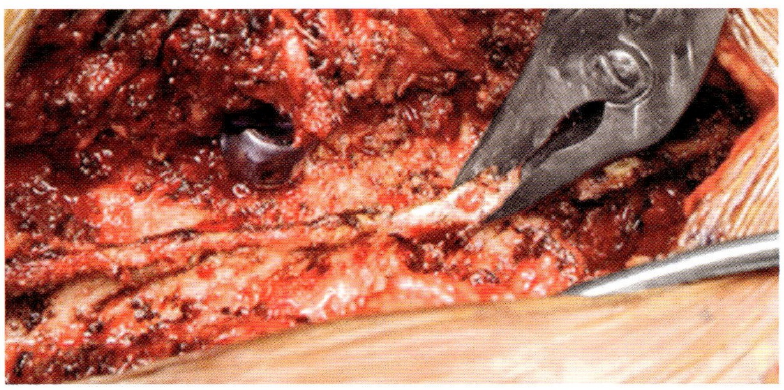

Fig. 13: Using a bone nibbler to remove the stumps of the remaining spinous process and also to thin out the lamina.

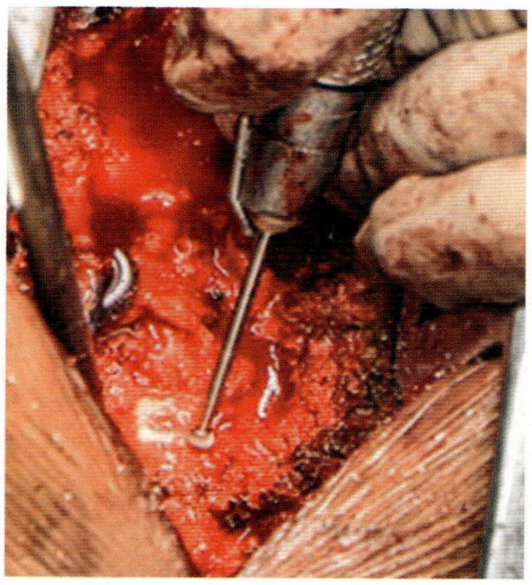

Fig. 14: In the thoracic level it is important to use a burr to thin the lamina and avoid Kerrison's ronguer.

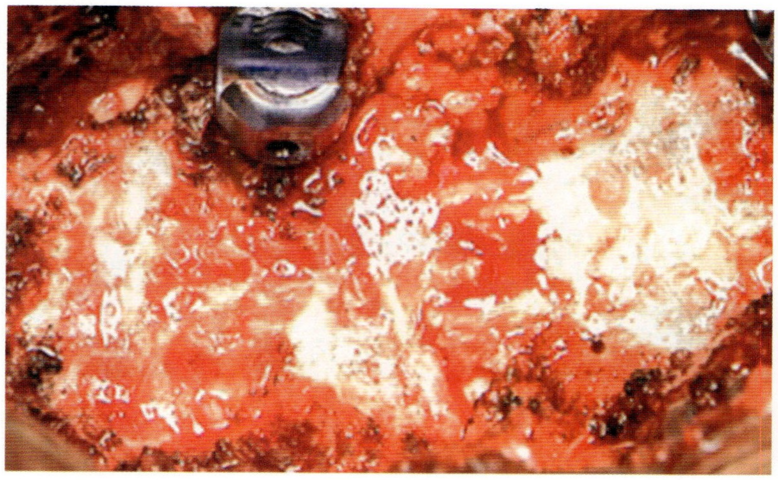

Fig. 15: Lamina after thinning out.

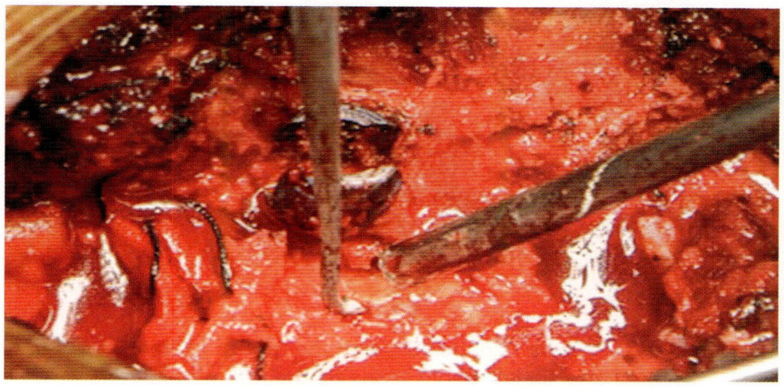

Fig. 16: A curved curette is hooked at the edge of the lamina and the thin layer of lamina is separated of the ligamentum flavum. The flavum is separated off.

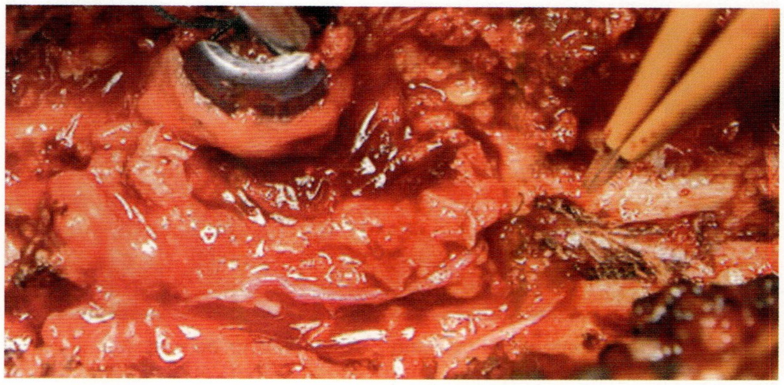

Fig. 17: Bipolar cautery tip point the distal extent of the epidural tumor with dura exposed.

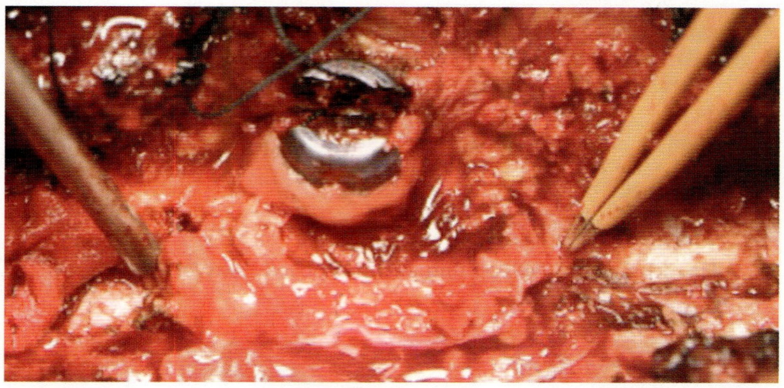

Fig. 18: Proximally the suction tip shows the extent of the tumor with the exposed normal dura. The tumor is yellow in color, soft in consistency easily separable from dura.

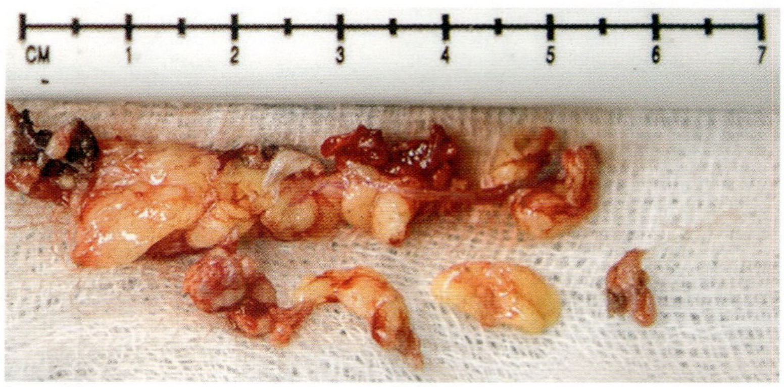

Fig. 19: Adipose tissue like soft friable tissue with engorged vessels. Histopathology report confirmed it later to be angiolipoma.

Defining the Extent of Tumor (Figs. 17 and 18)

With the help of preoperative study of MRI scans extend the laminectomy as distal and proximal as possible till the normal dura is seen. Normal dura looks bluish in color. Lateral demarcation of tumor may require facetectomy, pedicle osteotomy. Extraspinal extent of the tumor must be dealt with later after exposing the intradural part.

Removal of Tumor (Fig. 19)

It is pertinent to evaluate where the tumor is adherent too and whether there is any foraminal or bony extension. In our case, there was foraminal extension as evident on MRI but no bony or extraspinal extension. Be mindful of any vascular feeders and coagulate them in time to avoid retraction and uncontrollable bleeding. After defining its extent start gradually lifting of the tumor from the dura carefully separating adhesions if any with a dura retractor or microscissors. In our case, we were easily able to peel off the tumor from the dura. Tumor tissue had fat globules which coming off piece meal. We removed as much foraminal tissue as possible.

Completion of Procedure (Fig. 20)

When the dura is seen to be completely free posteriorly from its proximal most to distal most normal levels decompression is said to be complete.

Closure (Figs. 21 to 23)

After hemostasis and giving a thorough wash, a vacuum suction drain is placed beneath the muscle layer. First, the muscle and fascia are closed. It is important to have a watertight closure. A absorbable suture No. 1 is used for this layer in either continuous or interrupted manner. Muscles are always closed with interrupted stress to avoid ischemia. Subcutaneous layer is closed with absorbable suture No. 2-0 and skin can be closed with either an nonabsorbable suture 2-0 or skin staplers. Drain is fixed after confirming that it is not sutured mistakenly in the inner layers. We can infiltrate the muscle and subcutaneous layer with local anesthetic either lignocaine or a combination of lidocaine and sensorcaine.

Intraoperative blood loss was 700 mL which was anticipated. Drain output over next 48 hours was 150 mL. Total duration of surgery from incision to closure was 4 and 1/2 hours.

Postoperatively there was no neurodeficit. She was ambulatory in 48 hours with walker support and thereafter without any walking aid. There were no wound complications. Her feelings of heaviness and weakness in the lower limbs completely disappeared. Her joint position sense of both lower limbs was regained with crude touch sensation were still less. Hyperreflexia decreased, although Babinski's sign was still positive bilaterally.

COMPLICATIONS

- Direct cord injury
- Cord ischemia due to arteries supplying the cord
- Dural tear
- Wound infection
- Iatrogenic instability
- Pseudomeningocele.

Pseudomeningocele

Presenting a case of pseudomeningocele in a 16-year-old boy following dural leakage as a complication of surgical excision of epidural tumor. He had no neurological involvement. He presented with cystic swelling over back 6 months after surgery (Figs. 24 to 29 with head end on the left side of images).

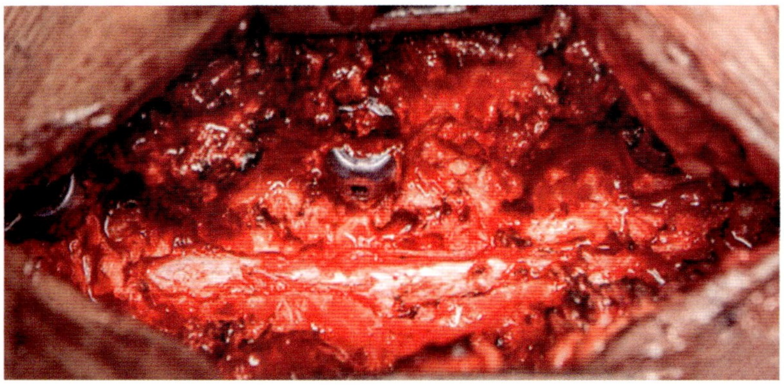

Fig. 20: The cord is decompressed completely when we see the dura free of any compression from cephalad to caudal direction. Dura was pulsatile after decompression.

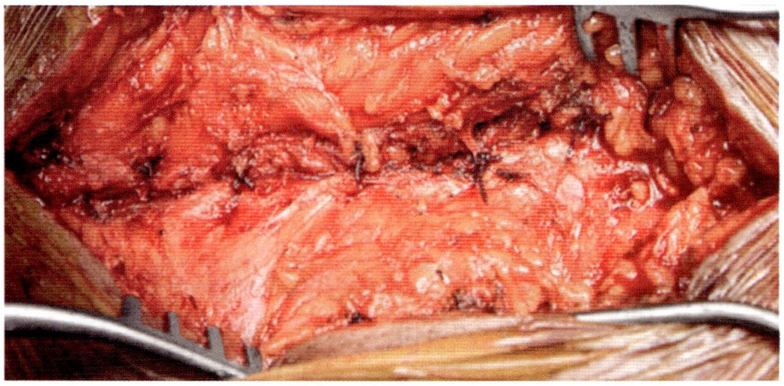

Fig. 21: Closure of fascia and muscles layer with interrupted sutures with absorbable suture No. 1.

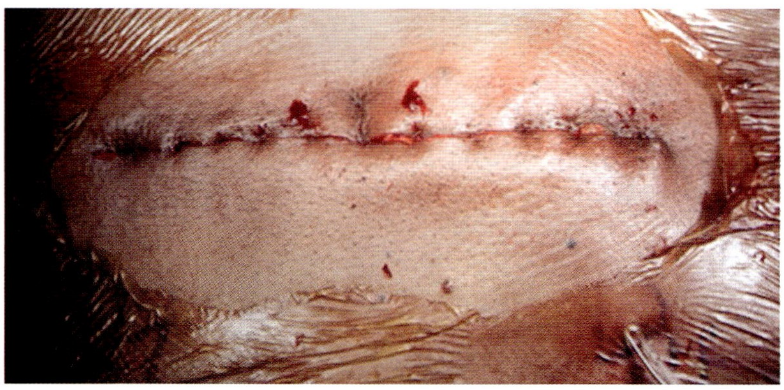

Fig. 22: Subcutaneous tissue was closed with absorbable suture No. 2-0.

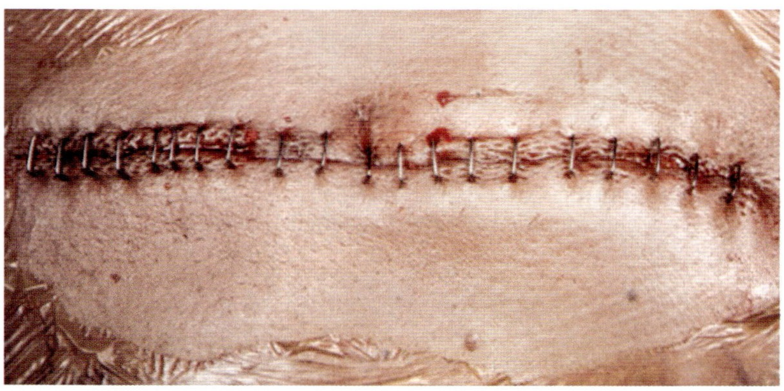

Fig. 23: Skin was closed with skin stapler.

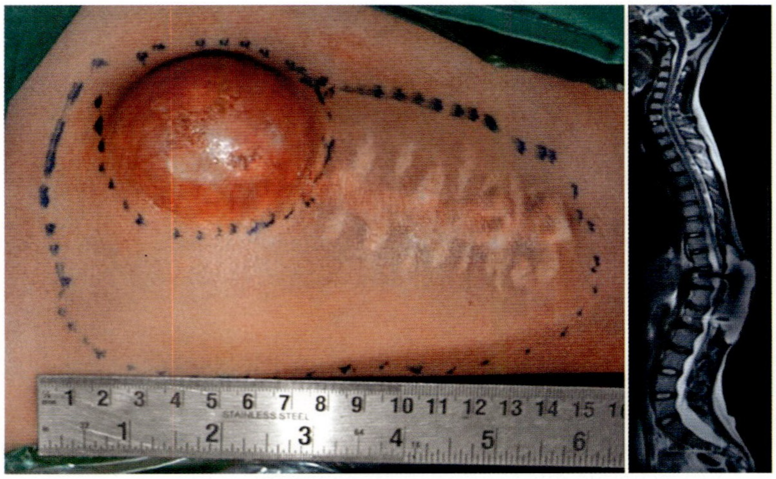

Fig. 24: Clinical and magnetic resonance imaging (MRI) picture of pseudo meningocele at thoracolumbar junction. Previous epidural tumor was removed from D11 region (left side of clinical picture is cephalad).

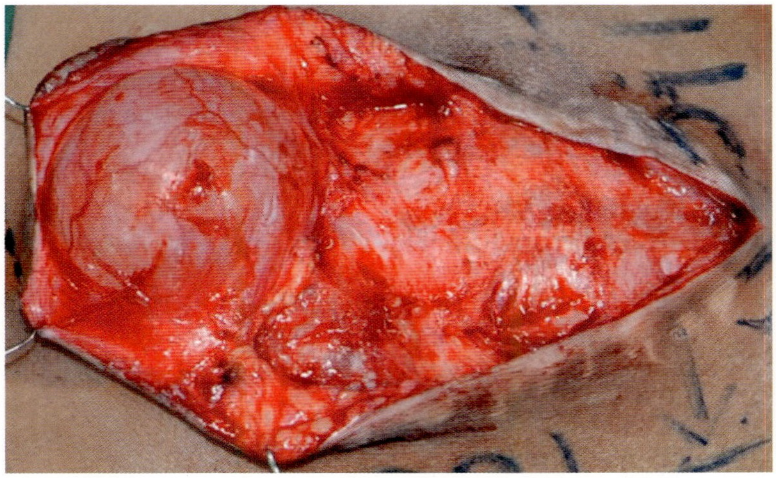

Fig. 25: Skin incision was taken in line of previous scar and extended proximally to include the cyst. Above figure shows the pseudo-meningocele after completely dissecting the cyst from subcutaneous tissue.

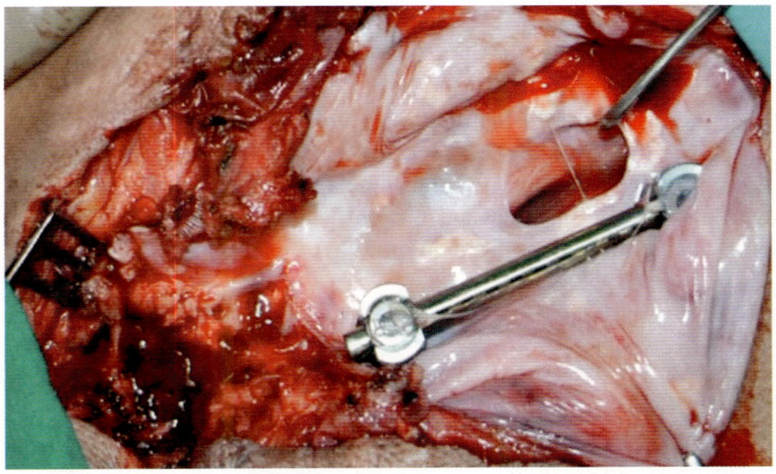

Fig. 26: After opening of the cyst, the opening within the dura is seen. The dural dissector is pointing towards the exposed cord.

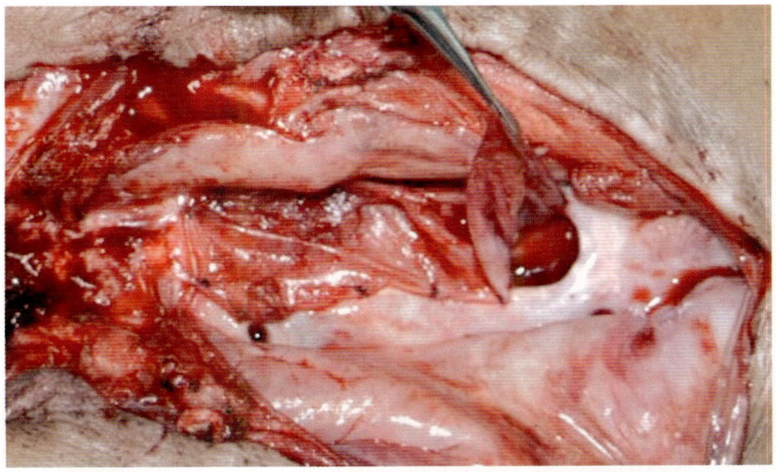

Fig. 27: The opening in the dura was sealed with synthetic dural patch and part of the cyst wall was cut and used as a patch to cover it up. Suturing was done intermittently with 4-0 prolene round body needle.

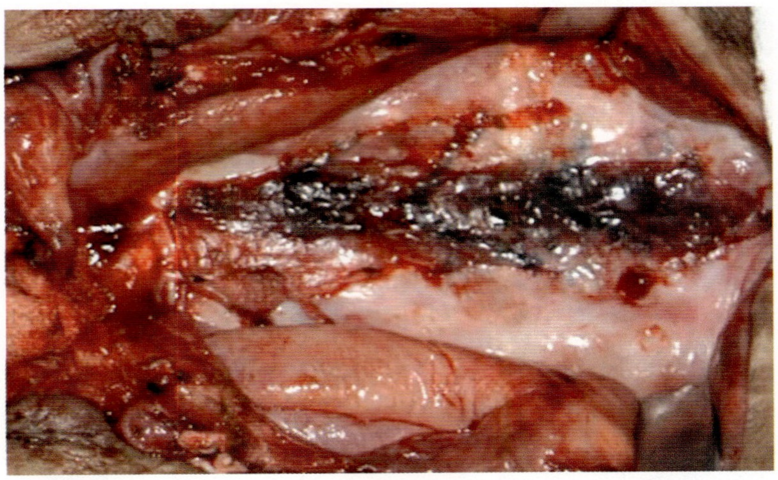

Fig. 28: After completely covering the rent edges of the suturing were additionally sealed with synthetic fibrin glue.

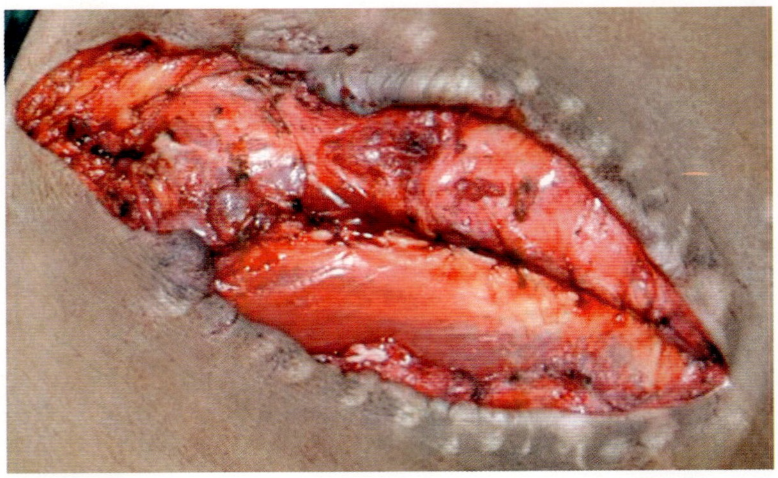

Fig. 29: Covering muscle and subcutaneous tissue was closed tightly with double breasting. Skin sutures were taken.

SUGGESTED READING

1. Surgery of Spinal Tumors. Jörg Klekamp, Madjid Samii.
2. Tumors of the Spine. Daniel Kim Ung-kyu Chang Se-Hoon Kim Mark Bilsky.
3. Spinal Cord and Spinal Column Tumors. Curtis A Dickman, Micheal G Fehlings, Ziya L Gokaslan.
4. Spine Oncology. Onder Ofluoglu.

CHAPTER 30

Cervical Interlaminar Epidural Steroid Injection

Uday Pote

INTRODUCTION

In general population, the prevalence of cervical radiculopathy is 3.5 per 1,000 population.[1]

The cervical radiculopathy results from nerve root dysfunction and is often due to mechanical compression. However radicular symptoms also result from inflammatory cytokines released from damaged intervertebral discs.[2] Cervical interlaminar epidural steroid injection (CIESI) is indicated for conservative management of axial neck pain, with or without radicular pain in shoulder, upper arm or up to fingers. In case of axial pain and/or bilateral radicular symptoms the position of the needle during the injection must be central. If the radicular pain is predominant then the position of the needle is paramedian toward the most affected side. The steroids have local anti-inflammatory and membrane stabilizing functions. CIESI is given to improve the symptoms of pain. They do not improve neurological deficits if any.[3]

INDICATIONS

- Neck pain
- Cervical radiculitis
- Post-laminectomy cervical pain
- Acute brachial plexitis
- Complex regional pain syndrome

CONTRAINDICATIONS

- Infective etiology
- Bleeding disorders
- Cervical malignancy

COMPLICATIONS

Minor

- Headache
- Increase in neck pain
- No relief in pain
- Nausea
- Facial flushing
- Dural puncture
- Local oozing of blood
- Superficial infection

Major

- Vasovagal reaction
- Vascular injury
- Epidural hematoma
- Epidural abscess
- Arachnoiditis
- Meningitis
- Neurodeficit.

PROCEDURE

We give all CIES injections under fluoroscopic guidance.

INSTRUMENT TABLE PREPARATION (FIG. 1)

The mentioned instruments must be ready. Be sure that you use different needles to withdraw anesthetic, Depo-medrol, dye and normal saline.

POSITION OF THE PATIENT (FIGS. 2 AND 3)

Marking: Under fluoroscopic guidance mark the space through which injection is to be given. Make sure that the neck is not tilted on either sides (Figs. 4A to E).

Landmarks to see on the C-arm images (Fig. 5)

- The spinolamellar line is the line where epidural space is expected to be.
- The lateral image is the safety image.
- Paint and drape the area marked for the injection and cover with the whole towel.

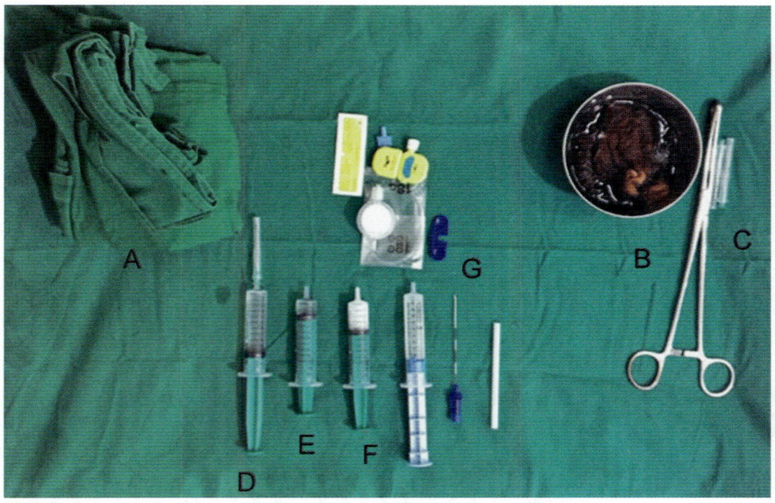

Fig. 1: Instruments on the table. (A) Hole sheet, (B) Sponge holder and betadine tray with gauzes, (C) 24G needles to withdraw saline and Depo-medrol and 16G to withdraw dye, (D) 10 cc syringe filled with 2% lignocaine with 21G 11/2 inch long needle attached, (E) Ionohexol dye, (F) Depo-medrol injection, (G) 18G epidural set with syringe filled with normal saline and air.

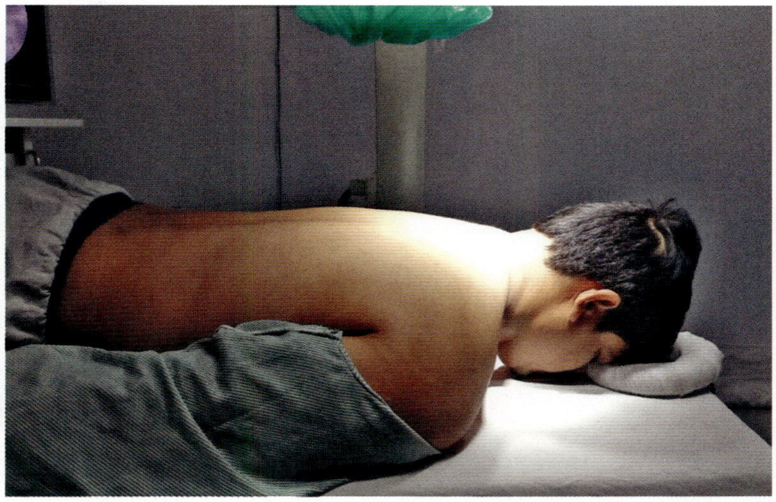

Fig. 2: Prone position. Head straight and resting with forehead on the ring pillow. Neck can be fully flexed with a pillow under chest. Both upper limbs must be by the sides.

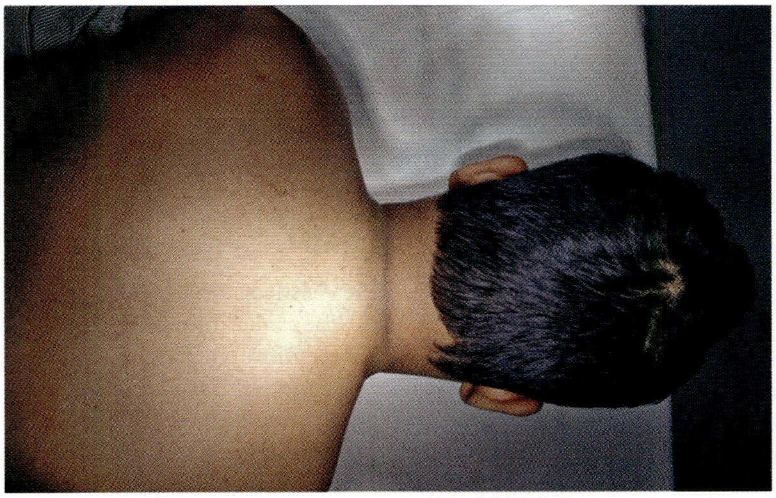

Fig. 3: Expose the entire neck with upper back. Look for any signs of local inflammation, infection or tattoos in the area to be injected.

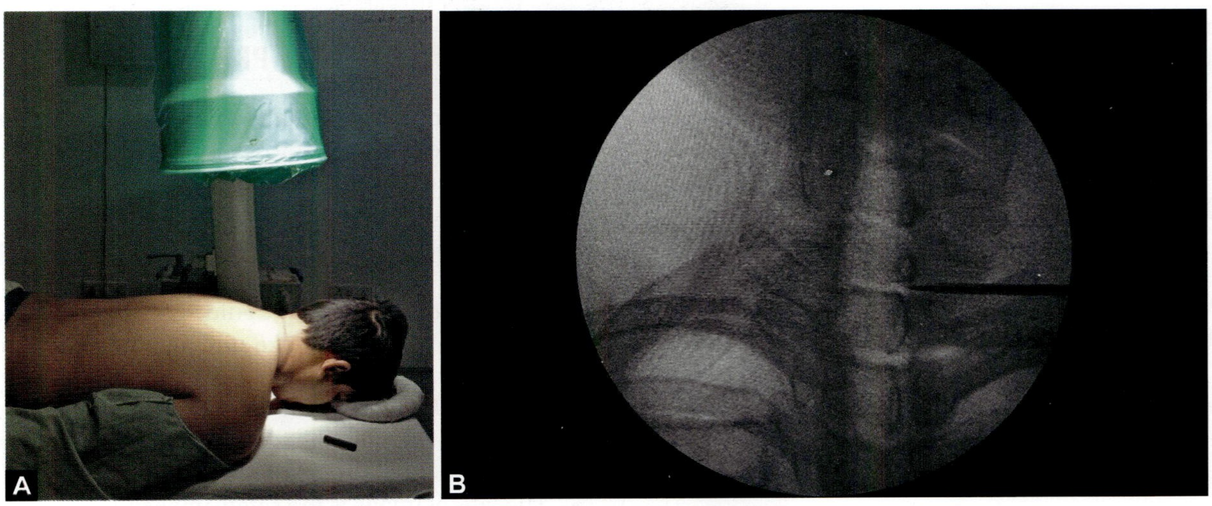

Figs. 4A and B: (A) Mark the C7-T1 level with C-arm tilted caudally 5°; (B) Anteroposterior view with 5° caudal tilt, with marker placed at C7-T1 space.

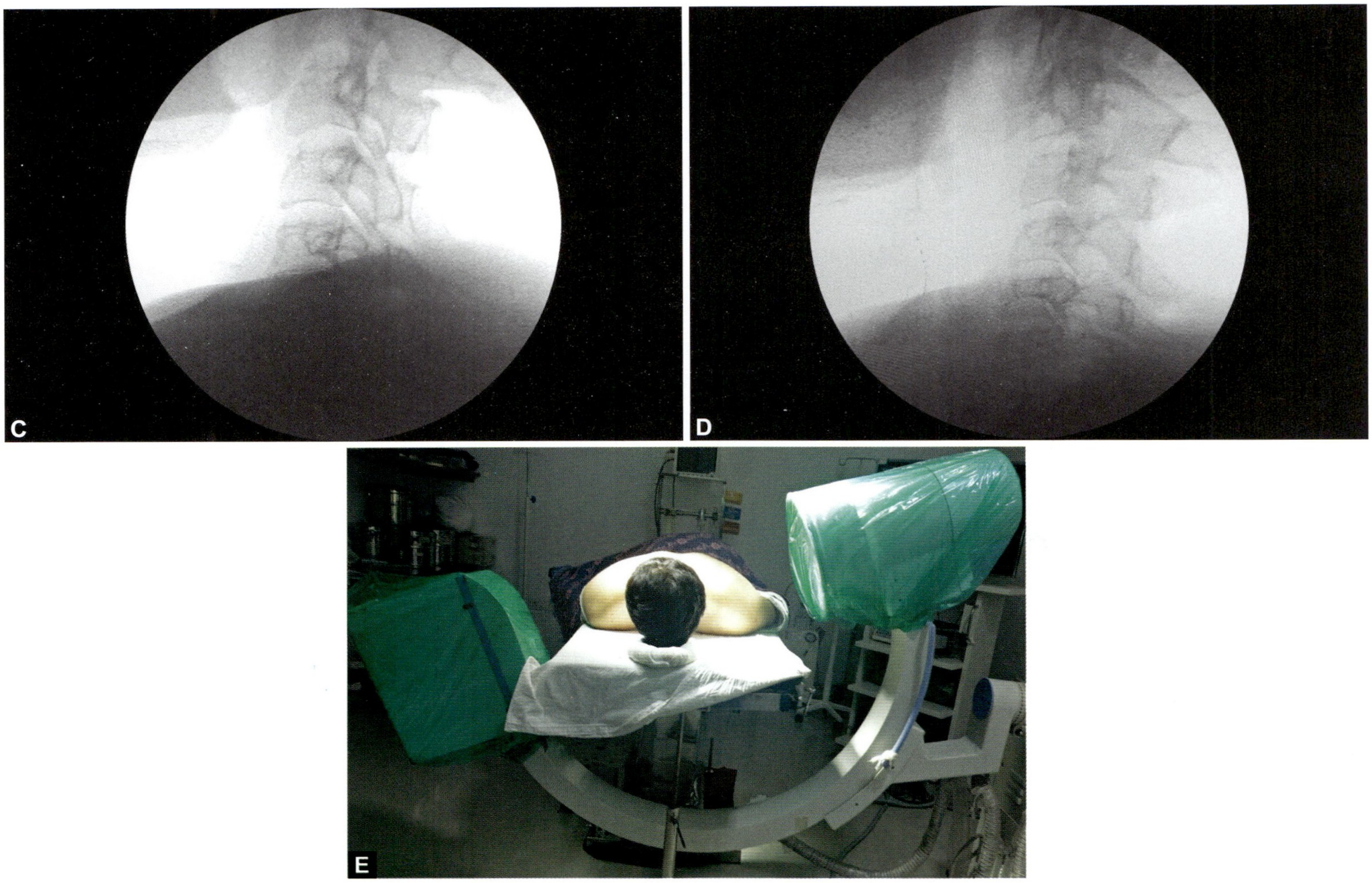

Figs. 4C to E: (C) True lateral view is the safety view. Pull the arms by the sides toward the feet by manual gentle traction to see the extent of the vertebrae visualized. Many times the C7/T1 space will not be visualized using a true lateral view; (D) Make the C-arm oblique till you at least visualize the C5-6 vertebral space; (E) Oblique tilt of the C-arm.

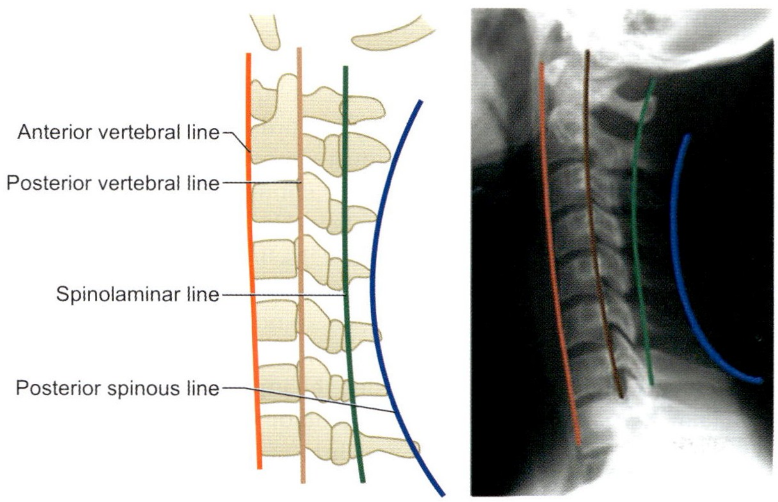

Fig. 5: Cervical spine trauma evaluation.
Source: https://www.orthobullets.com/spine/2012/cervical-spine-trauma-evaluation.

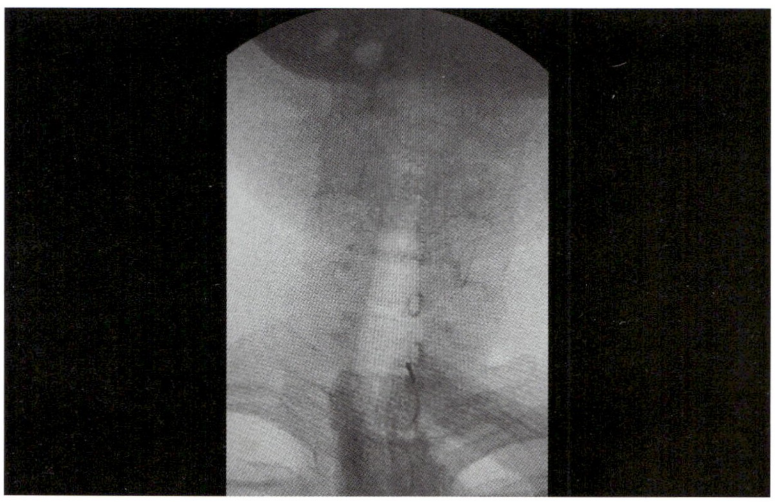

Fig. 6: Insert the Tuohy's needle while viewing in anteroposterior (AP) view.

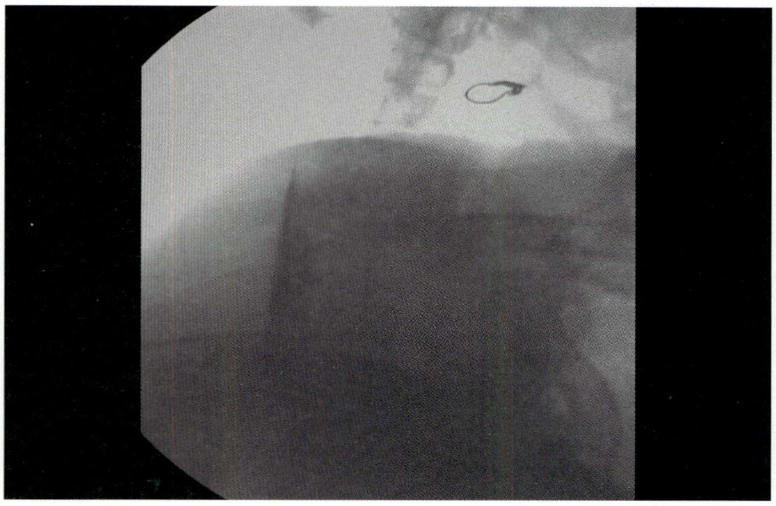

Fig. 7: Spread of the dye parallel to the cord.

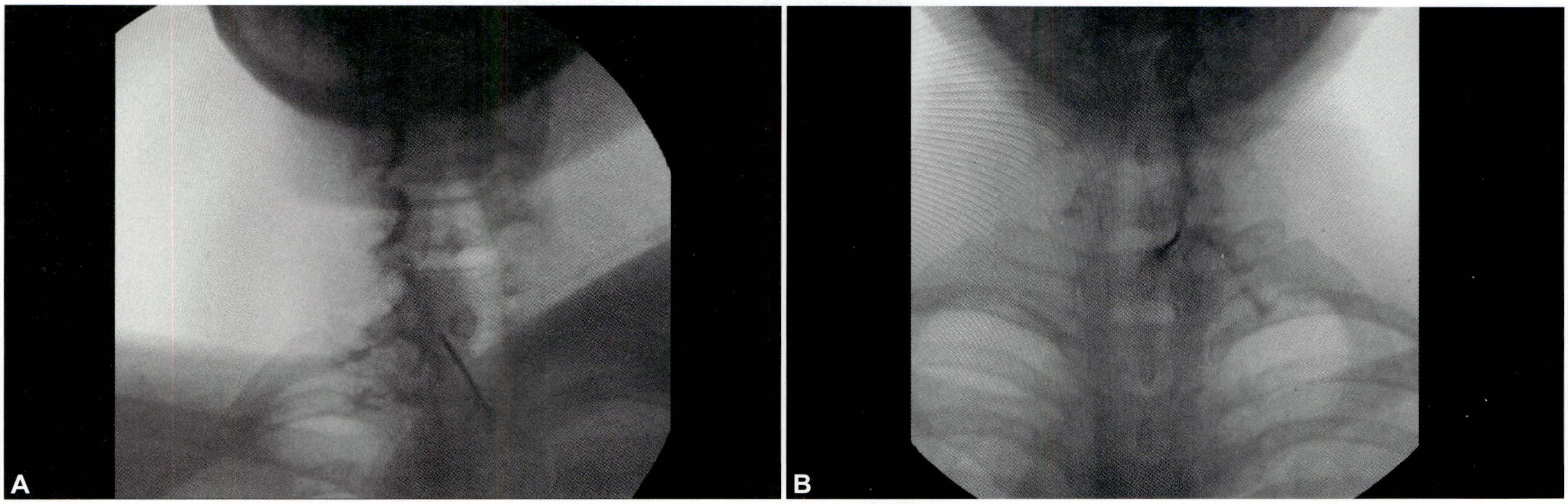

Figs. 8A and B: (A) Left-sided flow of the dye; (B) Right sided flow of the dye.

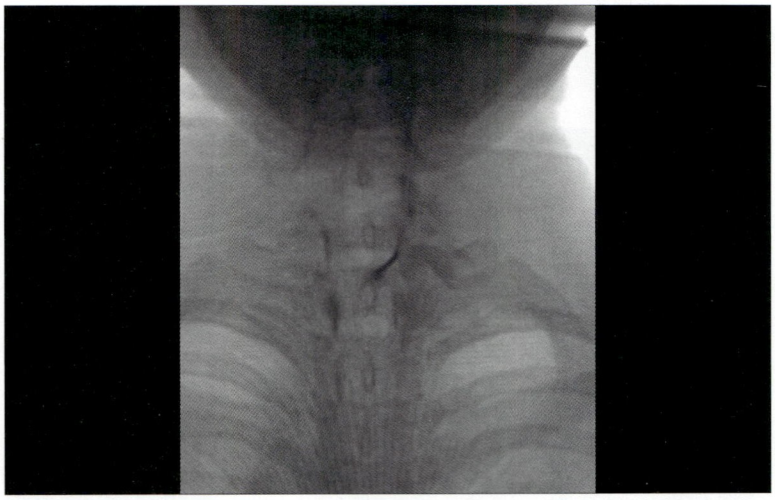

Fig. 9: Dye crossing the midline to the other side as the needle is in the space of Okada.

Inject 5–7 cc of anesthetic solution. Be careful not to penetrate too deep.

Use 18G Tuohy's needle to proceed. Constantly check AP and lateral views. If the pain is axial then direct the needle in the center and if the pain is unilateral direct the needle to the affected side (Fig. 6).

Make sure the needle is directed along the tip of the C7 spinous process. A resistance is felt when the interspinous ligament is pierced. This is the ligamentum flavum. Attach the loss of resistance syringe and check every millimeter you enter deeper. Once the resistance is lost and the saline from LOR syringe goes in smoothly, inject the dye and check the flow. If the epidural space is encountered the flow is parallel to the spinal cord in the lateral or oblique X-ray as in Figure 7. On AP view we can see it spread along the cord outline or if the needle is directed to any particular side of most symptoms then the flow will outline the nerve roots of the side. This confirms the positions and then appropriate dose of long acting steroid injection with or without diluting with normal saline is injected (Figs. 8A and B).

In case fluoroscopy is not available then, once the tip is of C7 is palpated direct the needle along the C7 spinous process toward the lamina and once the lamina is hit use the loss of resistance technique to identify the epidural space and then the injection is injected.

If at any time the patient feels any pain or tingling in the affected side or if the images show that the needle has penetrated deeper, abort the procedure and reinsert the needle after confirming the direction and location again. At times a space between the epidural space and ligamentum flavum is encountered and is called as the space of Okada wherein the dye will flow into the intervertebral joints and if needle is directed to one side then dye may cross over to the other side as well as shown in Figure 9. In such case very carefully and gently push the needle into epidural space, and reinject the dye to confirm.

POSTINJECTION

Local band aid is applied over the injection site and once the patient is supine, patient is asked to turn the head side-to-side. Patient is kept under observation for 1 hour and sent home with instructions against driving of vehicle for 48 hours and can resume all activities after 48 hours.

REFERENCES

1. Salemi G, Savettieri G, Meneghini F, et al. Prevalence of cervical spondylotic radiculopathy: a door-to-door survey in a Sicilian municipality. Acta Neurol Scand. 2009;93(2-3):184-8.
2. Ellenberg MR, Honet JC, Treanor WJ. Cervical radiculopathy. Arch Phys Med Rehabil. 1994;75(3):342-52.
3. Sternberg A, Kaadan M. Cervical epidural steroid injection for. Acta Anaesthesiol Scand. 1993;37:562-66.

CHAPTER 31

Lumbar Root Block

Uday Pote, Sharad M Hardikar

INTRODUCTION

The transforaminal epidural steroid injection is the most common and safe technique, to deliver the injectate in the ventral epidural space. The technique we use is slightly modified wherein we do not advance the needle completely on the ventral aspect of the vertebral body and thereby reducing the risk of vascular injection. We use the supraneural "safe triangle" location to inject the injectate. This diminishes the risk of intrathecal or vascular injection (Figs. 1A and B).

BASIC ANATOMY

The nerve root and dorsal root ganglion of the nerve root is situated anterior to the caudal superior articular process, caudal to the pedicle of the vertebral arch, and cranial to the inferior border of the vertebral body. The region of the safe triangle is defined by the inferior border of the pedicle, the anterior border of the nerve root, and the lateral border of the vertebral body. This is the target area where we have to inject.

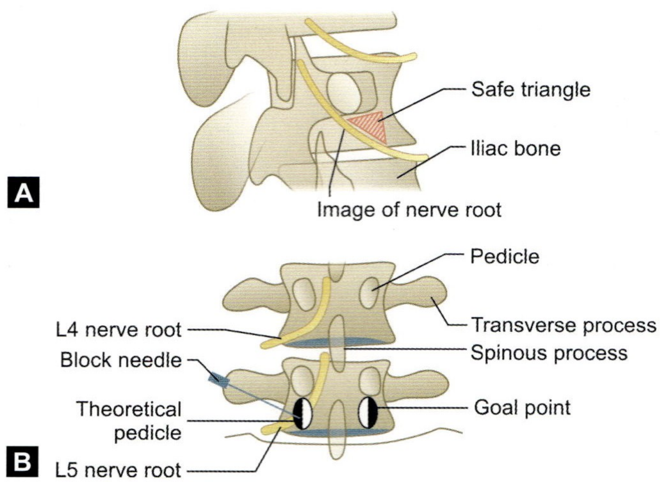

Figs. 1A and B: (A) Depicts the location of the safe triangle on oblique view; (B) Depicts the safe triangle location on the anteroposterior (AP) view.

The transforaminal steroid injections are also called as selective nerve root block (SNRB) or root block.

Indications for root block are radicular pain to the lower limb.

Complications are rare and includes increased back pain, radicular pain, nonpositional headaches, vasovagal reaction, intraoperative hypertension, nausea, dizziness, facial flushing, and transient leg paresis.

PROCEDURE

Things needed on the trolley.

POSITION

Patient is positioned prone. No Jacksons frame or bolsters needed. The hands are placed comfortable toward the head end.

Anteroposterior (AP), lateral and oblique fluoroscopic views are important.

On AP view, make sure that the end plates are parallel, the spinous processes are in straight line (not possible when scoliosis is present). In this view mark the midline along the spinous processes as shown in Figure 2.

In the lateral view we place the marker at the intervertebral disc up to the midpoint of the disc as shown in Figure 3.

The distance calculated on the lateral view from the skin is marked on the patients surface as shown in Figure 4 and that is the entry point to choose for the lumbar root block.

PROCEDURE

- The area marked is painted and draped.
- Lignocaine injection is injected locally and along the trajectory of the injection.
- Long 21G spinal needle is used and trajectory is again confirmed on AP images. The needle must be directed parallel to the iliac bones (Fig. 5).

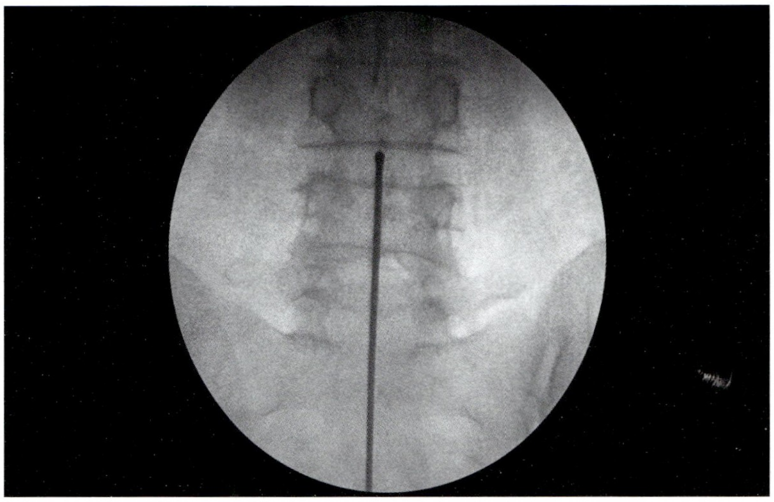

Fig. 2: Marking the midline.

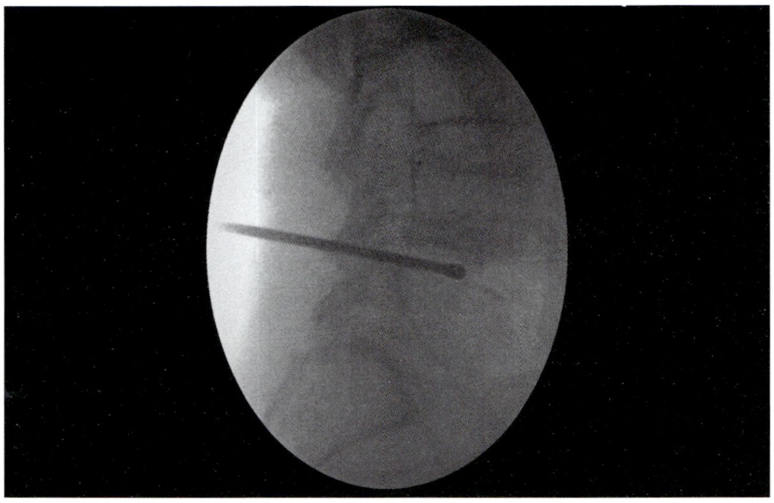

Fig. 3: Marker at the level of L4-5 disc space marking the mid-point in lateral view.

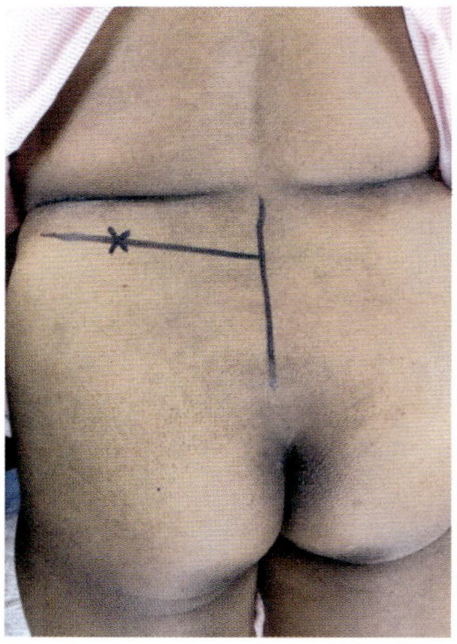

Fig. 4: Markings on the patients back where the markings done on the anterior and lateral fluoroscopic images intersect.

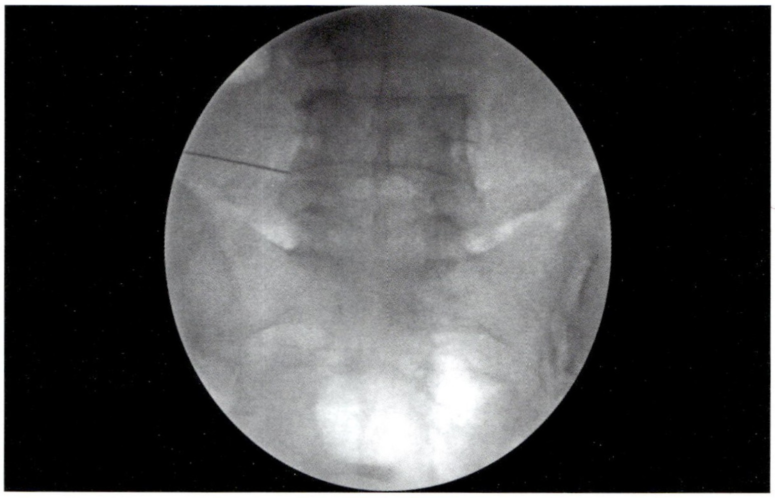

Fig. 5: Anteroposterior (AP) image showing the spinal needle parallel to the iliac crest and hitting the articular surface.

- The needle moves along the direction of the tip. The notch over the spinal needle marks the side of the bevel. Keeping these things in mind we can change the direction of the needle.
- Once the needle hits the articular surfaces check AP image.

Once the articular surface is hit, the needle is withdrawn a few millimeters and the reinserted with the tip pointed ventrally. This will negotiate the needle entering the safe triangle and confirm in the lateral image as shown in Figure 6. The patient will have radiating symptoms in this needle position which will indicate the proximity of the needle to the nerve root or the dorsal root ganglion.

The position is reconfirmed by injecting the dye. The dye delineates the nerve roots distinctly as shown in Figures 7 and 8.

Once the position is confirmed on both the AP and the lateral images, appropriate dose of long acting steroid mixed with lignocaine is injected at the site. The area of injection is cleaned and band aid dressing is applied.

Post injection patient is made supine and straight leg raise test is done to confirm the pain relief obtained. Patient is instructed to avoid driving or exercises for 2 days. Icing at the site of injection to reduce local inflammation.

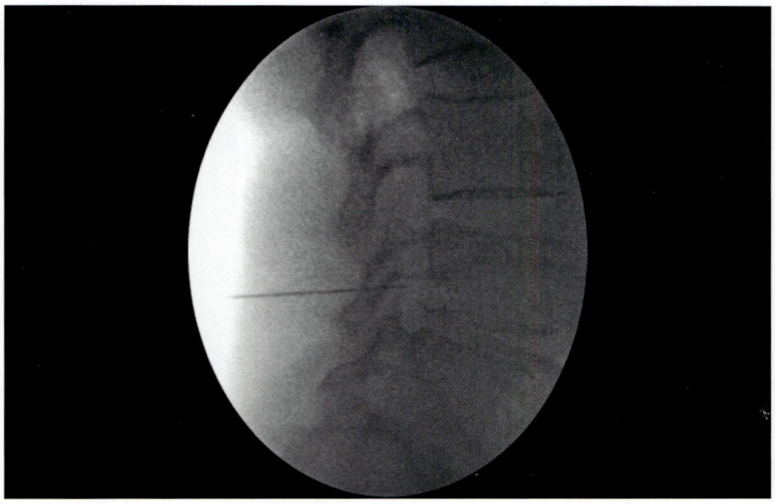

Fig. 6: Needle placement in the supraneural safe triangle.

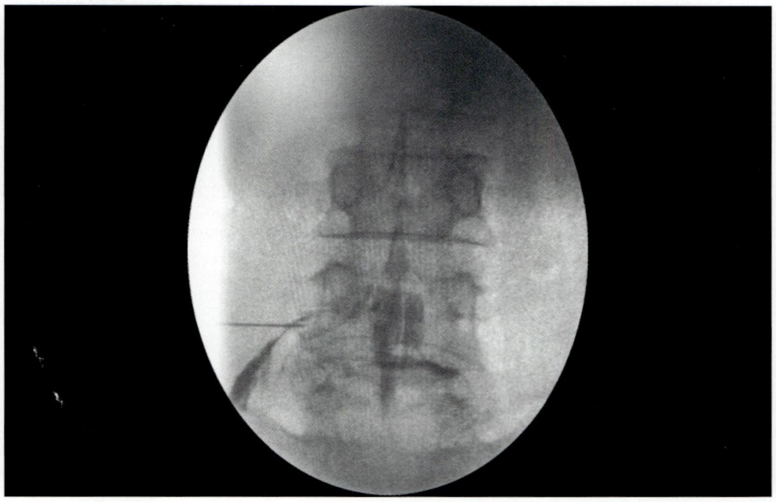

Fig. 7: Image is an anteroposterior (AP) view after the dye is injected. The injected part is seen flowing in the epidural space and along the course of the nerve root. The midline shows that the dye was in the disc space in the previous attempt when the needle is withdrawn and redirected.

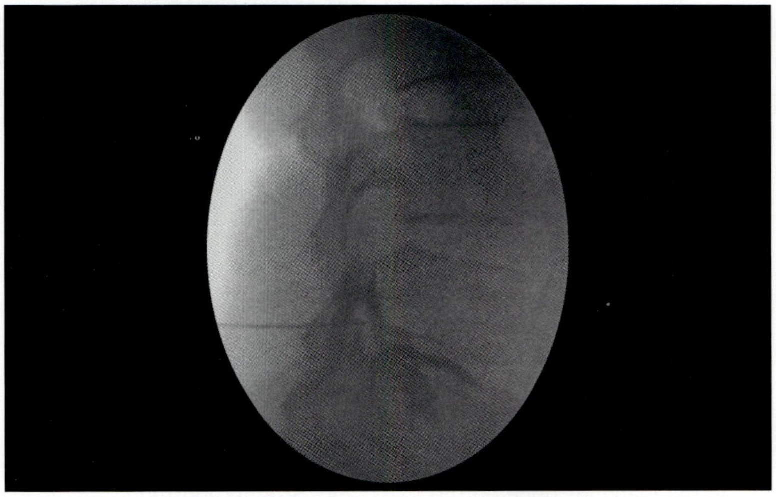

Fig. 8: Lateral view showing the dye flowing along the direction of the roots.

SECTION 4

WRIST AND HAND SURGERY

Section Editor: *Nilesh Dattatray Darawade*

CHAPTER 32

Flexor Tendon Injury

Abhijeet L Wahegaonkar, Satish A Mane, Anup S Bansode

INTRODUCTION

Treatment of flexor tendon injury is an arduous task for surgeon to achieve best possible functional outcome. Flexor tendon rupture can result from injury by sharp objects, from crush injury, and from sport injury.

ANATOMY AND CLASSIFICATION

There are nine flexor tendons, four of flexor digitorum superficialis (FDS), four of flexor digitorum profundus (FDP), and one of flexor pollicis longus (FPL). Flexor Tendon injury has been classified into five anatomical zones (Fig. 1).[1]

Zone II was also called as "no man's land" due to historic poor results in tendon repair in this zone. Flexor sheath consists of five annular and three cruciate pulleys (Fig. 2).[2]

CLINICAL FEATURES

Thorough physical examination of injured hand for tendons, nerve and vascular injury is necessary. In case of complete transection of tendon, no active flexion is seen and tenodesis effect is lost on passive wrist extension. Active flexion of finger may be present in partial rupture of tendon, but usually is painful. Examination for tendons should be performed individually in each finger.

INVESTIGATIONS

Thorough history taking and detailed physical examination is key for tendon injury and any neurovascular injury of hand.

Posteroanterior (PA), oblique, and true lateral X-ray views are taken to look for any bony injury.

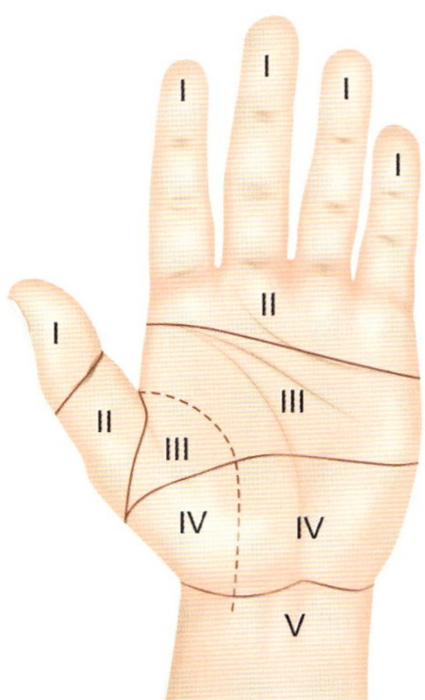

Fig. 1: Zone I—distal to flexor digitorum superficialis (FDS) insertion, zone II—from A1 pulley to FDS insertion, zone III—from transverse carpal ligament to A1 pulley (zone of lumbricals), zone IV—zone of carpal tunnel, and zone V—from proximal aspect of carpal tunnel to musculotendinous junction.

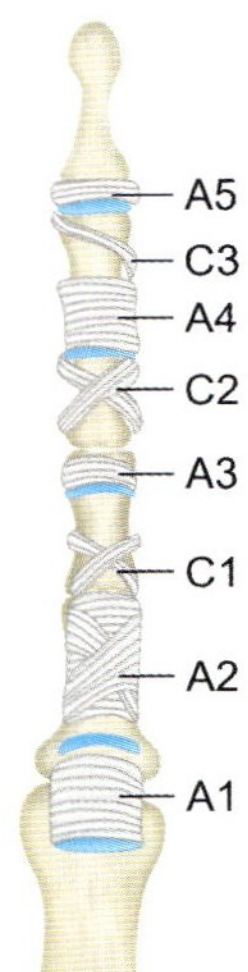

Fig. 2: A1, A3, and A5 pulleys take origin from volar plates of MP, PIP, DIP joints respectively; A2 pulley from proximal phalanx and A4 pulley from middle phalanx. C1 lies between A2 and A3, C2 between A3 and A4; while C3 between A4 and A5. (DIP: distal interphalangeal; MP: metacarpophalangeal; PIP: proximal interphalangeal)

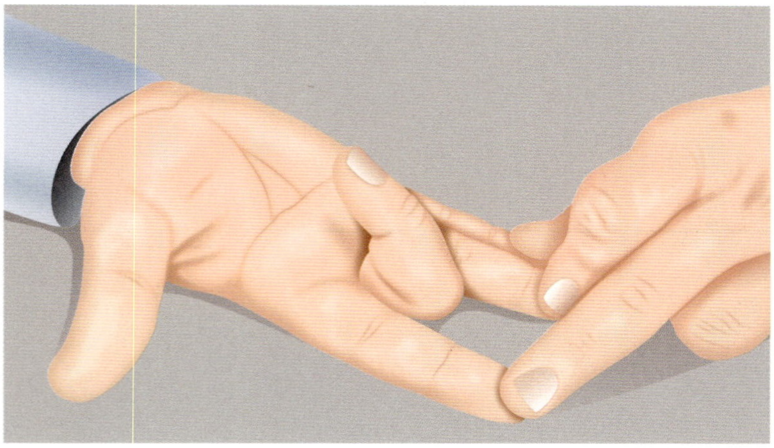

Fig. 3: FDS tendon is examined by asking patient to flex actively from PIP joint of involved finger while holding MP, PIP, and DIP joints of other uninvolved fingers in extension to eliminate FDP action. (DIP: distal interphalangeal; FDP: flexor digitorum profundus; FDS: flexor digitorum superficialis; MP: metacarpophalangeal; PIP: proximal interphalangeal)

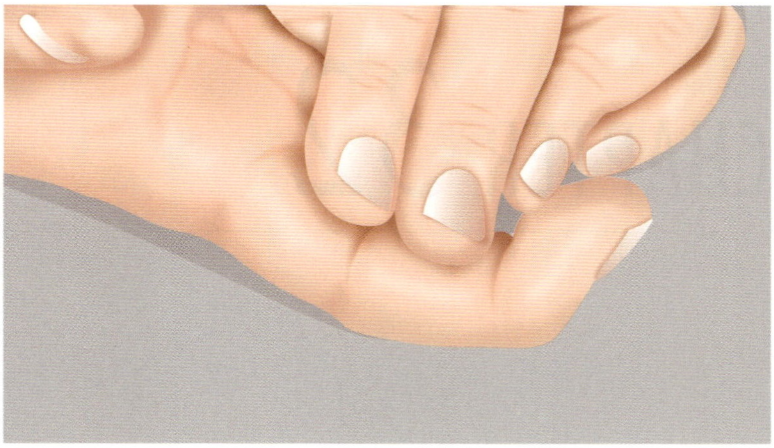

Fig. 4: FDP tendon injury is examined by holding middle phalanx firmly and asking patient to flex DIP joint actively. (DIP: distal interphalangeal; FDP: flexor digitorum profundus)

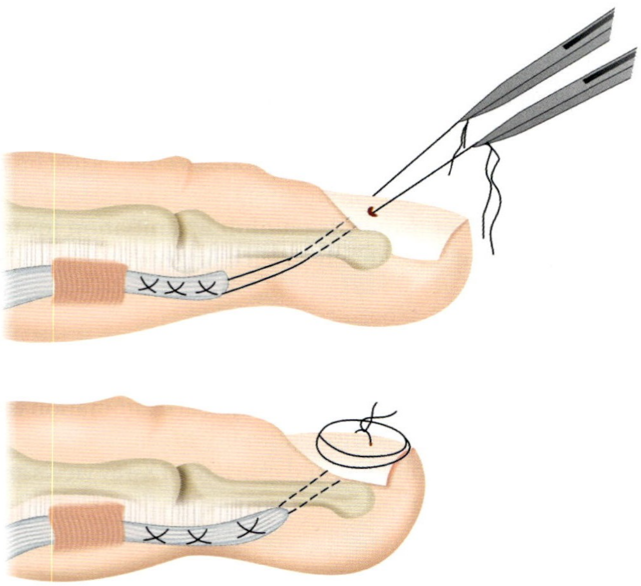

Fig. 5: "Pull-out technique" of tendon to bone repair. Core suture is taken in proximal end of tendon[4] and free ends of suture passed through or around distal phalanx and tied over dorsum of fingernail.

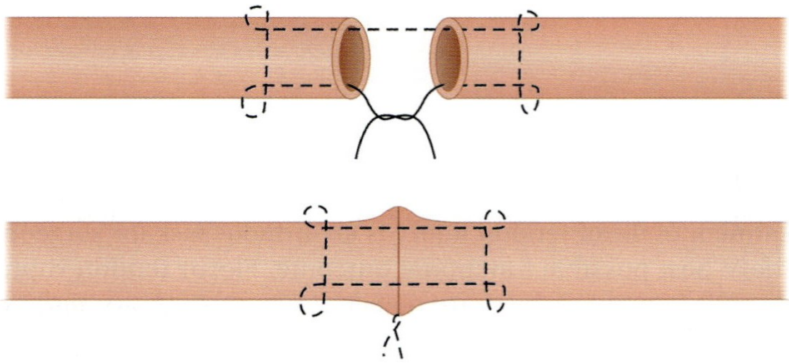

Fig. 6: Modified Kessler[6] method (two strand suture method).

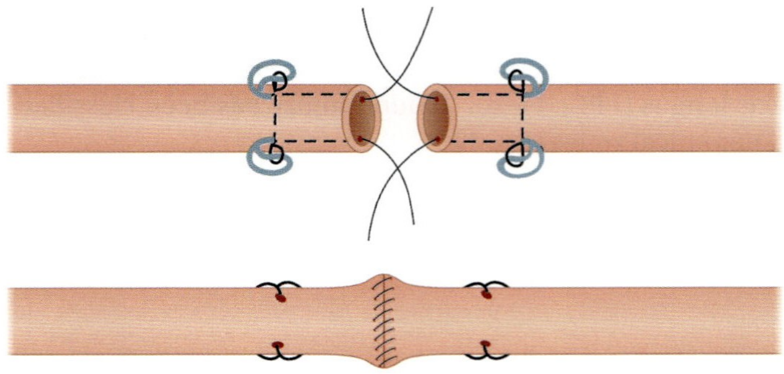

Fig. 7: Strickland core suture.

In chronic injury to tendon, dynamic ultrasound examination and or magnetic resonance imaging (MRI) will be required to locate two ends of tendon.

TREATMENT

Zone I Injury

- It includes injury to FDP tendon distal to FDS insertion or avulsion of FDP from its insertion.
- Primary tenorrhaphy is done if distal stump is more than 1 cm.
- Flexor digitorum profundus advancement and primary repair of FDP to bone is done if distal stump is less than 1 cm. FDP to bone repair can be done either by using anchor, miniscrew or by pull-out-technique.[3]

Zone II Injury

- Zone II includes the pulley system of flexor apparatus.
- Flexor tendons are repaired end to end by core suture and epitendinous sutures.
- Venting of pulley can be done in selected cases for easy passage of tendon.[5]

Zone III, IV, and V

- Technique of core and epitendinous sutures is same as zone II.
- Various techniques have been described for core suture of end to end tendon repair.
- Suture material commonly used for core suture is nonabsorbable suture 3-0 or 4-0 depending on tendon caliber.
- Prolene 5-0 or 6-0 is commonly used for epitendinous or circumferential suture.

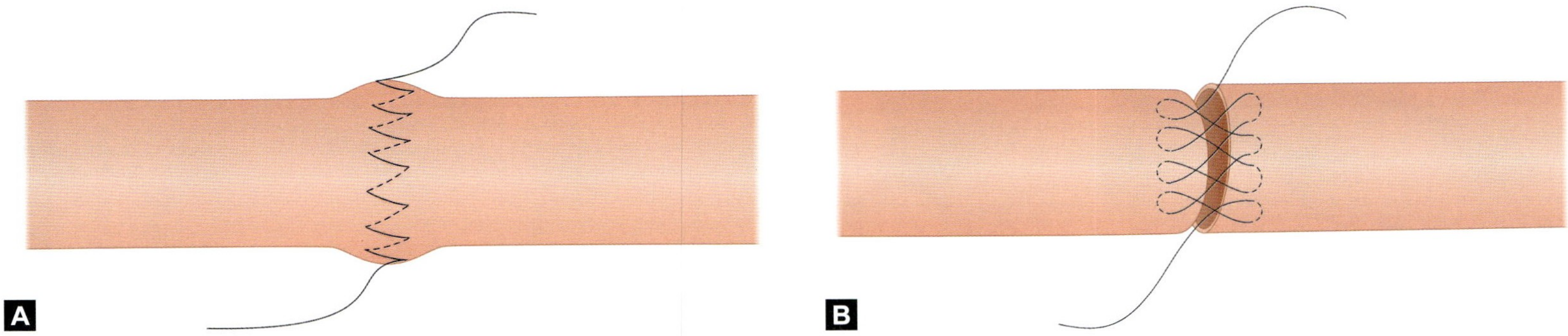

Figs. 8A and B: Epitendinous suture technique. (A) Simple running; (B) Cross stitch (Silfverskiold).[9]

SURGICAL STEPS

Simple running epitendinous and modified Kessler core suture technique in zone II flexor tendon injury.

Patient is in supine position on operating table with arm on side table. Tourniquet is applied to upper arm with proper padding. Under all aseptic precautions, cleaning, painting, and draping done.

Steps for flexor tendon repair are as follows:

Step 1: Brunner's incision is marked over palm and finger, incision is made with 15 No. blade (Fig. 9).

Step 2: After careful dissection with protection of neurovascular bundle, hematoma is seen at injury site (Fig. 10).

Step 3: Tendon sheath is empty, as tendon ends are retracted (Fig. 11).

Step 4: Identify tendon ends and bring them together by flexion of finger and wrist or by milking action. Tendon ends are held in position with needle No. 25 (Fig. 12).

Step 5: First back wall of tendon ends is sutured circumferentially with simple running suture method using prolene 5-0. This will facilitate easy core suture (Figs. 13A and B).

Step 6: In modified Kessler double strand core suture technique, first suture is passed longitudinally from cut end of tendon along the direction of tendon to come out dorsally using nonabsorbable suture 3-0 (Fig. 14).

Step 7: Then transverse suture is passed across the width of tendon (Fig. 15).

Step 8: Then longitudinal suture taken to come out from cut end of tendon (Figs. 16A and B).

Step 9: Longitudinal suture then taken through other cut end of tendon to come out through upper surface of tendon (Fig. 17).

Step 10: Transverse suture then passed across width of tendon (Fig. 18).

Step 11: Again this suture passed along the direction of tendon to come out through cut end of tendon (Fig. 19).

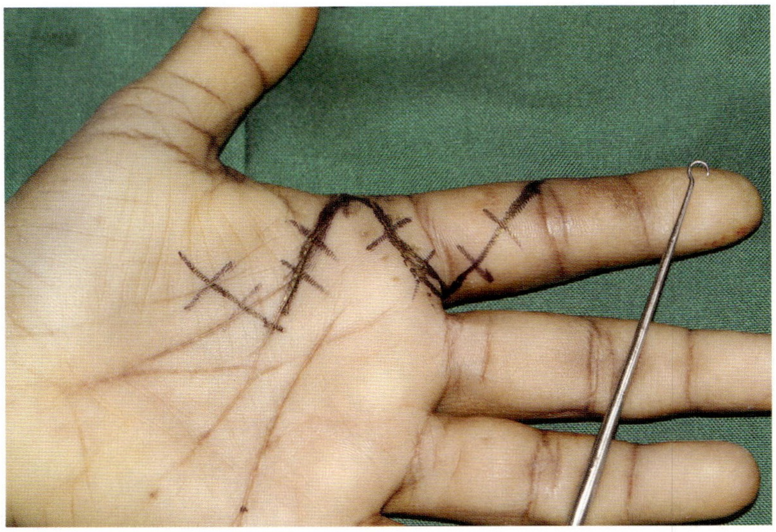

Fig. 9: Incision marking: Brunner's incision.

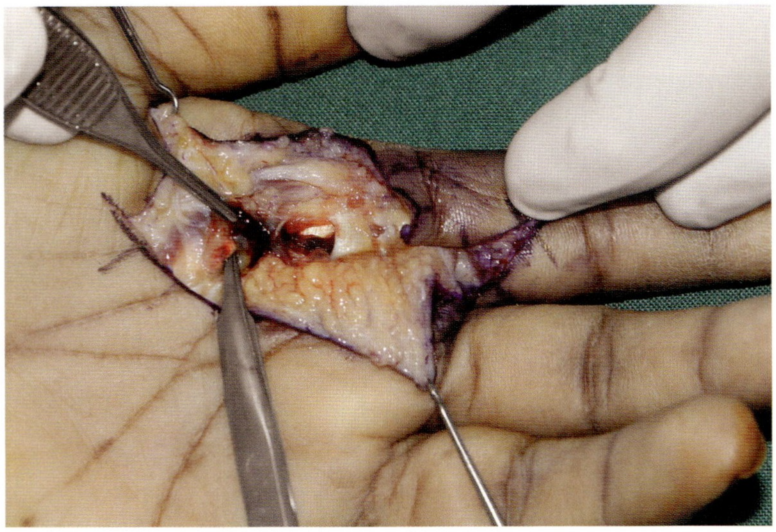

Fig. 10: Hematoma is seen at site of injury within sheath.

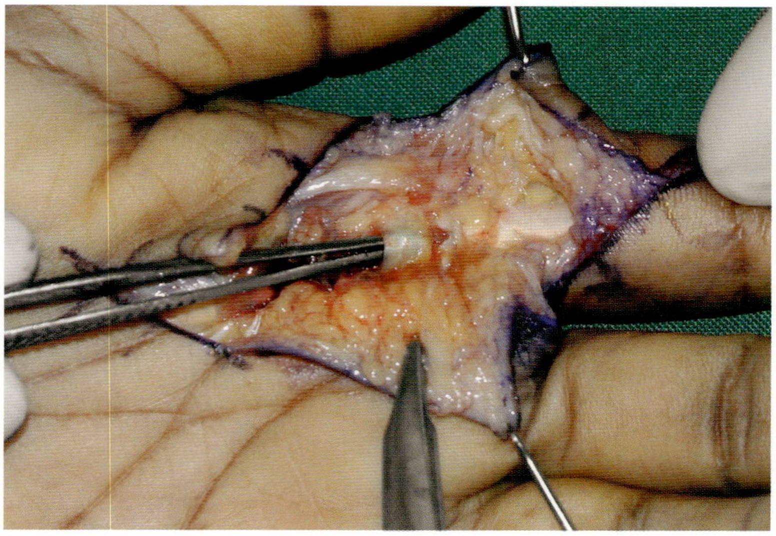

Fig. 11: Tendon sheath and pulleys are identified, empty sheath and pulleys are seen.

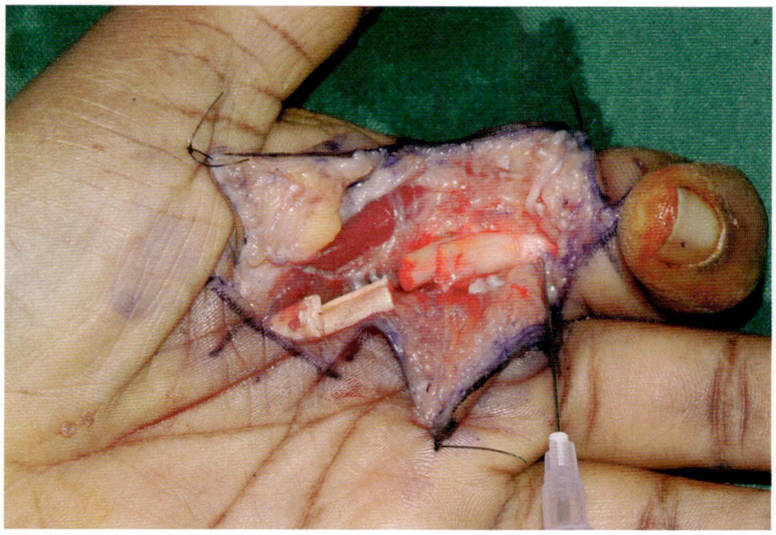

Fig. 12: Identification of proximal and distal ends of tendon by milking and hold in place by 25 No. needle.

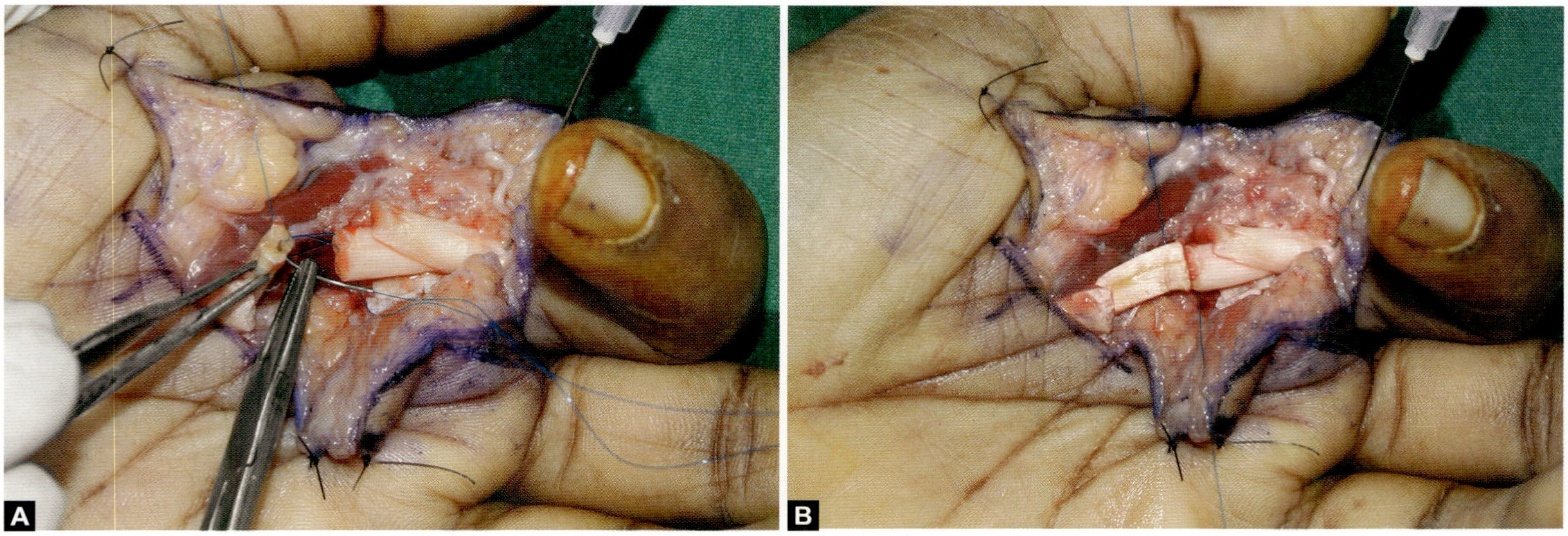

Figs. 13A and B: Simple running epitendinous technique using prolene 5-0; take dorsal aspect/wall suture first to facilitate easy core suture.

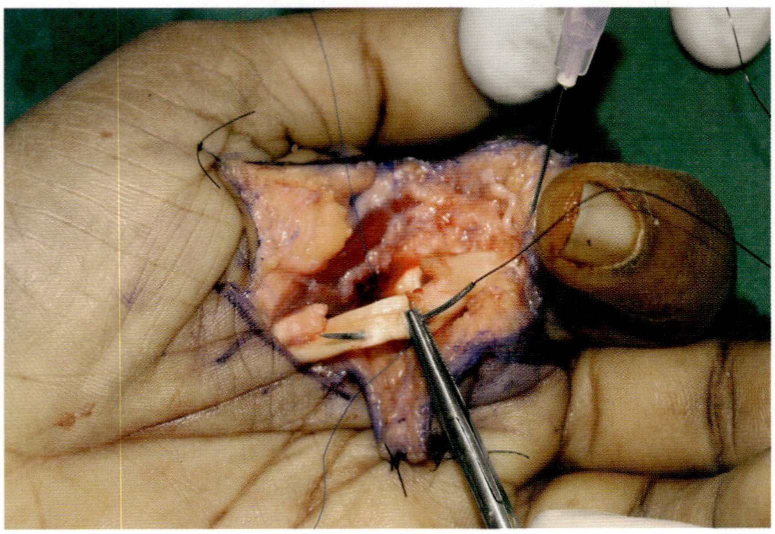

Fig. 14: First suture passing through cut end of tendon.

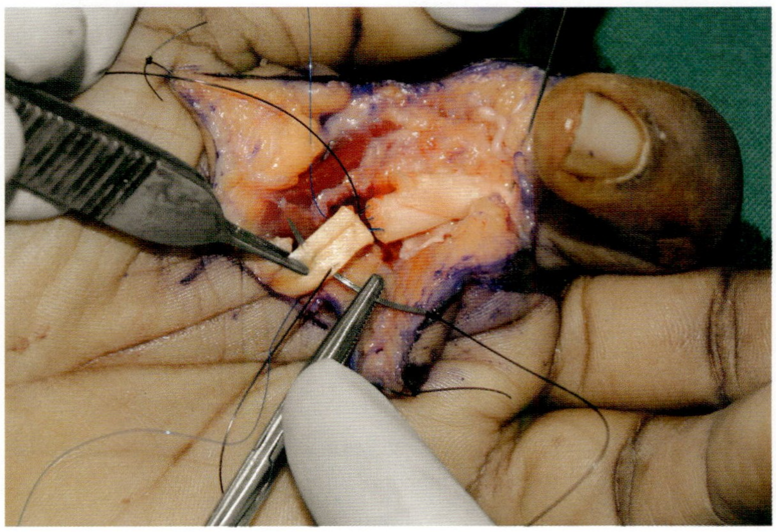

Fig. 15: Transverse suture.

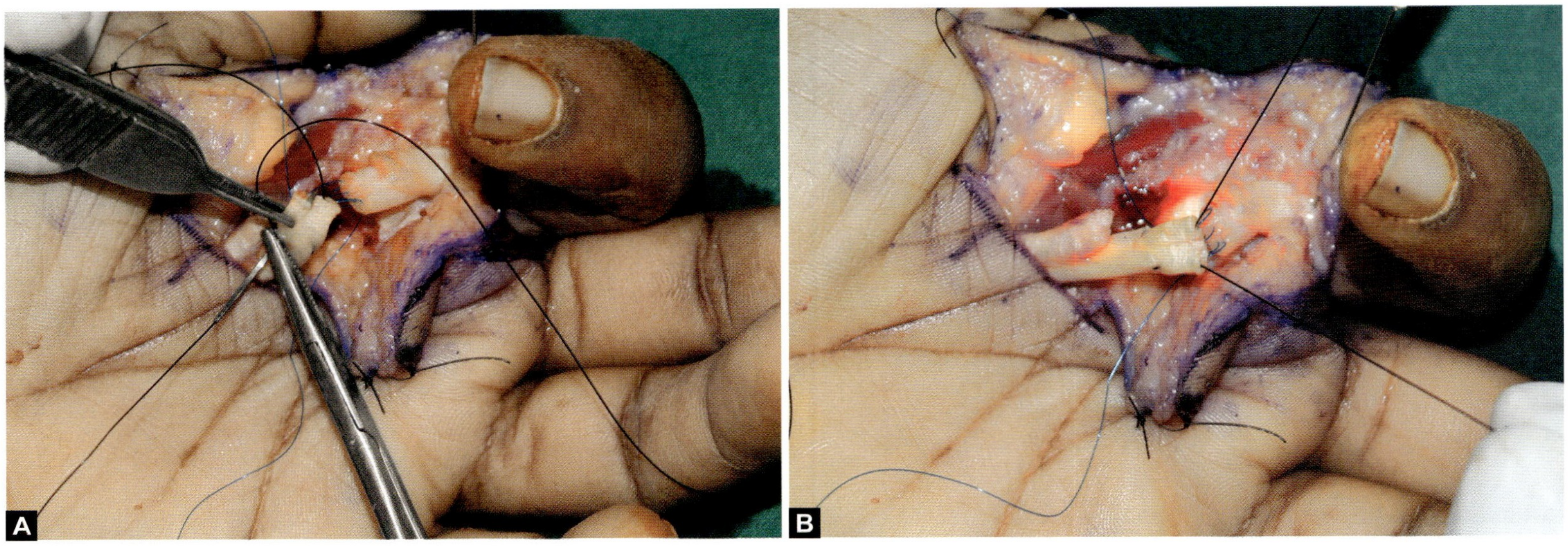

Figs. 16A and B: Longitudinal suture.

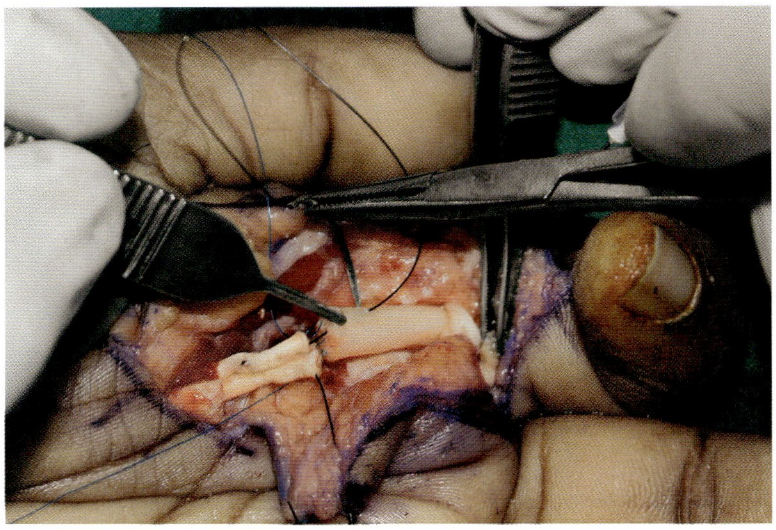

Fig. 17: Longitudinal suture through other end of tendon.

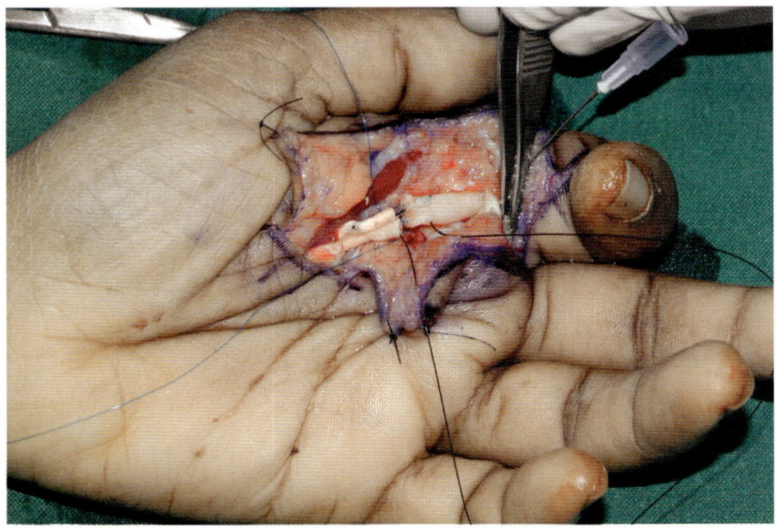

Fig. 18: Transverse suture.

Step 12: Two ends of suture tied to each other so that knot lies within substance of tendon at repair site (Fig. 20). It is important to note that contact between tendon cut surfaces is already achieved before even passing the core sutures with transfixing needles, positioning finger and wrist in flexion and epitendinous sutures. Trying to approximate tendon ends by tightening core sutures should be avoided and the core sutures should merely hold already opposed tendon ends together.

Step 13: Remaining epitendinous suture complete in front surface of tendon using prolene (Fig. 21).

Step 14: Final repair of tendon using modified Kessler two strand core suture and continuous running circumferential suture techniques (Fig. 22).

Step 15: In this case, venting of A2 pulley was done to facilitate easy passage/glide of tendon at repair site (Fig. 23). After repair finger should be passively mobilized through its complete range and gliding of repair confirmed through flexor sheath. If repair site is passing tight through sheath, sheath can be judicially opened. Every attempt should be made to keep A2 and A4 pulleys intact as much as possible.

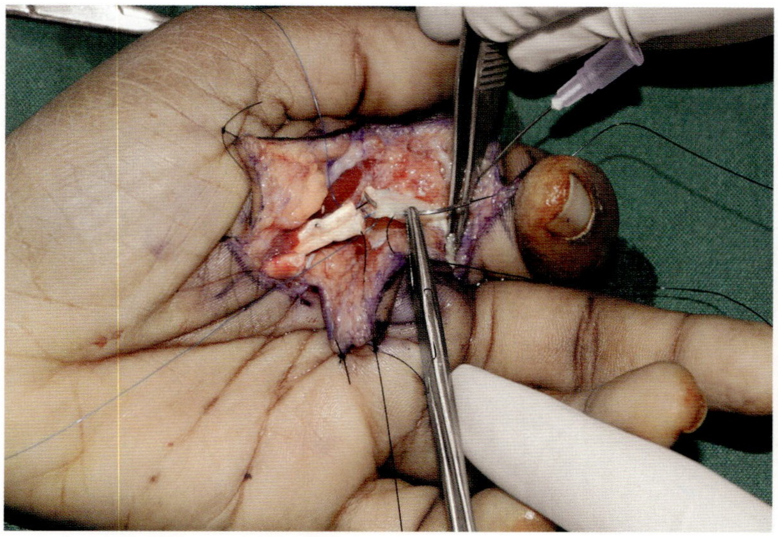

Fig. 19: Longitudinal suture coming out through cut end of tendon.

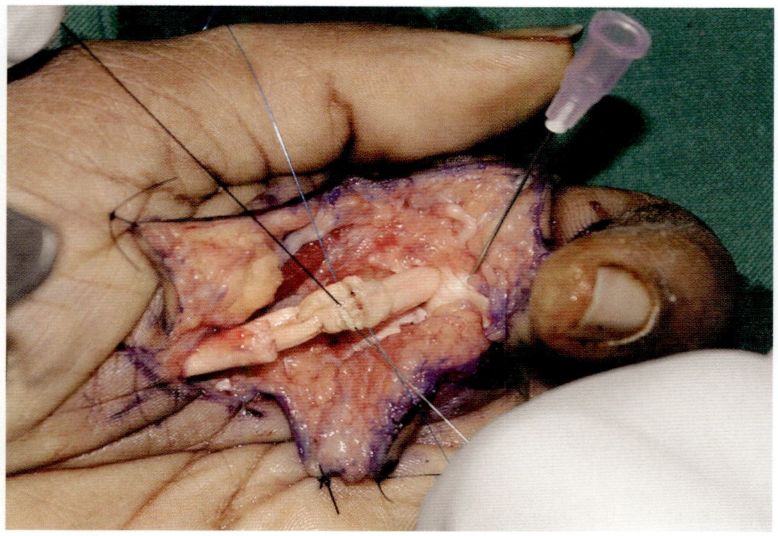

Fig. 20: Knot lies within tendon substance.

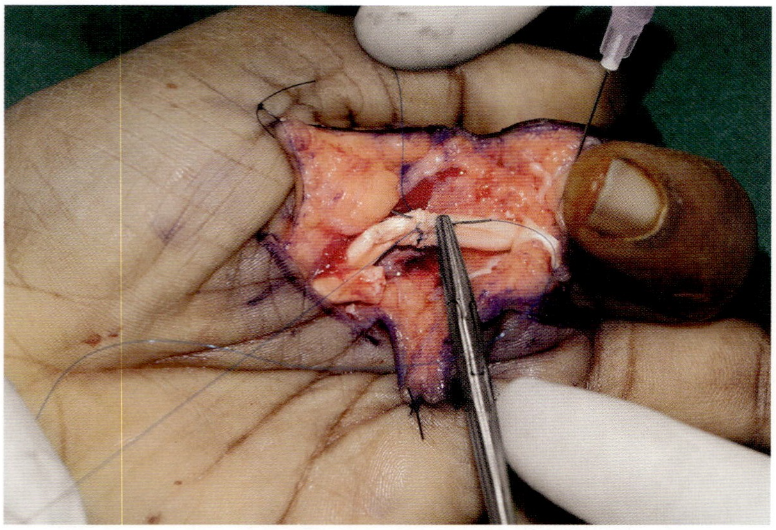

Fig. 21: Remaining epitendinous suturing.

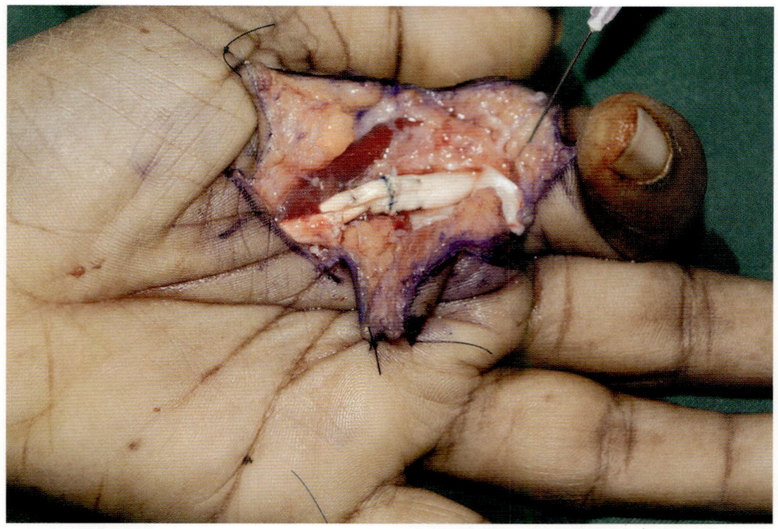

Fig. 22: Final repair.

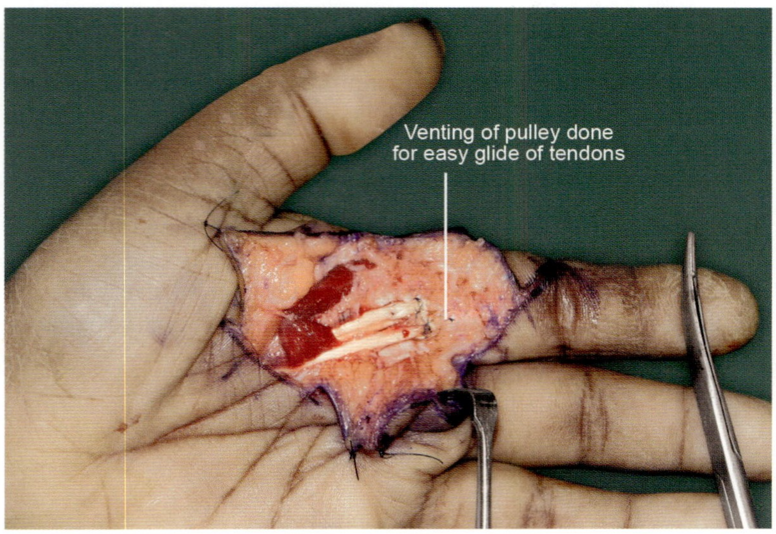

Fig. 23: Venting of A2 pulley.

POSTOPERATIVE REHABILITATION

Dorsal splint blocking extension is given to patient with wrist in neutral and metacarpophalangeal (MP) joint in 50–70° flexion.

Home-based exercise program should be taught to patient. Initially, passive flexion of fingers followed by active extension within the confines of splint.[10,11]

Splint removed after 4 weeks and isolated, active joint range of motion (ROM) started.

COMPLICATIONS

Following complications[12,13] can occur after tendon repair:

- Rupture or gaping of tendon repair
- Tendon adhesions
- Contractures of interphalangeal (IP) joints
- Skin flap necrosis
- Infection.

REFERENCES

1. Kleinert H, Kutz J, Ashbell T, et al. Primary repair of lacerated flexor tendons in "no man's land." J Bone Joint Surg Am. 1967;49:577.
2. Doyle JR. Anatomy of the finger flexor tendon sheath and pulley system. J Hand Surg Am. 1988;13:473-84.
3. McCallister WV, Ambrose HC, Katolik LI, Trumble TE. Comparison of pullout button versus suture anchor for zone I flexor tendon repair. J Hand Surg Am. 2006;31(2):246-51.
4. Brustein M, Pellegrini J, Choueka J, Heminger H, Mass D. Bone suture anchors versus the pullout button for repair of distal profundus tendon injuries: a comparison of strength in human cadaveric hands. J Hand Surg Am. 2001;26(3):489-96.
5. Kwai Ben I, Elliiot D. "Venting" or partial release of the A2 and A4 pulleys after repair of zone 2 flexor tendon injuries. J Hand Surg. 1998;23B: 649-54.
6. Kessler I. The "grasping" technique for tendon repair. Hand. 1973;5(3): 253-5.
7. Strickland JW. Flexor tendon injuries. I: Foundations of treatment. J Am Acad Orthop Surg. 1995;3:44-54.
8. Dona E, Turner AW, Gianoutsos MP, Walsh WR. Biomechanical properties of four circumferential flexor tendon suture techniques. J Hand Surg. 2003;28A:824-31.
9. Silfverskiöld KL, May EJ. Gap formation after flexor tendon repair in zone II: results with a new controlled motion programme. Scand J Plast Reconstr Surg Hand Surg. 1993;27:263-8.
10. Duran R, Houser R, Coleman C, et al. A preliminary report in the use of controlled passive motion following flexor tendon repair in zones II and III [abstract]. J Hand Surg [Am]. 1976;1:79.
11. Woo SL, Gelberman RH, Cobb NG, et al. The importance of controlled passive mobilization on flexor tendon healing: a biomechanical study. Acta Orthop Scand. 1981;52:615-22.
12. Mackin E. Flexor tenolysis. In: Hunter J, Schneider L, Mackin E (Eds): Tendon surgery in the hand, St. Louis, 1987, Mosby.
13. Winters SC, Seiler JG, 3rd, Woo SL, et al. Suture methods for flexor tendon repair: a biomechanical analysis during the first six weeks following repair. Ann Chir Main Memb Super. 1997;16:229-34.

CHAPTER 33

Scaphoid Fractures Screw Fixation for Delayed Union

Hitesh J Mangukiya, Shrinivas S Shintre

INTRODUCTION

The scaphoid is considered the worst bone to fracture in upper limb due to peculiar and poor blood supply. They occur most often due to fall on outstretched hand. These account for 10% of all hand fractures and 60–70% of all carpal fractures. 65% of scaphoid fracture involves waist, 25% involves proximal pole and 10% occurs in distal pole. Conservative treatment in the form of thumb spica splint is indicated in patient with acute stable fracture with minimal displacement for the period of 6–8 weeks. Internal fixation allows early joint motion and accelerates bone healing and leads to rapid functional recovery.

INDICATIONS FOR SURGERY

- Unstable scaphoid fracture with displacement more than 1 mm, scapholunate angle more than 60°, and radiolunate angle more than 15°.
- Indicated for patients with delayed unions or nonunions of scaphoid waist.

ANATOMY

Scaphoid is boat shaped. It is supplied with end arteries and flow is from distal to proximal hence fracture makes the bone avascular and prone to nonunion.

CLASSIFICATION

Herbert and Fischer described types of scaphoid fractures in his classification as follows:

Type A and B are acute fractures, type A is stable and type B is unstable. whereas Type C is delayed union and Type D established nonunion.

CLINICAL FEATURES

Patient usually presents with pain and swelling around anatomical snuff box following fall on outstretched hand. Tenderness is often present on scaphoid tubercle and anatomical snuffbox.

IMAGING

- Recommended radiographic views include anteroposterior (AP), lateral, scaphoid view (30° wrist extension and 20° ulnar deviation), and 45° pronation view.
- In presence of positive clinical findings; if radiograph is not showing fracture, then radiograph should be repeated in two to three weeks time.

Role of Magnetic Resonance Imaging

It is most sensitive for diagnosis of occult fractures of more than 24 hours duration.

Role of Computed Tomography Scan

It is useful for determining exact morphology of fractures, and post-operative situation to know about union of fractures.

MANAGEMENT OF SCAPHOID FRACTURE WITH OPEN REDUCTION AND INTERNAL FIXATION WITH HEADLESS CANNULATED CANCELLOUS SCREW: SURGICAL STEPS (FIGS. 1 TO 14)

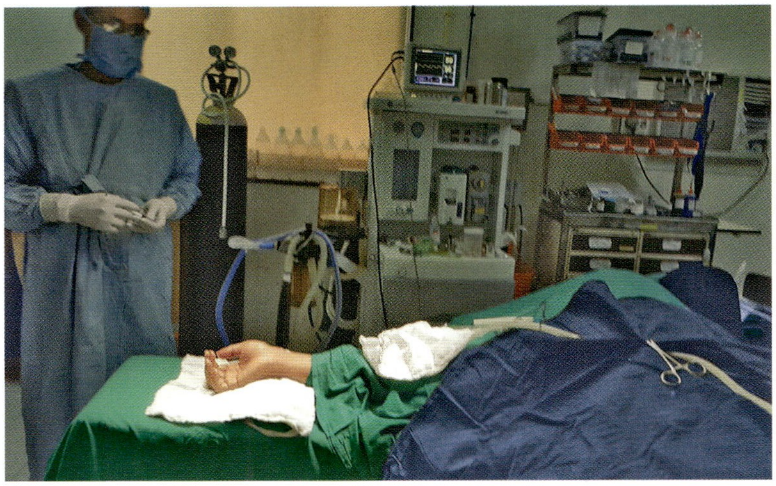

Fig. 1: Patient lies supine with affected extremity held in abduction, extension, and supination supported with hand rest.

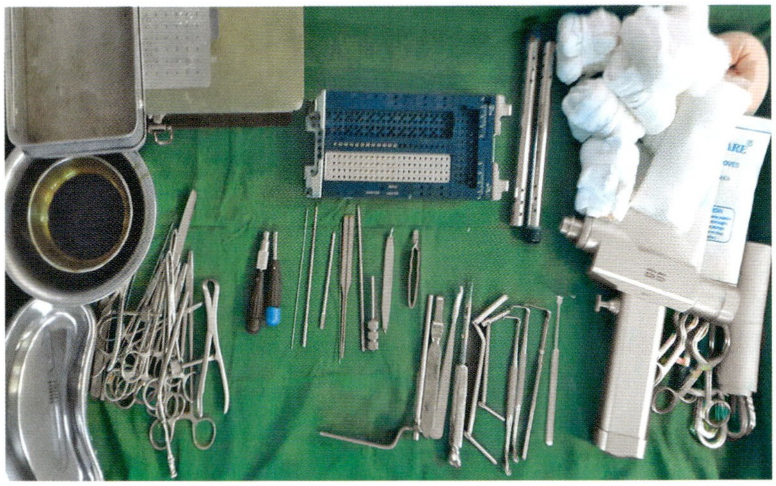

Fig. 2: Instrumentation and implants for the procedure.

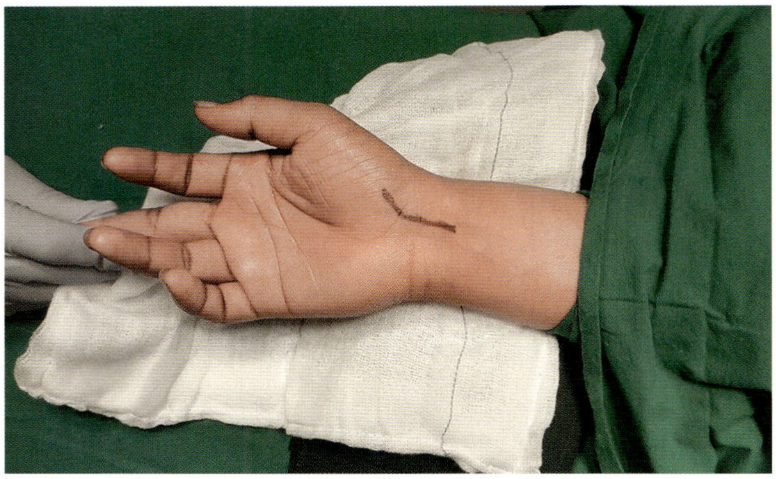

Fig. 3: Incision line mark running along flexor carpi radialis (FCR) tendon towards scaphoid tubercle and angled distally towards base of the thumb.

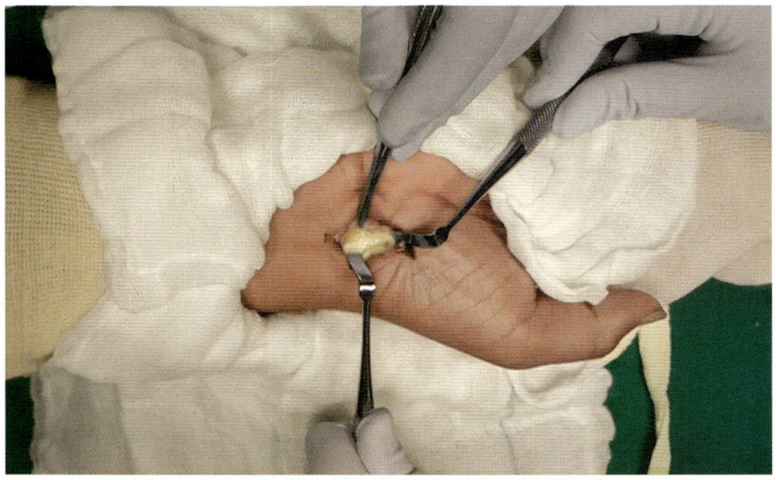

Fig. 4: Superficial dissection done along the incision line which shows superficial palmar branch of radial artery which runs close to scaphoid tubercle. This palmar branch can be ligated and divided if necessary.

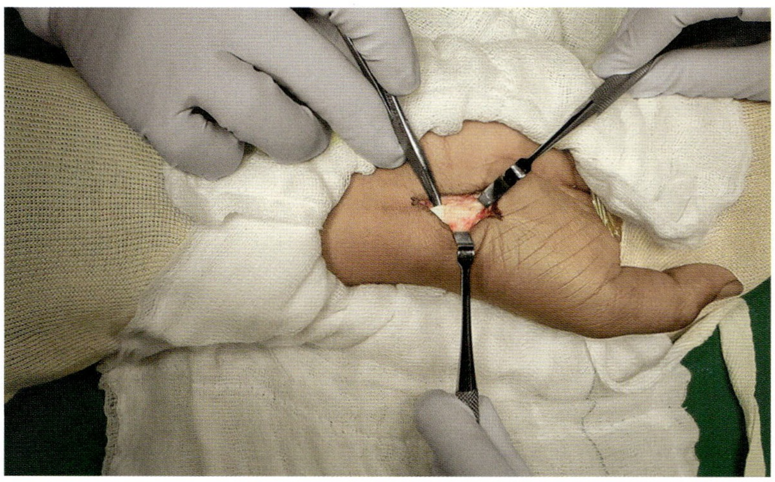

Fig. 5: Flexor carpi radialis (FCR) tendon sheath is opened and tendon is retracted towards the ulnar side.

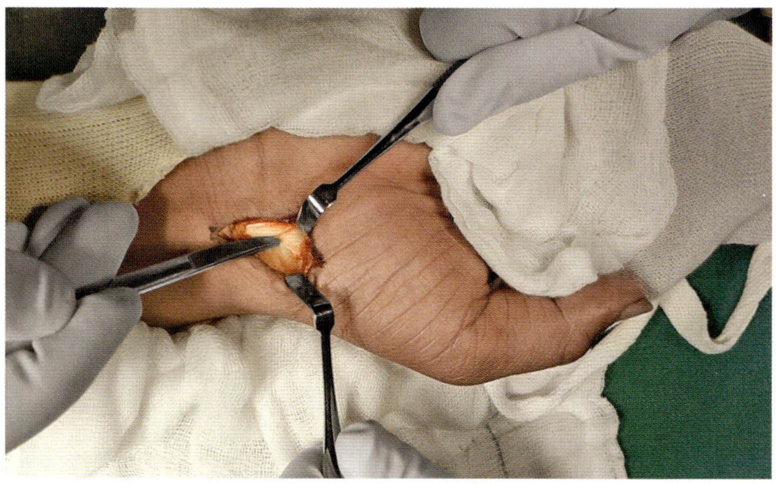

Fig. 6: Wrist capsule is exposed which is incised obliquely from tubercle towards volar rim of radius proximally.

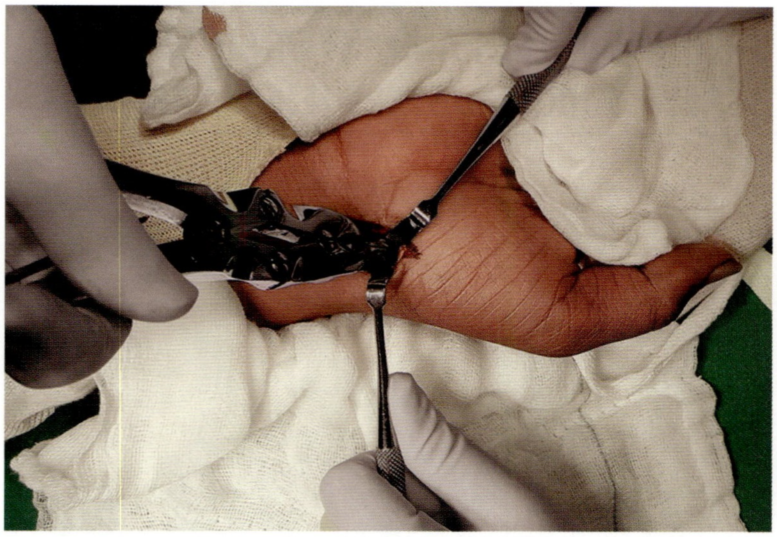

Fig. 7: Fracture site of scaphoid is exposed and intervening soft tissue is removed.

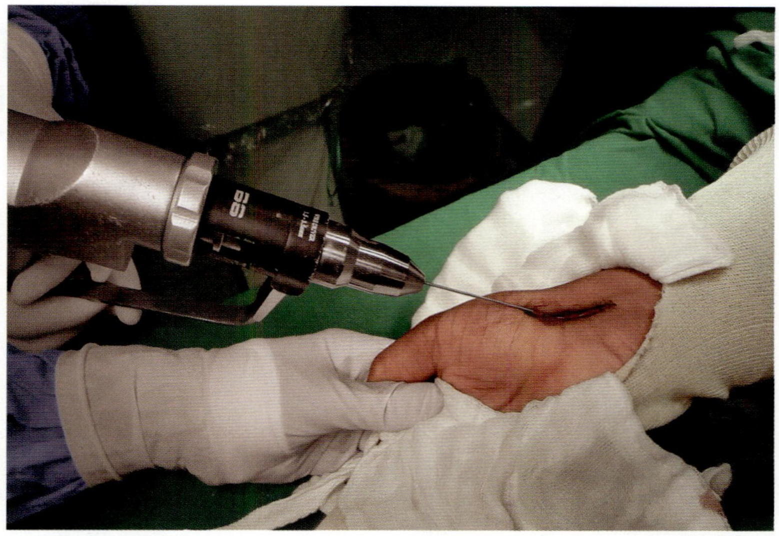

Fig. 8: Fracture is reduced using small reduction forceps and provisional K-wire fixation done to stabilize the fragments and to maintain rotational alignment during drilling and tapping.

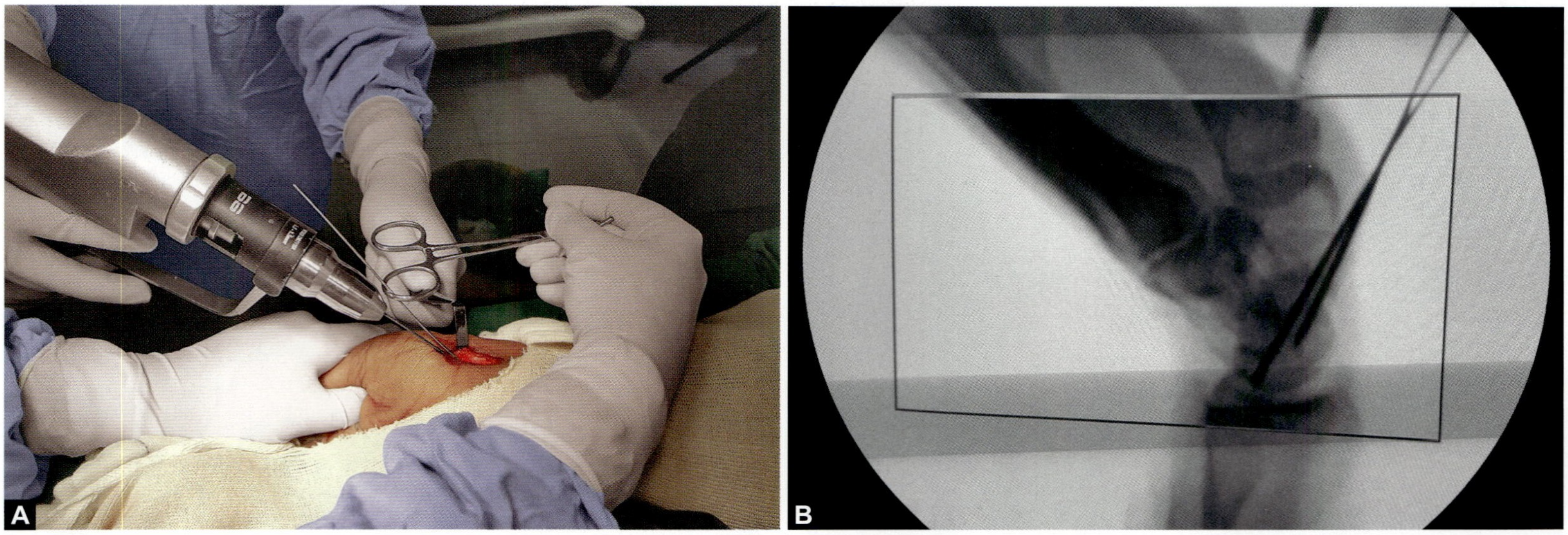

Figs. 9A and B: Guidewire is inserted perpendicular to fracture site and guidewire tract must be directed 45° medially and 45° dorsally along the mid-axis of the scaphoid.

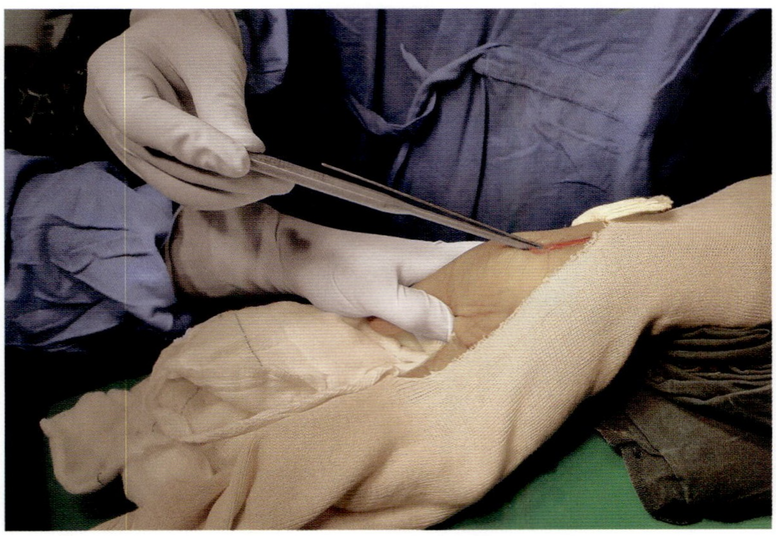

Fig. 10: Measuring the desired screw length.

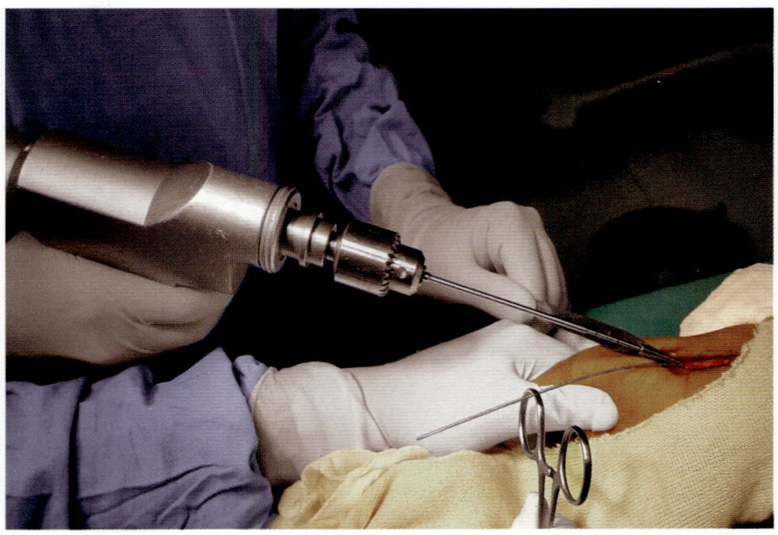

Fig. 11: Drilling over the guidewire in predetermined direction using a cannulated drill bit and power drill.

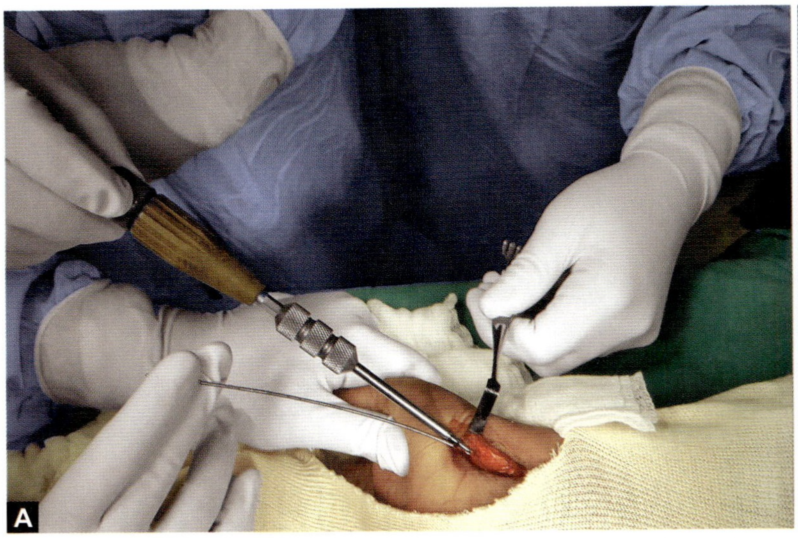

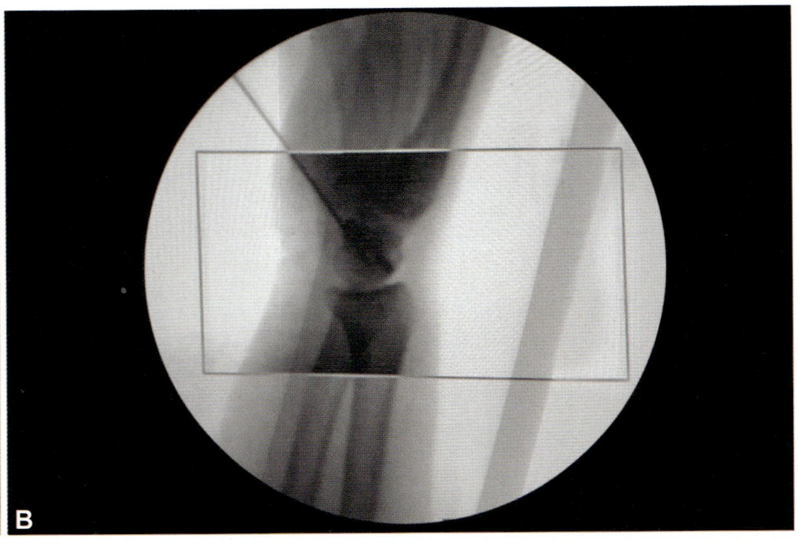

Figs. 12A and B: Appropriate length screw is tightened manually and near threaded portion is fully buried at insertion site.

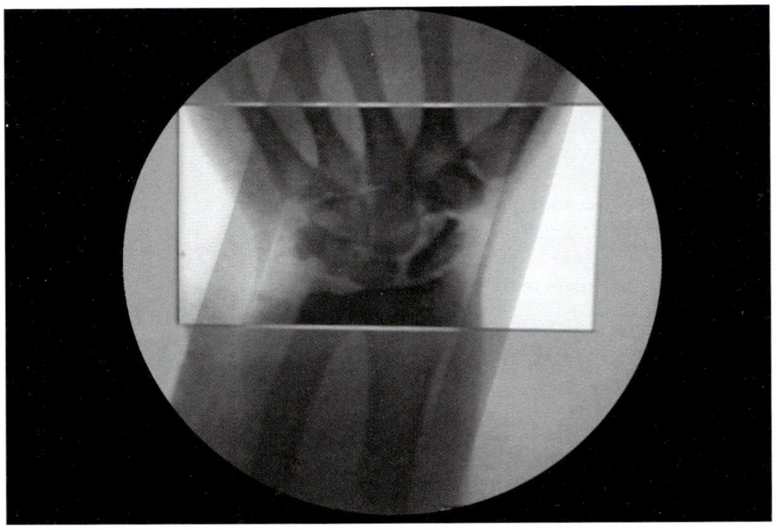

Fig. 13: Confirm screw position under C-arm guidance.

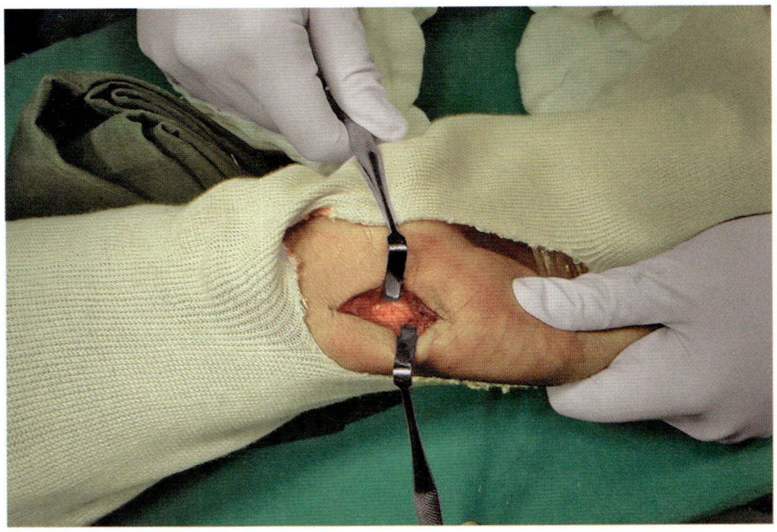

Fig. 14: Capsule is closed in continuous manner using absorbable suture.

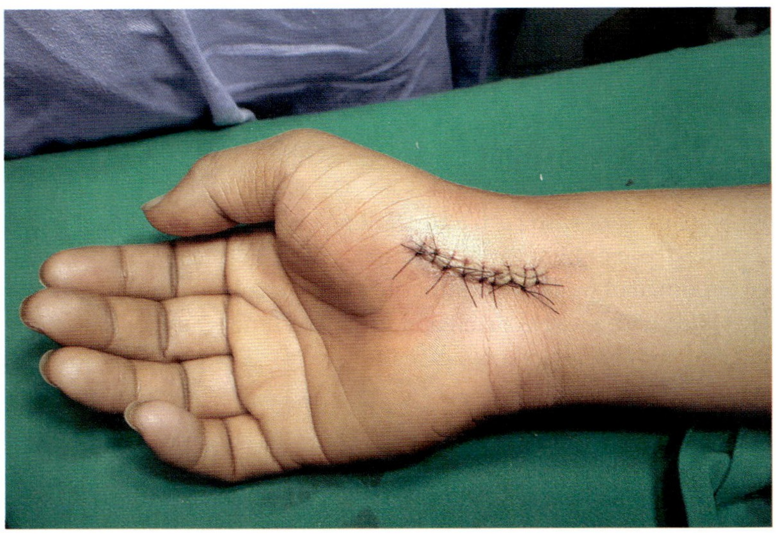

Fig. 15: Subcutaneous tissue and skin is closed with interrupted sutures.

POSTOPERATIVE MANAGEMENT

Elevate the operated extremity to reduce edema and encourage for active finger movements, but the wrist should be immobilized until wound healing. Once the wound is healed, begin with active wrist movements but patient should be warned against recurrent trauma and avoid contact sports for 3 months after surgery. Patient is followed up at regular interval to assess clinical and radiological union and identify any complication at earliest interval.

SUGGESTED READING

1. Davis EN, Chung KC, Kotsis SV, et al. A cost/utility analysis of open reduction and internal fixation versus cast immobilization for acute nondisplaced mid-waist scaphoid fracture. Plast Reconstr Surg. 2006;117(4):1223-35.
2. Geissler WB. Carpal fractures in athletes. Clin Sports Med. 2001;20(1): 167-88.
3. Grewal R, King GJ. An evidence-based approach to the management of acute scaphoid fractures. J Hand Surg Am. 2009;34(4):732-4.
4. Herbert TJ, Fisher WE. Management of the fractured scaphoid using a new bone screw. J Bone Joint Surg Br. 1984;66(1):114-23.

CHAPTER 34

Mallet Finger Repair

Abhijeet L Wahegaonkar, Satish A Mane, Anup S Bansode, Chaitanya Karande Patil

INTRODUCTION

Mallet finger is characterized by loss of extensor mechanism at distal interphalangeal (DIP) joint resulting in extensor lag, also known as drop finger or baseball finger.

Mallet finger injuries are described as "soft tissue mallet finger" or "bony mallet finger". Soft tissue mallet finger is result of discontinuity of terminal extensor tendon in zone I. Bony mallet finger injury results when terminal extensor tendon pulls away dorsal base of terminal phalanx resulting in fracture avulsion.

Closed injuries are most prevalent mainly resulting from sudden forceful passive flexion of an actively extended fingertip. Open injuries due to sharp injuries, crush or deep abrasions are relatively uncommon. Very rarely a forceful hyperextension at DIP may result in mallet injury.

It is commonly seen in athletes due to high velocity trauma and contact sports, but can be seen in minor injuries also.

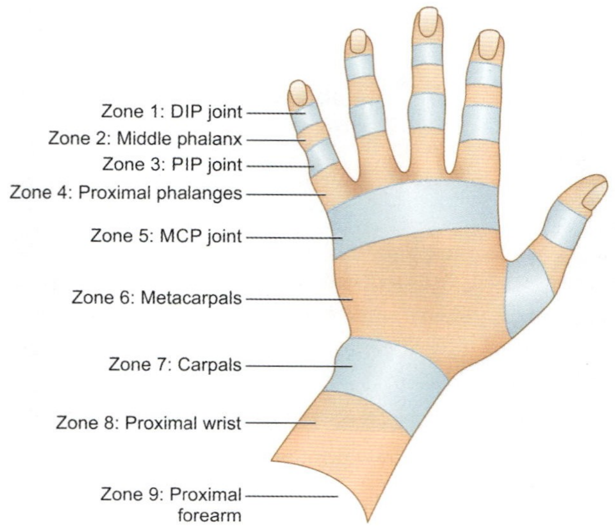

Fig. 1: Zones for extensor tendon injury. (DIP: distal interphalangeal; MCP: metacarpophalangeal; PIP: proximal interphalangeal)

ANATOMY AND CLASSIFICATION

Extensor tendon injuries are classified into nine zones (Fig. 1). Conjoined lateral bands on radial and ulnar side merge together over dorsum of middle phalanx to form terminal tendon which inserts over dorsal base of terminal phalanx. An area of avascularity in terminal tendon may predispose it to rupture.

Mallet fingers can be classified in various ways. The injuries less than 4 weeks are considered acute injuries while those presenting after 4 weeks are chronic injuries. Doyle proposed a classification of mallet fingers based on the mechanism of injury.

- *Type 1:* Closed injury, with or without small dorsal avulsion fracture
- *Type 2:* Open injury, laceration of tendon
- *Type 3:* Open injury with loss of skin, subcutaneous cover, and tendon substance
- *Type 4:* Mallet fracture
  - *A:* Transepiphyseal plate fracture in children
  - *B:* Hyperflexion injury with fracture of articular surface of 20–50%
  - *C:* Hyperextension injury with fracture of the articular surface more than 50% and with early or late volar subluxation of distal phalanx.

CLINICAL FEATURES

Patients present with pain and swelling over distal phalanx of finger with dropped or bent distal phalanx.

On range of motion examination, there is loss active extension at DIP joint with passive extension possible. Tenderness and swelling over DIP joint seen in acute cases.

INVESTIGATIONS

- Mallet finger is clinical diagnosis with thorough history taking and clinical examination.

- Radiographs posterioranterior (PA), oblique, and true lateral views are necessary to assess for bony avulsion injuries.
- Ultrasound examination may reveal closed mallet finger injuries.
- Magnetic resonance imaging (MRI) shows the rupture of terminal extensor tendon, but usually not required, as thorough clinical examination will give diagnosis.

TREATMENT

Type 1 Acute Mallet Injuries

These injuries can be treated with nonsurgical and surgical options.

Nonsurgical

DIP joint is immobilized in extension for nonoperative management. There are various commercially made splints available for DIP joint or one may cut and mould a simple aluminum splint and fix it with stickings. Splints can be applied dorsally or palmarly. It is recommended that splints should be used continuously for 6–8 weeks even during skin hygiene care followed by night splinting for another 4–6 weeks.

Surgical

- K-wire fixation across DIP joint with joint in extension without direct repair of ruptured tendon.
- Direct repair of ruptured extensor tendon with suture.

Type 2 and 3 Mallet Finger Injuries

Lacerations i.e. type 2 injury of extensor tendon are managed by debridement and tendon suture. Tendon may be repaired directly end-to-end or may be sutured incorporating the skin (tenodermodesis).

Type 3 injuries with skin loss and tendon substance may require skin coverage with or without tendon graft.

Type 4 Mallet Finger Injuries

These injuries with small bone fragment and without joint subluxation can be treated conservatively with splints as discussed earlier.

Operative: Fractures involving 30–50% of the joint surface are unstable and require surgery.

Several methods of closed reduction and K-wire fixation, extension block pinning are described for treating mallet fractures.

Open reduction and pull through suture, hook plate or anchor suture is an alternative method of treatment.

SURGICAL STEPS

Open surgical repair for rupture of terminal extensor tendon can be done under brachial plexus block or digital block.

We prefer transthecal digital block and digital tourniquet (Fig. 2).

Note: Open repair of a closed tendon rupture of mallet finger should be undertaken with extreme caution and when other options are not suitable. The skin over dorsum of DIP joint needs delicate handling and tendon tissue is very thin. For better handling magnifying loupes are highly recommended. Surgeon needs to be well versed in handling fine sutures and fine instruments are mandatory.

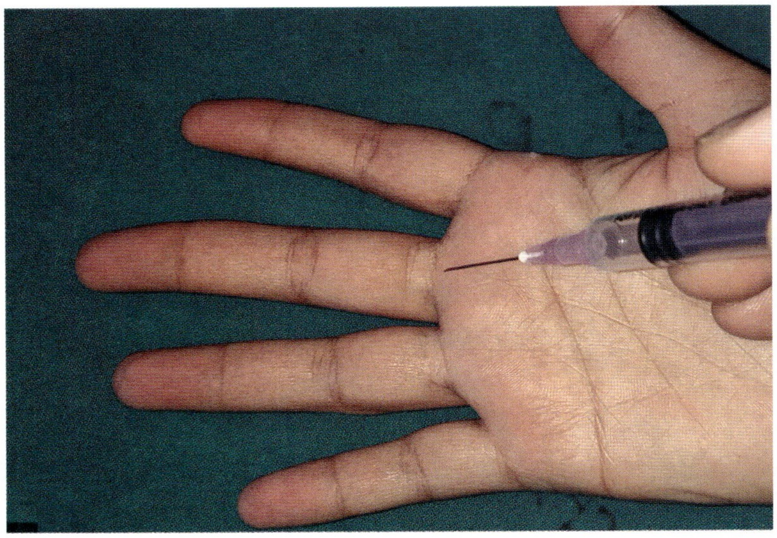

Fig. 2: Transthecal digital block.

Patient is in supine position on operating table with arm on side table. Underall aseptic precautions, cleaning, painting, and draping done.

STEPS

Step 1: Make L shaped or H shaped incision over dorsum of finger (Fig. 3).

Step 2: Raise the flaps proximally and distally to expose terminal extensor mechanism (Fig. 4).

Step 3: Any scar tissue if present, is excised with careful dissection to avoid tendon injury and to free tendon from scar tissue (Fig. 5).

Step 4: Periosteum over base of distal phalanx is peeled off and recipient area is prepared (Fig. 6).

Step 5: 1.2 or 1.5 mm K-wire is used across the distal interphalangeal (DIP) joint, which is held in 5–7° of hyperextension.

Step 6: Then hole is made over base of dorsum of distal phalanx for anchor with drill (Fig. 7).

Step 7: Anchor of 1.3 mm diameter along with its 4-0 suture is placed into base of distal phalanx (Fig. 8).

Step 8: Extensor tendon then repaired with 4-0 suture in horizontal mattress fashion tight enough so that tendon ends are in contact with bone surface.

Step 9: Skin closure is done using 5-0 nonabsorbable material.

Step 10: Sterile dressing applied.

Step 11: K-wire removal after 6 weeks and start gradual flexion-extension exercises. Continue night splinting for 4 more weeks.

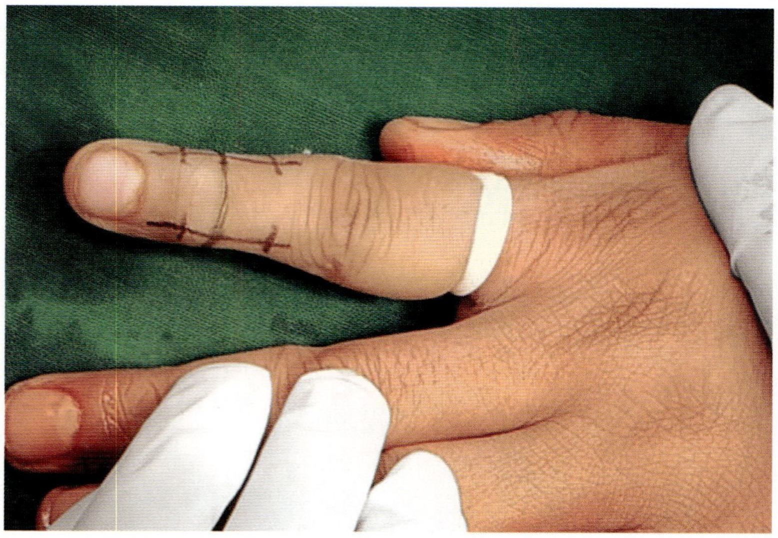

Fig. 3: H shaped incision over dorsum of finger.

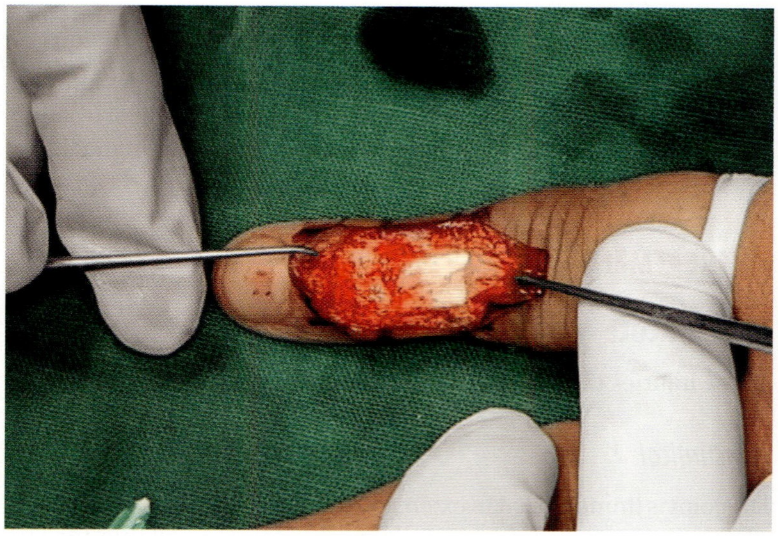

Fig. 4: Skin flaps are raised.

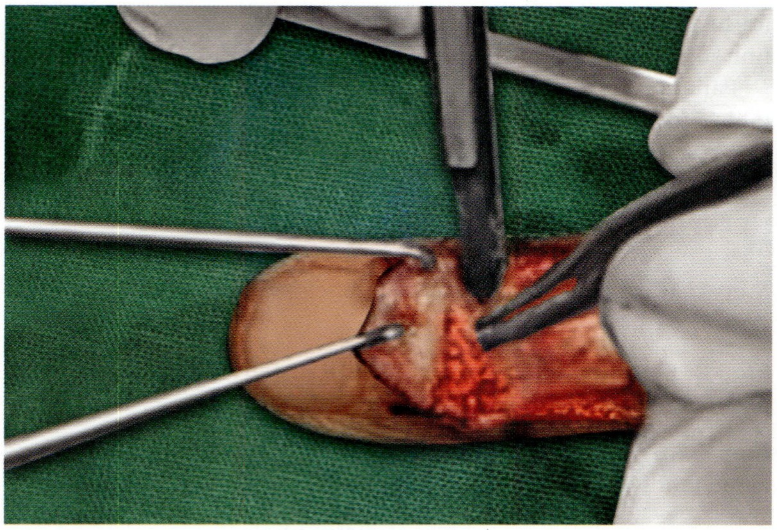

Fig. 5: Scar tissue excised and edges freshened.

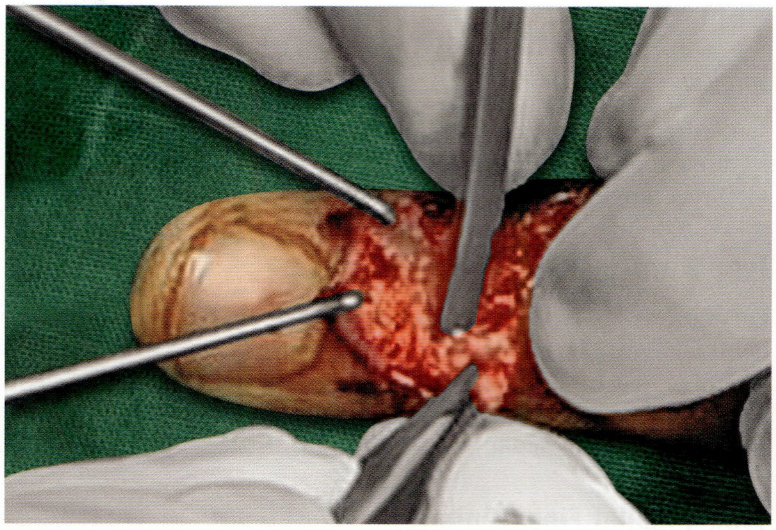

Fig. 6: Periosteum is removed and surface is prepared.

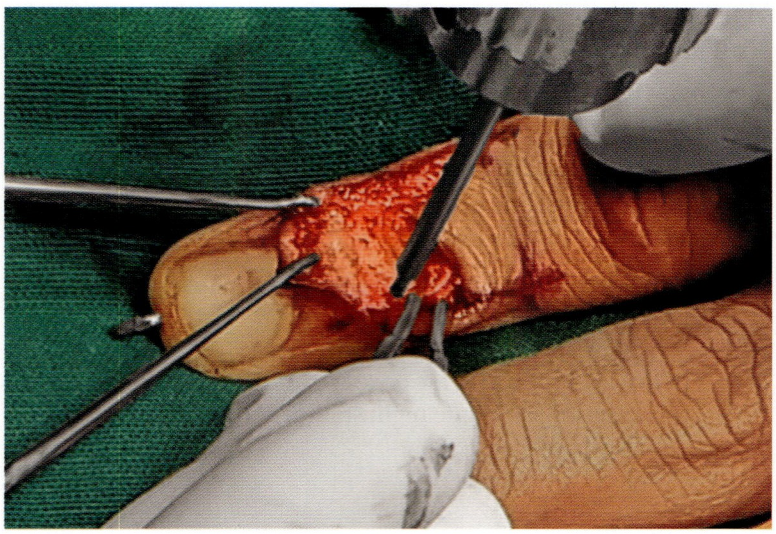

Fig. 7: Drill hole is made over base of dorsum of distal phalanx.

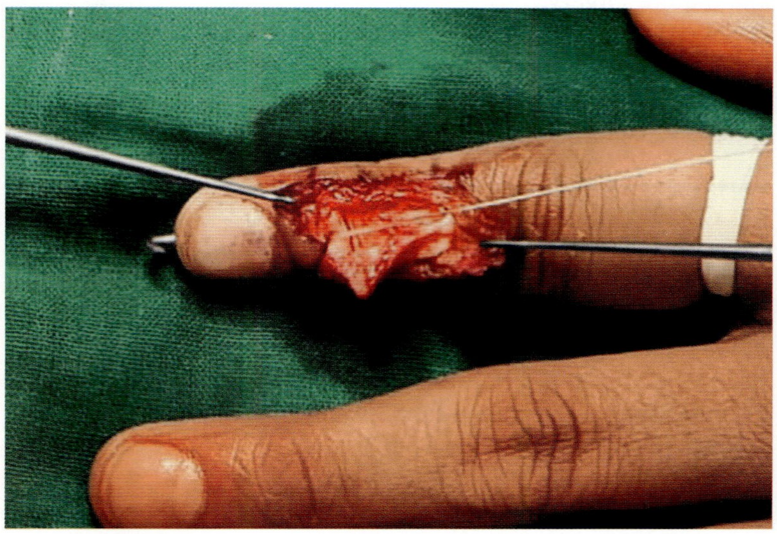

Fig. 8: Anchor is inserted into bone and tendon repair done.

POSTOPERATIVE PROTOCOL

Postoperatively K-wire removed after 6–8 weeks, and night splinting is recommended for 4 more weeks.

COMPLICATIONS

- Complications are seen with both methods of treatment i.e. conservative and surgical.
- Skin complications like dorsal skin ulceration and maceration.
- Other complications include nail deformity, infection, joint incongruity, implant failure, residual pain, and extensor lag.

SUGGESTED READING

1. Badia A, Riano F. A simple fixation method for unstable bony mallet finger. J Hand Surg Am. 2004;29(6):1051-5.
2. Bauze A, Bain GI. Internal suture for mallet finger fracture. J Hand Surg Br. 1999;24(6):688-92.
3. Doyle JR. Extensor tendons: acute injuries. In: Green DP, Hotchkiss RN, Pederson WC (Eds). Green's Operative Hand Surgery, 5th edition. New York: Churchill Livingstone; 1999.
4. Fritz D, Lutz M, Arora R, et al. Delayed single Kirschner wire compression technique for mallet fracture. J Hand Surg Br. 2005;30(2):180-4.
5. Garberman SF, Diao E, Peimer CA. Mallet finger: results of early versus delayed closed treatment. J Hand Surg Am. 1994;19(5):850-2.
6. Groth GN, Wilder DM, Young VL. The impact of compliance on the rehabilitation of patients with mallet finger injuries. J Hand Ther. 1994;7(1):21-4.
7. Hofmeister EP, Mazurek MT, Shin AY, et al. Extension block pinning for large mallet fractures. J Hand Surg Am. 2003;28(3):453-9.
8. Husain SN, Dietz JF, Kalainov DM, et al. A biomechanical study of distal interphalangeal joint subluxation after mallet fracture injury. J Hand Surg Am. 2008;33(1):26-30.
9. Kleinert HE, Verdan C. Report of the Committee on Tendon Injuries (International Federation of Societies for Surgery of the Hand). J Hand Surg Am. 1983;8:794-8.
10. Langer RH, Engber WD. Hyperextension mallet finger. Orthopedics. 1983;6:1426-31.
11. Nakamura K, Nanjyo B. Reassessment of surgery for mallet finger. Plast Reconstr Surg. 1994;93(1):141-9.
12. Okafor B, Mbubaegbu C, Munshi I, et al. Mallet deformity of the finger. Five-year follow-up of conservative treatment. J Bone Joint Surg Br. 1997;79(4):544-7.
13. Patel MR, Desai SS, Bassini-Lipson L. Conservative management of chronic mallet finger. J Hand Surg Am. 1986;11(4):570-3.
14. Pike J, Mulpuri K, Metzger M, et al. Blinded, prospective, randomized clinical trial comparing volar, dorsal, and custom thermoplastic splinting in treatment of acute mallet finger. J Hand Surg Am. 2010;35(4):580-8.
15. Stark HH, Boyes JH, Wilson JN. Mallet finger. J Bone Joint Surg Am. 1962;44:1061-8.
16. Stern PJ, Kastrup JJ. Complications and prognosis of treatment of mallet finger. J Hand Surg Am. 1988;13(3):329-34.
17. Theivendran K, Mahon A, Rajaratnam V. A novel hook plate fixation technique for the treatment of mallet fractures. Ann Plast Surg. 2007;58(1):112-5.
18. Ulker E, Cengiz A, Ozge E, et al. Repair of chronic mallet finger deformity using Miteck micro arc bone anchor. Ann Plast Surg. 2005;5:393-6.
19. Ulusoy MG, Karalezli N, Koçer U, et al. Pull-in suture technique for the treatment of mallet finger. Plast Reconstr Surg. 2006;118(3):696-702.
20. Warren RA, Norris SH, Ferguson DG. Mallet finger: a trial of two splints. J Hand Surg Br. 1988;13:151-3.
21. Wehbé MA, Schneider LH. Mallet fractures. J Bone Joint Surg Am. 1984;66(5):658-69.

CHAPTER 35

Ganglion Excision

Nilesh Dattatray Darawade

INTRODUCTION

Ganglions are the most common soft tissue tumors of hand. Their characteristic locations with relatively well-defined examination findings make the clinical diagnosis quite reliable. Treatment can be varied as per patient concerns from benign neglect to operative excision. Many times, simply alleviation of patient's anxiety by stating benign nature of the "tumor" is all patients want.

CLINICAL FEATURES

Patients usually present for the concern of new growth, pain or cosmetic issues. Incidence is more in women in 2nd to 4th decades. On palpation, a classical wrist ganglion is well-defined, firm to hard mass, usually nontender, and transilluminant. Overwhelming majority of ganglions are dorsal wrist ganglions. Next most common site is volar wrist. Ganglions have also been described originating from other joints of hand and from flexor sheath of finger. Uncommon variety of dorsal ganglion is so called "occult dorsal ganglion" which is difficult to diagnose clinically, may be evident only on wrist hyperflexion and commonly causes pain on forceful dorsiflexion of wrist.

PATHOANATOMY

Dorsal wrist ganglion is usually located distal to Lister's tubercle between tendons of second and third dorsal compartments. Its stalk usually originates from dorsal scapholunate ligament which needs to be exposed for a complete excision. A volar wrist ganglion may be at the level of scaphoid tubercle or proximal. In former location stalk usually can be traced to scaphotrapezial trapezoid joint, in latter situation to radiocarpal joint. On dissection there is well-defined single or multilobulated translucent sac filled with clear yellowish thick mucin.

ROLE OF IMAGING

For a typical case diagnosis can be reliably made clinically. In case of doubt or when any invasive modality of treatment is planned, radiograph and ultrasonogram are useful. Radiographs are usually normal barring rare intraosseous extension of ganglion in carpal bones. Ultrasonogram usually clinches the diagnosis. In difficult cases like occult dorsal ganglion magnetic resonance imaging (MRI) is helpful.

TREATMENT OPTIONS

Treatment may vary from benign neglect to surgical excision. When pain is the primary complaint then a trial of anti-inflammatory medications is warranted. Concerns of unsightly appearance need more invasive treatment. Aspiration with or without intralesional injections of steroid may be utilized while clearly stating possibility of recurrence. Surgical excision can be offered to chronically painful or unsightly ganglion. Arthroscopic excision of dorsal wrist ganglion is becoming increasingly popular, however at other locations open excision is the only surgical intervention available. It is important to trace and excise complete stalk of ganglion to minimize recurrence. Usually a cuff of capsule surrounding stalk from the joint ganglion needs to be excised and resultant gap is left open. Before attempting excision of a volar ganglion, it is important to evaluate palmar arch by performing Allen's test, as radial artery is at risk during dissection. Use of magnifying loupes is very helpful in volar ganglion excision.

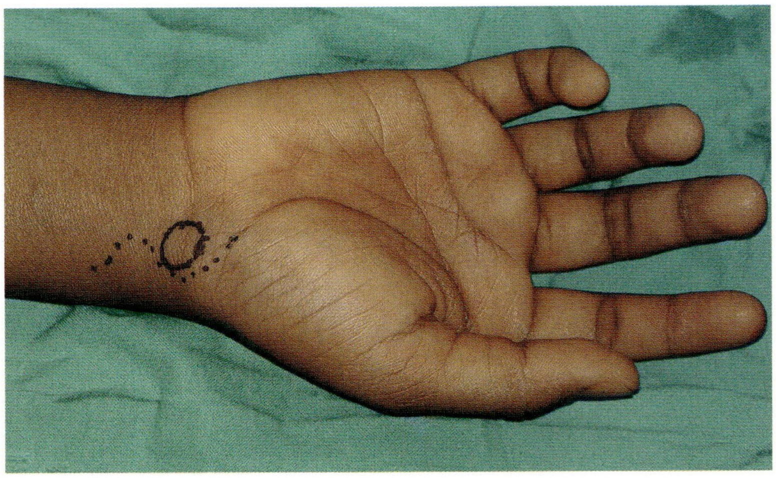

Fig. 1: Outline of ganglion marked with circle. Curvilinear dotted line represents surgical incision. Curvilinear incision minimizes chances of contracture across wrist joint. Incision should be planned for possible extension proximally, distally, towards carpal tunnel or even dorso-radially. Transverse incision is not amenable for such extensions.

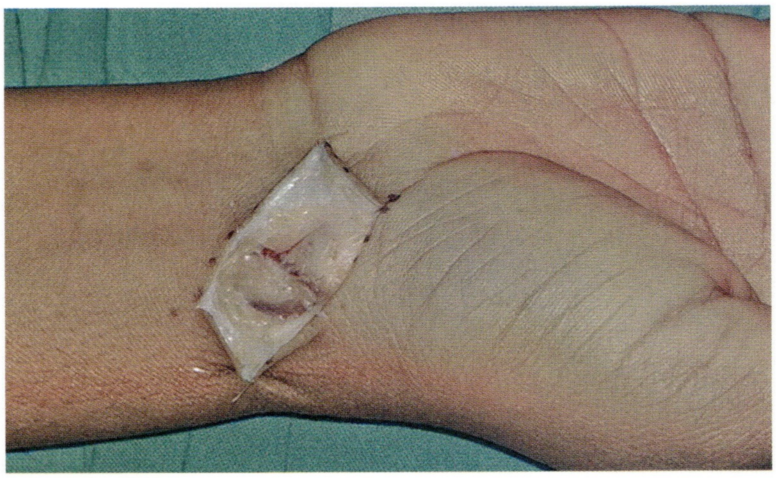

Fig. 2: Skin incision made and flaps retracted with stay sutures. Superficial veins are seen in subcutaneous tissue. Exsanguination only with moderate pressure allows veins to retain some blood, which makes way for easy identification and coagulation.

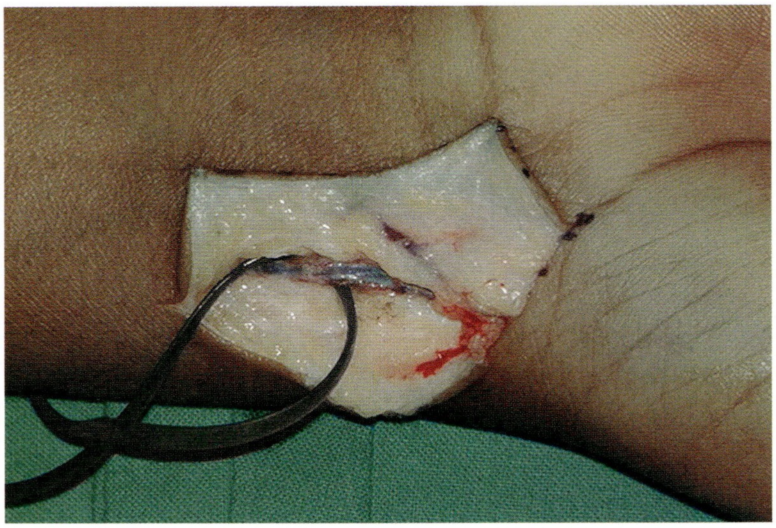

Fig. 3: It is prudent to isolate radial artery before dissection of ganglion begins. In proximal part of wound artery is identified and a vessel loop passed around it.

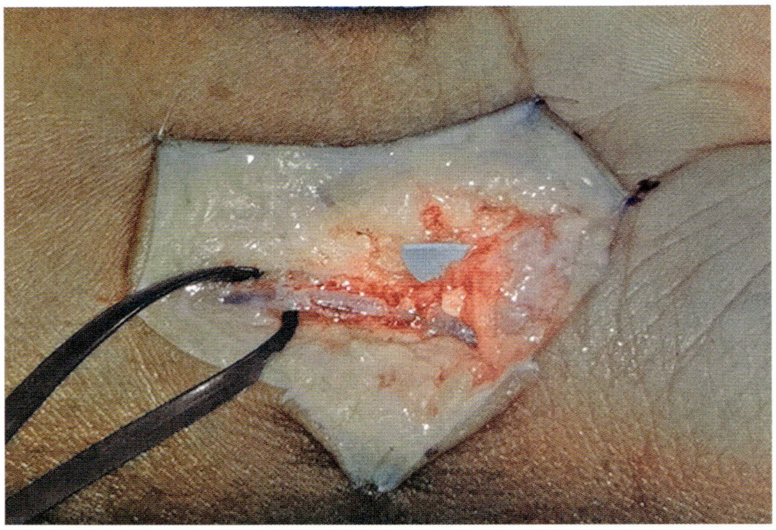

Fig. 4: After isolation of radial artery dissection around ganglion is begun. A branch of radial artery can be seen flush with ulnar aspect of ganglion. A blue background marker to highlight arterial branch.

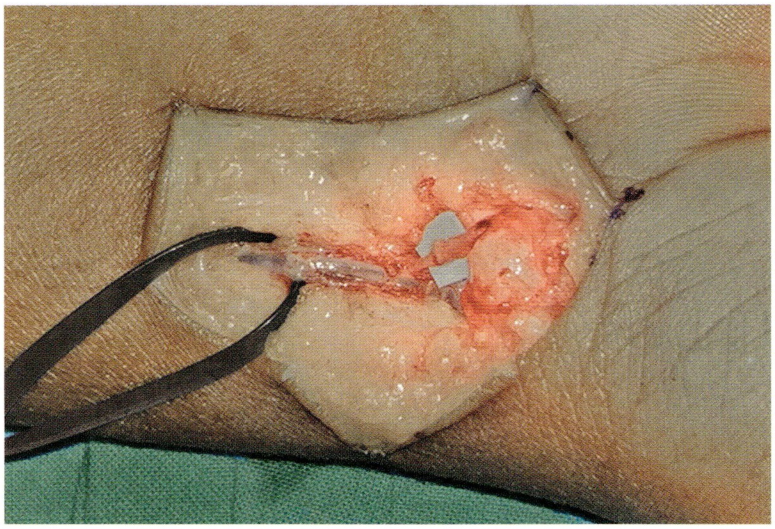

Fig. 5: Attempt should be made to dissect ganglion free from surrounding tissue while keeping arterial twig on ulnar aspect intact. If needed this branch may be sacrificed for excision of ganglion. A preoperative Allen test to confirm adequacy of palmar arch allays any fear while sacrificing any arterial branch.

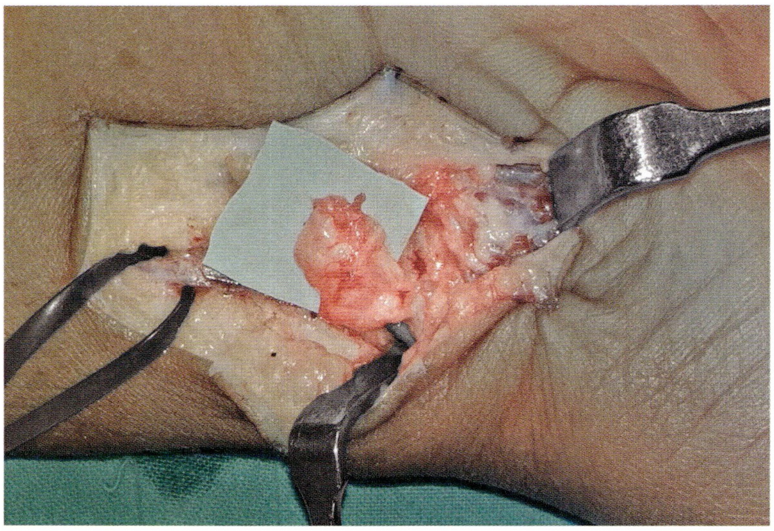

Fig. 6: Ganglion dissected towards its stalk distally. Upper right retractor exposes the thenar musculature. Lower right retractor demonstrates distal course of radial artery.

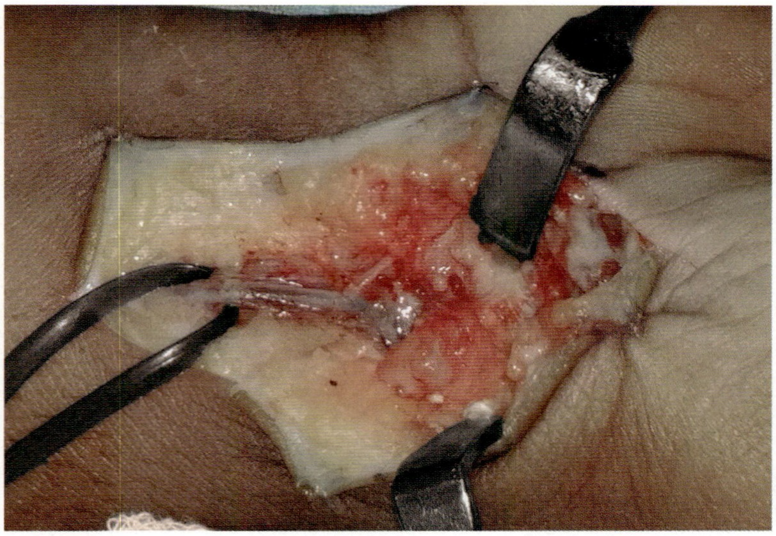

Fig. 7: Ganglion stalk traced to its origin, in this case scaphotrapezial trapezoid joint and excised with a cuff of capsule. Right lower retractor shows part of distal articular surface of scaphoid. Course of radial artery well seen after ganglion excision.

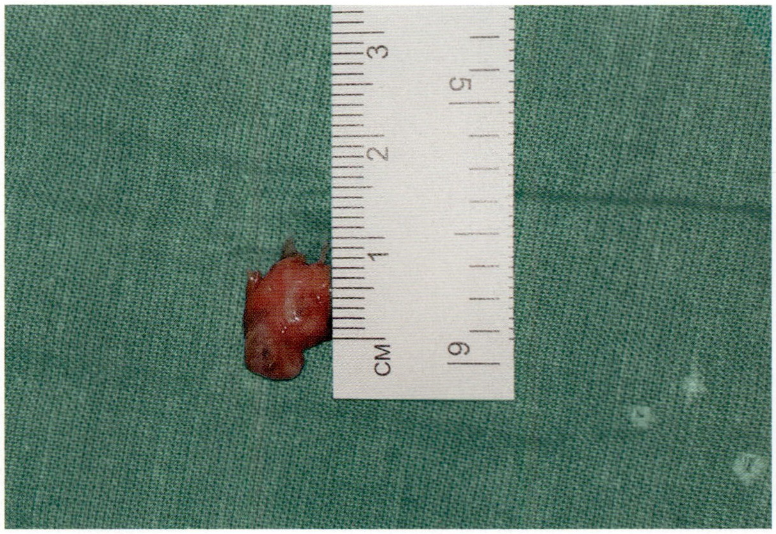

Fig. 8: Excised specimen sent for histopathological confirmation. It is common for ganglion to rupture during dissection, however dissection along its walls till base should give satisfactory result.

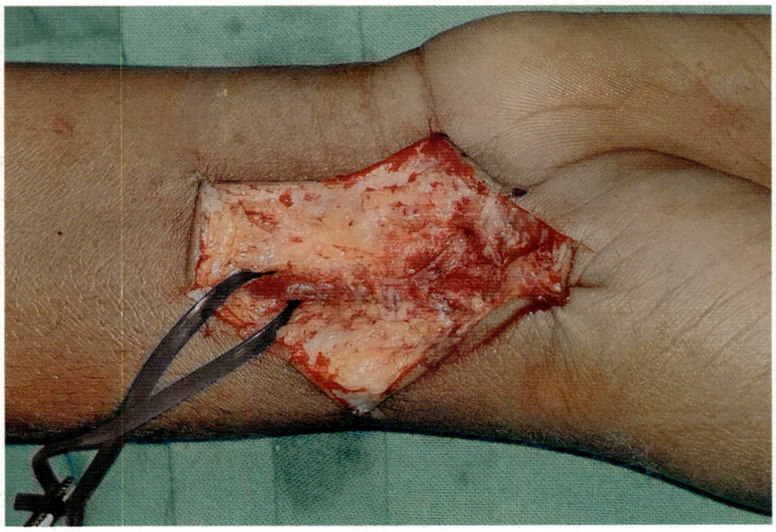

Fig. 9: Tourniquet deflated to confirm integrity of radial artery. Meticulous hemostasis is important for subcuticular sutures.

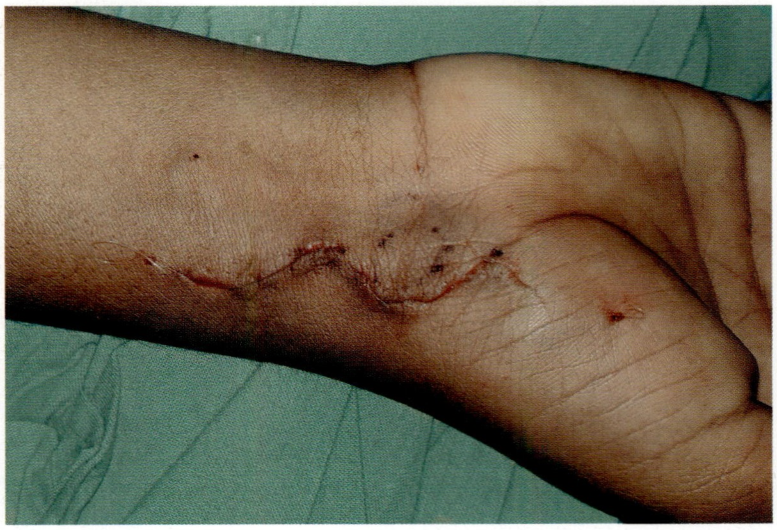

Fig. 10: Wound closed with 3-0 absorbable subcutaneous sutures and 4-0 monofilament synthetic subcuticular sutures. Sterile sticky strips applied to reinforce sutures.

SUGGESTED READING

1. Chang J, Neligan P. Plastic Surgery, 3rd edition. United States: Elsevier Saunders; 2012.
2. Wolfe S, Pederson W, Kozin SH. Green's Operative Hand Surgery, 6th edition. PA, USA: Elsevier Churchill Livingstone; 2010.

CHAPTER 36

De Quervains Disease Surgical Release

Onkar Lande, Mahaveer S Dugad, Nitish Agrawal, Sagar Gengaje

STENOSING TENOSYNOVITIS

Extensor pollicis brevis and the abductor pollicis longus tendons in the first dorsal compartment are affected, the condition is named after the Swiss physician Fritz de Quervain, who described this condition in 1895.

Adults of 30–50 years old especially women of childbearing age are affected. Radial sided wrist pain is commonly related in de Quervain tenosynovitis. Women are affected much more frequently than men. The cause is related to overuse, at home or at work, or maybe associated with rheumatoid arthritis. The presenting symptom is pain and tenderness at the radial styloid. Sometimes a thickening of the fibrous sheath is palpable. Finkelstein test usually is positive. Severe pain is elicited on grasping the patient's thumb and quickly abducting the hand ulnar ward. It is probably the most pathognomonic objective sign, though not confirmatory. The patient's history and occupation, the radiographs, and other physical findings also must be considered. Similar symptoms are present in arthritis in the scaphotrapeziotrapezoid, trapeziometacarpal and radiocarpal joints; superficial radial nerve entrapment or neuroma; and tenosynovitis at the crossing of the extensor pollicis brevis and abductor pollicis longus over the extensor carpi radialis longus and brevis (intersection syndrome).

Conservative management is initially offered and consists of splint wear and injection of a steroid preparation. Steroid injection may yield complete pain relief in majority of patients. When pain persists, surgery is the treatment of choice.

Anatomic variations in tendons are common in the first dorsal compartment and separate compartments have been noted in 21% of anatomic specimens. More than half of patients may have "aberrant" or duplicated tendons (usually the abductor pollicis longus), usually inserted more proximally and medially than usual, into the trapezium, the abductor pollicis brevis muscle, the opponens pollicis muscle, or the muscle fascia. Extensor pollicis brevis is absent in about 5% of wrists. Failure to identify and deal with these variations during surgery may account for any persistence of pain.

Failure to obtain complete relief after surgery may be due to following causes:

- Neuroma formation or neural adhesions
- Volar subluxation of tendon
- Failure to find and release of a separate aberrant tendon in a separate compartment
- Hypertrophy of scar
- Incorrect diagnosis such as a bone lesion in the distal radius, intersection syndrome, localized arthritic deformities, or more proximal nerve compression syndromes.

CLINICAL FEATURES

The patient presents with pain and restricted activity of wrist and difficulties in day-to-day household activities. Condition is common in women household worker and middle aged women.

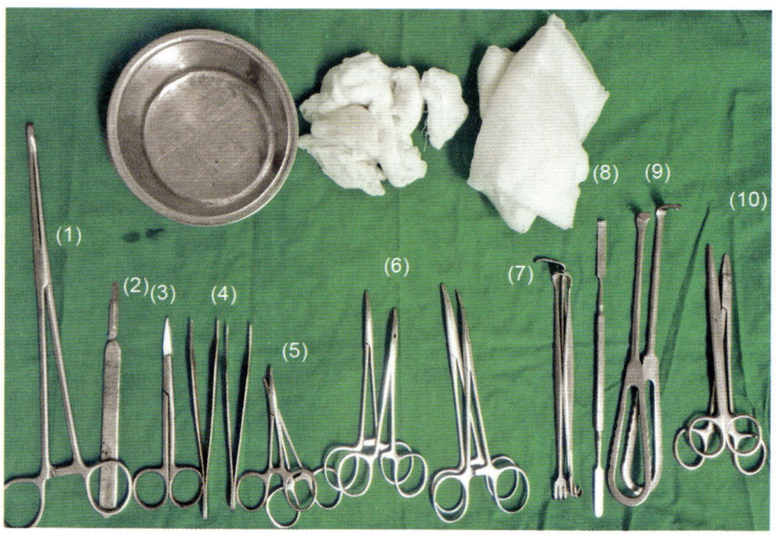

Fig. 1: (1) Sponge holding forceps, (2) Bard parker handle with blade 15, (3) Scissor, (4) Blunt forceps, (5) Mosquito forceps, (6) Artery forceps, (7) Catspaw retractor, (8) Dura protector, (9) Langenbeck retractor, (10) Needle holder with scissor.

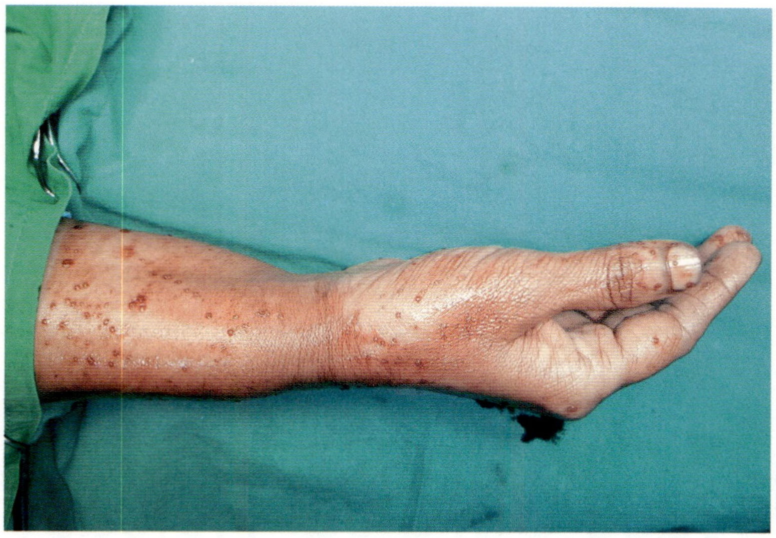

Fig. 2: Painting and draping done in standard manner. Forearm is kept in mid-prone position to assess dorsoradial aspect of wrist easily. Thumb is kept free to check movement of extensors tendons after release. Tourniquet inflated.

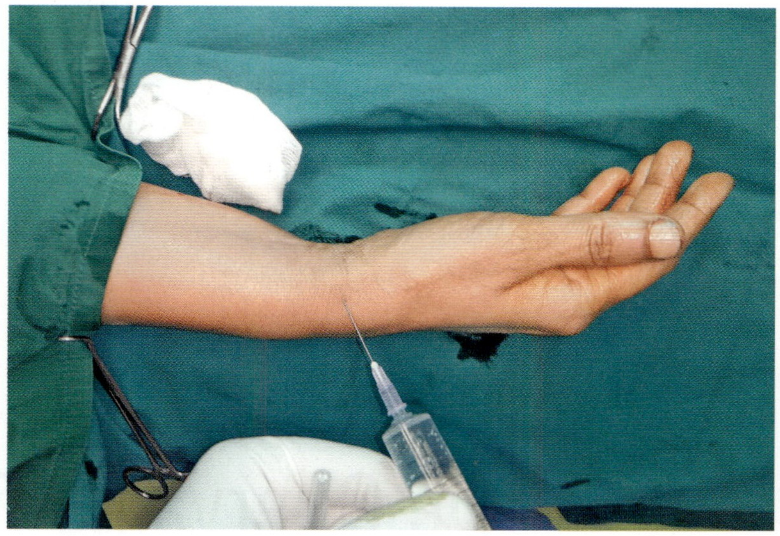

Fig. 3: Local anesthesia is infiltrated with aseptic precaution along proximal wrist crease centering over radial styloid.

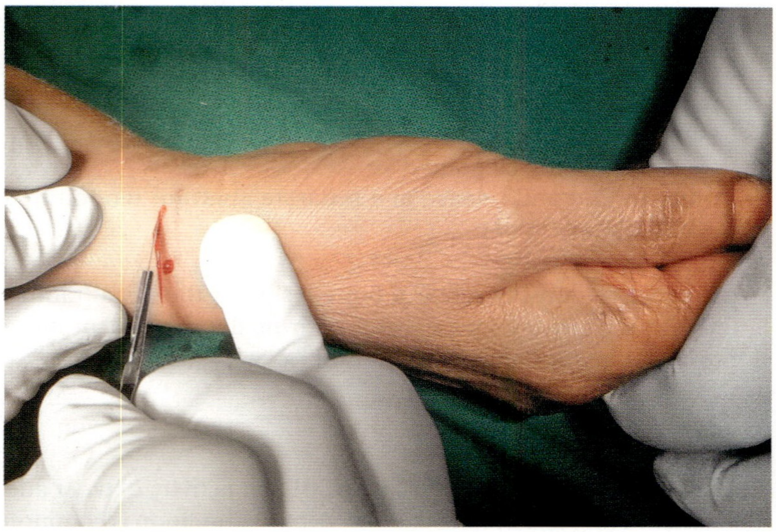

Fig. 4: Transverse incision centering over radial styloid is taken. Longitudinal and oblique incision is an option, the drawback being scar hypertrophy. In case of longitudinal incision one should take care that incision should not reach till anatomical snuff box to avoid injury to radial artery.

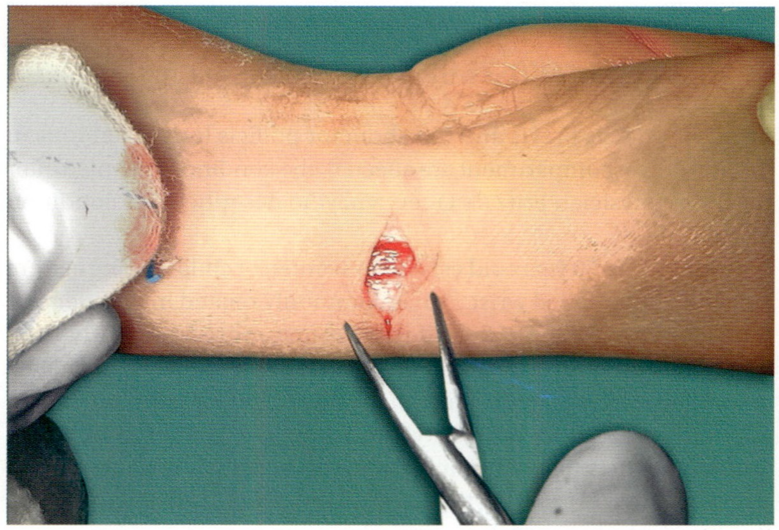

Fig. 5: Blunt dissection of subcutaneous tissue and fat pad done with artery forceps.

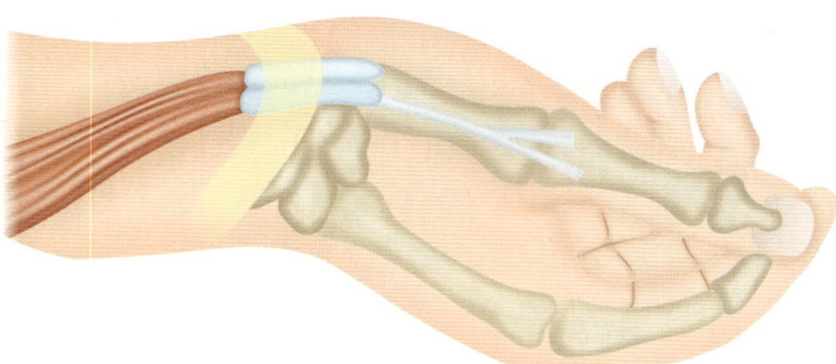

Fig. 6: Diagrammatic representation of tight tendon sheath of extensor pollicis brevis and the abductor pollicis longus causing De Quervain tenosynovitis.

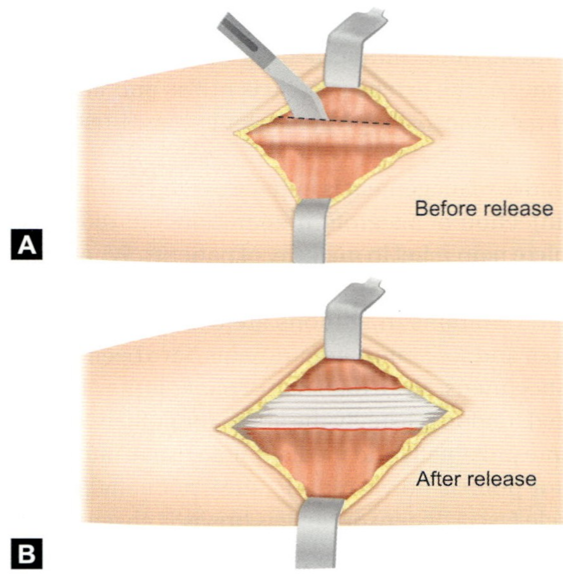

Figs. 7A and B: Diagrammatic representation of release of tight tendon sheath of extensor pollicis brevis and the abductor pollicis longus.

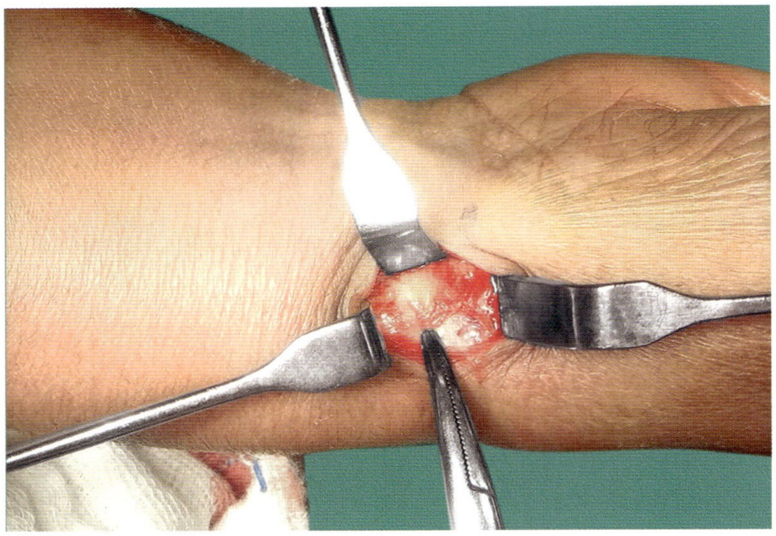

Fig. 8: Skin edges are retracted with right angle retractor to expose the sheath of first extensor compartment.

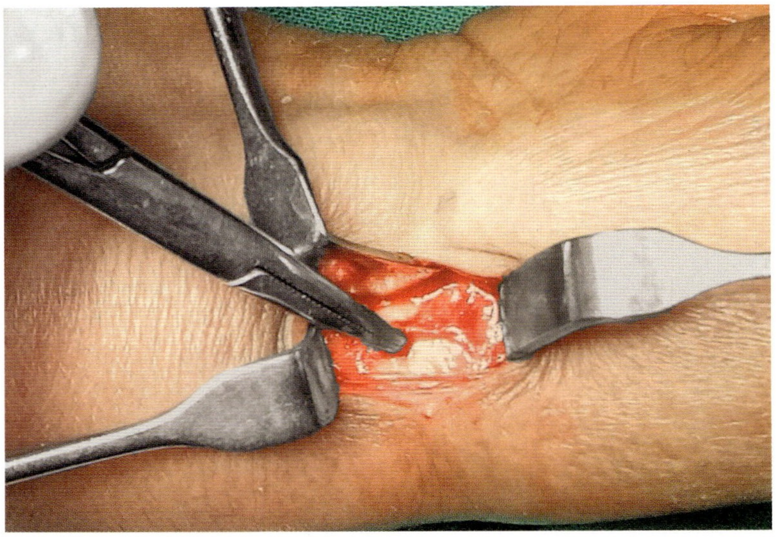

Fig. 9: Thickened retinaculum sheath felt around extensor pollicis brevis and abductor pollicis longus restricting their free movements.

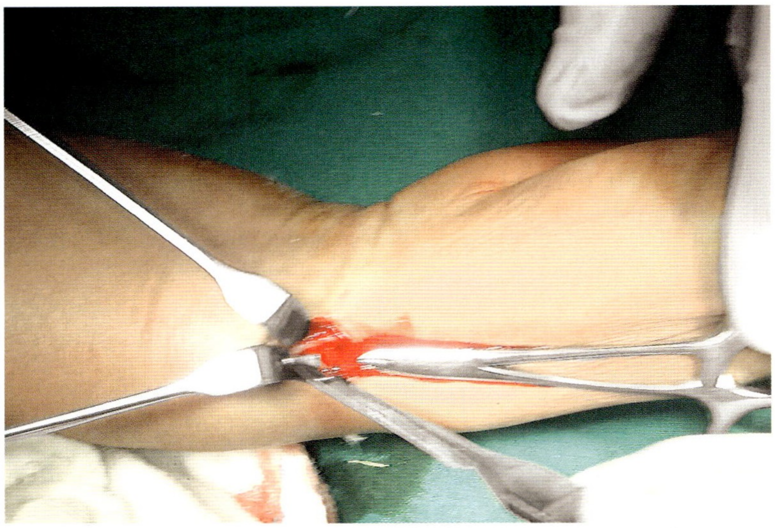

Fig. 10: Tight tendon sheath elevated with mosquito forceps to protect underlying tendons and sharply incised with knife on dorsoulnar aspect. Care should be taken not to incise volar side of sheath to avoid volar subluxation of tendons.

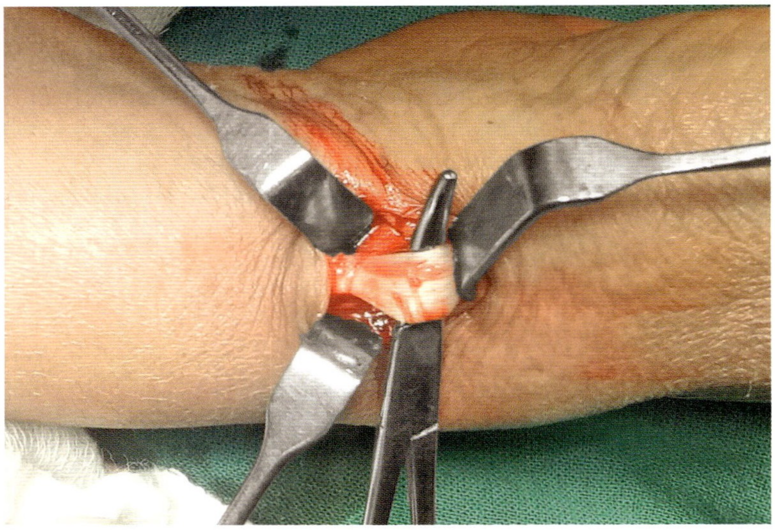

Fig. 11: Release of extensor pollicis brevis checked with mosquito forceps along with extension movement of thumb.

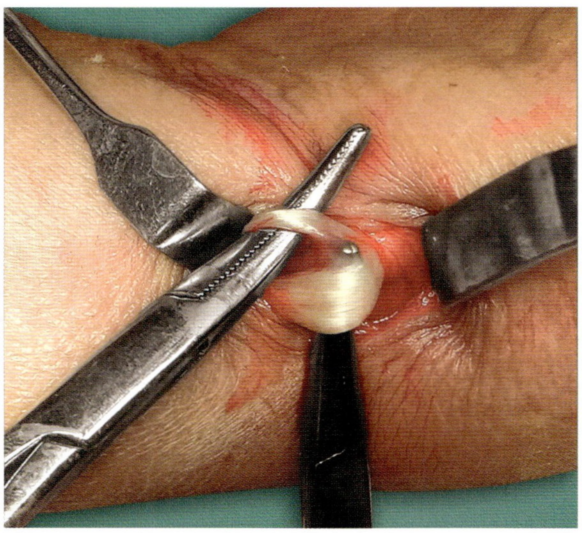

Fig. 12: Release of abductor pollicis longus checked with mosquito forceps along with abduction movement of thumb.

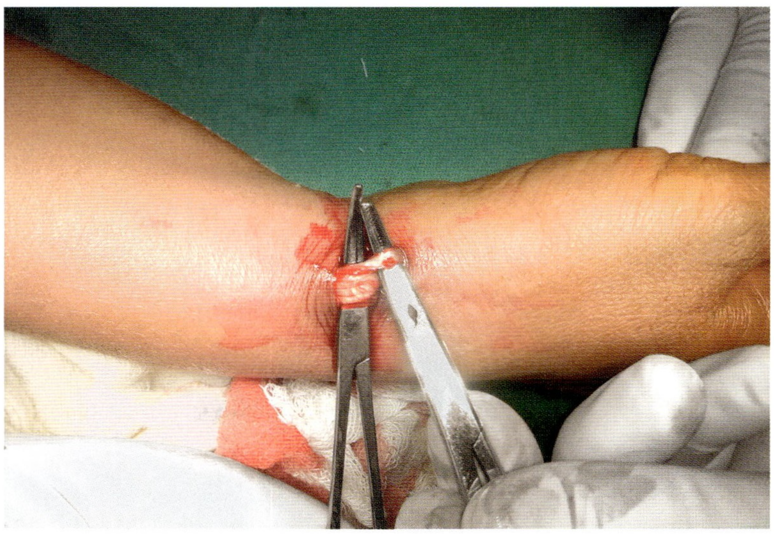

Fig. 13: De Quervain release completed.

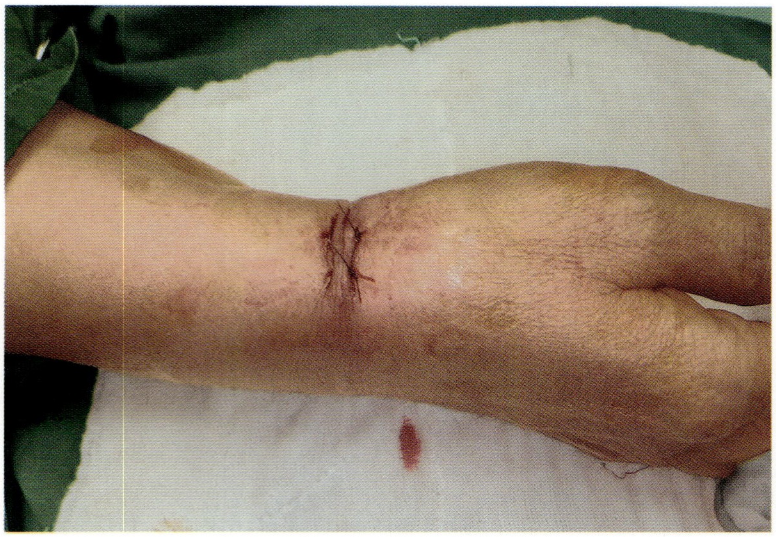

Fig. 14: Wash given with normal saline and direct skin suturing done.

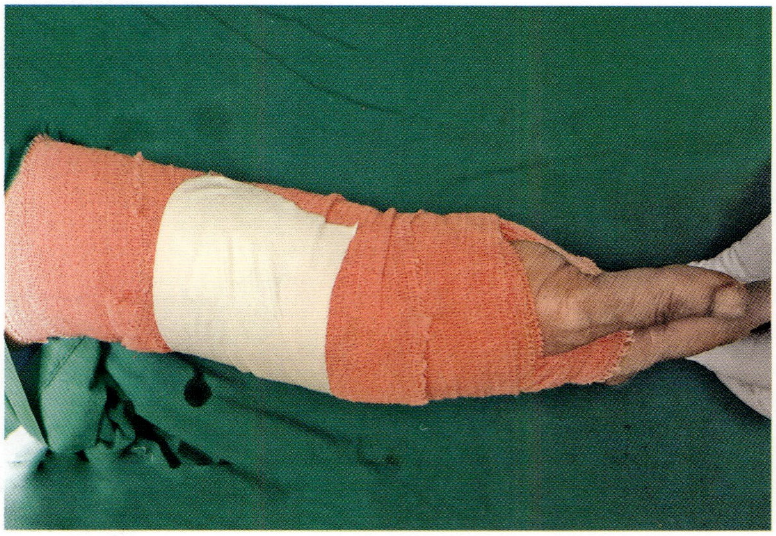

Fig. 15: Compression bandage given. Base of thumb left free to allow and encourage thumb movements. Tourniquet released.

POSTOPERATIVE MANAGEMENT

Abduction and extension movement started immediately and increased as tolerated:

- Hand elevation given for one day to avoid edema.
- Forceful wrist flexion is to be avoided to prevent volar subluxation of tendons.
- Suture removal done on day 14.

SUGGESTED READING

1. Ilyas AM. Nonsurgical treatment for de Quervain's tenosynovitis. J Hand Surg Am. 2009;34(5):928-9.
2. Ilyas AM, Ast M, Schaffer AA, et al. de Quervain tenosynovitis of the worst. J Am Acad Orthop Surg. 2007;15:757-64.
3. Mardani-kivi M, Karimi Mobarakeh M, Bahrami F, et al. Corticosteroids injection with or without thumb spica cast for de Quervain tenosynovitis. J Hand Surg Am. 2014;39:37-41.
4. Pensak MJ, Bayron J, Wolf JM. Current treatment of de Quervain tendinopathy. J Hand Surg Am. 2013;38(11):2247-9.
5. Scheller A, Schuh R, Honle W, et al. Long-term results of surgical release of de Quervain's stenosing tenosynovitis. Int Orthop. 2009;33(5): 1301-3.

CHAPTER 37

Trigger Finger Surgical Release

Trimbak Dapkekar, Onkar Lande, Devashish Raval, Nitish Agrawal

- Patients with more than 45 years age are more commonly affected. Collagen vascular disease is most common pathology.
- Stenosing tenosynovitis, leads to inability to extend and flex the flexed and extended digit respectively and and produces a palpable snap/triggering and most of the times it is painful.
- Nodule may be present in palm which may be the thickened area in the first annular pulley (A1) or a palpable or movable nodule or swelling of the flexor tendon just proximal to annulus at the metacarpophalangeal joint level may be present.
- A partially lacerated flexor tendon at this level may heal with a large nodule and causes triggering. Usually local tenderness can be elicited.
- Pressure increases the apparent snapping and triggering of the more distal joints. Triggering is seen in the proximal interphalangeal joint with trigger finger or in the interphalangeal joint with trigger thumb. Some other conditions, such as intra articular disorders (e.g. loose bodies, degenerative joint disease, and fractures) and common extensor tendon subluxation can also present as trigger finger.
- Nonoperative treatment includes stretching exercises, splinting of finger in extended position, dry needling and hot water fomentation. Single corticosteroid injection at local area is also effective.
- Persistence of triggering is more common than recurrence. Surgical management is done under local anesthesia to check release intraoperatively.
- Percutaneous trigger finger release is often associated with incomplete pulley release. There is substantial risk of damage to the flexor tendons and digital nerves.
- Trigger thumbs require release of the A1 pulley, whereas for trigger digits division of the A1 and A0, or proximal palmar pulley is necessary.

SURGICAL STEPS (FIGS. 1 TO 12)

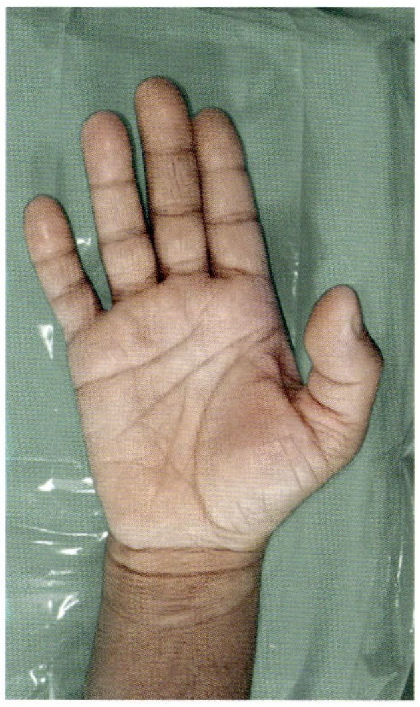

Fig. 1: Locking of thumb in flexed position.

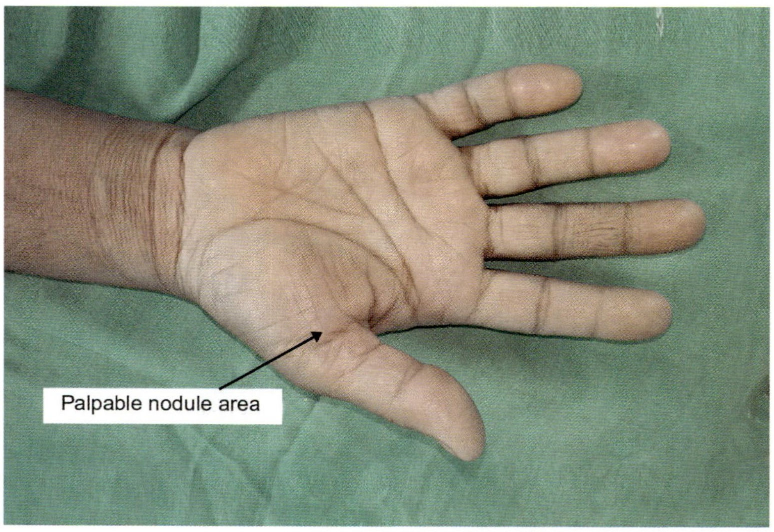

Fig. 2: Clinically nodule palpable over A1 pulley area. Tenderness and elicitable triggering present.

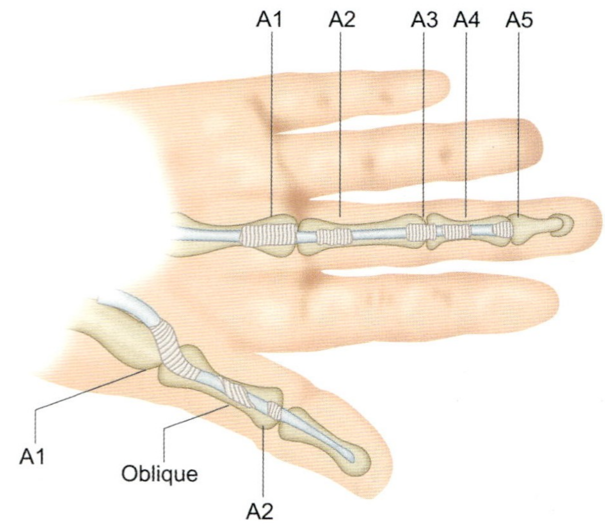

Fig. 3: Anatomy of pulleys of thumb and fingers.

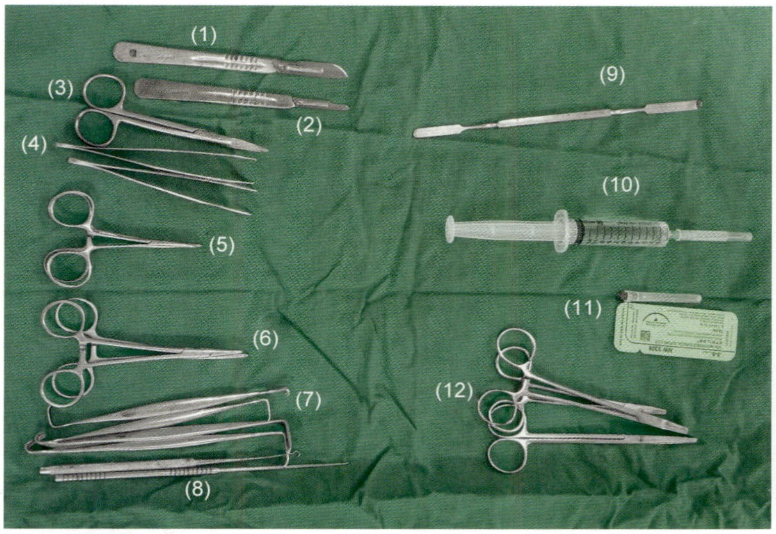

Fig. 4: (1) Bard-Parker handle with blade 21, (2) Bard-Parker handle with blade 15, (3) Dissecting scissors, (4) Forceps, (5) mosquito forceps, (6) Artery forceps, (7) Catspaw retractor, (8) Skin hook, (9) McDonalds dura protector, (10) Local anesthesia in syringe, (11) Nonabsorbable suture material, and (12) Needle holder with scissor.

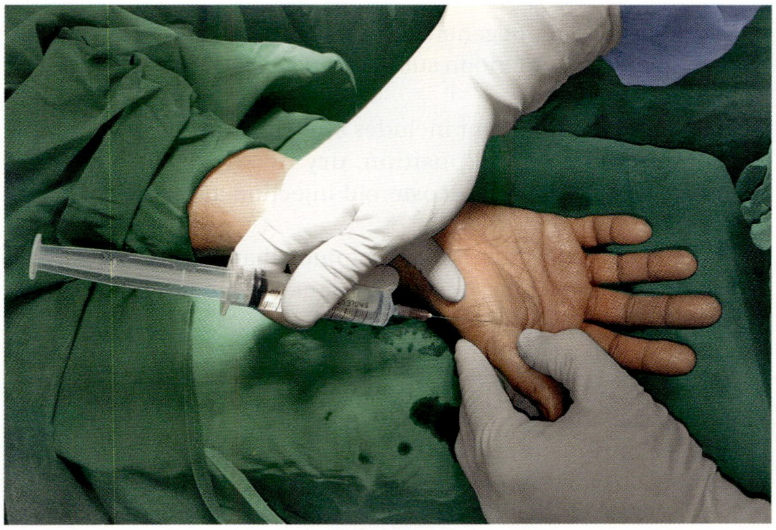

Fig. 5: Painting and draping done in standard manner. Hand rested on arm support in supination exposing palmar aspect of hand. Local anesthesia infiltrated parallel to proximal crease over base of thumb along the palpable nodule.

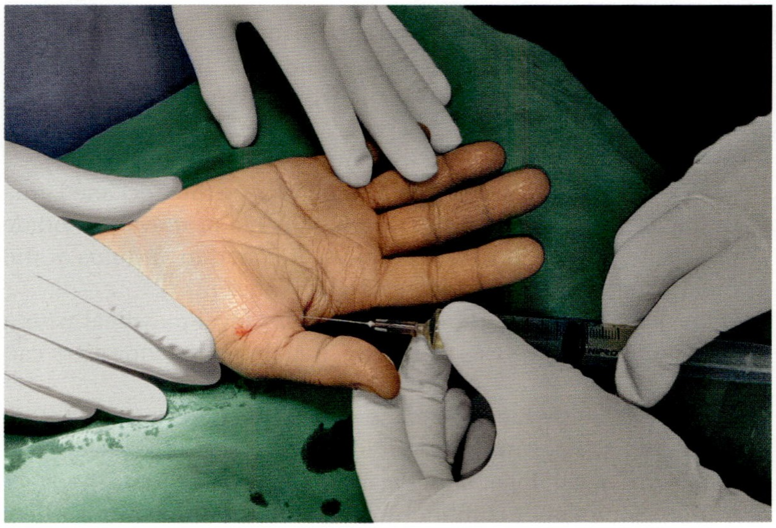

Fig. 6: Local anesthesia covering till first web space.

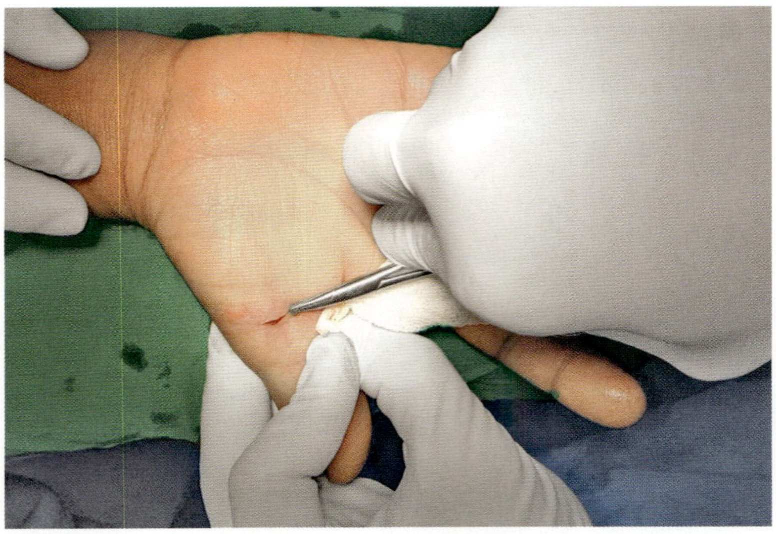

Fig. 7: Horizontal incision over proximal volar crease over head of first metacarpal area. Blunt dissection of subcutaneous soft tissue done with the help of mosquito forceps.

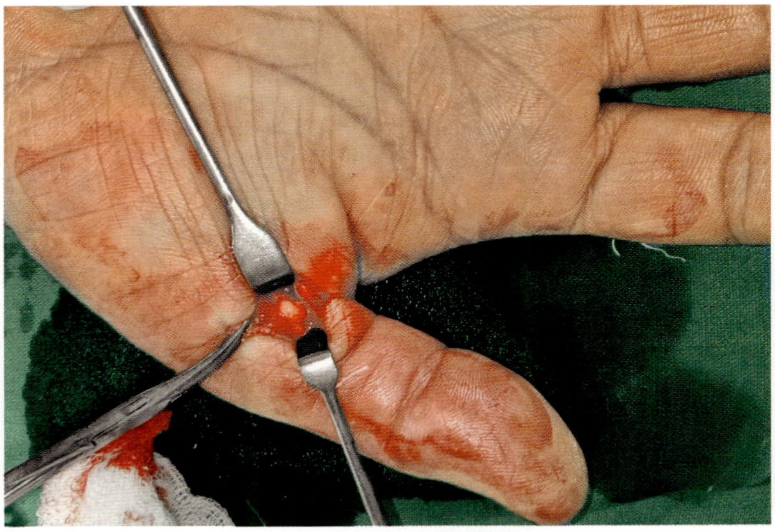

Fig. 8: Skin edges retracted with Langenbeck retractor. Tight A1 pulley identified.

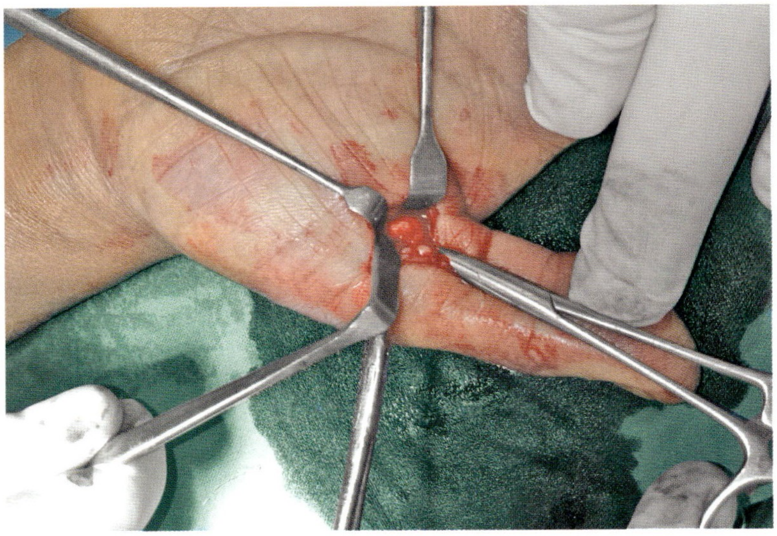

Fig. 9: Sharp incision to release the A1 pulley over flexor tendon made.

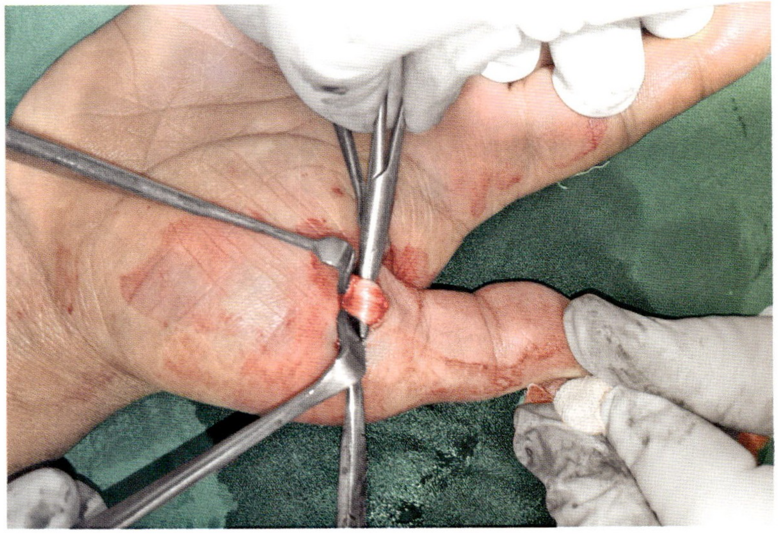

Fig. 10: Flexor tendon lifted with blunt instrument and flawless movements confirmed on table.

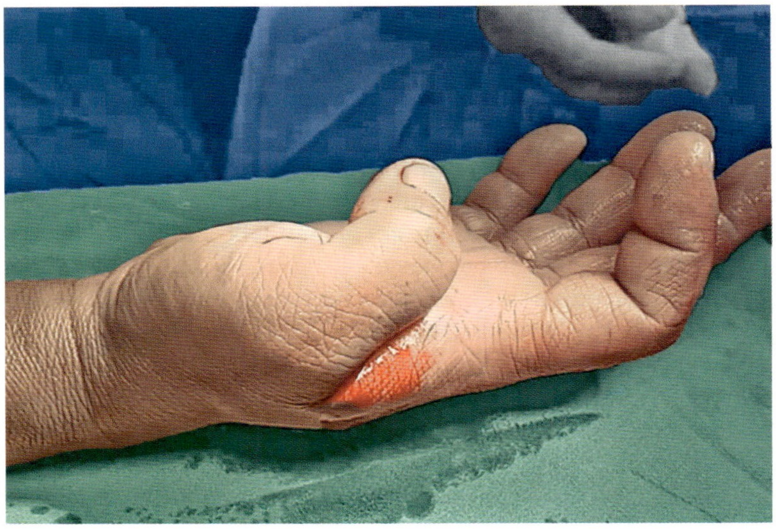

Fig. 11: Free active flexion of thumb confirmed on table.

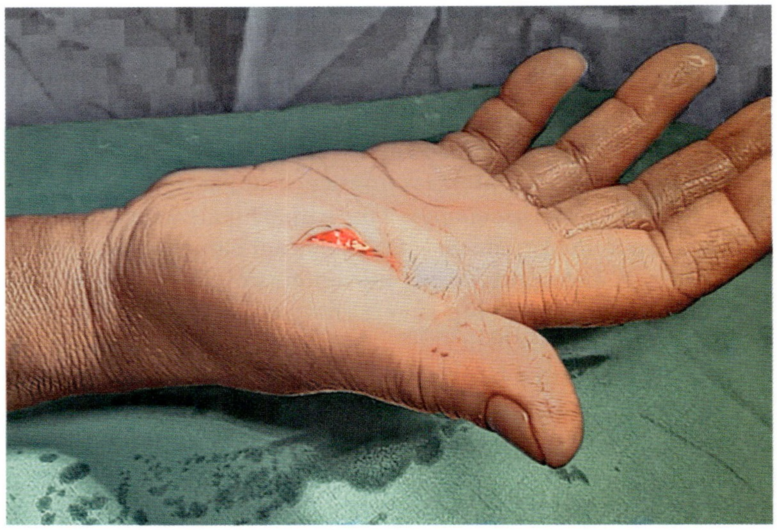

Fig. 12: Free active extension of thumb confirmed on table. Skin closure done. Dressing and pressure bandage applied.

POSTOPERATIVE MANAGEMENT

- Normal active flexion and extension of thumb allowed from evening as tolerated on day of surgery.
- Patient is advised to avoid heavy work for 2 weeks from operated hand. Sutures removed after 2 weeks.

SUGGESTED READING

1. Becker SJ, Braun Y, Janssen SJ, et al. Early patient satisfaction with different treatment pathway for trigger finger and thumb. J Hand Microsurg. 2015;7(2):283-93.
2. Brito JL, Rozental TD. Corticosteroids injection for idiopathic trigger finger. J Hand Surg Am. 2010;35(5):831-3.
3. Döring AC, Hagemen MG, Mulder FJ, et al. Trigger finger: assessment of surgeon and patient preference and priorities for decision making. J Hand Surg Am. 2014;39:2208-13.e2.
4. Everding NG, Bishop GB, Belyea CM, et al. Risk factors for complications or open trigger finger releases. Hand (N Y). 2015;10(2):297-300.
5. Schubert C, Hui-Chou HG, See AP, et al. Corticosteroids injection therapy for trigger finger or thumb: a retrospective review of 577 digits. Hand (NY). 2013;8(4):439-44.

CHAPTER 38

Radius Shortening in Kienbock's Disease

Pankaj Jindal, Madan Hardikar, Nitish Agrawal

- Kienbock's disease is avascular necrosis of carpal lunate presenting as pain in the wrist joint.
- The etiology remains unknown.
- It occurs more frequently in young active adults.
- It causes progressive collapse of the carpal lunate with associated alteration in the kinematics of the adjacent carpal bones leading to arthritis and restriction of movements of the affected wrist. Symptoms may develop several months before radiological changes become evident.
- Armistead reported occult lunate fractures on CT scan in some patients
- Incidence is common in young adult males [15-40 yrs] especially in heavy labourers.
- Natural course of untreated disease is fragmentation and sclerosis of lunate which progresses to carpal shortening, intercarpal malalignment and finally arthritis. Pain may present months before any radiographic evidence of disease and in such cases MRI or bone scan can make early diagnosis. Early diagnosis may possibly help in salvage of lunate. In young adults with seemingly nontraumatic onset of dorsal, central wrist pain and tenderness just distal and ulnar to Lister's tubercle should arouse suspicion of Kienbock's Disease and should be investigated thoroughly. Clinical correlation with MRI scan is important to differentiate from other disorders.
- Lichtman et al. proposed a classification of Kienbock disease based on the of radiographic changes.

Treatment considerations are based on Lichtman classification:

- *Stage I:* No visible changes are seen on radiograph; changes are seen on MRI. Treatment consists of immobilization and NSAIDs. If no improvement, to be treated as stage II.
- *Stage II:* Sclerosis of lunate seen on radiograph. Joint levelling procedures are advised: radial shortening or ulnar lengthening for patients who have ulnar negative variance. Radial wedge osteotomy or triple fusion in patients who are ulnar neutral. Distal radial core decompression to create local vascular healing response is also described.
- *Stage IIIA:* When lunate has collapsed, but scaphoid has not flexed and capitate has not migrated proximally. Joint leveling surgery like radius shortening in positive ulnar variance is recommended.
- *Stage IIIB:* While lunate has collapsed, scaphoid has flexed as well. Lunate starts to rotate and shows dorsal intercalated segment instability (DISI) pattern. Proximal row carpectomy or triple fusion is advised; must treat internal collapse pattern.
- *Stage IV:* Degeneration of adjacent intercarpal joints is seen. Wrist fusion, proximal row carpectomy, or limited intercarpal fusion is advised; must remove arthritic part of joint.

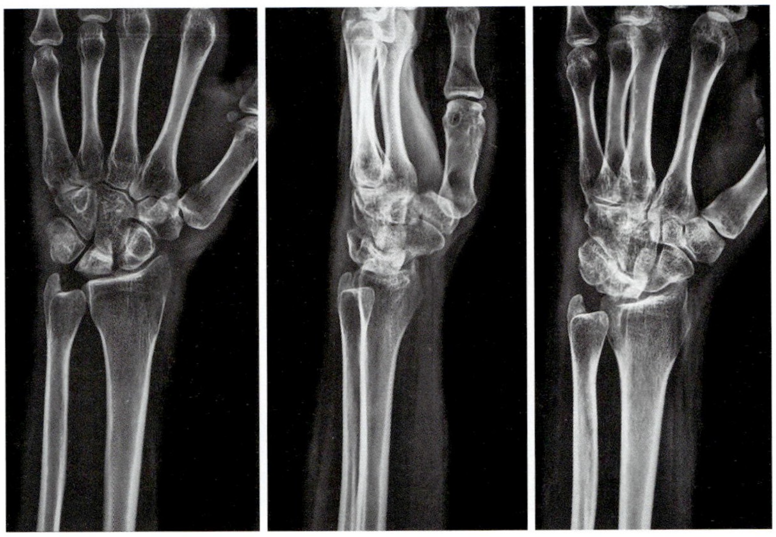

Fig. 1: X-ray posteroanterior view, and two oblique views show dense sclerotic lunate and caudal cephalad collapse of the lunate.

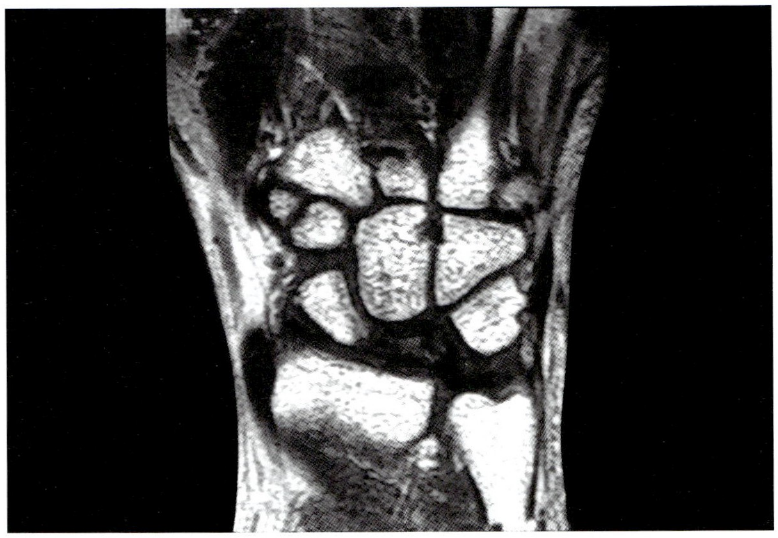

Fig. 2: MRI showing altered signal in the lunate.

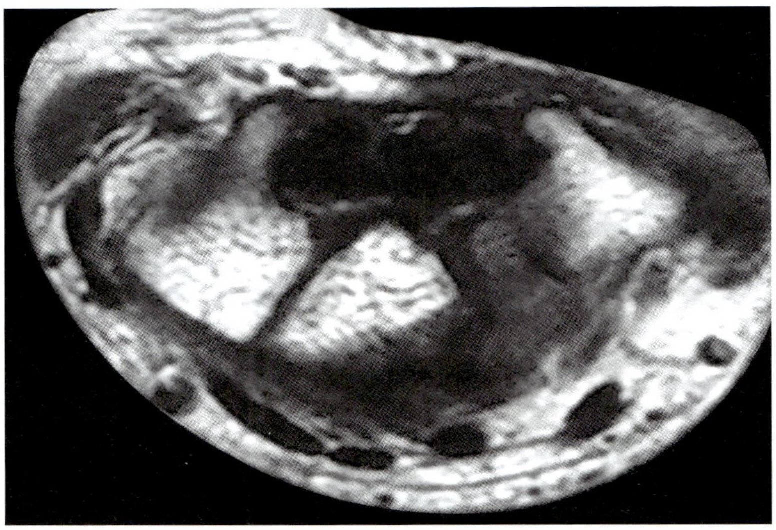

Fig. 3: Magnetic resonance imaging (MRI) axial view.

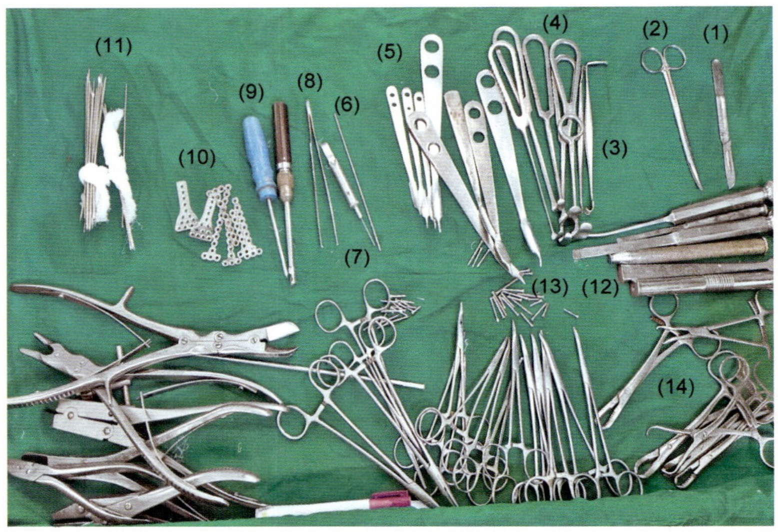

Fig. 4: (1) Bard-parker handle with blade, (2) Dissecting scissors, (3) Cat paw retractor, (4) Right angle retractor, (5) Hohmann bone lever/Hohmann retractor, (6) Drill bit, (7) Depth gauge, (8) Tooth forceps, (9) Screw driver, (10) 2.7 mm plate, (11) K-wires, (12) Osteotome, (13) Screws (2.7 mm), and (14) Bone clamps.

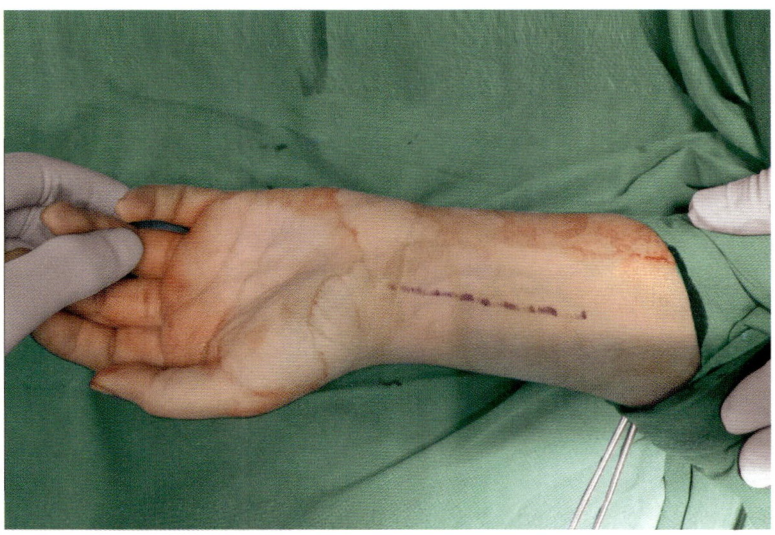

Fig. 5: Patient is positioned supine on operating table. Forearm kept in supination supported on hand rest. Painting and draping done in standard manner. Incision marked over palpable Flexor carpi radialis tendon.

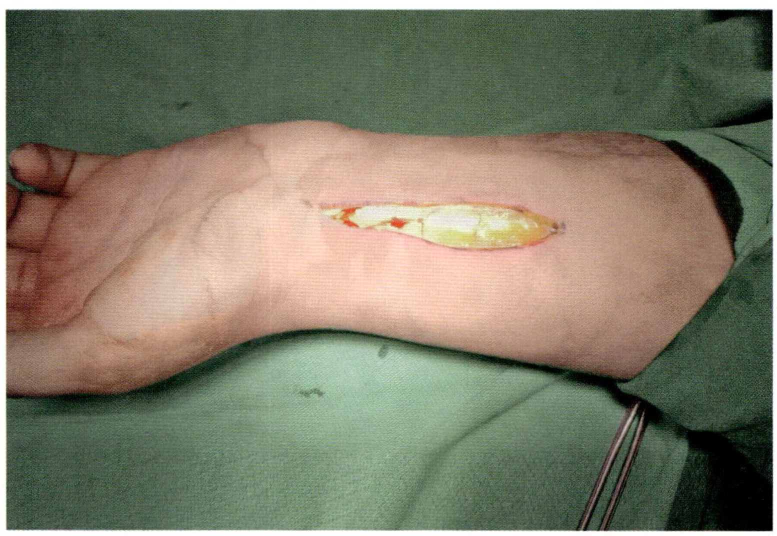

Fig. 6: Tourniquet is inflated. Incision made with skin knife over the marking.

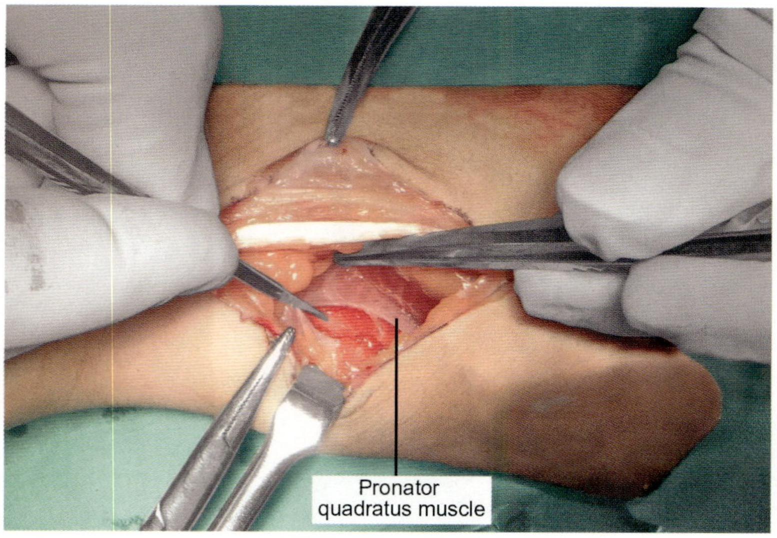

Fig. 7: Subcutaneous soft tissue, fascia dissected with dissecting scissors and retracted with right angle retractors. Small blood vessels caught with mosquito forceps. Pronator Quadratus muscle realeased from radius sharply.

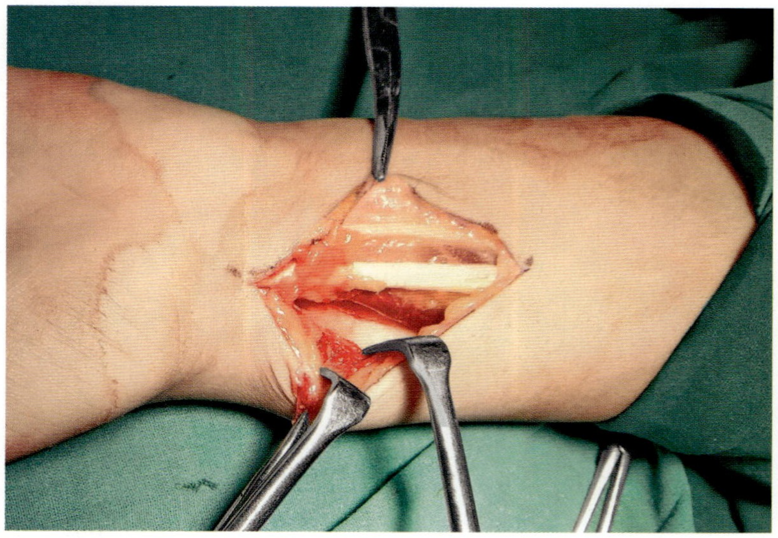

Fig. 8: Pronator quadratus muscle along with soft tissue and fascia retracted laterally and flexor carpi radialis and palmaris longus tendon retracted medially with right angle retractors.

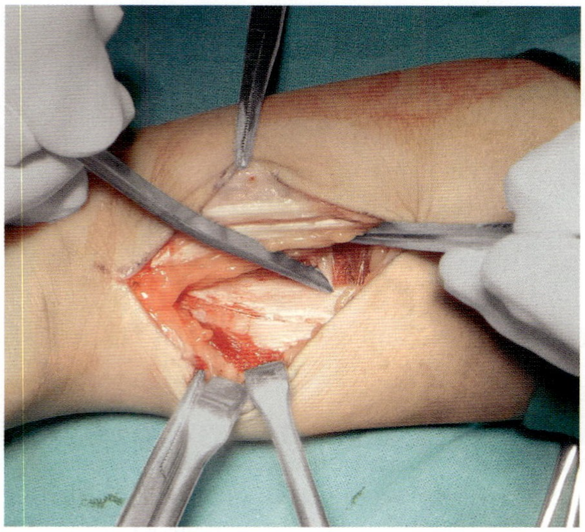

Fig. 9: Periosteum is separated with periosteum elevator on both proximally and distally.

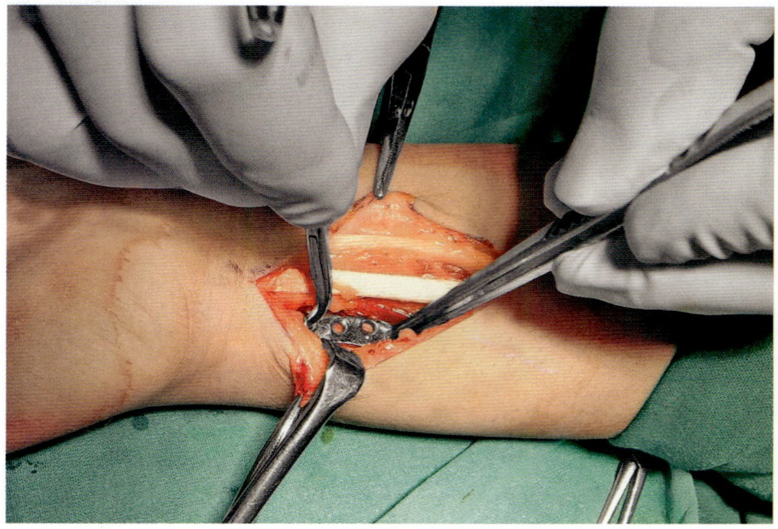

Fig. 10: 2.7 mm distal end radius precontoured plate is positioned temporarily over distal end of radius.

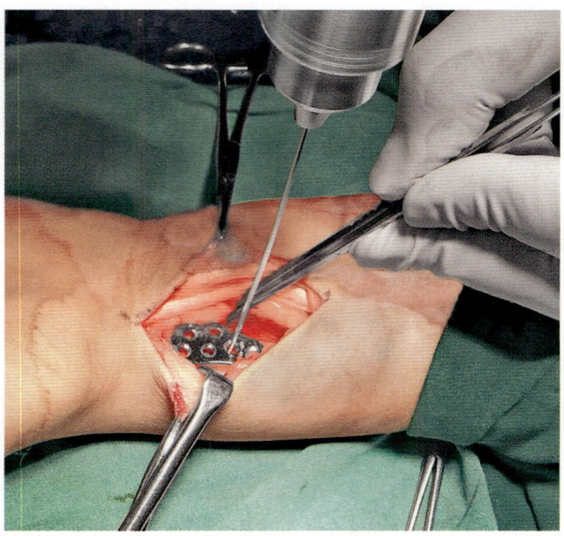

Fig. 11: Osteotomy site is identified and drilled with K-wires.

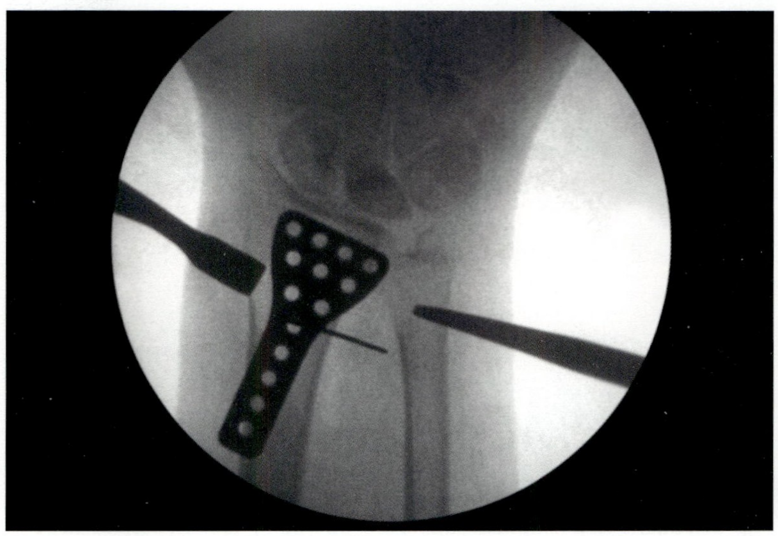

Fig. 12: Position of wire and osteotomy site confirmed on C-arm image intensifier.

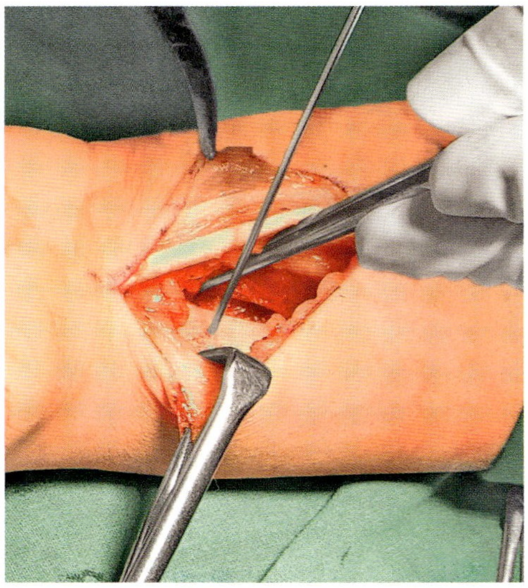

Fig. 13: Multiple holes made by K-wire at osteotomy site.

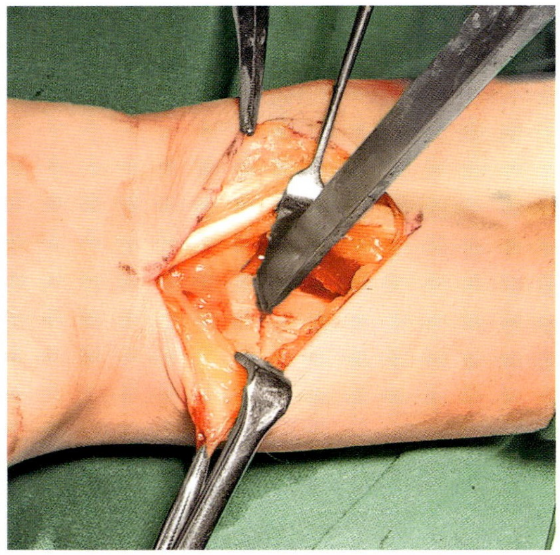

Fig. 14: Osteotomy done with osteotome and hammer.

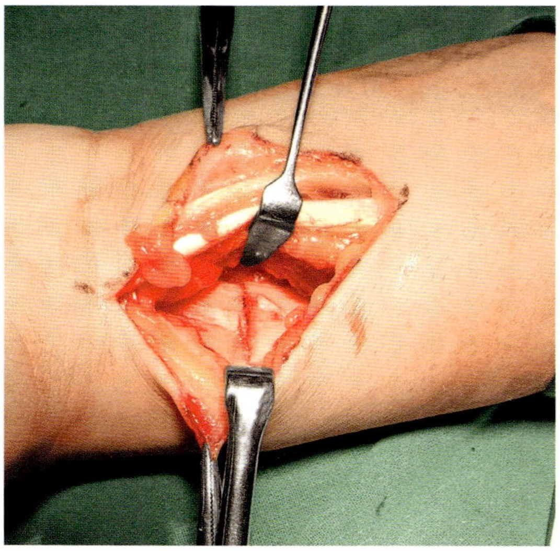

Fig. 15: Osteotomy completed.

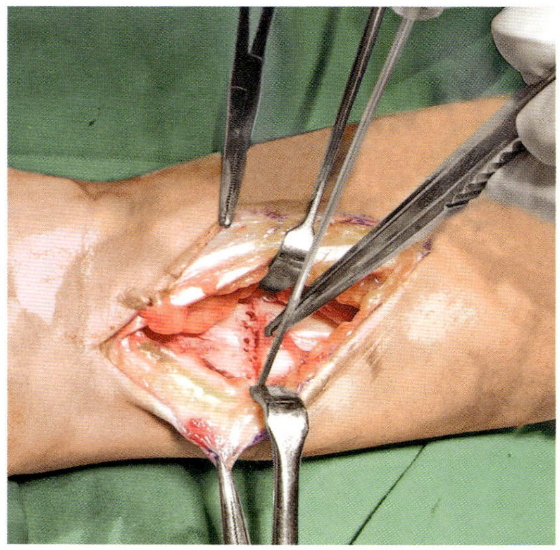

Fig. 16: Multiple holes made with K-wires 2 mm distal to osteotomy site, on distal fragment of radius for removal of 2 mm wide segment of radius.

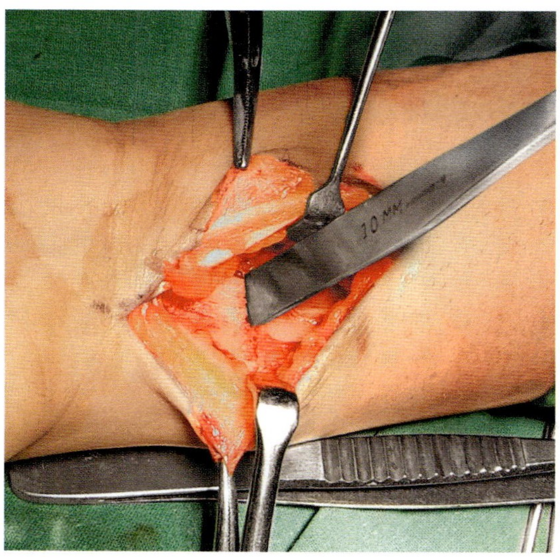

Fig. 17: Osteotomy done with osteotome and hammer.

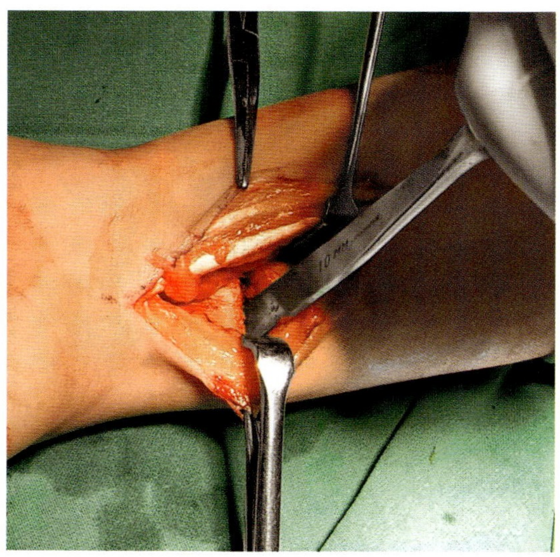

Fig. 18: Osteotomy completed with osteotome and hammer and 2 mm thickness bone segment removed.

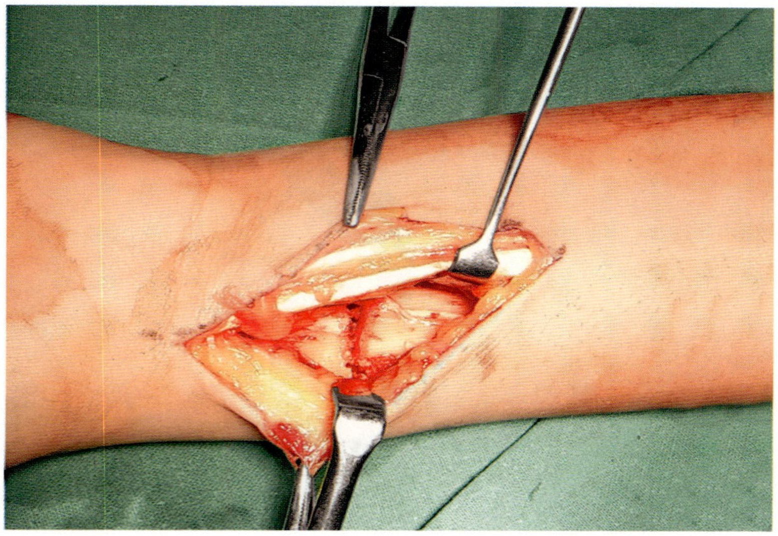

Fig. 19: Both distal and proximal ends are approximated for further fixation.

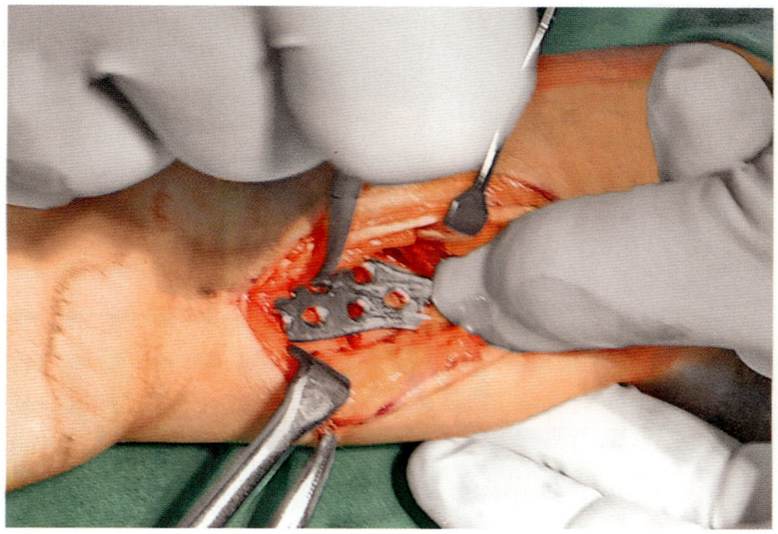

Fig. 20: 2.7 mm plate inserted for final fixation.

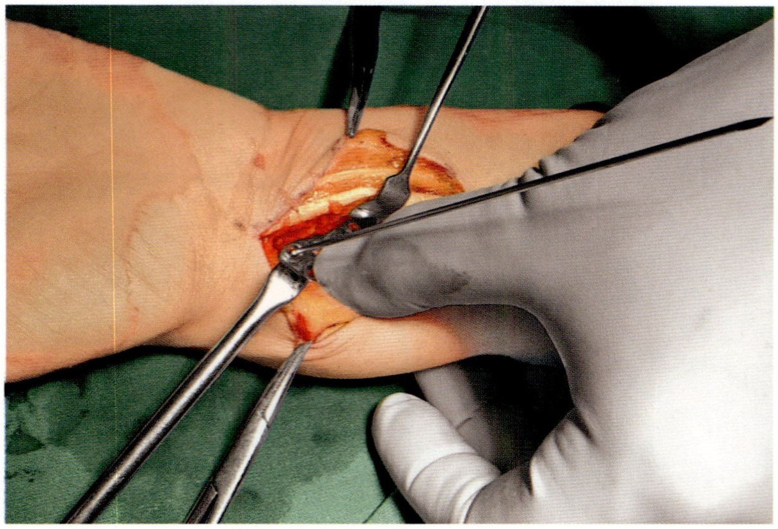

Fig. 21: Plate is temporarily fixed on distal fragment of radius with K-wire.

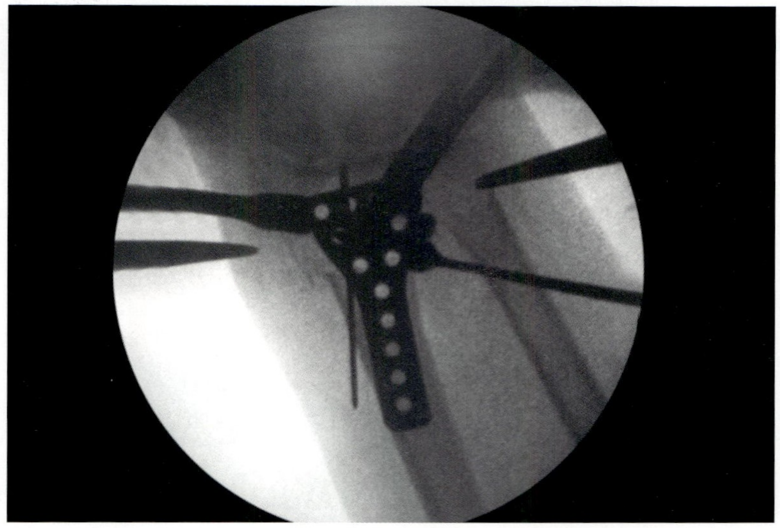

Fig. 22: Position of plate and K-wire confirmed over anteroposterior (AP) view on C-arm.

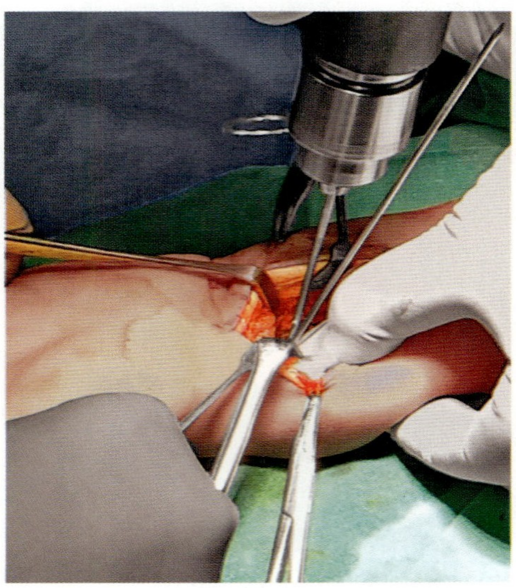

Fig. 23: Drilling for first distal screw on distal fragment of radius done.

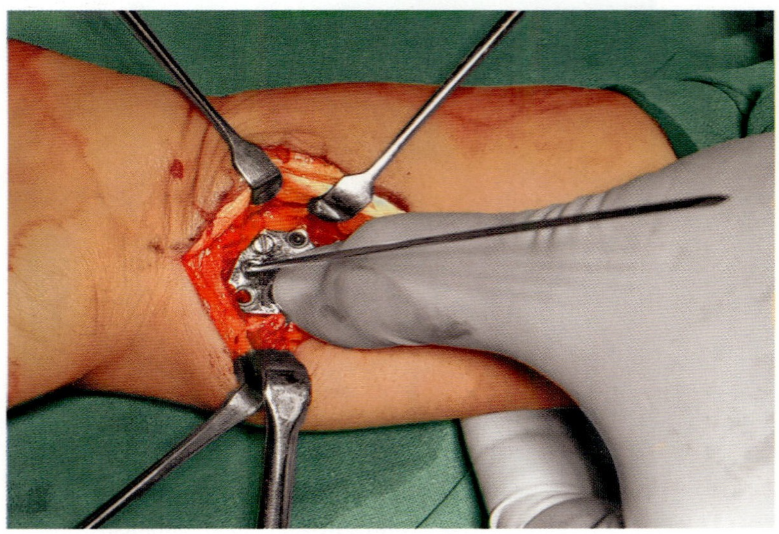

Fig. 24: 2.7 mm screw fixed on distal part of radius.

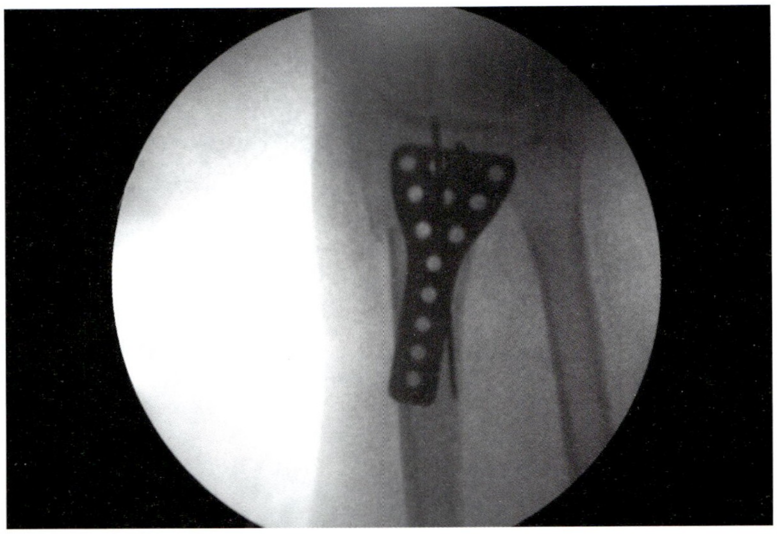

Fig. 25: Fixation of first screw confirmed over C-arm anteroposterior (AP) view.

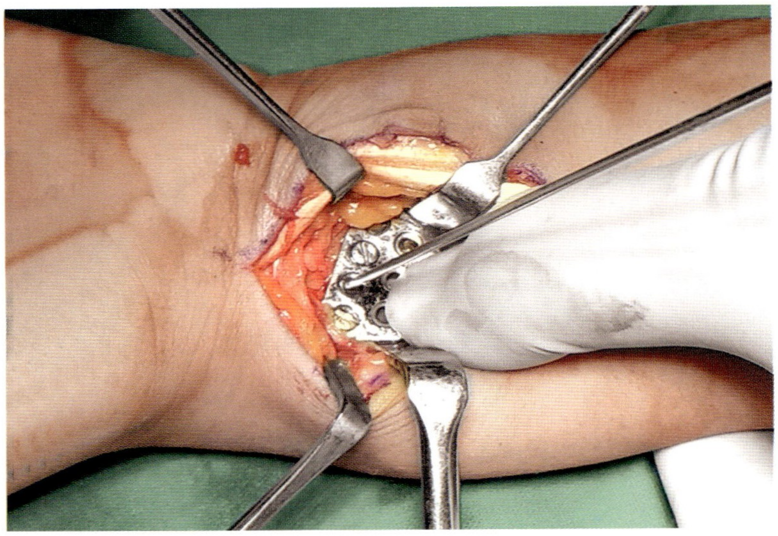

Fig. 26: Second distal screw fixation done.

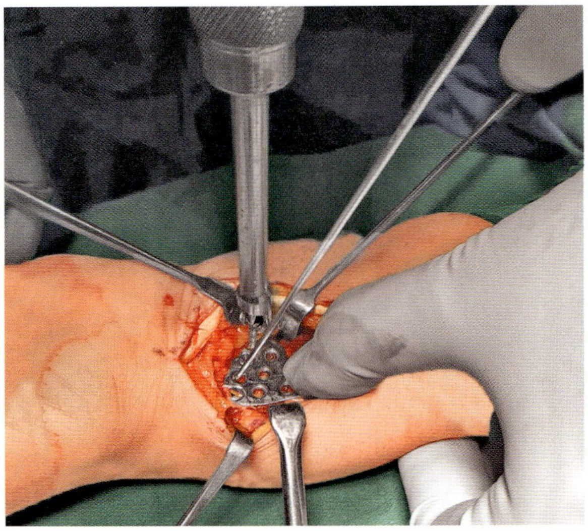

Fig. 27: Third distal screw fixation done.

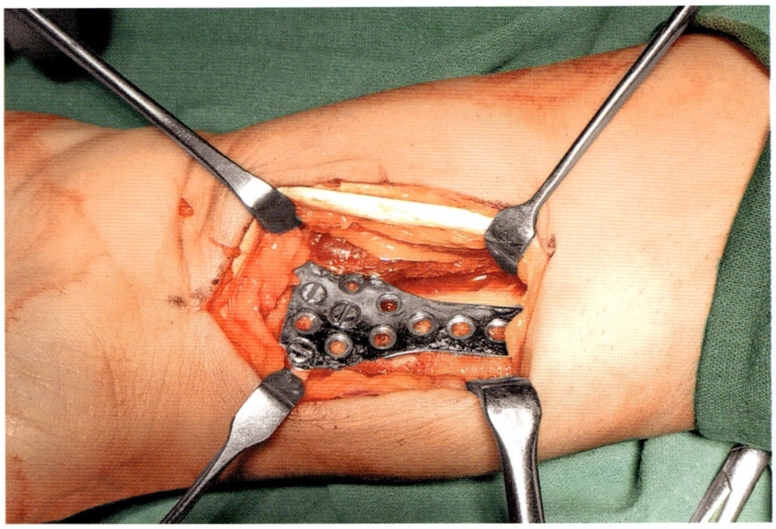

Fig. 28: K-wire removed and fourth distal screw fixation done.

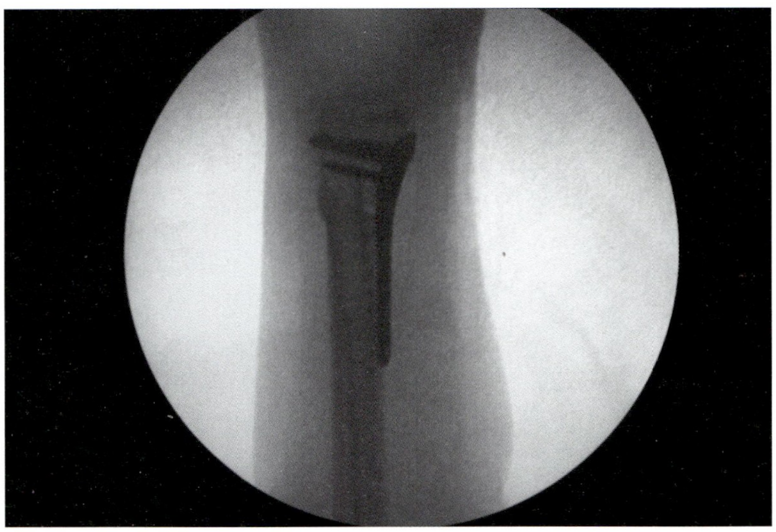

Fig. 29: Distally four screw fixation confirmed over C-arm on lateral view.

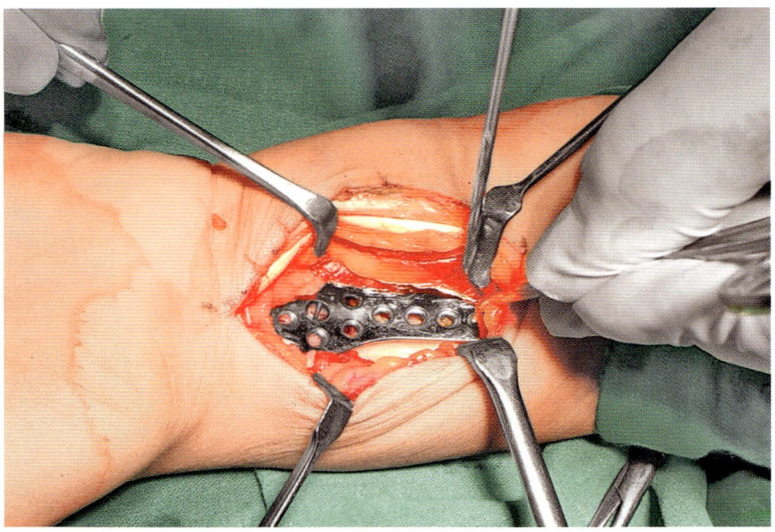

Fig. 30: Drilling for proximal plate fixation done.

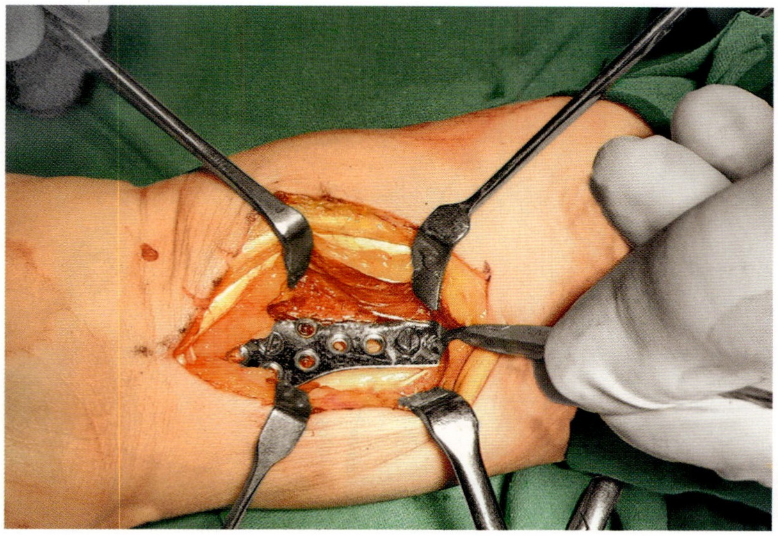

Fig. 31: Proximal first screw fixation done.

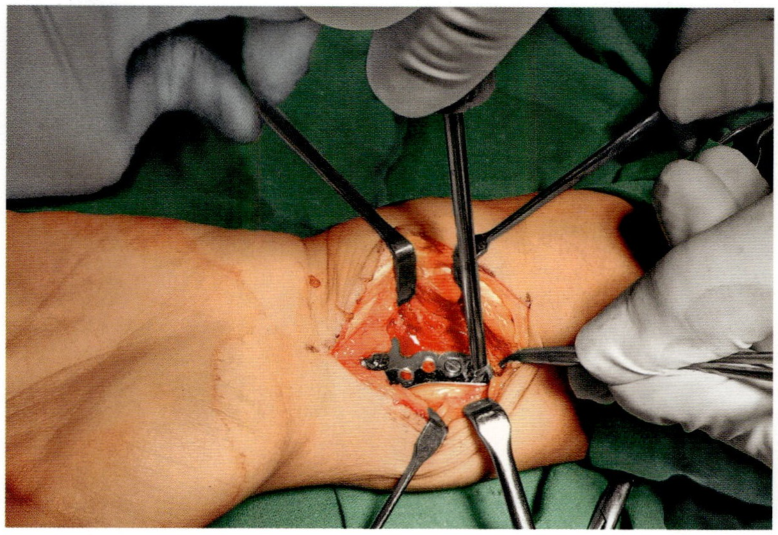

Fig. 32: Second proximal screw fixation done.

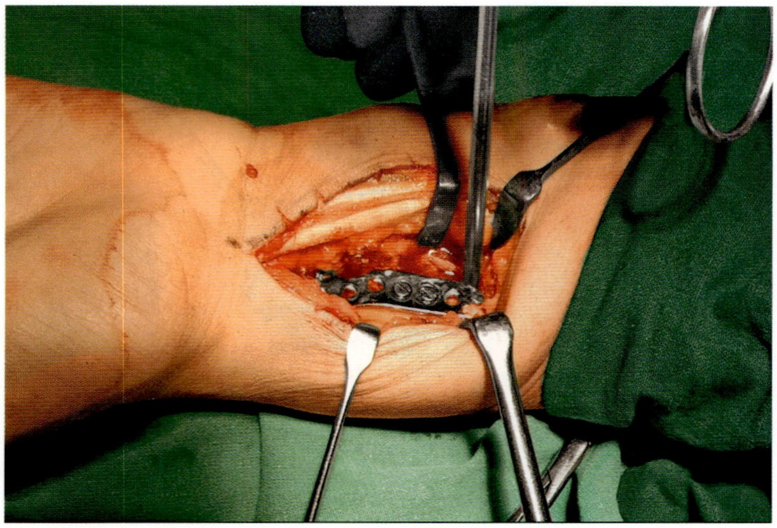

Fig. 33: Remaining proximal screw fixation done.

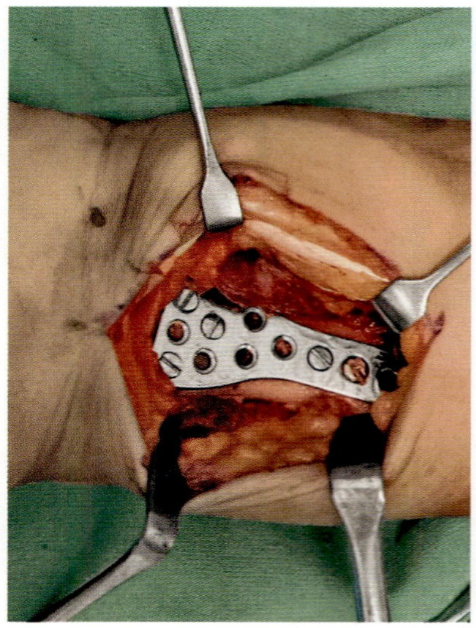

Fig. 34: Fixation complete with 2.7 mm plate and four distal and three proximal screws.

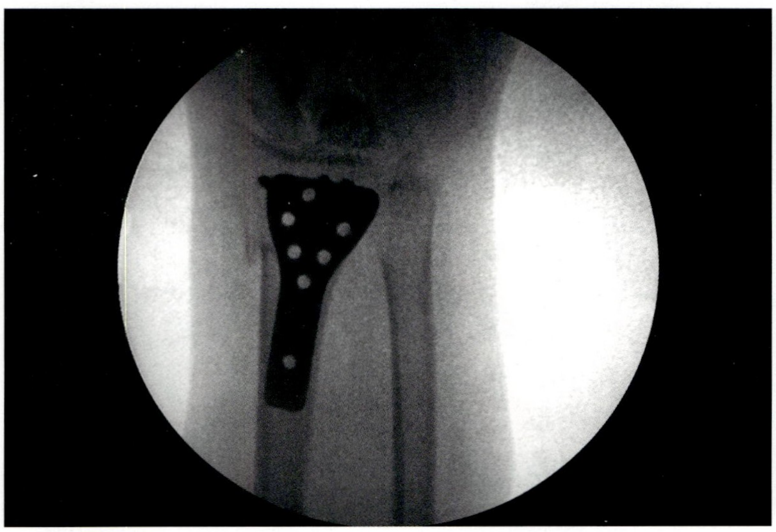

Fig. 35: Final fixation confirmed on anteroposterior view on C-arm.

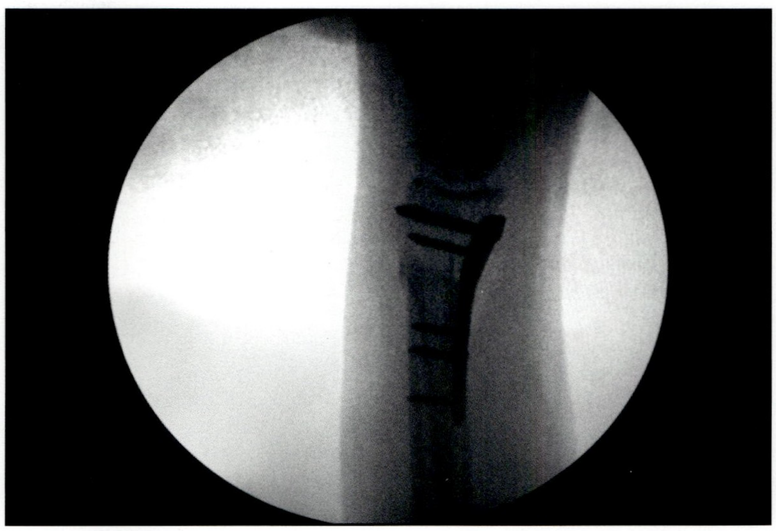

Fig. 36: Final fixation confirmed on lateral view on C-arm.

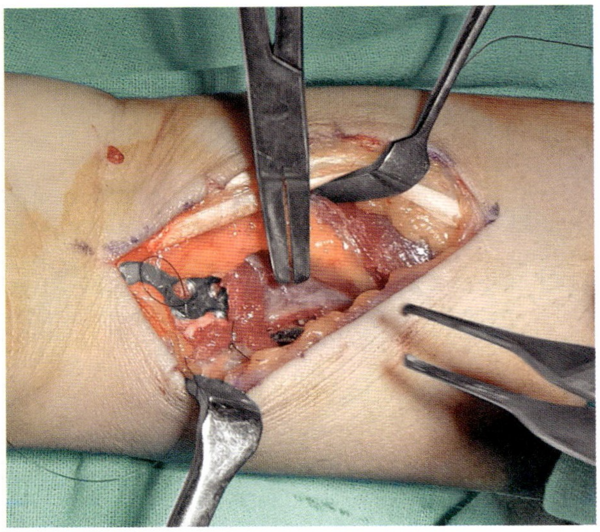

Fig. 37: Wash given with povidone iodine solution and normal saline and pronator quadratus sutured over plate with nonabsorbable suture material.

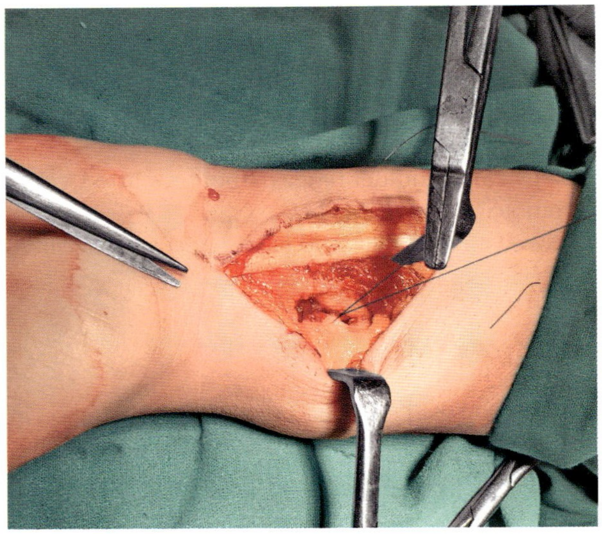

Fig. 38: Fascia and soft tissue suturing done.

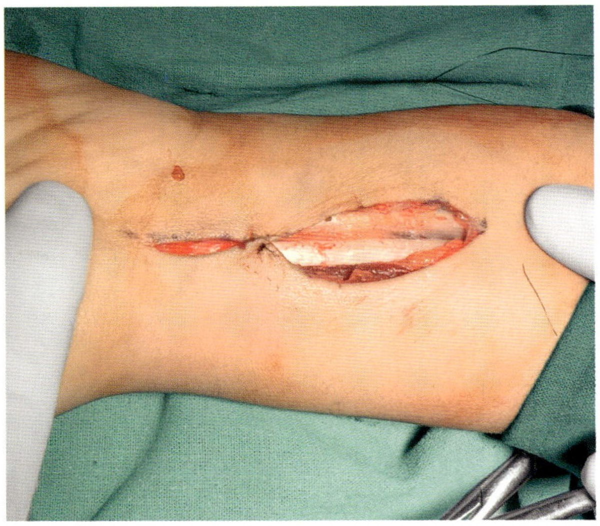

Fig. 39: Skin is approximated and suturing done with nylon suture material.

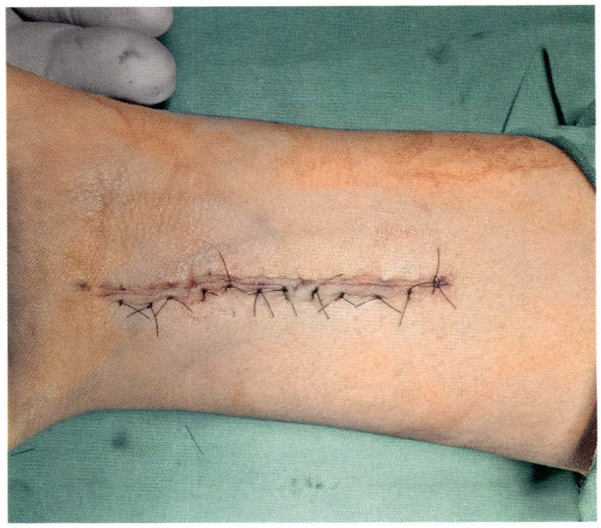

Fig. 40: Skin suturing completed.

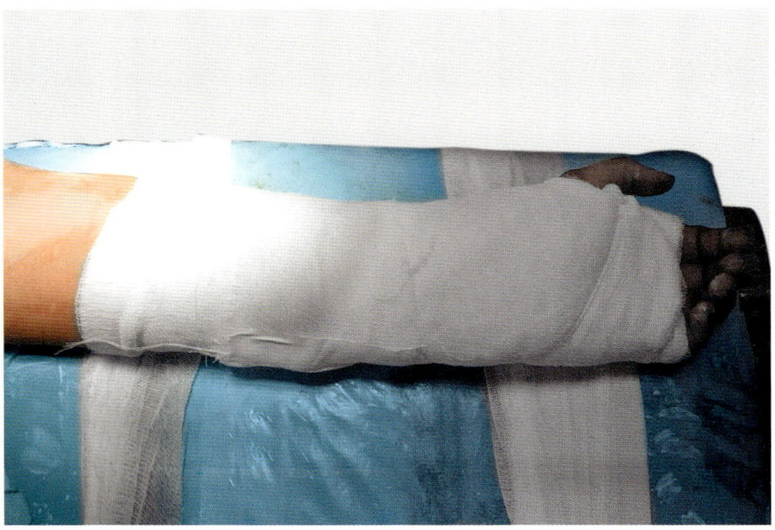

Fig. 41: Below elbow slab given for 21 days on volar aspect of forearm.

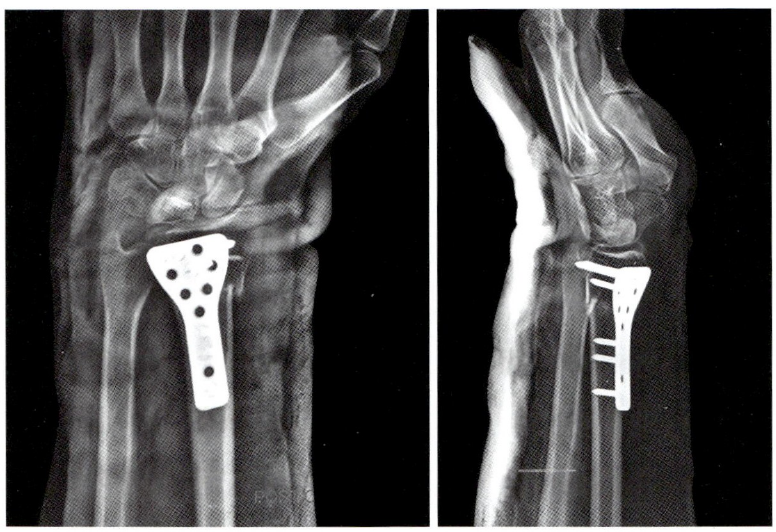

Fig. 42: Postoperative X-ray showing radial shortening and internal fixation done for Kienbock disease.

POSTOPERATIVE MANAGEMENT

- Active finger movements started from same day after anesthesia has worn off.
- Limb elevation given above heart level.
- Active elbow and shoulder range of motion started from day 1.
- Suture removal done on day 14.
- Slab removed after 21 days and passive/active range of motion of wrist started.

SUGGESTED READING

1. Bain GI, Yeo CJ, Morse LP. Kienbock disease: recent advances in the basic science, assessment and treatment. Hand Surg. 2015;20:352-65.
2. Lichtman DM, Lesley NE, Simmons SP. The classification and treatment of Kienbock's disease: the state of the art and a look at the future. J Hand Surg Eur Vol. 2010;35:549-54.
3. Matsui Y, Funakoshi T, Motomiya M, et al. Radial shortening osteotomy for Kienbock disease: minimum 10 year follow-up. J Hand Surg Am. 2014;39:679-85.
4. Saunders BM, Lichtman D. A classification-based treatment algorithms for Kienbock disease: current and future considerations. Tech Hand Up Extrem Surg. 2011;15:38-40.
5. Viljakka T, Tallroth K, Vastamaki M. Long-term outcome (20 to 33 years) of radial shortening osteotomy for Kienbock's lunatomalacia. J Hand Surg Eur Vol. 2014;39:761-9.

CHAPTER 39

Volar Barton Fracture Buttress Plate Fixation

Shrinivas S Shintre, Hitesh J Mangukiya, Vivek Mukund Badhe

INTRODUCTION

John Rhea Barton in 1838 described the fracture of the distal end of the radius that tends to involve the volar or dorsal rim of the distal end of the radius and has intra-articular extent. They make up around 1.3% of fractures of the distal radius. This injury is more common in young patient following high energy trauma.

FUNCTIONAL ANATOMY AND CLASSIFICATION

Rikli DA in 1996 described three column concept of distal end of radius.

1. The *radial column* comprises the radial styloid with the scaphoid facet. Only small loads are transmitted via this column. It serves primarily as a stabilizer, as an osseous buttress radially, limiting radial deviation.
2. The *intermediate column* comprises the lunate facet and the sigmoid notch. Serves primarily for load transmission.
3. The *ulnar column* is the ulnar head, with the distal radioulnar joint, the ulnar styloid and the triangular fibrocartilage. The ulnar column is the stabilizing pivot of the wrist.

Various classifications have been described in the past for distal end of radius fracture like Frykman, Fernandez, Melone, etc. in AO/ASIF classification system type B involves fracture due to shearing force and B3 particularly emphasize on volar barton fracture. According to the size of the Volar fragment, B3 fractures are further grouped as B3.1-small fragment fracture, B3.2-large fragment fracture and B3.3-comminuted fracture. Mehra et al in 1993, provided a classification for volar barton fracture which was based on the size of the fracture fragment and its associated comminution. Type 1 involves a single large fragment, Type 2 is a comminuted fracture with small as well as large fragments, and Type 3 involves a single large fragment with another additional cortical fragment inferior to it.

CLINICAL FEATURES

Patient typically presents with severe pain, swelling with restricted and painful movements of affected wrist. A thorough examination of surrounding neurovascular structure is must. A detailed history with status of median nerve and radial artery should always be documented.

IMAGING

A standard anteroposterior (AP) and lateral radiograph should always been done for initial evaluation. Computed tomography can be valuable in accurately defining anatomic disruption, particularly for intra-articular fractures with multiple components.

Standard radiographic parameters are used to assess the distal radius.

- Anteroposterior view
  - Radial height = 12 mm
  - Radial inclination = 23'
  - Ulnar variance = 0–2 mm
- Lateral view
  - Palmar tilt = 12'
  - Scapholunate angle = 30–80'

LaFontaine and Associates suggested five factors that indicate instability of distal radius fractures: (1) initial dorsal angulation greater than 20°, (2) dorsal metaphyseal comminution, (3) radiocarpal intra-articular involvement, (4) associated ulnar fractures, and (5) patient age older than 60 years. Abbaszadegan and colleagues suggested that instability is present if the initial radiograph reveals more than 4 mm of impaction or axial shortening.

TREATMENT OPTIONS

Various modalities of treatment are described in published works, including closed reduction and casting, percutaneous Kirschner wiring, and open reduction and internal fixation using either Kirschner wires or buttress plating. Closed reduction though easy to bring about, is not simple to maintain, with many patients suffering a loss of reduction. Early osteoarthritis, deformities, and instability of the fracture with or without subluxation are frequently seen complications with closed reduction and casting.

The advantage of plating is that it allows for more stable internal fixation with anatomic reduction done directly under vision producing better radiologic results. It is also shown to have a decreased period of immobilization and the return of wrist range of motion and function is quicker in these cases. Buttress plates provide reduction and an antiglide effect to intra articular fractures with a vertical shear. Modern locking plates themselves assist in reducing the intra-articular fracture. Tendon irritation, scar complications and the need for plate removal are associated complications.

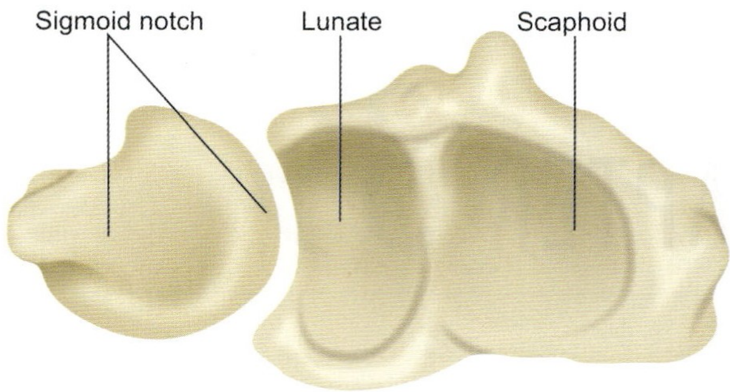

Fig. 1: The three-column concept.

SURGICAL STEPS (FIGS. 2 TO 17)

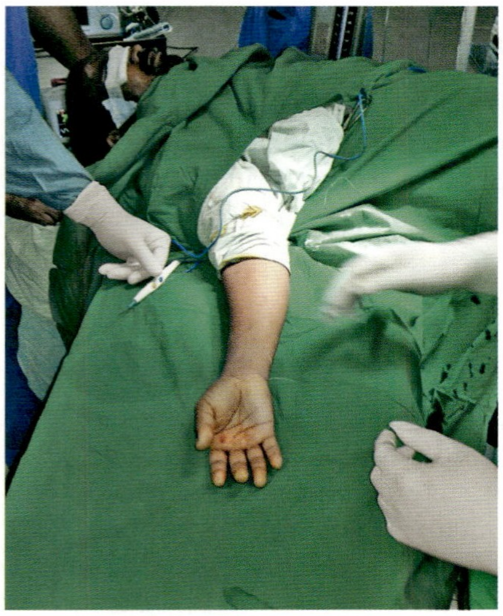

Fig. 2: Patient is lying supine with operated extremity is positioned in extension and forearm supination.

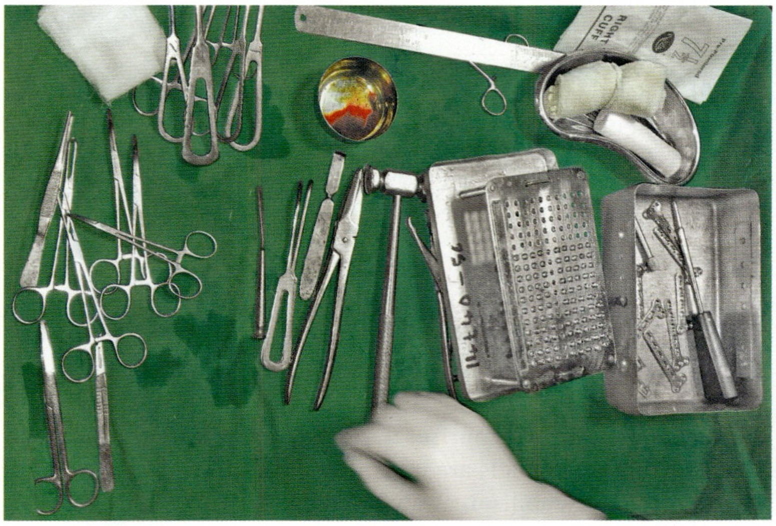

Fig. 3: Necessary surgical instruments and T plate set.

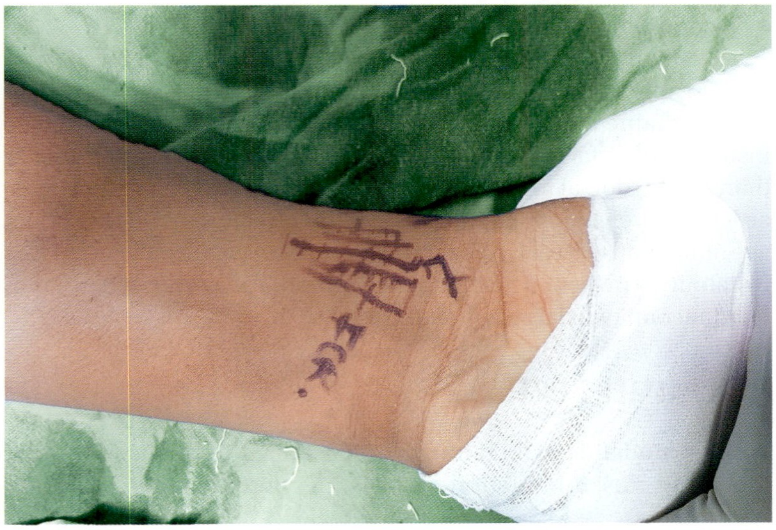

Fig. 4: Incision area is marked between flexor carpi ulnaris and radial artery.

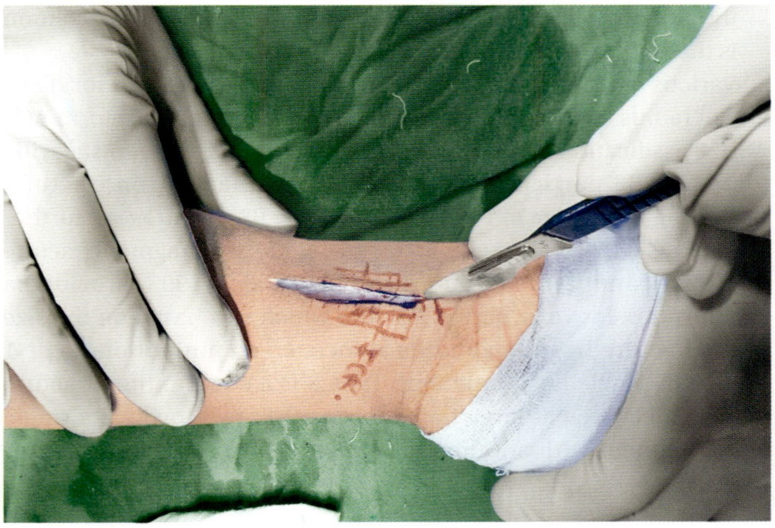

Fig. 5: Skin incision taken with 21 No. skin blade.

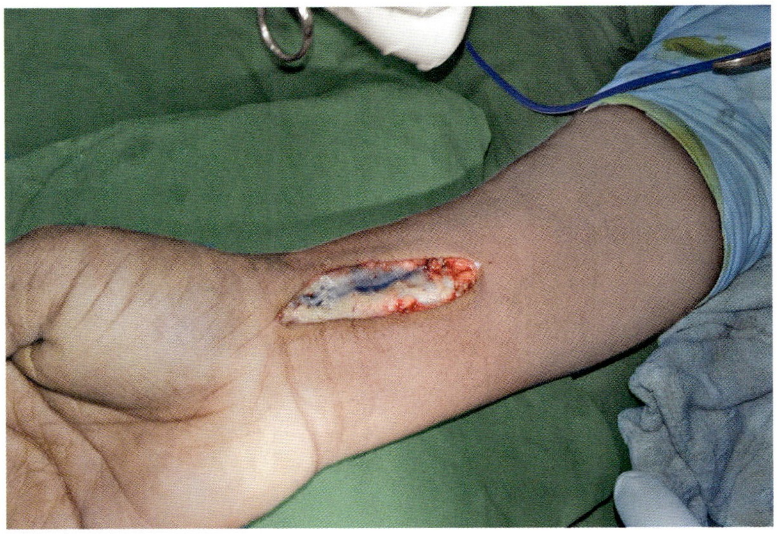

Fig. 6: Superficial dissection done.

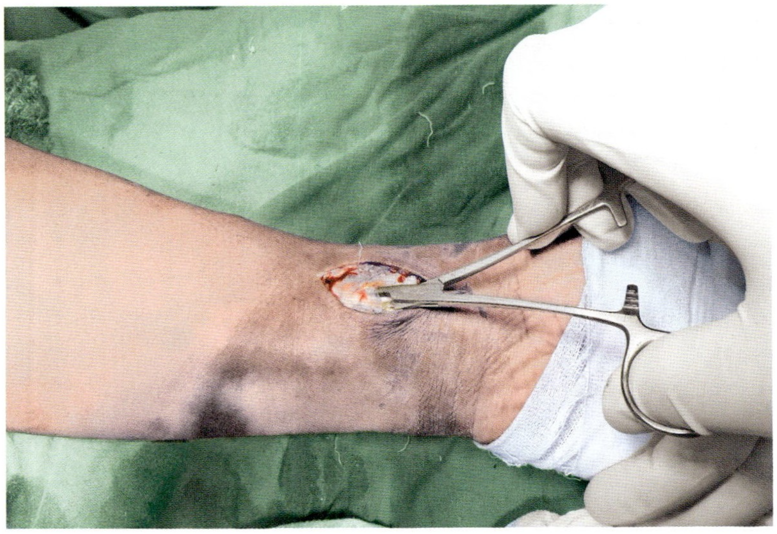

Fig. 7: Sharply incising the fascia overlying the flexor carpi radialis (FCR) tendon.

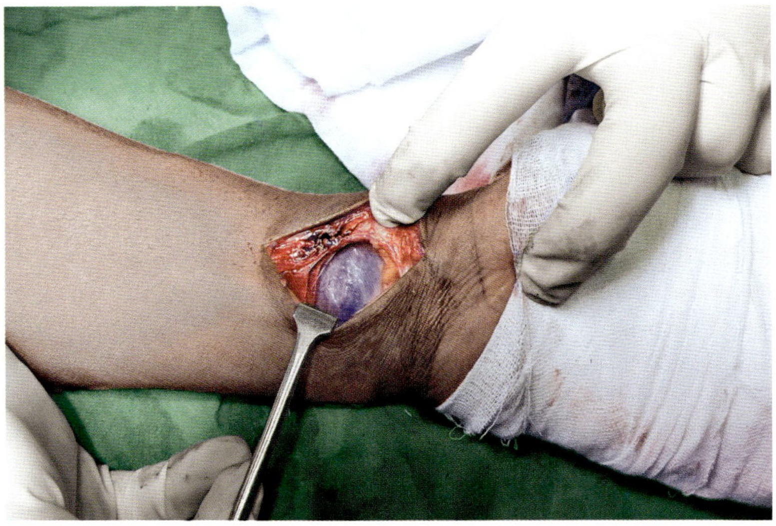

Fig. 8: Underlying pronator quadratus muscle.

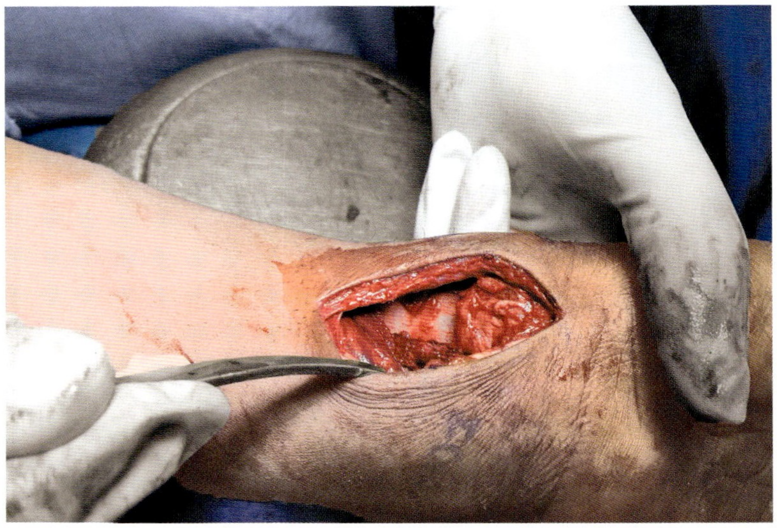

Fig. 9: Pronator quadratus is sharply incised from radial border of distal radius and retracted medially.

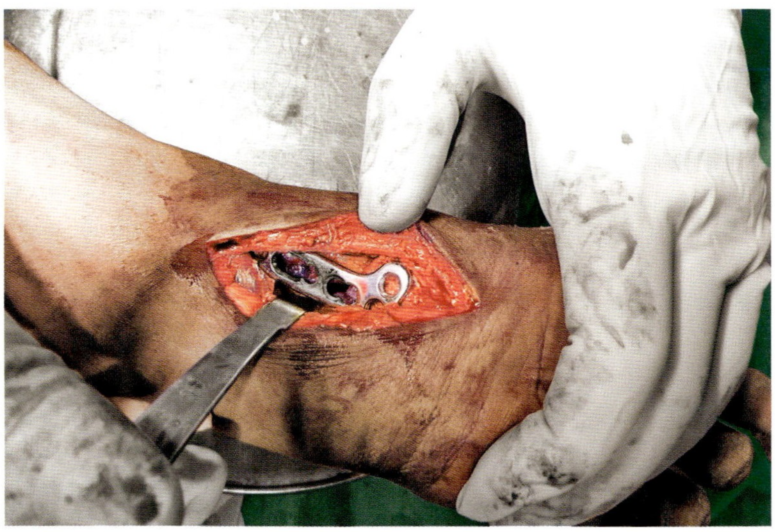

Fig. 10: Appropriate length T plate is placed on volar surface of distal radius.

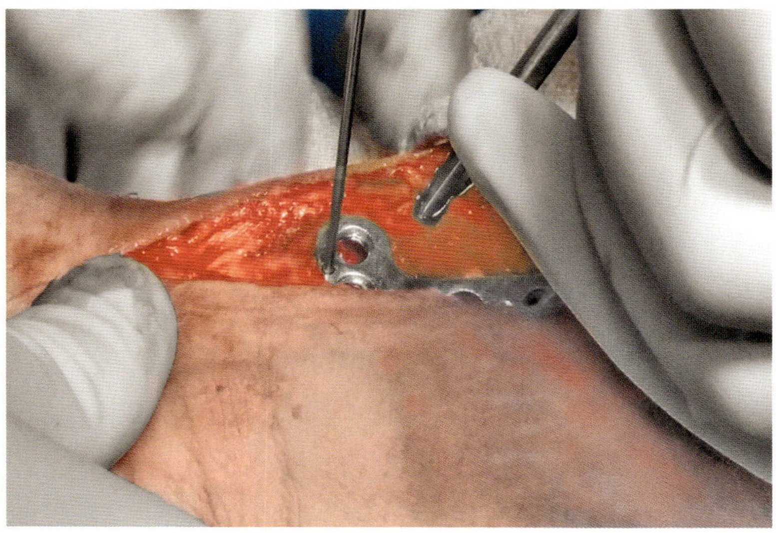

Fig. 11: Preliminary plate position done with K-wire.

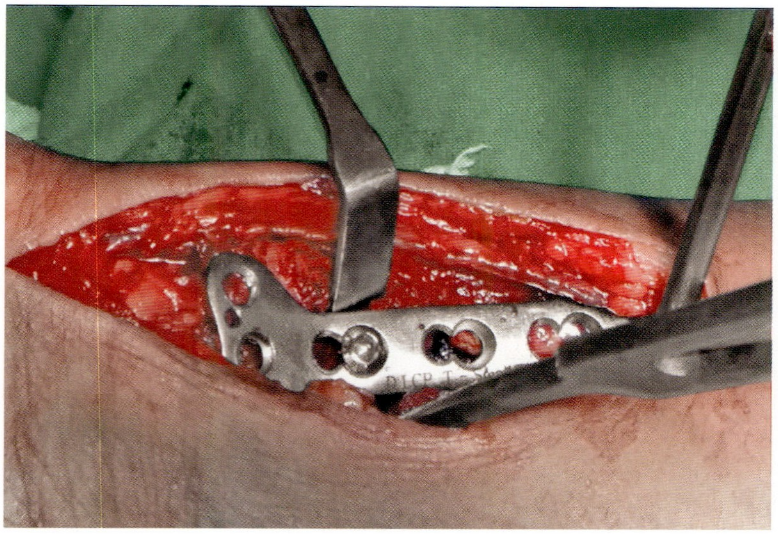

Fig. 12: After the satisfactory plate position, cortical screw is placed initially in diaphysis of radius.

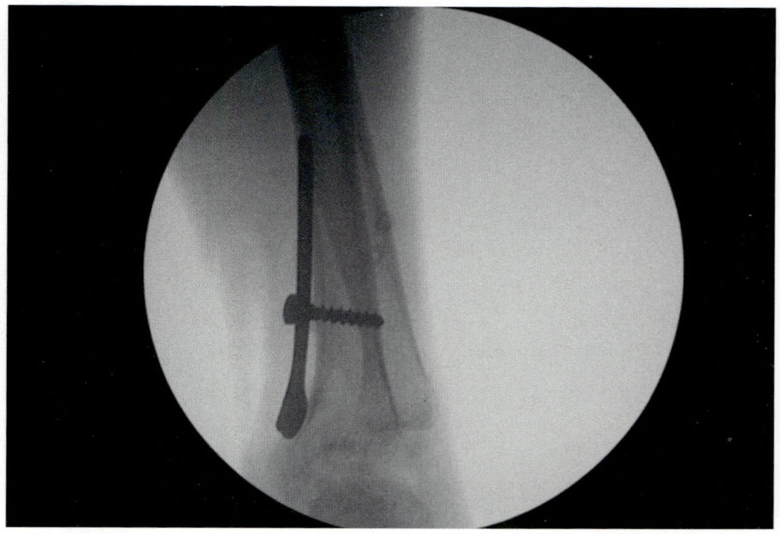

Fig. 13: C-arm lateral image of plate position with first cortical screw.

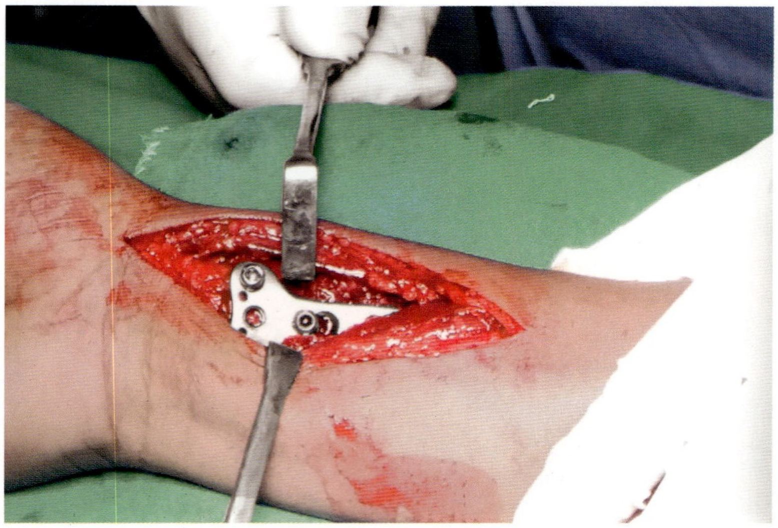

Fig. 14: Distal locking screws are placed in metaphysis of distal fragment.

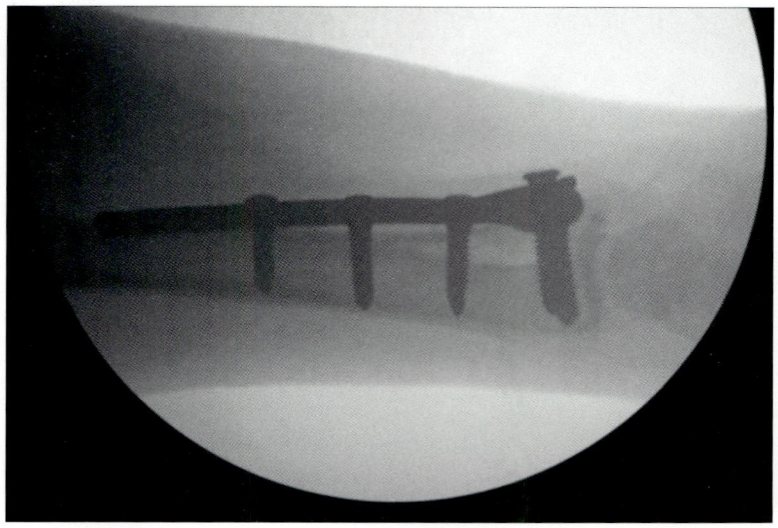

Fig. 15: C-arm lateral image showing final plate and screw construct.

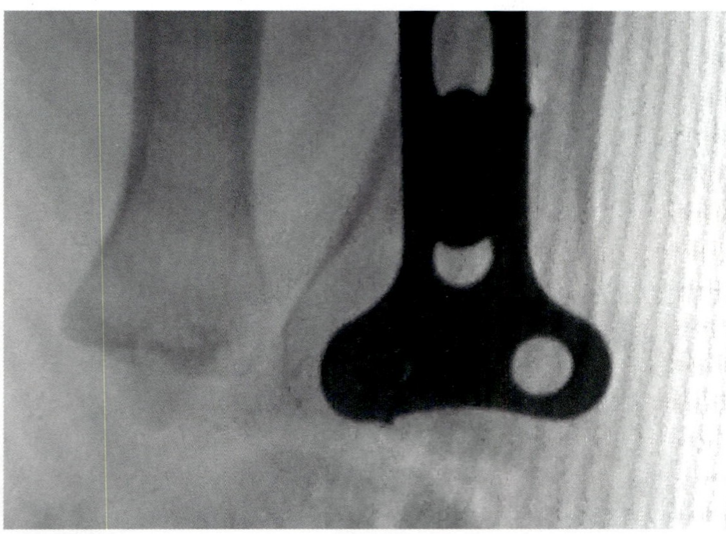

Fig. 16: C-arm posteroanterior (PA) view showing satisfactory fracture alignment and plate position.

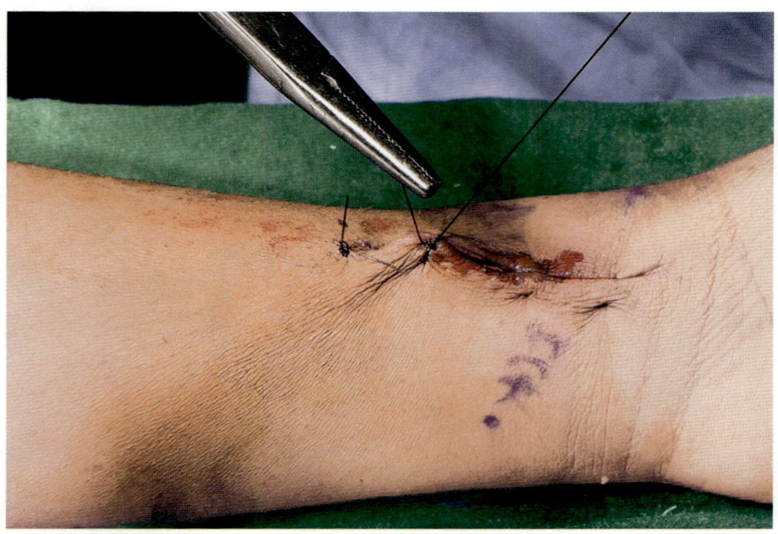

Fig. 17: After proper antiseptic wound wash, closure done in layers.

SUGGESTED READING

1. Abbaszadegan H, Johnsson U, von Sivers K. Prediction of instability of Colles' fractures. Acta Orthop Scand. 1989;60:646-50.
2. Barton JR. Views and treatment of an important injury to the wrist. Philadelphia Med Exam. 1838;1:365-8.
3. Illarramendi A, Gonzalez DV, Segal E, et al. Evaluation of simplified Frykman and AO classifications of fractures of the distal radius. Assessment of interobserver and intraobserver agreement. Int Orthop. 1998;22:111-5.
4. Kreder HJ, Hanel DP, Agel J, et al. Indirect reduction and percutaneous fixation versus open reduction and internal fixation for displaced intra-articular fractures of the distal radius: a randomised, controlled trial. J Bone Joint Surg Br. 2005;87(6):829-36.
5. LaFontaine M, Hardy D, Delince PH. Stability assessment of distal radius fractures. Injury. 1989;20:208-10.
6. Mackenney PJ, McQueen MM, Elton R. Prediction of instability in distal radial fractures. J Bone Joint Surg Am. 2006;88(9):1944-51.
7. Mehara AK, Rastogi S, Bhan S, et al. Classification and treatment of volar Barton fractures. Injury. 1993;24(1):55-9.
8. Rikli DA, Regazzoni P. Fractures of the distal end of the radius treated by internal fixation and early function. J Bone Joint Surg Br. 1996;78:588-92.
9. Thompson PW, Taylor J, Dawson A. The annual incidence and seasonal variation of fractures of the distal radius in men and women over 25 years in Dorset, UK. Injury. 2004;35(5):462-6.

CHAPTER 40

Carpal Tunnel Syndrome Surgical Release

Prahalad Kumar Singhi, Prateek Charuchandra Joshi

INTRODUCTION

It is the condition in which the median nerve is compressed in the "carpal tunnel", which is the interval between the carpal bones at a deeper level and the flexor retinaculum superficially. The flexor retinaculum (transverse carpal ligament) is a sheet of connective tissue between the hook of hamate and pisiform bone medially and the scaphoid tubercle laterally. The carpal tunnel is tightly packed with not only the median nerve, but also the flexor pollicis longus, flexor digitorum superficialis and flexor digitorum profundus tendons, with a normal intracompartment pressure of approximately 2.5 mm Hg. An increase in the pressure causes compression neuropathy to the median nerve. Obesity, diabetes, pregnancy, thyroid disorders, and glycogen storage disorders, especially in children, are the commonly implicated causes of carpal tunnel syndrome. In many patients there may be no obvious cause. It may be bilateral in many patients. The disorder generally presents as pain and paresthesias in the lateral 3½ digits on the palmar aspect; and with weakness of thenar musculature, especially thumb abductor. Clinically, diagnosis is made by considering the patient profile along with provocative tests such as Phalen's test. Electromyography (EMG) and nerve conduction studies may assist in diagnosis. Initial treatment is conservative. Surgery (carpal tunnel release) is offered to patients not responding to conservative treatment, and to those with gross weakness of the abductor pollicis brevis at presentation.

POSSIBLE COMPLICATIONS OF SURGERY

- Injury to underlying palmar cutaneous branch of median nerve.
- Inadvertent trauma to median nerve and the nearby tendons.
- Inadvertent trauma to palmar arch vessels.

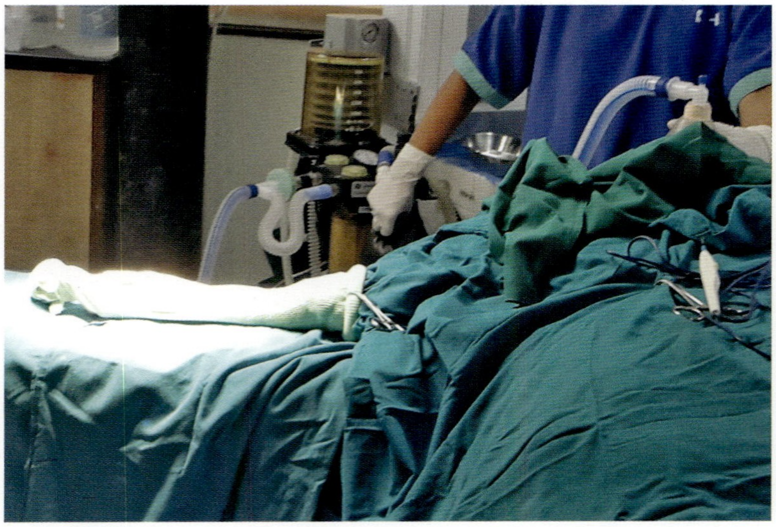

Fig. 1: Positioning of the patient. The patient is positioned supine with the arm in extension and supination on an arm rest. As per protocol, scrubbing of the limb, followed by painting with povidone iodine and draping with sterile drapes is done. A stockinette may be applied and a tourniquet may be used with exsanguination as per the surgeon's preference.

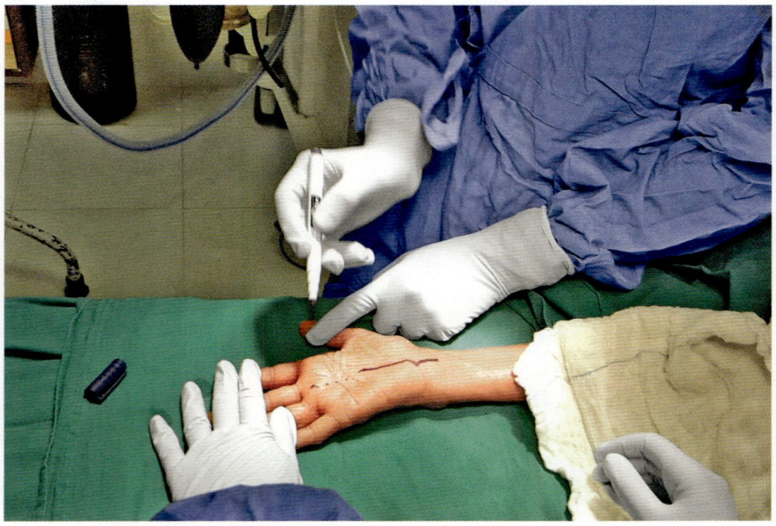

Fig. 2: The incision line being marked out using a sterile marker pen.

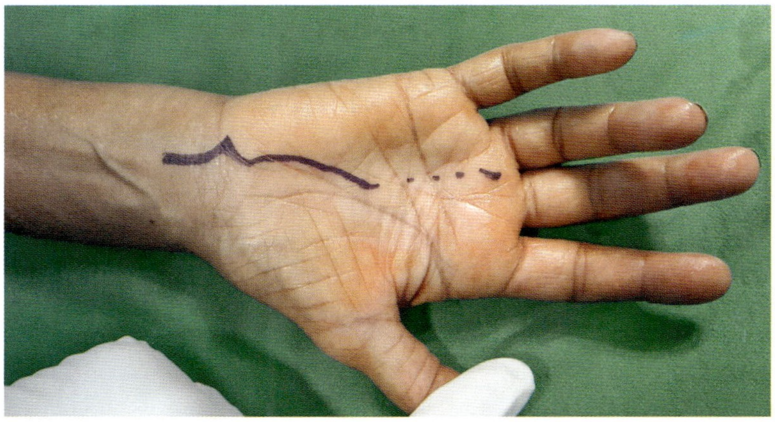

Fig. 3: The incision line starts proximal to the volar wrist crease. At the wrist, the incision is curved medially in order to avoid crossing the wrist crease at a right angle which would predispose to a hypertrophic scar limiting wrist motion. After crossing the wrist crease the incision is curved distally parallel to the thenar crease. The incision progresses distally till the proximal palmar crease.

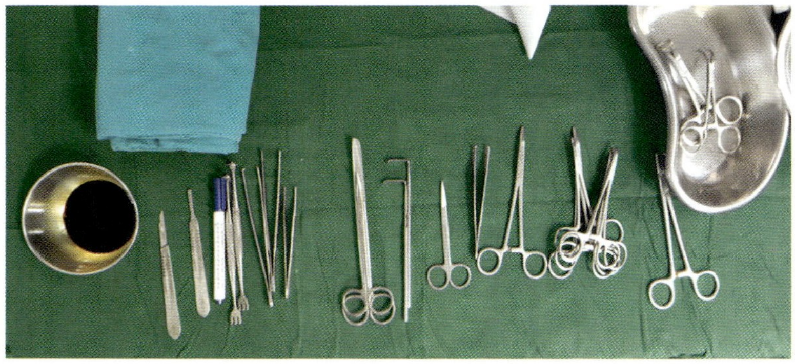

Fig. 4: The instrument trolley required for carpal tunnel release. General surgical instruments are sufficient for the procedure. In the image from left to right—povidone iodine for painting; small scalpel blades (No. 11 or 15) mounted on BP handles; sterile marker pen; cats paw retractors; toothed and plain forceps; stout scissors; right-angled retractors; tissue-cutting (dissecting) scissors; needle holders; artery forceps of all sizes; and towel clamps. Appropriate suture material for skin and subcutaneous tissue are required.

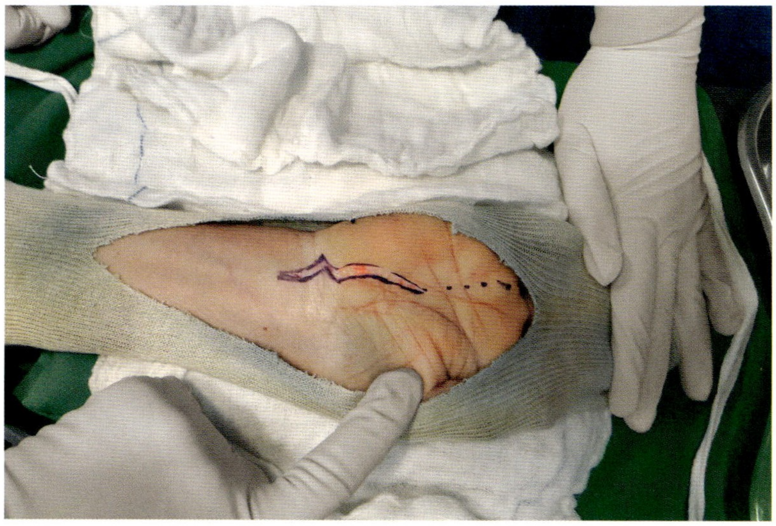

Fig. 5: Skin is incised along the line marked in Figure 3. Careful dissection should be undertaken to avoid iatrogenic injury to the palmar cutaneous branch of the median nerve which lies in close proximity to the incision. The tendon of palmaris longus is a subcutaneous landmark which can be used to appropriately place the incision.

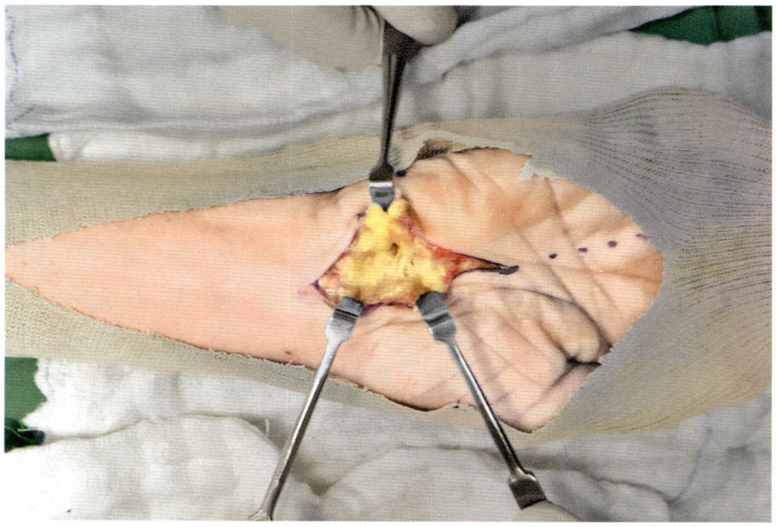

Fig. 6: The skin flaps are raised radially and ulnarly to expose the underlying subcutaneous fat, which is also dissected. The course of the palmar cutaneous branch of the median nerve is variable and hence dissection must be carried out meticulously.

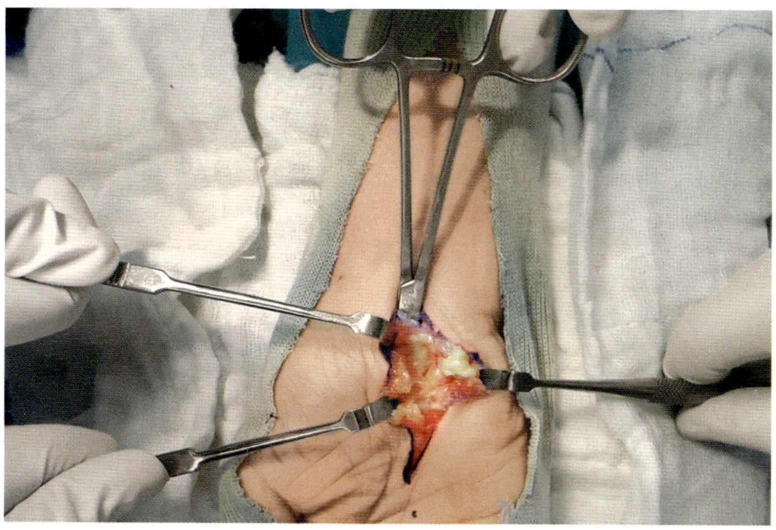

Fig. 7: Dissection is advanced to expose the insertion of the palmaris longus tendon into the transverse carpal ligament. Further dissection delineates the median nerve which lies between the tendons of palmaris longus and flexor carpi radialis. A blunt artery forceps is insinuated deep to the flexor retinaculum between the median nerve (deep) and the retinaculum which lies superficial to it.

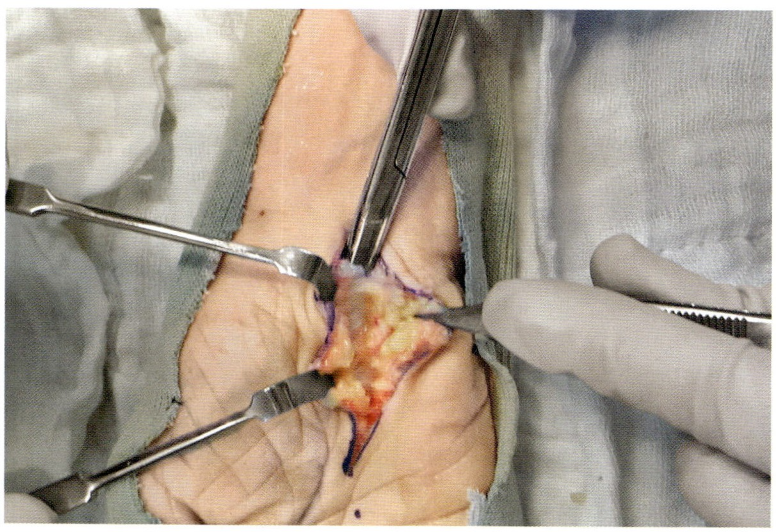

Fig. 8: The subretinacular plane created in Figure 7 is extended using a slender dissecting scissors.

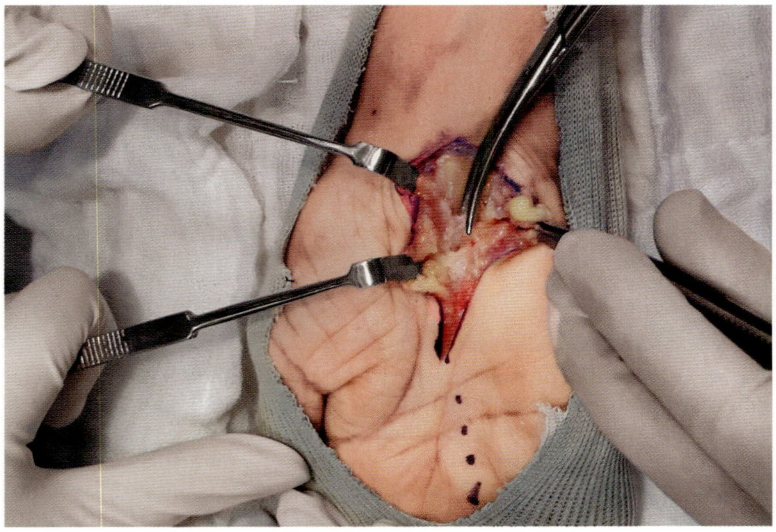

Fig. 9: The dissecting scissors is used to cautiously divide the flexor retinaculum throughout. The retinaculum should be divided longitudinally and ulnarly, in order to avoid the motor innervation to the thenar muscles.

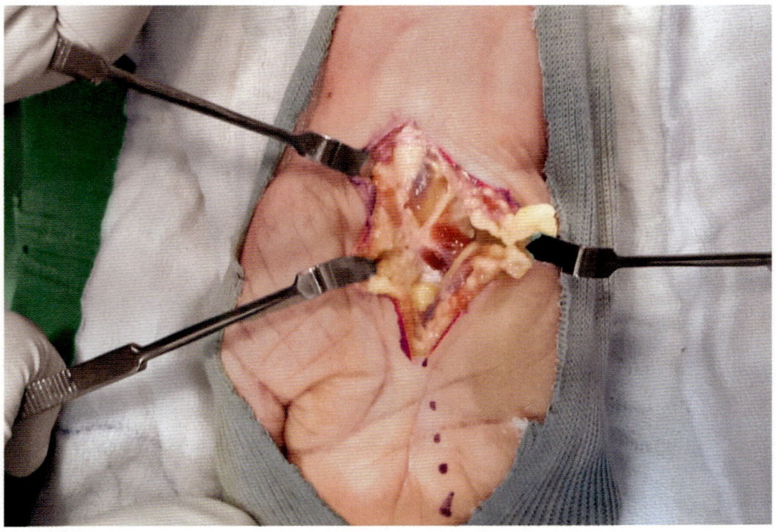

Fig. 10: The flexor retinaculum after being incised and retracted.

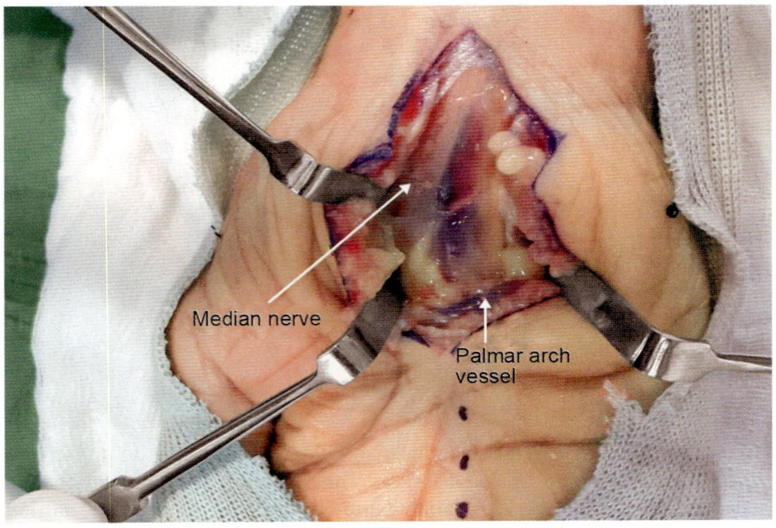

Fig. 11: Median nerve is now visualized after decompression. During division of the retinaculum, care should be taken to stop just short of the palmar arch vessels in order to prevent iatrogenic injury.

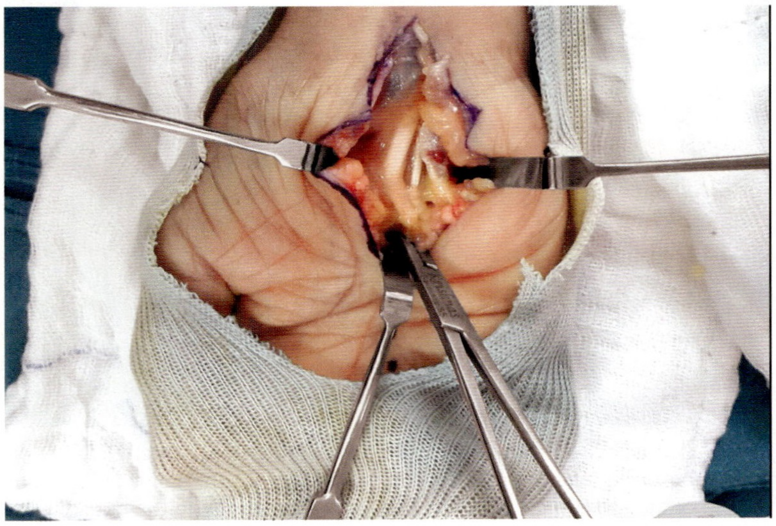

Fig. 12: After dissection is complete, median nerve lies free released from all the compressing fascia. Thorough wound wash is given. The retinaculum is not to be sutured back.

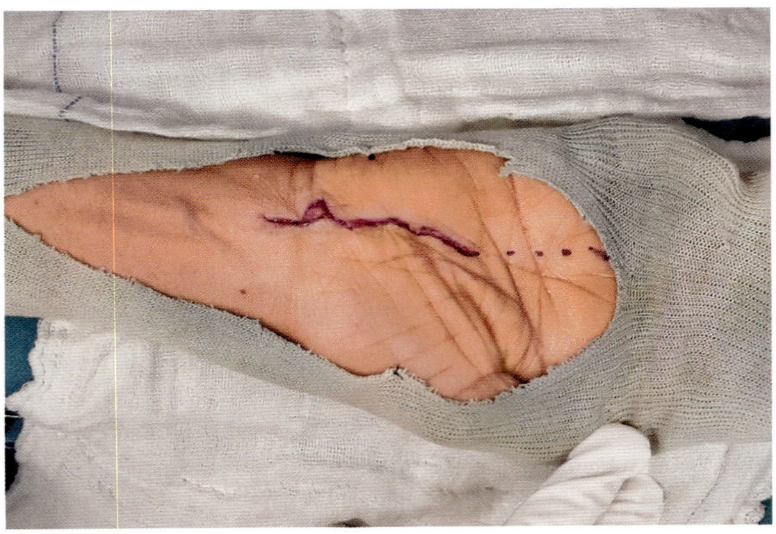

Fig. 13: Subcutaneous tissue is closed in line with the original incision.

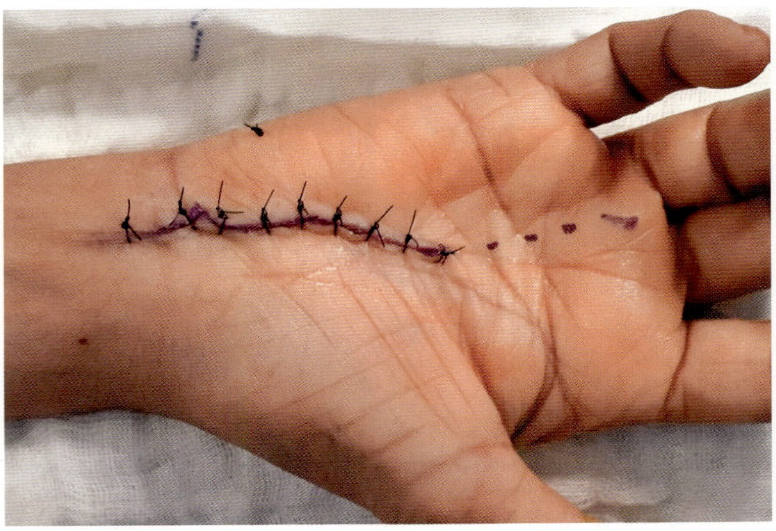

Fig. 14: Skin is closed using nonabsorbable sutures. Aseptic dressing is applied.

- Incomplete division of the flexor retinaculum, which may lead to recurrence.
- Surgical site infections and delayed wound healing which may be a complication of underlying comorbidities such as diabetes mellitus and thyroid disorders, which themselves predispose to carpal tunnel syndrome.
- In case the incision crosses the volar wrist crease at right angles, it may lead to hypertrophic scar later on, restricting wrist motion.

SUGGESTED READING

1. American Academy of Orthopaedic Surgeons. (2007). Clinical practice guideline on the diagnosis of carpal tunnel syndrome. [online] Available from http://www.aaos.org/Research/guidelines/CTS_guideline.pdf [Accessed October 2018].
2. Bland JDP, Rudolfer SM. Clinical surveillance of carpal tunnel syndrome in two areas of the United Kingdom, 1991–2001. J Neurol Neurosurg Psychiatry. 2003;74(12):1674-9.
3. Burton C, Chesterton L, Davenport G, et al. Developing agreed clinical criteria for the diagnosis of carpal tunnel syndrome in primary care—a clinical consensus exercise. Nottingham: Society of Academic Primary Care Annual Conference; 2013. p. 2E.2.
5. Ibrahim I, Khan WS, Goddard N, et al. Carpal tunnel syndrome: a review of the recent literature. Open Orthop J. 2012;6:69-76.
4. Latinovic R, Gulliford MC, Hughes RA. Incidence of common compressive neuropathies in primary care. J Neurol Neurosurg Psychiatry. 2006;77(2):263-5.

CHAPTER 41

Correction of Finger Contracture by Z-Plasty

Nilesh Dattatray Darawade

INTRODUCTION

Flexion contracture of fingers can result from myriad of causes both traumatic and nontraumatic. The list of possible pathological tissue responsible covers almost entire anatomy of finger starting from skin, deep fascia, flexor sheath, flexor tendons, collateral ligaments, and specialized capsular structures such as volar plate and bone itself. The structures missing from this list, the digital nerves and arteries although rarely responsible for contracture, tend to have a defining say during treatment of contracture by operative means, especially a severe contracture. The intention of this chapter is demonstration of correction of flexion contracture of fingers by Z-plasty and hence the discussion regarding pathophysiology will be limited to cases where Z-plasty is most appropriate choice.

PATHOLOGICAL ANATOMY AND CLINICAL EVALUATION

When dealing with a flexion contracture of finger, a surgeon should try and locate the structures contributing to contracture. History of trauma or its absence provides a broad pathway to possible pathogenesis. For example, absence of trauma in an elderly patient with prominent cords indicates pathology to be Dupuytren's contracture. History of trauma needs more work to narrow down structures involved. On examination, if the contracture of joint does not improve by change in position of adjacent joints e.g. proximal interphalangeal (PIP) contracture cannot be passively corrected at least partially by flexing metacarpophalangeal (MCP) joint, then joint capsule or bone itself is contributing to the pathology. If active range of motion is less than passive range, involvement of tendon should be suspected.

RADIOLOGICAL EVALUATION

For finger contracture, as in trauma cases true lateral radiograph should be taken for correct evaluation of bone. Bony changes are rarely seen such as in chronic contractures beginning in childhood when bone remodeling may be present or if there is arthrodesis or malunion. Presence of bony changes is indicative of compromised outcome. In cases where etiology lies in skin/subcutaneous tissue for contracture (cases where Z-plasty can correct contracture), bone should be normal apart from visible flexion attitude of the joint.

TREATMENT PHILOSOPHY

Z-plasty by itself can correct contractures primarily originating from skin and subcutaneous tissues only. Presence of palpable cord along volar aspect of finger with relative sparing of surrounding skin and rest of structures responds well to Z-plasty alone. This is commonly seen as after effect of a longitudinal wound over volar aspect of finger, rarely in post burn deformities as burns tend to involve wider surface area. Once a wider area of skin is involved and/or deeper structures are contributing substantially to contracture, Z-plasty tends to become an adjunct to the main surgery and sometimes may not be even useful to close the wounds. While treating a finger contracture, surgeon should be ready with further armamentarium namely skin grafting, flap cover to wounds, flexor tenolysis or tendon reconstruction, arthrolysis, etc.

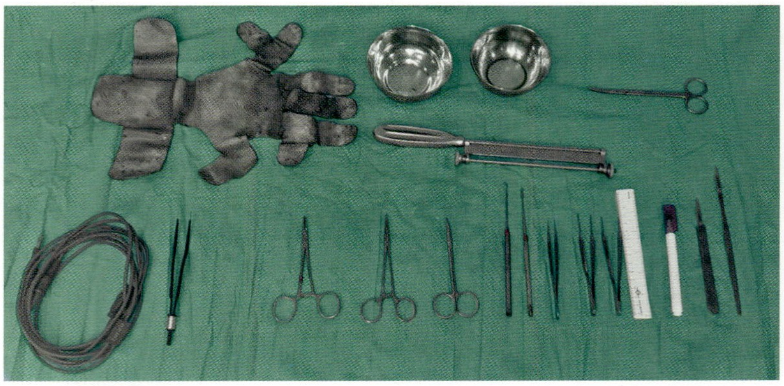

Fig. 1: Lead hand reduces need for one assistant and increases working space of surgeon. Bipolar cautery is essential in hand cases when important digital arteries are near dissection. A surgical marker should be considered an essential instrument and not using one creates unnecessary misery. Rest of instruments viz. toothed forceps, needle holders, dissecting scissors are finer than routine orthopaedic instrument set. In addition, use of pneumatic tourniquet is essential for safe and clear dissection.

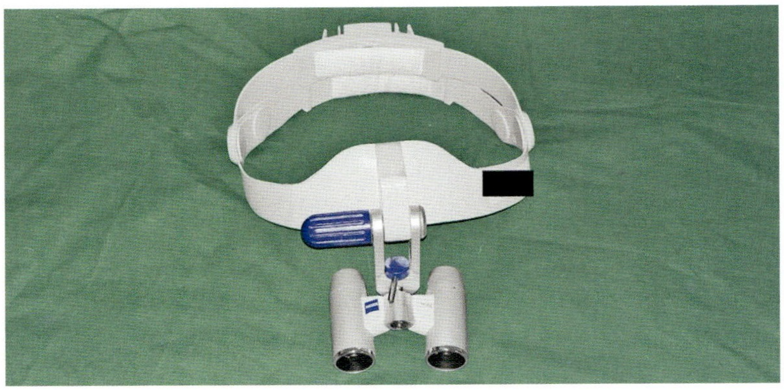

Fig. 2: Using magnifying loupes is essential when operating on hand.

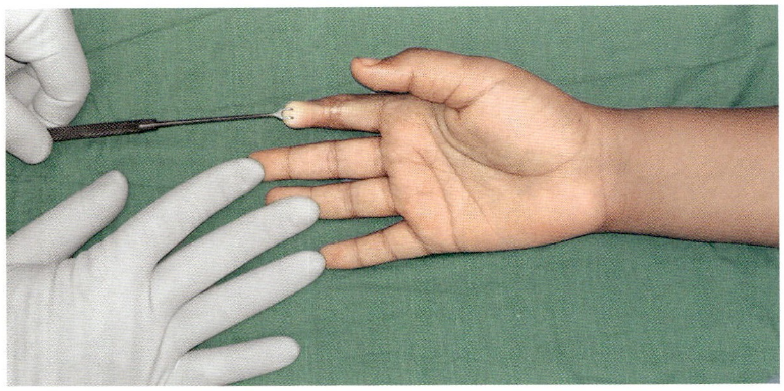

Fig. 3: Flexion contracture in index finger demonstrated. This was an old electric burn injury in a 10-year-old boy. Interphalangeal joints could be extended halfway from resting position after metacarpophalangeal joint flexion.

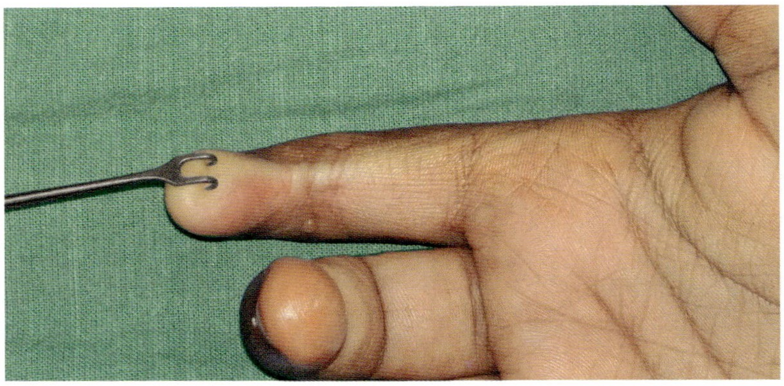

Fig. 4: A closer look at the volar cord primarily responsible for flexion contracture.

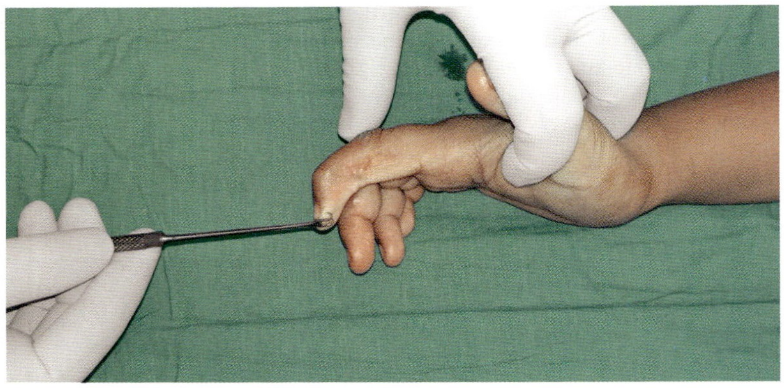

Fig. 5: Lateral clinical view demonstrating 40° flexion attitude at proximal interphalangeal (PIP) joint and 50° at distal interphalangeal (DIP) joint with attempted passive correction.

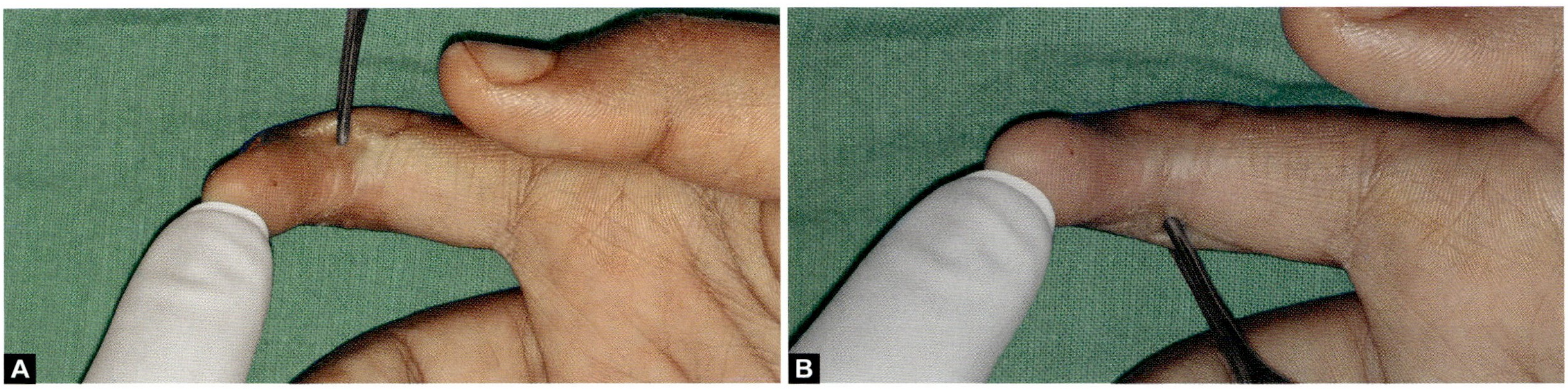

Figs. 6A and B: Pliability of skin on either side of cord demonstrated. If this region of skin is fibrotic and nonpliable, Z-plasty is unlikely to work. A Z-plasty utilizes lax skin adjacent to contracture and brings it along the line of contracture, Z-plasty will not close if there is adherent scar and effective shortening of skin in lateral region.

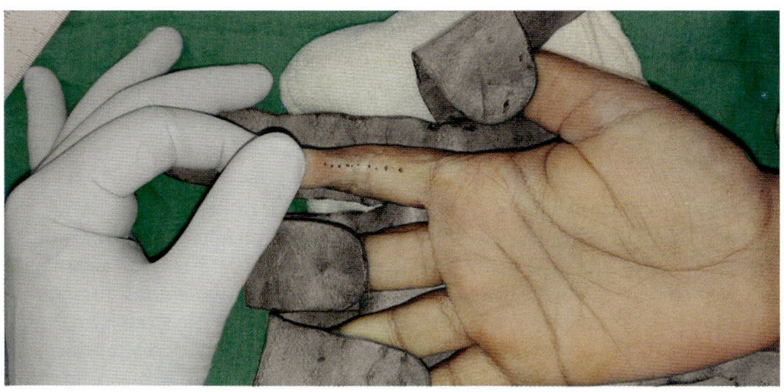

Fig. 7: Cord is marked along its length.

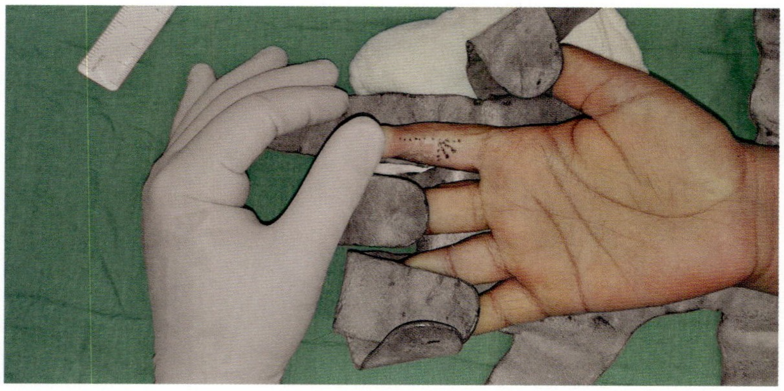

Fig. 8: Ideal angle of Z is 60°. This has been devised with experience as a good compromise between maximum length possible to gain in line of contracture and ability to get wound closure without undue tension on suture lines. Theoretically angles greater than 60° would gain more length along contracture, but the wound closure may become too tight. If the surgeon is more worried about wound closure then angles smaller than 60° will be safer. One way of ensuring angle in this case is to mark a perpendicular to longitudinal line and divide it into equal thirds. Two-thirds from longitudinal line should give us an angle of 60°. One can use small templates to mark angles if available.

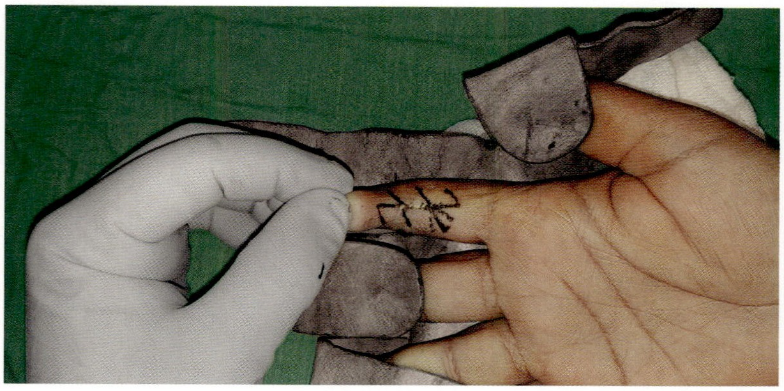

Fig. 9: Once the proximal Z has been marked, three Z-plasties are marked in series. It is very important to measure each arm of Z and keep all three arms of equal length. Making multiple Z-plasties in series distributes the tension in lateral soft tissues, after transposition of flaps across wider region ensures better closure and viability of tissues. Taking time to mark the flaps is first necessary part of surgery before making any incision.

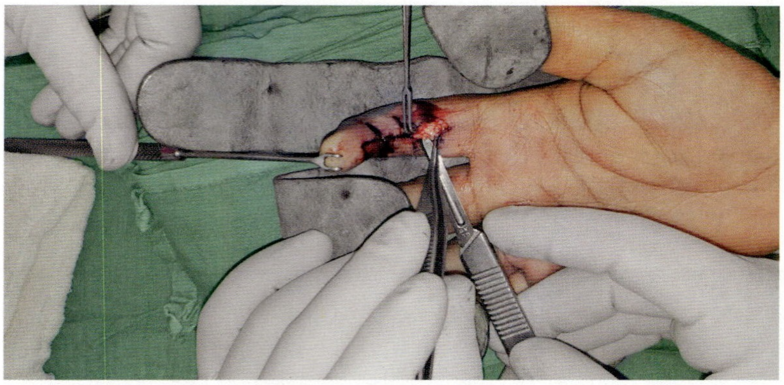

Fig. 10: Making the incision and raising flaps. Flaps are raised as thick as possible to ensure good blood flow till tip of flaps. However, once contracture band is released it is safer to prevent exposure of flexor tendon/sheath.

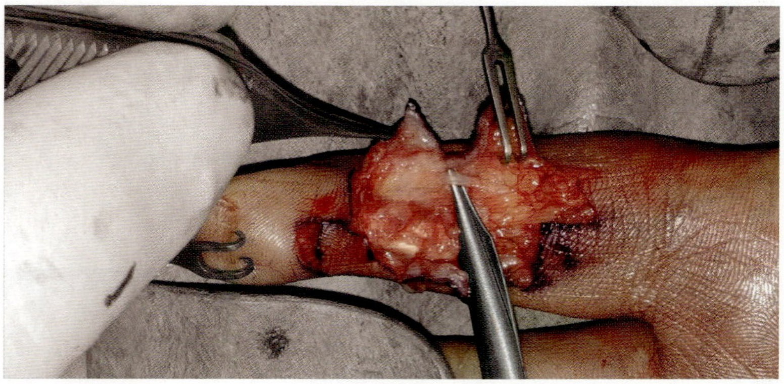

Fig. 11: Neurovascular bundles are quite close. It is safer to locate them to prevent inadvertent injury. Here radial digital nerve is isolated, digital artery lies directly beneath (dorsal) it.

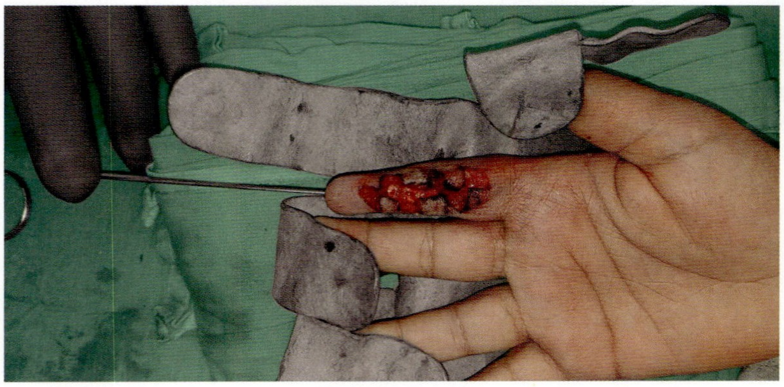

Fig. 12: Flaps from all three Z-plasties are raised. Notice the tendency of flaps to align themselves along the defects intended for transposition. Flexor sheath can be seen in midline. A 1.2 mm K-wire is used to transfix distal interphalangeal (DIP) joint. Use of K-wire is optional. The tourniquet has been deflated. Notice the discoloration of fingertip.

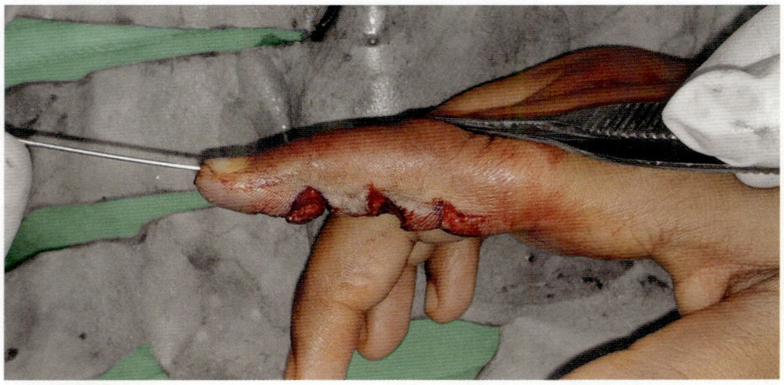

Fig. 13: Lateral clinical view of finger after release of contracture band. It is not necessary to get complete correction intraoperatively. In fact, sometimes it may to undesirable due to risk it poses on digital artery. It is author's practice to correct contractures more than 70–80° in two stages, first with a dynamic fixator and then Z-plasty to prevent excessive acute stretch on digital arteries. Despite such precautions it is usual to see a dysvascular fingertip at the time of release of tourniquet when finger is held with a K-wire in situ.

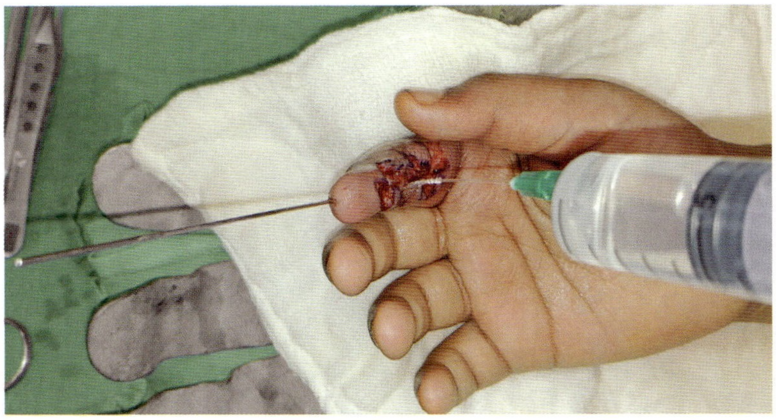

Fig. 14: In majority of cases, despite meticulous care of arteries they respond to acute correction by initial vasospasm. Thankfully this phenomenon is mostly transient and one needs to have patient and calm mind to tide over this period. Simply awaiting release of vasospasm is what is mostly needed. The process can be aided by increasing ambient temperature by switching off air conditioning if possible. It is handy to have mechanism to get warm sterile saline. In my practice before release of tourniquet I ask to keep couple of bottles of saline in hot water. Bathing the finger in warm saline helps in relief of vasoconstriction. In this figure, one can appreciate the pink fingertip after irrigation of finger with warm saline. Rarely, despite all these measures and waiting for 10–15 minutes if fingertip remains ischemic, I would remove K-wire and flex the finger. This will certainly relieve vasospasm. Then surgeon may choose to reinsert K-wire in new position with less extension than before or may forego it altogether. In this case, I did not attempt to transfix proximal interphalangeal (PIP) joint in extension to keep some pliability on vessels.

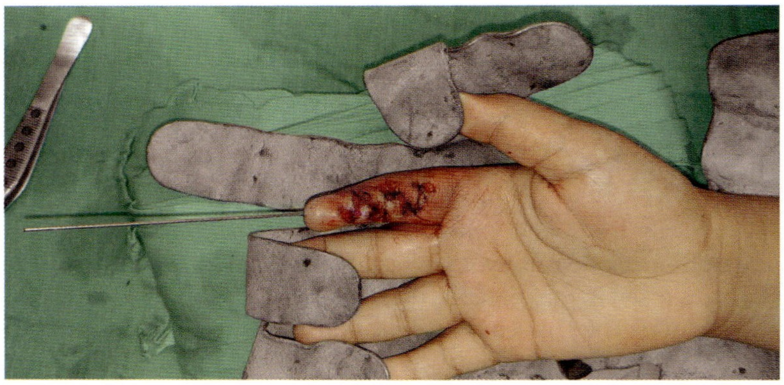

Fig. 15: Initial sutures are placed to assess relatively tension free transposition of flaps. If flaps are difficult to transpose one may reassess dissection at base of flap. If closure still seems tight, it is better to accept some gaping with secondary healing or application of split thickness skin graft than risking ischemia of flap by tight closure.

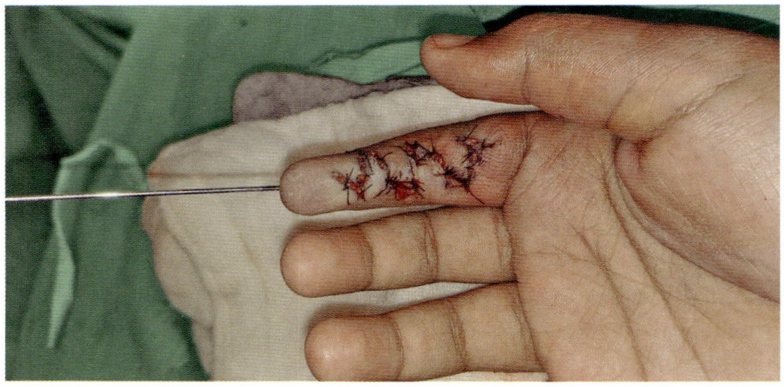

Fig. 16: Complete closure with transposition of flaps. In pediatric cases, I prefer use of absorbable suture material for skin closure 4-0 in this case. The K-wire was kept outside the skin and removed at 3 weeks. I prefer to apply a below elbow splint up to fingertips till suture removal for patient comfort and better compliance for limb elevation. I agree it is not mandatory and it is a matter of surgeon's choice.

SUGGESTED READING

1. McGregor A, McGregor I. Fundamental Techniques of Plastic Surgery and Their Surgical Applications, 10th edition. London, United Kingdom: Churchill Livingstone; 2000.
2. Wolfe S, Pederson W, Kozin SH. Green's Operative Hand Surgery, 6th edition. PA, USA: Elsevier Churchill Livingstone; 2011.

CHAPTER 42

Scaphoid Nonunion: Screw Fixation and Bone Grafting

Nilesh Dattatray Darawade

INTRODUCTION

Scaphoid is the most commonly fractured carpal bone. Due to oblique orientation of scaphoid in relation to both sagittal and coronal planes, it is difficult to evaluate scaphoid in standard orthogonal radiographs of wrist. Even with dedicated scaphoid views, e.g. wrist posteroanterior (PA) in ulnar deviation or oblique views of wrist, an undisplaced fracture may be missed due to cancellous bony composition of scaphoid. Unsurprisingly these fractures are commonly detected late and treatment of nonunion is fairly common.

PATHOANATOMY AND CLASSIFICATION

Scaphoid receives its blood supply in retrograde manner from dorsal carpal branch of radial artery (70–80%) and superficial palmar branch of radial artery (20–30%). There is some contribution from radioscapholunate ligament (ligament of Testut) as well. This retrograde blood flow increases the chances of avascular necrosis of proximal fragment after fractures. The more proximal the fracture line, higher is the risk of nonunion and avascular necrosis.

Scaphoid has been described as "tie-rod" of carpal joint. It is the only carpal bone bridging proximal and distal carpal rows. This unique role contributes to high forces at fracture site leading to nonunion and humpback deformity. In cases of nonunion, especially of waist fractures distal fragment tends to fall in palmar flexion and proximal tends to dorsiflex. This leads to resorption of volar margins of fractures leading to a dorsal apex convexity at nonunion, known as humpback deformity. Nonunion of scaphoid, if untreated will lead to progressive arthritis of radiocarpal and intercarpal joints, known as scaphoid nonunion advanced collapse (SNAC) wrist. Presence of SNAC element changes the approach to treat scaphoid nonunion. There are multiple classifications described for scaphoid nonunion. A practical way of classification is as follows:

- Nonunion of waist fracture, no arthritis or malalignment, and stable
- Nonunion of waist, no to minimal SNAC wrist (up to type 1), and humpback deformity
- Nonunion of proximal pole fracture and no arthritis
- Nonunion of waist fracture, SNAC type 2/3 arthritis
- Nonunion of proximal pole fracture, no arthritis, nonsalvageable (<5 mm fragment).

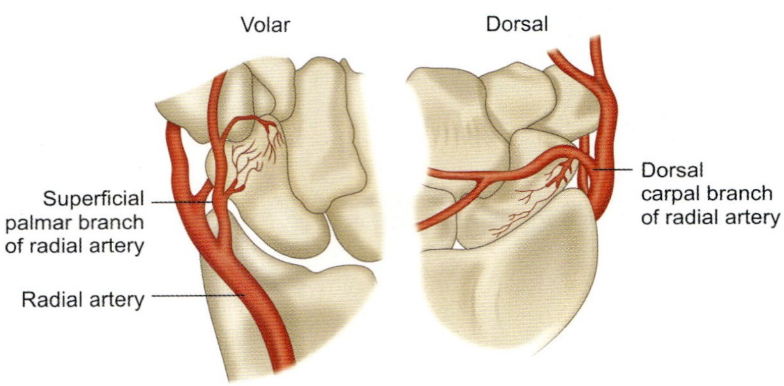

Fig. 1: Scaphoid blood supply.

CLINICAL FEATURES

Patients will commonly complain of radial sided wrist pain, difficulty in doing heavy activities with affected hand. In chronic cases patients may recognize restricted range of motion. On examination in addition to snuffbox tenderness and restricted range there may be decreased grip and pinch strength as compared to unaffected side.

INVESTIGATIONS

A scaphoid series, which includes wrist PA view in ulnar deviation, lateral view, pronation, and supination oblique views are utilized. Surgeon should assess for presence of dorsal intercalated segmental instability (DISI) deformity in lateral view. A computed tomography scan of wrist is especially useful to assess humpback deformity and plan surgical correction for same. In long standing nonunion or in nonunion of proximal pole fractures magnetic resonance imaging (MRI) is used to assess for avascular necrosis of proximal fragment.

TREATMENT OPTIONS

There is plethora of approaches for treatment of scaphoid nonunion depending on site of nonunion, presence/absence of humpback deformity, presence of avascular necrosis of proximal fragment, and presence of variable grades of SNAC arthritis of wrist. For detailed discussion of strategies, reader is directed to standard textbooks including Green's operative hand surgery. For sake of completion we will enumerate the strategies used—open reduction and internal fixation (ORIF) with nonvascularized bone graft by Matti-Russe technique (volar approach), ORIF with nonvascularized bone graft through dorsal approach, Fernandez wedge graft technique, vascularized bone graft, and fixation of scaphoid with 1–2 intercompartmental supraretinacular artery (ICSRA) pedicle/volar carpal artery pedicle/dorsal capsule pedicle/free medial condyle femoral graft. For cases of SNAC wrist in stage 1, one can reconstruct scaphoid nonunion with excision of radial styloid; for advanced SNAC however, excision of scaphoid with limited carpal fusion or formal wrist arthrodesis will be necessary.

In the following text we have demonstrated treatment of a stable scaphoid nonunion at waist without humpback deformity or DISI deformity or SNAC wrist.

This case demonstrates scaphoid waist nonunion in right wrist of 40 years old gentleman of 6 months duration. Nonunion was diagnosed with clinical suspicion and on computed tomography scan as radiographs were inconclusive. However, I would like to add this is an exception and good scaphoid and oblique views are usually enough to show nonunion. In this case there was no humpback deformity probably owing to relatively short course of nonunion and procedure was performed accordingly. In presence of a dorsal intercalated segmental instability (DISI) deformity and/or humpback deformity the procedure would need modifications from the following steps.

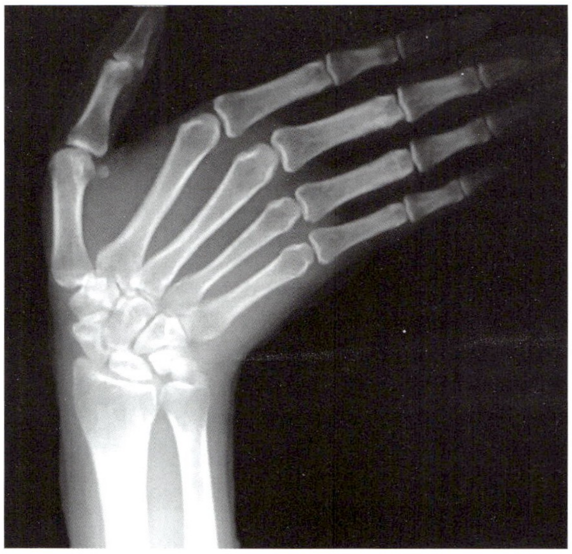

Fig. 2: Preoperative 1

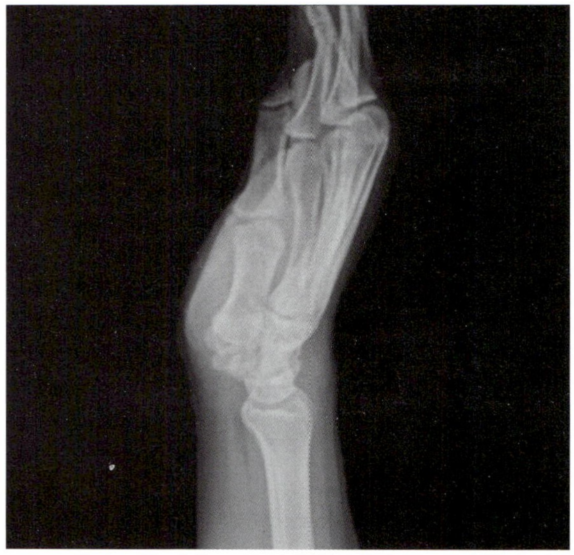

Fig. 3: Preoperative 2

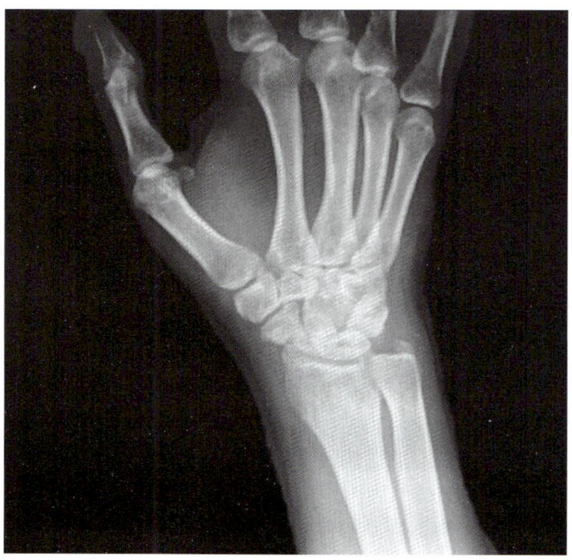

Fig. 4: Preoperative 3

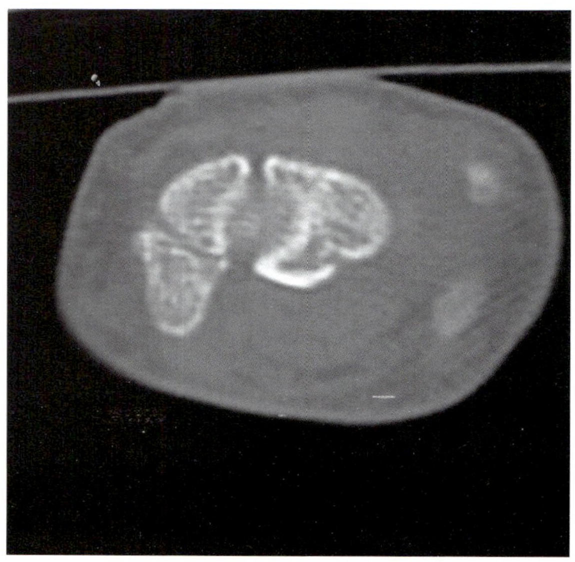

Fig. 5: Preoperative CT 2

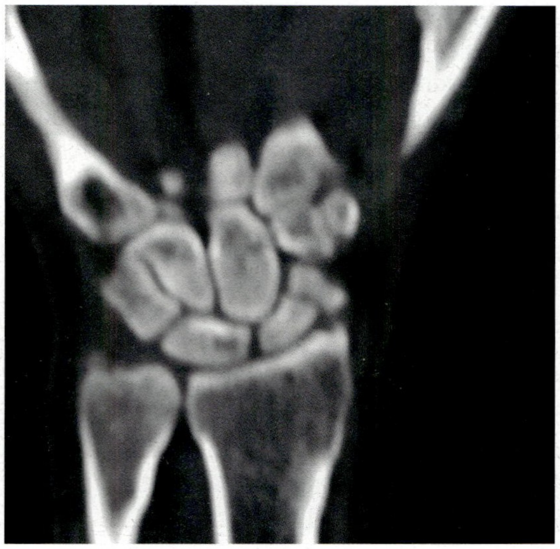

Fig. 6: Preoperative CT

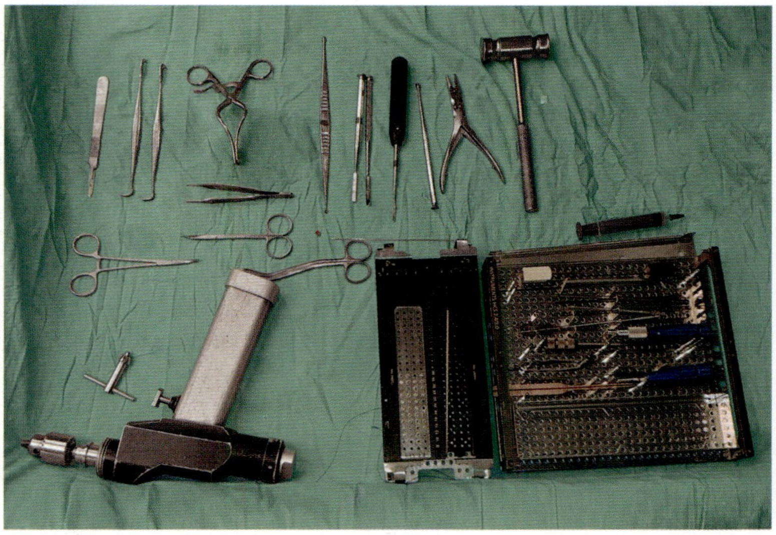

Fig. 7: A headless compression screw set, sharp small (0.5–1 cm) osteotome, power drill, and routine other orthopaedic instruments. I do use magnifying loupes, although one can do same surgery without one.

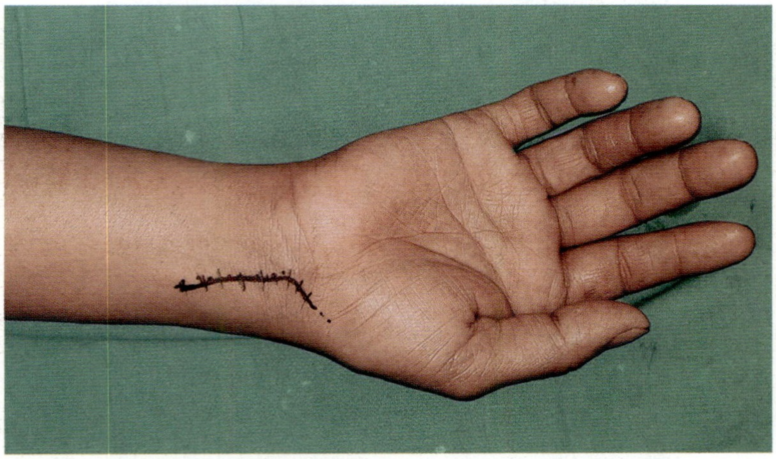

Fig. 8: Incision is marked in the shape of a hockey stick. Longitudinal arm is along flexor carpi radialis (FCR) tendon with a curve at distal wrist crease and incision continuing towards thumb. Limb exsanguinated gently and tourniquet raised.

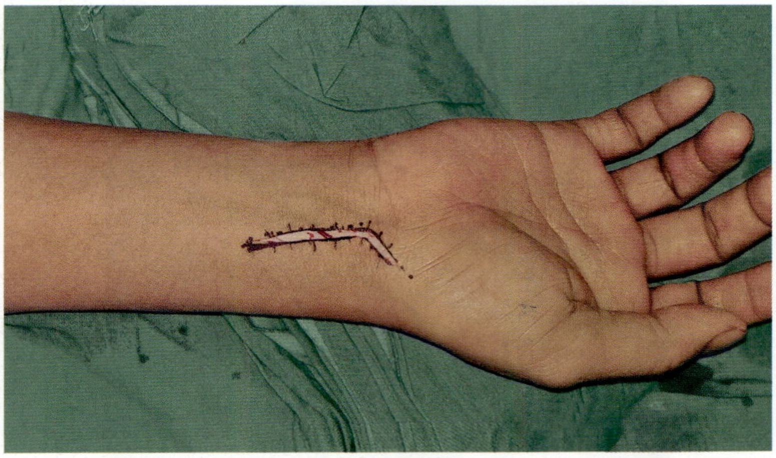

Fig. 9: Incision made along the marking. It is common to find superficial veins and I prefer to ligate vein as big as the one seen in this Figure. I prefer to apply Esmarch bandage lightly to try and retain some blood in veins before raising tourniquet. This makes identification and ligature/coagulation of veins much easier and control of bleeding after deflating tourniquet more manageable.

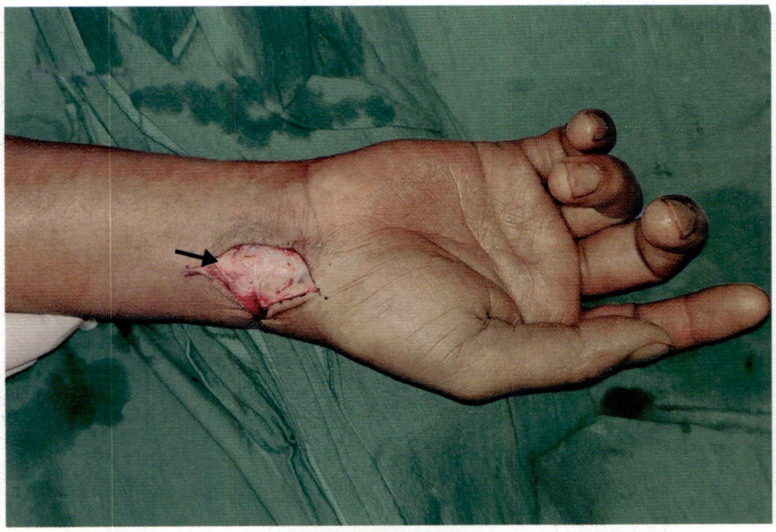

Fig. 10: Superficial dissection. Flexor carpi radialis (FCR) is seen under its sheath, marked by arrow here. Suturing the curved skin flap radially eases retraction.

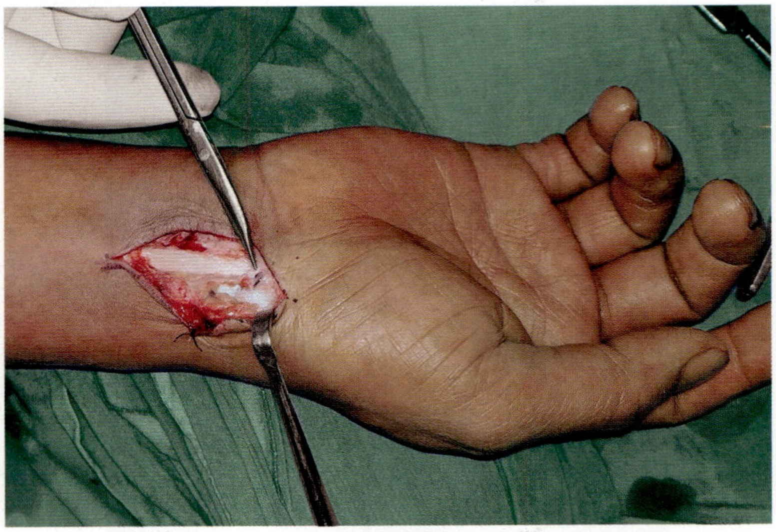

Fig. 11: Flexor carpi radialis (FCR) sheath is opened to expose the tendon. It is common to see superficial branch of radial artery in distal part of wound as shown here with a fine scissor. One can safely ligate it if it hampers exposure of scaphoid.

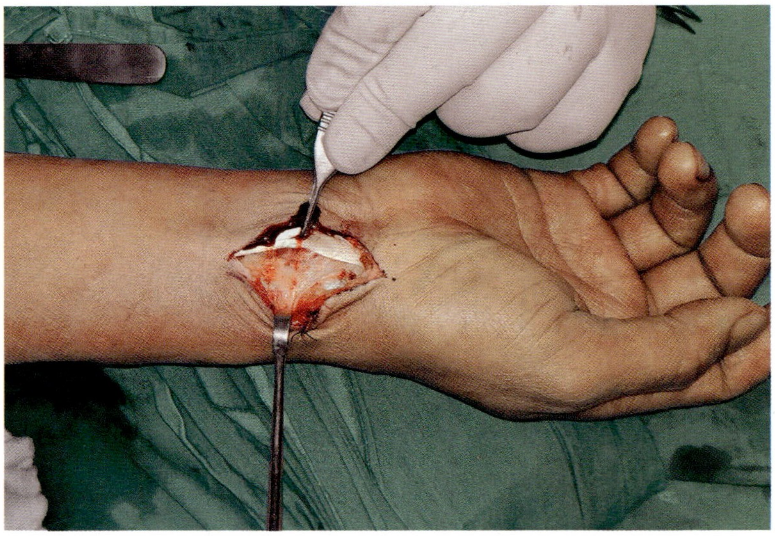

Fig. 12: Flexor carpi radialis (FCR) tendon retracted to expose subsheath. Subsheath is opened sharply.

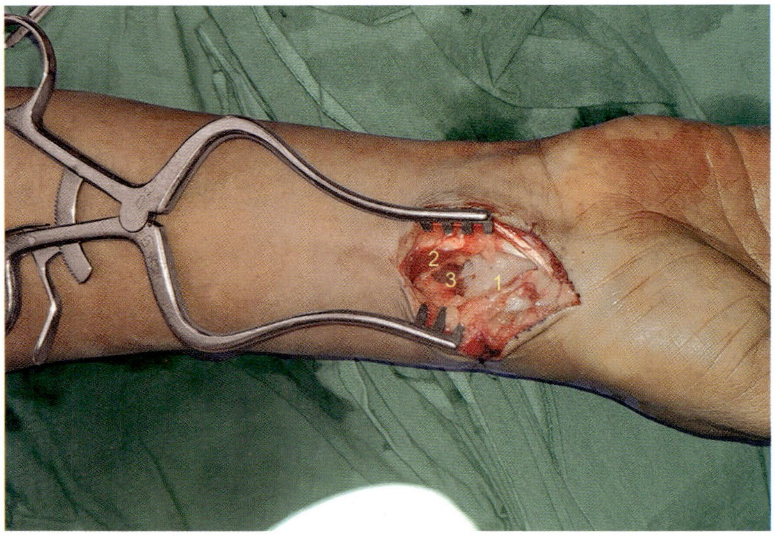

Fig. 13: After opening subsheath of flexor carpi radialis (FCR), fat is cleared off to expose wrist joint capsule (marked as 1). Numerical 2 denotes muscle tendon unit of flexor pollicis longus (FPL) and 3 denotes distal part of pronator quadratus muscle.

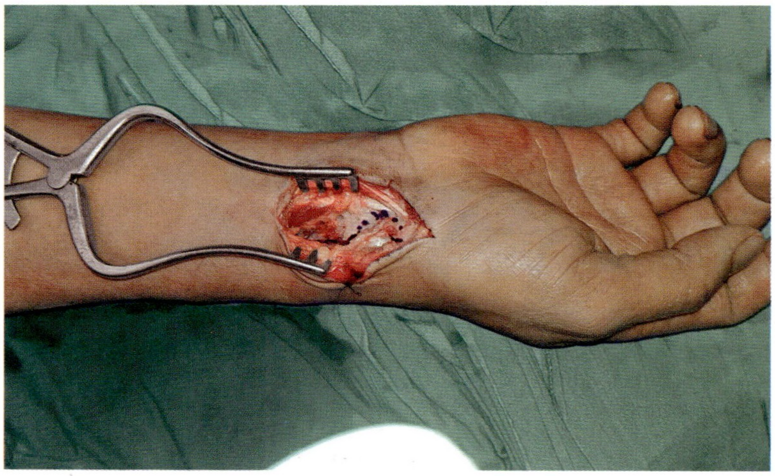

Fig. 14: Incision marked for capsulotomy. This curvilinear incision is described by Garcia Elias with the intention to split volar ligaments. One may divide capsule longitudinally along the long axis of scaphoid as well. In either situation, careful repair of ligament and capsule is very important.

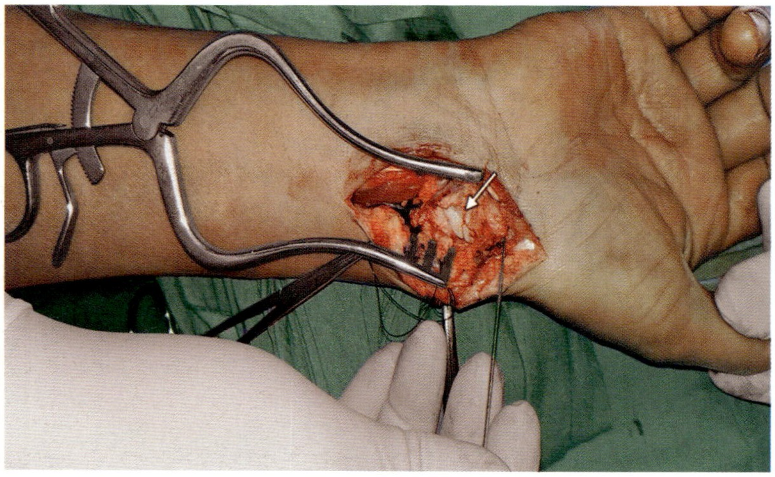

Fig. 15: The wrist capsule along with volar ligaments are sharply reflected off volar aspect of scaphoid. Arrow indicates nonunion site. A small K-wire indicates scaphotrapezial joint space.

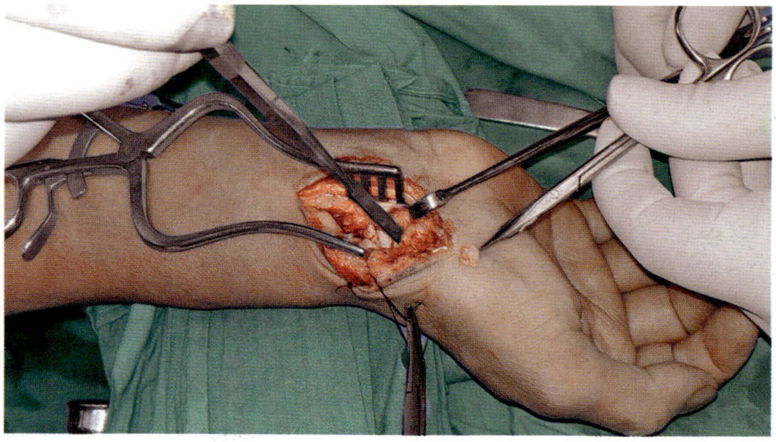

Fig. 16: Fracture surfaces of both fragments freshened with small osteotome to expose healthy bone. The scissor indicates removal of sclerotic margin of proximal fragment.

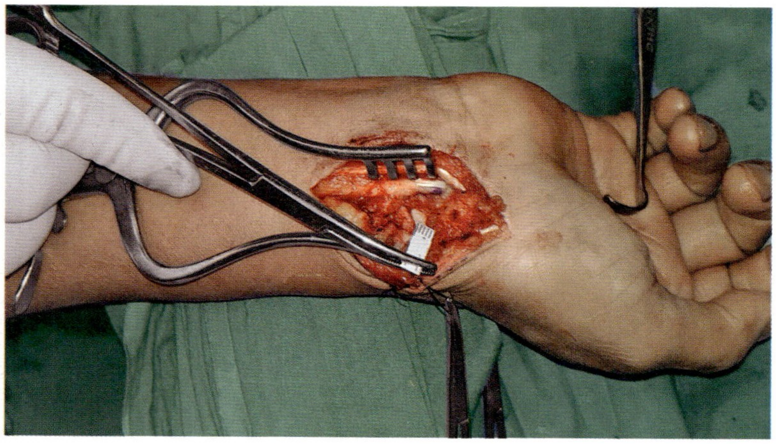

Fig. 17: Once the nonunion site is cleaned, the bony defect is measured. It is beneficial if dorsal cortex is not shaved off completely as this maintains the length of scaphoid.

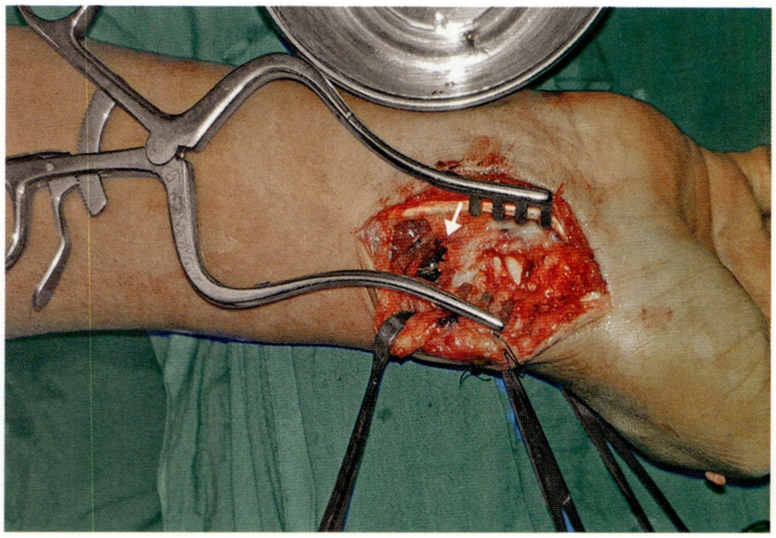

Fig. 18: Bone graft harvested from distal radius (arrow). I try to remove a single bone piece from volar radius with dimensions similar to the defect measured. I osteotomized only volar cortex, rest five surfaces are cancellous. After that more cancellous bone is harvested from residual window to pack in between both fragments. The gap at nonunion site after freshening of margins is seen well here.

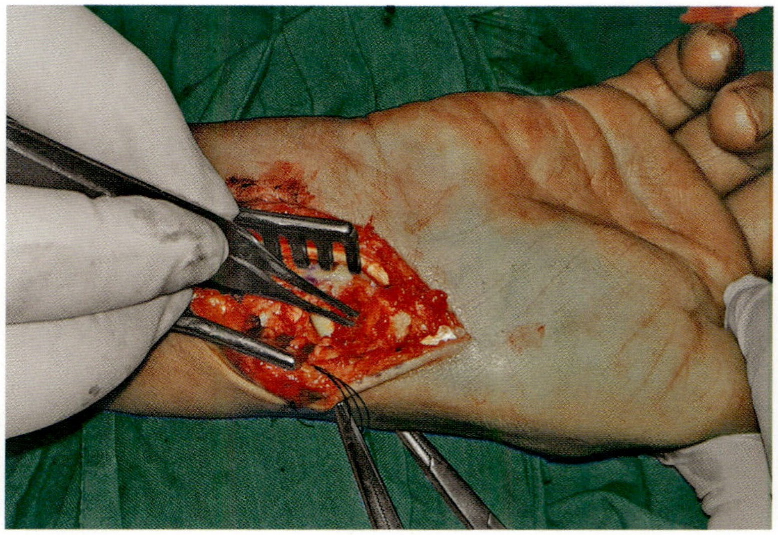

Fig. 19: Scaphoid fragments are aligned with wrist extension and ulnar deviation. A thick folded sheet under distal radius is immensely useful to achieve this position. This opens up nonunion site which is packed with bone graft.

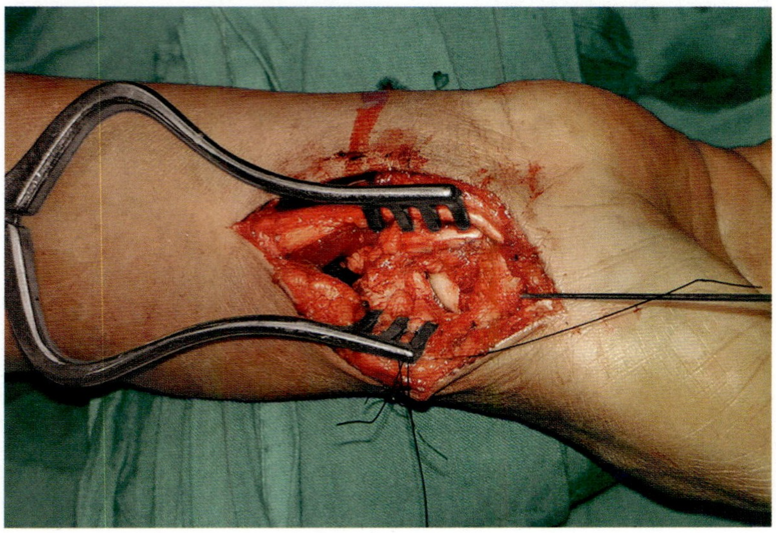

Fig. 20: If clinically alignment appears satisfactory, reduction is held with a guidewire along intended screw path. It is my practice to remove 2–3 mm bone of volar, proximal trapezium to get a more central location for guidewire. If surgeon would rather avoid this, one should hyperextend and ulnar deviate wrist to get trapezium out of way of guidewire. Extra precaution is needed afterwards to avoid bend in wire at this location. One useful guide for correct wire insertion is to aim towards radial tubercle in addition to visualization of proximal half of scaphoid.

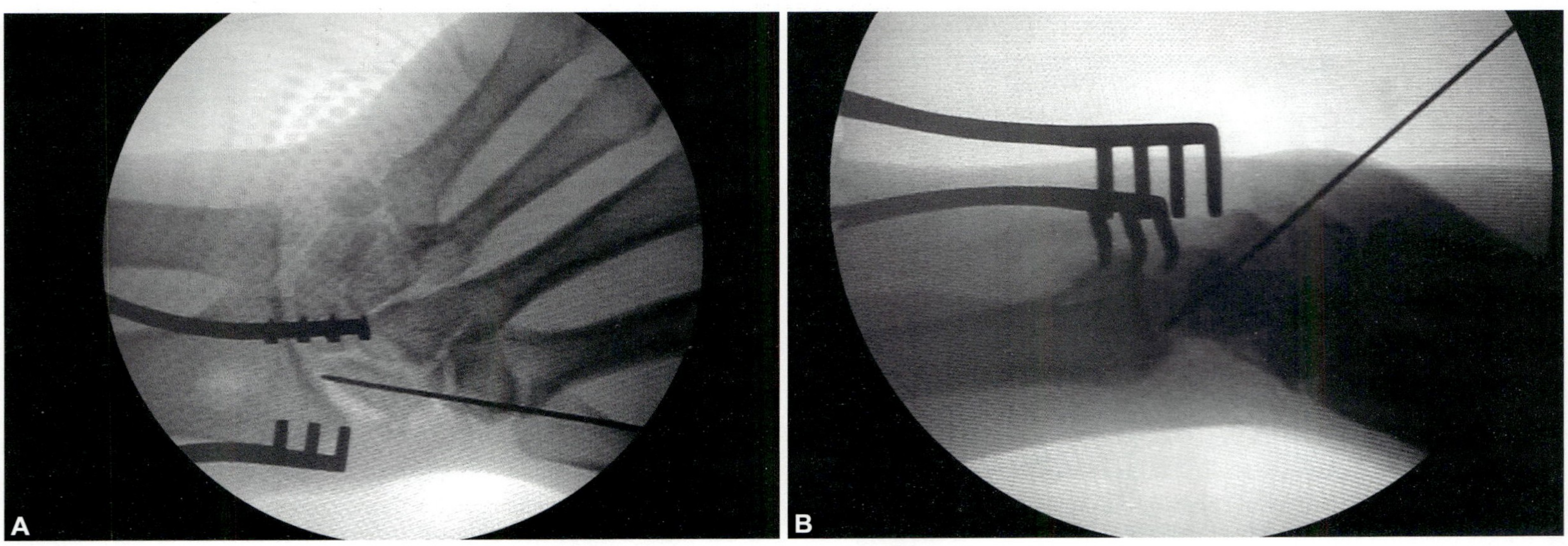

Figs. 21A and B: Intraoperative imaging to confirm adequate position of wire.

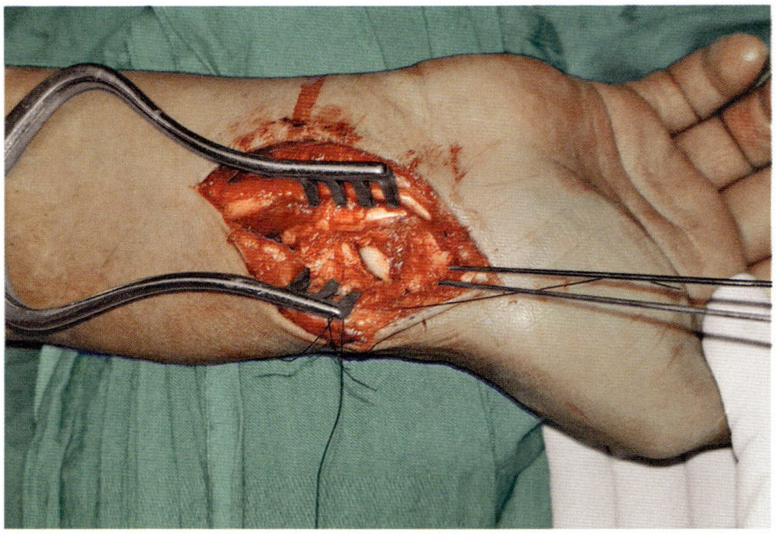

Fig. 22: Once a decision is made to accept the guidewire another K-wire (1.2 mm) inserted to act as a derotational wire. Care is taken to avoid getting this wire along the path of drill and screw.

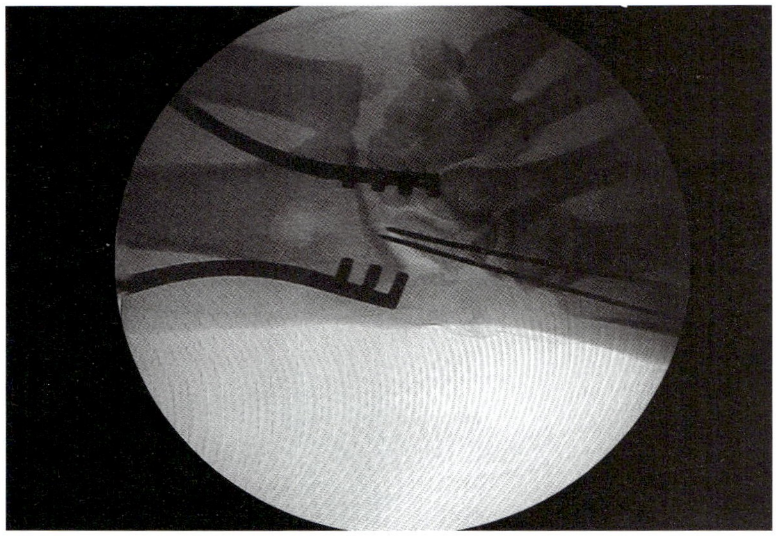

Fig. 23: Intraoperative imaging showing position of both wires. Most headless compression screw sets come with jigs to measure length of guidewire within bone. If not, one can calculate it with same length K-wire. To prevent screw protruding out from distal pole or avoid distraction at fracture site due to screw tip pushing at proximal pole, screw needs to be smaller by 3–4 mm than the length of guidewire in the bone.

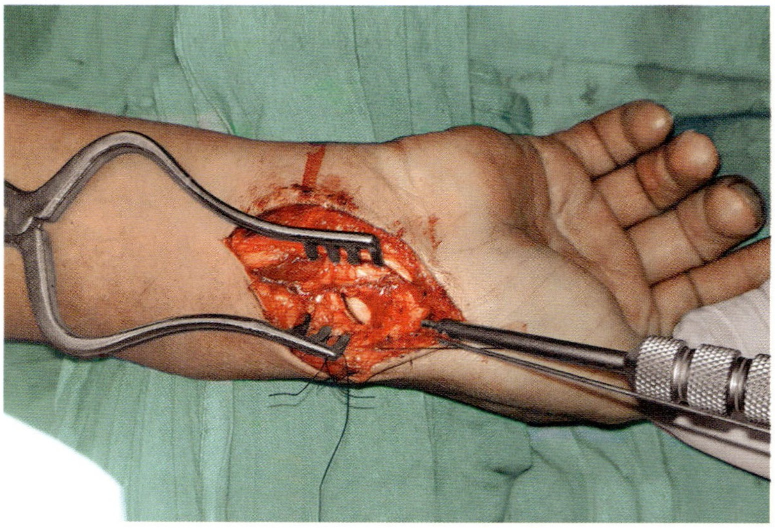

Fig. 24: The tract for screw was drilled over guidewire. It is prudent to familiarize oneself with instrumentation set before onset of surgery. Some headless screws need further drilling to countersink the proximal threaded portion of screw.

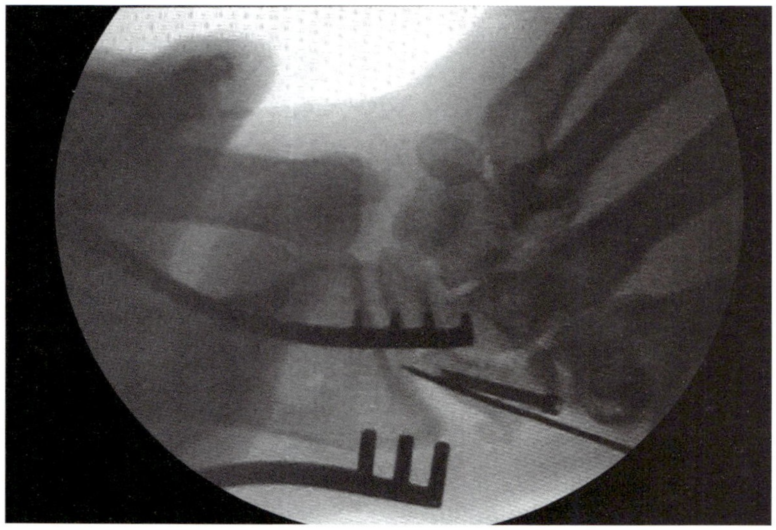

Fig. 25: Position of screw confirmed with intraoperative imaging. Note that despite screw head being driven deep to bone surface clinically, imaging appears as if part of head is still above surface of bone. This discrepancy is due to cartilage thickness not being appreciated in imaging. At this stage derotational wire was removed, stability of fixation checked by moving joint through its range of motion.

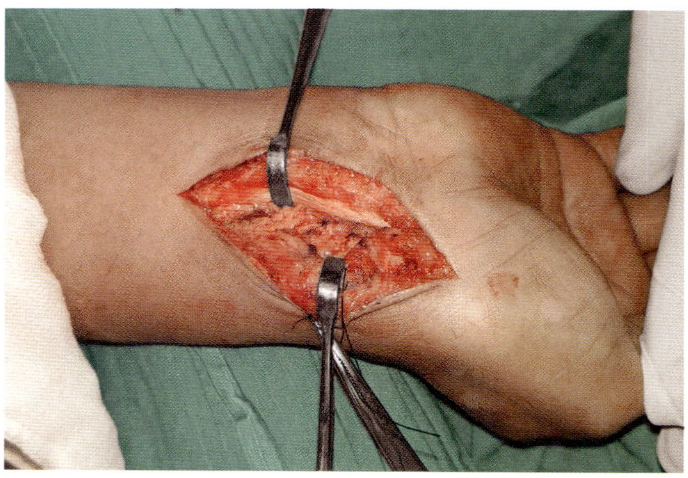

Fig. 26: Volar ligaments and capsule closed with 3-0 absorbable sutures, preferably with delayed absorption.

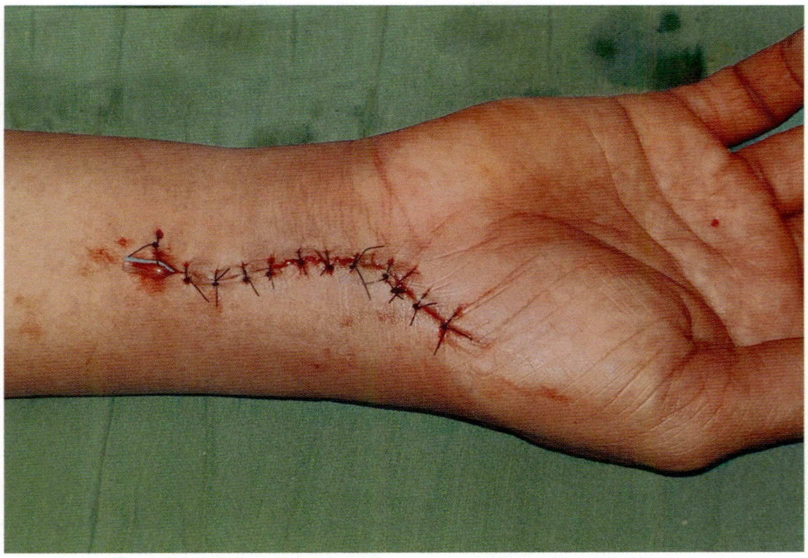

Fig. 27: After deflating tourniquet and achieving hemostasis wound closed with 3-0 nonabsorbable sutures with a drain kept in the wound. Placement of drain is optional as per surgeon's choice. Postoperatively I keep patients in below elbow thumb volar slab till suture removal. Afterwards I place the wrist in thumb spica cast keeping interphalangeal (IP) joint free for 8–12 weeks. Usually I get a computed tomography (CT) scan after this period to assess bone healing before mobilizing wrist.

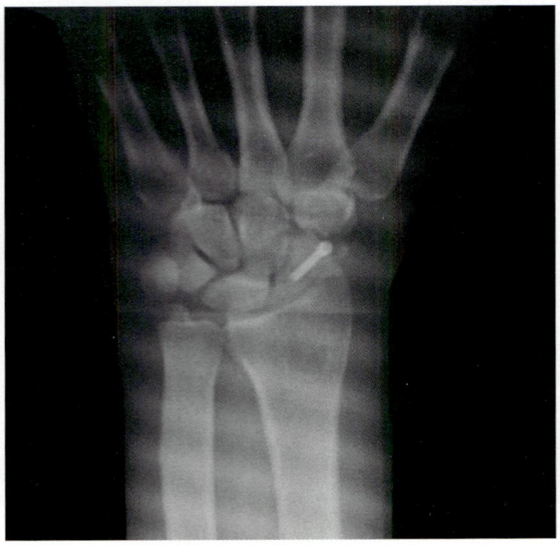

Fig. 28: Postoperative 1

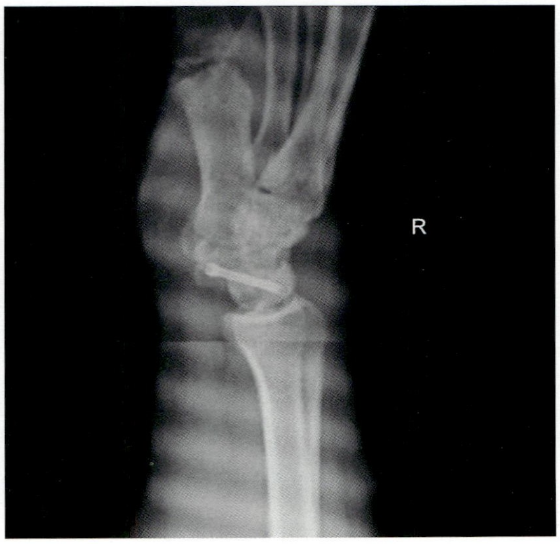

Fig. 29: Postoperative 2

SUGGESTED READING

1. Gelberman RH, Menon J. The vascularity of the scaphoid bone. J Hand Surg Am. 1980;5:508-13.
2. Slutsky DJ, Slade III JF. The Scaphoid. NY, USA: Thieme; 2011.
3. Wolfe S, Pederson Q, Kozin SH. Green's Operative Hand Surgery, 6th edition. PA, USA: Elsevier Churchill Livingstone; 2011.

CHAPTER 43

Epibasal Thumb Fracture/ Pseudo-Bennett Fracture: Plate Fixation

S Prakash, Madan Hardikar, Siddharth Jaiswal

INTRODUCTION

Among hand injuries metacarpal fractures are most common and they present to emergency departments and clinics frequently.

Fractures of first metacarpal are important as they have impact on overall function of hand. It is important to understand the morphology of fracture as treatment varies with morphology of fracture.

EPIDEMIOLOGY

Amongst fractures in hand, metacarpal injuries account for almost 30–40%. In all metacarpal fractures almost 25% account for first metacarpal fracture, second only to fifth metacarpal neck (i.e. "boxers") fractures in terms of frequency. Around 80% in fracture of first metacarpal involve the base.

Thumb fractures are commonly caused by falls and direct trauma secondary to accidents, sports and from punching solid objects. Thumb metacarpal fractures occur most often among younger males (10–29 years old). Thumb metacarpal epibasal fractures account for 16% of all metacarpal fractures.

CLASSIFICATION AND PATHOMECHANICS

Metacarpal fractures include:

- Intra-articular fractures
  - Bennett fracture dislocation
  - Rolando fracture
- Extra-articular
  - Epibasal thumb fracture (pseudo Bennett fracture)
- Transverse (including basilar and diaphyseal fracture)
- Oblique.

RADIOGRAPHIC EXAMINATION

In case of thumb fracture, posteroanterior, lateral, and oblique views should be done as a routine. A true lateral view is important to

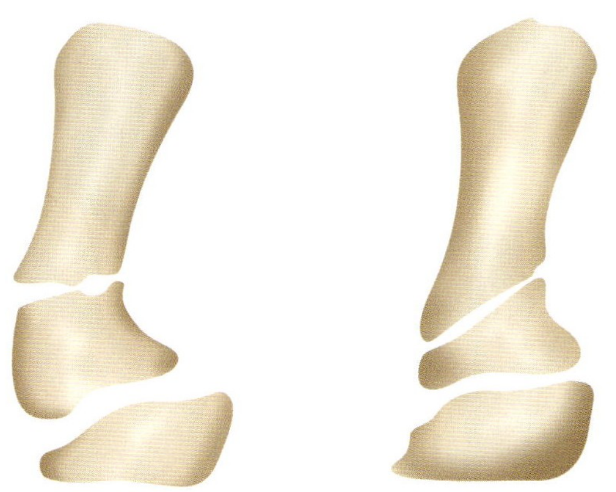

Fig. 1: Types of extra-articular fractures of thumb metacarpal according to morphology of fracture.

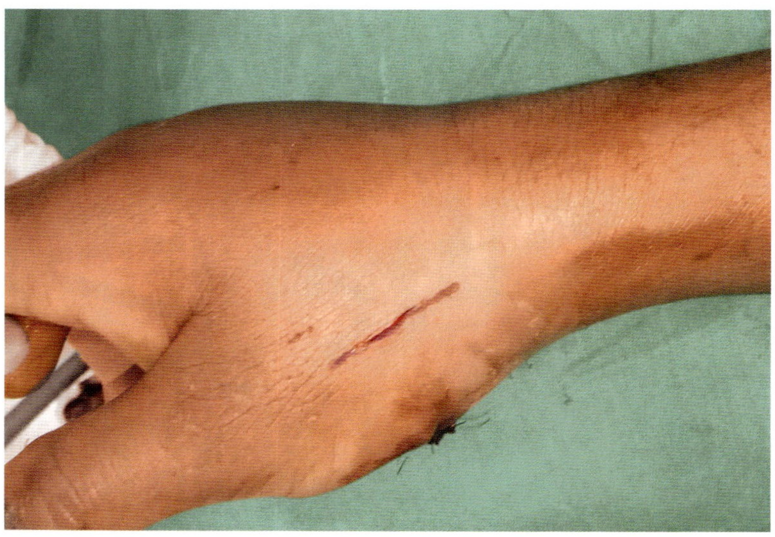

Fig. 2: Marking of surgical incision over dorsum of first metacarpal.

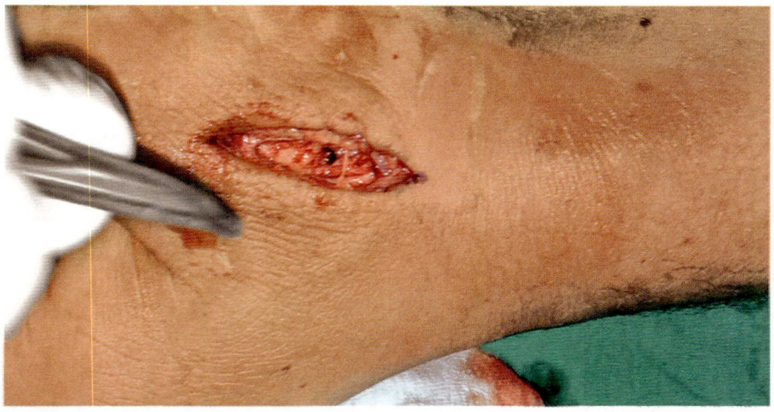

Fig. 3: Incision made over marking. After reaching subcutaneous fat it is important to identify and protect branches superficial radial nerve. To prevent inadvertent injury to nerve branches one may proceed with blunt dissection till bone is exposed.

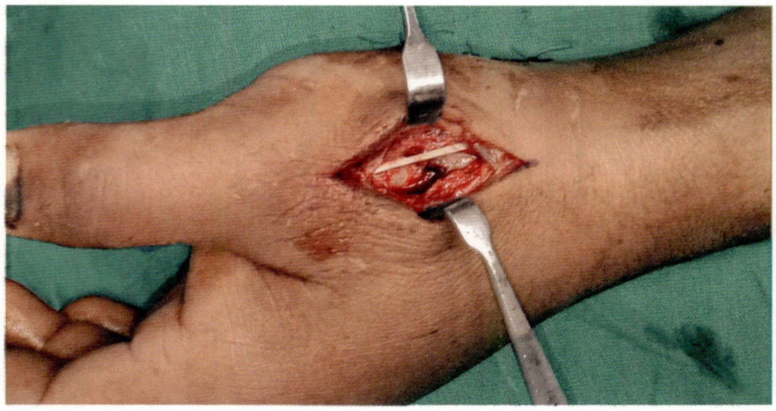

Fig 4: On retraction of skin and subcutaneous tissue the extensor pollicis brevis tendon seen. Bone is approached through interval between tendons of EPL and EPB.

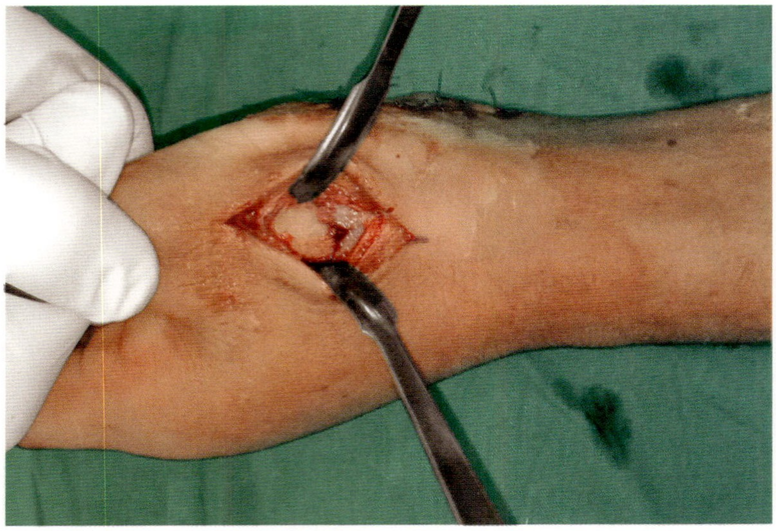

Fig. 5: With bone lever fracture site exposed.

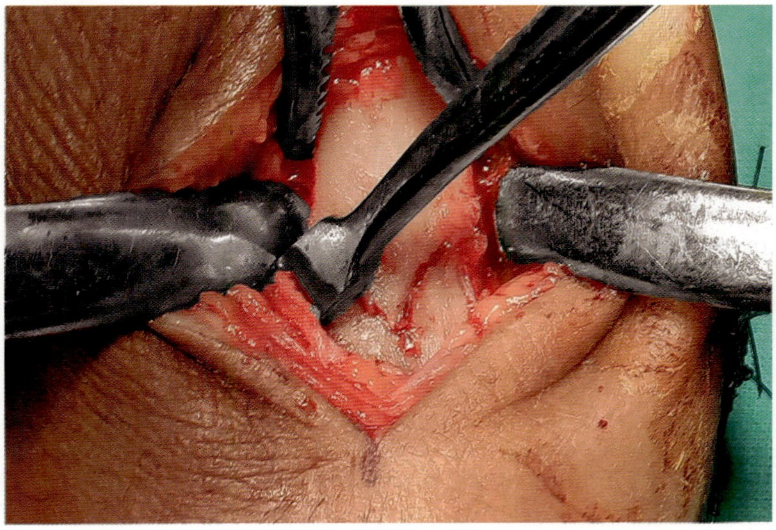

Fig 6: Fracture reduced with help of mini bone holder.

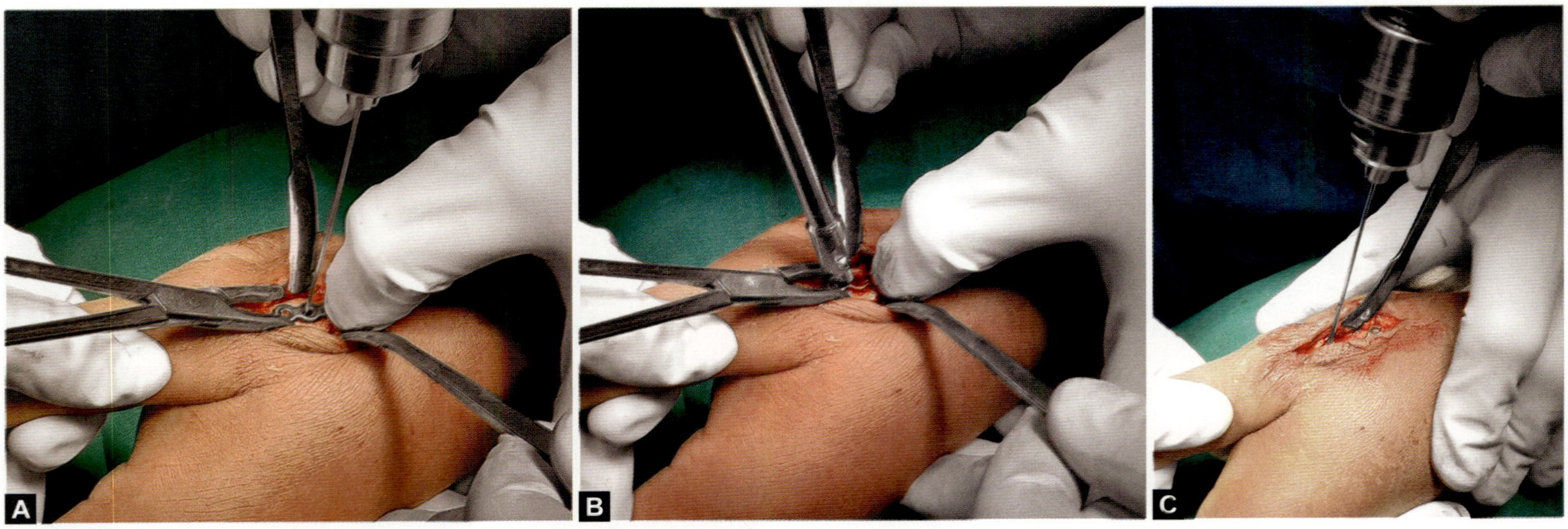

Figs. 7A to C: Reconstruction 2 mm T plate appropriately placed and fixed with 2 mm cortical screw appropriately directed. Dedicated implants for hand surgery provide with low profile 2/2.5 locking mini plates which are very useful for fixation in metaphyseal region of metacarpal.

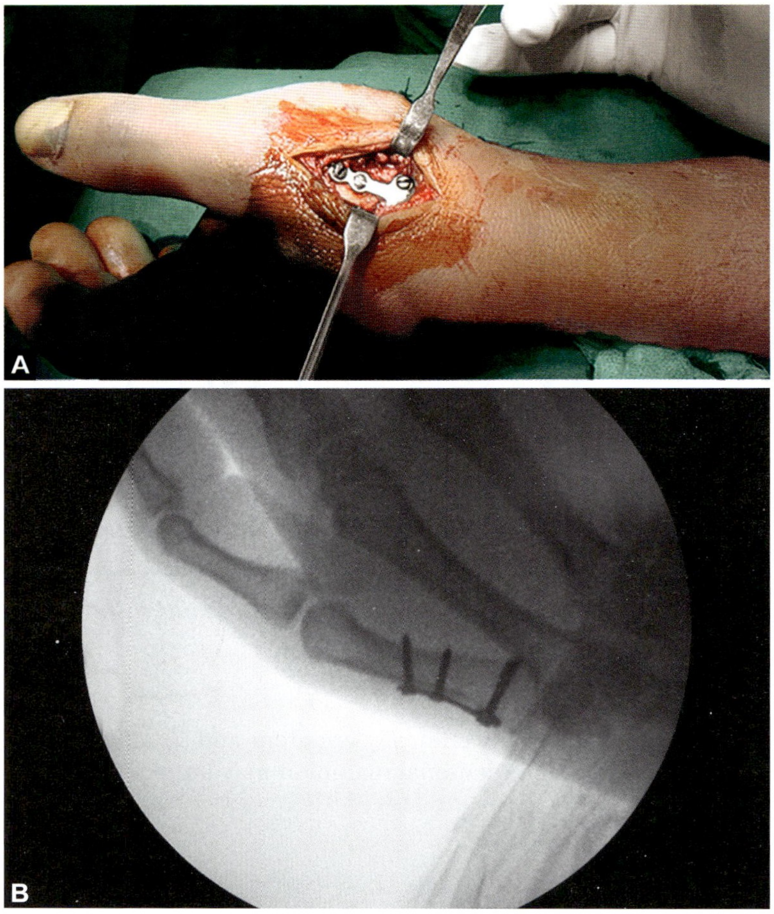

Figs. 8A and B: Clinical and radiological picture after fixation.

correctly demonstrate the base of the first metacarpal and the first carpometacarpal (CMC) joint. To obtain true lateral view of base of thumb, hand needs to be pronated around 20 degrees and X-ray beam directed 15–20 degrees distally.

TREATMENT

Extra-articular Fractures

Transverse and oblique are two main fracture patterns in extra-articular. Majority of fractures can be managed by conservative approach with closed reduction and thumb spica application. If fracture is unstable after closed reduction then percutaneous K-wire fixation is added. Up to 30° angulation can be accepted due to the compensatory movement at the CMC joint. Extra-articular fractures

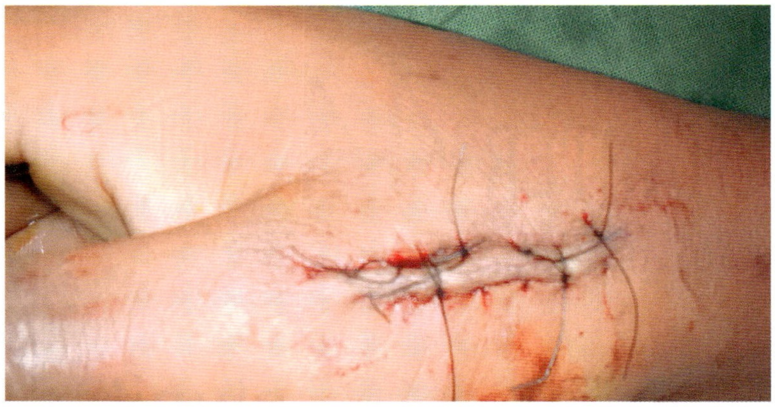

Fig. 9: Skin closure done.

rarely require open reduction. However delayed presentation with excessive angulation of fracture may necessitate open reduction as demonstrated here. In case of open reduction it is prudent to strive for rigid fixation so as to mobilize thumb early and minimize tendon adhesions in operative area.

COMPLICATIONS

There may be inadvertent injury to branches of superficial radial nerve which travel in close vicinity of dissection. This may lead to painful neuroma which is quite difficult to treat and best avoided.

Malunion is the most common complication with persistent dorsal apex angulation or rotational deformity.

Malunion with excessive angulation leads to loss of contour, excessive prominence of metacarpal head palmarly and attitude of MCP hyperextension and IP flexion [pseudo claw deformity].

Other complications could be tendon adhesions and stiffness of thumb which may necessitate tenolysis and implant removal.

SUGGESTED READING

1. Ashkenaze DM, Ruby LK. Metacarpal fractures and dislocations. Orthop Clin North Am. 1992;23:19-33.
2. Nakashian MN, Pointer L, Owens BD, et al. Incidence of metacarpal fractures in the US population. Hand (N Y). 2012;7:426-30.
3. Stanton JS, Dias JJ, Burke FD. Fractures of the tubular bones of the hand. J Hand Surg Eur Vol. 2007;32:626-36.
4. Fufa DT, Goldfarb CA. Fractures of the thumb and finger metacarpals in athletes. Hand Clin. 2012;28:379-88.
5. Cotterell IH, Richard MJ. Metacarpal and phalangeal fractures in athletes. Clin Sports Med. 2015;34:69-98.

CHAPTER 44

Malunited Finger Proximal Phalanx Corrective Osteotomy and Fixation

S Prakash, Sharad M Hardikar, Prashant Mall

INTRODUCTION

An overwhelming majority of fractures in hand especially in fingers are managed by nonoperative means. There are dynamic forces at work across fractures in fingers as in other areas of body. Due to this malunion at finger fractures is relatively common. Not all malunions need operative intervention though. In cases of articular incongruity, gross deviation or rotation at malunion resulting in scissoring of fingers on flexion causing functional and/or cosmetic impairment are indications for interventions.

Malunion is generally clinically apparent and usually seen on radiograph. However, rotational malunion may not be obvious on radiograph.

SURGICAL TREATMENT

The objective is to realign bone in a position that improves the function of the finger. Osteotomy is done at malunion site to achieve correction and fixed with K-wires or screws or plate and screws.

SURGICAL STEPS (FIGS. 1 TO 12)

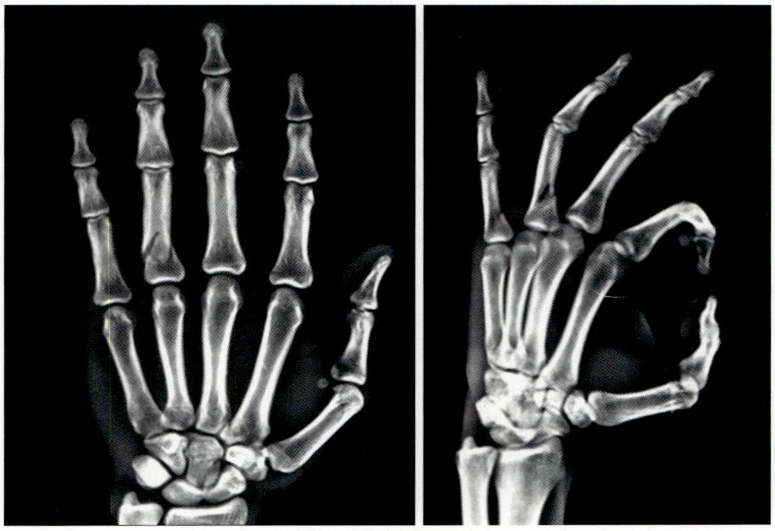

Fig. 1: Preoperative radiograph anteroposterior (AP) and oblique view showing angulation of fracture proximal phalanx.

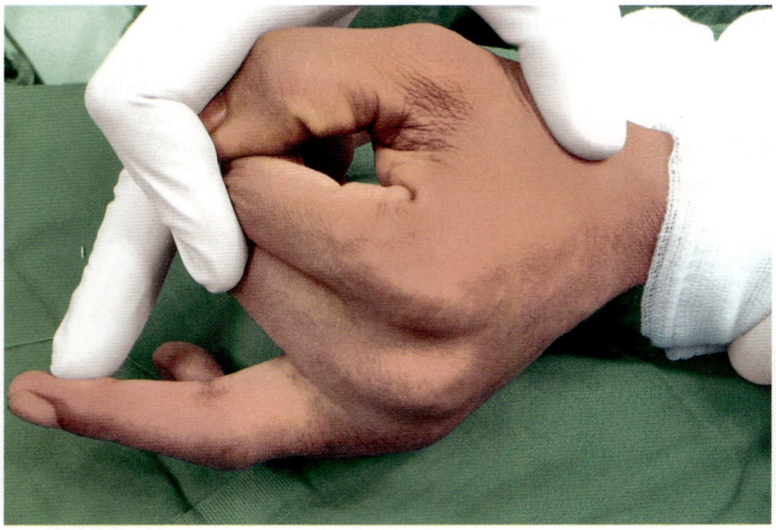

Fig. 2: Fixed flexion deformity at proximal interphalangeal (PIP) joint.

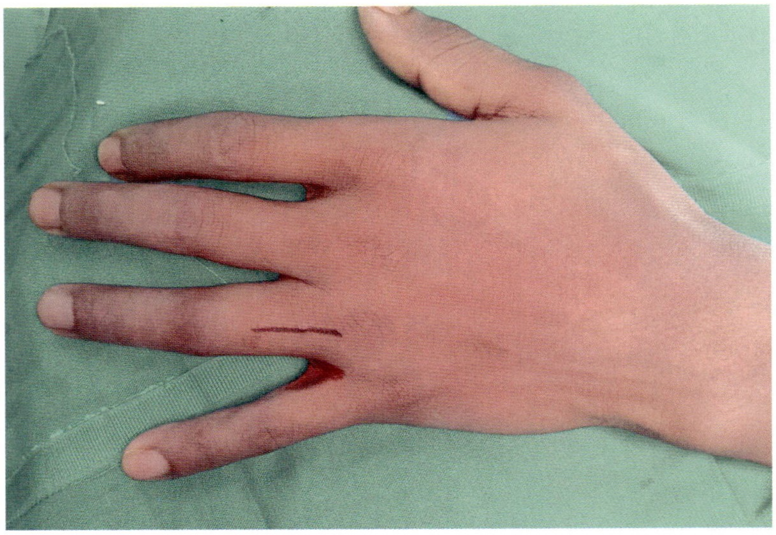

Fig. 3: Position, painting, and draping done, incision mark.

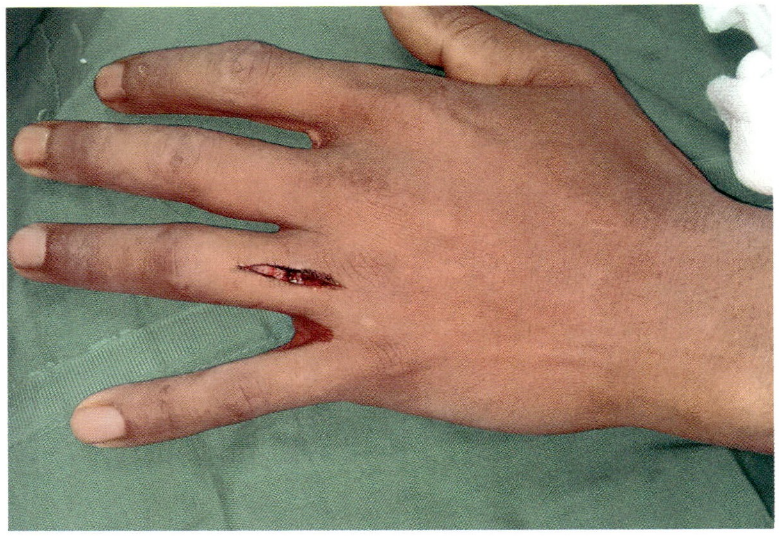

Fig. 4: Dorsal incision centered on the fracture site.

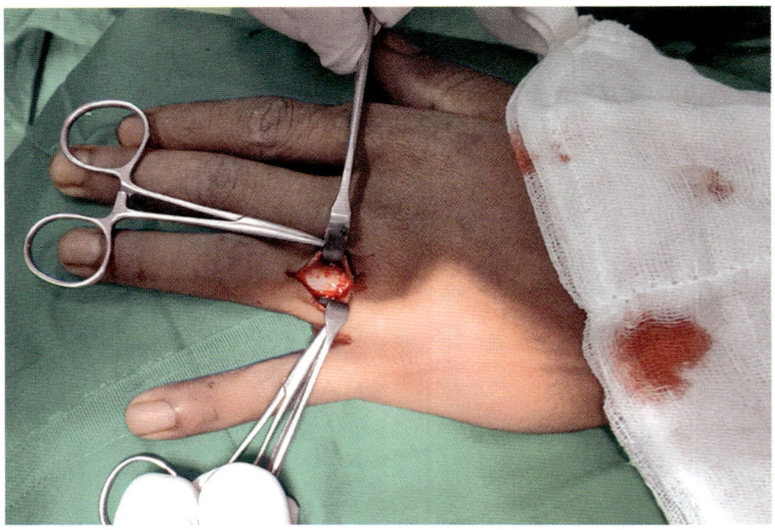

Fig. 5: Soft tissue exposed layer by layer, hood exposed.

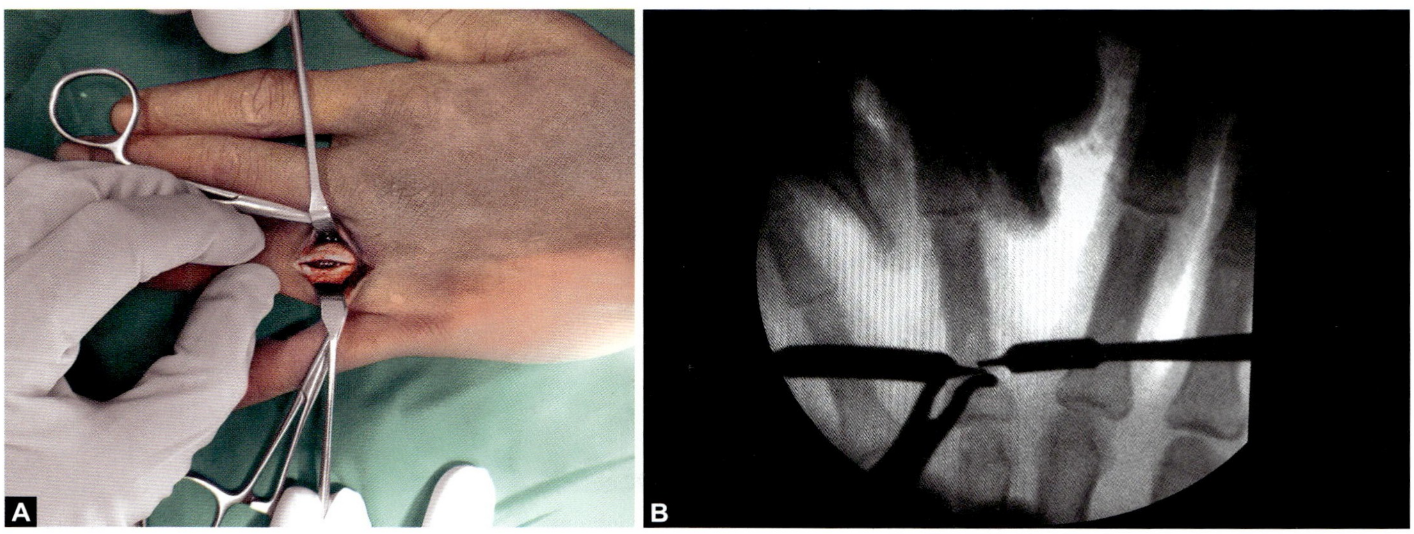

Figs. 6A and B: Extensor expansion split in midline with sharp incision to reach dorsum of bone underneath and corresponding C-arm image.

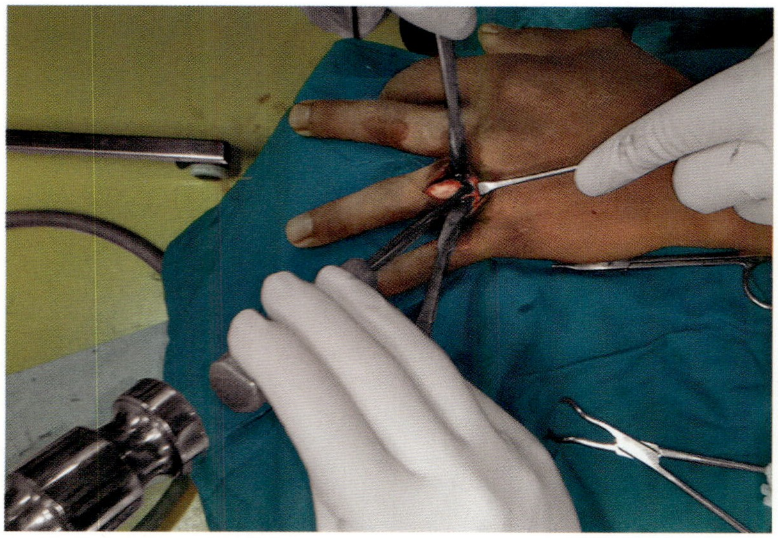

Fig. 7: Osteotomy done by osteotome at the malunited fracture site. Availability of small sharp osteotome of 3-6 mm is very important for this step.

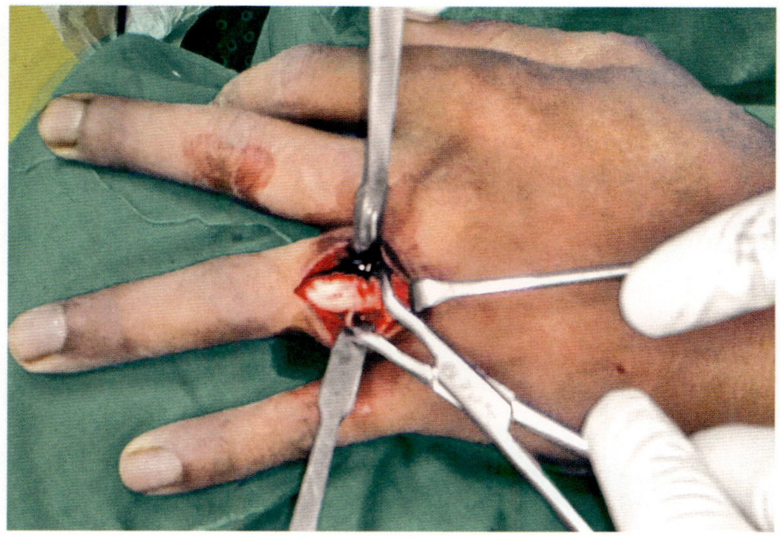

Fig. 8: Fracture reduced with bone holding forceps.

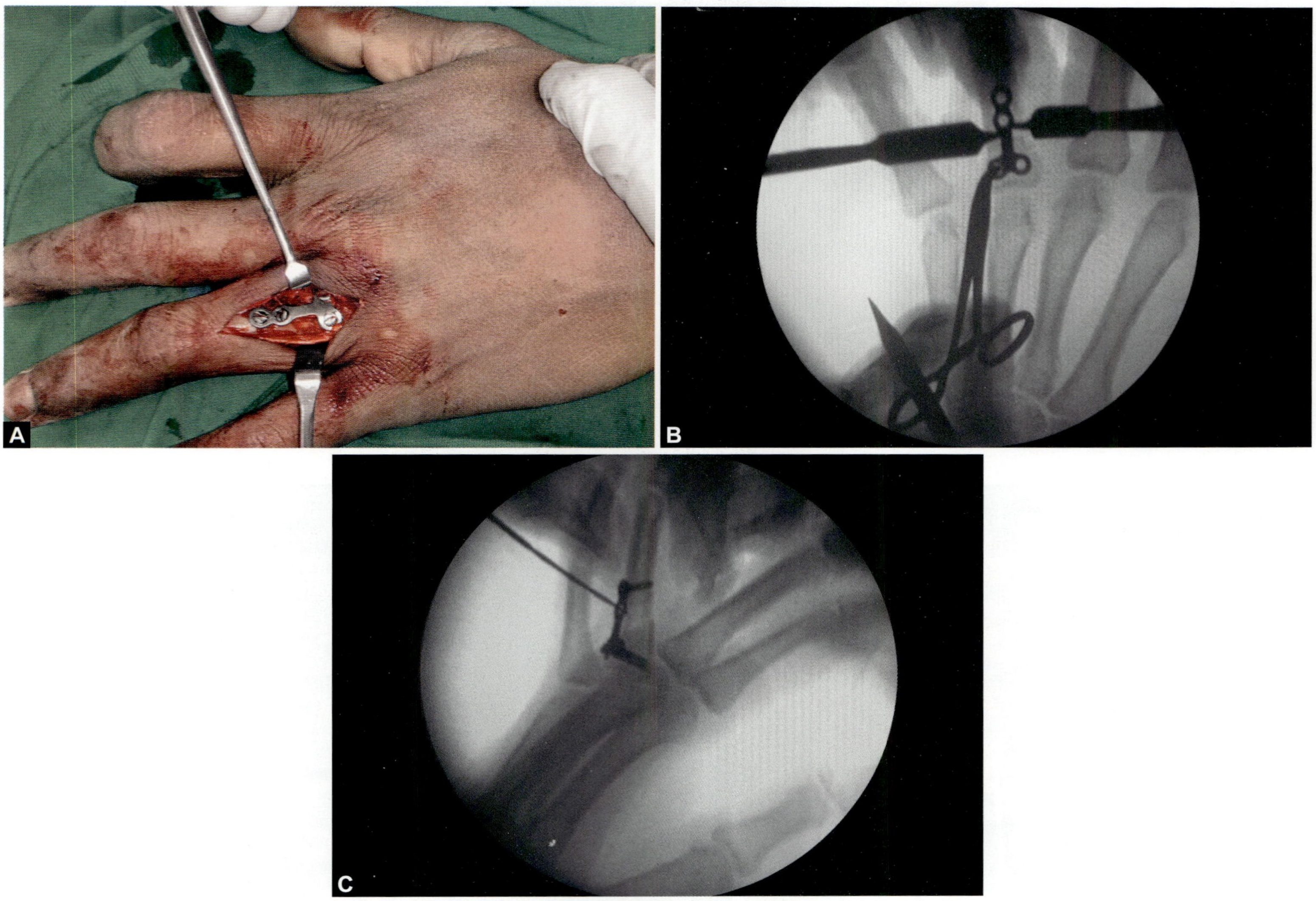

Figs. 9A to C: (A) Stabilized with 2 mm T shape reconstructive plate and (B and C) confirmed under C-arm. Implants are available with locking plates designed for small bones fixation with 1.3, 1.5, 2, 2.5 mm screws and low profile plates.

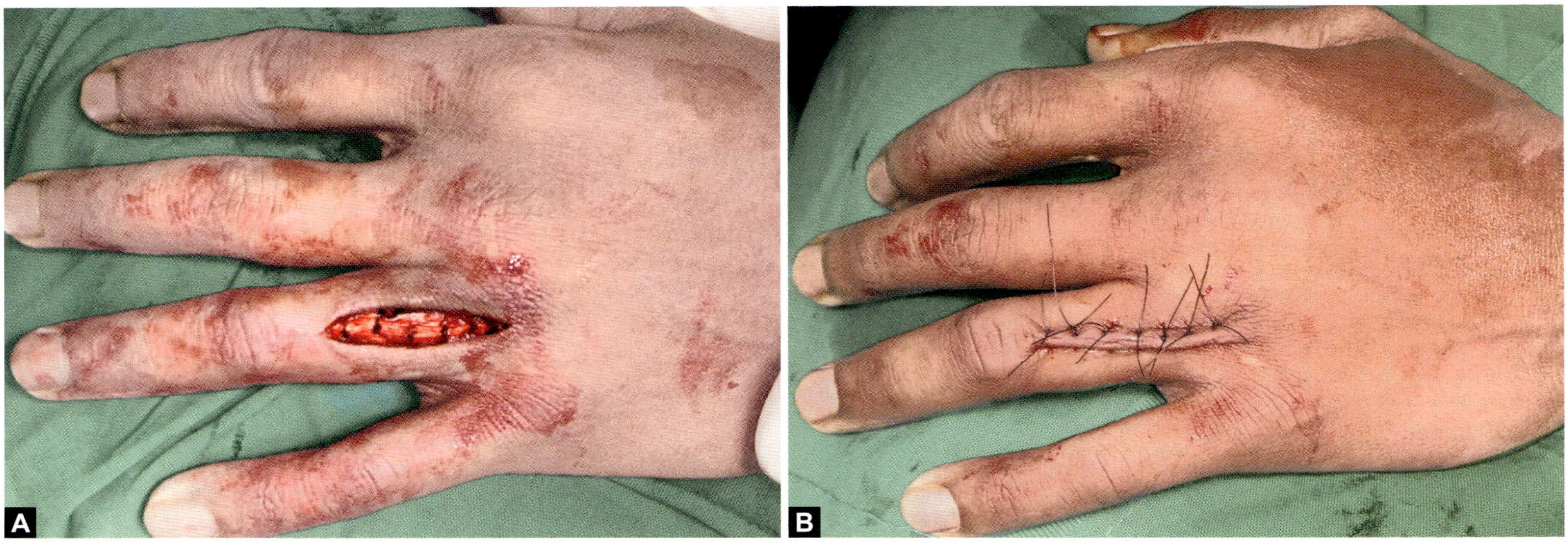

Figs. 10A and B: (A) Closure of extensor apparatus with fine nonabsorbable sutures; (B) Skin close with nonabsorbable suture.

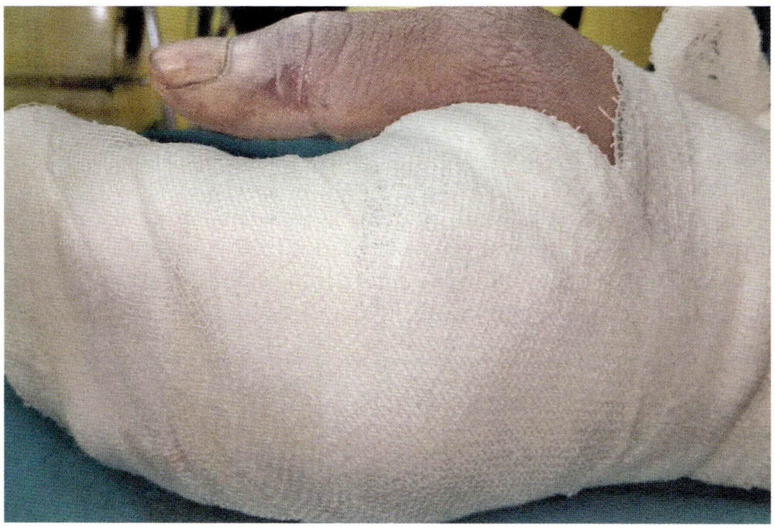

Fig. 11: Dressing done.

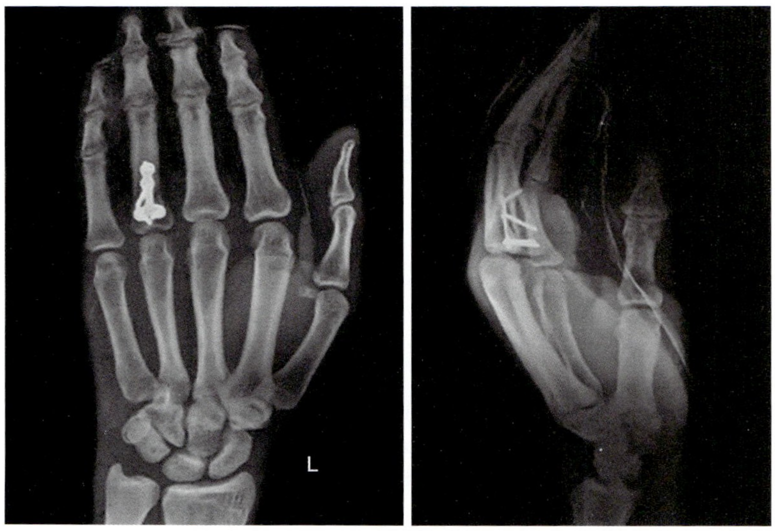

Fig. 12: Postoperative radiograph.

POSTOPERATIVE CARE

- After 2 weeks stitches will be removed. May need either a cast or a splint for a short period of 2–3 weeks. Immobilization for longer time may lead to fingers stiffness.
- Active and passive finger movements are started as pain subsides till full range is achieved.

SUGGESTED READING

1. Brei-Thoma P, Vögelin E, Franz T. Plate fixation of extra-articular fractures of the proximal phalanx: do new implants cause less problems? Arch Orthop Trauma Surg. 2015;135(3):439-45.

CHAPTER 45

Ulnar Nerve Decompression

Pankaj Jindal

ULNAR NERVE COMPRESSION

Anatomy

After median nerve compression in the carpal tunnel, the ulnar nerve compression at the elbow is the second most common site of nerve compression in the upper extremity. The ulnar nerve can also get compressed at the wrist in the region of the Guyon's Canal.

There are several sites on the medial side of the elbow where the ulnar nerve can be compressed. As the ulnar nerve travels from the anterior to the posterior compartment it is a potential site for the nerve compression. The ulnar nerve can be compressed when it is deep to the ligament between the medial epicondyle and the olecranon. The nerve can also be compressed when it is entering the belly of flexor carpi ulnaris. It can also get compressed within the belly of flexor carpi ulnaris. At times there may be an aberrant muscle called anconeus epitrochliaris.

Sometimes when the carrying the angle is significantly increased, like for example due to ununited lateral condyle of the humerus, the ulnar nerve at the elbow can get compressed.

When the elbow is acutely flexed, the ulnar nerve gets stretched, as it lies posterior to the axis of the elbow joint. In a person who is prone, the position of the elbow can predispose the ulnar nerve for compression.

There are various surgical options offered for decompression of the ulnar nerve. It is important to keep in mind, all the possible sites of compression of the ulnar nerve before undertaking decompression. All these sites needs to be considered and decompressed.

SURGICAL STEPS

A 40-year-old male physician presented with tingling and numbness in left small and ring fingers of 10 years duration. There was no weakness. There was no clawing. Froment sign was negative.

On examination, passive elbow flexion test was positive. The Tinel's sign was positive posterior to left medial epicondyle. There was no tenderness over the Guyon's canal. Costoclavicular compression test was negative ruling out compression due to a possibility of a cervical rib. Tinel's sign was absent over the median nerve at the wrist. Phalen test was negative.

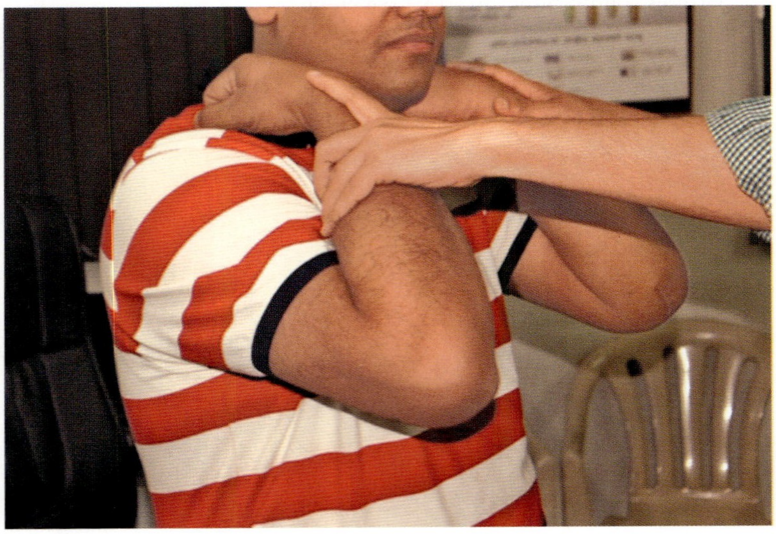

Fig. 1: Passive elbow flexion test. Both the elbows are passively flexed and held flexed for 2 minutes. A positive test indicates ulnar nerve compression at the elbow.

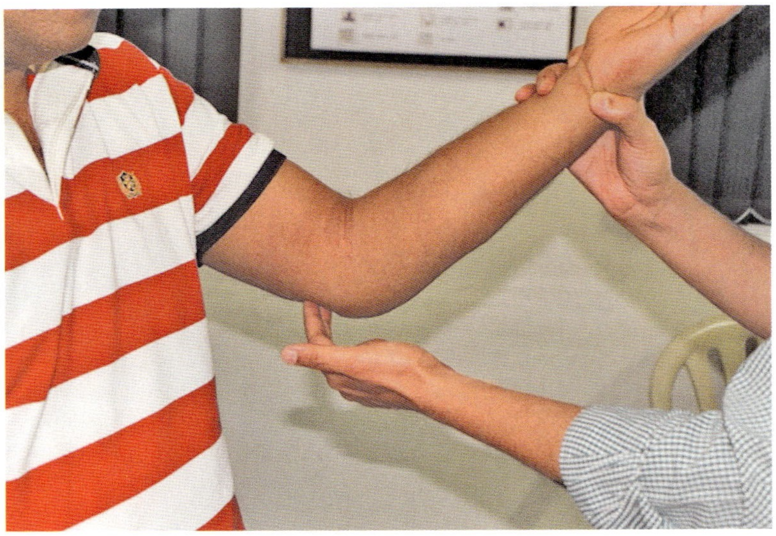

Fig. 2: The Tinel's sign is elicited by tapping gently along the surface anatomy of the ulnar nerve. A positive test is suggestive of ulnar nerve compression the elbow.

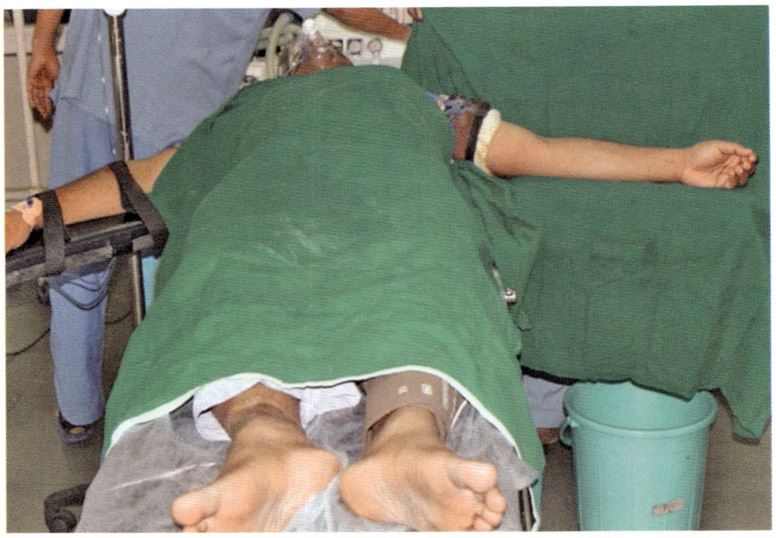

Fig. 3A: Patient is positioned supine and the affected arm is abducted on the arm rest. A pneumatic tourniquet is applied but not inflated.

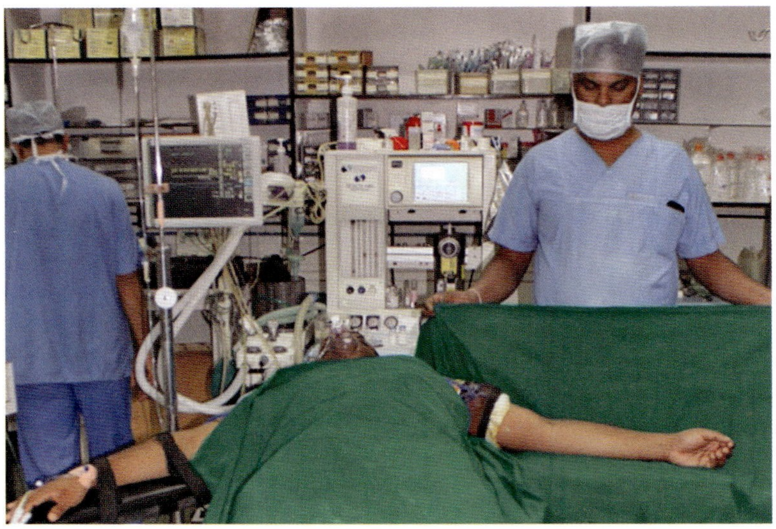

Fig. 3B: The unaffected arm rests on another narrow arm rest for anesthetist intravenous (IV) access.

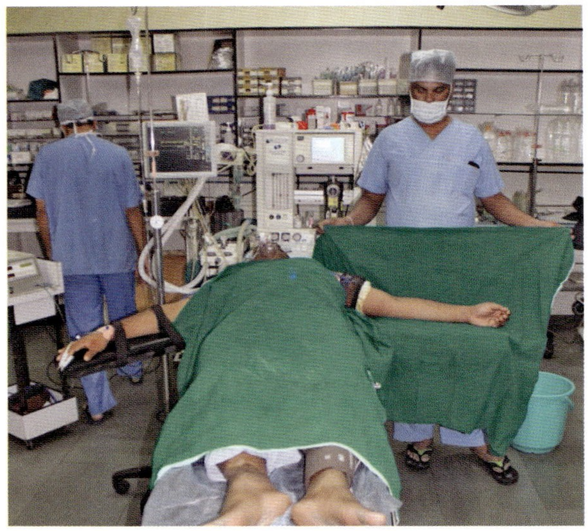

Fig. 3C: Noninvasive blood pressure cuff is applied on the leg.

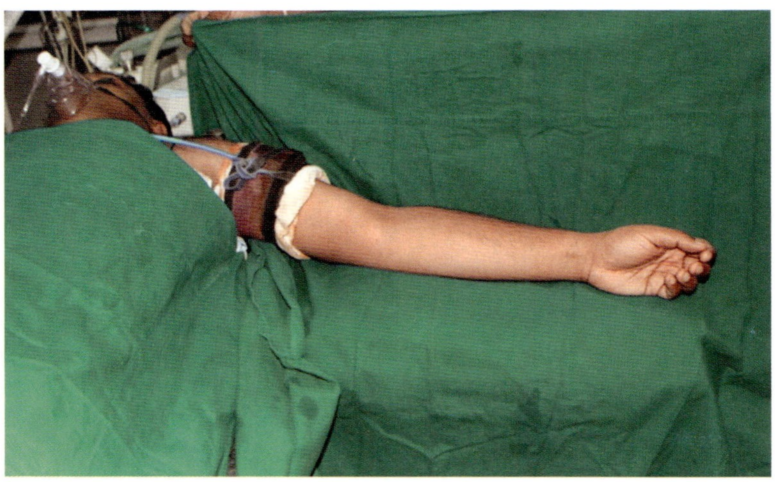

Fig. 3D: Close-up of pneumatic tourniquet position on the abducted arm on the arm rest.

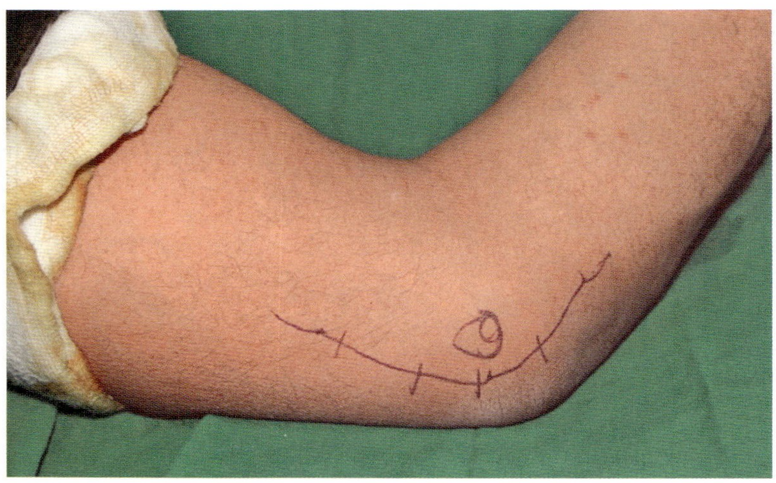

Fig. 4: An 10 cm incision is marked, posterior to medial epicondyle. The incision is parallel to surface anatomy of the ulnar nerve. The marking was done before the painting and draping to demonstrate the relation of the incision to the unsterile tourniquet. In the normal course the marking is done after painting, draping and the unsterile tourniquet is covered with sterile drapes.

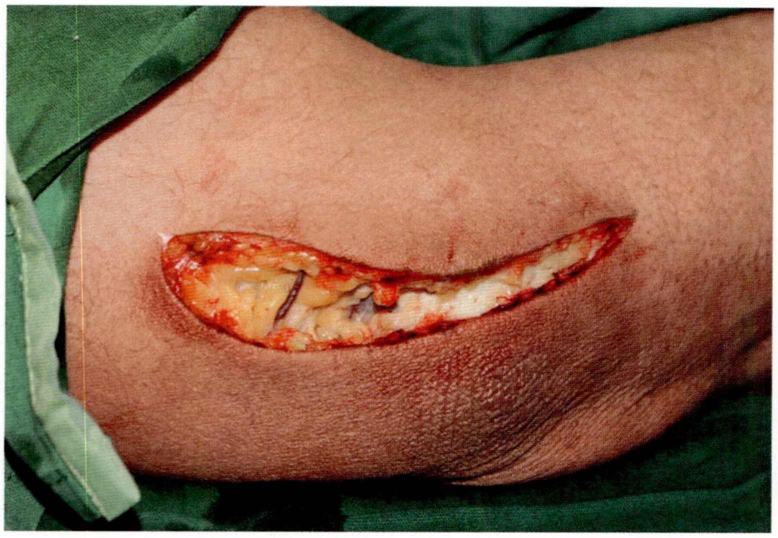

Fig. 5: After exsanguination and inflating the tourniquet to 100 mm above the systolic, the tourniquet is inflated. The skin incision is deepened. Bleeders are ligated or cauterized.

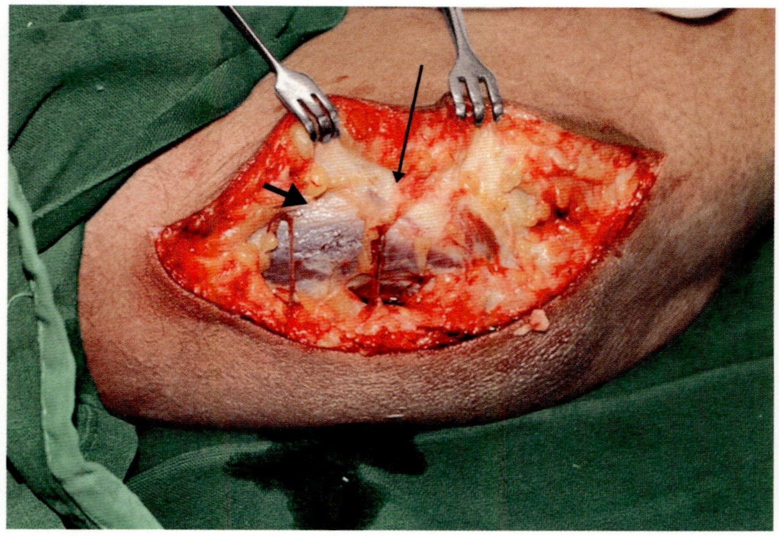

Fig. 6: Medial epicondyle is marked with a thin arrow. Ulnar nerve now visible is marked with a thick arrow.

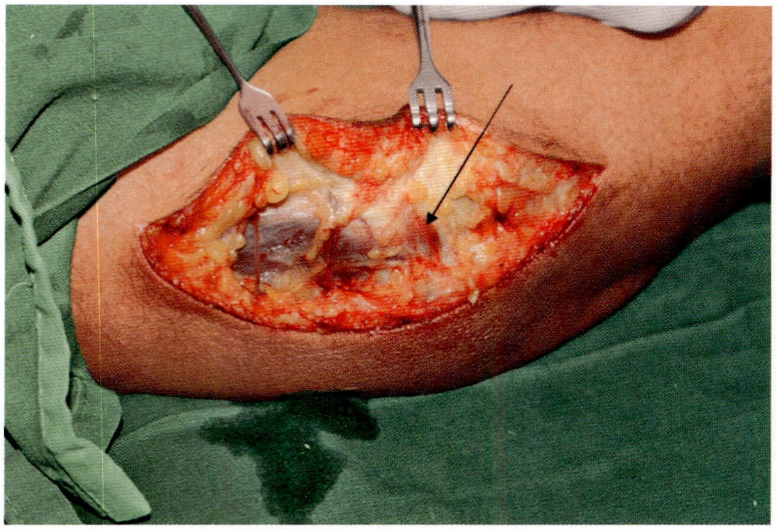

Fig. 7: Anconeus epitrochlearis (marked with an arrow) muscle is seen extending from the olecranon posteriorly to the medial epicondyle.

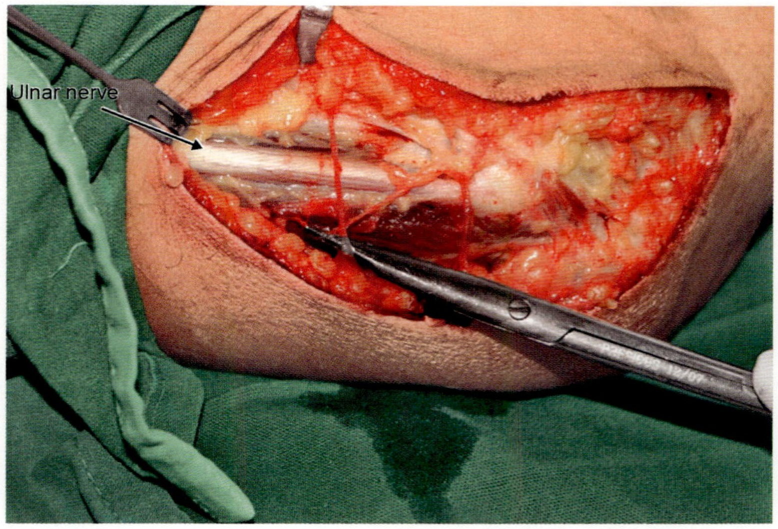

Fig. 8: Ulnar nerve seen distinctly.

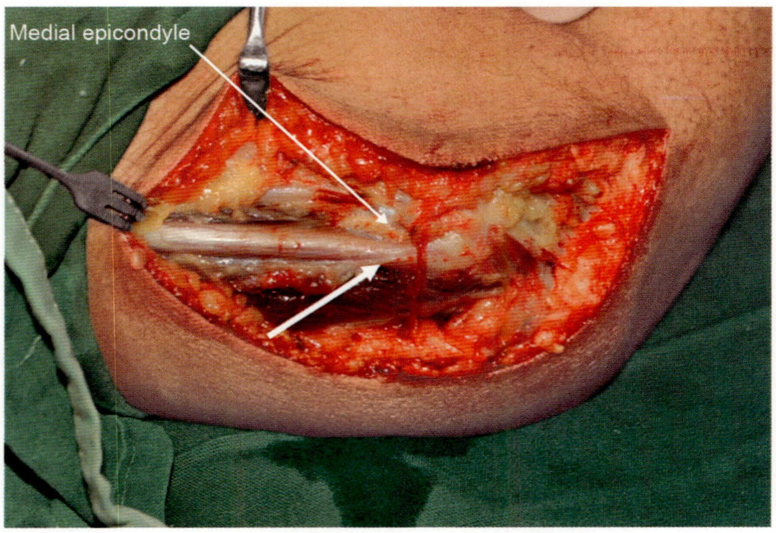

Fig. 9: Ulnar nerve traversing posterior to medial epicondyle as shown by thick arrow.

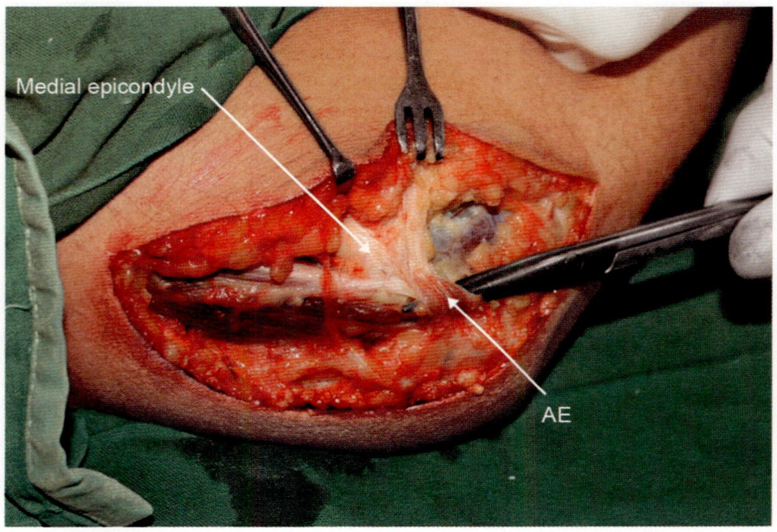

Fig. 10: Ulnar nerve traversing posterior to medial epicondyle and further in its course seen deep to anconeus epitrochlearis (AE) muscle, which is lifted up with a scissors.

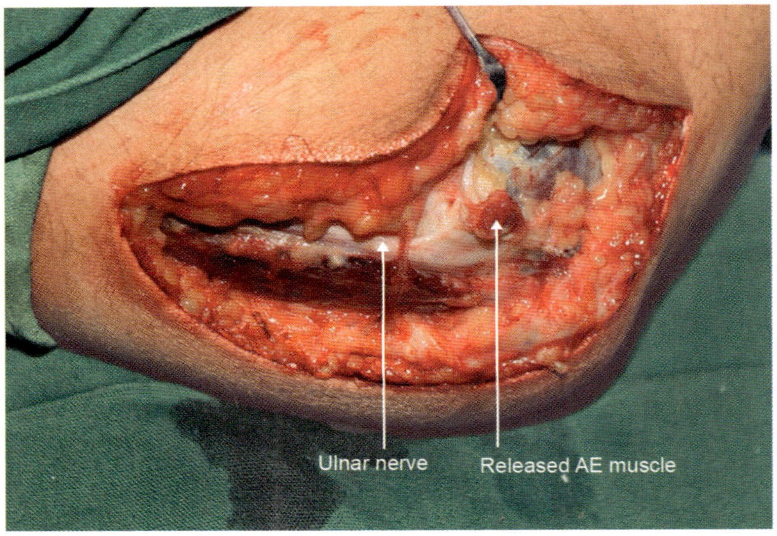

Fig. 11: Anconeus epitrochlearis (AE) muscle released, showing passage of ulnar nerve deep to it.

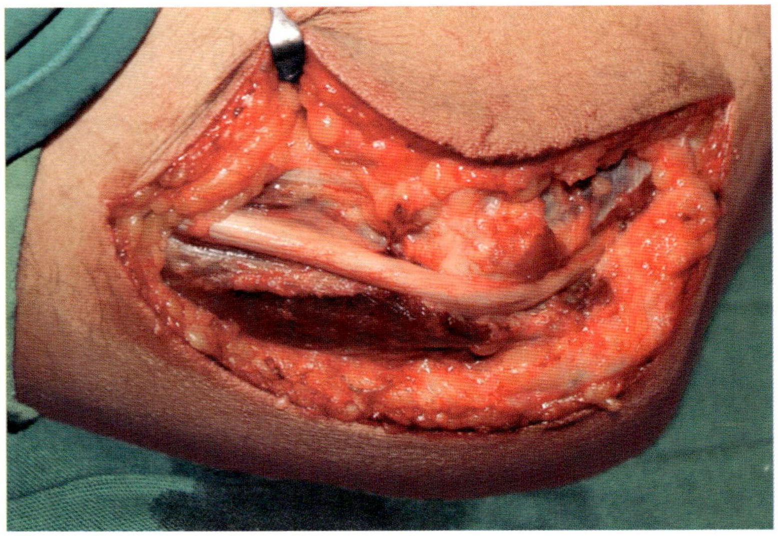

Fig. 12: Ulnar nerve showing a smooth passage posterior to medial epicondyle and entry into muscle of flexor carpi ulnaris.

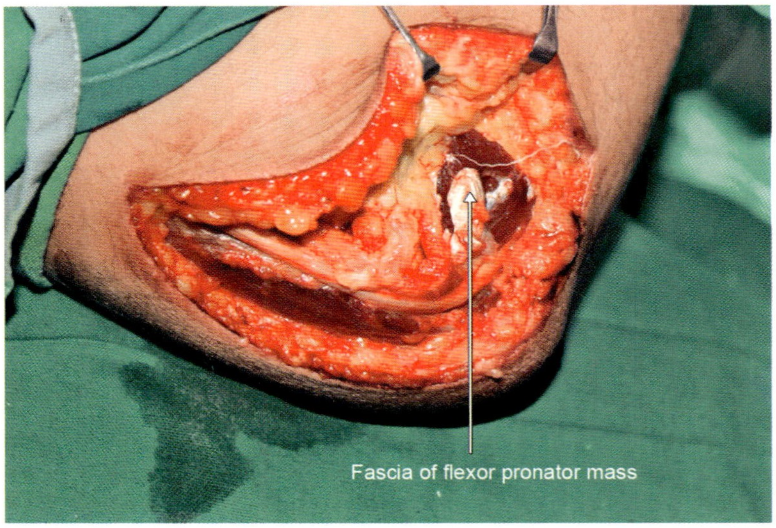

Fig. 13: Fascia of flexor pronator mass is reflected. This will be used to anchor the ulnar nerve after anterior transposition.

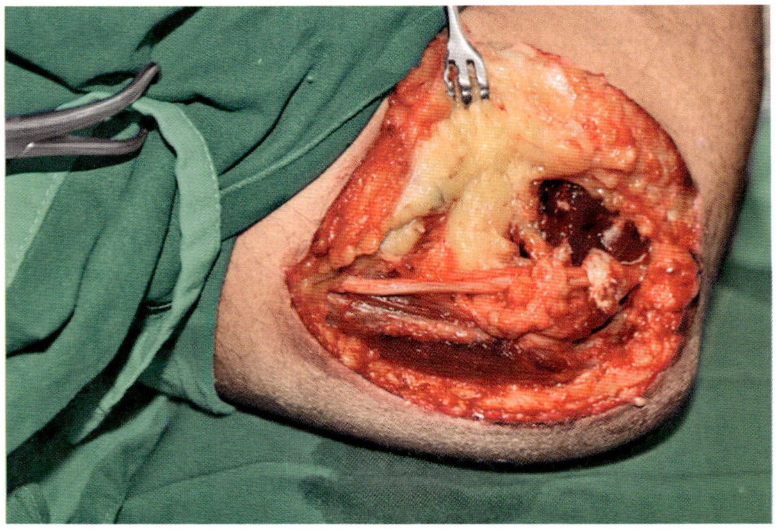

Fig. 14: Ulnar nerve transposed anteriorly. It is anchored in the new location within the fascia of flexor pronator mass.

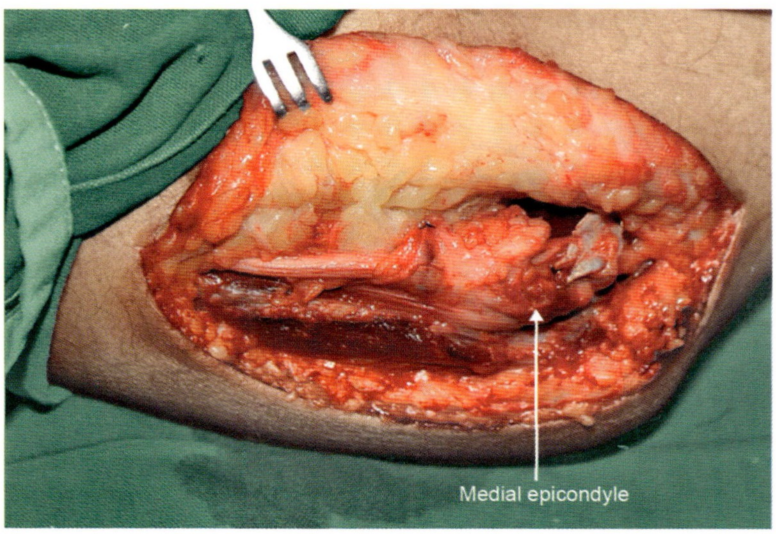

Fig. 15: Anchored ulnar nerve.

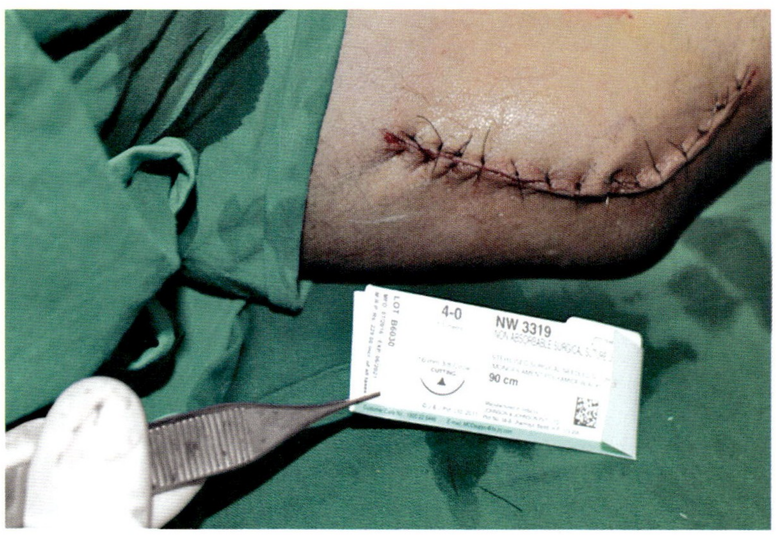

Fig. 16: Wound is closed with 4/0 polyamide in this particular case.

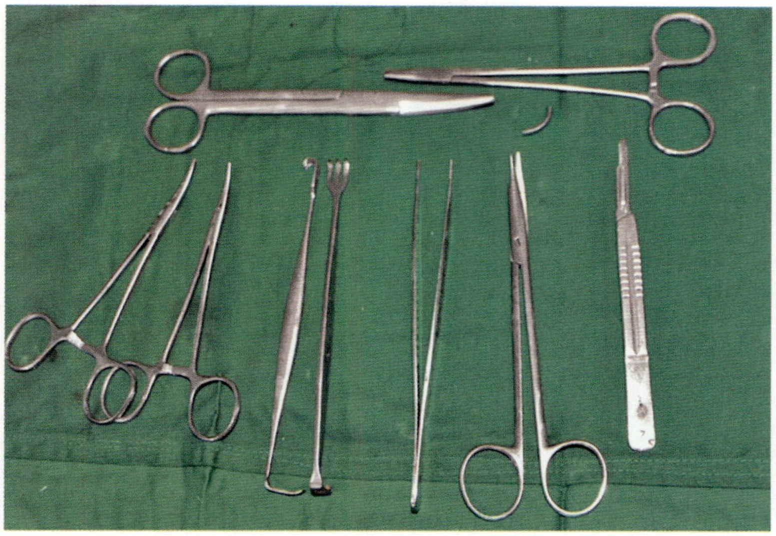

Fig. 17: The instruments used are shown. Most important is blade number 15 and 12.5 cm long Steven's scissors also called tenotomy scissors.

Electrophysiological study confirmed the clinical diagnosis of ulnar nerve compression.

SUGGESTED READING

1. Green's Operative hand surgery. Seventh edition. Elsevier Publication. 2017. pp. 940-6.

CHAPTER 46

Radial Tunnel Syndrome Decompression

Pankaj Jindal

Like median nerve compression causing carpal tunnel syndrome or ulnar nerve compression, motor branch of radial nerve is prone to compression in the upper part of the forearm. The patient presents with pain in the upper part of the forearm which may prevent the patient in doing day to day activities.

The deep tenderness is located about 3 finger breadth distal to lateral epicondyle over the belly of brachioradialis. It needs to to differentiated from tennis elbow where the pain is more proximal just anterior to lateral epicondyle.

Radial tunnel syndrome occurs due to compression of the motor branch of the radial nerve as the nerve passes between the two bellies of the supinator muscle.

Sometimes, the tennis elbow may coexist in these patients.

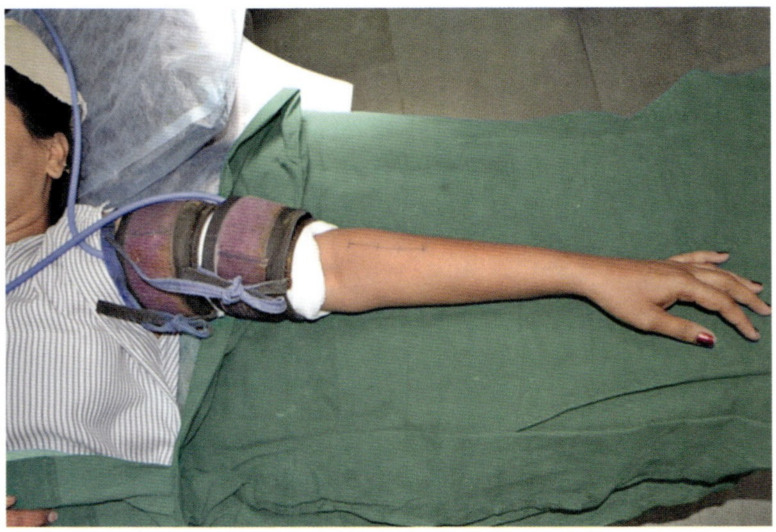

Fig. 1: Patient is positioned supine. Arm is extended. Double tourniquet in place. Surface marking of the proposed incision.

SURGICAL STEPS

40-year-old female had persistent localized pain over the mobile wad of Henry. Mobile wad of Henry is the three muscles outcropping from the lateral condyle of the humerus. She had no pain over lateral condyle of humerus and hence the diagnosis of tennis elbow was ruled out.

A diagnosis of radial tunnel syndrome was made. Radial tunnel syndrome is the compression of the motor branch of the radial nerve.

As she did not respond to rest, wait and watch for several months, it was decided to take her for surgical decompression of the motor branch of the radial nerve.

The patient was positioned supine on the operating table with the arm out stretched. Two pneumatic tourniquets were applied on the arm in preparation for regional Bier's block anesthesia (Fig. 1).

After painting and draping, intravenous catheter is inserted in a dorsal vein of the hand. Then upper of the two tourniquets is inflated to 250 mm of mercury. 6 mL of 2% Lignocaine without preservative is diluted with 18 mL of normal saline and injected (Fig. 2).

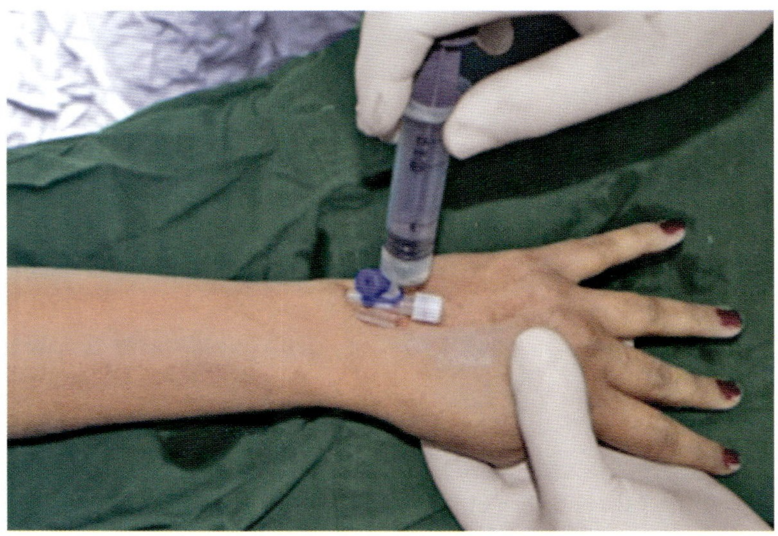

Fig. 2: Diluted lignocaine being injected after inflating the tourniquet.

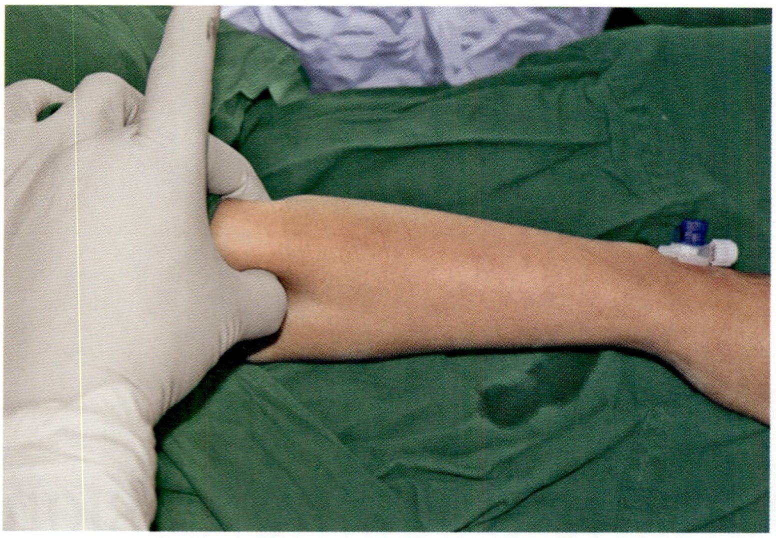

Fig. 3: The outcropping muscle on the lateral aspect of the upper arm is the brachioradialis.

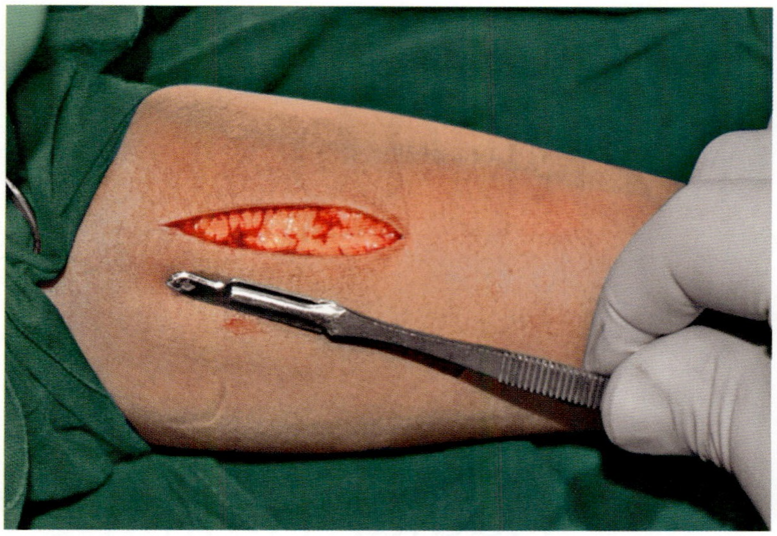

Fig. 4: 6 cm incision is made over brachioradialis muscle.

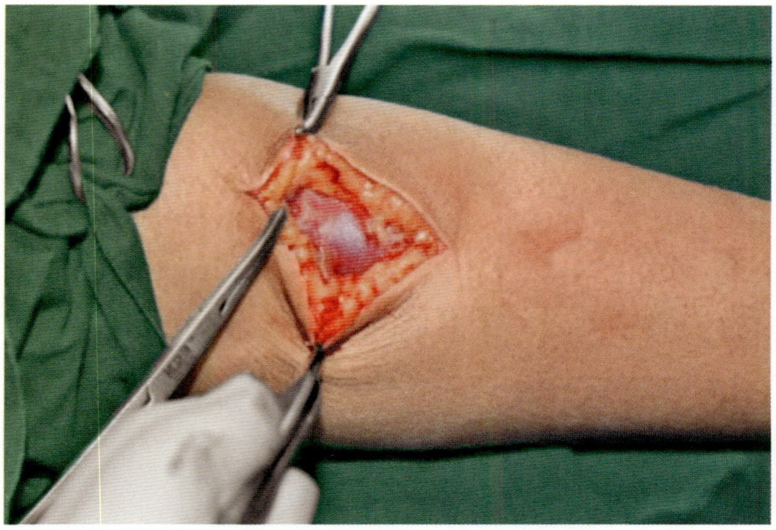

Fig. 5: The epimysium of the brachioradialis is incised.

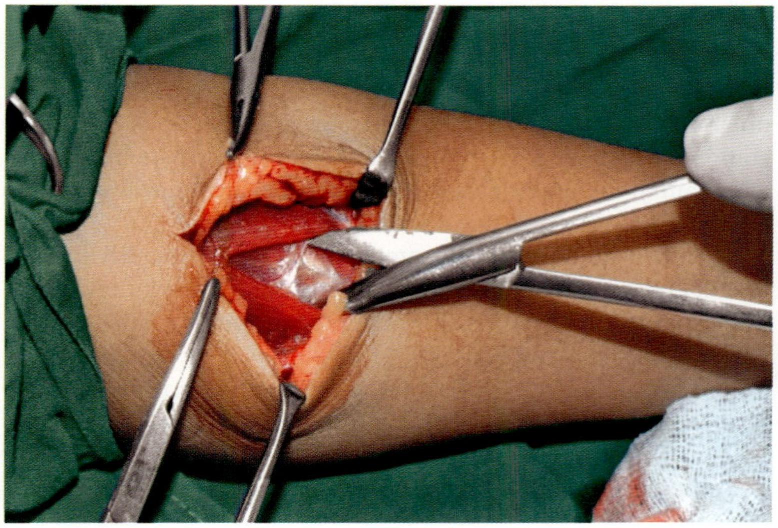

Fig. 6: The brachioradialis muscle is split along its fibbers.

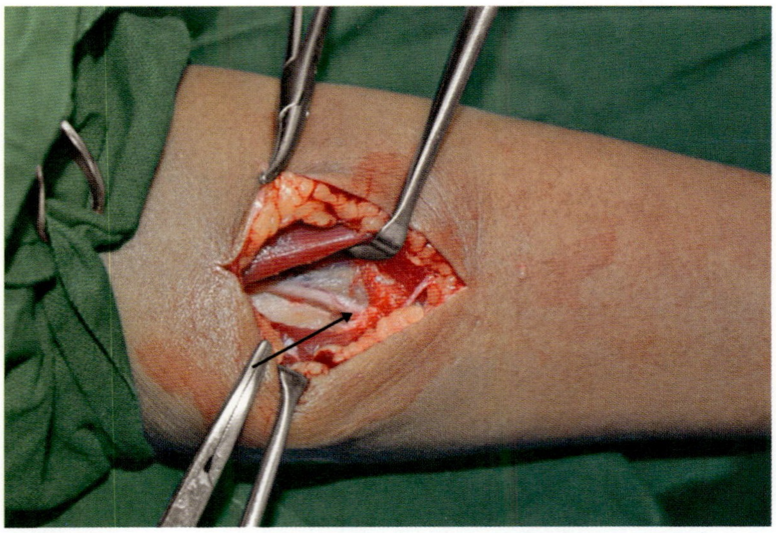

Fig. 7: The sensory branch of the radial nerve will be seen in the depth of the wound, deep to brachioradialis, marked by an arrow.

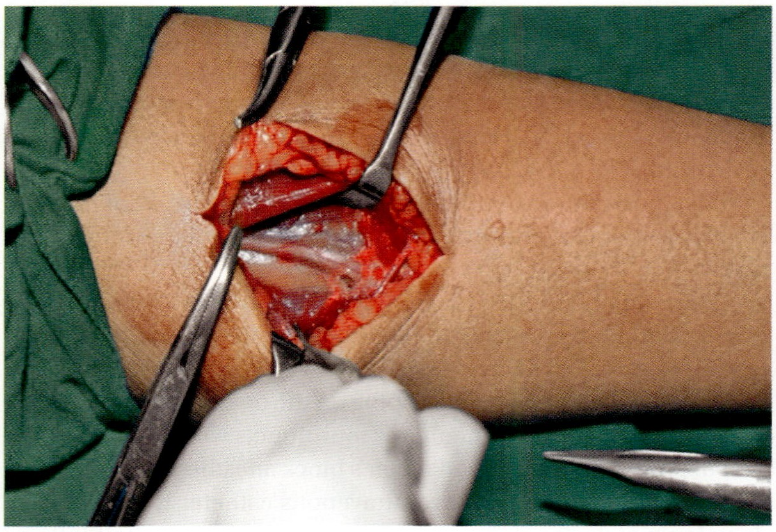

Fig. 8: As the sensory nerve is traced proximally, the motor branch of the radial nerve will be seen running distally and laterally deep to supinator muscle.

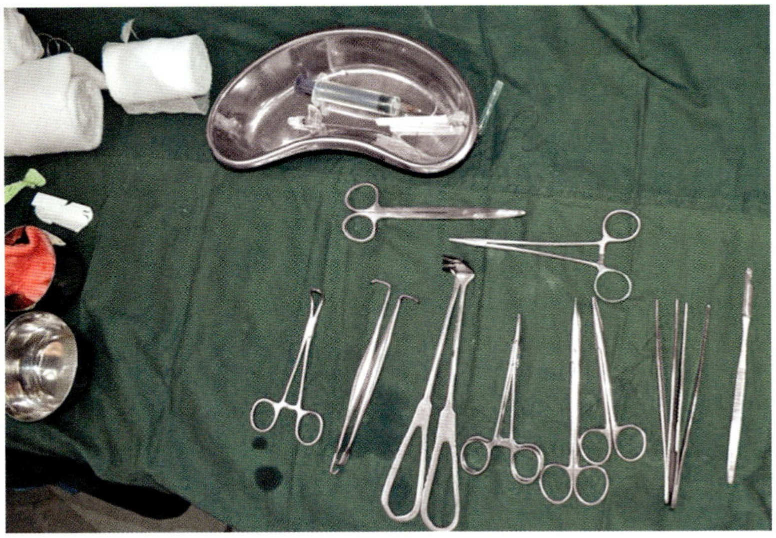

Fig. 9: Instruments necessary for surgery.

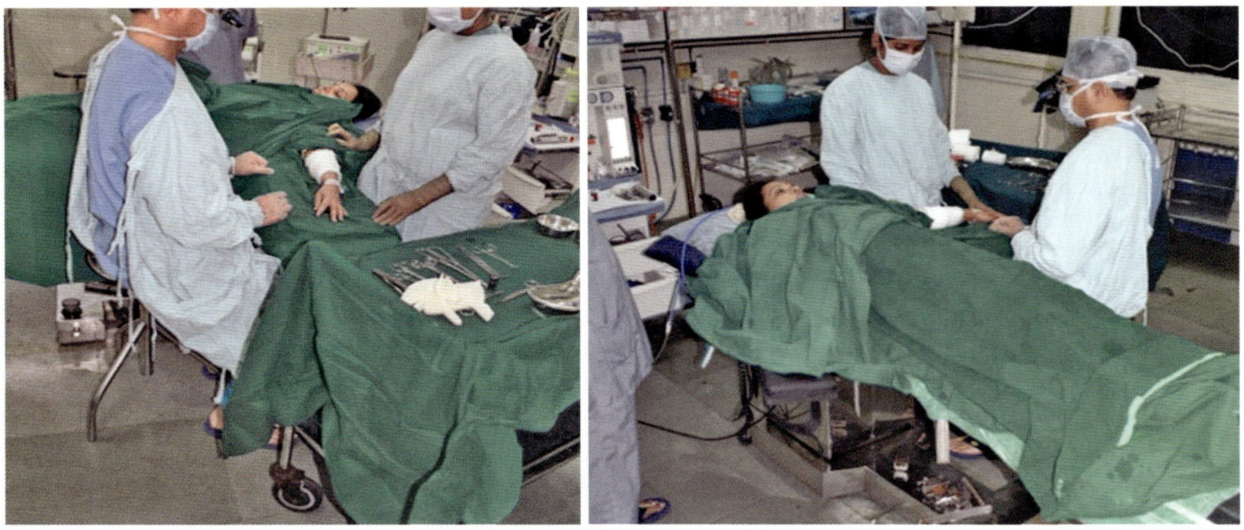

Fig. 10: Position of the surgeon, assisting nurse, patient and the instrument trolley at the end of the surgery.

SUGGESTED READING

1. Green's operative hand surgery. Seventh edition. Elsevier Publication. 2017;949-53.

CHAPTER 47

Excision of Soft Tissue Swelling of Thumb

S Prakash, Onkar Lande, Prashant Mall

INTRODUCTION

In benign tumors, tumors of soft tissue are more common than bone. These may originate in any tissue like subcutaneous tissue, muscles, blood vessels, ligaments and nerves.

Appearance of these is quite diverse. Some of the tumors can be quite aggressive. Adjacent soft tissue invasion increase the chance of inadequate excision therefore increasing the possibility of the recurrence of the tumor. For these reason, other treatment modalities like radiation are required.

Some examples of Benign tumors are as follows:

- Angiolipoma
- Lipoma
- Benign fibrous histiocytoma
- Neurofibroma
- Schwannoma
- Hemangioma
- GCT of tendon sheath
- Myxoma
- Neurilemmoma.

Few conditions like nodular fasciitis are not true tumors, but may need same treatment. A small number of these tumors may be related to an underlying inherited condition.

The majority of the tumors in this category are benign tumors of fat called lipomas. Lipomas frequently occur just beneath the skin as a soft painless mass and these grow slowly over a period of months to years. These soft tissue tumors are at very little risk so the patient and can be treated with marginal excision which is commonly called as "shelling out the tumor". Treatment has a high rate of success in this types. But not all of these lumps need to be Excised. We always wait and watch the lipoma,if symptomatic then go for treatment. Some of these lipomas are deep below the fascia or with the muscle group. Care should be exercised to distinguish these deep "lipomas" from cancers and lower grade cancers.

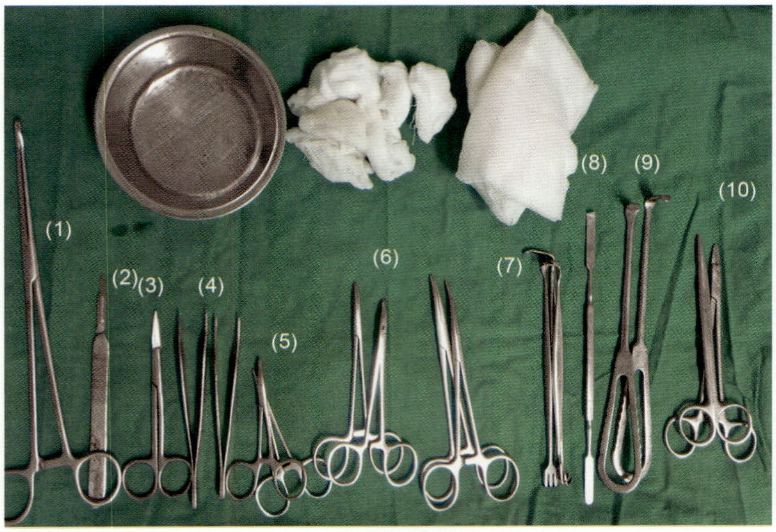

Fig. 1: *Instruments*: (1) Sponge-holding forceps, (2) Bard-Parker handle with blade 15, (3) scissor, (4) blunt forceps, (5) mosquito forceps, (6) artery forceps, (7) catspaw retractor, (8) dura protector, (9) Langenbeck retractor, and (10) needle holder with scissor.

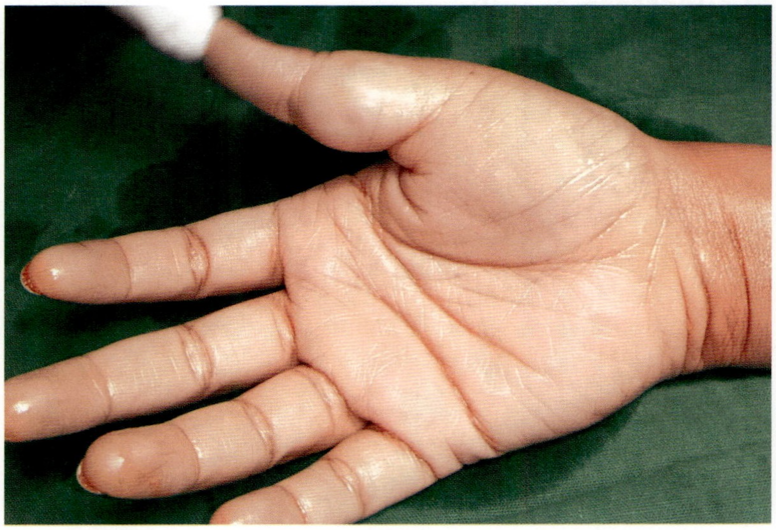

Fig. 2: Position given, painting and draping done.

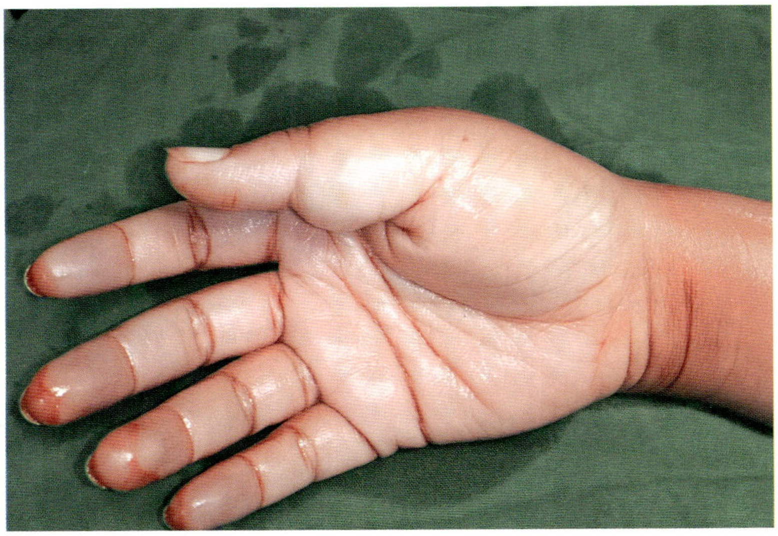

Fig. 3: Soft tissue swelling on the flexor aspect of the thumb.

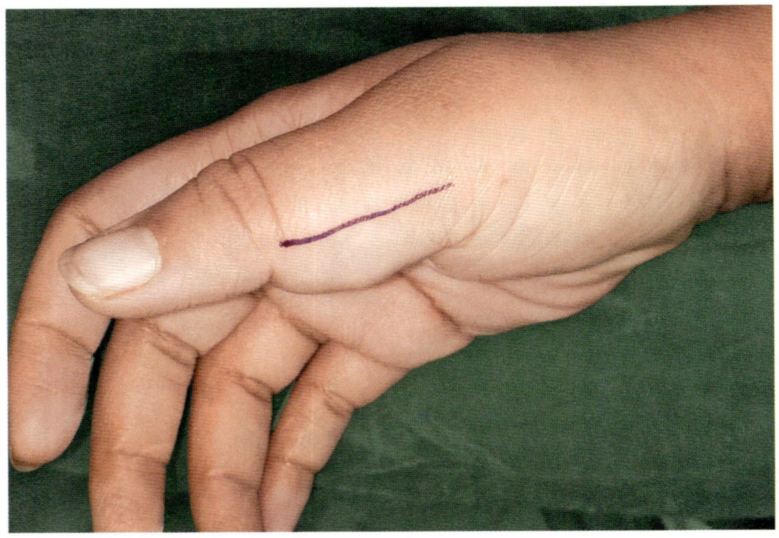

Fig. 4: Operative site marked.

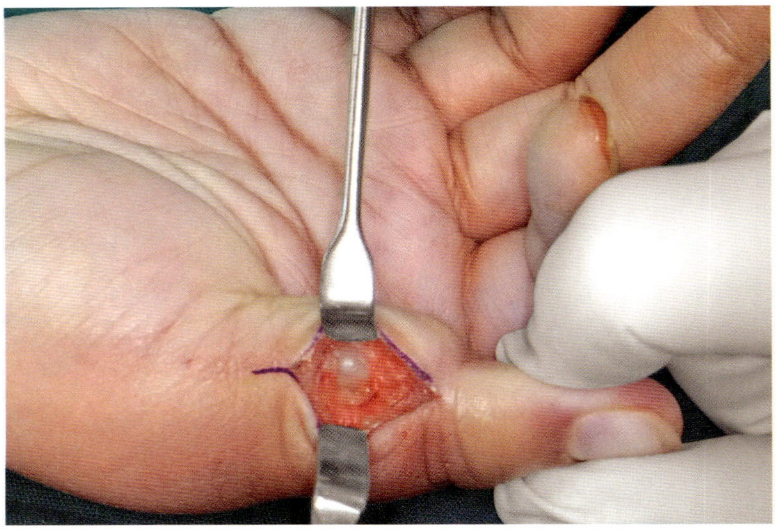

Fig. 5: Incision taken along the junction of the dorsal and volar aspect of thumb radially.

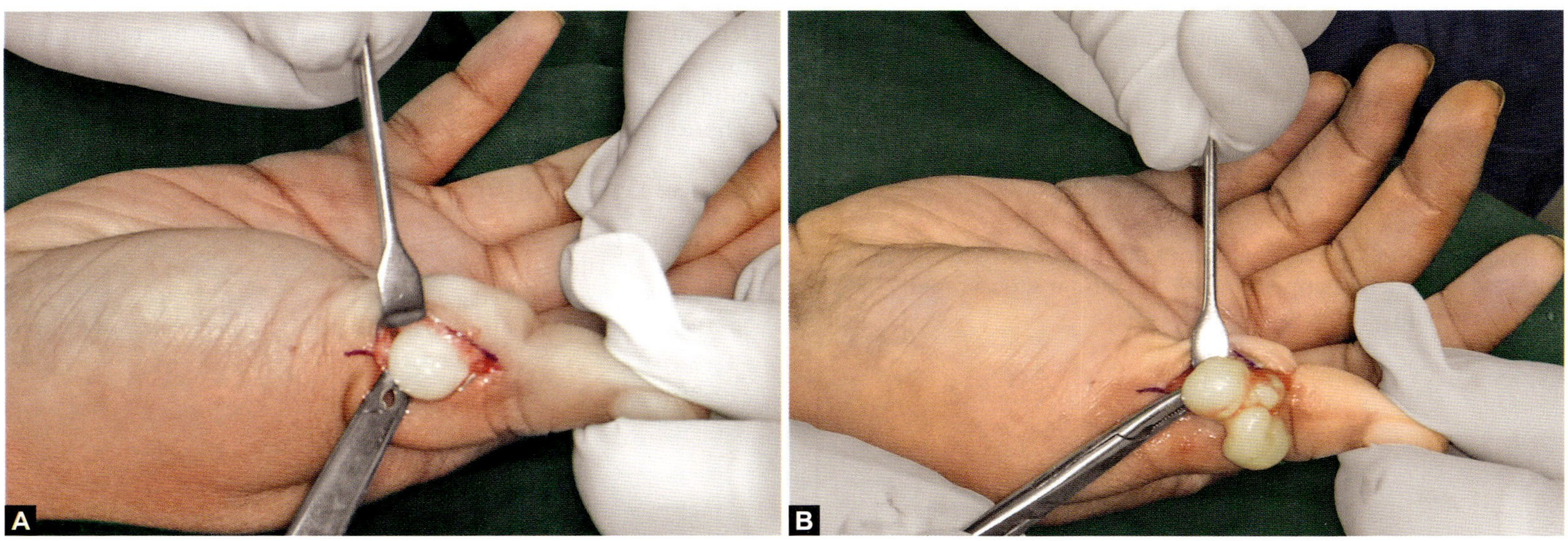

Figs. 6A and B: Soft tissue dissected layer by layer till swelling exposed.

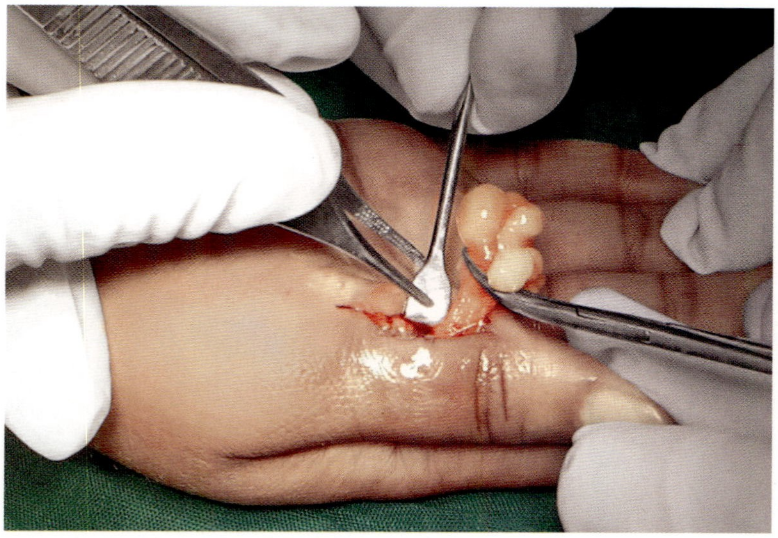

Fig. 7: With help of scissor soft tissue swelling incised with margin from the sheath of the flexor pollicis longus tendon.

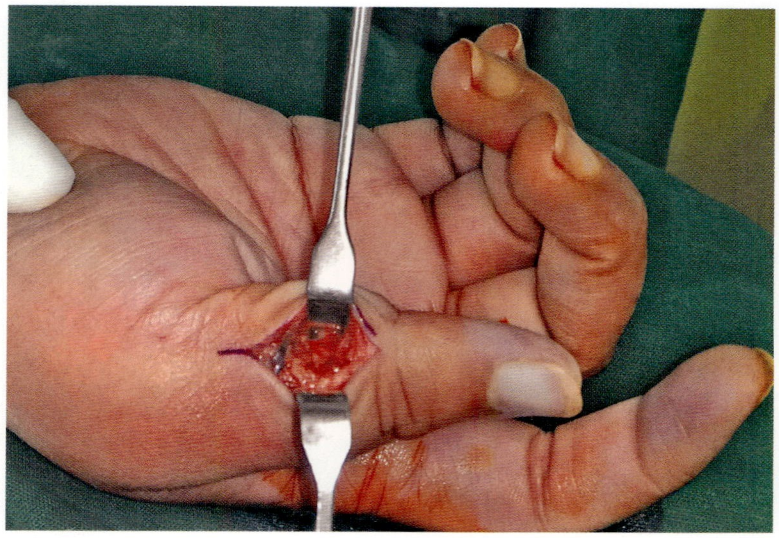

Fig. 8: Soft tissue swelling excised.

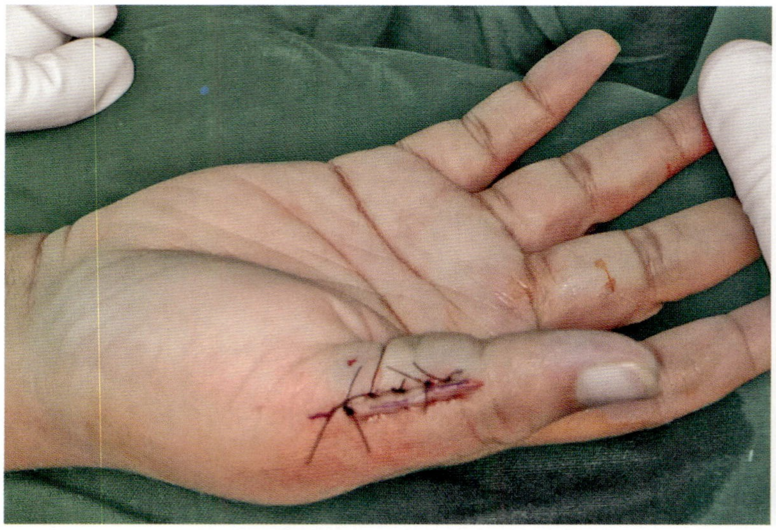

Fig. 9: Suturing done layer by layer.

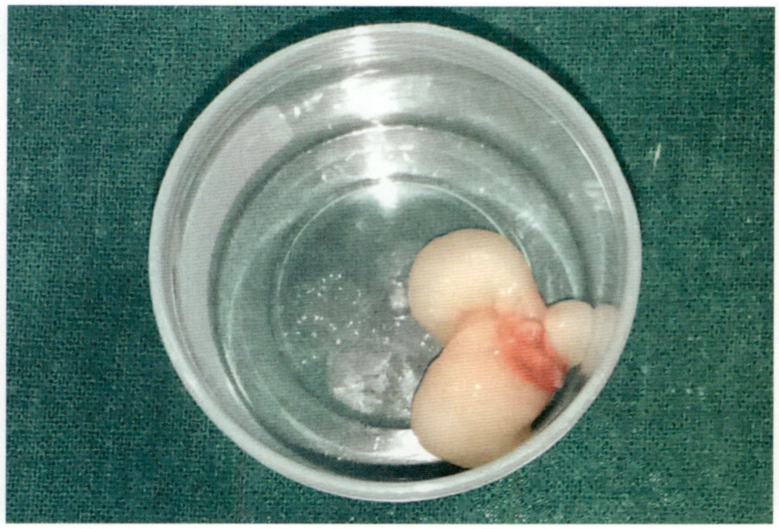

Fig. 10: Excised specimen.

Most of these tumors can be treated by a single procedure of marginal excision. Any large size tumor, any rapidly growing one or tumor with unusual presentation needs to undergo an adequate biopsy first. Magnetic resonance imaging scans though not totally reliable may offer a clue to the aggressive nature of the tumor.

SYMPTOMS

Benign soft tissue tumors sometimes may or may not be painful and widely distributed in appearance. If the tumor grows rapidly then it may cause pain.

TREATMENT

Depending on the type of tumor one may or, may not recommend surgery. Tumors are removed surgically while taking good care to avoid injury to surrounding normal blood vessels, nerves, muscle or bone.

SUGGESTED READING

1. Enzinger FM, Weiss SW. Soft Tissue Tumors. St Louis: CV Mosby Co.; 1983.
2. Hajdu SI. Differential Diagnosis of Soft Tissue and Bone Tumors. Philadelphia: Lea & Febiger; 1986.
3. Hajdu SI. Pathology of Soft Tissue Tumors. Philadelphia: Lea & Febiger; 1979.

CHAPTER 48

Fracture Neck of 5th Metacarpal K Wire Fixation

Ajit N Damle

SURGICAL STEPS (FIGS. 1 TO 6)

Use of a tourniquet, makes the procedure easy. The proximal end of the fifth metacarpal is palpated and the tip is located by palpation and confirmed by a C-arm image.

To make entry in the outer cortex of the metacarpal, either a small size Kuntscher Diamond Awl or a pointed device to locate a locking hole of an interlocking nail is used. It is used to penetrate the near cortex of the proximal metacarpal, by gentle rotation under pressure, till a small hole is made. This device is replaced by a 2 mm K-wire, held in a Jacob Chuck with T-handle, to make a track. Not more than 2 cm of K-wire is kept outside the chuck, or else, the wire bends, under pressure. The K-wire tip is stabilized in the cortex at right angle to the shaft and is then gently tilted, to be at an acute angle with the shaft, to be nearly parallel to the medullary cavity. By oscillating motion,

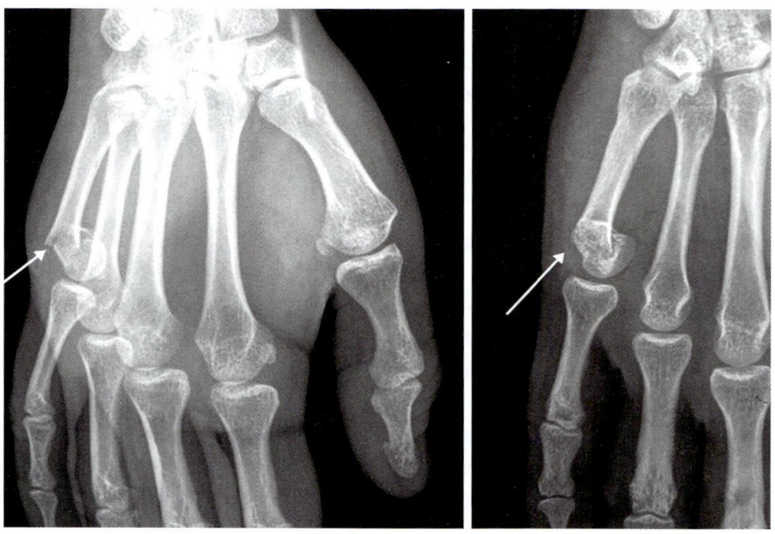

Fig. 1: Fracture neck of the fifth metacarpal.

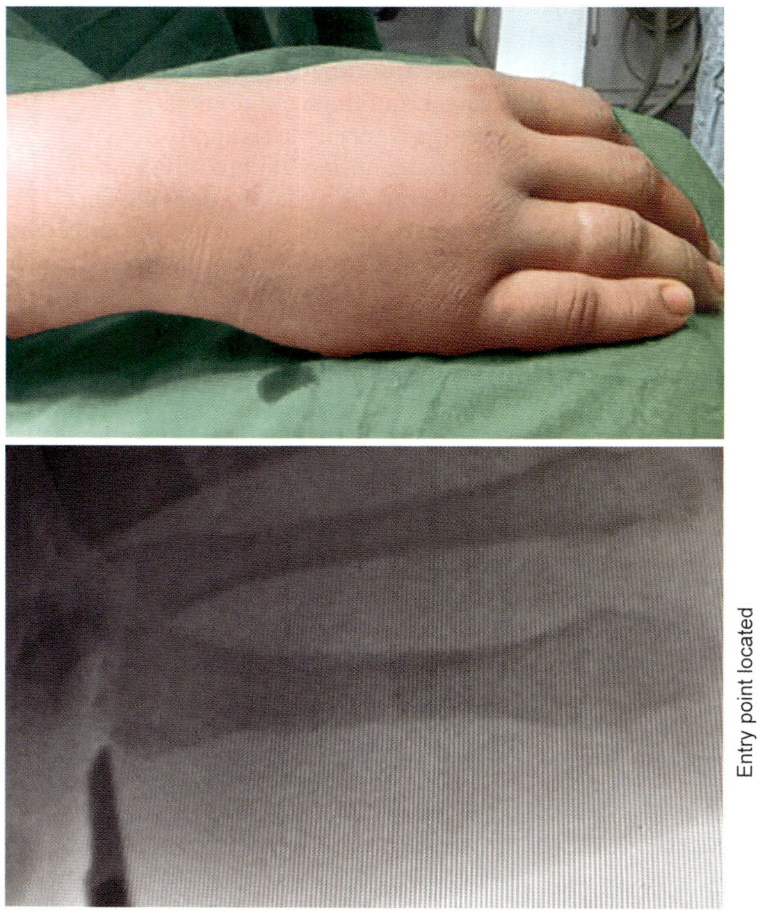

Fig. 2: One 2-mm K-wire and another 1.2 mm are selected. The later wire is bent at 4 mm from the trocar end to 30°. Keeping these two wires ready makes steps easy and expeditious. It is preferable to have two Jacob Chucks with T-handle, for each of these wires, to save time and make the procedure easy.

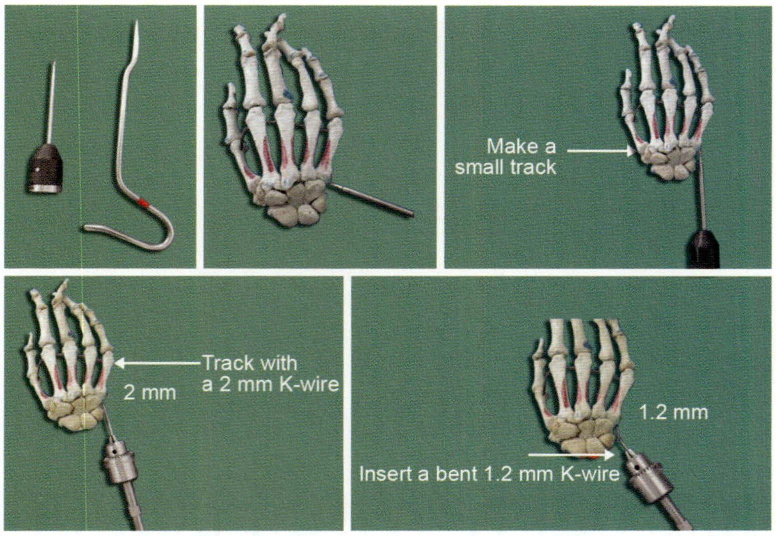

Fig. 3: Diagrams in insertion of K-wire.

an oblique track is made in the cortex. The other K-wire of 1.2 mm diameter mounted in a Jacob Chuck is taken and the tip is placed close to the first wire, as parallel to the shaft as possible, so it can be advanced proximal to distally (the first 2 mm K-wire is removed). As the 1.2 mm wire is advanced, it should glide along the endosteum and one gets a grating feel to hand, holding the chuck. This grating is a sure sign, that the wire is intraosseous. The chuck needs to be loosened, moved backwards on the wire, retightened, and the wire is gradually advanced.

The progress is monitored under C-arm, while traction is maintained on the little finger and the head of metacarpal is kept aligned to the shaft. The wire is advanced till it is approximately 4 mm from the subchondral area and confirmed in both the views under C-arm images. One should take care, that the wire does not penetrate the bone end and make a track in the bone, leading to the joint. One accepts, whatever good position of the wire, one can achieve, to confer stability to the fracture area.

Possible Problem during Insertion of the K-Wire

If the axis of the 1.2 mm K-wire insertion is incorrect, it abuts against the endosteum and can not be advanced, easily. Hence, it is slightly withdrawn till the entry site, angle of insertion is made more parallel to the shaft and advanced.

At this stage, one can have idea, if the cavity would accommodate another 1.2 mm K-wire. If so, another K-wire is passed in the same way. When it reaches, distal/three of the metacarpal, it is so placed, that the wire tip would be at 180°, compared to the first one, conferring a "bouquet" effect to the assembly. Both the wires are alternately advanced, till reach the subchondral bone. The tourniquet is released and wound closed.

Managing the Proximal End of the K-Wires

- Where to cut
- Whether to bury
- Whether to keep the end outside the skin.

All the three above different techniques are practiced by surgeons.

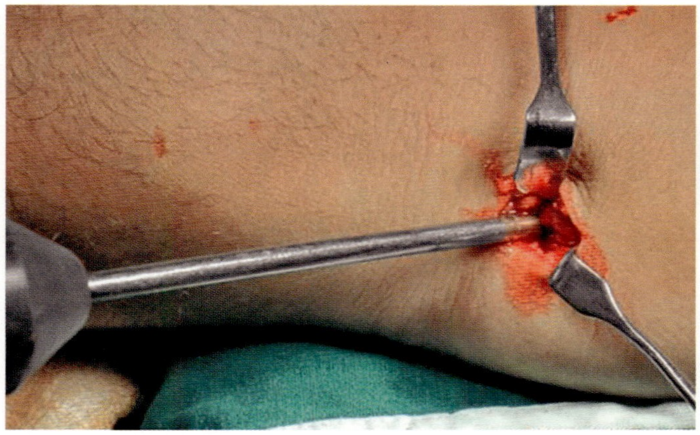

Entry track with an awl

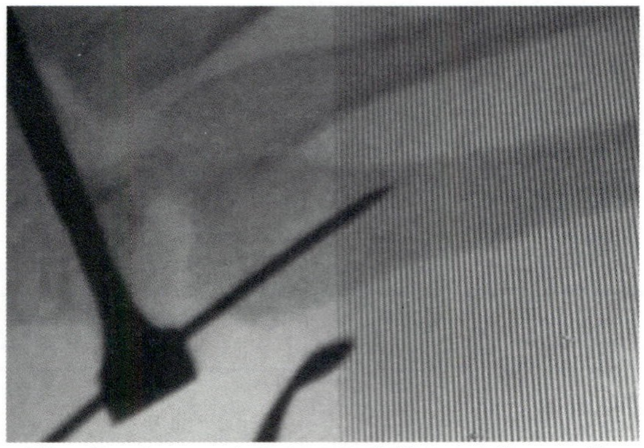

Wire direction needs to be parallel to medullary cavity, hence withdrawn

Fig. 4: Changing axis of K-wire entry.

Keeping the End Outside the Skin

- This offers ease in removal of the K-wire.
- However, after removal of the plaster support and mobilization of the hand, one needs to keep it dressed and covered to protect from causing injury to other limb.
- Such a fracture takes at least 2–3 months to consolidate.
- Removal of a K-wire, may lead to late reappearance of deformity at the fracture site and hence, one needs to continue to keep the wire in place, till the fracture consolidates.

Leaving the Tip of Wire Buried under the Skin

- I choose to slightly bend the wire near the entry track and cut-off at 4 mm from the track edge.
- This prevents migration of the wire.
- After removal of the plaster support, patient can have bath the same day.
- Since, the wire tips are buried under the skin, it is better accepted by the patient and gradually can mobilize the wrist and fingers well. The fracture continues to consolidate in the position achieved.

The wrist is immobilized by a cock up anterior plaster of Paris (POP) slab, till the proximal palmer crease and with a dorsal hood slab, till the proximal interphalangeal (PIP) joints, with metacarpophalangeal (MCP) in 90° flexion. The patient is encouraged to carry out active flexion of all fingers and keep them supple, with good range of motion.

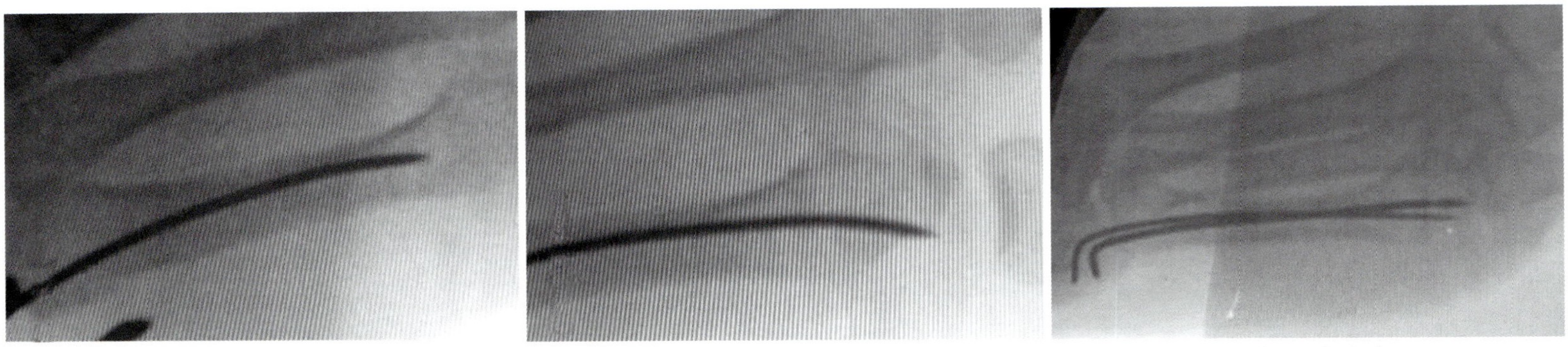

Wire advanced against endosterum — Final position — Insertion of IInd wire

Fig. 5: Second wire inserted.

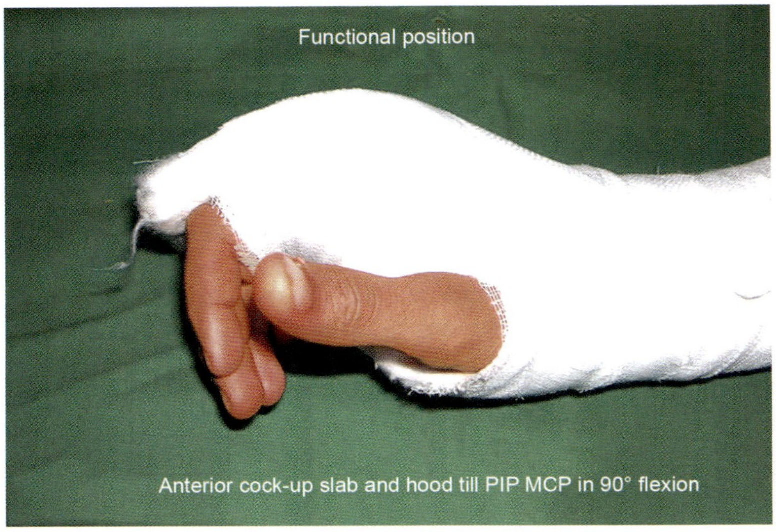

Fig. 6: Plaster slab support. (PIP: proximal interphalangeal; MCP: metacarpophalangeal)

CHAPTER 49

Glomus Tumor

Samrat K Taori

INTRODUCTION

Glomus tumor is considered as "hamartoma" developing from glomus body. Most of these tumors are found in hand and most commonly are located in fingertip, where it can be subungual (most common), parangual, palmar ulnar or palmar radial. Patients present with painful fingertip and there is classic triad of symptoms seen: (1) Cold hypersensitivity, (2) paroxysmal pain, and (3) pinpoint pain.

CLINICAL EXAMINATION

Clinical tests which suggest diagnosis are:

- *Love test*: Point tenderness assessed by head of pin (Figs. 1 and 2).
- *Hildreth's test*: Disappearance or absence of pain or tenderness on applying tourniquet (blood pressure cuff) after exsanguination of the limb and pain felt on releasing the tourniquet.
- *Cold test*: Pain on exposure to cold water or ice.
- Nail plate may show ridges, deformation or bluish discoloration in few cases (Figs. 2A to C).

INVESTIGATION

X-rays are mostly normal and few may show scalloping, erosive changes (Figs. 2D and E).

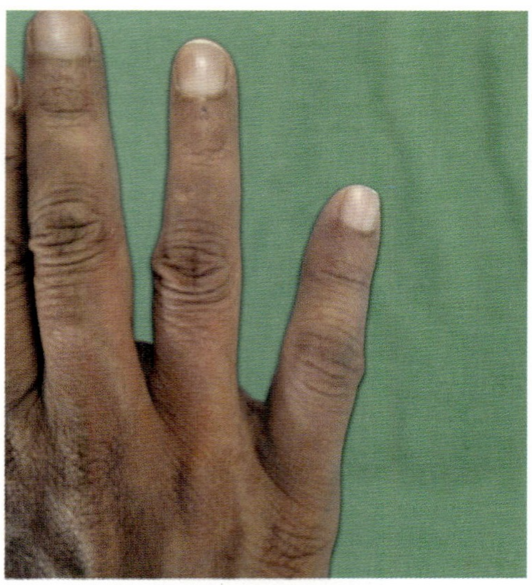

Fig. 1: Case A: Clinical examination showing pinpoint tenderness.

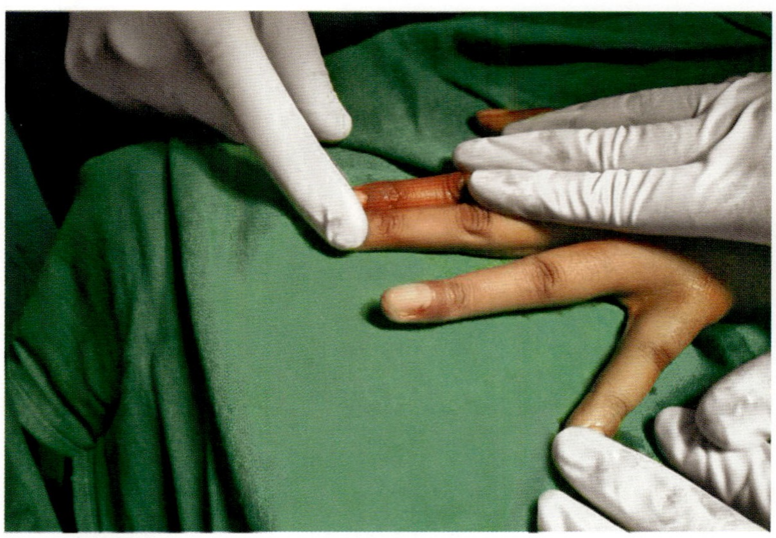

Fig. 2A: Case B: Clinical picture showing nail deformity due to subungual glomus tumor.

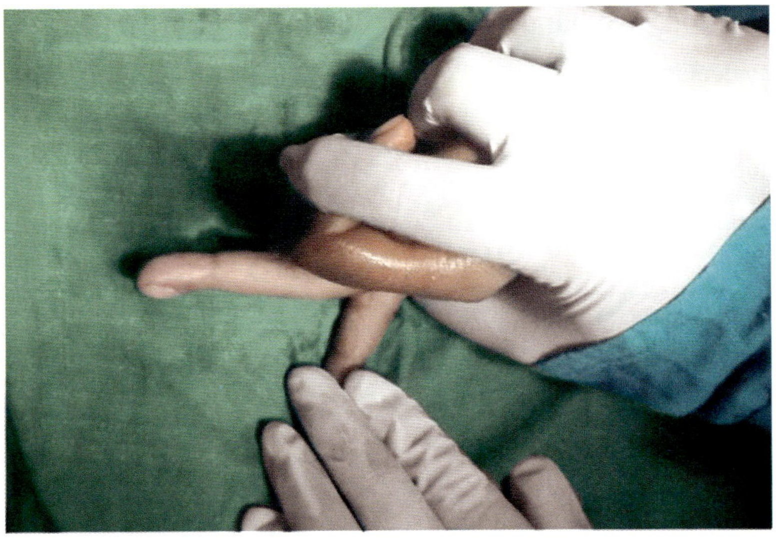

Fig. 2B: Case B: Clinical picture of nail deformity due to subungual glomus tumor.

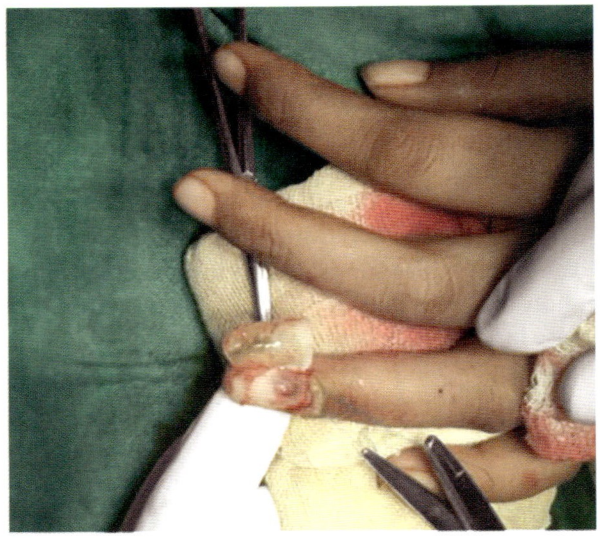

Fig. 2C: Intraoperative finding in case B.

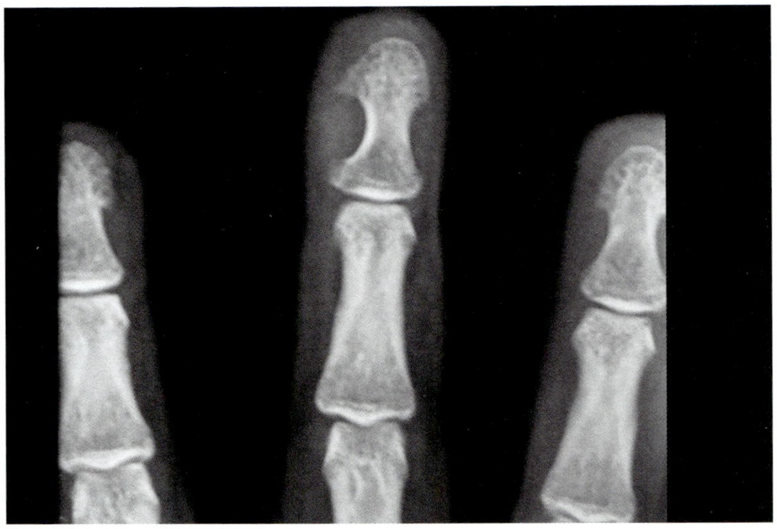

Fig. 2D: Case C: Scalloping seen on X-ray.

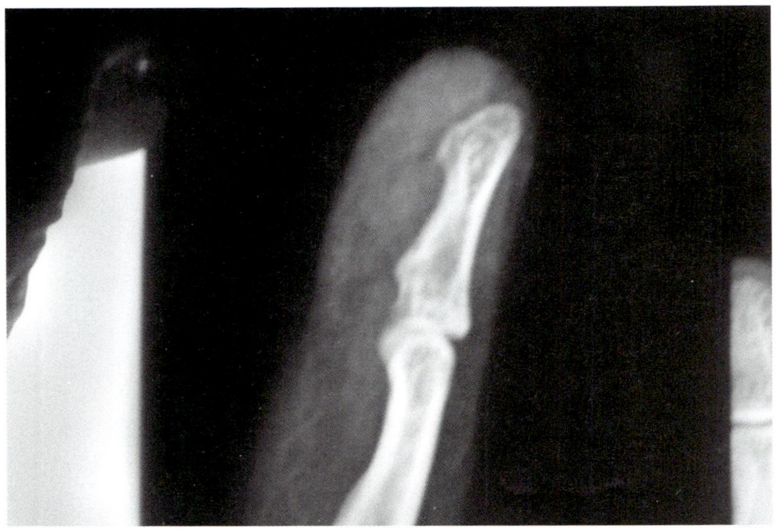

Fig 2E: Case C: Scalloping seen on X-ray

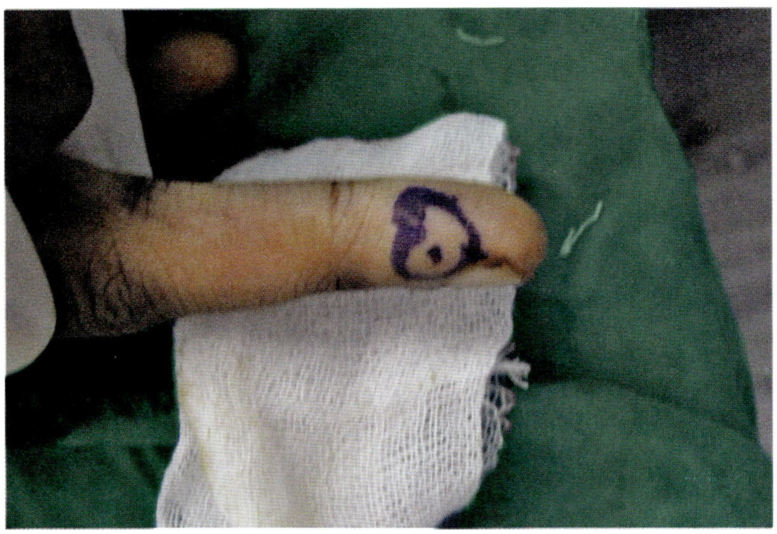

Fig. 2F: Clinical picture of case C.

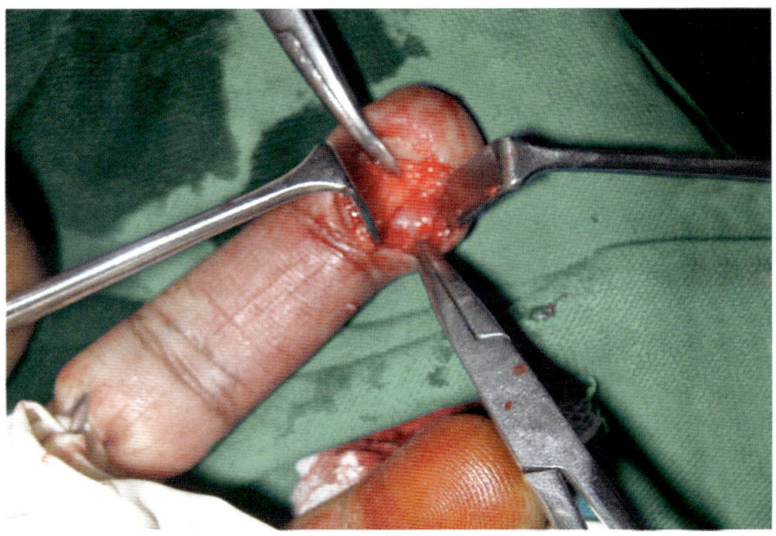

Fig. 2G: Intraoperative photograph of case (C) in Figures 2D and 2E volar ulnar lesion.

DIFFERENTIAL DIAGNOSIS

Differential diagnoses which should be considered and ruled out are:

- Subungual exostosis
- Osteoarthritis
- Pyogenic granuloma
- Hemangioma
- Chronic paronychia

There can be multiple lesions which may be painless. Recurrence is uncommon after complete excision but these painless lesions may later increase in size and become symptomatic and this can be cause of recurrence of pain at operated site.

TREATMENT

Surgical excision is the treatment of choice. Adequate illumination, tourniquet, magnification and meticulous technique are required.

OPERATIVE STEPS

We describe technique of excision of glomus tumor at subungual location since it the most common.

Case A is a 40 years old female who consulted for severe pain in finger tip at base of nail since 3 years. Diagnosis was based on classical clinical findings and X-ray was normal.

Excision of Subungual Glomus Tumor: Surgical Steps

Patient is operated under digital block or brachial block given as per discussion with the patient and as decided by anesthetist. Patient lying supine, affected limb is kept over hand table. Digital tourniquet/Arm tourniquet is applied.

SURGICAL STEPS

1. Short oblique incisions are taken at the base of nail and eponychium is gently reflected and sutured proximally by 4-0 nonabsorbable suture (Figs. 3 and 4)
2. Nail plate is elevated from the nailbed and kept attached to paronychium on one side. This requires a smooth and flat elevator. The plate is firmly attached at the hyponychium. I prefer to put a suture through the elevated nail plate which makes it convenient to retract (Figs. 3 and 4).
3. Subungual swelling is evident by subtle or significant elevation and color change. Vertical incision is made over the swelling incising the nailbed. This may be limited to sterile matrix or may extend proximally into the germinal matrix (Fig. 5).
4. The tumor is identified and gently separated from surrounding structures by sharp dissection (Figs. 6 and 7).

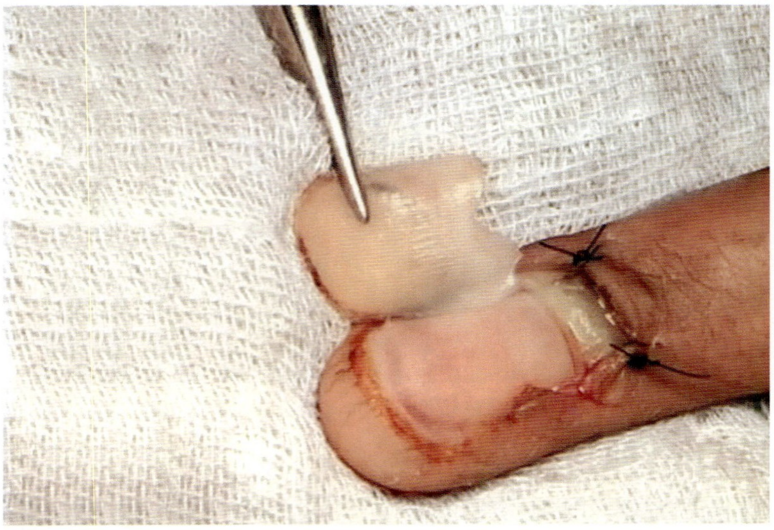

Fig. 3: Steps 1 and 2 case A.

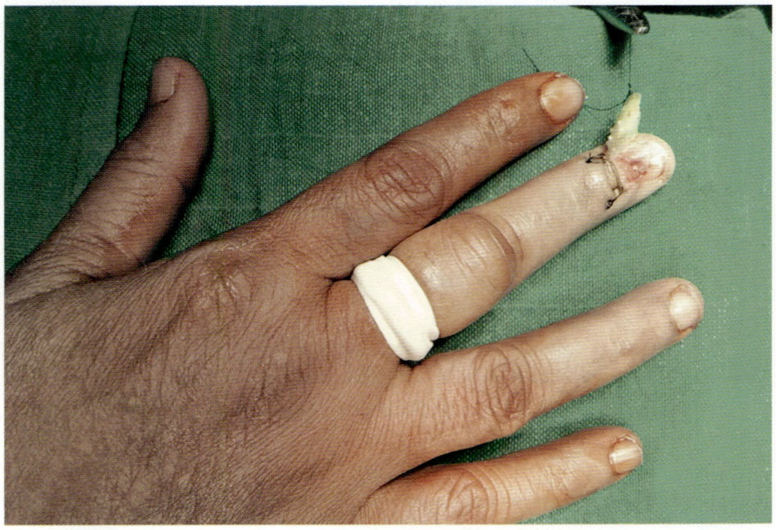

Fig. 4: Different case: Step 2 case D.

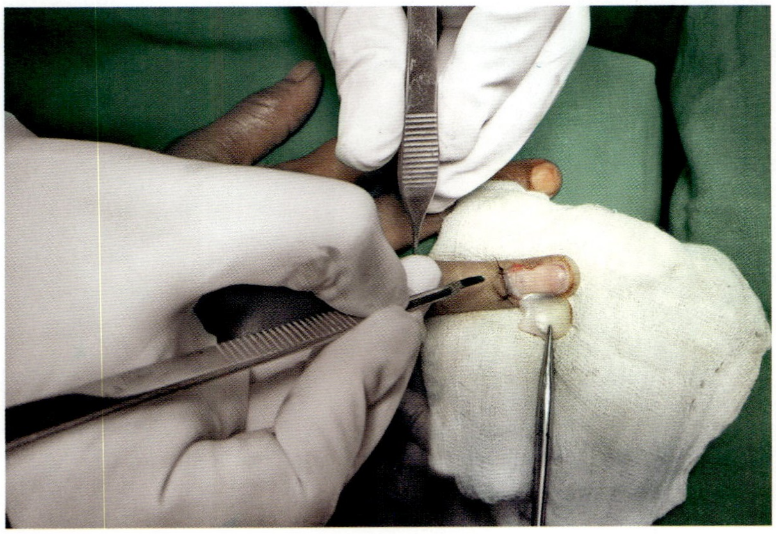

Fig. 5: Step 3.

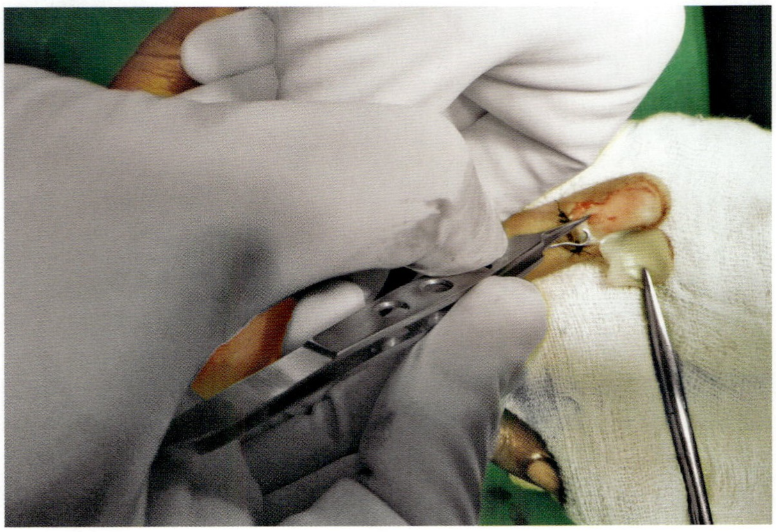

Fig. 6: Step 4.

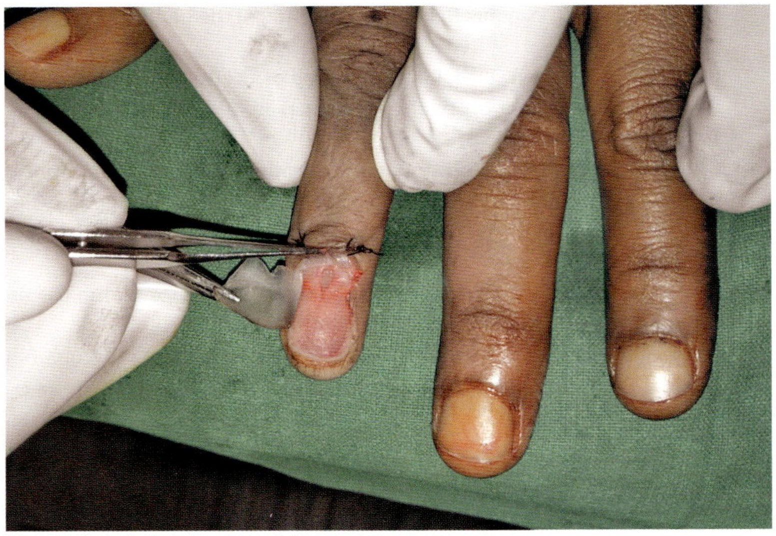

Fig. 7: Step 4.

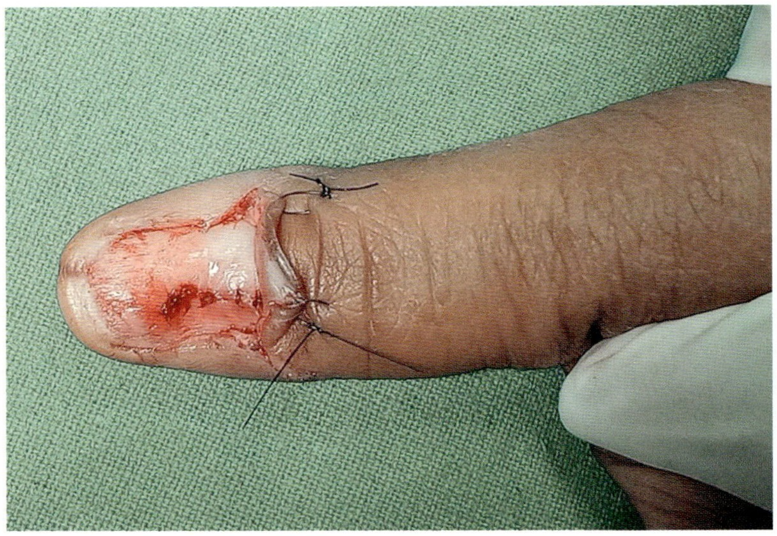

Fig. 8: Step 5: Different case D.

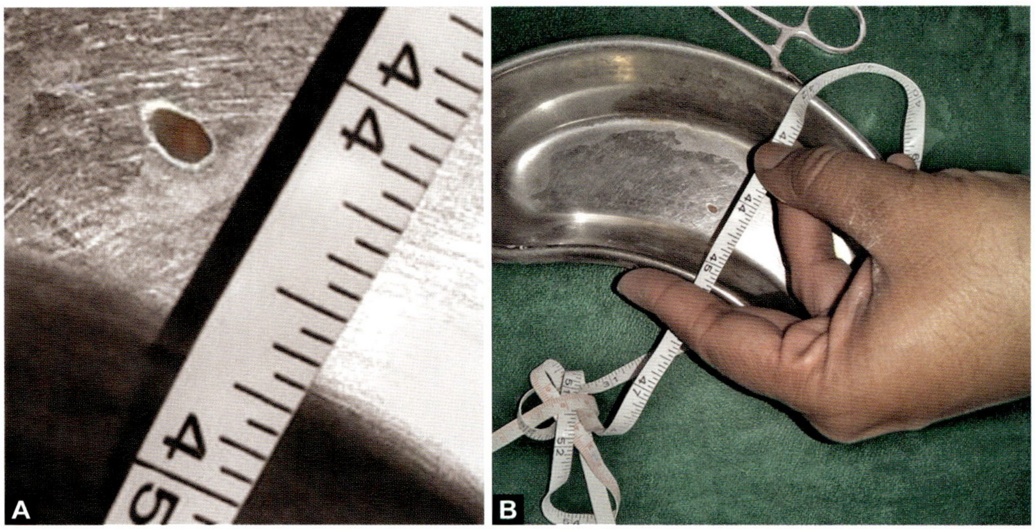

Figs. 9A and B: Specimen.

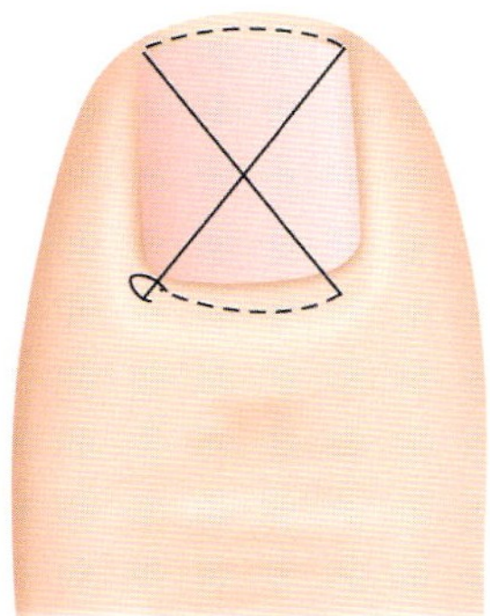

Fig. 10: Figure of 8 suture technique to stabilize the nail plate.

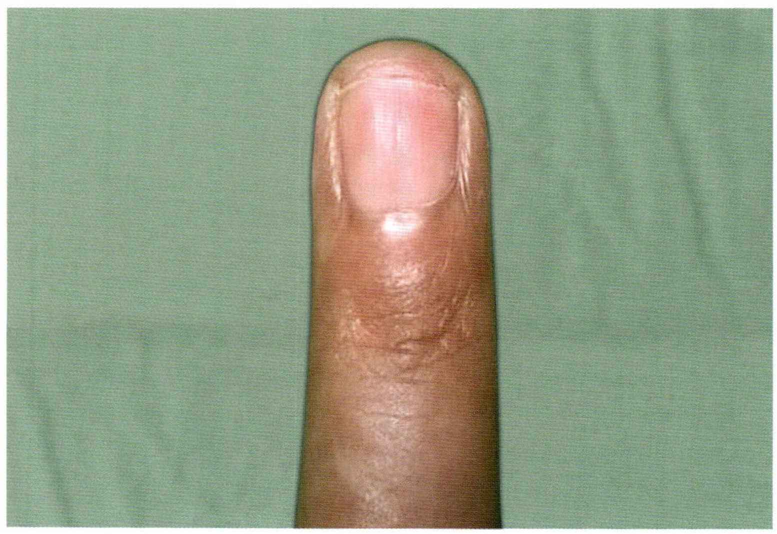

Fig. 11: Appearance of nail at the end of 1 year.

5. Nailbed is repaired by 6-0 absorbable or nonabsorbable suture material (Fig. 8).
6. Nail plate is fenestrated to allow drainage and repositioned in the nailfold. It is held in position by Figure of 8 sutures (Fig. 10).

POSTOPERATIVE PROTOCOL

Patient is advised strict limb elevation for initial 3 weeks padded aluminium splint is applied on finger on volar aspect for initial 3 weeks for rest to be operated part and to avoid accidental trauma. Gentle and complete movements are advised at regular intervals at all joints including distal interphalangeal joint by removing the splint.

SUGGESTED READING

1. Baek HJ, Lee SJ, Cho KH, et al. Subungual tumors: Clinicopathologic correlation with US and MR imaging findings. Radiographics. 2010;30:1621-36.
2. Bhaskaranand K, Navdag BC. Glomus tumors of the hand. J Hand Surg. 2002;27B:229-31.
3. Carroll RE, Berman AT. Glomus tumors of the hand: review of the literature and report on twenty-eight cases. J Bone Joint Surg Am. 1972;54:691-703.
4. Gandhi J, Yang SS, Hurd J. The anatomic location of digital glomus tumor recurrences. J Hand Surg Am. 2010;35:986-9.
5. Rettig AC, Strickland JW. Glomus tumor of the digits. J Hand Surg Am. 1977;2:261-5.
6. Van ruyssevelt CE, Vranckx P. Subungual glomus tumor: emphasis on MR angiography. Am J Roentgenol. 2004;182(1):263-4.
7. Wolfe S, Pederson W, Kozin SH. Green's Operative Hand Surgery, 6th Edition. London: Churchill Livingstone; 2010. p. 2392.

CHAPTER 50

Thenar Flap

Pankaj Jindal

An exposed bone needs to be covered with a flap. In case of finger tip injury, where the bone is exposed, various flaps are available, like cross finger flap, V to Y advancement flap to name just a few. The thenar flap offers a distinct advantage of having a perfect color match, without any donor site morbidity. The donor site can be approximated primarily.

SURGICAL STEPS

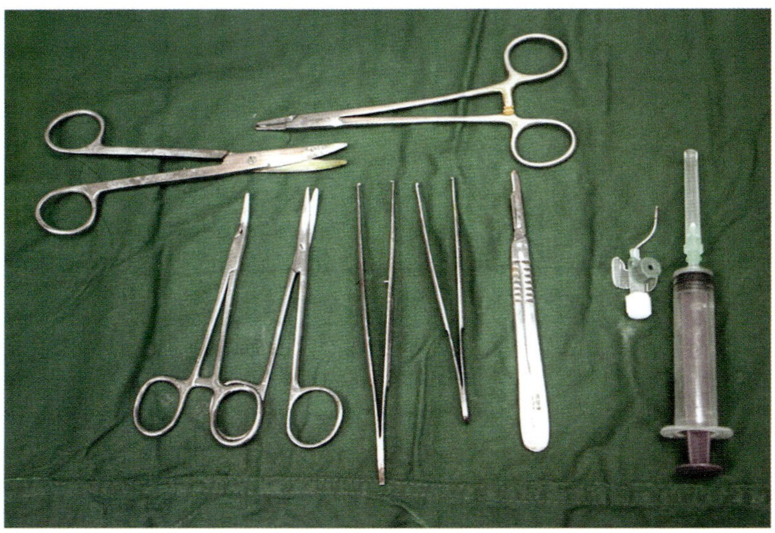

Fig. 1: Instrument trolley. Fine needle holder, fine toothed forceps, and tenotomy scissors are important for this surgery.

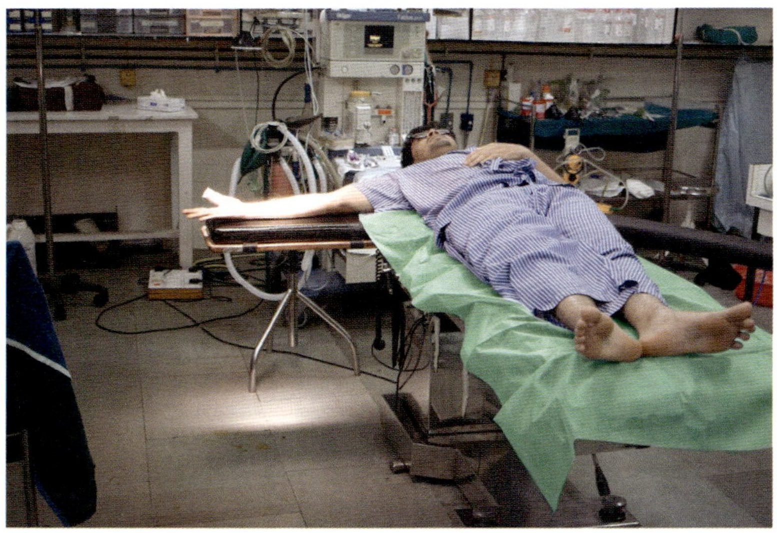

Fig. 2: Patient is supine on surgical table with hand on hand table in supine position.

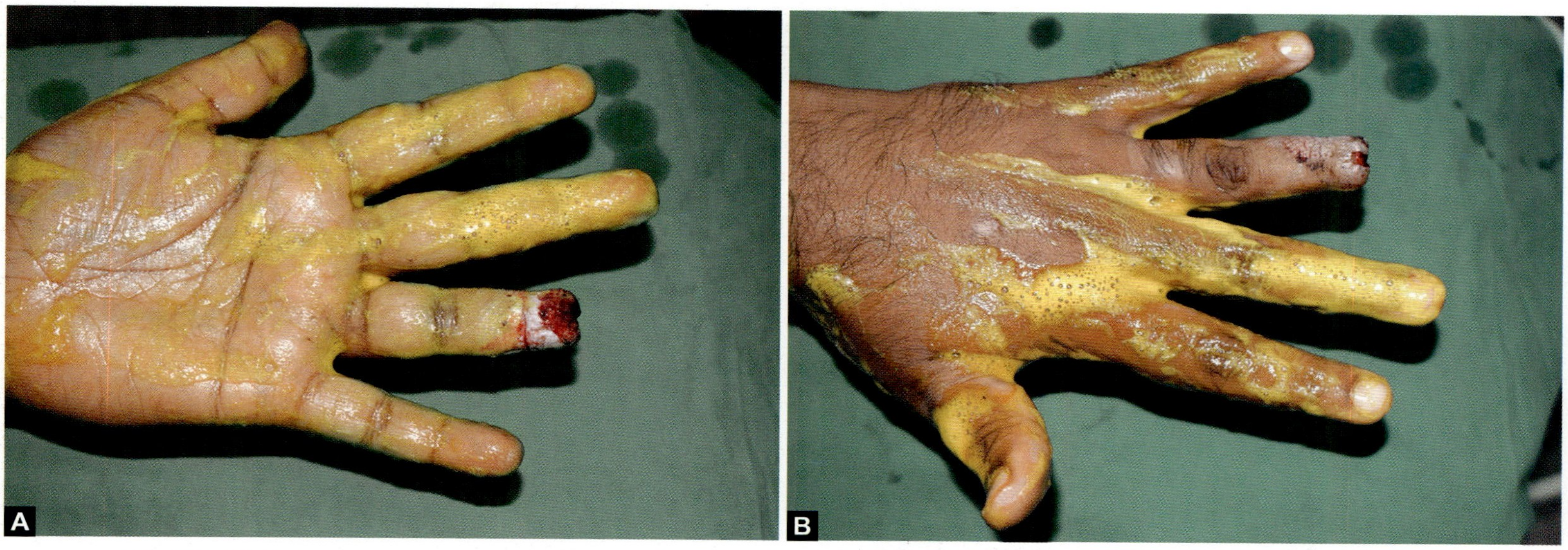

Figs. 3A and B: Figures showing traumatic loss of pulp of left ring finger. The wound was a transverse amputation of the fingertip. Thenar flap is best suited for transverse and volar oblique fingertip amputations.

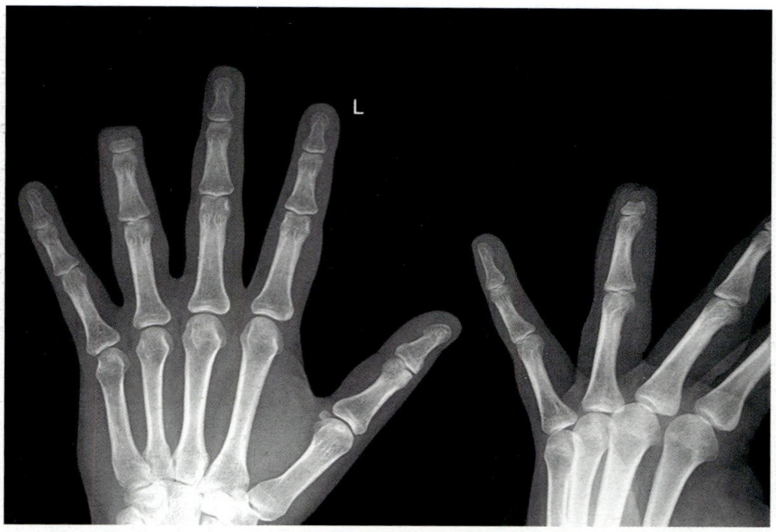

Fig. 4: Radiograph of injured finger showing loss of distal third-fourths of distal phalanx.

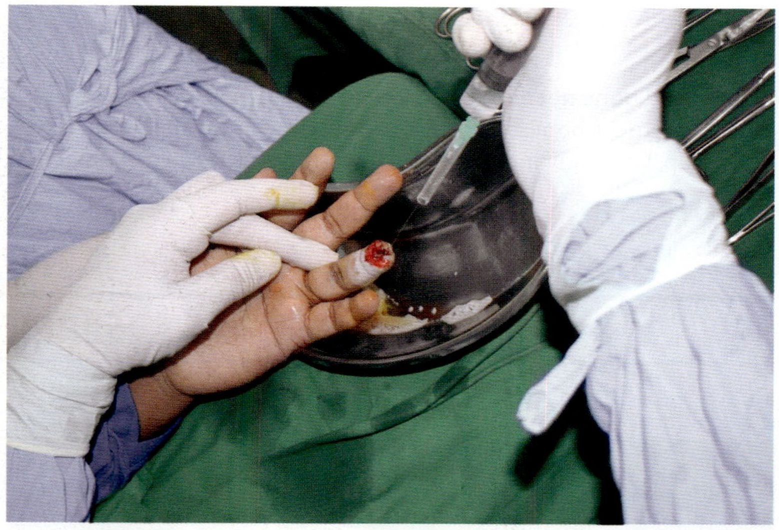

Fig. 5: Under Bier's block, wound is debrided well and washed with normal saline using 10 mL syringe with the needle. the hub covering the needle is cut at the close end with a bandage scissors. The hub over the needle provides the protection from accidental needle stick injury.

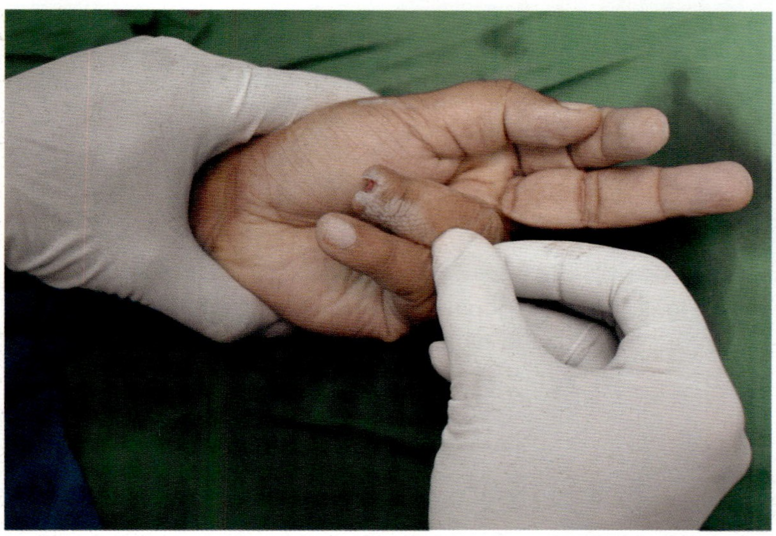

Fig. 6: Location of flap to be raised is determined by the comfortable reach of the recipient finger on the thenar area. This step is important as this position has to be maintained for 3 weeks.

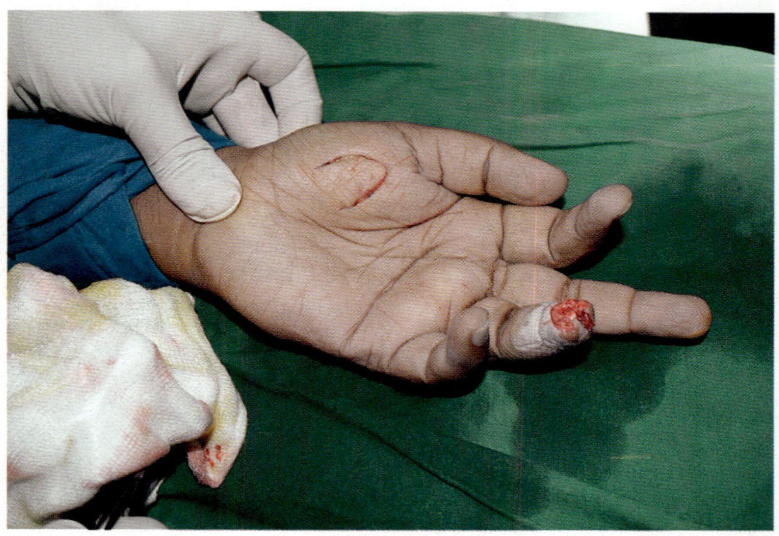

Fig. 7: Incision is made for an ulnarly-based random pattern flap of dimensions same or slightly larger than defect size.

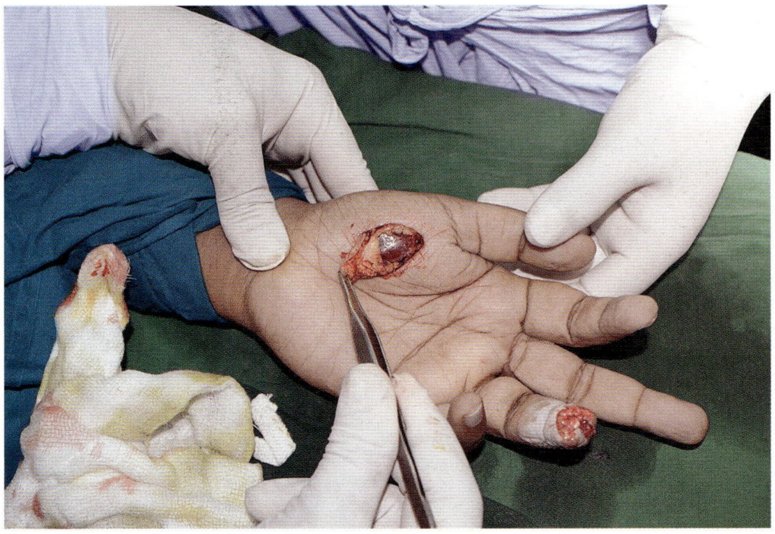

Fig. 8: Flap is raised in a plane superficial to thenar muscles so as to include skin, thenar fascia, and subcutaneous fat.

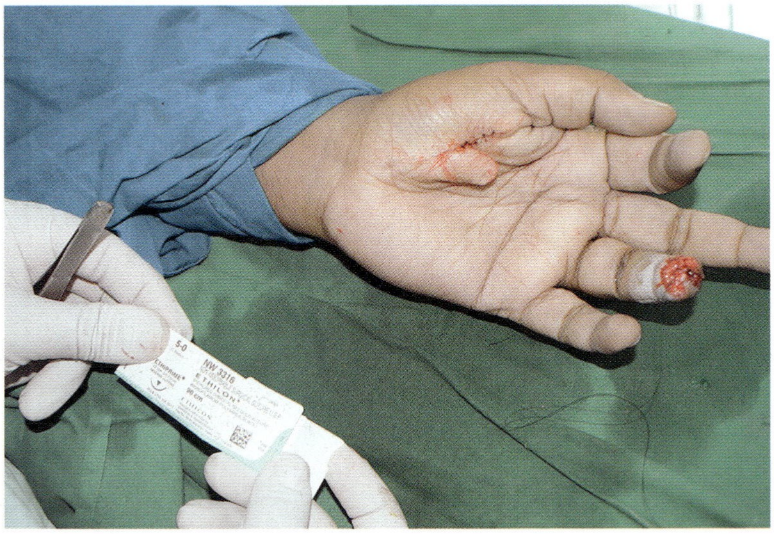

Fig. 9: Secondary defect is closed directly with fine nonabsorbable sutures.

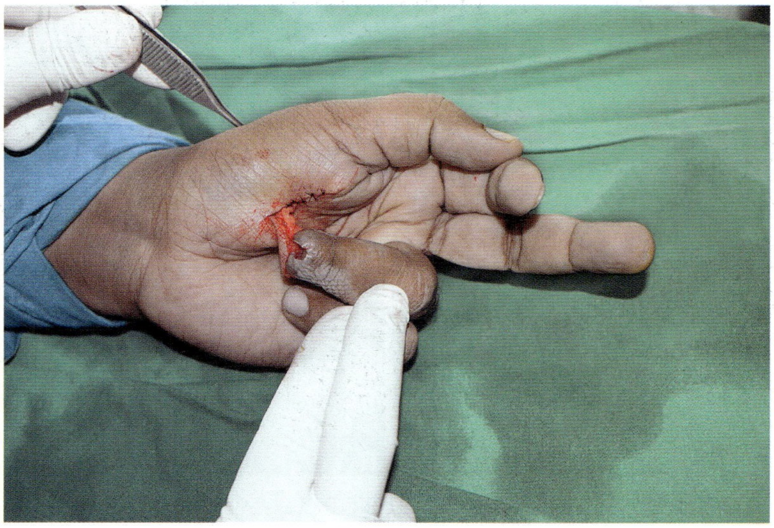

Fig. 10: Flap is rotated volarward for inset onto defect.

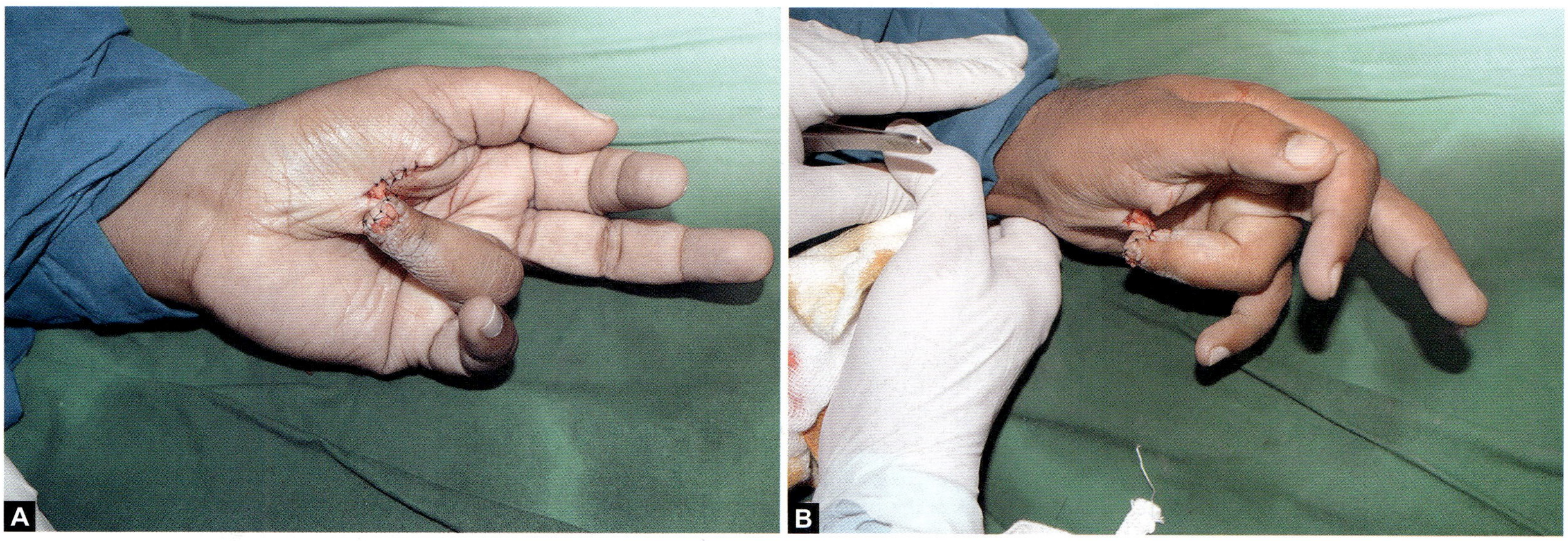

Figs. 11A and B: Inset completed with 5-0 nonabsorbable suture. Note raw area at base of flap which patient should be explained about. Raw area is likely to bleed in initial few hours and one should not be alarmed by persistent serous discharge from the same till wound is closed completely at second stage.

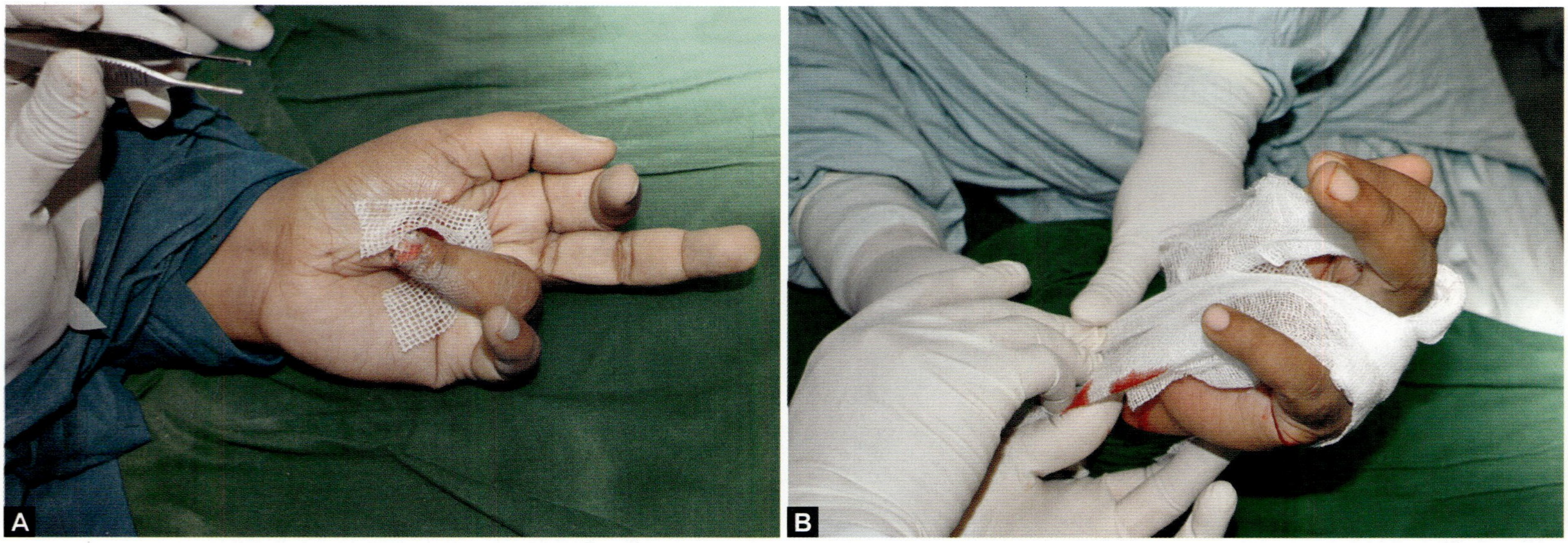

Figs. 12A and B: Dressing being applied. Surgeon may choose to protect the flap with a dorsal below elbow slab.

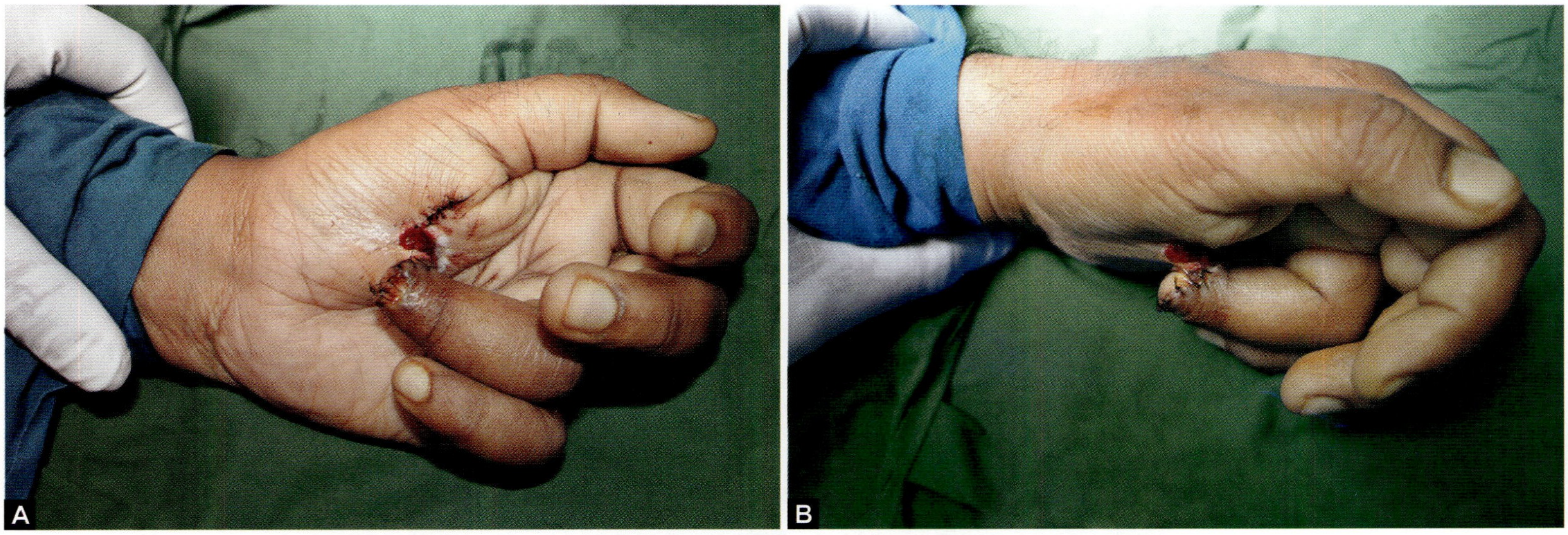

Figs. 13A and B: Appearance of flap at 3 weeks from index surgery. Note granulation tissue over raw area left at the end of index surgery. Position and anesthesia were similar to index procedure.

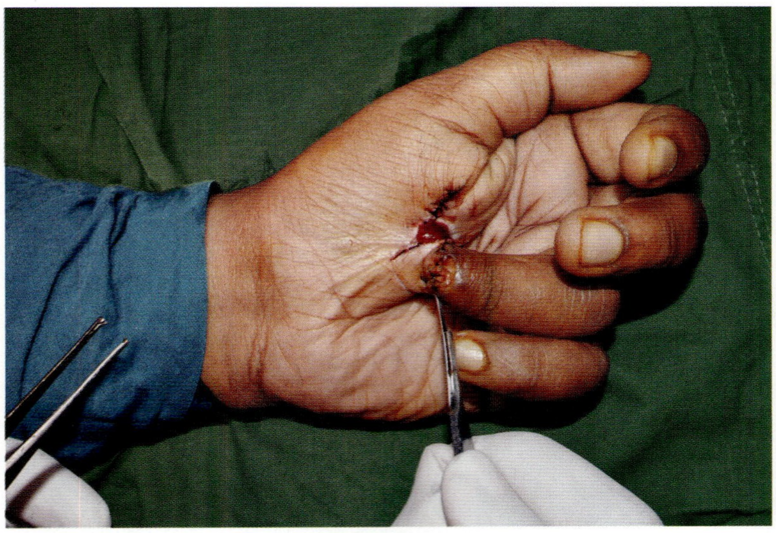

Fig. 14: An extended triangular tongue of skin of the thenar region, measuring about the same length as the base, is raised as an extension of the base of the flap. The depth of the skin incision should be just enough to include the subcutaneous fat. Care is needed to prevent damage to digital nerves lying in close proximity.

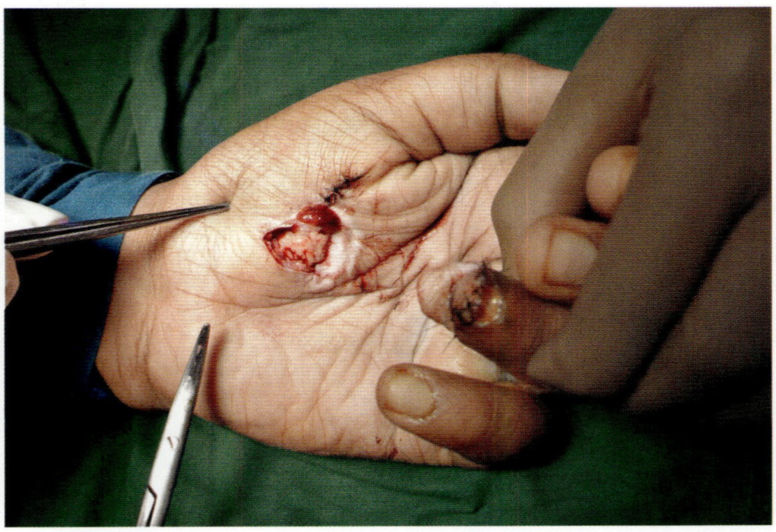

Fig. 15: Finger is detached from palm by dividing triangular extension of skin together with the flap.

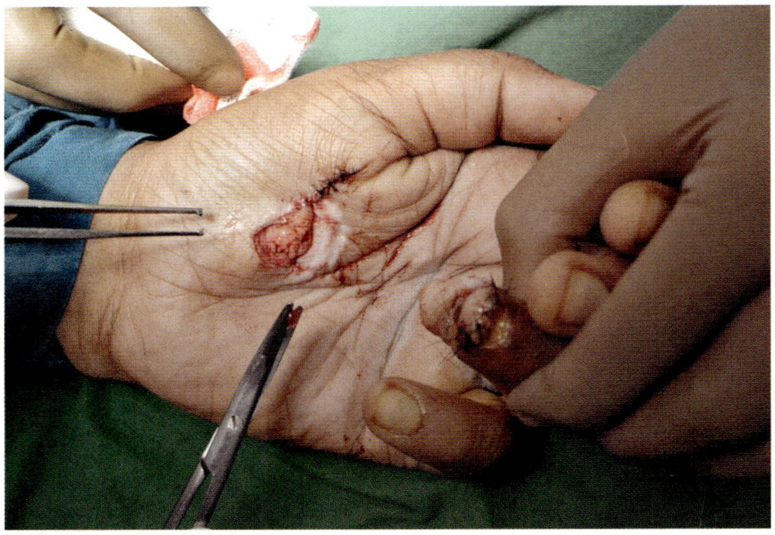

Fig. 16: Hypergranulation is removed from recipient site.

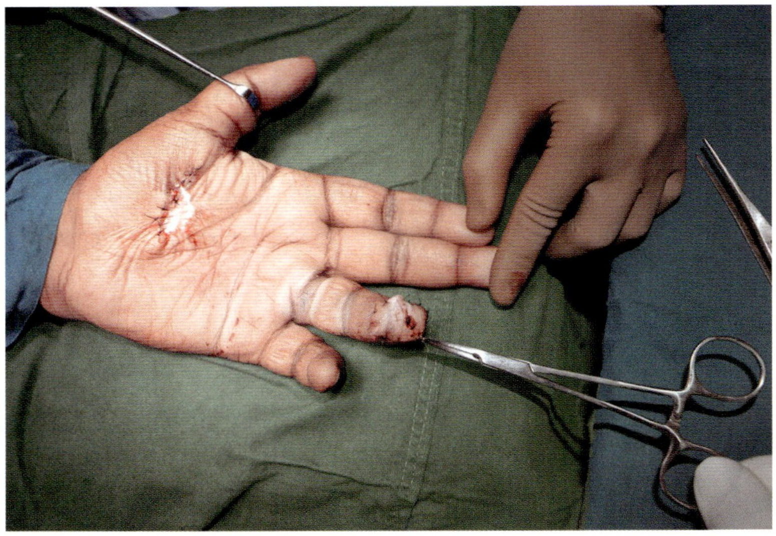

Fig. 17: Wounds over palm and finger is closed with 5-0 nonabsorbable sutures. Paraffin base dressing is applied.

SUGGESTED READING

1. Fingertip reconstruction with the laterally based thenar flap: indications and long-term functional results. Brian Rinker. Hand. 2006;1(1):2-8.

CHAPTER 51

Perilunate Dislocation

Pankaj Jindal

Perilunate dislocation occurs because of disruption of ligament around the lunate or fractures of the bones adjacent to lunate. When the ligaments fail, it is called lesser arc injury. When the injury occurs, with the fracture of that adjacent carpal, it is called greater arc injury. The injury occurs due to high velocity trauma and usually involves a young adult. As described in Mayfield's classification, the injury begins on the radial side of the lunate. The initial injury may be injury to the scapholunate ligament or fracture of the scaphoid bone. As the injury progresses, the injury will involve the ligament between the lunate and the capitate. In the further progression of the injury, the damage will involve the ligament between the lunate and the triquetrum.

SURGICAL STEPS (FIGS. 1 TO 26)

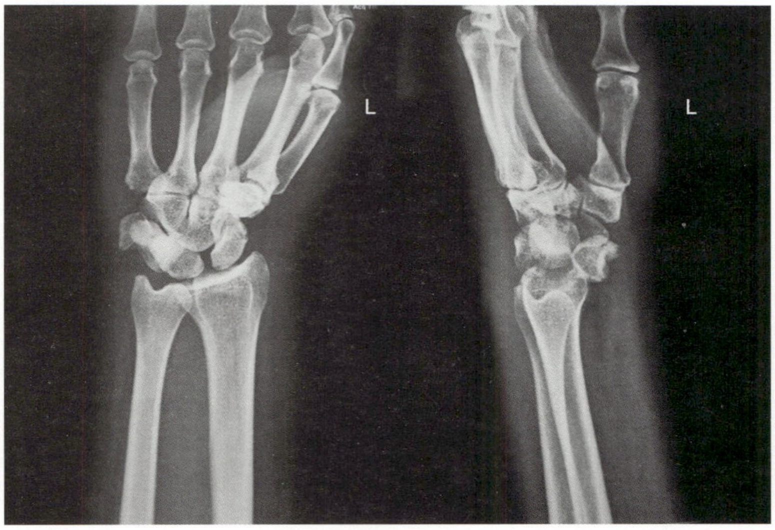

Fig. 1: Posteroanterior view of wrist in a 30-year-old patient with injury 6 weeks ago shows loss of concentric Gilula's lines. In lateral projection, the lunate is seen disengaged almost completely from distal radius with its distal articular surface pointing volarward, demonstrating "spilled teacup" sign. Clinically, the patient had symptoms of median nerve compression.

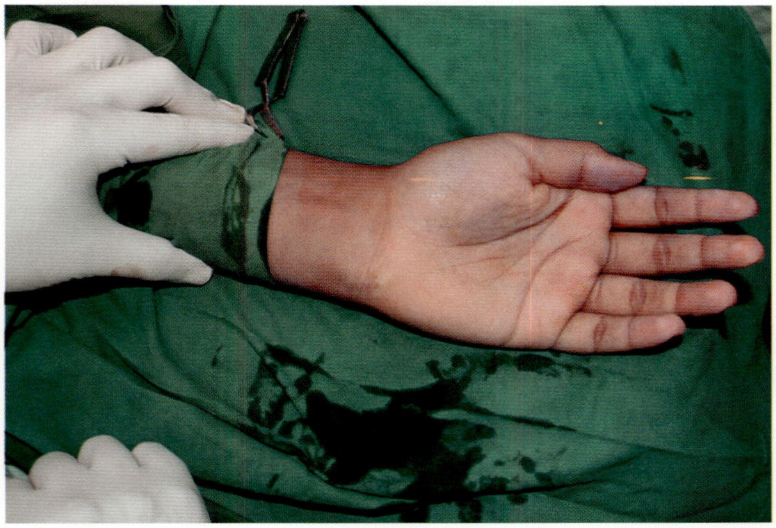

Fig. 2: Patient is supine on the operating table with the affected arm abducted to 90° on a radiolucent arm rest. Supraclavicular anesthesia is administered by the anesthetist. Tourniquet is applied on the upper arm.

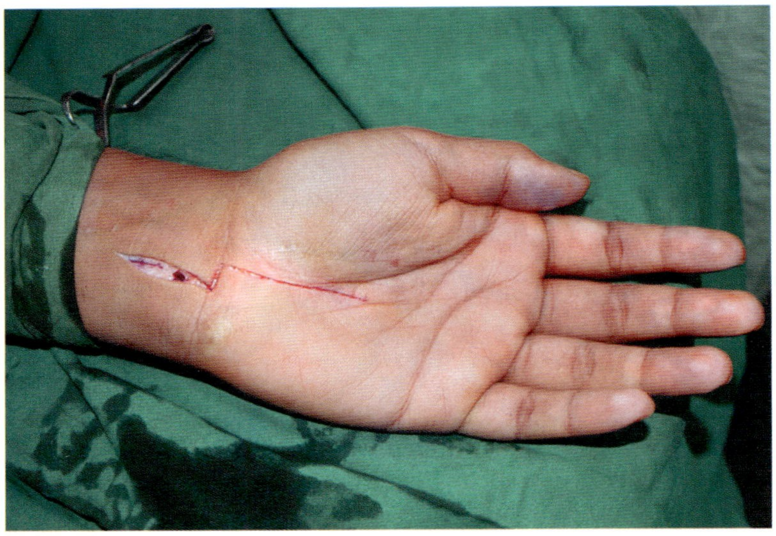

Fig. 3: Volar incision made in line with the ring finger, overlying the 4th metacarpal. At the level of the volar wrist crease, the incision curves parallel to the wrist crease and then proceeds proximally for another 2 cm.

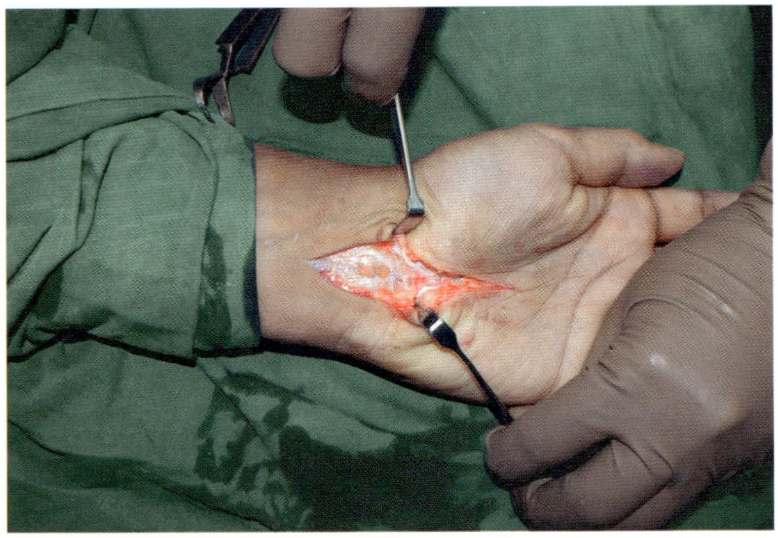

Fig. 4: As the incision is deepened, the median nerve is the first structure encountered in this case due to volar tenting of the median nerve by dislocated lunate.

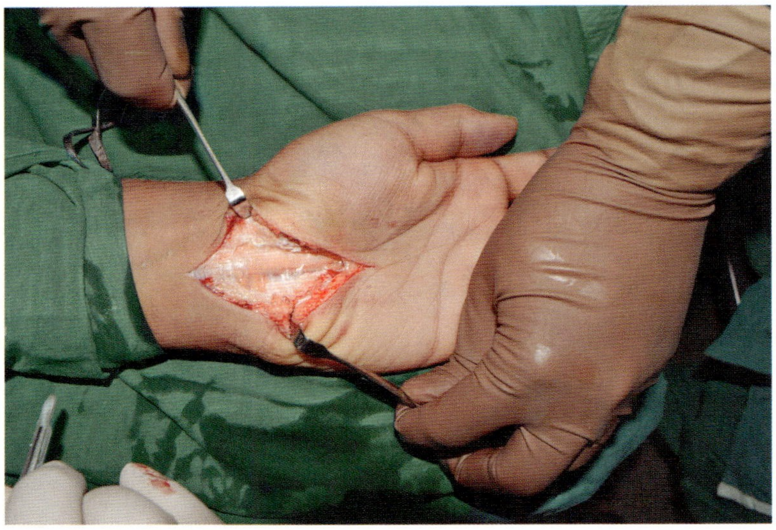

Fig. 5: Transverse carpal ligament divided to decompress the nerve and access carpus.

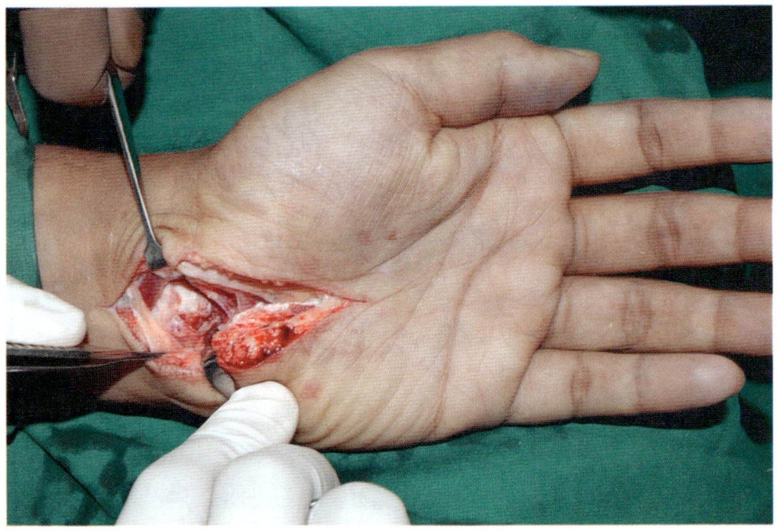

Fig. 6: Retracting the median nerve to the radial side reveals the lunate with its distal articular surface facing the surgeon.

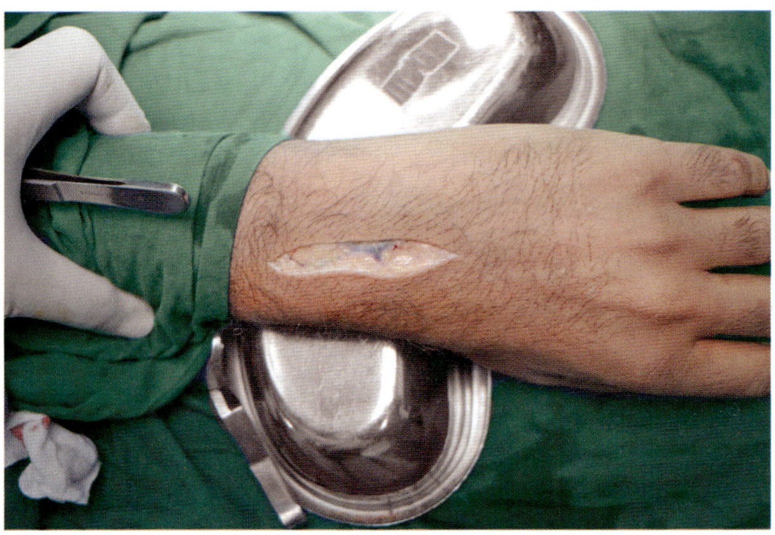

Fig. 7: Having completed decompression of the median nerve, we proceed to next part of the technique to relocate the lunate. Longitudinal dorsal incision is made over wrist just ulnar to Lister's tubercle.

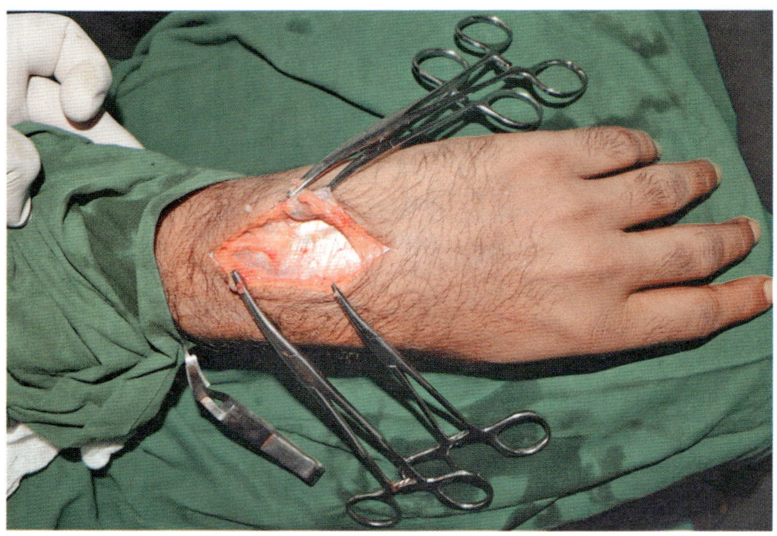

Fig. 8: The skin flaps are retracted exposing the extensor retinaculum (ER).

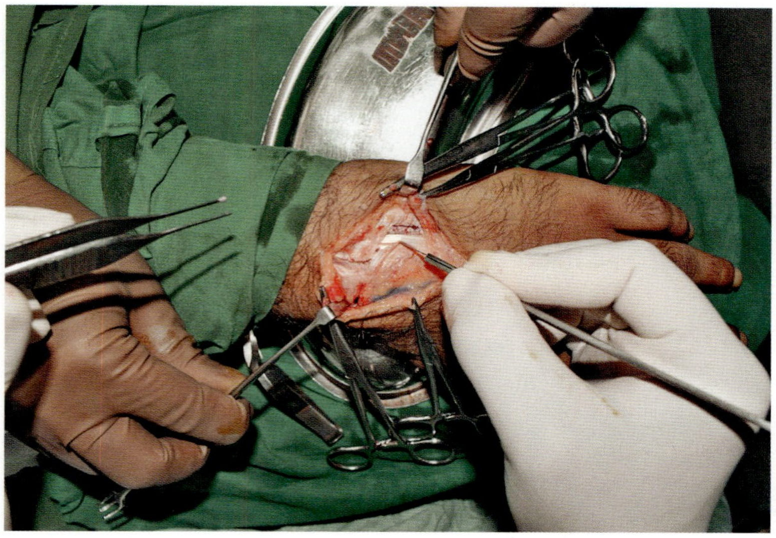

Fig. 9: The ER is incised in a step cut manner exposing the tendons of extensor pollicis longus (EPL).

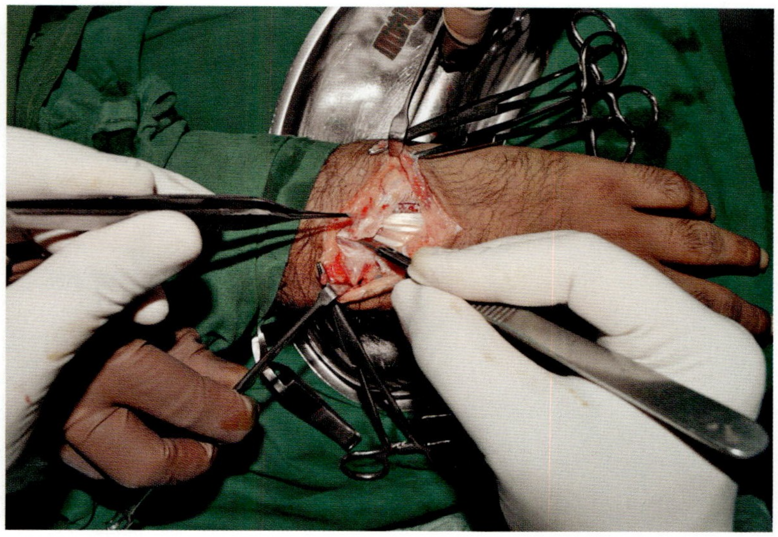

Fig. 10: Retinaculum flaps elevated to exposed extensor digitorum communis (EDC) tendons. The tendon of EPL is dissected out of its location from the ulnar aspect of the dorsal tubercle to the radial side.

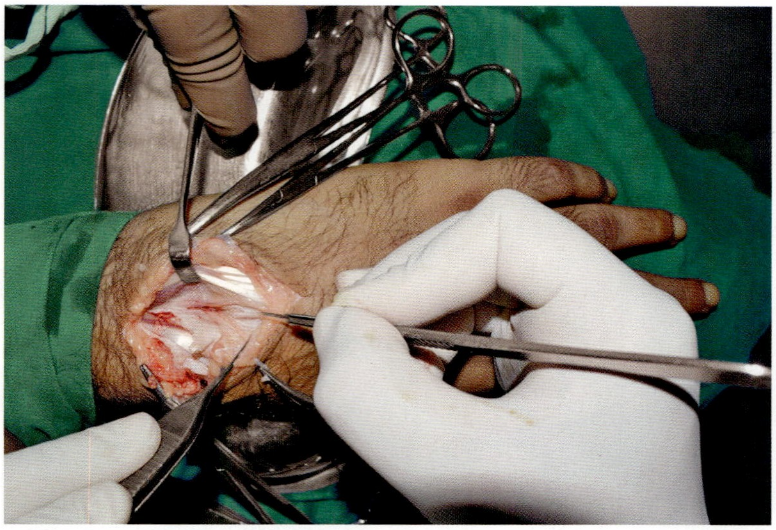

Fig. 11: There are multiple methods of approaching the radiocarpal joint described. The one method chosen here is described for its simplicity. After retracting extensor tendons, a longitudinal incision is made in the dorsal capsule of the radiocarpal joint.

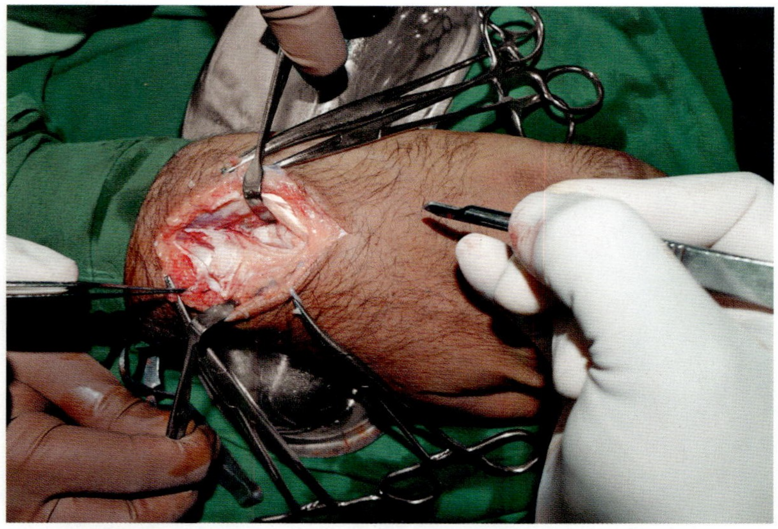

Fig. 12: Head of capitate bone is seen just deep to the capsule.

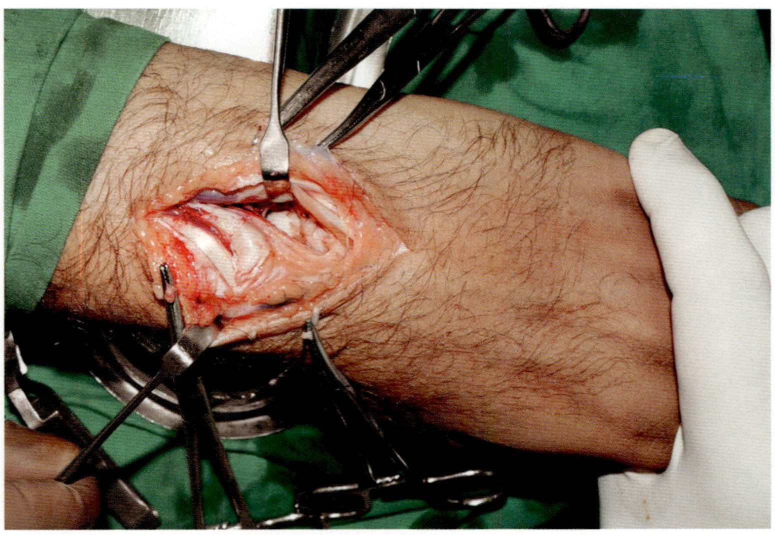

Fig. 13: Gentle longitudinal traction of the digits will expose a gap just proximal to the head of the capitate and the articular surface of the lower end of the radius.

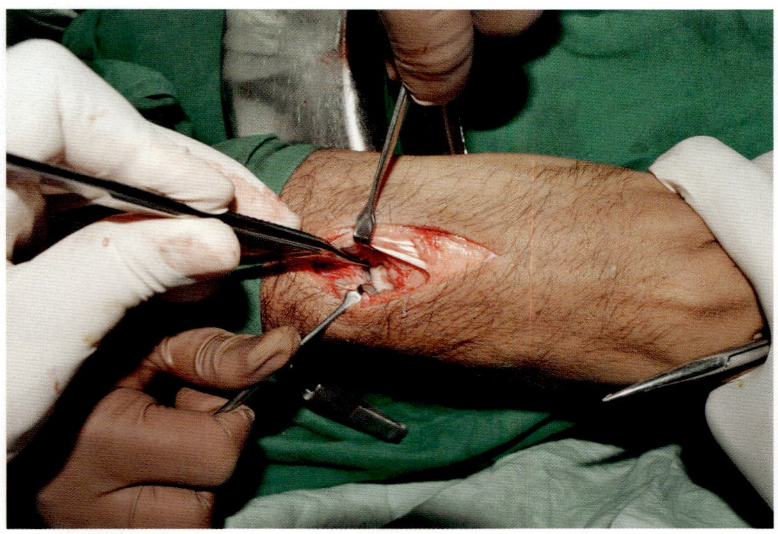

Fig. 14: While maintaining traction on the fingers, it is possible to see the lunate lying anteriorly in the gap between head of capitate and articular surface of radius.

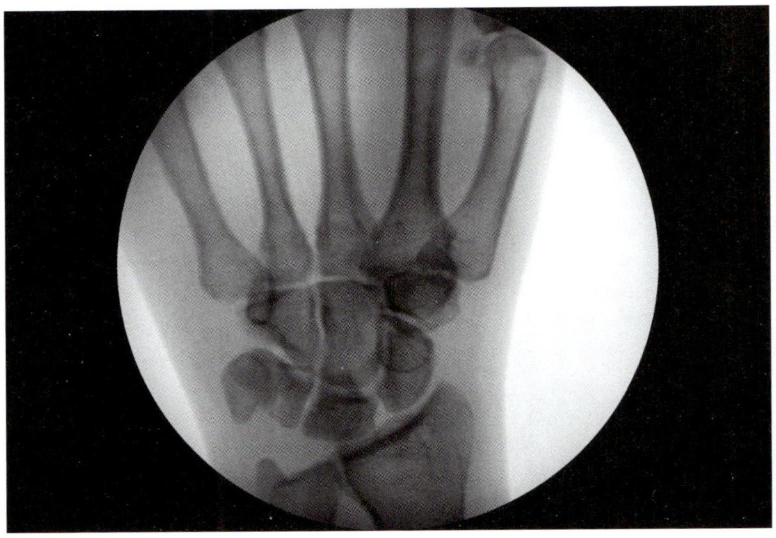
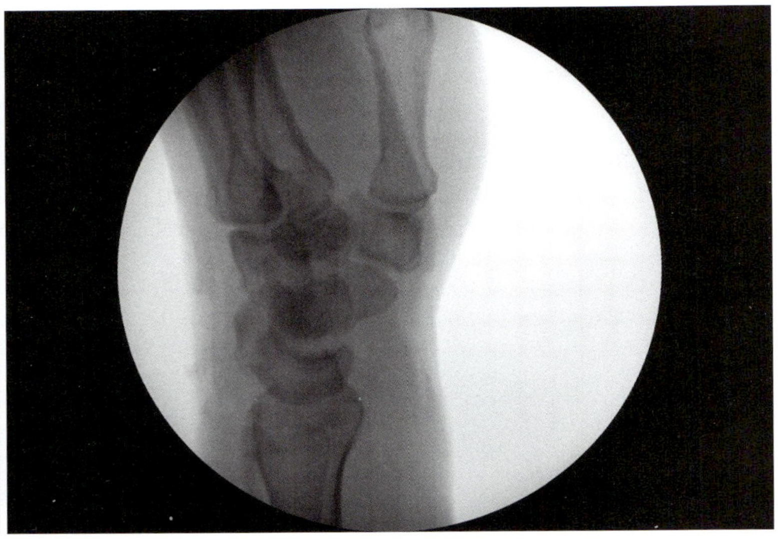

Figs. 15 and 16: Returning to the anterior aspect and providing persistent traction of fingers and dorsal push of lunate will smoothly glide the lunate back into its seat between radius and capitate. This is confirmed on the image intensifier. It is important to see if the lunate is dorsally angulated or palmarly angulated.

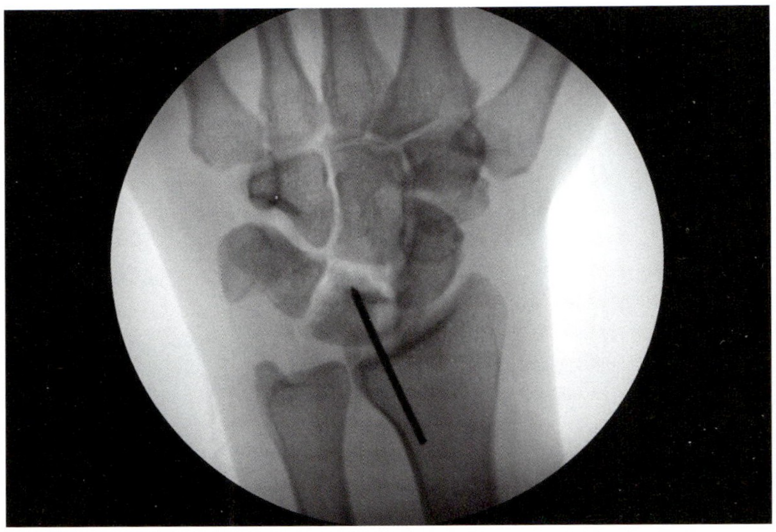
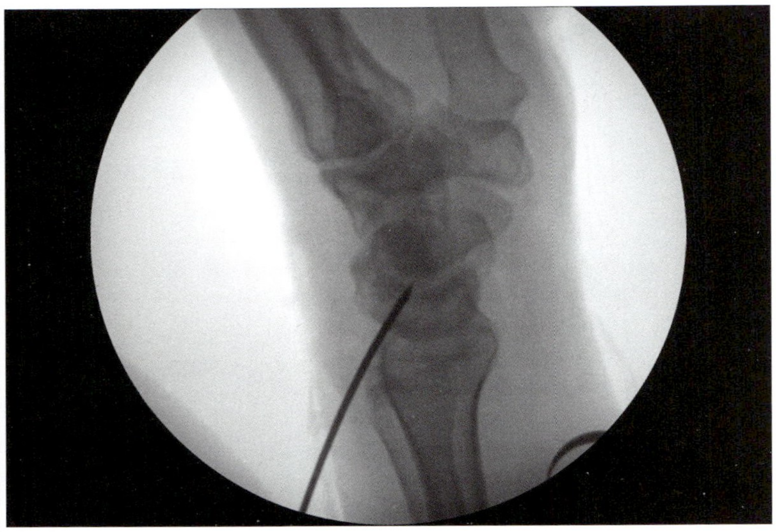

Figs. 17 and 18: A smooth 1.4-mm Kirschner wire is drilled in the lunate in posteroanterior direction, taking care that the leading edge of the wire does not penetrate the lunate on the anterior surface. This wire acts as a joystick to manipulate the lunate.

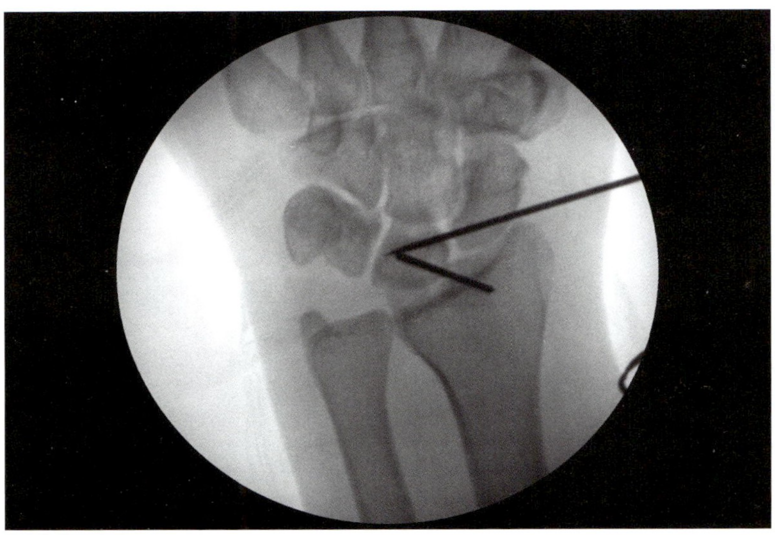
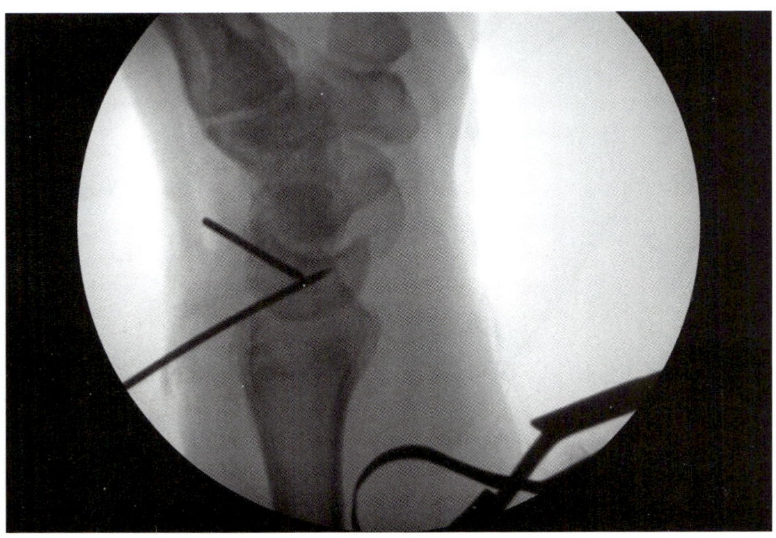

Figs. 19 and 20: A snug alignment of the ulnar surface of scaphoid and radial surface of the lunate is confirmed. The joystick in the lunate is used to ensure this snug fit. A 1.4-mm Kirschner wire is passed from the proximal pole of the scaphoid into the lunate.

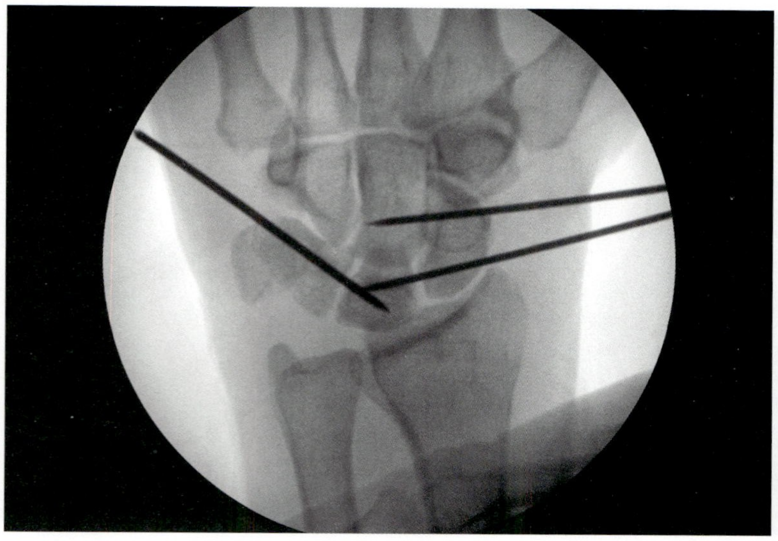

Fig. 21: Another Kirschner wire is passed from the distal pole of the scaphoid into the capitate. Third Kirschner wire is passed from the triquetrum into the lunate. Restoration of the three Gilula's lines is confirmed. Any loose remnant of the osteochondral pieces is removed.

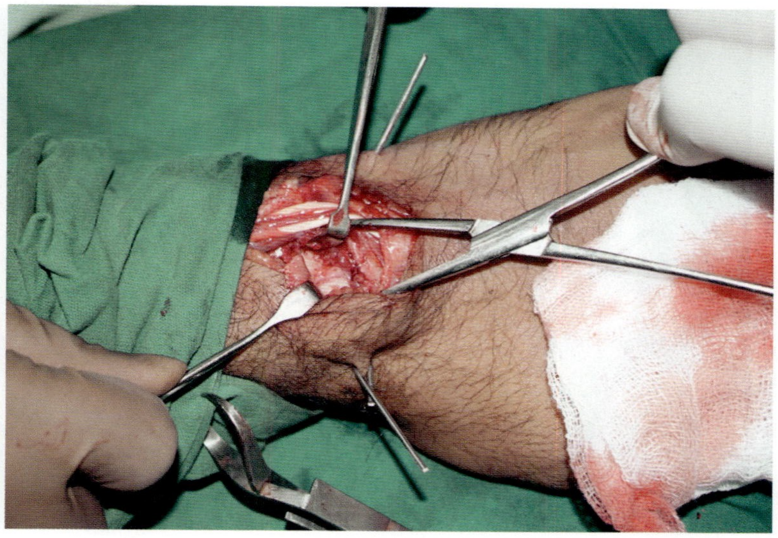

Fig. 22: Any remnant of ligament interposed is removed from between the capitate and lunate, from between the lunate and scaphoid.

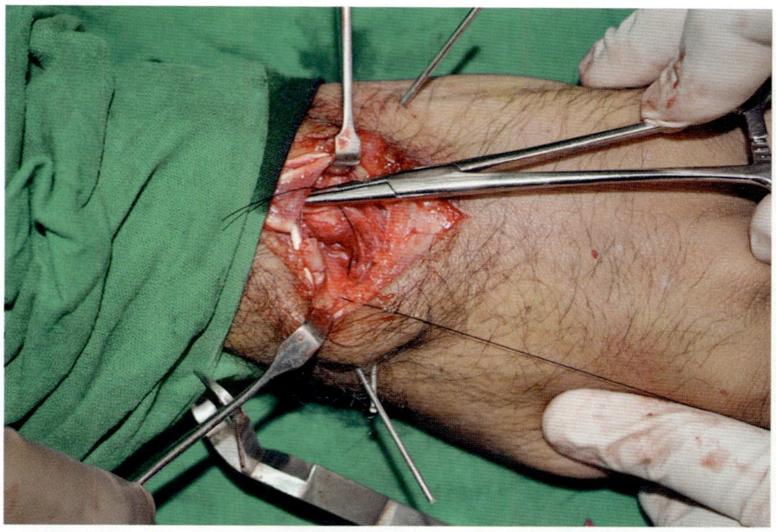

Fig. 23: The three Kirschner wires are cut short about 5 mm outside the skin. These are kept out for easy removal after the healing is completed. The joystick K wire inserted in the lunate is removed. Dorsal radiocarpal ligament is sutured using nonabsorbable suture material.

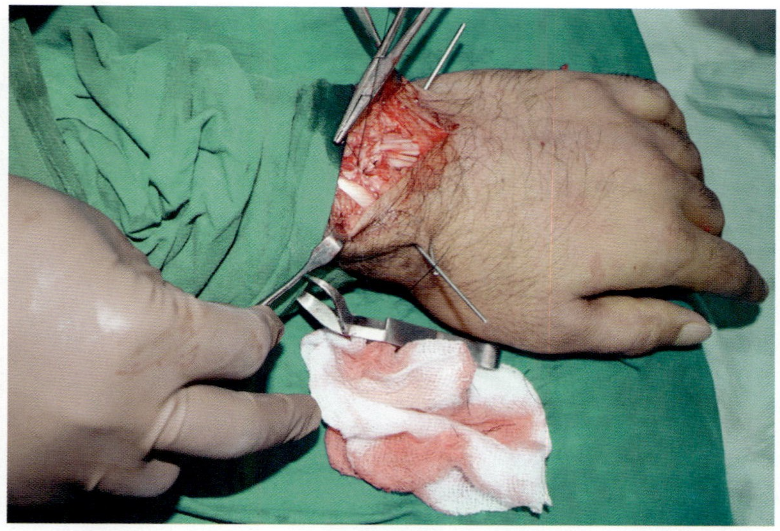

Fig. 24: extensor pollicis longus (EPL) tendon is placed radial to dorsal tubercle. ER is sutured back using nonabsorbable material tourniquet is deflated and hemostasis achieved.

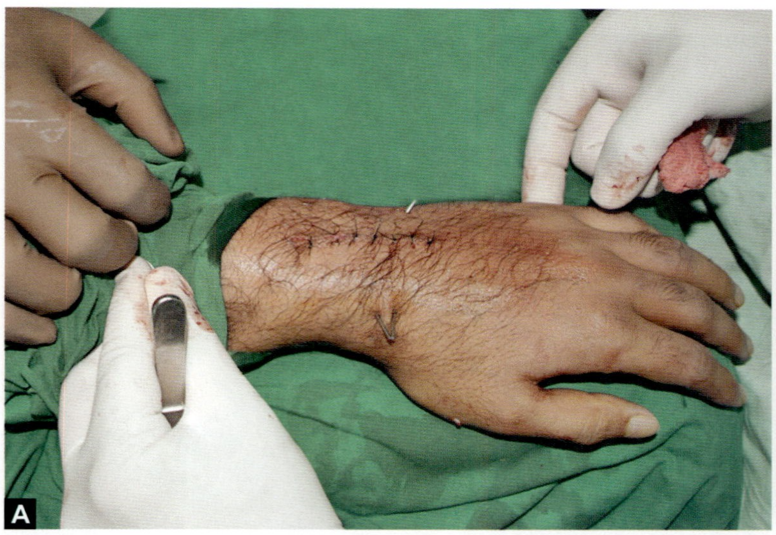

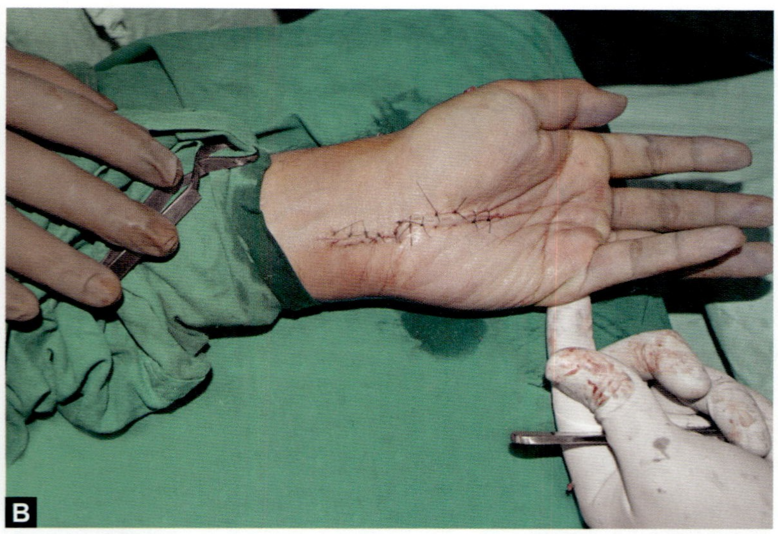

Figs. 25A and B: Volar and dorsal incisions closed with nonabsorbable sutures. A well-padded dorsal plaster splint is applied covering two-thirds of the forearm and keeping metacarpophalangeal joints free. The wrist is in about 15° extension.

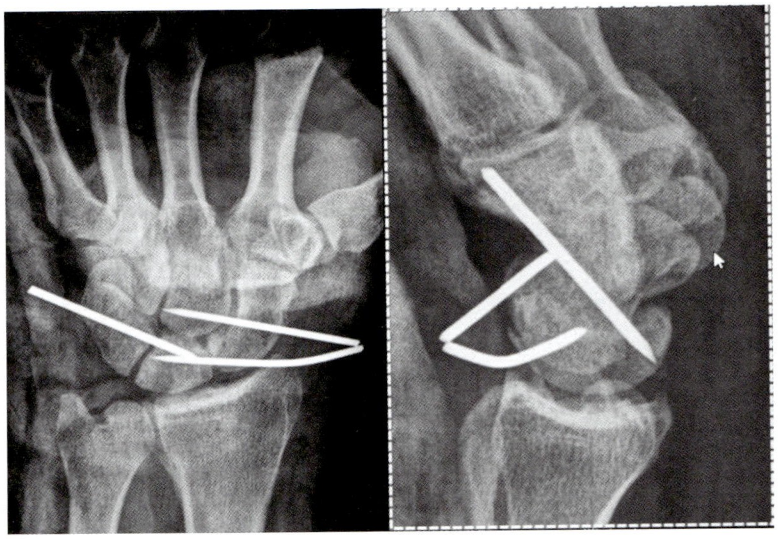

Fig. 26: Postoperative radiographs. The wrist is immobilized for 6–8 weeks after which K wires can be removed in office and gradual return to preinjury level of activity allowed over next 8 weeks.

SUGGESTED READING

1. David B. Jones Jr, Sanjeev Kakar. Perilunate Dislocations and Fracture Dislocations. J Hand Surg. 2012;37A:2168-74.

SECTION 5

ARTHROPLASTY

Section Editor: *Manoj Todkar*

CHAPTER 52

Primary Total Knee Replacement with Quadriceps Splitting Approach

Nakul Shah, Manoj Todkar, Shrinivas S Shintre

INDICATIONS OF TOTAL KNEE REPLACEMENT

Pain affecting daily activities of living because of arthritis or deformity due to osteoarthritis, rheumatoid arthritis, ankylosing spondylitis, gout, post-traumatic knee arthritis, osteonecrosis of distal femoral condyles.

CONTRAINDICATIONS OF TOTAL KNEE REPLACEMENT

Current or recent knee sepsis, remote source of ongoing infection, extensor mechanism discontinuity or dysfunction, recurvatum deformity because of muscle weakness, presence of well-functioning painless knee arthrodesis, poor skin condition, vascular compromise in the extremity, neuropathic arthropathy, morbid obesity, recurrent urinary tract infections.

RESULTS OF PRIMARY TOTAL KNEE REPLACEMENT

- *Functional and radiographic outcome measures:* Hospital for Special Surgery and the Knee Society Scoring System are commonly used scoring systems. These are preoperative and postoperative objective measurements recorded by the surgeon and patient-driven measures (pain, satisfaction, function) evaluated by patients.

  Total Knee Arthroplasty Radiographic Evaluation and Scoring System takes into account alignment of components, tibial surface coverage, radiolucency, signs of loosening, subluxation or dislocation.
- *Prosthesis survival:* Long-term series have documented the longevity of original total condylar prosthesis to be 95% at 15 years and 91% at 21 and 23 years.

COMPLICATIONS OF TOTAL KNEE ARTHROPLASTY

Deep venous thrombosis, pulmonary embolism, superficial or deep infections, periprosthetic fractures, patellofemoral instability, patellar clunk syndrome, extensor mechanism rupture, neurovascular injury, aseptic loosening of prosthesis.

SURGICAL STEPS (FIGS. 1 TO 17)

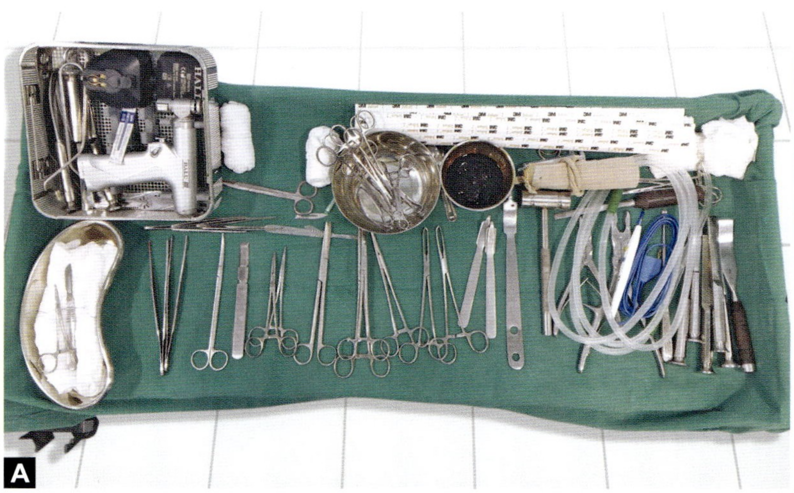

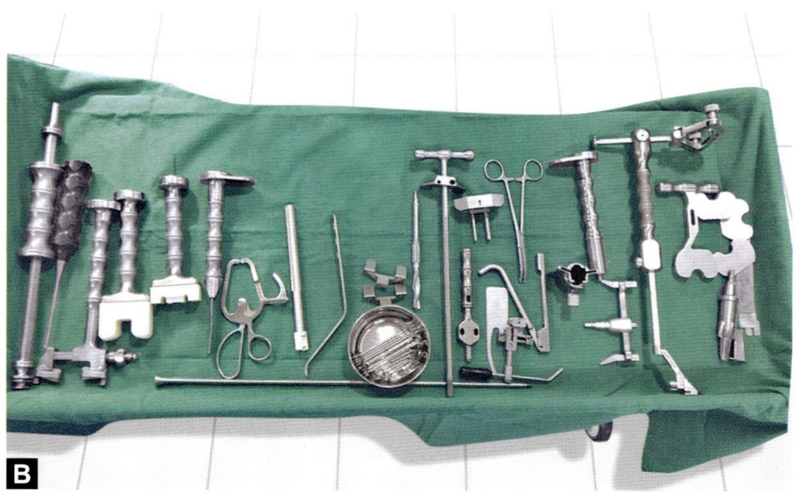

Figs. 1A and B: (A) General instrument trolley for total knee replacement (TKR); (B) Total knee replacement specific instrument trolley.

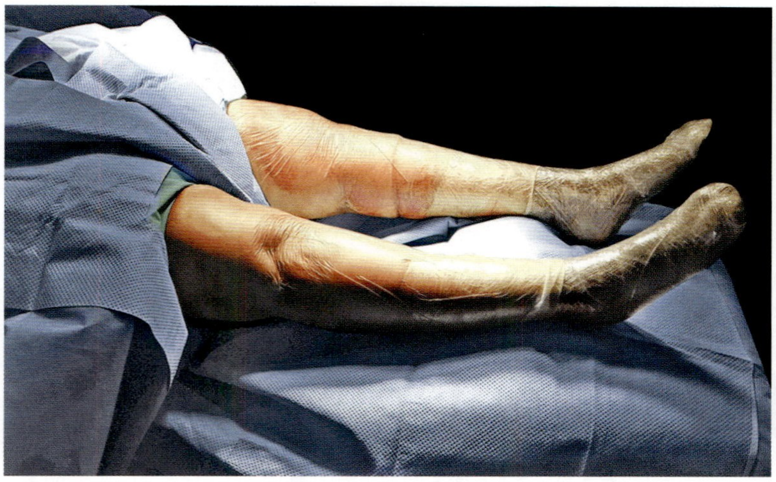

Fig. 2: Preparation and drape for bilateral total knee replacement.

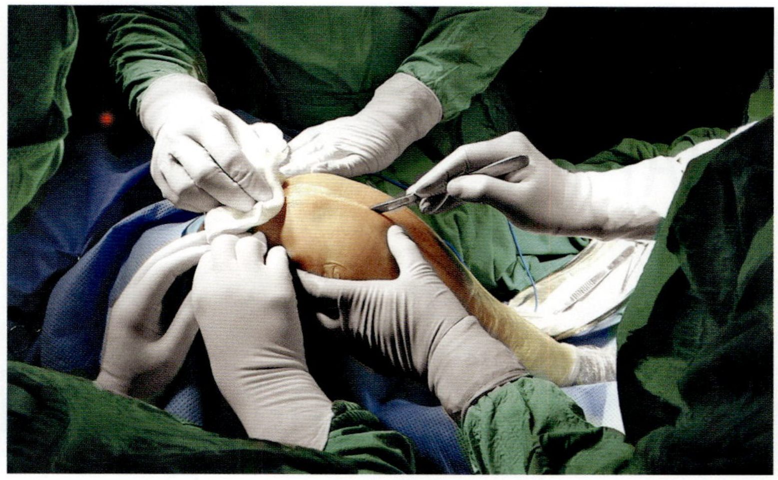

Fig. 3: Vertical midline incision.

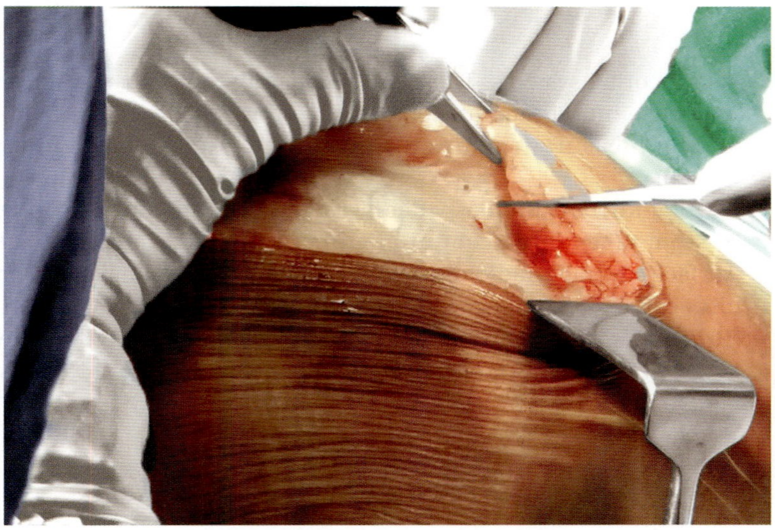

Fig. 4: Arthrotomy just medial to patellar tendon.

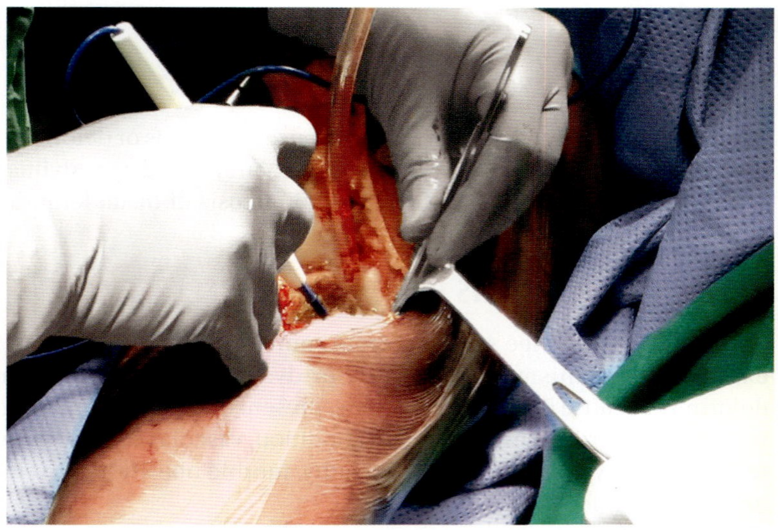

Fig. 5: Medial collateral ligament (MCL) release/elevation.

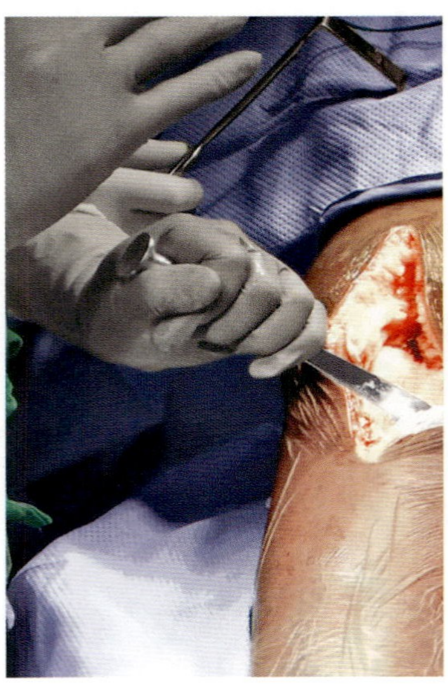

Fig. 6: Medial release.

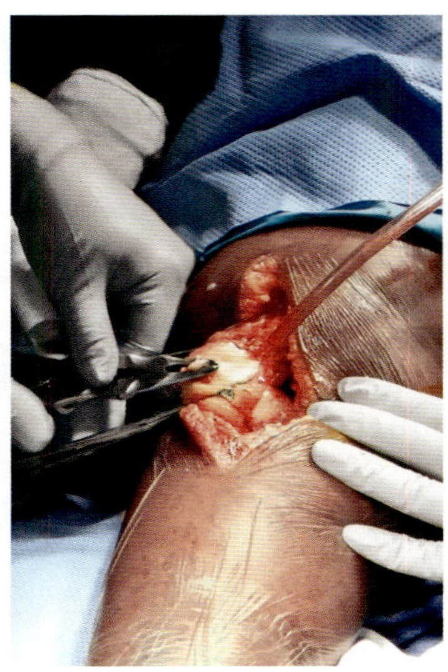

Fig. 7: Patellar osteophyte excision.

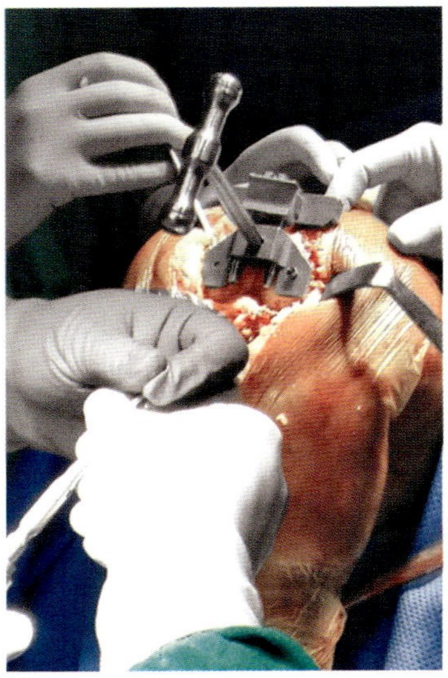

Fig. 8: Appropriate valgus guide and distal femoral cutting jig fixation.

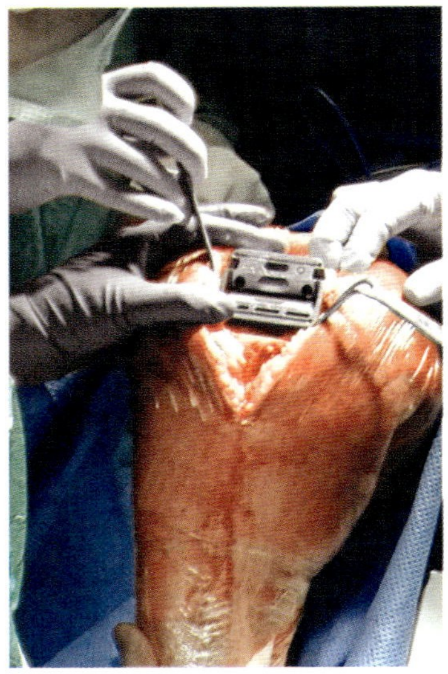

Fig. 9: Pinning of femoral cutting jig after taking distal femoral cut.

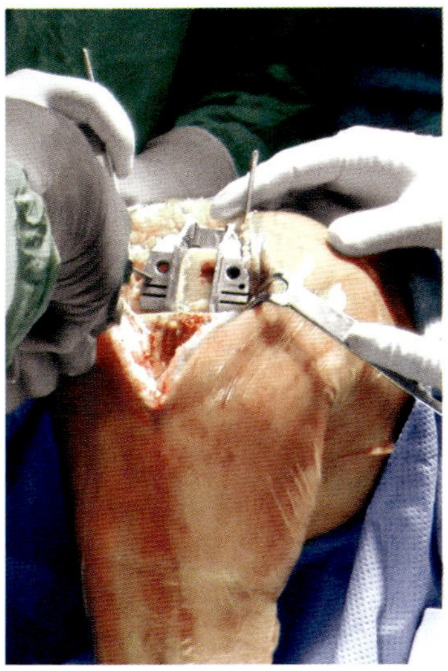

Fig. 10: Completed box cut.

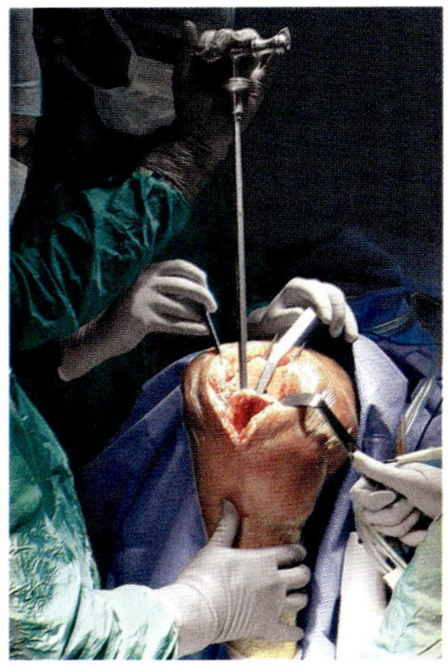

Fig. 11: Introduction of intramedullary rod in tibia.

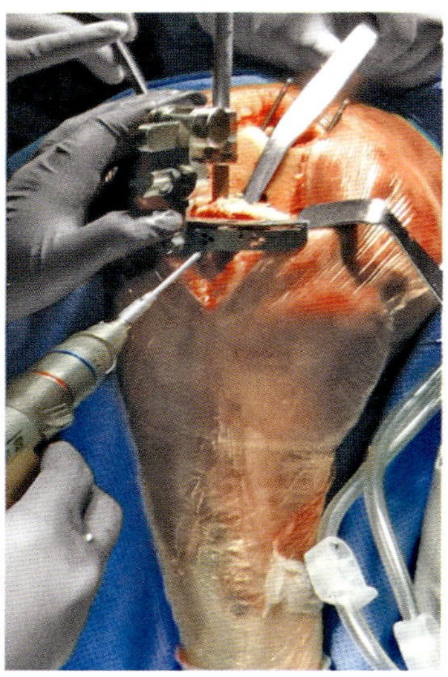

Fig. 12: Fixation of tibial jig with pins.

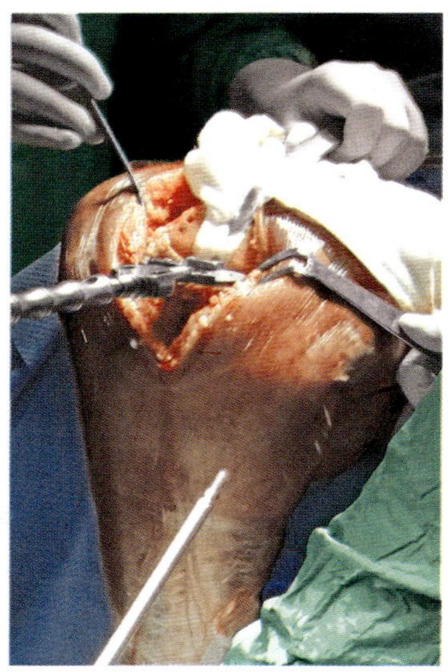

Fig. 13: Tibial base plate size selection and aligning to anterolateral tibial border.

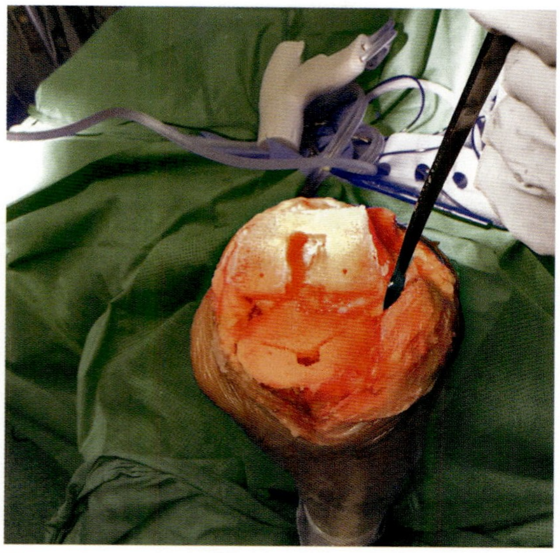

Fig. 14: Clean dry trabecular bone after pulse lavage.

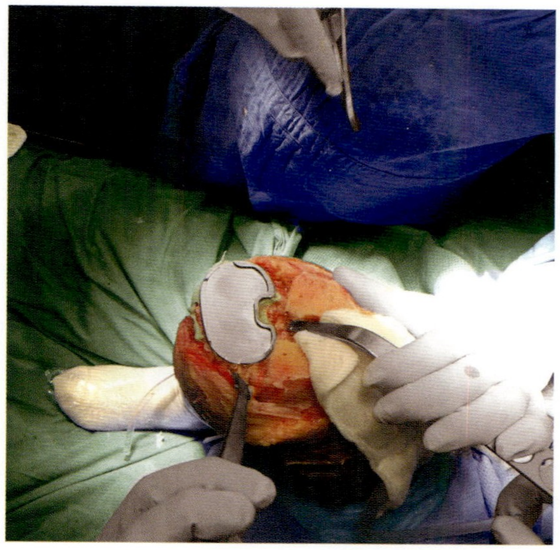

Fig. 15: Insertion of tibial base plate.

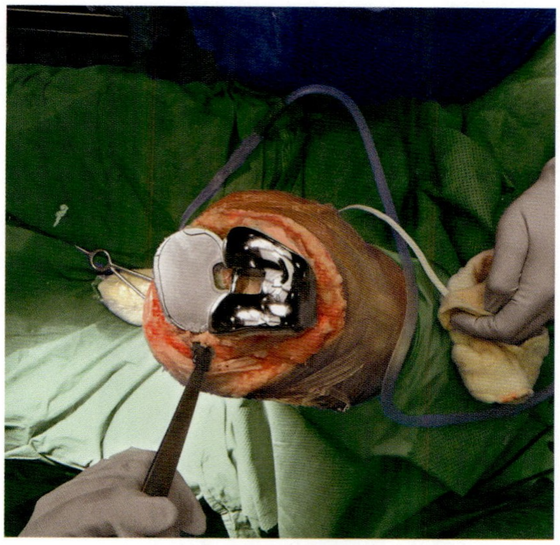

Fig. 16: Insertion of femoral component.

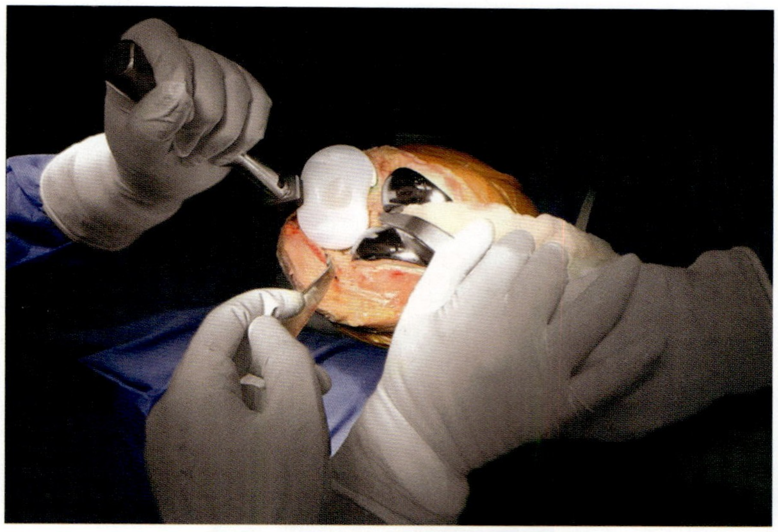

Fig. 17: Placement of polythene insert.

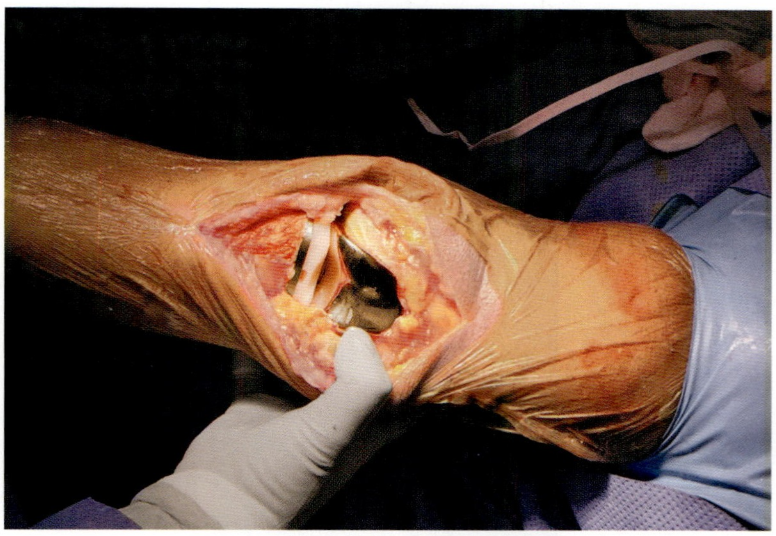

Fig. 18: Post-final implantation and cementation.

SUGGESTED READING

1. Baker PN, van der Meulen JH, Lewsey J, et al. The role of pain and function in determining patient satisfaction after total knee replacement: data from the National Joint Registry for England and Wales. J Bone Joint Surg Br. 2007;89-B:893-900.
2. Ethgen O, Bruyere O, Richy F, et al. Health-related quality of life in total hip and total knee arthroplasty. A qualitative and systematic review of the literature. J Bone Joint Surg Am. 2004;86:963-74.
3. Heck DA, Robinson RL, Partridge CM, et al. Patient outcomes after knee replacement. J Arthroplasty. 1998;13:229.
4. Jones CA, Voaklander DC, Suarez-Almazor ME. Determinants of function after total knee arthroplasty. Phys Ther. 2003;83:696-706.
5. Judge A, Cooper C, Williams S, et al. Patient-reported outcomes one year after primary hip replacement in a European collaborative cohort, Arthritis Care Res. 2010;62: 480-8.
6. Kennedy LG, Newman JH, Ackroyd CE, et al. When should we do knee replacements? Knee. 2003;10:161-6.
7. MacWilliam CH, Yood MU, Verner JJ, et al. Patient-related risk factors that predict poor outcome after total hip replacement. Health Serv Res. 1996;31: 623-38.
8. Nilsdotter AK, Petersson IF, Roos EM, et al. Predictors of patient relevant outcome after total hip replacement for osteoarthritis: a prospective study. Ann Rheum Dis. 2003;62:923-30.
9. Williams O, Fitzpatrick R, Hajat S, et al. Mortality, morbidity, and 1-year outcomes of primary elective total hip arthroplasty. J Arthroplasty. 2002; 17:165-71.
10. Wylde V, Dieppe P, Hewlett S, et al. Total knee replacement: is it really an effective procedure for all? Knee. 2007;14:417-23.

CHAPTER 53

Unicondylar Knee Arthroplasty

Pavan K Kohli

INTRODUCTION

Knee osteoarthritis is a leading cause of muscular disability and lower life expectancy. In recent times unicondylar knee arthroplasty has gained significant popularity. Several studies have shown that it is less invasive, more physiological, with larger and more functional postoperative range of motion (ROM), sustained pain relief, longer durability of implant compared to total joint arthroplasty.

PATHOANATOMY AND SURGICAL ANATOMY

Osteoarthritis is the most common form of arthritis in knee. Common symptoms include pain, swelling, deformity, decreased walking and exercises which affects all body functions finally affecting the life expectancy.

Knee osteoarthritis involves the progressive destruction of articular cartilage with exposure of underlying bone and associated pain along with cartilage ulcers, osteophyte formation, and bone erosion, etc. Although medial knee OA is the more prevalent variant of OA.

Surgical Anatomy

Standard incision for minimally invasive UKA is less than 3 inches (7–8 cm) and maintained below the vastus medialis obliques muscle.

CLINICAL FEATURES AND IMAGING

Physical Examination

Physical examination is a verification of the single condyle affliction, meniscal tests like Mcmurrays and ligament tests like Lachmann and medial collateral ligament test are useful adjuncts for supporting structures. The clinical deformity measurement viz. varus or valgus and fixed flexion deformity are noted. In addition it is also important to check for hyperlaxity syndrome.

It is extremely important to note the neurovascular status of the limb, many a L4 radiculopathy masquerade as knee pain. Clinical history and detail examination will provide correct answers.

Radiographic Assessment

Standard views are knee X-ray, AP in standing, weight bearing, lateral in 90° flexion, skyline patellar view, and varus and valgus stress views.

If required, magnetic resonance imaging (MRI) studies can be used to document cartilage status and concomitant spine pathology in suspected cases. The author is part of the team which has recently described a new radiological sign for "nonbone on bone OA principally involving femoral compartment in Indian patients" called the "Dervan ring sign" and the high prevalence of concomitant knee and spine pathologies as found on MRI studies. This clinical finding, often missed on cursory examination is further elucidated by the author and team as "Dervan dermatome syndrome".

The author would like to re-emphasize the importance of not treating just the X-ray. Rather the proper pain generator must be correctly identified before surgical decision, for a predictable result.

CONTRAINDICATIONS

To summarize, all contraindications except for rheumatoid or inflammatory arthritis and active infection are relative. Rheumatoid arthritis is progressive and will affect all compartments sooner or later.

Patient factors like concomitant comorbidities, high BMI, medium grade patellofemoral arthritis, chondrocalcinosis, ACL lesions are all relative. Unicompartmental knee replacement (UKR) is becoming the first choice of treatment of arthritis for properly selected Asian patients.

SURGICAL ALTERNATIVES TO UNICOMPARTMENTAL KNEE REPLACEMENT

Osteotomies Around the Knee

Although corrective knee osteotomies have been around for more than a century, problems with wound healing, bone union, delayed loss of reduction, recurrence of deformity and tendon injuries have placed it below arthroplasty in preference.

Joint Arthroplasty

It is now well accepted that joint arthroplasty is safe, and cost-effective method for treatment of advanced knee OA. With newer minimally invasive techniques, better engineering of polymers and spacers, and more affordable and available surgical procedures have made arthroplasty the first choice of treatment in arthritis. Out of total and partial knee arthroplasty, UKA is more minimally invasive, more functional, more durable, more Indian lifestyle friendly and can provide an important interval option for 15–20 years in younger patients and quicker recovery in older patients with comorbidities.

In fact many recent studies are proving longer survival with better functional results in patients of bicompartmental arthritis who undergo bicompartmental UKA vis-à-vis total knee replacement (TKR).

The secret probably lies in the preservation of the intercondylar notch and its components.

SURGERY

The principle is to restore natural alignment of the patient with well fixed and appropriately sized components.

The key for calculations of Bone cuts, both in the sagittal and coronal planes of the femur and the tibia, is that in the end the joint line and ligament stability are restored in both flexion and extension. On the average, the normal tibial plateau should be within 3° of varus to the tibial mechanical axis in the coronal view. In the sagittal plane, there is to be an average of 5–7° posterior slope of the tibial plateau. However, there is a wide individual variation, in the coronal plane from 0° to 5° varus and in the sagittal plane from 5° to 13° posterior slope. Hence for restoration of natural alignment and ligament tension, these variations should be taken into consideration and replicated.

1. Aim of surgery is a slight undercorrection of the deformity of the long leg axis. Medial UKA: 1–4° varus, lateral UKA: 3–7° valgus
2. In UKA, correct ligament balance is restored by accurate positioning the components and by insertion an appropriate thickness of bearing.
3. In patients with concomitant ACL tears, it is possible to reconstruct the ACL simultaneously in addition to UKA.

TECHNIQUES

Cemented versus Cementless

Internationally both cemented and cementless designs are in vogue with the latter making a comeback.

It has been proved that Cementation is an adequate fixation method for UKA and is therefore considered the standard technique. It results in high survivorship rates and good functional outcomes.

Fixed versus Mobile Bearing

UKA implants have run the full circle from fixed bearing to mobile bearing, back to fixed bearing as the primary choice of arthroplasty surgeons.

Lesser chances of insert dislocation, improved polymer survival and easily replicable surgeries have made fixed bearing Unicompartmental arthroplasty as the gold standard across most arthroplasty registries.

All Polyethylene versus Metal Backed

Mainly two fixed-bearing designs have been used for tibial resurfacing when performing a UKA: inlay (all-polyethylene) and onlay (metal-backed) ones. Studies for inlay versus onlay implants have concluded that there is superior load distribution over the tibial surface for the metal-backed onlay design.

Surgical Technique: Conventional versus Robot Assisted

Conventional manual techniques are routinely used in UKA surgery to achieve ideal implant position and alignment critical to short-term and long-term outcomes. Numerous studies have shown no additional benefit of robotic surgery and huge additional burden of costs. Conventional cutting guides have given precise results over a large follow-up.

SURGICAL STEPS (FIGS. 1 TO 15)

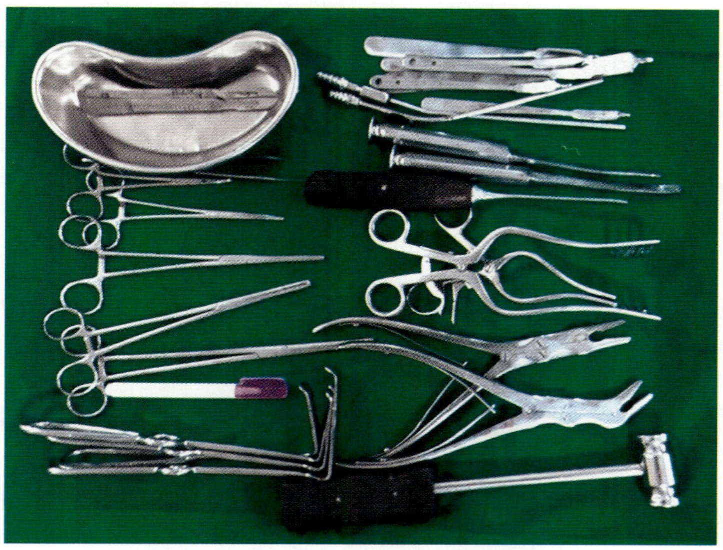

Fig. 1: Instrument trolley.

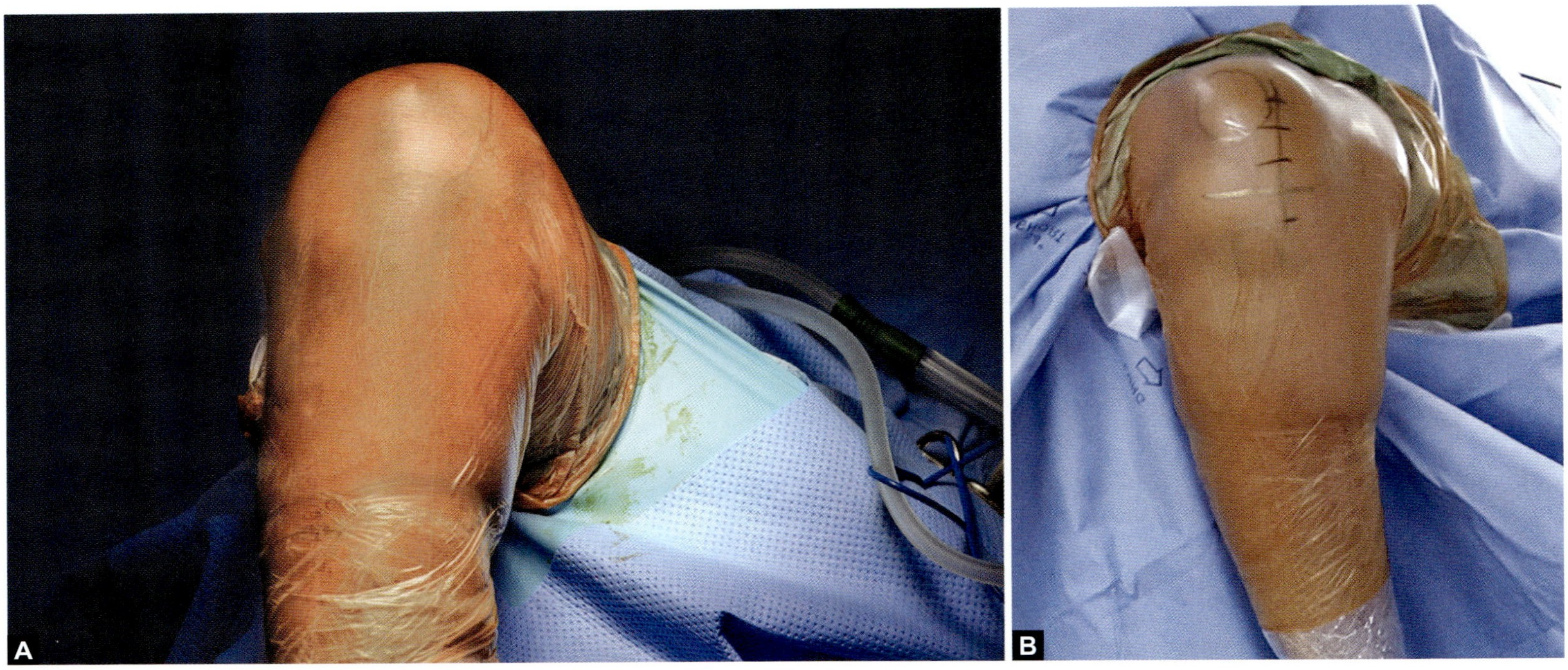

Figs. 2A and B: Preoperative position with draping in standard and leg holder position.

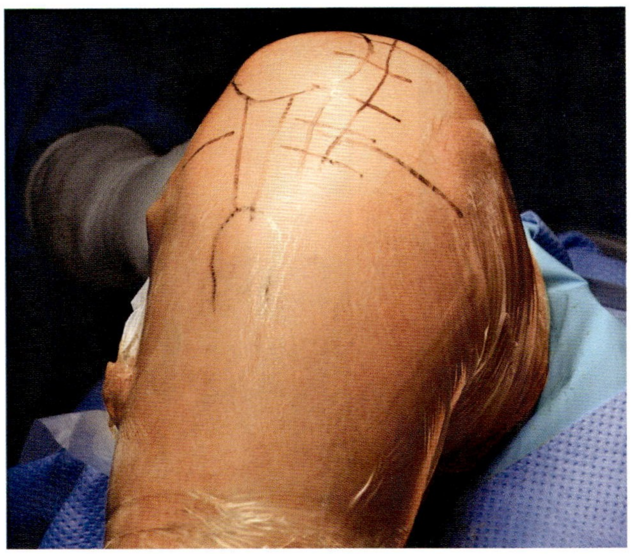

Fig. 3: Bony landmarks and incision marking.

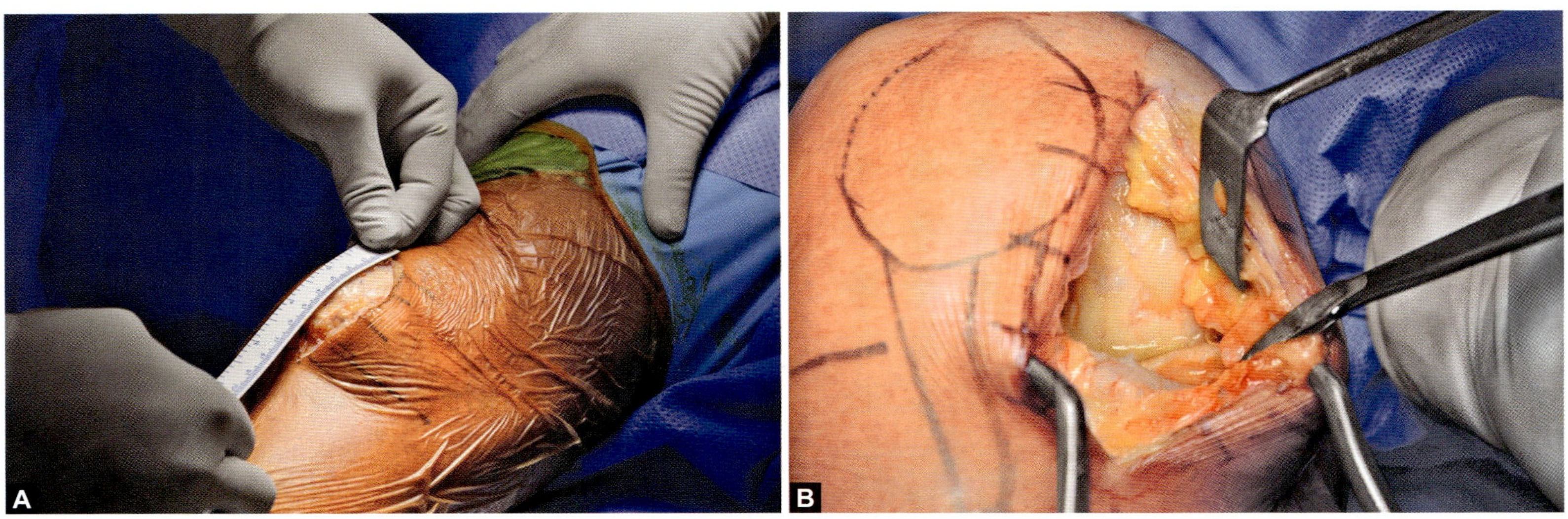

Figs. 4A and B: Soft tissue dissection and exposure of joint.

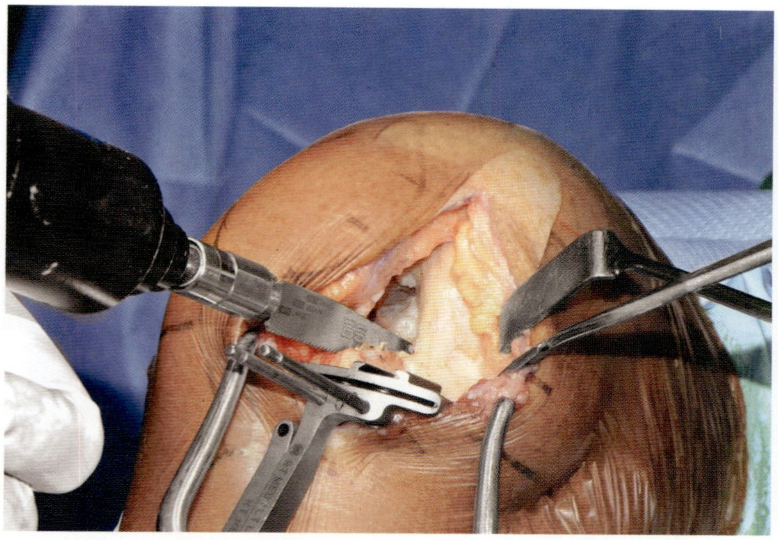

Fig. 5: Application of tibial cutting jig with sagittal and horizontal cuts.

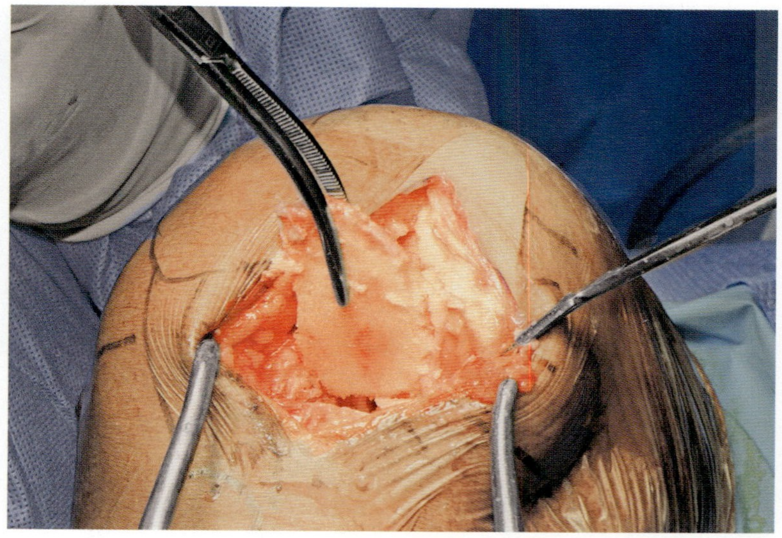

Fig. 6: Removal of tibial articular surface.

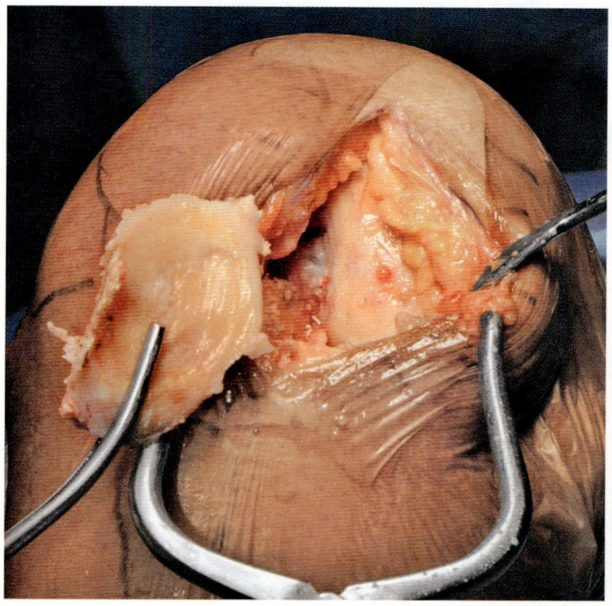

Fig. 7: Extensive erosion of cartilage seen on tibial surface.

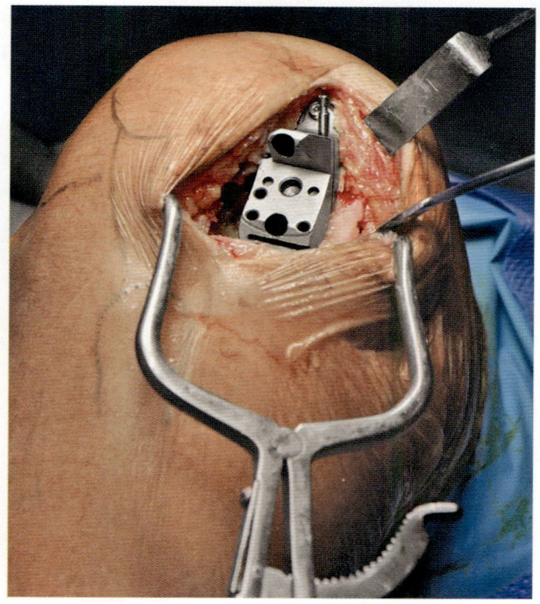

Fig. 8: Femur cutting jig applied.

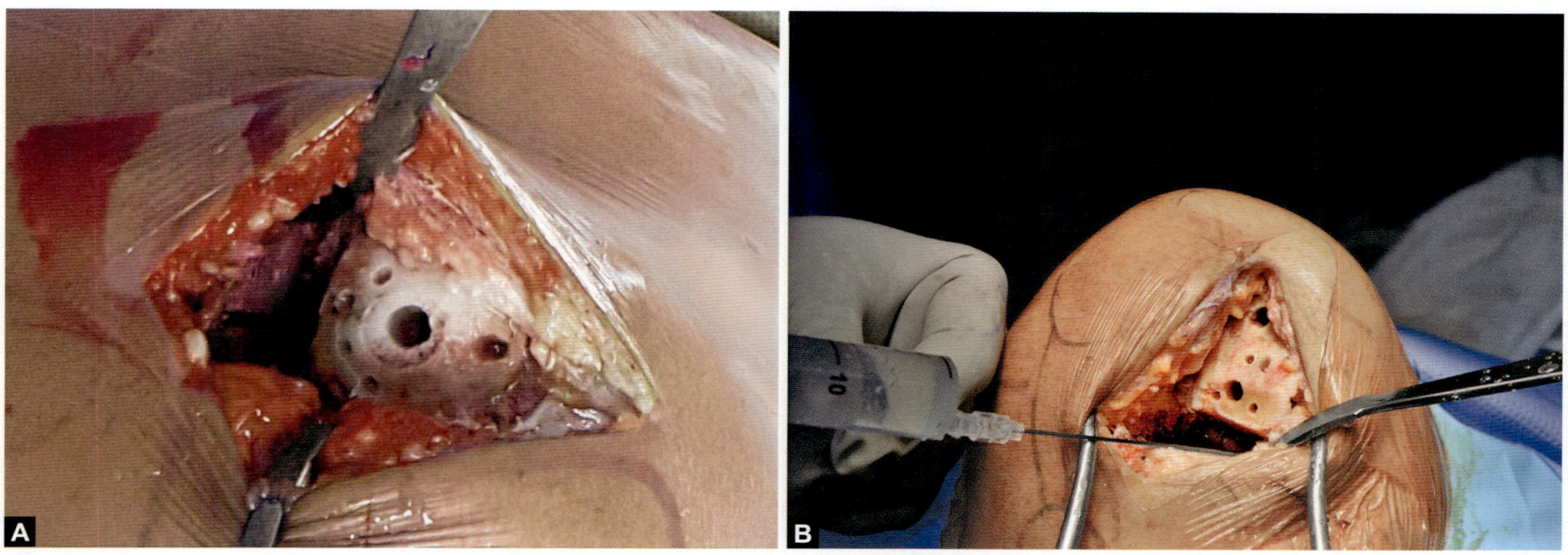

Figs. 9A and B: (A) Cut surface of femur after microplasty; (B) Standard Jig.

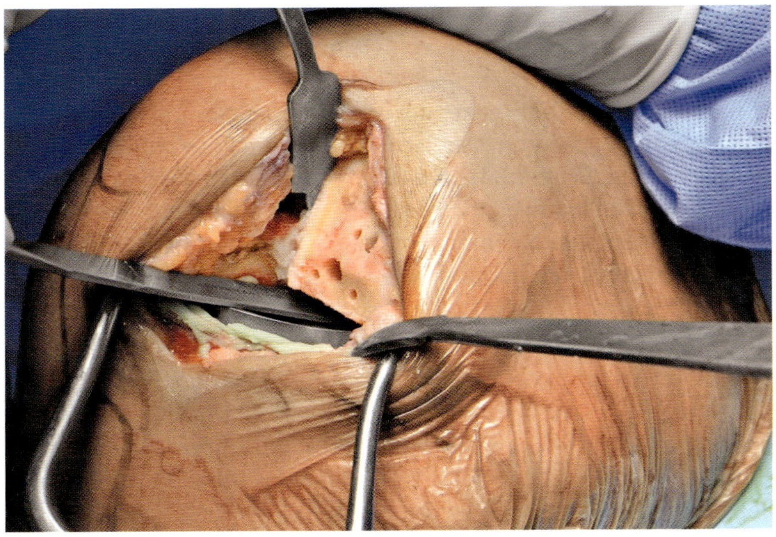

Fig. 10: Cement applied with pressurization.

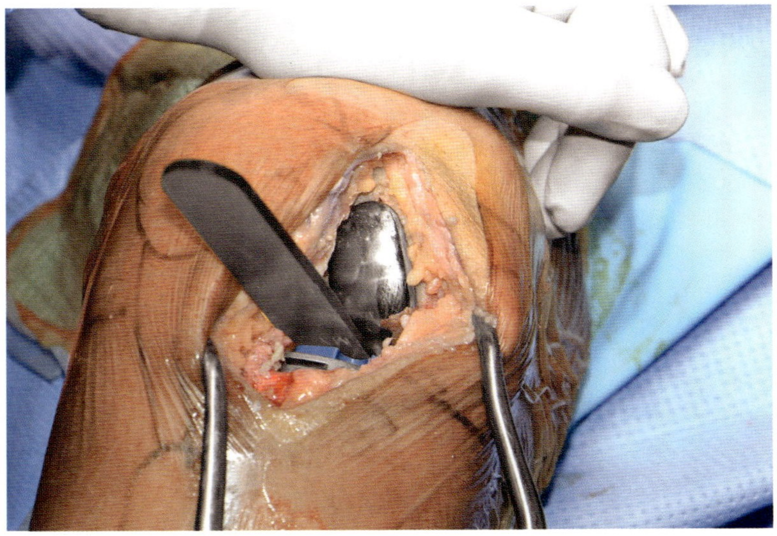

Fig. 11: Metal implants cemented with trial spacer and pressurizer.

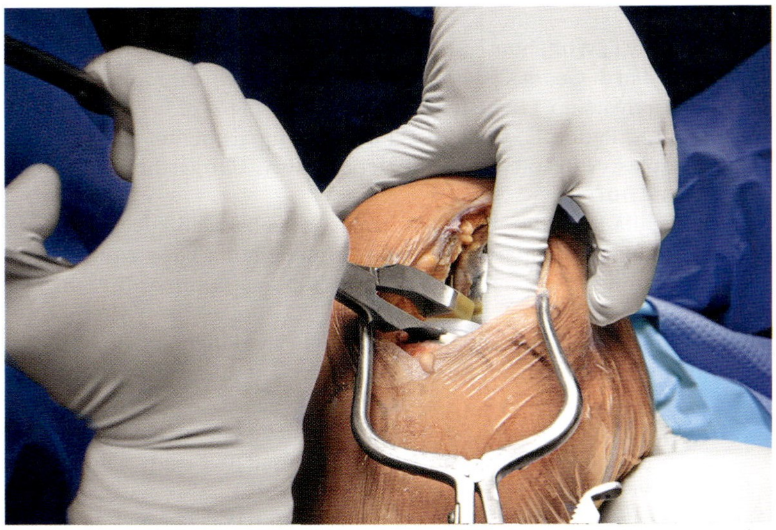

Fig. 12: Insertion of final polyethylene.

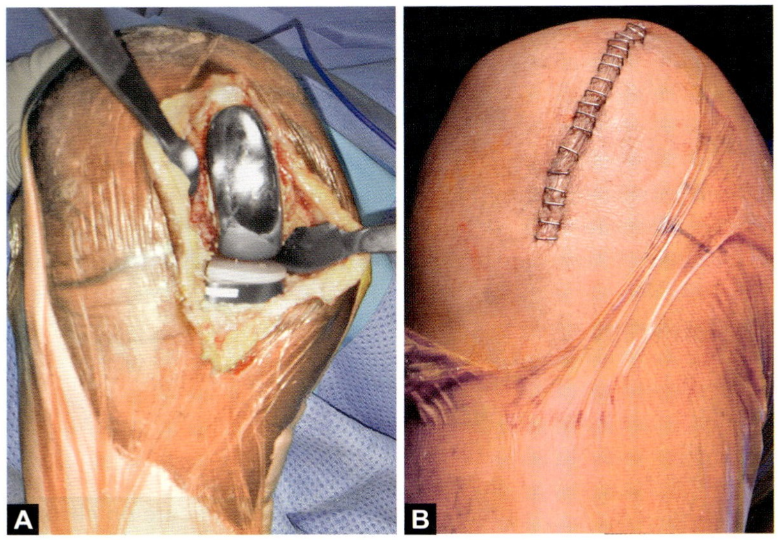

Figs. 13A and B: (A) Final implant before closure; (B) Final closure of incision.

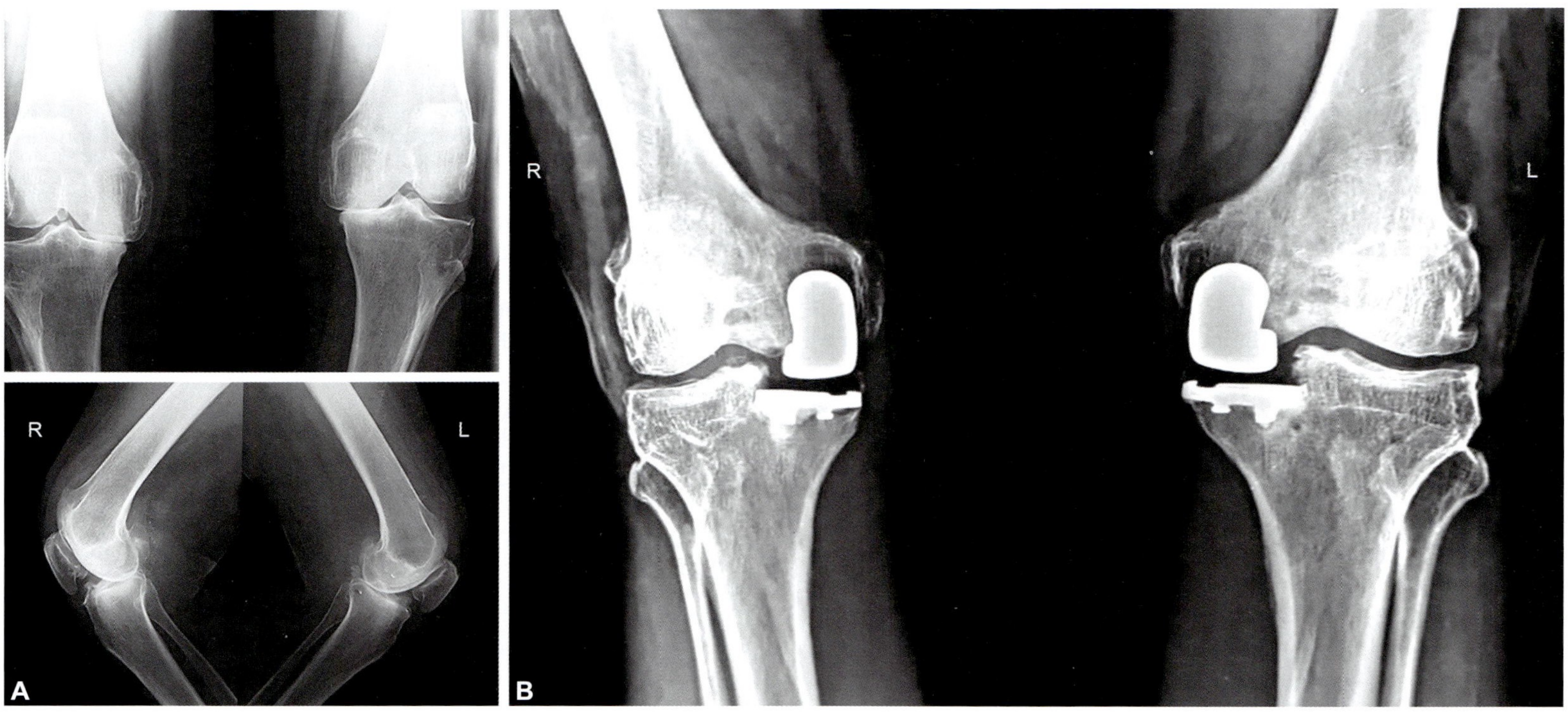

Figs. 14Aand B: Preoperative and postoperative X-ray showing medial compartment osteoarthritis and bilateral unicondylar knee replacement.

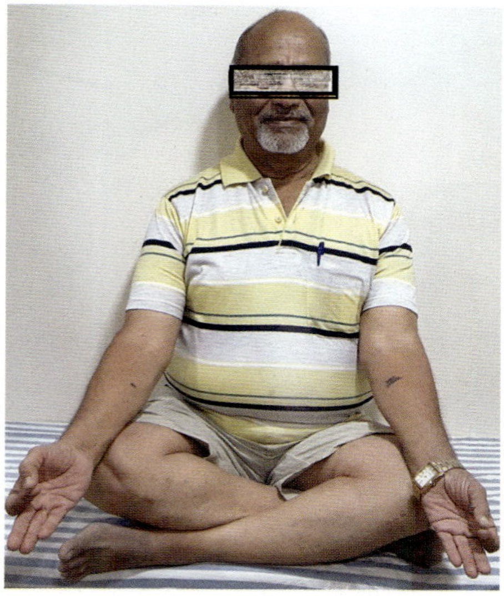

Fig. 15: Patient of bilateral unicondylar knee replacement (UKR) with full restoration of movement and resumption of normal lifestyle postoperatively.

POSTOPERATIVE CARE

Wound Care

Wound closure is done in layers. Recent trends avoid drains and use Trenexamic acid (IV) intra-articularly and allow same day mobilization. Sutures are removed on the 12/14 days postoperatively.

Physiotherapy

Physiotherapy is important for postoperative rehabilitation. The patient is made to stand on his legs just and walk a few steps about 6–7 hours postsurgery.

Care must be taken to preserve proper ergonomics and prevent undue loading of the spine and prevent acute or acute on chronic axial and appendicular musculoskeletal injuries.

COMPLICATIONS

- *Aseptic loosening*: Aseptic loosening remains an important cause of failure with most cases presenting in the first 2 years. RLLs must be specifically looked for and treated in early stages.
- *Progression of osteoarthritis*: Progression of OA in the contralateral compartment—the restoration of normal kinematics with a slight undercorrection of the deformity is the aim.
- *Polyethylene wear*: Better polymer engineering with better cutting guides has decreased the prevalence of early polyethylene wear. It is interesting to note that biomechanical studies have shown more wear with the same polyethylene, if implanted in TKR mode, vis-à-vis bicompartmental unicondylar mode.
- *Pain*: With modern investigative techniques, and sound theoretical backing, the true pain generator can and should be identified. Many a radiculopathy come disguised as persistent knee pain and many a hip arthritis is referred to the knee. Proper protocols for persistent pain must be followed in investigation and treatment.
- Other complications infection, malalignment, fracture and tibial subsidence are technique-related complications resulting in early failure.

ACKNOWLEDGMENT

The author would like to acknowledge the contribution of Dr Sidharth Hardikar, Medical Officer BKL Walawalkar Hospital, Dervan for his help in preparing the manuscript.

SUGGESTED READING

1. Ackroyd CE, Whitehouse SL, Newman JH, et al. A comparative study of the medial St Georg sled and kinematic total knee arthroplasties. Ten-year survivorship. J Bone Joint Surg Br. 2002;84:667-72.
2. Amin AK, Patton JT, Cook RE, et al. Unicompartmental or total knee arthroplasty? Results from a matched study. Clin Orthop Relat Res. 2006;451:101-6.
3. Hassaballa MA, Porteous AJ, Newman JH. Observed kneeling ability after total, unicompartmental and patellofemoral knee arthroplasty: perception versus reality. Knee Surg Sports Traumatol Arthrosc. 2004;12:136-9.
4. Komistek RD, Allain J, Anderson DT, et al. In vivo kinematics for subjects with and without an anterior cruciate ligament. Clin Orthop Relat Res. 2002;404:315-25.
5. Laurencin CT, Zelicof SB, Scott RD, et al. Unicompartmental versus total knee arthroplasty in the same patient. A comparative study. Clin Orthop Relat Res. 1991;273:151-6.
6. Lombardi AV Jr, Berend KR, Walter CA, et al. Is recover faster for mobile-bearing unicompartmental than total knee arthroplasty? Clin Orthop Relat Res. 2009;467:1450-7.
7. Morris MJ, Molli RG, Berend KR, et al. Mortality and perioperative complications after unicompartmental knee arthroplasty. Knee. 2013;20:218-20.
8. Newman J, Pydisetty RV, Ackroyd C. Unicompartmental or total knee replacement: the 15-year results of a prospective randomised controlled trial. J Bone Joint Surg Br. 2009;91:52-7.
9. Price AJ, Oppold PT, Murray DW, et al. Simultaneous in vitro measurement of patellofemoral kinematics and forces following Oxford medial unicompartmental knee replacement. J Bone Joint Surg Br. 2006;88:1591-5.
10. Repicci JA, Eberle RW. Minimally invasive surgical technique for unicondylar knee arthroplasty. J South Orthop Assoc. 1999;8:20-7.

CHAPTER 54

Primary Uncemented Total Hip Replacement with Mini Posterior Approach

Manish R Dastane, Umesh Birole

INTRODUCTION

Posterior approach to hip offers good visualization of hip joint for total hip replacement.

Mini approach to hip offers additional advantage in terms of early mobilization, less blood loss, minimal soft tissue damage and improved confidence of the patient in the surgical procedure.

Also, it minimizes the need of multiple instruments obscuring operative field, and decreased tension on neurovascular structures.

PLANE

- *Internervous plane*: There is no internervous plane.
- *Intermuscular plane*: Through the gluteus maximus.

POTENTIAL COMPLICATIONS

Possible complications are nerve and vascular injuries.

Intraoperative:
- Injury to sciatic nerve
- Bleeding from superior gluteal artery

Postoperative:
- Trochanteric bursitis

SURGICAL PROCEDURES

Mini Posterior Approach to Hip

Indications

- Total hip replacement
- Removal of loose bodies
- Posterior wall of acetabulum fracture fixations
- Partial hip replacement
- Drainage of septic hip.

Here, we are describing steps of mini posterior approach to hip:

Structures at Risk

1. Sciatic nerve during manipulation
2. Superior gluteal artery
3. Inferior gluteal artery.

Steps

Lateral position is given to the patient. Tip of shoulder and greater trochanter should be in same line in lateral decubitus. Mark the greater trochanter and the incision line with a marker (Fig. 1). Sterile adhesive drape is applied over the operative field (Fig. 2). Fascia of gluteus maximus along with tensor fascia lata is released for an adequate exposure distally (In arthritic/stiff hips, the gluteus maximus tendon insertion is split as well for better exposure). Split the gluteus maximus fibers proximally and place Charnley's retractors underneath the fascia. A Hohmann spike is placed under the abductor muscles and the tip of the spike is gently tapped on the iliac bone to avoid the slip off of the retractor tip. This gives optimal visualization of the rotators and the joint capsule directly. Short external rotators are tagged and resected to expose the capsule. Arthrotomy is performed and the head is delivered out. Head osteotomy is done using an oscillating power saw at the correct (preferably templated) neck length.

Ligamentum teres and the adherent capsule needs resection. Arthritic and calcified labrum needs complete removal. Femoral canal is prepared first for the combined anteversion technique especially for the uncemented total hips. The redundant tissues in the pyriform fossa are resected and the entry area is cleared. Femoral canal entry is made using a box type chisel to create a lateral most entry point. The femoral canal is opened using graduated hand reamers. Broaching is done in progressive manner for an optimal fit. The broach should snugly fit in the femoral canal and the whole leg should move on gentle rotatory attempts to rotate the inserted broach handle (Fig. 15). At this point, the native anteversion can be calculated using the posterior condylar plane.

(Ask the assistant to flex knee 90° and check the broach plane in relation to the posterior condylar plane)

After the femoral preparation, place a Charnley's pin superior to the acetabulum to tent away the proximal tissues (Fig. 18). A strong curved retractor is placed anterior to the anterior acetabular wall to keep the femoral neck away from the exposed acetabular field. All the osteophytes are nibbled out especially the one in the bottom of cotyloid notch underneath this lies the true depth of the cavity. Serial reaming of the acteabular cavity is done until subchondral bleeding bone is obtained maintaining the correct acetabular anteversion and inclination (Fig. 19). Trial cup placement is done at this point. Good indication of optimal press-fit is gentle shaky movement of the whole pelvis on attempts to pull out this trial cup. Scoop out the bone slurry from the last few reams and this slurry can be placed between the back side off the cup and the acetabular floor for better osteointegration (Fig. 20).

Place a blunt retractor under transverse acetabular ligament to keep the soft tissues away and the metallic acetabular cup is tapped snugly in the reamed cavity (Fig. 21). Tapping helps in the press-fit grip of the metal cup. Acetabular liner is fitted over the metallic cup using the ball shaped tap provided by the company. (Various manufacturers have different liner locking mechanisms for the cups) Femoral prosthesis is implanted in the previously prepared femoral canal whose femoral anteversion was estimated earlier. Reduce the femoral prosthesis into the acetabular cup and check the combined angle of anteversion by doing the coplanar test. For this test the leg should be slightly flexed, abducted and internally rotated till the cup rim, liner rim and the bottom flat surface of the prosthetic femoral head are in the same plane (Fig. 25). Measure the angle between the leg and the table. The hip should be stable in all movements and free of bony or metal impingement. Suture the tagged short external rotators back to their insertion site or the posterior edge of the greater trochanter (Fig. 26)

Close the fascia in layers after hemostasis is achieved. Skin closure done.

SURGICAL STEPS

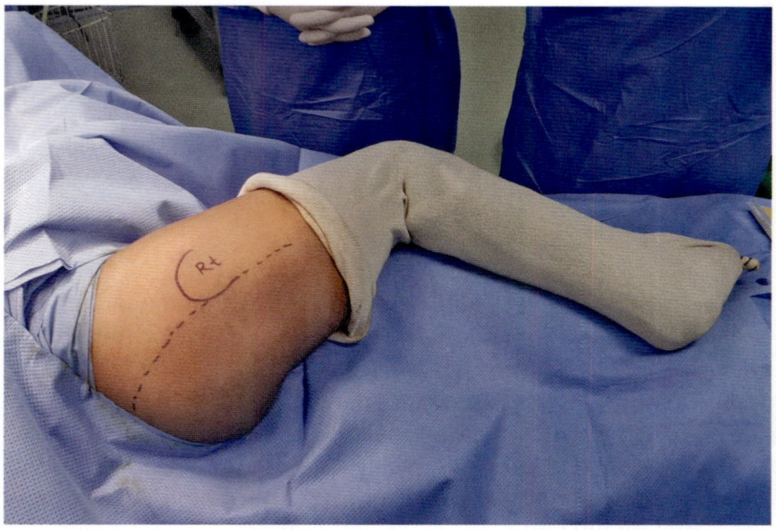

Fig. 1: Lateral position of the patient. Mark the greater trochanter.

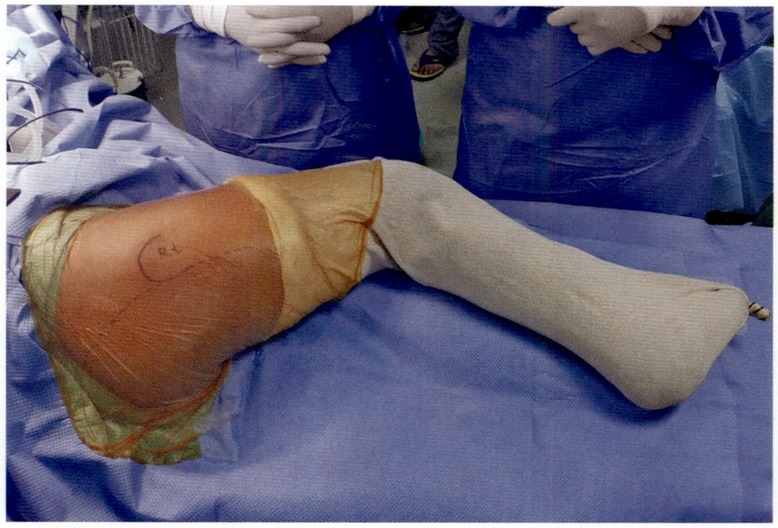

Fig. 2: Sterile sticky drape over operative site to create an additional sterile field.

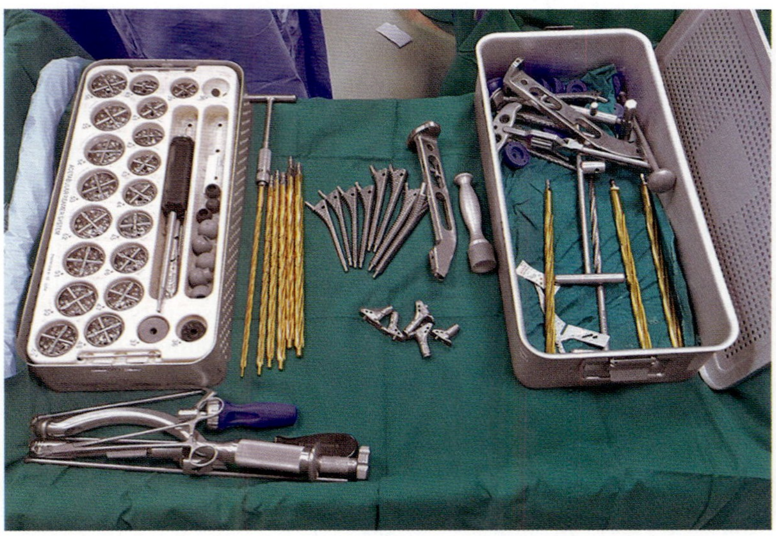

Fig. 3: Instrument trolley with acetabular reamers and broach of different sizes.

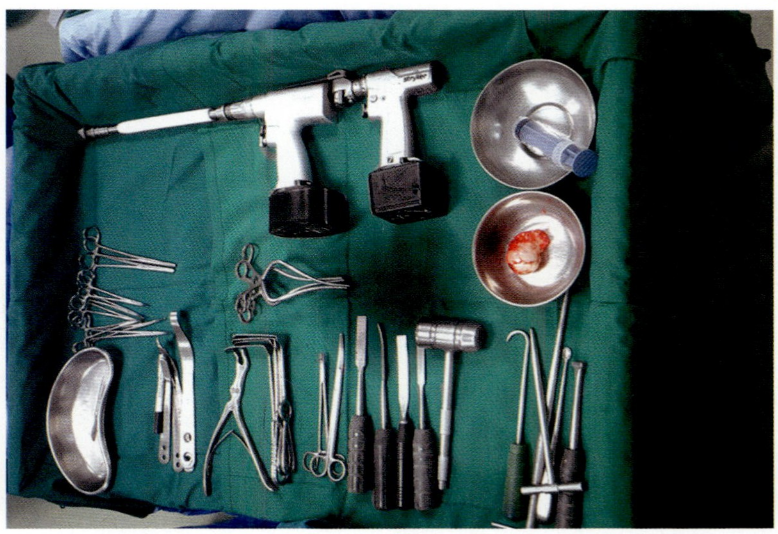

Fig. 4: General orthopaedic instruments including blunt retractor and bone hook.

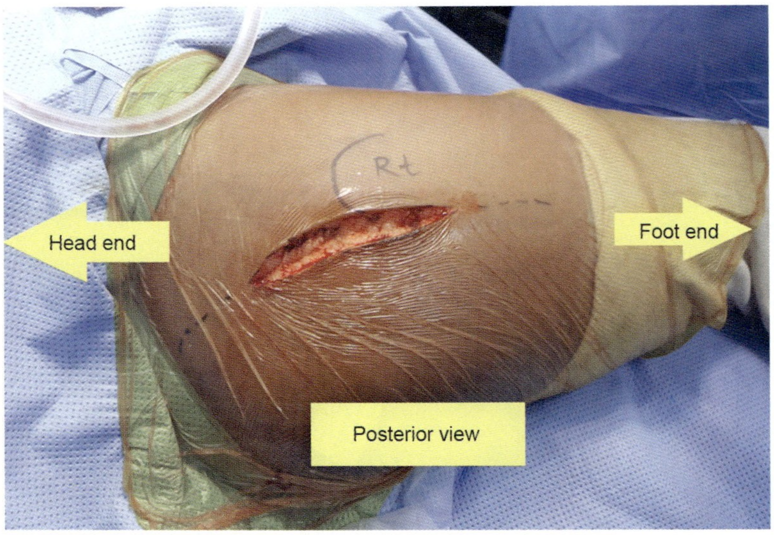

Fig. 5: Mini posterior incision.

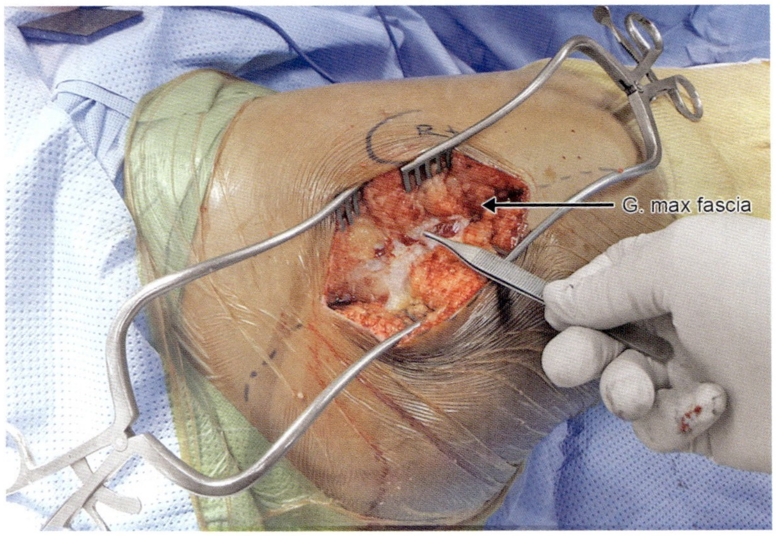

Fig. 6: Fascia of gluteus maximus (GMax) is partially released for adequate exposure.

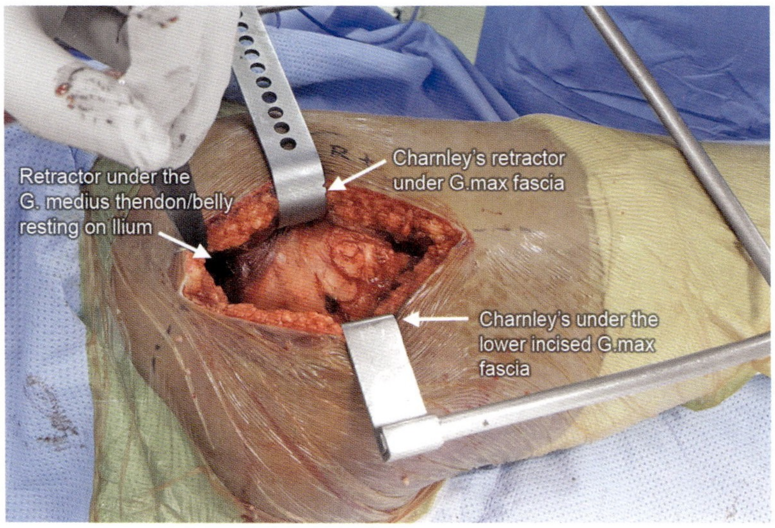

Fig. 7: After tensor fascia lata (TFL) is split, Charnley's retractors are placed underneath GMax fascia.

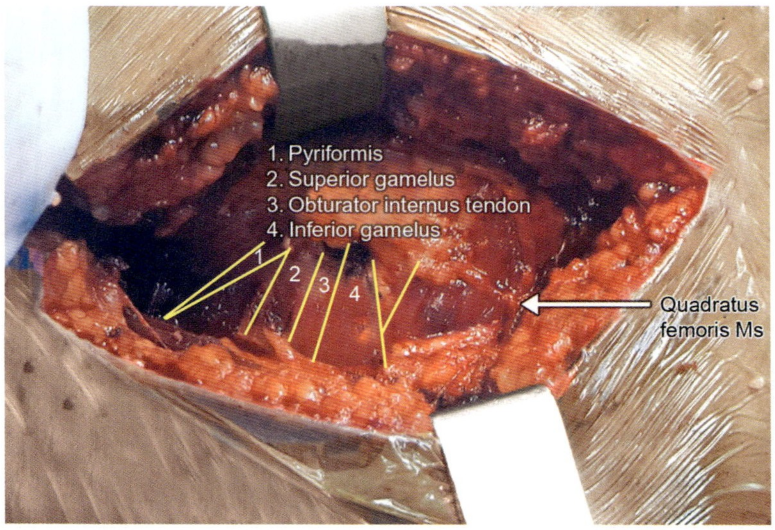

Fig. 8: Short external rotators are tagged and split away from their insertion.

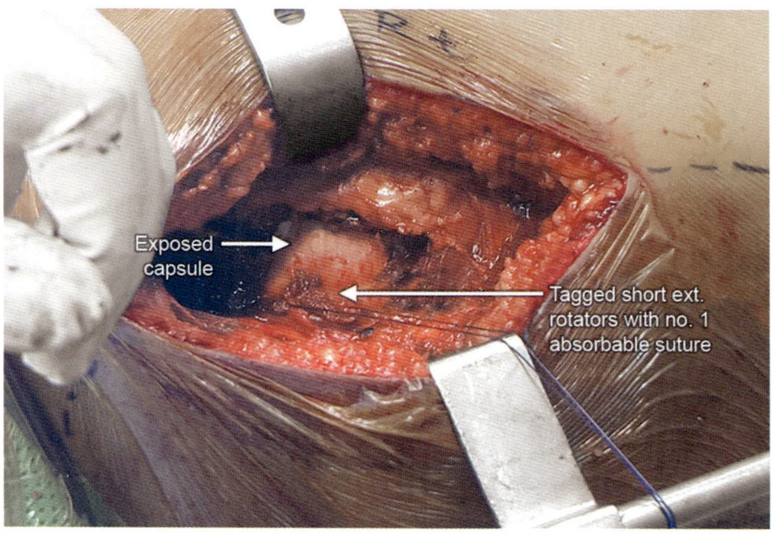

Fig. 9: Capsule of the hip joint is exposed after retracting short external rotators.

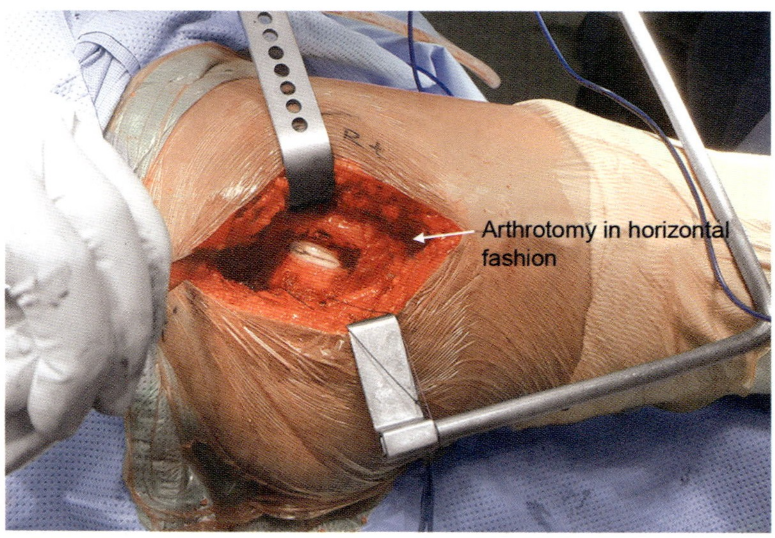

Fig. 10: Mark the arthrotomy site on the exposed capsule more towards the femoral metaphysis side.

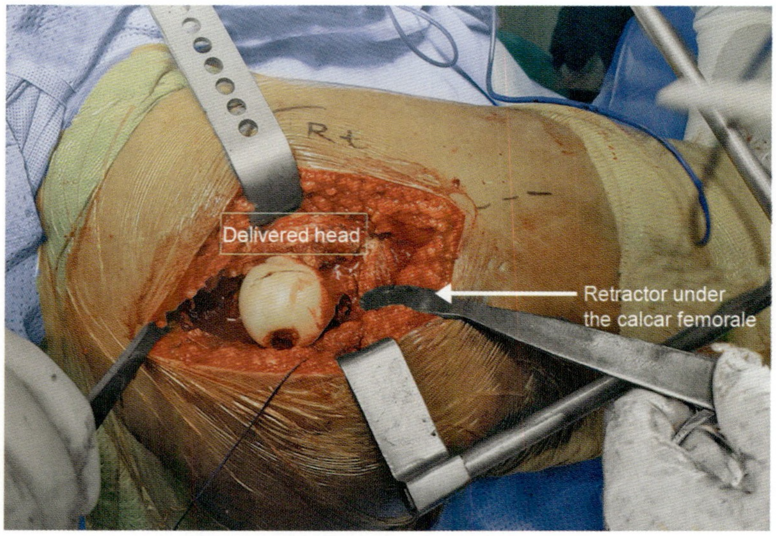

Fig. 11: Place retractor under calcar and deliver the head. Alternatively, cork screw can be used to deliver the head.

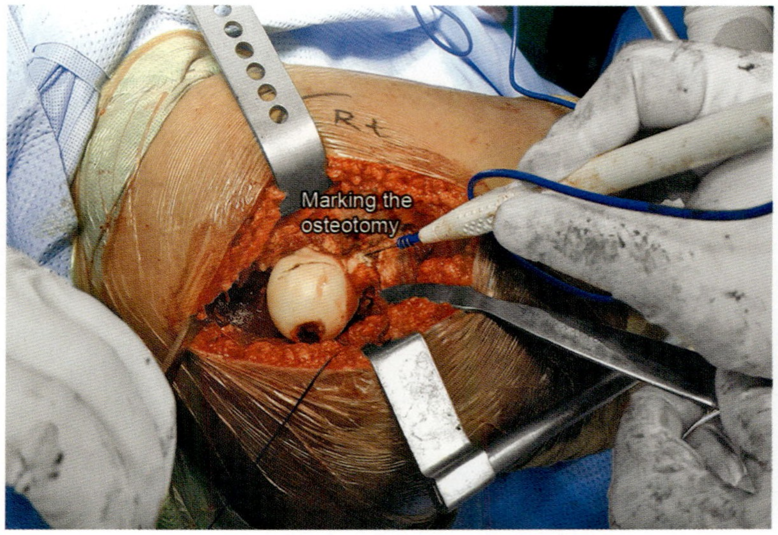

Fig. 12: Mark the site of osteotomy as per the intended leg length correction.

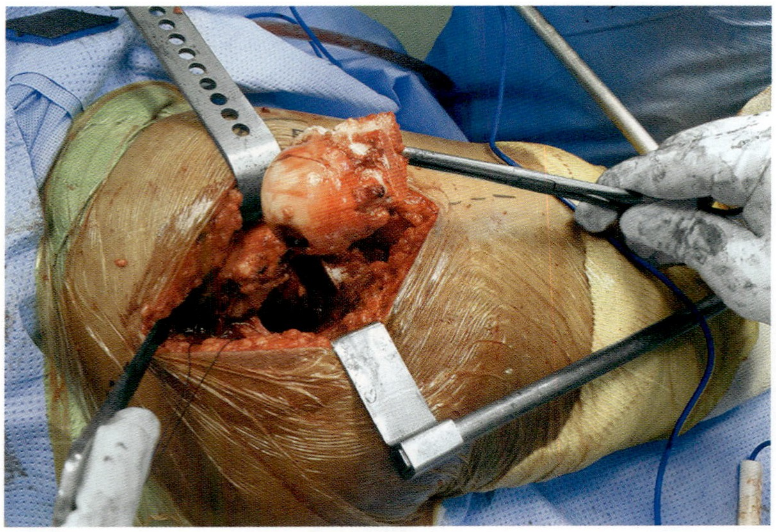

Fig. 13: Deliver the head. Ligamentum teres need to be cut using stout scissors.

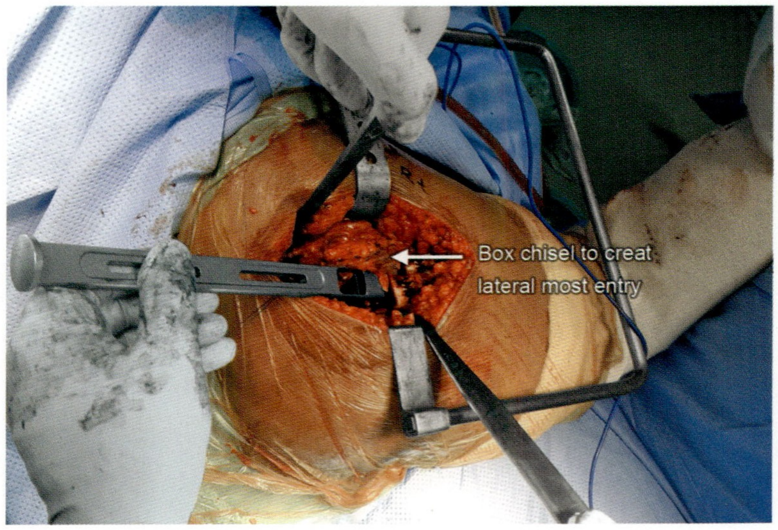

Fig. 14: Entry is made using a box chisel to create a lateral most entry point.

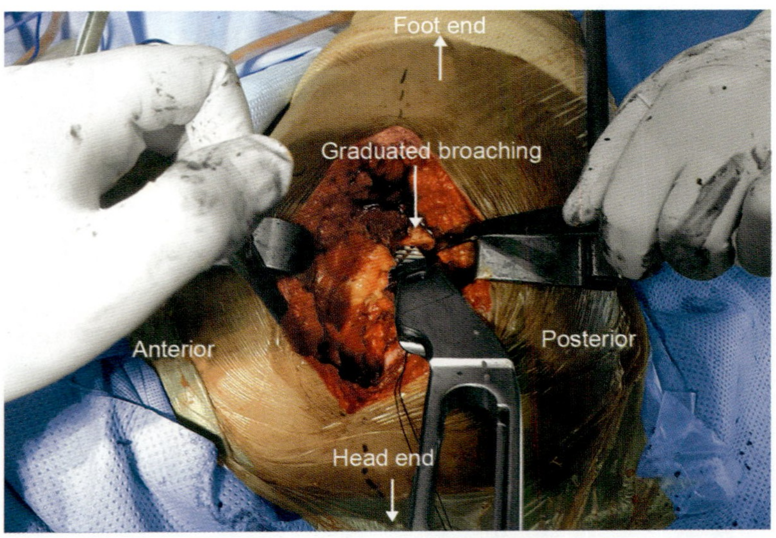

Fig. 15: Broaching is done gradually. Broach should be snugly fitting the femoral canal.

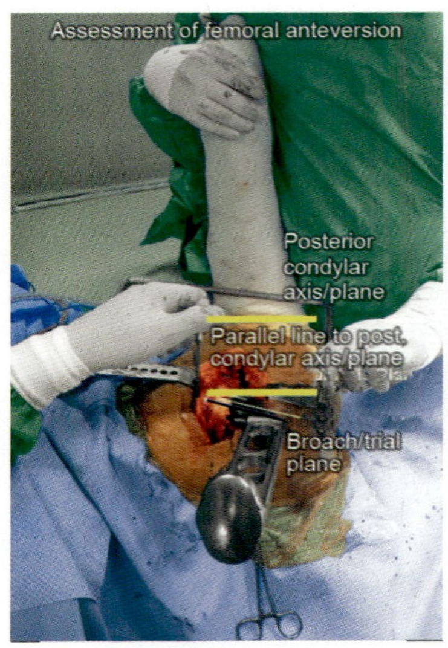

Fig. 16: Ask the assistant to flex knee at 90 degrees and compare the plane of the broach with the posterior condylar plane to determine the anterversion.

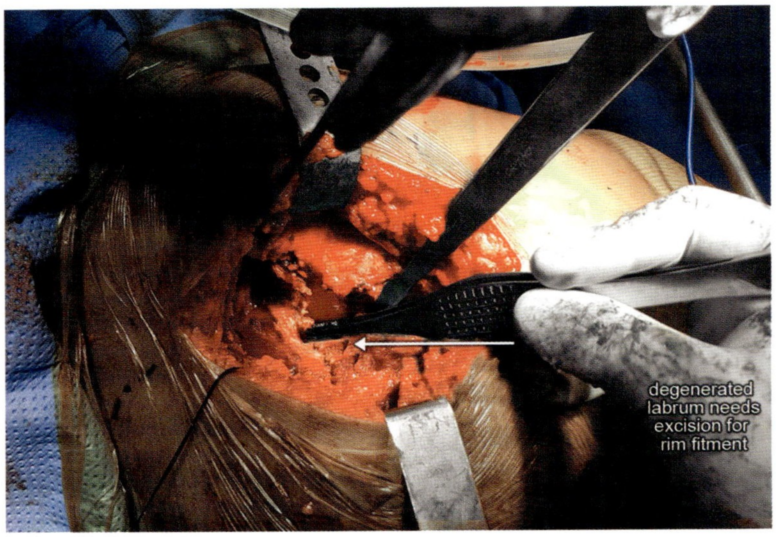

Fig. 17: Excise the acetabular labrum, which prevents bony fitment of implant.

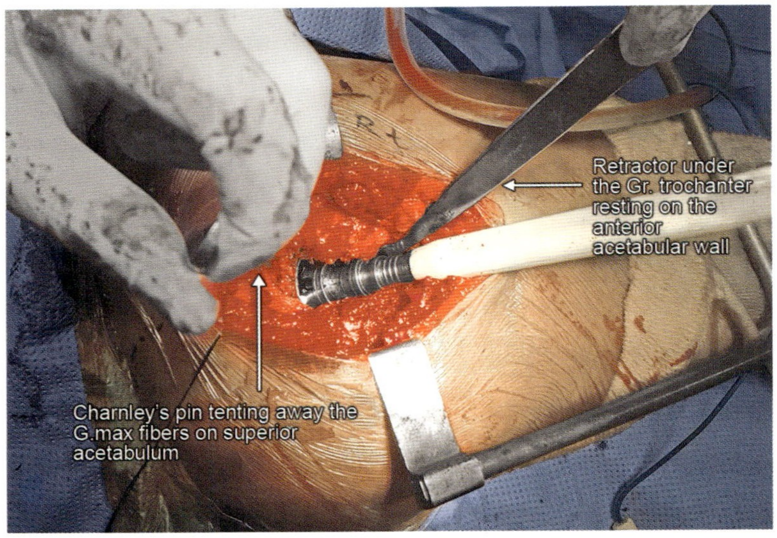

Fig. 18: Place Charnley's pin proximal to superior acetabulum and a retractor over anterior acetabular wall. This exposes the acetabular cavity well.

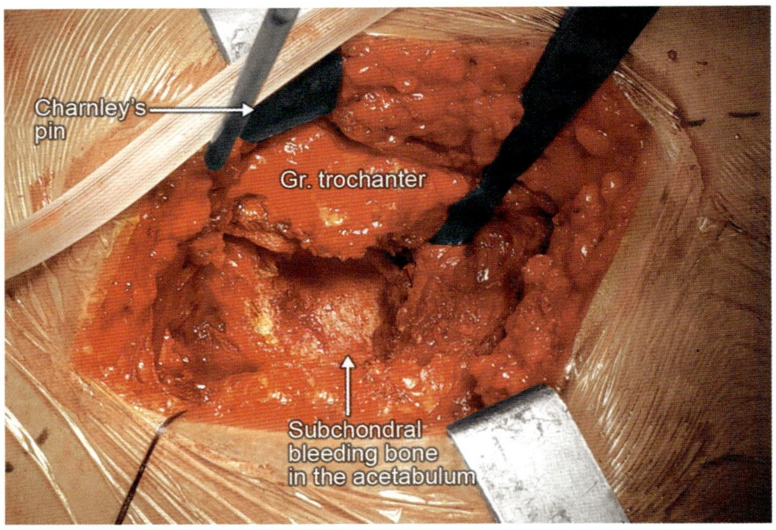

Fig. 19: Graduated reaming is done till bleeding subchondral bone is exposed

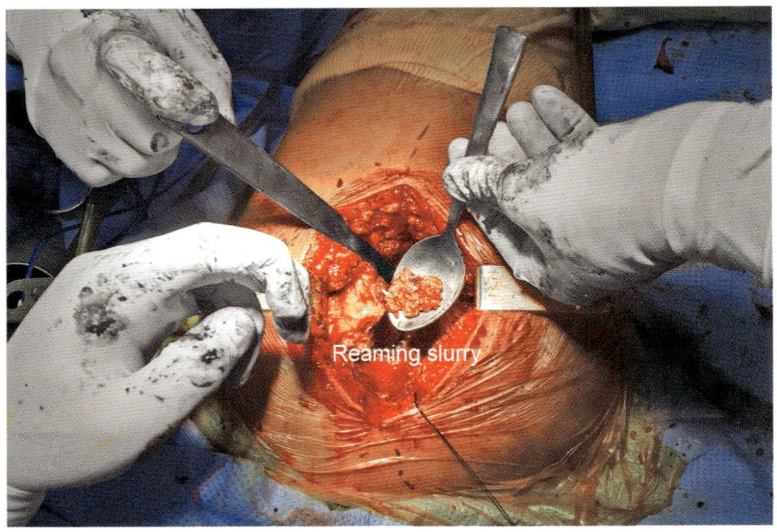

Fig. 20: Scoop out the reaming slurry. This acts as bone graft substitute for osteointegration.

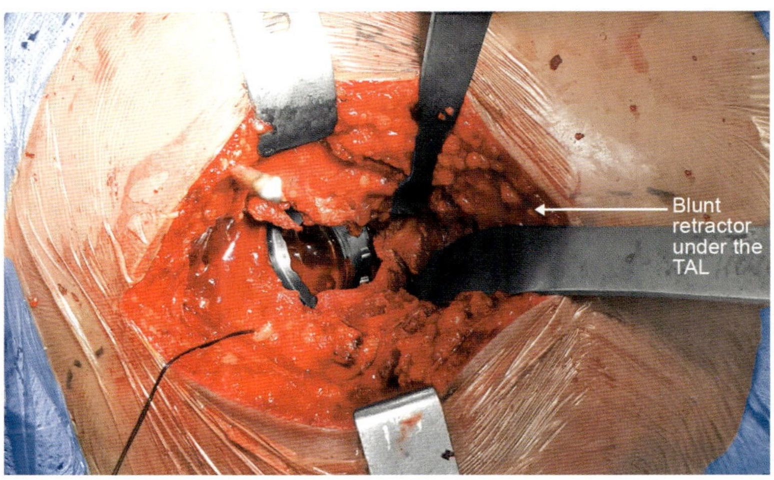

Fig. 21: Place blunt retractor under transverse acetabular ligament and metallic acetabular cup is tapped snugly in the reamed cavity to acheive the press-fit..

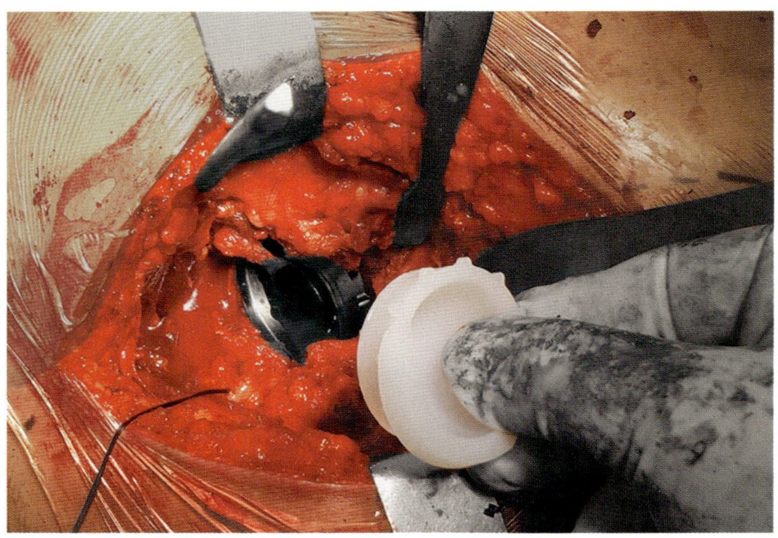

Fig. 22: Ultra-high molecular weight polyethylene (UHMWPE) liner being is fitted inside the metallic cup.

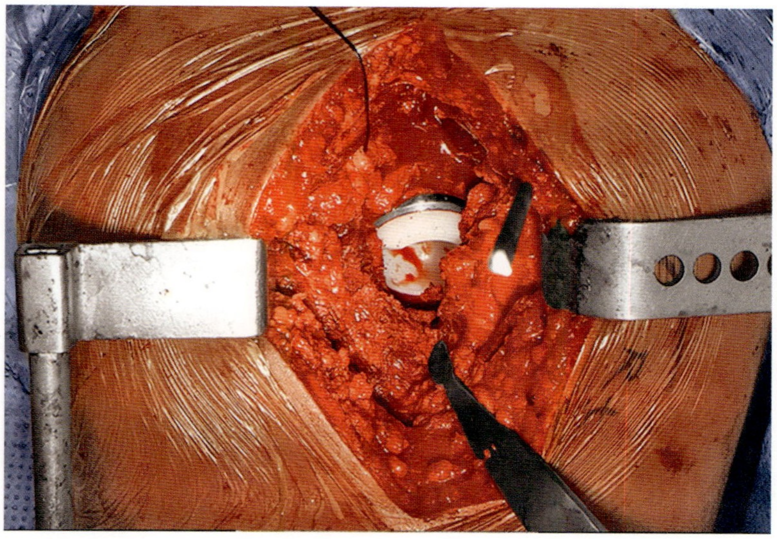

Fig. 23: Check the cup position in correct saggital and coronal plane.

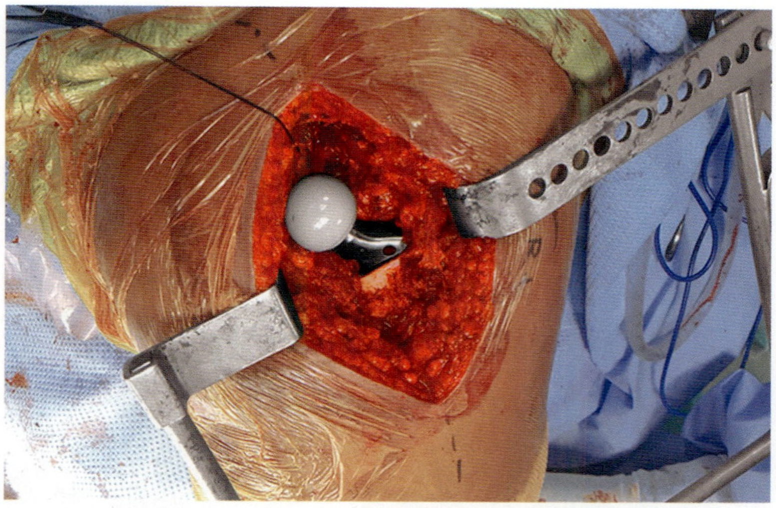

Fig. 24: Femoral prosthesis takes the same orientation as per the earlier broaching. Here ceramic head is gently tapped on the taper.

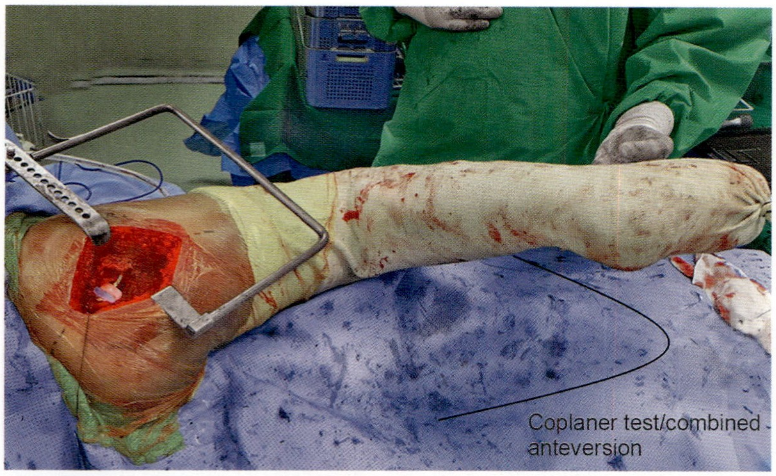

Fig. 25: Reduce the femoral prosthesis into the acetabular cup and check the combined angle of anteversion. For this the leg should be slightly flexed, abducted and internally rotated till the cup rim, liner rim and the bottom flat surface of the prosthetic femoral head are in the same plane. Measure the angle between the leg and the table.

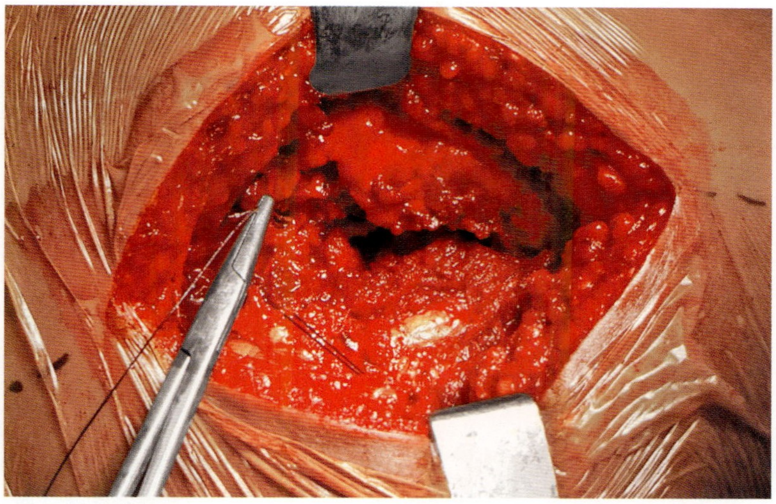

Fig. 26: Suture the tagged short external rotators back to their insertion site or through the holes in the posterior edge of the greater trochanter.

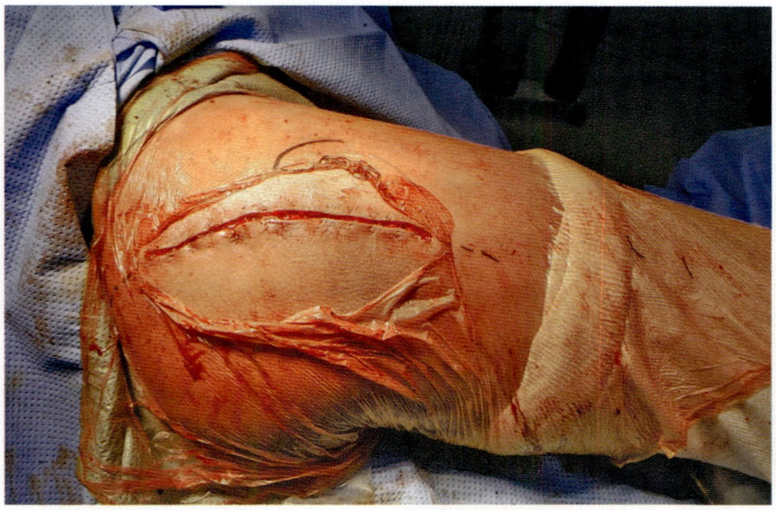

Fig. 27: Close the fascia in layers using absorbable sutures.

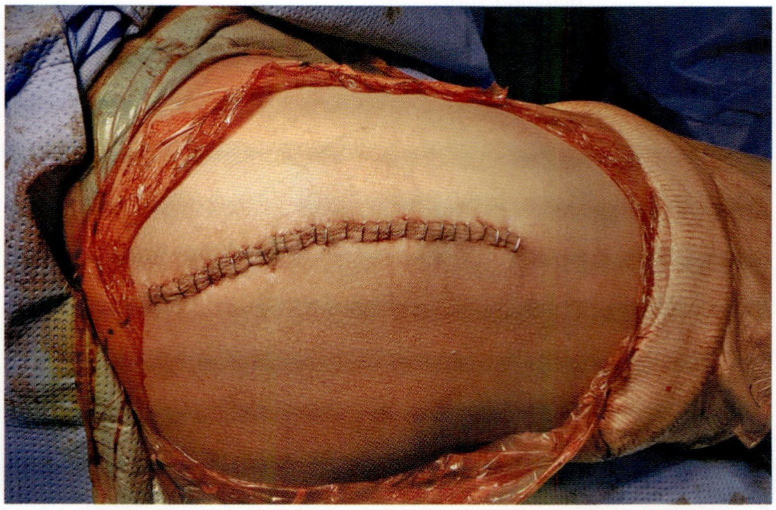

Fig. 28: Skin is closed using skin staplers or non absorbable sutures.

SUGGESTED READING

1. Berstock JR, Blom AW, Beswick AD. A systematic review and meta-analysis of the standard versus mini-incision posterior approach to total hip arthroplasty. J Arthroplasty. 2014;29(10):1970-82.
2. Dorr LD, Dastane MR, et al. Combined Anteversion Technique for Total Hip Arthroplasty Clin Orthop Relat Res. 2009;467(1):119-27.
3. Procyk S. Initial results with a mini-posterior approach for total hip arthroplasty. Int Orthop. 2007;31(Suppl 1):17-20.

CHAPTER 55

Total Hip Replacement with Anterolateral Approach

Kiran Kharat

KEY POINTS TO NOTE

- It can be done supine with a sandbag under the buttock with the patient of the edge of the table or in the lateral decubitus using bolsters and padded supports.
- The skin incision is above the tip of the trochanter and below in a line along the femoral shaft.
- The tensor is split in line but posteriorly in the proximal part along the gluteus maximus to prevent a tight posterior sling.
- With the leg in external rotation, the medius and minimus are released sharply leaving a cuff near the trochanter edge.
- Acetabular exposure is helped by releasing the reflected head of the rectus femoris.

HISTORICAL ASPECTS

- Kocher described it first in 1903.
- Hardinge made it popular in 1982.
- Lester Borden described the anatomy of the gluteus medius and minimus and provided the basis for anatomical repair.

ADVANTAGES

As some of the posterior capsule is retained, the chances of dislocation are reduced. The acetabular exposure is excellent and as there is no iatrogenic flexion of the pelvis this results in appropriate component placement.

INDICATIONS AND CONTRAINDICATIONS

It can be used for the majority of hip replacements and is also extensile.

It is contraindicated in patients who have had old femoral fractures malunited in flexion. It cannot be considered when there are limb length inequality issues of more than 2 cm as repair cannot be adequate.

OVERALL PLANNING

1. Any pre-existing hardware?
2. Previous scars?
3. Limb length issues?
4. Previous malunited femoral fractures?
5. Aim to medialize the acetabulum to the floor of the fovea to reduce the body weight lever arm and reduce demand on the abductor mechanism.
6. The inferior edge of the socket should correspond with the acetabular outlet to restore the center of rotation and also the working length of the abductors.
7. The cup abduction should be 45° using the inferior cotyledons as a guide.
8. The version should correspond with the native acetabulum.

SURGICAL STEPS (FIGS. 1 TO 20)

1. Lateral decubitus. Stable supports to align the two anterior superior iliac spines vertical when viewed from the ends or sides.
2. Skin incision is over the trochanter angled slightly posterior.
3. Tensor fascia lata incised and extended proximally curving into the gluteus maximus and distally along the line of the femoral shaft. A tight posterior sling is avoided by the curved incision.
4. The underlying abductors are preserved using a blunt instrument.
5. The leg is held in gentle external rotation stretching the gluteus medius showing its fan-like extent.
6. Mark to remove a third or half of the medius from the femur in a distal to proximal fashion. It is imperative to leave a cuff behind.
7. The release is carried up to the anterosuperior corner of the greater trochanter and direction changed in line with the muscle belly.
8. The minimus is exposed and dissected and a cuff left behind to repair.
9. The capsule is now seen and the retractors are placed on either side.
10. The capsule is released in a T or circumferentially.

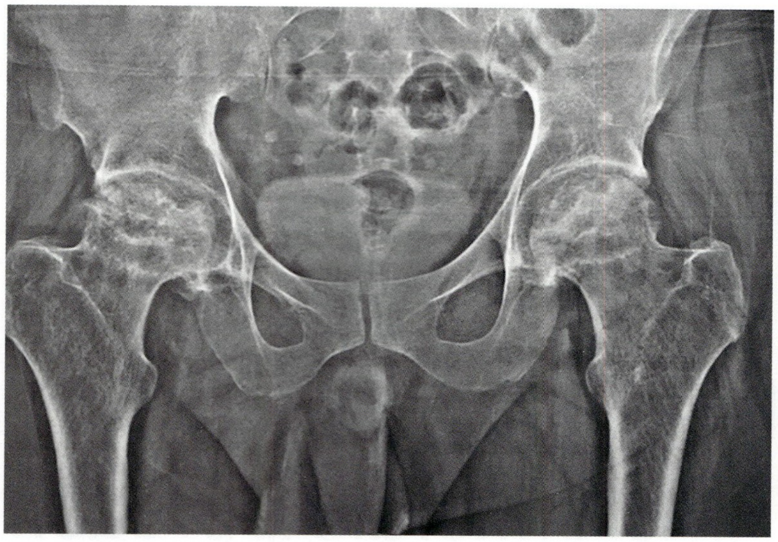

Fig. 1: X-ray pelvis both hips anteroposterior (AP) view showing post-avascular necrosis (AVN) collapse and subsequent arthritis changes.

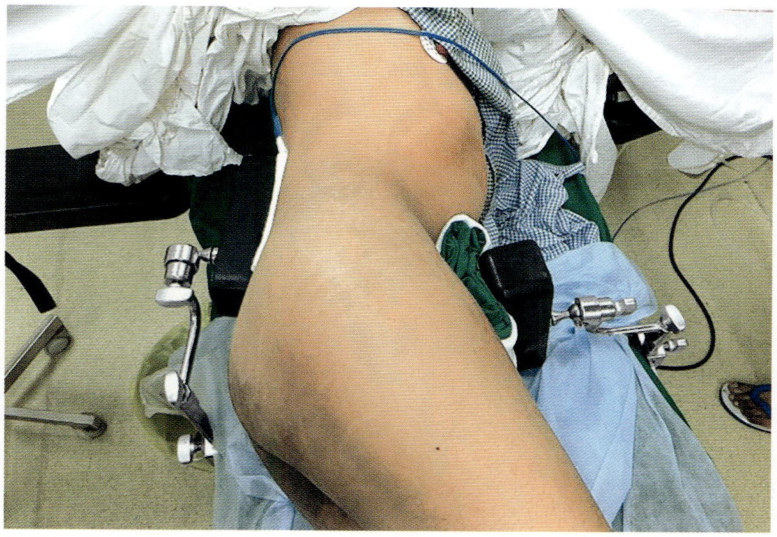

Fig. 2: Lateral decubitus showing padded bolsters attached to table keeping the operative area without obstruction and allowing free excursion of the limb with the pelvis perpendicular to the horizontal plane.

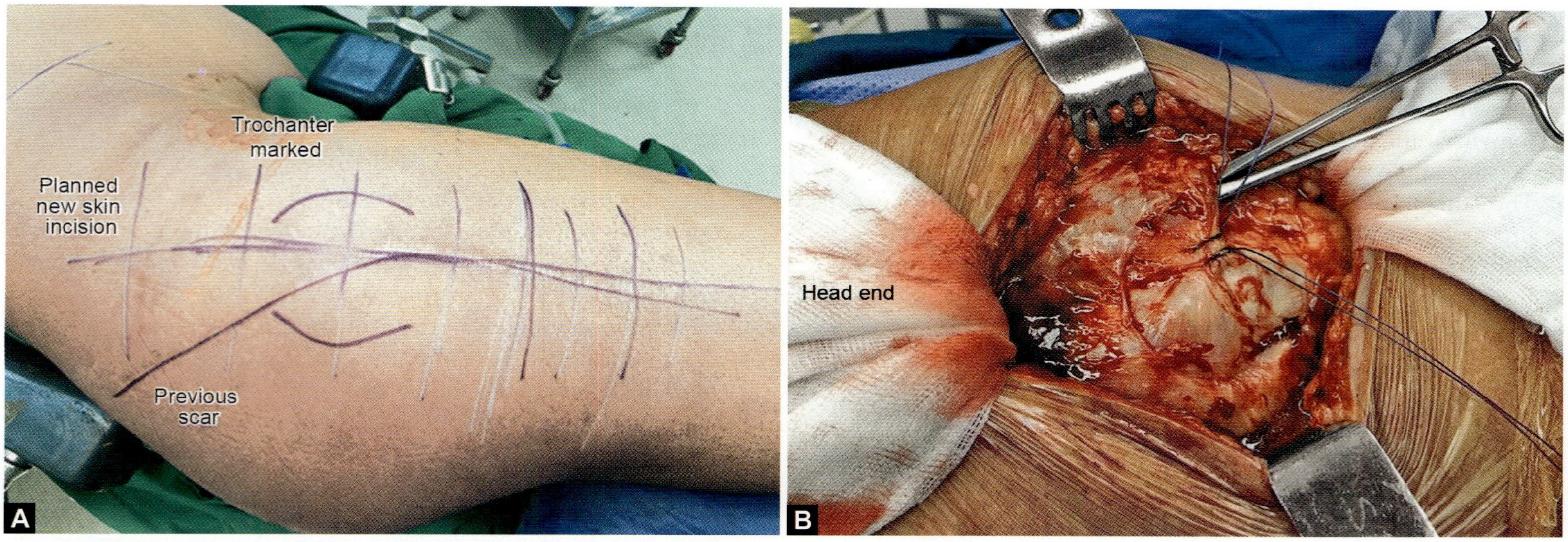

Figs. 3A and B: (A) Top view showing previous scars and the new planned scar; (B) Identifying the starting point of gluteus medius dissection using stay sutures. A curved artery is under the fan-shaped gluteus medius to stretch it and also to give a visual limit to the proximal end of the straight limb of dissection before turning in the direction of the muscle fibers. The superior gluteal nerve is 3–5 cm above the tip of the greater trochanter and this awareness is important to protect it by avoiding straying into that area.

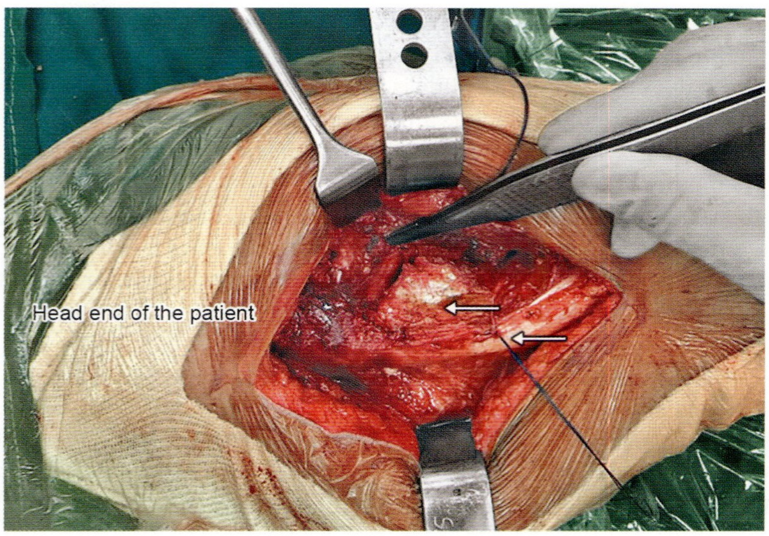

Fig. 4: Stay sutures in the inferior pole of the gluteus medius (arrow) with retracted muscle showing the anterior part of the neck (arrow). The proximal dissection into the muscle at an angle like a hockey stick blade avoids damage to the superior gluteal nerve.

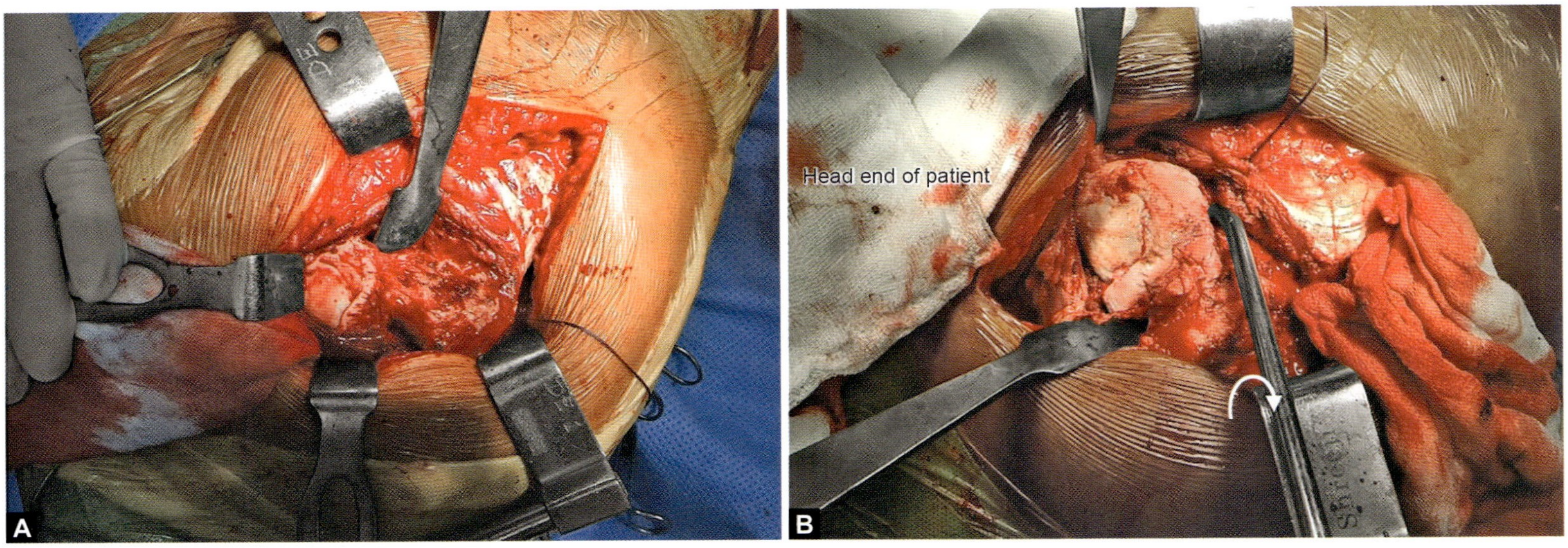

Figs. 5A and B: (A) The femoral head delivered by a gentle flexion external rotation and adduction movement of the limb by the assistant; (B) Sometimes a hook can be used to help deliver a deformed large head in conjunction with the flexion, external rotation and adduction maneuver.

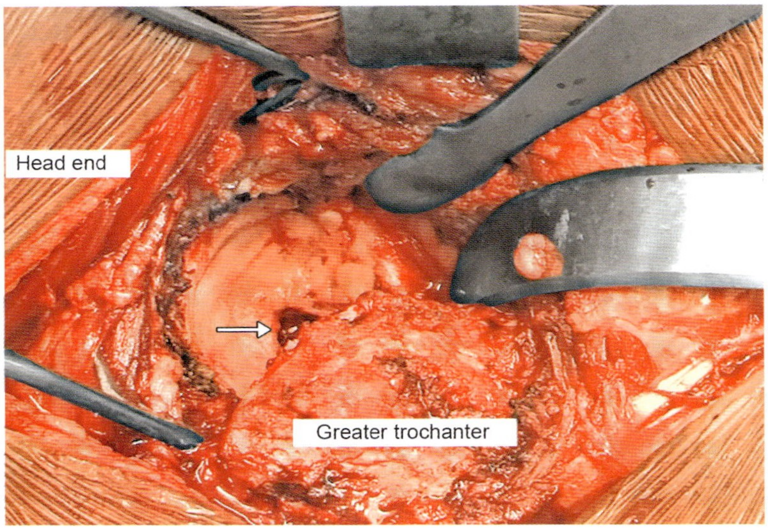

Fig. 6: Acetabulum exposed with strategic curved long retractors. Part of fovea seen (arrow).

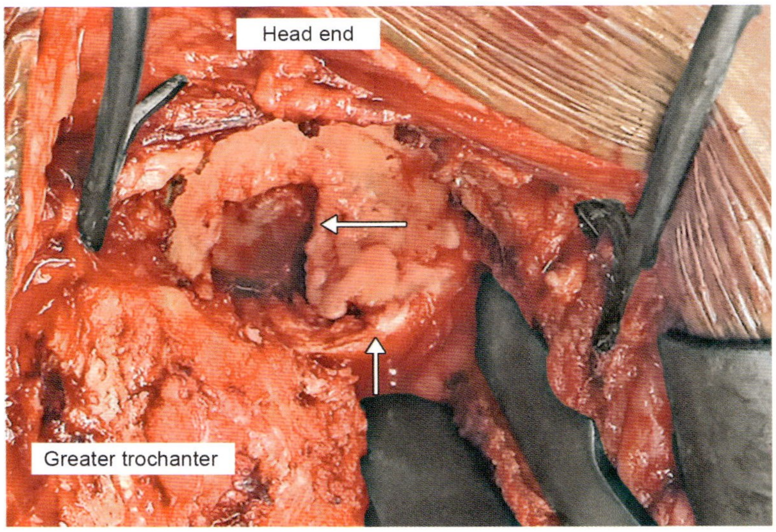

Fig. 7: Overhead view showing complete circumferential view of the acetabulum. Central fovea with overhanging osteophytes (arrow). The transverse acetabular ligament (TAL) (arrow).

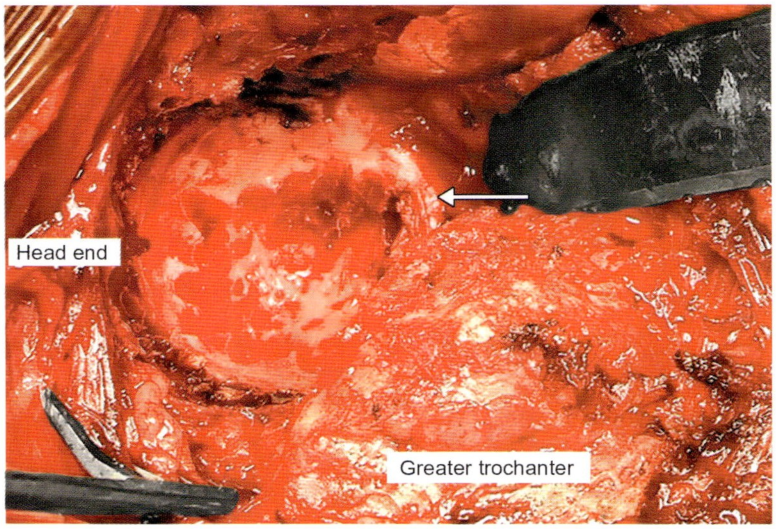

Fig. 8: Medialization by controlled removal of floor osteophytes using a gouge. The TAL (arrow).

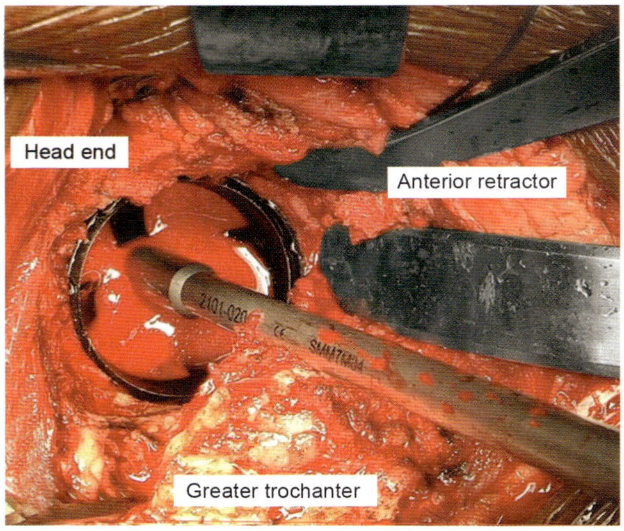

Fig. 9: Overhead view showing trial acetabular shell insert in place to get orientation of final abduction and version.

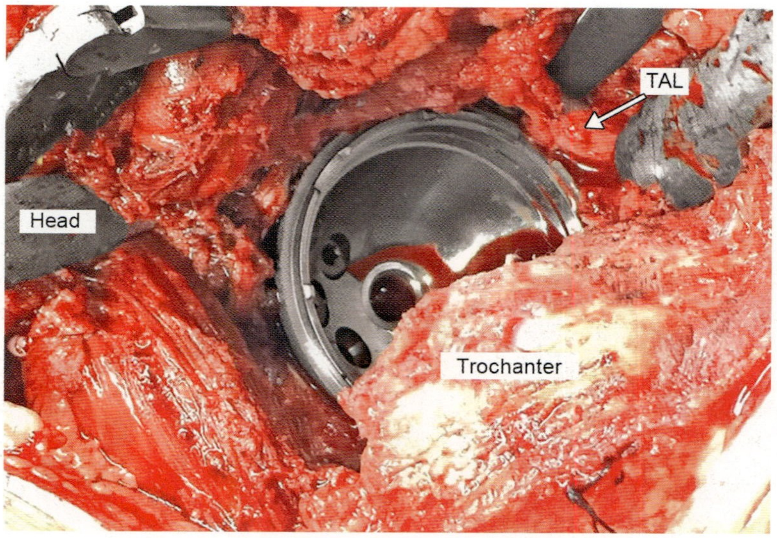

Fig. 10: Final uncemented cup in place. TAL retractor (arrow).

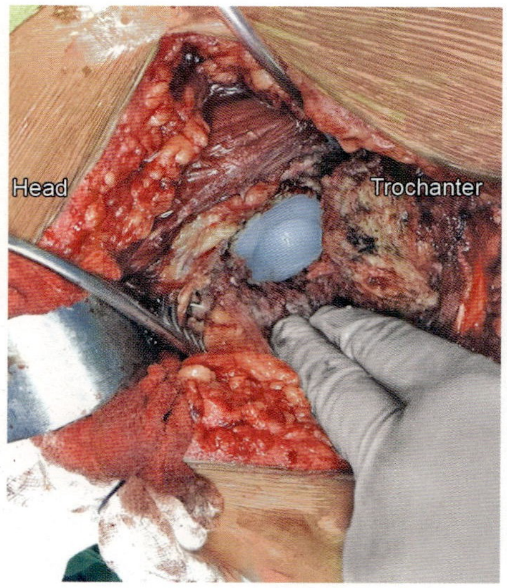

Fig. 11: Overhead view showing cemented cup in place.

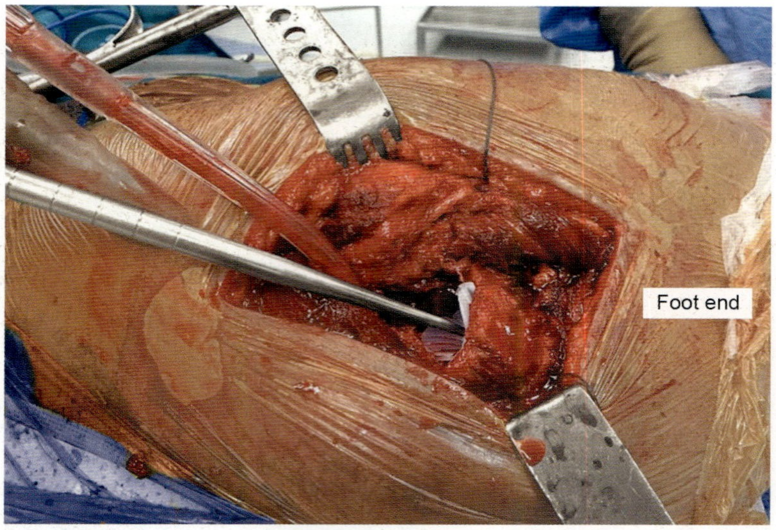

Fig. 12: After femur broaching, a cement restrictor being inserted.

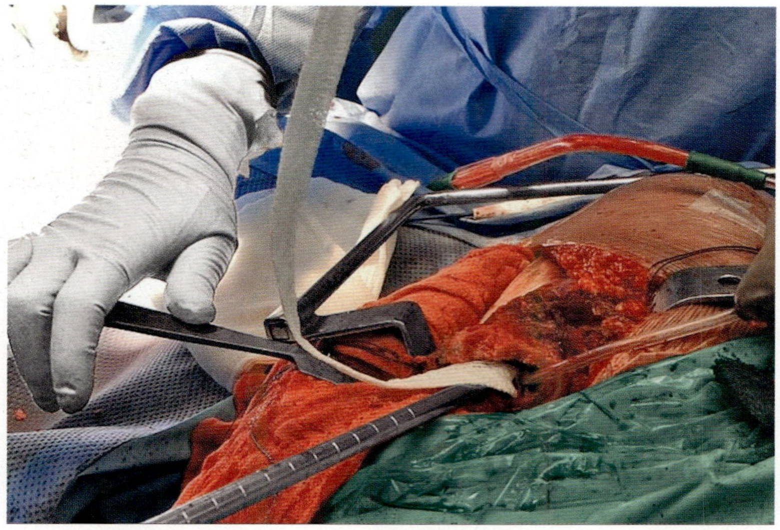

Fig. 13: After plugging at the correct length distally with a cement restrictor, the canal is cleaned and vented and packed with a roller gauze dipped in peroxide or saline mixed with adrenaline.

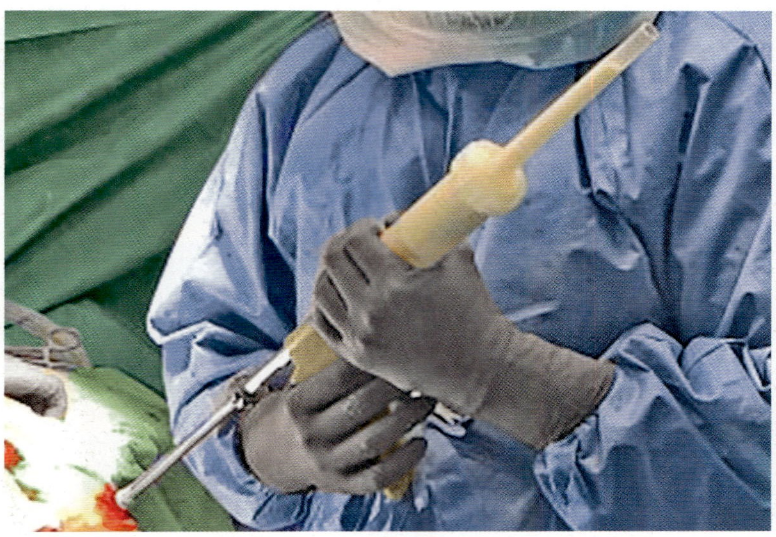

Fig. 14: Low viscosity cement in a cement gun.

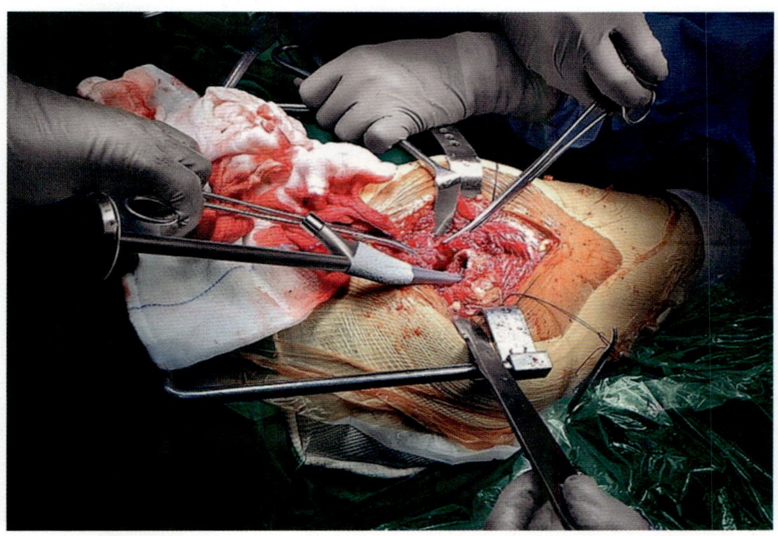

Fig. 15: Tapered wedge proximally-coated stem being inserted in prepared canal. One option depending on patient characteristics.

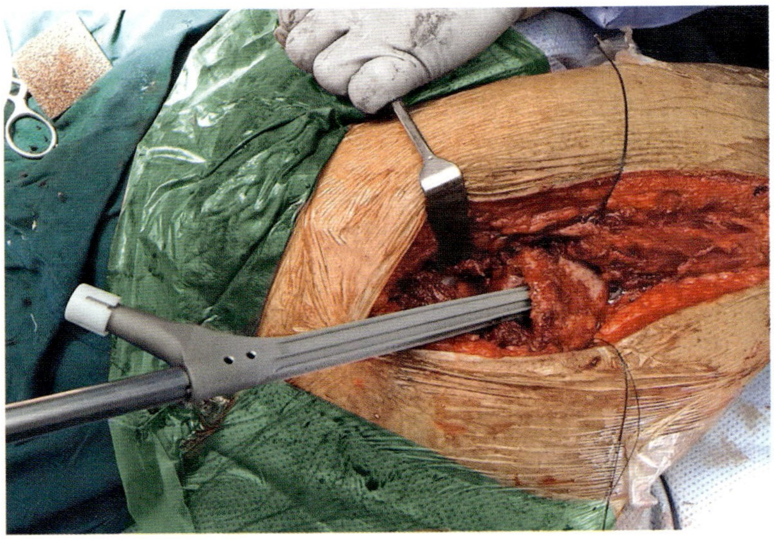

Fig. 16: A grit-blasted fluted titanium conical stem being inserted in prepared canal. The exposure allows excellent visualization of the femur. Another option depending upon patient characteristics.

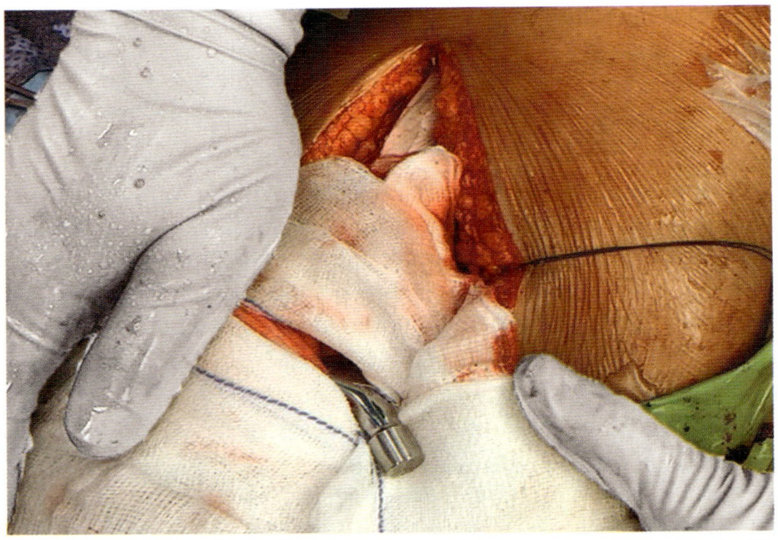

Fig. 17: The taper being prepared with due care to accept the femoral head. It should be completely clean and dry.

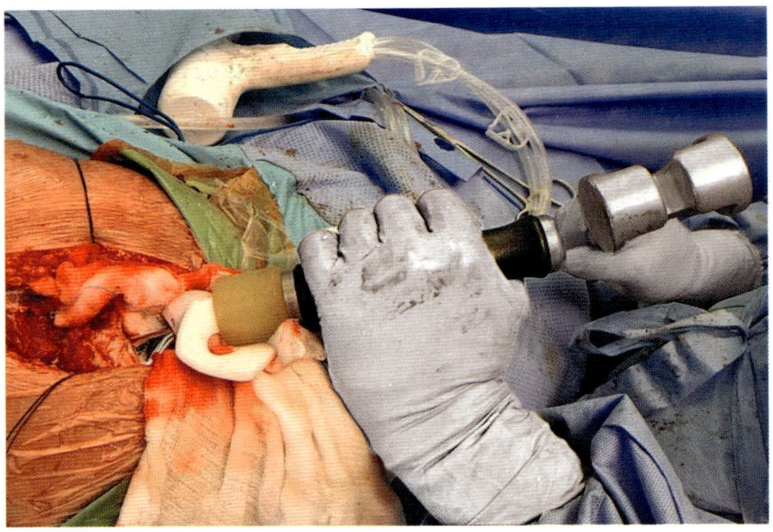

Fig. 18: The ceramic head protected with a clean sponge foam before impacting firmly with a mallet.

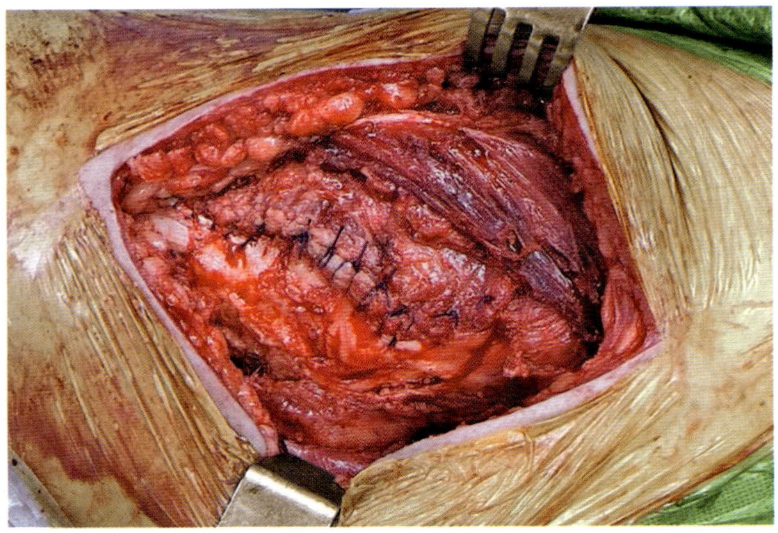

Fig. 19: A watertight abductor closure using No. 1 Absorbable suture. Intermittent sutures are taken through the trochanter bone using drill holes if necessary to ensure more strength to the repair.

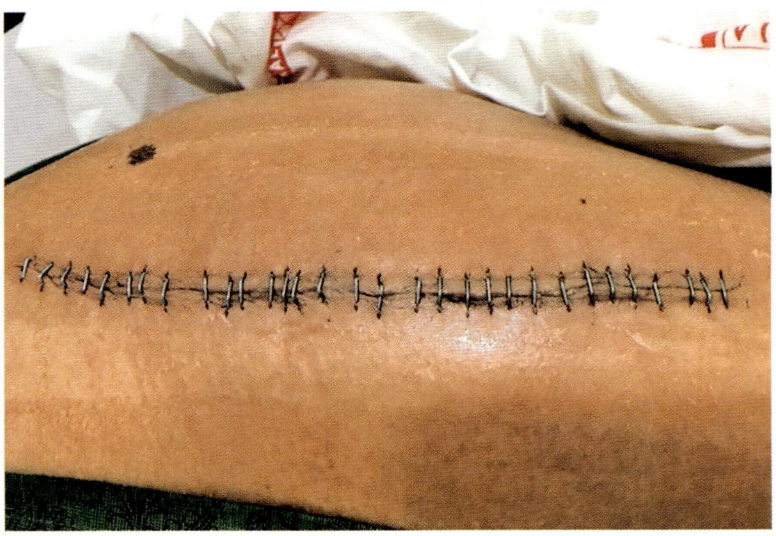

Fig. 20: Skin closure with staples without drain.

11. The hip is flexed and slowly rotated externally along with controlled adduction. A hook can be used to deliver the head and the leg placed in a prepared sterile pouch anteriorly.
12. Appropriate neck osteotomy is done keeping in mind the length and offset.
13. Hip replacement steps are performed according to the philosophy of the system chosen.
14. Watertight closure in layers—first minimus and then medius. The repair should be cuff to cuff and bone drill holes through the trochanter should be used for further augmentation.

KNOWN COMPLICATIONS

- Heterotopic ossification
- Limp-abductor lurch
- Nerve injury
- Fractures

- Limb length inequality
- Instability.

SUMMARY

This approach gives excellent access to the hip in the majority of pathologies. The acetabular exposure requires less force on the soft tissue retraction aspect. The retained posterior capsule gives more stability. Meticulous soft tissue repair using a good cuff to cuff repair augmented with transosseous sutures ensures good outcomes.

SUGGESTED READING

1. Asayama I, Chamnongkich S, Simpson KJ, et al. Reconstructed hip joint position and abductor muscle strength after THA. J Arthroplasty. 2005;20:414-20.
2. Barber TC, Roger DJ, Goodman SB, et al. Early outcome of THA using the direct lateral approach versus the posterior surgical approach. Orthopedics. 1996;19:873-5.
3. Damm P, Zonneveld J, Brackertz S, et al. Gluteal muscle damage leads to higher in vivo hip joint loads 3 months after total hip arthroplasty. PLoS One. 2018;13(1):e0190626.
4. Delanois RE, Sultan AA, Albayar AA, et al. The Röttinger approach for total hip arthroplasty: technique, comparison to the direct lateral approach and review of literature. Ann Transl Med. 2017;5(Suppl 3):S31.
5. Demos HA, Rorabeck CH, Bourne RB, et al. Instability in primary total hip arthroplasty with the direct lateral approach. Clin Orthop Relat Res. 2001;393:168-80.
6. Downing ND, Clark DI, Hutchinson JW, et al. Hip abductor strength following THA: a prospective comparison of the posterior and lateral approach in 100 patients. Acta Orthop Scand. 2001;72:215-20.
7. Hardinge K. The direct lateral approach to the hip. J Bone Joint Surg Br. 1982;64:17-9.
8. Jameson SS, Mason J, Baker P, et al. A comparison of surgical approaches for primary hip arthroplasty: a cohort study of patient reported outcome measures (PROMs) and early revision using linked national databases. J Arthroplasty. 2014;29:1248-55.
9. Masonis JL, Bourne RB. Surgical approach, abductor function and THA dislocation. Clin Orthop Relat Res. 2002;405:46-53.
10. Moskal JT, Mann JW 3rd. A modified direct lateral approach for primary and revision THA: a prospective analysis of 453 cases. J Arthroplasty. 1996;11:255-66.
11. Mulliken BD, Rorabeck CH, Bourne RB, et al. A modified direct lateral approach in total hip arthroplasty: a comprehensive review. J Arthroplasty. 1998;13:737-47.
12. Peters RM, van Beers LW, van Steenbergen LN, et al. Similar superior patient-reported outcome measures for anterior and posterolateral approaches after total hip arthroplasty: postoperative patient-reported outcome measure improvement after 3 months in 12,774 primary total hip arthroplasties using the anterior, anterolateral, straight lateral, or posterolateral approach. J Arthroplasty. 2018;33(6):1786-93.
13. Ugland TO, Haugeberg G, Svenningsen S, et al. Less periprosthetic bone loss following the anterolateral approach to the hip compared with the direct lateral approach. A subgroup analysis from a randomized trial in patients with a femoral neck fracture. Acta Orthop. 2018;89(1):23-8.
14. Yue C, MD, Kang P, Pei F, et al. Comparison of direct anterior and lateral approaches in THA. A systematic review and meta-analysis (PRISMA). Medicine (Baltimore). 2015;94(50):e2126.

CHAPTER 56

Radial Head Replacement for Fracture Head Radius

Shrikant Sagane, Raghav Barve, Madan Hardikar

INTRODUCTION

Radial head fractures are very common among elbow injuries. It is more often found in females than males. The prevalence is more in 20–60 years of age. Minimally displaced fractures are isolated injuries while comminuted fractures are associated with soft tissue injuries and may be associated with elbow dislocation.

MECHANISM OF INJURY

1. *Valgus loading*: It causes impaction of radial head against capitellum.
2. Axial loading of forearm.

CLASSIFICATION

There are two classification systems.

1. *Mason classification*:
   - Type 1—radial head fracture without displacement
   - Type 2—marginal sector fracture with displacement
   - Type 3—comminuted fracture involves whole radial head
   - Type 4—radial head fracture with elbow dislocation.
2. *Broberg and Morrey classification*:
   - Type 1—fracture less than 2 mm displacement
   - Type 2—fracture more than 2 mm displacement
   - Type 3—comminuted fracture.

   Smith and Hotchkiss defined safe zone for plating the radial head.

CLINICAL FEATURES

These patients present with pain, swelling, stiffness, of elbow and tenderness over lateral epicondyle and tenderness over medial epicondyle. Forearm rotation is affected and there is loss of terminal extension. It may be associated with distal radioulnar joint tenderness.

RADIOLOGICAL IMAGING

Anteroposterior (AP) and lateral view of elbow and distal radioulnar joint are required which may determine size, location and amount of comminution of radial head. CT scan will determine exact location of fracture fragments.

TREATMENT

Vast majority of undisplaced fractures with no restriction of rotation of forearm are treated with simple immobilization. Fractures of radial head involving more than 30% of articular area or more than 2 mm of displacement with block to rotation of forearm need surgical treatment. Severely comminuted fractures may need radial head replacement.

- *Fracture fragment less than 25% of articular diameter*: Excision of fragment
- *Displaced noncomminuted fracture of radial head limits forearm rotation (involve more than 30% of articular area)*: Open reduction and internal fixation of radial head.
- *Displaced fracture of radial head with severe comminution*: Excision of radial head
- *Unconstructable comminuted fracture of radial head with bony and ligamentous injury*: Radial head replacement.

SURGICAL PROCEDURE OF RADIAL HEAD REPLACEMENT

Surgical Approach

The Kocher approach between extensor carpi ulnaris and anconeus muscle is used most often.

SURGICAL STEPS (FIGS. 1 TO 22)

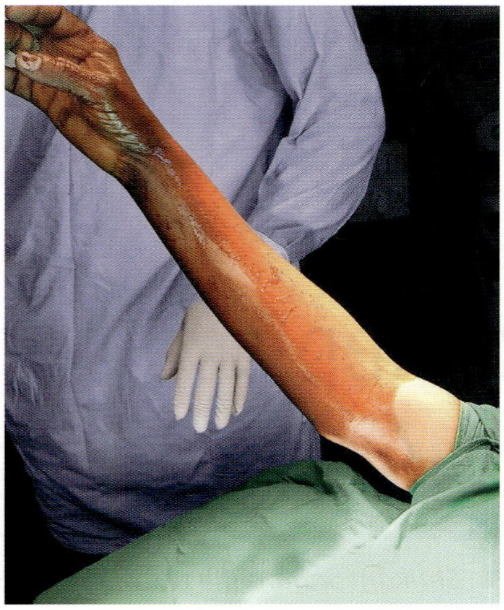

Fig. 1: Position—under general anesthesia supine position on operating table.

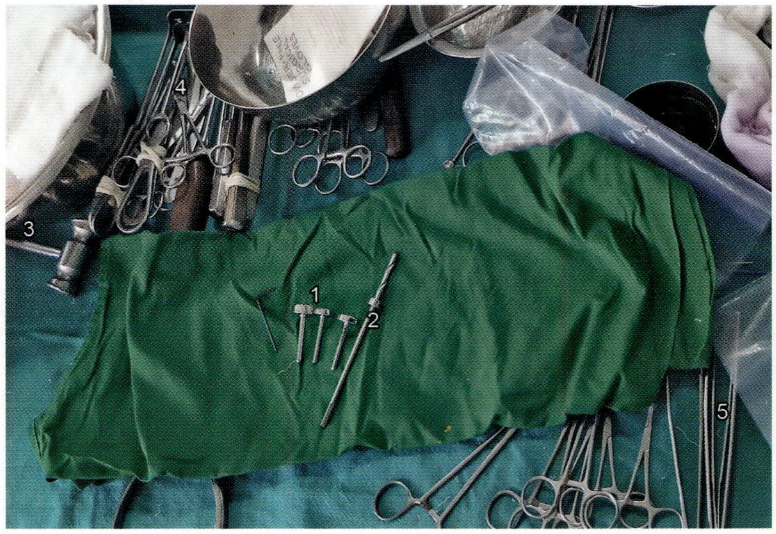

Fig. 2: Instruments: 1. Radial head prosthesis of various sizes; 2. Reamer; 3. Mallet; 4. General orthopaedic instruments including retractors, spikes, periosteum elevator, osteotome, bone hook, scissors, artery forceps; 5. Tissue holding forceps.

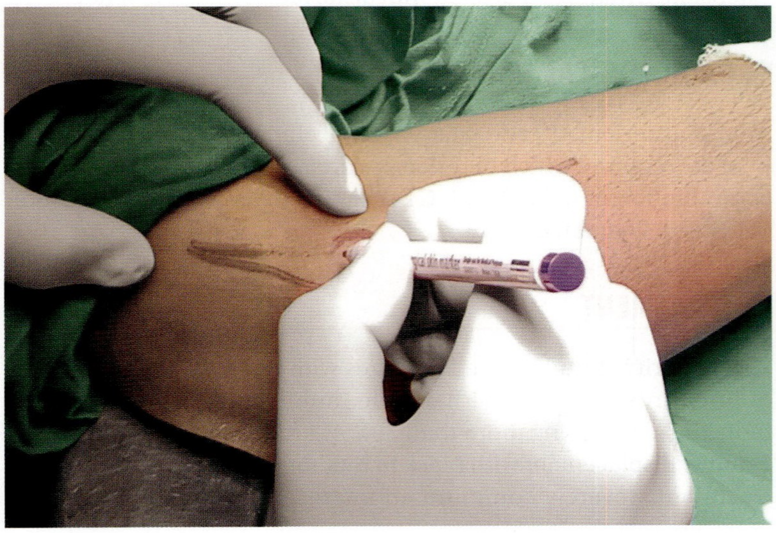

Fig. 3: Draping of patient, skin incision starting just above lateral condyle humerus.

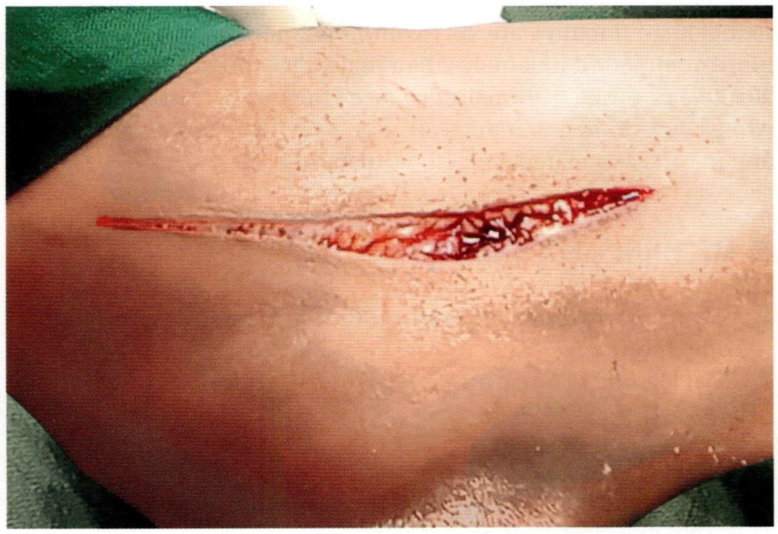

Fig. 4: Skin incision is taken with 22 No. blade.

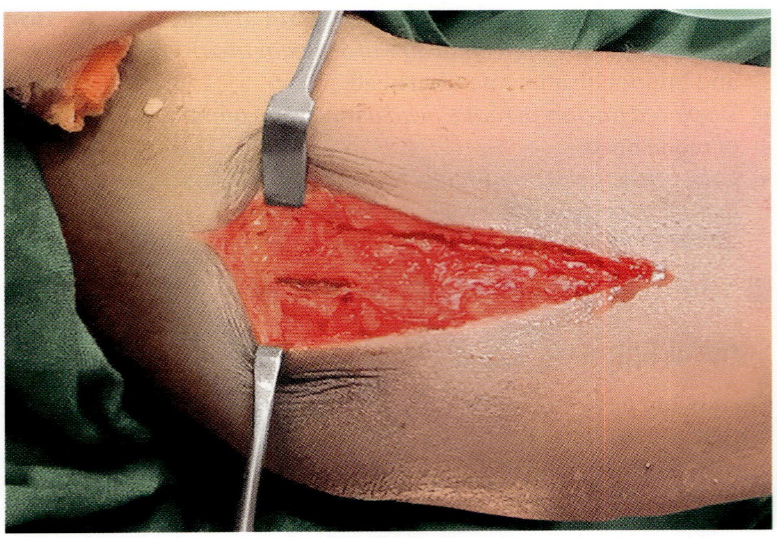

Fig. 5: Blunt dissection through subcutaneous plane.

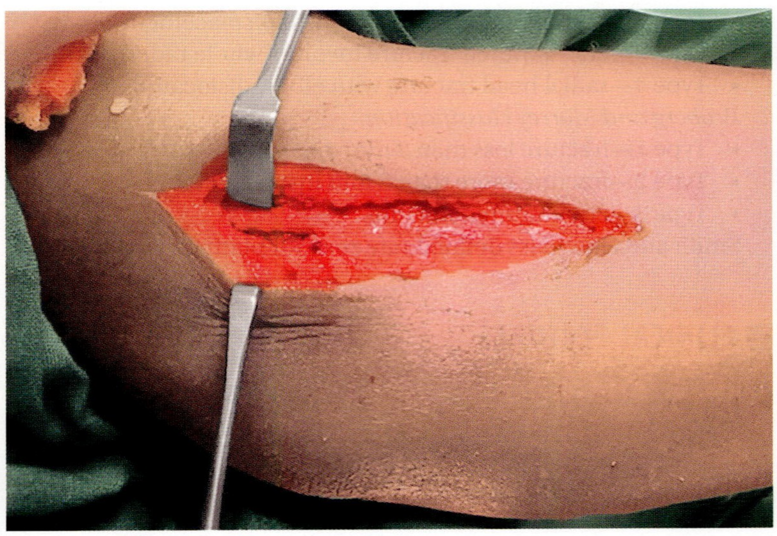

Fig. 6: Subcutaneous dissection showing common extensor origin.

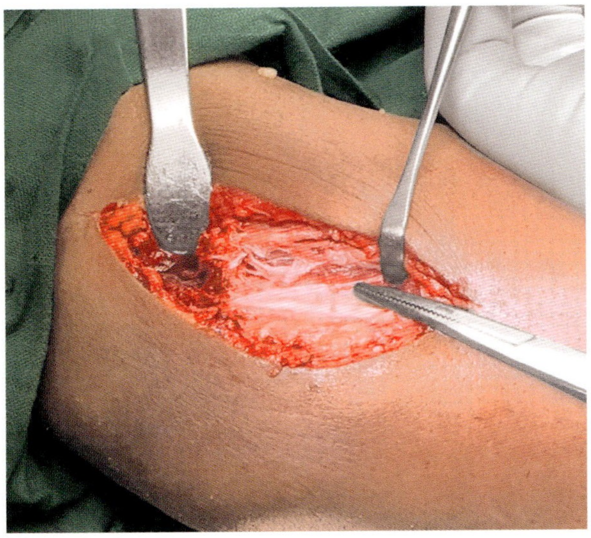

Fig. 7: Common extensor origin separated and secured.

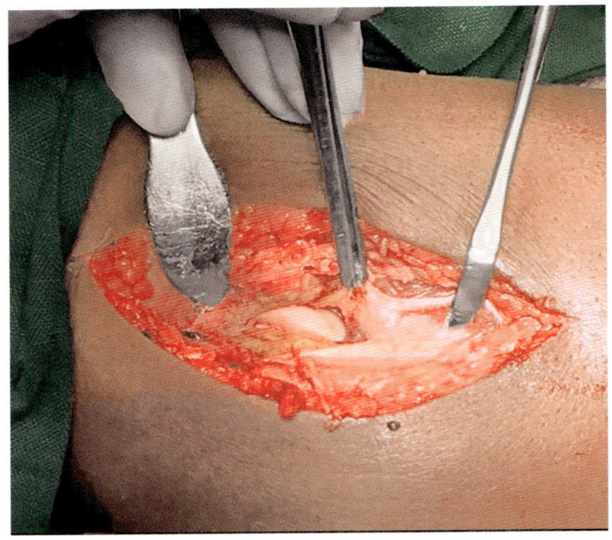

Fig. 8: Fractured head of radius reached after dissection.

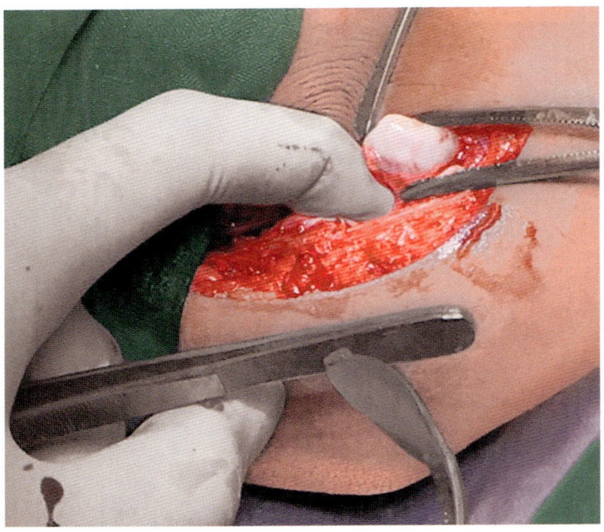

Fig. 9: Radial head excised and separated.

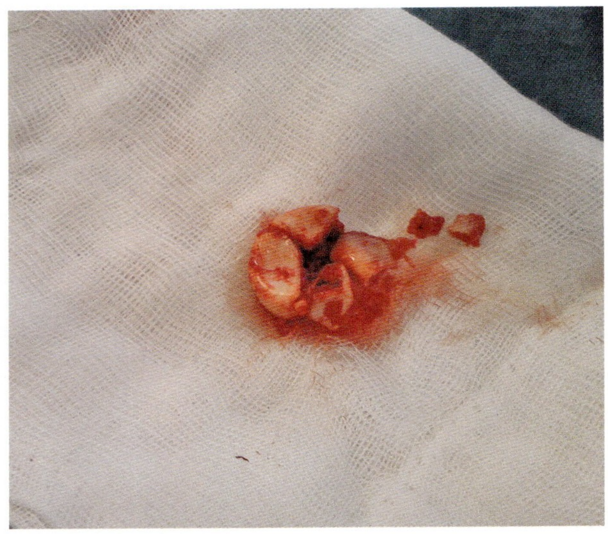

Fig. 10: Excised head of radius.

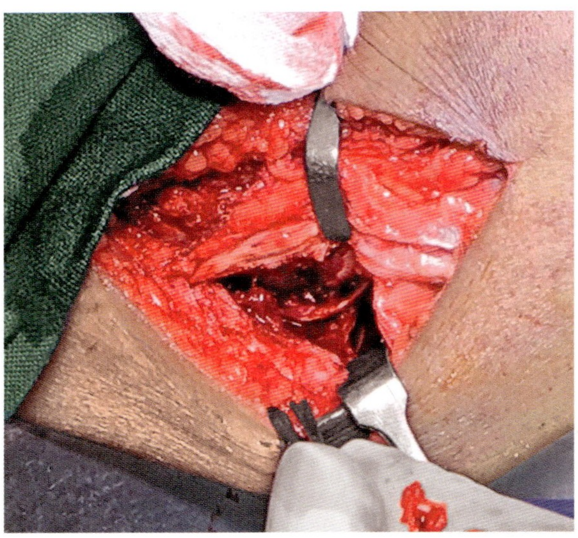

Fig. 11: Demonstration of the medullary canal of the radius with head excised.

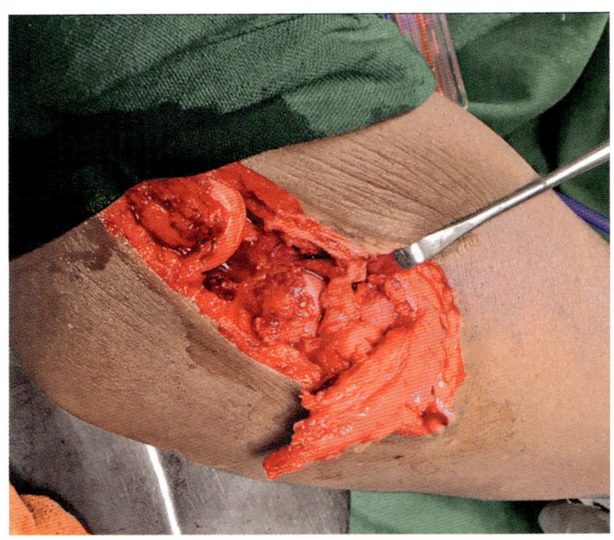

Fig. 12: Canal to be reamed after dissection.

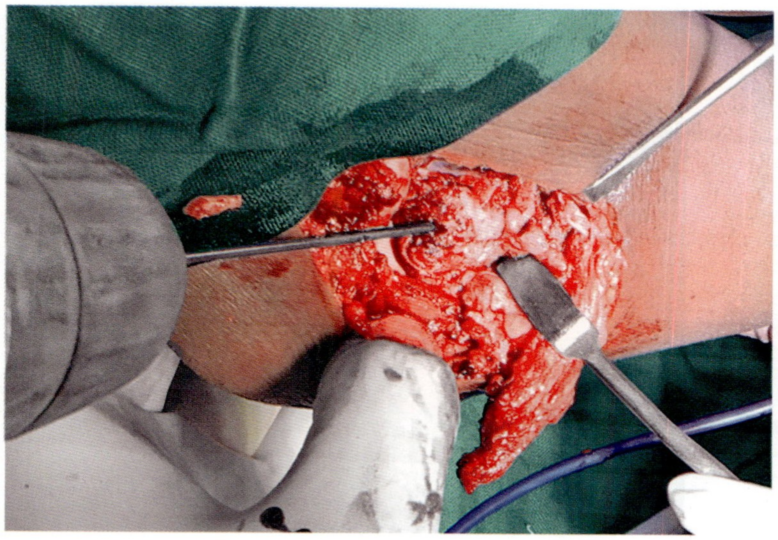

Fig. 13: Canal drilled using K-wire.

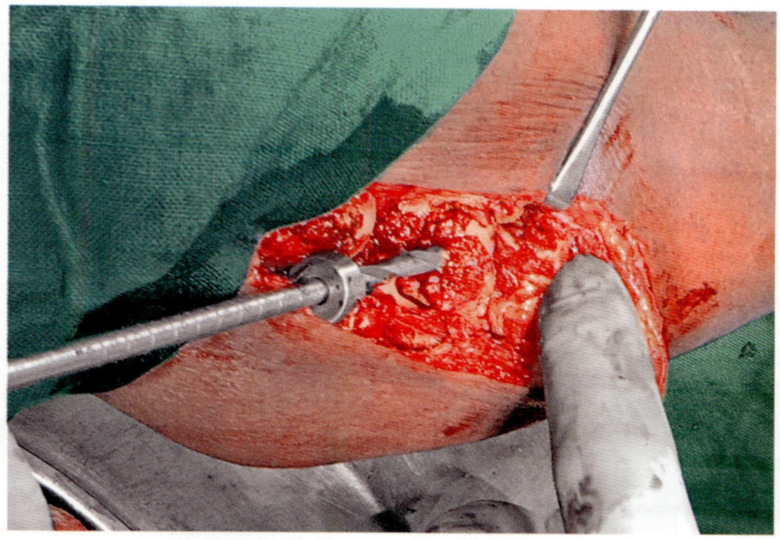

Fig. 14: Reaming of medullary canal done.

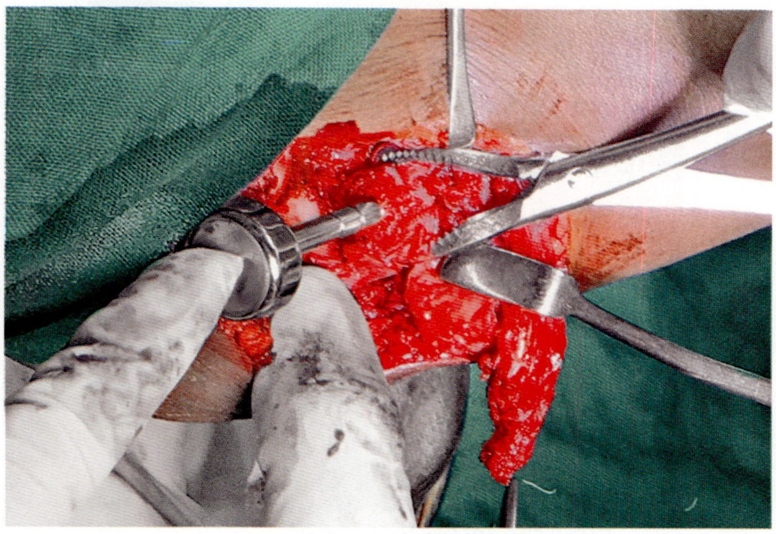

Fig. 15: Radial head prosthesis introduced into the canal.

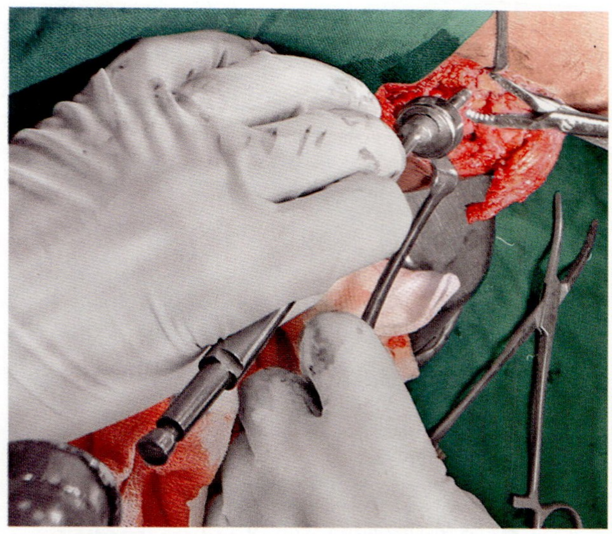

Fig. 16: Radial head prosthesis is hammered and pushed inside further.

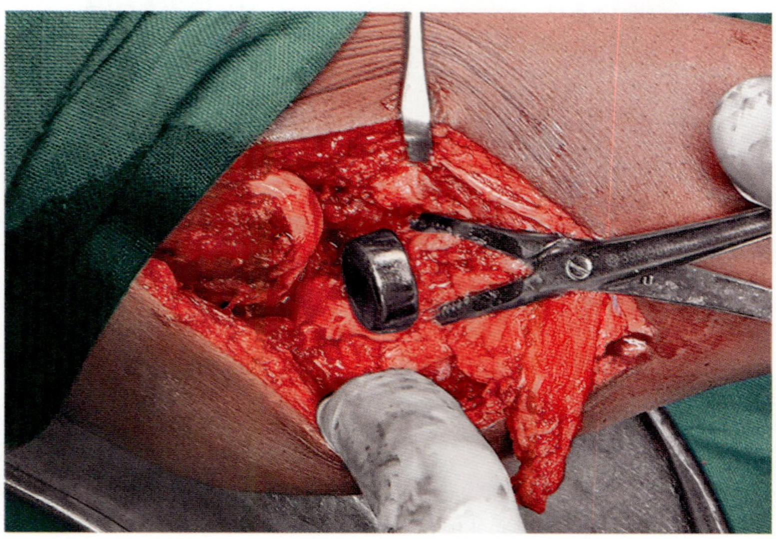

Fig. 17: Radial head prosthesis after complete hammering.

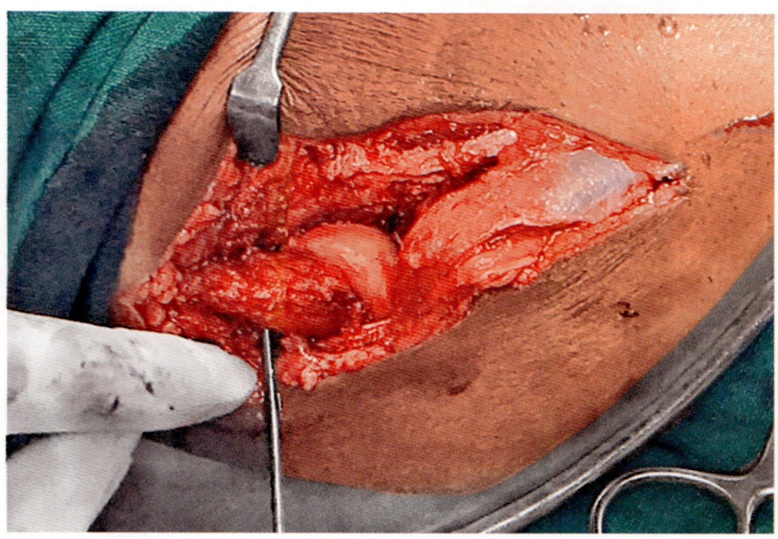

Fig. 18: Using K-wire distal humerus is drilled with forearm in flexion.

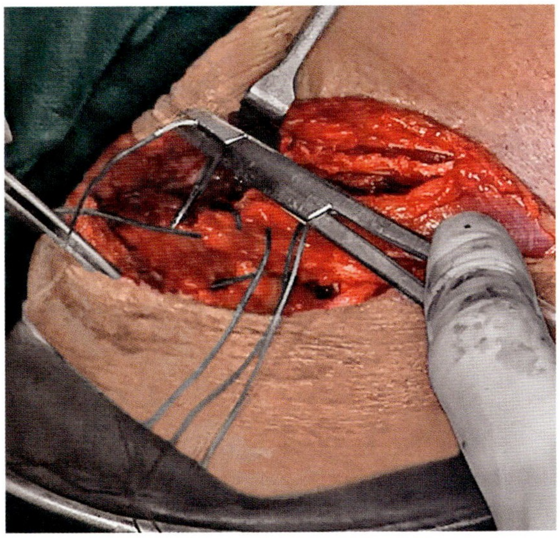

Fig. 19: Suturing common extensor origin to the hole drilled in distal humerus earlier.

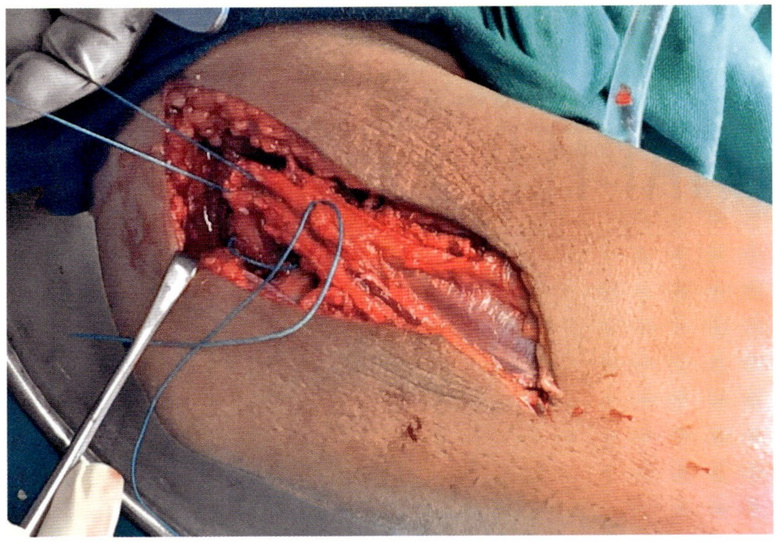

Fig. 20: Suturing of common extensor origin to distal humerus in flexed forearm completed.

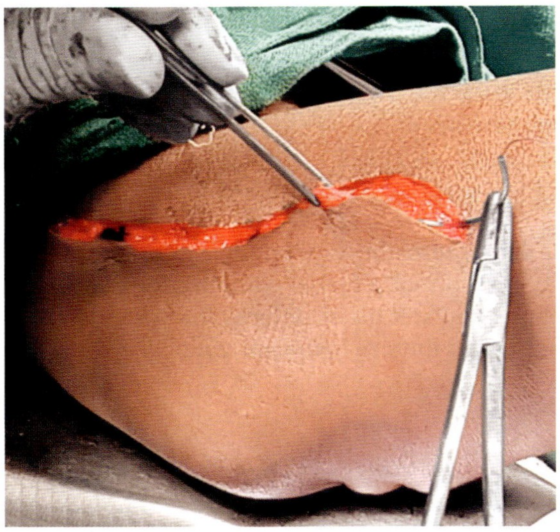

Fig. 21: Subcutaneous suturing done with absorbable suture material.

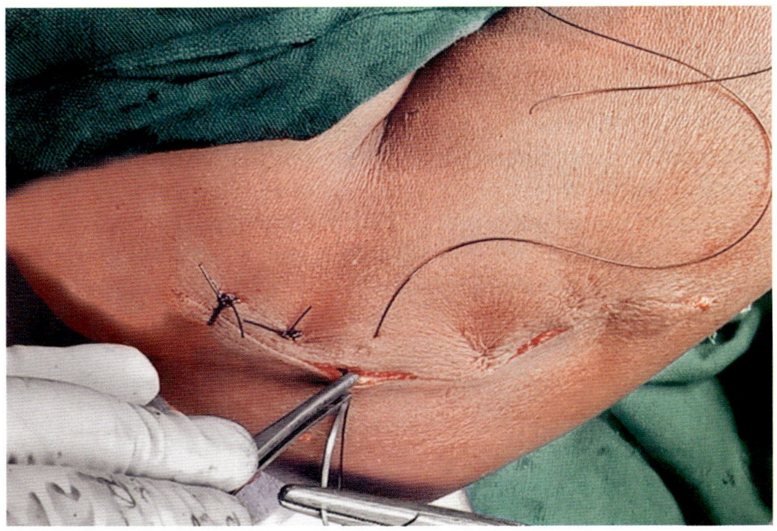

Fig. 22: Skin closure with nonabsorbable suture material.

COMPLICATIONS

Vascular and nerve injury mainly posterior interosseous nerve (PIN).

SUGGESTED READING

1. Amis AA, Dowson D, Unsworth A, et al. An examination of the elbow articulation with particular reference to variation of the carrying angle. Eng Med. 1977;6:76-80.
2. Amis AA, Dowson D, Wright V, et al. The derivation of elbow joint forces, and their relation to prosthesis design. J Med Eng Technol. 1979;3:229-34.
3. Carn RM, Medige J, Curtain D, et al. Silicone rubber replacement of the severely fractured radial head. Clin Orthop Relat Res. 1986;209: 259-69.
4. Cherry JC. Use of acrylic prosthesis in the treatment of fractures of the head of the radius. J Bone Joint Surg Br. 1953;35(1):70-1.
5. Coleman DA, Blair WF, Shurr D. Resection of the radial head for fracture of the radial head: long-term follow-up of seventeen cases. J Bone Joint Surg Am. 1987;69(3):385-92.
6. Goldberg I, Peylan J, Yosipovitch Z. Late results of excision of the radial head for an isolated closed fracture. J Bone Joint Surg Am. 1986;68(5): 675-9.

CHAPTER 57

Megaprosthetic Total Knee Replacement

Manoj Todkar, Vishal Patil, Shrinivas S Shintre

INDICATIONS

Reconstruction of bone defects caused by resection of bone tumors with modular megaprostheses plays a key role in the treatment of bone tumors. Other indications for megaprosthesis replacement surgery are primary malignant tumors, extensive metastatic disease, major trauma or end-stage revision arthroplasty to reconstruct large skeletal defects, or replace bone of low quality. The advances in the medical treatment of sarcoma patients have improved outcomes and limb-preserving surgery has proved to have comparable patient survival rates to amputation. The functional recovery after reconstruction with megaprostheses is often very satisfactory and the patient can enjoy a good quality of life.

RESULTS

The results of megaprostheses are poor as compared to primary total hip or knee arthroplasty. A higher complication rate is because of the extended bone and soft tissue defects, the complex biomechanical reconstruction and the size of the implants.

SURGICAL STEPS (FIGS. 1 TO 25)

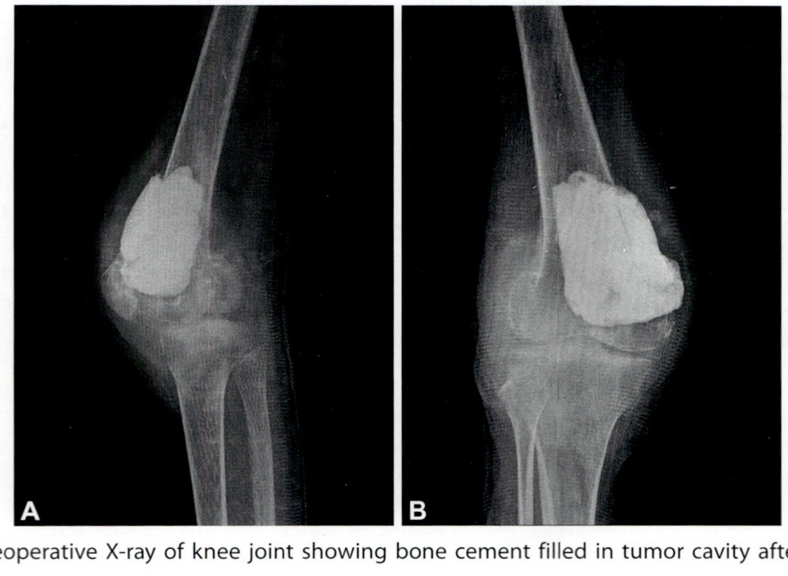

Figs. 1A and B: Preoperative X-ray of knee joint showing bone cement filled in tumor cavity after excision of tumor.

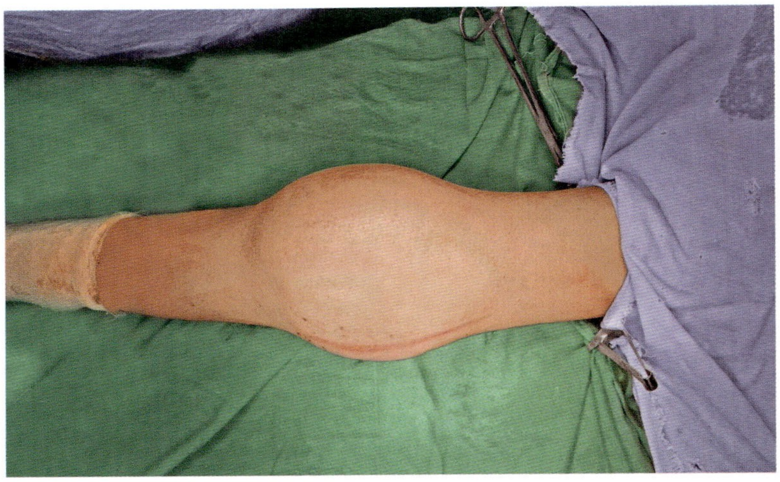

Fig. 2: Photograph showing knee joint with previous healed scar.

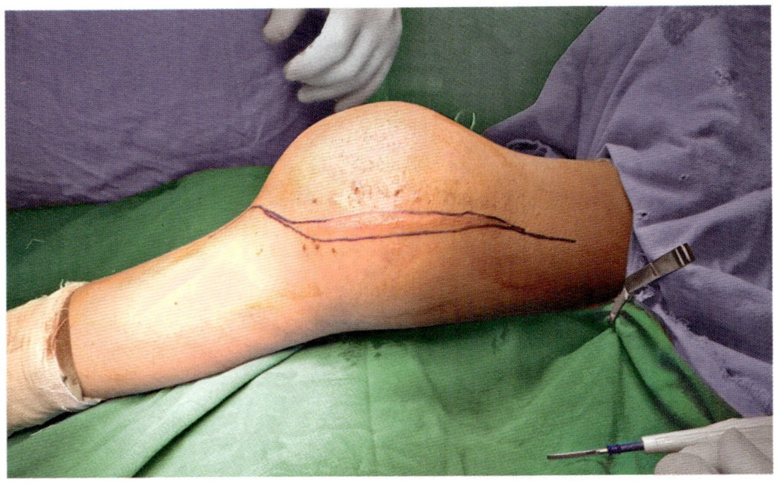

Fig. 3: Skin incision marked over old scar.

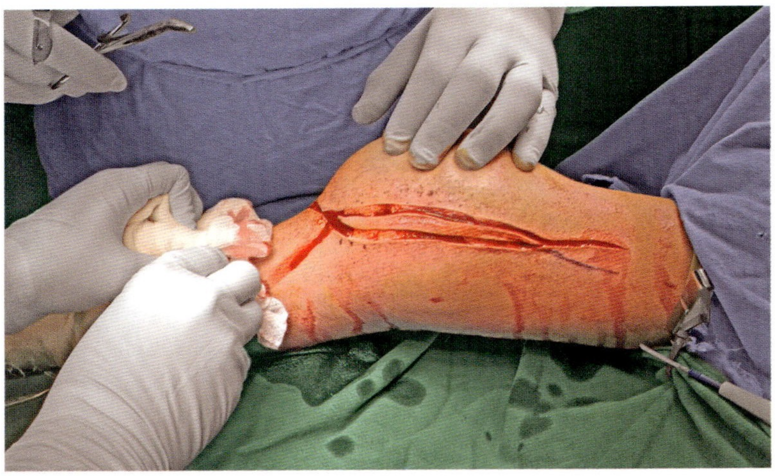

Fig. 4: Old scar excised with incision.

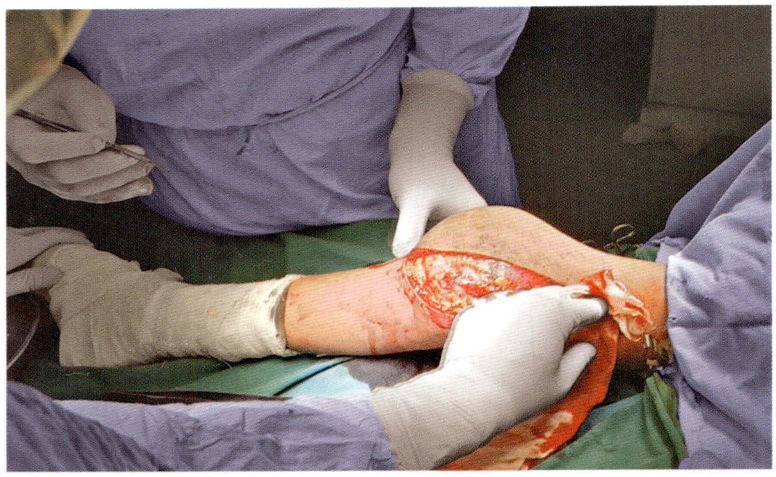

Fig. 5: Subcutaneous dissection.

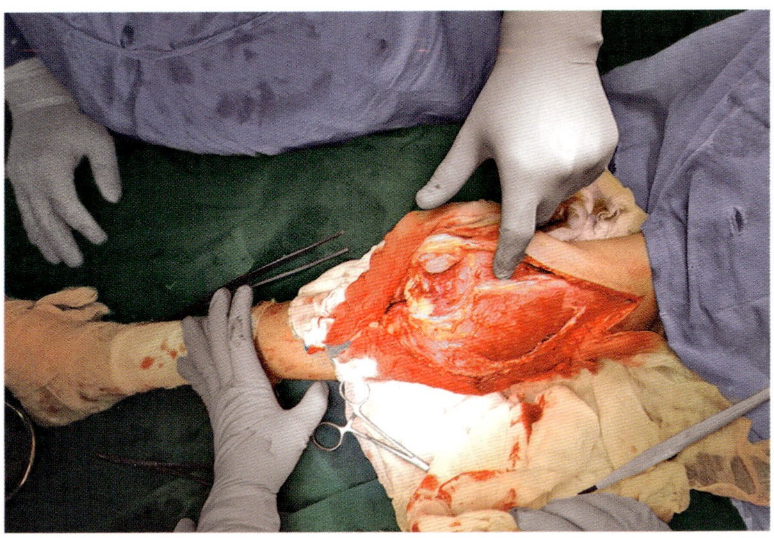

Fig. 6: Medial parapatellar approach to knee joint. Patella retracted laterally.

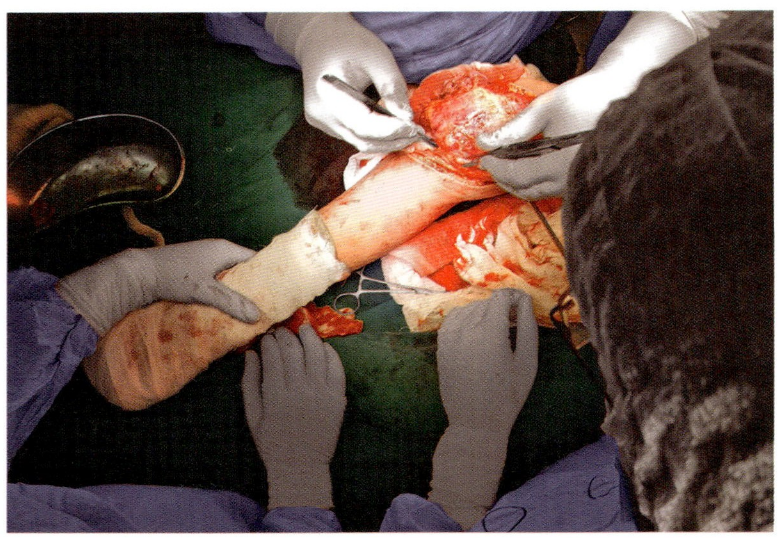

Fig. 7: Knee joint and distal femur exposed.

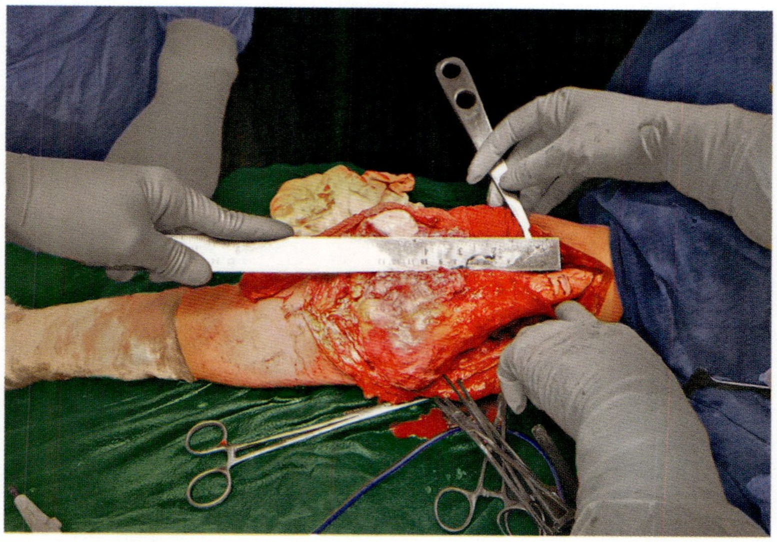

Fig. 8: Length of distal femur to be resected measured.

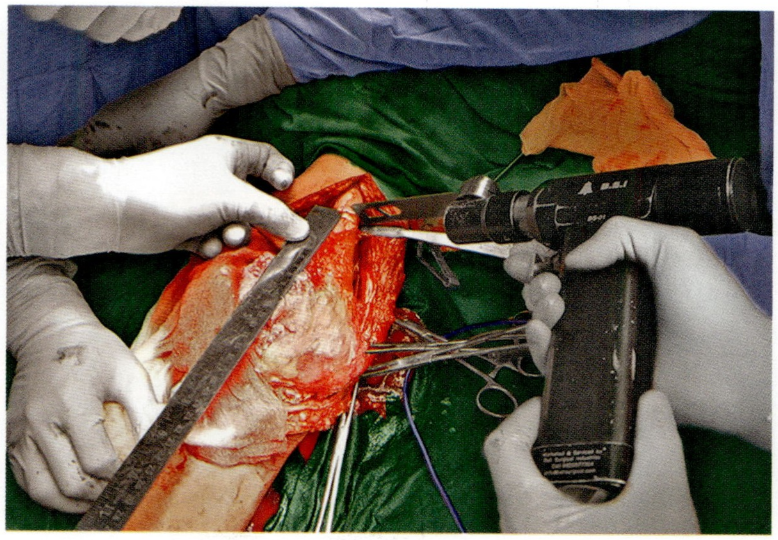

Fig. 9:. Gigli saw used to cut femur.

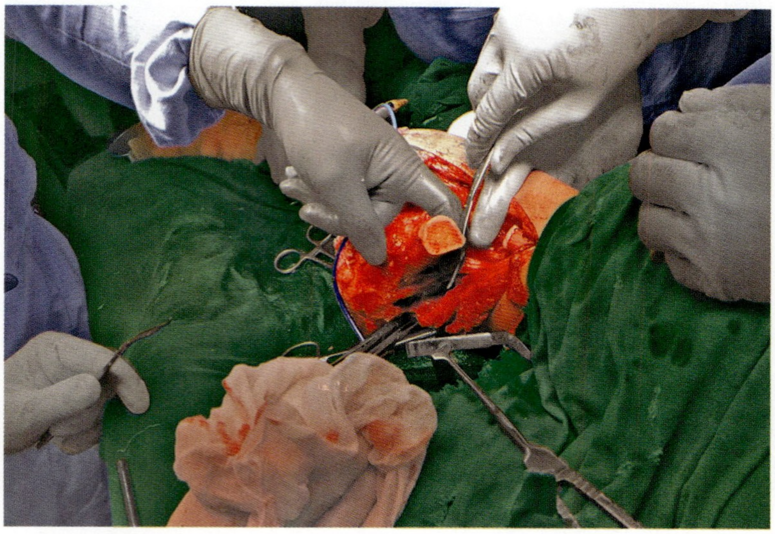

Fig. 10: Distal femur dissected from muscle and ligamentous attachments.

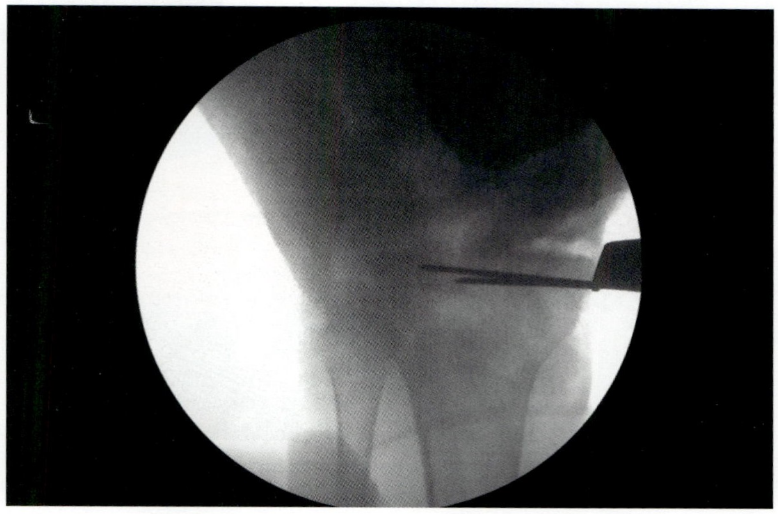

Fig. 11: K-wires inserted in proximal tibia under C-arm control to decide resection level.

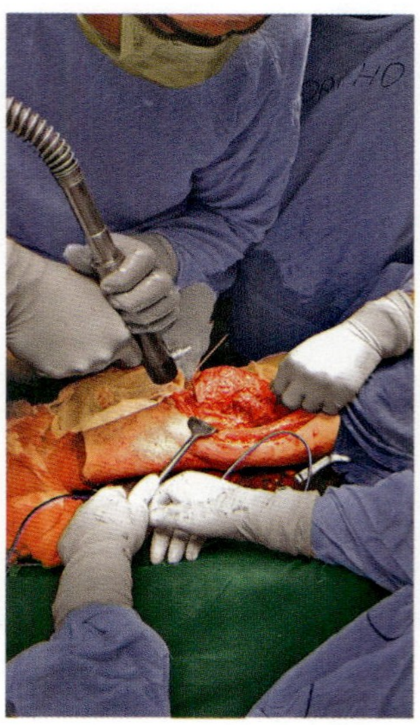

Fig. 12: Saw used to take tibial cut at desired level.

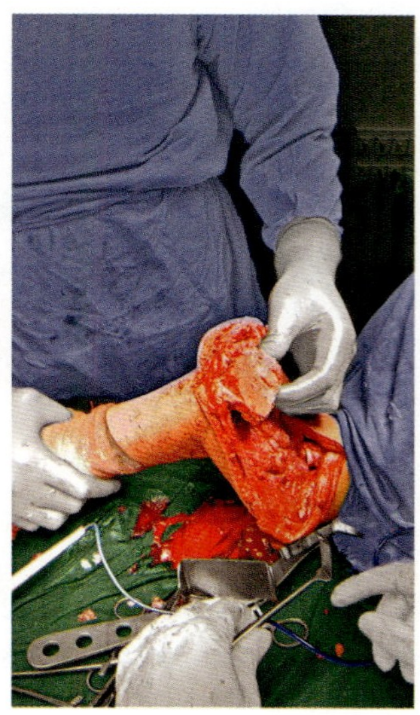

Fig. 13: Resected proximal tibia and distal femur removed.

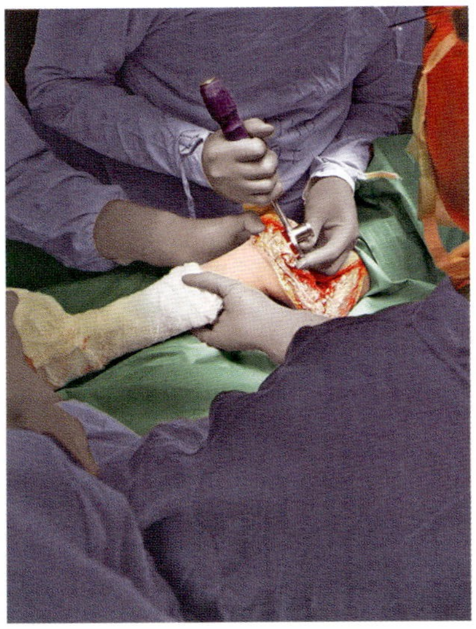

Fig. 14: Tibia prepared using jig. Intramedullary reaming and broaching done.

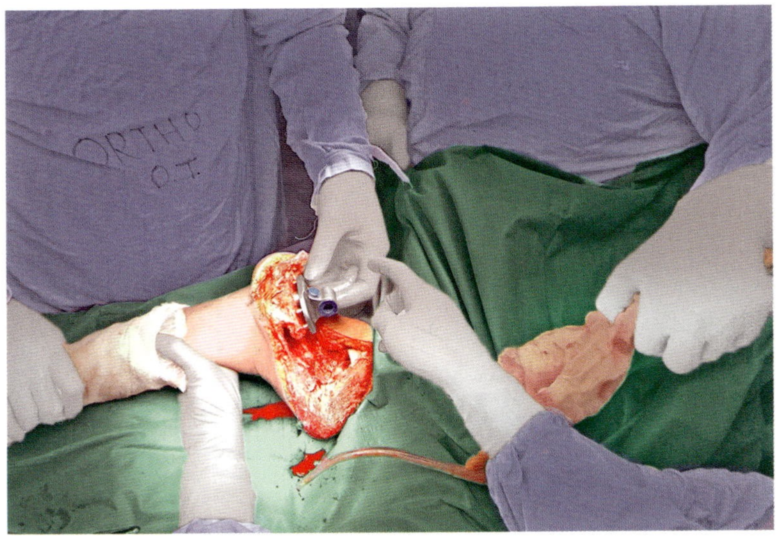

Fig. 15: Trial tibial component inserted in prepared tibia.

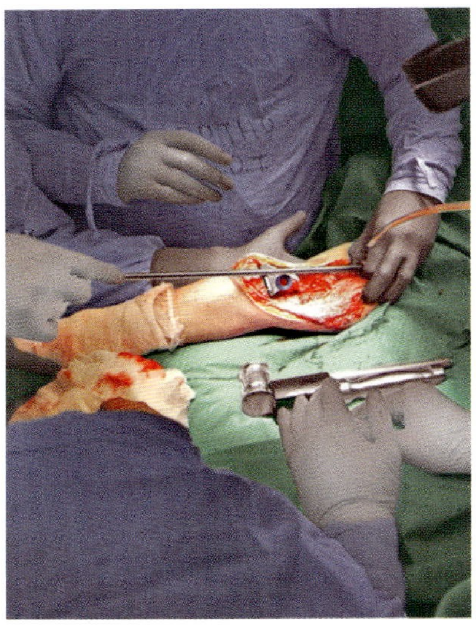

Fig. 16: Femoral canal prepared with intramedullary reamers.

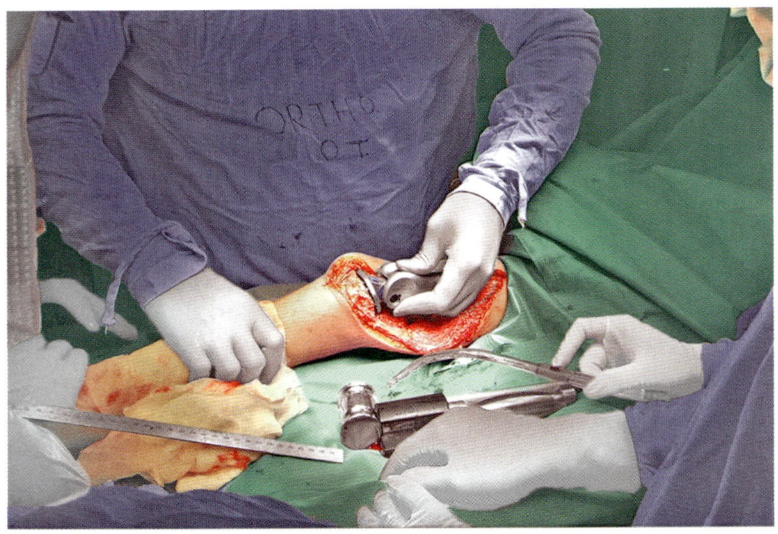

Fig. 17: Trial femoral component inserted in femur.

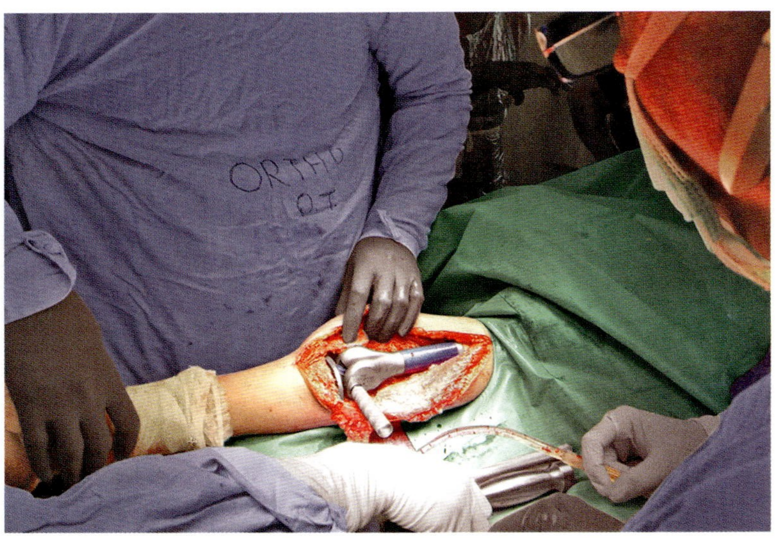

Fig. 18: Hinge assembled and trial of prosthetic joint taken.

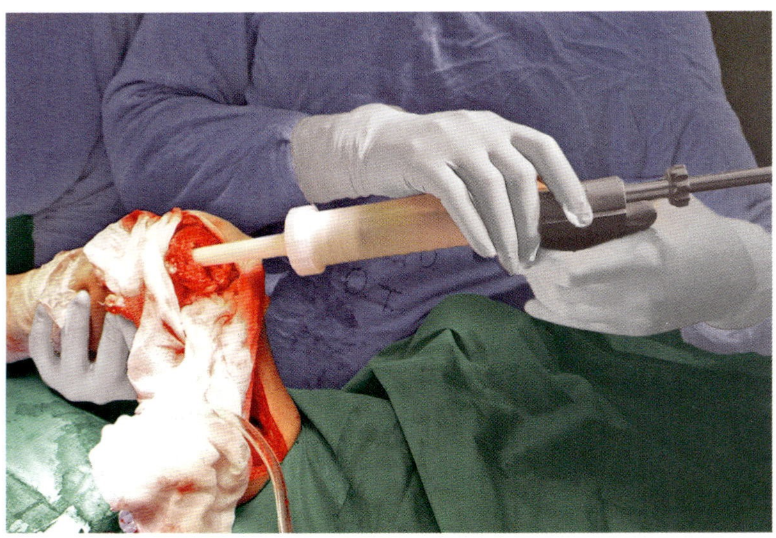

Fig. 19: After preparation of canal, bone cement introduced in tibial canal using cement gun.

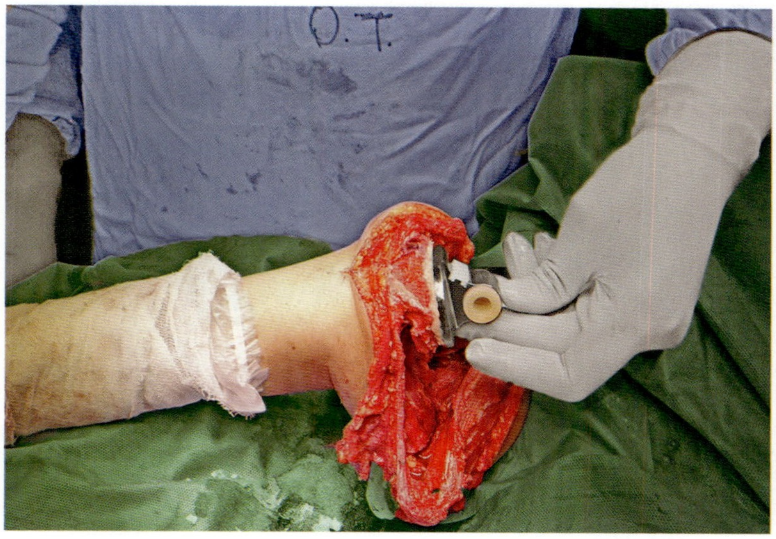

Fig. 20: Tibial component inserted in tibia and pressurized.

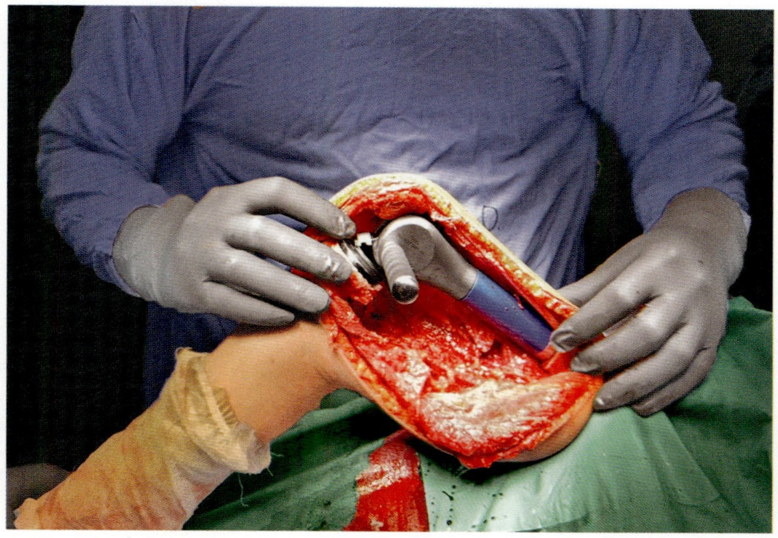

Fig. 21: Trial femoral component inserted in femur and trial of range of motion checked.

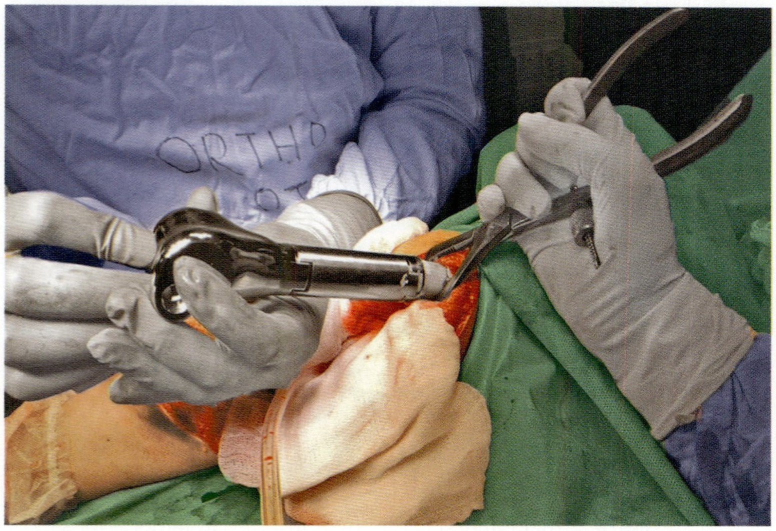

Fig. 22: Femoral canal prepared and femoral component cemented in.

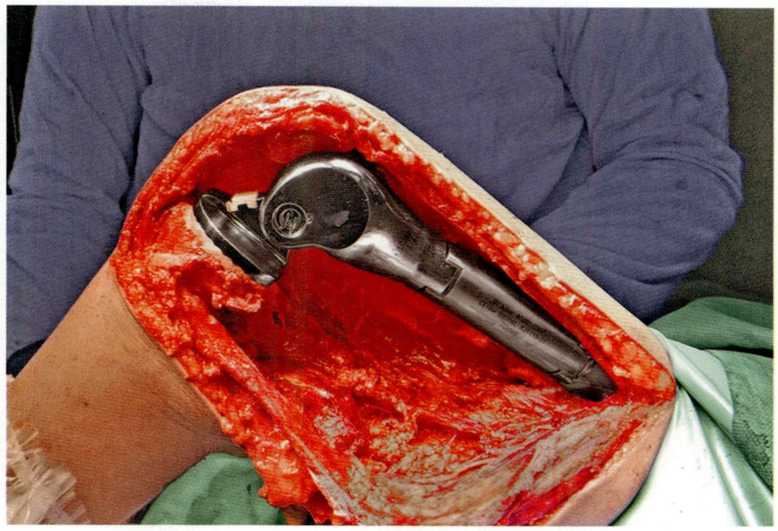

Fig. 23: Hinge of megaprosthesis assembled and range of motion checked.

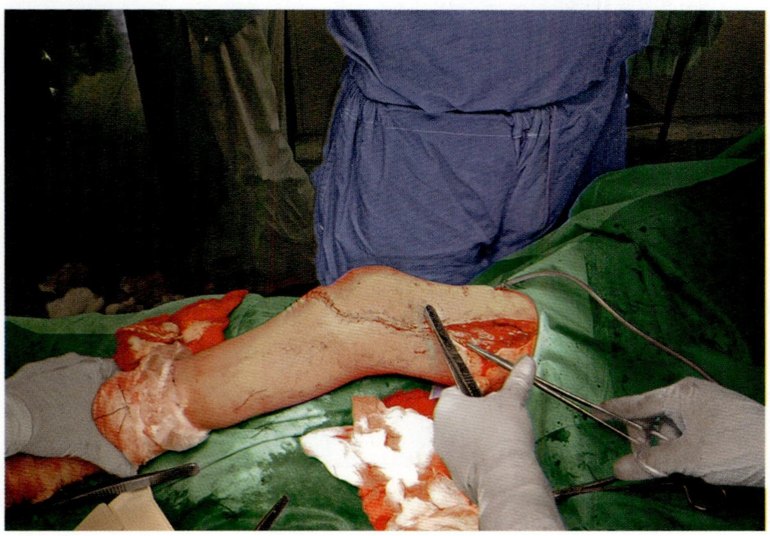

Fig. 24: Closure of wound done in layers over drain.

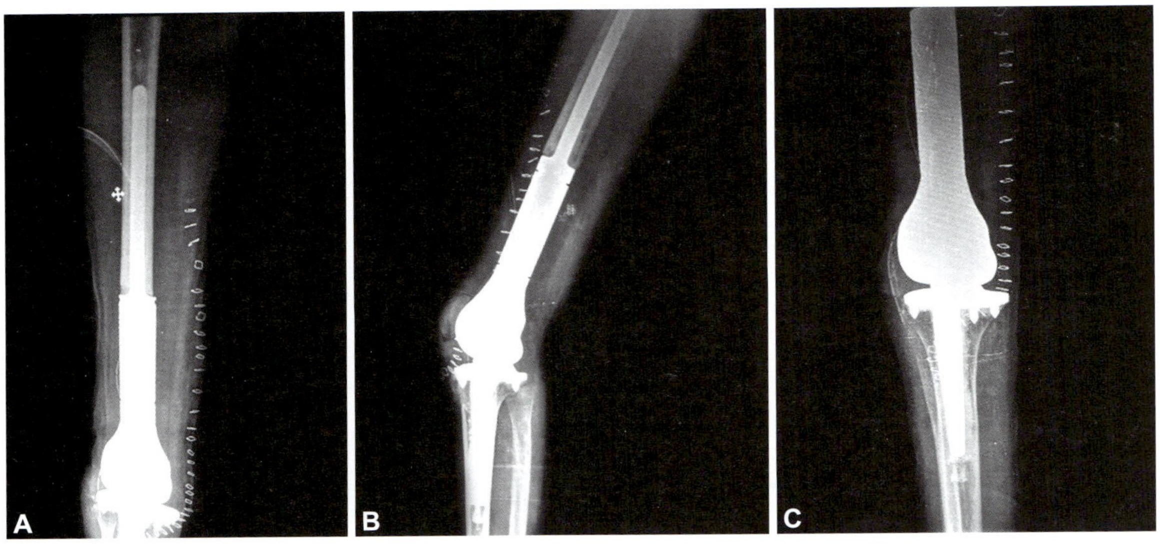

Figs. 25A to C: Postoperative X-ray showing megaprosthesis.

COMPLICATIONS

Megaprostheses have high complication rates for wound dehiscence, deep infection, mechanical failure and loosening, local recurrence of tumor and they are extremely difficult to revise. The complication rates reported in the literature range from 25% to 92%. Aseptic loosening as a complication is reported to range from 0% to 31%.

SUGGESTED READING

1. Blunn GW, Briggs TW, Cannon SR, et al. Cementless fixation for primary segmental bone tumor endoprostheses. Clin Orthop Relat Res. 2000;372:223-30.
2. Bradish CF, Kemp HB, Scales JT, et al. Distal femoral replacement by custom-made prostheses: clinical follow-up and survivorship analysis. J Bone Joint Surg Br. 1987;69:276-84.
3. Capanna R. Modular Kotz prosthesis: the Rizzoli experience. In: Yamamuro T (Ed). New Developments for Limb Salvage in Musculoskeletal Tumors. Tokyo: Springer; 1989. pp. 37-44.
4. Capanna R, Morris HG, Campanacci D, et al. Modular uncemented prosthetic reconstruction after resection of tumours of the distal femur. J Bone Joint Surg Br. 1994;76:178-86.
5. Choong PF, Sim FH, Pritchard DJ, et al. Megaprostheses after resection of distal femoral tumors: A rotating hinge design in 30 patients followed for 2–7 years. Acta Orthop Scand. 1996;67:345-51.
6. Enneking WF, Dunham W, Gebhardt MC, et al. A system for the functional evaluation of reconstructive procedures after surgical treatment of tumors of the musculoskeletal system. Clin Orthop Relat Res. 1993;286: 241-6.
7. Gerrand CH, Currie D, Grigoris P, et al. Prosthetic reconstruction of the femur for primary bone sarcoma. Int Orthop. 1999;23:286-90.
8. Griffin AM, Parsons JA, Davis AM, et al. Uncemented tumor endoprostheses at the knee: root causes of failure. Clin Orthop Relat Res. 2005;438:71-9.
9. Heisel C, Breusch SJ, Schmid G, et al. Lower limb salvage surgery with MUTARS endoprostheses: 2 to 7 year results. Acta Orthop Belg. 2004;70:142-7.

CHAPTER 58

Modified Direct Lateral Approach to Hip

YJ Mahale

INTRODUCTION

The various approaches to the hip are:

1. Anterior—Smith-Petersen
2. Anterolateral—Watson-Jones
3. Lateral—McFarland and Osborne, Hardinge
4. Posterolateral—Gibson
5. Posterior—Osborne, Moore
6. Medial—Ludloff, Ferguson.

The direct lateral approaches are:

1. McFarland and Osborne—1954.

Hardinge (1982) was the first to modify this approach.

Other modifications:

1. McLauchlan (1984)
2. Dall (1986)
3. Learmonth (1996)
4. Mulliken (1998)
5. Pai (2002)
6. Present modification is since 1991.

McFarland and Osborne who first described the direct lateral approach to the hip aimed at preserving the gluteus medius muscle. Their observation was that the vastus lateralis and gluteus medius work together through the thick periosteum of the greater trochanter. Mcfarland and Osborne's (1954) direct lateral approach has gone through several changes and modifications. All the approaches have good results. The approach described here may seem strenuous but with time it becomes easier.

INDICATIONS

Following operative procedures can be done through this approach

- Excision arthroplasty
- Excision arthroplasty and Pelvic supportive osteotomy
- Joint clearance for Tuberculosis
- Arthrodesis
- Austin Moore prosthesis insertion
- Bipolar prosthesis insertion
- Total hip replacement.

SURGICAL STEPS TO DEMONSTRATE MODIFIED DIRECT LATERAL APPROACH TO HIP IN HEMIARTHROPLASTY OPERATION USING AUSTIN MOORE PROSTHESIS FOR FRACTURE NECK OF FEMUR

1. Patient is given a true lateral position in such a way that the limb to be operated is at the top.
2. Of the total length of the incision, approximately one-third should be above and two-thirds should be below the greater trochanter in line with femoral shaft.
3. A lateral longitudinal incision is taken. Fat and the underlying deep fascia is cut in line with skin incision. Retract the cut edges of the fascia.
4. Tensor fasciae lata along with part of gluteus maximus is pulled anteriorly and remaining gluteus maximus posteriorly.
5. The cut edges of the fascia are retracted and tensor fasciae latae along with part of gluteus maximus is pulled anteriorly and remaining gluteus maximus posteriorly.
6. Gluteus medius, greater trochanter and vastus lateralis are identified and seen. The bursa on the greater trochanter is excised.
7. Divide gluteus medius muscle in the direction of their fibers at the region of posterior two-thirds and anterior one-third of the superior border of the greater trochanter.
8. The superior gluteal neurovascular bundle is protected by keeping the upper limit of the split to less than 4–5 cm above the upper border of the greater trochanter.
9. Stay suture in the gluteus medius, 4–5 cm above the greater trochanter is taken to prevent accidental upward prolongation of the split.
10. The periosteum of the greater trochanter is dissected in line with skin incision. The periosteum is dissected and elevated anteriorly and posteriorly with further reflection of the anterior part along with the anterior wall. Reflected posterior part will allow suture of anterior flap to periosteum during closure.
11. The fibers of the vastus lateralis muscle overlying on the lateral aspect of the proximal part of femur are split.
12. After splitting the gluteus medius, retract the underlying fat to expose the gluteus minimus muscle. Now divide the gluteus

minimus in the line with the fibers along with the underlying capsule up to the bone.

13. Develop an anterior flap that consists of gluteus medius anterior part along with underlying gluteus minimus muscle and capsule proximally, thick periosteum of the greater trochanter and anterior capsule in the middle and vastus lateralis muscle anterior part distally, i.e. gluteus medius—Vastus lateralis flap (G-V flap).
14. The anterior flap is further enlarged following the greater trochanter anterior part and the neck while externally rotating the hip. Then the fracture neck of femur is made visible or the hip dislocated by further externally rotating the hip in adduction and flexion.
15. Neck of femur is cut to increase the exposure to extract the head and to fit the prosthesis later.
16. Femoral head is extracted with the cork screw. Complete the exposure of the acetabulum by inserting appropriate retractors around the acetabulum.
17. Placement of the prosthesis after reaming of the proximal femur.
18. The wound is thoroughly irrigated and closed in a layered manner with drain in situ.
19. Gluteus minimus along with underlying capsule is closed at the split and to the greater trochanter where it is inserted with 1-0 absorbable suture.
20. Suturing of the middle of the anterior flap to the greater trochanter consisting of thick periosteum of the greater trochanter with the underlying anterior capsule with three transosseous sutures using 5-0 strong nonabsorbable suture is done.
21. Closure of gluteus medius split, middle anterior flap consisting of anterior capsule with overlying thick periosteum of the greater trochanter and vastus lateralis with 1–0 absorbable sutures is done.
22. The fascia lata incision is closed along with the fascia covering the gluteus maximus with 1-0 absorbable sutures.
23. Subcutaneous layer is closed with 2-0 absorbable sutures.
24. Skin is closed as desired with 2-0 nylon sutures.

SURGICAL STEPS (FIGS. 1 TO 16)

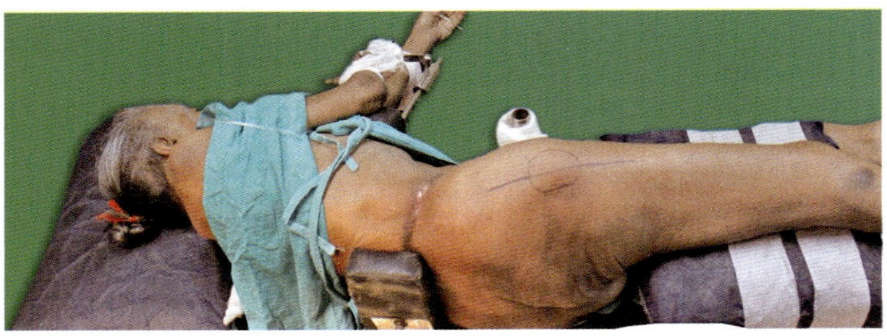

Fig. 1: Patient in lateral position.

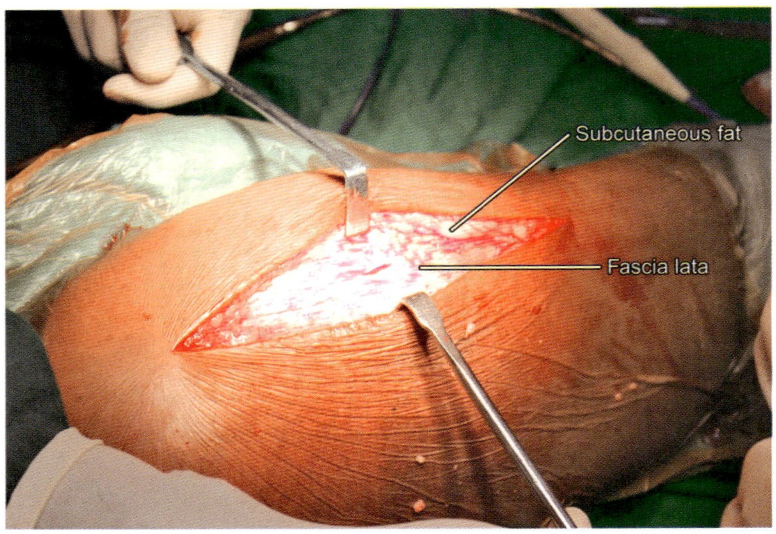

Fig. 2: Skin incised longitudinally over greater trochanter.

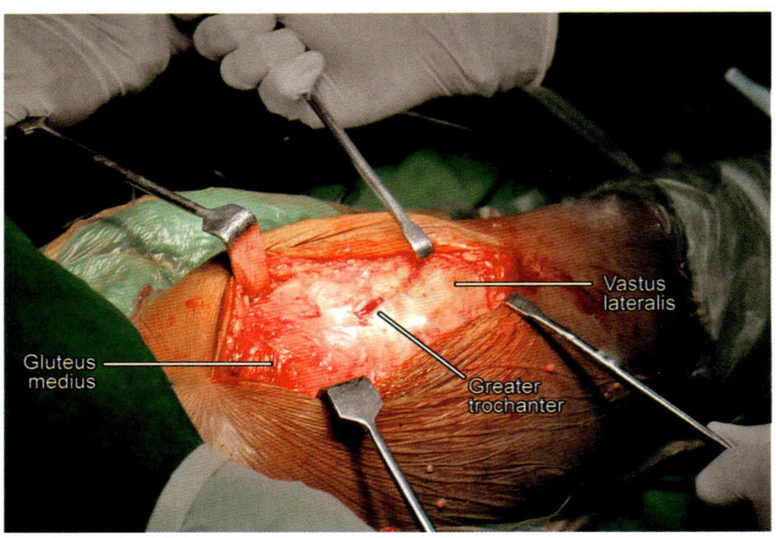

Fig. 3: Fascia lata incised.

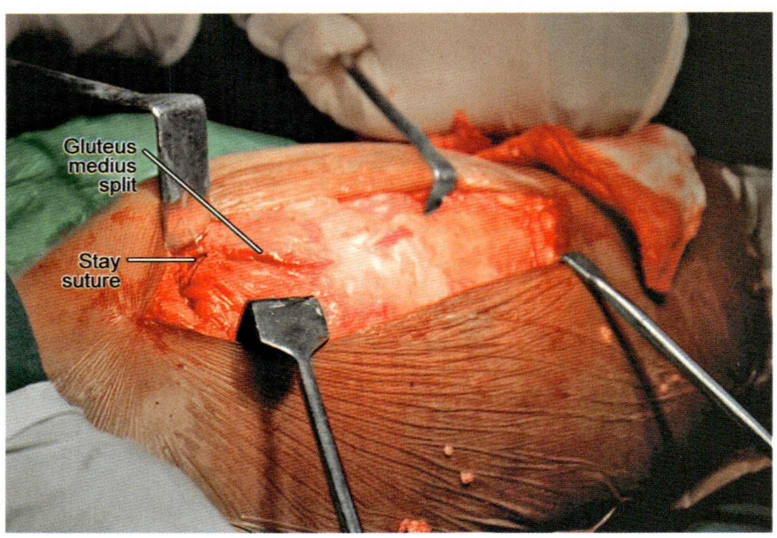

Fig. 4: Gluteus medius split in direction of muscle fibers.

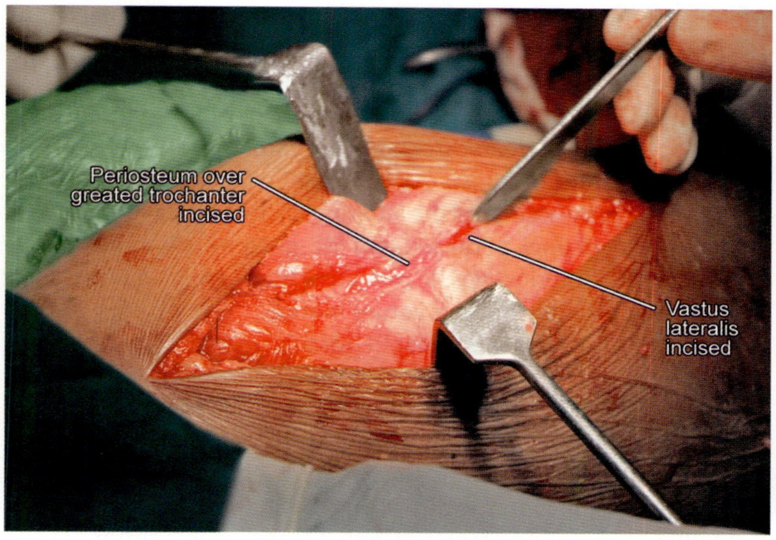

Fig. 5: Periosteum over greater trochanter incised.

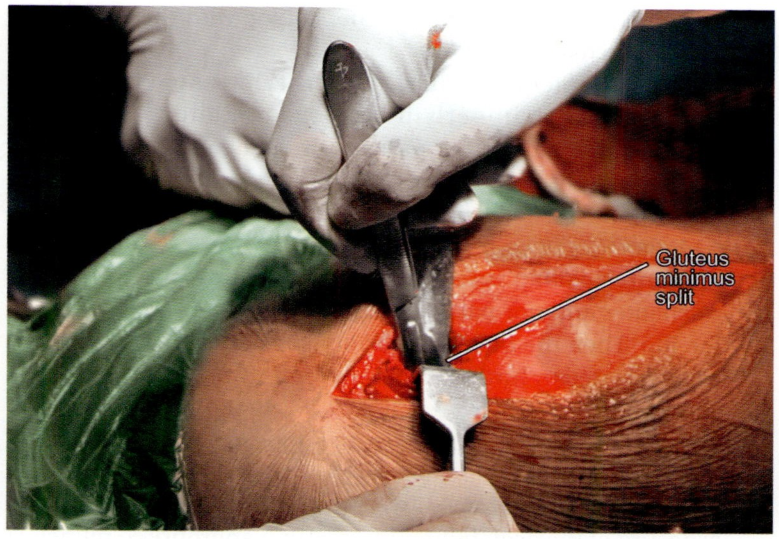

Fig. 6: Gluteus minimus split.

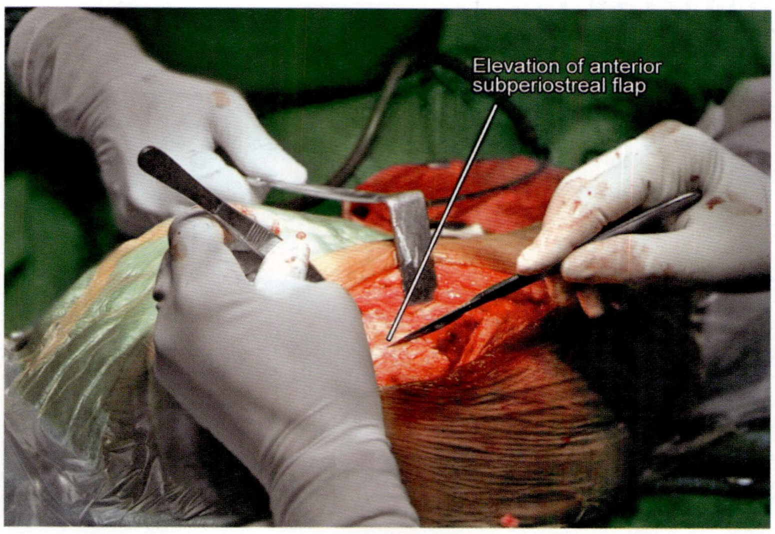

Fig. 7: Anterior subperiosteal flap elevated.

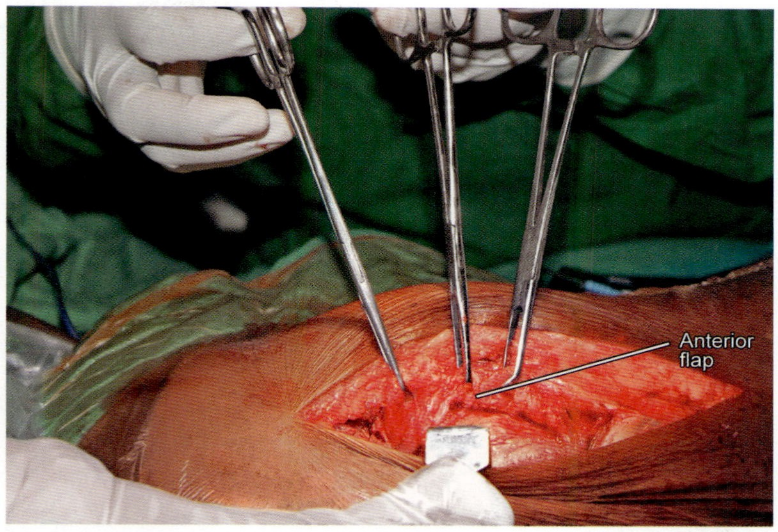

Fig. 8: Anterior flap created.

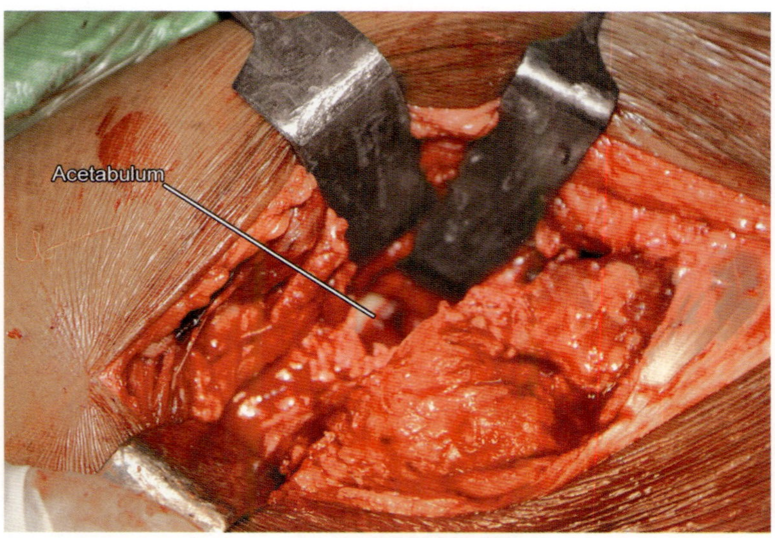

Fig. 9: Head extracted and acetabulum exposed.

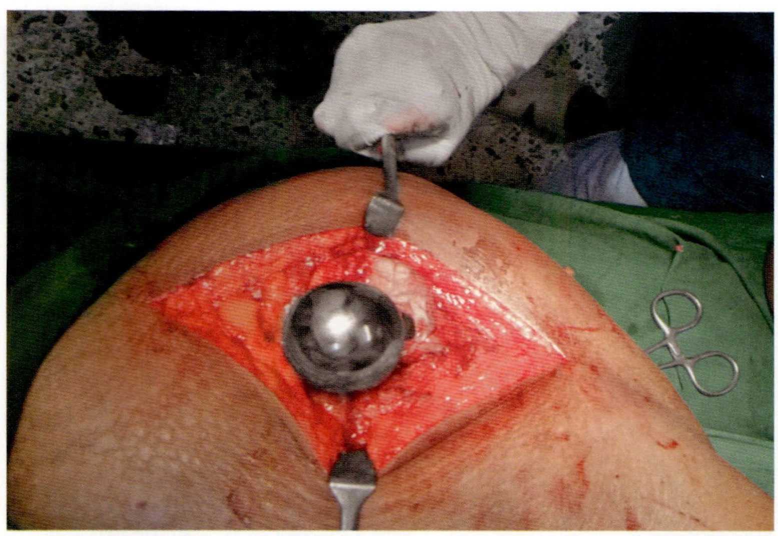

Fig. 10: Hemiarthroplasty done.

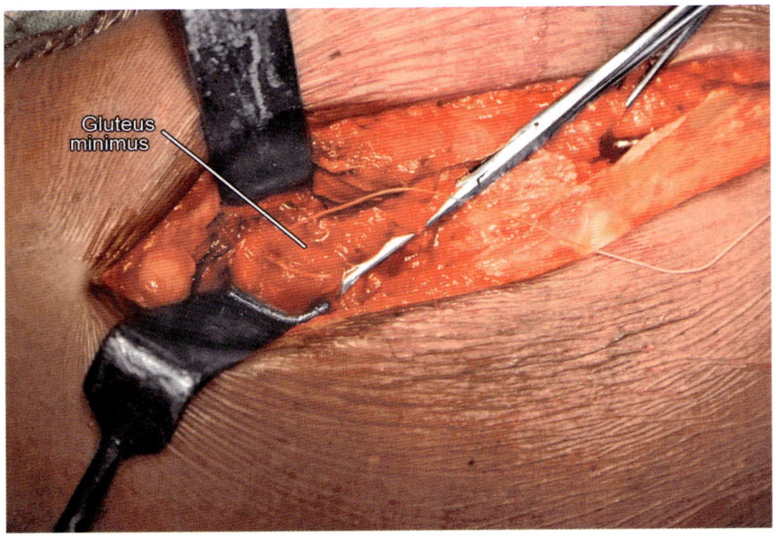

Fig. 11: Gluteus minimus muscle repaired.

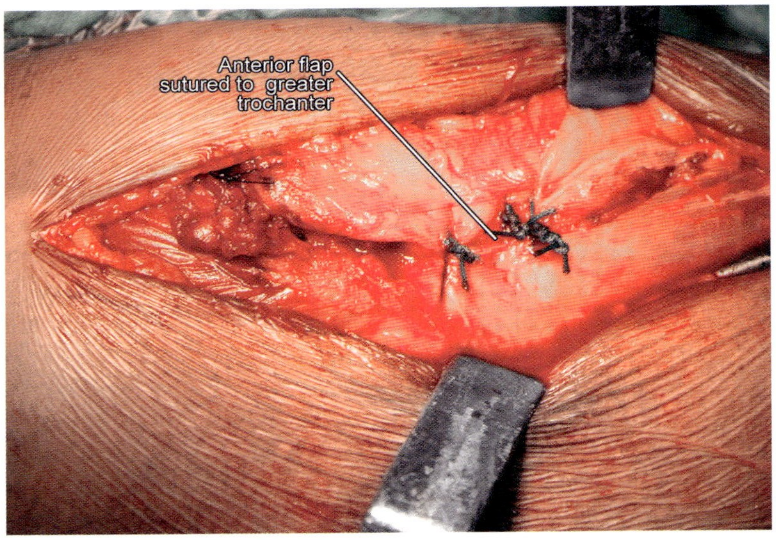

Fig. 12: Anterior flap reposed.

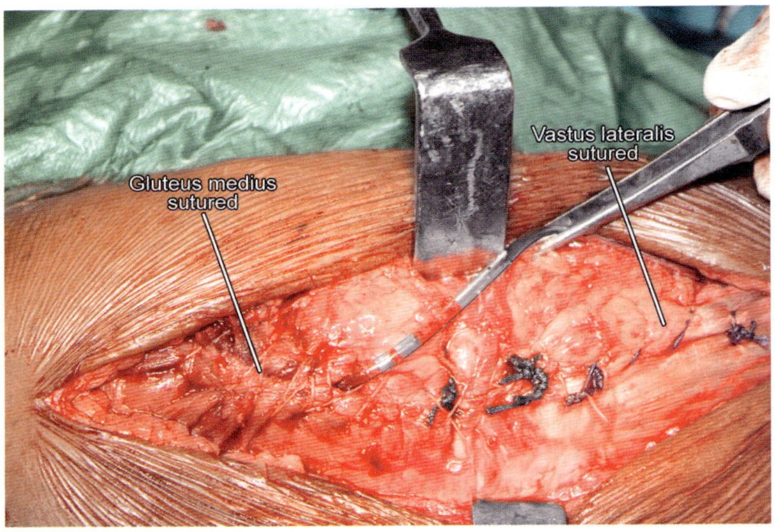

Fig. 13: Gluteus medius and vastus lateralis repaired.

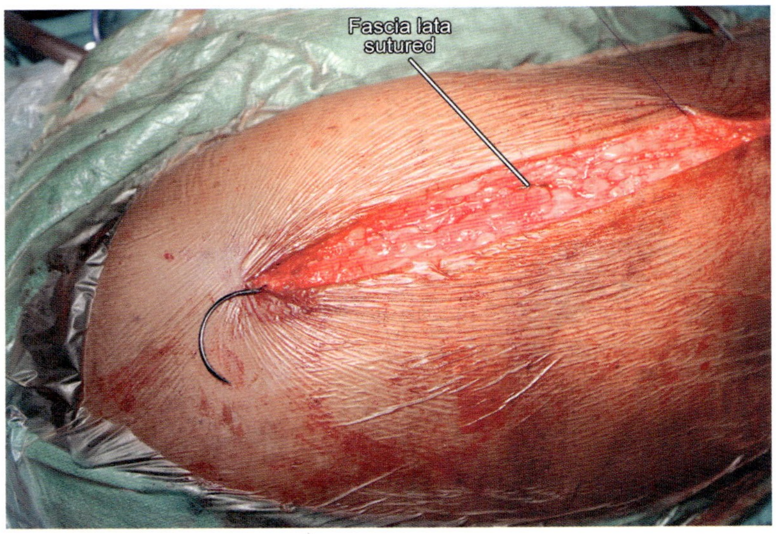

Fig. 14: Fascia lata sutured.

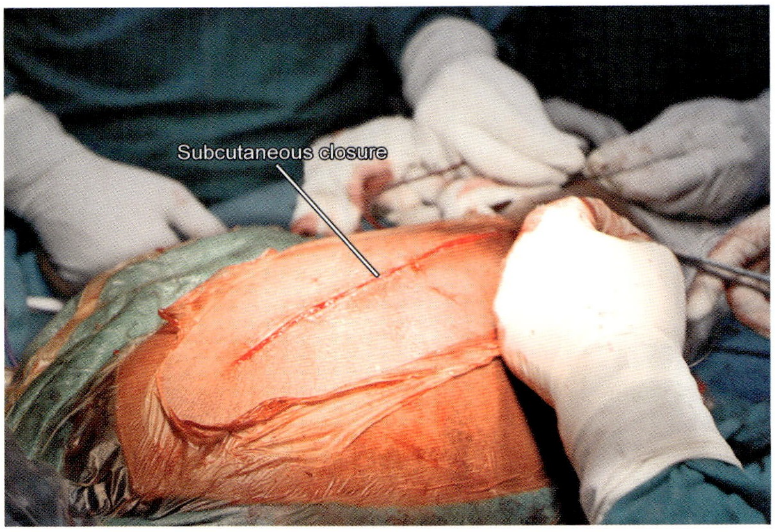

Fig. 15: Subcutaneous closure.

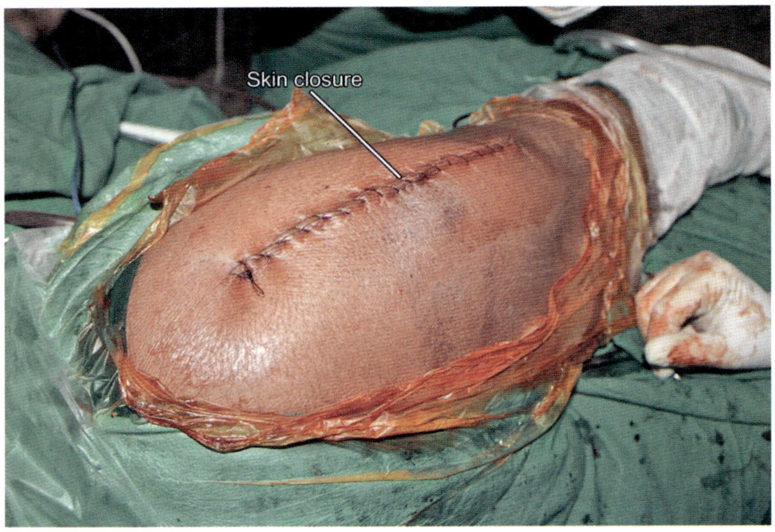

Fig. 16: Skin closure.

FOLLOWING COMPLICATIONS CAN OCCUR

- The superior gluteal neurovascular bundle injury—due to accidental upward prolongation of the split more than 4–5 cm above the upper border of the greater trochanter.
- Trendelenburg gait—due to G-V flap avulsion.

ADVANTAGES

- Lateral position so that the gluteal fat gets retracted posteriorly and anteriorly due to gravity.
- Gluteus medius—major bulk preserved as it is divided in the region of posterior two-thirds and anterior one-third.
- No trochanteric osteotomy.
- Away from perineal region which decreases chances of infection.
- G–V flap and capsule sutured to greater trochanter by transosseous sutures.
- No major neurovascular structure encountered because of stay suture.
- Can be converted to anterior or posterior approach intraoperatively if needed.
- Blood loss is minimum.
- Posterior capsule intact and anterior capsule sutured to minimize the chances of dislocation.
- Abductor strength retained.

DISADVANTAGES

- Initially the approach is difficult but with experience it gets easier.
- Extension of approach distally is easy but proximally is difficult.
- Wide exposure not possible.

SUGGESTED READING

1. Asayama I, Chamnongkich S, Simpson KJ, et al. Reconstructed hip joint position and abductor muscle strength after THA. J Arthroplasty. 2005;20:414-20.
2. Barber TC, Roger DJ, Goodman SB, et al. Early outcome of THA using the direct lateral approach versus the posterior surgical approach. Orthopedics. 1996;19:873-5.
3. Damm P, Zonneveld J, Brackertz S, et al. Gluteal muscle damage leads to higher in vivo hip joint loads 3 months after total hip arthroplasty. PLoS One. 2018;13(1):e0190626.
4. Delanois RE, Sultan AA, Albayar AA, et al. The Röttinger approach for total hip arthroplasty: technique, comparison to the direct lateral approach and review of literature. Ann Transl Med. 2017;5(Suppl 3):S31.
5. Demos HA, Rorabeck CH, Bourne RB, et al. Instability in primary total hip arthroplasty with the direct lateral approach. Clin Orthop Relat Res. 2001;393:168-80.
6. Downing ND, Clark DI, Hutchinson JW, et al. Hip abductor strength following THA: a prospective comparison of the posterior and lateral approach in 100 patients. Acta Orthop Scand. 2001;72:215-20.
7. Hardinge K. The direct lateral approach to the hip. J Bone Joint Surg Br. 1982;64:17-9.
8. Jameson SS, Mason J, Baker P, et al. A comparison of surgical approaches for primary hip arthroplasty: a cohort study of patient reported outcome measures (PROMs) and early revision using linked national databases. J Arthroplasty. 2014;29:1248-55.
9. Masonis JL, Bourne RB. Surgical approach, abductor function and THA dislocation. Clin Orthop Relat Res. 2002;405:46-53.
10. Moskal JT, Mann JW 3rd. A modified direct lateral approach for primary and revision THA: a prospective analysis of 453 cases. J Arthroplasty. 1996;11:255-66.
11. Mulliken BD, Rorabeck CH, Bourne RB, et al. A modified direct lateral approach in total hip arthroplasty: a comprehensive review. J Arthroplasty. 1998;13:737-47.
12. Peters RM, van Beers LW, van Steenbergen LN, et al. Similar superior patient-reported outcome measures for anterior and posterolateral approaches after total hip arthroplasty: postoperative patient-reported outcome measure improvement after 3 months in 12,774 primary total hip arthroplasties using the anterior, anterolateral, straight lateral, or posterolateral approach. J Arthroplasty. 2018;33(6):1786-93.
13. Ugland TO, Haugeberg G, Svenningsen S, et al. Less periprosthetic bone loss following the anterolateral approach to the hip compared with the direct lateral approach. A subgroup analysis from a randomized trial in patients with a femoral neck fracture. Acta Orthop. 2018;89(1):23-8.
14. Yue C, MD, Kang P, Pei F, et al. Comparison of direct anterior and lateral approaches in THA. A systematic review and meta-analysis (PRISMA). Medicine (Baltimore). 2015;94(50):e2126.

SECTION 6

ANKLE AND FOOT

Section Editors: *Amit Swamy, Amit R Kale*

CHAPTER 59

Medial Malleolar Fracture Fixation

Shrinivas S Shintre, Prateek Charuchandra Joshi

TENSION BAND WIRING

INTRODUCTION

Medial malleolus fractures are a very common outcome of blunt trauma to the ankle. Isolated medial malleolus fractures are not as common as fracture of medial and lateral malleoli, termed as bimalleolar fracture (Pott's fracture).

Medial malleolus fractures may result from low-energy trauma such as a fall from standing height associated with a twisting injury or with high-energy trauma such as road traffic accidents.

INDICATIONS

K-wire fixation/screw fixation is indicated for closed stable fractures of the medial malleolus with minimal or no comminution. Buttressing by a plate may be needed for unstable varieties.

Associated conditions such as wound infection, compound fracture or neurovascular injury may necessitate temporary external fixation before the patient can be optimized for definitive fixation.

For the often-associated fracture of the lateral malleolus (lower end of the fibula), either plating with a 3.5-mm dynamic compression plate or a one-third tubular plate may be undertaken. Alternatively, lateral malleolar fractures may be fixed with a long Kirschner wire passed into the intramedullary canal of the fibula.

POSTOPERATIVE PROTOCOL

Patient can be mobilized on a walker non-weightbearing on the operated limb. Range of motion exercises for the knee and hip may be initiated provided, there is no associated injury to these joints.

SURGICAL STEPS (FIGS. 1 TO 26)

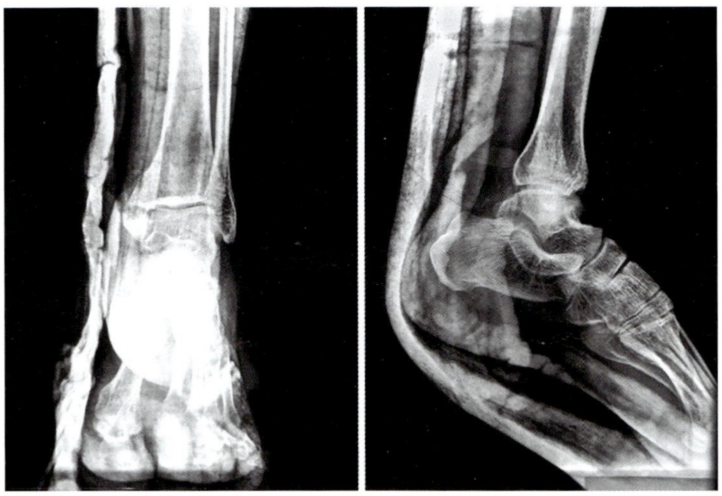

Fig. 1: Preoperative radiograph of the patient with medial malleolar fracture (closed) without any neurovascular injury.

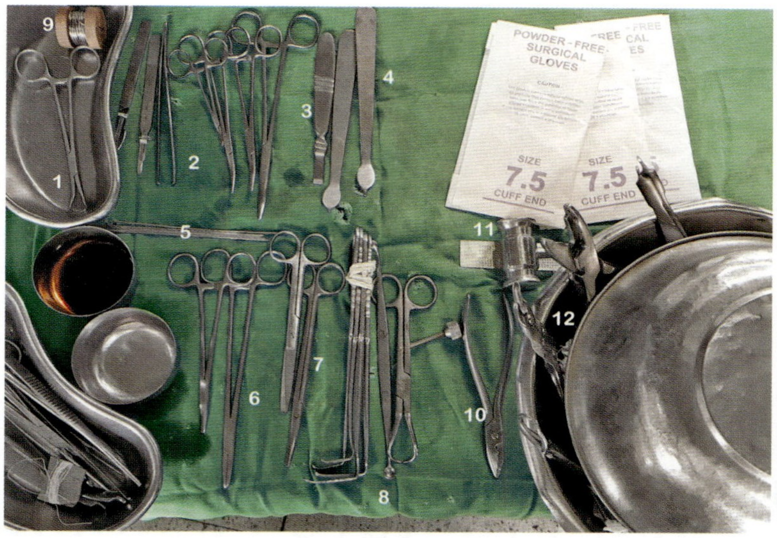

Fig. 2: Sterile instrument trolley as arranged for K-wire fixation of medial malleolus. (1) Towel clip, (2) General surgical instruments including surgical blades, artery forceps, toothed and plain forceps, (3) Sharp periosteum elevator, (4) Bone spikes, (5) Kirschner wires of varying thickness (0.5 mm to 3.0 mm), (6) Needle holders, (7) Cutting and dissecting scissors, (8) Retractors and scoop, (9) Stainless steel wire (for tension band wire application), (10) Plier, (11) Mallet, (12) Bone nibbler and stout plier. In addition, general orthopaedic instruments, sterile drapes, and dressing and drill machine with 3.2 mm and 2.7 mm drill bits should be available.

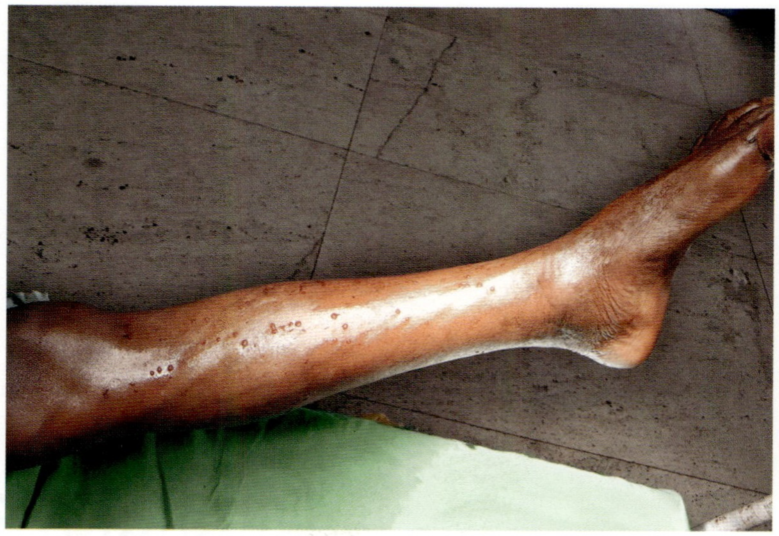

Fig. 3: After pneumatic tourniquet application in mid thigh, operative limb is cleaned with povidone–iodine scrub and wiped down with surgical spirit.

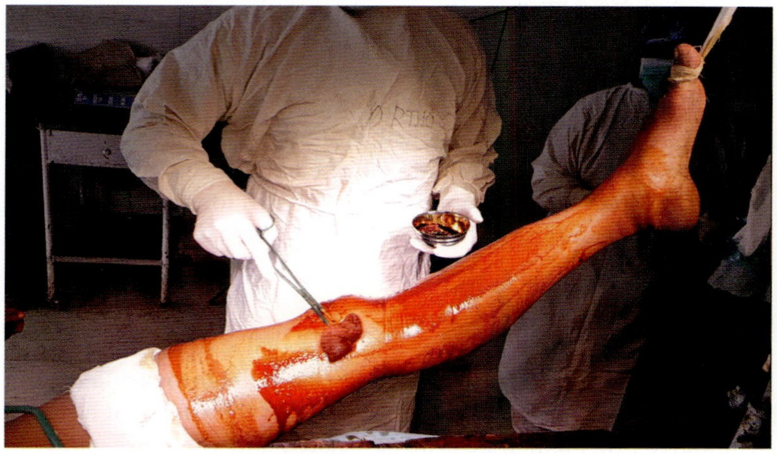

Fig. 4: Painting with povidone–iodine.

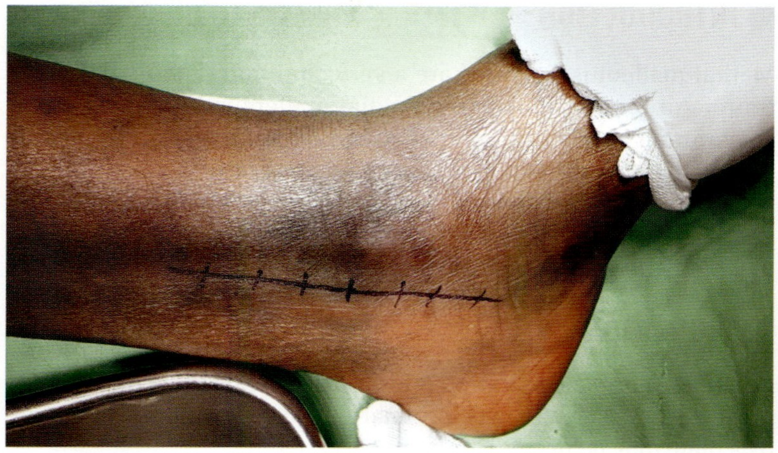

Fig. 5: The limb ready for surgery after inflation of tourniquet to a pressure of approximately 300 mm Hg. Skin should be incised either just posterior to medial malleolus for better skin flap (or over the medial malleolus to avoid underlying neurovascular structures as per surgeon's choice).

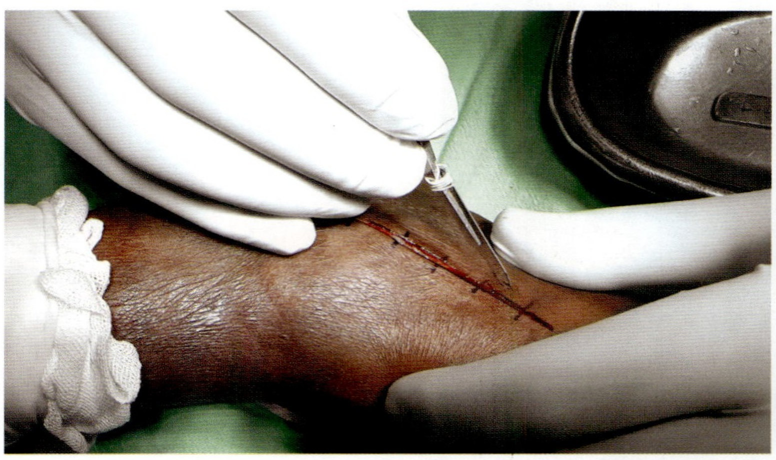

Fig. 6: Superficial and deep fascia is incised in line with the skin incision.

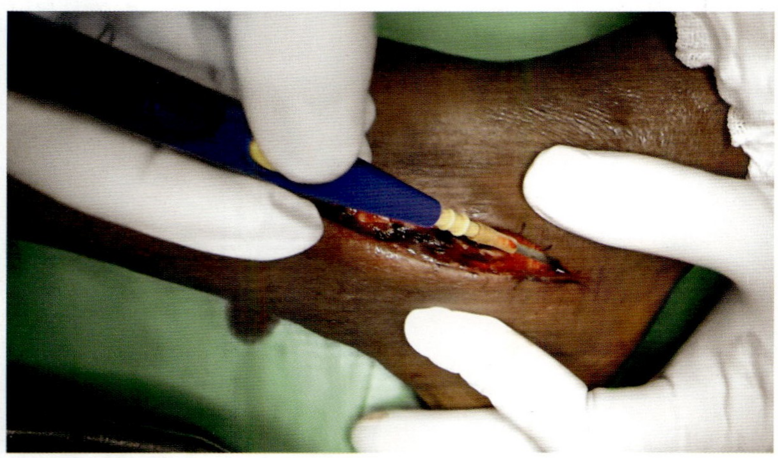

Fig. 7: Cautery may be used in deeper planes to reduce chances of postoperative hematoma.

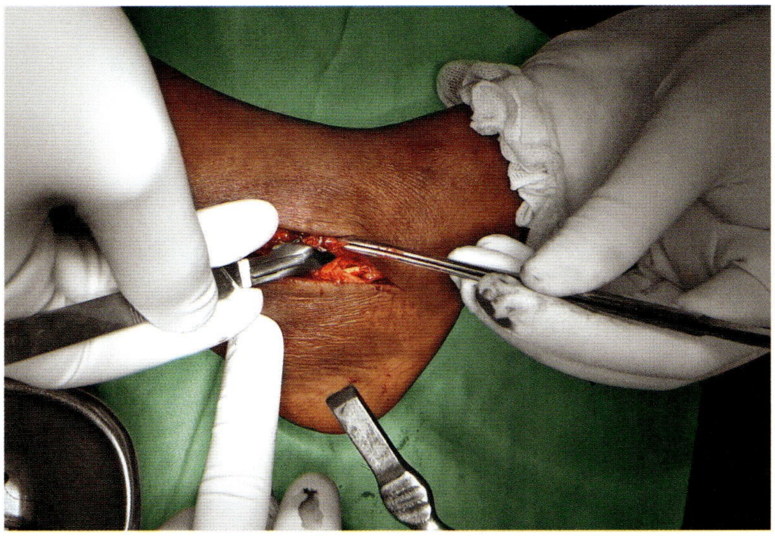

Fig. 8: Care is taken to avoid separating skin from deeper tissues so as to raise the full thickness flap over the malleolus for protecting the vascularity.

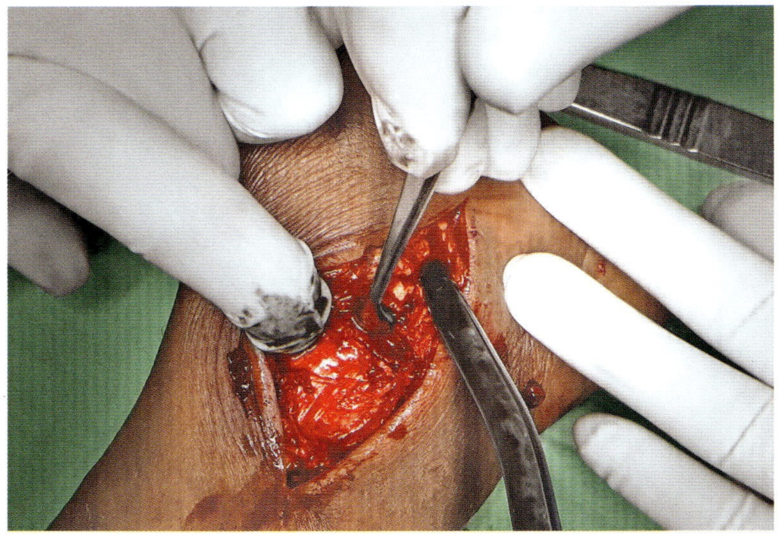

Fig. 9: The fracture site is cleaned. Blood clot and debris are removed using a sharp curette and artery forceps. Opposing surfaces of the bone at the fracture site are freshened.

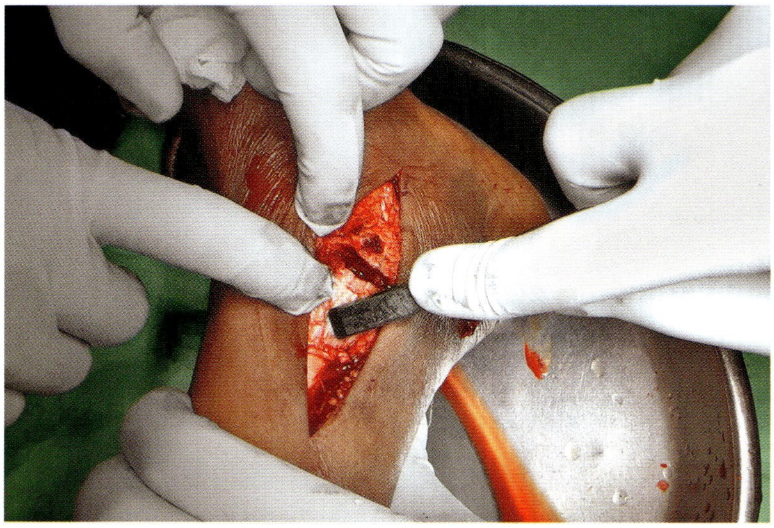

Fig. 10: Periosteum on either fragment is elevated just sufficient to prevent its inversion at fracture site (about 2–3 mm).

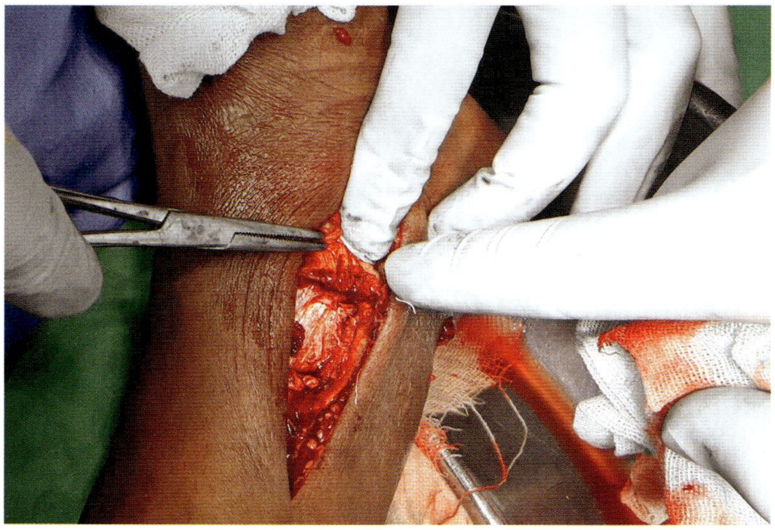

Fig. 11: The intervening soft tissue and bony debris further cleared from the fracture site by washing using saline-filled syringe. Then check reduction is done to see the accurate approximation of the fragments.

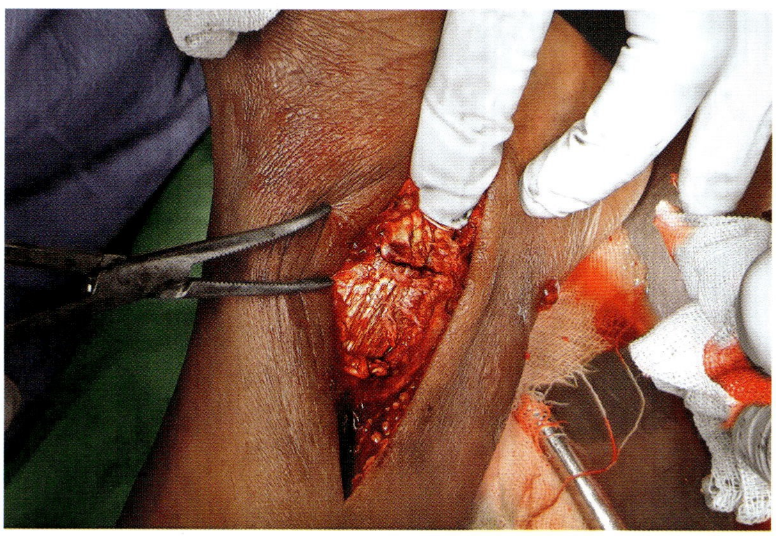

Fig. 12: Fracture fragments are held together with a pointed reduction clamp showing anatomical reduction.

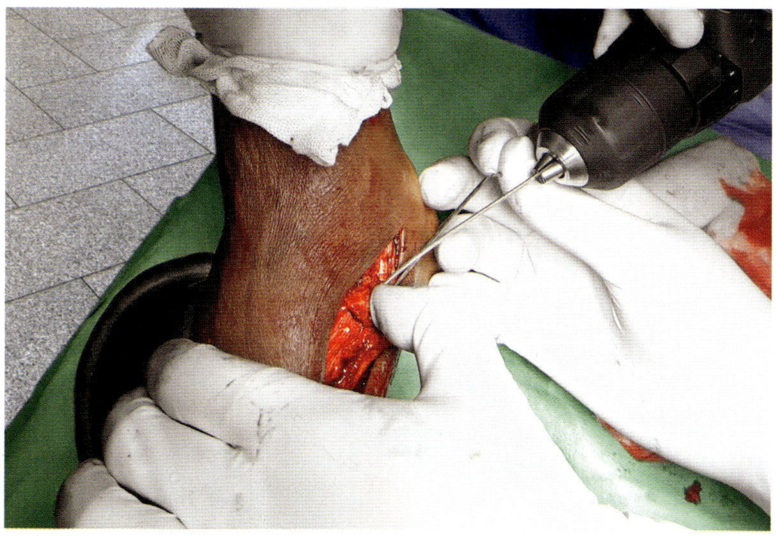

Fig. 13: By surgeon's judgment or under fluoroscopic guidance, parallel Kirschner wires are inserted into the medial malleolus at inclination of 5–10° from the bony surface, across the fracture site into the opposite cortex.

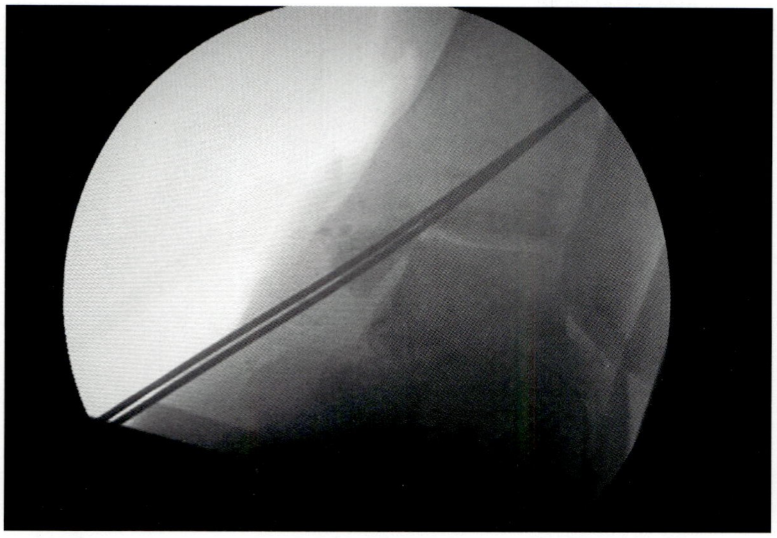

Fig. 14: Fluoroscopic view to confirm hold on the fracture fragments as well as bicortical purchase into the bone, but care should be taken to prevent intra-articular insertion of the wire.

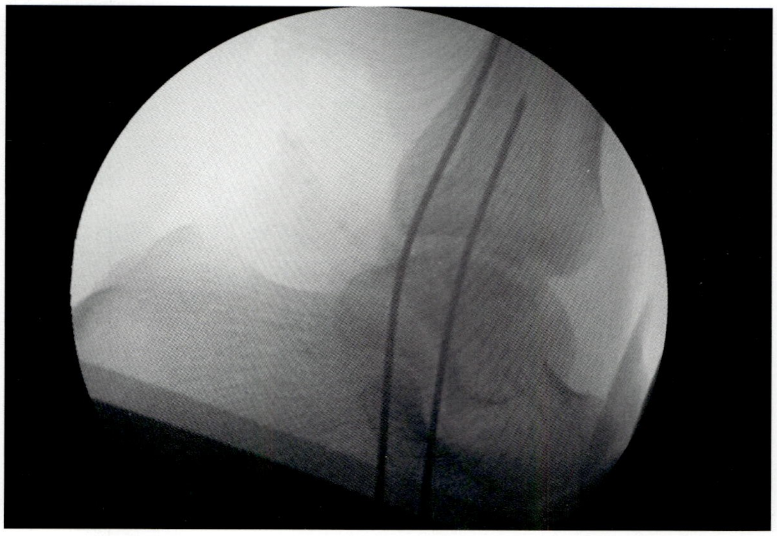

Fig. 15: The corresponding lateral view on intraoperative fluoroscopy. Wires should be parallel or divergent but not convergent.

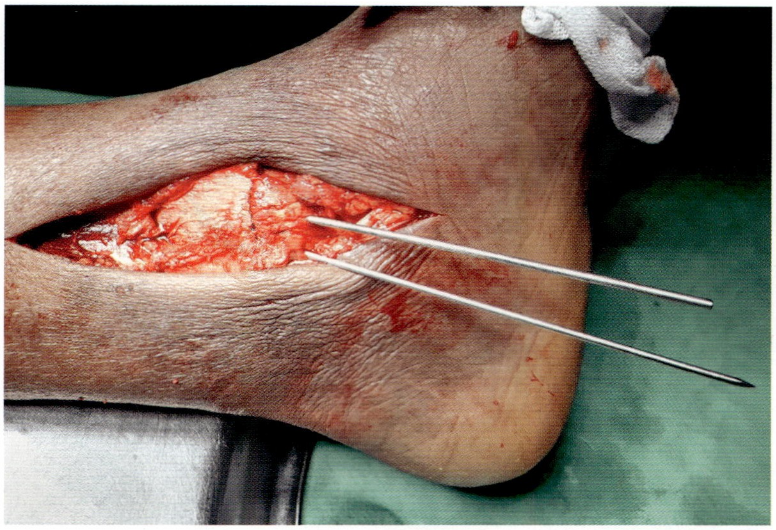

Fig. 16: Clinical photograph of the Kirschner wires in situ. Fracture has been held in anatomic reduction.

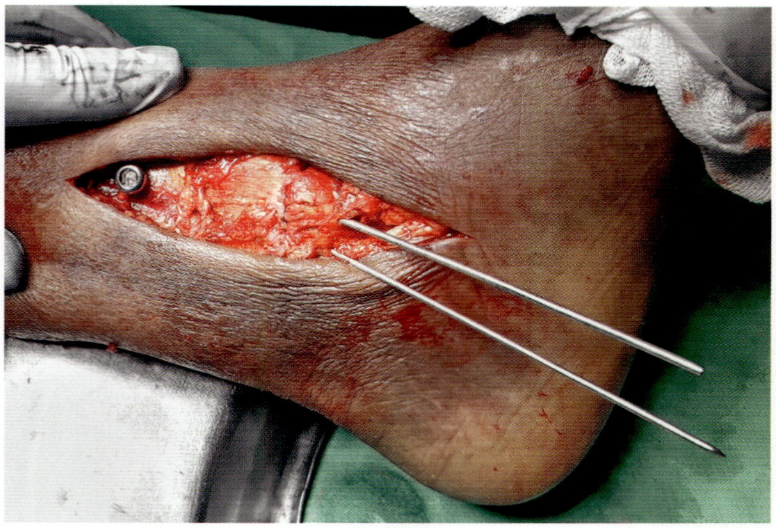

Fig. 17: A drill hole is made about 5 cm from the fracture site mediolaterally into the shaft of the tibia in the coronal plane. The screw should be partially tightened and have bicortical purchase in the bone. As an alternative to screw anteroposterior drill hole may be made in metaphysis and stainless steel wire is anchored in it.

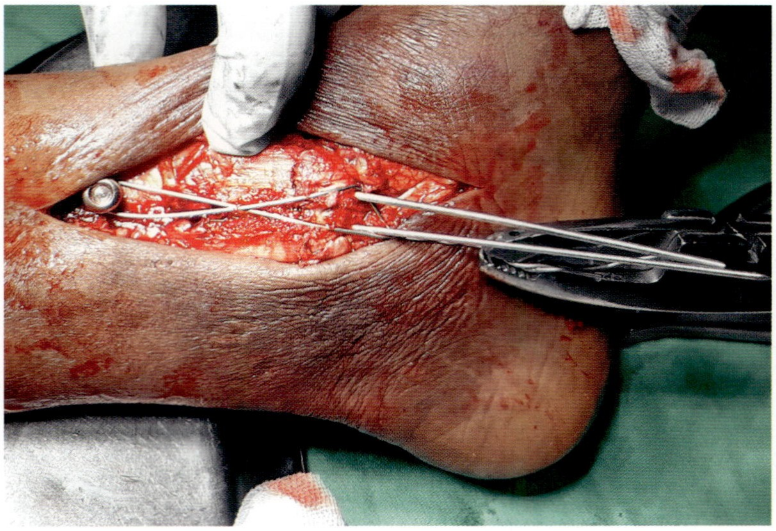

Fig. 18: A stainless steel tension band wire (TBW) is wound over the screw and then over ends of Kirschner wires in a figure-of-eight pattern. The ends are twisted around each other and tightened with a small plier.

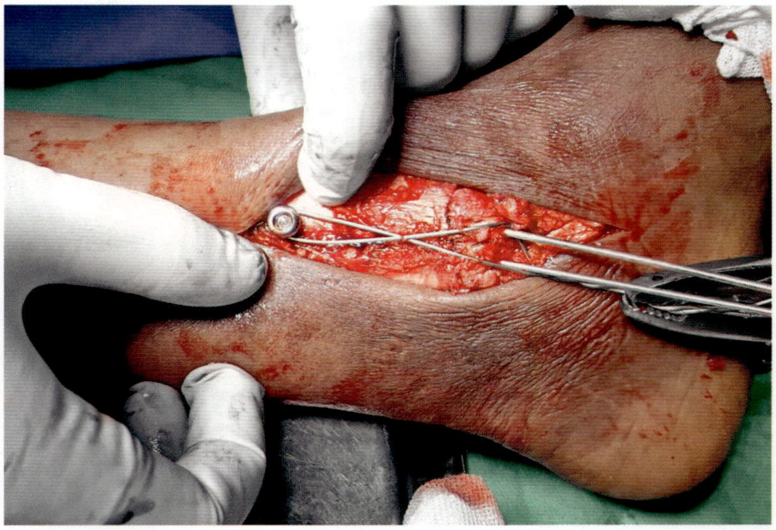

Fig. 19: The figure-of-eight construct being further tightened, producing compressive forces at the fracture site. After sufficient tightening, the end of the tension band wire (TBW) is cut and buried into the adjacent soft tissue.

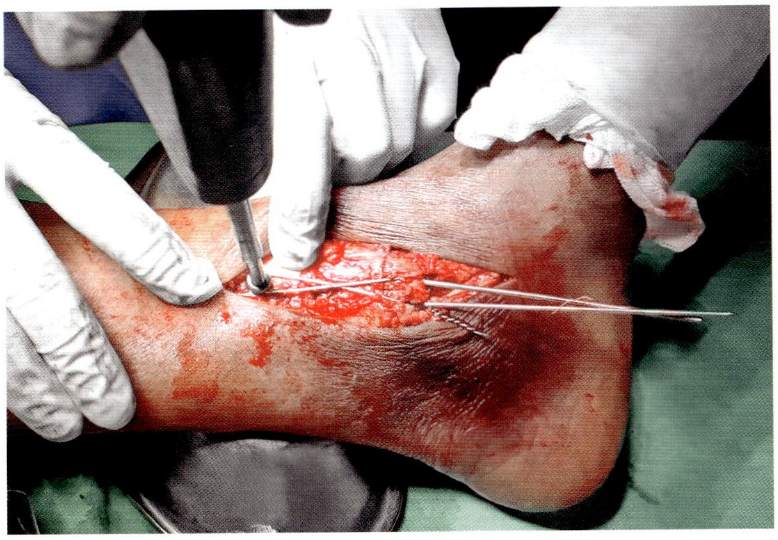

Fig. 20: After the figure-of-eight construct has been fully tightened, the anchoring screw is also tightened to the full extent in order to provide sufficient grip on the tension band wire.

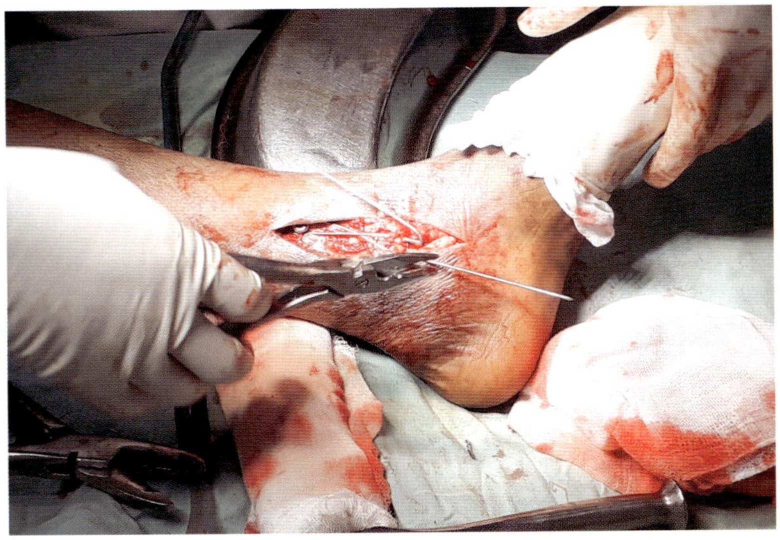

Fig. 21: After tightening the anchor screw, the Kirschner wires are bent to an acute angle and cut. The cut ends of the wire are to be buried into the adjacent soft tissue to prevent subsequent skin irritation to the patient.

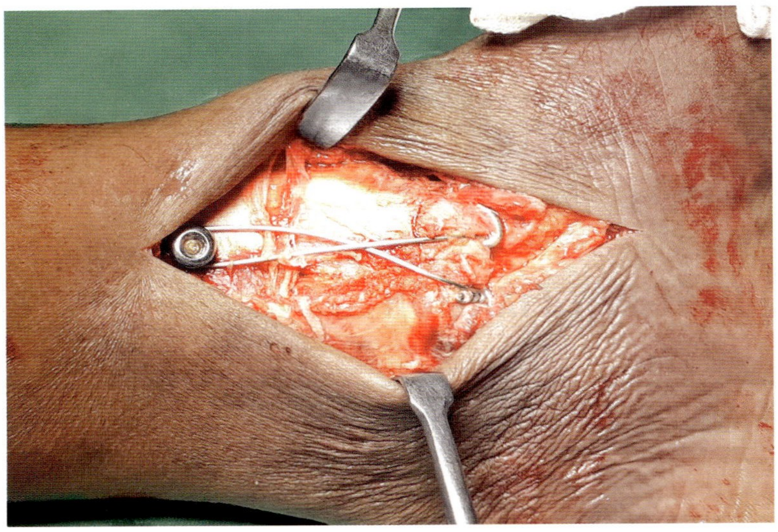

Fig. 22: The final construct before closure. Anatomic reduction at the fracture site with compression and figure-of-eight tension band construct with the anchoring screw in situ and ends of the Kirschner wires bent and buried into surrounding soft tissue.

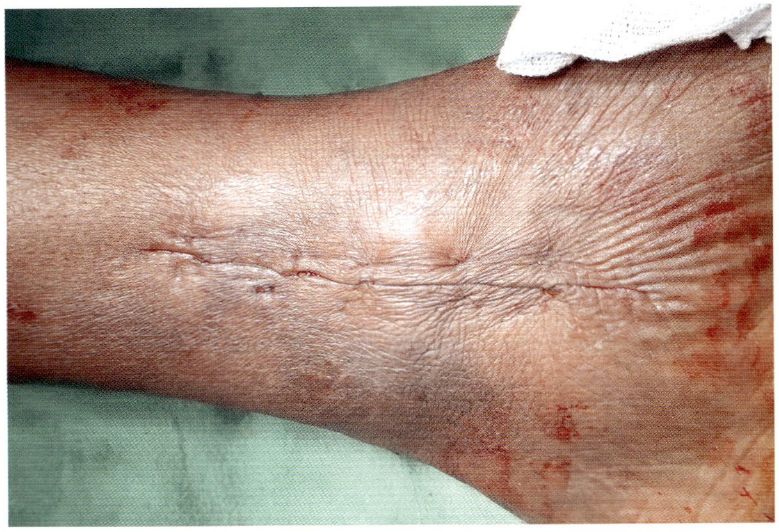

Fig. 23: Subcutaneous tissue is sutured using interrupted polyglactin sutures (2-0).

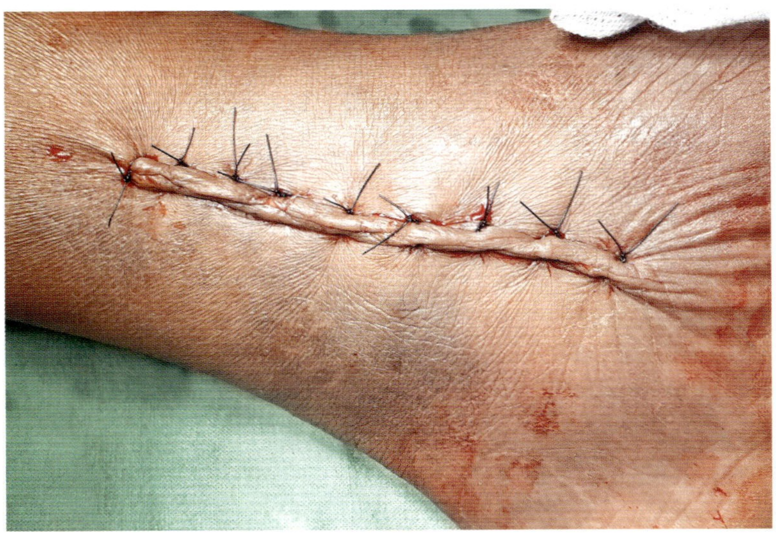

Fig. 24: Skin is closed using nonabsorbable nylon sutures taken in mattress fashion.

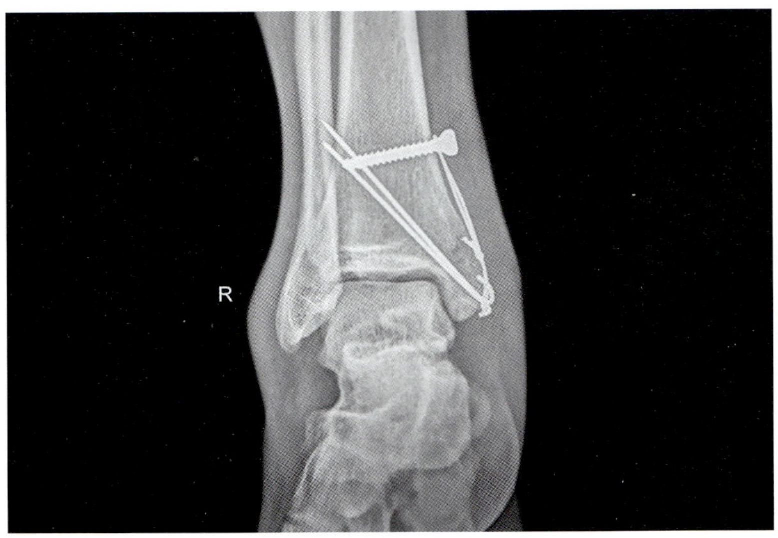

Fig. 25: Postoperative radiograph in anteroposterior view showing tension band construct and Kirschner wires in situ. Anchoring screw is seen to hold the wire construct in place.

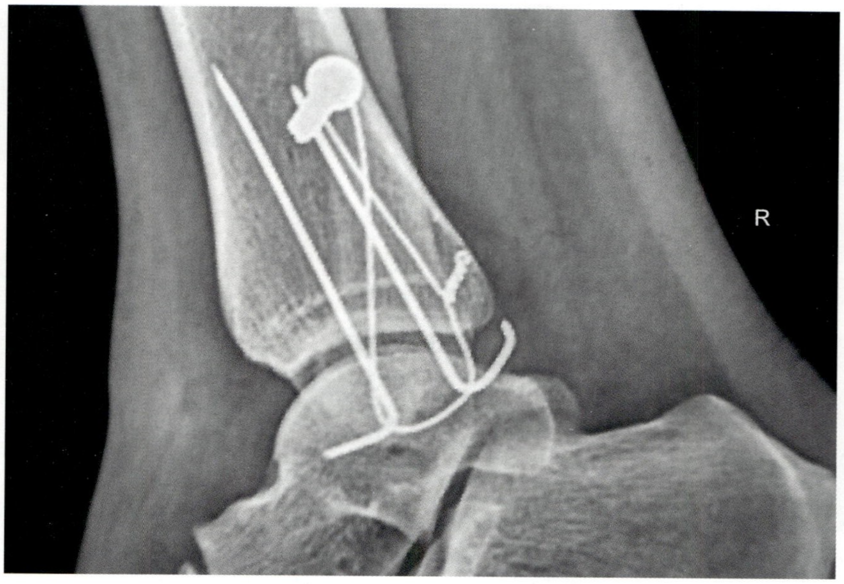

Fig. 26: Postoperative lateral radiograph of the same patient.

Regular wound dressing and cleaning should be done to minimize the chances of wound infection.

Suture removal can be done after 12–15 days postoperatively.

After radiological evidence of fracture healing, the patient can be given trial of partial weight bearing.

CANNULATED CANCELLOUS SCREW FIXATION

SURGICAL STEPS (FIGS. 27 TO 38)

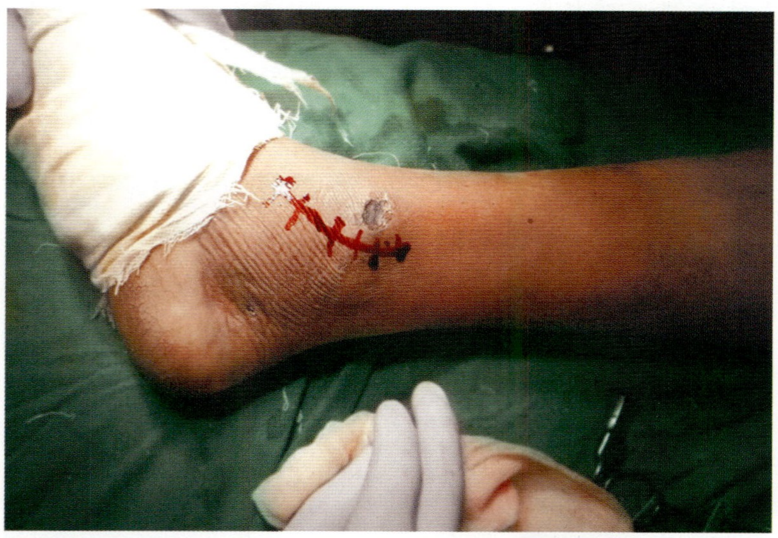

Fig. 27: Patient is positioned supine on the operating table, under appropriate anesthesia, the operative limb is scrubbed with povidone iodine and sterile painting and draping is done. The incision is marked over the bony prominence of medial malleolus with an anterior curve at the distal end (inverted J-shaped incision). This anterior curve of incision helps to visualize anteromedial corner of ankle joint.

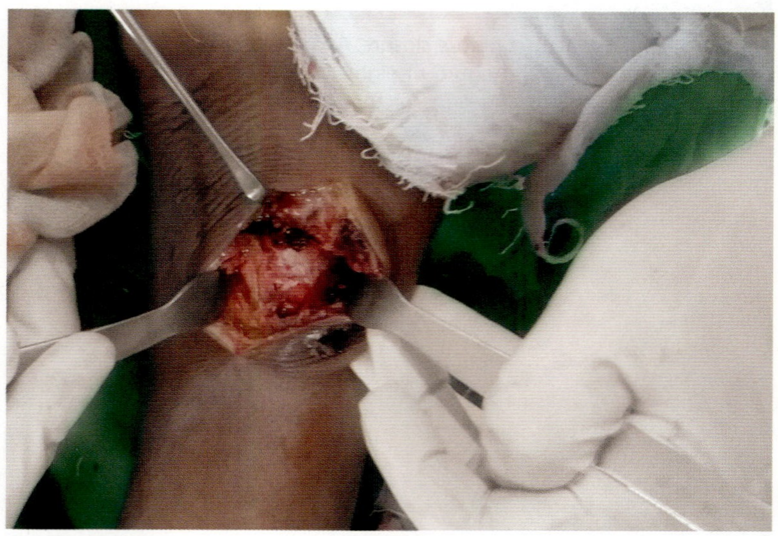

Fig. 28: Skin and soft tissue overlying the malleolus are dissected to expose the underlying bone. Care should be taken to not traumatize the posterior tibial artery and the saphenous vein which lie in close proximity to the malleolus. The fracture site is exposed and cleaned.

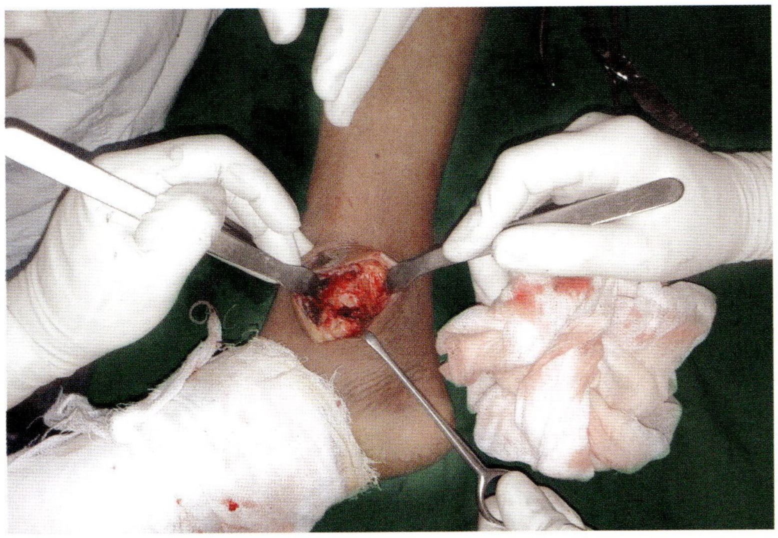

Fig. 29: Bone spikes are used to expose the proximal and distal fracture fragments and the fracture edges are freshened, soft tissue and debris removed.

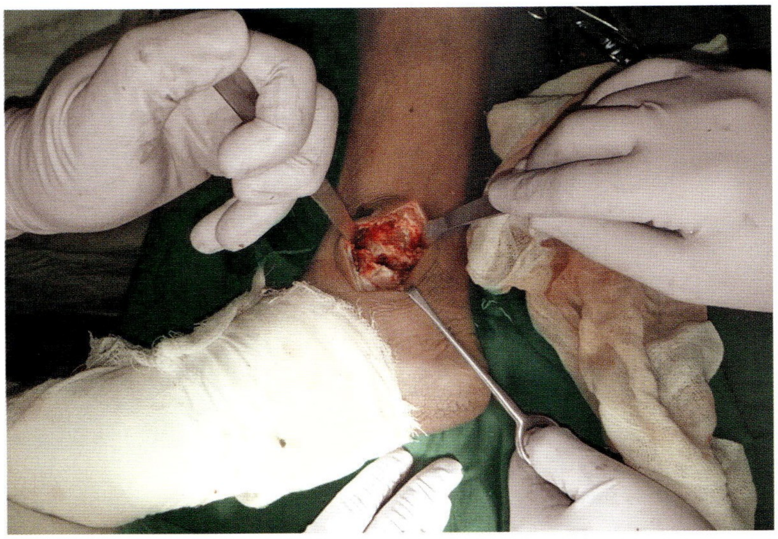

Fig. 30: Reduction is achieved using bone holding forceps or spikes.

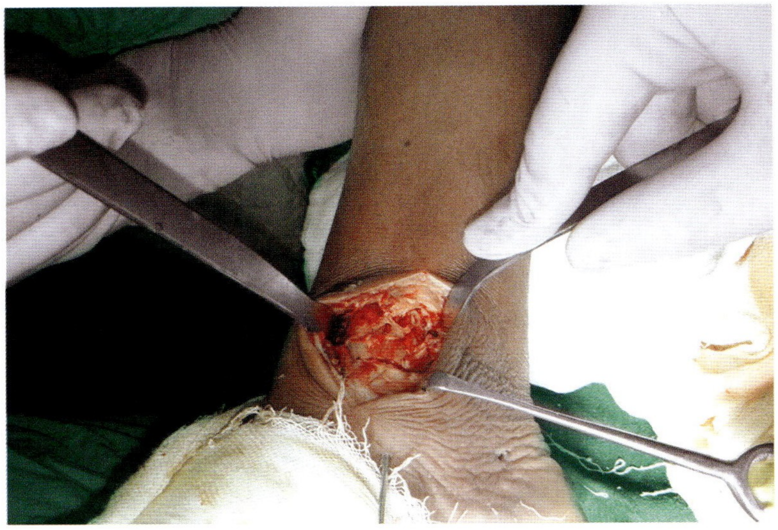

Fig. 31: A guidewire is passed from the tip of the malleolus, directed supero-laterally in the coronal plane, across the fracture site, into the distal tibia and advanced until it achieves a hold in the lateral tibial cortex.

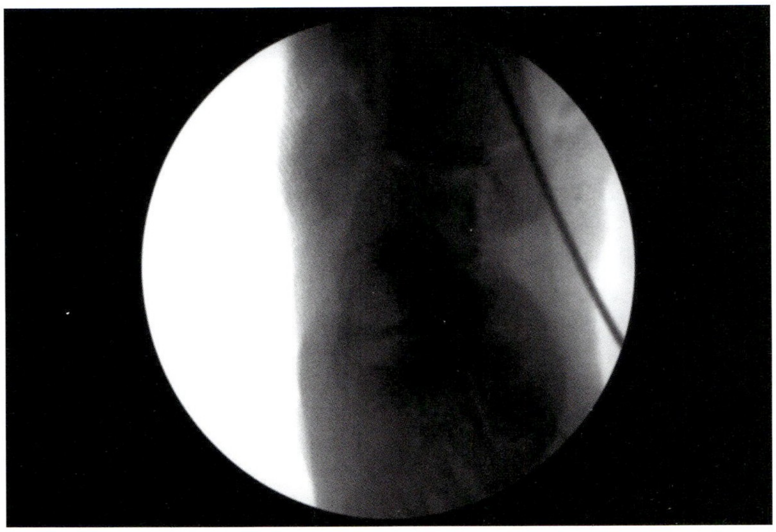

Fig. 32: Direction of the wire and reduction of the fracture are confirmed under fluoroscopy. Anteroposterior, lateral and mortise views are obtained.

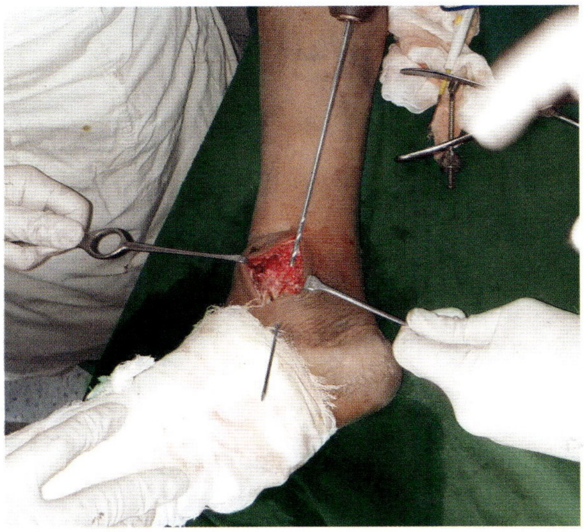

Fig. 33: A small depression is drilled into the medial tibial cortex (need not be through the entire cortical thickness) in order to provide a site to anchor the sharp reduction clamp.

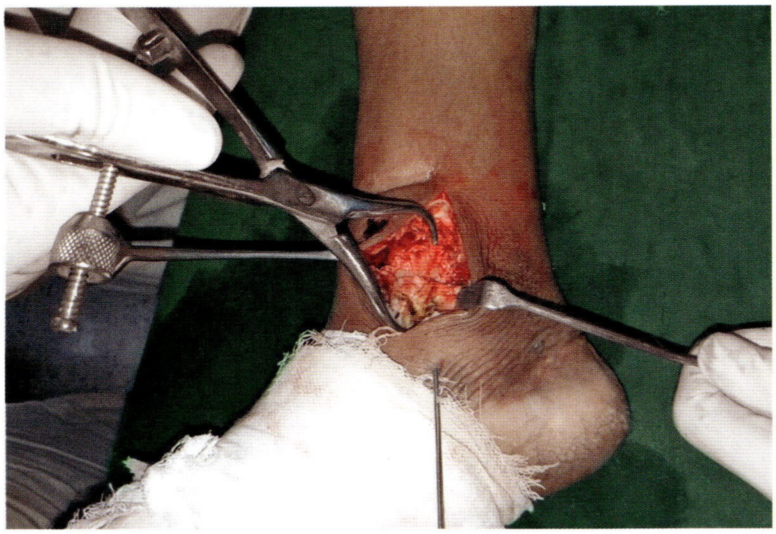

Fig. 34: Pointed reduction clamp is applied across the fracture site by inserting one prong into the hole made in the previous step, and the other prong at the inferior tip of the medial malleolus.

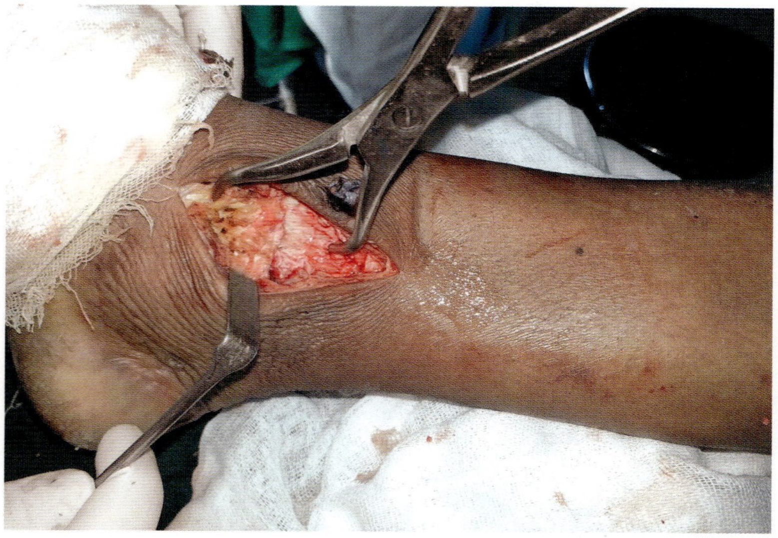

Fig. 35: Compression is achieved at the fracture site by tightening the pointed reduction clamp.

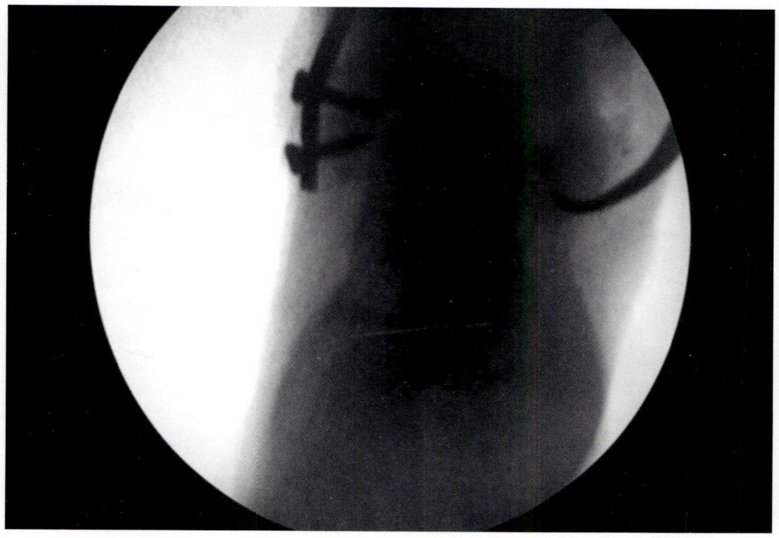

Fig. 36: Reduction is confirmed on fluoroscopy. Anteroposterior, lateral and mortise views are obtained.

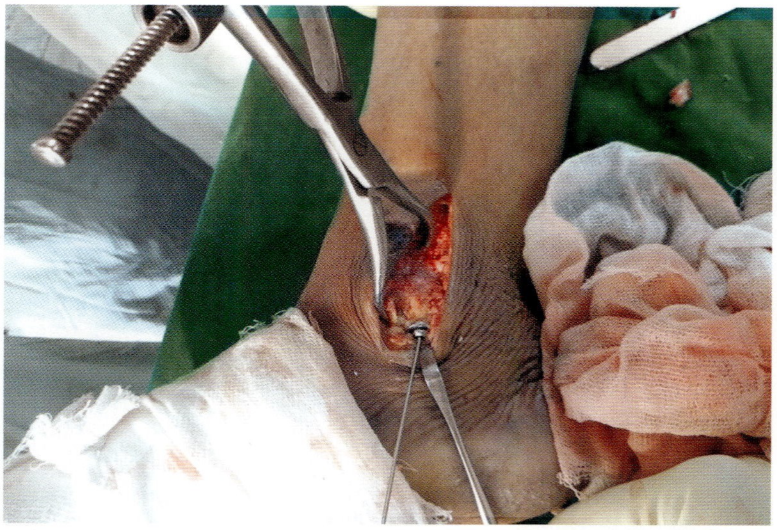

Fig. 37: A cannulated drill bit is passed over the guidewire and the bone is drilled over the guidewire, through distal fragment, across the fracture site and into the proximal fragment till the lateral tibial cortex. A partially threaded cannulated cancellous (CC) screw of appropriate length and with its washer is passed over the guidewire and tightened. Purchase of screw is improved if the threads engage the far cortex.

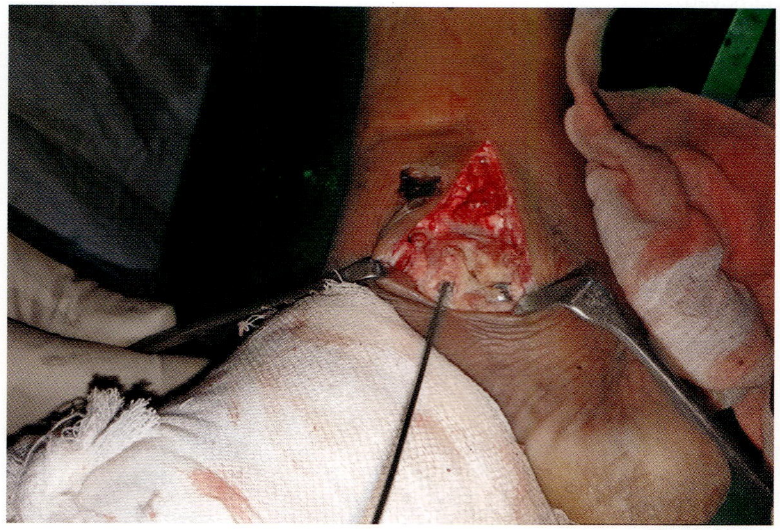

Fig. 38: Another guidewire is drilled into the distal fragment, across the fracture site into the proximal fragment, parallel to the first one in both anteroposterior and lateral planes. Some surgeons prefer a divergent configuration of screws, however convergent screws are not acceptable. Drilling and screw insertion is done as per the previous step. Second screw or K wire is inserted depending upon the size of the fragment and these act as derotation screw/wire.

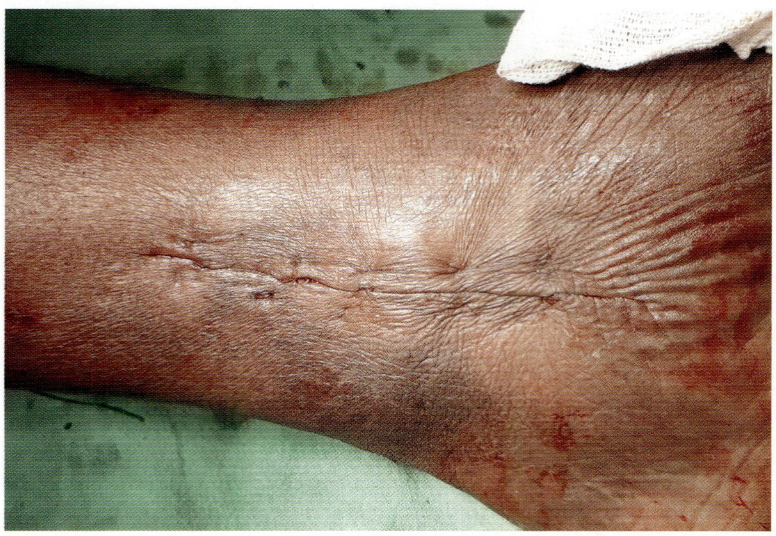

Fig. 39: Soft tissue is closed with absorbable sutures and skin incision is sutured using mattress sutures of non-absorbable nylon.

POSSIBLE COMPLICATIONS

Apart from anesthetic complications, this surgery may be complicated by inadvertent injury to posteromedial neurovascular structures during surgical dissection. Intraoperative fluoroscopy should be utilized to ensure that the Kirschner wires do not enter the ankle joint which could lead to postoperative arthropathy and septic arthritis in the setting of infection. Postoperative surgical site infections and suture line gaping can be prevented by proper wound care. Appropriate weight bearing and physiotherapy will reduce the probability of non-union or malunion.

SUMMARY

Medial malleolus fractures are commonly encountered as a result of blunt trauma to the ankle.

Kirschner wire fixation and compression using tension band construct or screw fixation is seen to produce good results. Meticulous wound care, limb elevation and physiotherapy will minimize postoperative complications.

SUGGESTED READING

1. Fowler TT, Pugh KJ, Litsky AS, et al. Medial malleolar fractures: a biomechanical study of fixation techniques. Orthopedics. 2011;34(8): e349-55.
2. Johnson BA, Fallat LM. Comparison of tension band wire and cancellous bone screw fixation for medial malleolar fractures. J Foot Ankle Surg. 1997;36(4):284-9.
3. Lendemans S, Nast-Kolb D, Täger G. Aitken grade III fracture of the medial malleolus: operative technique. Unfallchirurg. 2009;112(2):202-6.
4. Ricci WM, Tornetta P, Borrelli J Jr. Lag screw fixation of medial malleolar fractures: a biomechanical, radiographic, and clinical comparison of unicortical partially threaded lag screws and bicortical fully threaded lag screws. J Orthop Trauma. 2012;26(10):602-6.
5. Wendsche P, Dráč P. Are malleolar fractures easy to treat? Acta Chir Orthop Traumatol Cech. 2012;79(6):540-8.

CHAPTER 60

Achilles Tendon Rupture Repair

Gautam Salunkhe

INTRODUCTION

Rupture of the Achilles tendon is a common injury occurring as an occupational hazard in farms and industry, in strenuous sports, in daily walking due to unexpected strains, and in degenerative conditions.

PATHOANATOMY

An open injury due to a sharp object (sickle, blades, and burrs) cutting the tendon is seen in farmers, carpenters, and factory workers, respectively. The tendon is cut at the site of skin injury, depending on the state of plantar flexion the leg was in at that time. These are usually mid-substance tears.

A sports injury is also in mid-substance, resulting from forced contraction of the gastrocnemius-soleus muscle against an unexpected dorsiflexion. This can also occur in domestic life following a mis-step, by the same mechanism. It is characteristically accompanied by an audible snap at the time of occurrence.

Degenerative tears are seen in the predisposed; that is elderly, those with associated with diabetes mellitus, and those who have had been administered ill-advised steroid injections locally for their symptoms. These are mostly insertional by location.

CLINICAL EXAMINATION

Features seen are:

- High-stepping gait
- Inability to raise the heels from the ground
- *Thomson's test*: In prone position, squeezing the calf muscle will not transmit plantar flexion at the ankle.
- The site of rupture is easily located on palpation, the gap being felt and the edges of rupture being tender.

INVESTIGATIONS

- *X-rays*: These are helpful in degenerative tears and will show calcific tendinitis.
- *Ultrasonography and magnetic resonance imaging (MRI)*: These will identify the site of rupture.

However, none of these are required to reach a diagnosis, which can be done on clinical examination alone.

TREATMENT OPTIONS

- *Conservative treatment*—by cast immobilization and commercial static and functional braces.
- *Surgery*—open repair
- *Surgery*—minimally invasive or percutaneous repair.

Warning: An absolute contraindication for surgery is a limb with vascular compromise. Thromboangiitis obliterans, atherosclerosis obliterans, and venous thrombosis exclude the patients from any surgery and cast treatment.

DECISION MAKING

- Open repairs are more precise in approximation, but have a high rate of wound complications.
- Closed repairs give good to average approximation, and have an extremely low rate of wound complications.
- Since immobilization is required in both, a minimally invasive or percutaneous approach has great advantages over open surgery.

INSTRUMENTS

Open Repair (Figs. 1 to 19)

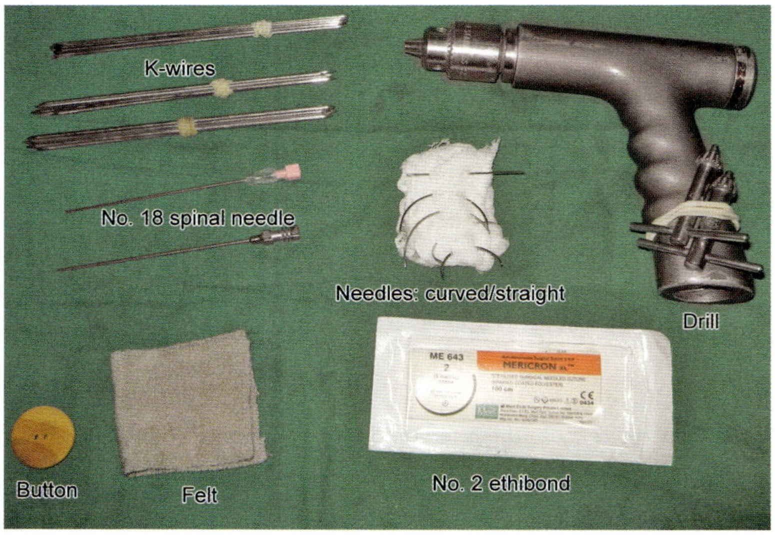

Fig. 1: Other than general instruments, a few simple instruments are required: K-wires, No. 18 spinal needles, wooden curtain button, felt, straight and curved needles, and drill.

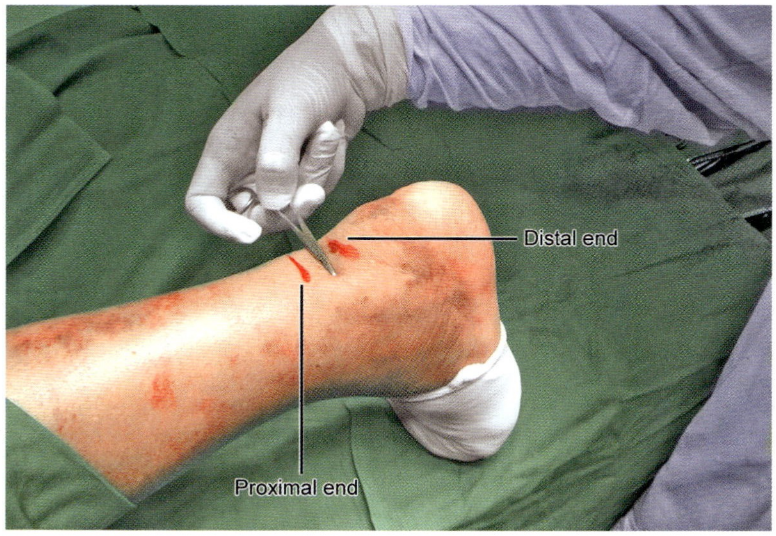

Fig. 2: In prone position, with tourniquet inflated, the proximal and distal edges are palpated and marked.

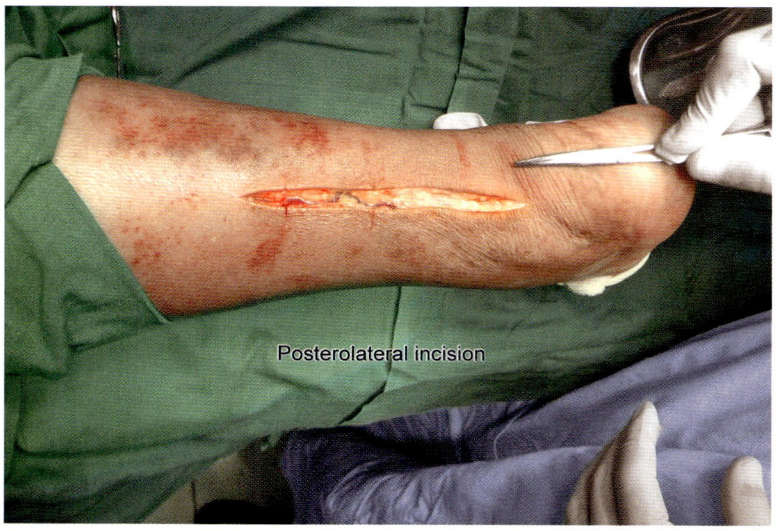

Fig. 3: A long posterolateral straight incision is taken from proximal to the rupture till the calcaneal tuberosity. The incision is taken deep, with the skin, subcutaneous fat and fascia cut in a single layer. The incision may be varied to posteromedial, lazy S, or posterocentral.

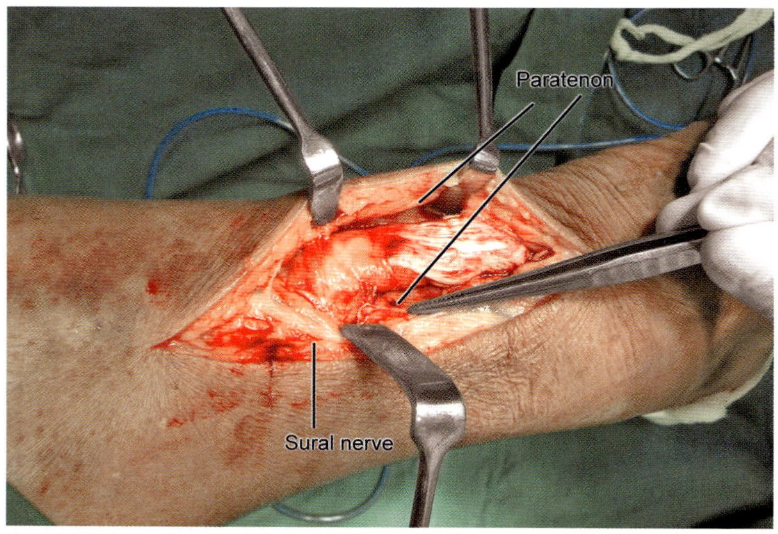

Fig. 4: The sural nerve is easily identified and retracted. The paratenon over the Achilles-tendon is cut longitudinally to expose the rupture.

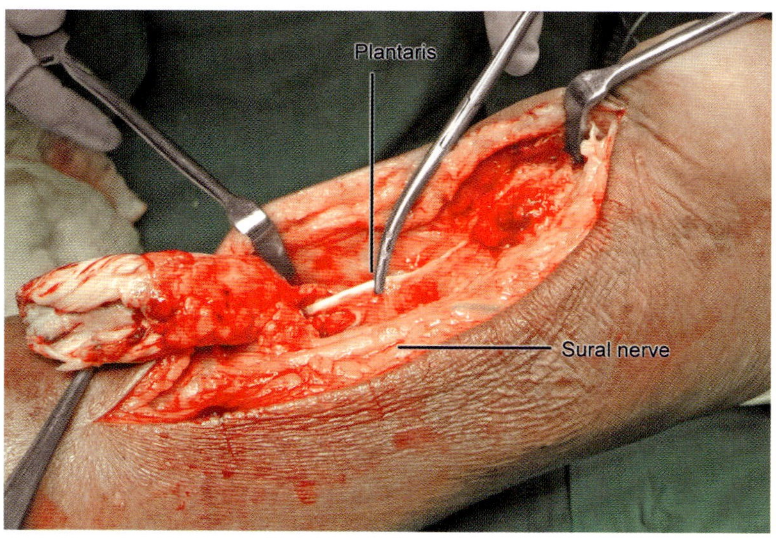

Fig. 5: The plantaris is seen in the medial limit of the incision, the sural nerve on the lateral limit.

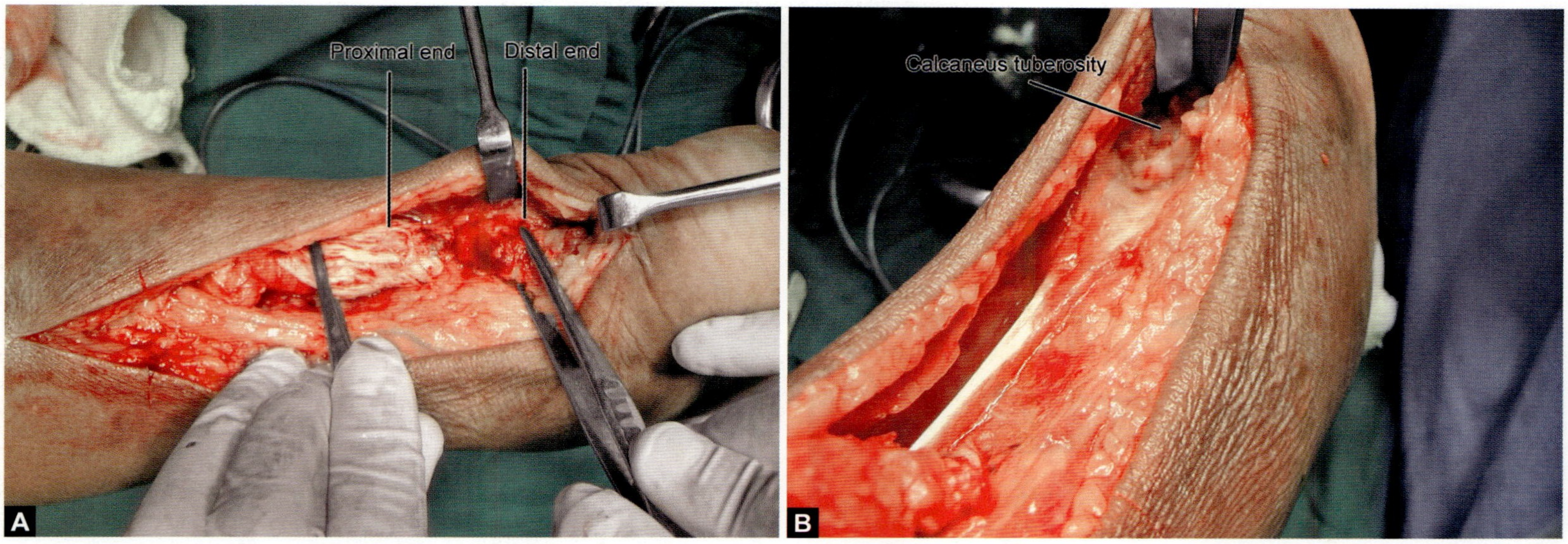

Figs. 6A and B: The degenerative distal element of the Achilles tendon is debrided to expose the insertion on the calcaneal tuberosity.

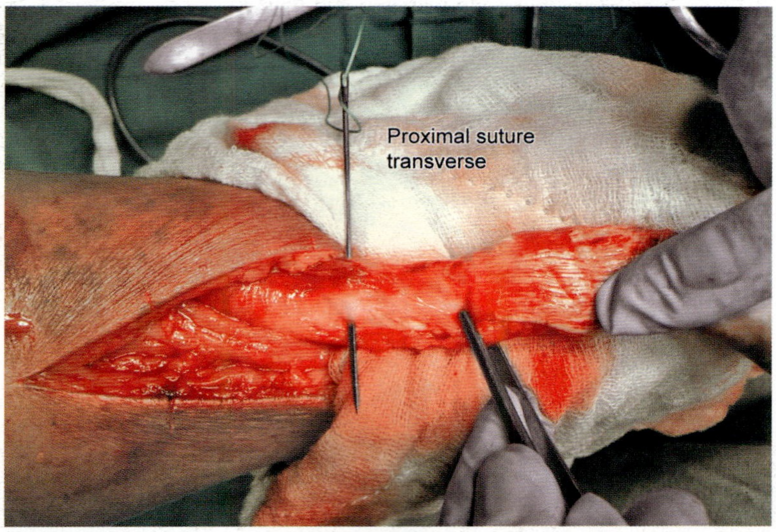

Fig. 7: A Bunnell stitch is fashioned of No. 2 strong nonabsorbable material. The suture is first passed transversely in the proximal tendon, away from the rupture.

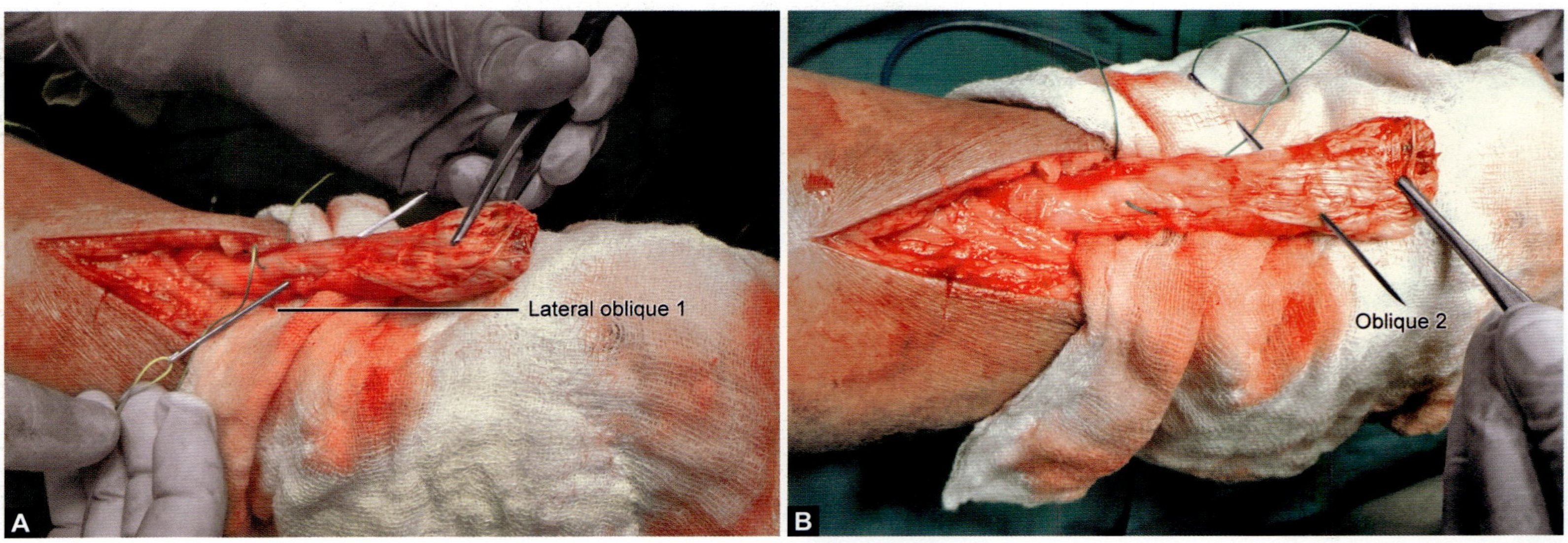

Figs. 8A and B

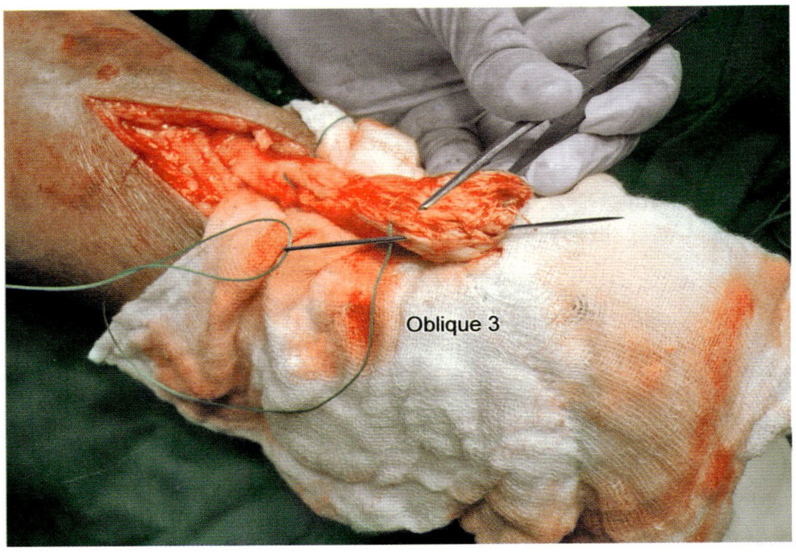

Fig. 8C

Figs. 8A to C: The lateral end of the suture is passed obliquely through the proximal tendon in two stages, till it appears out of the ruptured end of the tendon.

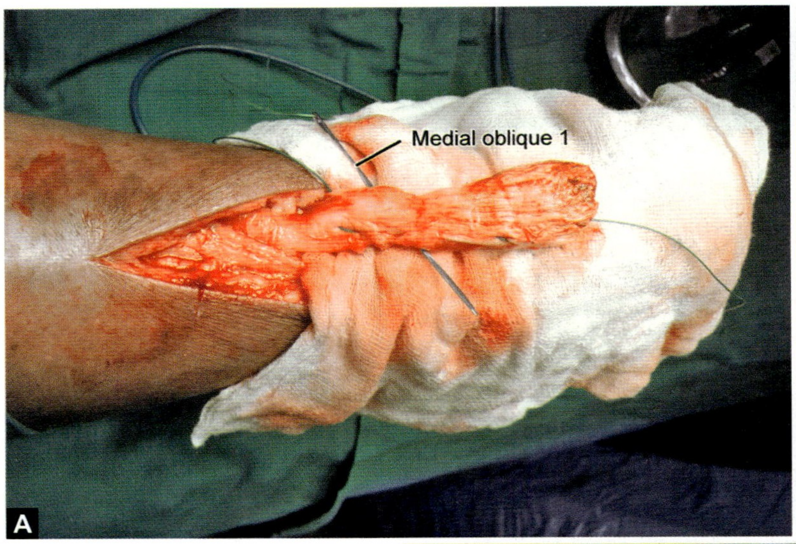

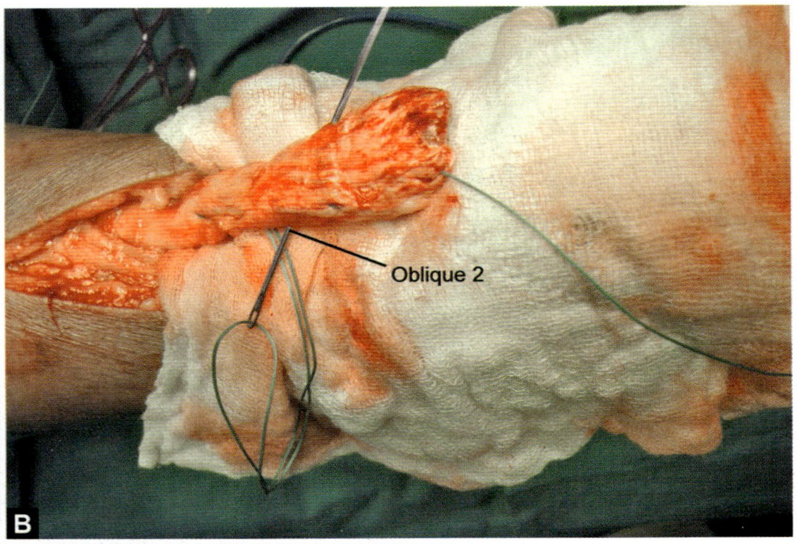

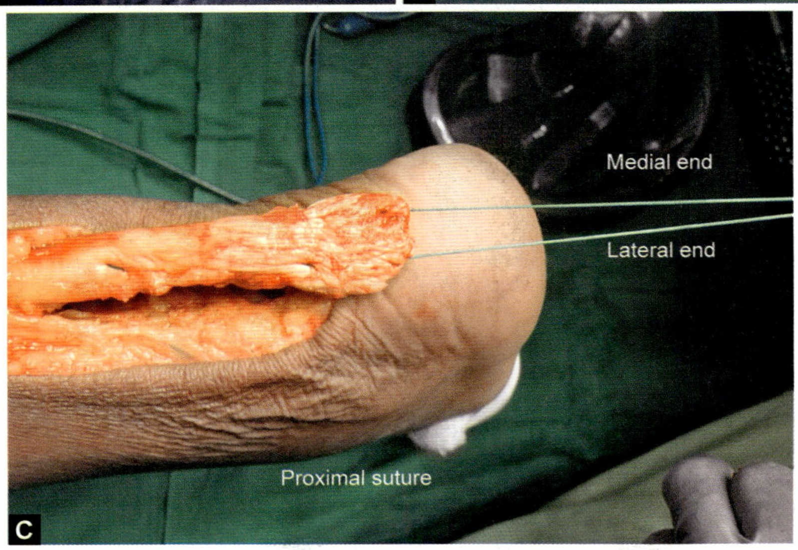

Figs. 9A to C: The medial end of the suture is similarly passed obliquely down the proximal tendon, till it exits from the rupture.

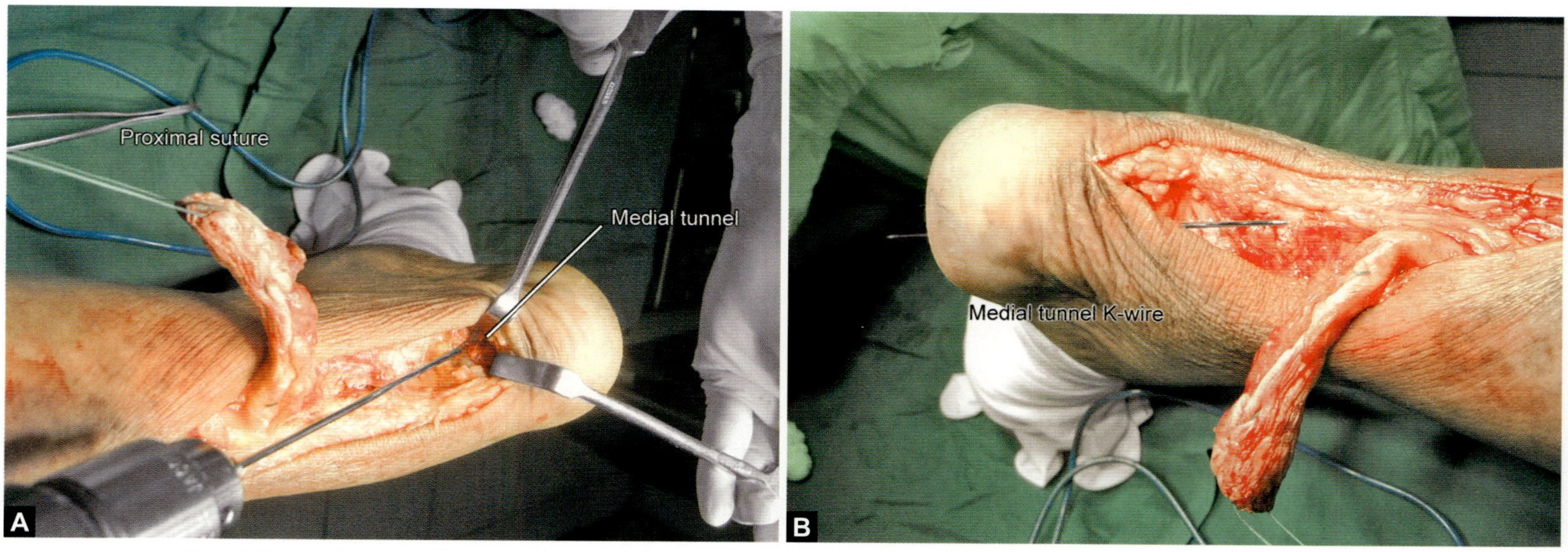

Figs. 10A and B: A tunnel is created in the calcaneum using a K-wire, drilling from the tuberosity to exit from the heel.

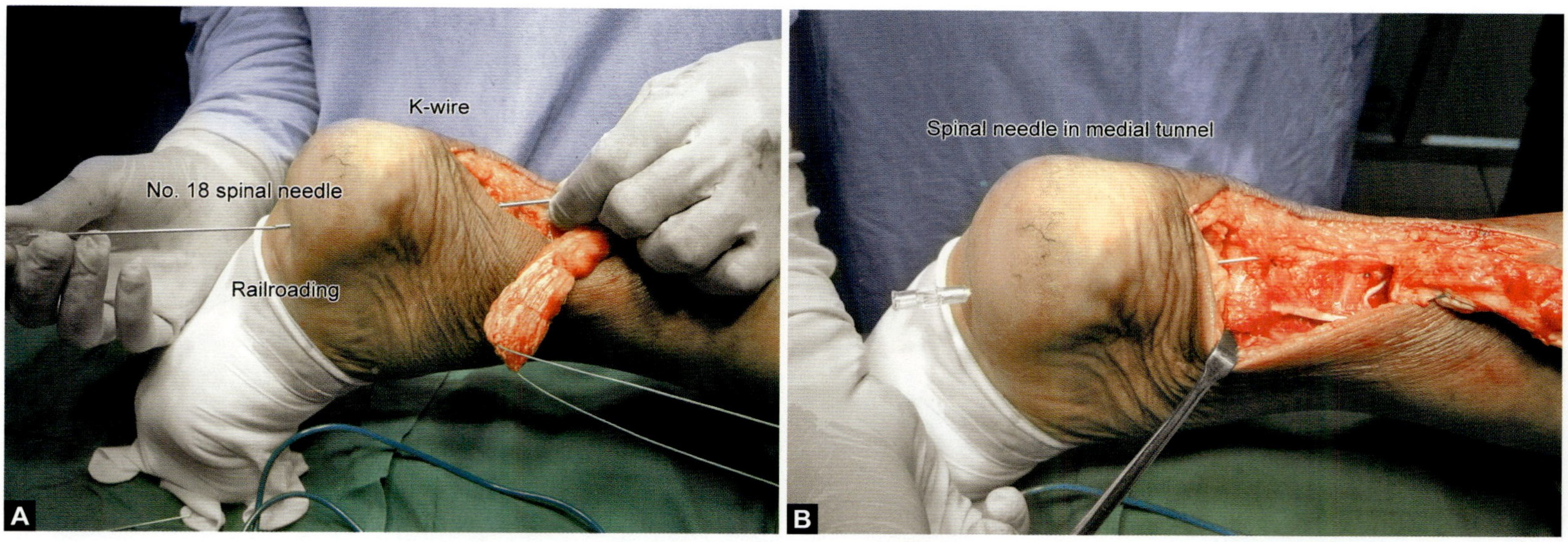

Figs. 11A and B: A No. 18 spinal needle is introduced from the heel into the tuberosity, by railroading over the K-wire.

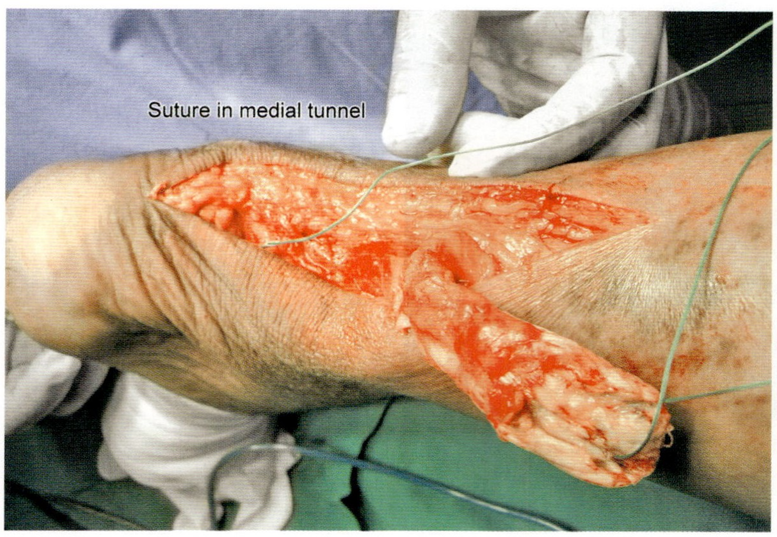

Fig. 12: The medial end of the suture is introduced into the spinal needle to enter the medial tunnel.

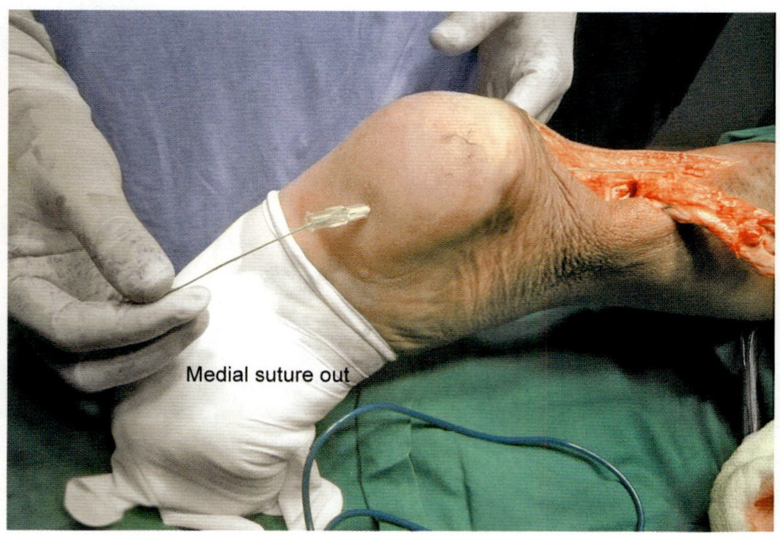

Fig. 13: As the suture exits from the heel, the spinal needle is withdrawn.

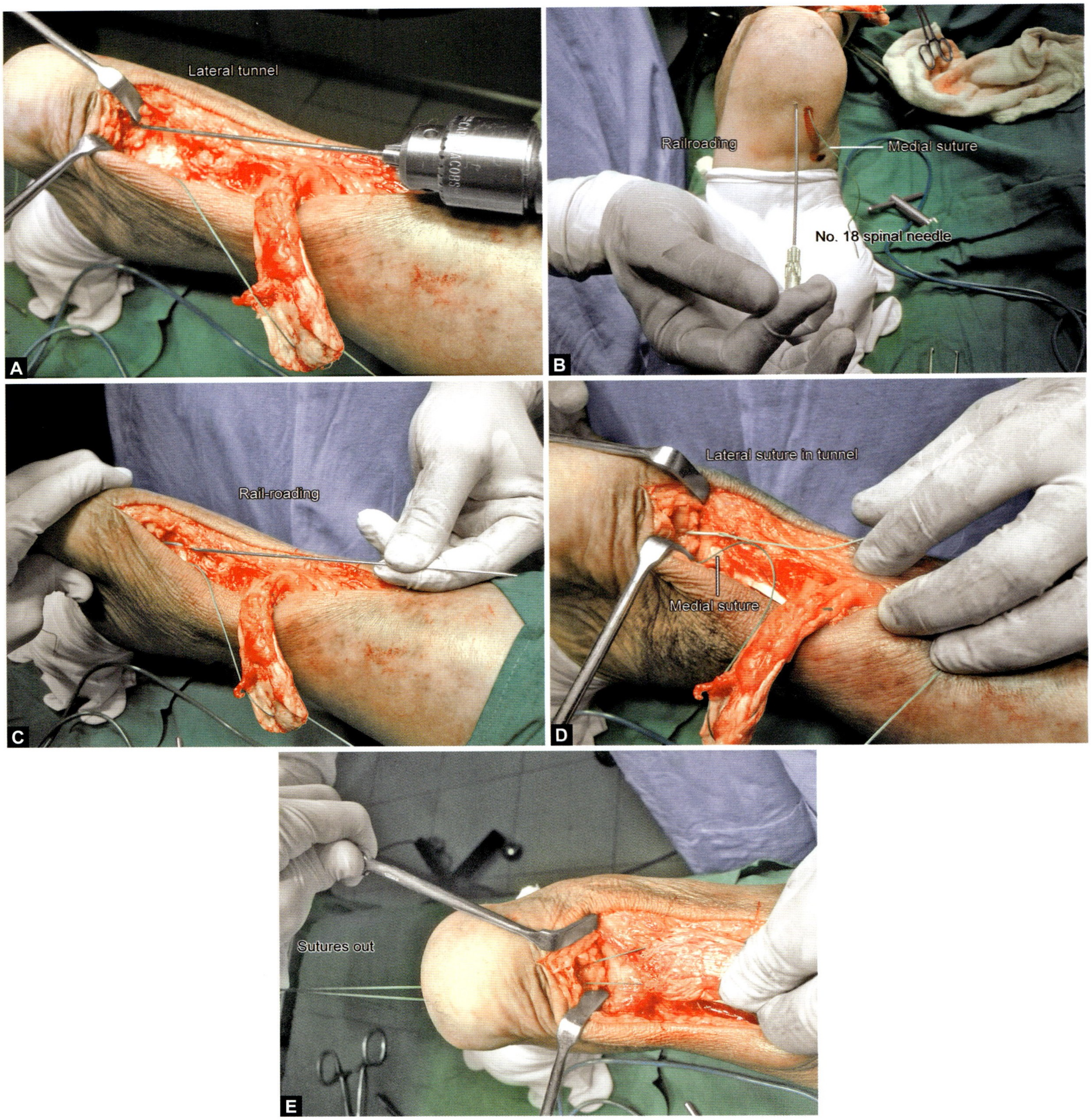

Figs. 14A to E: Similarly, the lateral tunnel is created and the lateral end of the suture is withdrawn from the heel.

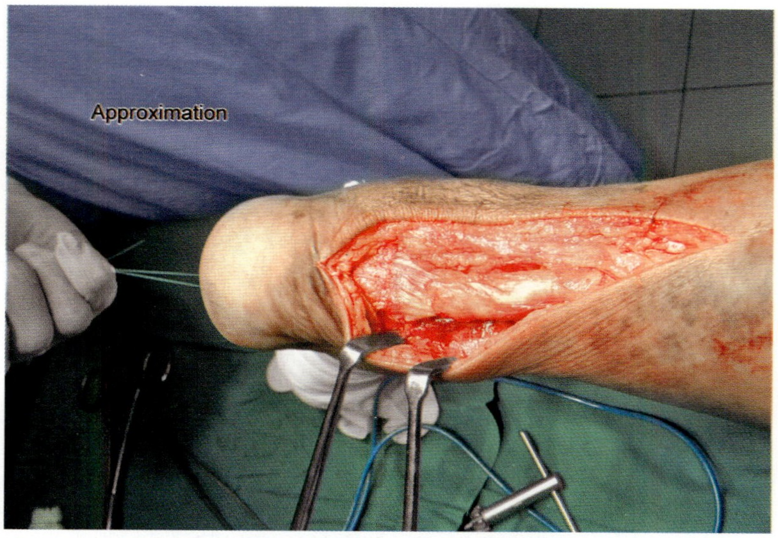

Fig. 15: Approximation of the tendon is achieved by traction on the sutures at the heel.

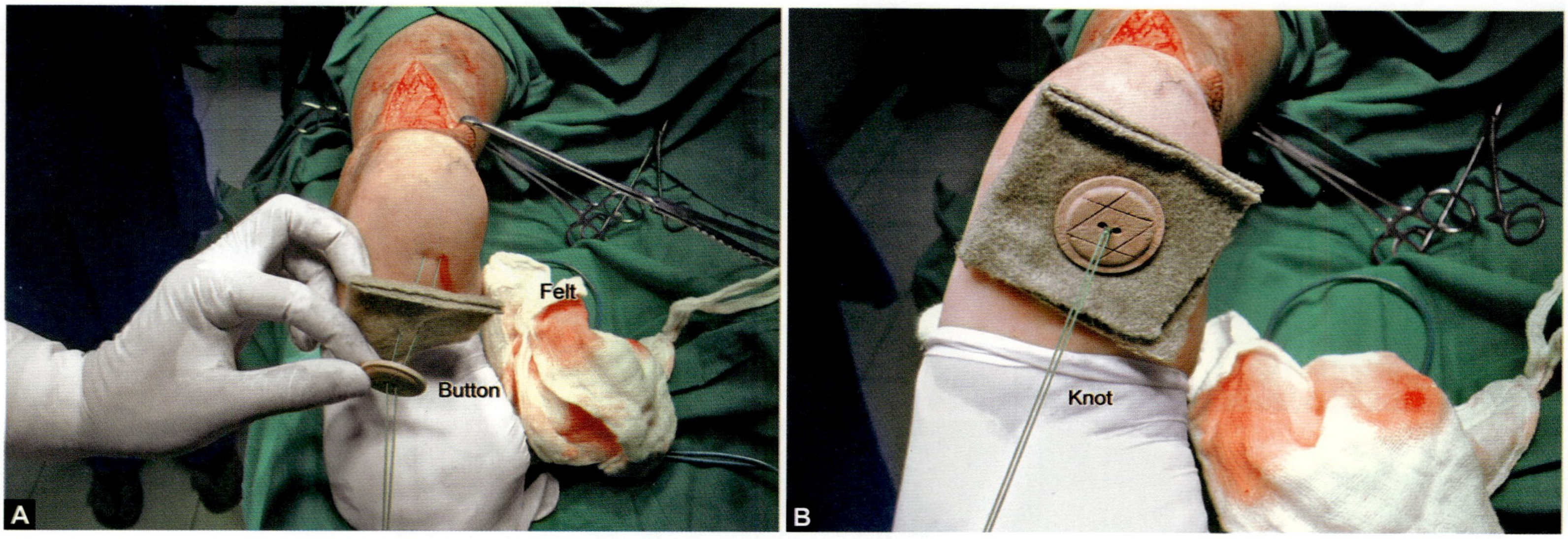

Figs. 16A and B: The sutures are passed through a protective felt into a button, and the knot is tied with the ankle in plantar flexion.

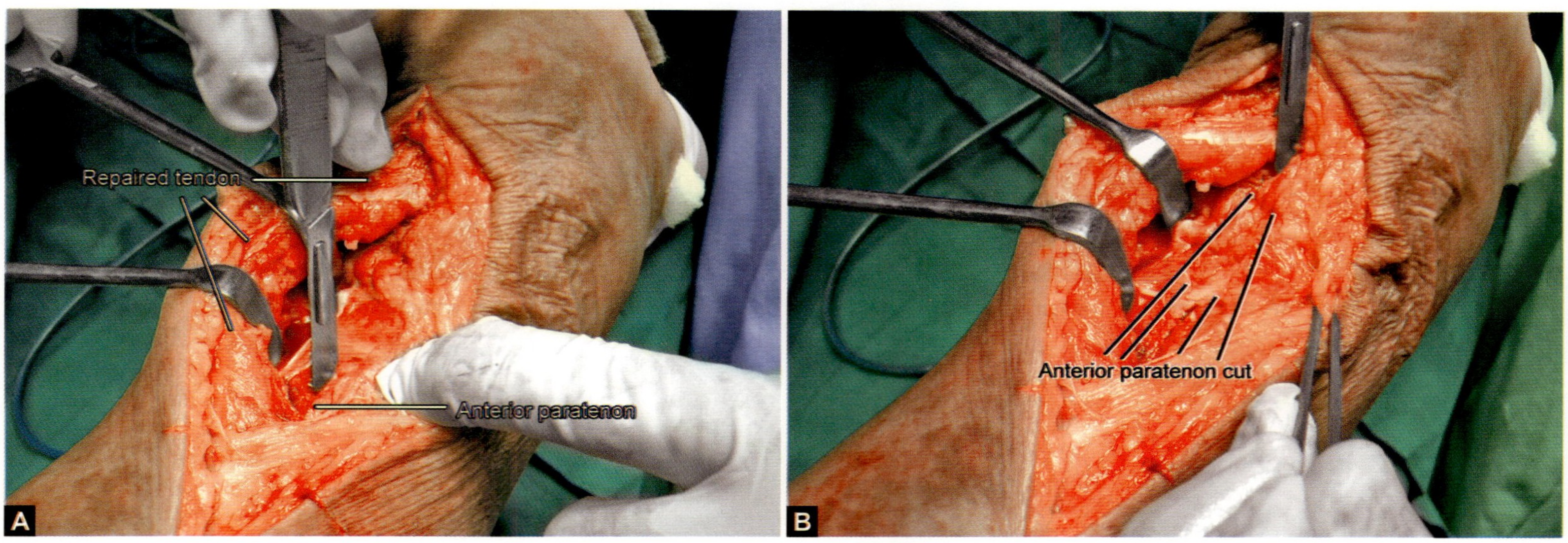

Figs. 17A and B: The repaired tendon is retracted, and a longitudinal cut is taken on the anterior paratenon. This is done to aid repair of the paratenon posteriorly.

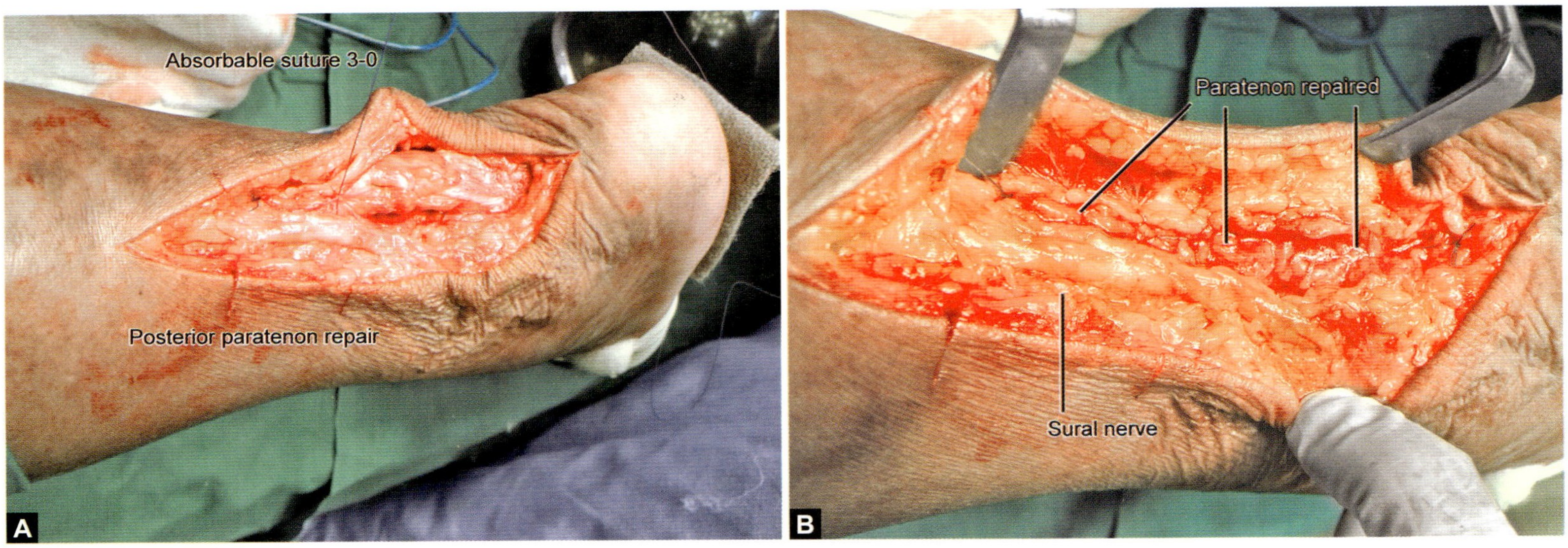

Figs. 18A and B: The posterior paratenon is repaired using a continuous 3-0 absorbable suture. The tourniquet is released and hemostasis is attended to.

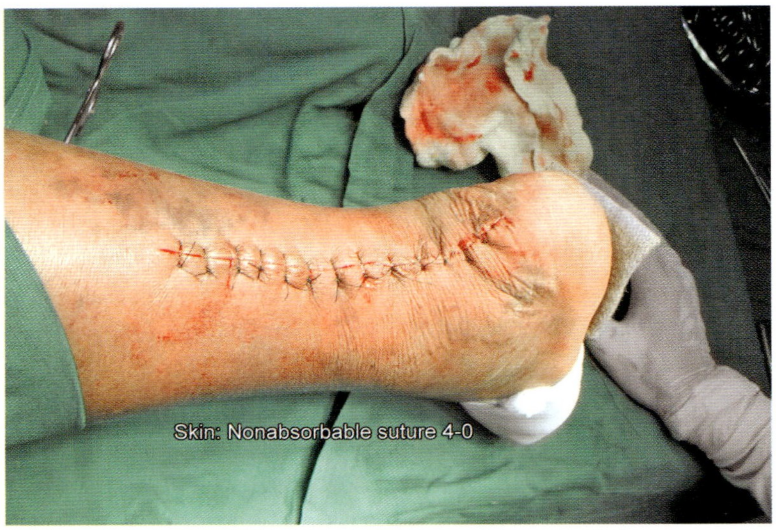

Fig. 19: The skin is sutured using 4-0 monofilament nylon sutures.

An above knee cast is applied.

Variations

The sutures were originally described to be taken outside the cast and tied. This required final closure of the wound, and tensioning of the suture after the cast is applied. The approximation of the repair cannot be verified this way.

Suture anchors can be used to fix into the calcaneum. Here, the fixation would be in reverse order; i.e. calcaneal fixation, followed by suture into the proximal tendon. Approximation would be by tensioning proximally. Many other suture fixation devices have been tried.

Complications

- Wound dehiscence is the most common complication.
- Infection and joint stiffness can occur.
- The operative scar may be adherent to the repaired tendon.

Minimally Invasive Repair (Figs 20 to 27)

- As the Achilles tendon is a percutaneous structure, the suture can be passed through stab incisions over the tendon. In old, compound, and insertional tears, the suture can be passed into the distal tendon or heel using a transverse incision along the Langers lines. This wound has no difficulties in healing, and is barely visible later.
- The anatomy of the sural nerve, as shown previously, should be kept in mind while passing these sutures.
- The above knee cast is applied and kept for 6 weeks.
- For open and minimally invasive repairs, the cast is removed at 6 weeks. The button and felt are released by cutting the suture. The nonabsobable suture is cut close to the skin. It retracts inside as the ankle position is brought to neutral.
- Further protocol is described later.

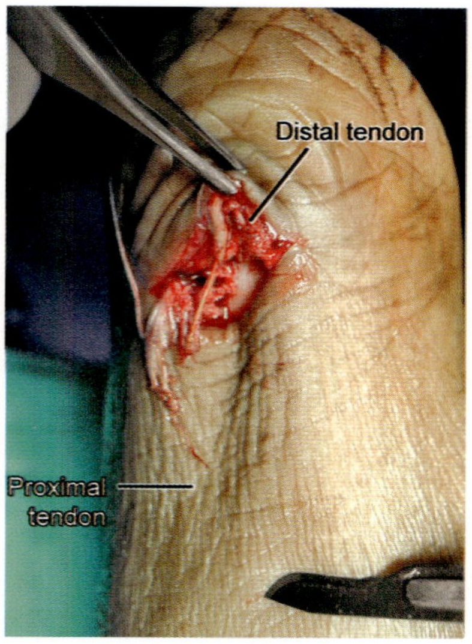

Fig. 20: Compound insertional rupture.

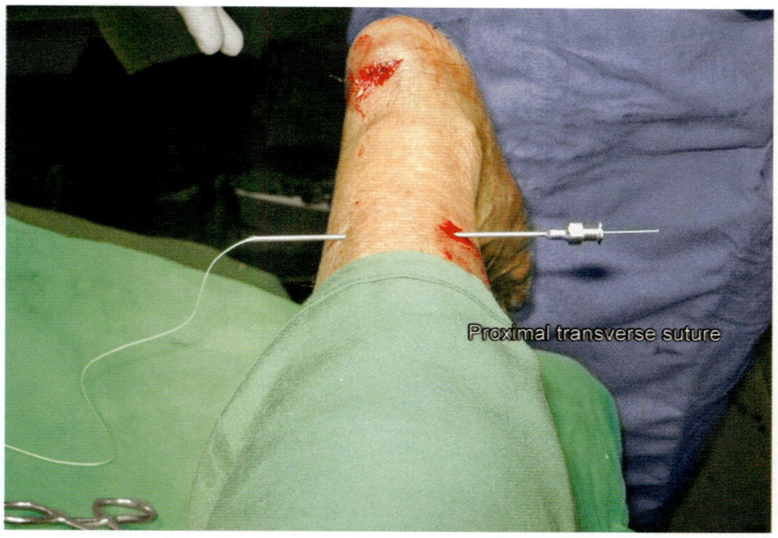

Fig. 21: No. 18 spinal needle inserted after stab incisions, used to pass the No. 2 nonabsobable suture transversely through the proximal tendon.

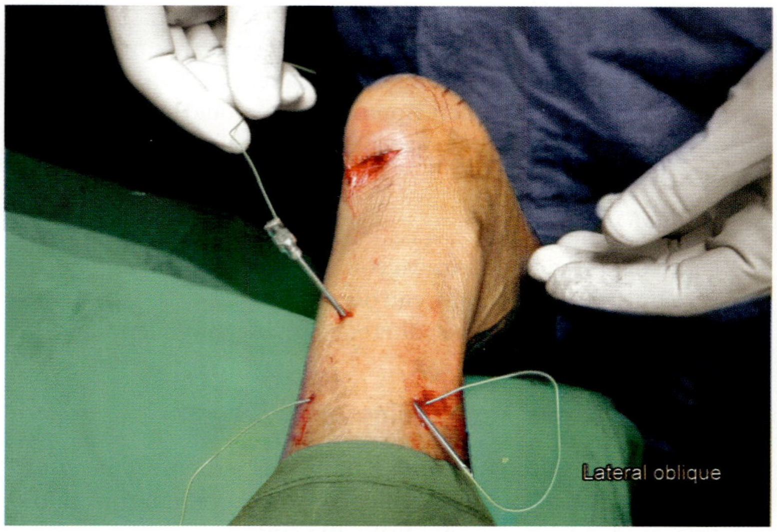

Fig. 22: Lateral end oblique suture is taken distally into the proximal tendon.

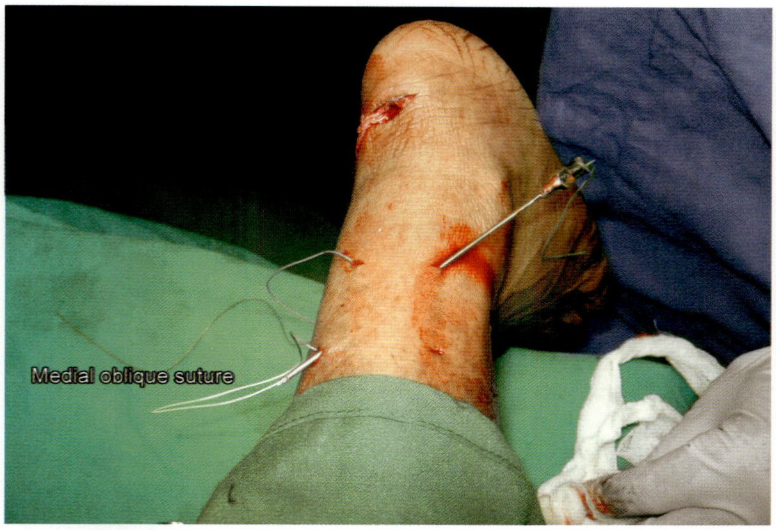

Fig. 23: Medial end oblique suture is taken into the proximal tendon.

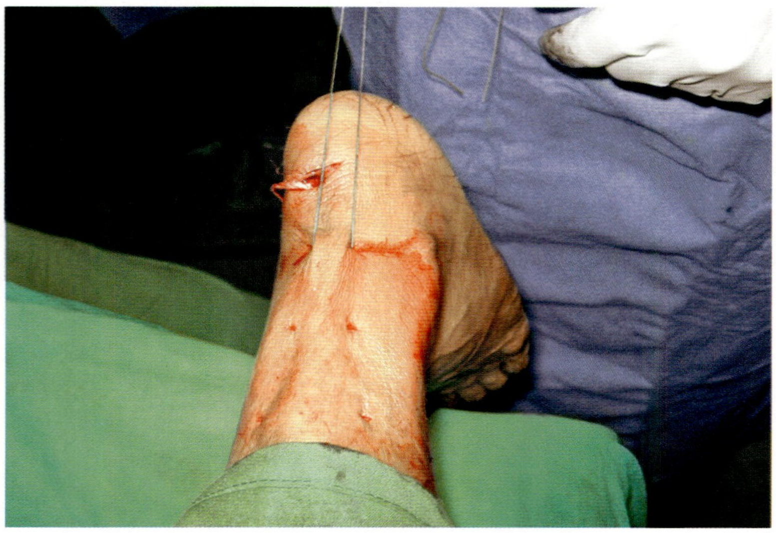

Fig. 24: Repeating steps shown in figures 22 and 23 carries the suture further distally into the tendon.

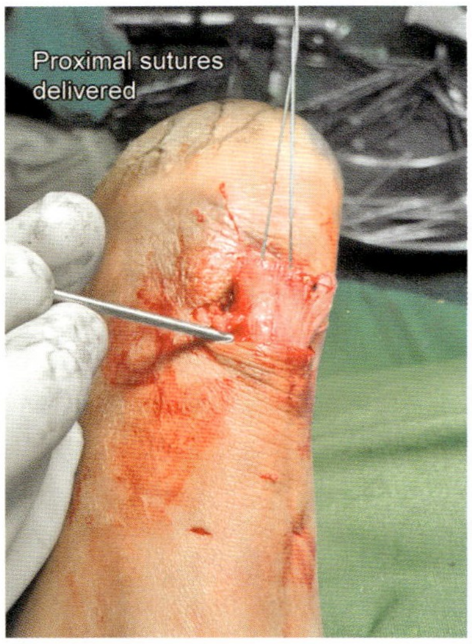

Fig. 25: The suture ends are retrieved and the tendon delivered into the wound. In closed insertional closed tears, a transverse incision is taken proximal to the calcaneal tuberosity to retrieve the suture ends.

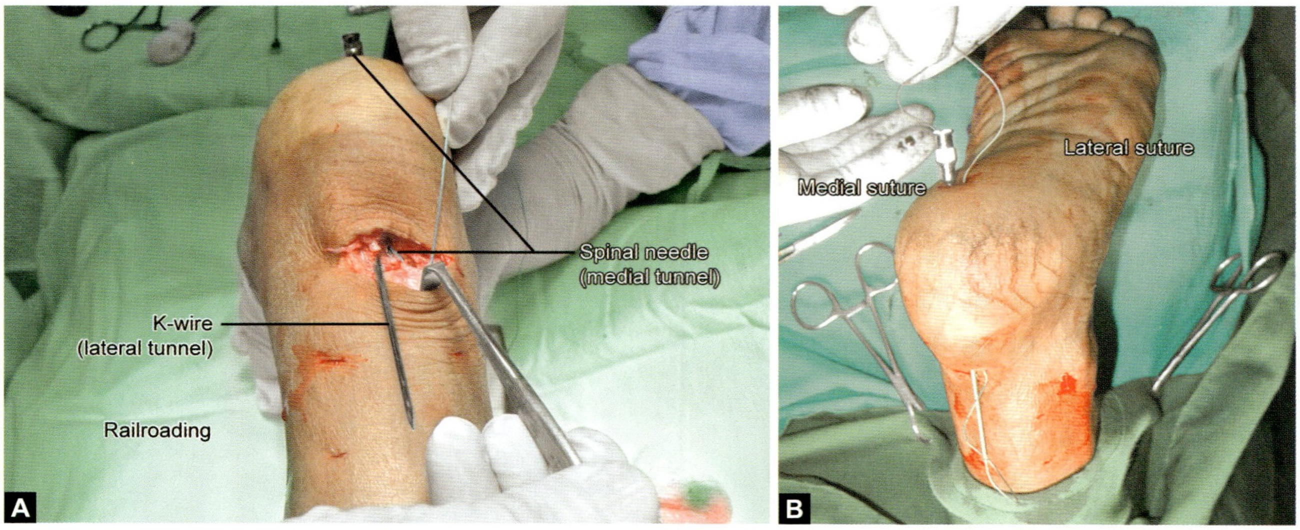

Figs. 26A and B: Using the K-wire needle railroading technique, the sutures are passed into medial and lateral tunnels to exit from the heel.

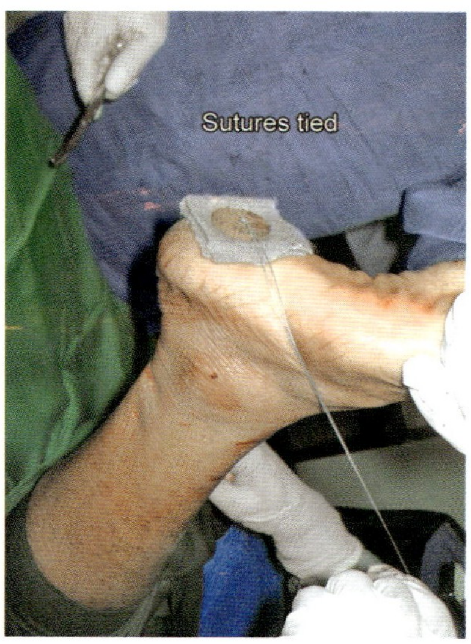

Fig. 27: The sutures are passed through protective felt, sutured over a button over the heel. The knee is flexed and the ankle plantar flexed while tying the suture. The approximation can be checked by palpation at this time. The transverse incision is closed using 4-0 nonaborbable suture material. The stab incisions need not be sutured.

Percutaneous Repair (Figs. 28 to 45)

Midsubstance tears are ideally suited for percutaneous repairs. The technique of Ma and Griffith is used.

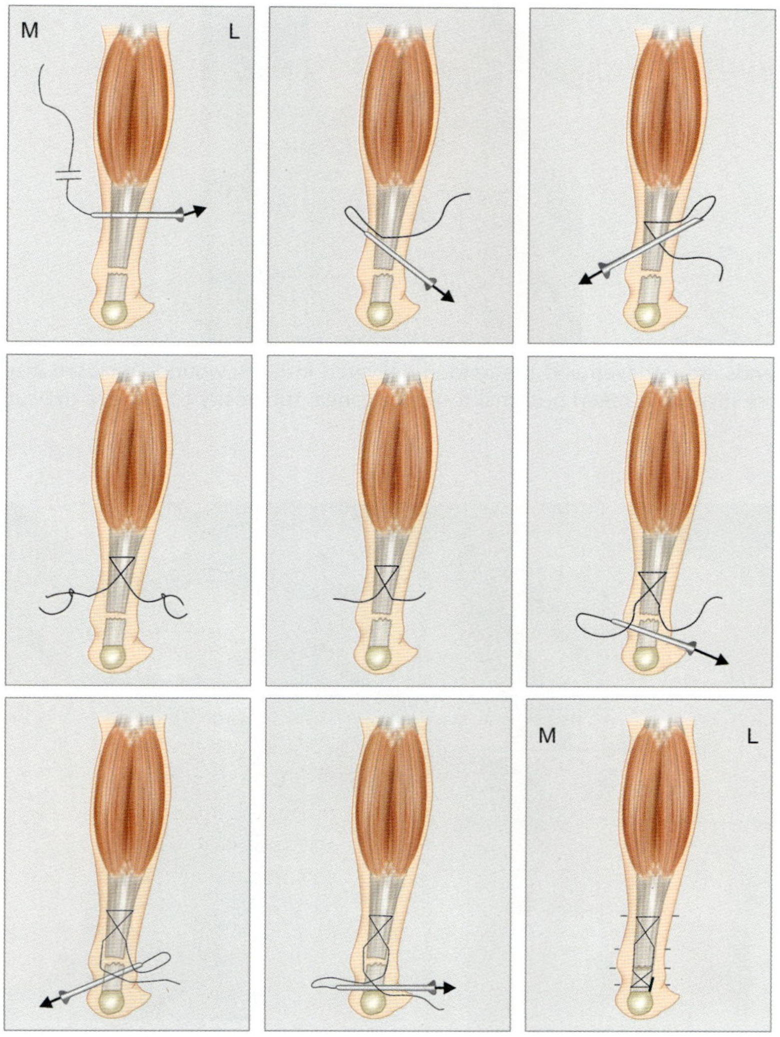

Fig. 28: The Ma Griffith technique for closed midsubstance rupture repair.

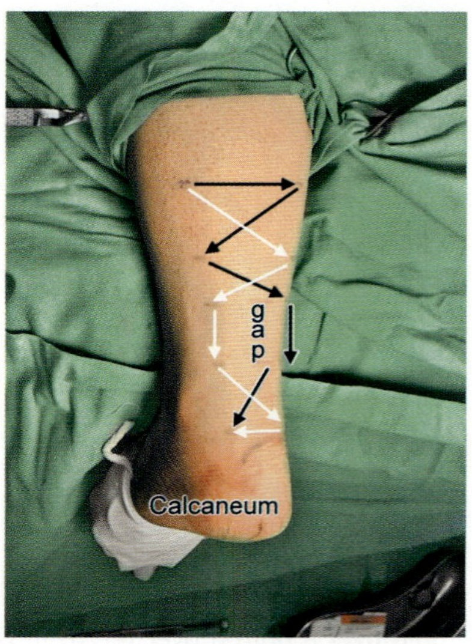

Fig. 29: Planning of the surgery: landmarks marked as calcaneum, gap, and suture entry by marking ink. Arrows show the planned path of suture.

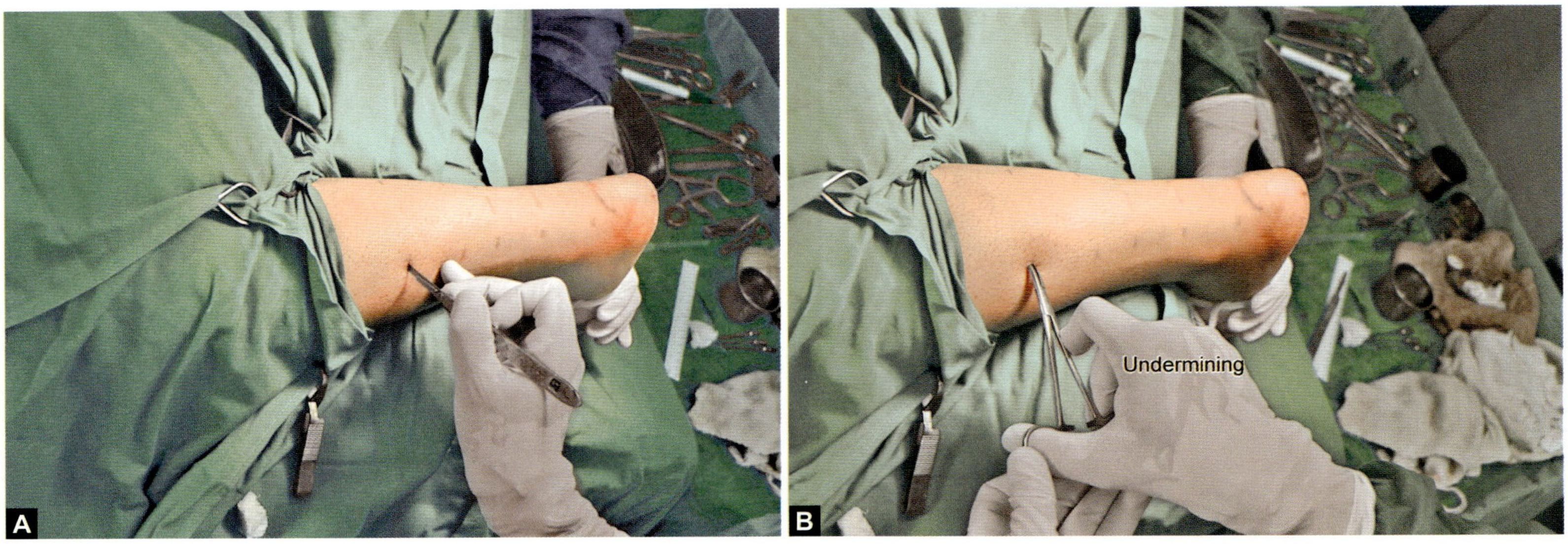

Figs. 30A and B: Incision and undermining.

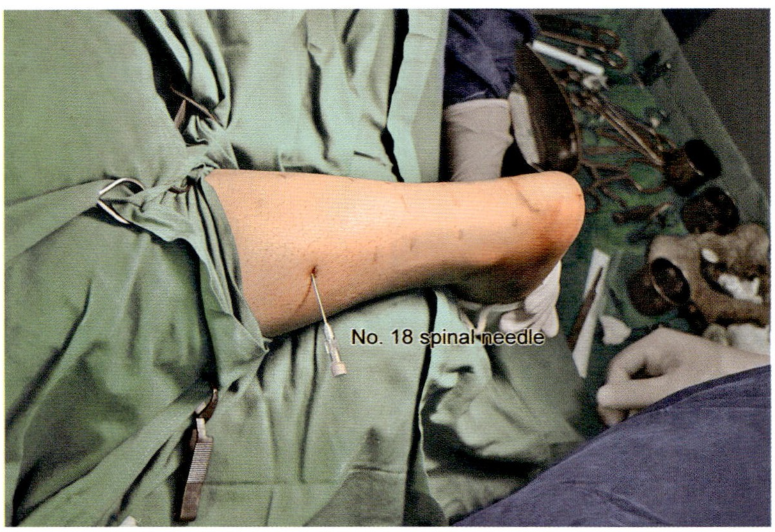

Fig. 31: Passage of spinal needle.

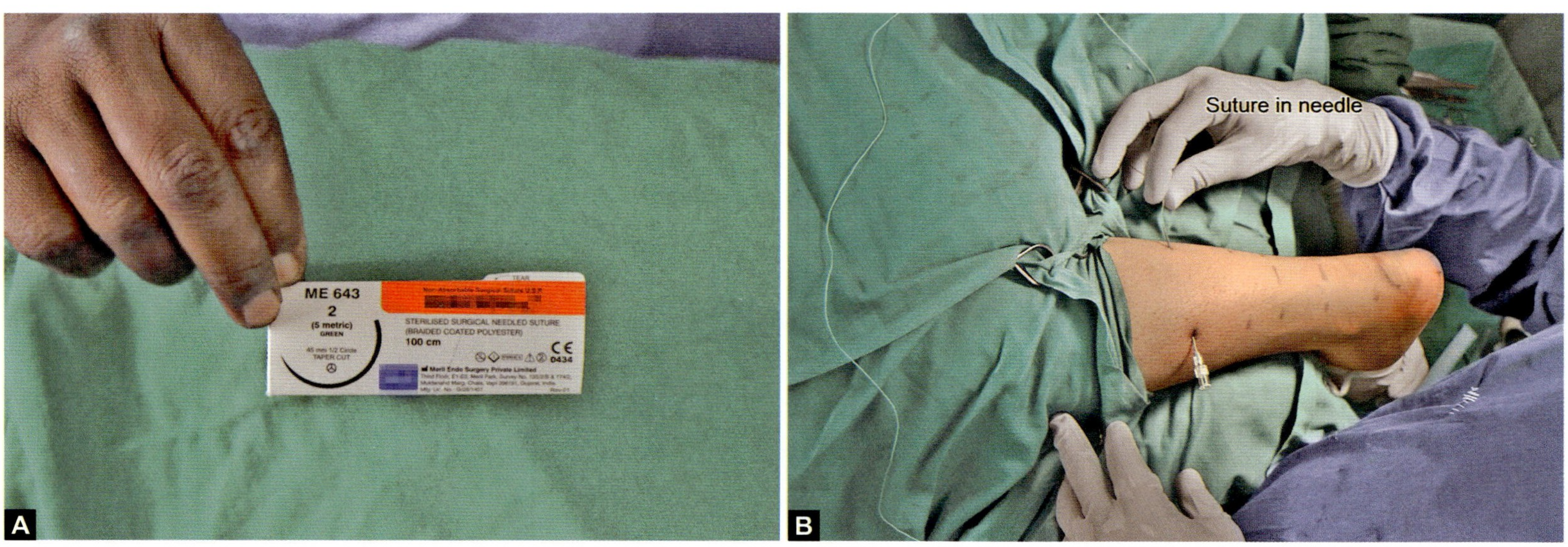

Figs. 32A and B: Nonabsorbable suture No. 2 polyester introduced in needle.

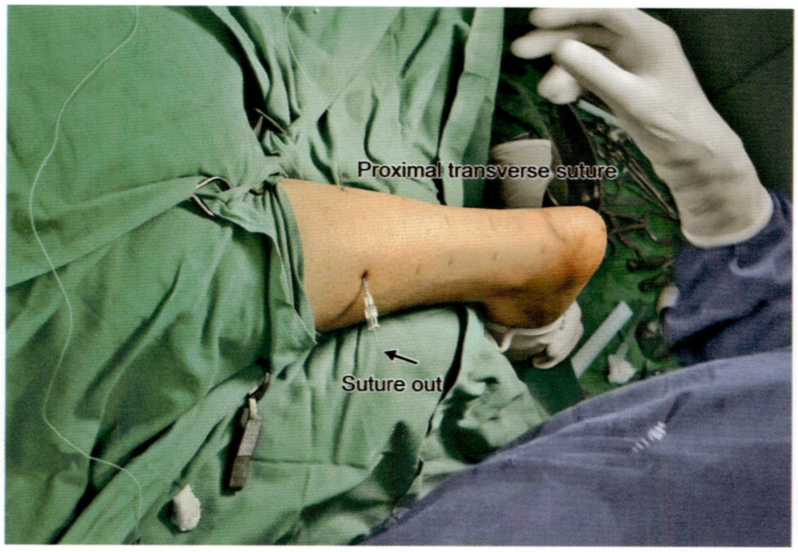

Fig. 33: Proximal transverse suture passed.

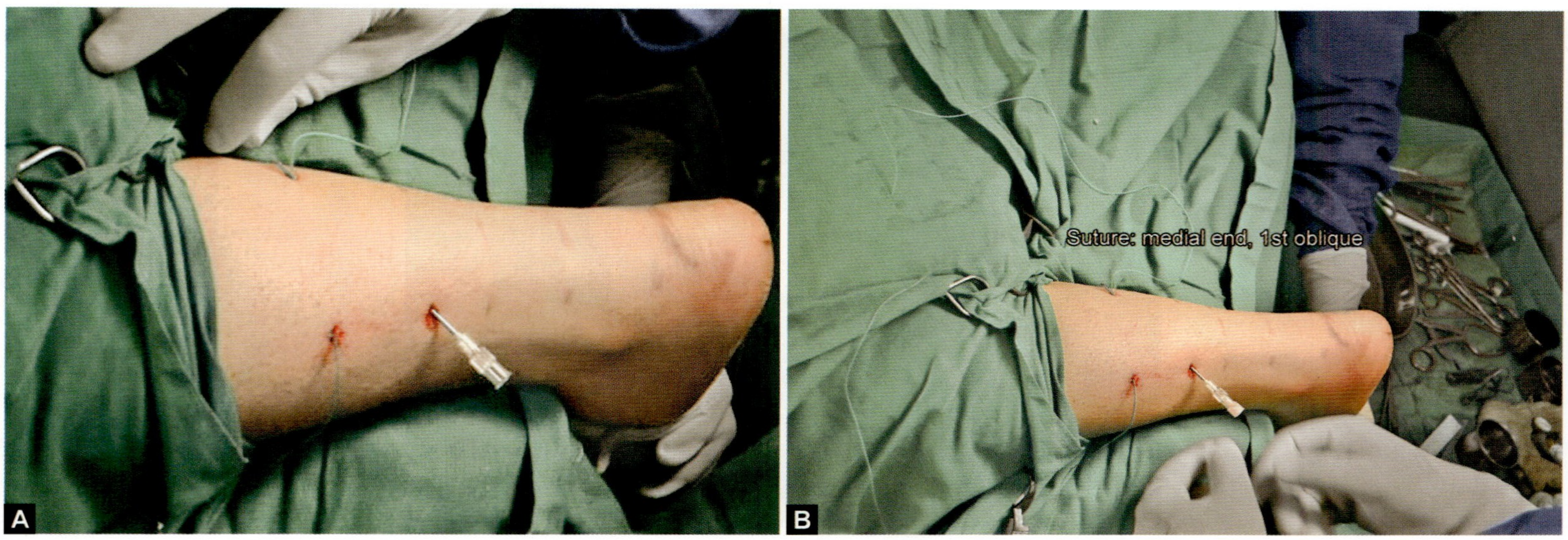

Figs. 34A and B: Passing the medial end, 1st oblique suture.

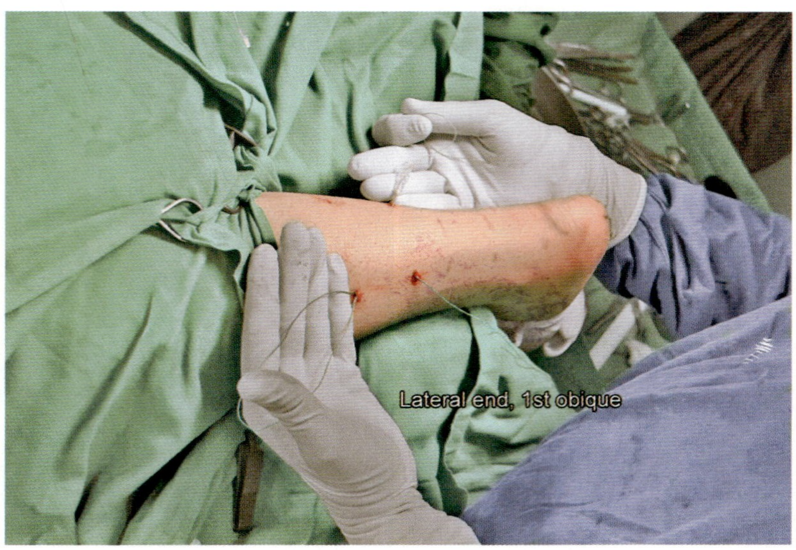

Fig. 35: Lateral end, 1st oblique suture passed.

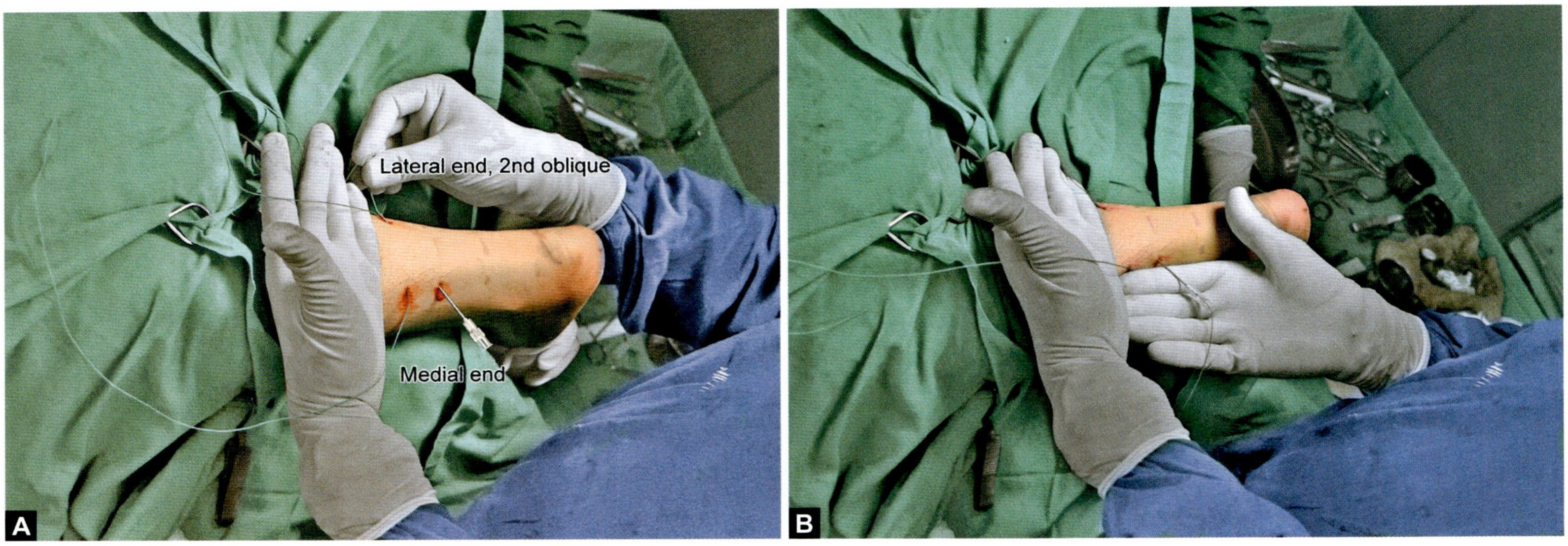

Figs. 36A and B: Lateral end of suture, 2nd oblique suture passed.

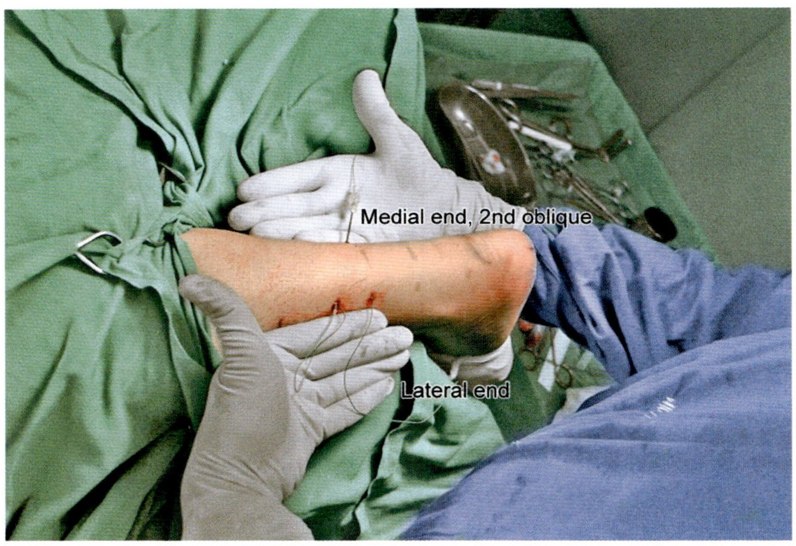

Fig. 37: Medial end 2nd oblique suture passed.

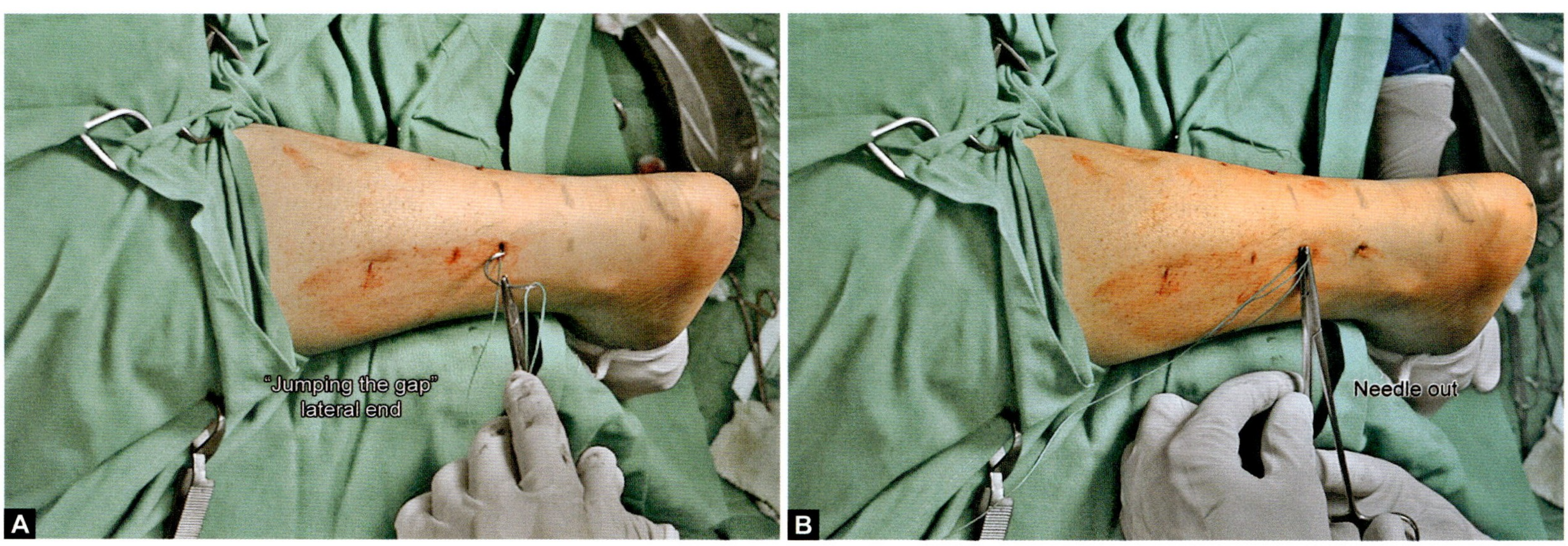

Figs. 38A and B: The suture is brought percutaneously as described till the rupture site. It is then mounted on a large curved needle, and used to "jump the gap".

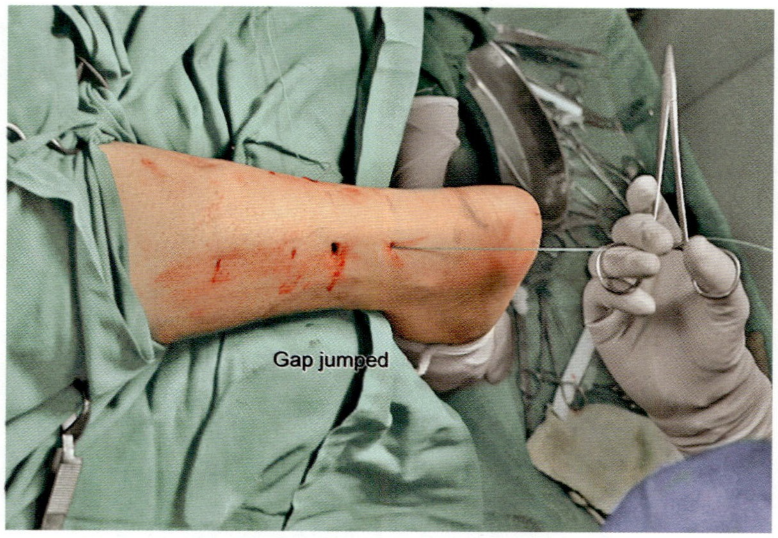

Fig. 39: Gap jumped lateral side.

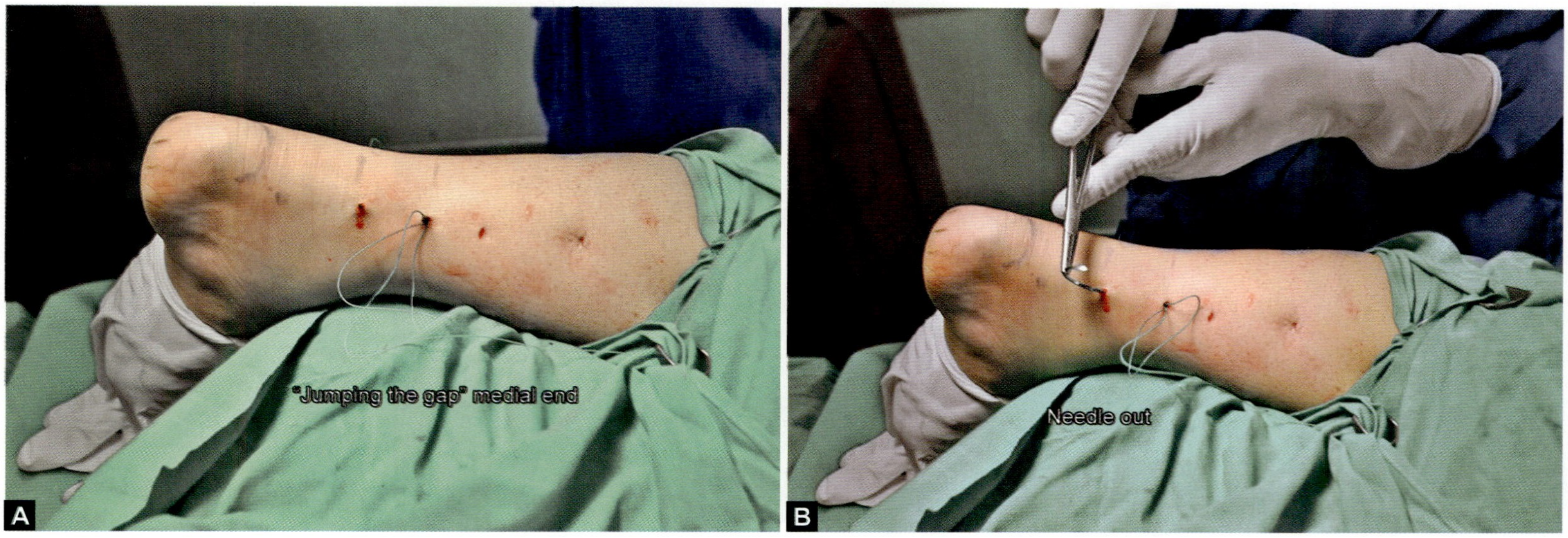

Figs. 40A and B: Gap jumped on medial side.

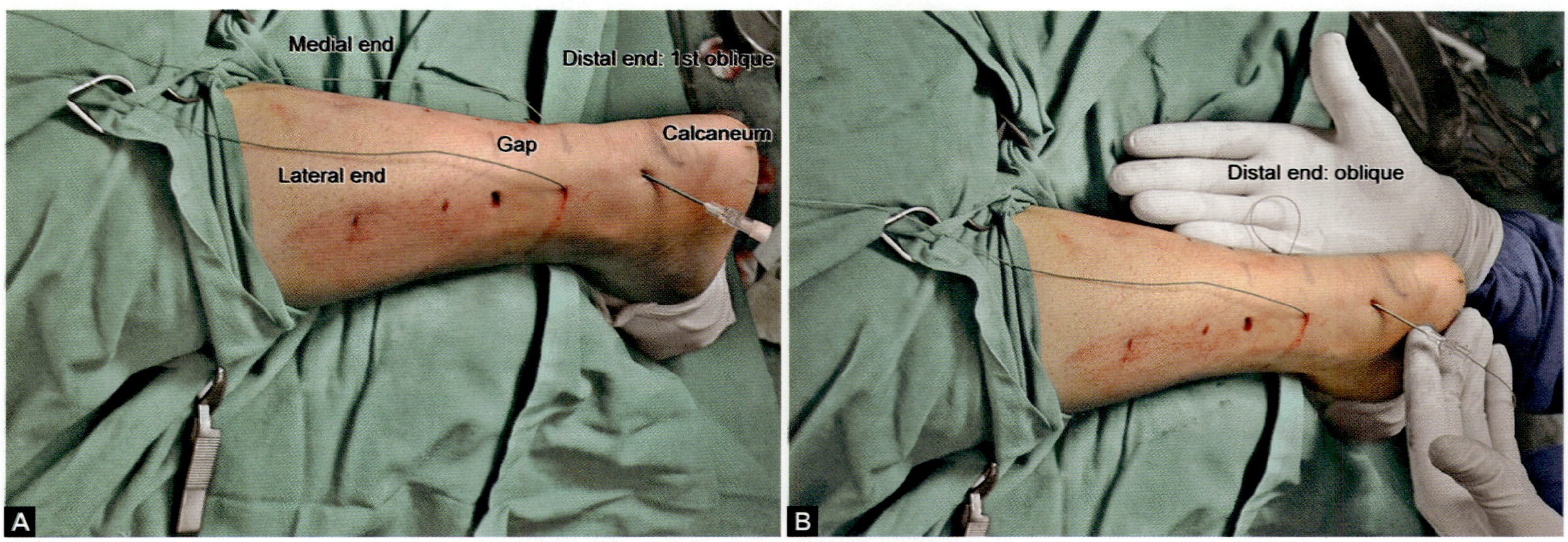

Figs. 41A and B: First distal oblique suture passed.

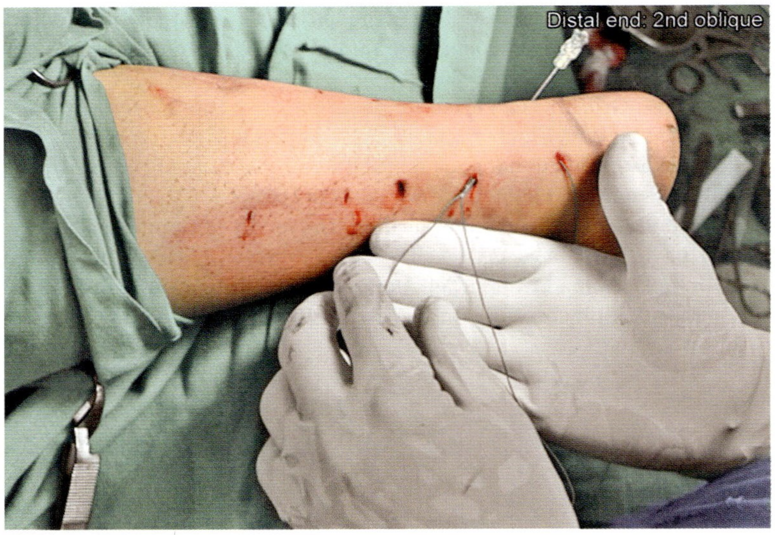

Fig. 42: 2nd distal oblique suture passed.

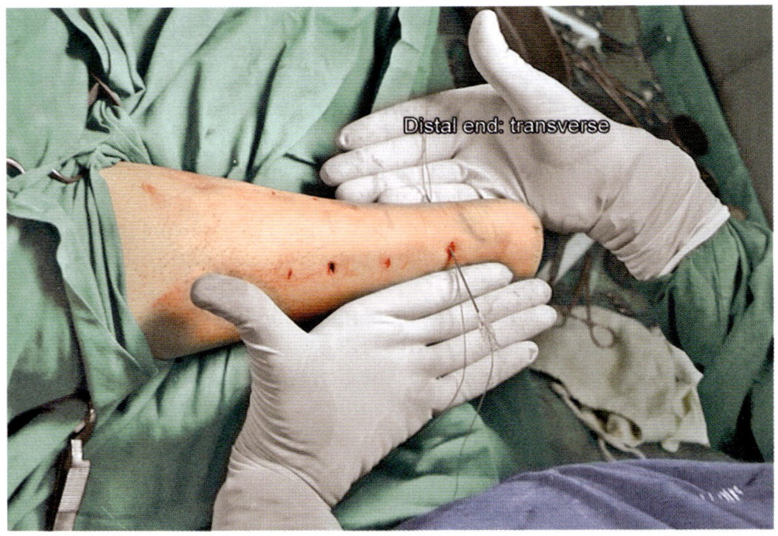

Fig. 43: Distal transverse suture passed.

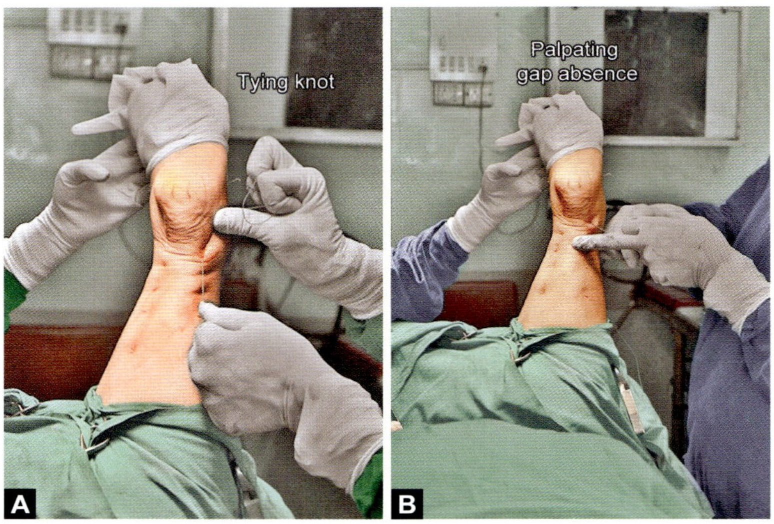

Figs. 44A and B: The knot is tied, and the absence of gap is palpated.

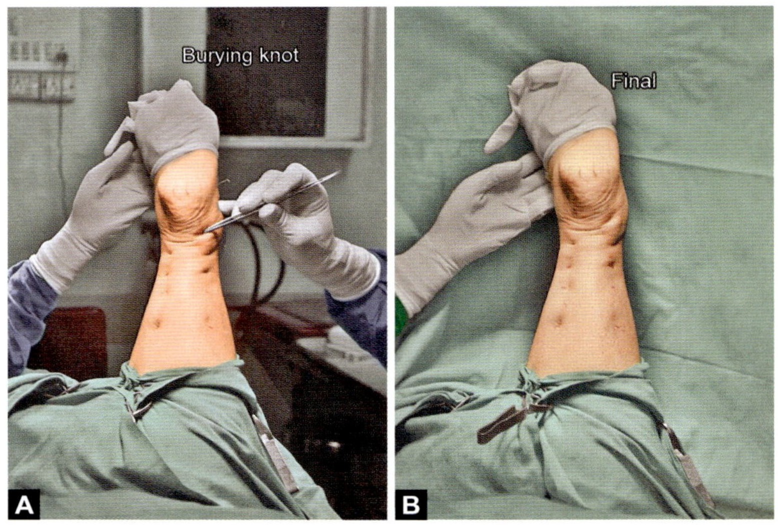

Figs. 45A and B: The knot is buried subcutaneously.

An above knee cast is applied and kept for 6 weeks.

Variations

- Various authors describe different suture patterns. This is a personal choice.
- No 2 absorbable suture can be used. This is to reduce the effect of a possible sural nerve injury.

Complications

- Sural nerve injury with resultant hypoesthesia is the most common complication.
- There are hardly any complications related to wound healing.

FURTHER POSTOPERATIVE PROTOCOL AND REHABILITATION

- After 6 weeks, the cast is removed and a below knee walking cast is applied, incorporating a heel filler of 1-1.5-inch height. The patient bears weight on this cast for 4-6 weeks.
- After this cast is removed, the patient is advised a 1 inch heel-raise in shoes, to be used for 1 month.
- Thereafter, the patient wears normal footwear and does active dorsiflexion exercises.

Photo credits: Dr Navinkumar Yadav, Tanvi Salunkhe

SUGGESTED READING

1. Azar FM, Canale ST, Beaty JH. Chapter 46: Traumatic Disorders. Campbell's Operative Orthopedics, 10th edition. USA: Mosby Inc. [Elsevier]; 2003. pp. 2459-64.
2. Bradley JP, Tibone JE. Percutaneous and open surgical repairs of Achilles tendon ruptures—a comparative study. Am J Sports Med. 19901;8(2): 188-95.
3. Brumann M, Baumbach SF, Mutschler W, et al. Accelerated rehabilitation following Achilles tendon repair: development of an evidence based protocol. Injury. 2014;45(11):1782-90.
4. Cretnik A, Kosanovic M, Smrkolj V. Percutaneous vs open repair of the ruptured Achilles tendon. Am J Sports Med. 2005;33(9):1369-79.
5. Ding WG, Li H, Zhu YP, et al. Comparison between tenocutaneous suture and Kessler suture techniques in treating acute closed Achilles tendon rupture. Foot Ankle Surg. 2014;20(2);105-8.

6. Fu C, Qu W. Mini incision repair with double-Tsuge loop suture vs. open repair with modified kessler suture. Surgeon. 2015;13(4):207-12.
7. García-Germán D, Rubio-Quevedo R, Lopez-Goenaga J, et al. Achilles tendon recurrent rupture following surgical repair. Foot Ankle Surg. 2009;15(3):152-4.
8. Guillo S, Del Bono A, Dias M, et al. Percutaneous repair of acute ruptures of the tendo Achilles. Surgeon. 2013;11(1):14-9.
9. Henriquez H, Munoz R, Carcuro G, et al. Is percutaneous repair better than open repair in acute Achilles tendon rupture? Clin Orthop Rel Res. 2012;470(4):988-1003.
10. Kou J. AAOS clinical practice guideline: acute Achilles tendon rupture. J Am Acad Orth Surg. 2010;18(8):511-3.
11. Labib SA, Rolf R, Dacus R, et al. Gift box repair of the Achilles tendon: a modification of the Krackow technique. Foot Ankle Int. 2009;30(5): 410-14.
12. Lim J, Dalai R, Waseem M. Percutaneous vs open repair of the ruptured Achilles tendon—a prospective randomized controlled study. Foot Ankle Int. 2001;22(7):559-65.
13. Ma GW, Griffith TG. Percutaneous repair of acute closed ruptures Achilles tendon. Clin Orth Rel Res. 1977;(128):247-55.
14. Salunkhe GD. Percutaneous repair for the treatment of rupture of the Achilles tendon. J Foot Ankle Soc. 2014;2(2):51-9.
15. Sathe VM. Personal communication. University of Connecticut; USA; 2010.
16. Young J, Sayana MK, McClelland D, et al. Techniques in foot & ankle surgery. Lippincott, Williams & Wilkins. 2006;5(1):9-14.

CHAPTER 61

Fracture of Neck of Talus: Open Reduction and Internal Fixation

Milind Modak, Neelkamal Sourav

INTRODUCTION

Among tarsal bones, talus is second largest tarsal bone consisting of head, neck, body, lateral process, and posterior process. The posterior process is divided into the medial and lateral tubercle by a groove, which corresponds to flexor hallucis longus (FHL) tendon. About 60% of surface area has articular cartilage covering. Talus fracture is rare type of fracture. Incidence of talus fracture is less than 1% of all fractures. It is second most common tarsal fracture after calcaneus fracture.

MECHANISM OF INJURY

The most common cause of talus fracture is motor vehicle accidents and fall from heights. Most common mechanism of talus neck fracture is axially transmitted force in dorsiflexion and high-energy trauma with hypersupination or pronation of foot cause talar body fracture. About 25% of talar neck fracture have concomitant medial malleolus fracture (hind foot supination injury).

Blood Supply

The arterioles that enter the talus pass through articular cartilage and synovial membrane in which they are vulnerable to trauma. Major blood supply is by three main vessels—(1) posterior tibial artery, (2) anterior tibial artery, and (3) perforating peroneal artery through sinus tarsi. The talus has a very rich intraosseous blood supply.

CLASSIFICATION

Anatomical Classification

- Lateral process fracture
- Posterior fracture
- Talar head fracture
- Talar body fracture
- Talar neck fracture.

Hawkins Classification (1970)

It is used for talar neck fracture (reported rates of osteonecrosis).

- *Type 1*: Nondisplaced (0–30%)
- *Type 2*: Fracture + subtalar subluxation or dislocation (20–50%)
- *Type 3*: Fracture + subtalar + tibiotalar dislocation (83–100%)
- *Type 4 (added by Canale and Kelly, 1978)*: Fracture + subtalar + tibiotalar + talonavicular dislocation.

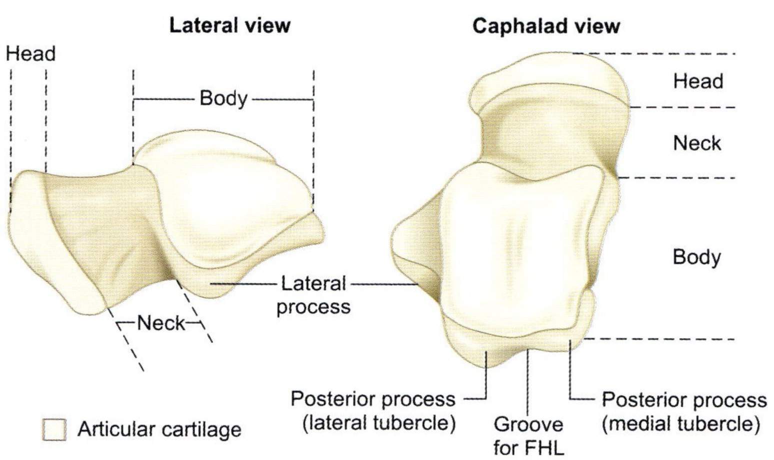

Fig. 1: Anatomy of talus.

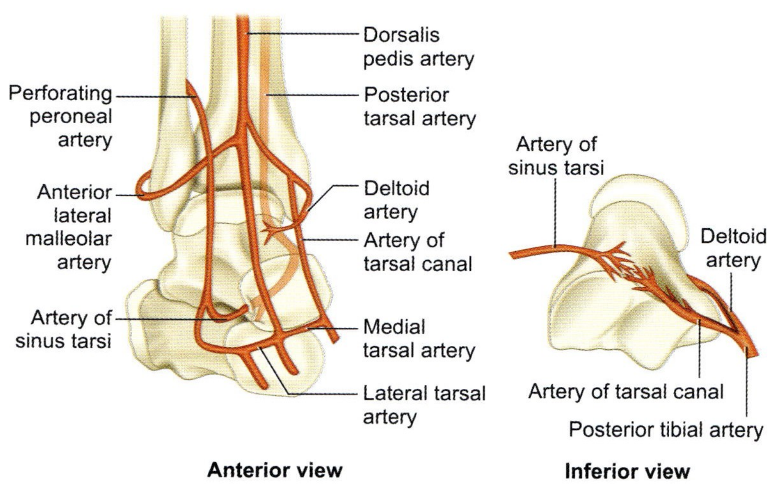

Fig. 2: Blood supply of talus bone.

Sneppen Classification

For body of talus fracture:
- *Group 1:* Transchondral dome fracture:
  - Horizontal
  - Sagittal
  - Coronal
- *Group 2:* Shear fracture
- *Group 3:* Posterior tubercle fracture
- *Group 4:* Lateral process fracture
- *Group 5:* Crush fracture.

Mullers AO/OTA Classification

In this system of classification, fractures are grouped according to increasing severity with increasing treatment difficulty and worst prognosis:
- *C1:* Osteochondral injuries with ankle joint involvement
- *C2:* Subtalar joint involvement
- *C3:* Ankle and subtalar joint involvement.

CLINICAL PRESENTATION

Patients present with severe pain associated with gross swelling at ankle joint, unable to move ankle, and ecchymosis is present. Shape of hindfoot and ankle joint is distorted, if associated dislocation is present.

RADIOGRAPHIC EVALUATION

Plane X-ray with anteroposterior, lateral, and mortise view is required for evaluation of neck in addition we use canale view. In canale view, foot is in 15° pronation and plantigrade on an X-ray film and angle of the beam at 75° to the horizontal.
- Computed tomography (CT) scan with 3D reconstruction gives excellent visualization of the congruity of the subtalar joint and comminution and displacement of the fracture fragment as well as associated adjoining fracture.
- Magnetic resonance imaging (MRI) scan is important to diagnose osteonecrosis.

TREATMENT OPTIONS

Talar Neck Fracture

Hawkins Type 1

Generally, nonoperative management is opted for by nonweight-bearing cast with ankle in slight equinus for 1 month then short leg walking cast is applied for 2 more months till clinical and X-ray signs of healing appear.

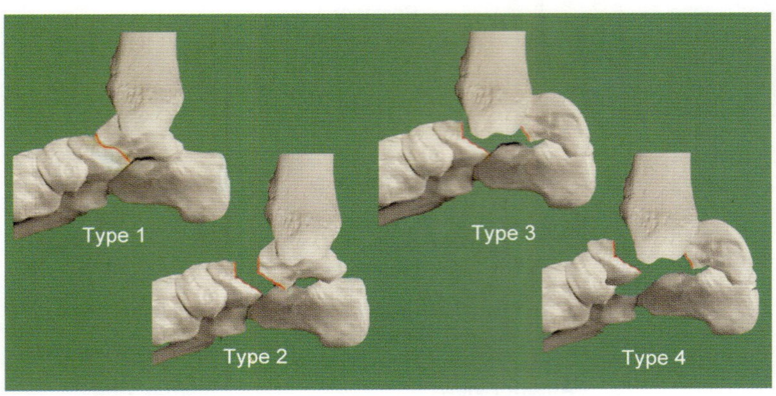

Fig. 3: Hawkins classification.

Hawkins Types 2, 3, and 4

These intra-articular displaced fractures must be reduced anatomically and fixed securely. Surgical intervention is in form of screw fixation by either anterior to posterior or posterior to anterior direction. In case of comminution to maintain the length of talus, mini plates may be used.

These fractures are approached by either anteromedial or anterolateral incision.

Talar Body Fracture

As it is weight-bearing area and forms joint surface of ankle, anatomical reduction is important. Anteromedial approach with medial malleolus osteotomy is used most commonly.

Talectomy alone or talectomy with calcaneotibial fusion may be used in comminuted talar body fracture that can not be reconstructed.

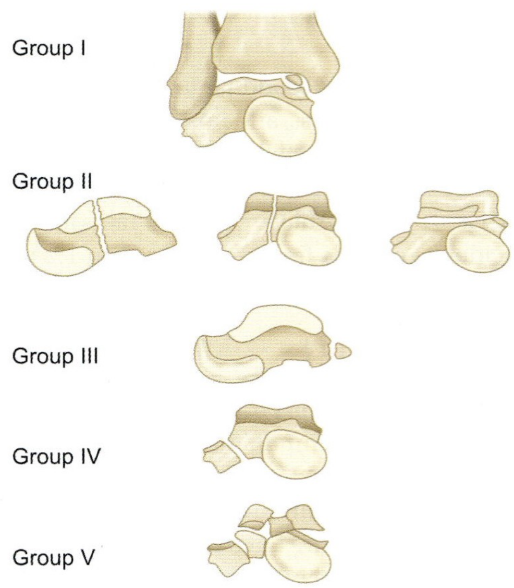

Fig. 4: Sneppen classification.

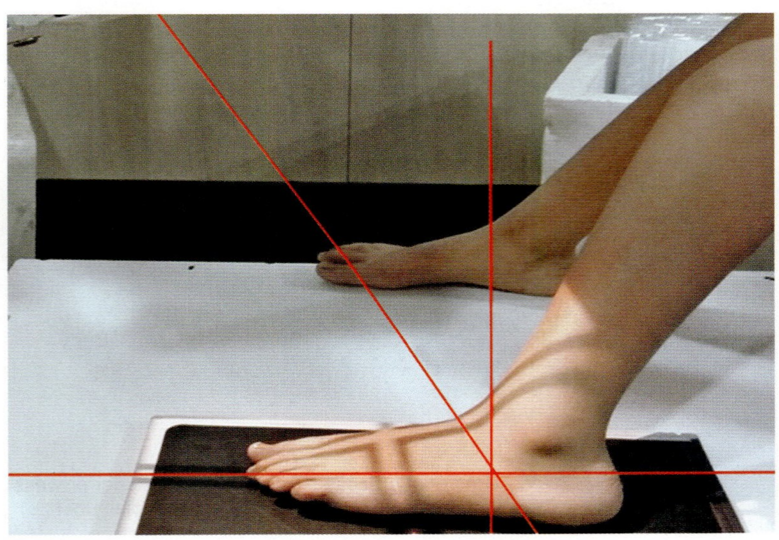
Fig. 5: Canale view positioning of foot.

SURGICAL STEPS

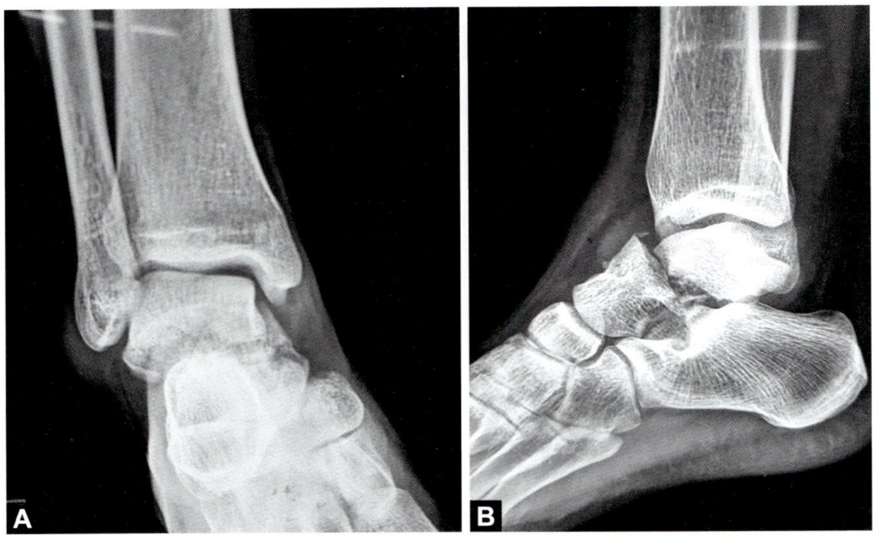

Figs. 6A and B: *X-rays*: Routine ankle and foot anteroposterior (AP) and lateral radiograph necessary, including AP, mortise, and lateral view. Lateral view shows neck of talus, and talonavicular, tibiotalar, and talocalcaneal joint incongruencies can be evaluated. Mortise view for tibiotalar and AP view of foot for talonavicular joint incongruencies.

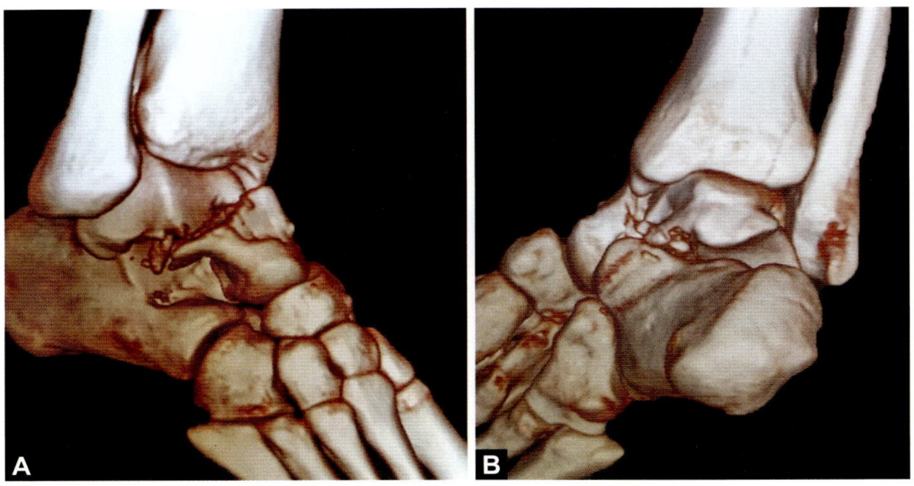

Figs. 7A and B: *Computed tomography (CT) scan*: Look for associated fracture and evaluate comminution and displacement of talus fracture.

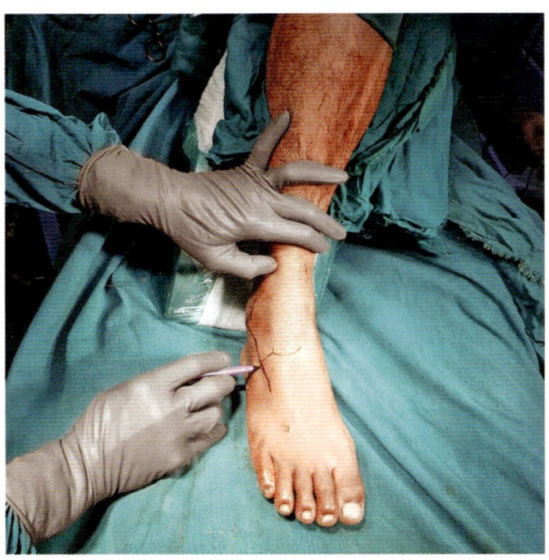

Fig. 8: *Positioning and lateral incision marking*: Supine position with bump over ipsilateral buttock with lower extremity either extended or flexed at knee to facilitate C-arm imaging during surgery. Radiolucent table top is necessary. Start at the anteroinferior part of the lateral malleolus and proceed in line with the 4th ray of the foot up to the base of 4th metatarsal.

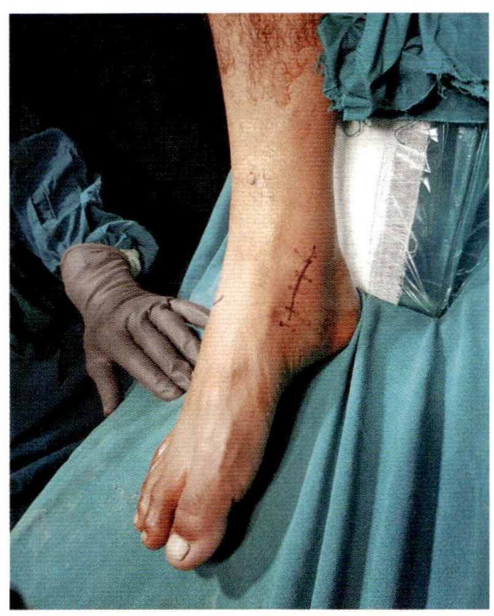

Fig. 9: *Position and medial incision marking*: Start at medial malleolus and extend up to the tuberosity of the navicular. Dissection should be least traumatic, being careful of the blood supply and soft tissue.

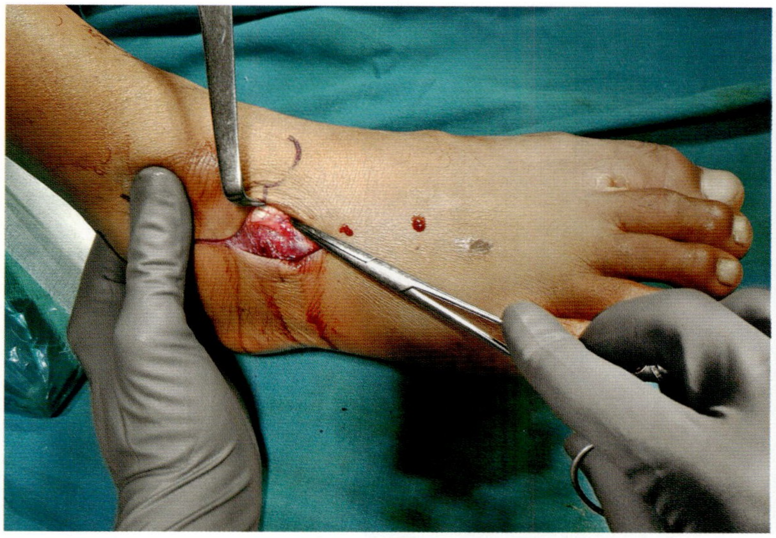

Fig. 10: *Incisions deepened and fracture seen:* In case of comminuted fractures it is better to expose from both sides to ensure accurate reduction of fracture. Skin flaps are to be maintained as thick as possible around ankle area.

- On lateral side dissection, preserve superficial peroneal nerve in proximal part of incision. Interval between extensor digitorum longus tendon and extensor brevis muscle is used. Fat pad of sinus tarsi is incised to visualize the lateral talar neck, lateral process, lateral talar head, and lateral dome.
- On anteromedial dissection, care to be taken to protect long saphenous vein and saphenous nerve.

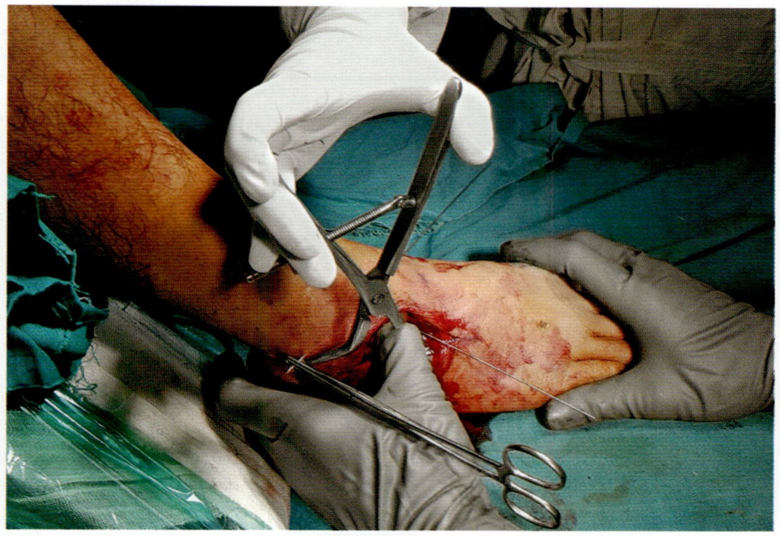

Fig. 11: Reduction clamp seen holding reduction of fracture. K-wires used as joysticks and external fixator to distract fracture are useful reduction aids.

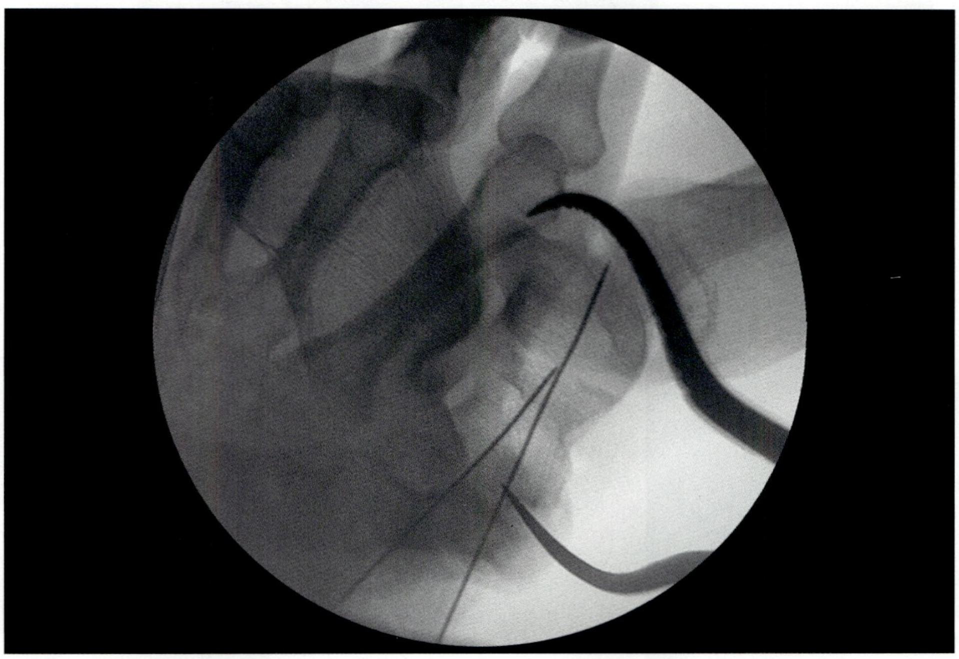

Fig. 12: *Intraoperative C-arm picture*: Satisfactory reduction and alignment hold by reduction clamp and provisional fixation by K-wire.

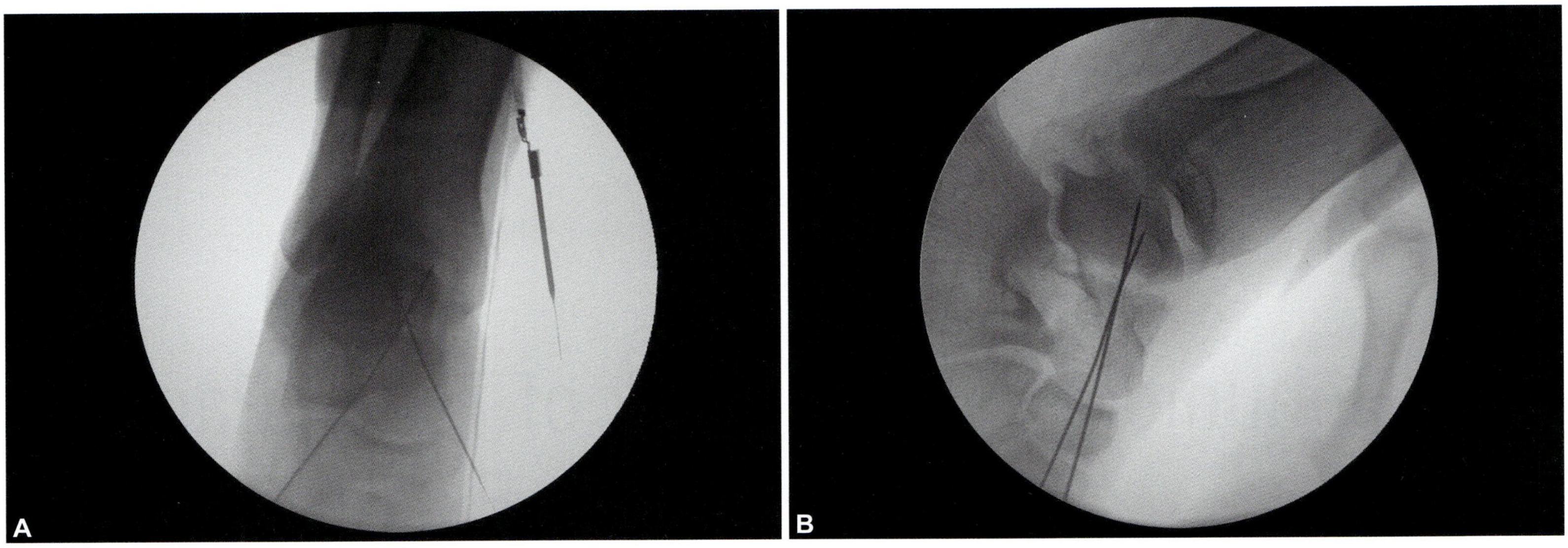

Figs. 13A and B: *Intraoperative C-arm picture:* (A) Anteroposterior (AP) view showing provisional fixation by K-wire (guidewire used for cannulated screw). (B) Lateral view showing the provisional fixation by K-wire (guidewire).

- Cannulated screws are passed over K-wires/guidewires. On noncomminuted side, which is usually lateral one, half-threaded compression screw is applied and on comminuted side, which is usually medial full-threaded position screw is used. Length of screw and screw position should be adequate. Countersinking of head is required when entry is through articular cartilage. At times, contoured mini plates are required to bridge severe comminution and prevent shortening.
- Closure is performed in layers in a standard routine manner.

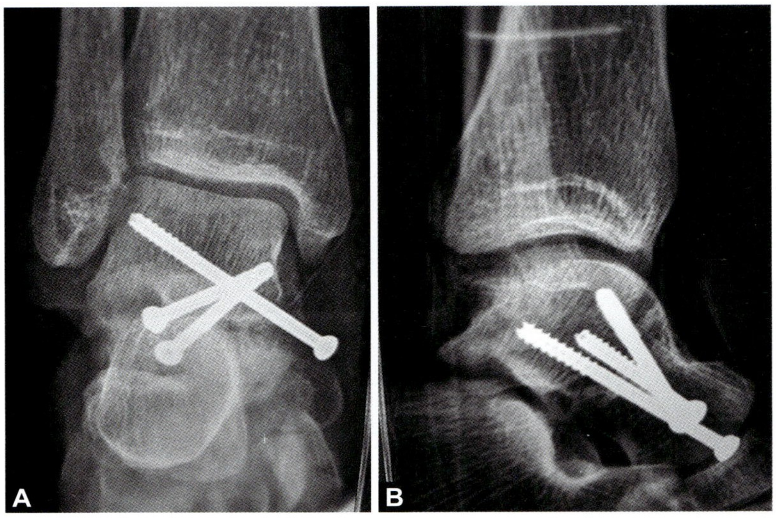

Figs. 14A and B: *Postoperative X-ray* showing good position of implant and fracture: (A) Anteroposterior view; and (B) Lateral view.

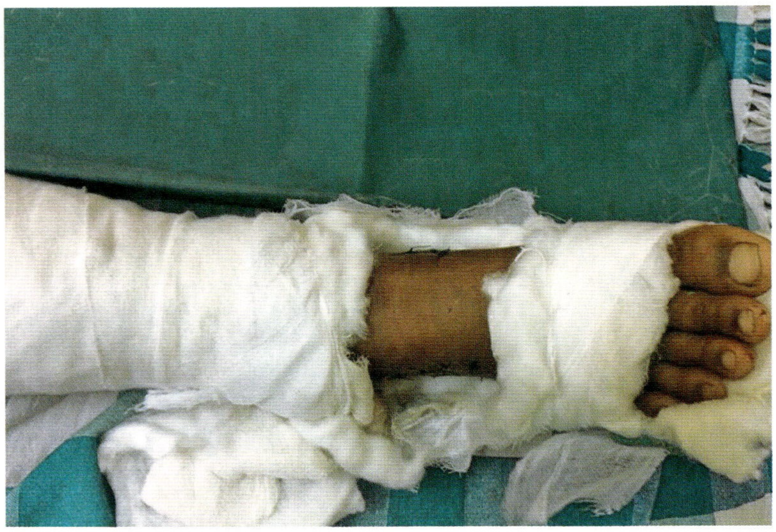

Fig. 15: *Postoperative care and rehabilitation:* After fixation, closure is performed. Suction drain is used, if oozing is expected. Short limb posterior splint is applied. If the fixation is stable, ankle mobilization can be commenced after 6 weeks. However, if the fracture is comminuted and there is extensive soft tissue injury, the posterior splint is continued for 12 weeks. The patient is advised progressive weight-bearing after 12 weeks.

COMPLICATIONS

Avascular necrosis (AVN) of talus is the most common complication seen after talus fracture. On X-ray, Hawkins sign (seen at 8 weeks), a subchondral lucency on mortise view is indicative of intact blood supply and indicates good prognosis. It suggests viability of bone.

Malunion, nonunion, and subtalar arthritis are rare complication.

PEARLS

- To look for and manage associated fractures—as evident on CT scan
- Plan approach in view of blood supply and soft tissue injury
- Displaced neck fracture should be approached, reduced and fixed from medial and the lateral side, simultaneously and not sequentially
- If a medial malleolus osteotomy is planned, take care of the posterior tibial tendon.

SUGGESTED READING

1. Canale ST, Kelly FB Jr. Fractures of the neck of the talus: long-term evaluation of 71 cases. J Bone Joint Surg Am. 1978;60:143-56.
2. Coltart WD. Aviator's astragalus. J Bone Joint Surg. 1952;34B:545-66.
3. Hawkins LG. Fractures of the neck of the talus. J Bone Joint Surg Am. 1970;52:991-1002.
4. Swanson TV, Bray TJ, Holmes GB Jr. Fractures of the talar neck. A mechanical study of fixation. J Bone Joint Surg Am. 1992;74:544-51.

CHAPTER 62

Nonunion Fracture Neck of Talus, Pantalar Fusion using External Fixator

Chandan V Bhole, Jignesh Yeshwant Tandel, Rachit Vipul Shah

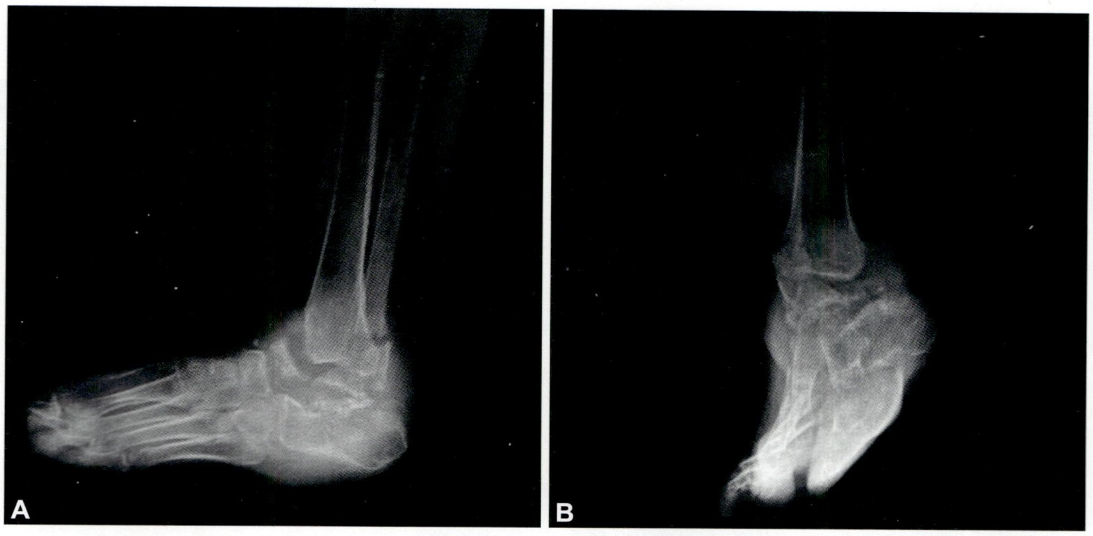

Figs. 1A and B: Lateral and AP X-rays of ankle joint showing arthritic changes secondary to nonunion of fracture talus.

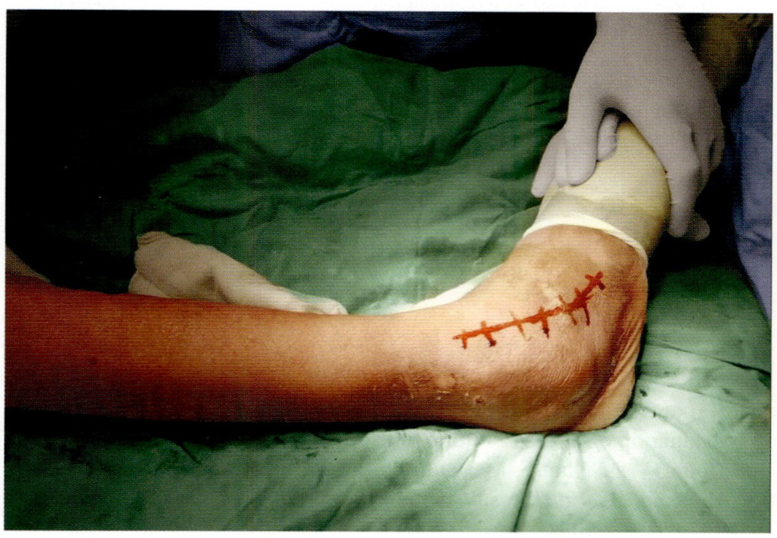

Fig. 2: Incision marked at anterolateral aspect of ankle.

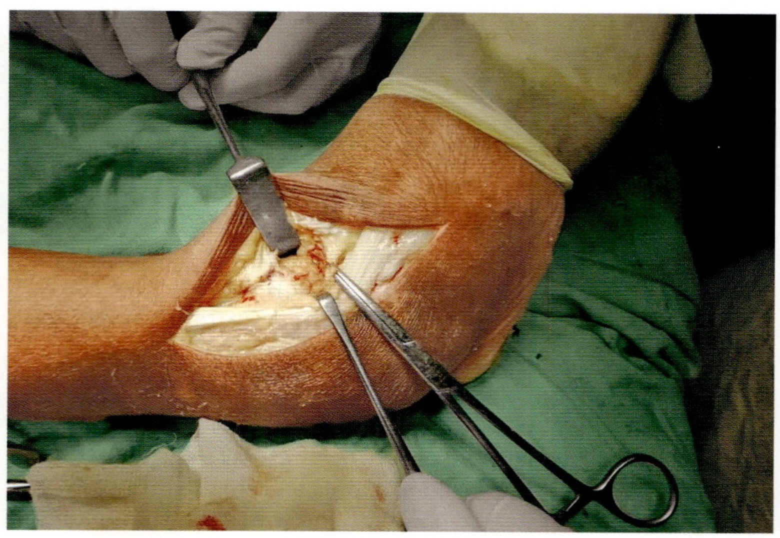

Fig. 3: Skin and subcutaneous tissue incised, extensor digitorum tendons retracted, sinus tarsi fat exposed.

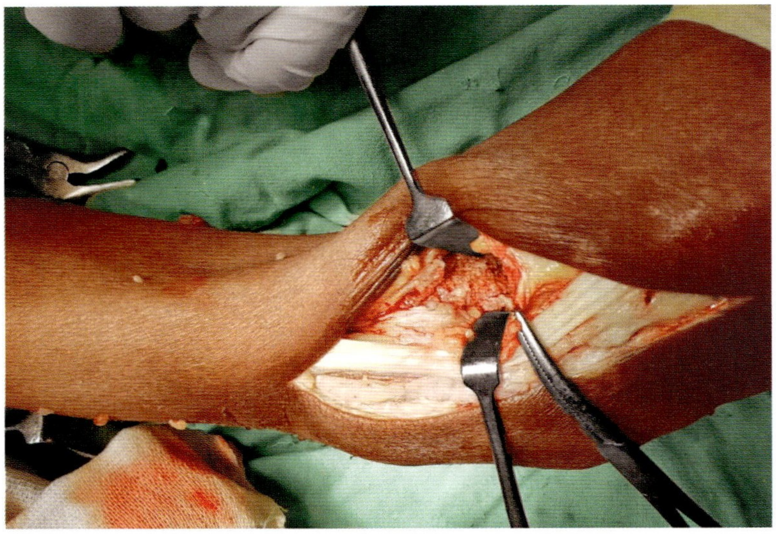

Fig. 4: Ankle capsule opened to complete arthrotomy.

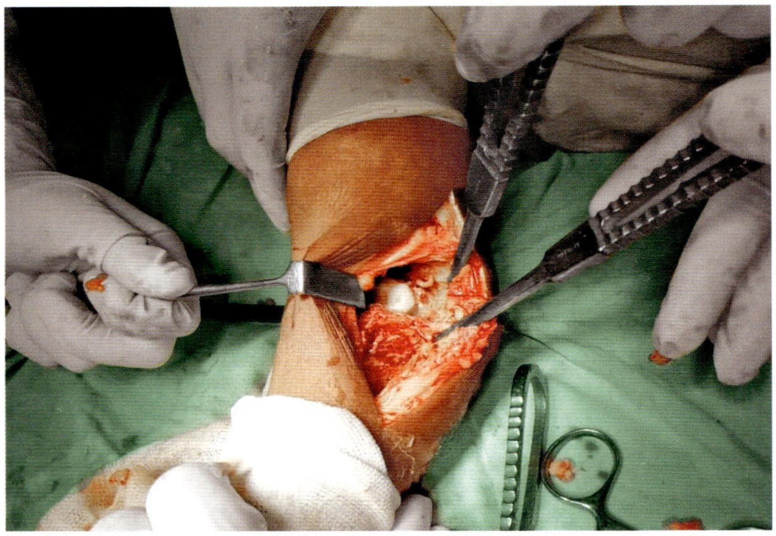

Fig. 5: Joint debridement done.

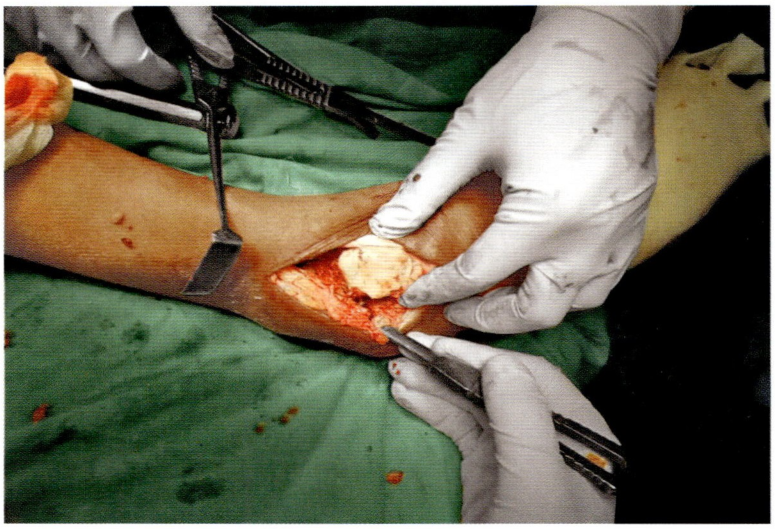

Fig. 6: Talus fracture fragments exposed.

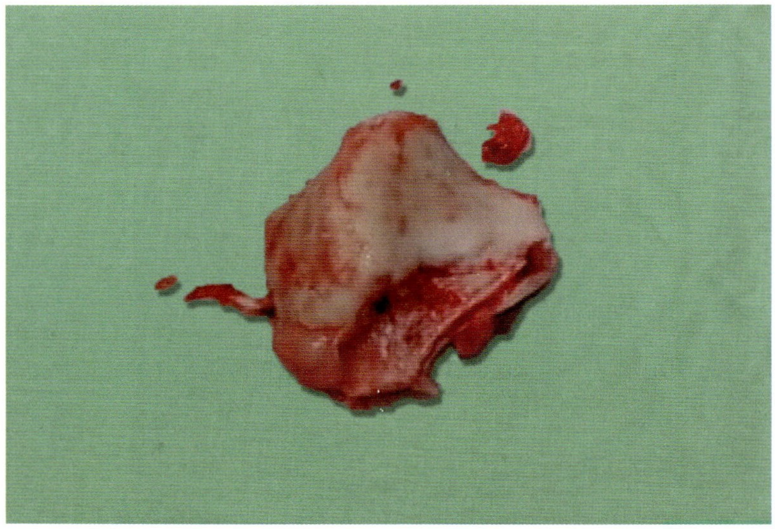

Fig. 7: Excised talar fragment.

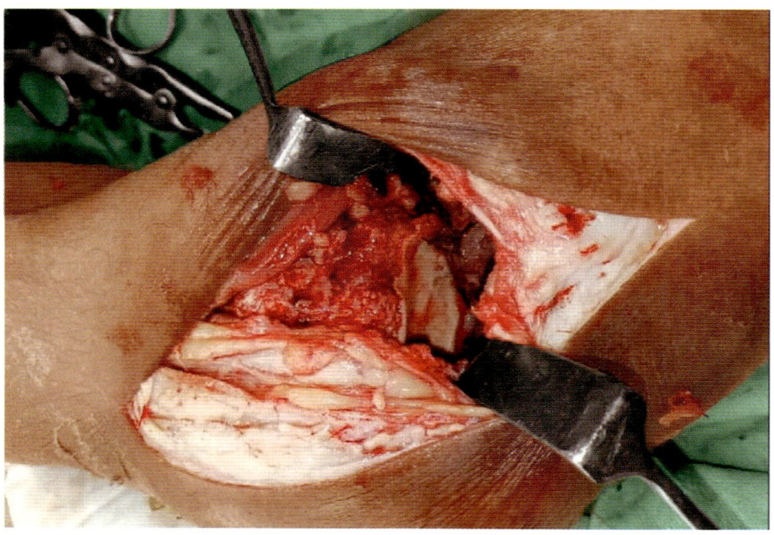

Fig. 8: Exposure of undersurface of tibia for removal of cartilage.

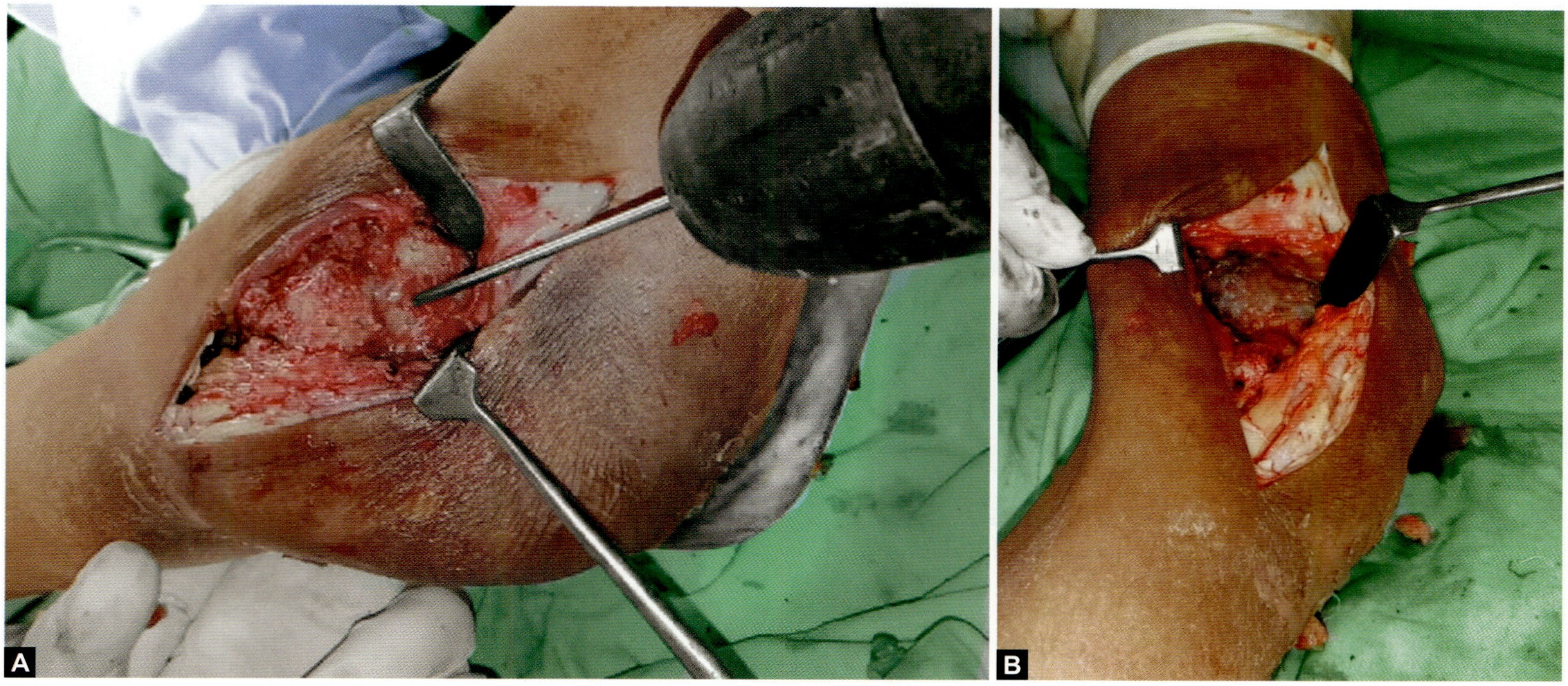

Figs. 9A and B: Bone graft and temporary K-wire fixation.

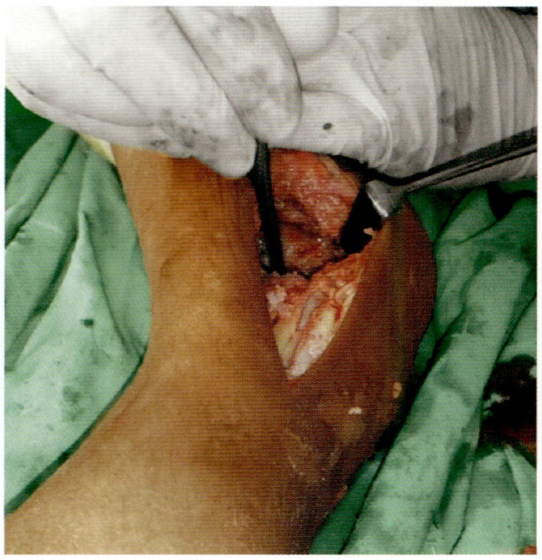

Fig. 10: Graft packed into ankle and subtalar joint area.

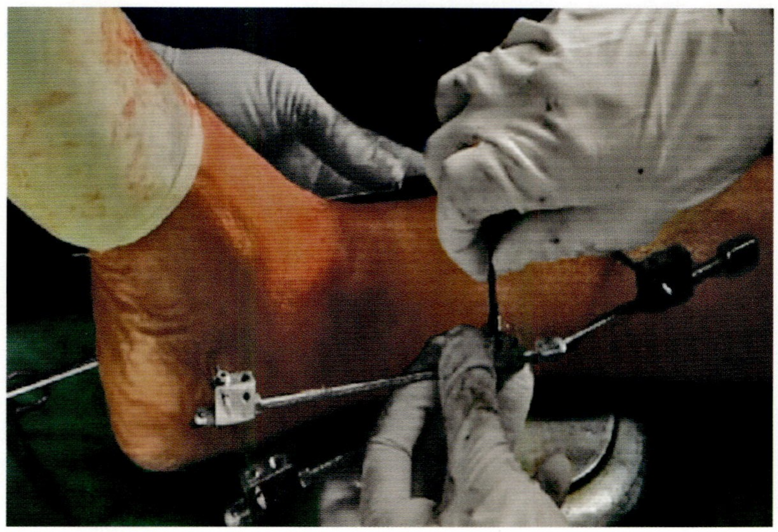

Fig. 11: External fixator applied.

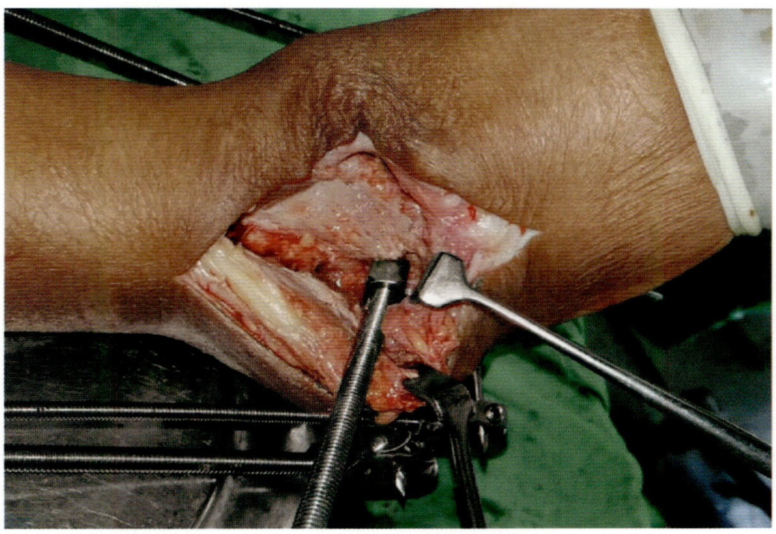

Fig. 12: Bone graft punched in space between tibia and calcaneum.

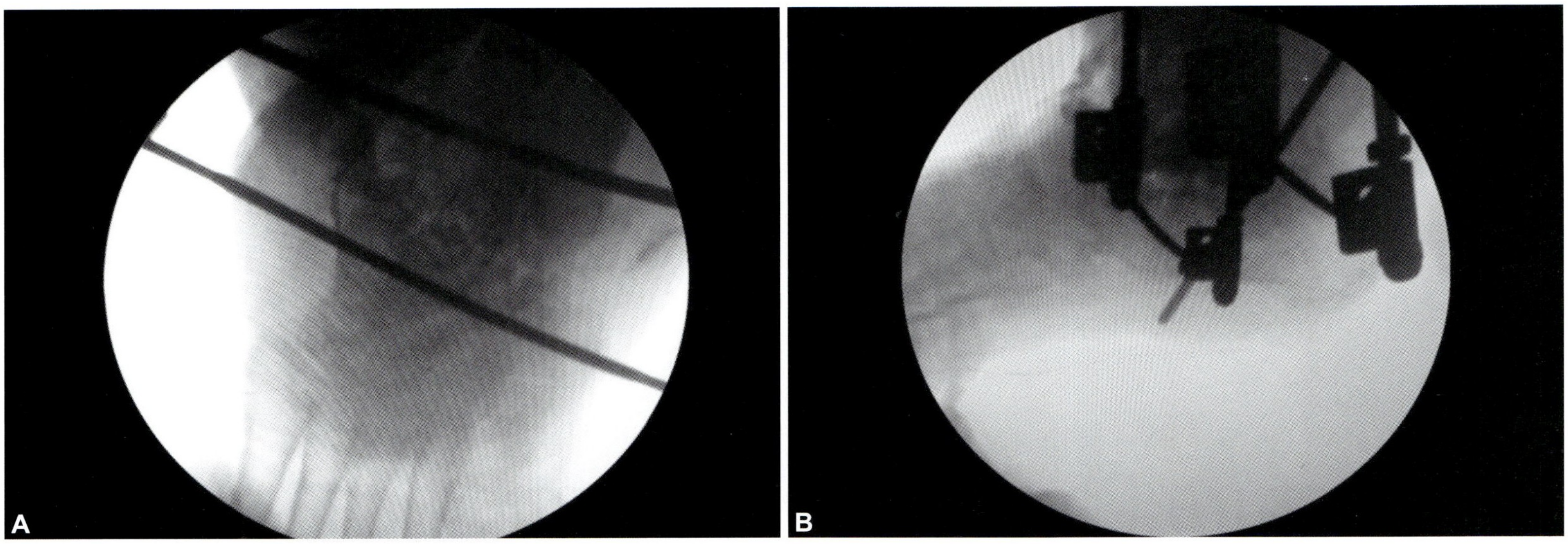

Figs. 13A and B: AP and Lateral C-arm image of tibiocalcaneal fusion.

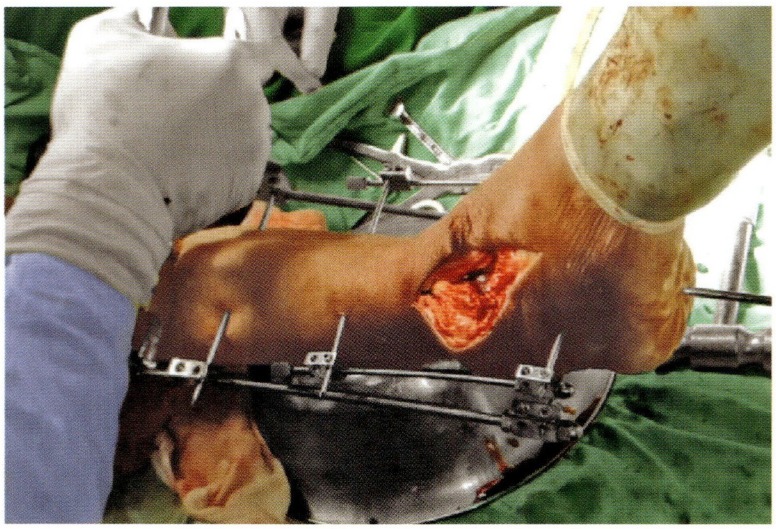

Fig. 14: Final external fixator positioning.

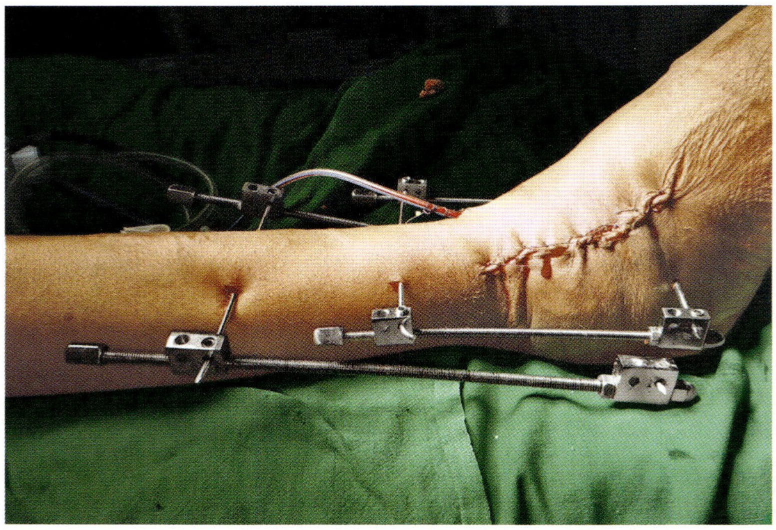

Fig. 15: Wound closure.

CHAPTER 63

Fracture Calcaneum Reduction and Fixation

S Prakash, Amit R Kale, Nitish Agrawal, Vijay M Panchanadikar, Anurag Daxini, Nagesh Naik, Rajkumar Ekambaram, Siddharth Hardikar

FRACTURE CALCANEUM CC SCREW FIXATION

S Prakash, Amit R Kale, Nitish Agrawal

INTRODUCTION

Calcaneum is most frequently fractured tarsal bone. Peak incidence of fracture is in males aged 20–29 years. Displaced intra-articular fractures comprise vast majority of all calcaneus fractures. Approximately, 10% of calcaneus fractures are open injuries. 70% of calcaneal fractures occur due to fall from height. Bilateral calcaneus fractures are present in 5–10% of cases.

MECHANISM OF INJURY

- Axial loading due to fall from height is responsible for most intra-articular fractures.
- Twisting forces are responsible for extra-articular calcaneus fractures like sustentaculum, anterior and medial processes fractures.

CLINICAL FEATURES

Severe heel pain, tenderness, swelling, heel widening, and shortening are typical presenting features. Ecchymosis of heel and blistering of skin may also be present.

- Compartment syndrome of foot may happen, which results in clawing of the lesser toes.
- Concomitant injuries like lumbar spine fractures and lower limb fractures found in 50% of patients of fracture calcaneus and associated with high energy injuries.

RADIOGRAPHIC EVALUATION

- Lateral view of the hindfoot, anteroposterior (AP) view of the foot, a Harris axial view, and an ankle series.
- On lateral radiograph, decrease in Bohler angle (normally between 20° and 40°) indicates that the weight-bearing posterior facet of the calcaneus has collapsed and increase in the Gissane (crucial) angle (normal between 105° and 135°), indicates collapse of the posterior facet.
- In Harris axial view, joint surface, loss of height, increase in width, and angulation of the tuberosity fragment are visualized.

Computed tomography (CT) scan images are taken in axial, 30° semicoronal plane, and sagittal planes and are taken 2–3 mm slices.

- *The axial view*—calcaneocuboid joint, the anteroinferior aspect of the posterior facet, and the sustentaculum tali.
- *Sagittal reconstruction*—posterior facet, calcaneal tuberosity, and its anterior process.

CLASSIFICATION

Extra-articular Fractures

- Anterior process fractures
- Tuberosity fractures
- Medial process fractures
- Sustentacular fractures
- Body fractures without involving the subtalar joint.

Intra-articular Fractures

Essex–Lopresti Classification

Primary fracture line: The fracture line exits anterolaterally at the crucial angle or as far distally as the calcaneocuboid joint. Posteriorly, the fracture moves from plantar medial to dorsal lateral, producing two main fragments. The sustentacular (anteromedial) and tuberosity (posterolateral) fragments.

Secondary fracture line:

- *Tongue-type fracture*: A secondary fracture line appears beneath the facet and exits posteriorly through the tuberosity.
- *Joint depression fracture*: A secondary fracture line exits just behind the posterior facet.

Sanders' Classification Based on CT scan

- Type 1: Nondisplaced posterior facet.
- Type 2: One fracture alone in the posterior facet.
- Type 3: Two fracture lines in posterior facet.
- Type 4: Comminuted fractures.

TREATMENT

Nonoperative Treatment

- Initially, a plaster slab is given for one to two weeks till edema subsides. Then a plaster cast is applied for another two to three weeks till pain reduces following which a removable splint in neutral flexion is given and range of motion (ROM) exercises are started. Patients are mobilized non weight bearing early on and continued for 10–12 weeks.
- *Indications of nonoperative treatment are*:
  - Nondisplaced intra-articular fractures
  - Nondisplaced or minimally displaced extra-articular fractures
  - Fractures in patients with severe peripheral vascular disease, insulin-dependent diabetes
  - Open fractures, fractures with gross swelling and doubtful skin viability and unstable patients.
  - Anterior process fractures with less than 25% involvement of the calcaneocuboid articulation.

Operative Treatment

Indications of operative treatment are:

- Anterior process of the calcaneus fractures with more than 25% involvement of the calcaneocuboid articulation.
- Displaced intra-articular fractures involving the posterior facet.
- Displaced fractures of the calcaneal tuberosity, with or without skin compromise
- Open fractures of the calcaneus
- Fracture dislocations of the calcaneus.

EXTRA-ARTICULAR FRACTURES

- In anterior process fractures, definitive fixation involves small or mini-fragment screws fixation.
- In tuberosity fracture, lag screw fixation with or without cerclage wiring is done.
- Calcaneus body fractures are true extra-articular fractures. Open reduction and internal fixation is done in severe displaced fractures.
- *Medial process fractures*: Nondisplaced fractures are treated with short leg weight-bearing cast.

INTRA-ARTICULAR FRACTURES

Operative goals comprise of restoration of congruity of the subtalar articulation, Bohler angle, normal width and height of the calcaneus, maintenance of the normal calcaneocuboid articulation and neutralization of the varus deformity of the fracture.

- Open reduction and internal fixation is done through lateral L-shaped incision.
- For tongue-type fractures, percutaneous reduction and leg screw fixation are preferred. Closed reduction with percutaneous fixation carries minimal risk of wound complications and less operative time. It ensures faster healing because of less soft tissue trauma. This approach is good in patient with significant comorbidity, soft tissue compromise, and polytrauma cases. The goals of this approach include improvement of the heel alignment and adequate reduction of the posterior facet.
- In selective high-energy injuries (type 4), primary subtalar or triple arthrodesis may be performed.
- In postoperative management, patient is kept non-weight-bearing for 8–12 weeks and full weight-bearing started after 12 weeks.

FRACTURE CALCANEUM CCS OPERATIVE STEPS (FIGS. 1 TO 27)

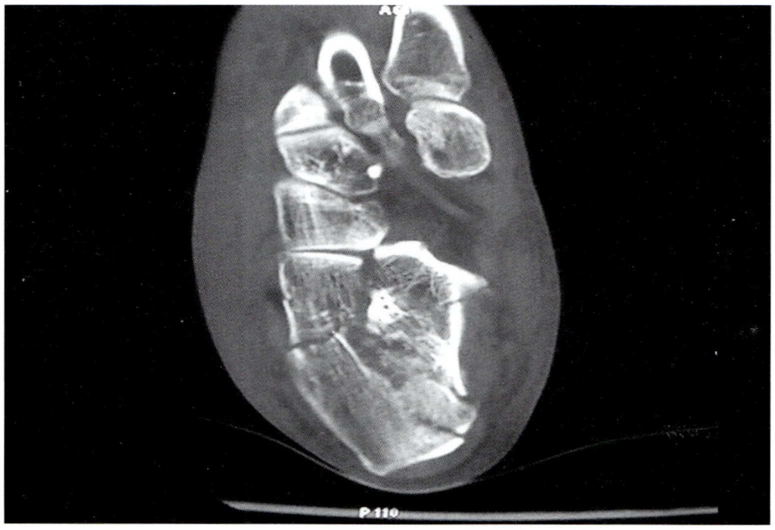

Fig. 1: Computed tomography (CT) scan of right ankle with foot axial view showing fracture line exiting anterolaterally on calcaneocuboid joint and posteriorly plantar medial to dorsal lateral side.

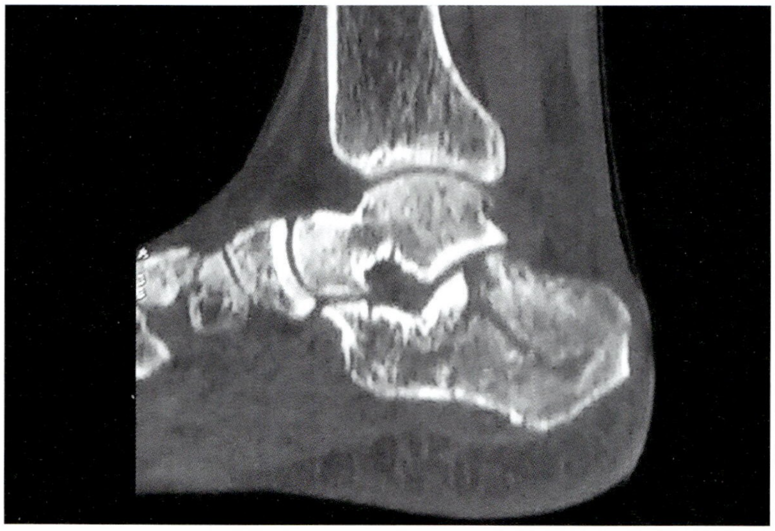

Fig. 2: Sagittal view showing secondary fracture line below posterior facet and exits posteriorly through tuberosity.

- Diagnosis—tongue type fracture of right calcaneum.

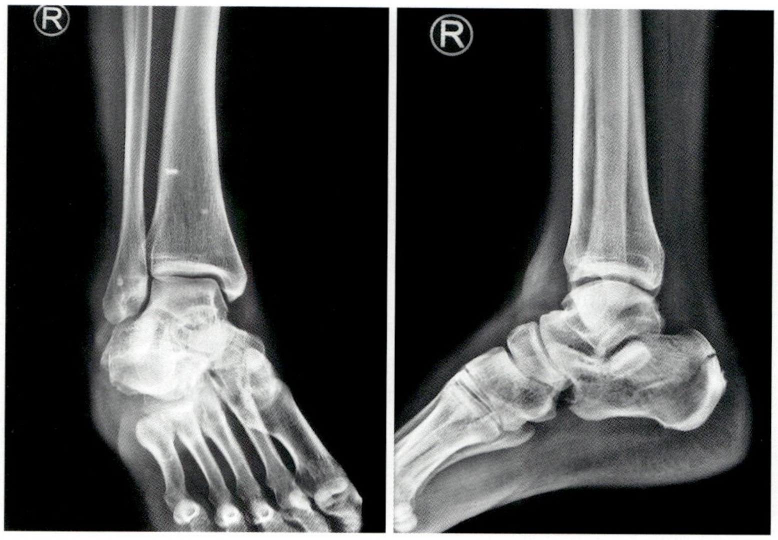

Fig. 3: Anteroposterior and lateral X-ray of right ankle and foot showing tongue type fracture of calcaneum.

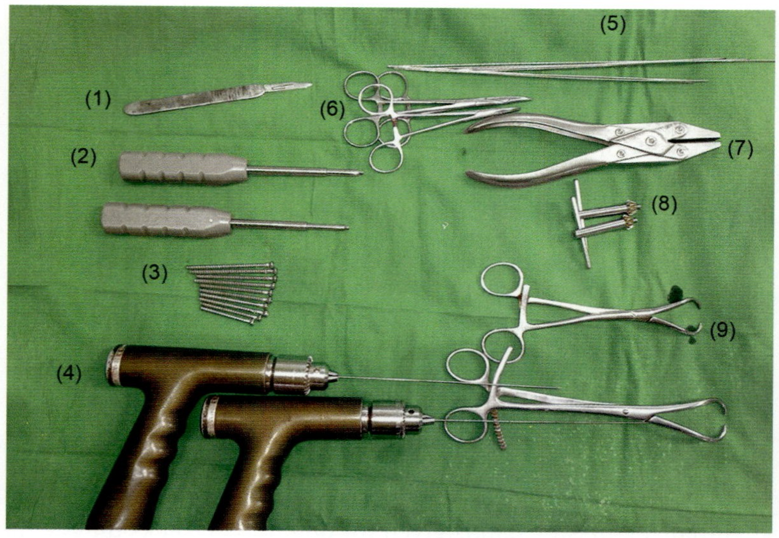

Fig. 4: Instrument trolly. (1) Stab knife, (2) Screw driver, (3) 4.0 mm cannulated cancellous screws of different sizes in difference of 5 mm, (4) Drill, (5) Guidewires (1.5 mm) of similar length, (6) Artery and mosquito forceps, (7) Pliar, (8) Chuck key, (9) Bone holding forceps—for reduction.

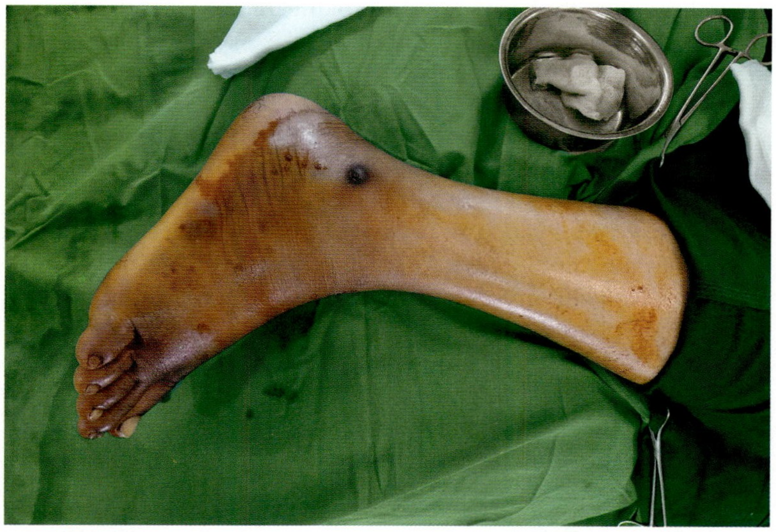

Fig. 5: Lateral position given on operating table. Scrubbing, painting, and draping done in standard manner in left lateral position.

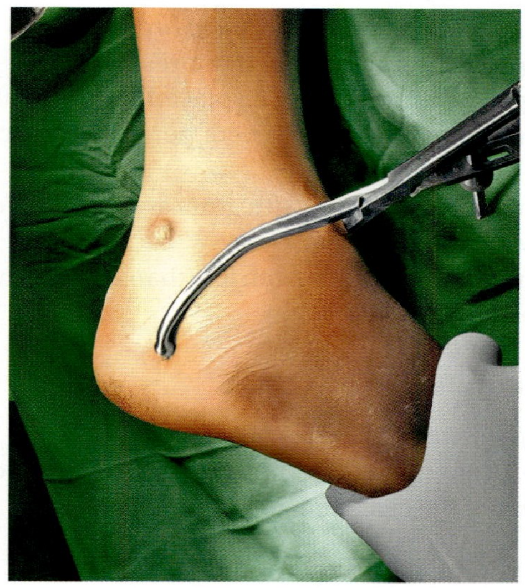

Fig. 6: Reduction of fracture done with pointed bone holding forceps.

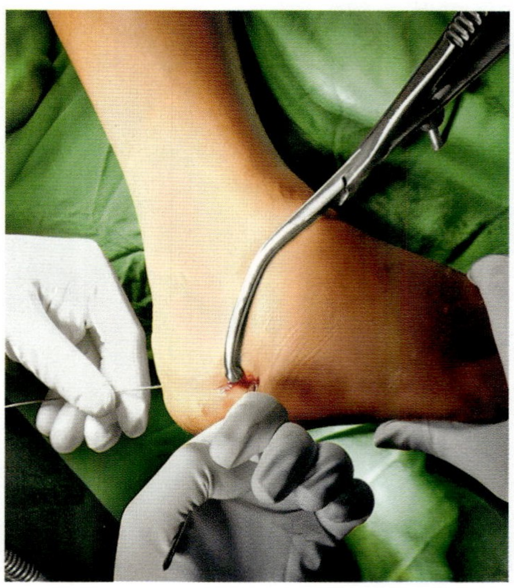

Fig. 7: Depressed posterior articular facet elevated with thick wire entering from lateral side to maintain subtalar articular surface and reduction held with bone holding forceps.

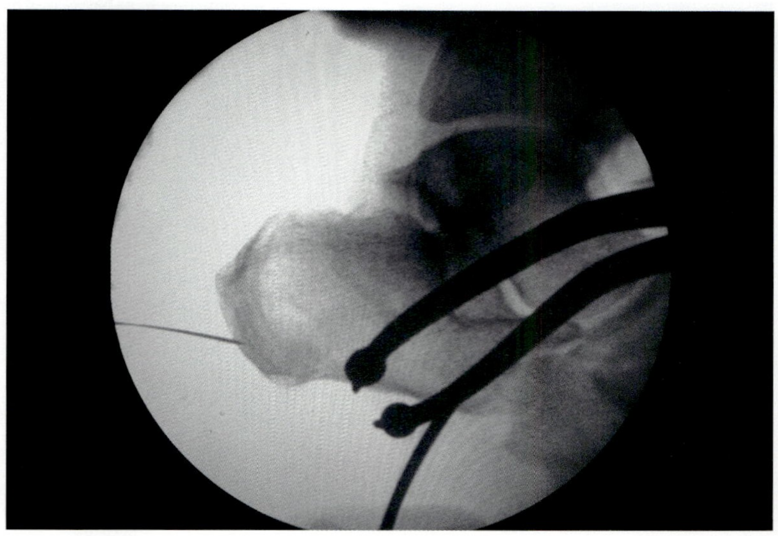

Fig. 8: Reduction of fracture confirmed under C-arm image intensifier.

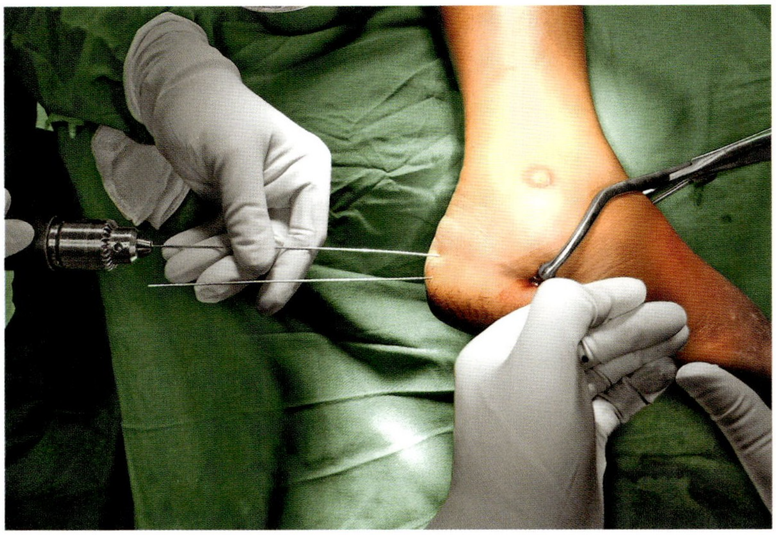

Fig. 9: First guidewire is inserted from lateral side of posteroinferior part of tuberosity to hold primary fracture line. Second guidewire is inserted from just below attachment of Achilles tendon laterally to hold primary fracture line anterolaterally. Third guidewire inserted just below attachment of Achilles tendon medially and passes up to anteromedially side to hold primary fracture line anteromedially.

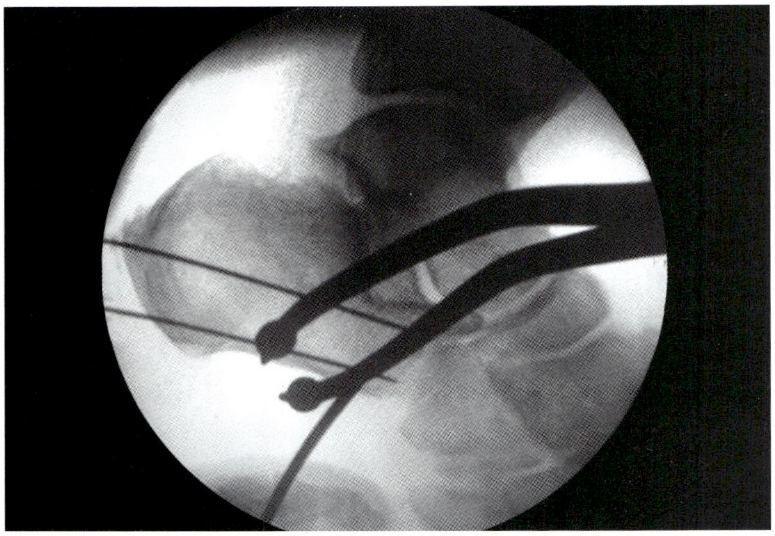

Fig. 10: Position of first, second, and third wire confirmed over lateral view of C-arm.

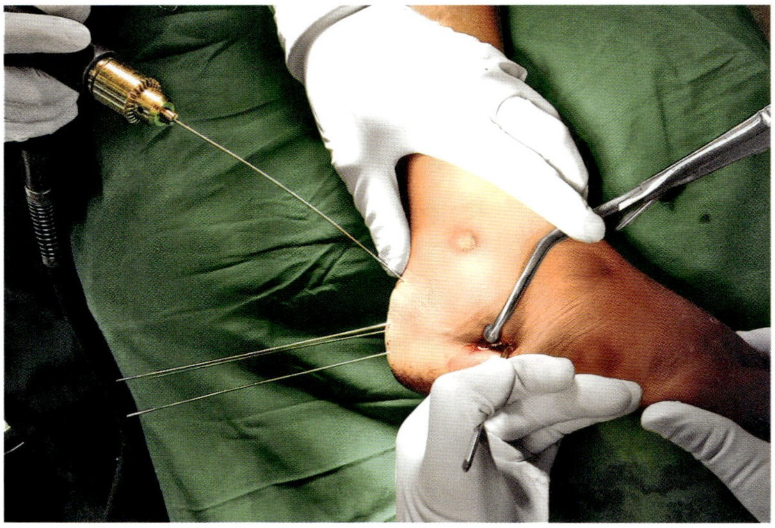

Fig. 11: Fourth guidewire inserted from superior pole of tuberosity (posterolateral side) to body of calcaneum to hold tongue type fracture line.

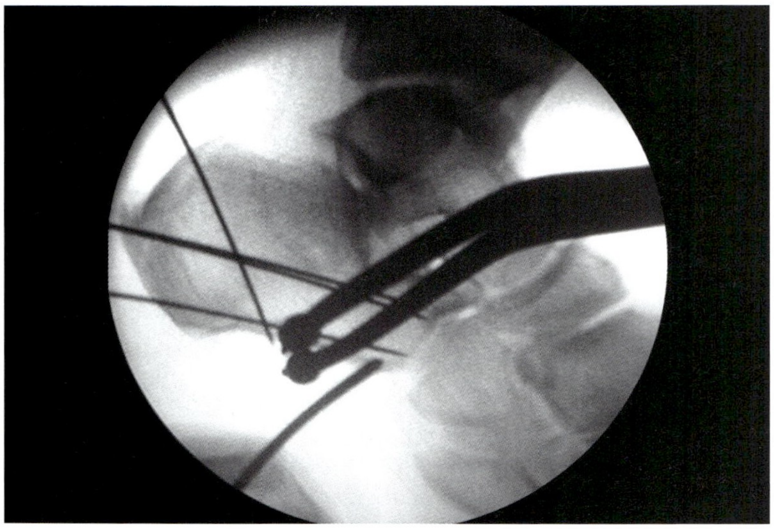

Fig. 12: Position of fourth guidewire confirmed over lateral view of C-arm.

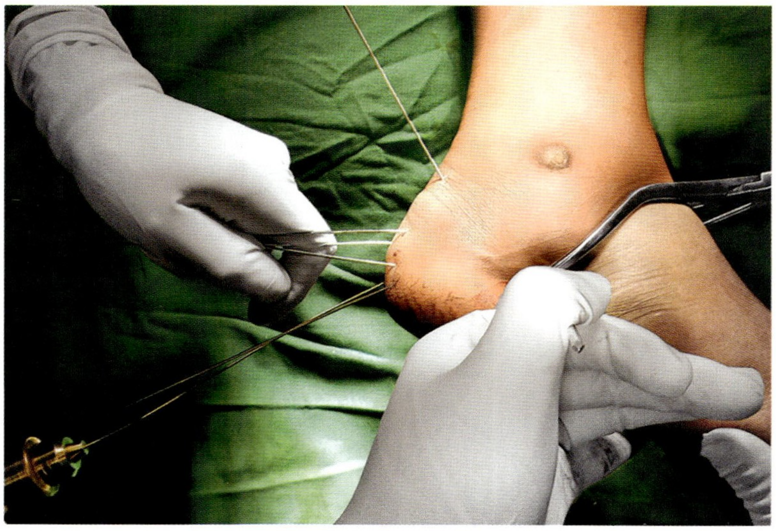

Fig. 13: Fifth and sixth guidewire inserted from posteroinferior part of calcaneum toward posterior talar articular surface to hold depressed posterior talar articular surface in position.

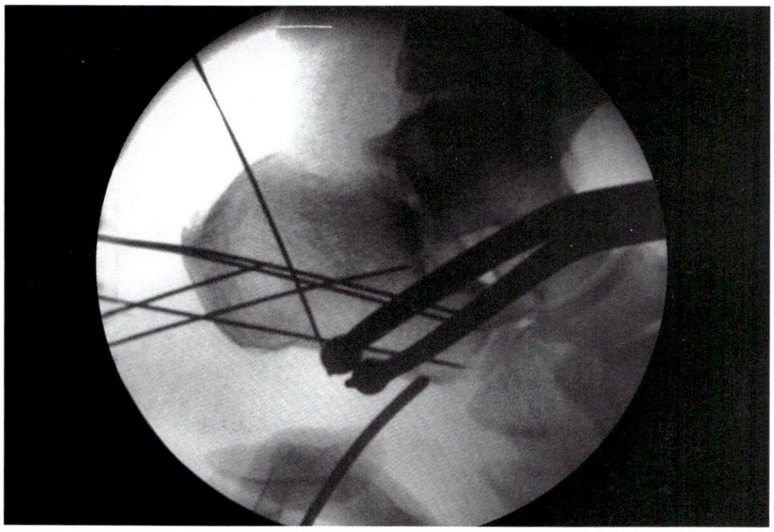

Fig. 14: Position of fifth and sixth wire confirmed over lateral view of C-arm.

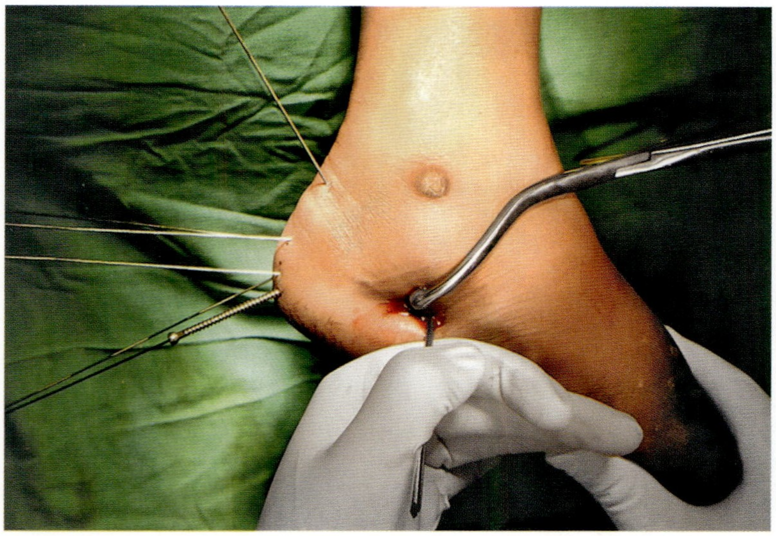

Fig. 15: Screw length is measured with same length guidewire and stab incision taken with stab knife and 4 mm fully threaded self-tapping CC screw inserted in fifth guidewire.

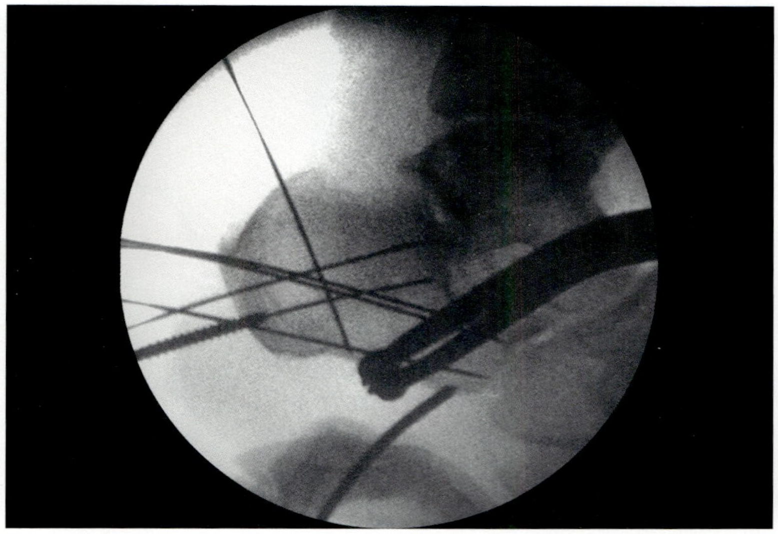

Fig. 16: Screw fixation done under lateral X-ray on C-arm.

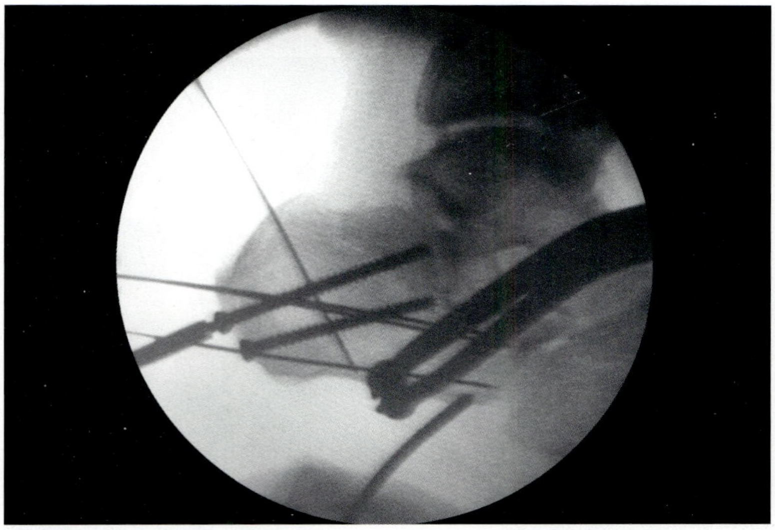

Fig. 17: CC screw fixation done under C-arm to hold depressed posterior talar articular surface in position.

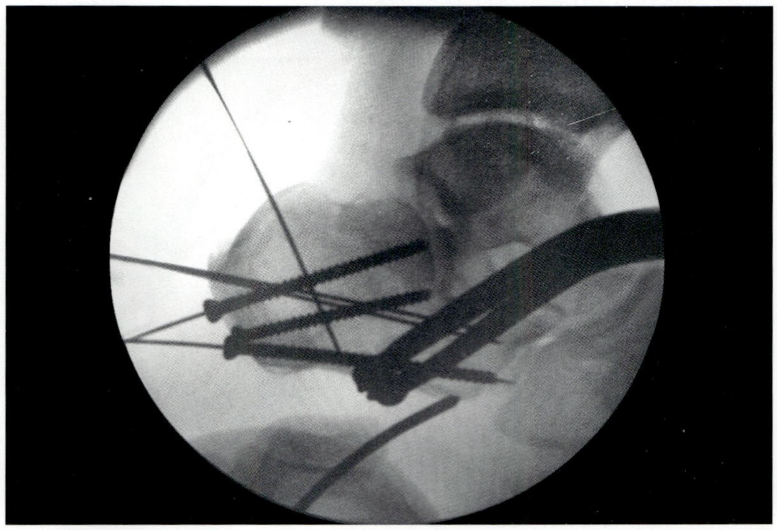

Fig. 18: Third CC screw fixation done under C-arm in first guidewire to hold primary fracture line.

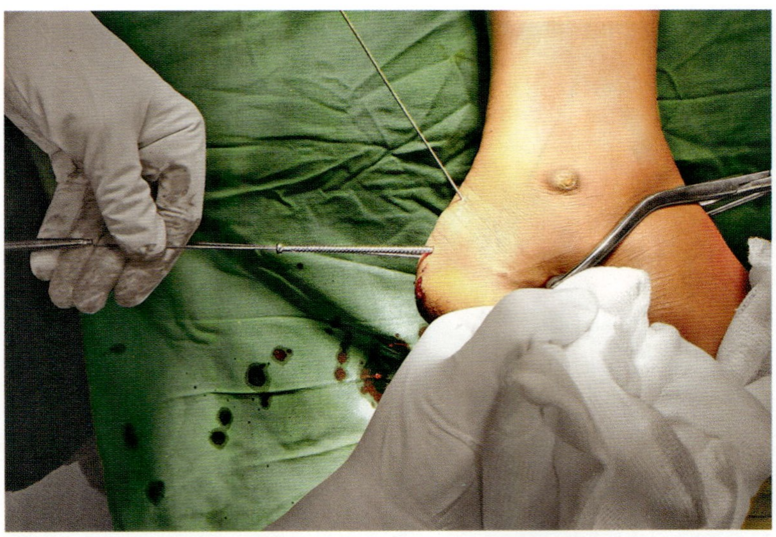

Fig. 19: Fourth CC screw inserted in second guidewire is from just below attachment of Achilles tendon laterally to hold primary fracture line anterolaterally.

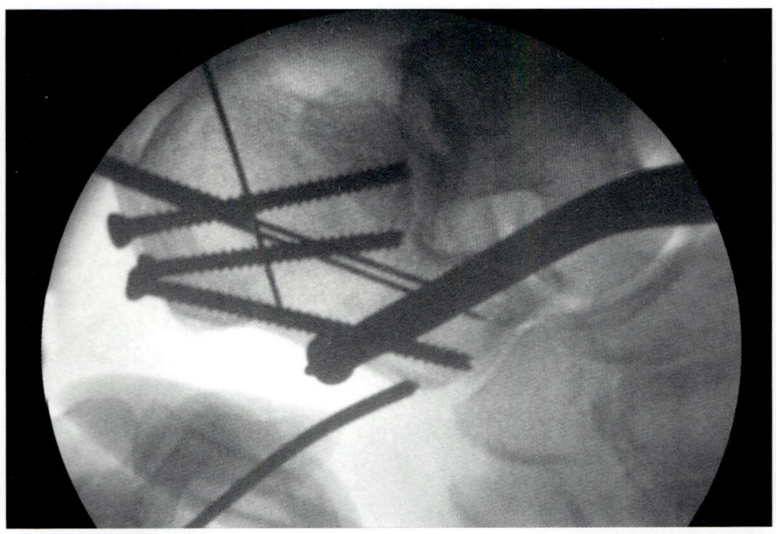

Fig. 20: Fixation of fourth screw confirmed in C-arm.

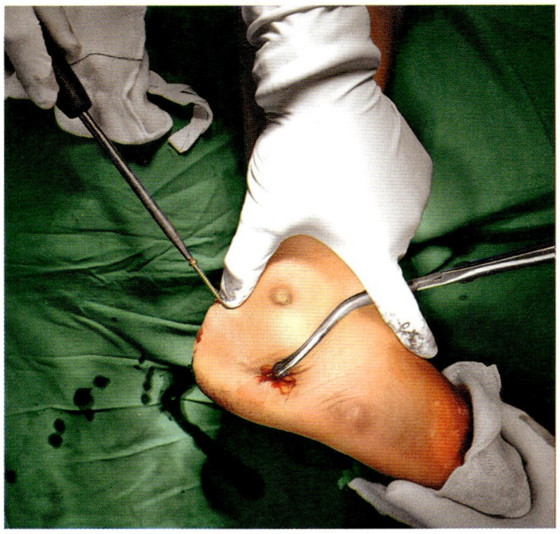

Fig. 21: Fifth screw fixation done in third guidewire from just below attachment of Achilles tendon medially and passes up to anteromedially side to hold primary fracture line anteromedially.

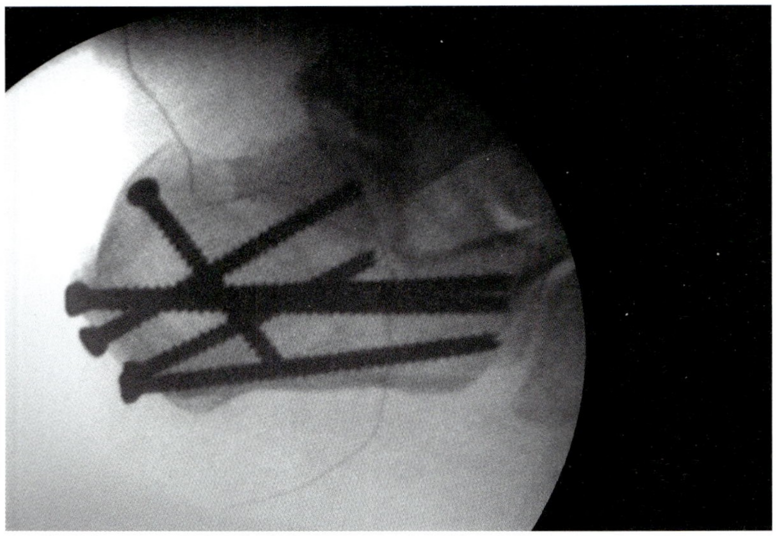

Fig. 22: Sixth CC screw fixation done under C-arm in fourth guidewire from superior pole of tuberosity (posterolateral side) to body of calcaneum to hold tongue type fracture line.

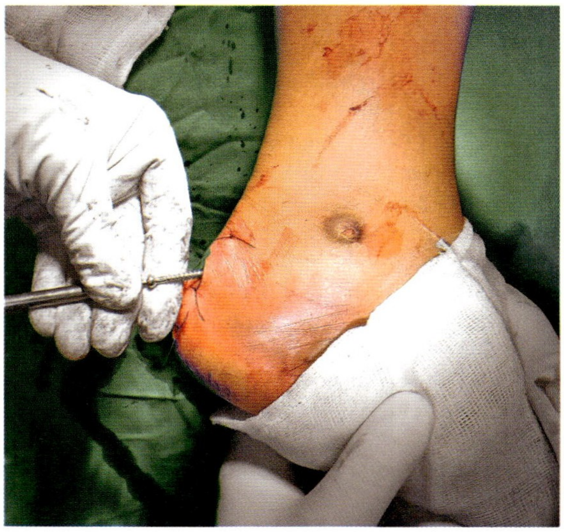

Fig. 23: Additional seventh CC screw fixation done from posterosuperior part toward posterior talar articular surface to hold depressed posterior talar articular surface.

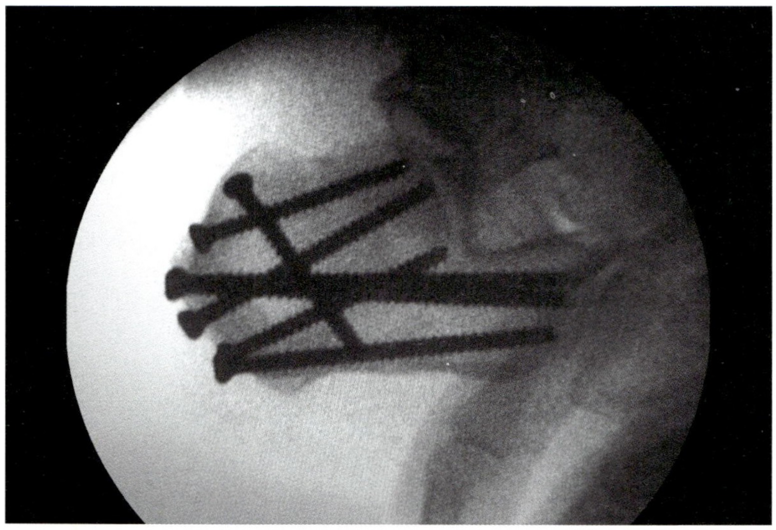

Fig. 24: Final seventh CC screw fixation confirmed under C-arm image intensifier in lateral view.

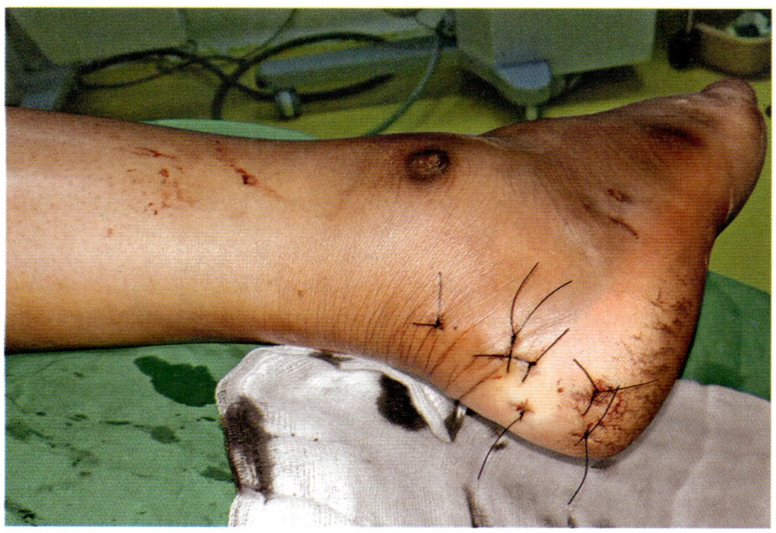

Fig. 25: Suturing of all stab skin incision done with 2.0 nylon suture material.

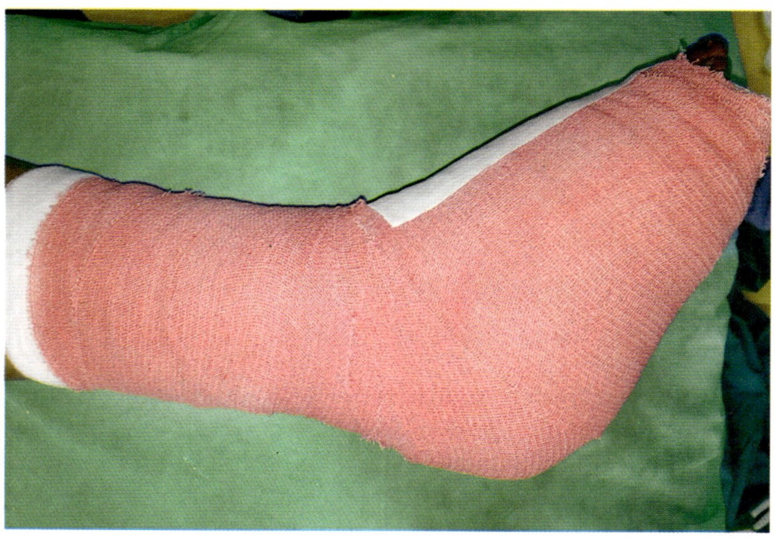

Fig. 26: Compression bandage given after dressing and limb elevation given.

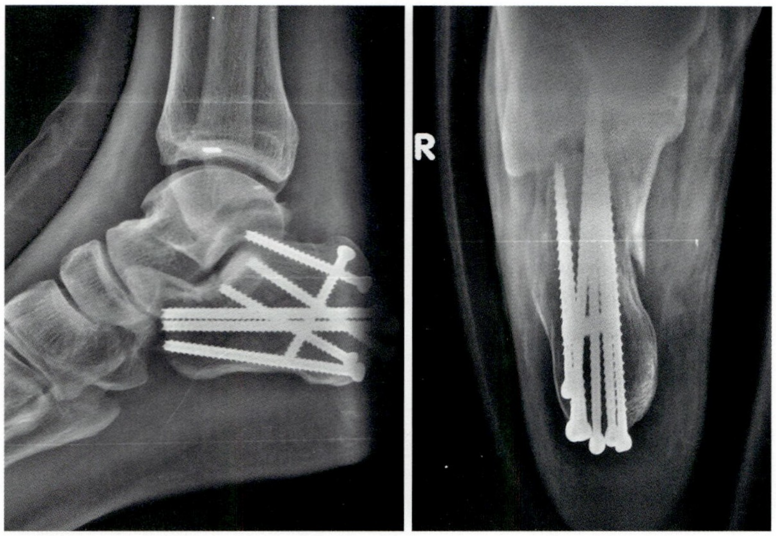

Fig. 27: Postoperative X-ray showing percutaneous CC screws fixation in tongue type calcaneum fracture.

POSTOPERATIVE MANAGEMENT

Active toe movements initiated from day of surgery:
- Ankle dorsiflexion and plantar flexion exercises started from 1st day.
- Hamstring strengthening exercises and static quadriceps exercise started from 1st day.
- Non-weight-bearing mobilization with walker support started from 2nd day.
- Suture removal done on day 14. Non-weight-bearing is kept for 10–12 weeks.

COMPLICATIONS

- Calcaneal osteomyelitis
- Wound dehiscence
- Increase heel width
- Peroneal tendonitis
- Post-traumatic arthritis (subtalar or calcaneocuboid)
- Sural nerve injury
- Chronic heel pain
- Loss of subtalar motion
- Complex regional pain syndrome.

SUGGESTED READING

1. De vroome SW, van Der linden FM. Cohort study on the percutaneous treatment of displaced intra-articular fractures of the calcaneus. Foot Ankle Int. 2014;35(2):156-62.
2. Epstein N, Chandran S, Chou L. Current concept review: intra-articular fractures of the calcaneal. Foot Ankle Int. 2012;33(1):79-86.
3. Rammelt S, Amlang M, Barthel S, et al. Percutaneous treatment of less severe intra-articular calcaneal fractures. Clin Orthop Relat Res. 2010;468(4):983-90.
4. Stulik J, Stehlik J, Rysavy M, et al. Minimally invasive treatment of intra-articular fractures of the calcaneum. J Bone Joint Surg. 2006;88(12):1634-41.
5. Tomesen T, Biert J, Frolke JP. Treatment of displaced intra-articular calcaneal fractures with closed reductions and per cutaneous screw fixation. J Bone Joint Surg. 2011;93(10):920-8.
6. Wiersema B, Brokaw D, Weber T, et al. Complications associated with open calcaneal fractures. Foot Ankle Int. 2011;32:1052.

FRACTURE CALCANEUM MINIMALLY INVASIVE PLATE OSTEOSYNTHESIS

Vijay M Panchanadikar, Anurag Daxini

MINIMALLY INVASIVE PLATE OSTEOSYNTHESIS THROUGH SINUS TARSI APPROACH

Calcaneal fractures are known as one of the most difficult intra-articular fractures to treat. Displaced malunited calcaneal fractures can be a source of significant residual pain and disability to the patient and many times the clinical outcome does not satisfy the surgeon and the patient. Both operative and nonoperative management have its own advantages and disadvantages. Most surgeons prefer operative treatment for displaced fractures, which can be via extensile lateral approach or mini incision sinus tarsi approach, which needs especially designed mini plates. Here we describe sinus tarsi mini incision approach with a technical trick, wherein the standard length plate is slid through the incision and locking screws are inserted through stab incisions. The elevated thalamic fragment is supported prior to plate fixation with cancellous screws. Though uncommon possible complications include sural nerve or peroneal tendon injury and infection.

SURGICAL STEPS (FIGS. 28 TO 47)

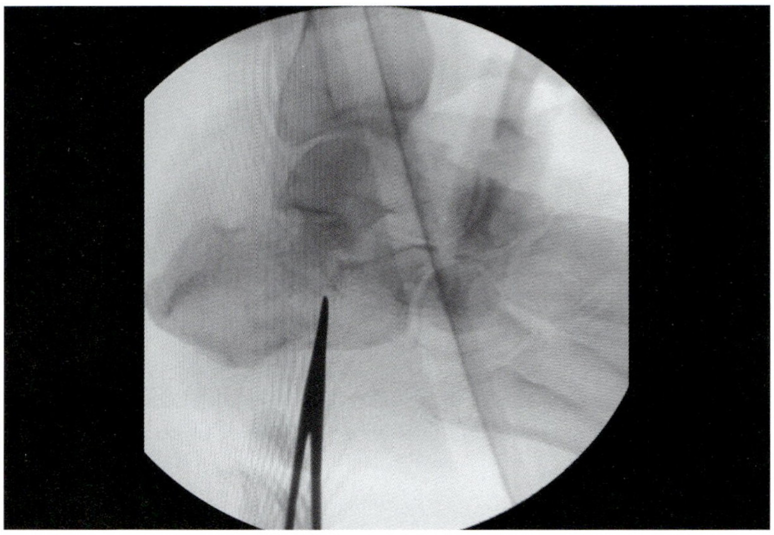

Fig. 28: Lateral view of intraoperative C-arm image showing fracture pattern.

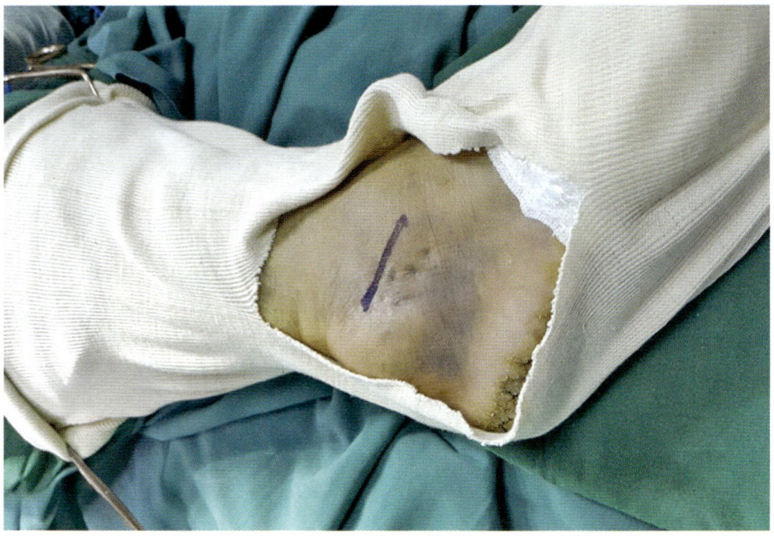

Fig. 29: Skin incision marked for sinus tarsi approach.

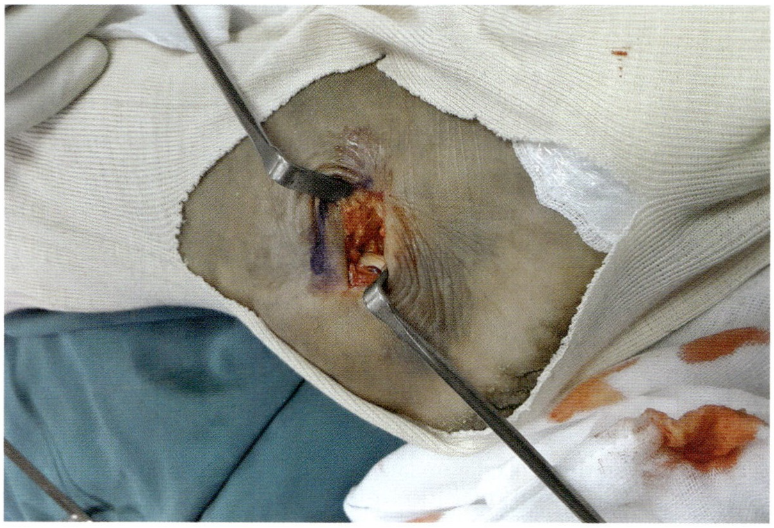

Fig. 30: Skin incision deepened. Sural nerve and peroneal tendons carefully protected and retracted at posterior corner of incision.

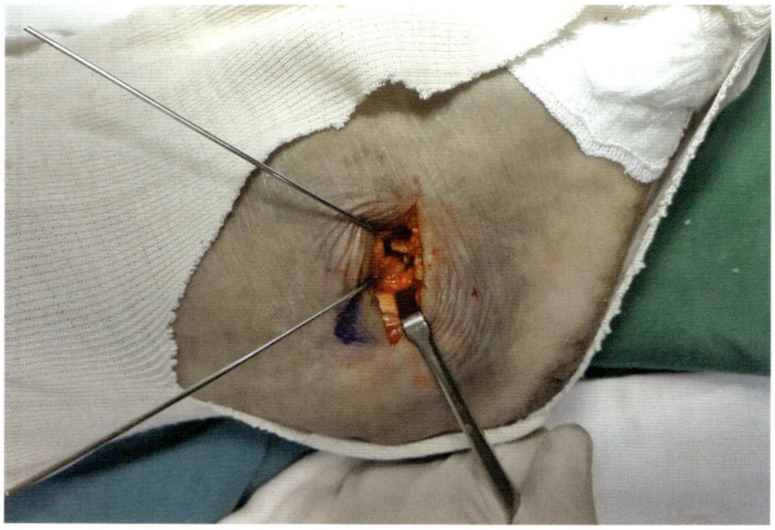

Fig. 31: K-wires are drilled and used as retraction tools at proximal part.

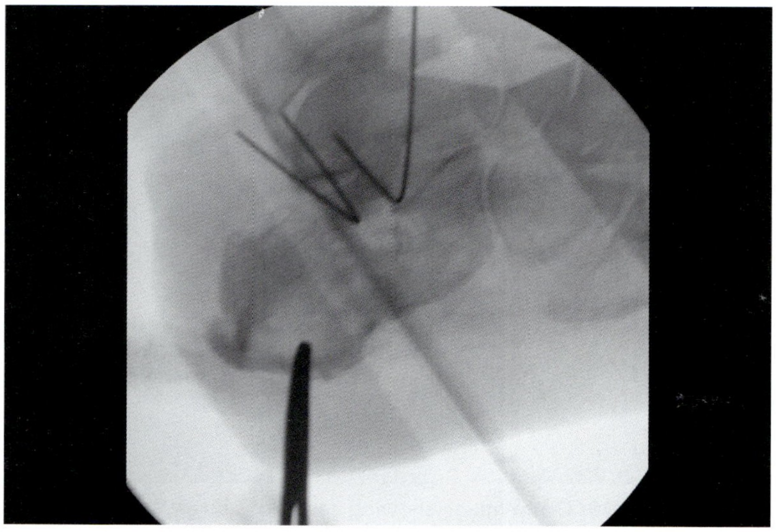

Fig. 32: C-arm image post-K-wire insertion.

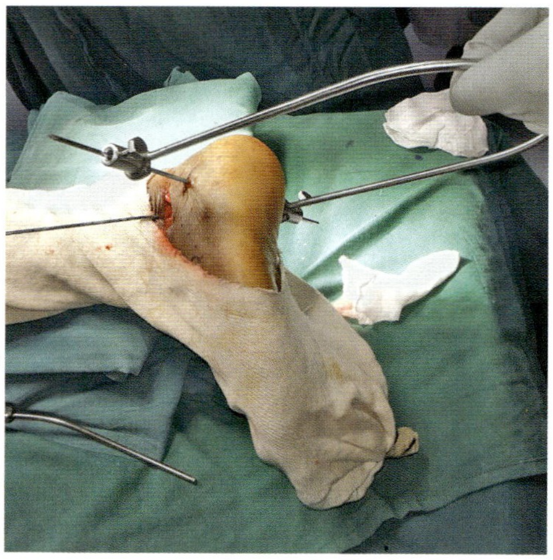

Fig. 33: Steinmann pin inserted into calcaneum and Bohler stirrup fixed over the pin. This is used as hand grip to assist in reduction of fracture (Image from a different surgery).

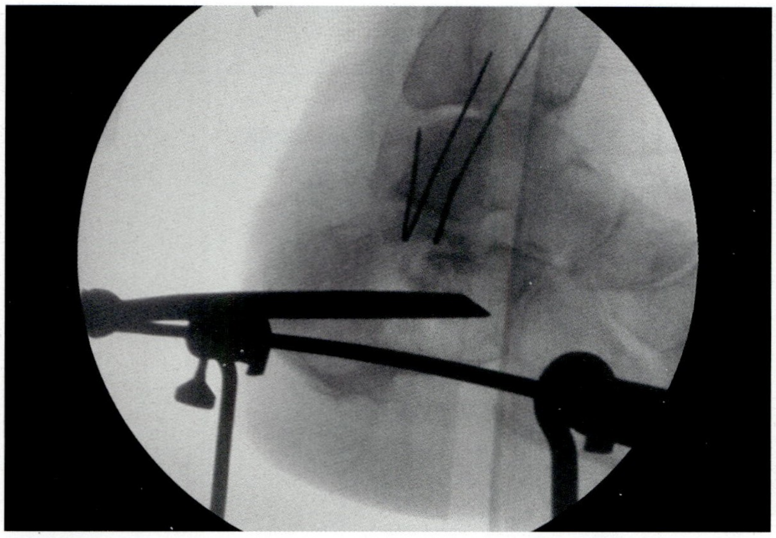

Fig. 34: Reduction done by manipulating the Bohler stirrup and use of periosteum elevator/osteotome for elevation of depressed intra-articular fragment.

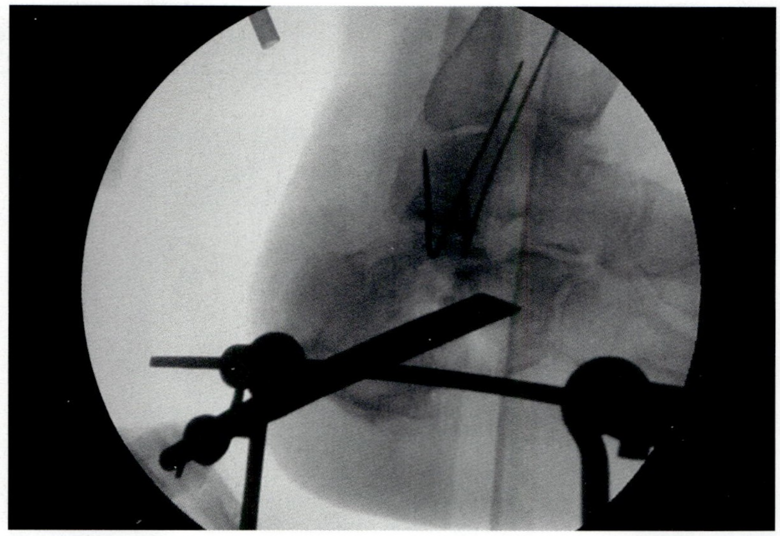

Fig. 35: C-arm image showing final acceptable reduction of the fracture.

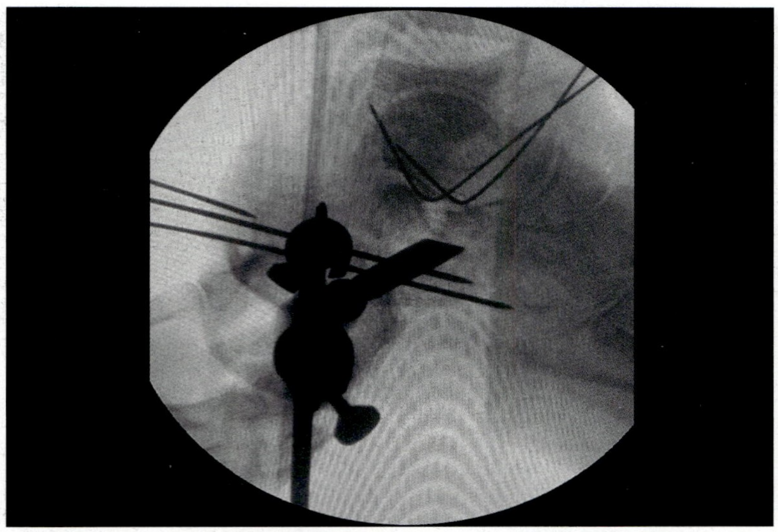

Fig. 36: K-wires are provisionally inserted across the fracture site.

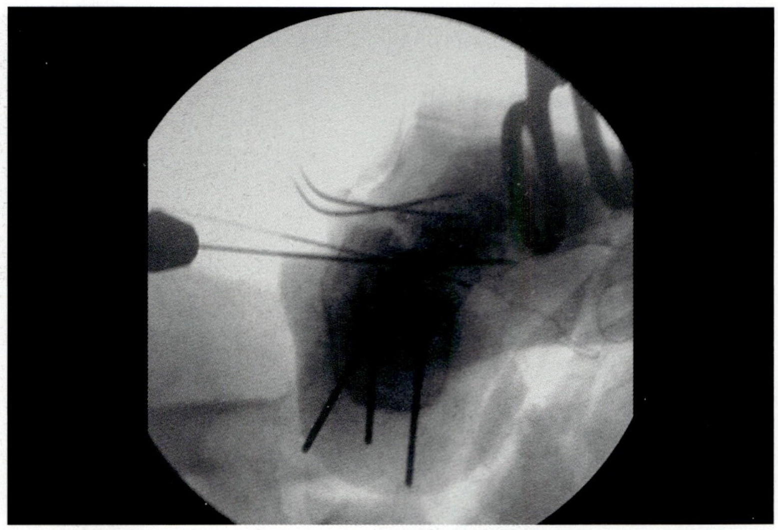

Fig. 37: Guidewires drilled from lateral to medial side to hold reduced intra-articular fragment.

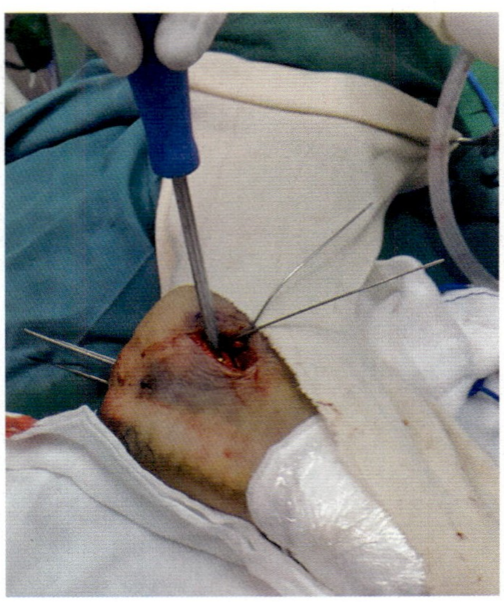

Fig. 38: Cancellous screws are inserted over the guidewire into and across the intra-articular fragment for better hold and stability and prevent subsequent collapse.

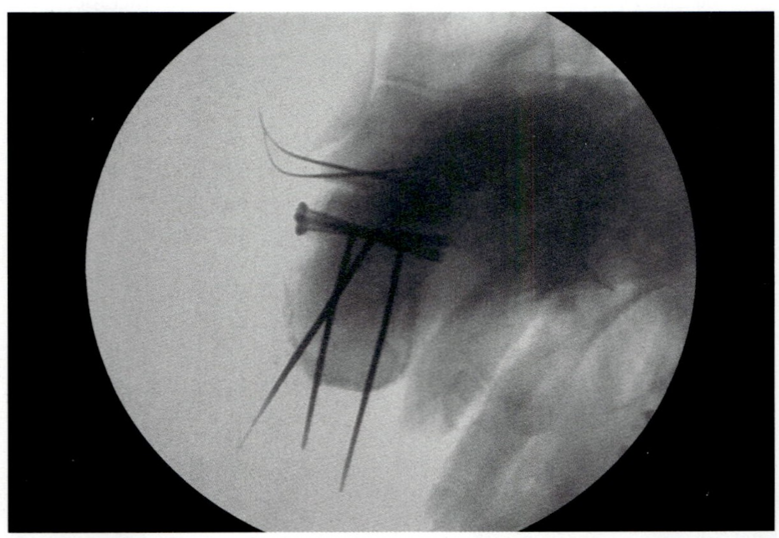

Fig. 39: C-arm image showing cancellous screw with good purchase in opposite cortex.

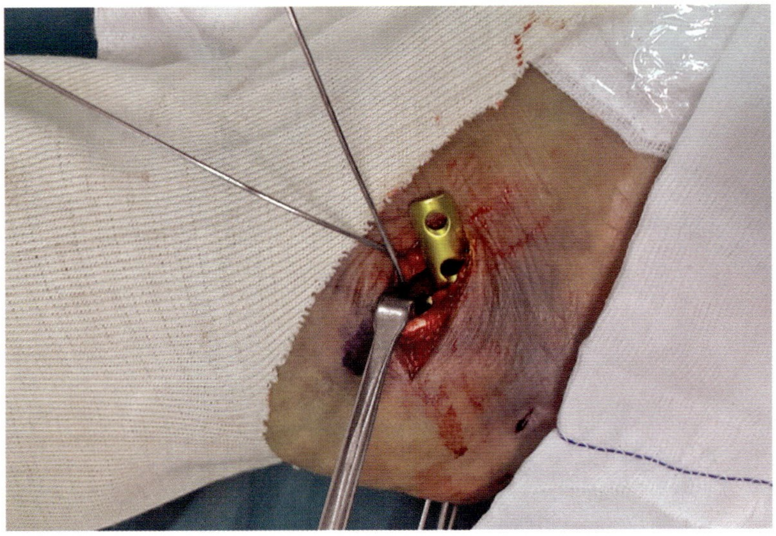

Fig. 40: Standard one-third tubular plate slided through the mini incision.

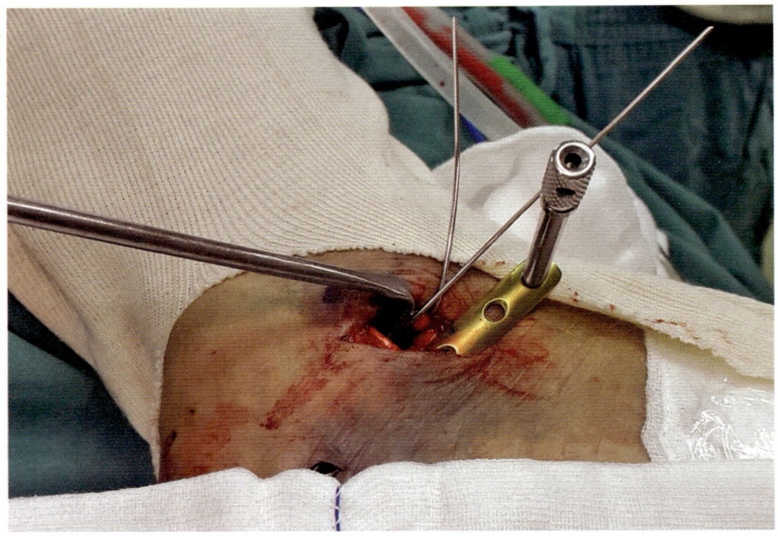

Fig. 41: Locking drill sleeve used to control placement of plate.

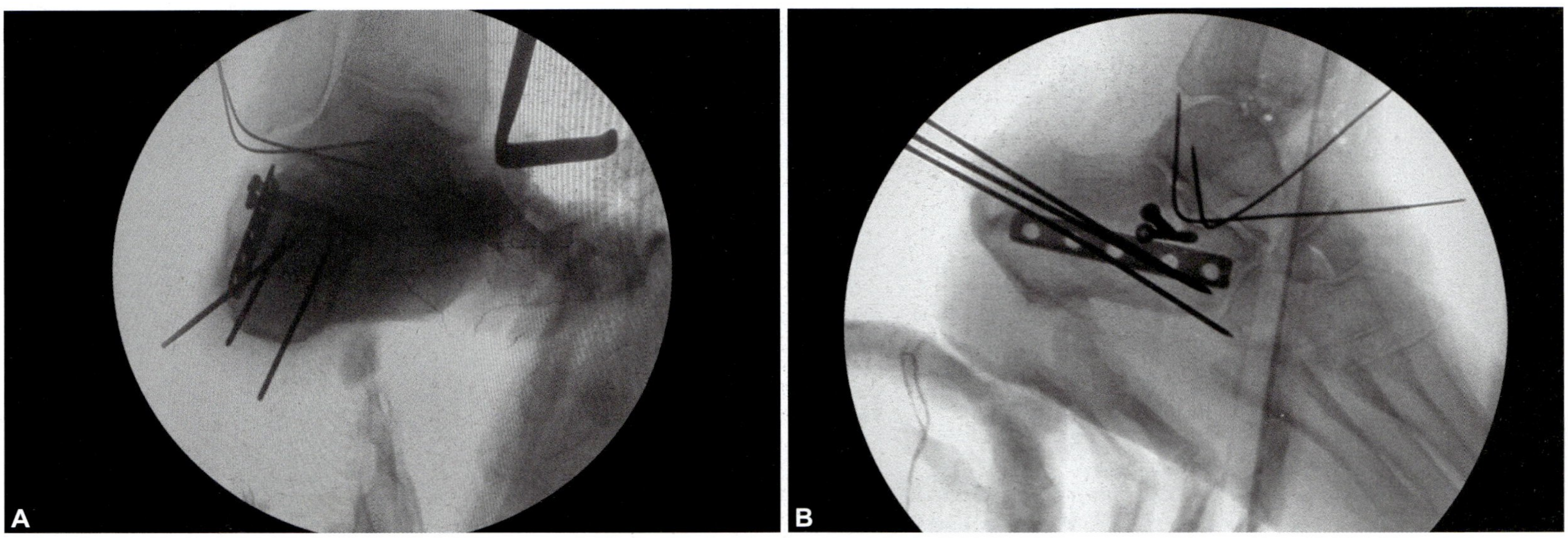

Figs. 42A and B: C-arm images showing provisional plate position.

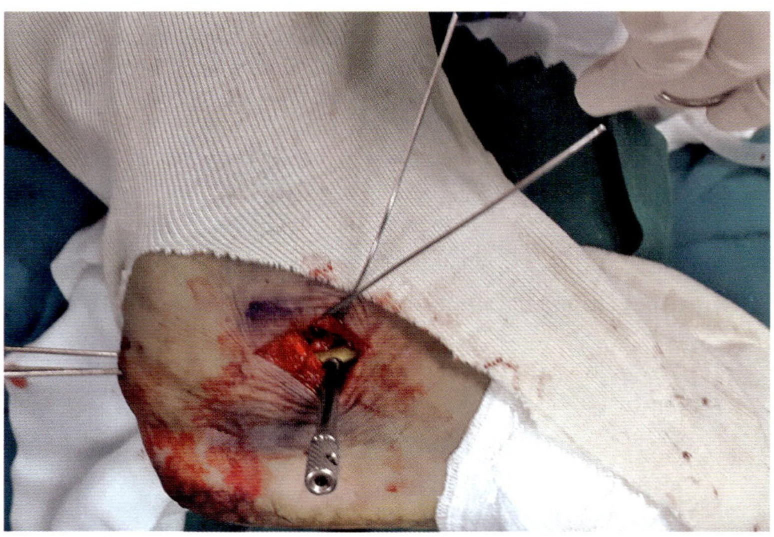

Fig. 43: The plate is placed over the lateral surface of calcaneum.

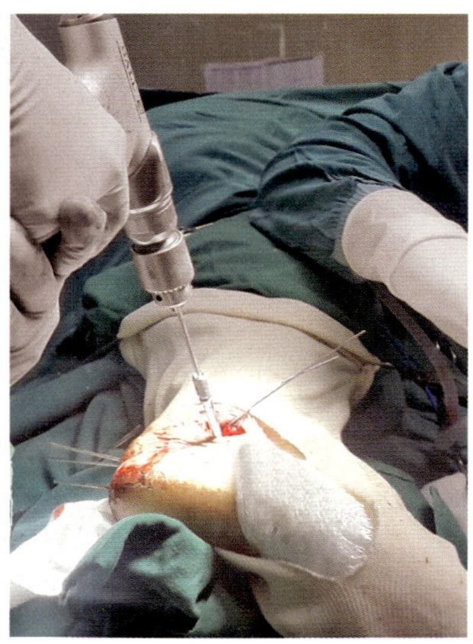

Fig. 44: Cortex is drilled through locking sleeve and locking screw applied.

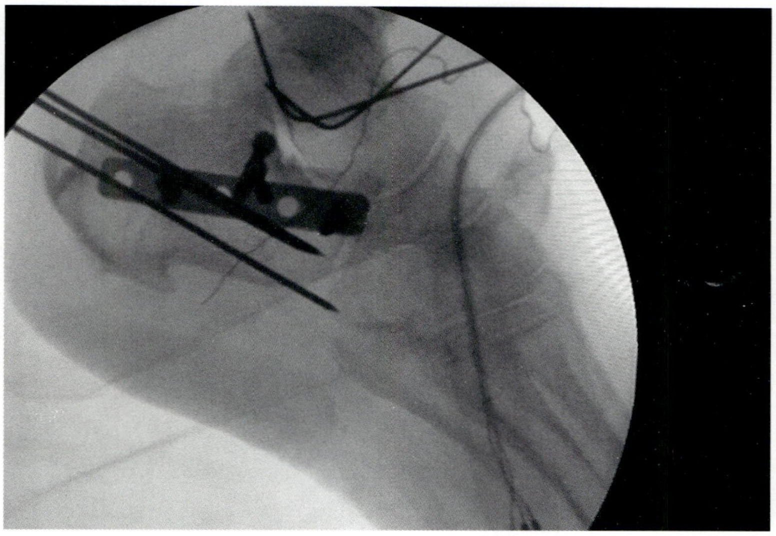

Fig. 45: Remaining locking screws fixed to plate, one-by-one, through stab incisions away from main incision, by C-arm assisted locating of holes.

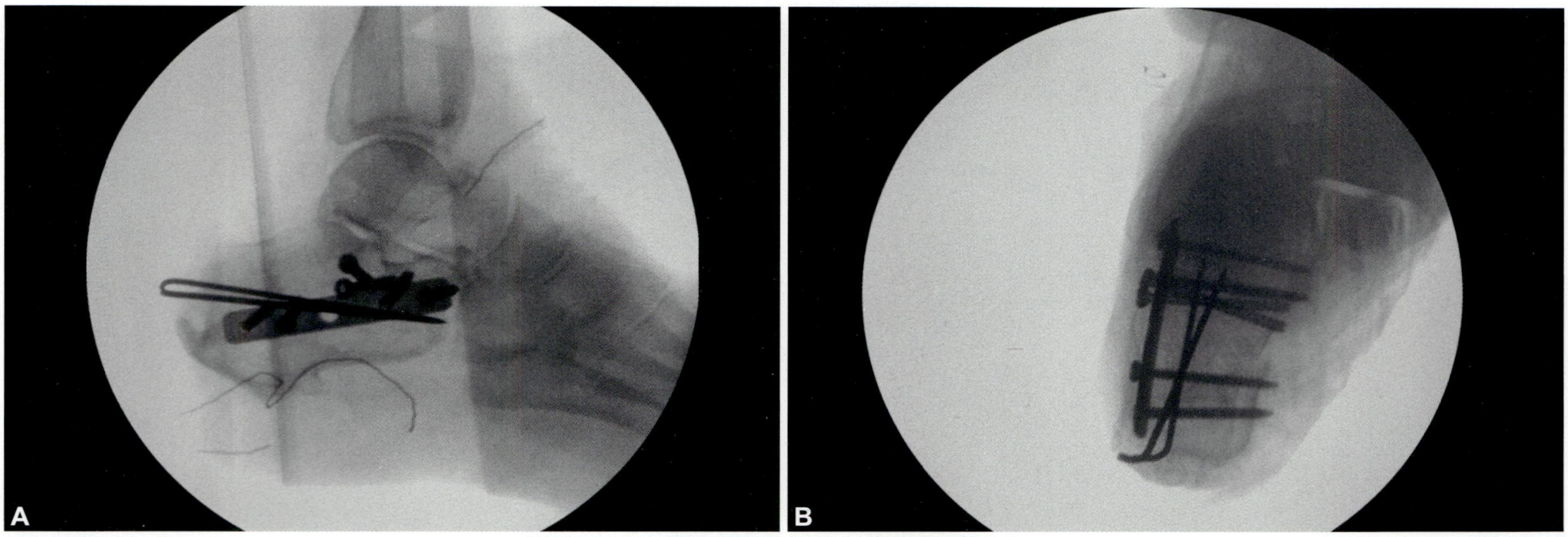

Figs. 46A and B: Final C-arm images of position of plate.

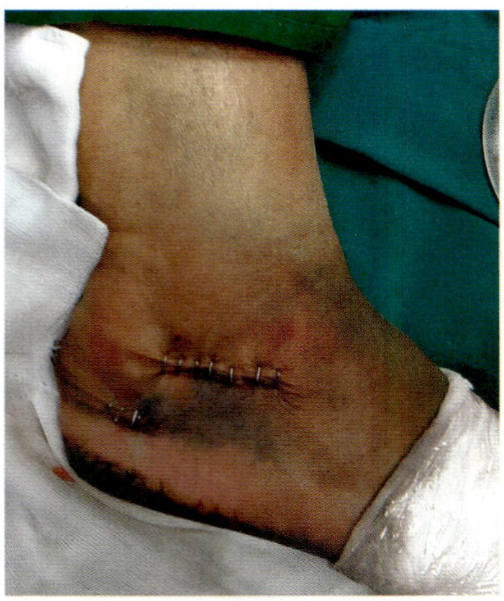

Fig. 47: Skin closed in layers.

SUGGESTED READING

1. Basile A. Comparison between sinus tarsi approach and extensile lateral approach for treatment of closed displaced intra-articular calcaneal fractures: a multicenter prospective study. J Foot Ankle Surg. 2016;55(3):513-21.
2. Jordaan P. Open reduction and internal fixation of calcaneus fractures through a sinus tarsi approach. SA Orthop J. 2016.
3. Femino JE, Vaseenon T, Levin DA, et al. Modification of the Sinus tarsi approach for open reduction and plate fixation of intraarticular calcaneus fractures: The limits of proximal extension based upon the vascular anatomy of lateral calcaneal artery. Iowa Orthop J. 2010;30:161-7.

FRACTURE CALCANEUM K-WIRE FIXATION

Nagesh Naik, Rajkumar Ekambaram, Shrinivas S Shintre

INTRODUCTION

- Calcaneus or os calcis is the most common tarsal bone to be fractured, its incidence being 60% of all tarsal bones.
- Most of the calcaneus fractures are often intra-articular.
- The mechanism of injury is due to fall from height.
- It may also be associated with spinal traumas and pelvic fractures. Proper examination should be made to rule it out.

CLINICAL FEATURES

- Pain over the heel, swelling, and tenderness associated with heel widening and shortening.
- Ecchymosis and blisters over the heel are typical.
- Open fractures are less common.
- Examination of soft tissue structures and neurovascular structures is mandatory.
- Although compartment syndrome of the foot is less common in calcaneum fractures, it should be carefully ruled out.
- Spine examination is must and so is checking the neurology.

INVESTIGATIONS

- Anteroposterior (AP) and lateral views of hindfoot, Harris axial view (foot in dorsiflexion and beam directed from 45° cephalad).
- Bohler angle (20–40°) and Gissane crucial angle (105–135°) have to be checked for in lateral views.
- Fracture extension to calcaneocuboid joint is checked.
- Computed tomography (CT) images to know about the articular surface, sustentaculum, overall shape of heel.

TREATMENT

- Minimally displaced extra-articular fractures are managed conservatively with slab/cast and physiotherapy started.
- Operative intervention is initiated for intra-articular fractures.

SURGICAL STEPS (FIGS. 48 TO 59)

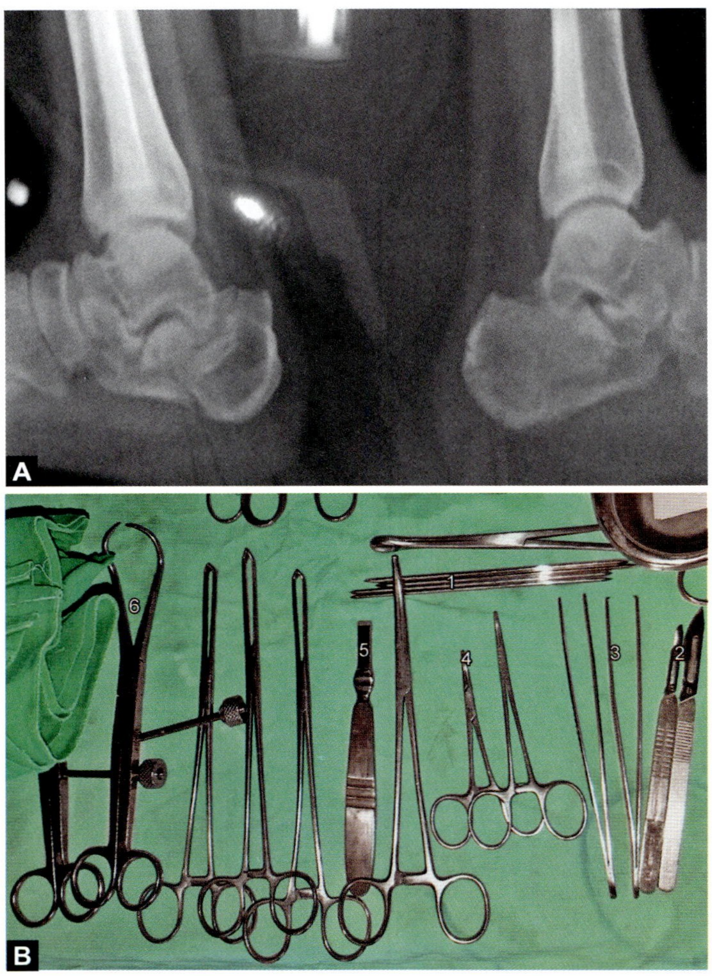

Figs. 48A and B: (A) Preoperative radiograph of the patient with fracture calcaneum; (B) Instrument trolley showing: (1) K-wires, (2) Skin knife, (3) Tissue-holding forceps, (4) Artery forceps, (5) Periosteum elevator, (6) Pointed reduction forceps.

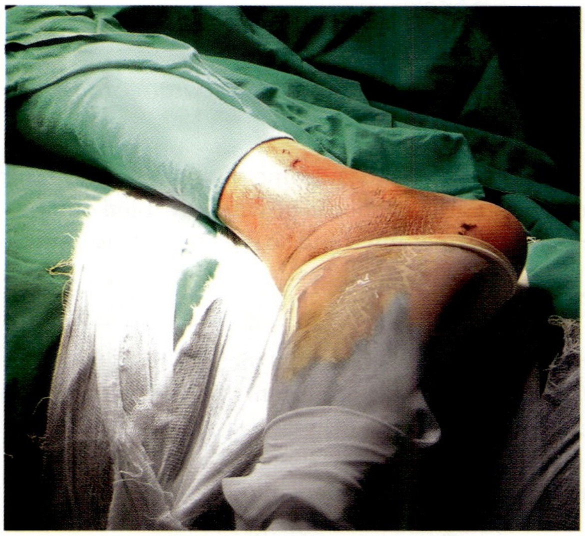

Fig. 49: Painting and draping of the limb are done with povidone–iodine.

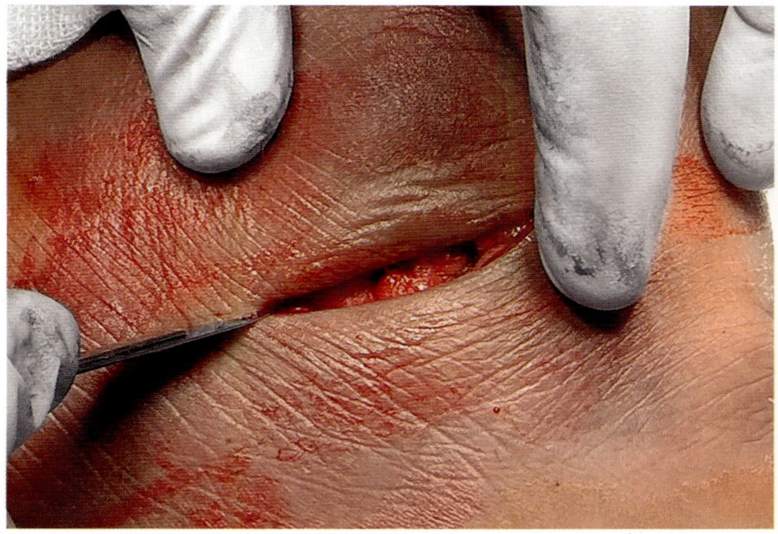

Fig. 50: Skin incision of 4–7 cm is taken on lateral aspect of foot over talus.

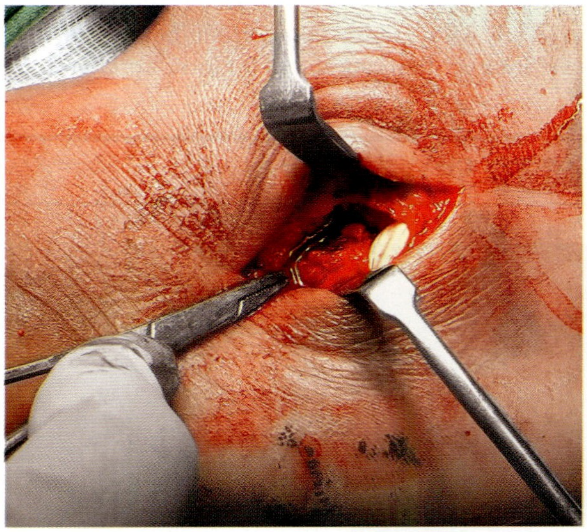

Fig. 51: Deep dissection done and bone reached.

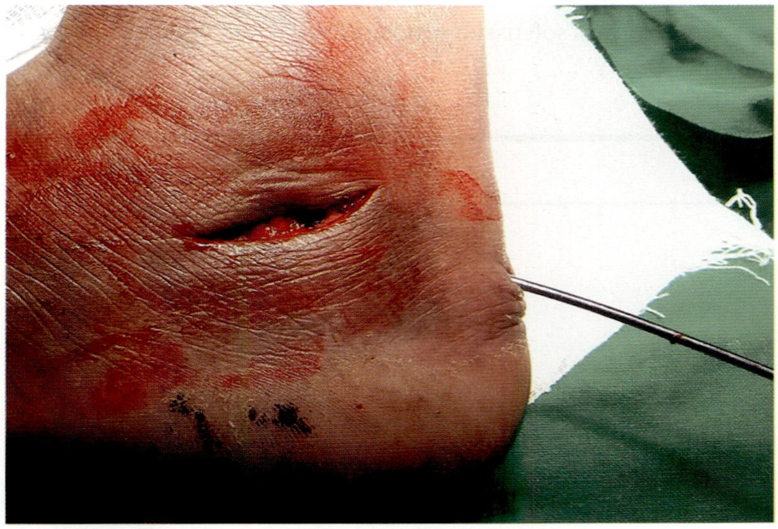

Fig. 52: Reduction is attempted and then a K-wire is introduced posteromedial to Achilles tendon to attain the articular congruity of calcaneum.

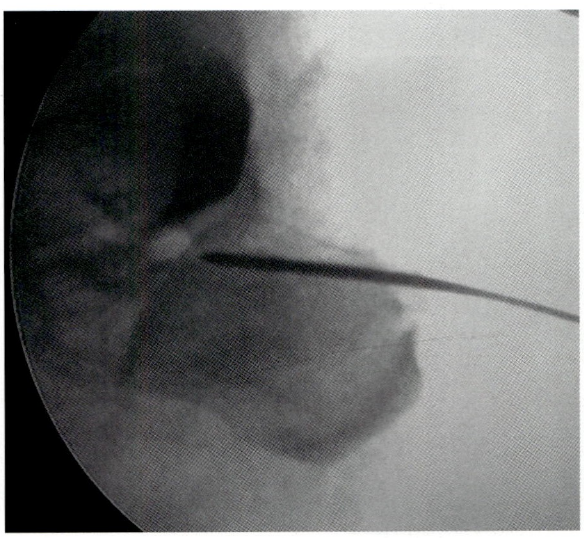

Fig. 53: C-arm confirmation of K-wire in calcaneum.

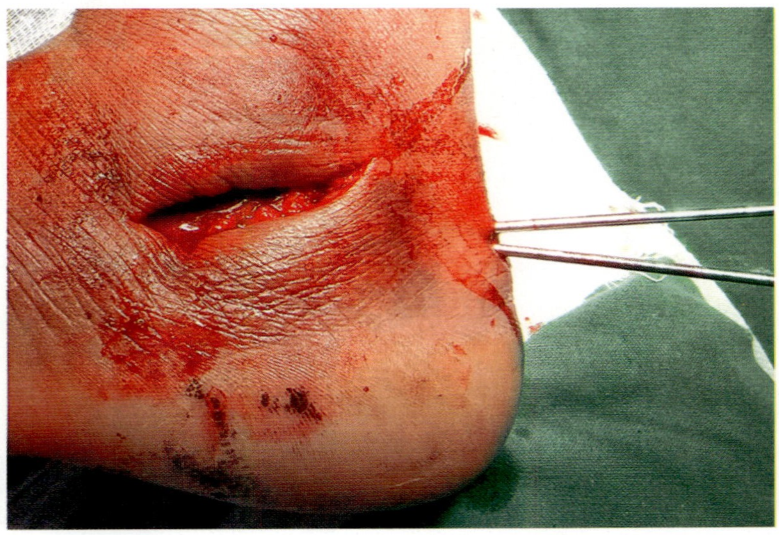

Fig. 54: Another K-wire is introduced through calcaneal tuberosity and fixed to cuboid bone that maintains reduction.

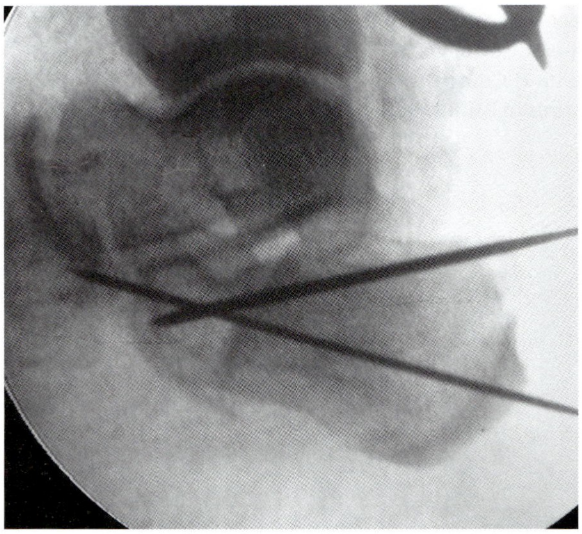

Fig. 55: C-arm image showing both K-wires.

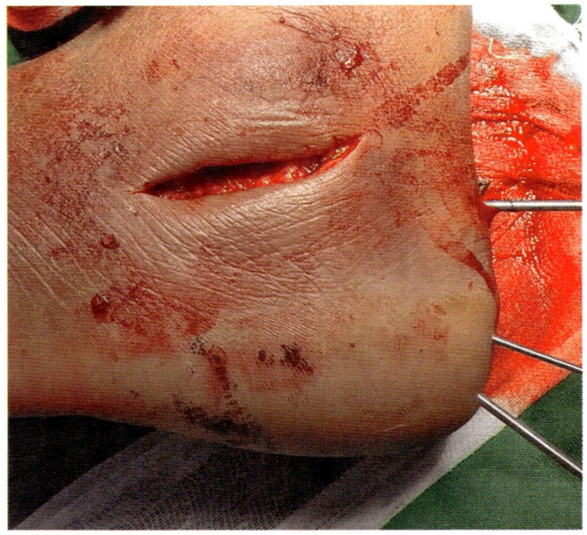

Fig. 56: Another K-wire is introduced inferior to the second K-wire and fixed to cuboid.

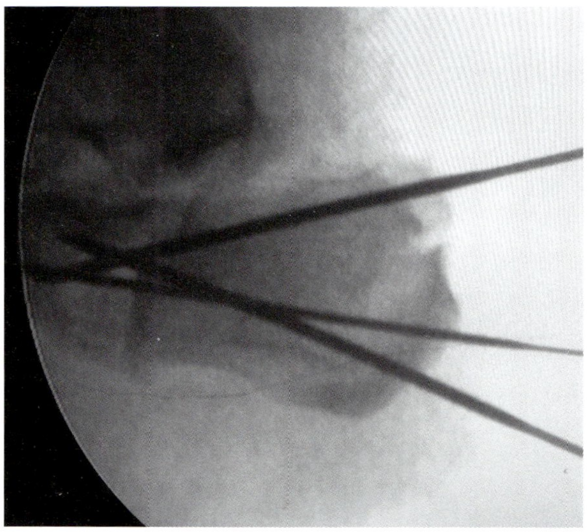

Fig. 57: C-arm image showing reduction of calcaneum using K-wires.

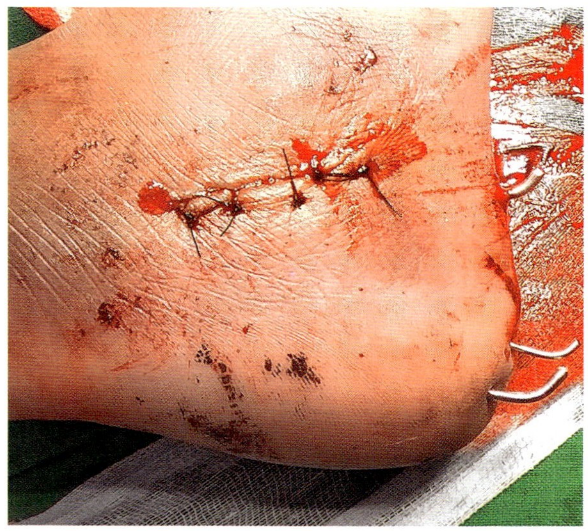

Fig. 58: Wash is given with povidone–iodine. Skin is closed with nonabsorbable suture material 2-0.

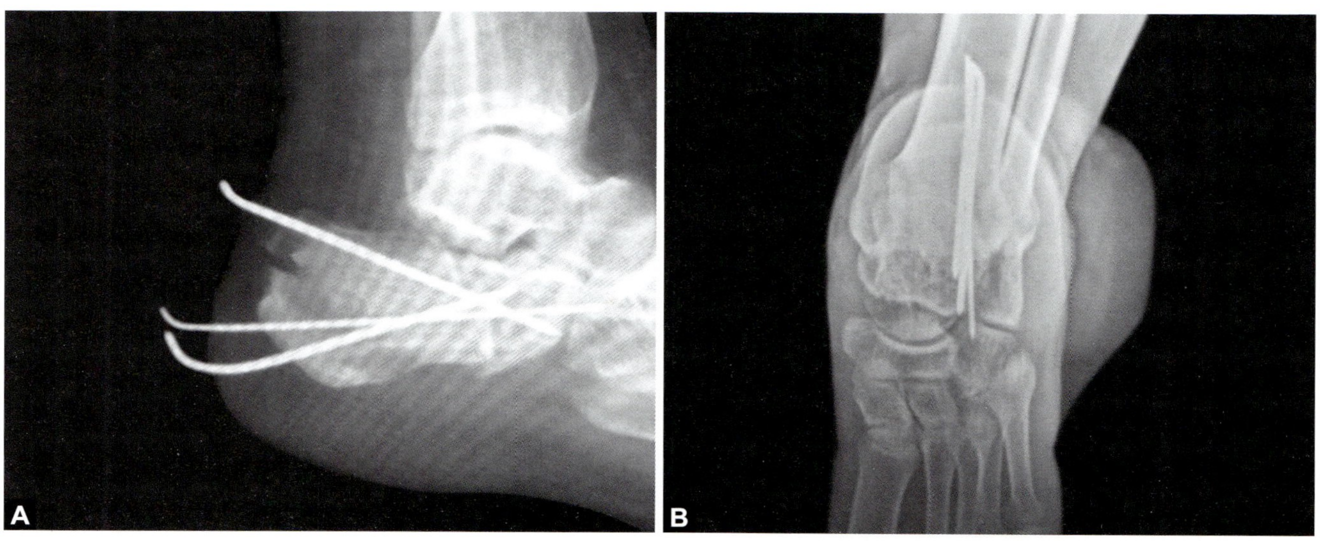

Figs. 59A and B: Postoperative radiographs.

SUGGESTED READING

1. Azar FM, Canale ST, Beaty JH. Campbell's Operative Orthopaedics, 13th edition. Canada: Elsevier; 2016.
2. Blom A, Warwick D, Whitehouse M. Apley and Solomon's System of Orthopaedics and Trauma, 10th edition. Boca Raton, Florida, United States: CRC Press; 2017.
3. Miller MD, Thompson SR. Miller's Review of Orthopaedics, 7th edition. Canada: Elsevier; 2016.
4. Tornetta P, Court-Brown C, Heckmen JD, et al. Rockwood and Green's Fractures in Adults, 8th edition. USA: Wolters Kluwer; 2014.

CHAPTER 64

Metatarsal Fractures Fixation

S Prakash, Siddharth Jaiswal

INTRODUCTION

Metatarsal bone is located between the tarsal bones and the phalanges of the toes in our feet. When we are standing, walking, or running, these bones bear most of our body weight. Metatarsal fractures are common across all ages and occur equally in men and women.

Each metatarsal is divided into segments, i.e. the head, neck, shaft, and base.

March fracture is an unusual type of fracture of the distal third of metatarsal occurring because of recurrent stress. More common in soldiers, also occurs in hikers, and even those, like hospital doctors, whose duties require long standing. March fractures commonly seen in second and third metatarsal bones of the foot.

EPIDEMIOLOGY

- In adults fracture is seen most commonly in fifth metatarsal.
- Peak incidence is between 20–50 years of age.
- Commonly associated with second and fourth metatarsal fractures. Isolated third metatarsal fractures are rare.

MECHANISM

These fractures occur as a result of direct hit or by indirect mechanism when hindfoot and leg rotate on fixed forefoot.

Associated conditions:
- *Lisfranc injury*:
  - Lisfranc like injuries are seen when multiple proximal metatarsals fracture.
- In ballet dancer, fracture at base of second metatarsal seen.

CLASSIFICATION

Classification of metatarsal fractures depends on:
- Location
- Fracture pattern
- Displacement
- Angulation
- Articular involvement.

IMAGING

- *Radiographs*:
  - Anteroposterior (AP), lateral and oblique views of foot
  - *Optional*: Stress views to be ordered in both anteroposterior and lateral planes.
- CT scan advised to rule out Lisfranc fracture and periarticular injuries.
- MRI or bone scan to rule out stress or occult fracture.

CLINICAL PRESENTATION

Patients typically presents with pain, swelling and tenderness in the midfoot to forefoot.

Swelling and tenderness is noted over the affected metatarsal. Patients usually can bear weight though with limp.

TREATMENT

Nonsurgical Treatment

Most undisplaced fractures can be managed conservatively. Treatment includes rest and unloading of the foot. Plaster cast is usually sufficient. In some cases, several weeks of crutches may be required; 2–3 months are required for complete recovery.

Surgical Treatment

Surgery is indicated for a displaced metatarsal fractures or in case of nonunion. Surgery involves fixation with a plate and screws or K-wires and at times a bone graft in case of nonunion.

SURGICAL STEPS (FIGS. 1 TO 12)

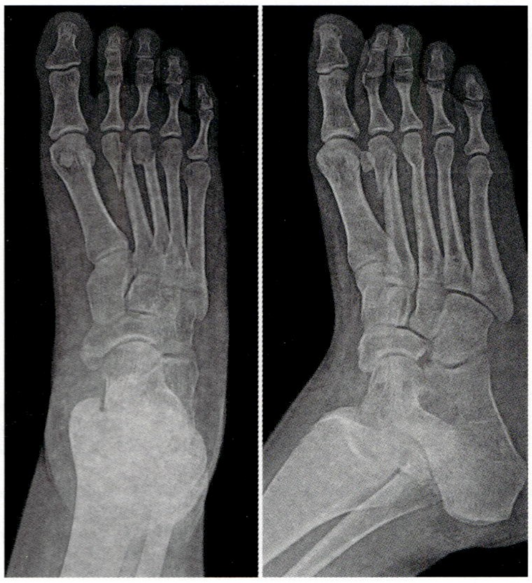

Fig. 1: Preoperative X-ray: fracture distal shaft of second metatarsal and fracture third neck metatarsal.

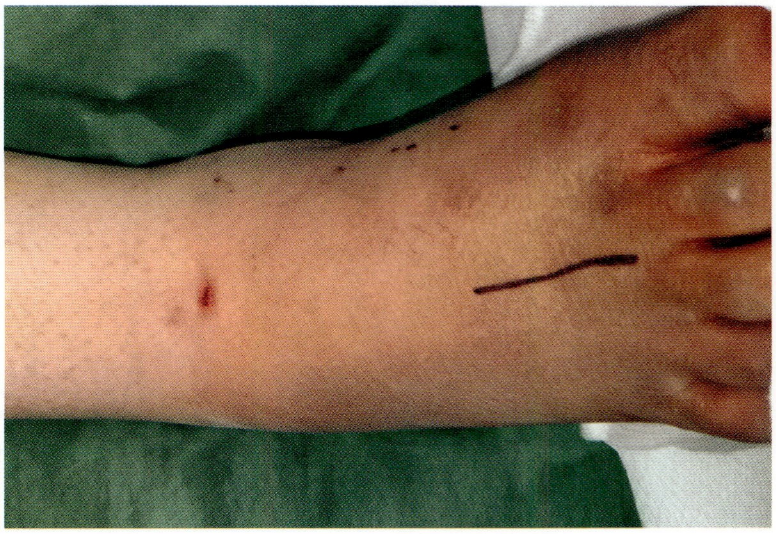

Fig. 2: Incision (1 inch in length): Surface marking inch in length between second and third metatarsal distally.

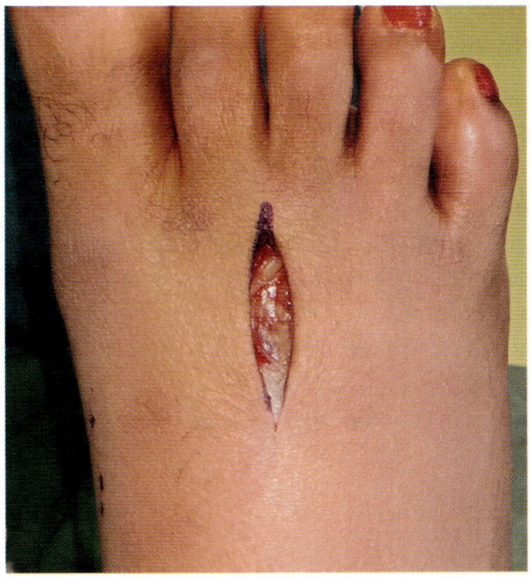

Fig. 3: Incision taken over marking.

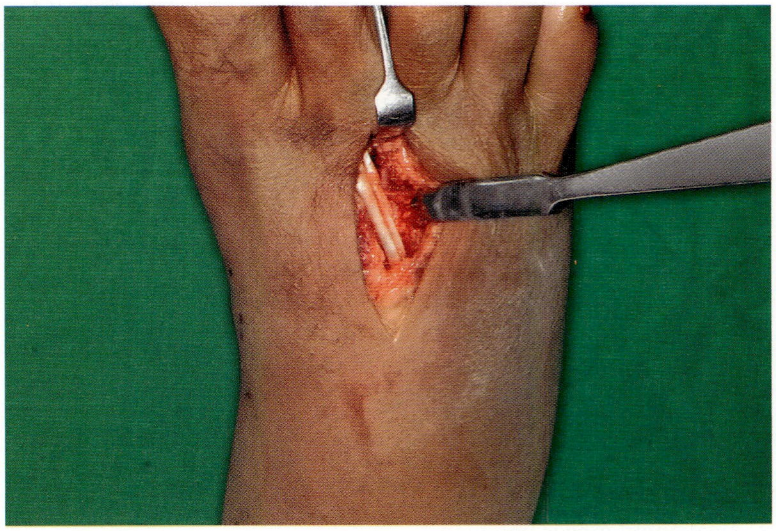

Fig. 4: Extensor digitorum longus and brevis over second metatarsal exposed.

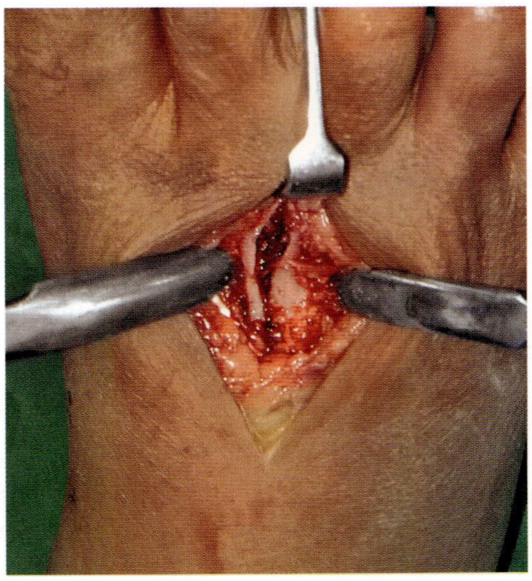

Fig. 5: Fracture site exposed with bone lever.

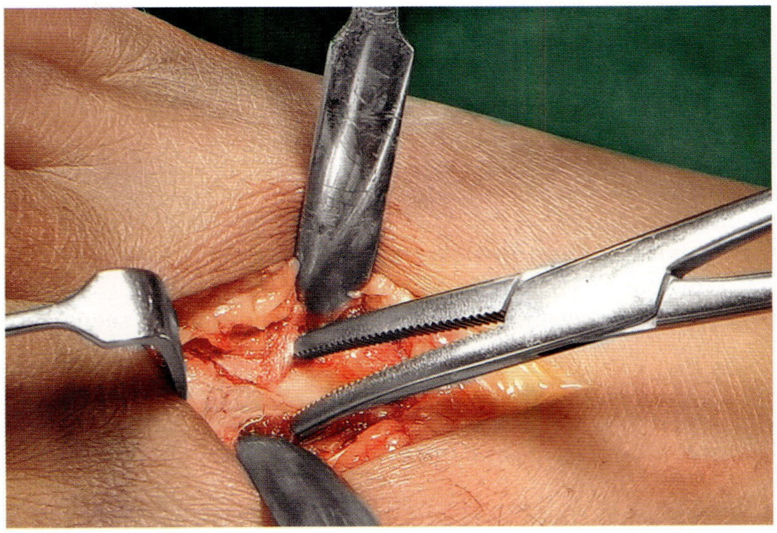

Fig. 6: Fracture reduction done with help of bone-holding forceps.

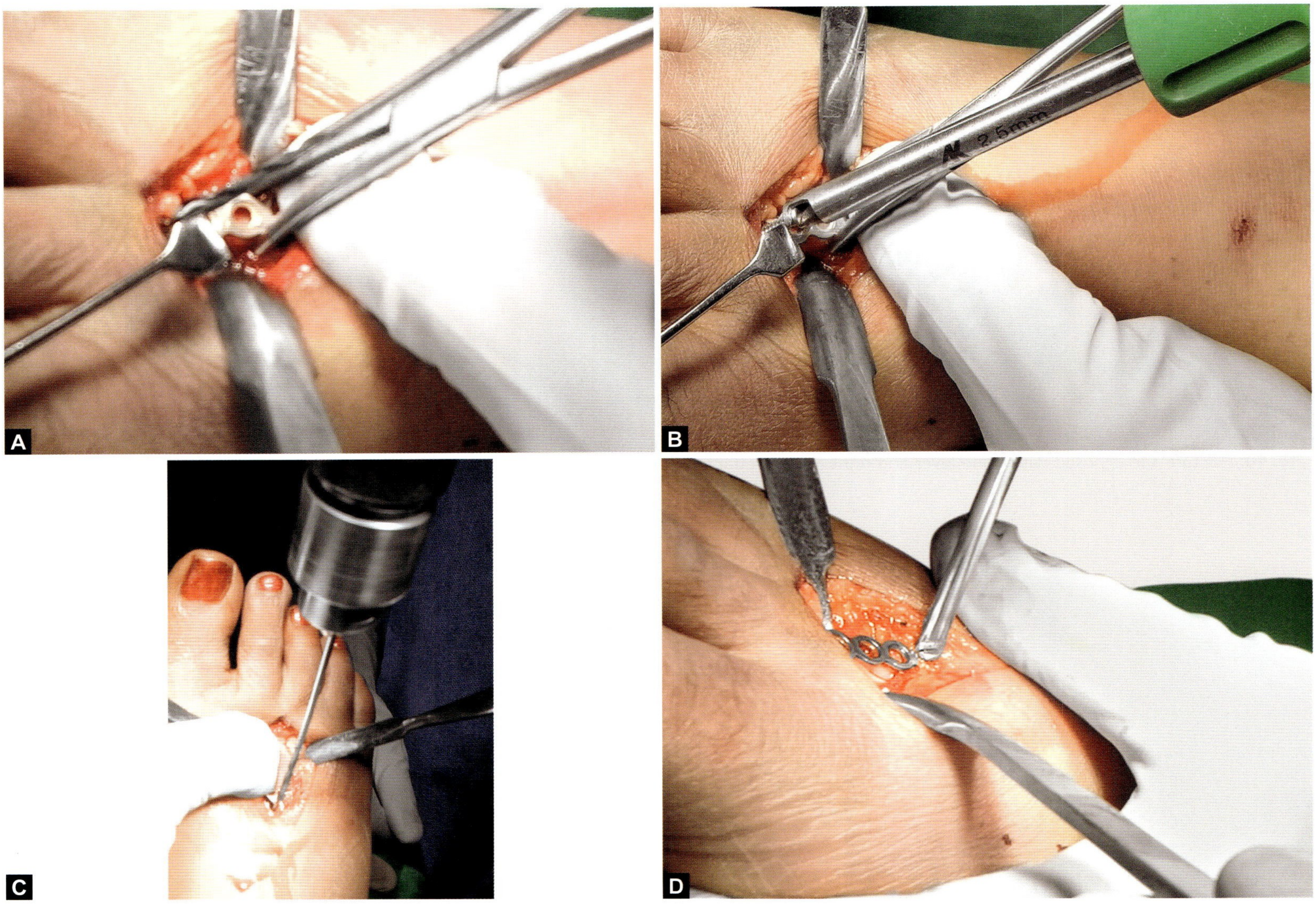

Figs. 7A to D: 2.5 mm reconstruction plate placed across fracture and fixation done with screw.

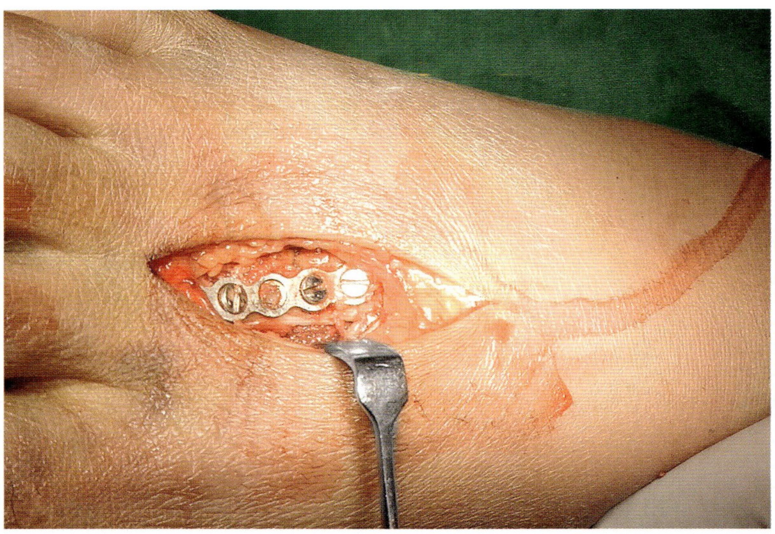

Fig. 8: Clinical photo after fixation of fracture shaft second metatarsal.

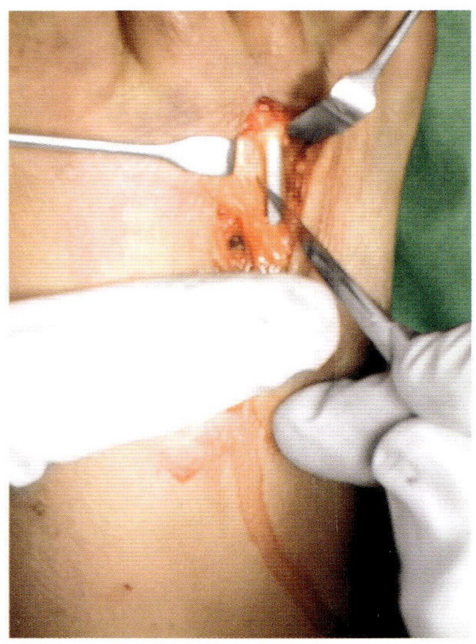

Fig. 9: Extensor digitorum longus over third metatarsal exposed.

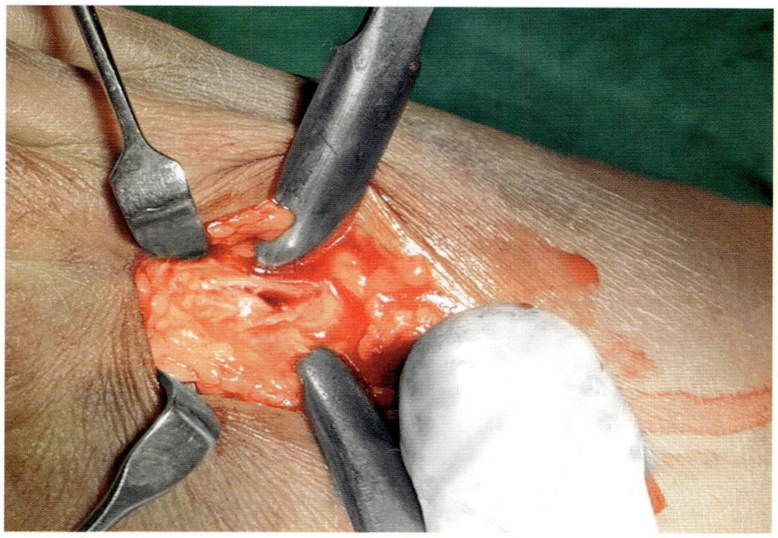

Fig. 10: Fracture site exposed with bone lever and right-angled retractor.

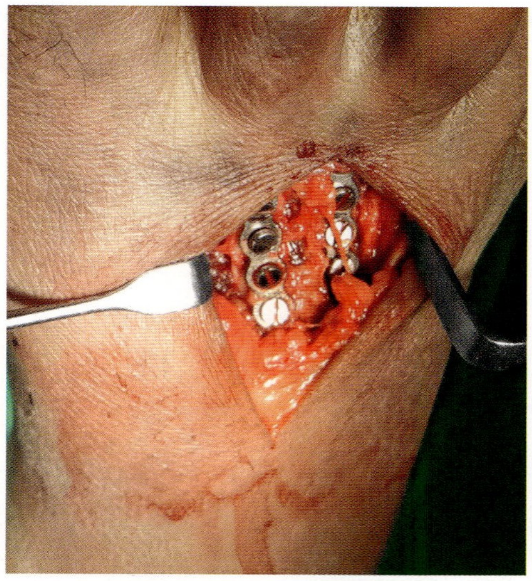

Fig. 11: Reconstruction 2.5-mm plate placed across fracture and fixation done with cortical screws.

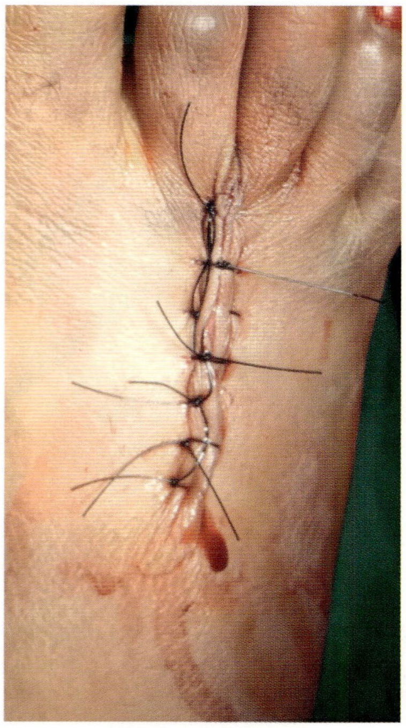

Fig. 12: Skin closure.

POTENTIAL COMPLICATIONS OF METATARSAL FRACTURES

Though uncommon following complications are noted.

- Vascular injury.
- Delayed healing and nonunion (mainly proximal fifth metatarsal fractures distal to styloid)
- Malunion
- Compartment syndrome
- Infection and osteomyelitis in case of open fracture.

SUGGESTED READING

1. Eiff MP, Hatch RL, Calmbach WL. Fracture Management for Primary Care, 2nd edition. Philadelphia, PA: Saunders; 2003: pp. 331-52.
2. Eiff MP, Saultz JW. Fracture care by family physicians. J Am Board Fam Pract. 1993;6:179-81.
3. Hatch RL, Rosenbaum CI. Fracture care by family physicians. A review of 295 cases. J Fam Pract. 1994;38:238-44.
4. O'Malley MJ, Hamilton WG, Munyak J. Fractures of the distal shaft of the fifth metatarsal. "Dancer's fracture". Am J Sports Med. 1996;24:240-3.
5. Zenios M, Kim WY, Sampath J, et al. Functional treatment of acute metatarsal fractures: a prospective randomised comparison of management in a cast versus elasticated support bandage. Injury. 2005;36:832-5.

CHAPTER 65

Diabetic Foot: Midfoot Amputation

Sachin Nagapurkar, Nitish Agrawal, Abhishek Ranjan

INTRODUCTION

Incidence of diabetic foot ulceration is uncommon in diabetic foot patients and is about 15%. The most common reason for nontraumatic lower limb amputation is diabetic foot. The risk of lower extremity amputation is increased by 15–46 times in diabetics as compared to healthy individuals. About 3–5% of diabetic foot patients are amputees.

About 85% of amputations can be prevented by early detection and appropriate management of these ulcers.

RISK FACTORS FOR LOWER EXTREMITY AMPUTATION IN THE DIABETIC FOOT

- Peripheral neuropathy
- Arterial insufficiency
- Autonomic neuropathy
- Foot deformity and callosity formation
- Limited joint mobility
- History of foot ulcer or lower extremity amputation.
- Obesity
- Impaired vision
- Poor footwear
- Poor glucose control.

WAGNER–MEGGITT CLASSIFICATION OF DIABETIC FOOT ULCER

- *Grade 0*: No ulcer
- *Grade 1*: Superficial skin ulcer
- *Grade 2*: Deep ulcer extending through ligament, tendon, joint capsule, or deep fascia without abscess or osteomyelitis
- *Grade 3*: Deep ulcer with abscess or osteomyelitis or joint sepsis
- *Grade 4*: Localized gangrene of forefoot or heel
- *Grade 5*: Gangrene involves whole foot.

DIAGNOSIS OF DIABETIC FOOT ULCER

Blood test like blood glucose level and urine for glucose and ketones, full blood count, erythrocyte sedimentation rate (ESR), C-reactive protein (CRP), blood urea, electrolytes, and creatinine levels, glycosylated hemoglobin (HbA1C), hepatic, and renal function tests.

- X-ray
- Magnetic resonance imaging
- Technetium or white blood cell (WBC)-labeled indium-111 bone scan
- Culture and sensitivity examination of cultures from the deeper tissue.

TREATMENT

Nonsurgical Treatment

- Strict control of blood glucose levels should be done with strict diabetic diet, the use of oral hypoglycemic drugs and insulin
- Negative pressure wound therapy
- Hyperbaric oxygen therapy
- Orthotics and braces can be used for healing of diabetic foot ulcer
- Mechanical offloading.

Surgical Treatment

- Surgery for debridement of foot ulcer and preventing new ones can help people recover from diabetic foot ulcers.
- Debridement for grade 2 ulcer with intravenous antibiotics.
- For grade 3, emergency drainage of acute infection is necessary.
- For grade 4 and 5, amputation at appropriate level.

AMPUTATIONS

Removal of part of or an entire limb through one or more bones. It is called disarticulation when it is performed through a joint. It is not a failure of surgery but a reconstructive procedure. Goal is surgical reconstruction that retains most function of the limb.

Classification

- Emergency or traumatic or elective
- Provisional and definitive
- Open and closed
- End bearing and cone bearing.

Indications of Amputation

Congenital Conditions

Hemimelia, polydactyly, congenital pseudarthrosis, proximal femoral focal deficiency (PFFD), gross congenital malformations.

Acquired

- *Trauma*: Mangled limb, crush injury
- *Vascular*: DM (diabetic) angiopathy, peripheral vascular disease (PVD)
- *Infective*: Methicillin resistant *Staphylococcus aureus*, clostridia
- *Neoplasm*: Osteosarcoma
- Frost bite
- Burns.

Goals of Amputations

- To get rid of all necrotic infected and painful tissue
- To have a wound that heals successfully
- To have an appropriate remnant stump that is able to accommodate a prosthesis.

Preoperative Assessment

- To ascertain indication
- Site of amputation
- General medical condition
- Rehabilitation potential
- Counseling
- Written consent
- Optimization.

Assessment of whole patient including affected limb and unaffected limb is conducted thoroughly.

Assessment of social, physical and psychological status of the patient is important.

Preoperative Evaluation

Investigation

- To confirm diagnosis:
  - Doppler, X-ray, FBS (fasting blood sugar), and technetium-99 bone scan
- Ability of wound healing:
  - Trans cutaneous oxygen measurement hemoglobin, serum albumin, and absolute lymphocyte count.

Ideal Amputation Stump

- It should be of optimum length
- The end of stump should be smooth and rounded
- It should be firm
- The opposing group of muscles should be sutured together over the end of the bone
- The muscles are sutured in such a way that they will be converted into firm fibrous tissue and serve as an effective cushion
- Vascularity of the flaps should be normal
- There should be no projecting spur of bone
- The position of the scar should be away from pressure points and should be transverse to avoid pulling up between two bones in amputation scar
- In case of upper limb, the scar can be terminal, but in lower limb an anterior or posterior scar is desirable to avoid pressure of weight of artificial limb.

SURGICAL STEPS (FIGS. 1 TO 23)

A 60-year-old male presented with complaints of blackening of left foot with nonhealing ulcer since 4 months. Color Doppler study of left lower limb showed diminished circulation of dorsalis pedis and posterior tibial artery with atherosclerotic changes. Patient is a known case of diabetes mellitus.

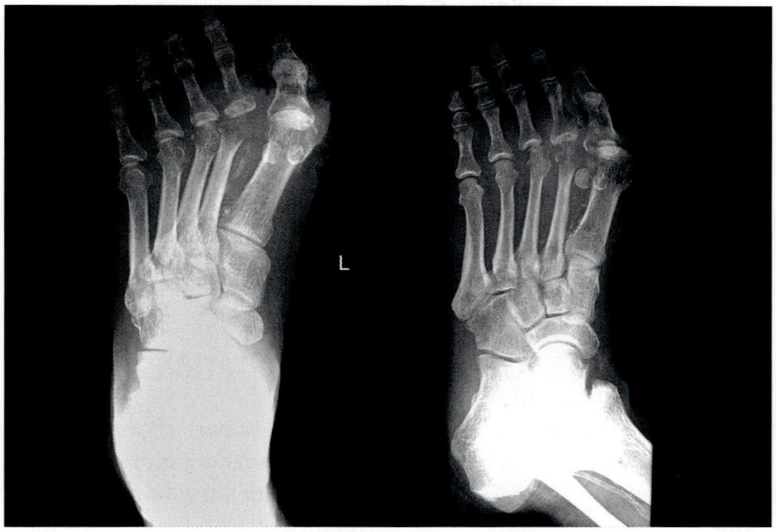

Fig. 1: Preoperative X-ray.

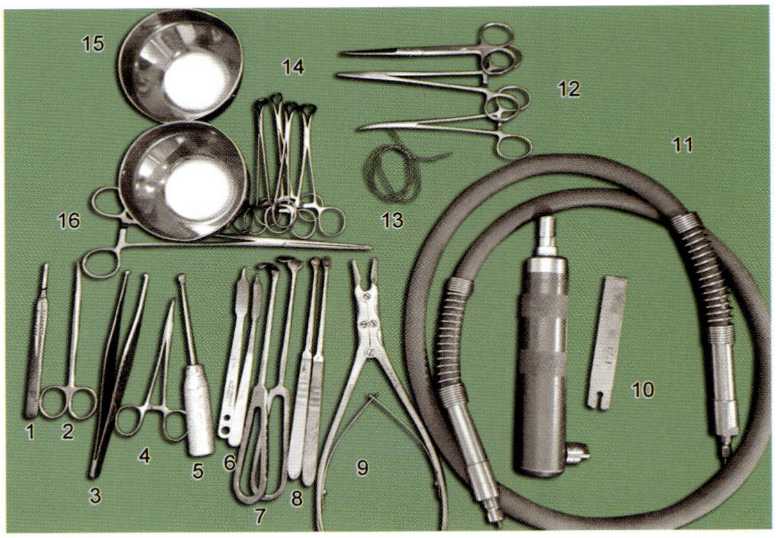

Fig. 2: (1) Bard Parker handle knife, (2) Dissecting scissor, (3) Tooth forceps, (4) Mosquito forceps, (5) Periosteum, (6) Hohmann bone lever, (7) Right angle retractor, (8) Curettes, (9) Bone nibbler, (10) Saw blade, (11) Drill, (12) Scissors, (13) Linen thread, (14) Towel clip, (15) Sterile container, (16) Sponge holding forceps.

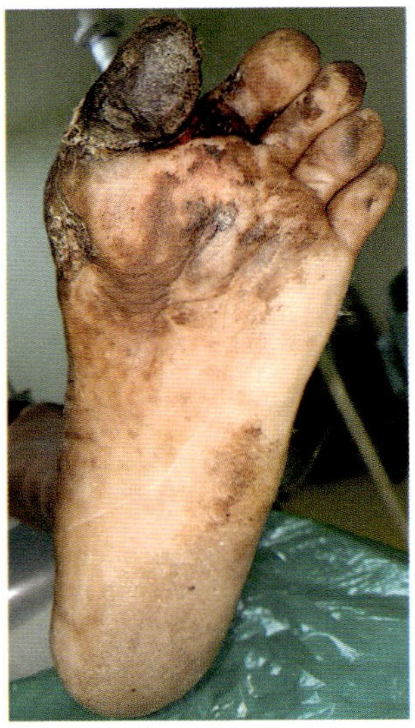

Fig. 3: Plantar aspect of foot showing dry gangrene of great toe.

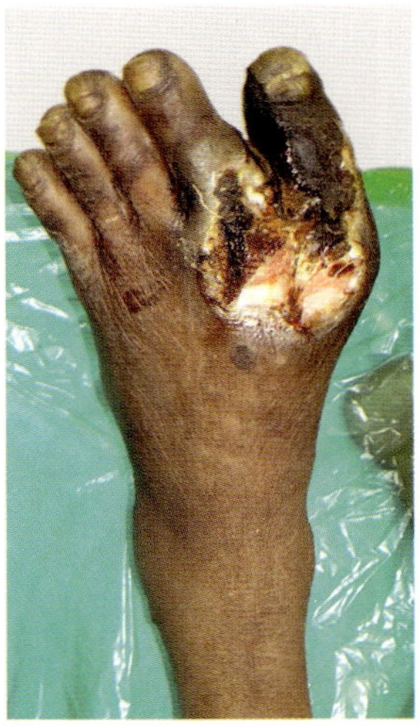

Fig. 4: Dorsum of foot showing dry gangrene of great toe with nonhealing ulcer around first and second metatarsal region with diminished blood supply to all other toes.

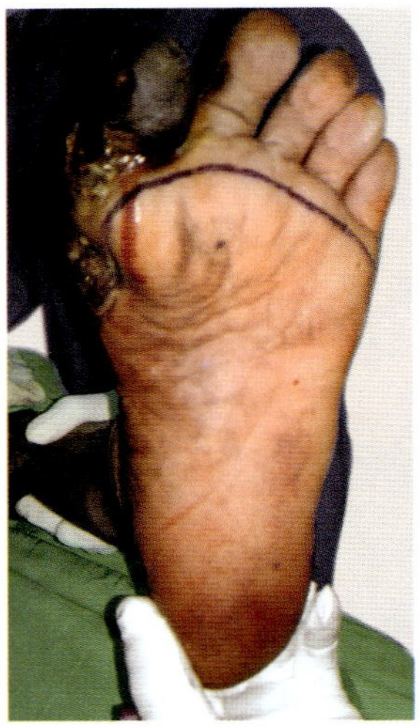

Fig. 5: Incision site was marked on plantar aspect of foot on metatarso-phalangeal joint area 3–4 cm distal to bone level of amputation.

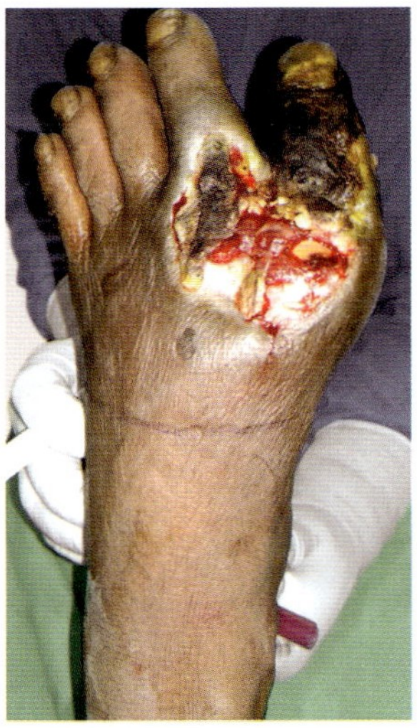

Fig. 6: Incision site was marked on dorsum of foot on metatarsal shaft region (transmetatarsal region) proximal to ulcer 1–2 cm distal to bone level of amputation.

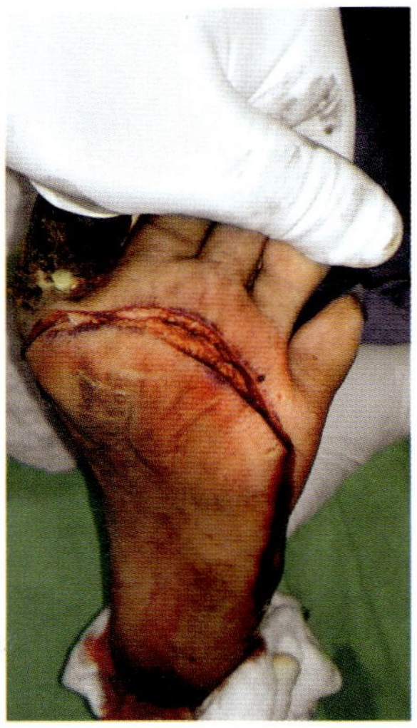

Fig. 7: A racquet incision is taken on plantar aspect of foot 3–4 cm distal to bone level of amputation to create flap for amputation stump. If muscle and skin are viable, plantar flap is preferred. If viability is doubtful then both plantar and dorsal concave open fish mouth incision are preferred.

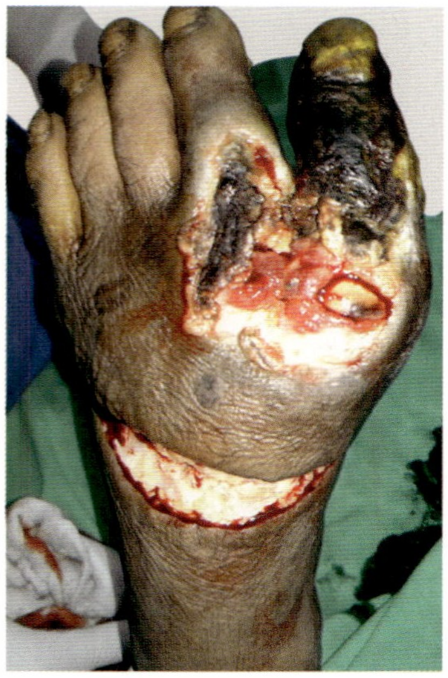

Fig. 8: Incision taken on dorsal aspect of foot at transmetatarsal region.

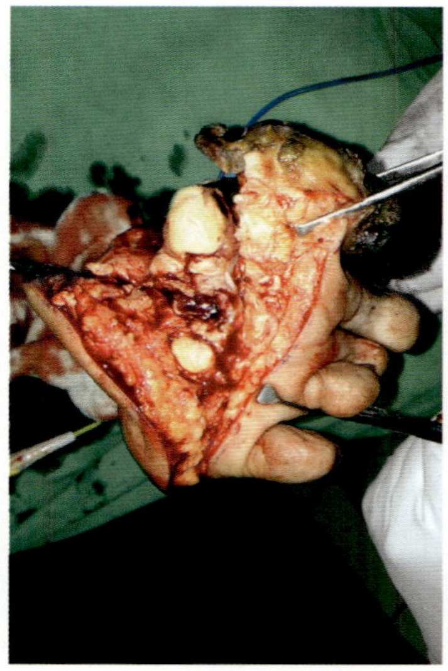

Fig. 9: Soft tissue, superficial fat, fascia, and capsule of joint were dissected with cautery. Tendons are retracted distally and sharp cut taken on proximal end to allow retraction of tendon ends proximally into stump. Soft tissue retracted with Allis tissue forceps. Disarticulation done at metatarsophalangeal joints and all toes along with ulcer are discarded.

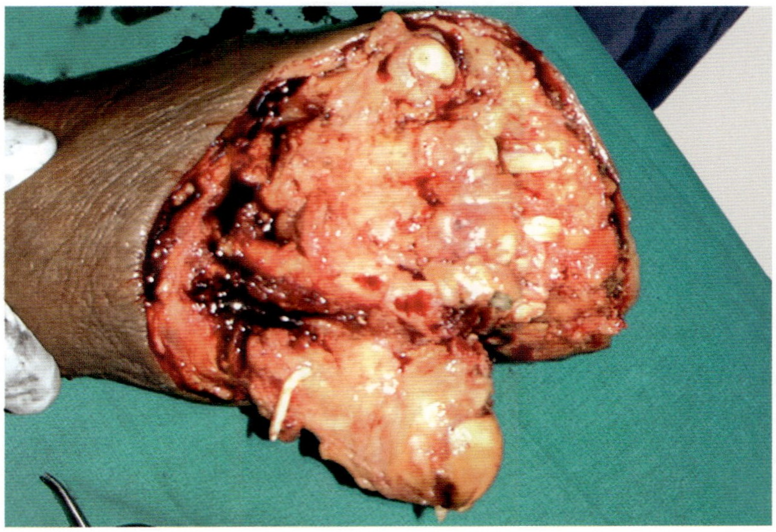

Fig. 10: All metatarsals are now exposed with minimal soft tissue.

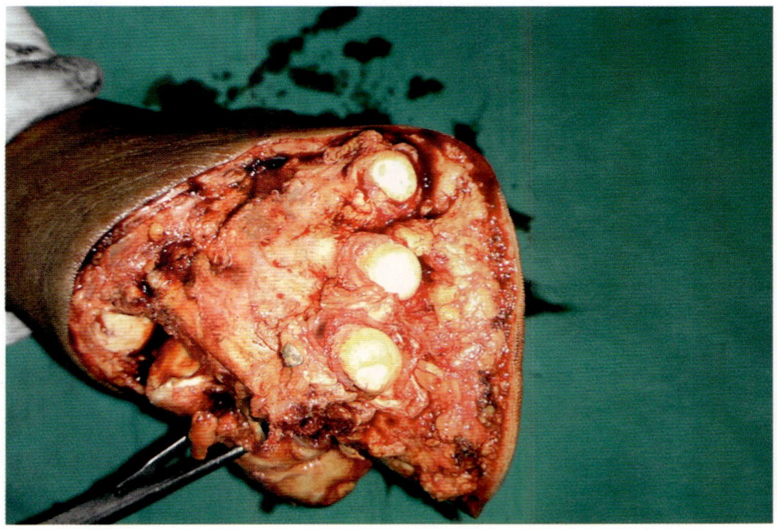

Fig. 11: Disarticulation of first tarsometatarsal joint is done and first metatarsal amputated.

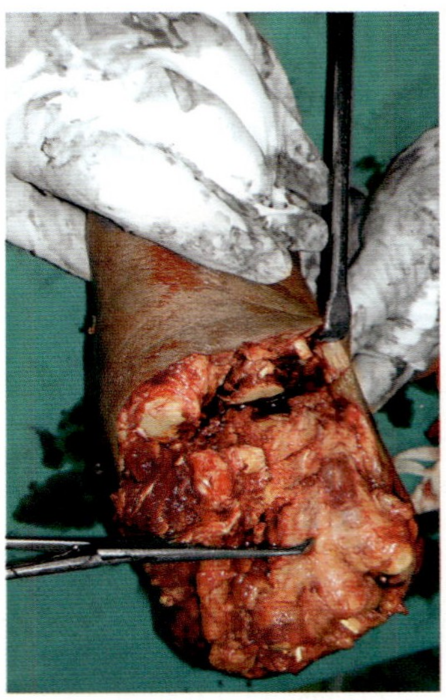

Fig. 12: Disarticulation of second, third, fourth, and fifth tarsometatarsal joint is done and metatarsals amputated.

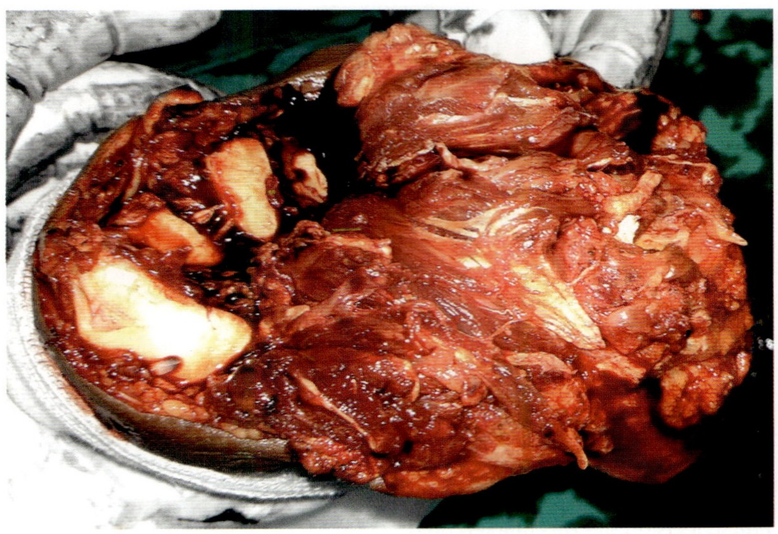

Fig. 13: All three cuneiform along with cuboid bones were exposed. There should be no projecting spur of bone. Tourniquet is released. Ample capillary bleeding is noted.

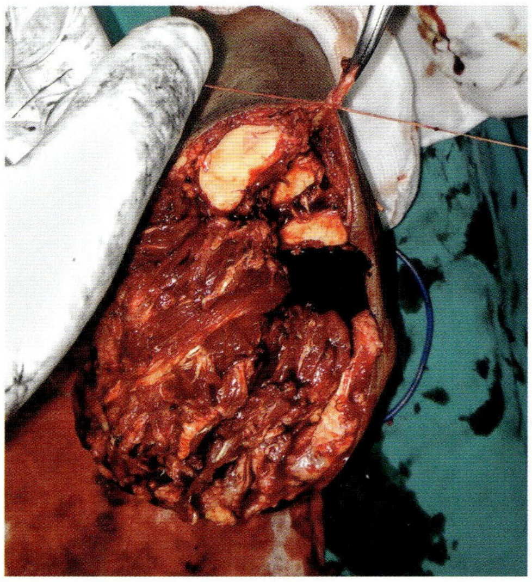

Fig. 14: Dorsalis pedis artery is tied with linen thread.

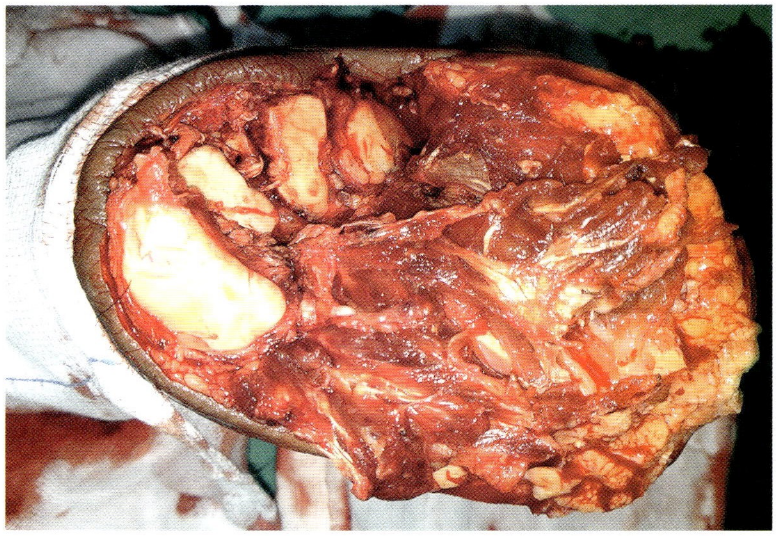

Fig. 15: Plantar flap is created.

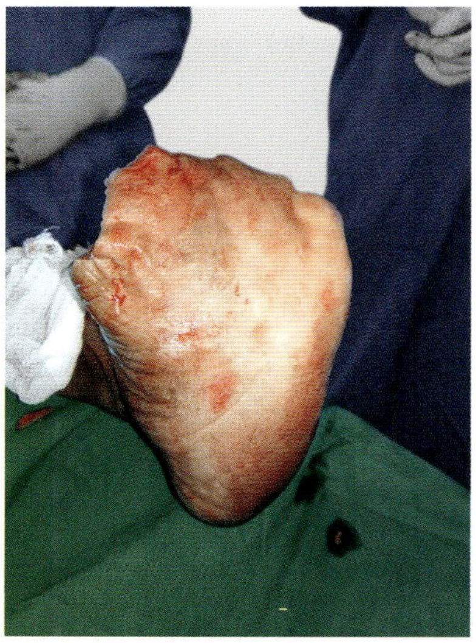

Fig. 16: Opposite group of muscles are sutured together over the end of bones by pulling over of plantar side muscles. Muscles are sutured in such a way that they will serve as an effective cushion.

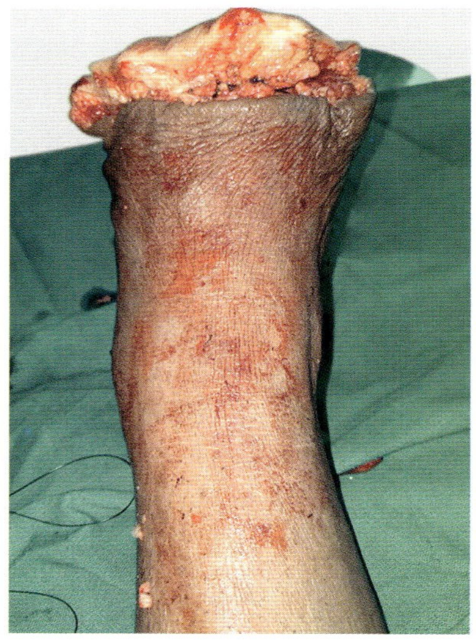

Fig. 17: Fascia and subcutaneous tissue suturing done with absorbable suture material.

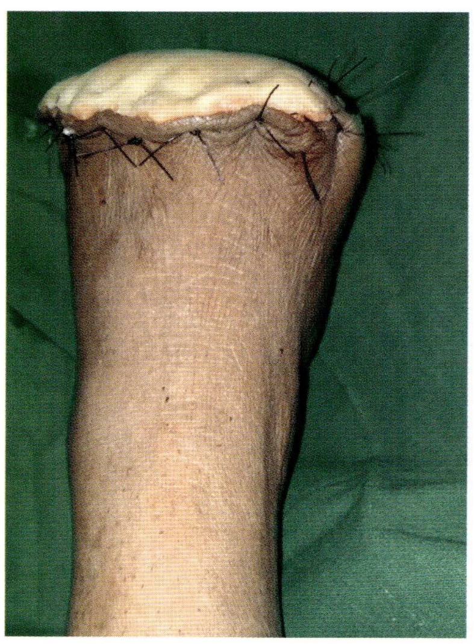

Fig. 18: Skin sutured in interrupted manner by nonabsorbable suture material. Dog ear should be avoided at the suture ends. Approximation of skin is achieved with minimum tension to prevent necrosis of skin at suture line. A corrugated drain may be kept depending on oozing to prevent hematoma formation.

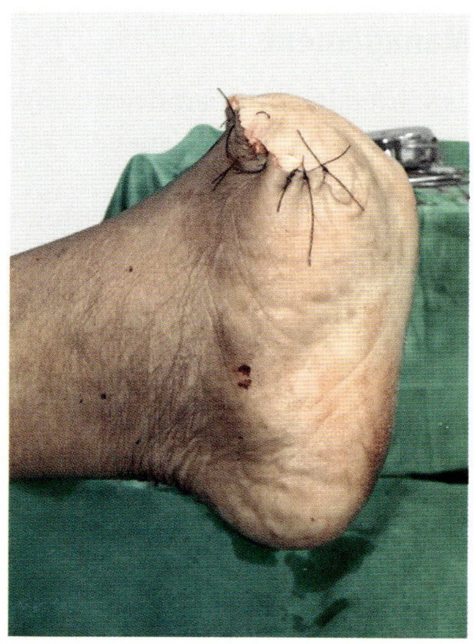

Fig. 19: Medial side.

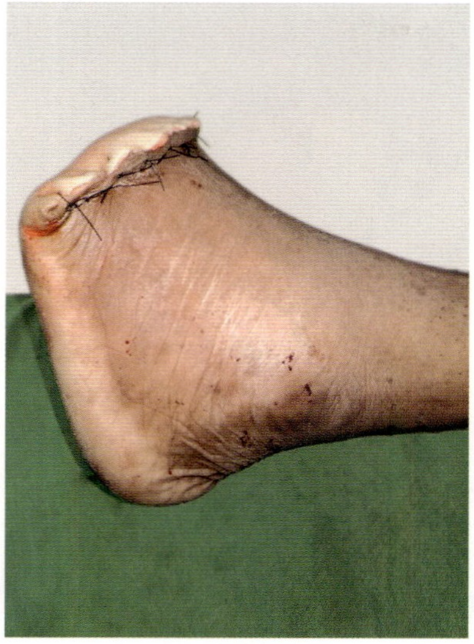

Fig. 20: Lateral side.

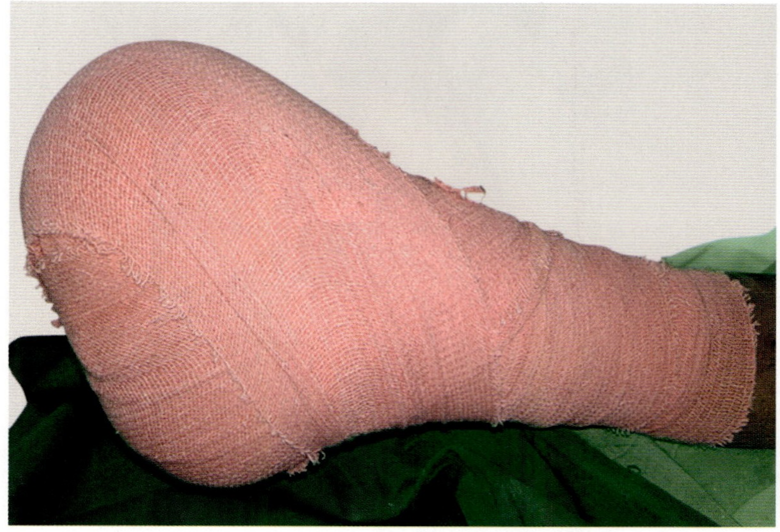

Fig. 21: Light compression dressing was done.

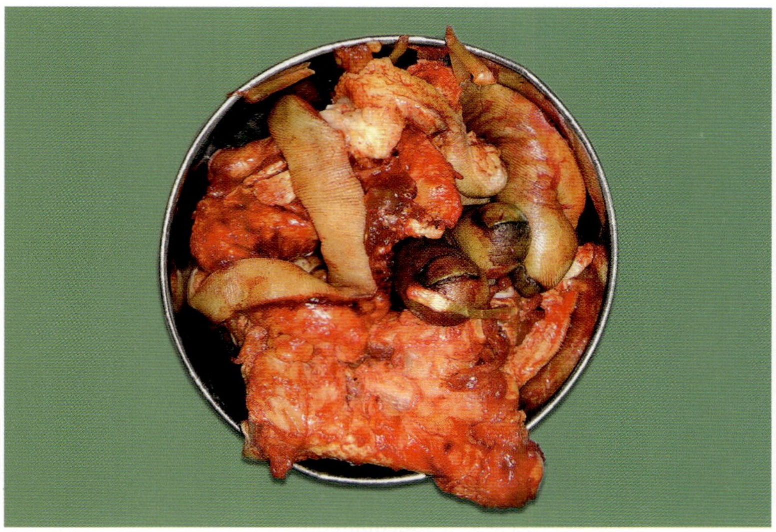

Fig. 22: Amputated tissue was discarded.

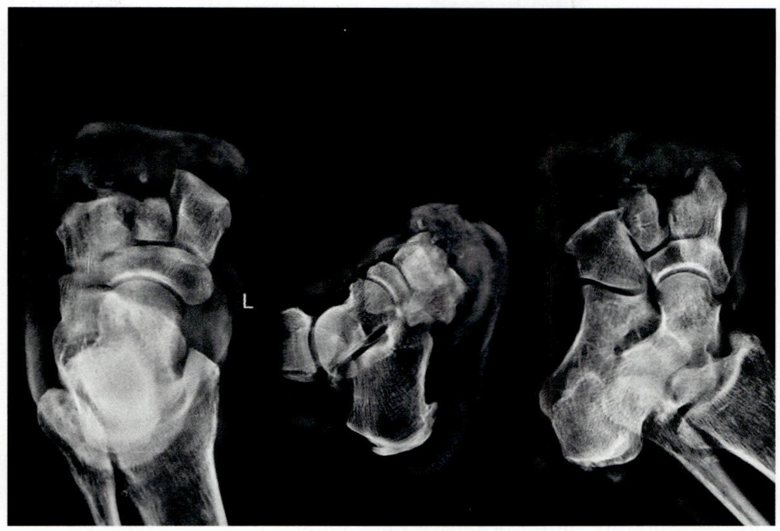

Fig. 23: Postoperative X-ray.

Postoperative Management

- Pentoxifylline is started in postoperative management to increase peripheral circulation to improve success rate and survival of stump.
- Drain is removed after 48 hours and dressing was changed and wound checked for any soakage or edema.
- Suture removal is planned after 3–4 weeks when maximum healing noticed.

SUGGESTED READING

1. Brown M, Tang W, Patel A, et al. Partial foot amputation in patient with diabetic foot ulcers. Foot Ankle Int. 2012;33(9):707-16.
2. Capobianco CM, Stapleton JJ, Zgonis T. Soft tissue reconstruction pyramid in diabetic foot ulcers. Foot Ankle Spec. 2010;3(5):241-8.
3. Edwards J, Stapley S. Debridement of diabetic foot ulcers. Cochrane Database Syst Rev. 2010;(1):CD003556.
4. Loldahl M. Hyperbaric oxygen therapy as adjunctive treatment of diabetic foot ulcers. Med Clin North Am. 2013;97(5):957-80.

SECTION 7

GENERAL ORTHOPAEDICS

Section Editor: *Santosh Jeevannavar*

CHAPTER 66

Nonunion of Fracture Clavicle: Plate Fixation and Bone Grafting

Yash K Shah

INTRODUCTION

Nonunion of the fractures of the clavicle has an incidence of 1% to 4%. The risk factors are inadequate immobilization, severity of the trauma, gross displacement, location of fracture, re-fracture and initial open reduction.

The rate of nonunion following primary internal fixation is 0.1% to 4%.

Various techniques have been successfully used to treat nonunions and the success rate reported by Jupiter et al is 90%.

RISK FACTORS

Old age, female sex, displacement and comminution are important risk factors for nonunion. Yet most of the fractures are more common in young males, hence more cases of nonunions are seen in them.

SYMPTOMS

Nonunions of clavicle fractures may have a wide variety of symptoms, e.g. pain, clicking sensation, weakness, restriction of movement, neurological symptoms, cosmetic deformity, thoracic outlet syndrome and subclavian vein compression. Other reported symptoms include disturbed sleep, difficulty in doing daily activities, sporting activities and reduction in sexual activities.

INVESTIGATIONS

- X-ray clavicle anteroposterior (AP) view is advised.
- Computed tomography (CT) scan (in equivocal cases).

MANAGING NONUNION OF FRACTURES

For asymptomatic nonunion no treatment is advised. However patient should be willing to accept some cosmetic deformity and functional restriction.

However if he is symptomatic, then he can be treated with either a plate, or an intramedullary device with or without bone grafting. The success of this intervention is around 90%.

The treatment options are:

- Plating and autograft
- Plating and allograft
- Plating and vascular fibular graft
- Intramedullary fixation
- External fixator
- Bone morphogenic proteins
- Electrical stimulation.

Plating and Autograft

Iliac crest grafts are used in majority of the cases. The drawbacks of this modality are limited supply of autograft and donor site morbidity.

Plating and Allograft

Allografts are an option, but have limited osteoinductive capacity and may transmit diseases, also they have a limited capacity to incorporate.

Plating and Vascular Fibular Graft

Vascularized fibular and medial femoral condyle grafts are mostly indicated only in revision cases in which the primary treatment of nonunion has failed.

Intramedullary Fixation and External Fixation

These two modalities are rarely used. Intramedullary fixation although gives a more cosmetically acceptable scar, it is not as rigid. External fixation has been used to treat pseudoarthroses along with Papineau technique.

NONUNION OF LATERAL-END CLAVICLE FRACTURES

Lateral end clavicle fractures have a higher rate of nonunion as compared to mid shaft varying between 18% to 40%.

If nonunion lateral end clavicle is symptomatic, excision is usually done if the fragment is small and the coracoclavicluar ligaments are intact. If the fragment is large, then it is treated with open reduction and internal fixation, similar to the treatment of acute fractures of the clavicle. A bone graft may be added.

NONUNION OF LONG BONES CLAVICLE—SURGICAL STEPS

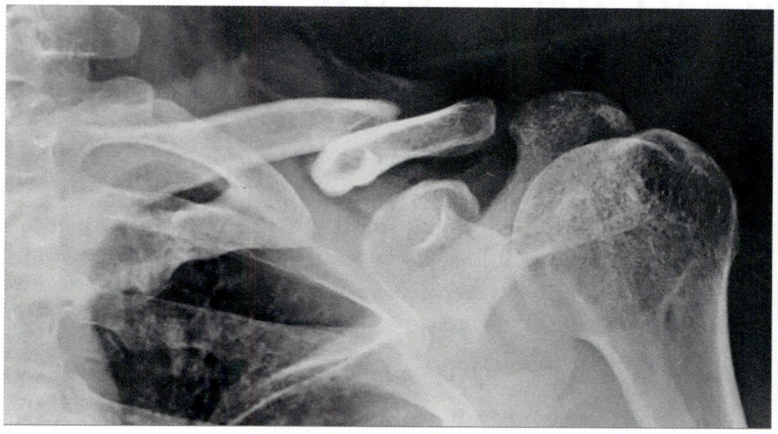

Fig. 1: X-ray showing a nonunion of the shaft of clavicle. Sclerosis can be observed at the ends of the clavicle.

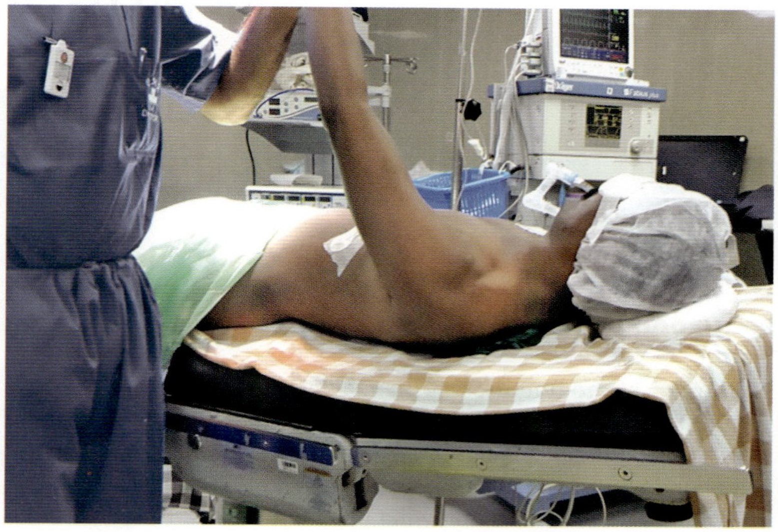

Fig. 2: Position of the patient. Head can be slightly elevated or patient can be fully supine. Make sure that if the patient is intubated the endotracheal tube is on the opposite side of the fracture.

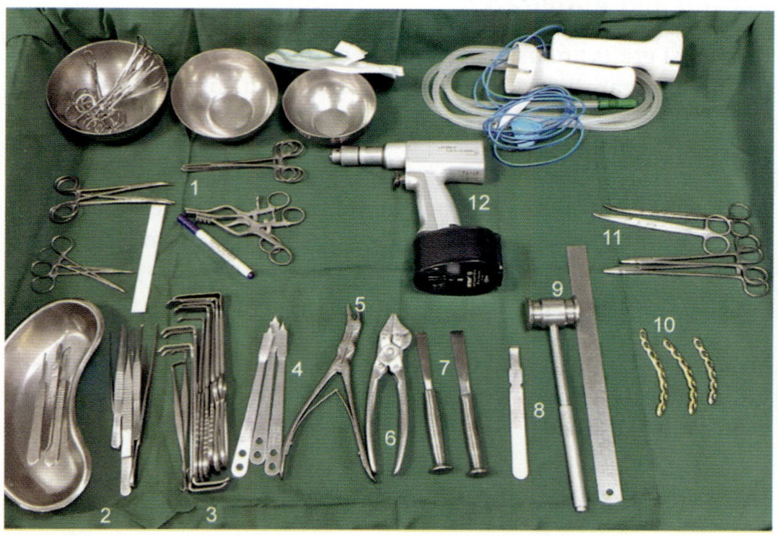

Fig. 3: Instruments required for clavicle plating. In addition, the instruments needed for iliac crest bone graft harvesting must be there. And if the bone graft harvest is planned simultaneously, we must have two sets of mastoid retractors, forceps, osteotomes, etc. (1) General surgical instruments (artery forceps, Allis forceps, Mollison mastoid retractor), (2) Toothed and plain forceps, and No. 15 and No. 23 sterile surgical blades on Bard Parker handles, (3) Right angle retractors of various sizes, (4) Bone spikes, (5) Bone nibbler, (6) Plier, (7) Sharp osteotomes, (8) Periosteum elevator, (9) Mallet, (10) Clavicle dynamic compression (DC) plates, (11) Needle holders and dissecting scissors, (12) Cordless power drill.

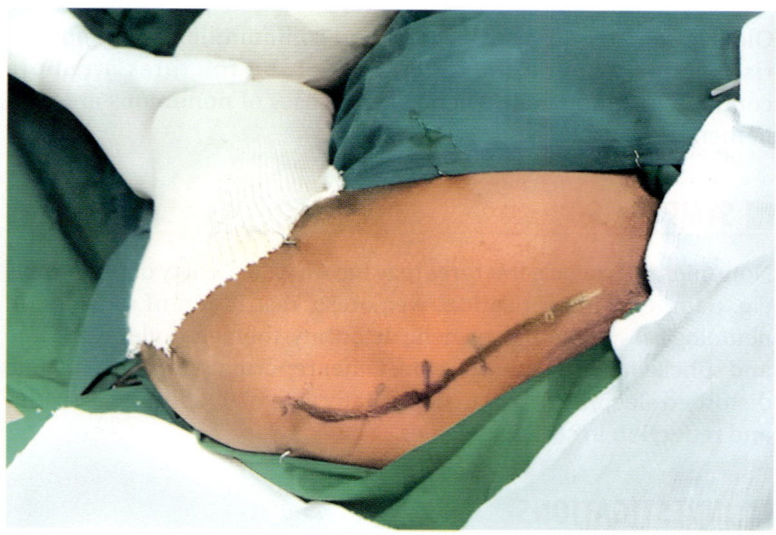

Fig. 4: After painting and draping, skin incision is marked with a sterile skin marking pen.

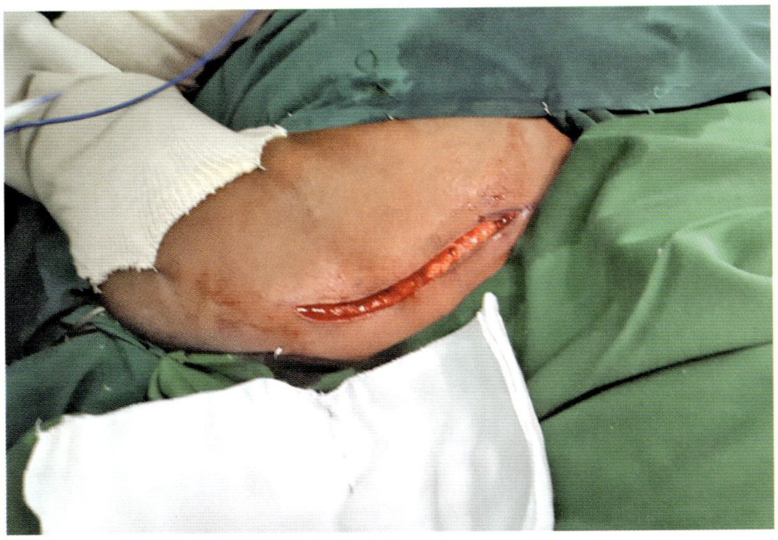

Fig. 5: Skin incision of about 8–10 cm is made.

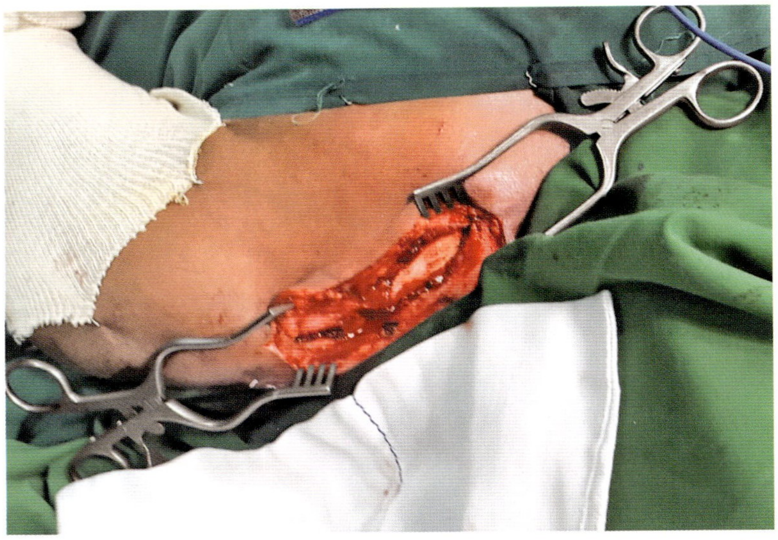

Fig. 6: Two self-retaining retractors reduce the work of the assistant. Care should be taken to relieve the pressure on the skin in case the surgery is taking too much time.

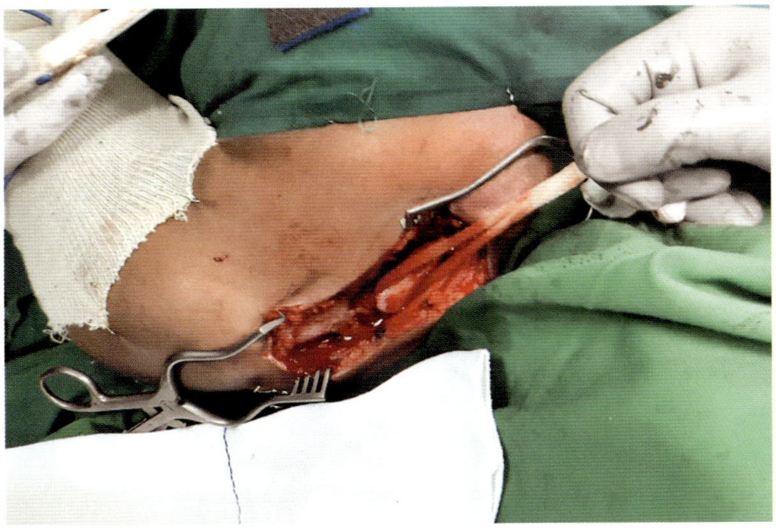

Fig. 7: One of the fragments may be hooked out with a roller bandage and lifted up, so that it becomes easy to curette and clean the sclerotic ends of the fracture.

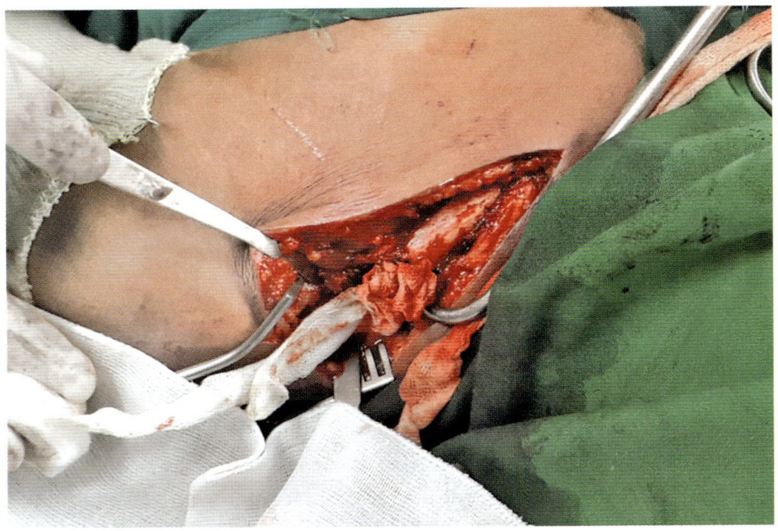

Fig. 8: Identify the fractured ends and freshen the edges.

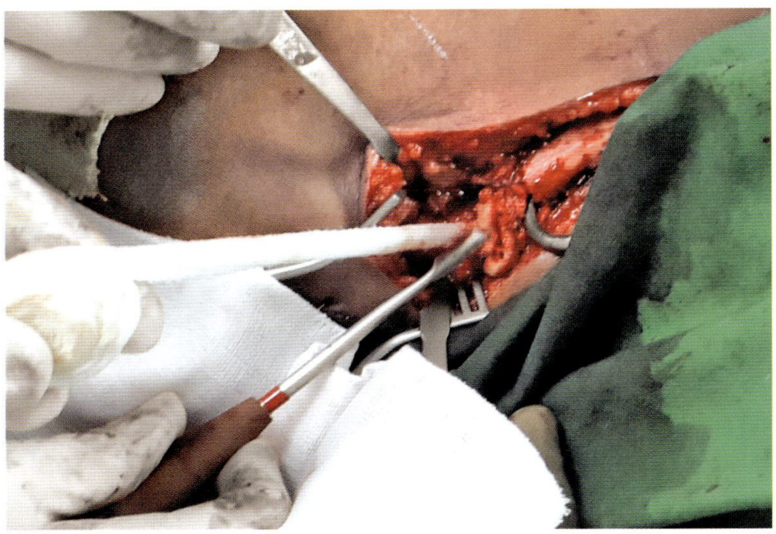

Fig. 9: Freshening of fracture edges done.

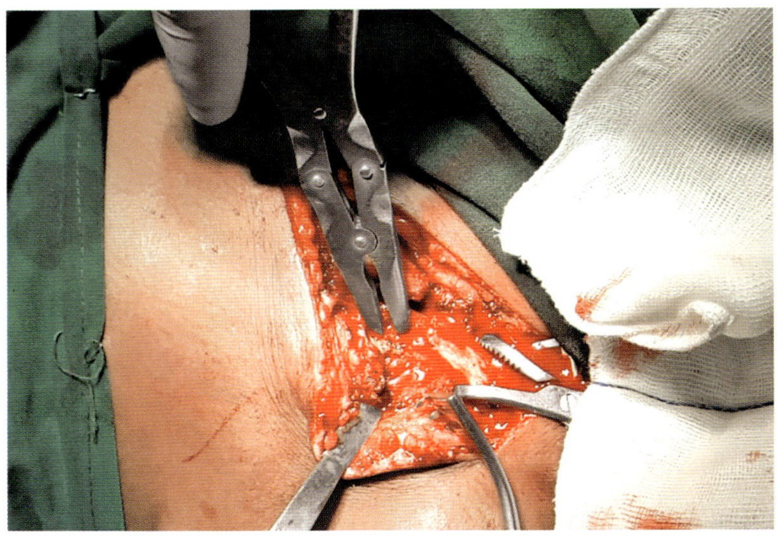

Fig. 10: Use a bone nibbler to nibble out the sclerotic bone ends.

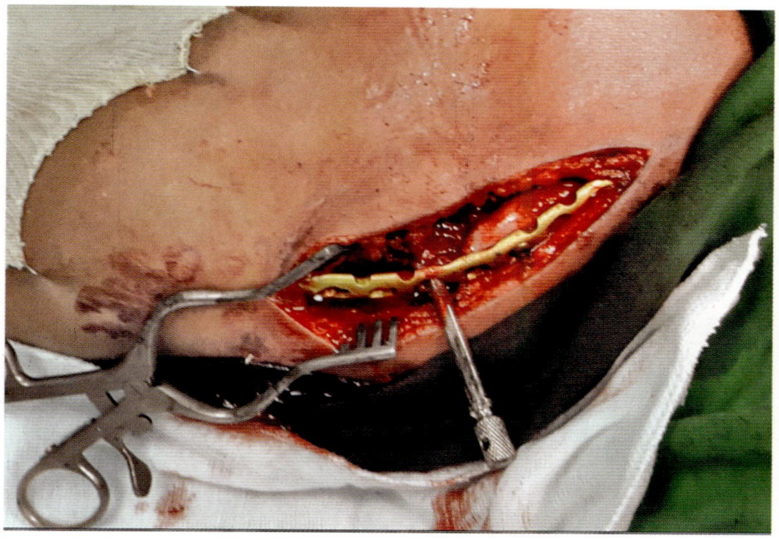

Fig. 11: Apply the plate with sleeve on the clavicle.

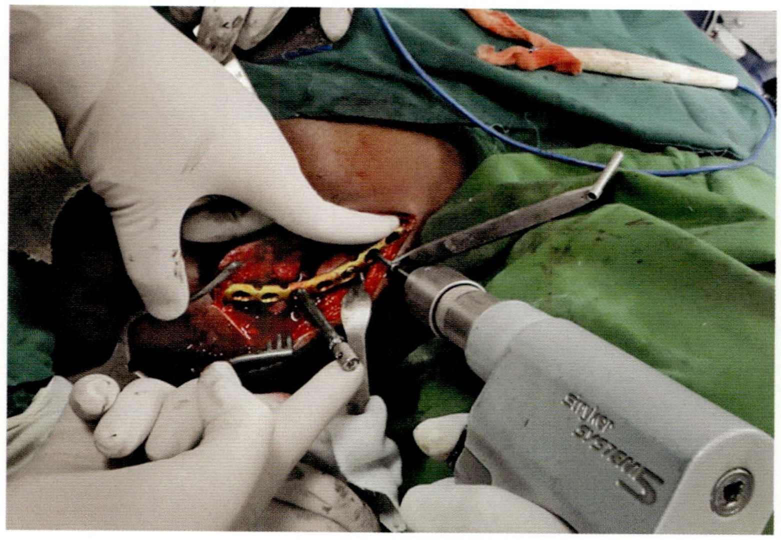

Fig. 12: One-by-one apply the locking screws.

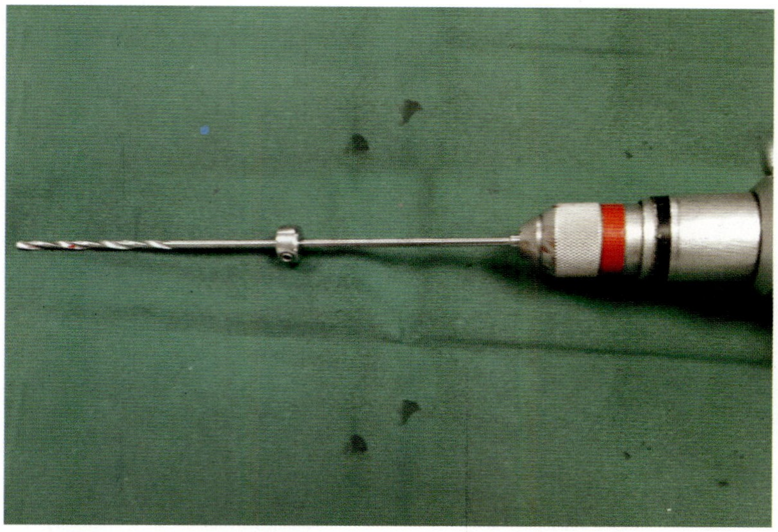

Fig. 13: It is always better to use such a drill bit where you can control the depth, so as to avoid injury to the nerves and vessel inferior to the clavicle. Care should be taken to avoid slippage of drill guard.

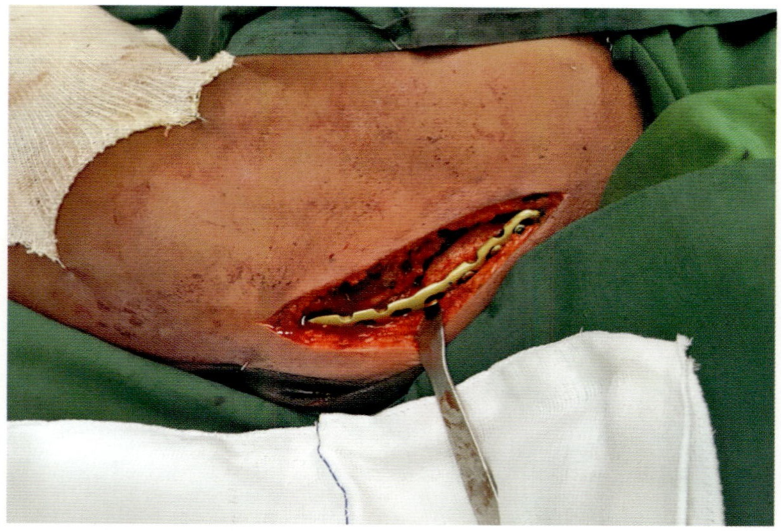

Fig. 14: After inserting all the screws, yet a gap can be seen.

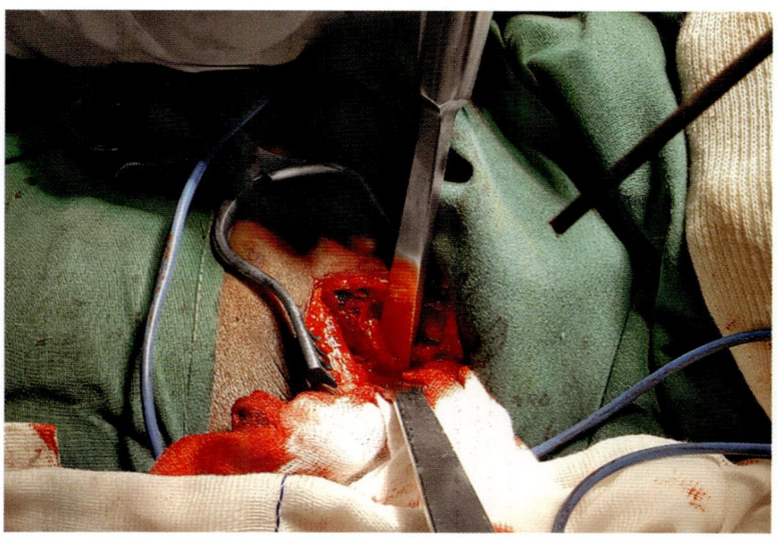

Fig. 15: An Iliac crest bone graft is harvested.

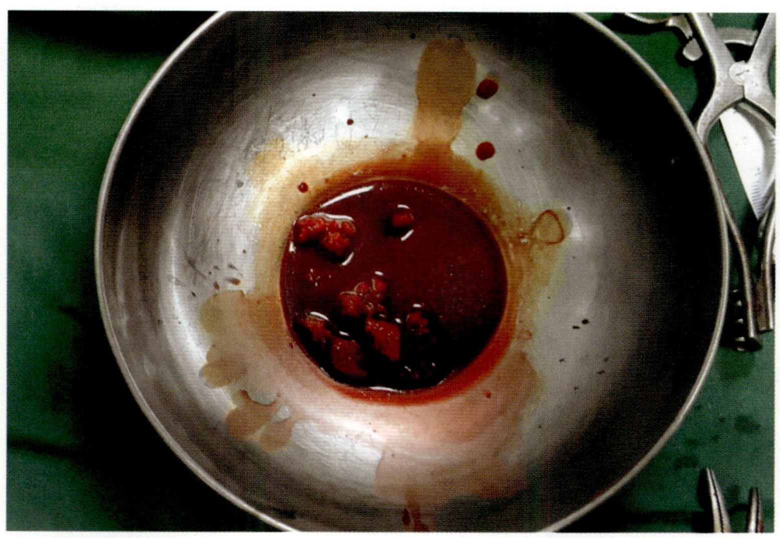

Fig. 16: Bone graft, which is harvested from the Iliac crest. Blood, which oozes should also be inserted at the fracture site as it has a lot of osteoprogenitor cells.

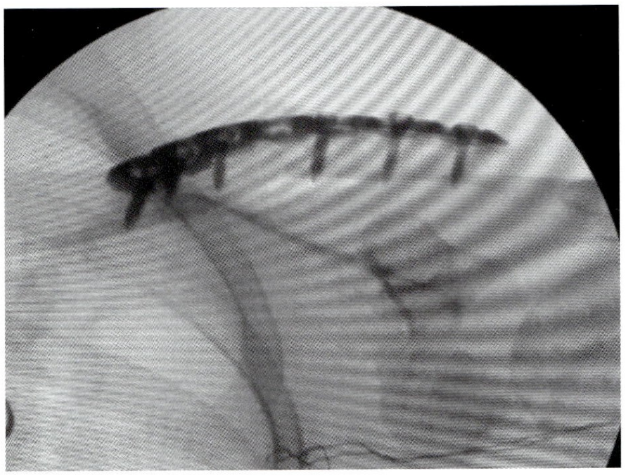

Fig. 17: Intraoperative C-arm picture before inserting the bone graft at the fracture site.

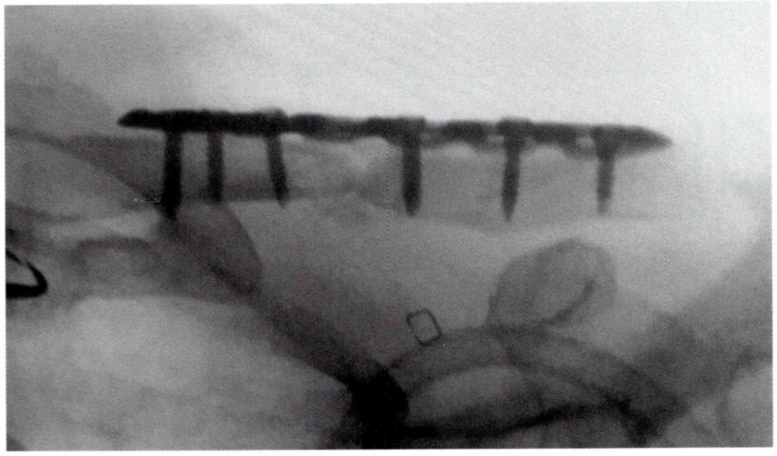

Fig. 18: Intraoperative C-arm picture after inserting the bone graft at the fracture site.

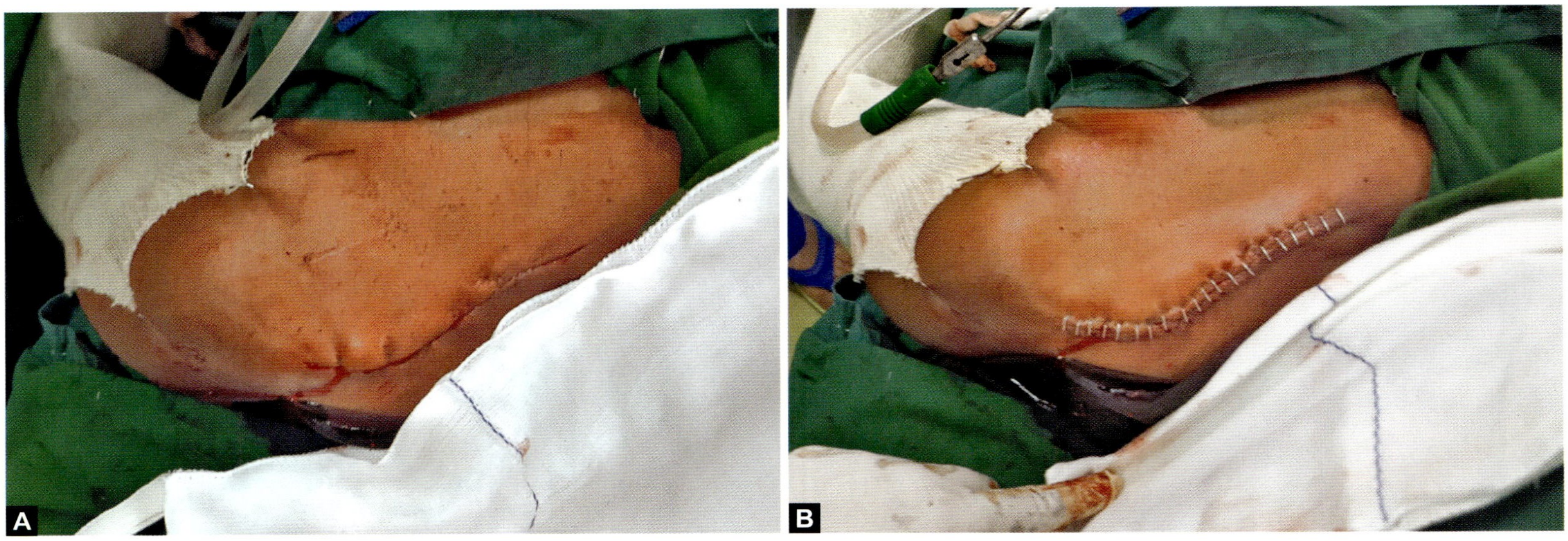

Figs. 19A and B: (A) After suturing the subcutaneous layer with absorbable suture (polyglactin); (B) Skin can be closed with either staples or sutures.

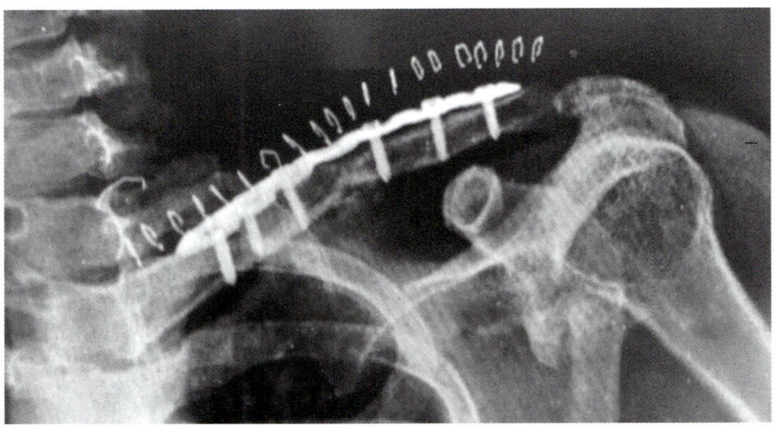

Fig. 20: Final postoperative X-ray showing the bone graft in place.

SUGGESTED READING

1. Cook SD, Baffes GC, Wolfe MW, et al. Recombinant human bone morphogenetic protein-7 induces healing in a canine long-bone segmental defect model. Clin Orthop Relat Res. 1994;301:302-12.
2. Eskola A, Vaianionpaa S, Myllynen P. Surgery for ununited clavicular fracture. Acta Orthop Scand. 1986;57:366-7.
3. Fukuda E, Yasuda I. On the piezoelectric effect of bone. J Physiol Soc Jpn. 1957;12:1158-62.
4. Gazdag AR, Lane JM, Glaser D, et al. Alternatives to autogenous bone graft: efficacy and indications. J Am Acad Orthop Surg. 1995;3:1-8.
5. Heiple KG, Chase SW, Herndon CH. A comparative study of the healing process following different types of bone transplantation. J Bone Joint Surg. 1963;45A:1593-616.
6. Johnson EW Jr, Collins HR. Nonunion of the clavicle. Arch Surg. 1963; 87:963-6.
7. Jupiter JB, Leffert RD. Nonunion of the clavicle. J Bone Joint Surg. 1987;69A:753-60.
8. Lente RW. Cases of un-united fracture treated by electricity. N Y State J Med. 1850;5:317-9.
9. Manske DJ, Szabo RN. The operative treatment of mid-shaft clavicular non-unions. J Bone Joint Surg. 1985;67A:1367-71.
10. Mazet R. Migration of a Kirschner wire from the shoulder region on to the lung: report of two cases. J Bone Joint Surg. 1943;25A:477-83.
11. Mulder DS, Greenwood FA, Brooks CE. Post-traumatic thoracic outlet syndrome. J Trauma. 1973;13:706-13.
12. Neer CS II: Nonunion of the clavicle. JAMA. 1960;172:1006-11.
13. Nogi J, Heckman JD, Hakala M, et al. Nonunion of the clavicle in the child: A case report. Clin Orthop Relat Res. 1975;110:19-21.
14. Rockwood CA. Treatment of the outer clavicle in children and adults. Orthop Trans. 1982;6:472.
15. Rowe CR. An atlas of anatomy and treatment of mid-clavicular fractures. Clin Orthop Relat Res. 1968;58:29-42.
16. Schwartz N, Leixnering M. Technik und Ergebnisse der Klavikula-Markdrahtung. Zentralbl Chir. 1986;111:640-7.
17. Urist MR, Mikulski A, Lietze A. Solubilized and insolubilized bone morphogenetic protein. Proc Natl Acad Sci USA. 1979;76(4):1828-32.

CHAPTER 67

Nonunion Patella Fixation by Tension Band Wiring and Bone Grafting

Shrinivas S Shintre, Chittanand Mendhe, Rajkumar Ekambaram

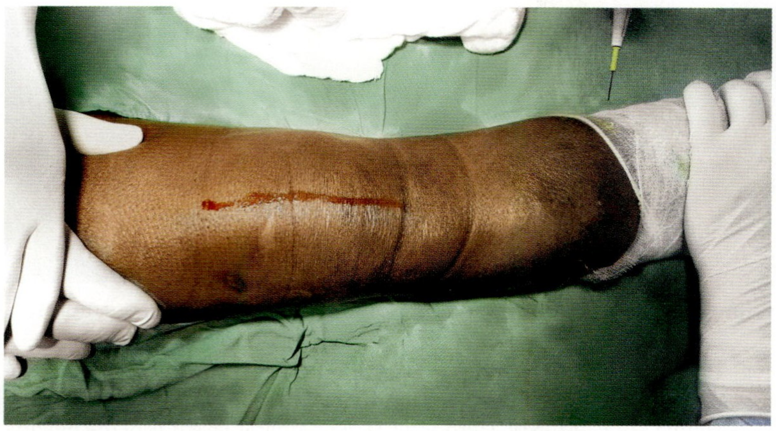

Fig. 1: Position of patient is supine. Painting and draping done, knee flexed to 30–40°. Incision site is marked over anterior aspect of knee 4–5 cm above superior patella border to tibial tuberosity.

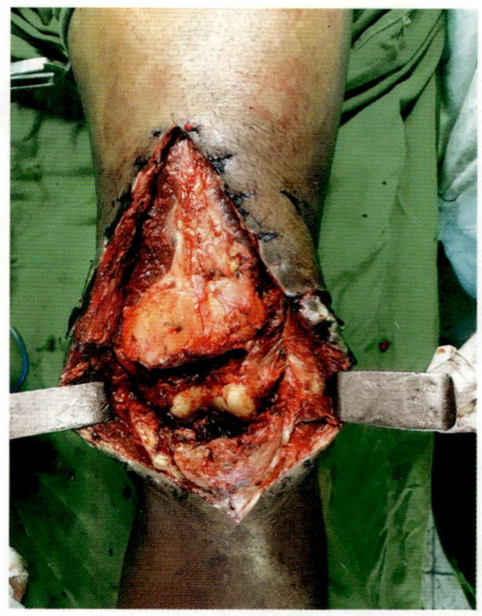

Fig. 2: Take a vertical incision, subcutaneous layer is dissected and fracture site identified. There is nearly 3–4 cm gap between two fracture fragments when knee is extended. Fracture site freshened.

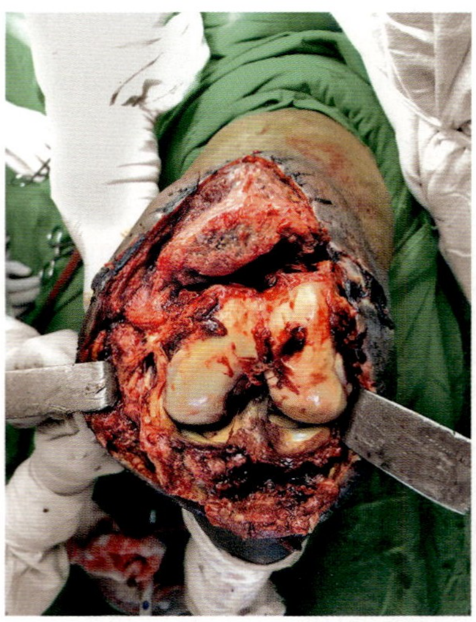

Fig. 3: After knee is flexed, underlying femoral condyles and tibial condyles are exposed and proximal fragment is pulled superiorly.

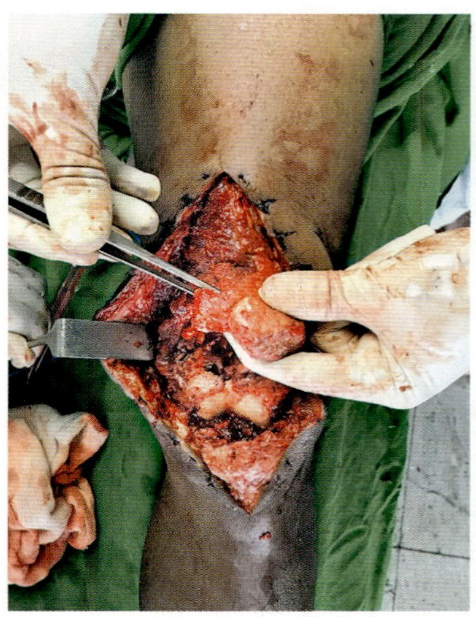

Fig. 4: Retinaculum attachment from medial and lateral side of patella is released and some part of quadriceps tendon is detached.

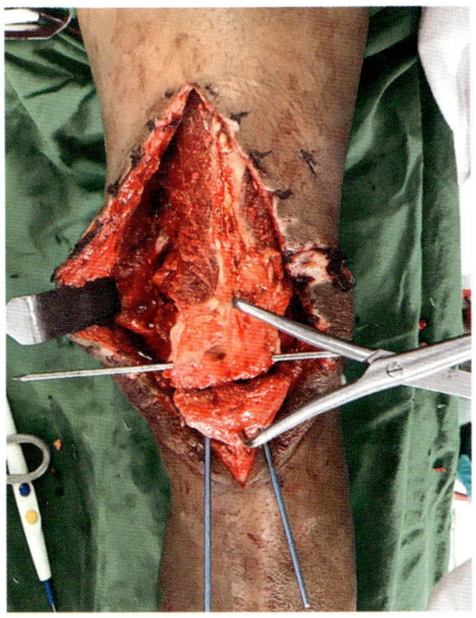

Fig. 5: One thick K-wire is passed transversely from superior fragment of fracture so that it helps to pull that fragment, pointed reduction clamp is applied after reducing both fragments and reduction is maintained. Two parallel K-wires are passed perpendicular to the fracture site.

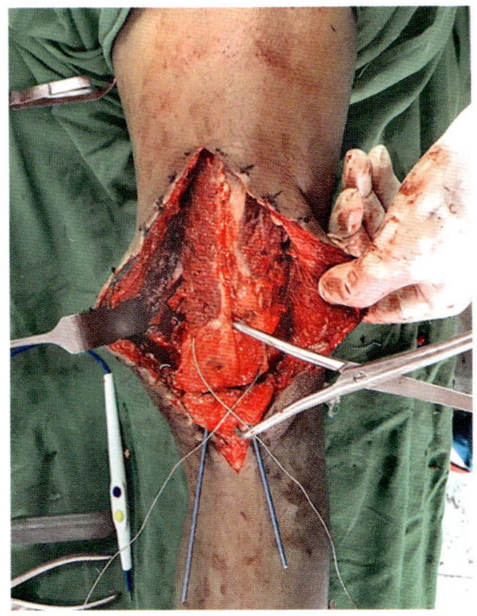

Fig. 6: Stainless steel (SS) wire is passed through quadriceps tendon. Crossed in a figure-of-eight pattern over front of patella and then passed through patellar tendon.

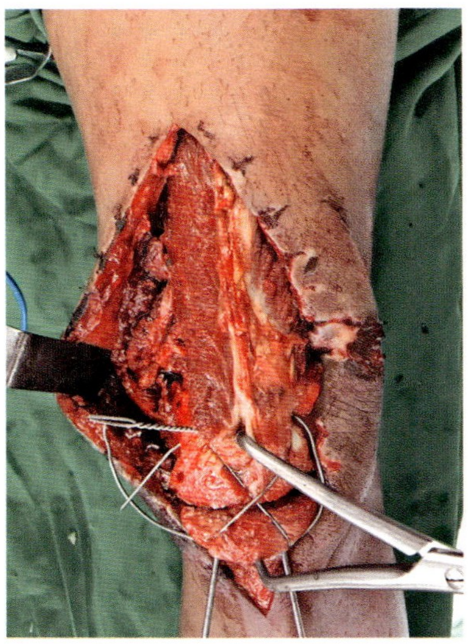

Fig. 7: Stainless steel (SS) wire ends are twisted till fracture site is compressed. One has to make sure that wire should not break due to over twisting. Another SS wire is passed in such way that it forms a circle around patella.

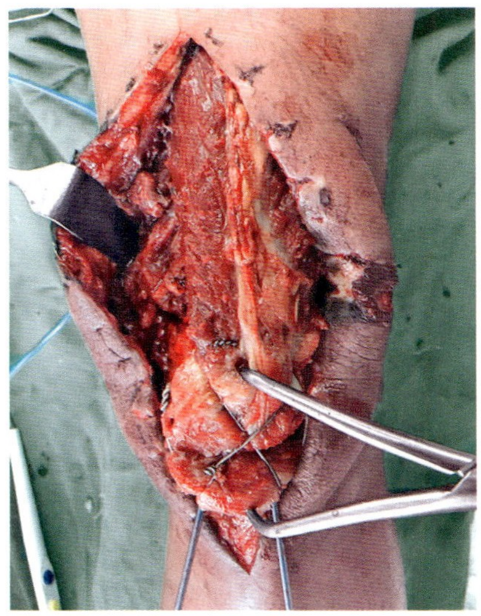

Fig. 8: A circlage wire is passed and its ends are also twisted and cut keeping minimum 4–5 twists and buried in muscles.

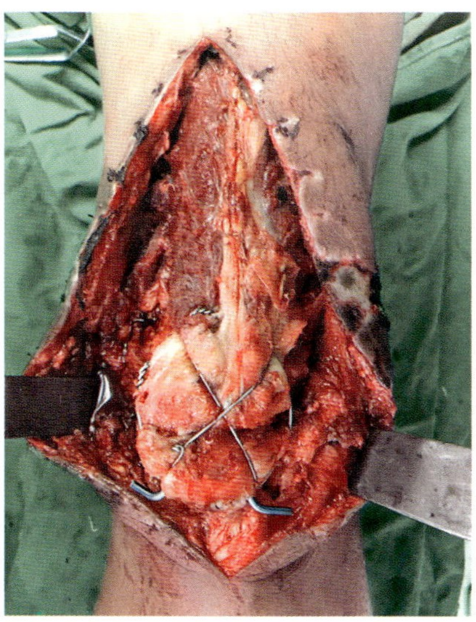

Fig. 9: Both K-wire ends are cut and bent.

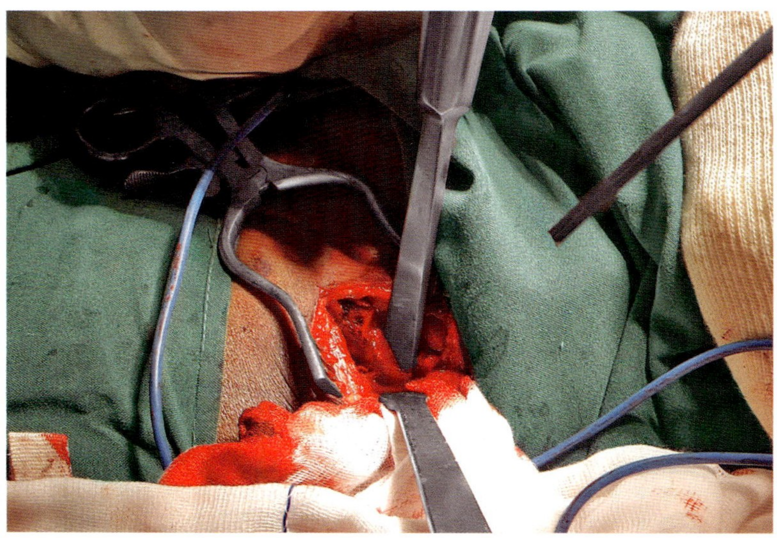

Fig. 10: Bone graft from iliac crest is harvested.

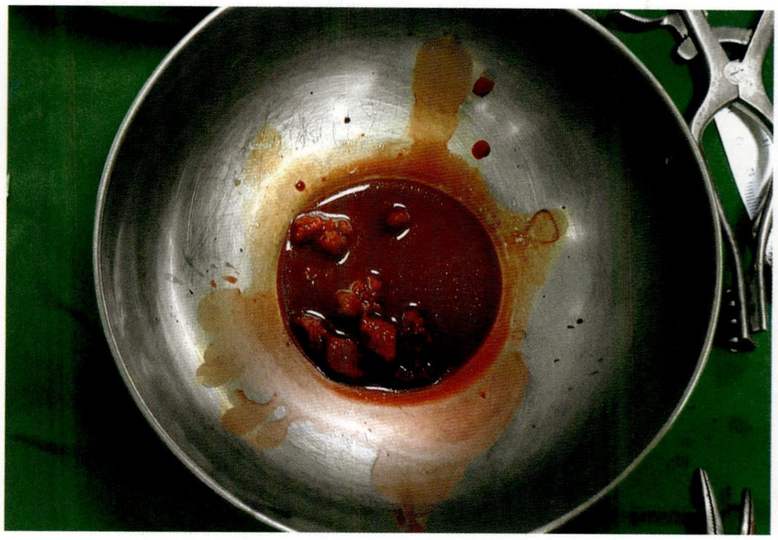

Fig. 11: Bone graft from iliac crest has to be kept in fracture site after giving proper wash with normal saline and wound is closed in layer.

CHAPTER 68

Nonunion Tibia-Fixation and Bone Grafting

S Prakash, Sharad M Hardikar, Nitish Agrawal

INTRODUCTION

Nonunion is considered established when minimum of 9 months have elapsed since fracture with no visible progressive sign of healing for 3 months.

Tibia is most common adult bone in nonunion.

TYPES OF NONUNION BASED ON VASCULARITY

- *Hypervascular nonunion*: Due to excessive movement over fracture site:
  - Elephant foot
  - Horse hoof
  - Oligotrophic.
- *Avascular nonunion*:
  - Torsion wedge
  - Comminuted
  - Defect
  - Atrophic.

CAUSES OF NONUNION

- Open
- Comminuted
- Infection
- Insecurely fixed means the two ends are not apposed properly
- Soft-tissue imposition
- Immobilized for insufficient time
- Irradiated bone.

RISK FACTORS

- Poor general health
- Smoking
- Nonsteroidal anti-inflammatory drugs (NSAIDs) and steroid drugs
- Metabolic and nutritional disorders.

DIAGNOSIS

- Inability to bear weight
- Abnormal motion in two dimensions
- White blood cell (WBC), erythrocyte sedimentation rate (ESR), and C-reactive protein (CRP) to rule out infection
- X-ray
- Computed tomography (CT) scan
- Magnetic resonance imaging (MRI)
- Indium-111 based WBC bone scan.

TREATMENT

Nonoperative Treatment

- Low-intensity ultrasound
- Electrical and electromagnetic stimulation.

Operative Treatment

- For previous intramedullary nailing exchange reamed nailing, plate and screws fixation and external fixator with or without bone graft can be done.
- Removal of all scar tissue between the fracture fragments and freshening of edges is important and can be fixed with plate and screws fixation or external fixator.
- In Ilizarov external fixator affected area of the bone can be removed and ends are docked and the remaining bone is lengthened with corticotomy.

SURGICAL STEPS

- Supine position.
- Painting and draping of iliac crest and nonunion tibia site done.

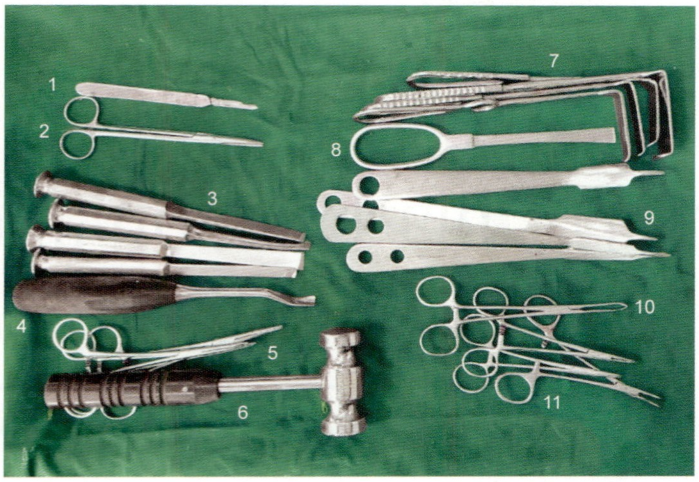

Fig. 1: (1) Bard-Parker handle with blade, (2) Scissor, (3) Osteotome, (4) Curette, (5) Artery forceps, (6) Hammer, (7) Right angle retractor, (8) Periosteum elevator, (9) Hohmann bone lever, (10) Tissue forceps, (11) Mosquito forceps.

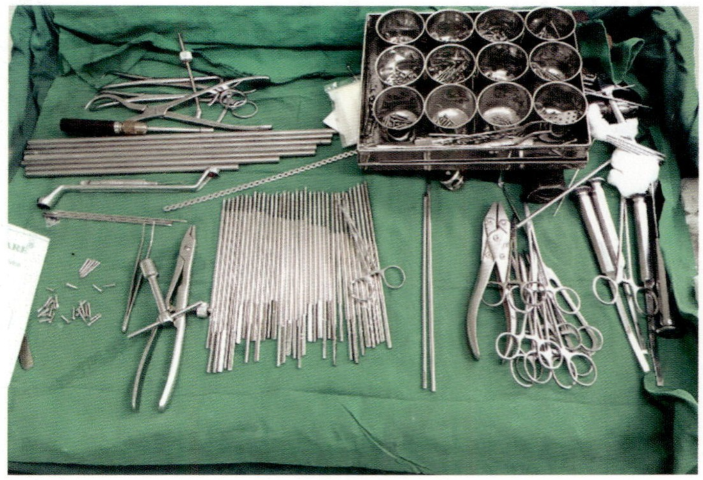

Fig. 2: External fixator set and cortical screws.

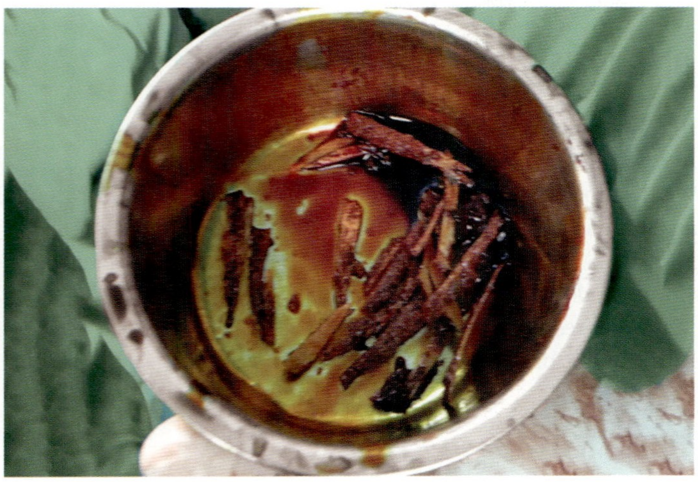

Fig. 3: Cortical and cancellous bone graft harvested from iliac crest.

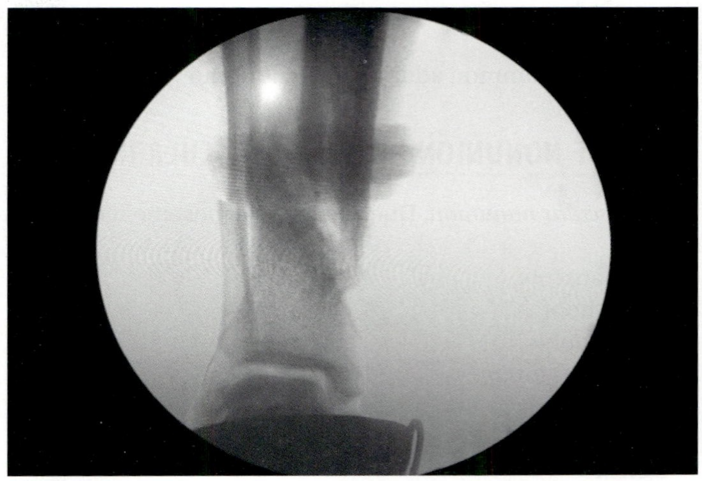

Fig. 4: Fracture site identified over C-arm image intensifier.

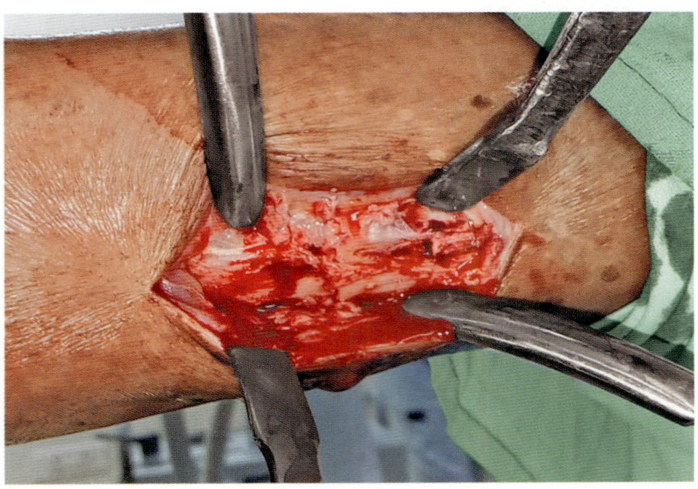

Fig. 5: Incision taken on posterolateral aspect over nonunion fibula site. Soft tissue retracted with bone lever and nonunion site of fibula exposed.

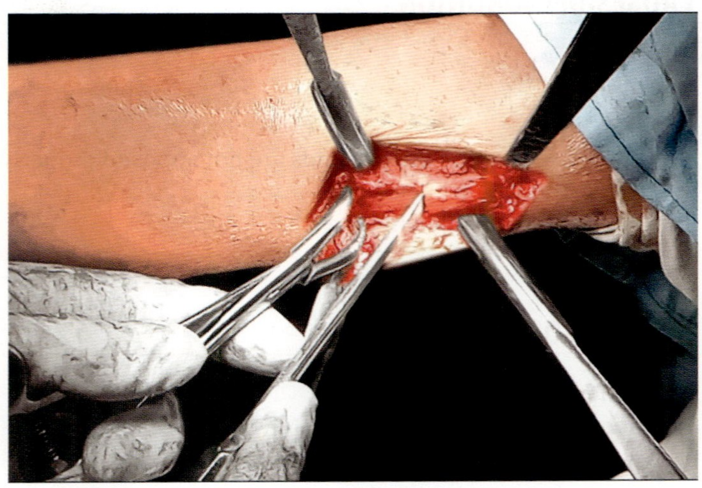

Fig. 6: Fibrosis removed and edges freshened from nonunion site by osteotome, hammer, and other instruments like nibbler.

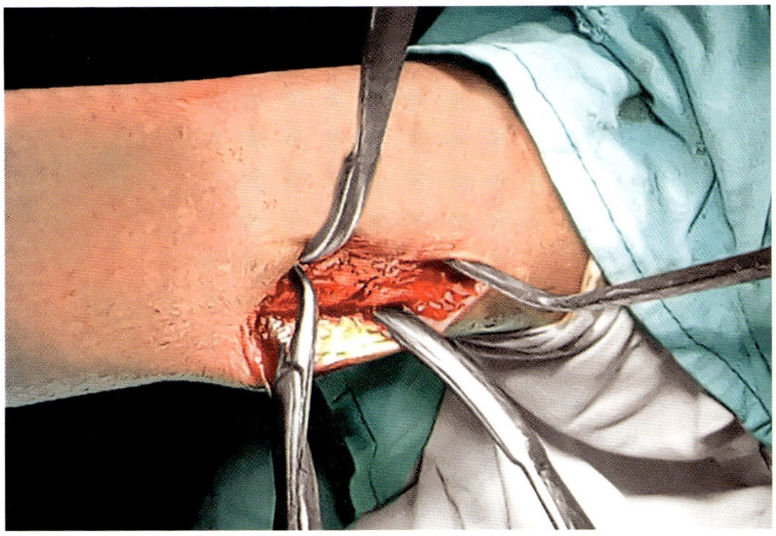

Fig. 7: Bone graft inserted at nonunion site.

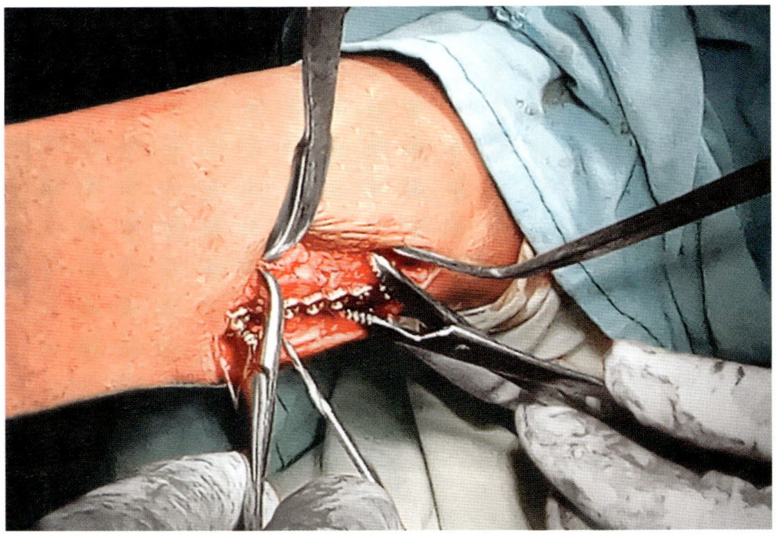

Fig. 8: Eight hole 2.7 mm reconstruction plate used for fixation. Proximal screw fixation is done.

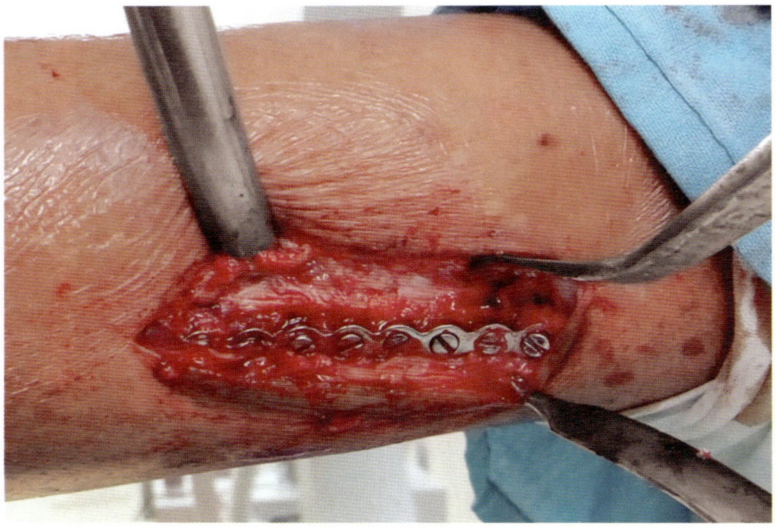

Fig. 9: Fibula nonunion fixed with eight hole plate and eight screws.

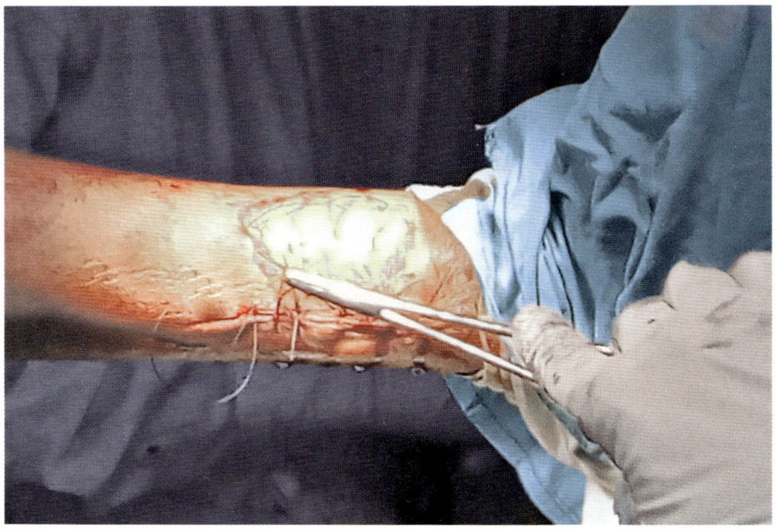

Fig. 10: Skin suturing done with nonabsorbable suture material.

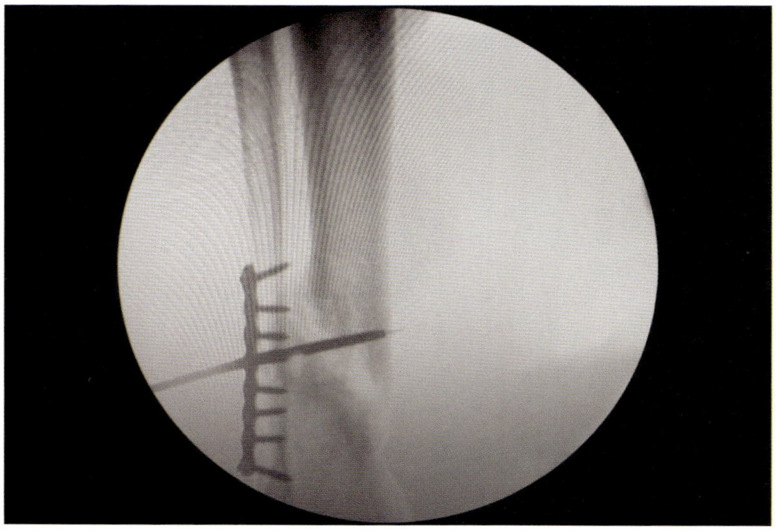

Fig. 11: Nonunion tibia site identified over C-arm anteroposterior view.

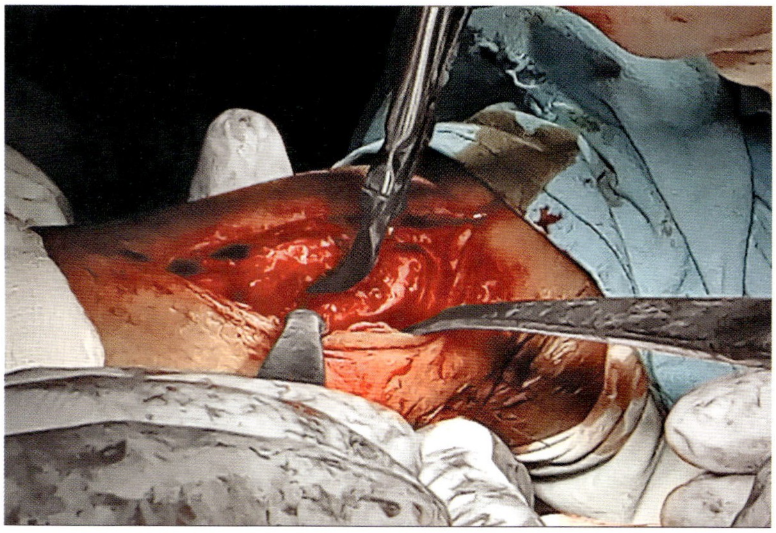

Fig. 12: Skin incision taken over anterolateral aspect of tibia over nonunion site.

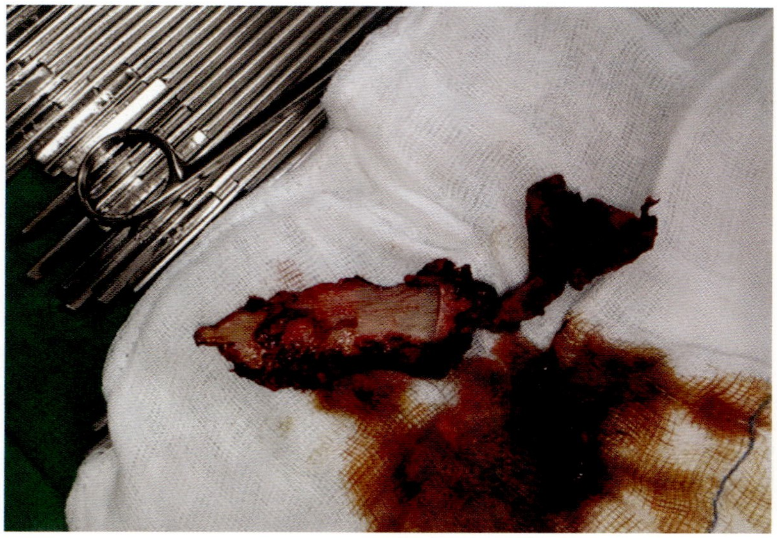

Fig. 13: Fibrotic tissue removed from nonunion site.

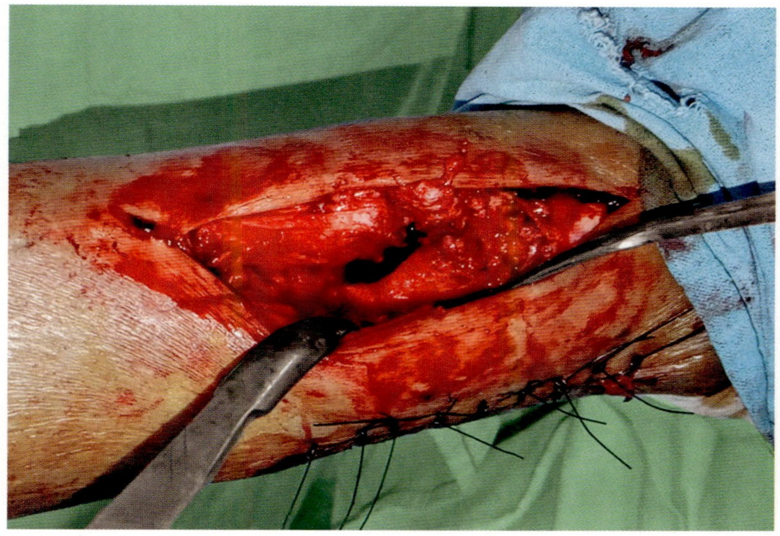

Fig. 14: Nonunion of distal third tibia exposed. Bone graft inserted at nonunion site.

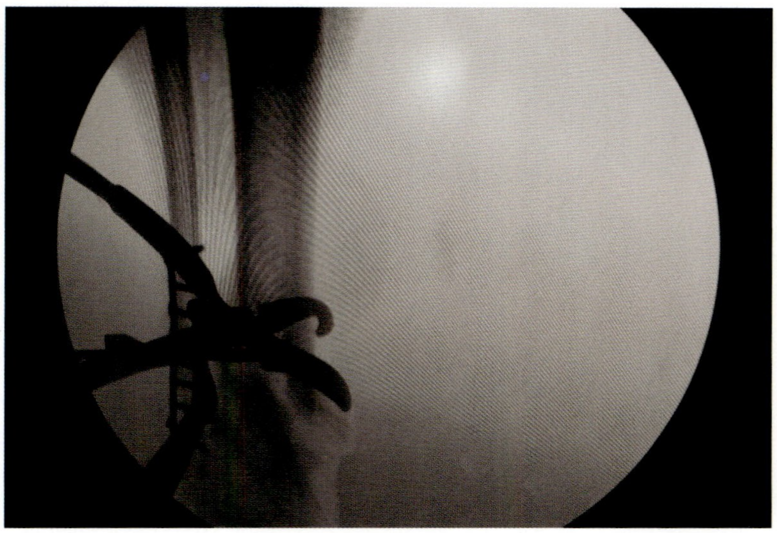

Fig. 15: Proximal segment of nonunion held with bone holding forceps.

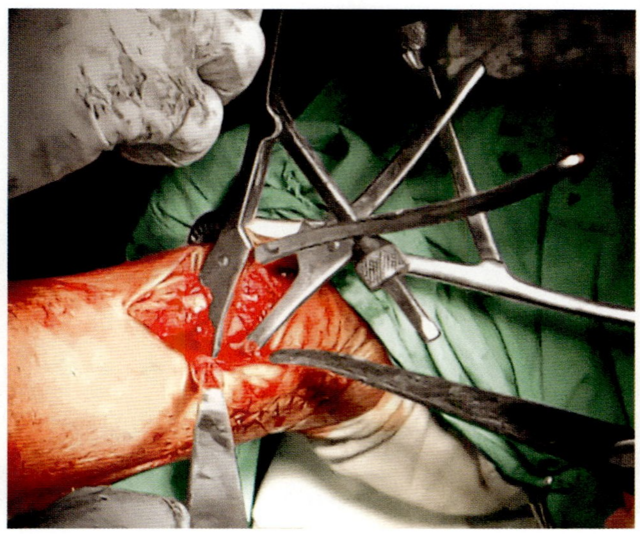

Fig. 16: Reduction of fracture attempted with bone holding reduction clamps or forceps.

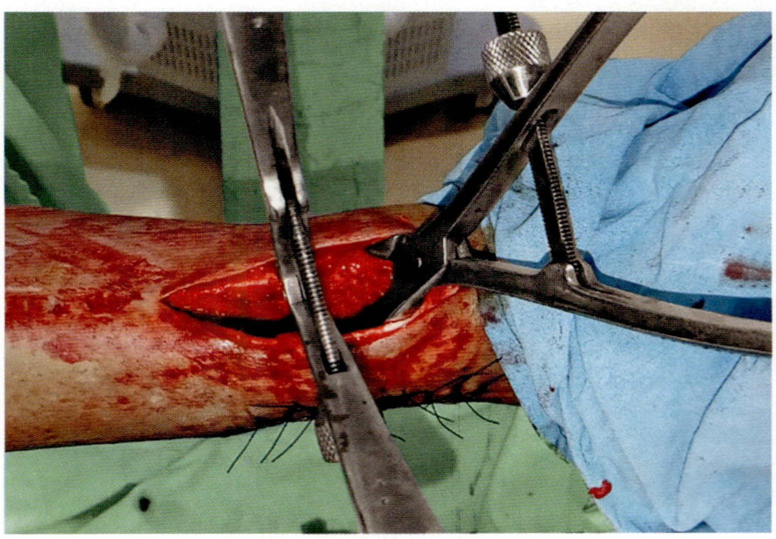

Fig. 17: Reduction achieved.

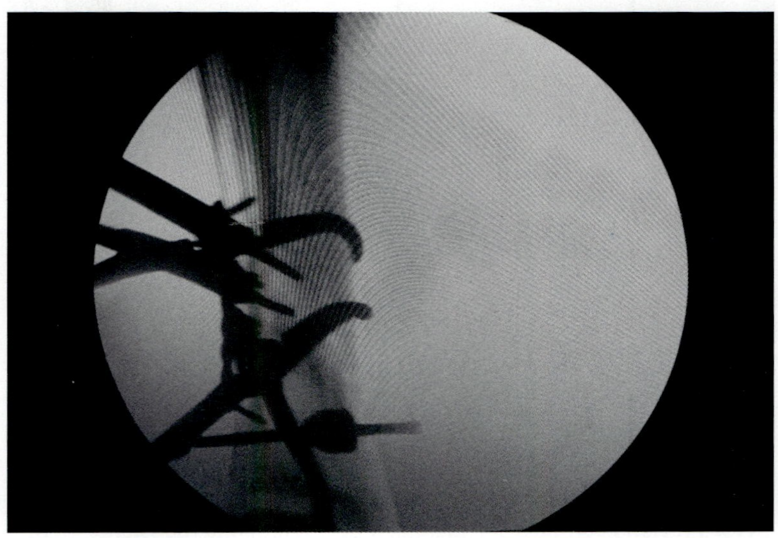

Fig. 18: Reduction confirmed over C-arm image intensifier.

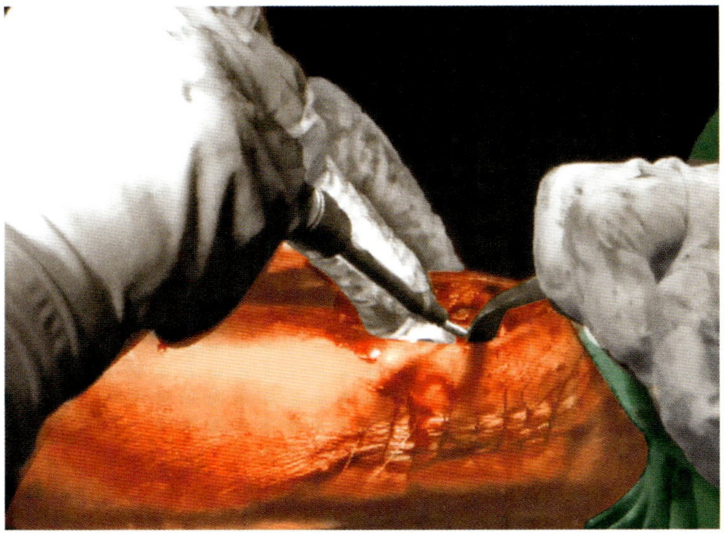

Fig. 19: Interfragmentary lag screw inserted across fracture site after drilling and tapping.

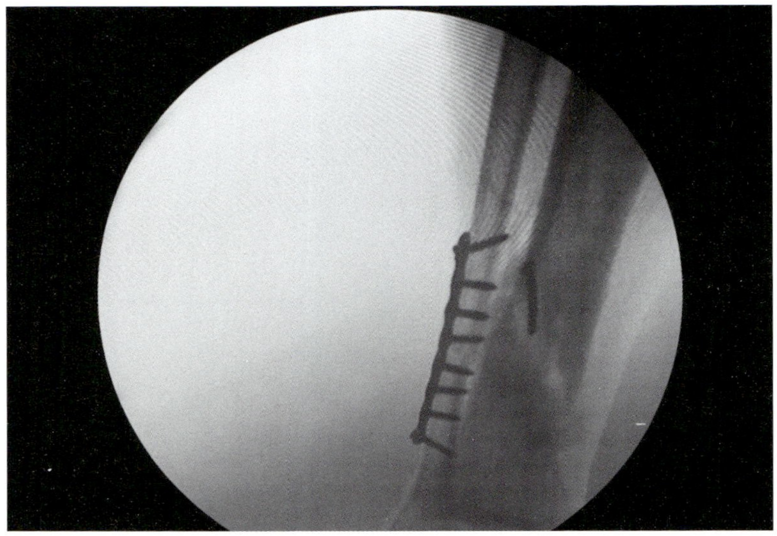

Fig. 20: Lag screw fixation confirmed over C-arm anteroposterior (AP) view.

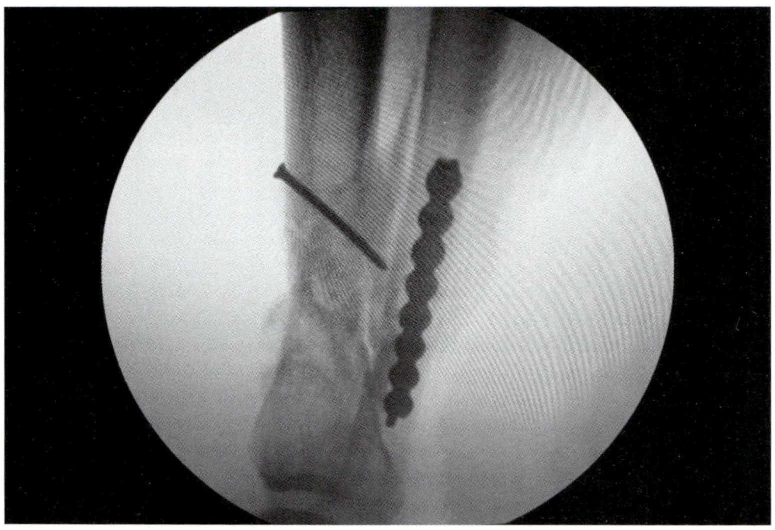

Fig. 21: Lag screw fixation confirmed over C-arm lateral view.

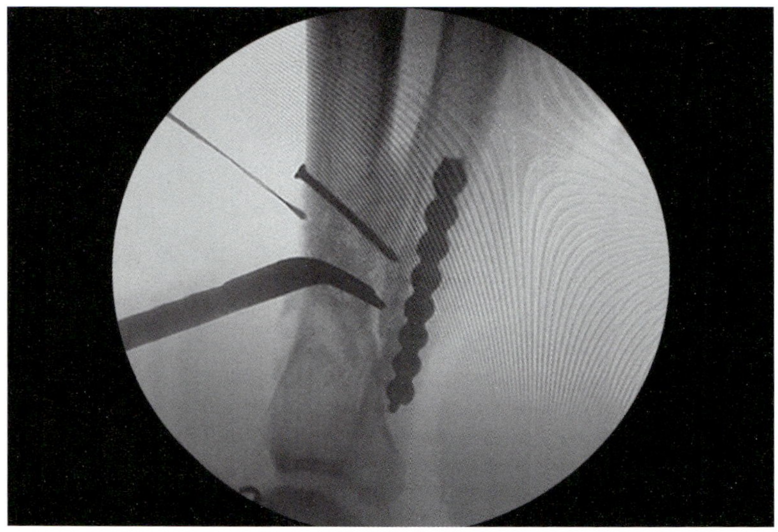

Fig. 22: Drilling for second lag screw done.

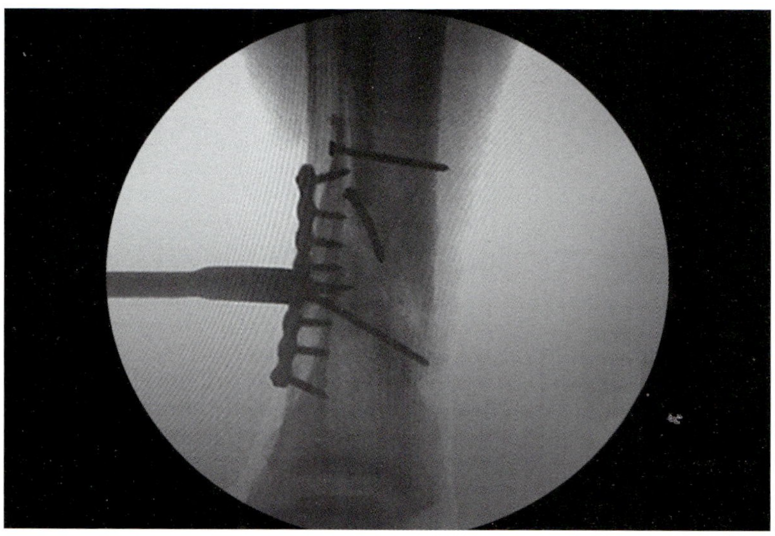

Fig. 23: Total three lag screw fixation done and confirmed under C-arm anteroposterior (AP) view.

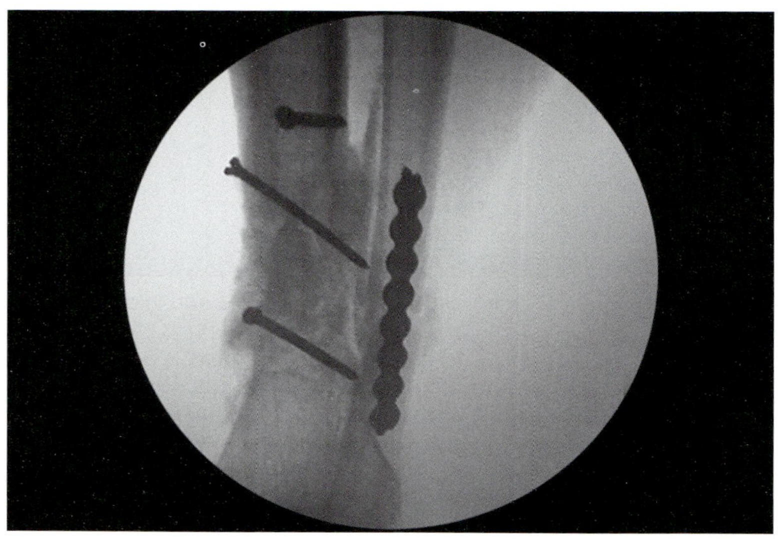

Fig. 24:
- Lag screw fixation confirmed over C-arm lateral view.
- Closure of wound in layers done.

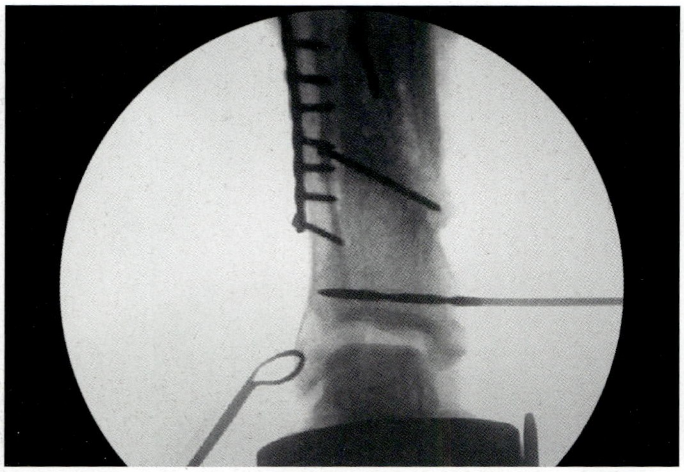

Fig. 25: Drilling for most distal Schanz pin done under C-arm anteroposterior (AP) view.

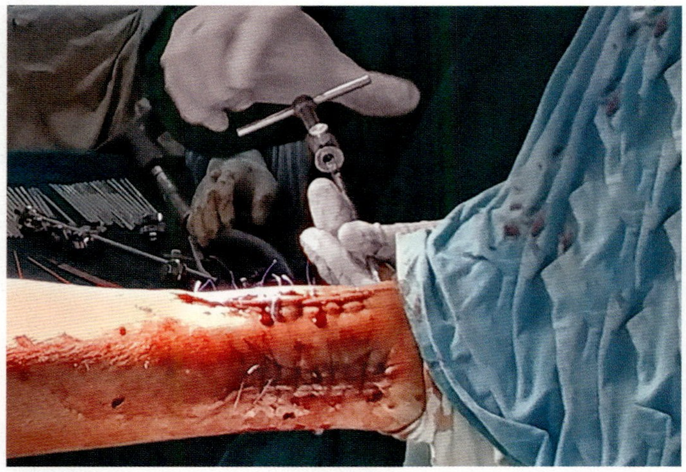

Fig. 26: Most distal Schanz pin inserted in subchondral bone.

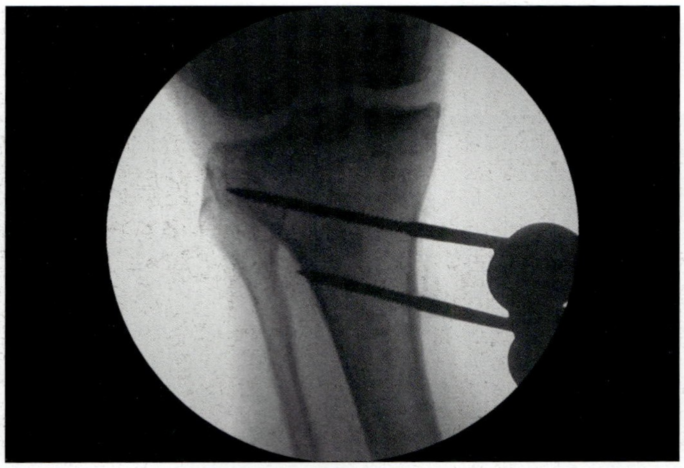

Fig. 27: Two Schanz pin fixation done in proximal tibia and confirmed over C-arm.

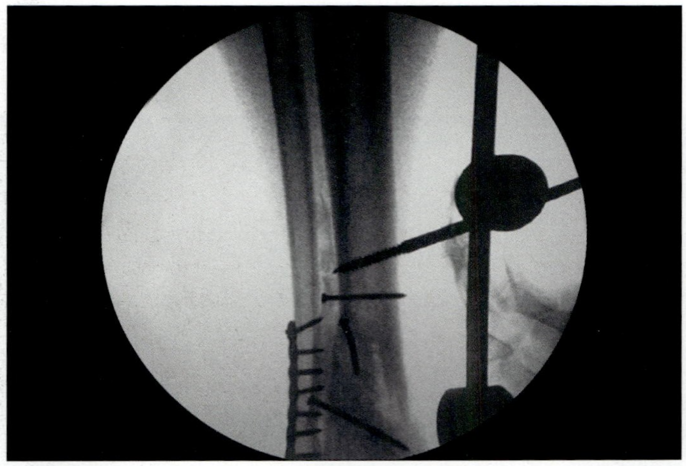

Fig. 28: One more Schanz pin fixation done proximal to nonunion site.

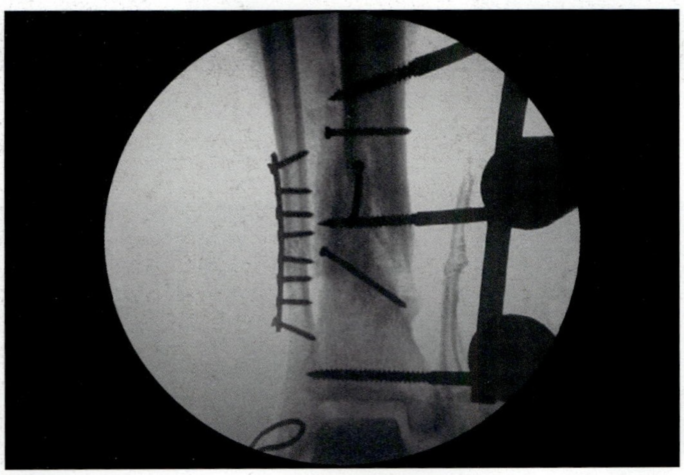

Fig. 29: Another Schanz pin fixation done across nonunion site.

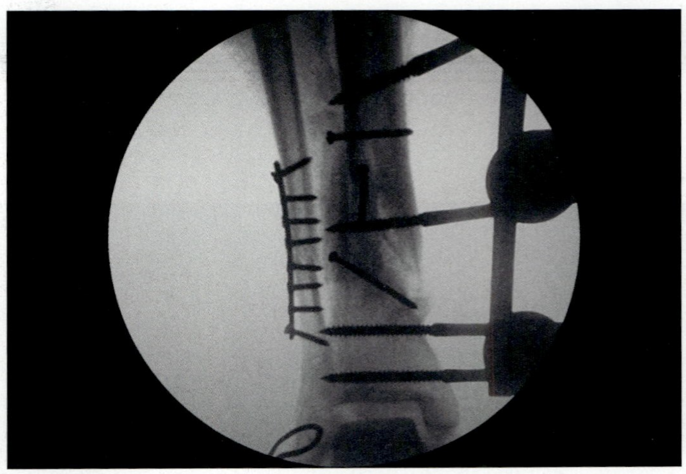

Fig. 30: One more Schanz pin fixation done distal to nonunion site.

Final fixation of nonunion distal third tibia fibula done with open reduction internal fixation (ORIF) with plate and screws with bone grafting for fibula, and ORIF with interfragmentary lag screw with bone grafting with external fixation done for tibia.

SUGGESTED READING

1. Antonova E, Burge R, Mershon J. Tibial shaft fracture: costly burden of nonunion. BMC Musculoskelet Disord. 2013;14:42.
2. Fong K, Truong V, Foote CJ. Predictors of nonunion and reoperation in patient with fracture of tibia: an observational study. BMC Musculoskelet Disord. 2013;14:103.
3. Ryzewicz M, Morgan SJ, Linford E. Central bone grafting for nonunion of fracture of tibia: a retrospective series. J Bone Joint Surg. 2009;91(4): 522-9.

CHAPTER 69

Bone Graft Harvesting

S Prakash, Trimbak Dapkekar, Siddharth Jaiswal

INTRODUCTION

Bone grafting is a surgical procedure through which damaged and diseased bone rebuild and repair by using transplanted bone.

The first recorded bone implant was performed in 1668.

INDICATION

Indications for bone graft are:

- Filling cavities and defects resulting from infections, tumors, cyst, etc.
- Arthrodesis of destroyed joints
- As a bone block to limit joint motion
- For treatment of nonunion, delayed union.
- Occasionally for fresh fractures to promote union.

BIOLOGICAL MECHANISM

Osteoconduction

- Provides a scaffold on which bone growth takes place.

Osteoinduction

It involves the stimulation of progenitor cells to differentiate into osteoblasts that help in formation of new bone. Bone morphogenic proteins are the cell mediators of osteoinduction. A bone graft material that is osteoconductive and osteoinductive will trigger the formation of new osteoblasts, that promote faster integration of the graft.

Osteogenesis

It occur when osteoblasts from the bone graft material contribute to new bone growth along with bone growth via other mechanism.

STRUCTURE AND TYPES OF GRAFT

Cortical and cancellous bone grafts are used for structural support and for osteogenesis respectively.

Autograft

Autologous (autogenous) bone grafting involves harvesting the graft from the same individual receiving the graft.

Allograft

Allograft bone is derived from humans like autogenous bone, difference is that it harvested from an individual other than one receiving the graft. It can be taken from cadaver and sourced from a bone bank.

Heterogeneous Grafts

- Bone from another species.

Cancellous Bone Substitutes

Hydroxyapatite and tricalcium phosphate, synthetic and naturally occurring materials are nowadays used as substitutes for cancellous bone graft.

Xenograft

Xenograft is a bone graft harvested from a species other than human, such as bovine.

GROWTH FACTORS

Growth factor consist of either human growth factors or bone morphogenitic proteins (BMPs) that help in osteogenesis. It can be produced by using recombinant DNA technology.

Sources of Cancellous Bones

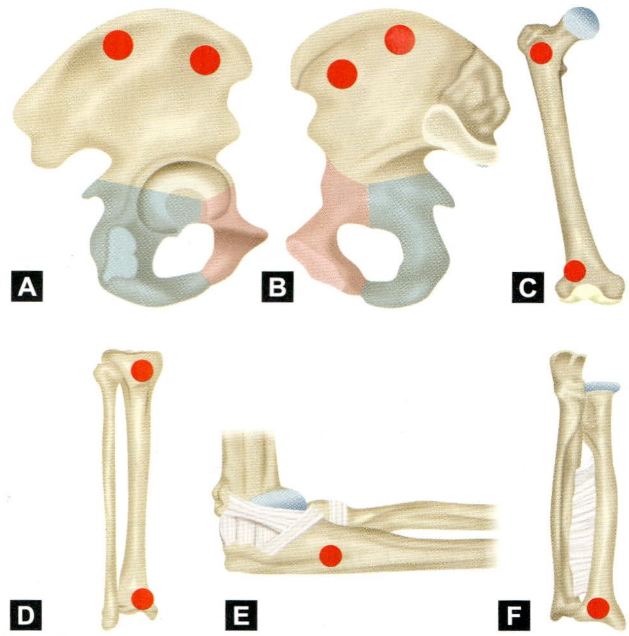

Figs. 1A to F: (A and B) Inner and outer lip of iliac crest; (C) Anterior aspect of greater trochanter and distal femoral condyle; (D) Proximal and distal tibia; (E) The olecranon; (F) The radial styloid.

COMPLICATIONS

A) Anterior Ilium

Pain

It can result from dissection, hematoma, neuropraxia of cutaneous nerve or from infection.

Wound Healing

Wound healing complications are common after harvesting bone graft, having mutilple origins including infection, hematoma and wound dehiscence.

Nerve Damage

Incision to be placed at least 2 cm away from ASIS so as to avoid injury to lateral femoral cutaneous nerve.

Hernia

Herniation of abdominal contents can be a potentially serious complication reported at a bone graft site.

Pelvic Fracture

Avulsion fracture from the ASIS have been reported from the origin of sartorius and tensor fascia lata. Older females and osteoporotic bones are found to be at a higher risk for this complication.

B) Proximal Tibial Graft

Fracture: The most common complication while taking graft from proximal tibial.

SURGICAL STEPS

A) ILIAC CREST GRAFT HARVESTING

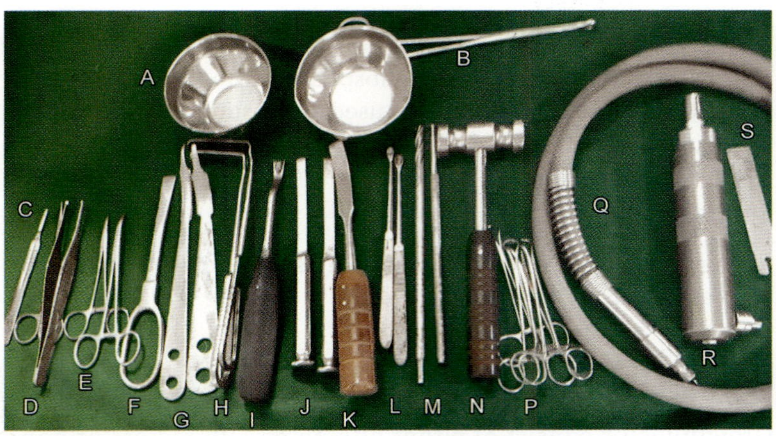

Fig. 2: (A) Bowl, (B) sponge holding forceps, (C) BP handle, (D) tooth forceps, (E) curved artery forceps, (F) periosteum elevator, (G) bone lever, (H) right-angled retractor, (I) gouge, (J) osteotome, (K) curved osteotome, (L) bone curettage, (M) drill bit, (N) hammer, (P) towel clip, (Q) oscillatory drill, (R) oscillatory bone saw, and (S) saw blade.

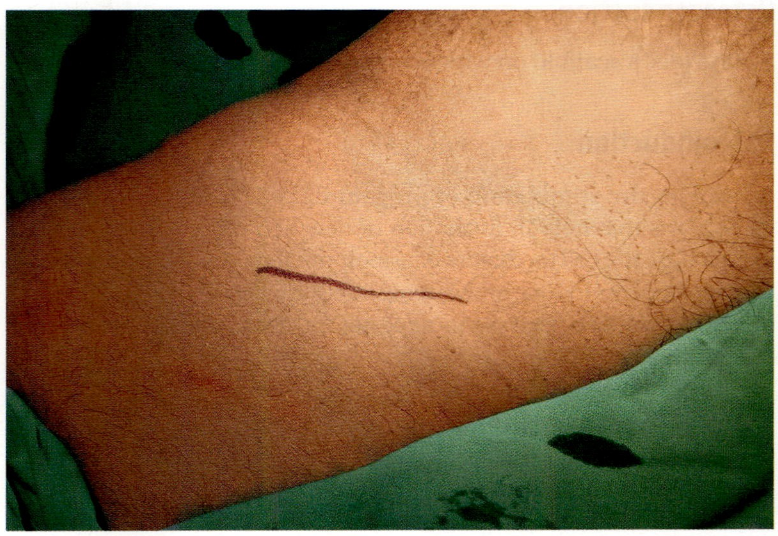

Fig. 3: Mark along anterior fourth of iliac crest up to iliac tubercle.

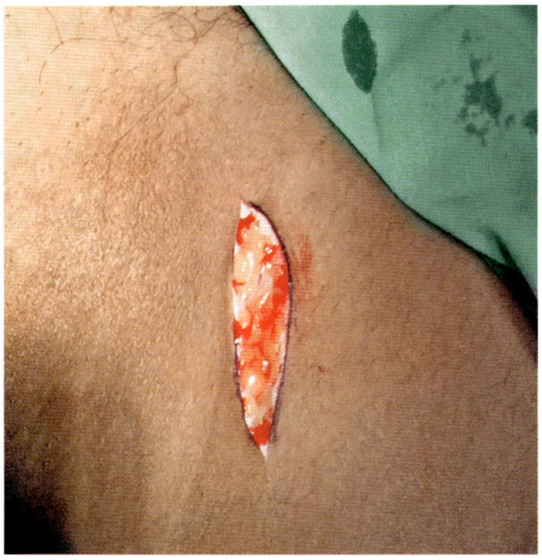

Fig. 4: Incision taken with knife over marking to expose iliac crest.

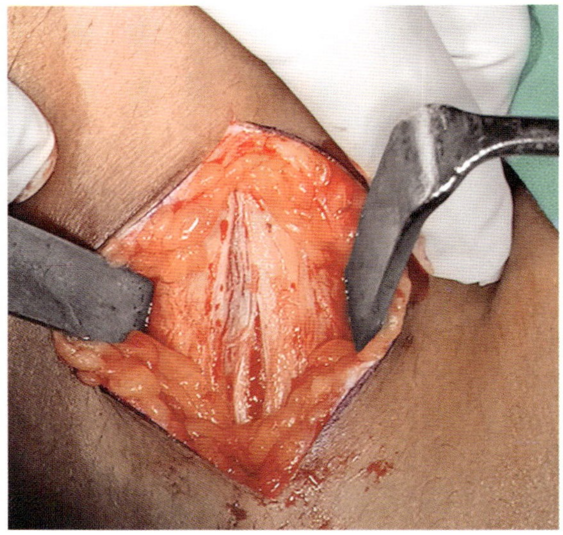

Fig. 5: Retracting soft tissue with help of right angle retractor.

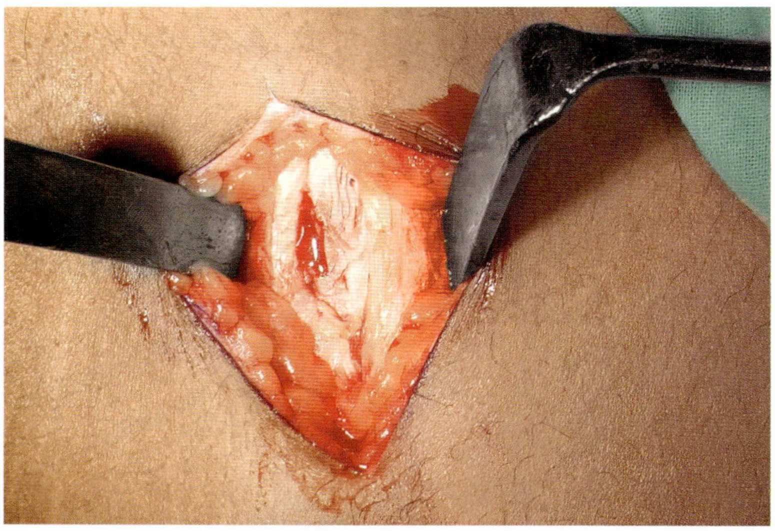

Fig. 6: Subperiosteally stripping of tensor fascia lata and gluteus minimus and part of gluteus medius.

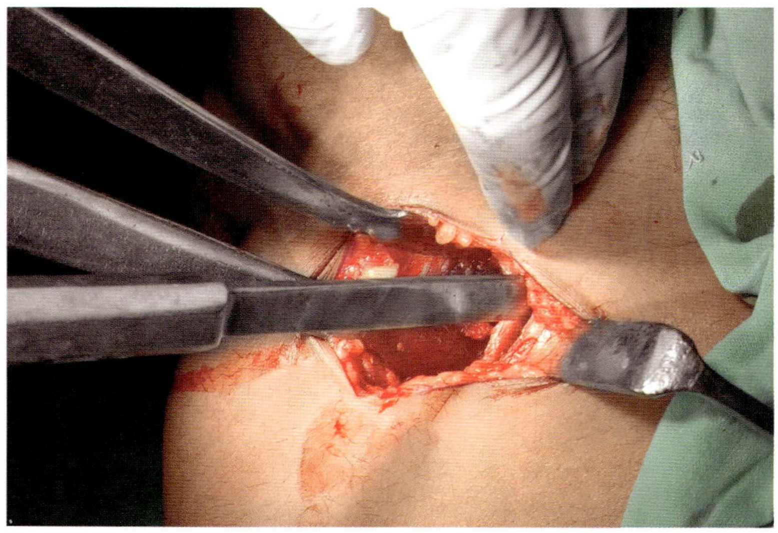

Fig. 7: With help of straight osteotome, osteotomy done along outer lip of iliac crest from anterior superior iliac spine (ASIS) to iliac tubercle.

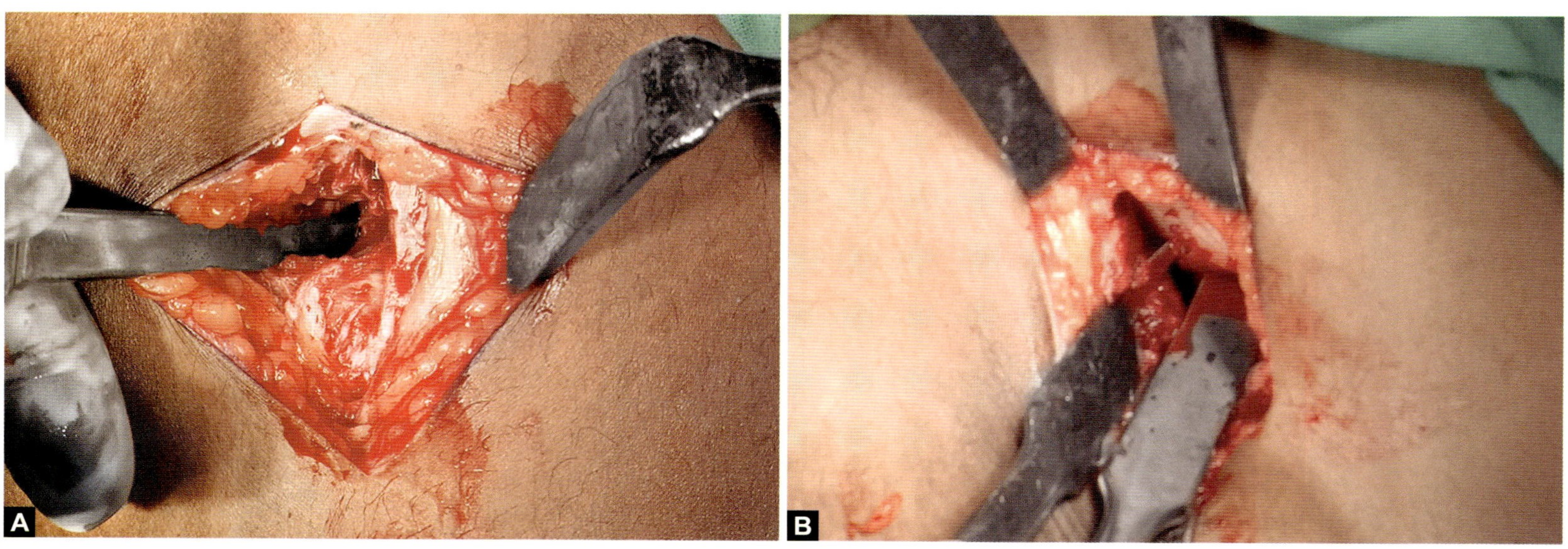

Figs. 8A and B: Vertically down cut though anterior superior iliac spine (ASIS) and iliac tubercle.

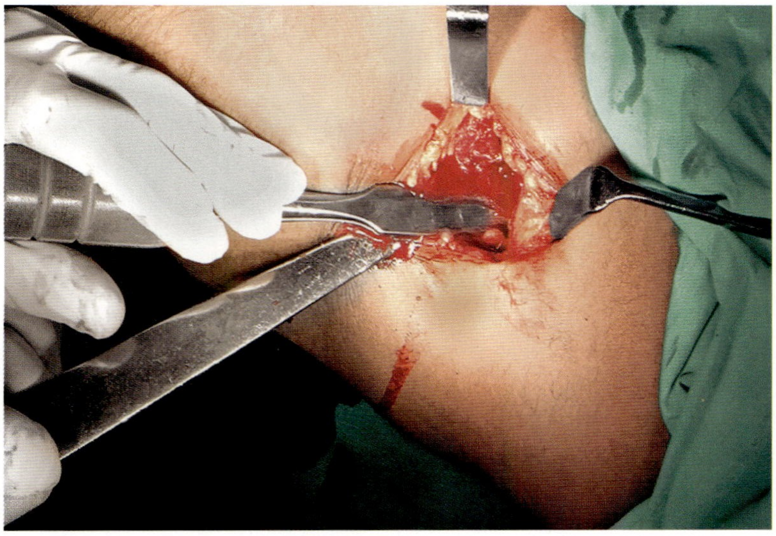

Fig. 9: With curved osteotome joining, the two vertical cut as distal as possible.

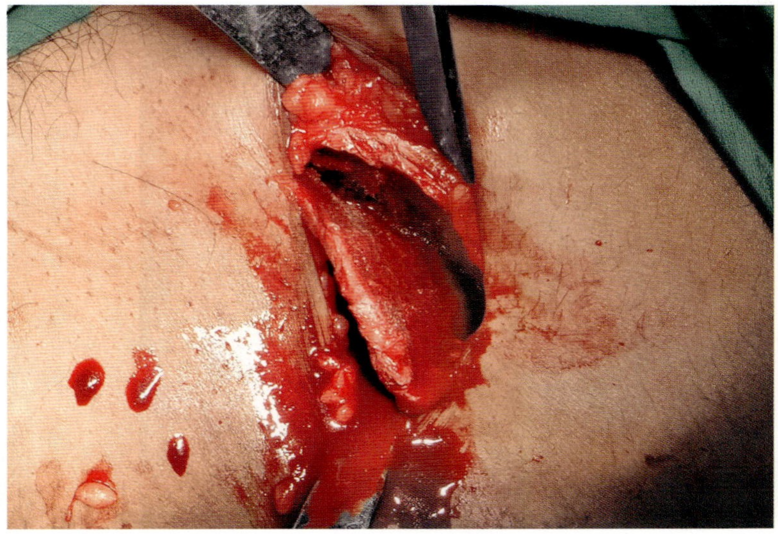

Fig. 10: Graft harvested.

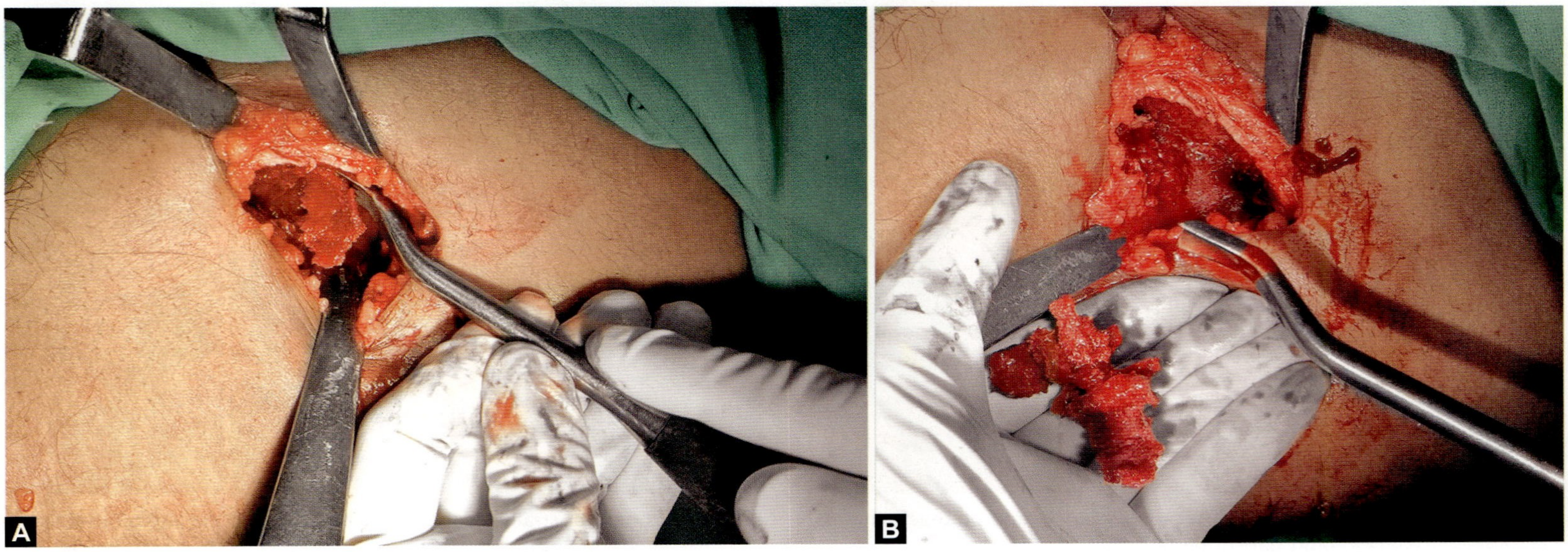

Figs. 11A and B: Removing cancellous bone of inner table with gouge.

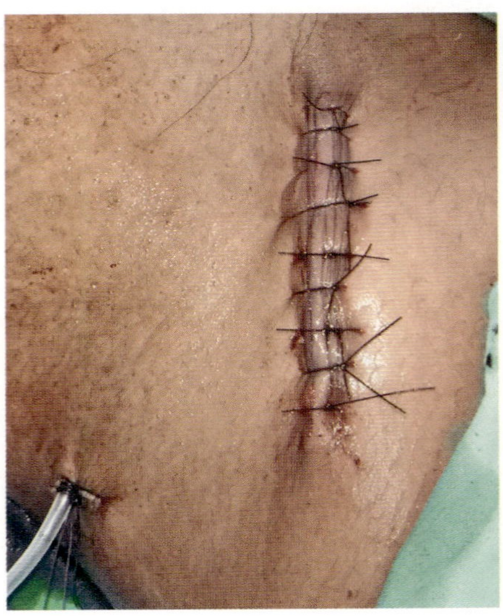

Fig. 12: Muscle and skin closure with drain in situ.

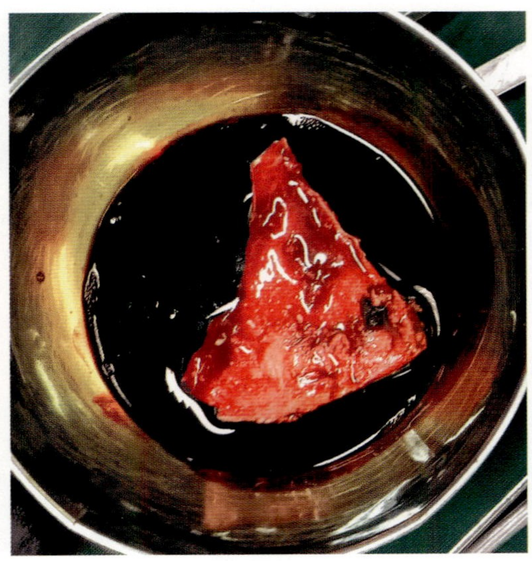

Fig. 13: Unicortical iliac crest graft in povidone–iodine.

B) FIBULAR BONE GRAFT HARVESTING

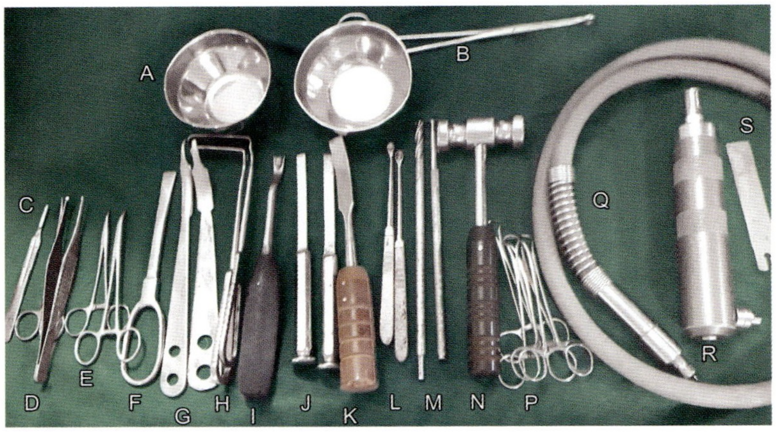

Fig. 14: (A) Bowl, (B) sponge holding forceps, (C) BP handle, (D) tooth forceps, (E) curved artery forceps, (F) periosteum elevator, (G) bone lever, (H) right-angled retractor, (I) gouge, (J) osteotome, (K) curved osteotome, (L) bone curettage, (M) drill bit, (N) hammer, (P) towel clip, (Q) oscillatory drill, (R) oscillatory bone saw, (S) saw blade.

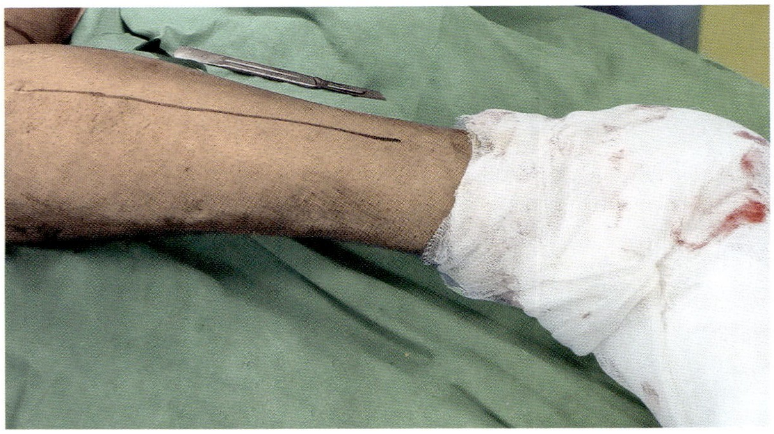

Fig. 15: Mark along fibular shaft from fibular head to junction of lower one-fourth and upper three-fourth.

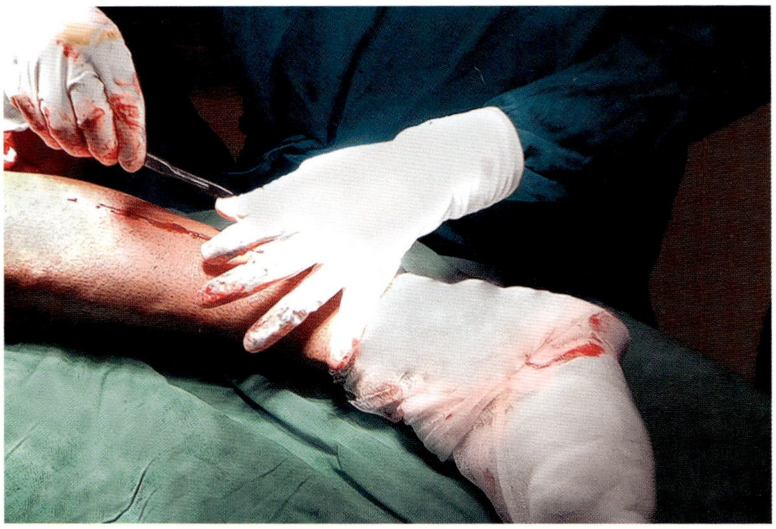

Fig. 16: Incision taken with knife over marking.

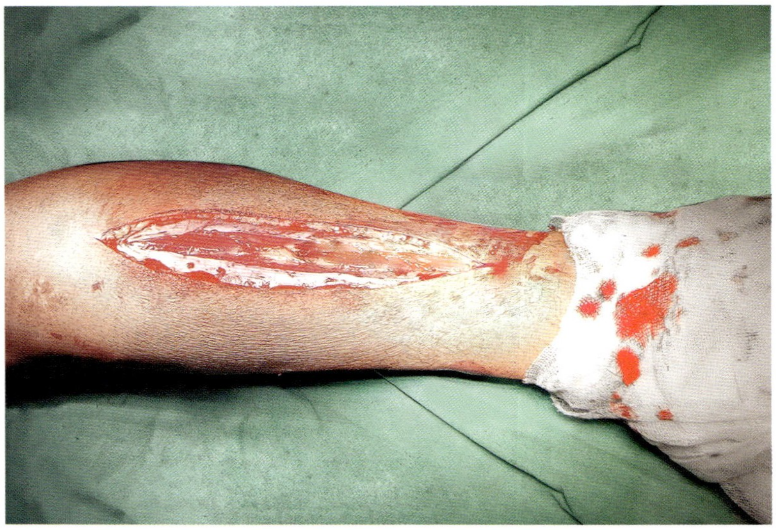

Fig. 17: Skin and fascia separated and peroneus longus muscle exposed.

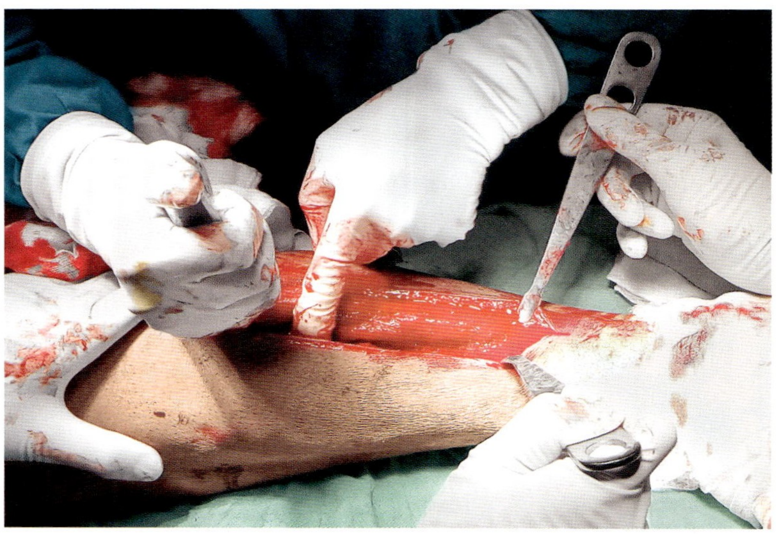

Fig. 18: Peroneus longus muscle retracted anteriorly, soleus retracted posteriorly, and proximally and flexor hallucis longus posteriorly and distally with help of bone lever. Fibula exposed.

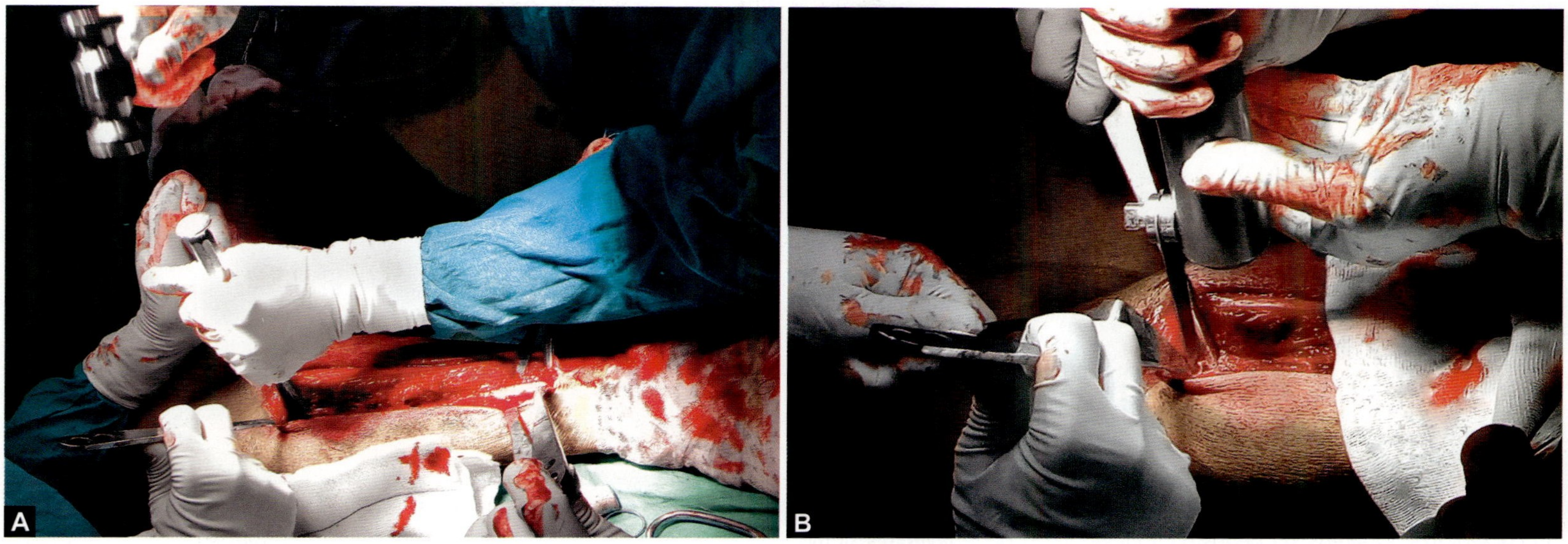

Figs. 19A and B: Defining the site with osteotome proximally and cutting the fibula with help of oscillatory bone saw.

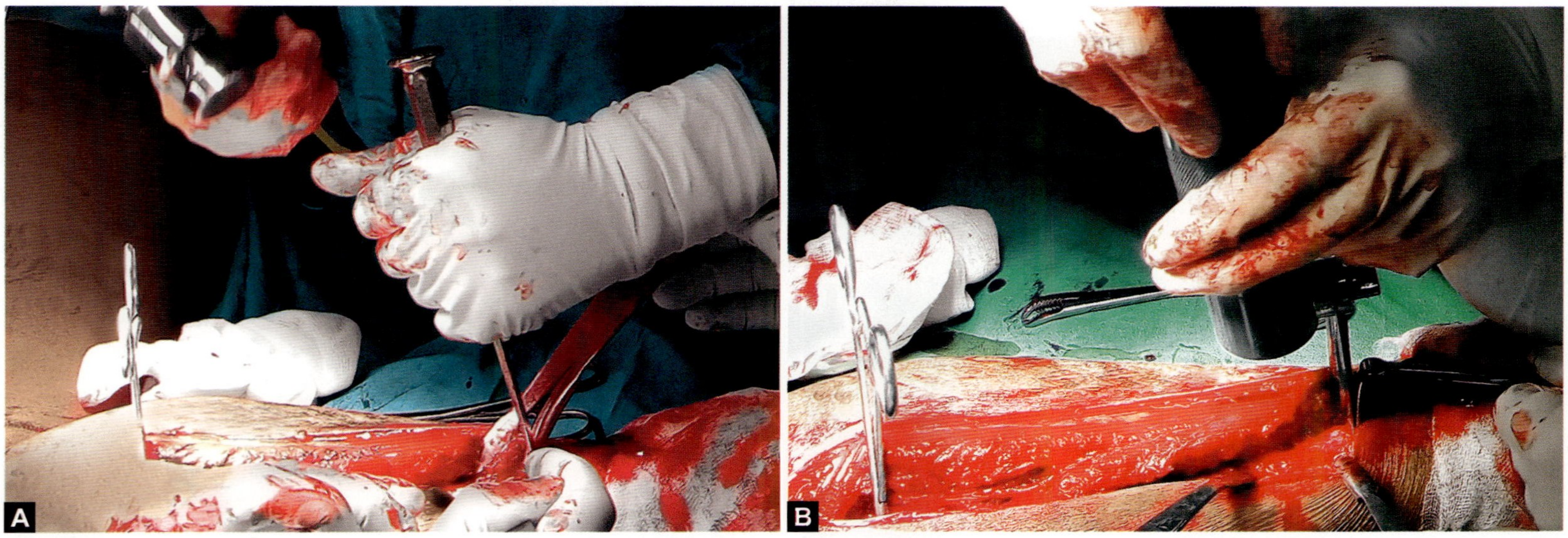

Figs. 20A and B: Defining the site with osteotome distally and cutting the fibula with help of oscillatory bone saw.

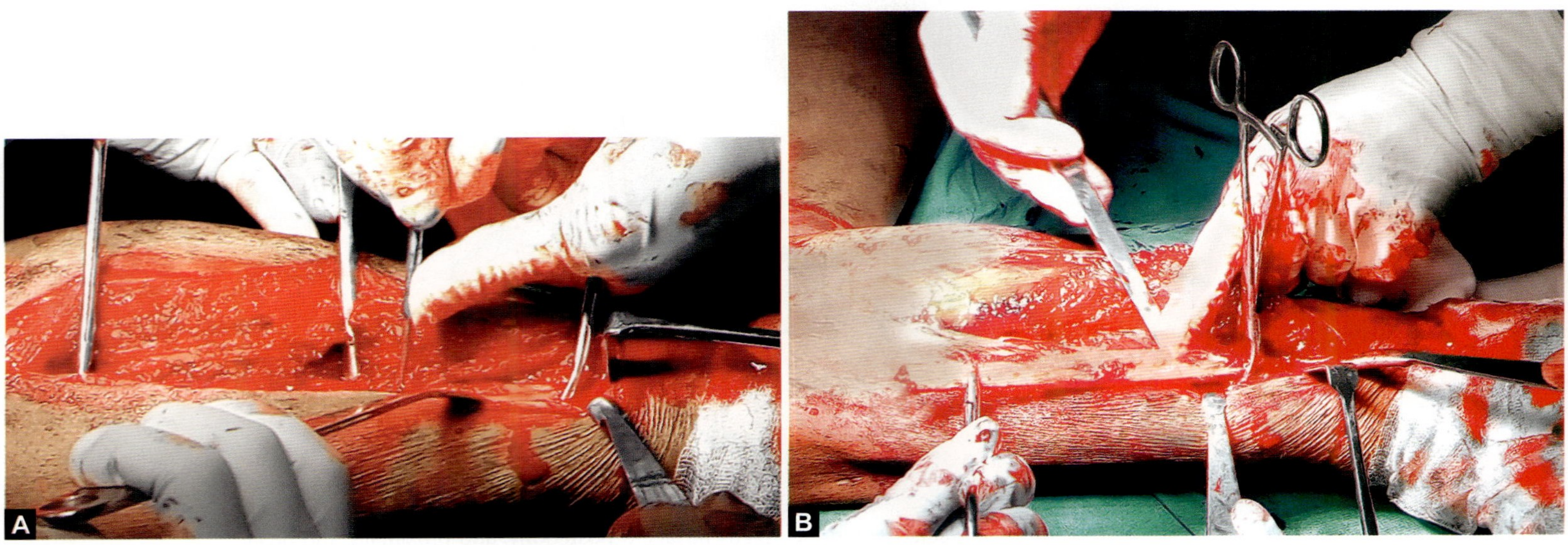

Figs. 21A and B: Fibular graft held with bone holding forceps and harvesting with periosteum elevator.

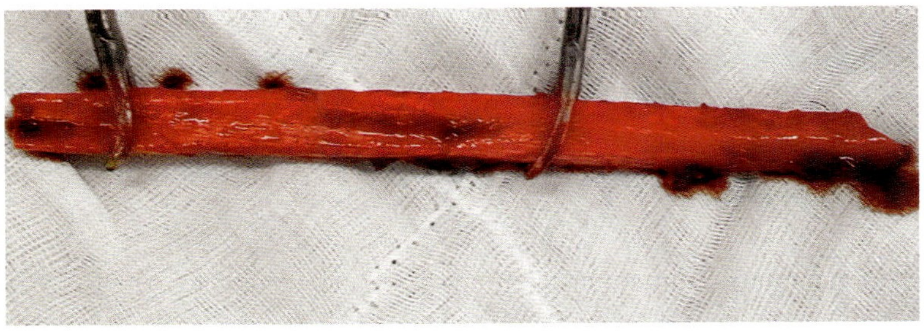

Fig. 22: Harvested fibular bone graft.

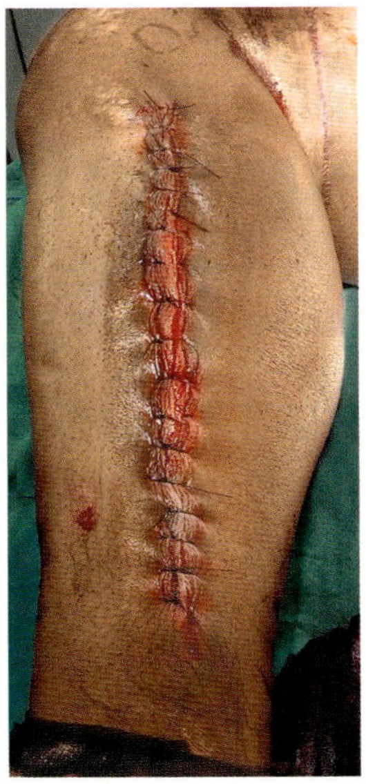

Fig. 23: Skin closure.

Fibular Graft

While removing the fibular graft, these points should be considered:

- Peroneal nerve to be protected.
- The distal fourth of the bone must be left intact to maintain a stable ankle.

Complication of Allograft

- Nonunion
- Fracture
- Infection
- Graft disease transmission.

SUGGESTED READING

1. Abbott LC, Schottstaedt ER, Saunders JB, et al. The Evaluation of Cortical and Cancellous Bone as Grafting Material. A Clinical and Experimental Study. J Bone Joint Surg. 1947;29:381-414.
2. Alt V, Nawab A, Seligson D. Bone grafting from the proximal tibia. Trauma. 1999;47:555-7.
3. Arora BK, Laskin DM. Sex Chromatin as a Cellular Label of Osteogenesis by Bone Grafts. J Bone Joint Surg. 1964;46-A:1269-76.
4. Burchardt H, Glowczewskie FP, Enneking WF. Allogenic Segmental Fibular Transplants in Azathioprine-immunosuppressed Dogs. J Bone Joint Surg. 1977;59-A:881-94.
5. Chase SW, Herndon CH. The fate of autogenous and homogenous bone grafts: A historical review. J Bone Joint Surg. 1955;37-A:809-41.
6. Delloye C, Verhelpen M, d'Hemricourt J, et al. Morphometric and Physical Investigations of Segmental Cortical Bone Autografts in Canine Ulnar Defects. Clin Orthop. 1992;282:273-885.
7. Dick HM, Strauch RJ. Infection of massive bone allografts. Clin Orthop Relat Res. 1994;306:46-53.
8. Ebraheim NA, Yang H, Lu J, et al. Anterior iliac crest bone graft: anatomic considerations. Spine. 1997;22:847-49.
9. Enneking WF, Burchardt H, Puhl J, et al. Physical and Biologic Aspects of Repair in Dog Cortical Bone Transplants. J Bone Joint Surg. 1975;57-A:237-52.
10. Enneking WF, Morris JL. Human Autologous Cortical Bone Transplants. Clin Orthop. 1972;87:28-39.
11. Harkins HN, Phemister DB. Simplified technic of onlay grafts. JAMA. 1937;109:1501.
12. Kurz LT, Garfin SR, Booth RE. Harvesting autogenous iliac bone grafts: a review of complications and techniques. Spine. 1989;14:1324-31.
13. Ottolenghi CE. Massive Osteoarticular Bone Grafts. Technique and Results of 62 Cases. Clin Orthop. 1972;87:156-170.
14. O'Keeffe RM, Riemer BL, Butterfield SL. Harvesting of autogenous cancellous bone graft from the proximal tibial metaphysis: a review of 230 cases. J Orthop Trauma. 1991;5:469-74.
15. Phemister DB. The Fate of Transplanted Bone and regenerative Power of its Various Constituents. Surg Gynecol Obstet. 1914;19:303.
16. Ray RD, Sabet TY. Bone Grafts: Cellular Survival versus Induction. J Bone Joint Surg. 1963;45-A:337-44.
17. Ray RD. Vascularization of Bone Grafts and Implants. Clin Orthop. 1972;87:43-51.
18. Weikel AM, Habal MB. Meralgia paresthetica: a complication of iliac bone procurement. Plast Reconstr Surg. 1977;60:572-4.

CHAPTER 70

Brodie's Abscess Decompression

S Prakash, Ashish Ratnani, Nitish Agrawal, Nikhil Mamoria

INTRODUCTION

Brodie's abscess is a form of subacute osteomyelitis. The abscess is surrounded by dense fibrous tissue and sclerotic bone. The disease is develops by accumulation of the pathogenic organisms in the terminal arterioles and capillaries of the bone's metaphysis. The increasing pressure due to edema and an increase in granulation will initiate the process of bone necrosis and abscess formation, known as "Brodie's abscess".

CLINICAL PRESENTATION

Localized pain, severe at night and relieved by aspirin. The symptoms are similar to that of osteoid osteoma.

LOCATION OF TYPICAL BRODIE'S ABSCESS

Metaphysis of tubular bones are ordinarily involved, so also carpal and tarsal bones. Other possible areas are pelvis, the vertebrae, calcaneus, the clavicle, and talus are affected less often. Most common area involved is at the proximal/distal tibia metaphysis. Femur is next commonly involved site. Lower limb is affected more frequently than upper limb.

DIAGNOSIS AND PROGNOSIS

Diagnosis is a challenge as the signs and symptoms of the acute (osteomyelitis) form of the disease are absent. There may be delay in diagnosis ranging from a few months to many years. The prognosis is good with a 100% cure rate.

IMPACT TO FUNCTIONING

The disease will affect normal functioning of the limb and gait cycle. There is some loss of function due to protective guarding of the limb. Shorter unilateral weight-bearing moments in the gait cycle of the involved extremity are noted.

COMPLICATIONS

- Epidermoid carcinoma
- Pathological fractures
- Amyloidosis
- Contractures of adjacent joints.

RADIOGRAPHIC FEATURES

Oval, elliptical, or serpentine radiolucency is normally more than 1 cm encompassed by a vigorously reactive sclerosis, granulation tissue, also, a nidus less then 1 cm. The edges frequently seem scalloped on radiograph.

Computed tomography (CT) scan is best to visualize Brodie's abscess. Related decay of delicate tissue close to the site of contamination and shortening of the influenced bone might be present.

BEST IMAGING MODALITY

Magnetic resonance imaging (MRI) is the most sensitive investigation to evaluate a Brodie's abscess. Nuclear bone scan is a more sensitive test to detect early disease. Computed tomography (CT) can be used to differentiate a Brodie's abscess from osteoid osteoma.

Role of Imaging in Diagnosis and Management

Magnetic resonance imaging, using the combination of dark focus on T1-weighted images and a bright signal on T2-weighted images typically indicates osteomyelitis. Sonogram is helpful to localize the site of underlying infection when drainage is planned.

RADIOLOGICAL CLASSIFICATION

Radiological classification in 1982, Roberts et al., modified and expanded Gledhill's classification:

Radiological classification	*Location*	*Features*
Type I	Metaphyseal	Type Ia is a punched-out central metaphyseal lesion. Type Ib is an eccentric metaphyseal cortical erosion.
Type II	Diaphyseal	Type IIa is a localized cortical and periosteal reaction. In Type IIb medullary abscess present in the diaphysis without cortical destruction but with onion skin periosteal reaction.
Type III	Epiphyseal	Type IIIa is a primary epiphyseal osteomyelitis. In Type IIIb lesion crosses the epiphysis and involves both the epiphysis and the metaphysic.
Type IV	Metaphyseal equivalent	Type IVa involves the vertebral body with an erosive or destructive process. Type IVb involves the flat bones of the pelvis. Type IVc involves the small bones, such as the tarsal bones.

TREATMENT

Surgical treatment is required. In small abscesses, surgical evacuation and curettage is performed under antibiotic cover. After evacuation, packing with cancellous bone chips is advisable in large abscesses.

SURGICAL STEPS (FIGS. 1 TO 33)

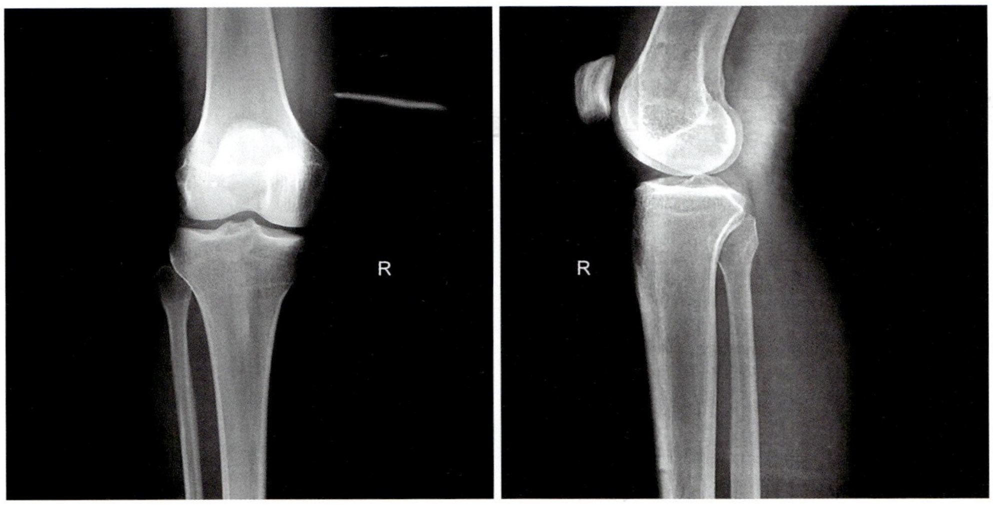

Fig. 1: X-ray right knee (anteroposterior/lateral view) showing well-defined lytic lesion with sclerotic rim in medial aspect of distal end of femur.

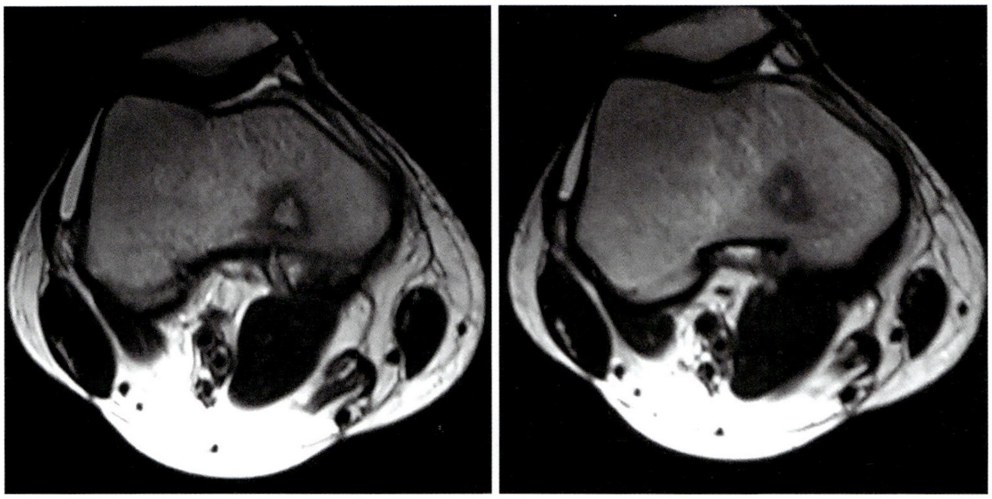

Fig. 2: Computed tomography (CT) scan of right knee joint with femur:

- There is 10 × 7 mm sized well-defined lytic lesion with narrow zone of transition is noted involving the medial aspect of distal end of femur. Subtle sclerotic rim is noted. Tiny subcentimetric bone island is noted in the lateral femoral condyle. Two subchondral cysts are noted in the lateral tibial condyle. Tiny bone island is noted in the patella.
- *Impression:* CT scan of right knee joint reveals well-defined lytic lesion with narrow zone of transition and subtle sclerotic rim involving the medial aspect of distal end of femur—in view of history of pain relieved on medication, likely suggestive of osteoid osteoma. Suggest magnetic resonance imaging (MRI) correlation.

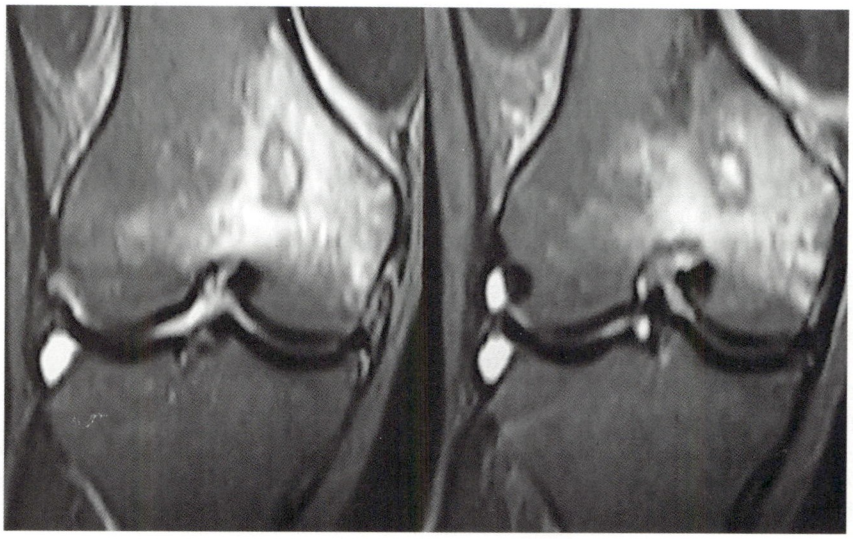

Fig. 3: Computed tomography (CT) scan postcontrast.

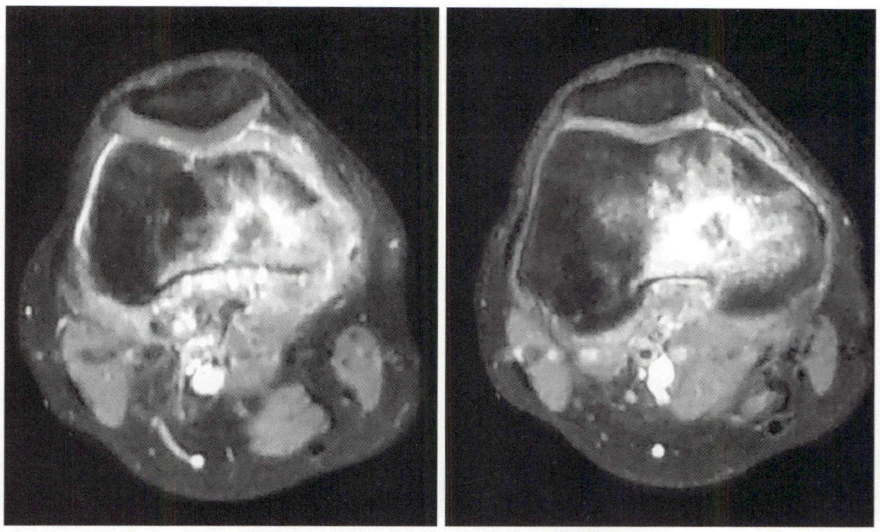

Fig. 4: T1 axial postcontrast image:

- *Magnetic resonance imaging (MRI) right knee joint*: There is fairly well-defined lesion noted in the metaphyseal region of medial condyle of femur, posteriorly and near to the intercondylar ridge measuring approximately 1 cm x 1.4 cm x 2.1 cm. This lesion appears hyperintense on T2W/STIR (T2-weighted short-tau inversion recovery) and hypointense on T1W images. This lesion shows peripheral T2W/STIR hypointense rim. This lesion shows heterogeneous postcontrast enhancement.
- Hyperintense signal intensity on T2W/PDFS (proton density fat saturated) images is noted in medial femoral condyle and intercondylar region surrounding this lesion, which appears hypointense on T1W images likely suggestive of marrow edema. Surrounding soft-tissue shows edema.
- *Impression*: Heterogeneously enhancing fairly well-defined lesion in the medial condyle of femur likely suggestive of osteoid osteoma.

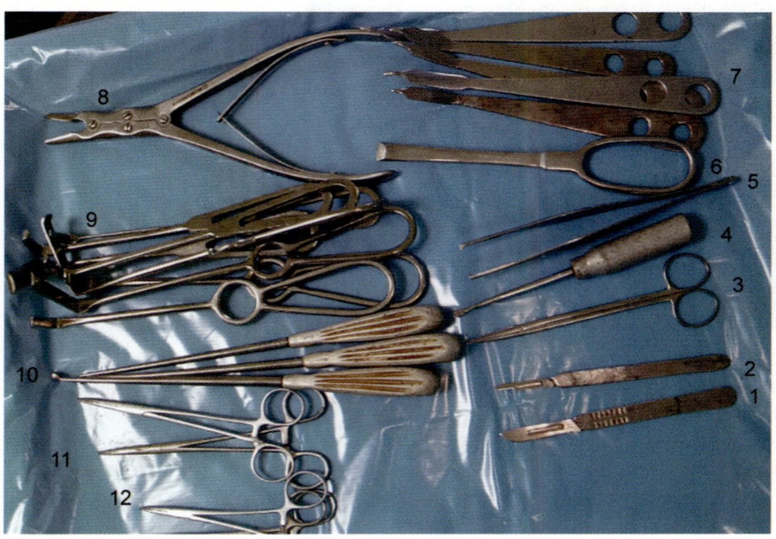

Fig. 5:

1. Bard–Parker handle with blade number 21
2. Bard–Parker handle with blade number 15
3. Dissecting scissor
4. Periosteum
5. Tooth forceps
6. Periosteum elevator
7. Hohmann bone lever
8. Bone nibbler
9. Right angle retractor
10. Curette
11. Artery forceps
12. Mosquito forceps.

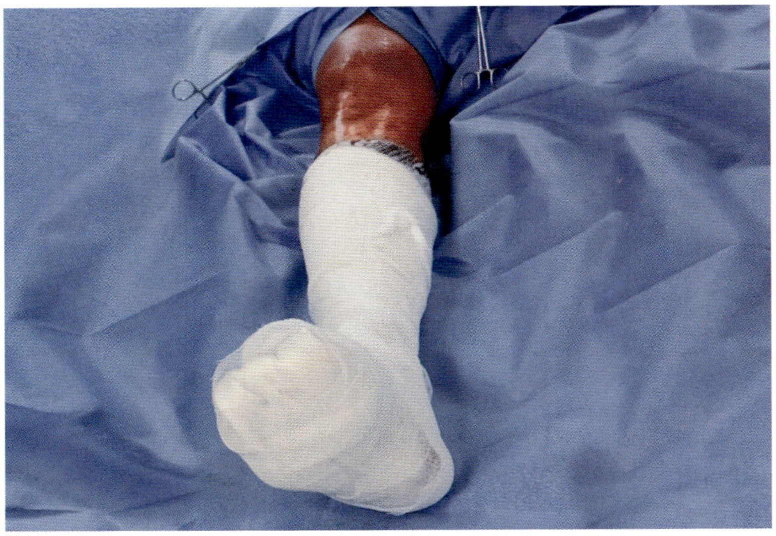

Fig. 6: Supine position given on operating table right lower limb kept in extension exposing knee and distal femur. Painting and draping done in standard manner.

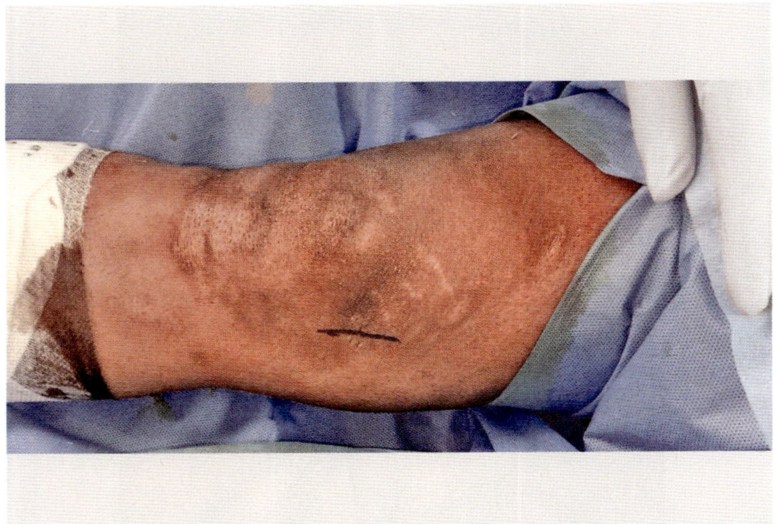

Fig. 7: Incision site marked over medial side of distal femur at supracondylar femur level.

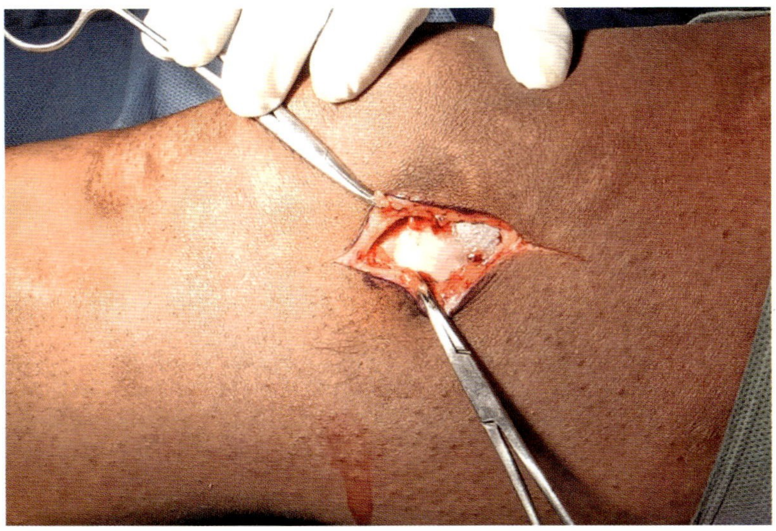

Fig. 8: Incision taken with knife, small blood vessels are caught with artery forceps. Subcutaneous tissue, fat pad, and fascia dissected with stab knife. Skin, subcutaneous tissue, and fascia retracted with right angle retractor.

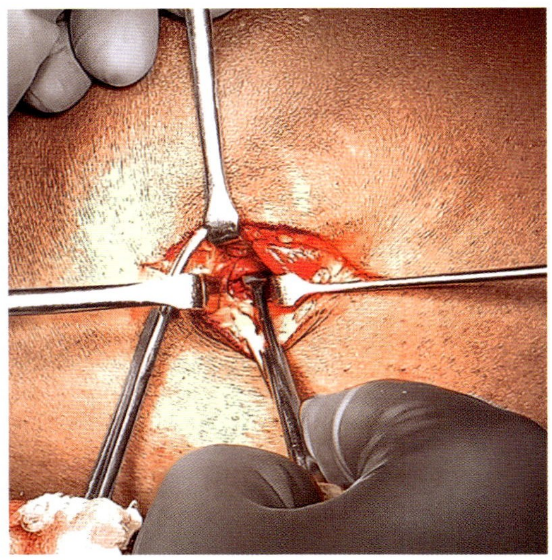

Fig. 9: Muscle fibers are separated along the length with periosteum.

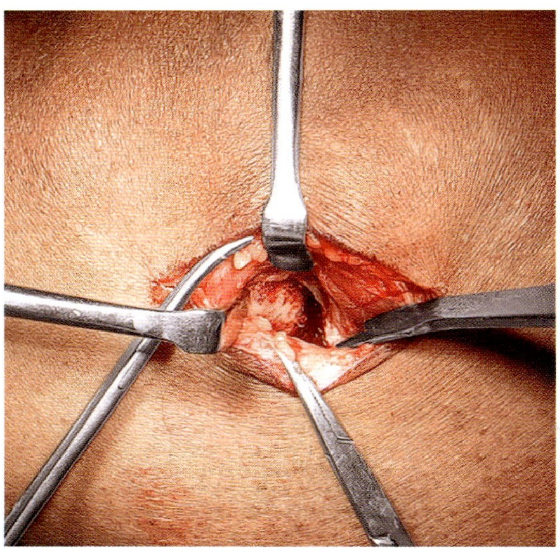

Fig. 10: Muscle with other soft tissue retracted with right angle retractor and bone is exposed.

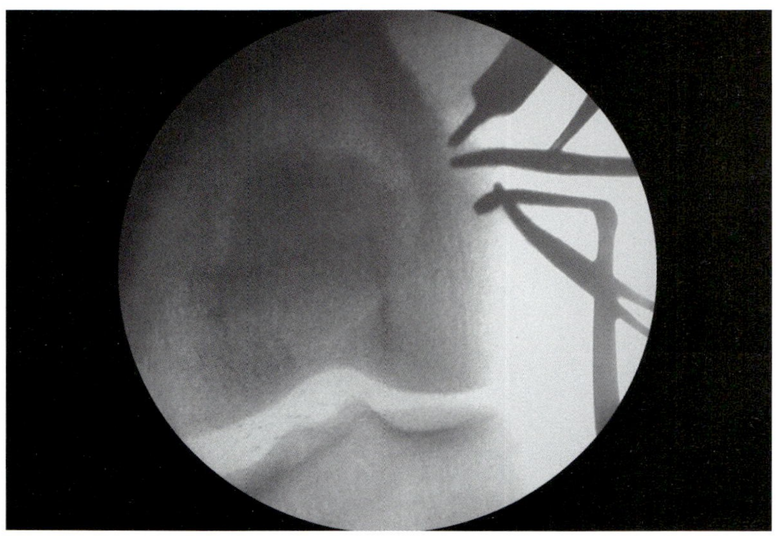

Fig. 11: Entry site for drainage identified over C-arm image intensifier.

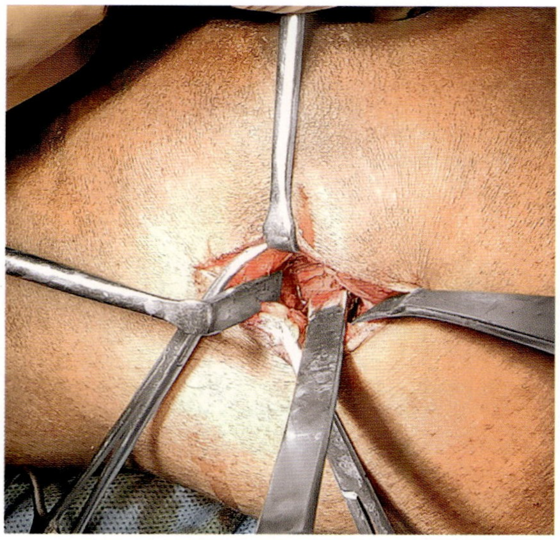

Fig. 12: Small window done with osteotome and hammer in cortical bone at the level of lesion. Cortical window completed with osteotome and hammer.

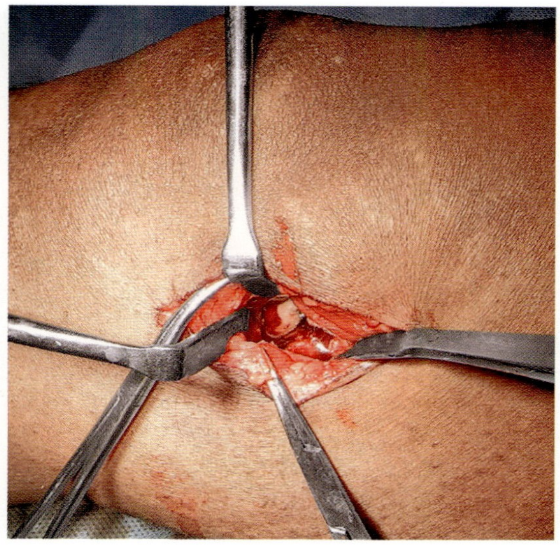

Fig. 13: Infected tissue with pus found in cavity of lesion.

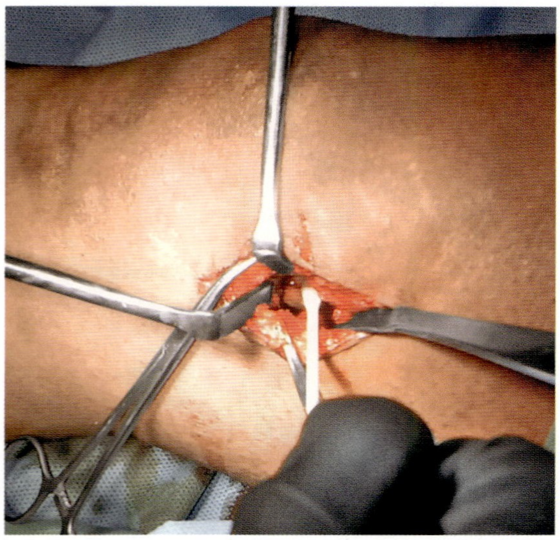

Fig. 14: Swab culture was taken from infected tissue from the lesion.

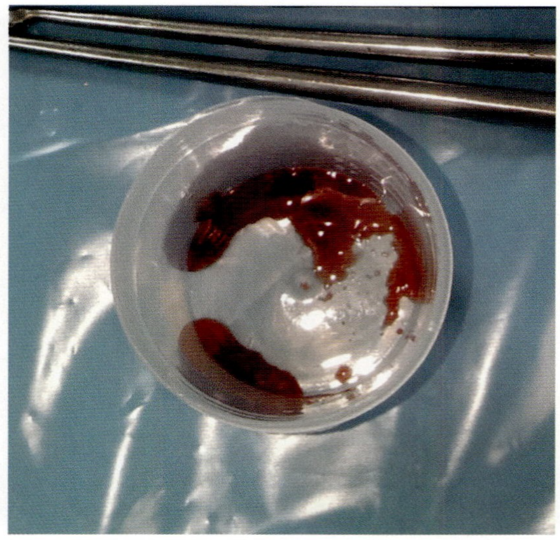

Fig. 15: Infected fluid from cavity collected in sterile container.

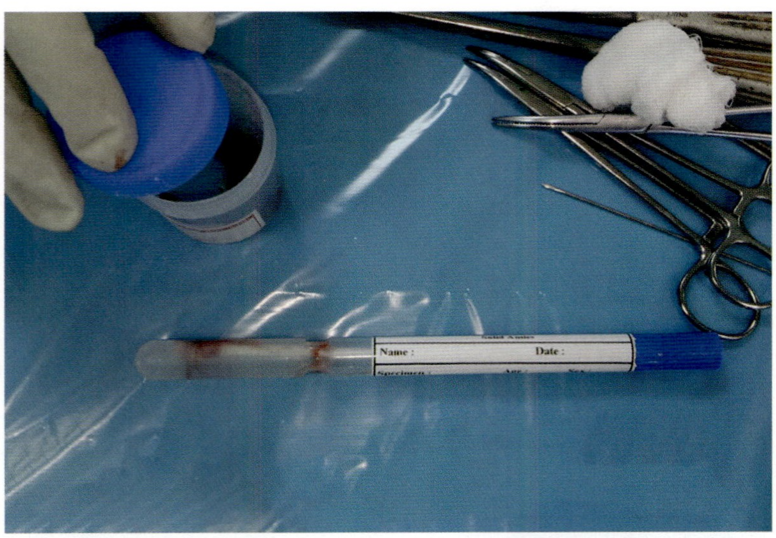

Fig. 16: Swab culture and fluid collected in sterile container send for Gram stain, Zn stain, culture sensitivity, TB PCR (tuberculosis polymerase chain reaction) and histopathological examinations.

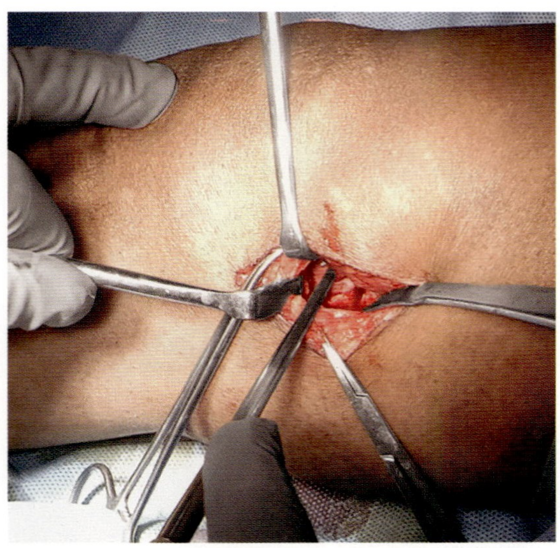

Fig. 17: Curettage of infected cavity done with curette.

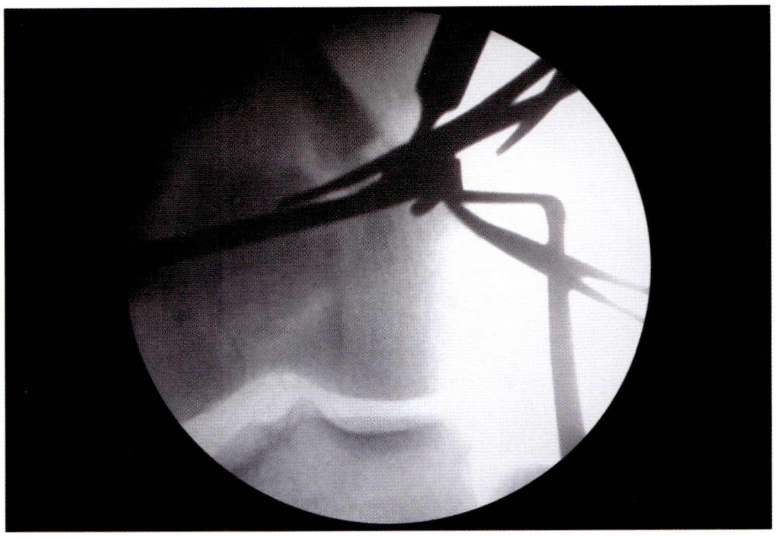

Fig. 18: Curettage of cavity confirmed in C-arm image intensifier.

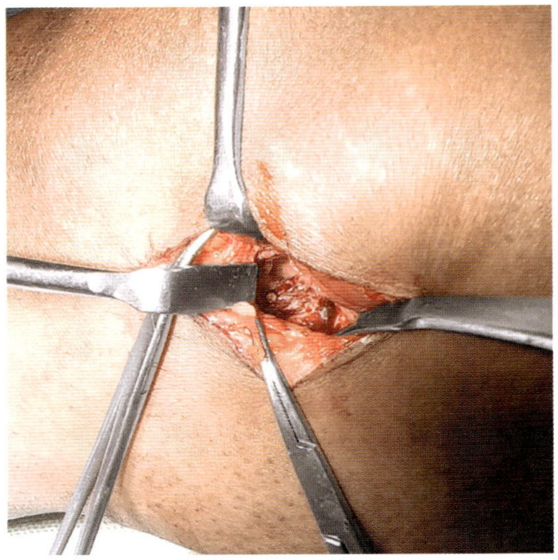

Fig. 19: Sequestrum or dead bone tissue removed from infected cavity.

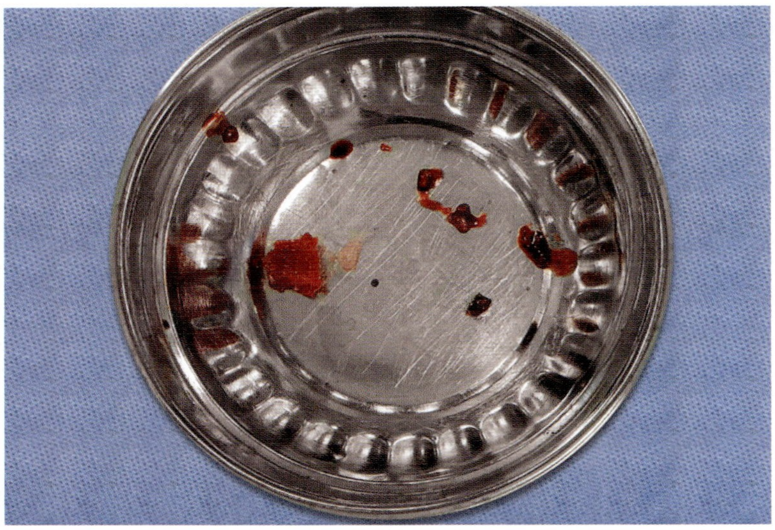

Fig. 20: Infected bone tissue sent for histopathological examination.

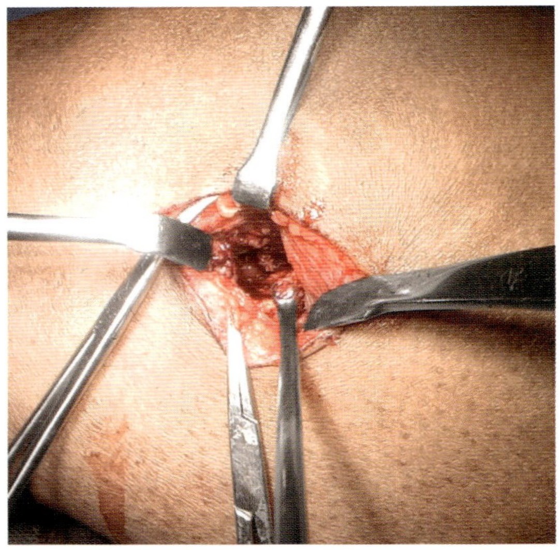

Fig. 21: Further curettage of lesion cavity done with curette.

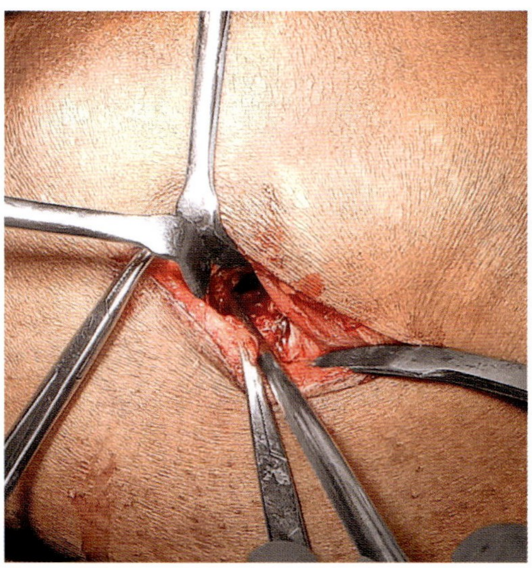

Fig. 22: Curettage complete.

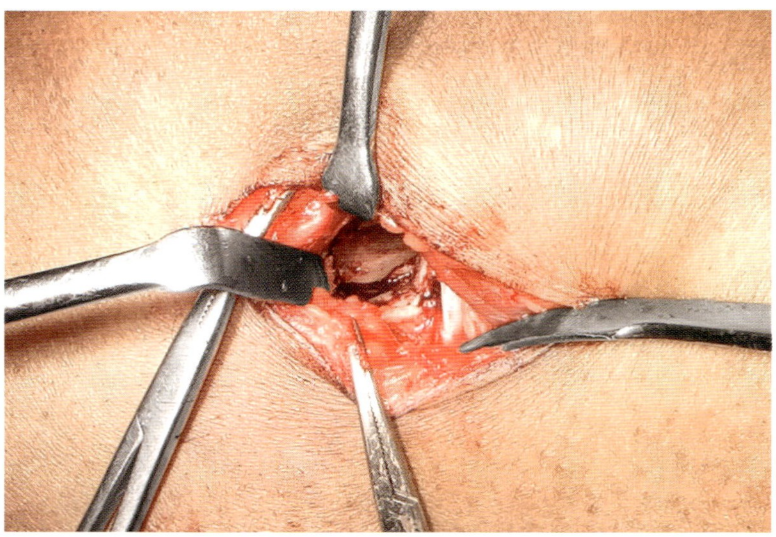

Fig. 23: Sclerotic rim seen covering lesion.

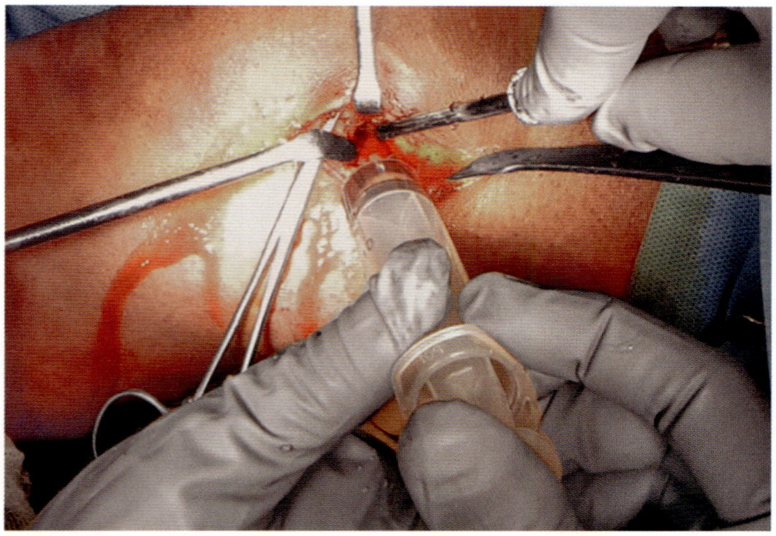

Fig. 24: Wash in cavity given with normal saline and povidone–iodine.

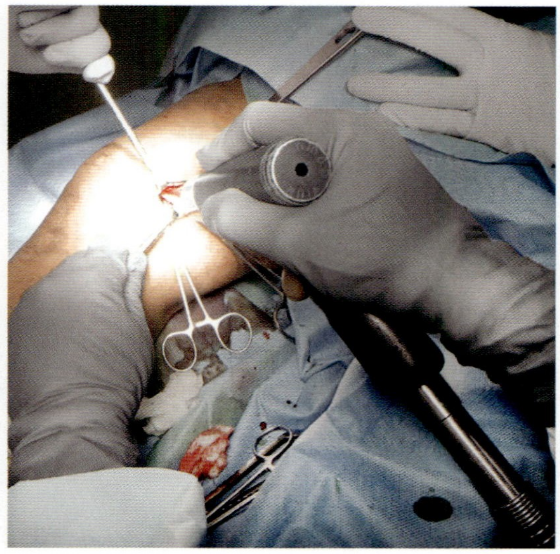

Fig. 25: Small hole made in wall of cavity for enhancing bone formation in cavity.

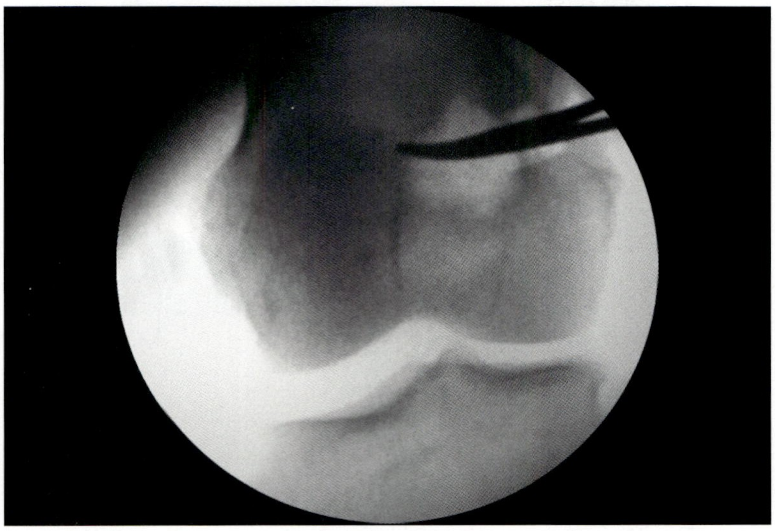

Fig. 26: Curettage and drainage completed and confirmed over C-arm on anteroposterior (AP) view.

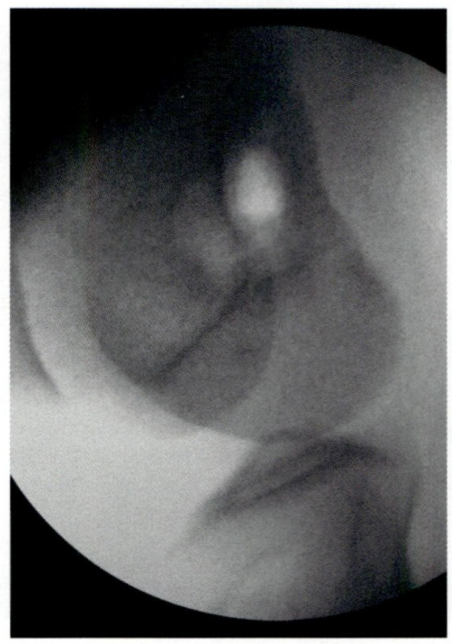

Fig. 27: Curettage and drainage completed and confirmed on C-arm lateral view.

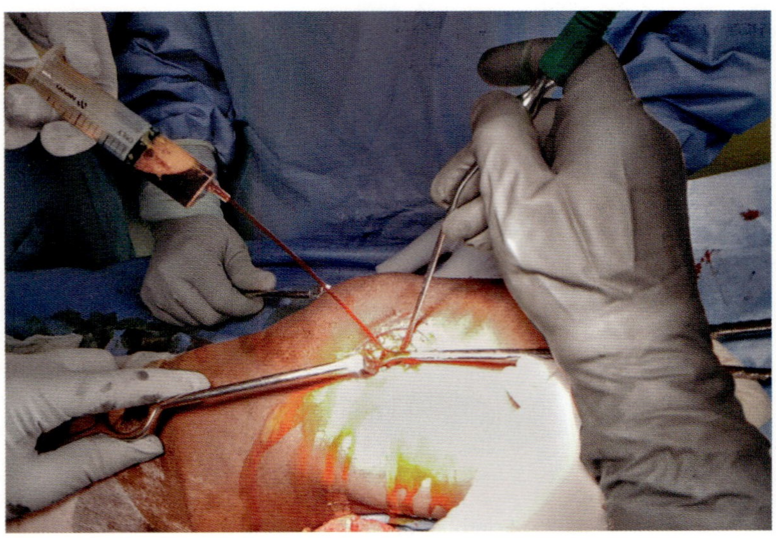

Fig. 28: Again cavity washed with normal saline and povidone–iodine solution.

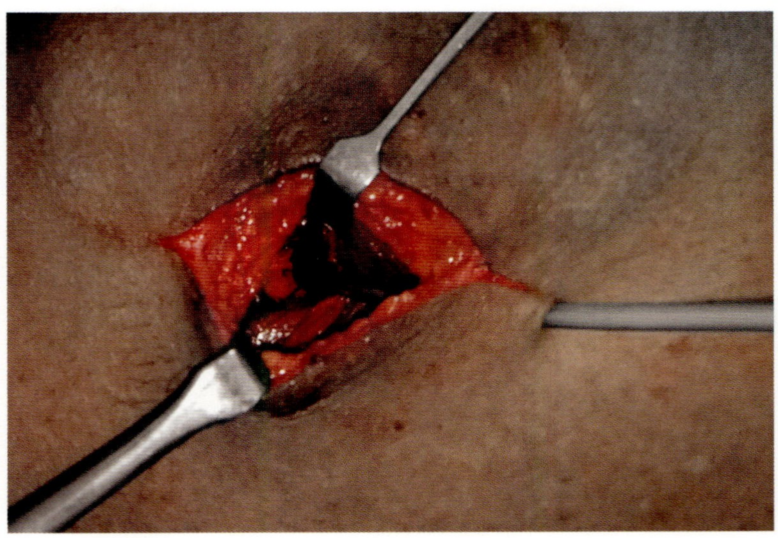

Fig. 29: Suction drain was put in infected cavity.

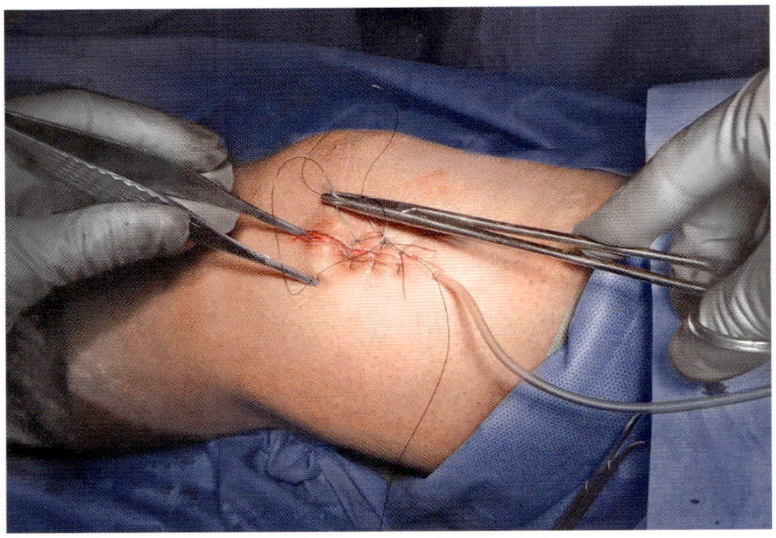

Fig. 30: Fascia and soft tissue sutured done with absorbable suture material.

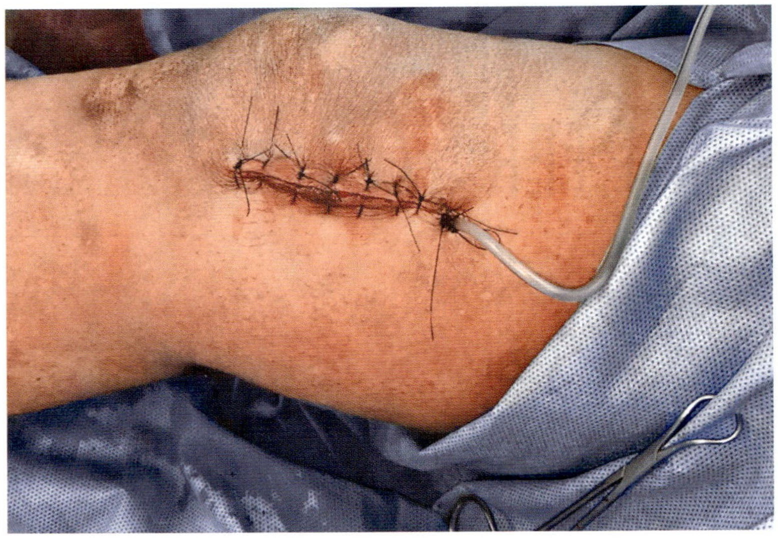

Fig. 31: Skin suturing done with Nonabsorbable material.

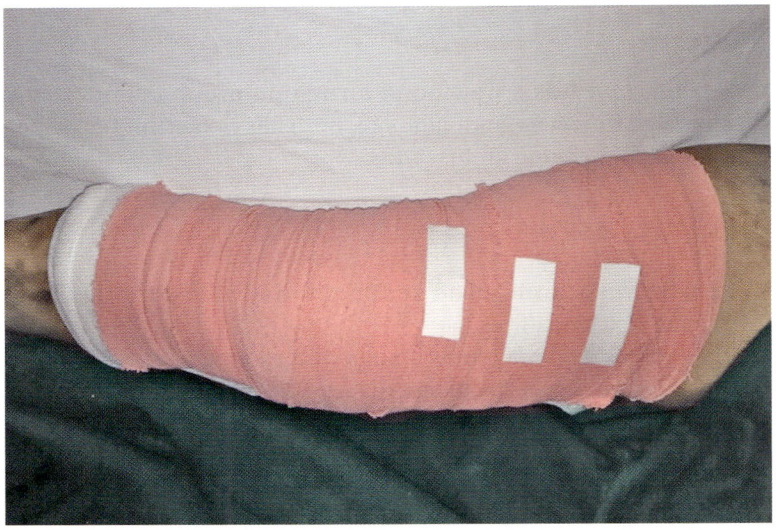

Fig. 32: Tight compression bandage was given after dressing.

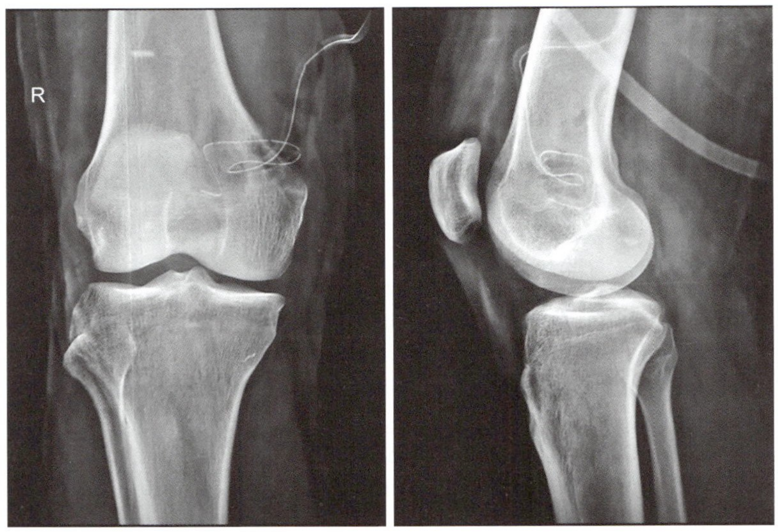

Fig. 33: Postoperative X-ray [anteroposterior (AP)/lateral view] showing complete curettage and drainage of lesion cavity with suction catheter in situ.

POSTOPERATIVE MANAGEMENT

- Active toe movement started from day 0. Ankle dorsiflexion, plantar flexion, hamstring strengthening, quadriceps strengthening, hip range of motion exercises started from day 1.
- Nonweight-bearing (NWB) mobilization with walker support started from day 2.
- Suture removal done on day 21.
- Patient was kept NWB for 21 days.
- Partial toe touch weight-bearing mobilization started after 3 weeks.
- Full weight-bearing mobilization started after 10–12 weeks.
- Polymerase chain reaction (PCR) for tuberculosis (TB)—*Mycobacterium tuberculosis* complex DNA detected.
- Antitubercular drugs started after 1 week.

SUGGESTED READING

1. Afshar A, Mohammadi A. The "Penumbra Sign" on Magnetic Resonance Images of Brodie's Abscess: A Case Report. Iran J Radiol. 2011;8(4): 245-8.
2. Brant WE, Helms CA. Fundamentals of diagnostic radiology. Philadelphia: Lippincott Williams & Wilkins; 2007.
3. Dähnert W. Radiology review manual. Philadelphia: Lippincott Williams & Wilkins; 2007.
4. McHugh CH, Shapeero LG, Murphey FL. Case for diagnosis. Brodie abscess. Mil Med. 2007;172(7):viii-xi.
5. Schlur C, Bachy M, Wajfisz A, et al. Osteoid osteoma mimicking Brodie's abscess in a 13-year-old girl. Pediatr Int. 2013;55(2):e29-31.

CHAPTER 71

Sequestrectomy and Saucerization for Chronic Osteomyelitis

Rajeev Nene, Mahaveer S Dugad, Rajkumar Ekambaram

INTRODUCTION

- Chronic osteomyelitis is the infection of the bone persisting more than 3 weeks
- It is a sequel to acute osteomyelitis following hematogenous spread
- The metaphyseal end of the bone is the common site where infective organisms lodge particularly due to the hairpin configuration of blood vessels leading to vascular stasis
- May also occur following inadequate treatment of primary infections, compound fractures, peri-implant infections
- Acute exacerbations of chronic osteomyelitis occur in recent trauma, immunosuppressed individuals, and extremes of age.

CLINICAL FEATURES

Symptoms are less marked than signs in chronic osteomyelitis.

Fever, swelling, discharge of tiny bone spicules over the sinuses present over the bone, and irregular thickening of bone are characteristic. Acute exacerbation produces symptoms like fever, bony tenderness on palpation.

- *Sequestrum*: It is a piece of dead bone that has separated due to necrosis of normal bone surrounded by infective granulation tissue. It has rough outer surface and smooth sclerotic inner surface
- *Involucrum*: It is a new bone formation around sequestrum separated from it by granulation tissue. It has cloaca through which pus inside the bone drains out.

INVESTIGATIONS

- Leukocytosis and raised sedimentation rates are the main hematological features
- Plain radiograph may show involucrum as irregular thickening of the bone and sequestrum as a dense sclerotic bone
- Sinogram by injecting radio-opaque dye in the sinus tract may help to visualize its extent
- Gallium-67 and indium-111–labeled leukocyte scan gives more precision of diagnosis of infection.

TREATMENT

- Antibiotics are started according to culture sensitivity
- Sequestrectomy and saucerization are planned only after proper visualization of sequestrum in radiograph. Once done, it leaves a bony defect, which can be closed by bone graft, myoplasty, and antibiotic beads
- Hyperbaric oxygen therapy
- Amputation may be used as salvage for severe life-threatening infections.

SURGICAL STEPS (FIGS. 1 TO 26)

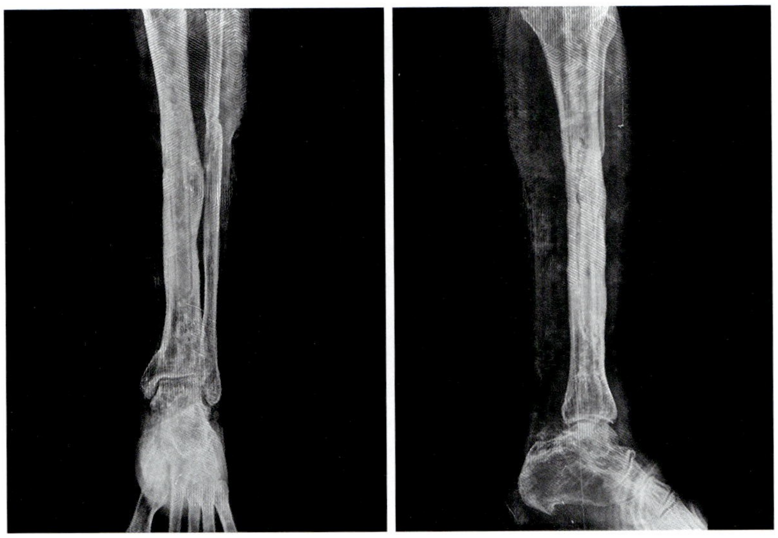

Fig. 1: Preoperative X-ray showing osteomyelitis changes over left distal shaft tibia.

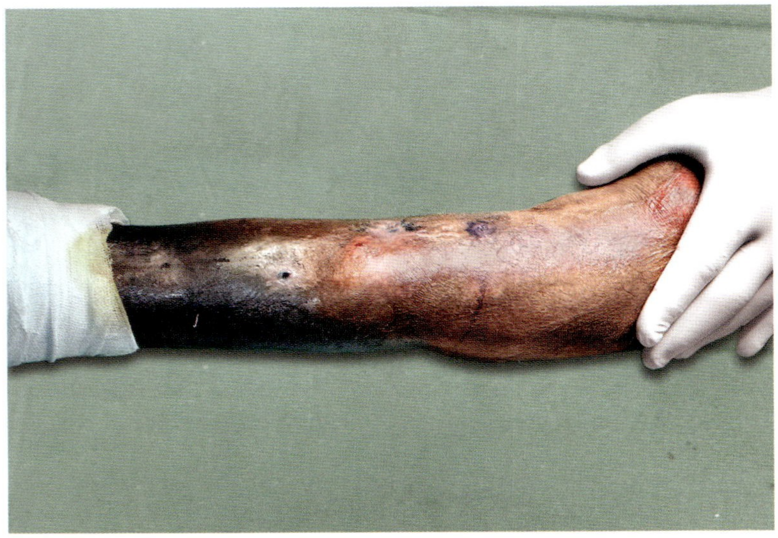

Fig. 2: Supine positioning of the limb after painting and draping.

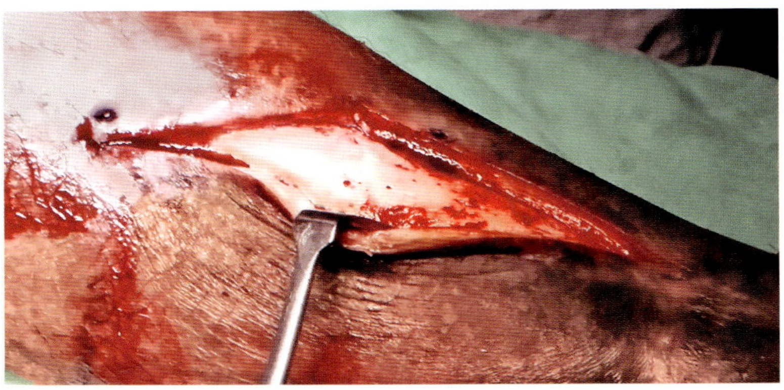

Fig. 3: Skin is incised and retracted.

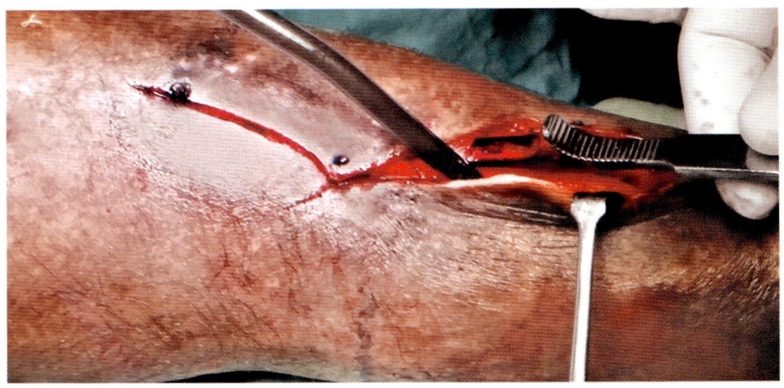

Fig. 4: Periosteum elevator is used to elevate full thickness flap of the bony surface.

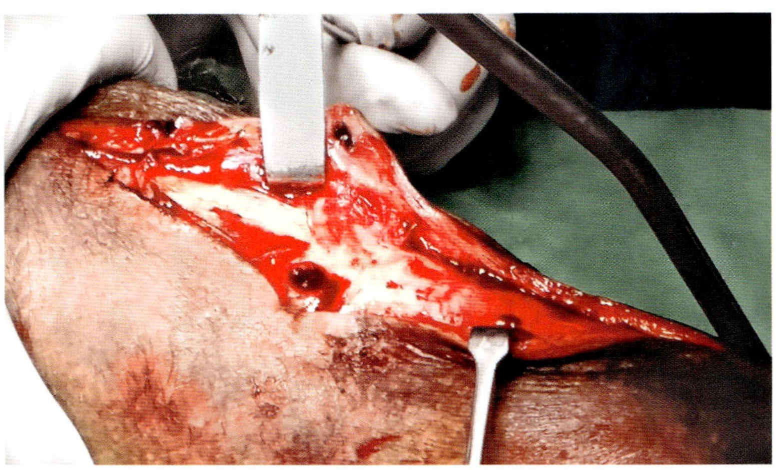

Fig. 5: Deep dissection is done and bone is exposed. Note the presence of thickened bone (involucrum).

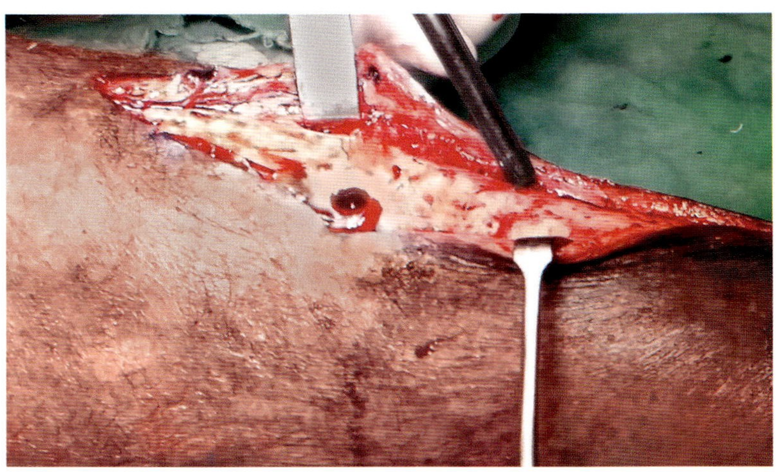

Fig. 6: Skin and deep tissue are retracted. Cloaca is seen with pus oozing through it.

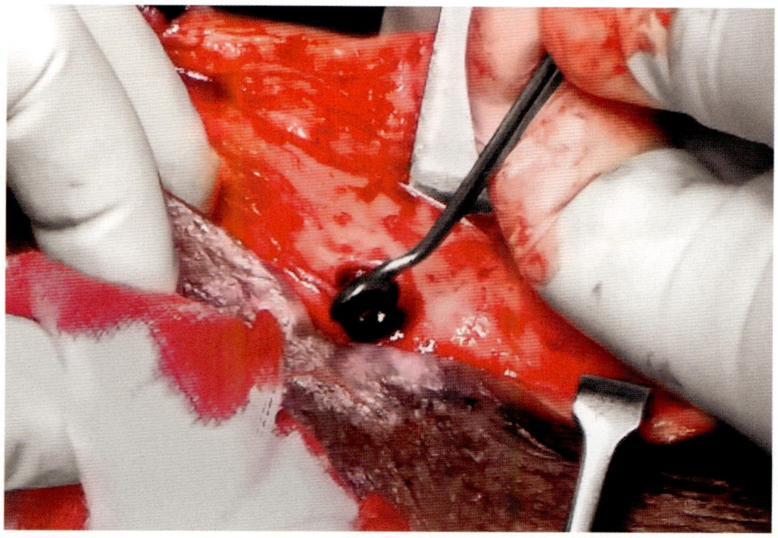

Fig. 7: Pus and infective material from the cloaca is scooped out.

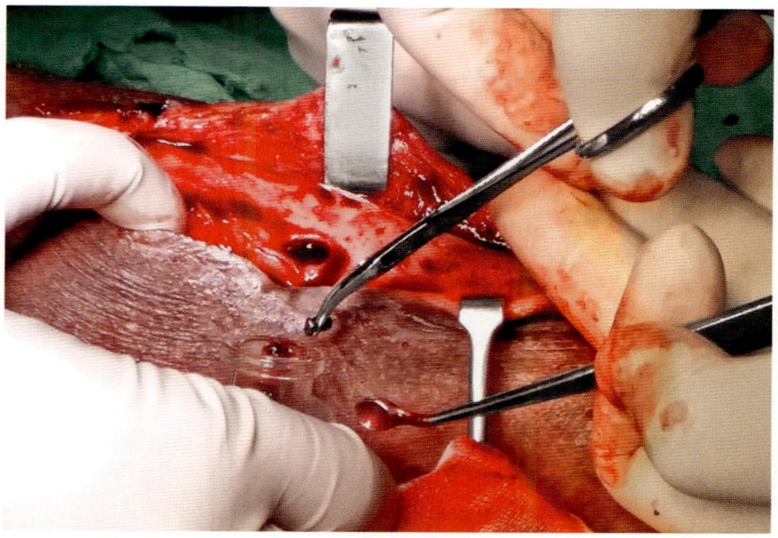

Fig. 8: The scooped out necrotic material is collected for culture sensitivity.

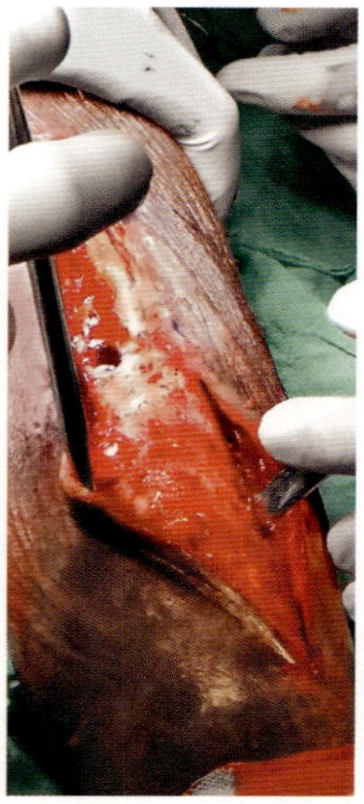

Fig. 9: Margins of the thickened bone are further delineated to prepare it for making the bone window.

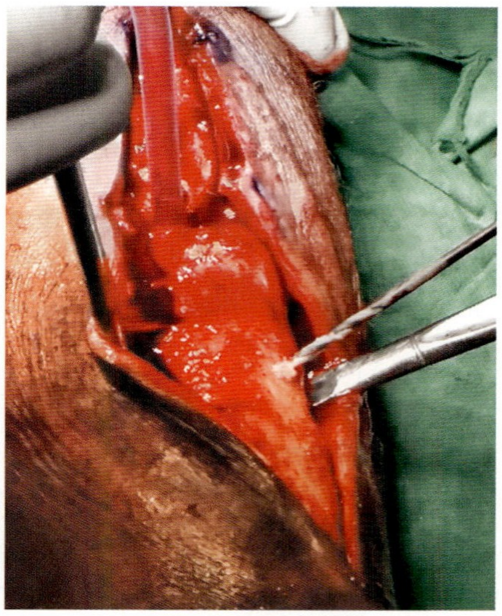

Fig. 10: Bone drilling is started over the margin of the bone window.

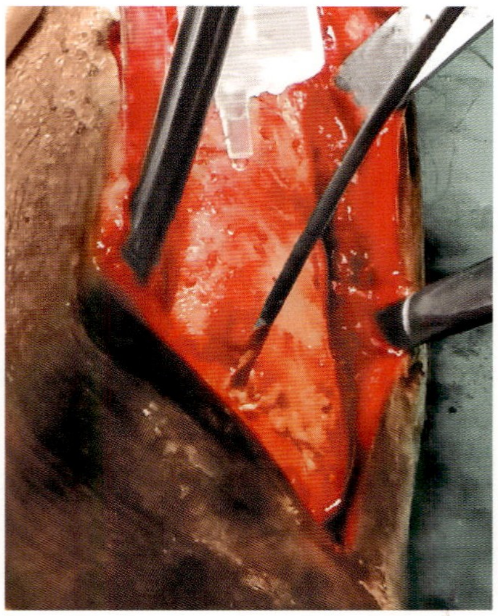

Fig. 11: Multiple unicortical drill holes are made to ensure controlled osteotomy of the bone window.

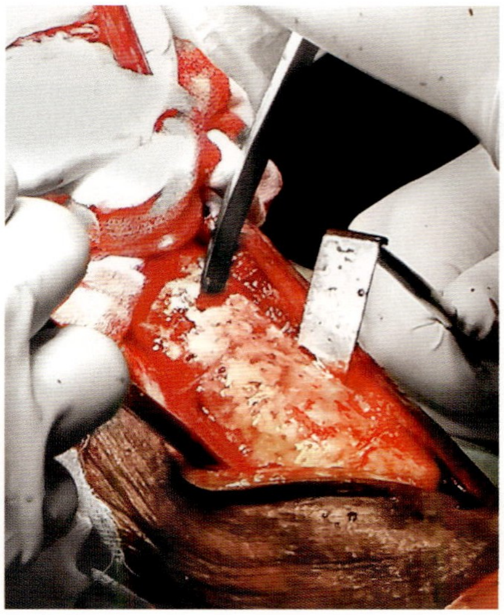

Fig. 12: Using osteotome bone is removed by connecting the previously made drill holes to each other.

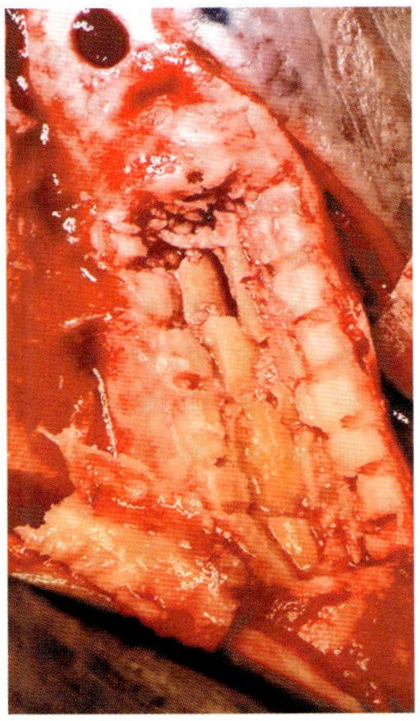

Fig. 13: Osteomyelitic cavity of the bone is seen filled with multiple sequestra and unhealthy granulation and pus.

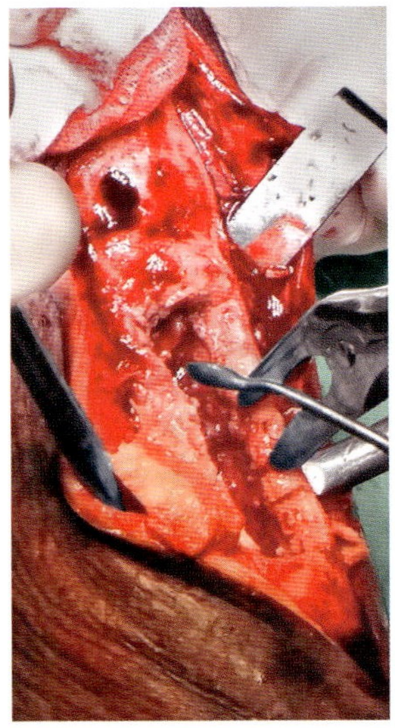

Fig. 14: After removing all the sequestra, the infective granulation tissue is scooped out.

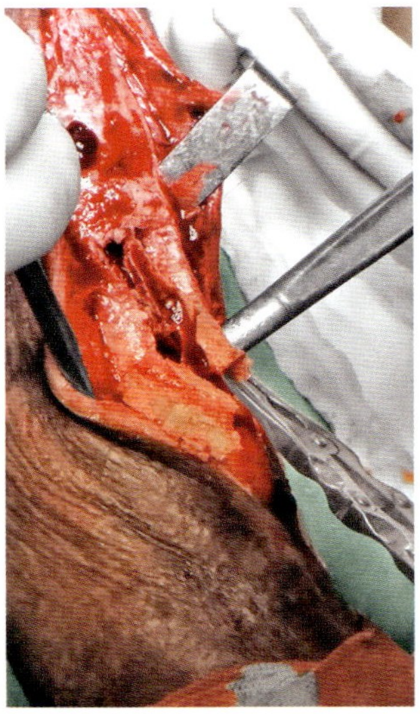

Fig. 15: End of sequestrum protruding through proximal medullary canal is identified and removed by holding carefully with nibbler.

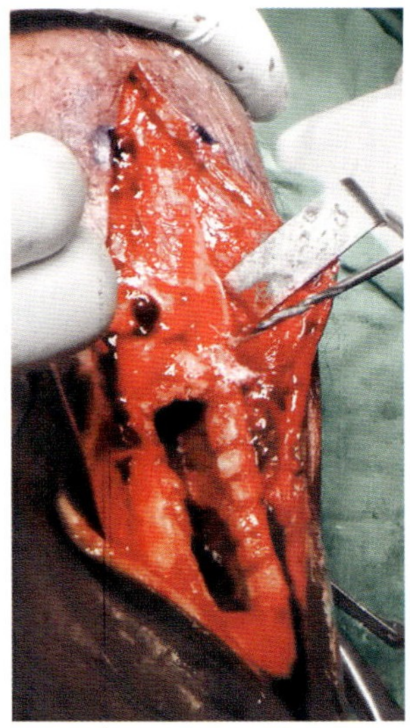

Fig. 16: For more proximal sequestra proximal cortex is drilled around the sinus to extend the bone window.

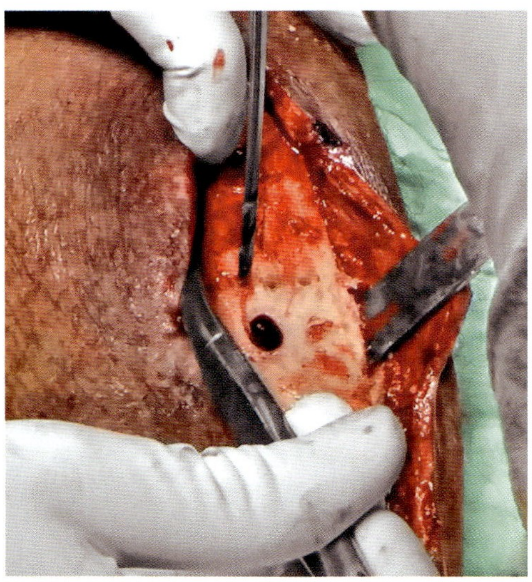

Fig. 17: Making multiple drill holes to mark the proximal extent of the window.

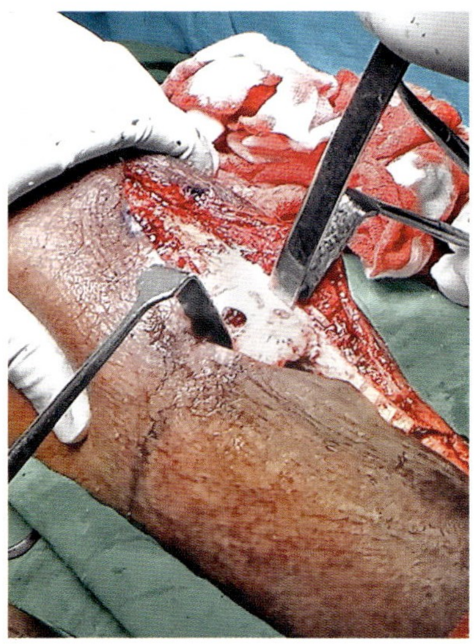

Fig. 18: Cortex is removed using osteotome.

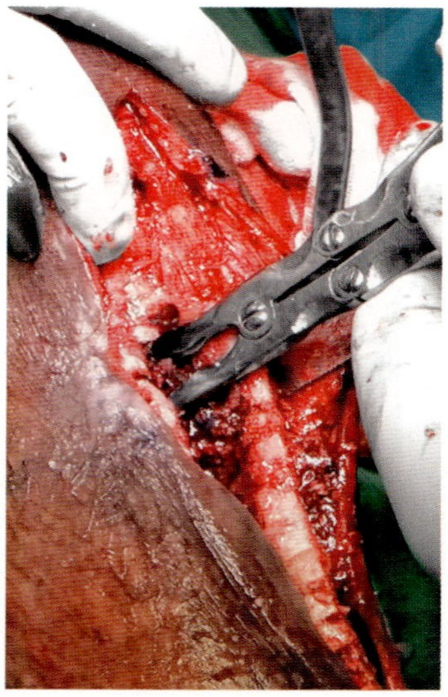

Fig. 19: Sequestrum inside is removed again with nibbler.

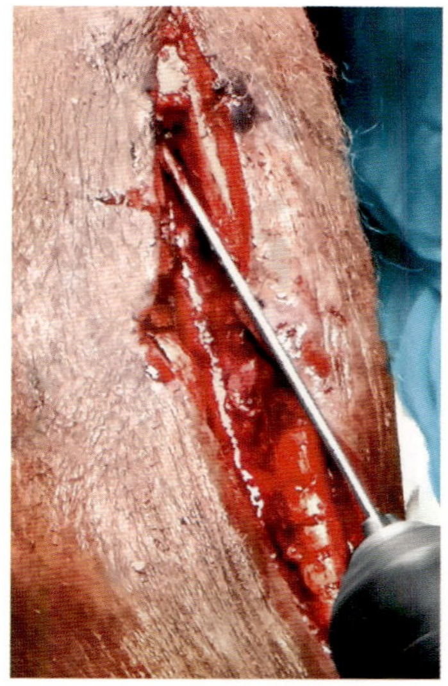

Fig. 20: After sequestrectomy, medullary canal is opened with drill bit.

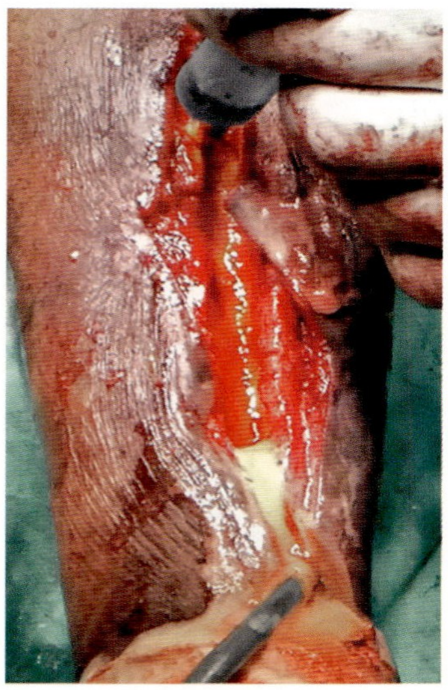

Fig. 21: Wash with povidone iodine solution and hydrogen peroxide is given and kept for a minute.

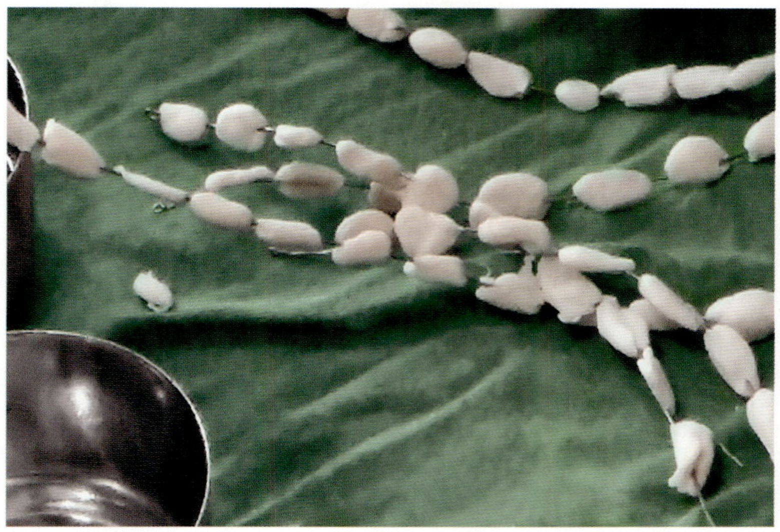

Fig. 22: Antibiotic beads made of vancomycin are prepared.

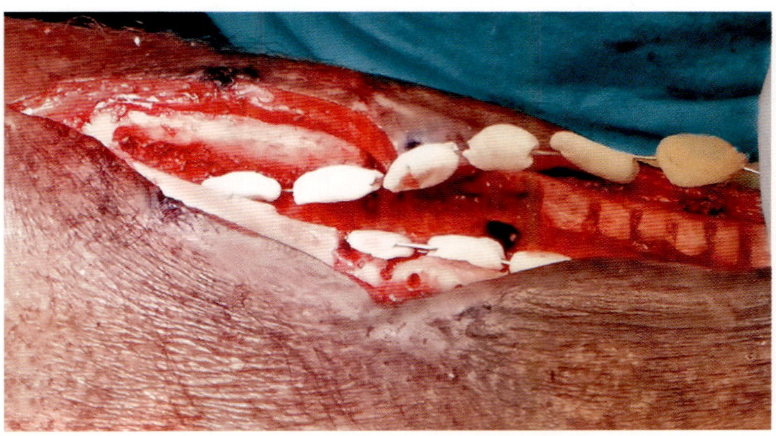

Fig. 23: Vancomycin beads are introduced into the canal.

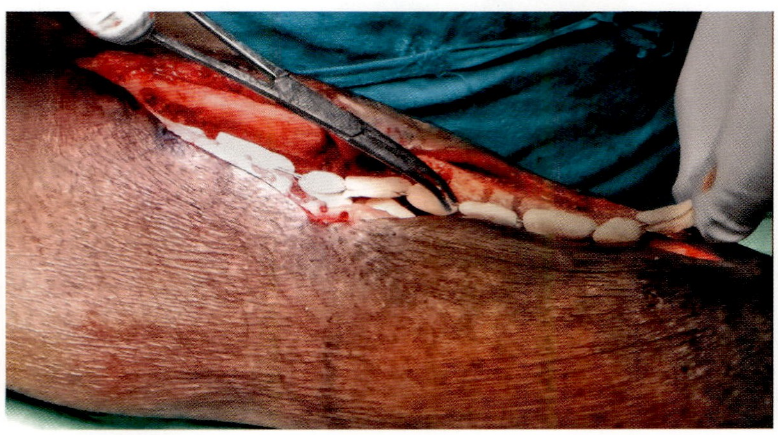

Fig. 24: Some more vancomycin beads are introduced further to pack the bony cavity.

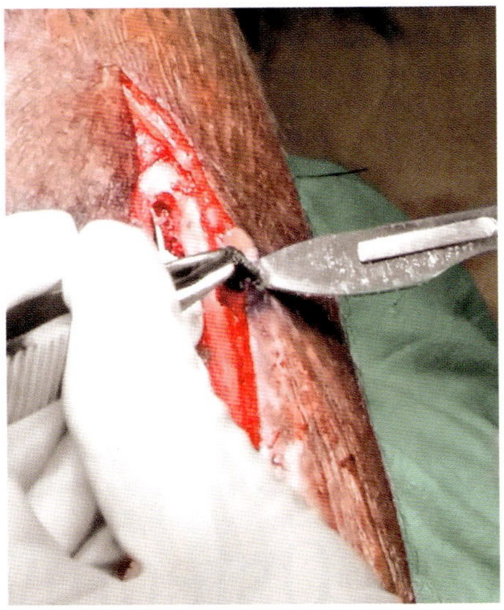

Fig. 25: Sinus tract excision is done.

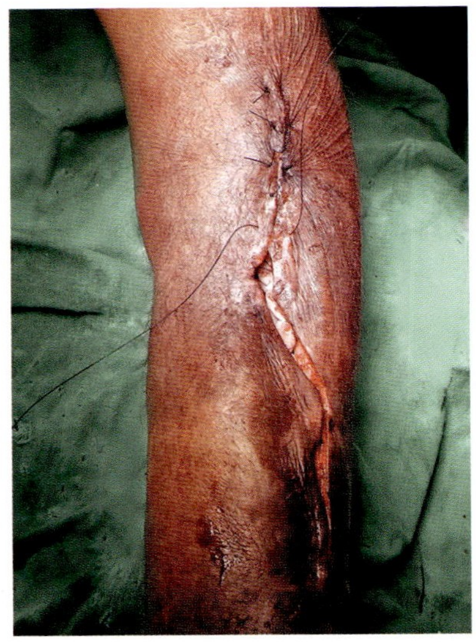

Fig. 26: Skin closure done with nonabsorbable 2-0 suture.

COMPLICATIONS

Growth disturbances like shortening of the limb or deformities pathological fractures, squamous cell carcinoma of the sinus tract are to be watched for.

SUGGESTED READING

1. Blockey NJ, Watson JT. Acute osteomyelitis in children. J Bone Joint Surg. 1970;52-B:77.
2. Cole WG, Dalziel RE, Leitl S. Treatment of acute osteomyelitis in childhood. J Bone Joint Surg. 1982;64-B:218.
3. Jackson MA, Nelson JD. Etiology and medical management of acute suppurative bone and joint infections in pediatric patients. J Pediatr Orthop. 1982;2:313.
4. Learmonth ID, Dall G, Pallock DJ. Acute osteomyelitis and septic arthritis in children: A simple approach to treatment. S Afr Med J. 1984;65:117.
5. Orr HW. The treatment of acute osteomyelitis by drainage and rest. J Bone Joint Surg. 1927;9:733.
6. Trueta J. Acute haematogenous osteomyelitis: Its pathology and treatment. Bull Hosp Joint Dis. 1993;145.

CHAPTER 72

Metaphyseal Drill Hole for Acute Osteomyelitis

Amit R Kale, Kumar Kanishk

INTRODUCTION

Osteomyelitis is an infection and inflammation of the bone and the bone marrow with involvement of surrounding tissue. It can be due to bacterial or fungal infection of bones. Long bones of extremity are involved in children while spine and hip involvement is common in adults. *Staphylococcus aureus* is most common bacteria causing acute osteomyelitis.

CAUSES

Microorganisms may infect bone through one or more of three basic methods:
1. Hematogenous spread
2. Adjacent infected areas
3. Penetrating trauma, postsurgical infection.

DIAGNOSIS

Blood tests:
- Hemogram
- C-reactive protein
- Erythrocyte sedimentation rate (ESR).

X-rays and computerized tomography (CT) scan:
- Radiographs and CT are method of diagnosis.

Magnetic resonance imaging (MRI):
- Confirmation is with MRI
- Edema on T2 sequence is sensitive but not specific. Bone marrow and cortical destruction on T1 sequence is more specific.

Bone biopsy:
- Bone biopsy is gold standard as it provides information about causative organism.

TREATMENT

The treatment for osteomyelitis is surgery to remove dead and necrotic bone portion, followed by antibiotics.

The principles for surgery of osteomyelitis are as follows:
- Drain the infected area.
- Remove diseased bone and tissue of infected area.
- Restore blood flow to the bone and infected area.
- Remove any foreign objects/substance in infected area.

Medical Therapy

Surgery is the most important modality at present, but it has to be supported by antibiotic treatment.

DESCRIPTION

Causative microorganisms in osteomyelitis are *S. aureus, Enterobacter* species, and group A and B *Streptococcus* species, *Haemophilus influenzae Salmonella,* etc. Different organisms are found in different age groups.

COMPLICATIONS

- Dead bone (osteonecrosis)
- Septic arthritis
- Impaired growth
- Skin cancer

SURGICAL STEPS (FIGS. 1 TO 13)

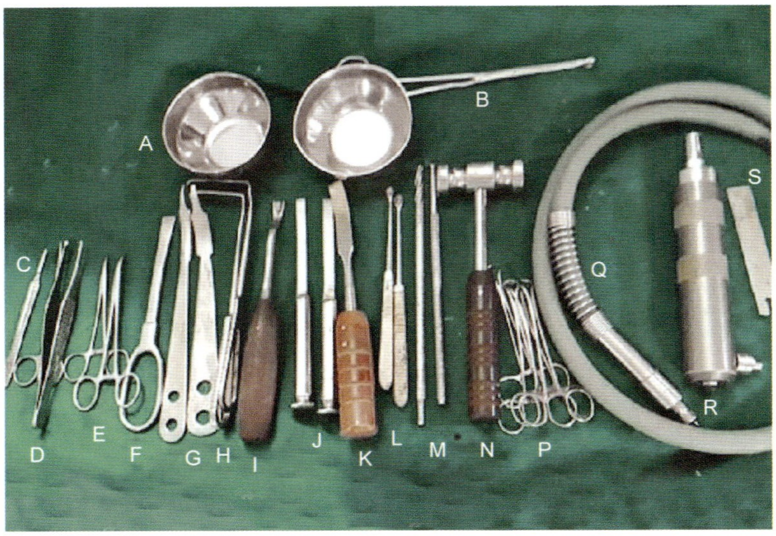

Fig. 1: (A) Bowl, (B) sponge-holding forceps, (C) BP handle, (D) tooth forceps, (E) curved artery forceps, (F) periosteum elevator, (G) bone lever, (H) right-angled retractor, (I) gouge, (J) osteotome, (K) curved osteotome, (L) bone curettage, (M) drill bit, (N) hammer, (P) towel clip, (Q) electric cable of drill, (R) oscillatory bone saw, (S) saw blade.

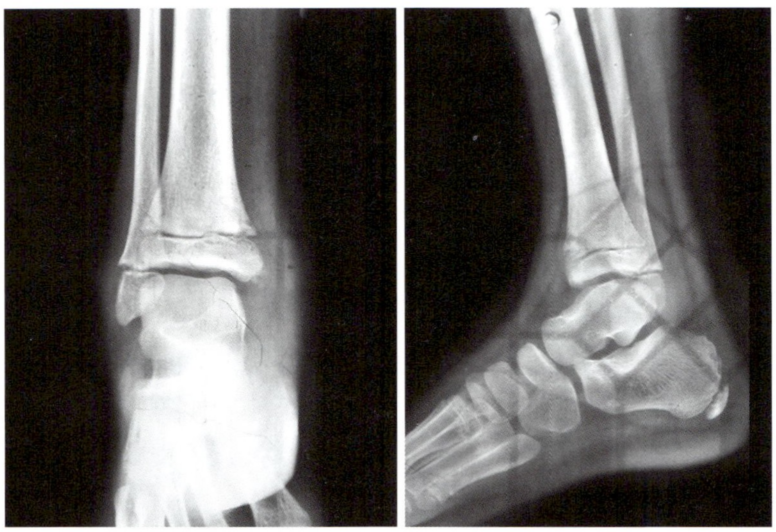

Fig. 2: X-ray of right ankle joint anteroposterior (AP)/lateral view of 15-year-old male patient.
- Tibia fibula distal end with talus and calcaneus bone.
- Epiphysis space is reduced over medial aspect.
- Sclerosis appearance noted.
- Early stage of necrotic bone.

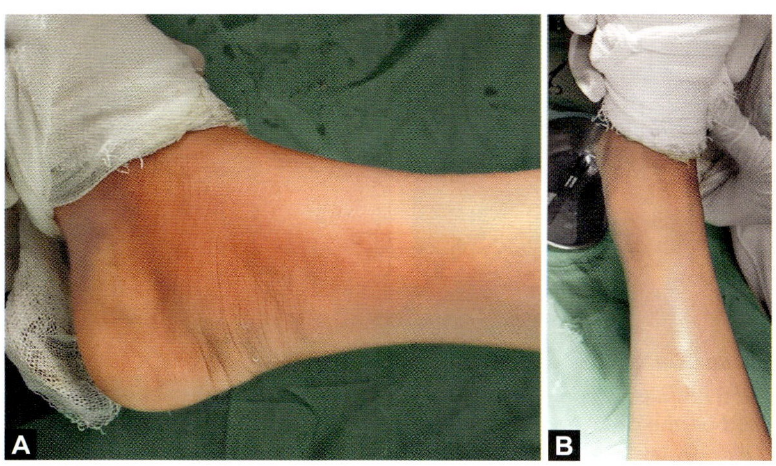

Figs. 3A and B: (A) Lateral view—swelling with erythema over medial aspect of ankle 10 cm × 8 cm; (B) Anterior view asymmetry in ankle joint—with swelling over medial aspect of ankle.

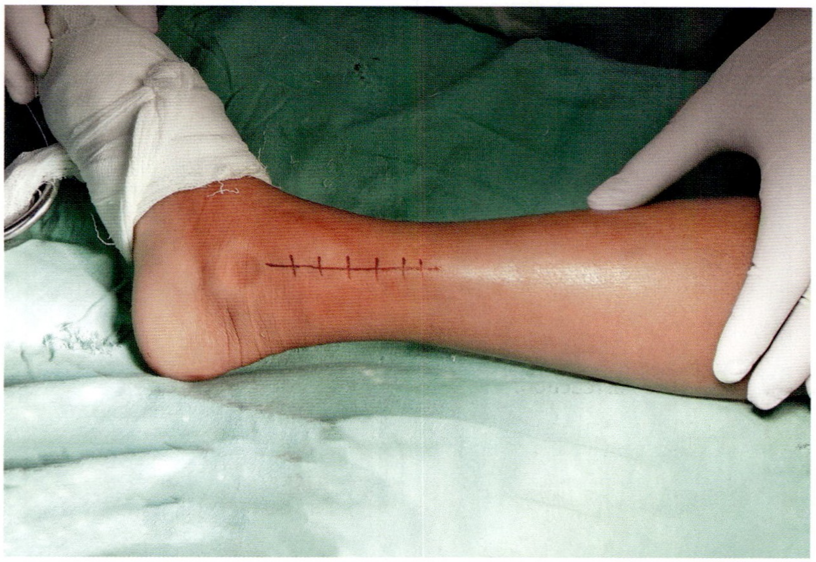

Fig. 4: Marking done over the medial malleolus of right ankle—10 cm of length marked for incision over medial aspect from distal end of malleolus to distal end of tibia. Incision will be taken over this marked portion.

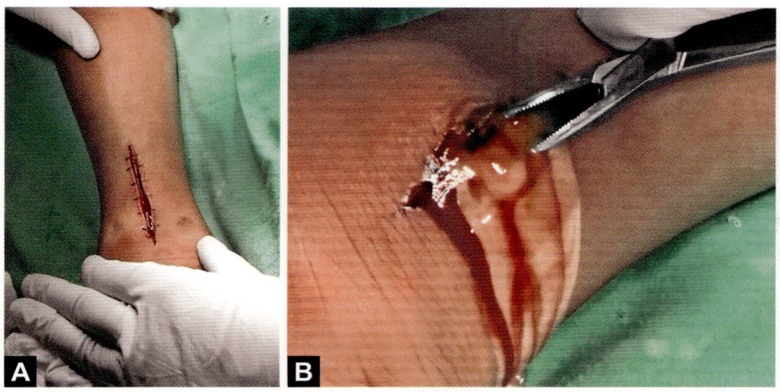

Figs. 5A and B: Incision taken over skinmark and deepened through subcutaneous tissue. As subcutaneous tissue was retracted, purulent discharge is evident.

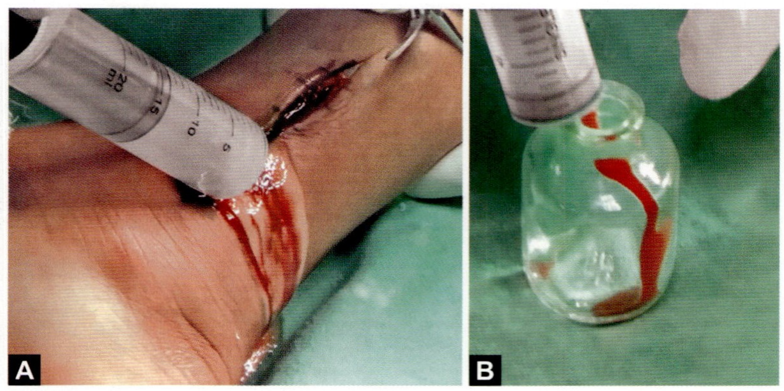

Figs. 6A and B: Purulent discharge is extracted in syringe and sent for histopathological examination studies and culture sensitivity in a container.

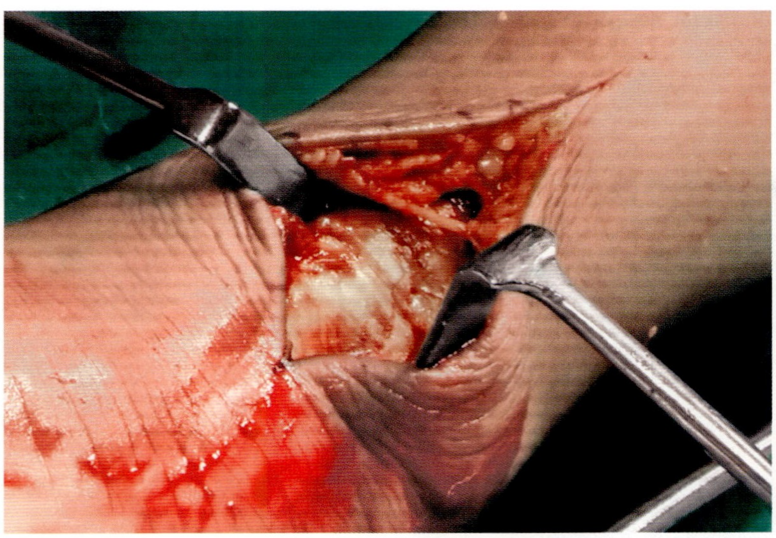

Fig. 7: Further dissection of soft tissues and muscles is done and medial surface of tibial bone is exposed on the distal end.

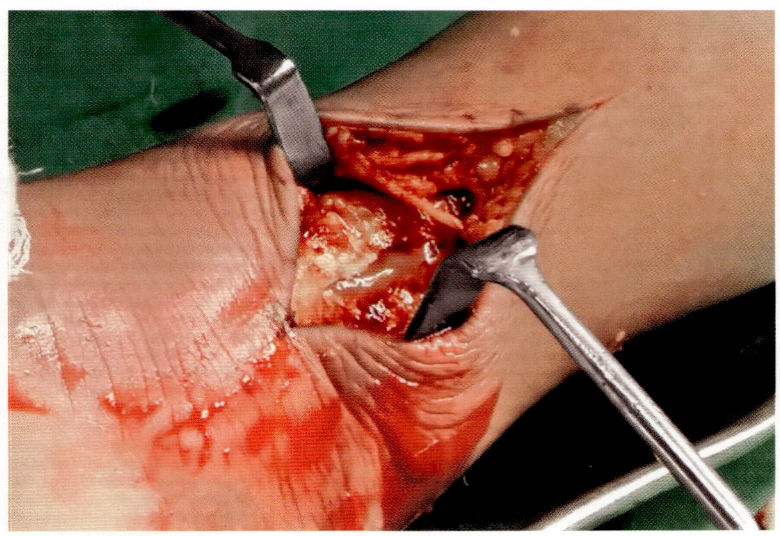

Fig. 8: Distal end of tibia is exposed with medial malleolus.

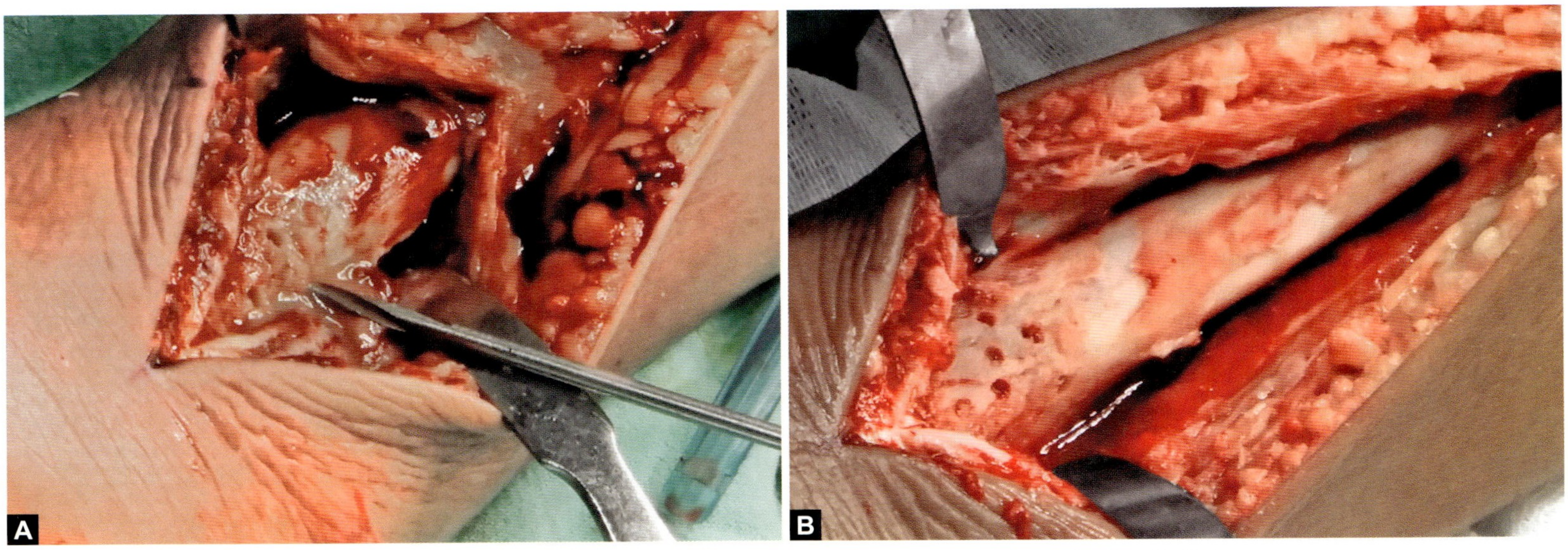

Figs. 9A and B: Multiple drill holes done in cortex over medial aspect of distal end of tibia.

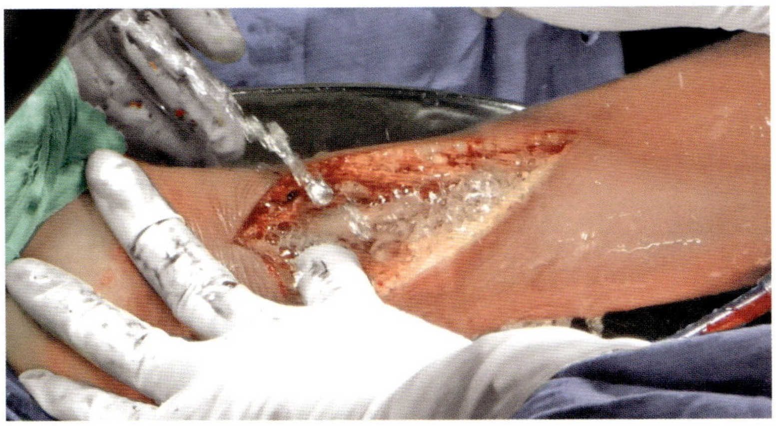

Fig. 10: Wash given with saline, hydrogen peroxide and povidone iodine.

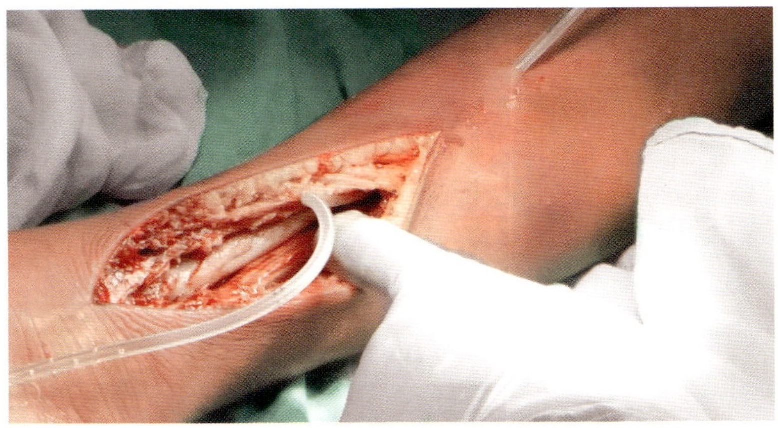

Fig. 11: Drain inserted in the operated site and sutured.

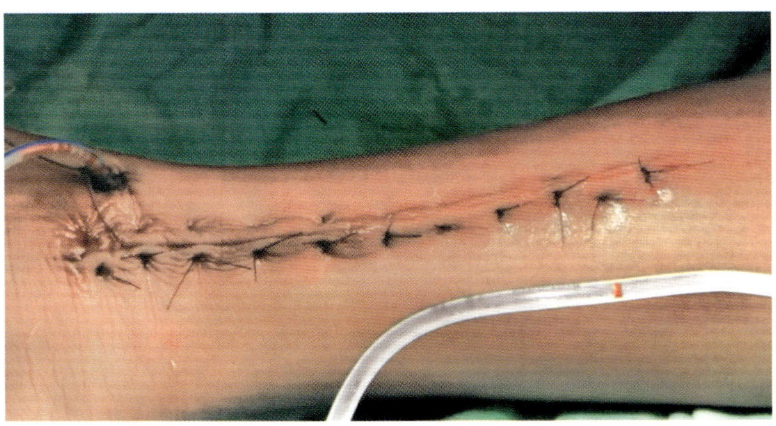

Fig. 12: Closure of incision done with nonabsorbable suture 2.0 in single layer with two drains.

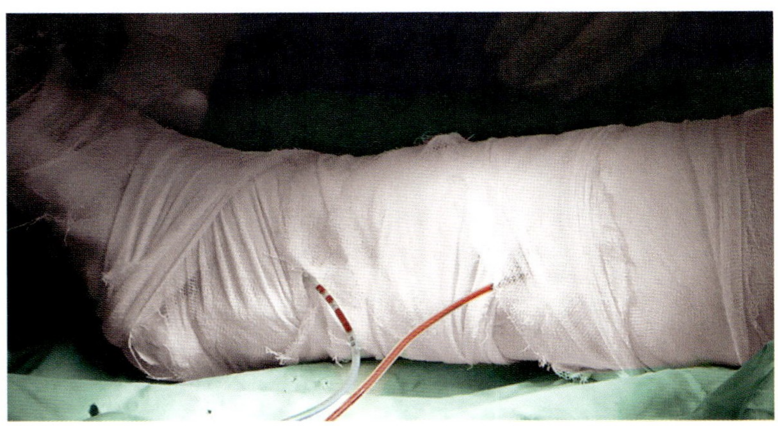

Fig. 13: Dressing done over operated site with below knee slab given.

SUGGESTED READING

1. Bennett JE, Raphael D, Blaser MJ. Principles and Practice of Infectious Diseases. Canada: Elsevier Health Sciences; 2014.
2. Brackenridge RDC, Croxson RS, Mackenzie R. Medical Selection of Life Risks, 5th edition Swiss Re branded. Berlin, Germany: Springer; 2016.
3. Burnett MW, Bass KW, Cook BA. Etiology of osteomyelitis complicating sickle cell disease. Pediatrics. 1998;101(2):296-7.
4. Ferri FF. Ferri's Clinical Advisor 2018 E-Book: 5 Books, 1st edition. London: Elsevier Health Sciences; 2018.
5. Genetic and Rare Diseases Information Center (GARD). (2016). Osteomyelitis. [online] Available from https://rarediseases.info.nih.gov/diseases/7286/osteomyelitis. [Accessed, October, 2018].
6. Kumar V, Abbas AK, Nelson F, et al. Robbins Basic Pathology, 8th edition. Philadelphia: Saunders Elsevier; 2007.
7. Maureen H. Streptococcal Infections. Gale Encyclopedia of Medicine. The Gale Group. 2002.
8. NORD (National Organization for Rare Disorders). (2005). Osteomyelitis. [online] Available from https://rarediseases.org/rare-diseases/osteomyelitis/. [Accessed, October, 2018].
9. Schmitt SK. Osteomyelitis. Infect Dis Clin N Am. 2017;31(2):325-38.
10. Silman AJ, Smolen JS, Weinblatt ME, et al. Rheumatology E-Book. USA. Elsevier Health Sciences; 2014. .

CHAPTER 73

Valgus Intertrochanteric Osteotomy

Wasudeo M Gadegone

INTRODUCTION

The reported incidence of non union in fracture neck of the femur is 15–30% inspite of emergence of newer implants and techniques.[1,2] The main cause of non-union, is the shearing force acts on the vertically oriented fracture line producing fibrous tissue leading to eventual non-union.[3,4]

In India, a patient may come 3–6 months after an injury, untreated or treated by a bone-setter hence neglected fracture of the neck of the femur is seen with more frequency. It always present as a non-union and shortening. Many a times in spite of a well performed osteosynthesis non-union may develop.

The treatment options can be categorized as either improving biology or biomechanics. A valgus intertrochanteric osteotomy with or without bone grafting reorients the fracture site into a more horizontal position. This restores the limb length and buttresses the head neck fragment from below to improve stability when used with internal fixation device. The axial loading in this situation helps achieve union.[5,6]

The proximal femoral Pauwel's valgus osteotomy is mostly fixed by an angled blade plate, but it produces medialization of the distal shaft producing a valgus strain on the knee joint (Fig. 1). This article aims to propose an alternative method of fixing a valgus osteotomy using a sliding hip screw with or without bone grafting instead of a blade plate. Dynamic hip screw fixation helps to achieve the lateral translation. The lateralization of the distal shaft of femur restores the mechanical axis and prevents the degenerative changes in the knee joint (Fig. 2).[7]

Valgus osteotomy mainly indicated in:

1. Non-union of fracture neck of femur after failed primary osteosynthesis.
2. Neglected and delayed presentation [Sandhu's type I and II non-union]
3. Primary or secondary coxa vara.
4. Fresh fracture neck femur with vertical shear pattern.
5. Malunited trochanteric fracture.

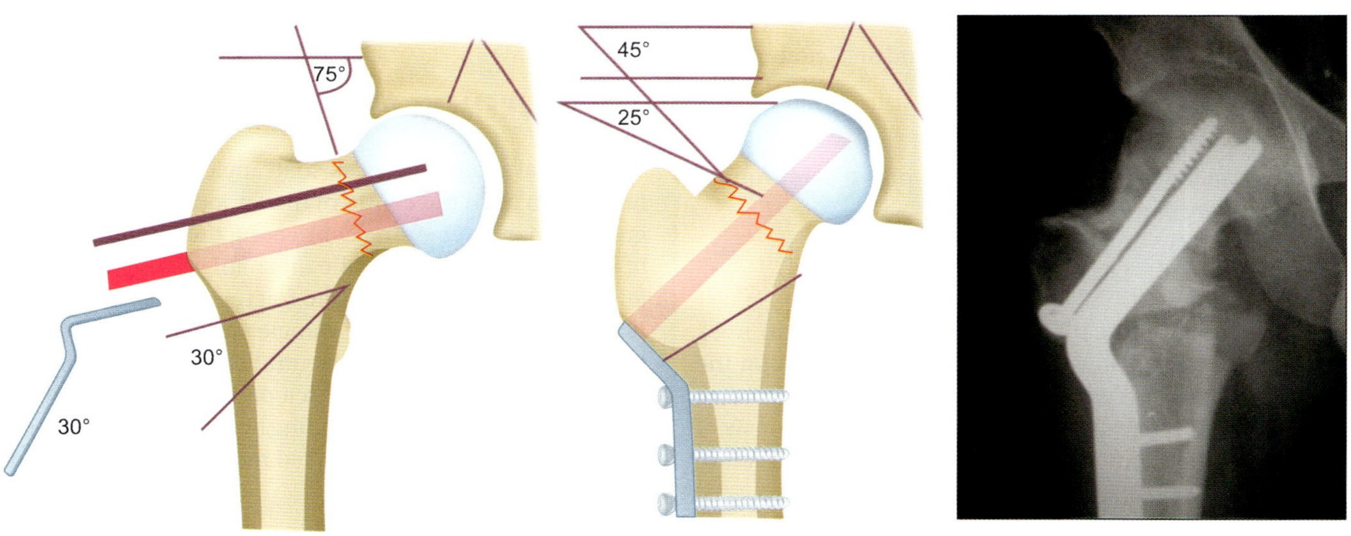

Fig. 1: Pauwel's osteotomy; medialization of distal fragment

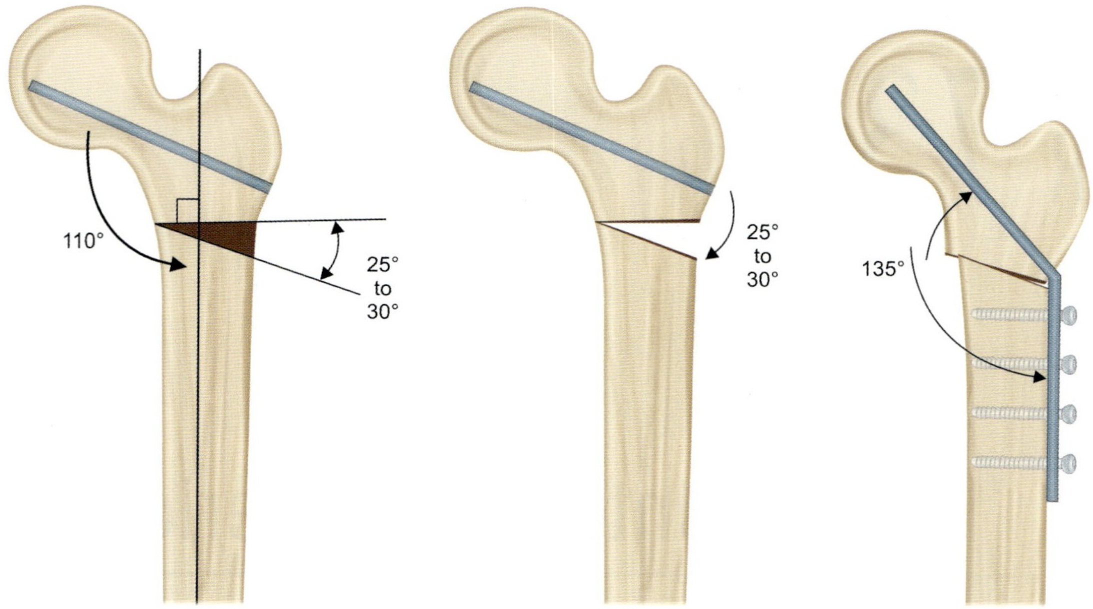

Fig. 2: Modified Pauwel's osteotomy; Lateralization of distal shaft.

INDICATIONS FOR VALGUS OSTEOTOMY WITH FIBULAR GRAFTING

- Fracture surfaces are smooth and sclerosed.
- Resorption of the neck is more than 1 cm (Sandhu's type II non-union) and the head of the femur looks viable on the X-ray.[8]

INVESTIGATIONS

Apart from routine investigation, radiograph, computed tomography (CT) scan, and magnetic resonance imaging (MRI) are required for the assessment of non-union and avascular necrosis (AVN) before planning of surgery.

Radiograph

Anteroposterior (AP), lateral, and frog leg view of pelvis are essential to measure the neck-shaft angle and assess the hip joint integrity.

Computed Tomography Scan or Bone Scan

A CT scan is extremely helpful to diagnose a femoral neck non-union.

Magnetic Resonance Imaging

The MRI scanning can help to confirm the presence of a non-union and AVN. The possibility of AVN should be

Pauwel's Angle

In 1935, the first biomechanical classification for femoral neck fractures was introduced by Pauwel's taking in to consideration the fracture line. Pauwel's observed that the obliquity of the fracture line with the horizontal plane significantly affects the prognosis of the fracture neck fracture. Pauwel's classified the angle of fracture inclination into three types.

Pauwel's Classification (Fig. 3)

Type I: Pauwel's angle less than 30° [Compressive forces are maximum.]

Type II: Pauwel's angle between 30° and 50° [Shearing forces occurs and may have a negative effect on bone healing].

Type III: Pauwel's angle more than 50° [Shearing forces which are dominant creates a significant amount of varus force which will more lead to fracture displacement and varus collapse].

PREOPERATIVE PLANNING

The pre-operative planning and drawing is of utmost importance. It should include the following: Pauwel's angle as ascertained by radiographs, position and the type of implant to be used, the entry point on the lateral cortex and the end point of the screw in the head of femur. It should also include the calculations of wedge angle, the site and type of wedge (closing or open wedge, half closed and half opens called as neutral wedge) and lateral translation of the distal femur (Figs. 4 to 6).

MEASUREMENT OF PAUWEL'S ANGLE

The normal anatomical neck-shaft angle ranges from 124° to 136°. The line drawn from the center of the femoral head bisects the tip of the greater trochanter. A line connecting these 2 points makes an angle of 90° (range 85–95°) with the mechanical axis of the femur. Pauwel's angle is the angle made by the fracture line with the horizontal line. It is preferred to measure the angle after the reduction of the fracture by traction, abduction and neutral or internal rotation as this angle may be difficult to calculate in a patients with delayed presentation and in patients with long-standing non-union. The Pauwel's angle can only be confirmed when a closed reduction is performed on fracture table (Fig. 7).

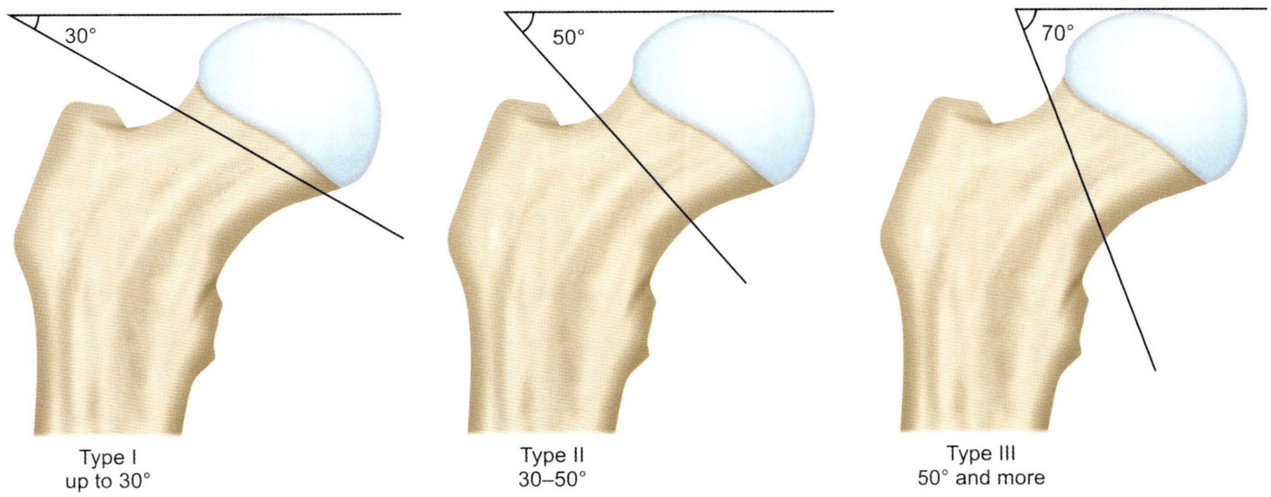

Fig. 3: Pauwel's classification.

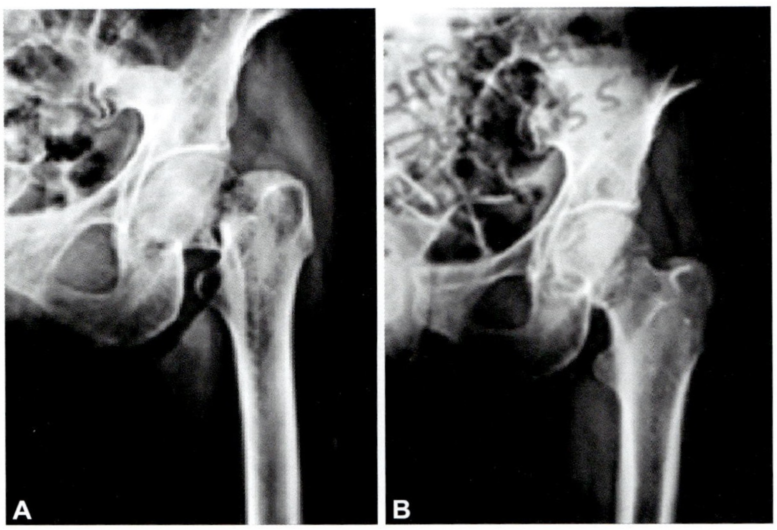

Figs. 4A and B: (A) Preoperative X-ray; (B) X-ray after reduction.

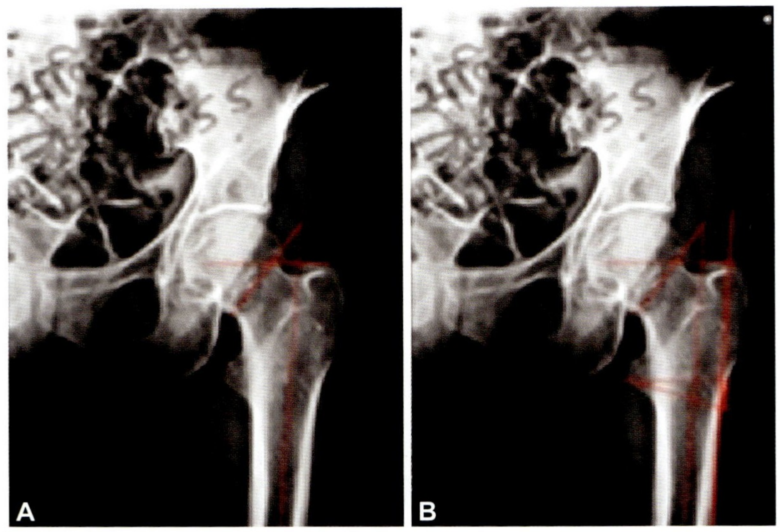

Figs. 5A and B: (A) Pauwel's angle; (B) Planning of osteotomy at lesser trochanter level.

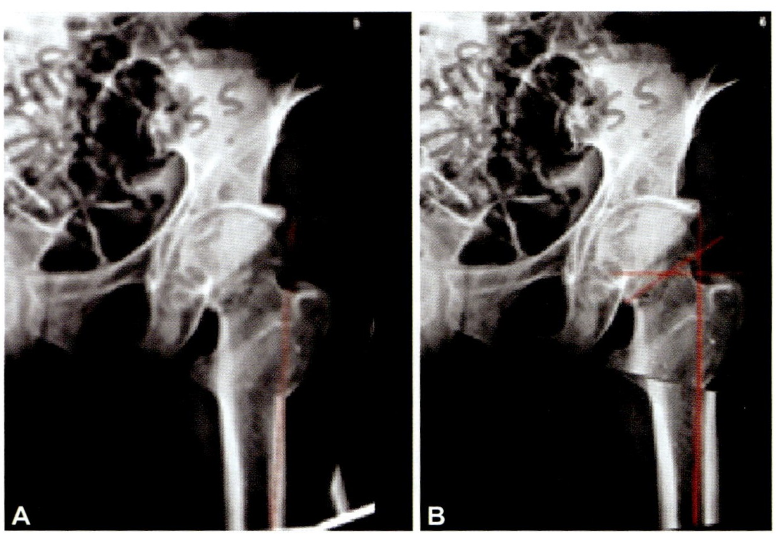

Figs. 6A and B: (A) Valgus osteotomy with medialization; (B) Valgus osteotomy with laterlization.

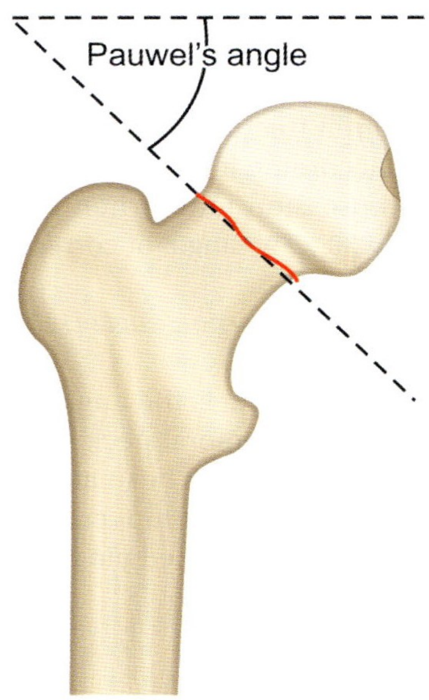

Fig. 7: Pauwel's angle is the angle made by fracture line with the horizontal line.

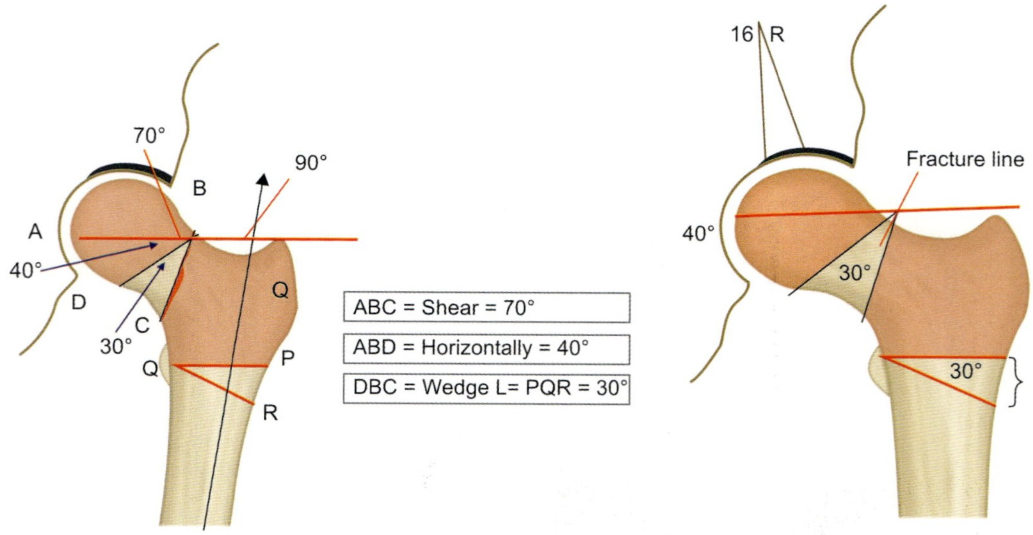

Fig. 8: A calculation of Pauwel's angle and osteotomy wedge.

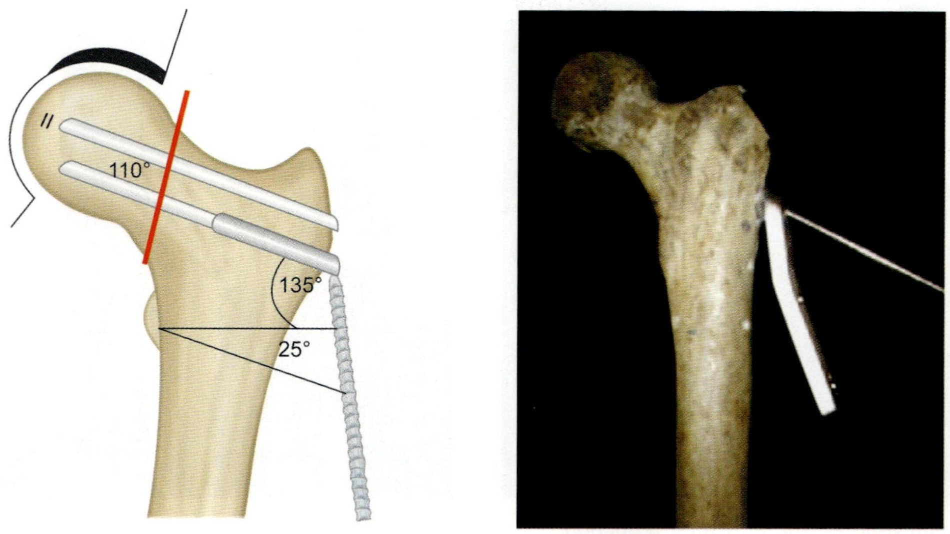

Fig. 9: DHS fixation site. Guidewire pin insertion angle is the angle created between the borders of the pin which is placed slightly inferior of femoral head at the start of operation from lateral femoral cortex.

Calculation of the Wedge Angle

To achieve a final desired fracture plane, osteotomy angle of less than 30° is desirable. According to Pauwel's principles a non-union will come under compression force when the shearing angle is changed from >70° to <30°. The angle of correction or wedge angle is calculated as:

Implant angle [135°] -pin insertion angle [110°] = osteotomy angle [25°] (Fig. 8)

Guidewire pin insertion angle is the angle created between the borders of the pin within the femoral neck (which is placed at the center or slightly inferior of femoral head at the start of operation) and lateral femoral cortex. The sliding hip screw is placed towards the center of the head at the predetermined pin insertion angle (Fig. 9).

PROCEDURE

In a case of preoperative limb shortening, preoperative upper tibial skeletal traction is used for 1–2 weeks with weights up to 8–10 kg to bring the shaft of the femur as distal as possible. Fracture gap is determined as per Sandhu classification in all patients with prior limb shortening.[8] The fracture reduction is obtained on a fracture table accurately by gentle traction in external rotation followed by internal rotation and abduction by about 15°–20° and confirmed under an image intensifier in AP and lateral views.

The surgery is performed on a fracture table with fluoroscopic control, with the patient in supine position (Figs. 10 to 12). The fracture site is not exposed unless reduction is not achieved by closed methods. The implants used for previous osteosynthesis, if present, is removed. The two guidewires are passed. The one superior guidewire is for derotation screw and inferior guidewire for the dynamic hip screw. In a relatively fresh fracture derotation screw may not be required if the stability is good with the DHS alone. A lateral approach is used and the vastus lateralis muscle is released in the 'L' shape manner and lifted subperiosteally (Figs. 13 to 15). Temporary stabilization of fracture is done by 3 mm K-wire. The inferior guidewire is passed at an angle of 110° from the base of GT to the lower quadrant of the femoral head in AP view and central in lateral view.

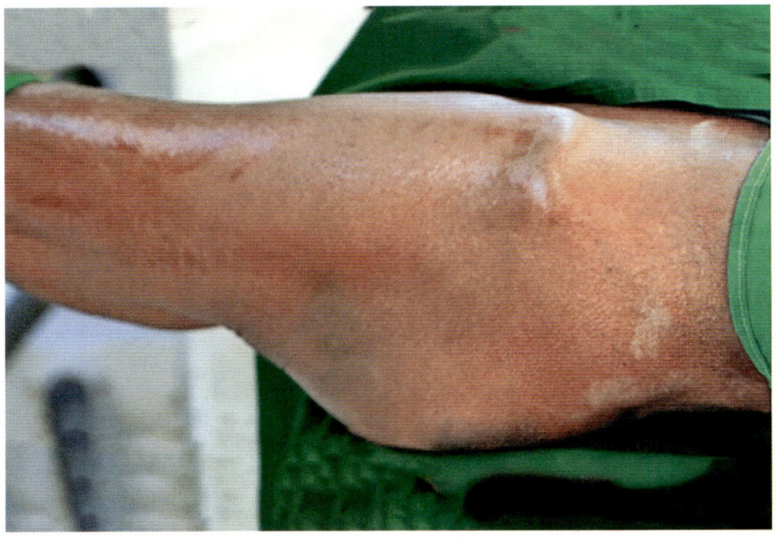

Fig. 10: Position of the patient on fracture table.

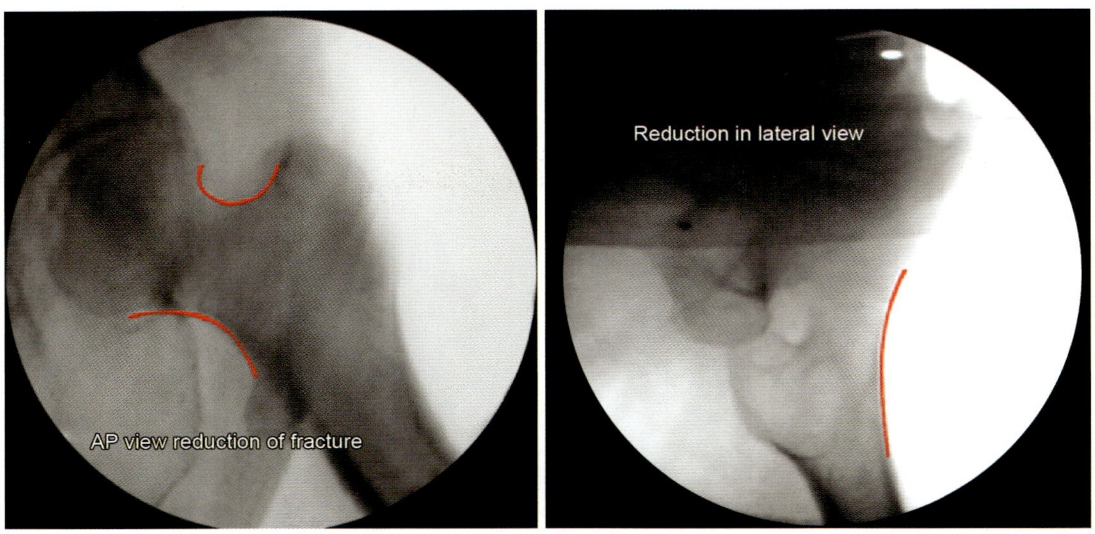

Fig. 11: Closed reduction of fracture.
(AP: anteroposterior)

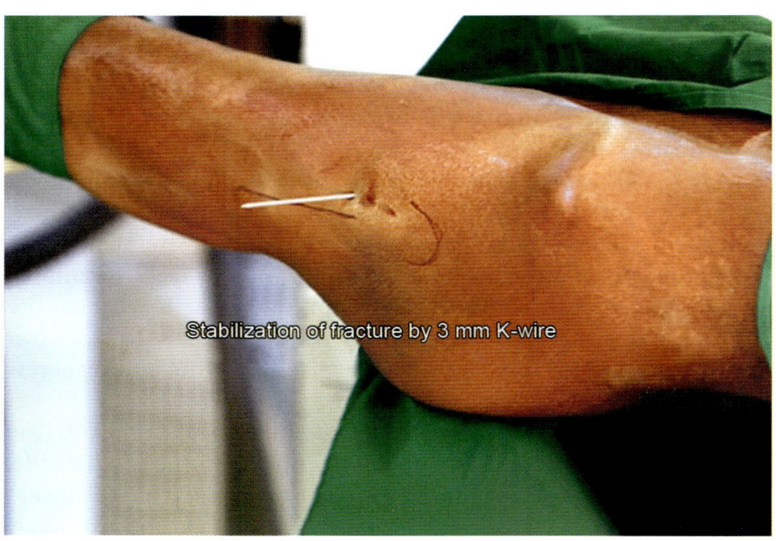

Fig. 12: Stabilization of fracture.

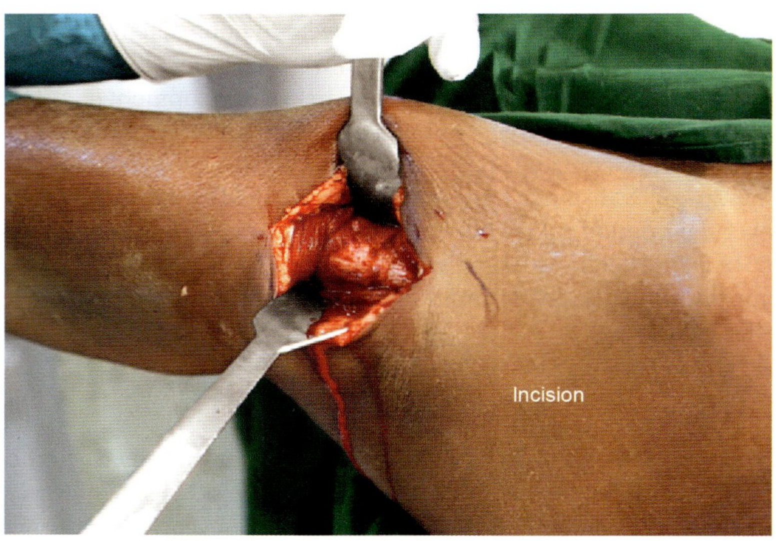

Fig. 13: Incision.

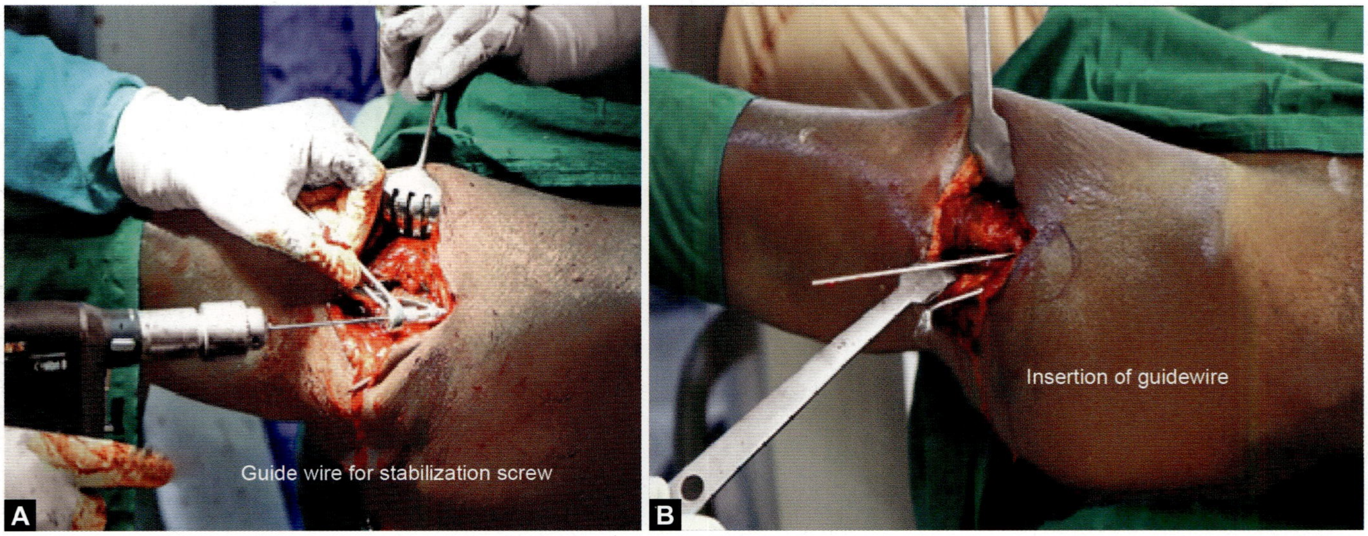

Figs. 14A and B: Insertion of guidewire.

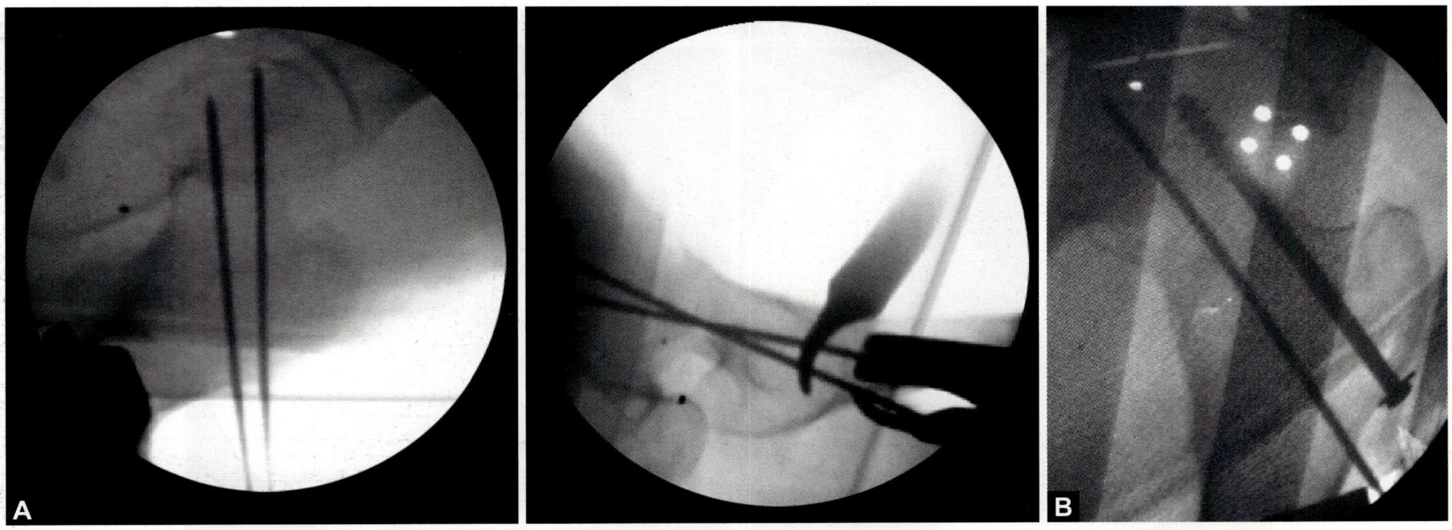

Figs. 15A and B: (A) Guidewire insertion; (B) The derotation CC screw insertion.

The second guidewire is passed superiorly for derotation screw, and parallel to the previous inferiorly placed wire. A 6.5 cancellous screw is inserted over it to stabilize the fracture to prevent displacement during the subsequent manipulations (Fig. 16). The derotation CC screw insertion is recommended to prevent rotation of femoral head which might further jeopardize the precarious blood supply to the femoral head and thereby increase the risk of development of AVN.

Reaming is done to accommodate the screw, after tapping under fluoroscopic control (Figs. 17 to 20). After due consideration of the tip- apex distance, appropriate length of DHS screw is passed over the inferior guidewire at an angle of 110°. A side plate of 135° DHS is inserted over the screw leaving the side plate at an angle of approximately 25°-30° from the lateral aspect of the femoral shaft site (Fig. 21).

Intertrochanteric Osteotomy (Figs. 9A to F)

If 25°-30° of wedge is to be removed, the base of the wedge should be on the lateral cortex and apex towards the medial side of lesser trochanter. A V shaped piece of bone from the lateral cortex measuring 2 to 2.5 cm is removed. Removing a large wedge of bone is not advisable. Pauwel's devised Y- osteotomy which closes on lateral side and opens on medial side. The wedge of the bone removed is morcellized and used as bone graft for the medial defect.

Now 1 cm below the level of the elbow of the plate (which is usually at or just proximal to the level of the lesser trochanter (LT) a femoral osteotomy is performed by creating space for the oscillating saw. Using a template a pre-determined wedge usually of 25–30° is removed and the shaft of the femur abducted and fixed to the plate by cortical screws.

This 25–30° wedge allowed accurate apposition of the proximal femur. The procedure included an intertrochanteric osteotomy, removal of a lateral wedge, subsequent valgization, lateral displacement of the distal fragment and internal fixation by DHS. Rotational misalignment is prevented by placing marks or K-wire on the lateral cortex of femur before performing an osteotomy. After the osteotomy 135° barrel plate is inserted over the sliding screw (Figs. 22 and 23).

When the plate is pushed to the lateral cortex of the femur, the lateral side is closed and the osteotomy opens on the medial side. This results in more horizontal fracture line of neck of femur. Pauwel's angle or shear angle, which was 70 ° may come close to approximately 30–40°.

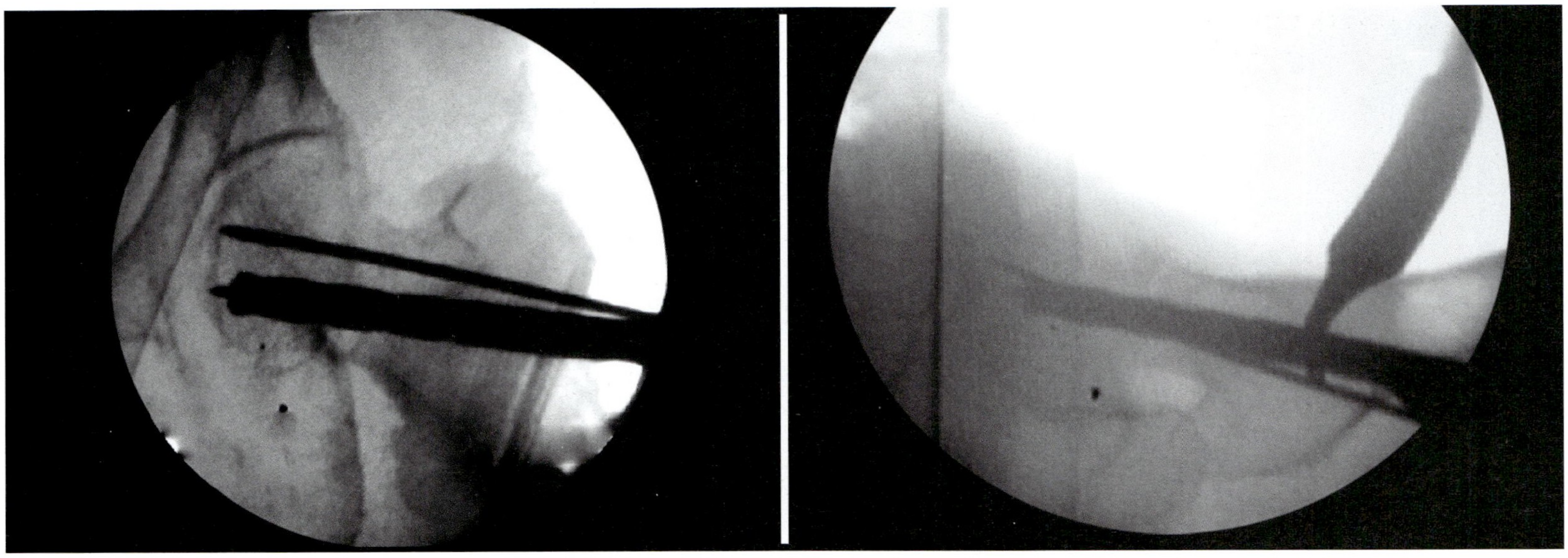

Fig. 16: Insertion of DHS reamer.

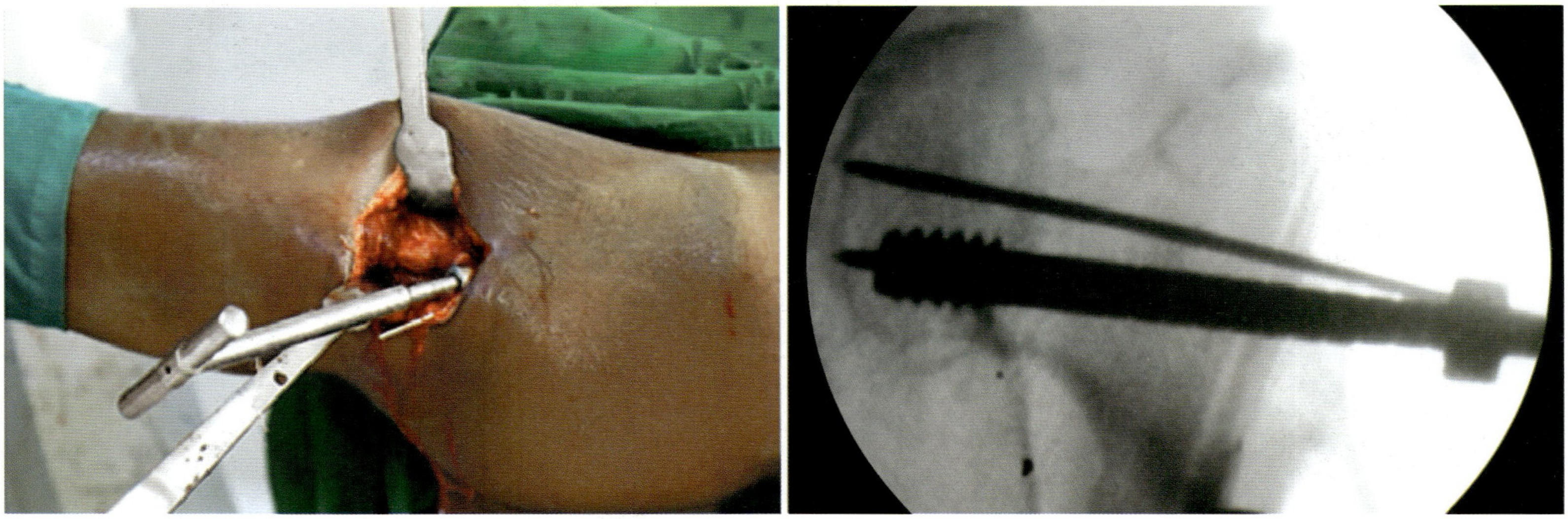

Fig. 17: Tapping for DHS screw.

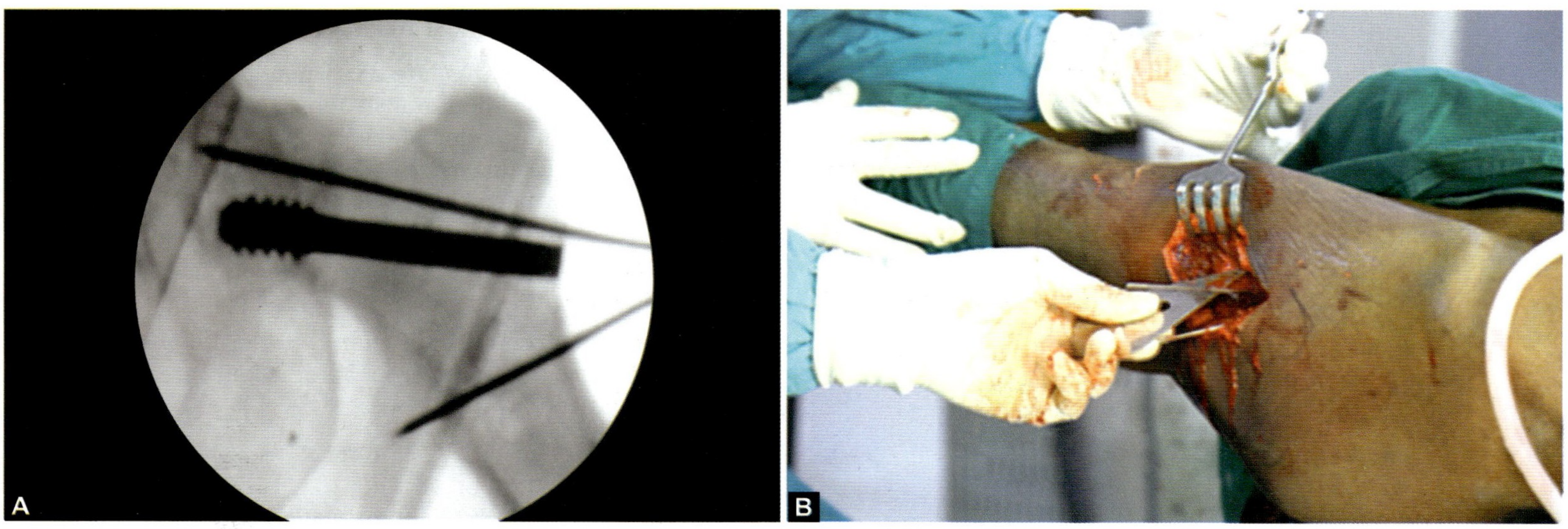

Figs. 18A and B: (A) Insertion of DHS screw and osteotomy guidewire; (B) Marking for removal of osteotomy wedge.

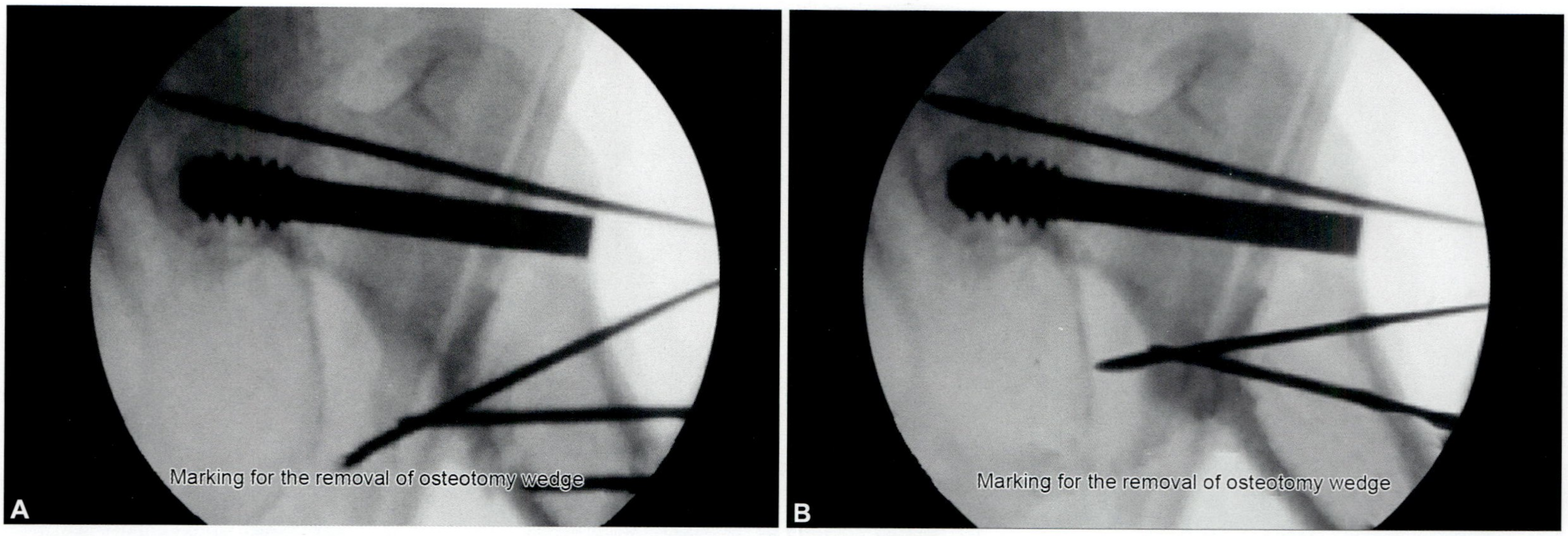

Figs. 19A and B: (A) At the level of lesser trochanter; (B) Above the level of lesser trochanter marking for the removal of wedge.

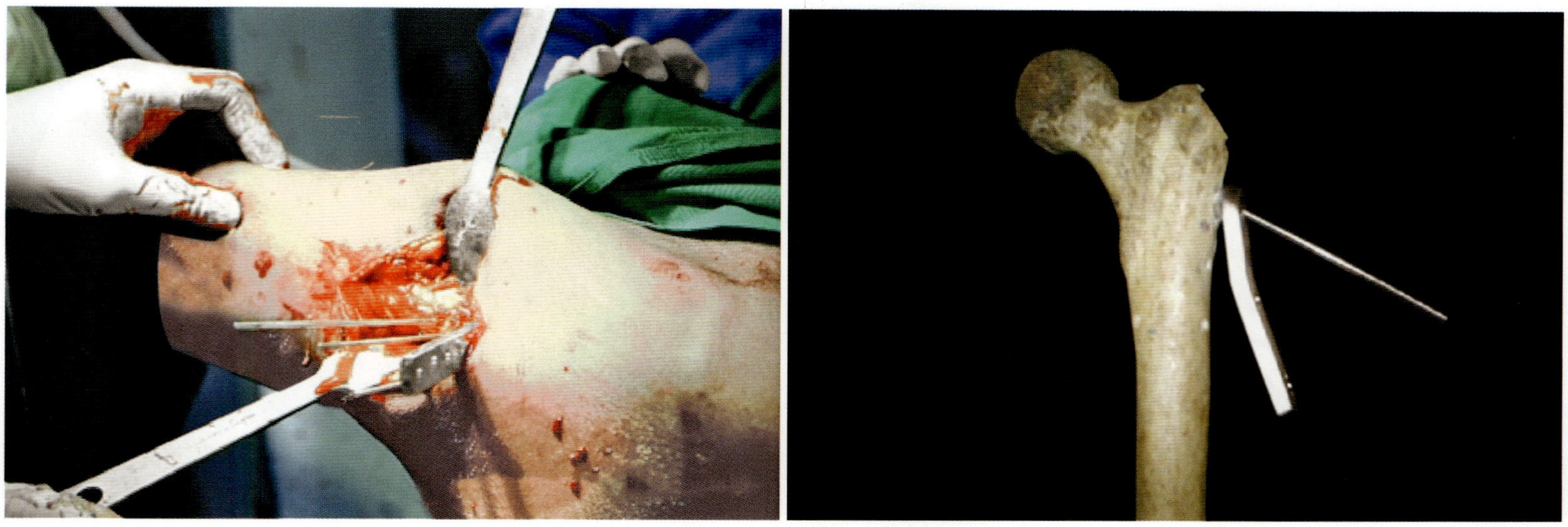

Fig. 20: Insertion of 135° DHS barrel.

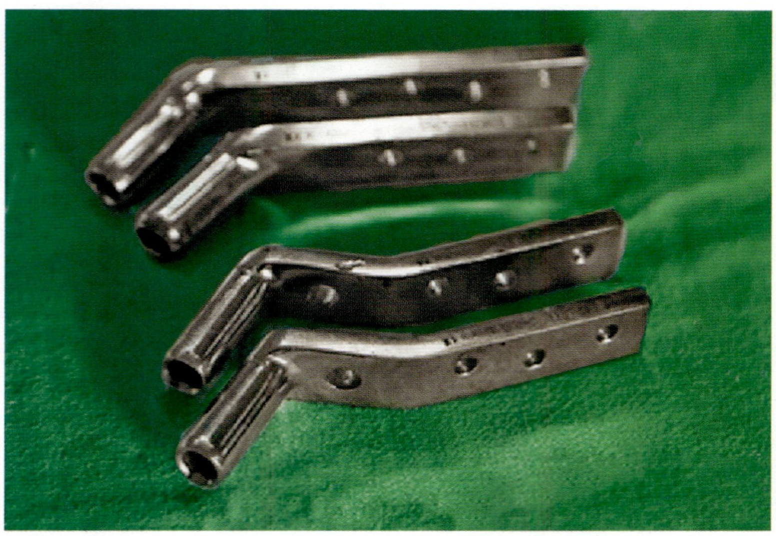

Fig. 21: DHS and angled DHS

Restoration of Mechanical Axis of Lower Limb

The mechanical axis shifts laterally when a valgus osteotomy is done and stabilized without translation. The mechanical axis gets restored by lateral translation of the shaft (distal fragment). Double angled plate is not useful for correction of mechanical axis. Standard dynamic hip screw barrel plate will automatically translate distal fragment laterally and restore mechanical axis (Fig. 24).

Limb Length

Limb length equalization is difficult in neglected and nonunited femoral neck fracture however it can be taken care of by careful planning the osteotomy.

Fibular Grafting

Length of the superior screw approximates the length of the fibular graft. The outer part of the fibula of adequate length is harvested by

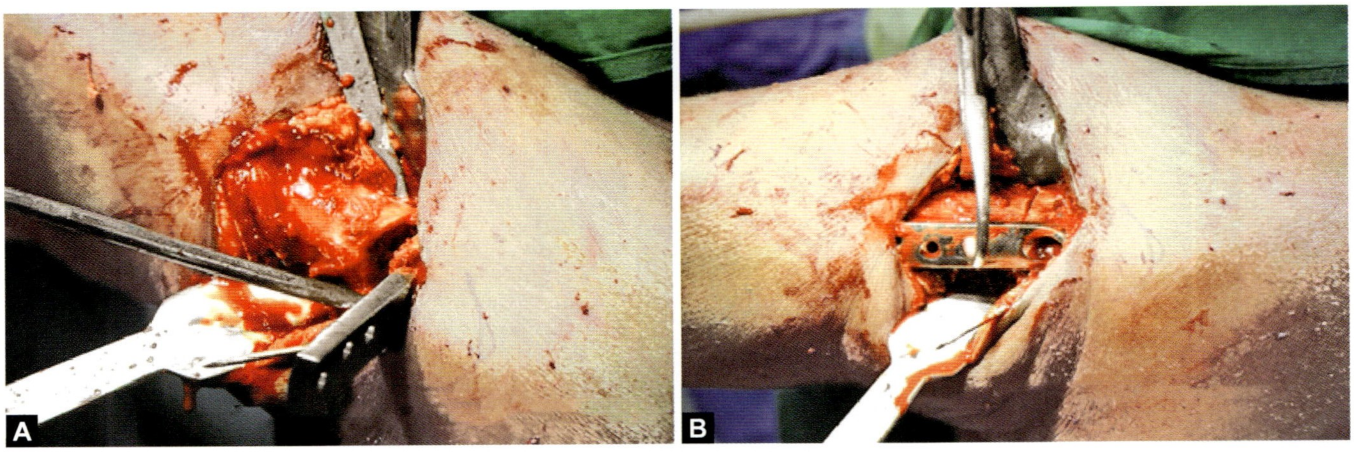

Figs. 22A and B: (A) Removal of osteotomy wedge; (B) Closure of osteotomy.

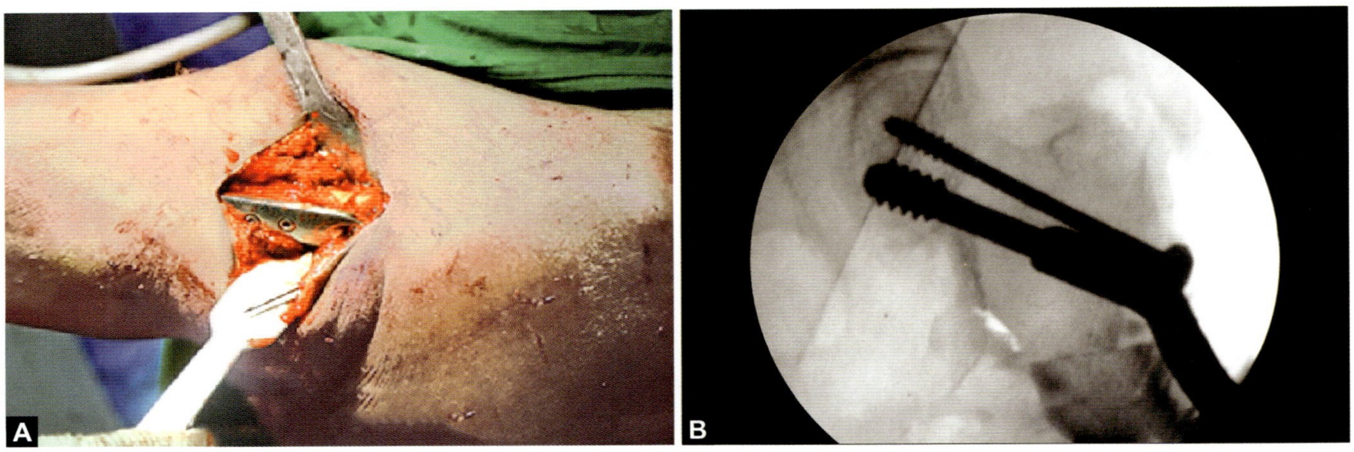

Figs. 23A and B: (A) Fixation of osteotomy; (B) Insertion of stabilization screw.

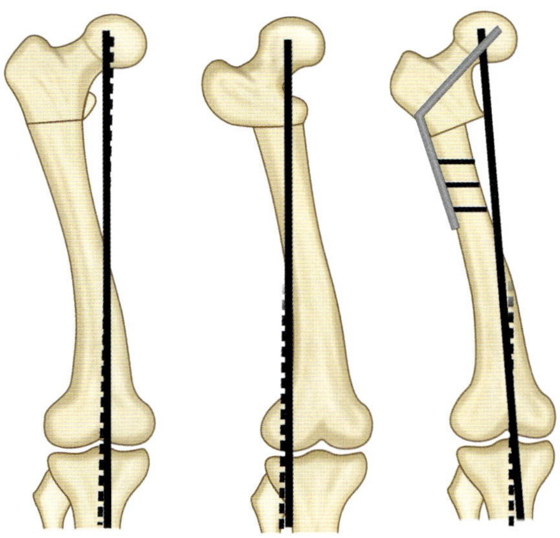

Fig. 24: Alignment mechanical axis after osteotomy.

an oscillating saw from the middle third of the ipsilateral leg. The interosseous border is kept intact. The superior screw is now removed. The fibular graft is inserted in the tunnel of the cancellous screw. It is impacted up to the subchondral part of the femoral head under an image intensifier guidance. Closure is performed in layers over a negative suction drain (Fig. 25).

POSTOPERATIVE CARE

The isometric quadriceps exercises and knee bending are initiated on the second postoperative day. Non-weight-bearing ambulation on crutches is encouraged as soon as tolerated. Weight bearing is permitted after 6 weeks as per tolerance. Regular follow-up is ensured postoperatively at monthly intervals until radiographic union and at 3 months, 6 months and 1 year since surgery and yearly after that. Radiographs are evaluated for signs of union and appearance of signs of AVN. Radiographic union is established by the presence of bridging trabeculae across the fracture and the osteotomy site in both AP and lateral views. Full weight bearing is allowed after radiographic union of the fracture (Figs. 26 and 27).

DISCUSSION

Patient who presents with fracture neck femur 3 to 4 weeks after the injury, has variable degrees of neck absorption, proximal migration of the greater trochanter and disuse osteoporosis with the ensuing co-morbidities.[9-12] Therefore three weeks or older fractures of the neck of femur are considered as neglected and should be treated as non-union.

In the non-union or neglected fracture neck of the femur in patients is less than >60 years of age preservation of the femoral head which is so essential for daily activities of sitting and squatting in our

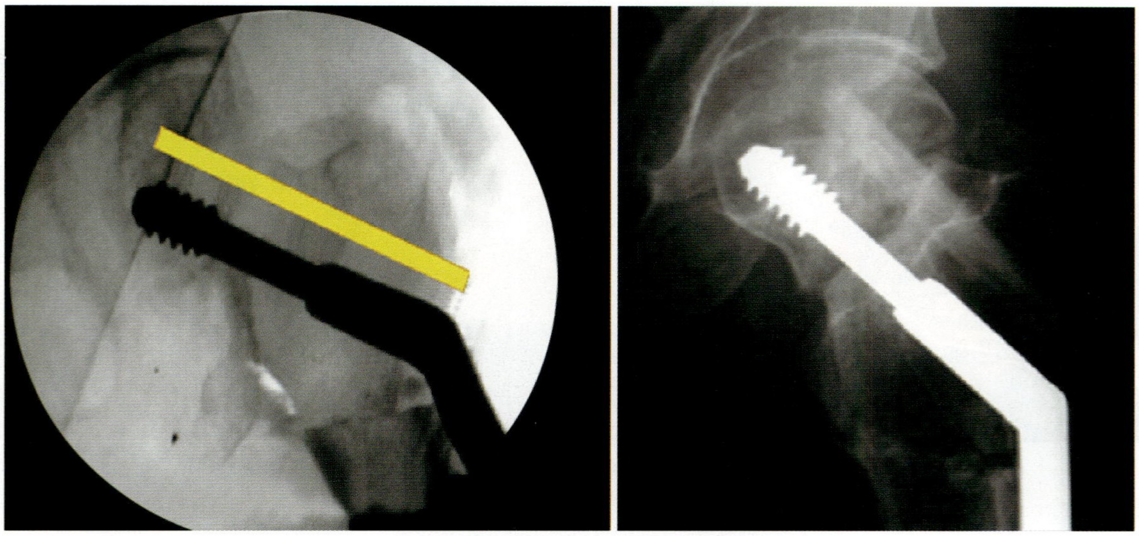

Fig. 25: Insertion of fibular graft.

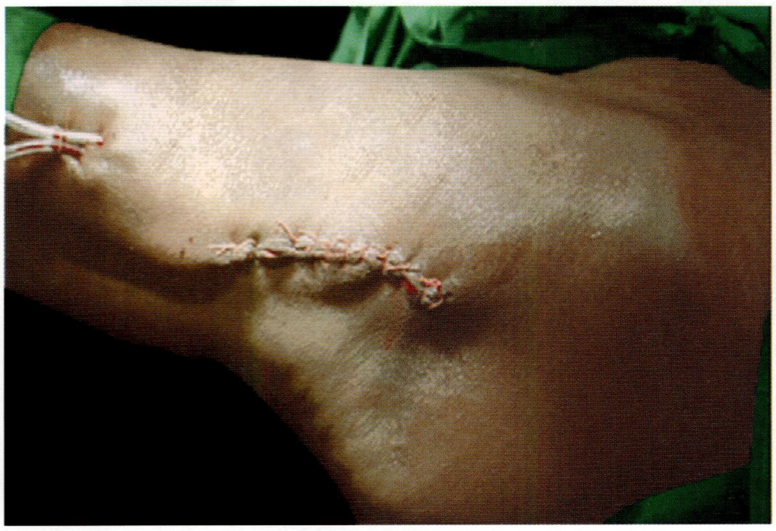

Fig. 26: Closure of wound.

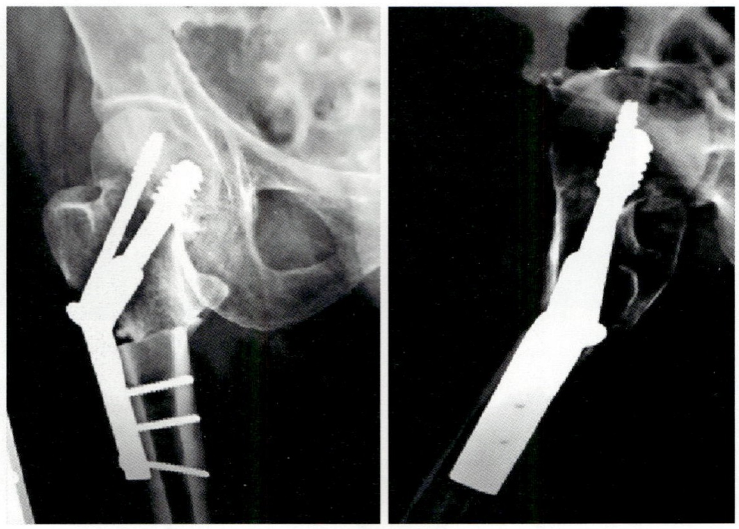

Fig. 27: Postoperative X-ray

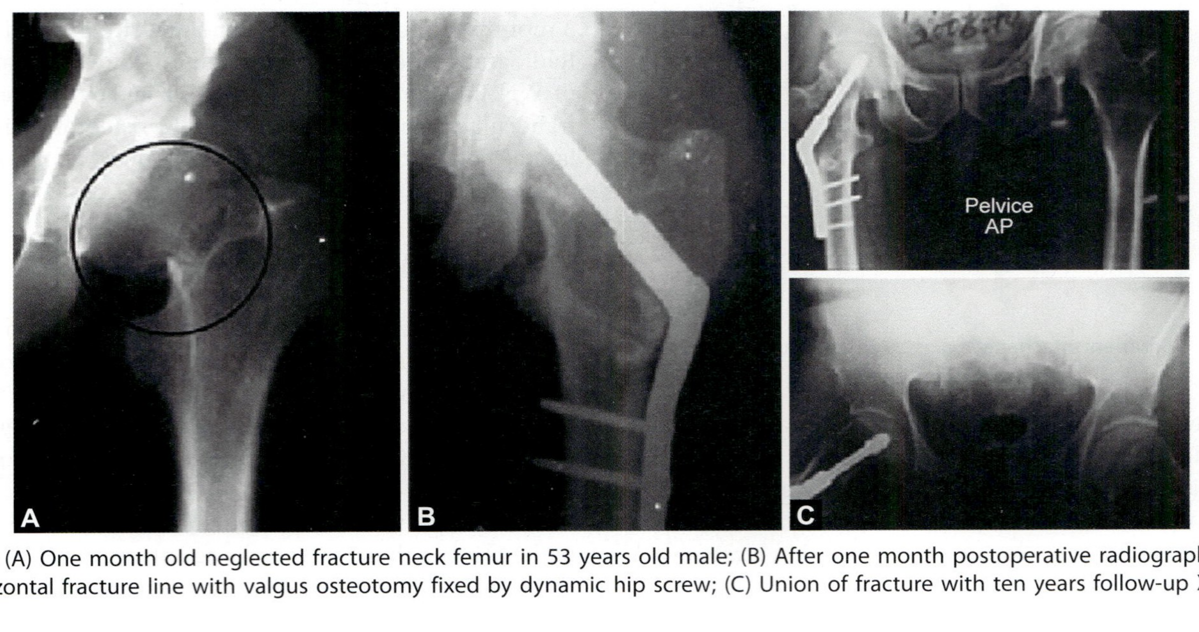

Figs. 28A to C: (A) One month old neglected fracture neck femur in 53 years old male; (B) After one month postoperative radiograph showing more horizontal fracture line with valgus osteotomy fixed by dynamic hip screw; (C) Union of fracture with ten years follow-up X-ray.

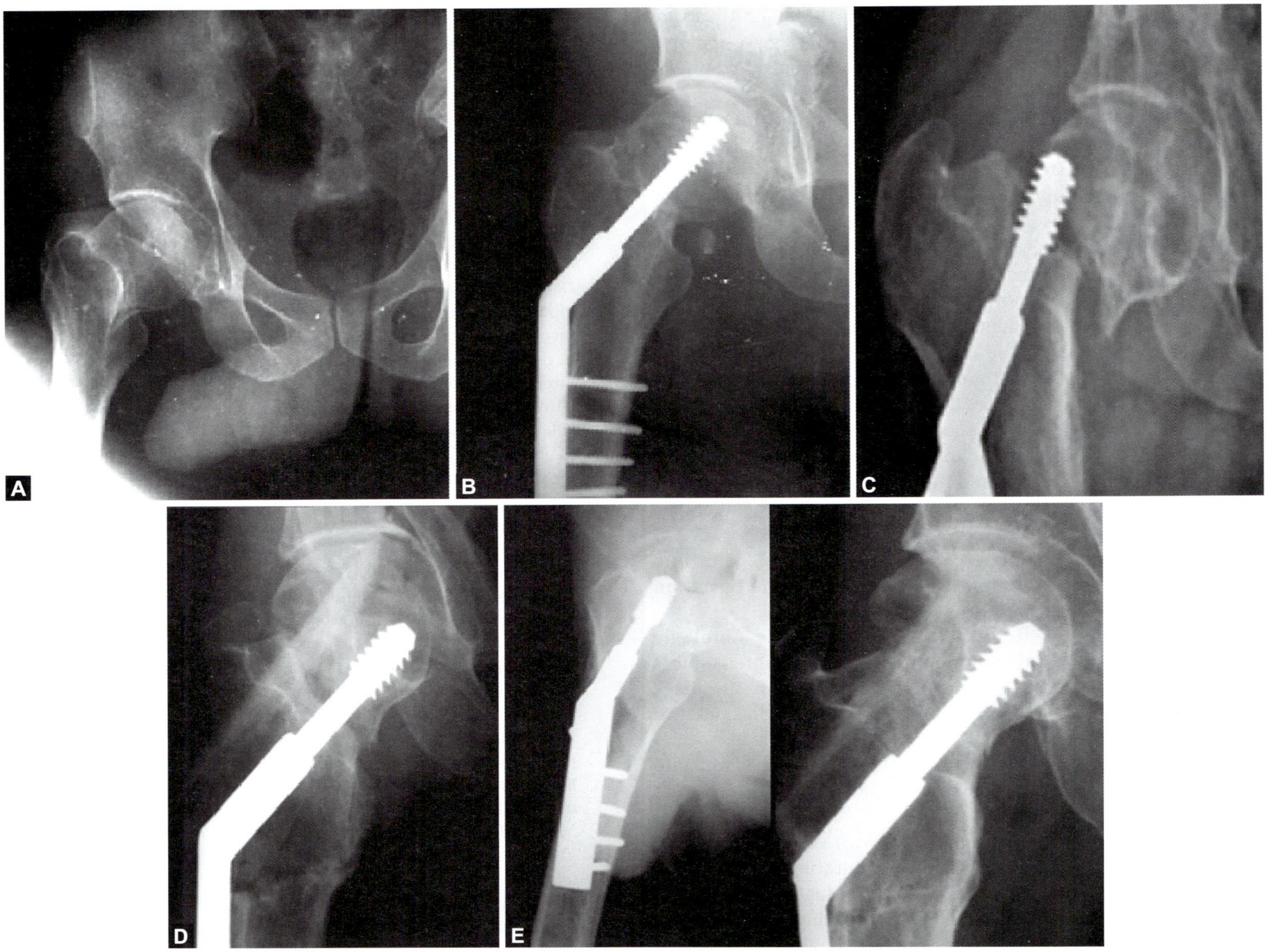

Figs. 29A to E: (A) Vertical fracture line intracapsular fracture neck femur; (B) The fracture is stabilized with DHS; (C) Screw cut out of DHS; (D) Valgus osteotomy with fibular graft osteotomy; (E) Final image showing union of fracture and a valgus- osteotomy with incorporation of fibular graft.

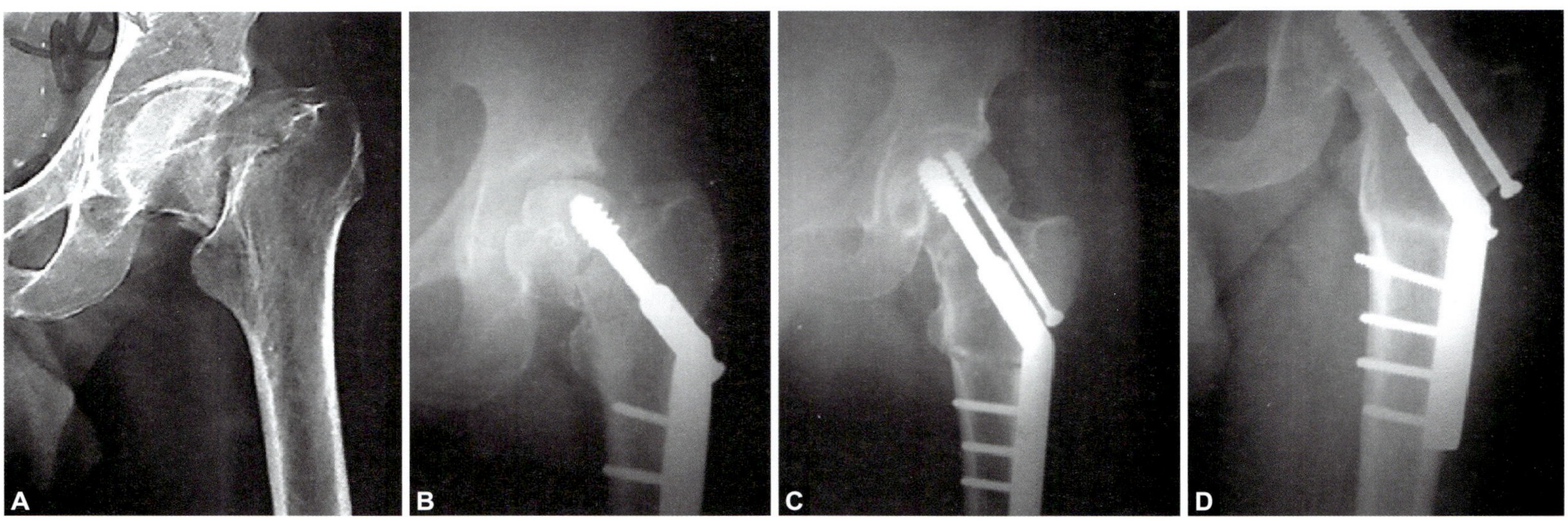

Figs. 30A to D: (A) This severe vertical fracture line through the femoral neck is a high-risk for nonunion; (B) DHS fixation after one month follow-up; (C) Postoperative radiograph showing more horizontal fracture line with valgus osteotomy fixed by dynamic hip screw; (D) One year follow-up X-ray union of fracture as well as osteotomy.

population. The types of procedures to preserve the femoral head are (1) osteosynthesis with or without bone grafting (2) valgus osteotomy (2) valgus osteotomy + fibular graft. (3) Free or vascularized fibular graft (4) quadratus femoris muscle pedicle graft.[13-15]

Osteotomy at the intertrochanteric level is advantageous because, the osteotomy is easier to execute as it is through the cancellous bone and bone healing is faster.

Pauwels Y-osteotomy avoids a large wedge from lateral cortex hence preferred. This is a lateral closed wedge and medially open wedge osteotomy. In valgus osteotomy medialization of the shaft takes place and the mechanical axis is shifted lateral to the knee joint. Use of an angled blade plate does not lead to any translation and mechanical axis is not corrected. The patient may develop severe osteoarthrosis of the lateral compartment of the knee because of medialization of the shaft of the femur. The lateral translation of the shaft is achieved with use of simple DHS and it restores the mechanical axis.[16]

The osteotomy is a biologic procedure that has been described in various studies. The surgical technique under an image intensifier is simple and can be completed in an average setup. The image intensifier allows closed reduction and completion of the operative procedure through a smaller incision.

A 25 to 30° wedge is sufficient to place the head of femur into valgus and larger intertrochanteric wedges of bone based on Pauwel's angle are not required.

Various studies have described the osteotomy as a biologic procedure. The surgical technique under an image intensifier is simple to perform. It can be executed in any average setup. The image intensifier enables closed reduction and completion of the operative procedure through a smaller incision.

A 25° to 30° wedge is mostly enough to place the head of femur into valgus. Large intertrochanteric wedges of bone based on Pauwel's angle are not necessary.

The femoral neck fracture nonunion with variable degree of resorption of neck is a mechano-biological problem. Addressing, just a mechanical (fixation) or biological (grafting) problem is not enough, and a combination of the two approaches must be used. Valgus osteotomy with fibular bone grafting is most successful in a absorbed neck in neglected and non-united fracture where the replacement surgery is not indicated.[6,17] Valgus osteotomy reorients the fracture angle and fibular graft act as a strut graft which helps as mechanical support and its incorporation helps in union. The successful fracture healing needed some components: osteogenic cells, osteoinductive factors, a stable osteoconductive scaffold and mechanical stability, which was acknowledged as a diamond concept which is provided by valgus osteotomy, bone grafting and osteosynthesis by DHS. Very rarely requires an open reduction and freshening of edges of fracture when closed reduction is not achieved. In physiologically older patients replacement arthroplasty by bipolar or total hip replacement (THR) is the treatment of choice.

While performing the operation an excessive valgus should be avoided as it leads to (1)limb length discrepancy. (2) excessive pressure on the head resulting in pain and osteoarthrosis, (3) avascular necrosis, (4) persistent limp, and (5) Trendelenburg gait.

We therefore conclude that valgus osteotomy with or without bone grafting is excellent option for non-union and neglected fracture of neck of femur in young adults <60 years of age.

REFERENCES

1. Mathews V, Cabanela ME. Femoral neck nonunion treatment. Clin Orthop Relat Res. 2004;419:57-64.
2. Damany DS, Parker MJ, Chojnowski A. Complications after intracapsular hip fractures in young adults. A meta-analysis of 18 published studies involving 564 fractures. Injury. 2005;36:131-41.
3. Parker MJ. Prediction of fracture union after internal fixation of intracapsular femoral neck fractures. Injury. 1994;25.
4. Pauwels F. Biomechanics of the normal and diseased hip. Springer Science and Business Media; 1976.
5. Marti RK, Schüller HM, Raaymakers EL. Intertrochanteric osteotomy for non- union of the femoral neck. J Bone Joint Surg Br. 1989;71: 782-7.
6. Gadegone WM, Ramteke AA, Lokhande V, Salphade Y. Valgus intertrochanteric osteotomy and fibular strut graft in the management of neglected femoral neck fracture. Injury. 2013;44:763-8.
7. Kulkarni SG, Kulkarni GS, Babhulkar S, Kulkarni MG, Kulkarni RM Injury. Accuracy of valgus osteotomy using dynamic hip screw. 2017;48 Suppl 2:S2-S7.
8. Sandhu HS, Sandhu PS, Kapoor A. Neglected fractured neck of the femur: A predictive classification and treatment by osteosynthesis. Clin Orthop Relat Res. 2005;14-20.
9. Viju Daniel Varghese, Abel Livingston, PR Boopalan, and Thilak S JepegnanamWorld J Orthop. 2016;7(5):301-7.
10. Jain AK, Mukunth R, Srivastava A. Valgus osteotomy for nonunion and neglected neck of femur fractures. Treatment of neglected femoral neck fracture. Indian J Orthop. 2015;49:17-27.
11. Kalra M, Anand S. Valgus intertrochanteric osteotomy for neglected femoral neck fractures in young adults. Int Orthop. 2001;25:363-6.
12. Roshan A, Ram S. The neglected femoral neck fracture in young adults: review of a challenging problem. Clinical Medicine and Research 2008;6(1):33-9.
13. LeCroy CM, Rizzo M, Gunneson EE, Urbaniak JR. Free vascularized fibular bone grafting in the management of femoral neck nonunion in patients younger than fifty years. J Orthop Trauma. 2002;16:464-72.
14. Meyers MH, Harvey JP, Moore TM. Delayed treatment of subcapital and transcervical fractures of the neck of the femur with internal fixation and a muscle pedicle bone graft. Orthop Clin North Am. 1974;5:743-56.
15. Magu NK, Rohilla R, Singh R, Tater R. Modified Pauwels' intertrochanteric osteotomy in neglected femoral neck fracture. Clin Orthop Relat Res. 2009;467:1064-73. [PMC free article]
16. Varshney MK, Trikha V. Intertrochanteric osteotomy using a dynamic hip screwfor femoral neck nonunion. Journal of Orthopaedic Trauma 2005;19(10):751.
17. Sen RK, Tripathy SK, Goyal T, Aggarwal S, Tahasildar N, Singh D, Singh AK. Osteosynthesis of femoral-neck nonunion with angle blade plate and autogenous fibular graft. IntOrthop. 2012;36:827-32.

CHAPTER 74

High Tibial Osteotomy for Varus Deformity

Shrinivas S Shintre, Chittanand Mendhe, Rajkumar Ekambaram

SURGICAL STEPS (FIGS. 1 TO 17)

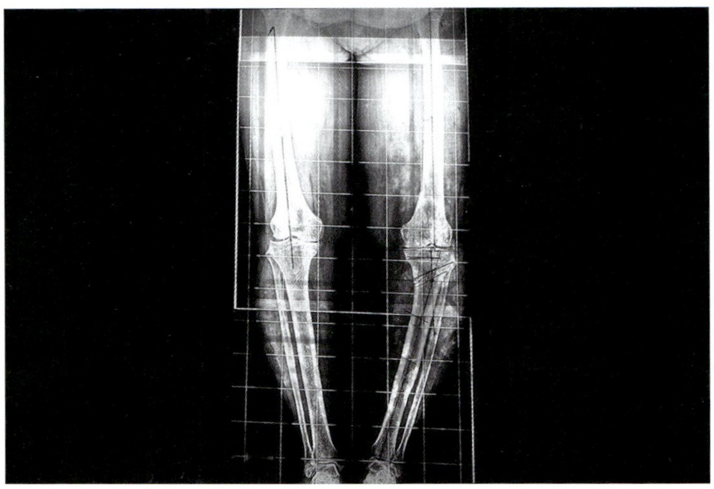

Fig. 1: Scanogram showing varus deformity in left tibia with markings on the osteotomy site.

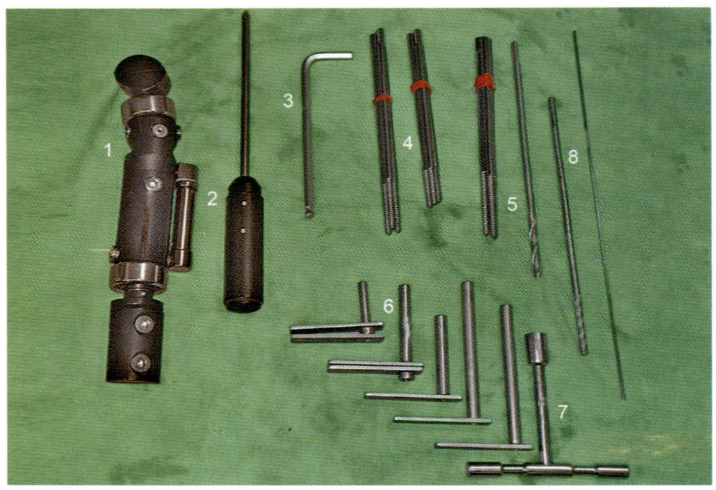

Fig. 2: Instrument trolley showing (1) High tibial osteotomy (HTO) clamp as external fixator, (2) Awl, (3) Allen key, (4) Schanz pin, (5) Drill bits, (6) Sleeves, (7) T-handle, and (8) K-wire.

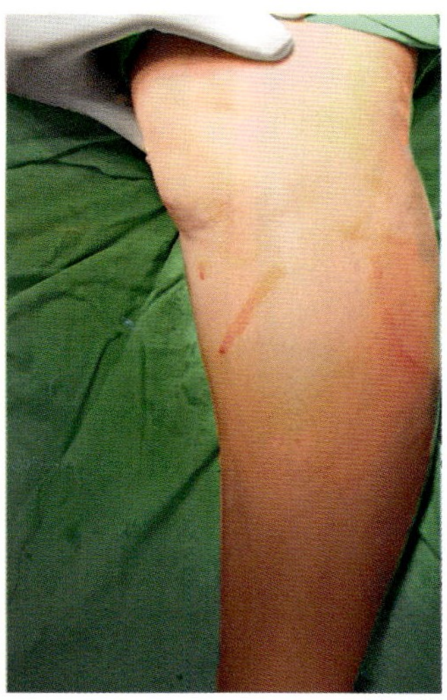

Fig. 3: Operative limb is painted and draped. Marking is made on medial side of leg for Schanz pin insertion.

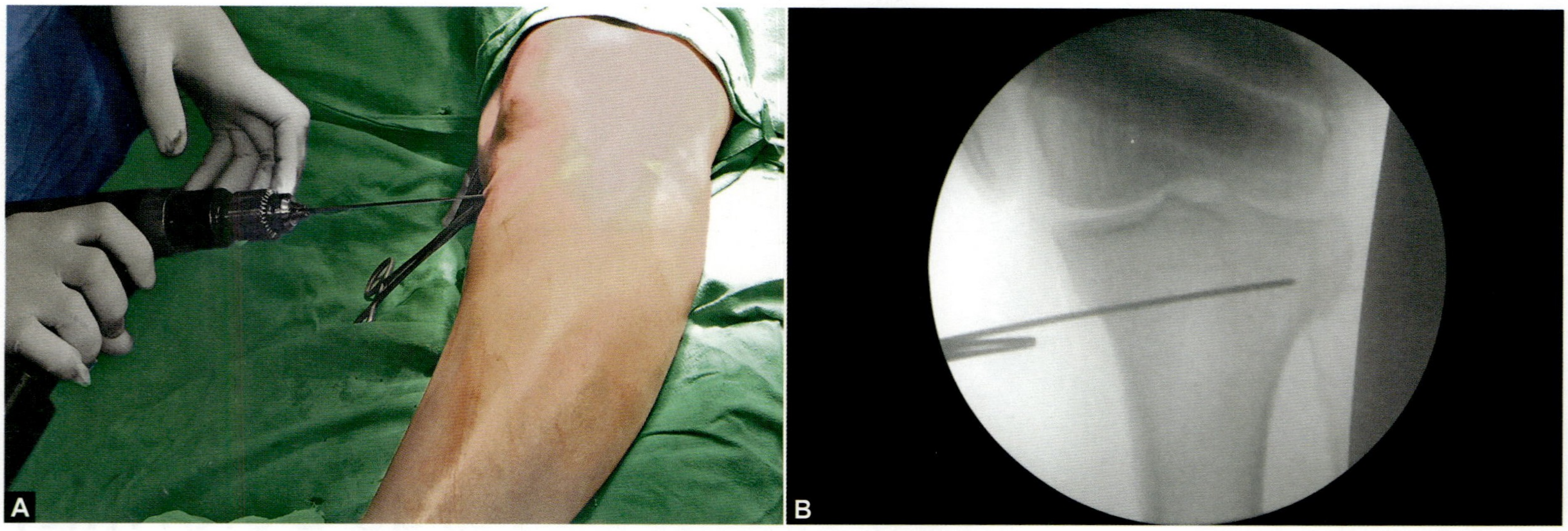

Figs. 4A and B: A guidewire to be introduced 4 cm below joint line starting posteromedially and directed laterally toward the tip of fibula (A) and confirmed with C-arm (B).

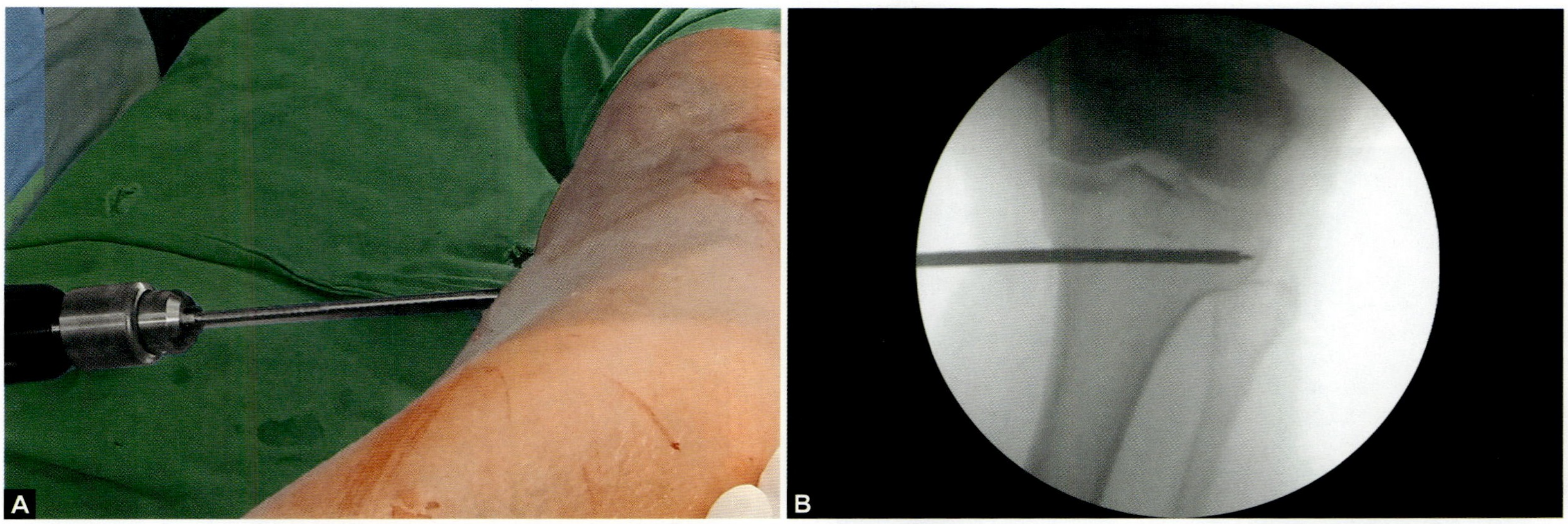

Figs. 5A and B: Incision is taken and drilling with cannulated drill bit is done over the guidewire (A) and confirmed with C-arm (B).

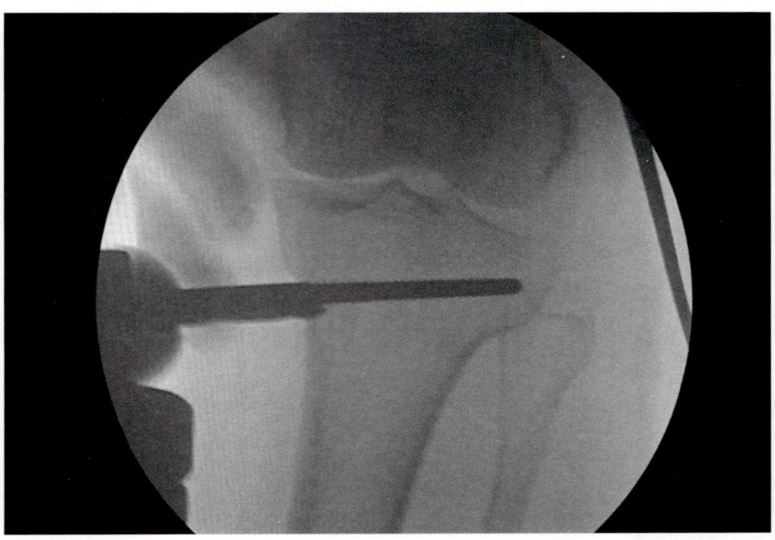

Fig. 6: Fluoroscopic image showing Schanz pin is inserted in proximal tibia.

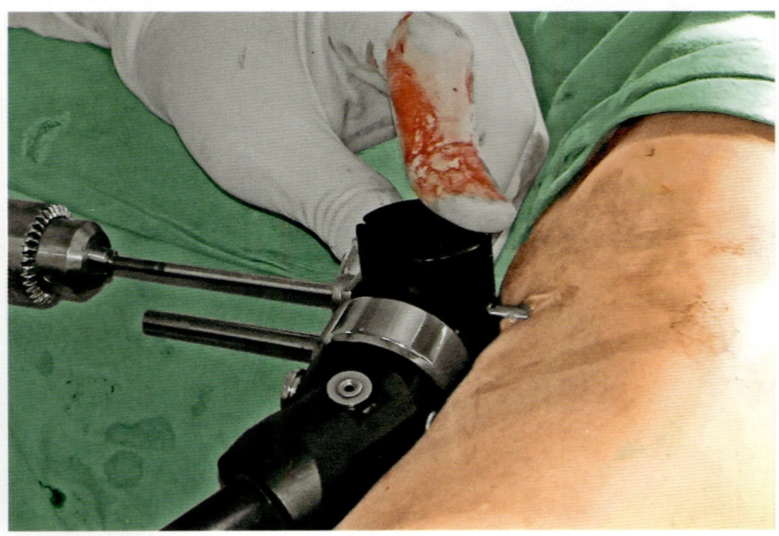

Fig. 7: Second Schanz pin is inserted through external fixator clamp just anterior to the previously introduced pin.

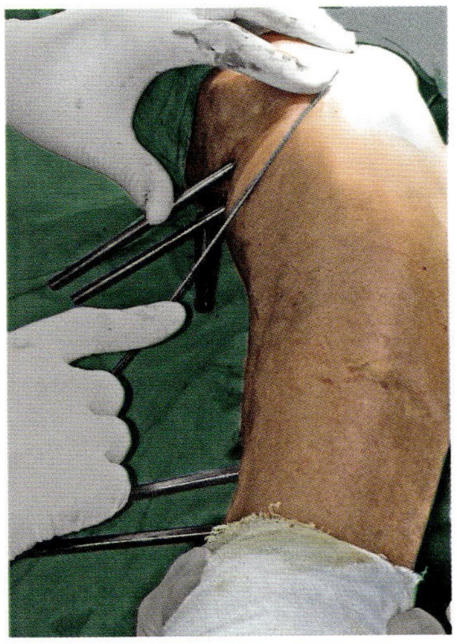

Fig. 8: Another two Schanz pins are introduced in distal tibia along the same plane medially.

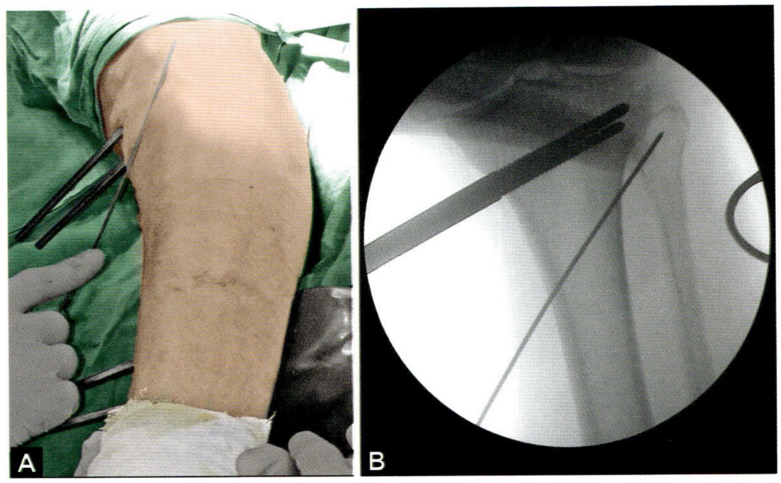

Figs. 9A and B: A guidewire is placed externally 5 cm inferior to the Schanz pin with tip pointing laterally toward head of fibula (A) and confirmed with C-arm (B) to determine the osteotomy angle.

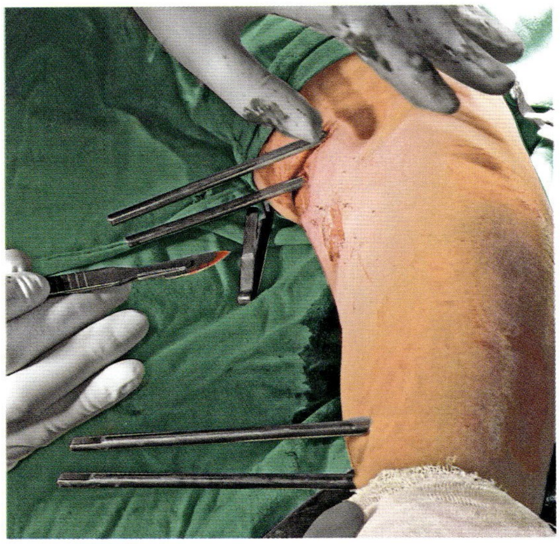

Fig. 10: An incision of 4 cm on the anteromedial aspect for the osteotomy site.

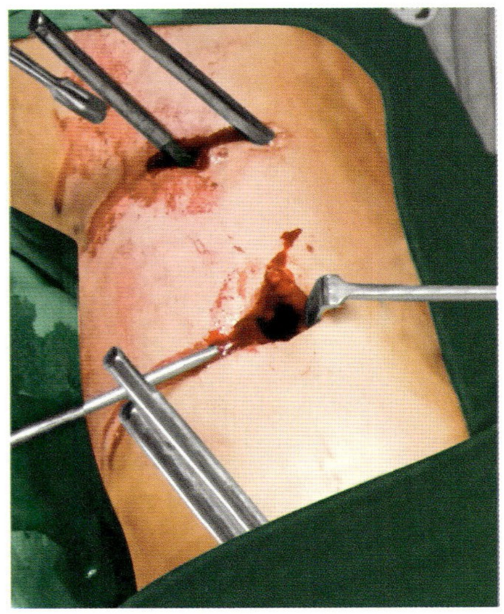

Fig. 11: Further deep dissection is done and tissue is retracted.

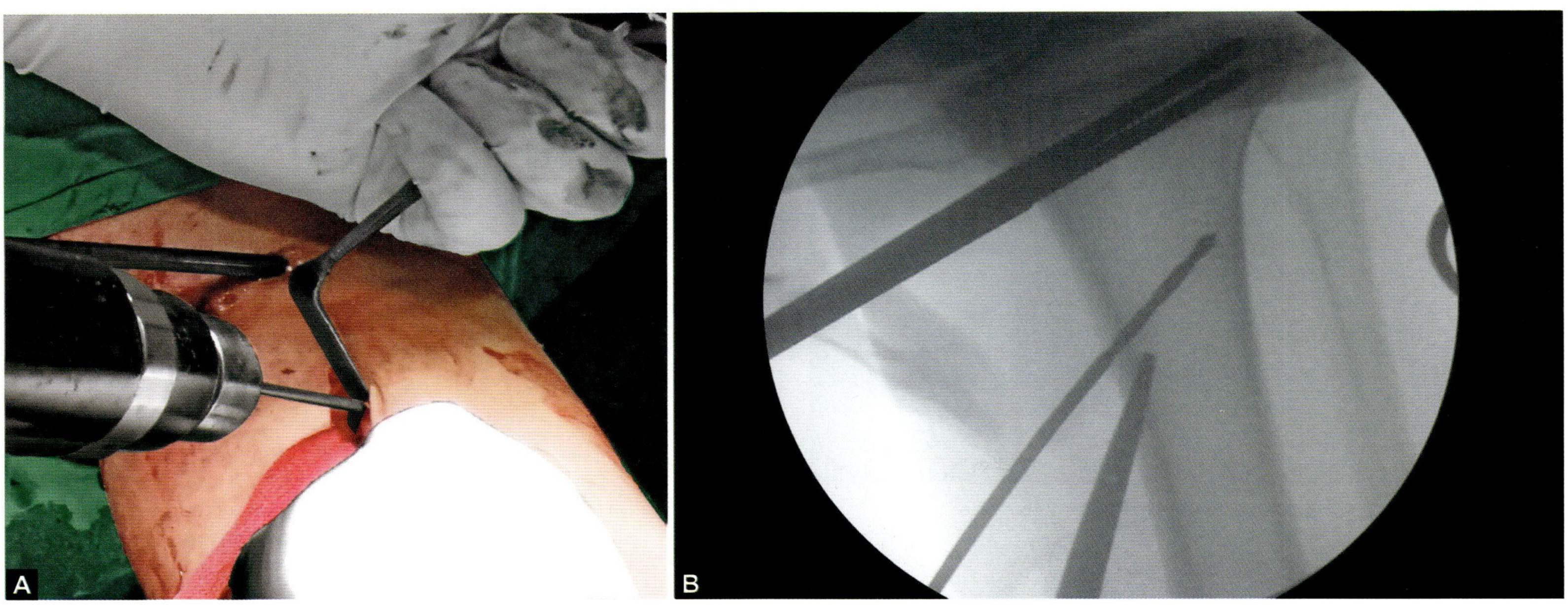

Figs. 12A and B: A drill hole is made in near cortex for osteotomy (A) and confirmed with C-arm image (B).

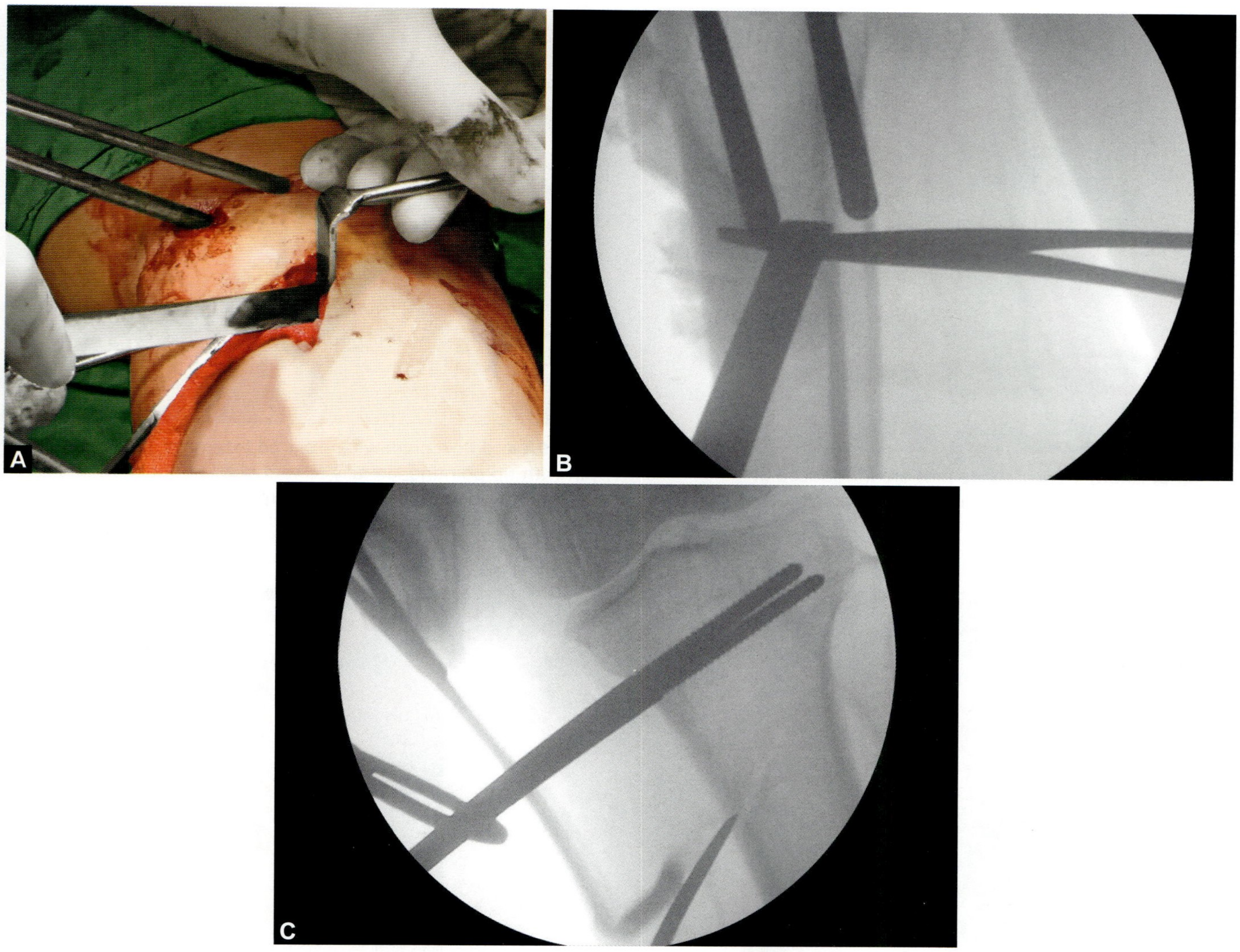

Figs. 13A to C: The drilled cortex is osteotomized with osteotome (A) and the corresponding C-arm image (B and C).

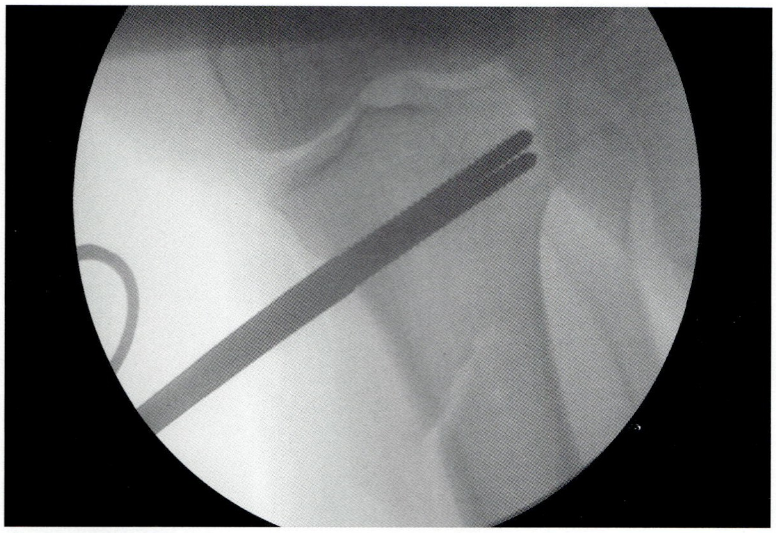

Fig. 14: C-arm image after osteotomy is done.

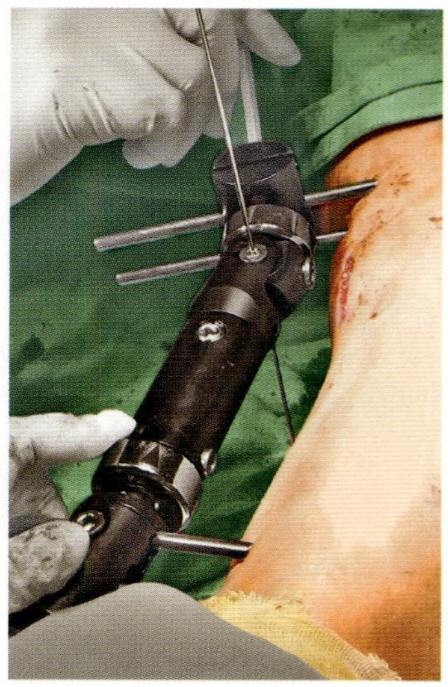

Fig. 15: Proximal and distal Schanz pins are connected by high tibial osteotomy (HTO) clamp (external fixator).

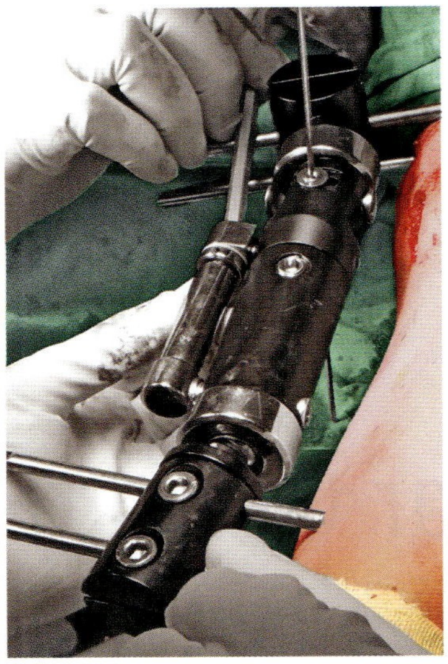

Fig. 16: External fixator assembly is tightened with valgus tension applied.

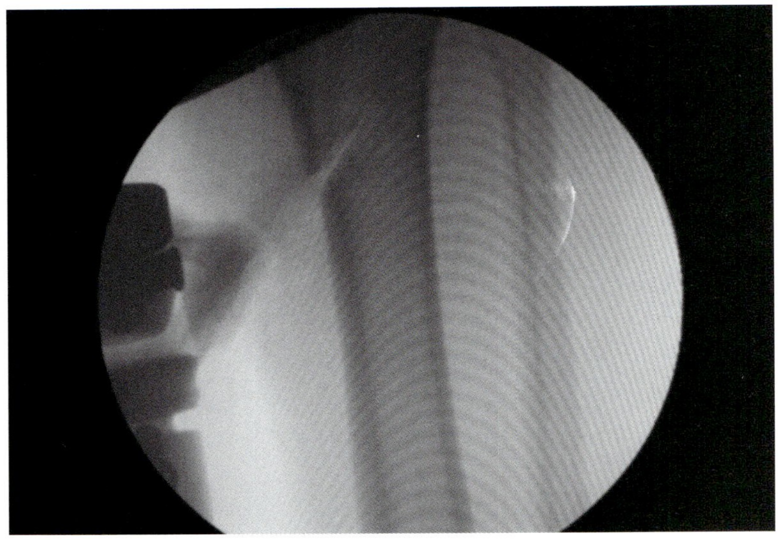

Fig. 17: Confirmation with C-arm. Valgus correction obtained. Incision is closed in layers.

CHAPTER 75

Proximal Fibular Osteotomy for Knee Osteoarthritis

Sachin Nagapurkar, Sharad M Hardikar, Siddharth Jaiswal, Mahaveer S Dugad

INTRODUCTION

In todays world knee osteoarthritis (OA) is one of the most common joint disorder which cause severe pain and difficulty in movement. For advanced knee osteoarthritis total knee arthroplasty (TKA) is very effective for relieving pain and improves joint function. However, it is complex and expensive and in some patient revision surgery may be required. For young patient with OA knee, hightibial osteotomy (HTO) is the surgical treatment of choice.

In 2015 Zhang et al. reported that proximal fibular osteotomy (PFO), a new surgery for OA knee. In severe genu varus, PFO increases the medial joint space and also the axial alignment of the lower extremity in some patient.

METHODS

To analyze the ratio of knee joint space (medial/lateral compartment) and the alignment of the lower extremity, preoperative and postoperative weight bearing and whole lower extremity radiograph should be obtained.

The medial joint space is obtained by drawing a vertical line (A) between two horizontal lines (C and D) that are drawn from the lowest point of the medial condyle of the femur and medial plateau of the tibia, respectively. The lateral joint space is obtained by drawing a vertical line (B) between two horizontal lines (E and F) that are drawn from the lowest point of the lateral condyle of the femur and lateral plateau of the tibia, respectively. The ratio of the knee joint space (medial/lateral) is calculated by the ratio of A/B (Fig. 1).

Figure 2 on the whole lower extremity radiograph the hip-knee-ankle angle was measured. Line A is drawn from the center of the femur to the center of the knee and line B is drawn from the center of the knee to the center of the ankle. The intersection angle α between lines A and B represents the hip-knee-ankle angle.

Figure 3 mechanism of pain relief and joint space improvement after PFO:

A. In the normal condition, equal loads were distributed on the medial and lateral tibia plateau.
B. In osteoarthritis, a greater load was shifted to the medial tibia plateau.
C. After PFO, abnormal load was corrected.

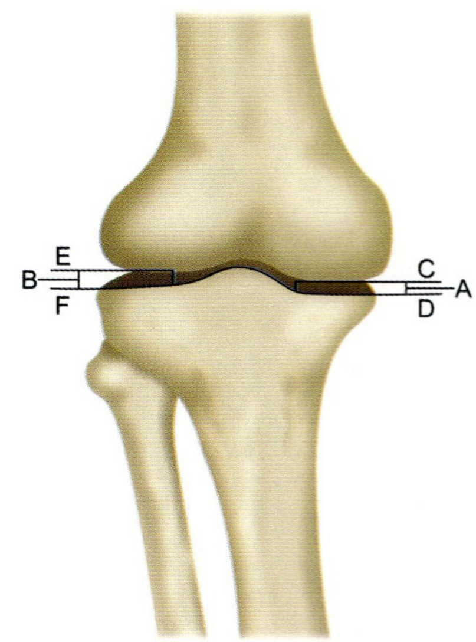

Fig. 1: Ratio of the knee joint space (medial/lateral).

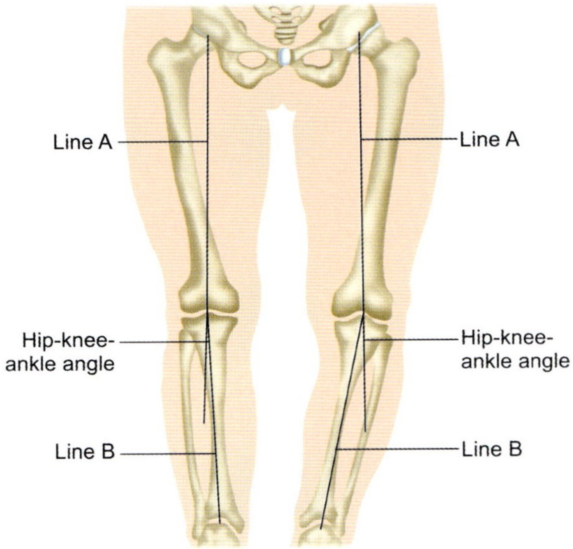

Fig. 2: The hip-knee-ankle angle.

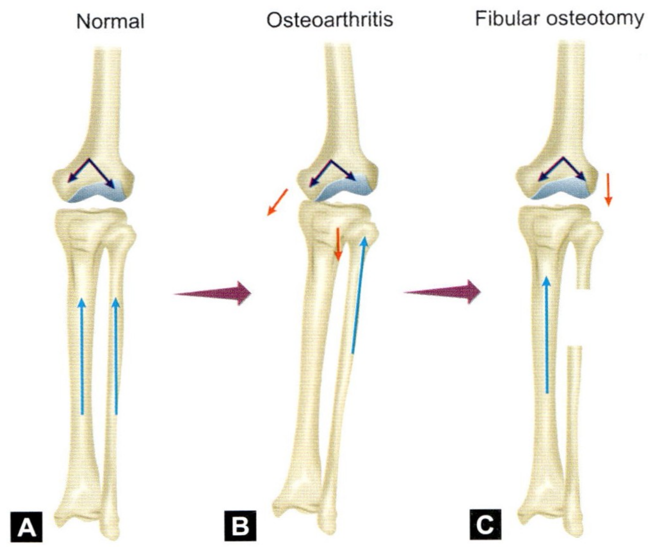

Fig. 3: Proximal fibular osteotomy.

SURGICAL STEPS (FIGS. 4 TO 15)

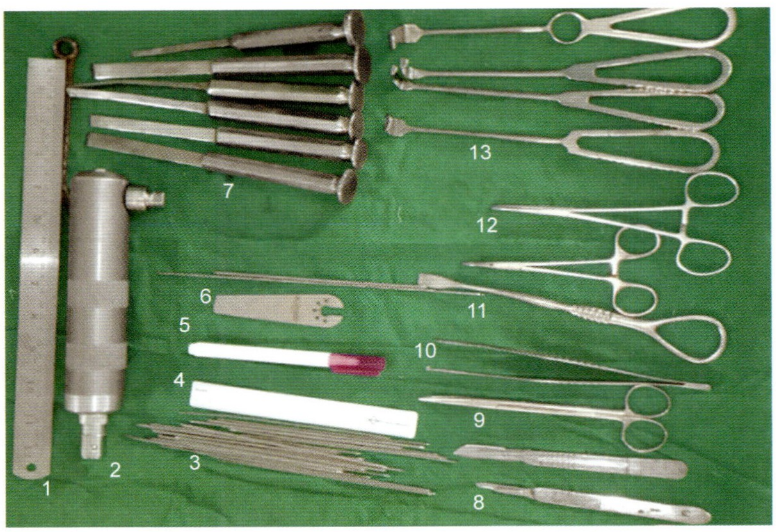

Fig. 4: (1) Measuring scale; (2) oscillatory bone saw; (3) K-wire; (4) disposable scale; (5) marker; (6) saw blade; (7) Osteotome; (8) blade with BP handle; (9) Scissor; (10) tooth forceps, (11) periosteum elevator; (12) artery forceps; (13) right-angled retractor.

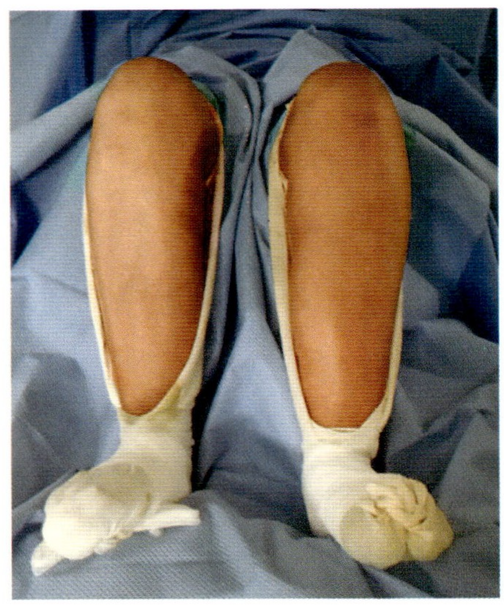

Fig. 5: Position of limb.

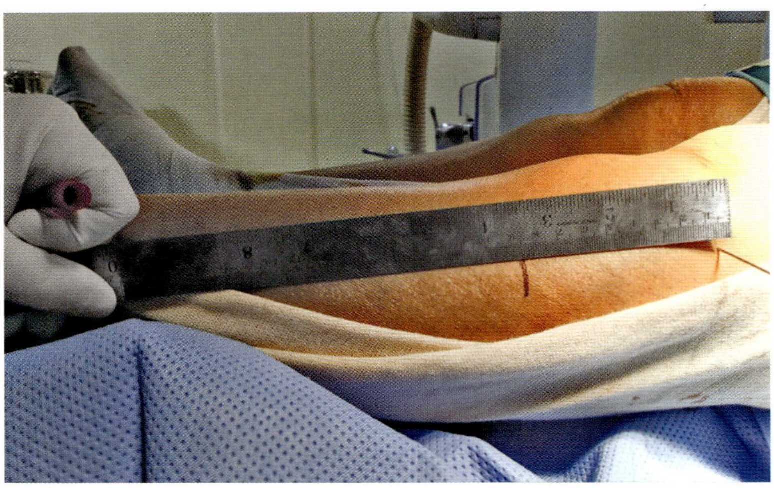

Fig. 6: Marking 8.5 cm from fibular head.

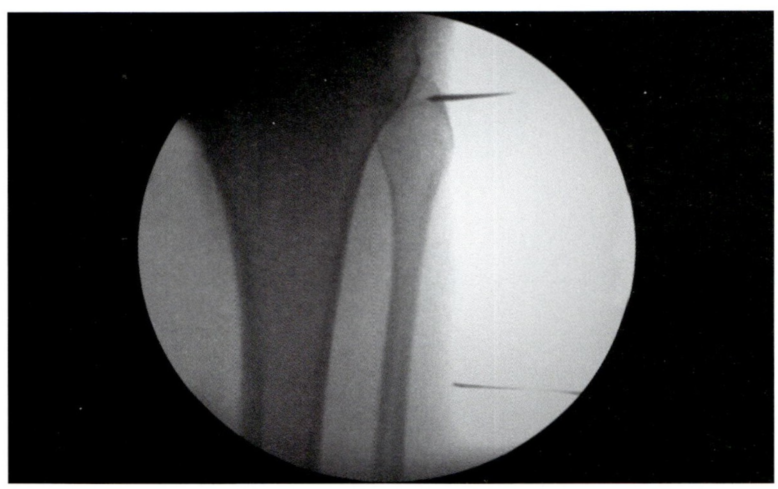

Fig. 7: On C-arm position of fibular marking confirmed.

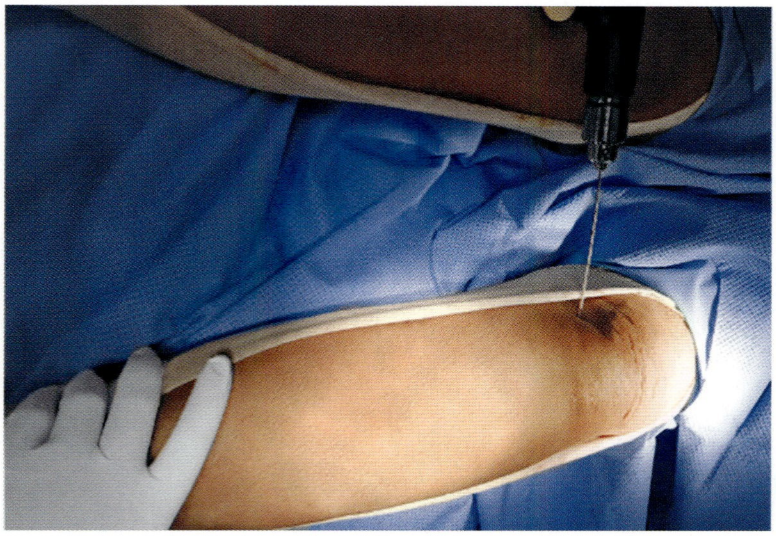

Fig. 8: Medial condyle of femur core decompression.

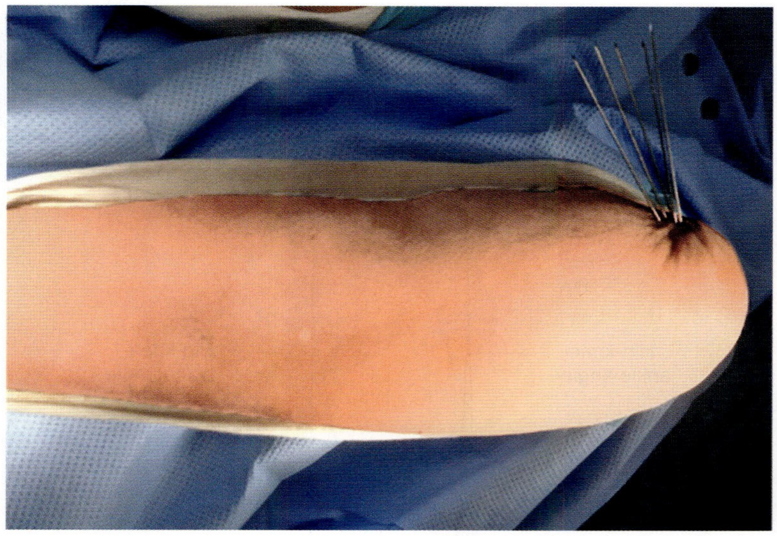

Fig. 9A: Medial condyle of femur decompression with multiple K-wire.

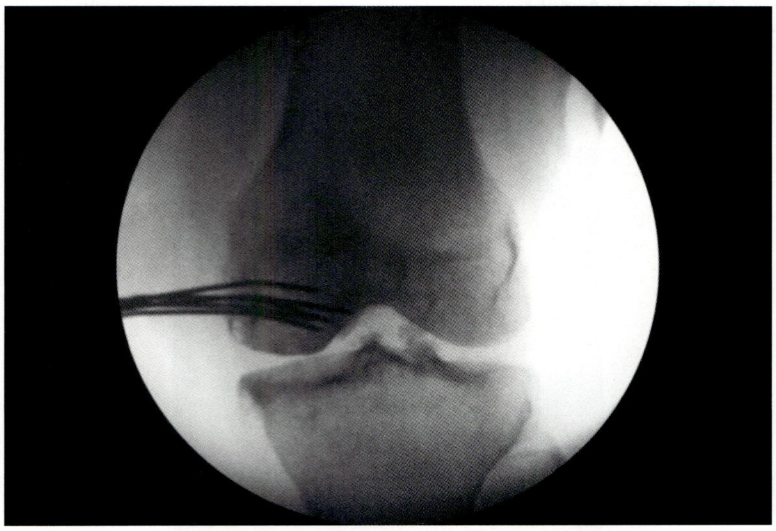

Fig. 9B: Medial condyle of femur decompression confirmed on C-arm.

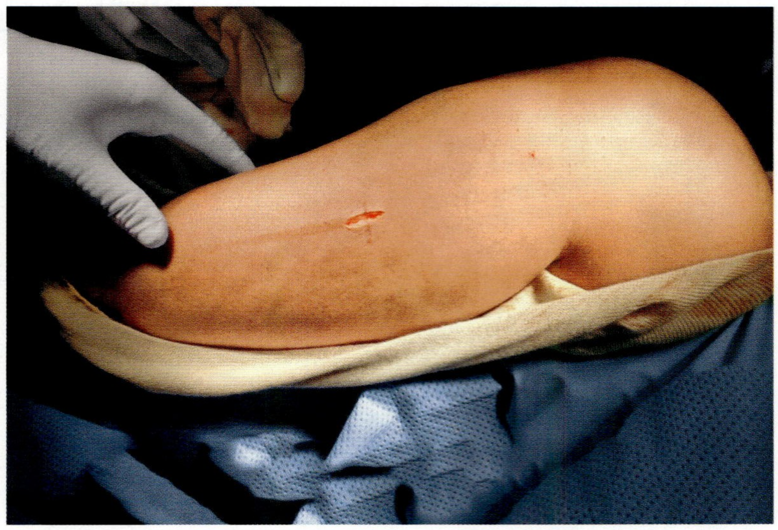

Fig. 10: Incision made over lateral surface of leg at 8.5 cm below the fibular head.

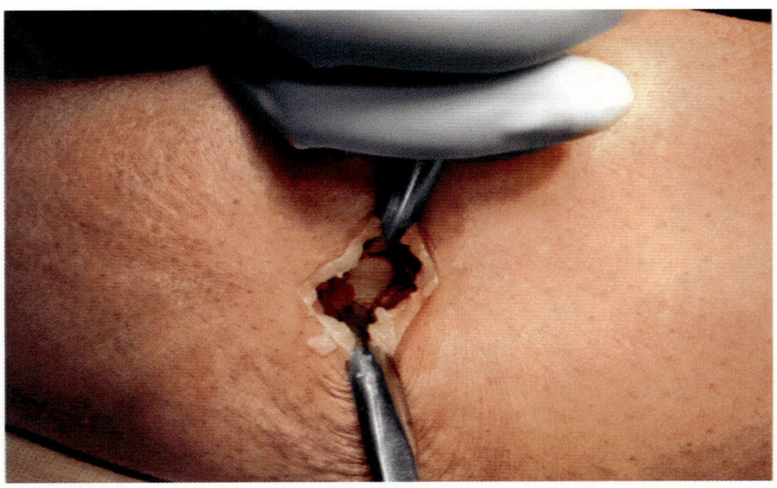

Fig. 11: Fibular bone exposed.

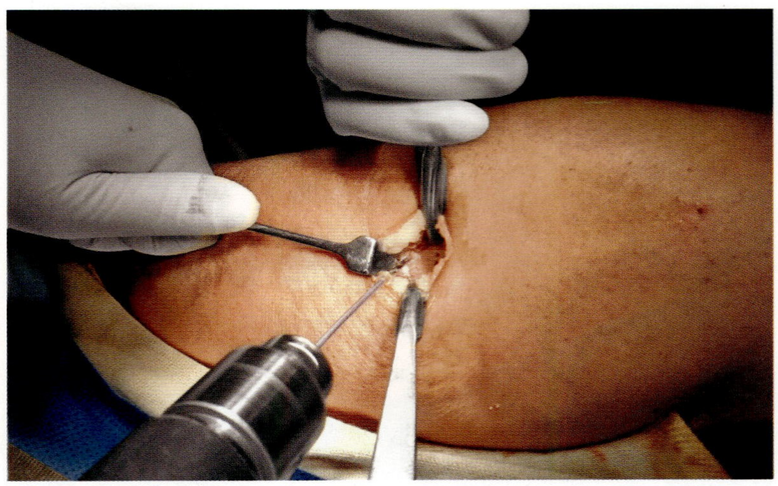

Fig. 12: Length of 1 cm marked over fibular shaft at 8.5 cm from fibular head.

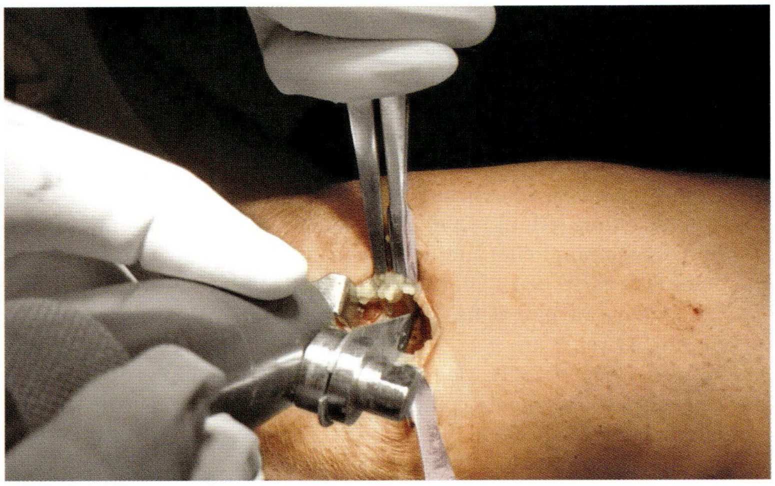

Fig. 13: Fibular osteotomy of length 1 cm done with help of bone saw.

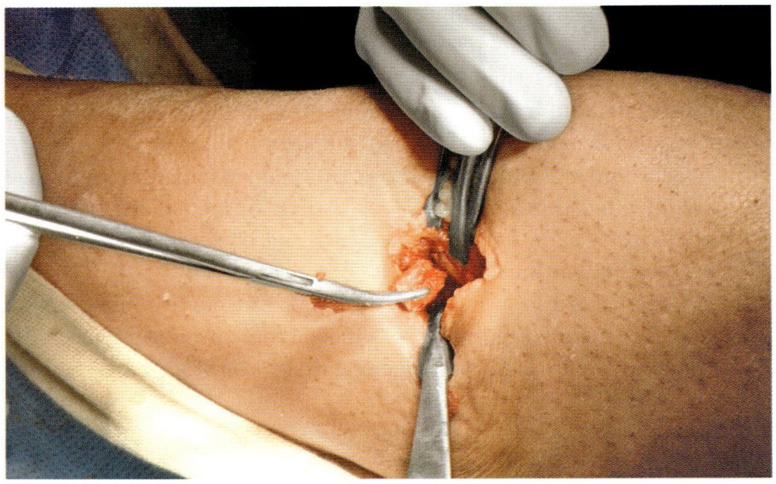

Fig. 14A: Removal of resected piece of fibula.

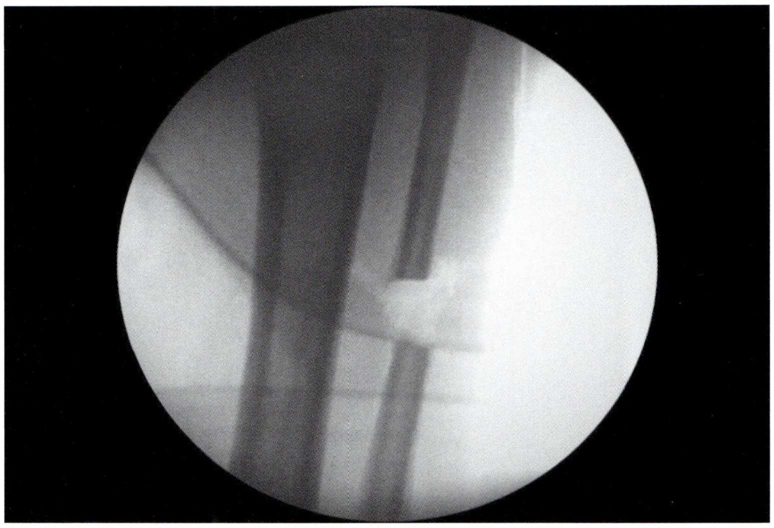

Fig. 14B: Confirmation of osteotomy of fibula with help of C-arm.

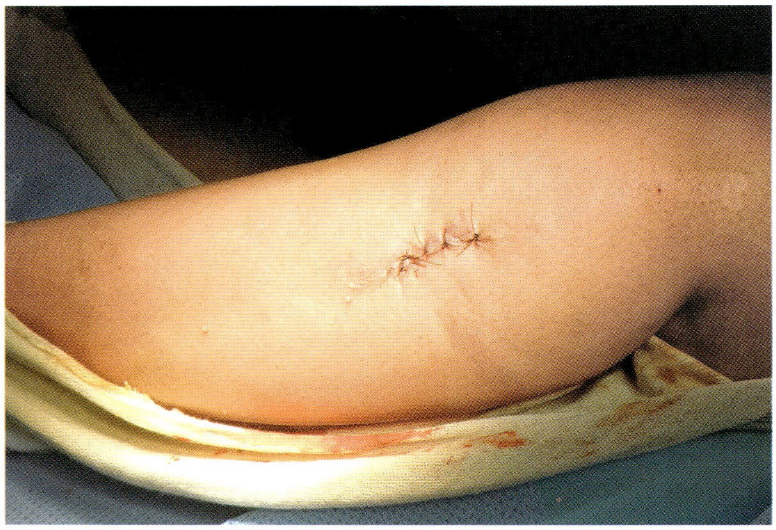

Fig. 15A: Skin closure.

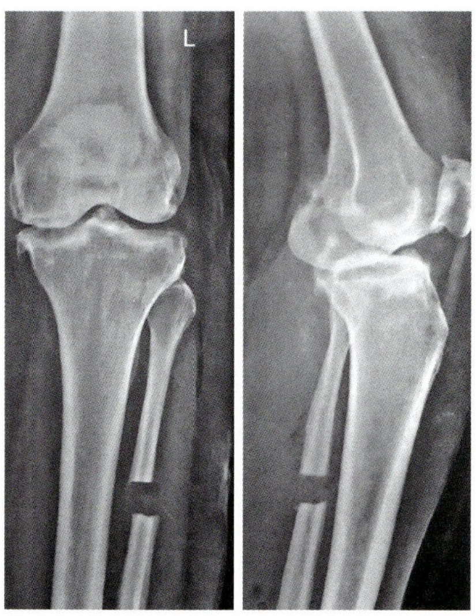

Fig. 15B: Postoperative X-ray of proximal fibular osteotomy.

COMPLICATION

In PFO, higher incidence of peroneal nerve palsy is noted. This can be lowered by performing fibular osteotomy in an area 4–7 cm away from the fibular head.

CONCLUSION

The PFO demonstrates that this osteotomy technique postoperatively improves joint function and relieves pain in patient of medial compartment osteoarthritis.

SUGGESTED READING

1. Altman R, Asch E, Bloch D. Development of criteria for the classification and reporting of osteoarthritis. Classification of osteoarthritis of the knee. Diagnostic and therapeutic criteria committee of the American rheumatism association. Arthritis Rheum. 1986;29:1039-49.

2. Burnett RS, Bourne RB. Indications for patellar resurfacing in total knee arthroplasty. J Bone Joint Surg. 2003;85:728-45.
3. Chen HW, Liu GD, Ou S, et al. Open reduction and internal fixation of posterolateral tibial plateau fractures through fibula osteotomy-free posterolateral approach. J Orthop Traum. 2014;28:513-7.
4. Duivenvoorden T, Brouwer RW, Baan A. Comparison of closing-wedge and opening-wedge high tibial osteotomy for medial compartment osteoarthritis of the knee: a randomized controlled trial with a six-year follow-up. J Bone Joint Surg Am. 2014;96:1425-32.
5. Laprade RF, Spiridonov SI, Nystrom LM. Prospective outcomes of young and middle-aged adults with medial compartment osteoarthritis treated with a proximal tibial opening wedge osteotomy. Arthroscopy. 2012;28:354-64.
6. Ogbemudia AO, Umebese PF, Bafor A, et al. The level of fibula osteotomy and incidence of peroneal nerve palsy in proximal tibial osteotomy. J Surg Tech Case Rep. 2010;2:17-9.
7. Simkin PA. Bone pain and pressure in osteoarthritic joints. Novartis Found Symp. 2004;260:179-86; discussion 186-190, 277-179.
8. Sprenger TR, Doerzbacher JF. Tibial osteotomy for the treatment of varus gonarthrosis. Survival and failure analysis to twenty-two years. J Bone Joint Surg Am. 2003;85-A(3):469-74.
9. W-Dahl A, Robertsson O, Lidgren V. Surgery for knee osteoarthritis in younger patients. Acta Orthop. 2010;81:161-4.
10. Wei XC, Wang XH, Li PC, et al. Proximal Fibular Osteotomy, A New Surgery for Pain Relief and Improvement of Joint Function in Human Knee Osteoarthritis: a Short-Term Clinical Study. Poster #: 1071. ORS 2016 Annual Meeting at the Disney's Coronado Springs Resort in Orlando, Florida, March 5–8.
11. Yang ZY, Chen W, Li CX. Medial compartment decompression by fibular osteotomy to treat medial compartment knee osteoarthritis: a pilot study. Orthopedics. 2015;38:e1110-4.
12. Zhang YZ. Innovations in Orthopedics and Traumatology in China. Chin Med J (Engl). 2015;128:2841-2.

CHAPTER 76

Titanium Elastic Nail Removal from Tibia

Sachin Nagapurkar, Rajkumar Ekambaram, Rachit Vipul Shah

INDICATIONS FOR TENS REMOVAL

Closed fractures of tibia in children within 13–15 years of age are mostly treated by titanium elastic nailing system (TENS) technique under proper guidance of C-arm.

Usually TENS nail can be removed after radiological confirmation of proper union usually after 16–20 months.

But it can be also removed in case of situations from infection, revision surgery required, nonunion, malunion, and nail tip exposed (Fig. 1).

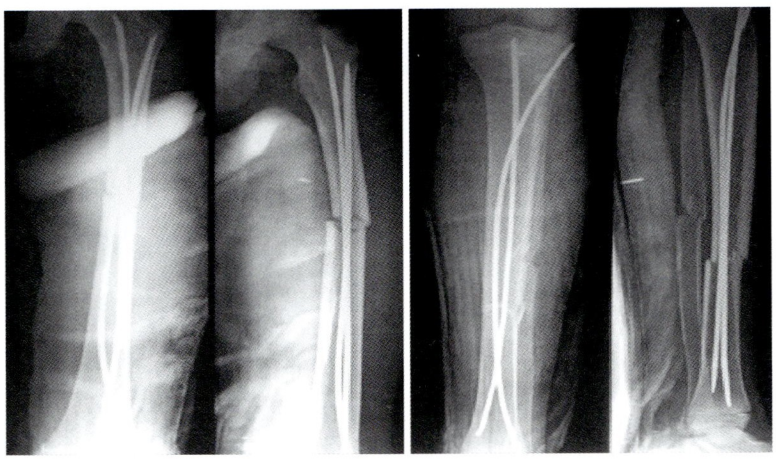

Fig. 1: Postoperative X-ray of 12-year-old boy with femoral and tibial fracture treated with TENS nail.

INSTRUMENTS NEEDED

Sterile instrument trolley containing 22 size scalpel blade, artery forceps of required sizes, tissue holding forceps, extraction pliers, nibbler, osteotome, if necessary bevelled impactor, and hammer (Fig. 2).

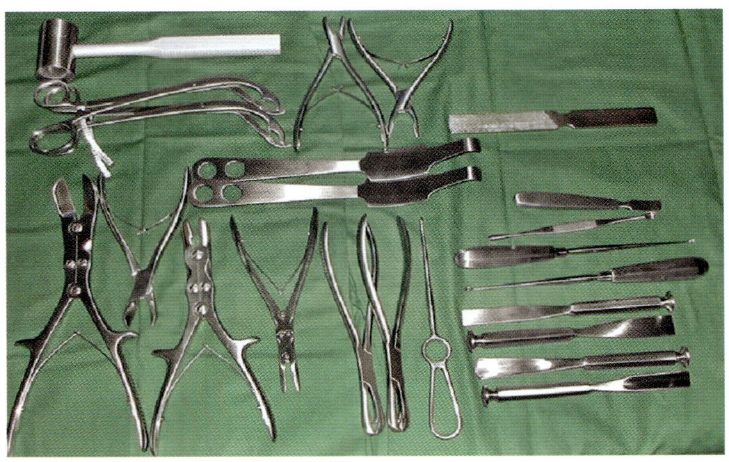

Fig. 2: Instrument trolley for removal of titanium elastic nailing system (TENS).

SURGICAL STEPS

STEP 1

Do proper painting and draping of the limb with proper exposure of the same. Under proper aseptic precautions with adequate local or regional block with lignocaine, especially over the entry point of the nail inserted previously. Now using scalpel blade gently take a skin incision is made over the skin at palpated tip of the nail or near the old scar of insertion surgery, if tip cannot be palpated. Sometimes it is wise to use C-arm assistance to locate the incision exactly over the tip.

STEP 2 (FIG. 3)

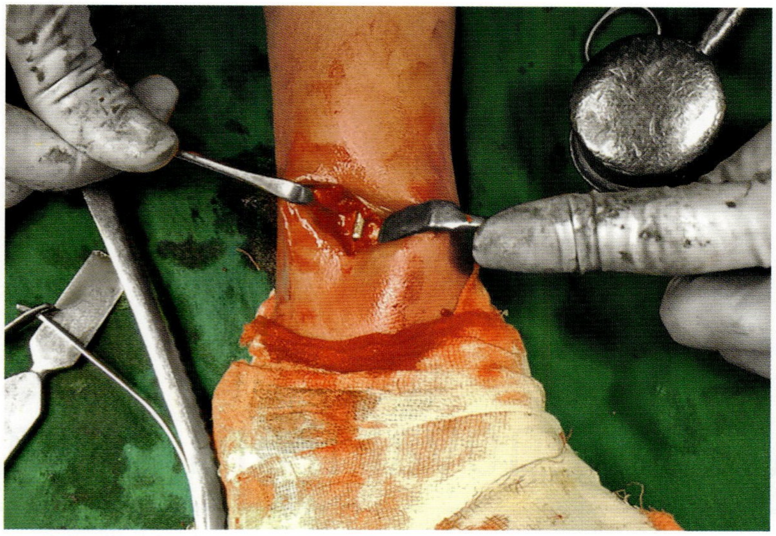

Fig. 3: By dissection, identify the tip of the nail introduced. If that seems difficult C-arm guidance is advised.

STEP 3 (FIG. 4A)

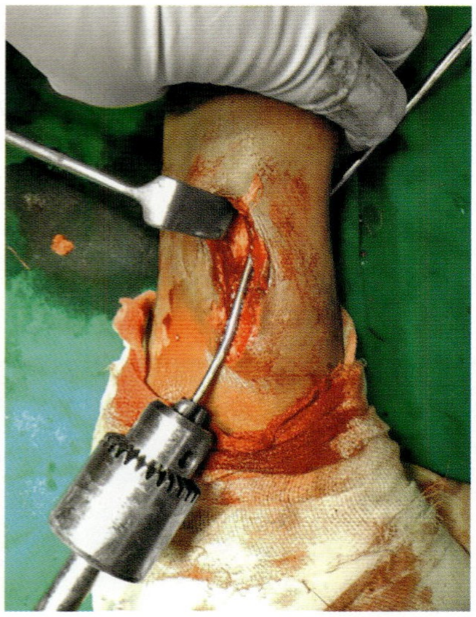

Fig. 4A: Retract the soft tissues and gently pull the TENS (Titanium Elastic Nailing System) nail by holding with extraction plier or chuck, it may be tapped lightly in reverse direction over T handle of chuck in order to facilitate the removal.

STEP 4 (FIG. 4B)

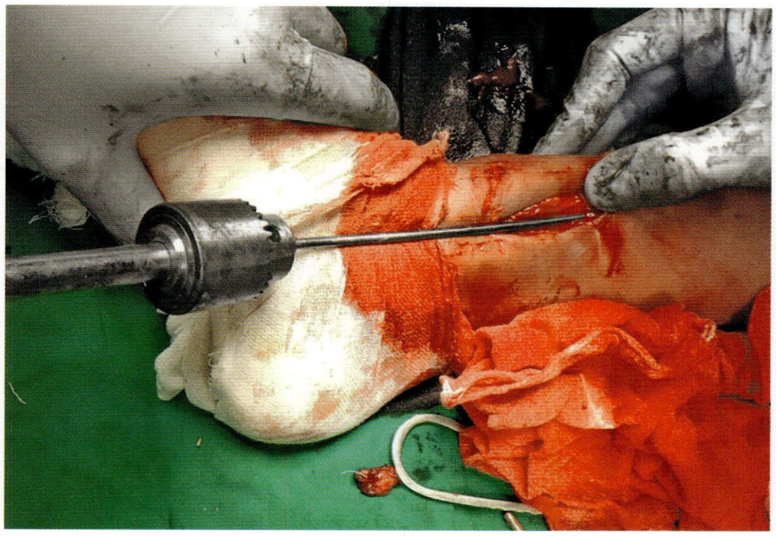

Fig. 4B: The nail is removed by above procedure.

STEP 5

Give adequate wash using normal saline and povidone–iodine. Use hydrogen peroxide, if grossly infected and start skin closure with nonabsorbable 2-0 sutures.

CHAPTER 77

Open Repair of Rotator Cuff Tear

Milind Modak, Snehal Dantkale, Neelkamal Sourav

INTRODUCTION

A group of four muscles arising from the scapula and surrounding the shoulder joint forms the rotator cuff. The tendons of each of the four muscles then blend with the joint capsule and stabilize the shoulder as they attach to humeral tuberosity. The muscle tendons that form the cuff are subscapularis, supraspinatus, infraspinatus and teres minor. Rotator cuff can be torn following trauma or wear and tear of tendons.

ANATOMY

The musculotendinous cuff is formed by the fusion of the short, flat, broad, tendons of the four rotators, as along with the fibrous capsule. The fusion occurs 12–20 mm lateral to the point of insertion of tendons onto the humerus. The distance between the articular cartilage to medial footprint of rotator cuff is 1.6–1.9 mm. Rotator cuff provides dynamic stability to the shoulder joint by balancing the opposing forces acting on the joint.

Rotator cuff is differentiated into five histologic areas (five layers). This is important to understand why most tears are on the articular side, as it is weaker than the bursal side.

- *Layer I* (1 mm thick):
  - Most superficial layer and composed of fibers from the coracohumeral ligament, which extends posteriorly and obliquely.
- *Layer II* (3–5 mm thick):
  - Composed of densely packed fibers that parallel the long axis of the tendon.
- *Layer III* (3 mm thick):
  - Smaller loosely organized bundles of collagen at 45° angle to the long axis of the tendon.
- *Layer IV* (1–2 mm thick):
  - Loose connective tissue and thick collagen bands and merges with fibers from coracohumeral ligament.
- *Layer V* (2 mm thick):
  - Shoulder capsule.

PATHOPHYSIOLOGY

An understanding of the pathophysiology is important to be able to manage a case of rotator cuff injury. Traumatic and degenerative tears are actually a spectrum of overlap.

Rotator cuff fiber failure has at least four adverse effects:

1. Increased load neighboring fibers, which are intact and these start failing sequentially giving rise to a zipper phenomenon.
2. Detached cuff fiber diminishes the fiber force the cuff fiber can exert.
3. Anatomy distortion compromises the blood supply of tendon fiber and there is progressive local ischemia.
4. Torn surface of the cuff tendon is exposed to the joint synovial fluid. This fluid contains lytic enzymes. These enzymes remove the hematoma. The hematoma assists the healing process.

These four mechanisms and an attempt of healing give rise to scar tissue which does not have the normal resilience and fails with subsequent loading.

In the absence of repair, the degenerative process continues through the supraspinatus tendon. If not repaired this would lead to the continued degeneration of the anterior portion of the supraspinatus tendon.

Following four mechanisms come into play as the defect advances. This gives rise to a defect in the supraspinatus. At first the defect propagates posteriorly from supraspinatus to the infraspinatus.

Because of the loss of the spacer effect of the rotator cuff there is superior displacement of the humeral head. This affects the biceps tendon. This puts a strain on the biceps tendon which becomes thicker and broader initially but later on it may lead to the rupture of the long head of biceps brachi. The tendon of long head of biceps can rupture in chronic situation.

The subscapularis tendon is the next to be involved as the defect extends anteroinferiorly from the lesser tuberosity which may lead to the rupture of transverse humeral ligament medially.

With destabilized humeral head with proximal migration, there is progressive cuff degeneration due to abrasion which leads to the development of a traction spur in the coracoacromial ligament.

There is wear and tear of the superior labrum and glenoid allowing the damaged tendons of rotator cuff to slide below the humeral head. So now these tendon try to elevate the head of humerus instead of keeping it down in its normal position.

After failure of full thickness of the rotator cuff, it may progress into what is known as cuff tear arthropathy. It is a secondary degenerative joint disorder caused due to the pressure of the humeral head against the coracoacromial arch.

Chronic cases may end up in irreversible damage leading to loss of movement, retraction fatty degeneration and atrophy of the involved structures. Following the tear in tendons muscles undergo variable changes. Muscles may be atrophied which is more prominent near the fascia or may undergo fatty change near their origin from scapula.

It is important to know the pathophysiology of cuff tear to deal with the problem in a better way as damage evolves over time.

Mechanisms of tear include:

- *Chronic degenerative tear*:
  - Primary etiology is intrinsic degeneration, mainly seen in older patients.
- *Chronic impingement*:
  - Tear starts within the tendon or on bursal surface.
- *Acute avulsion injuries*:
  - Acute subscapularis tears are common in younger patients following a fall.
  - Acute supraspinatus muscle, the infraspinatus muscle and teres minor muscle tears are seen in patients more than 40 years with a shoulder dislocation.
- *Iatrogenic injuries*:
  - Due to failure of surgical repair.

PROGNOSIS

Almost half of the asymptomatic tears would develop the symptoms in 2–3 years.

CLINICAL FEATURES

The clinical manifestation includes shoulder stiffness, weakness, instability, and arthritis. Progressive pain in the anterolateral aspect of the shoulder aggravates on overhead activities. There is increase in intensity of pain at night and restriction of movements of shoulder. The shoulder may or may not weak. On clinical examination, supraspinatus and infraspinatus are seen to be atrophied. Tenderness is present along anterolateral aspect of proximal arm. Palpable subacromial crepitus is present. Neers and Hawkins–Kennedy signs are positive. Lift-off or Napoleon test is positive. Occasionally in a patient with full thickness tear, passive range motion is normal.

IMAGING

X-rays

Anteroposterior (AP) view, internal and external rotation AP views, axillary view, outlet view, and 30° caudal tilt view. Some findings on X-ray present as small fragment of the greater tuberosity, sclerosis of under surface of the acromion (eyebrow sign), tendon spur of the coracoacromial ligament. And associated findings are acromioclavicular arthritis, chronic calcific arthritis, and displacement tuberosities.

Ultrasonography

It is useful for diagnosis of cuff pathology and biceps tendon evaluation but examiner dependent. Being real time, dynamic, and interactive, the information is helps to make treatment plan, decision in primary as well as postsurgical rotator condition.

Magnetic Resonance Imaging Scans

Specificity 95% and sensitivity 100% for full thickness rotator cuff tear, also provides information on tear size, tear configuration, tendon involvement, tear chronicity in terms of fatty infiltration and muscle atrophy.

Atrophy can be interpreted on the basis of occupation ratio and the tangent sign. Changes suggestive of atrophy and fatty infiltration, difficult to return function of rotator cuff.

TREATMENT

Treatment modality depends on the multiple factors like activity and age of patient, mechanism of tear either degenerative or traumatic avulsion, characteristics of tear, dimension of tear, associated with muscle atrophy, partial thickness tears versus complete tear, articular sided versus bursal sided, bursal-sided tears are treated more aggressively.

Nonsurgical

- *Physical therapy, nonsteroidal anti-inflammatory drugs (NSAIDs), subacromial corticosteroid injections*: It is first line of treatment for most tears, mainly for partial tears. Avoid forceful overhead activity. Aggressive rotator cuff and scapular-stabilizer strengthening over a 3–6-month is recommended. Subacromial injections are suggested, if impingement is thought to be major cause of symptoms.
- Nonoperative treatment is suggested for chronic full thickness cuff tears. When a possibility of achieving a durable cuff repair is doubtful as in atraumatic tears, supraspinatus atrophy, repeated injury, smokers, and debilitated.

Surgery

Prognostic factor related to the durability of the rotator cuff repair is assessed before embarking on surgery and patient and the relatives are explained the overall outcome possibilities.

The favorable prognostic factors are a young patient (age less than 55 years of age), with an acute traumatic episodes unrelated to work, a short duration of weakness, a nonsmoker with no comorbidities.

Subacromial Decompression and Rotator Cuff Debridement

Indicated in patients with a low-grade partial articular sided rotator cuff tear.

Rotator Cuff Repair (Arthroscopic or Mini-open)

Open Rotator Cuff Repair

It is preferred in condition where the quality of the remaining tissue is poor and significant tendon retraction and adhesions, which make arthroscopic rotator cuff repair more difficult.

Open rotator cuff repair: surgical technique:

The first open rotator cuff repair was done by Dr Codman (1911) modified by Neer (1972) and included 5 basic principles of rotator cuff repair: (1) Very careful repair of deltoid origin, (2) Subacromial release, (3) To obtain freely mobile muscle tendon units surgical release as much as needed, (4) Confirm tendon to tuberosity transosseous fixation, (5) Rehabilitation with early range of motion exercise under supervision.

Following is the step-by-step approach for open rotator cuff repair and detailed surgical procedure.

(Please post pictures and pictures description here step-by-step).

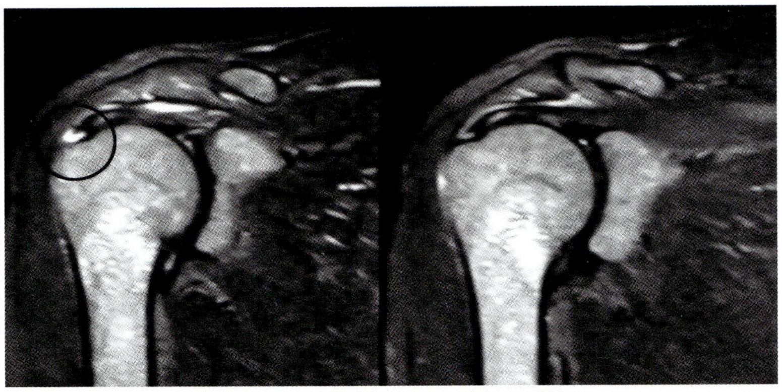

MRI showing full thickness rotator cuff tear

Fig. 1: MRI images of elderly patient suggestive of full thickness rotator cuff tear.

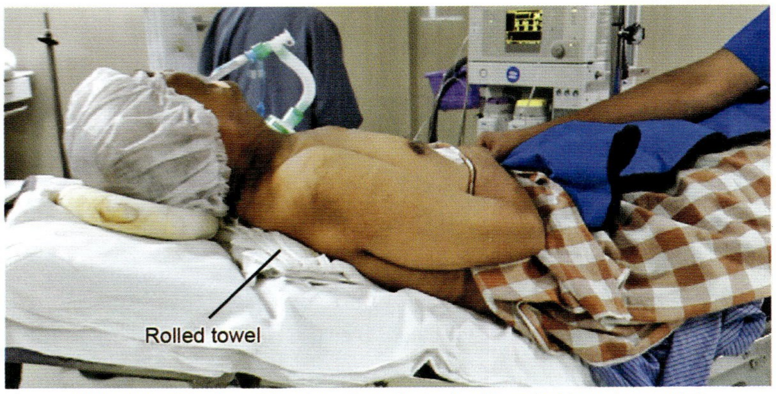

Patient positioning side view (beach chair with rolled towel scapula)

Fig. 2: Positioning of patient: Place the patient in a beach chair position with rolled towel under scapula to elevate it under anesthesia. Patient's head should be secured with straps.

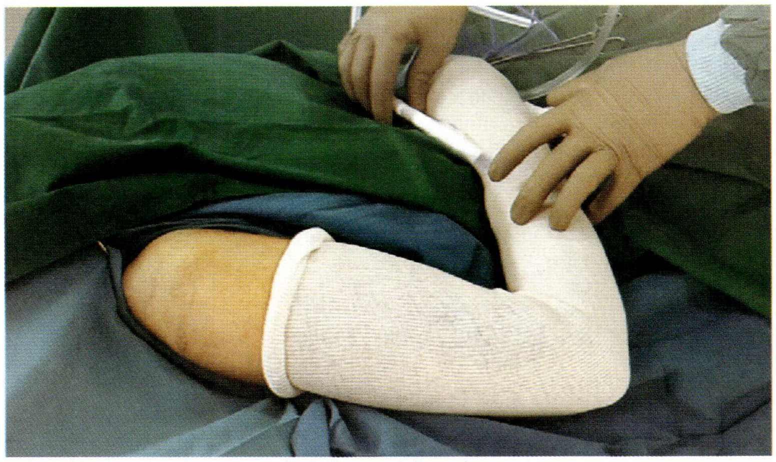

Painting and drapping

Fig. 3: Painting and draping should be done in standard fashion after primary scrubbing the parts.

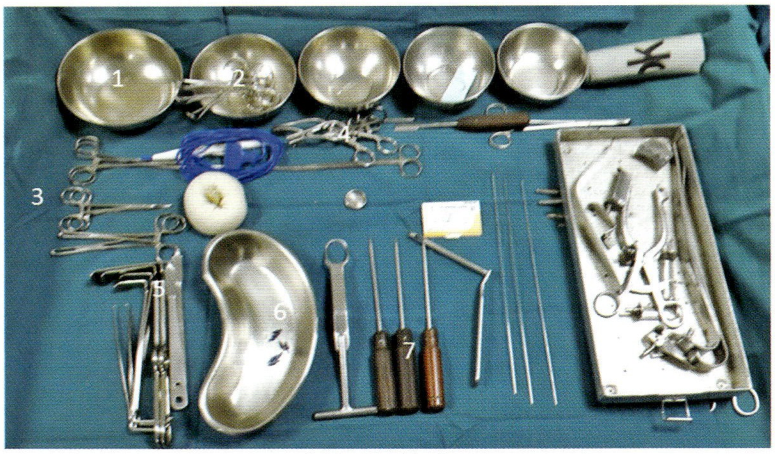

Instrument trolley

Fig. 4: General set of instruments with specific instruments for rotator cuff repair should be arranged and ready before start of the procedure.

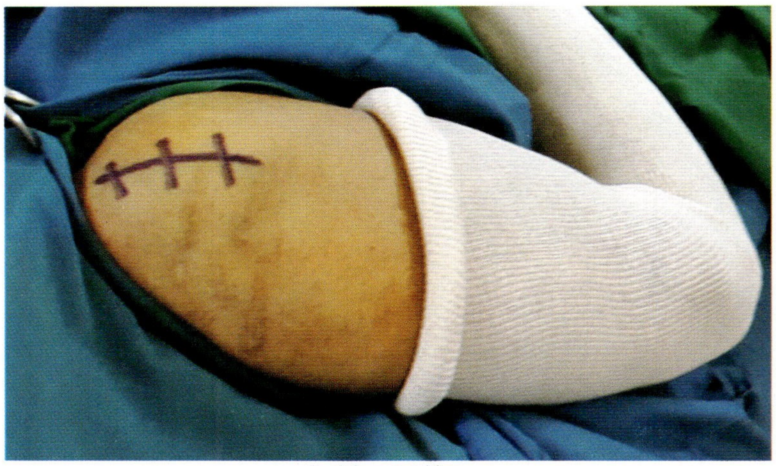

Incision marking

Fig. 5: Incision marking: Various approaches can be used. Extensile approach, sabre cut, anterior approach through the acromioclavicular joint. Palpate lateral border of acromion and head of humerus. Mark the incision 5–6 cm approx as shown in picture.

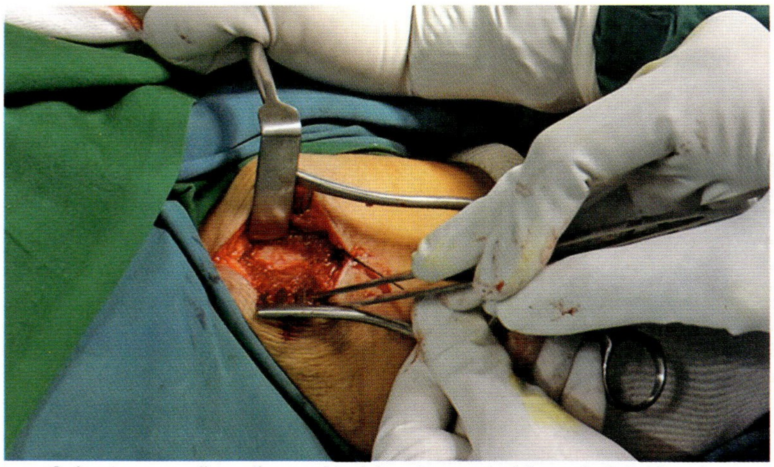

Subcutaneous dissection and incision deepended through deltoid raphe

Fig. 6: Subcutaneous dissection and incision deepened through Deltoid Raphe.

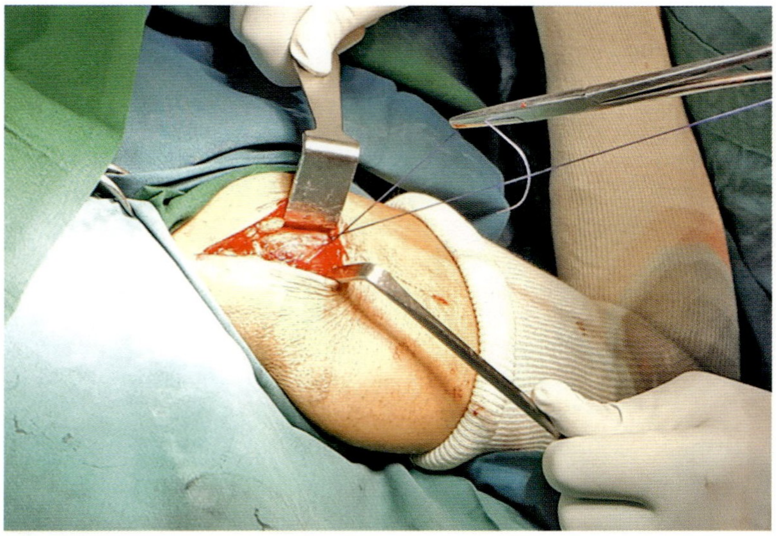

Stay suture in deltoid

Fig. 7: Protective stay suture should be put in Deltoid to prevent accidental Axillary nerve Injury. This is 5 cm distal to acromial origin of deltoid (deltoid split).

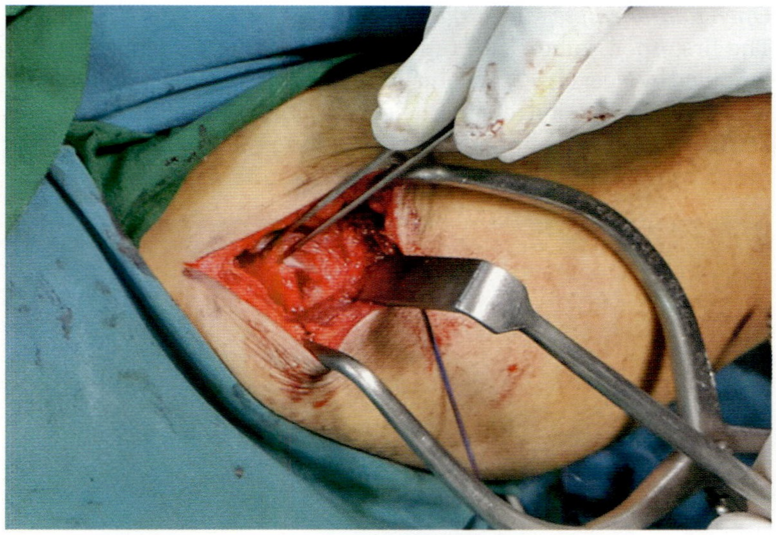

Visualize the cuff defect

Fig. 8: Visualize the cuff defect: The deltoid is split beginning at the acromioclavicular joint. The anterior deltoid is detached about 2 cm off the anterior surface of the acromion from the acromioclavicular joint to the anterolateral corner of acromion. Bursectomy is performed. The subacromial bursa is differentiated from the cuff by rotating the humerus. On internal rotation the posterior margin of the cuff and the edge of the bursa can be identified. Two heads of Deltoid muscle retracted and humeral head exposed and defect Identified. Defect Identification is facilitated by internal and external rotation that brings posterior and anterior edge of defect into view. Identify the shape of the tendon tear, the tendon which are involved in the extent of retraction and presence of intratendinous tears/split. The split is repaired prior to commencement of cuff tear repair. The torn cuff is mobilized by suture through the torn cuff rather than using clamps. The biceps tendon is examined and dealt with appropriately tendons if excessively frayed or torn and incorporated in cuff tear defect repair if the defect is significant.

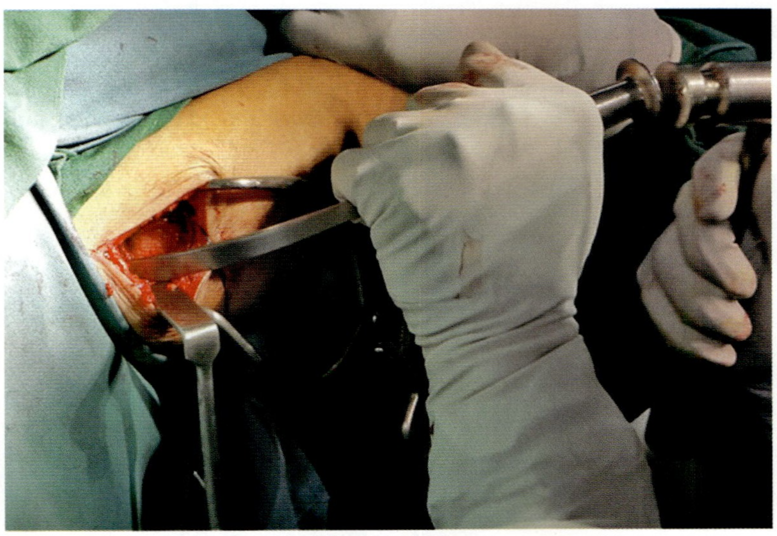

Acromioplasty

Fig. 9: Acromioplasty: Acromioplasty should be done by using nibbler and osteotome. During decompression the coracoacromial bands are identified. Traction on the arm opens the subacromial place. The undersurface of the acromion is palpated to identify shape of the acromion, slope, irregular surface and osteophytes, subacromial adhesion are broken by a sweeping finger and removed. The acromioplasty is done by an osteotome levering down the humeral head. The acromion protruding from anterior portion of acromioclavicular joint is removed. The thickness of the anterior wedge of the acromion can be upto 1 cm depending on the thickness of the spur and the acromion. A file is used if required, to smoothen the undersurface of acromion. Adequacy of acromioplasty is confirmed by forward elevation of arm. More extensive AC joint excision (shaving off of inferior surface of AC joint) is done if there is associated AC arthritis with inferior osteophyte or increased exposure for a massive rotator cuff tear with retraction is required.

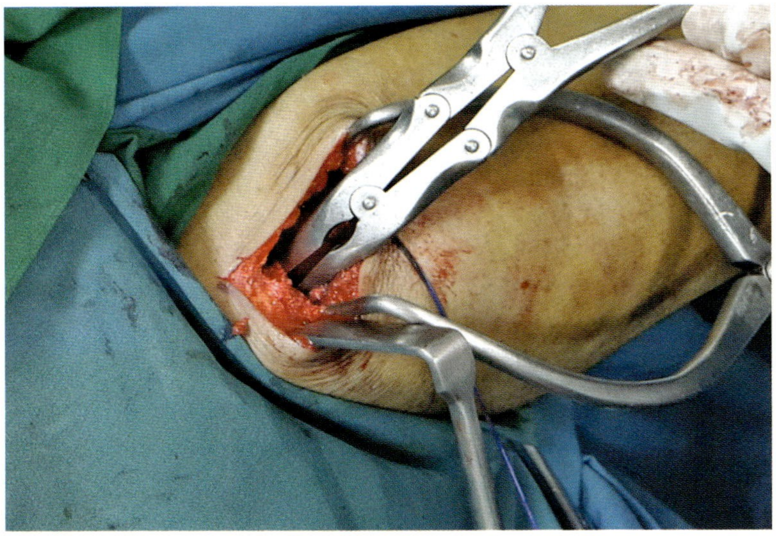

Foot print preparation

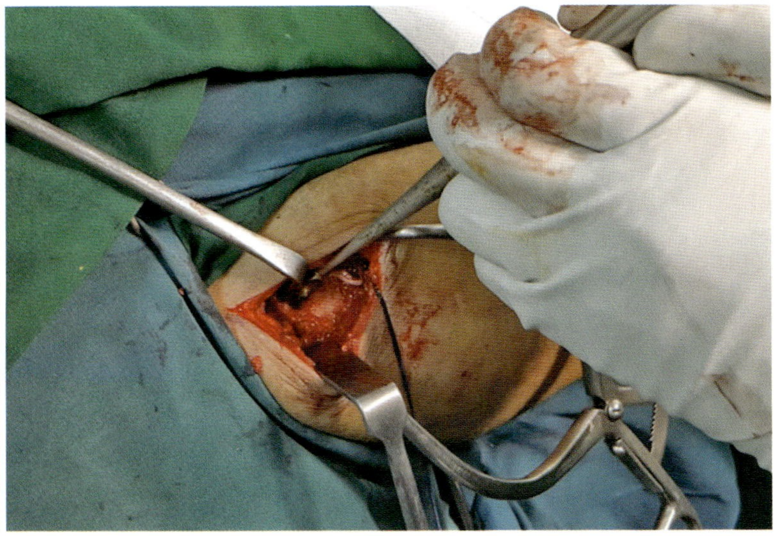

Foot print preparation

Figs. 10 and 11: Footprint preparation: Footprint is identified and decorticated. A trough about 2–3 mm, deep is prepared. After the bony trough is made, any bony projection on the greater tuberosity are nibbled/trimmed with nibbler, drill, and osteotome, etc. taking care to maintain the cortical bridge of greater tuberosity. Torn edges of Rotator Cuff brought into field by humeral rotation and stay sutures taken. Using stay sutures torn edges pulled forward and adhesions released by blunt dissection. Avoid too deep dissection inferiorly near teres minor and near spinoglenoid notch to avoid nerve injuries.

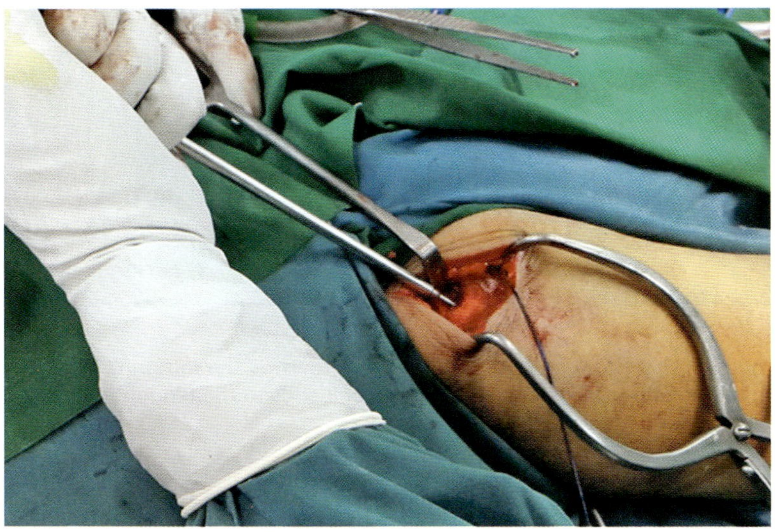

Suture anchor introduction

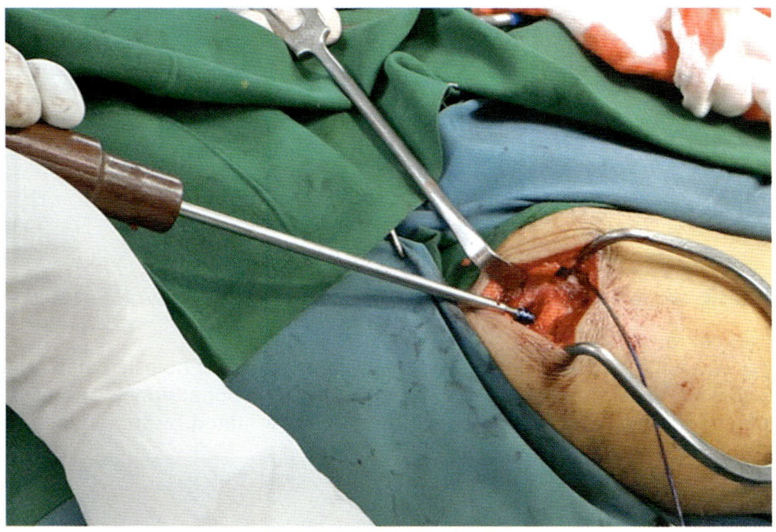

Suture anchor introduction

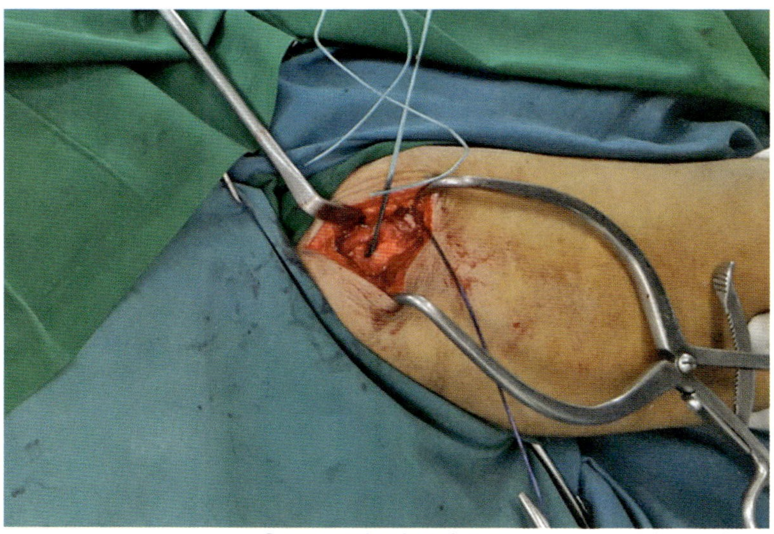

Suture anchor introduction

Figs. 12 to 14: Suture anchors Introduction: Suture anchor combined with bone tunnels and lateral row repair create a more secure repair. Suture anchor are inserted in the decorticated greater tuberosity. Suture anchor are inserted 1 cm apart. (Here titanium bone anchors with No. 2 Nonabsorbable suture material is used.)

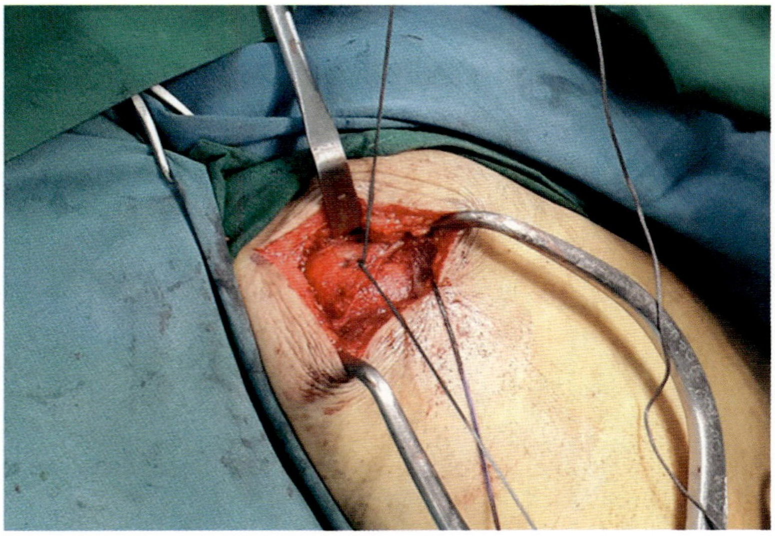

Fig. 15: Repair of rotator cuff is done by suturing the torn edges together.

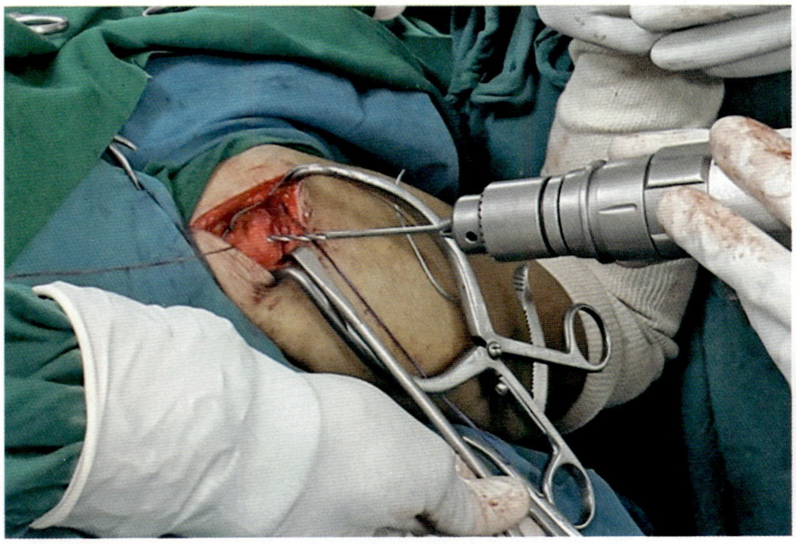

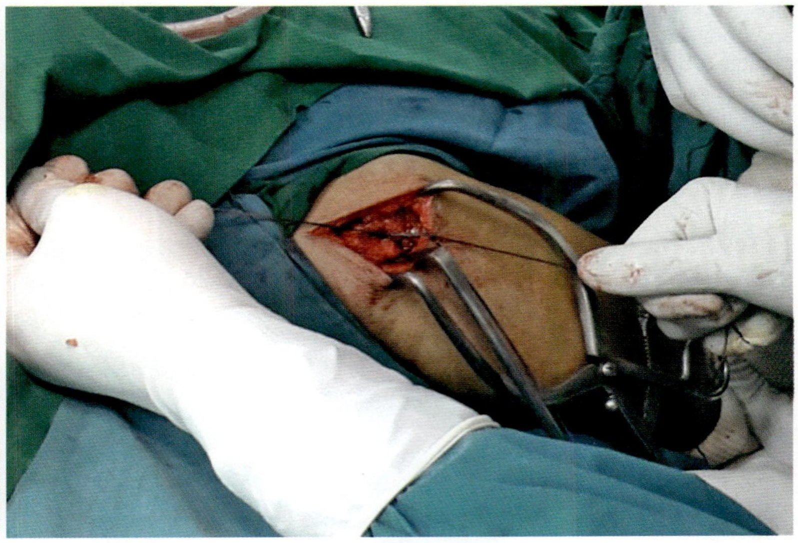

Figs. 16 and 17: Lateral row repair: As an alternative drill holes created over outer aspect of greater tuberosity aiming towards the footprint, 1 cm apart and 2–3 cm distal to the footprint. The initially placed bone tunnels and passing the nonabsorbable suture in a figure of 8 adds to the tendon-bone surface contact ending a more secure repair. This step is facilitated by some type of suture passer.

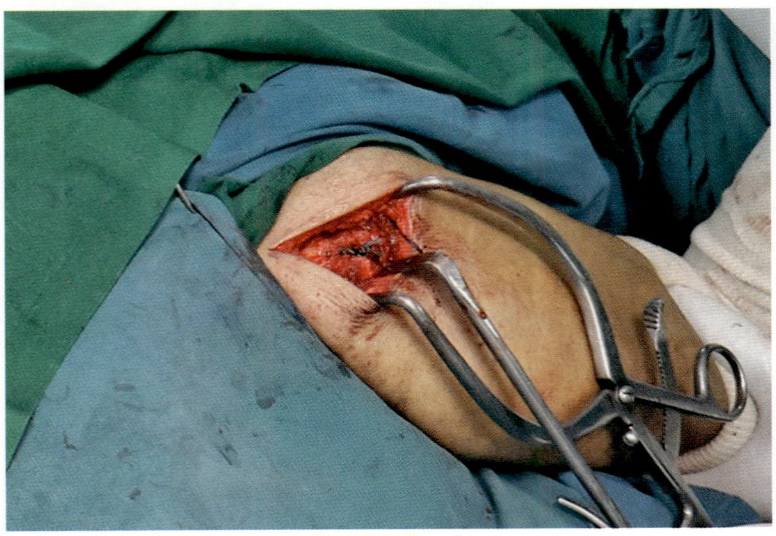

Fig. 18: Complete repair: After the repair is completed with the arm in neutral position and neutral rotation the joint is cautiously flexed and the humerus externally rotated to asses the tightness of the repair and adequacy of decompression. The wound is thoroughly irrigated, the deltoid split is repair.

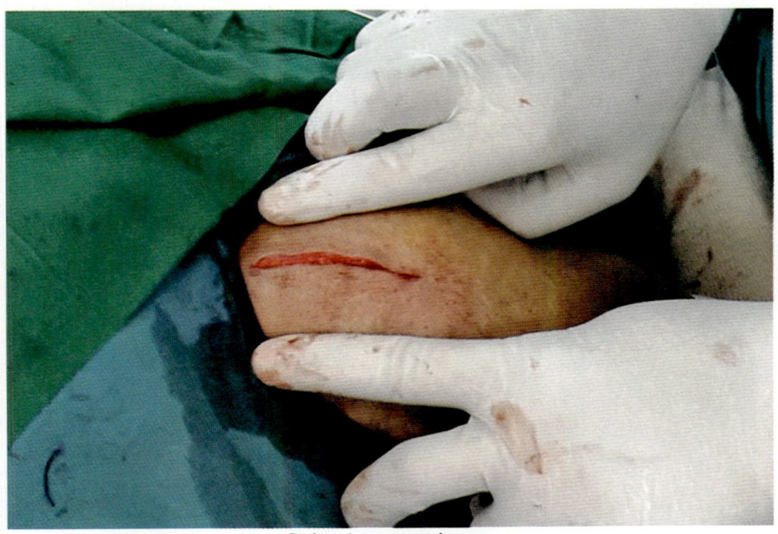

Fig. 19: Subcutaneus closure.

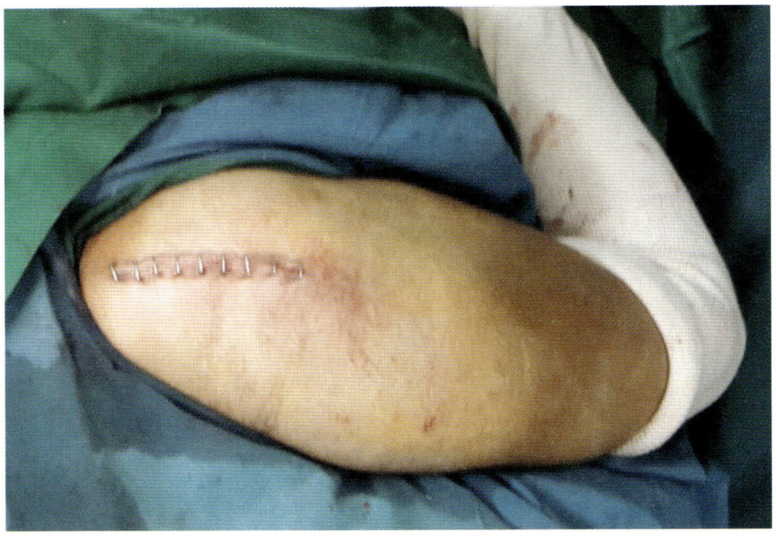

Skin closure

Fig. 20: Skin closure.

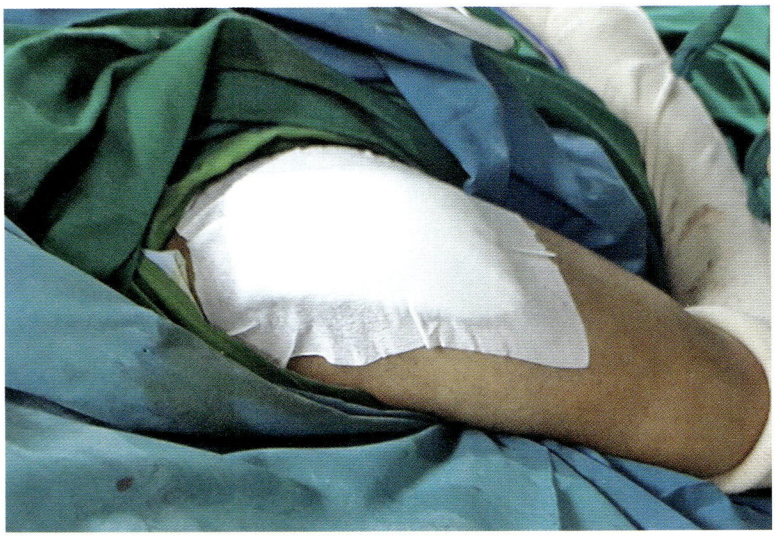

Dressing

Fig. 21: Dressing.

REHABILITATION

We keep upper limb in shoulder RH immobilizer for 3 weeks with early start of elbow, wrist, and hand range of motion (ROM), shoulder shrugs, and scapular retraction. After 3 weeks, we start with pendulum exercises, active and active-assisted ROM till 6–8 weeks. Once full range of motion is achieved, one can begin strengthening exercises for rotator cuff.

COMPLICATIONS

- Recurrence or repair failure
- Deltoid detachment
- Axillary nerve injury
- Suprascapular nerve injury
- Infection
- Stiffness.

SUGGESTED READING

1. Duquin TR, Buyea C, Bisson LJ. Which method of rotator cuff repair leads to the highest rate of structural healing? A systematic review. Am J Sports Med. 2010;38:835-41.
2. Morse K, Davis AD, Afra R, et al. Arthroscopic versus mini-open rotator cuff repair: a comprehensive review and meta-analysis. Am J Sports Med. 2008;36:1824-8.
3. Nho SJ, Shindle MK, Sherman SL, et al. Systematic review of arthroscopic rotator cuff repair and mini-open rotator cuff repair. J Bone Joint Surg Am. 2007;89:127-36.
4. Verma NN, Dunn W, Adler RS, et al. All-arthroscopic versus mini-open rotator cuff repair: a retrospective review with minimum 2-year follow-up. Arthroscopy. 2006;22:587-94.
5. Yamaguchi K, Ball CM, Galatz LM. Arthroscopic rotator cuff repair; transition from mini-open to all-arthroscopic. Clin Orthop Relat Res. 2001;390:83-94.
6. Yamaguchi K. Mini-open rotator cuff repair: an updated perspective. Instr Course Lect. 2001;50:53-61.

CHAPTER 78

Distal Biceps Tendon Rupture Repair

Vijay M Panchanadikar, Anurag Daxini, Snehal Dantkale

INTRODUCTION

Distal biceps rupture is a rare condition as compared to proximal ones. It occurs in young adults due to eccentric extension load applied to a flexed elbow. Patients usually present with mild pain, history of popping sound, and bulge in affected arm. Diagnosis is clinical with easy to diagnose clinical tests, such as Hook test and Popeye sign and confirmed by ultrasonography (USG) or magnetic resonance imaging (MRI). The condition is a challenging entity to an orthopaedic surgeon; different surgeons prefer different techniques each having its own merits and demerits. Results of surgical repair of this injury are better than conservative treatment. No clear advantage is credited to either one incision suture anchor or two incision technique. With two incision technique, the retracted end of the tendon is brought down and braided with heavy nonabsorbable suture, the tendon is then pulled through the posterolateral incision and the tendon stump buried in a trap door made over the radial tuberosity. Prompt diagnosis and surgical repair ensure superior functional outcomes.

ACUTE DISTAL BICEPS RUPTURE: OPERATIVE STEPS (FIGS. 1 TO 21)

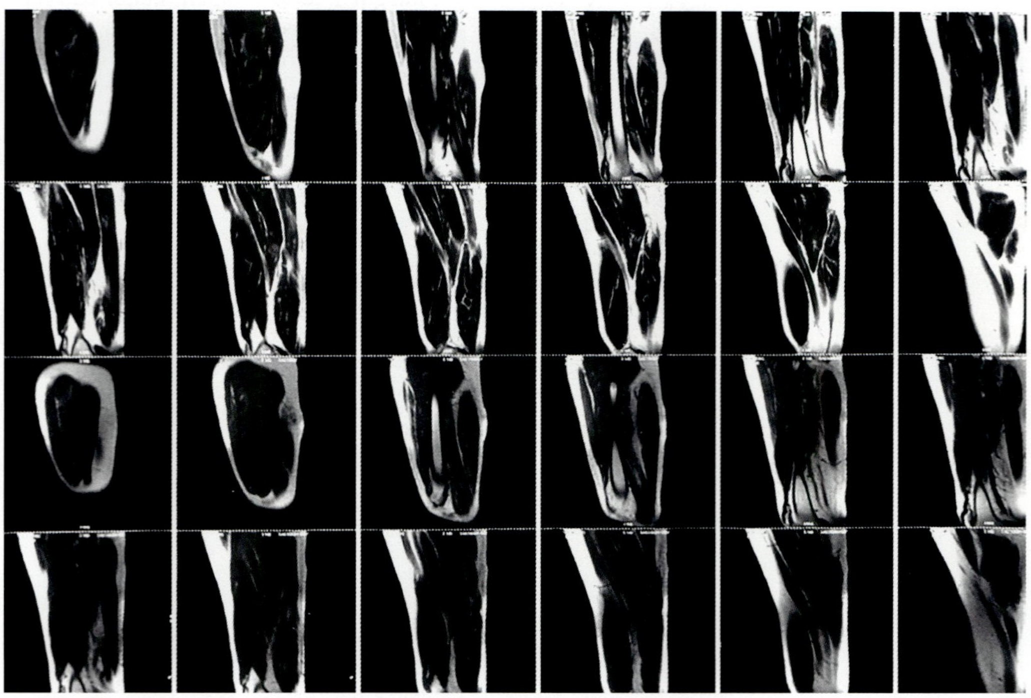

Fig. 1: Magnetic resonance imaging (MRI) report showing complete tear of distal biceps.

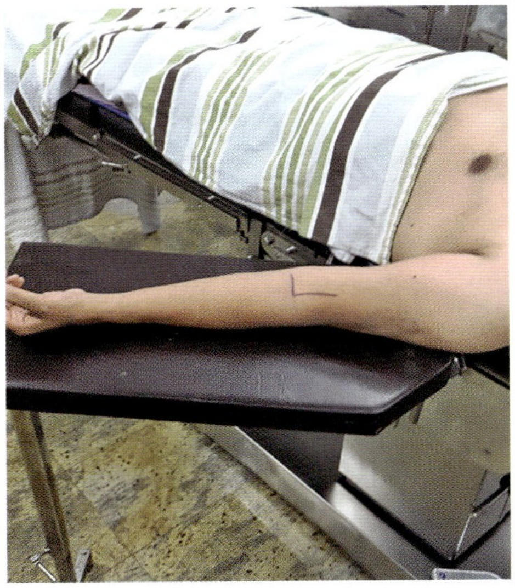

Fig. 2: Position of the patient on table.

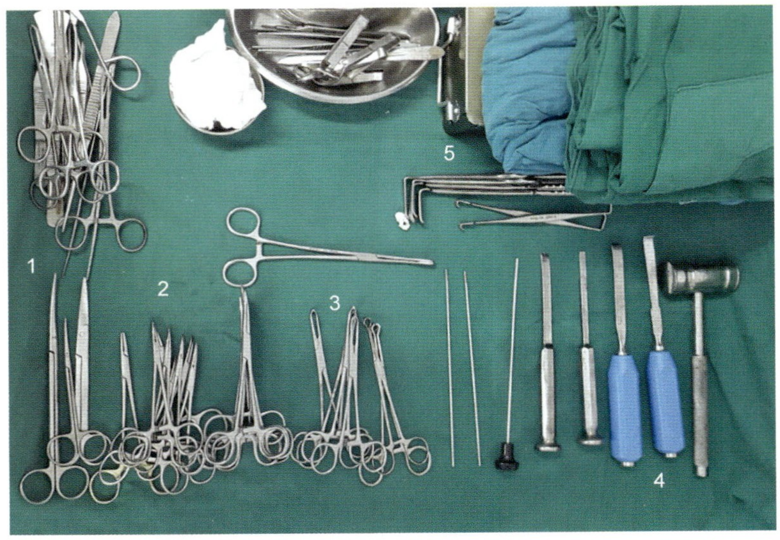

Fig. 3: Trolley with various sets of instruments required (1—curved and straight scissors, 2—artery hemostat, 3—Allis and Babcock forceps, 4—osteotome hammer, 5—retractors). Small curved Mayo needles are also required.

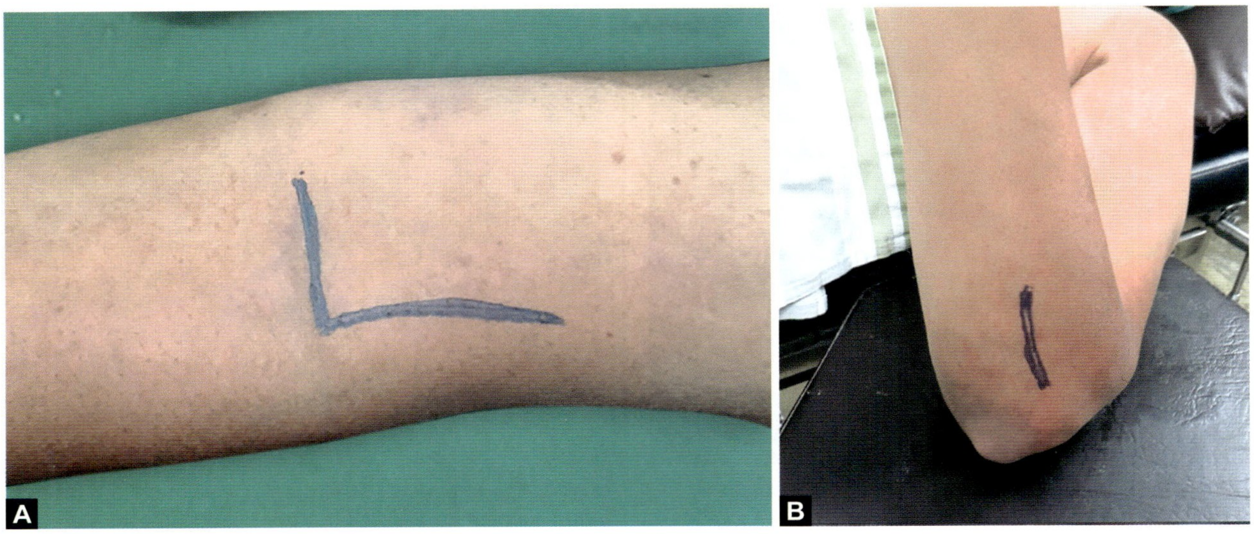

Figs. 4A and B: Double skin incision technique used and skin incision marked. While deepening the anterior L incision take care to avoid injury to the lateral antebrachial cutaneous nerve.

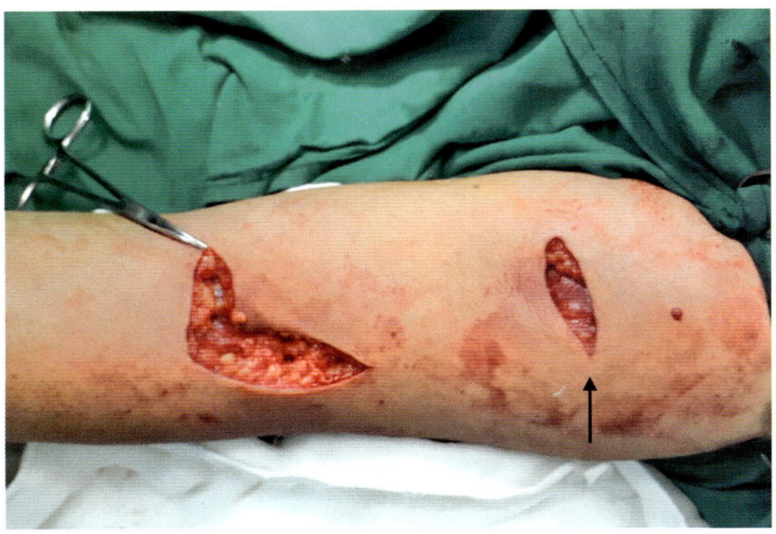

Fig. 5: Another incision taken proximally to locate the retracted end of the ruptured biceps tendon.

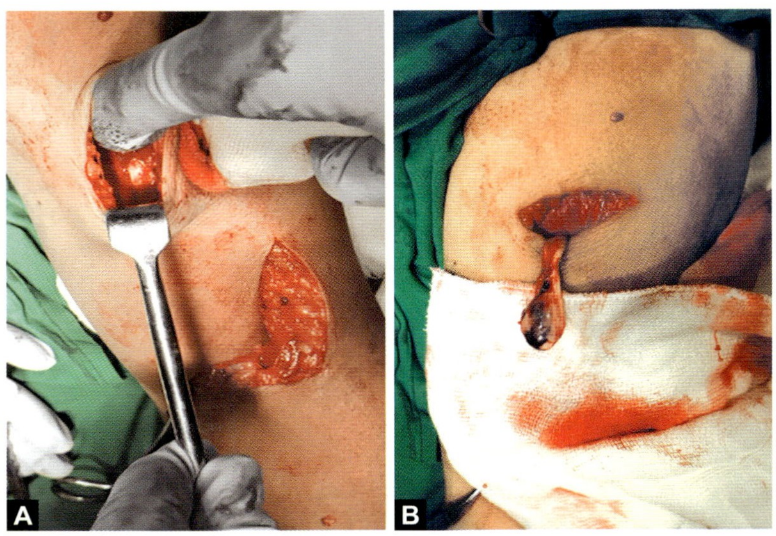

Figs. 6A and B: Retracted tendon located.

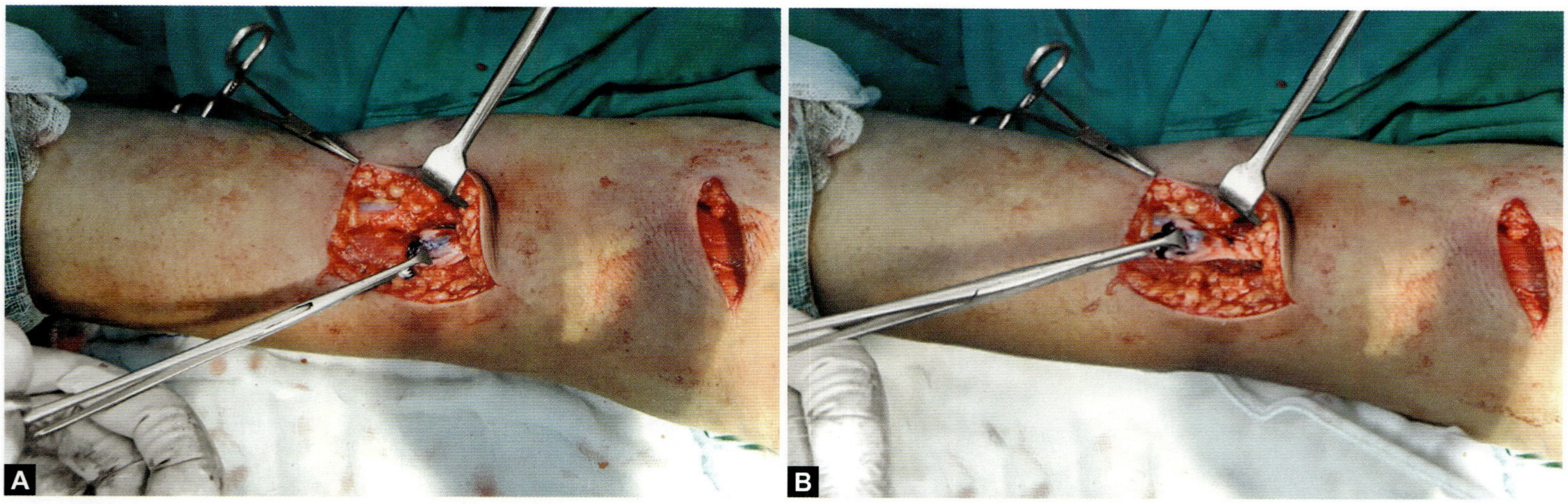

Figs. 7A and B: Ruptured tendon brought out through the anterior L-shaped incision over elbow.

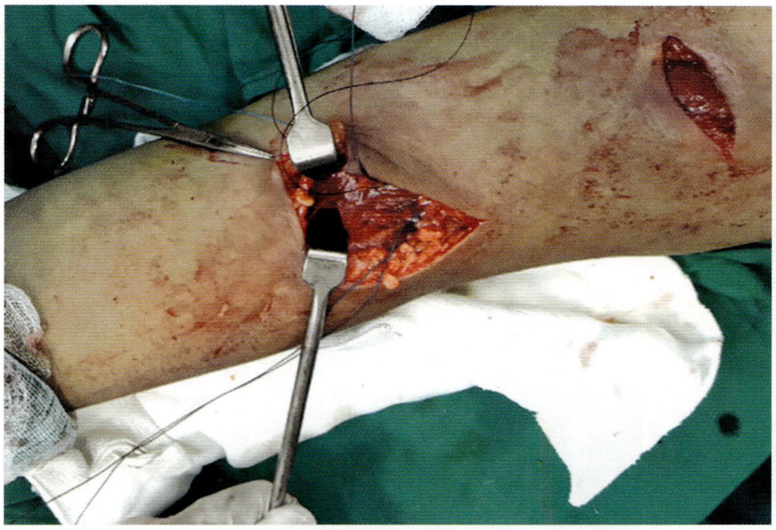

Fig. 8: The ruptured tendon braided with nonabsorbable suture material to facilitate its fixation.

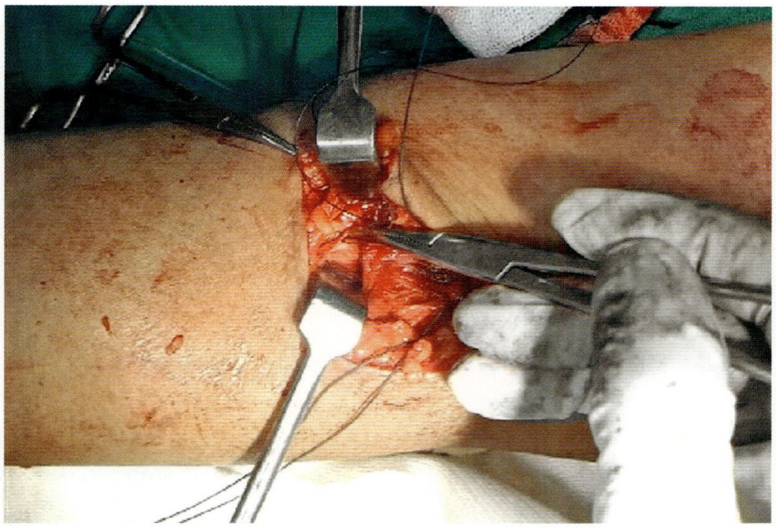

Fig. 9: The interval between radius and ulna identified by blunt dissection with hemostat and radial tuberosity located. Carefully avoid adjacent neurovascular structures.

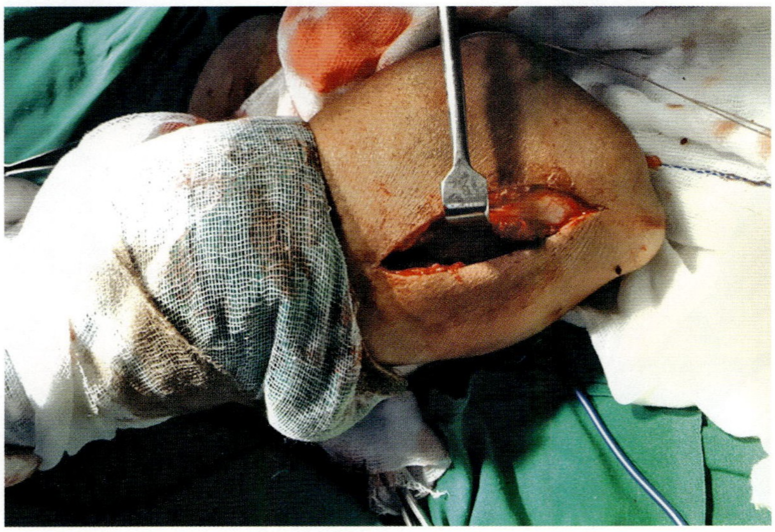

Fig. 10: The second incision taken over the posterolateral surface of proximal forearm.

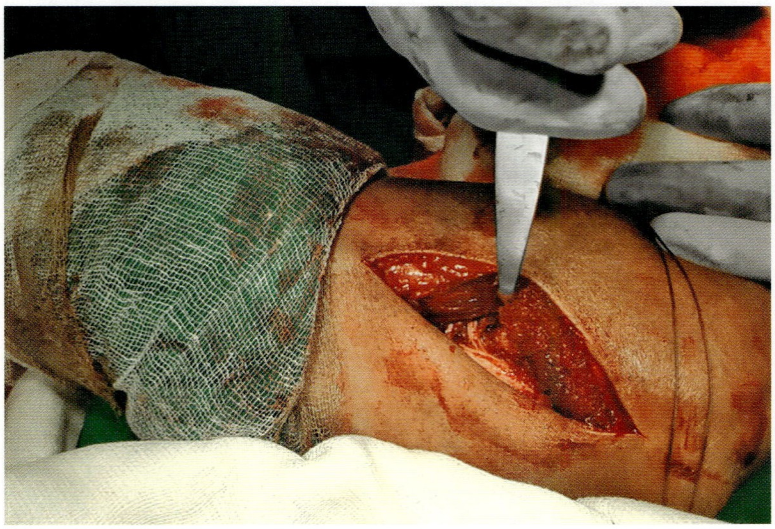

Fig. 11: Anconeus muscle is elevated off ulna.

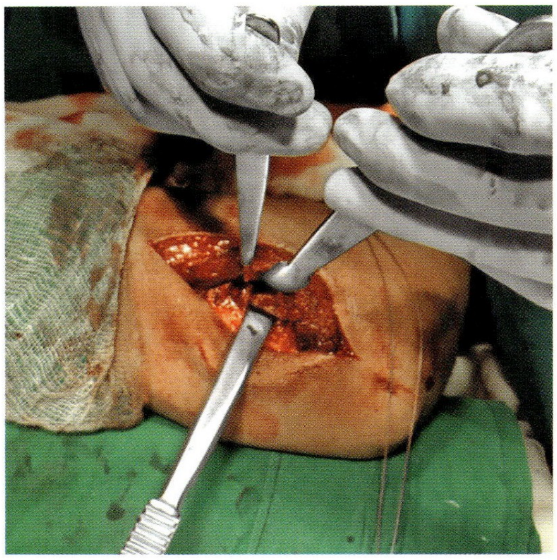

Fig. 12: Judicious use of spike retractors exposes this area well, which is otherwise difficult.

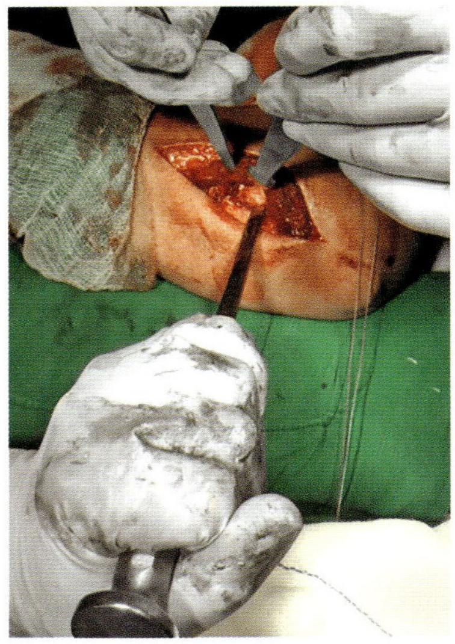

Fig. 13: With forearm fully pronated to bring radial tuberosity in view trap door is made over tuberosity by use of narrow osteotome. Drill bit use to be avoided for fear of raising bone dust that may later contribute to radioulnar synostosis.

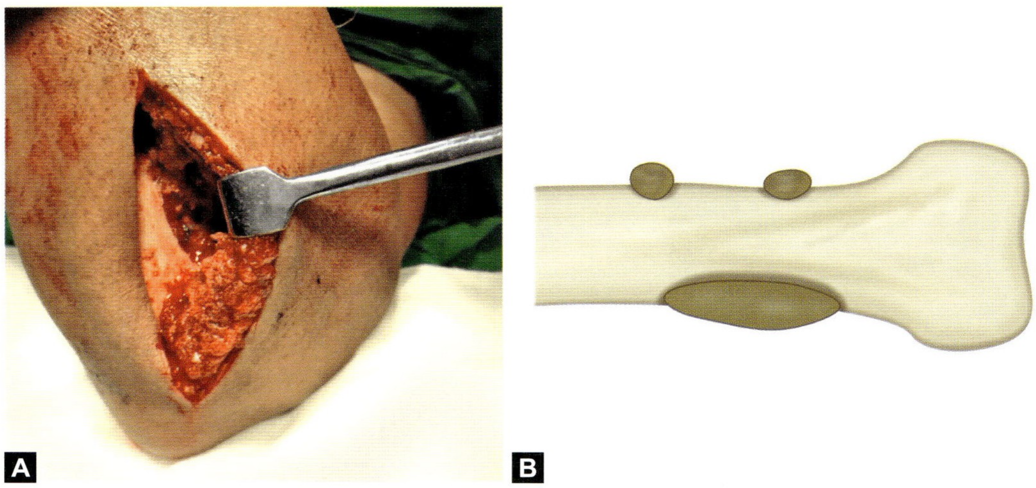

Figs. 14A and B: The trapdoor is clearly seen. (A) Two holes are made opposite trapdoor preferably with K-wires with forearm in supination; (B) Ensure wide bone bridge.

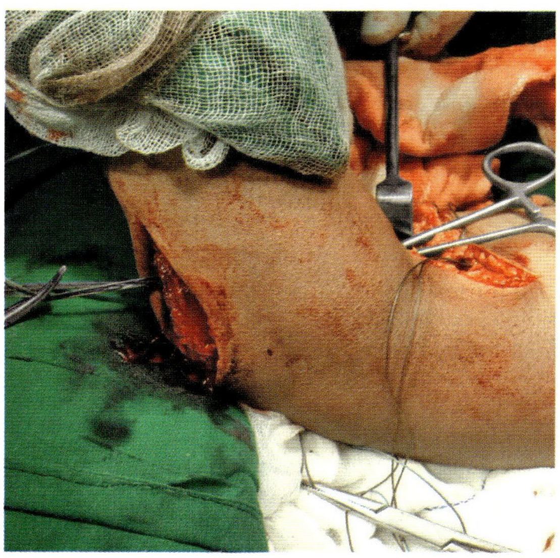

Fig. 15: The braided nonabsorbable sutures of the tendon are delivered bluntly by a hemostat into the second incision and kept aside.

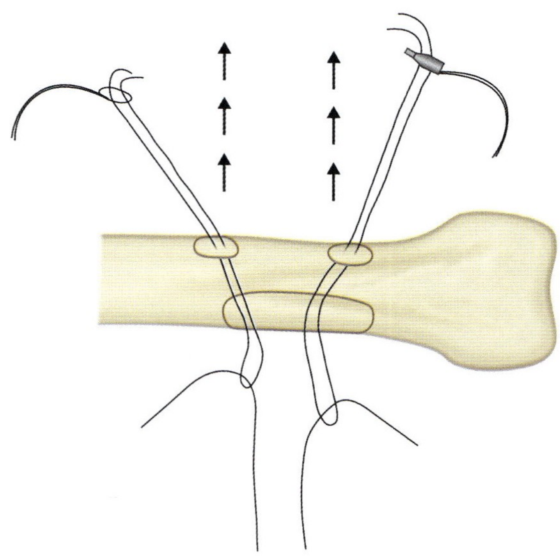

Fig. 16: Two nylon loops on small curved needles (various sizes to be kept available on table) passed from trapdoor out through holes, one loop through each hole. Straight suture passers are not useful in this narrow cramped area. Alternatively, small curved hemostats are used to "push" or "retrieve" the loops.

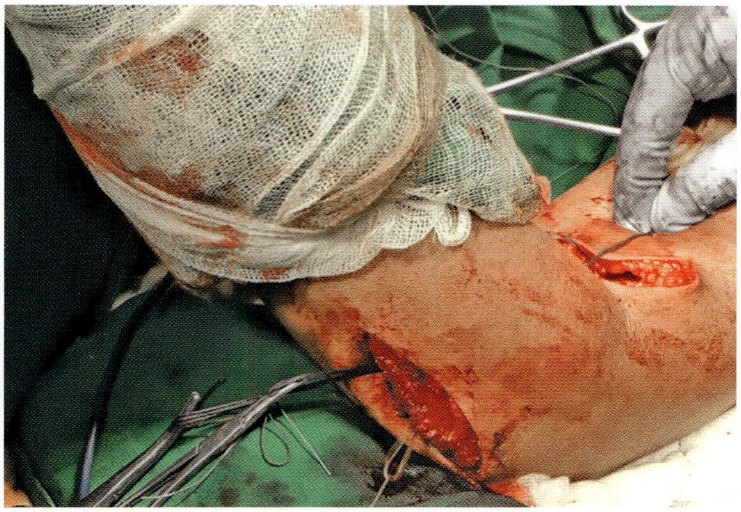

Fig. 17: The previously kept aside braided nonabsorbable sutures of the biceps tendon are now fed to the nylon loops, each into one loop.

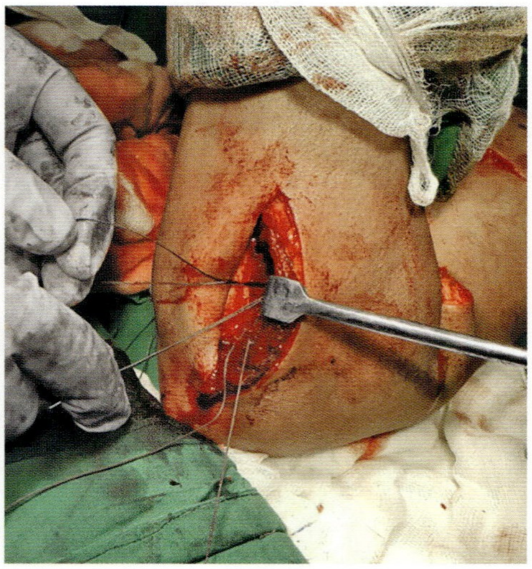

Fig. 18: Suture ends are brought out through the holes by pulling out nylon loops. Care is taken to ensure that tendon stump is buried in trapdoor and nonabsorbable sutures are pulled out taut.

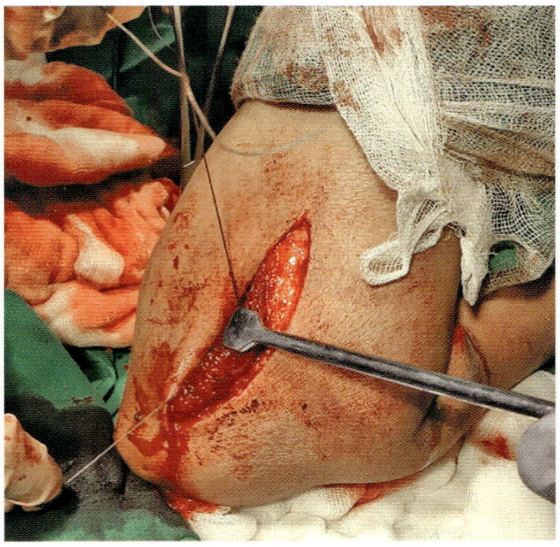

Fig. 19: Knots are tied in full supination and partial flexion, and position secured. The trapdoor is then closed.

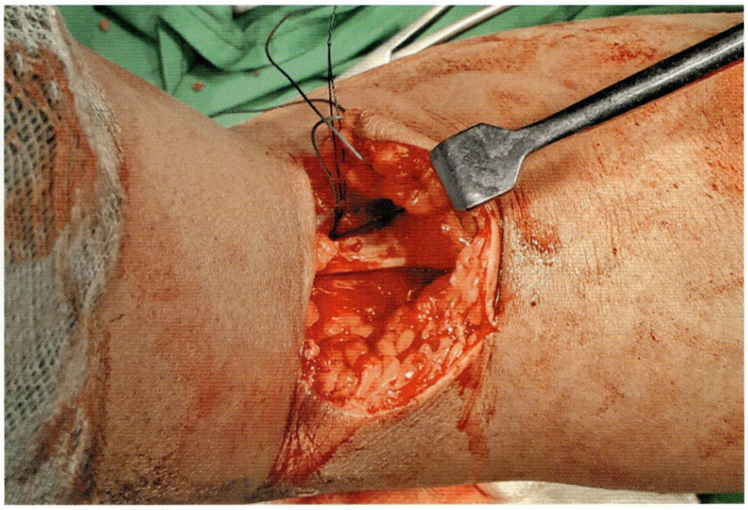

Fig. 20: The taut refixed biceps tendon is seen.

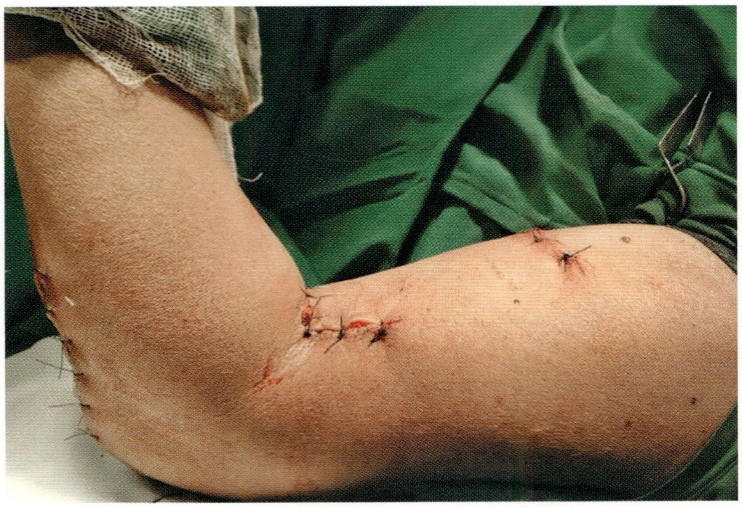

Fig. 21: Final skin closure with nonabsorbable suture material.

COMPLICATIONS

- Infection
- Rerupture
- Neurovascular injury, more specifically lateral antebrachial cutaneous nerve palsy more common after one incision technique
- Loss of strength of supination and flexion
- Proximal radioulnar synostosis is reportedly more common after two-incision technique.

POSTOPERATIVE PROTOCOL

Patient's arm is immobilized in above elbow slab with elbow in 90° for a period till sutures removed. After that, a hinged brace is given to be worn for a month and intermittent passive flexion and active extension exercise is allowed. Full range of motion (ROM) is usually achieved in 4–6 weeks. Return to normal activity is restricted till 4 months.

SUGGESTED READING

1. Failla JM, Amadio PC, Morrey BF, et al. Proximal radioulnar synostosis after repair of distal biceps brachii rupture by the two-incision technique. Report of four cases. Clin Orthop Relat Res. 1990;(253):133-6.
2. Kelly EW, Morrey BF, O'Driscoll SW. Complications of repair of the distal biceps tendon with the modified two-incision technique. J Bone Joint Surg Am. 2000;82-A(11):1575-81.
3. Ward JP, Shreve MC, Youm T, et al. Ruptures of the distal biceps tendon. Bull Hosp Jt Dis. 2014;72(1):110-9.

CHAPTER 79

Core Decompression for Avascular Necrosis of Femoral Head

Chandrashekhar Dixit, Vinay Gautam

INTRODUCTION

Avascular necrosis (AVN), many a times called as osteonecrosis, as there is necrosis of bone cells because of ischemia, is a relatively common disease described by death of cellular elements of bone or marrow. Femoral head is one of the most common sites of involvement. Treatment of earlier stage of AVN of hip is debatable. Hip core decompression surgery is one of the options for early stages of AVN of hip.

CLASSIFICATION OF AVASCULAR NECROSIS HIP

Ficat and Arlet classification of avascular necrosis of femoral head:

- *Stage 0*:
  - *Plain radiograph*: Normal
  - *Magnetic resonance imaging (MRI)*: Normal
  - *Clinical symptoms*: Nil.
- *Stage I*:
  - *Plain radiograph*: Normal or minor osteopenia
  - *MRI*: Edema
  - *Bone scan*: Increased uptake
  - *Clinical symptoms*: Pain typically in the groin.
- *Stage II*:
  - *Plain radiograph*: Mixed osteopenia and/or sclerosis and/or subchondral cysts, without any subchondral lucency (crescent sign)
  - *MRI*: Geographic defect
  - *Bone scan*: Increased uptake
  - *Clinical symptoms*: Pain and stiffness.
- *Stage III*:
  - *Plain radiograph*: Crescent sign and eventual cortical collapse
  - *MRI*: Same as plain radiograph
  - *Clinical symptoms*: Pain and stiffness ± radiation to knee and limp.
- *Stage IV*:
  - *Plain radiograph*: End-stage with evidence of secondary degenerative change
  - *MRI*: Same as plain radiograph
  - *Clinical symptoms*: Pain and limp.

CLINICAL FEATURES

Patient is typically asymptomatic in early stage. Patient usually presents with pain in groin and hip. There may be limited range of motion and limp. Associated risk factors should be looked into. Osteoncrosis should always be suspected when patient has pain but his X-rays are normal.

Unilateral cases should always be looked for opposite hip involvement.

RADIOLOGICAL FEATURES

In earlier stage of AVN hip, X-ray [anteroposterior (AP) and frog leg lateral] will look normal and require further imaging. MRI of hip will suggest about involvement of hip and also conclude area of involvement. Both X-rays and MRI help for staging and grading of disease, and bilateral involvement.

Few salient feature which confirms the diagnosis of AVN are:

- Collapse of femoral head
- Sequestrum in subchondral area in weight bearing area (crescent sign)
- Double line sign on T2 image
- Histological confirmation

Bone marrow biopsy, venography and barometric measurement are few invasive test which are rarely used.

TREATMENT OPTIONS

Whatever may be the etiology of the disease, aim of treatment is to prevent subchondral collapse.

It includes:

- *Pharmacological treatment*: Bisphosphonates, lipid-lowering agents, vasoactive substances, and anticoagulants.
- *Biophysical treatment*: Extracorporeal shockwave therapy (ESWT), pulse electromagnetic therapy, and hyperbaric oxygen (HBO) therapy.

- *Surgical treatment*:
  - *Femoral head-sparing procedures*:
    - Core decompression alone
    - Core decompression with bone grafting, biological agents, and tantalum implant
    - Rotational osteotomies (Sugioka).
  - *Femoral head-replacing procedures*:
    - Hip resurfacing procedure
    - Total hip replacement.

SURGICAL STEPS (FIGS. 1 TO 37)

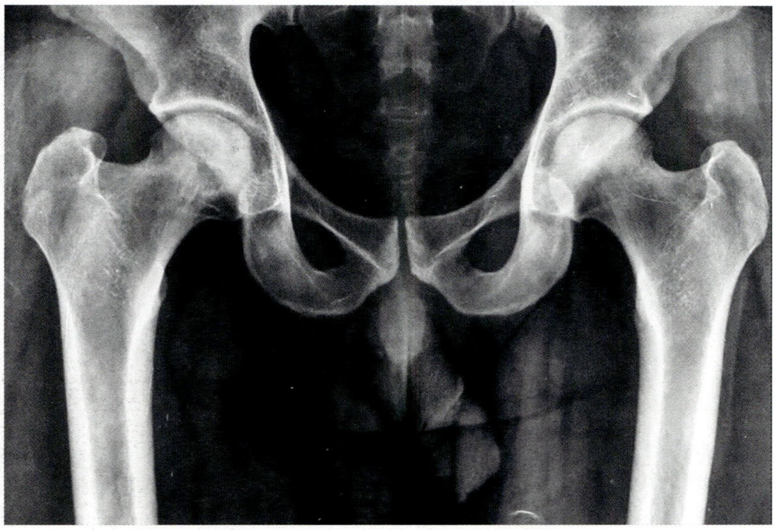

Fig. 1: X-ray pelvis with both hips (PBH) showing bilateral sclerosis of femoral head without flattening or collapse.

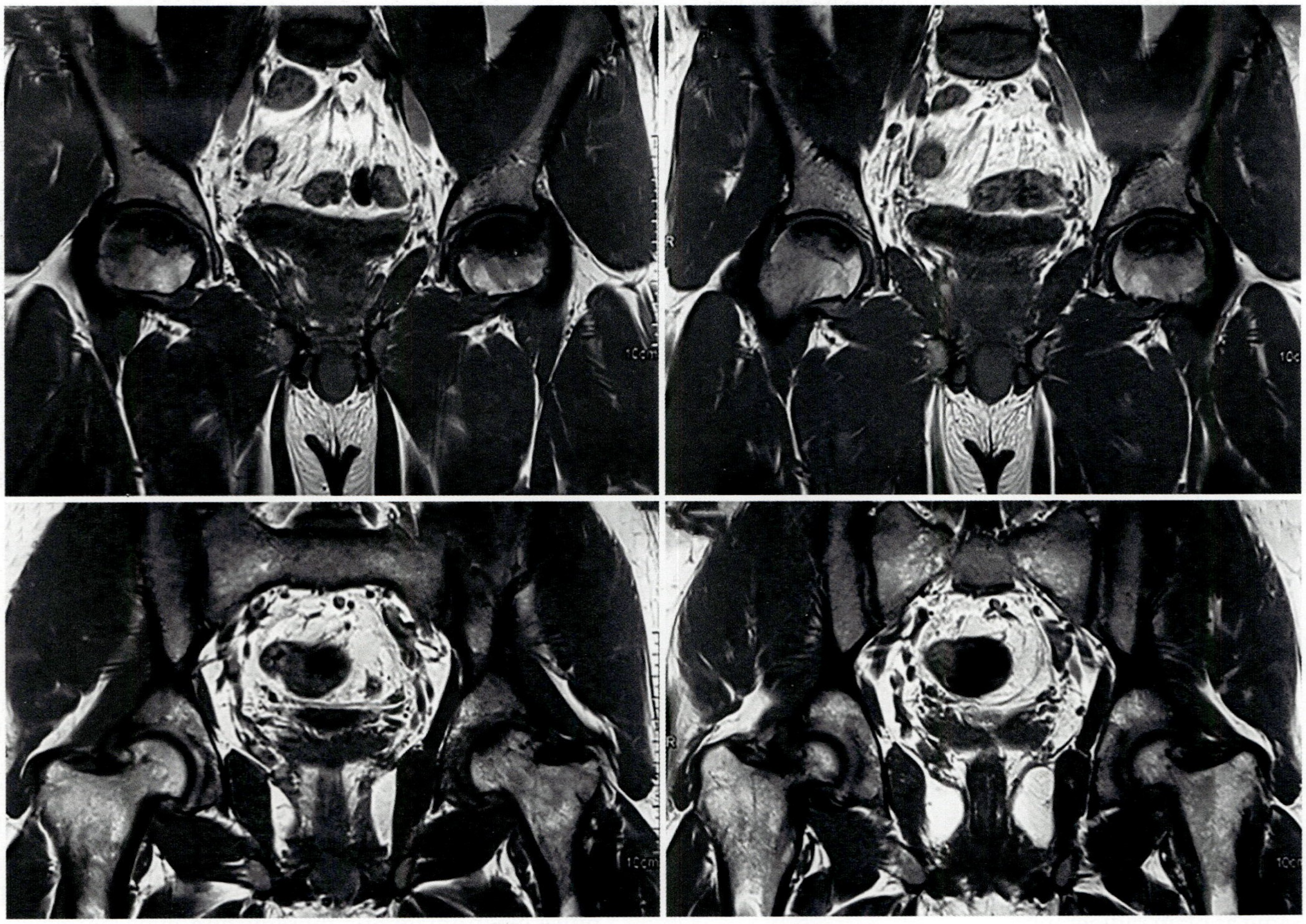

Fig. 2: T1 MRI (magnetic resonance imaging)—coronal section showing hypointense signal in superior area of both femoral heads.

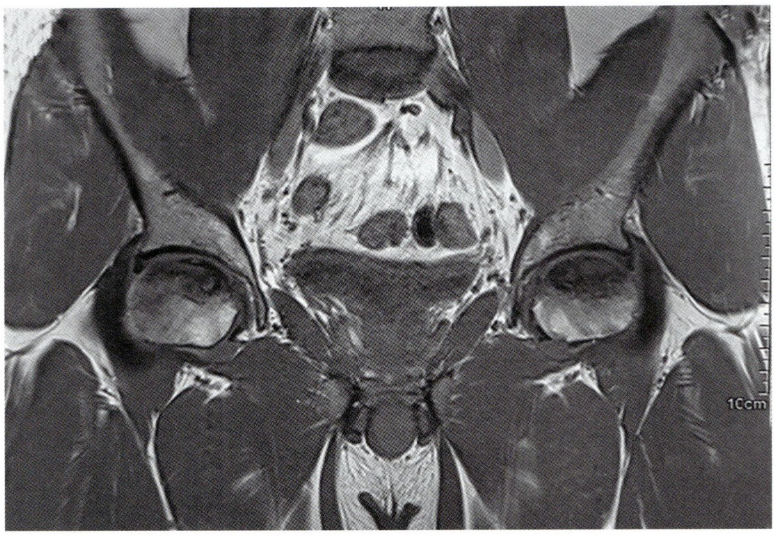

Fig. 3: T1 coronal MRI (magnetic resonance imaging) (zoom).

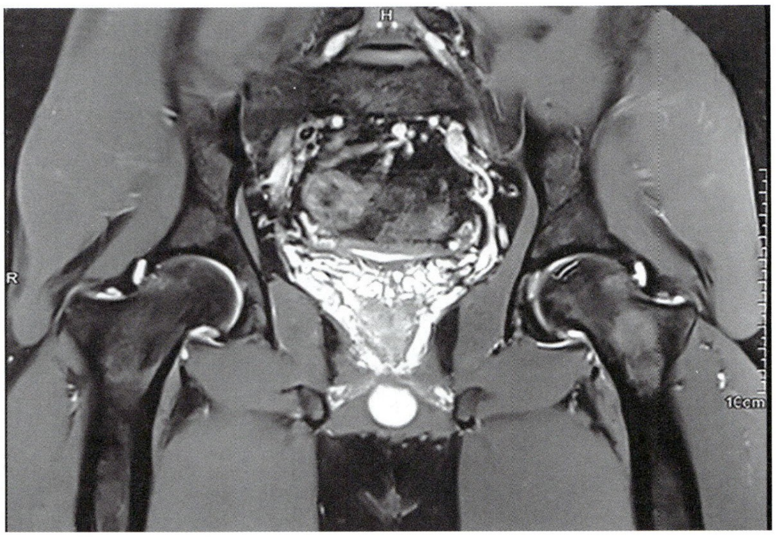

Fig. 4: T2 coronal MRI showing peculiar "double rim sign" in subchondral area left side.

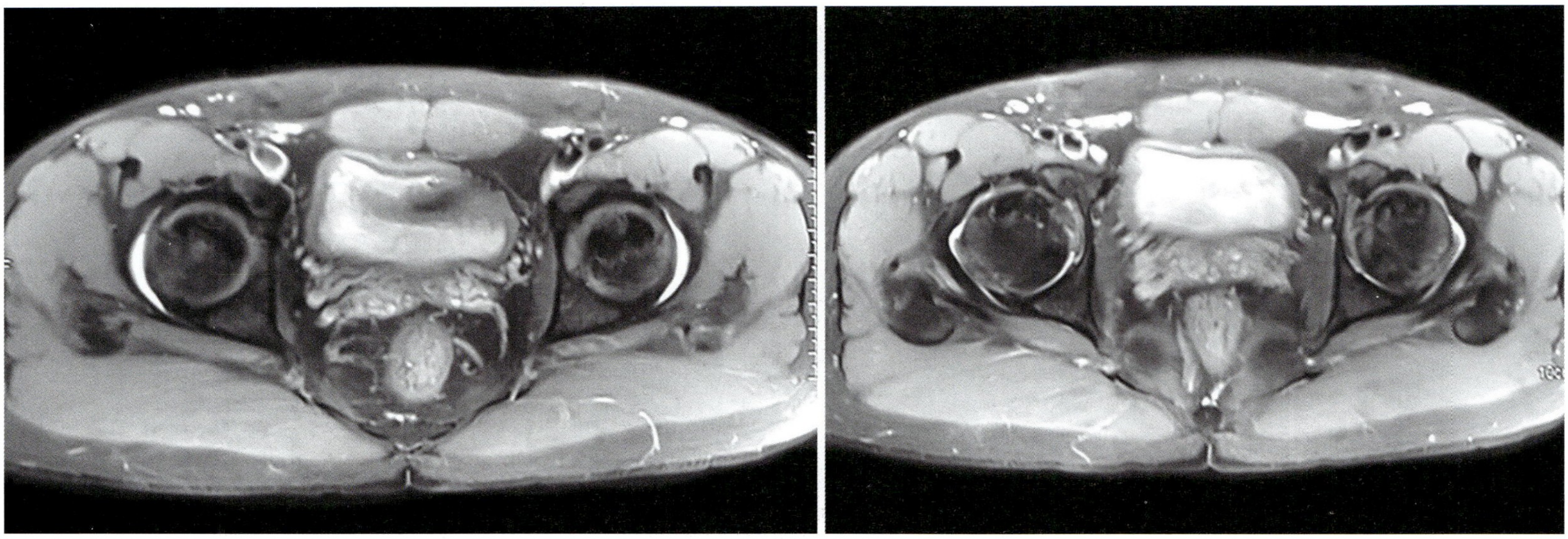

Fig. 5: T2 axial MRI showing hypointense signal in anterior sector of femoral head.

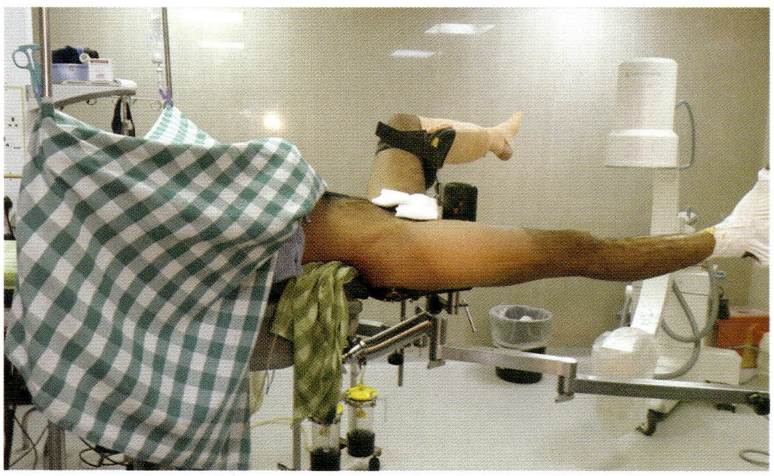

Fig. 6: Position of patient on fracture table after appropriate anesthesia.

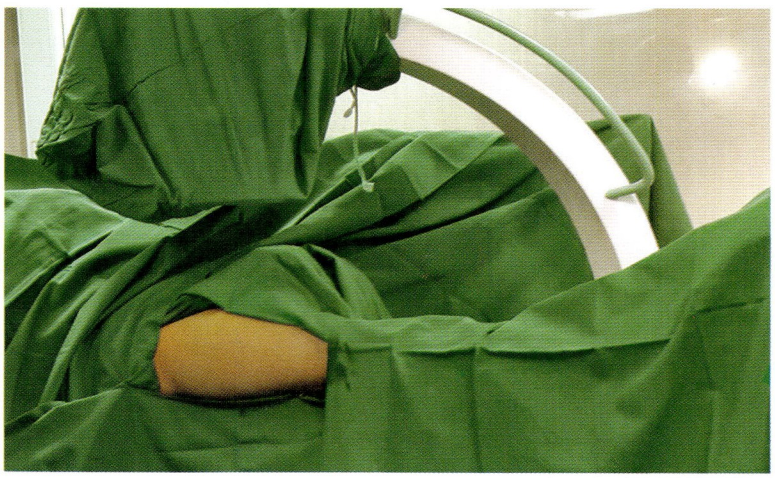

Fig. 7: Position of patient after draping.

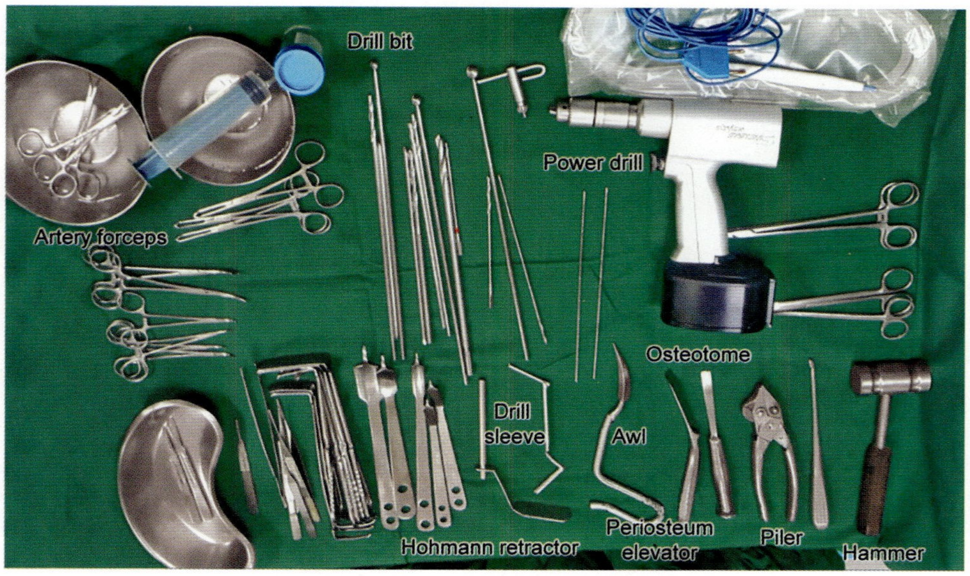

Fig. 8: Complete instrument set required.

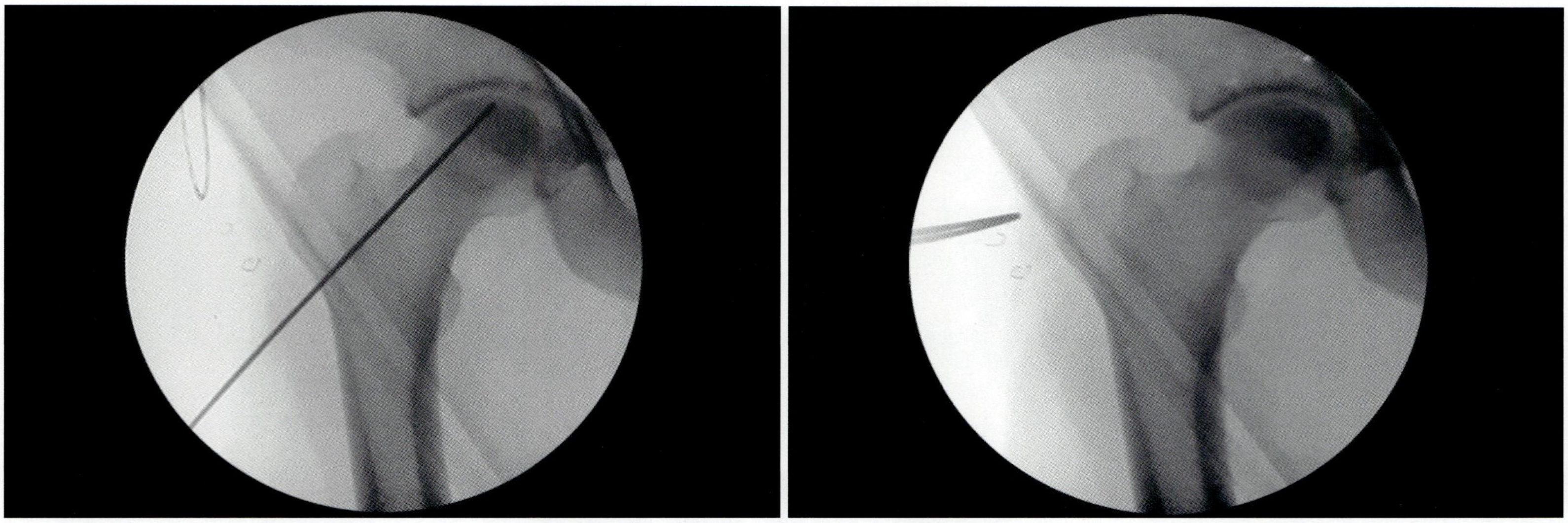

Fig. 9: Check the level of skin incision over image intensifier using guidewire over the anterior body surface.

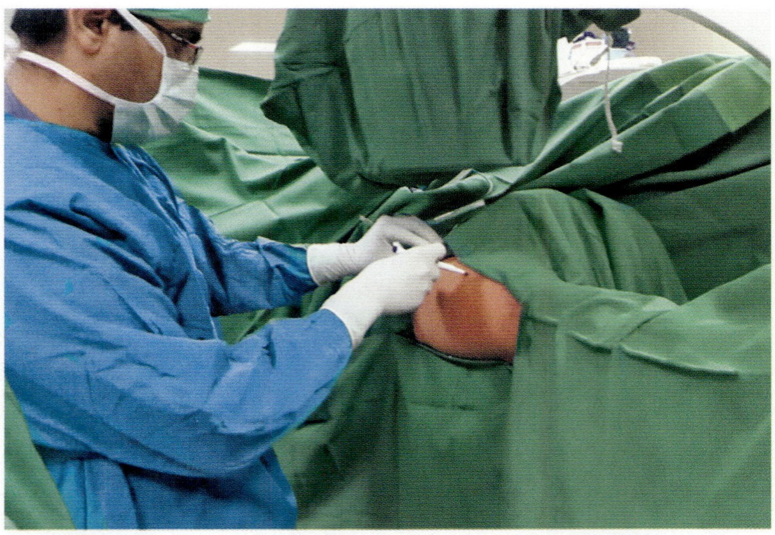

Fig. 10: Check the level of skin incision over image intensifier using guidewire over the anterior body surface.

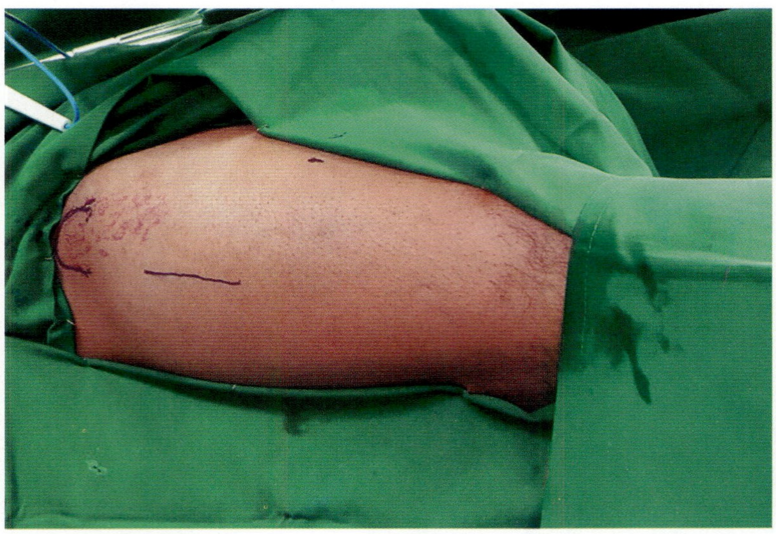

Fig. 11: Marking the skin incision.

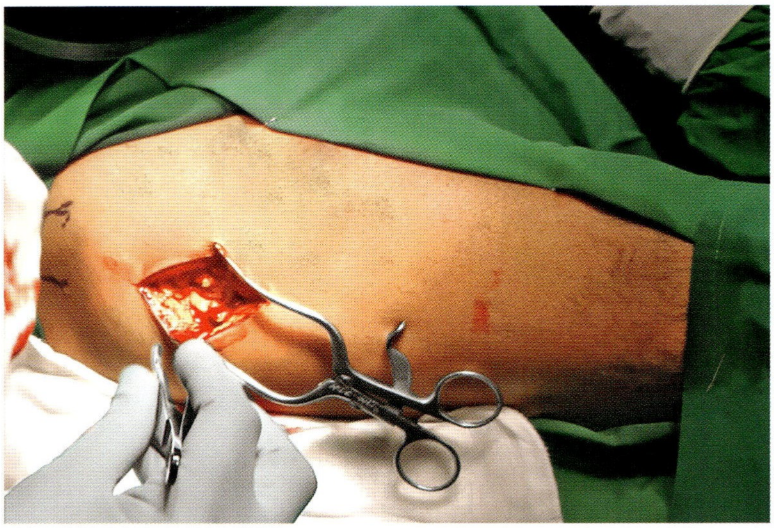

Fig. 12: Skin and superficial fascia incised.

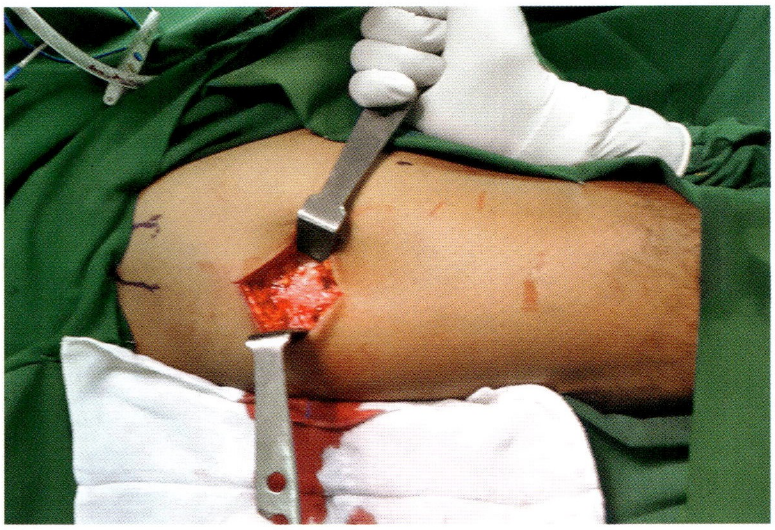

Fig. 13: Tensor fascia lata exposed.

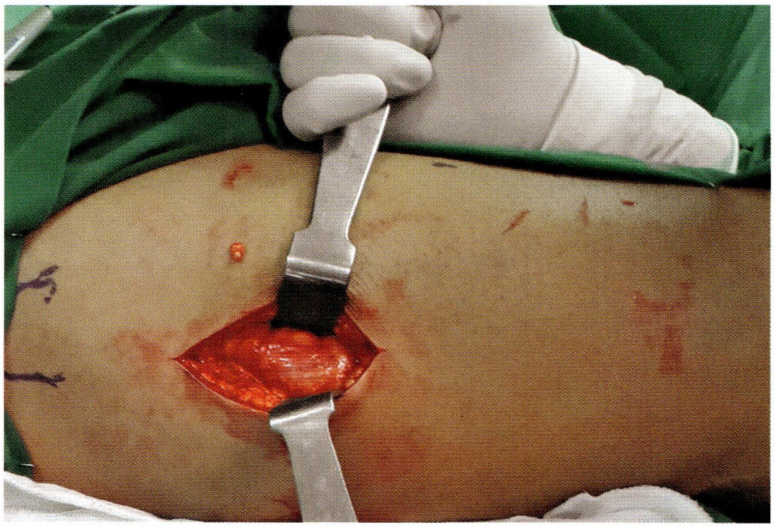

Fig. 14: Tensor fascia lata incised and vastus lateralis exposed.

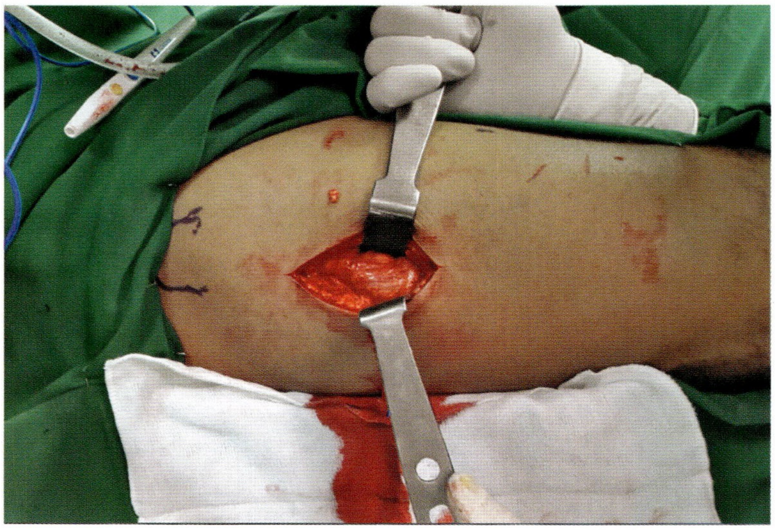

Fig. 15: Attempts made to separate posterior border of vastus to elevate it anteriorly.

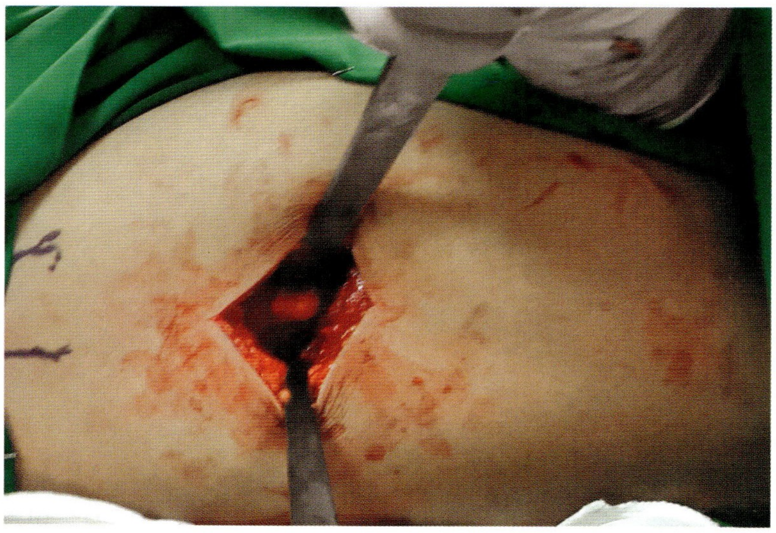

Fig. 16: Lateral aspect of femur reached after elevating vastus.

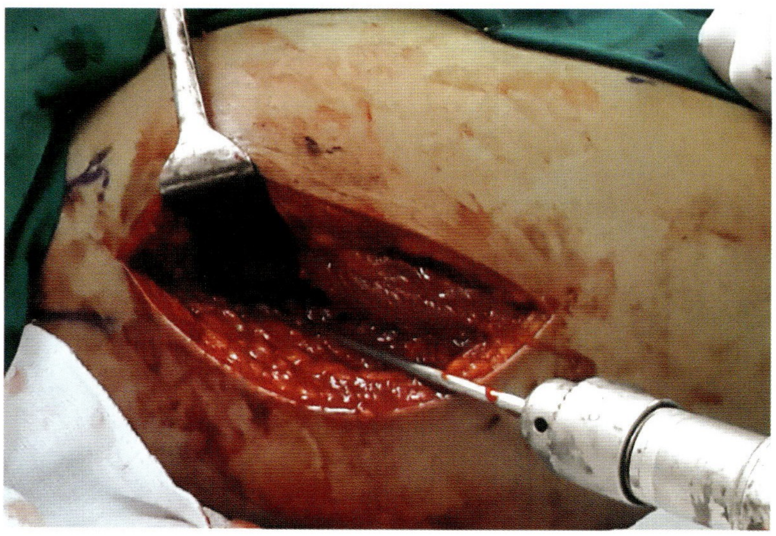

Fig. 17: 3.5-mm long drill bit at starting point.

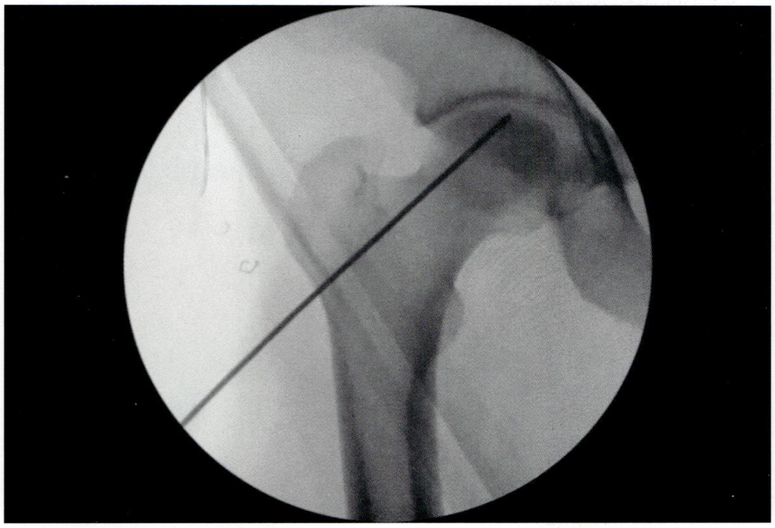

Fig. 18: Adequacy of starting point on lateral cortex is again confirmed with guidewire over the anterior body surface on fluoroscopy.

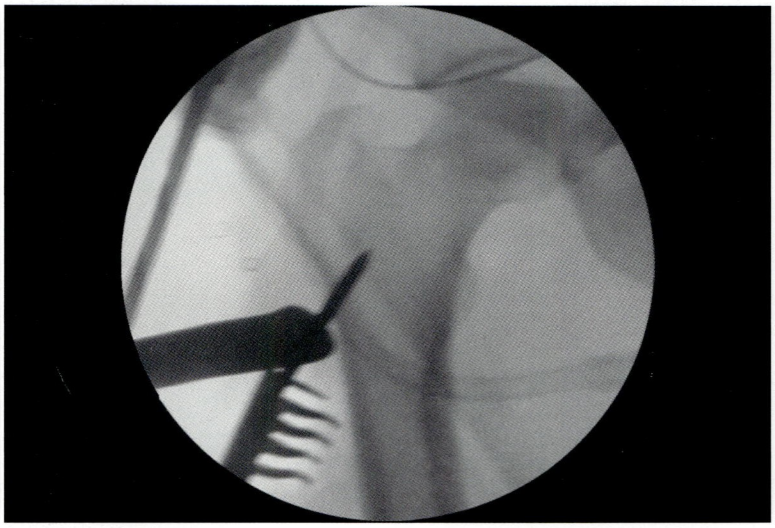

Fig. 19: Drill bit/Steinmann pin advanced in desired direction.

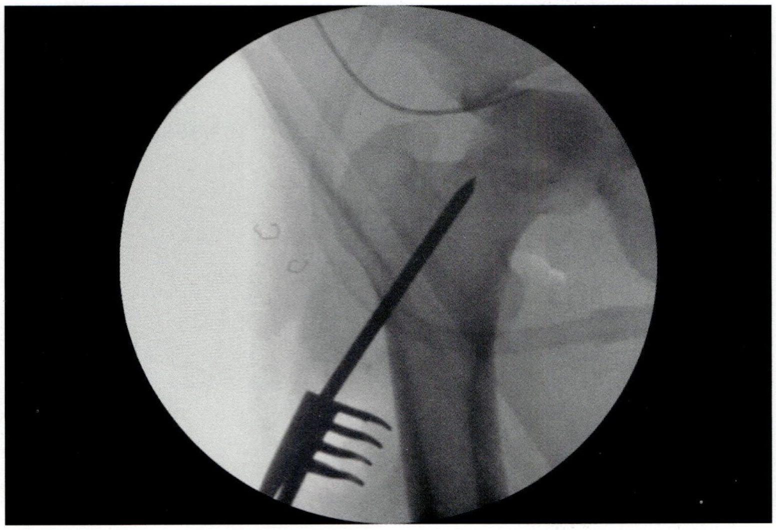

Fig. 20: Drill bit/Steinmann pin aimed in superior sector of head in anteroposterior (AP) view.

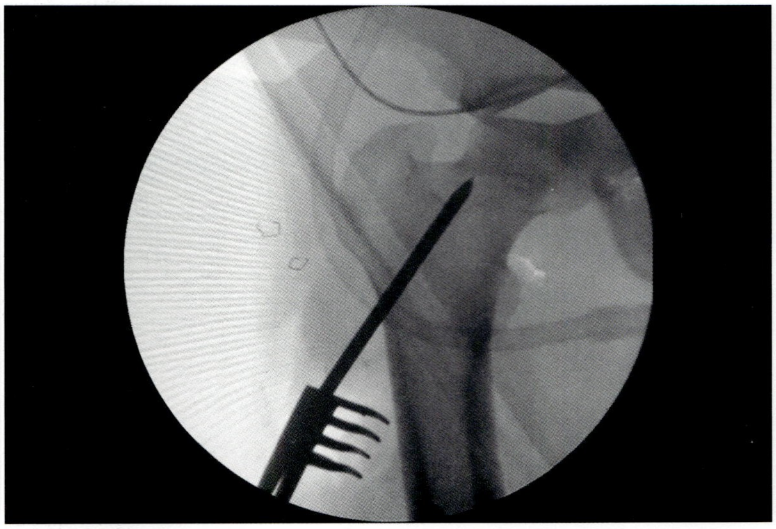

Fig. 21: Drill bit/Steinmann pin advanced till neck. Stop at this point to check the projection in lateral view.

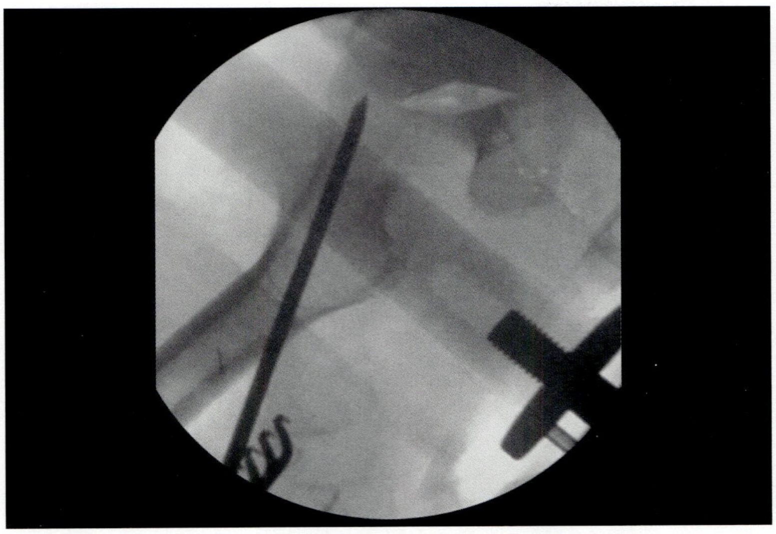

Fig. 22: Lateral view aiming drill bit/Steinmann pin toward anterior sector of head.

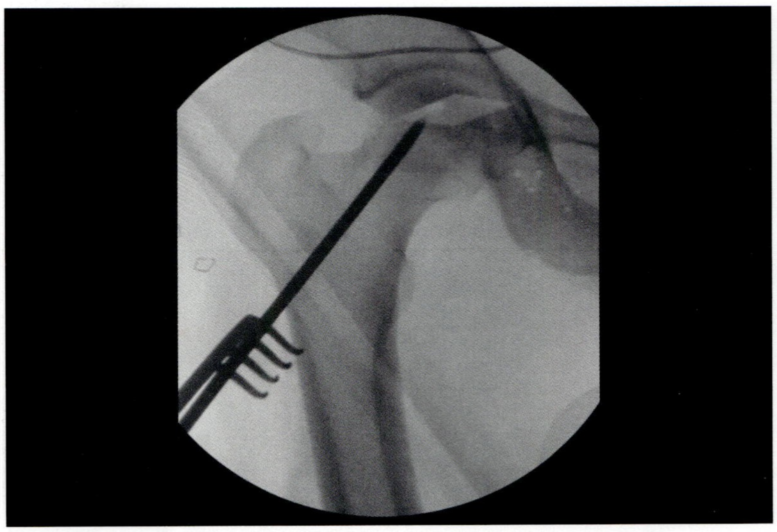

Fig. 23: Advancing the drill bit/Steinmann pin in same direction.

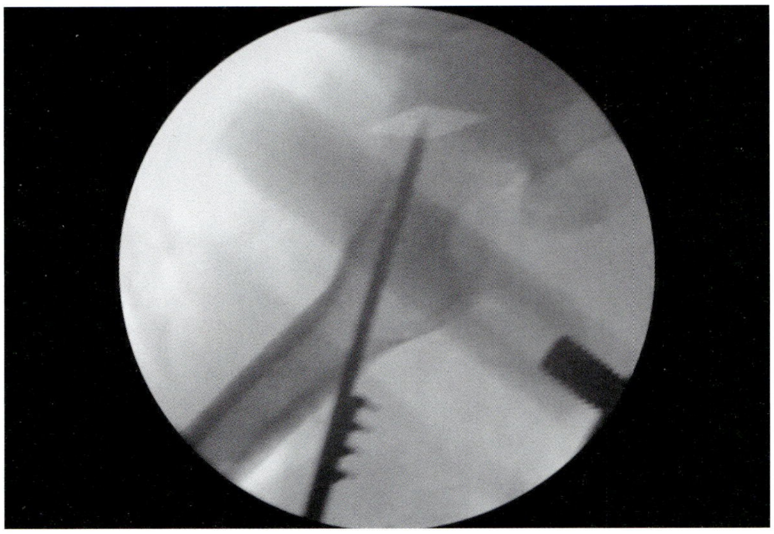

Fig. 24: Reconfirming the projection in lateral view after advancement.

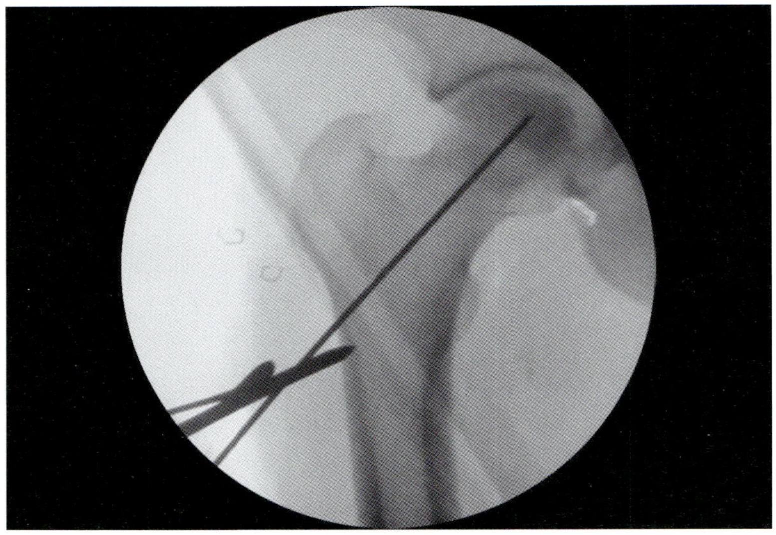

Fig. 25: New entry point for centro-superior sector decompression confirmed using guidewire over the anterior body surface.

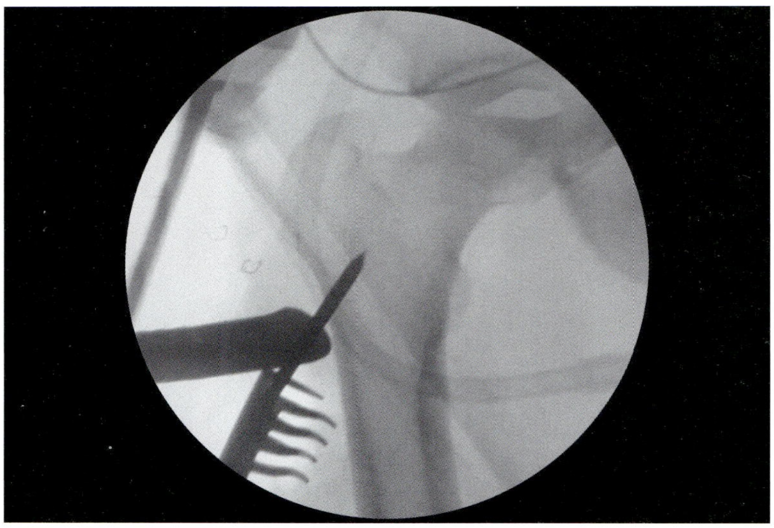

Fig. 26: Drill bit/Steinmann pin entry made and advanced.

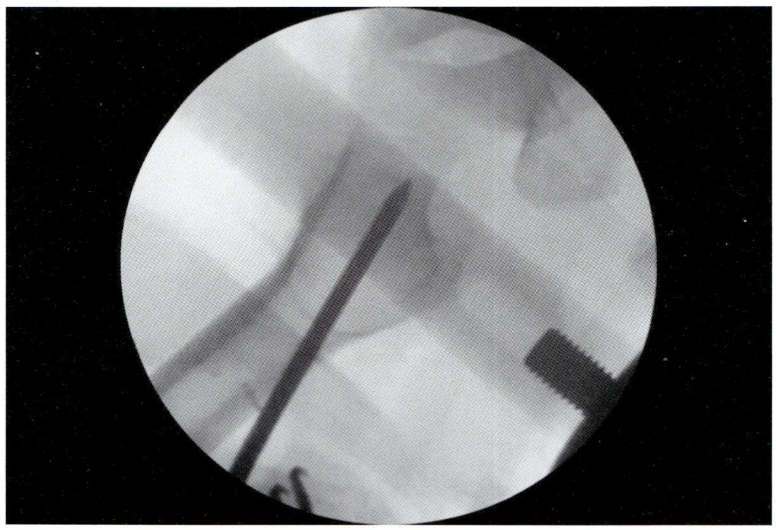

Fig. 27: Projection checked in lateral view to aim at central sector of head.

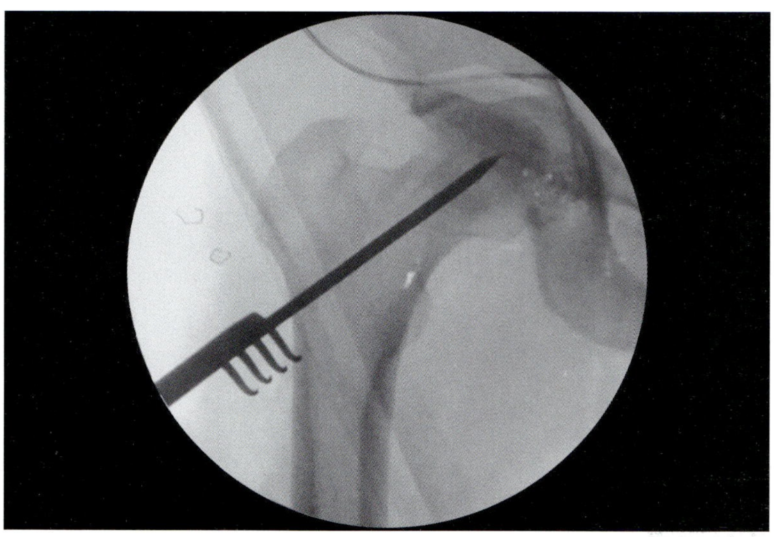

Fig. 28: Anteroposterior (AP) view showing decompression of centro-superior sector of head.

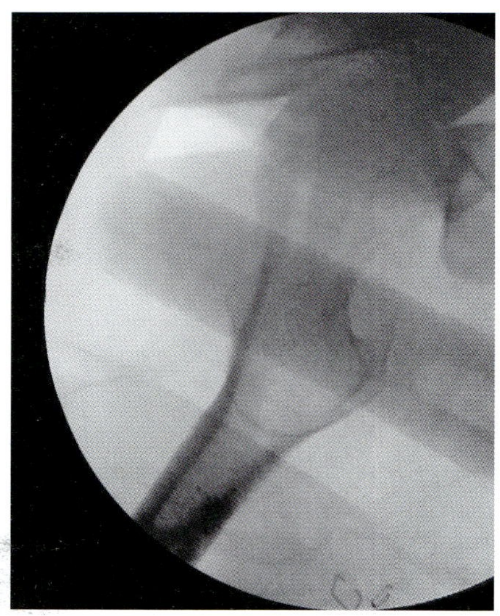

Fig. 29: Lateral view showing drill bit path in anterior and central sector of femoral head.

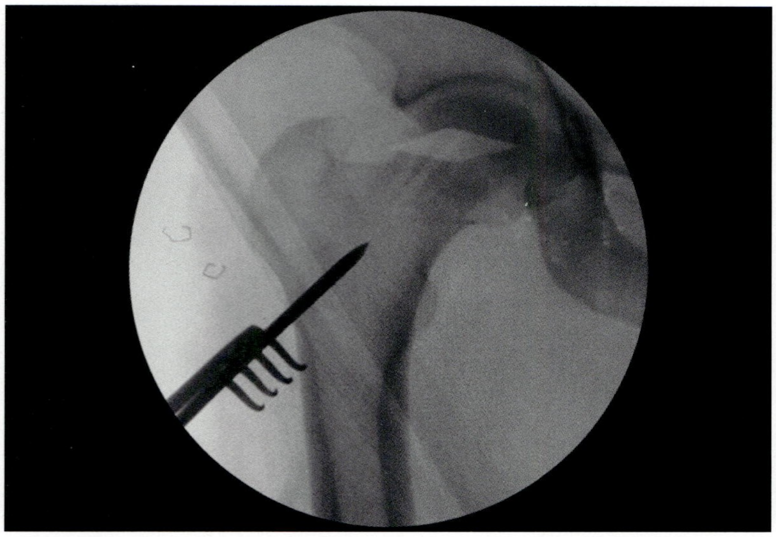

Fig. 30: Anteroposterior (AP) view showing drill bit path decompressing superior and central sector.

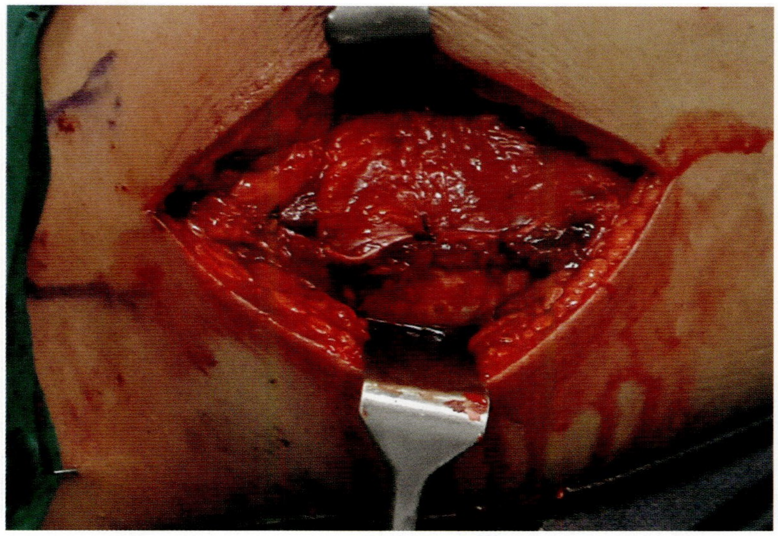

Fig. 31: As vastus is only elevated, tensor fascia lata is sutured with intermittent suture.

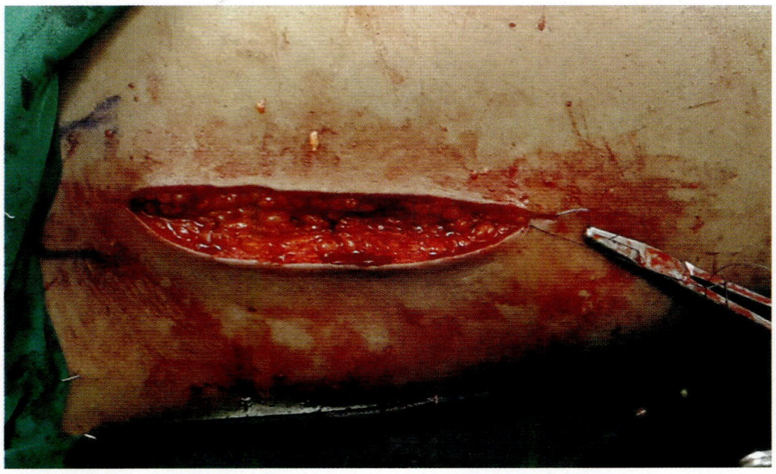

Fig. 32: Subcutaneous layer sutured.

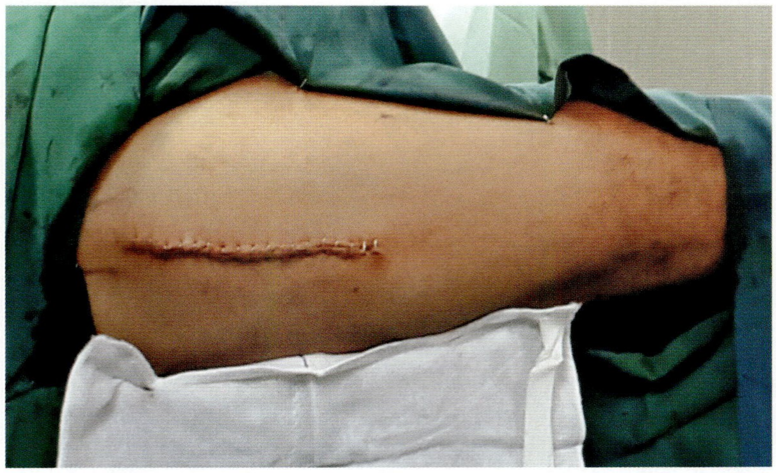

Fig. 33: Closure of skin with staples.

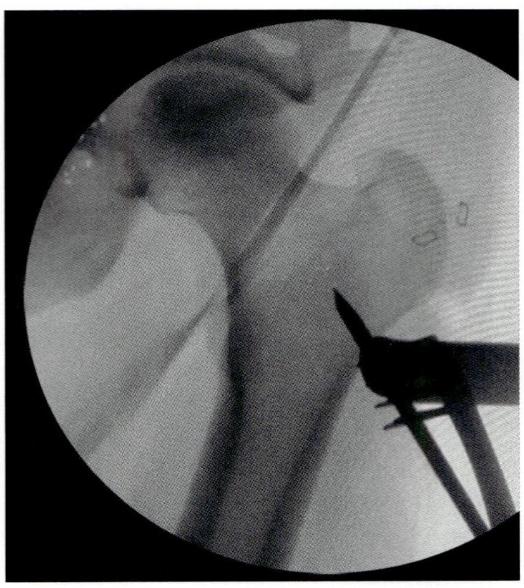

Fig. 34: Similar process done on opposite hip: entry made with drill bit.

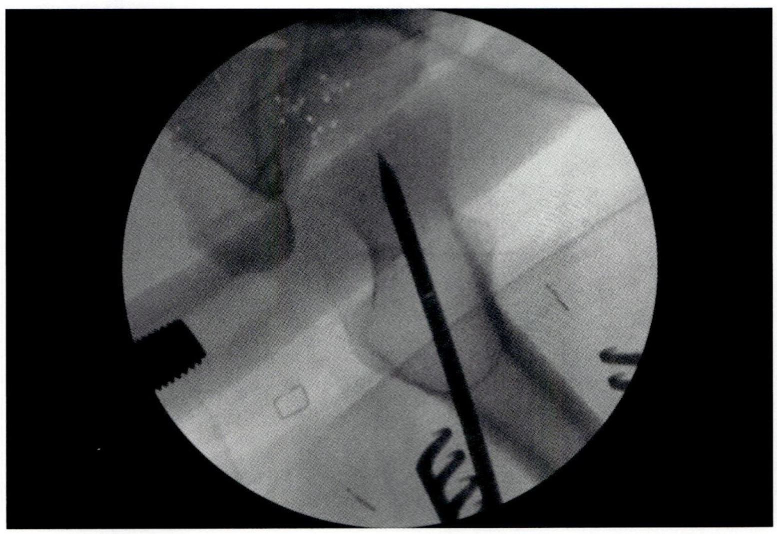

Fig. 35: Projection checked in lateral view to confirm decompression of anterior sector of head.

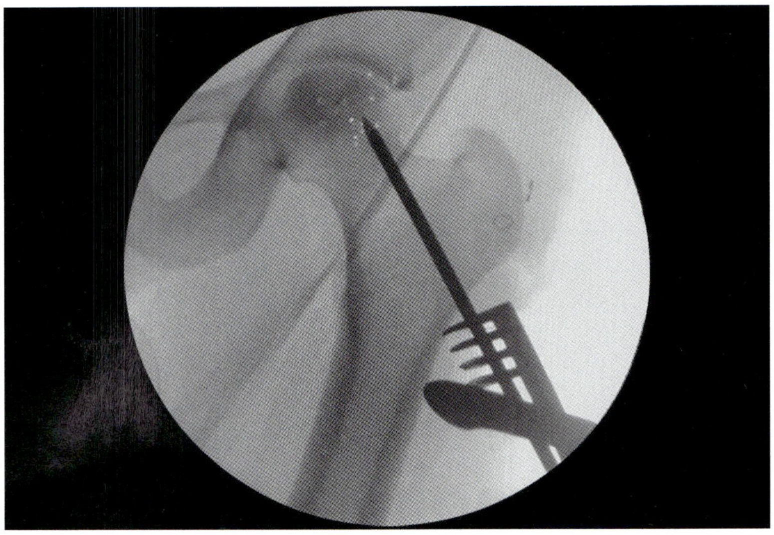

Fig. 36: Anteroposterior (AP) view of same confirming decompression of superior sector of head.

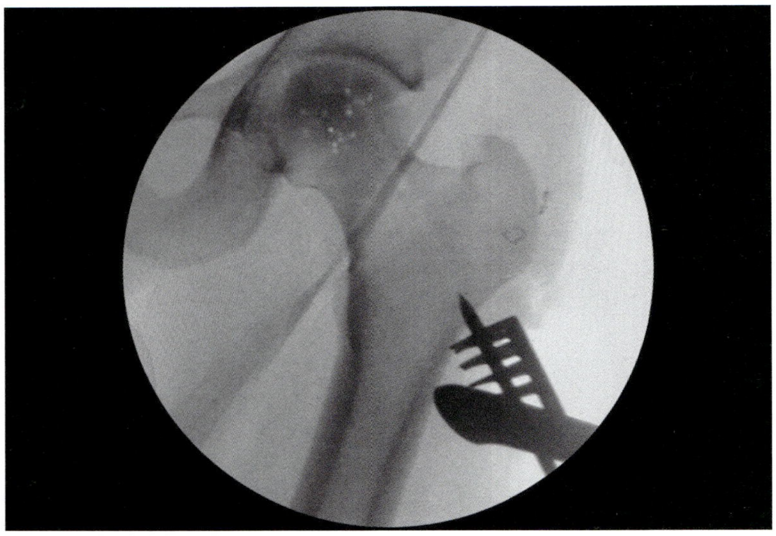

Fig. 37: Similar process is repeated with aim of decompression of central sector of head.

SUGGESTED READING

1. Ficat RP. Idiopathic bone necrosis of the femoral head. Early diagnosis and treatment. J Bone Joint Surg Br. 1985;67(1):3-9.
2. Lieberman JR, Berry DJ, Mont MA, et al. Osteonecrosis of the hip: management in the 21st century. Instr Course Lect JBJS. 2003;52:337-55.
3. Mont MA, Carbone JJ, Fairbank AC. Core decompression versus nonoperative management for osteonecrosis of the hip. Clin Orthop Relat Res. 1996;324:169-78.
4. Petrigliano FA, Lieberman JR. Osteonecrosis of the hip: novel approaches to evaluation and treatment. Clin Orthop Relat Res. 2007;465:53-62.
5. Song WS, Yoo JJ, Kim YM, et al. Results of multiple drilling compared with those of conventional methods of core decompression. Clin Orthop Relat Res. 2007;454:139-46.
6. Steinberg ME. Diagnostic imaging and role of stage and lesion size in determining outcome in osteonecrosis of the femoral head. Tech Orthop. 2001;16:6-15.

CHAPTER 80

Compression Arthrodesis of Ankle

Manoj Todkar, Hardik Shah

INDICATIONS OF ANKLE FUSION

Ankle fusion is carried out for relief of pain and instability due to disabling tibiotalar arthritis.

BIOMECHANICAL PRINCIPLES

- Patient selection should be done carefully for ankle fusion. Chopart's and Lisfranc's joints should have enough range of movement to compensate for loss of ankle motion during gait cycle.
- Patient should be willing to wear modified shoes after fusion.
- The optimal position for ankle fusion is neutral flexion, varus, valgus, and dorsiflexion should be avoided.

SURGICAL STEPS (FIGS. 1 TO 25)

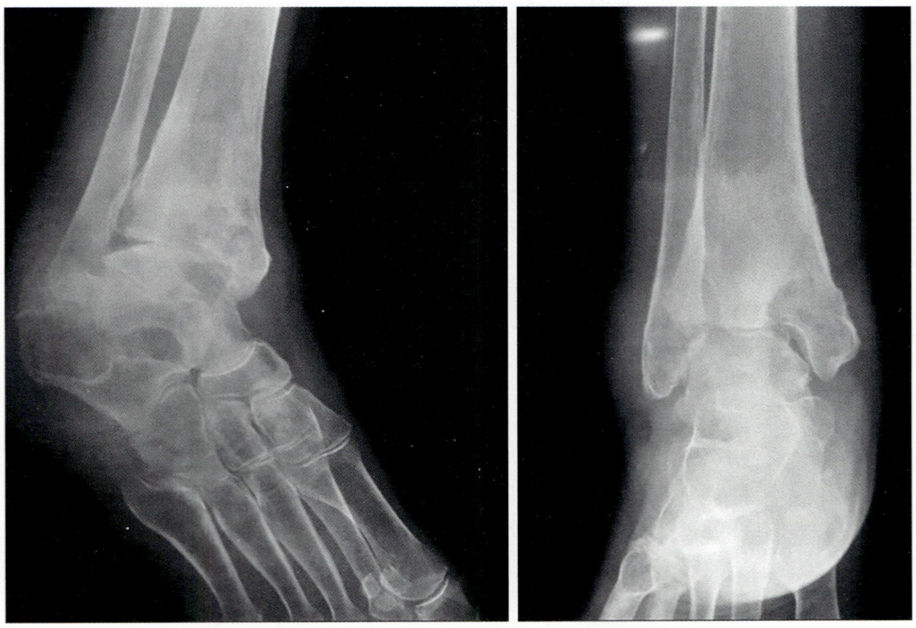

Fig. 1: Radiograph of ankle showing arthritic changes due to infection.

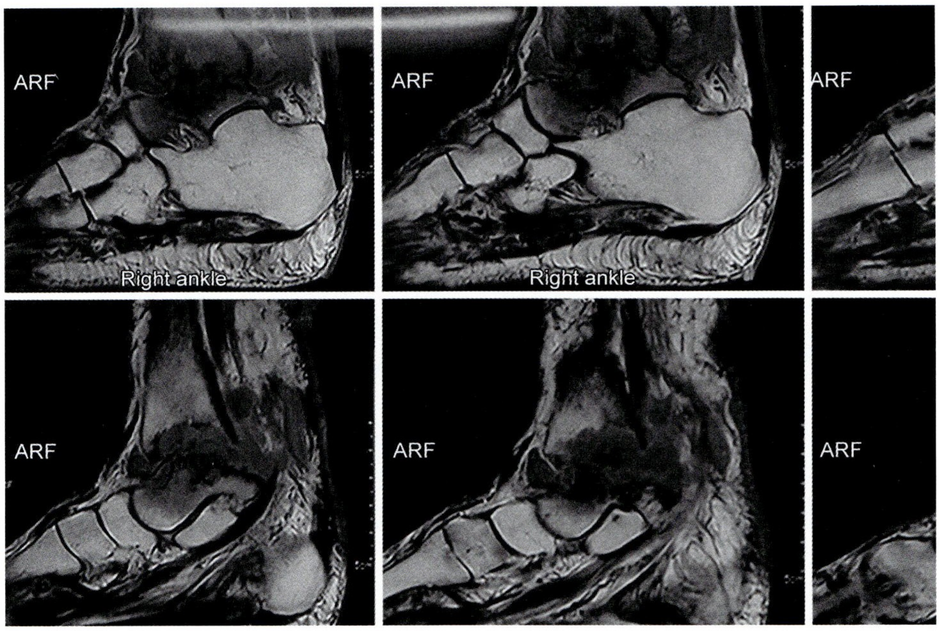

Fig. 2: Magnetic resonance imaging (MRI) of ankle showing arthritic changes.

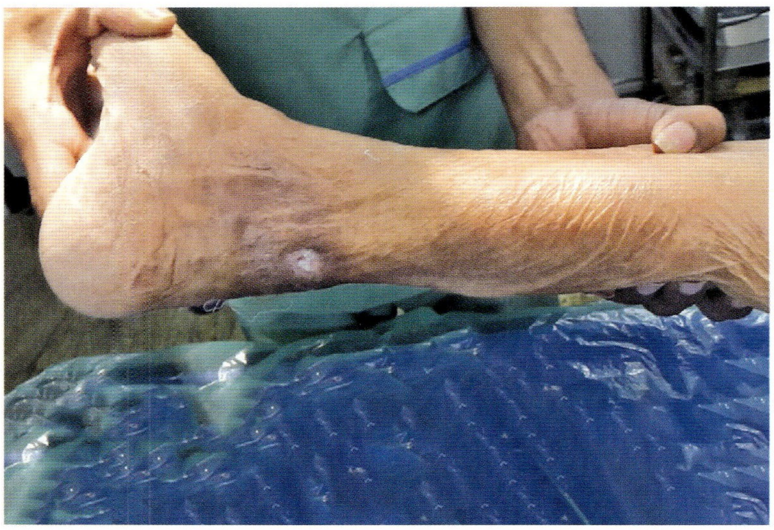

Fig. 3: Clinical photograph of stiff ankle. Note sinus tract posteriorly.

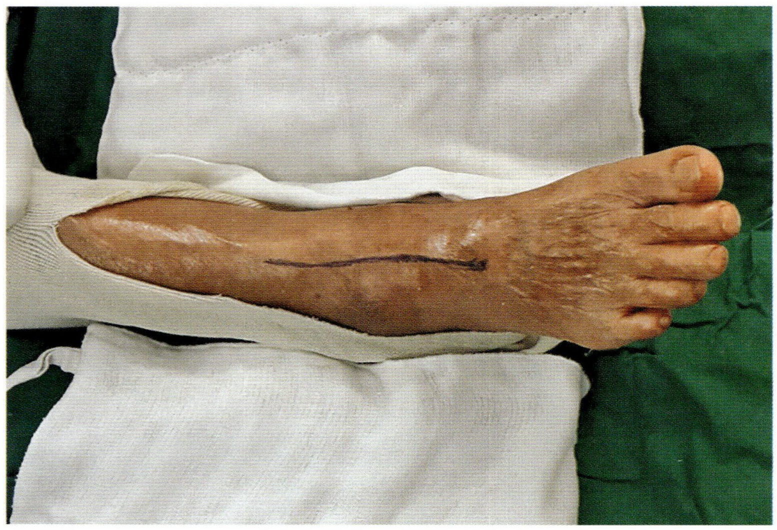

Fig. 4: Skin marking for anterior approach to ankle joint. Incision is made immediately lateral to anterior tibial tendon extending to the level of talonavicular joint.

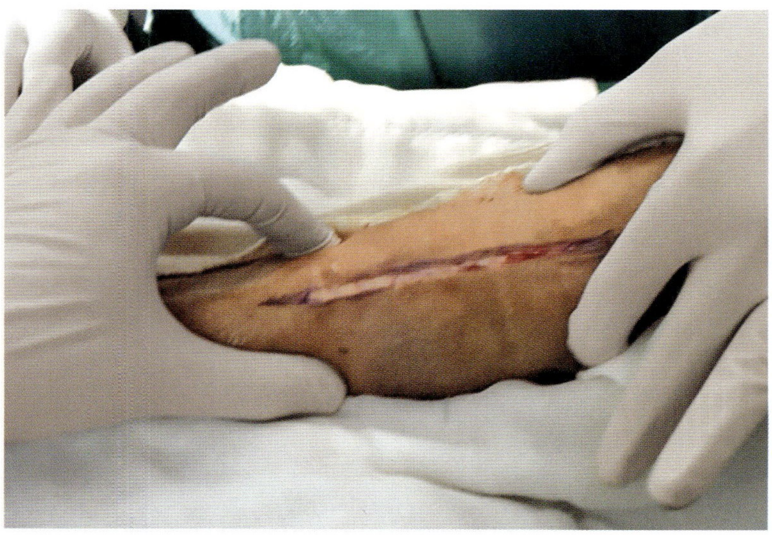

Fig. 5: Skin incision.

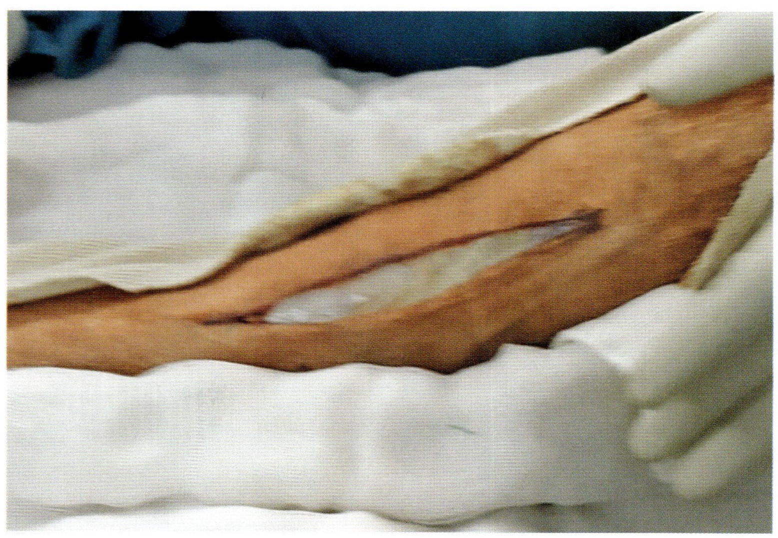

Fig. 6: Superficial dissection.

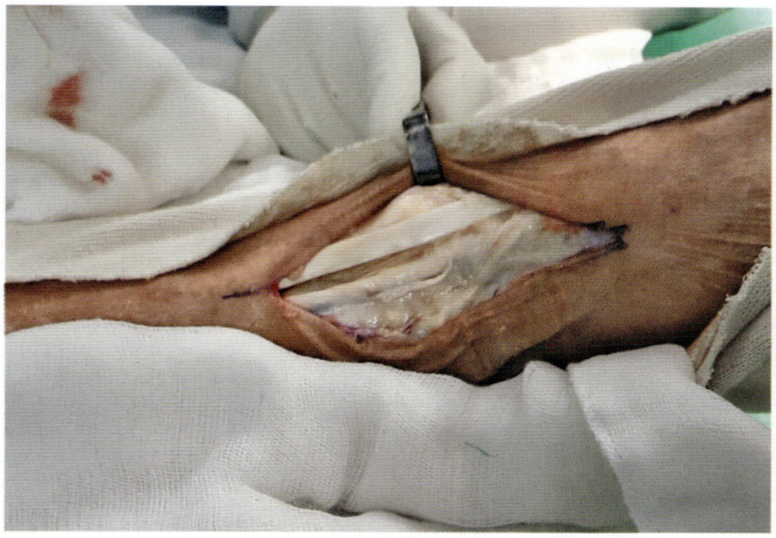

Fig. 7: Superficial perineal nerve is protected in distal part of incision. Extensor retinaculum is incised longitudinally.

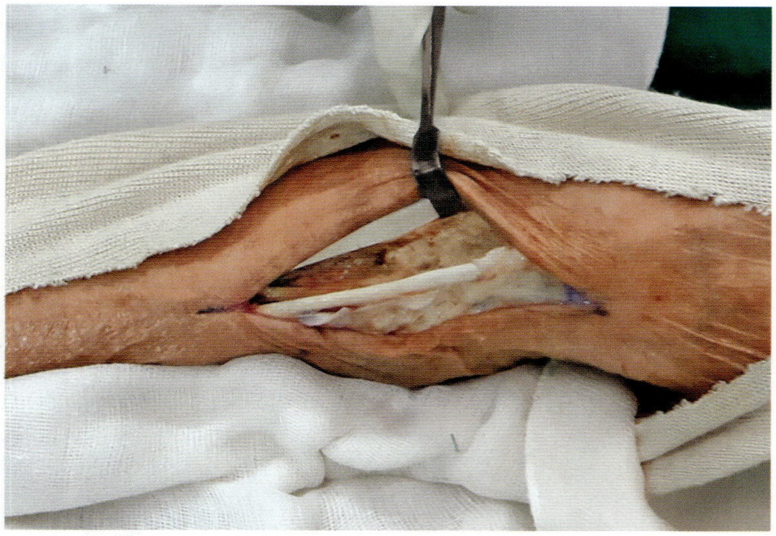

Fig. 8: Deep dissection is done through the anterior tibial tendon or through extensor hallucis longus (EHL). The neurovascular bundle is directly posterior to EHL at the level of ankle joint.

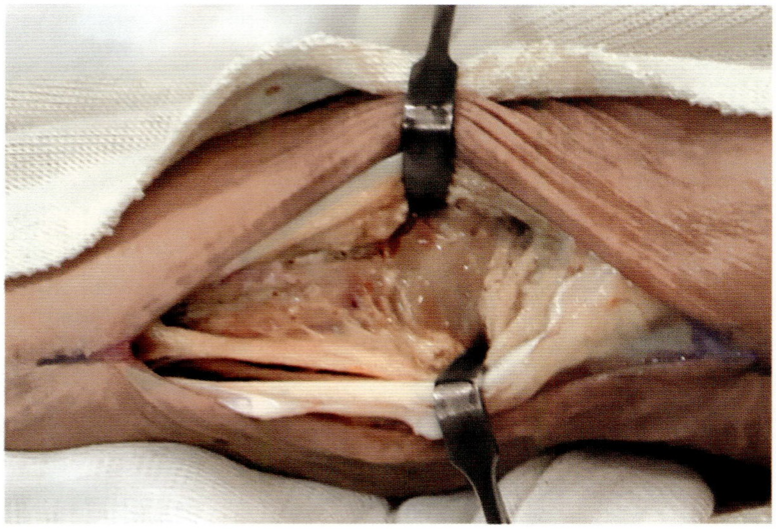

Fig. 9: Ankle joint capsule is exposed.

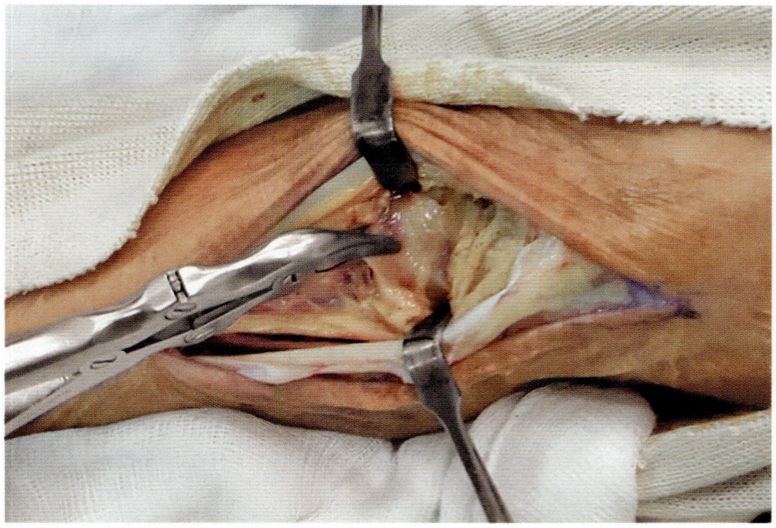

Fig. 10: Removal of tibial and talar osteophytes and synovium and debris with nibbler.

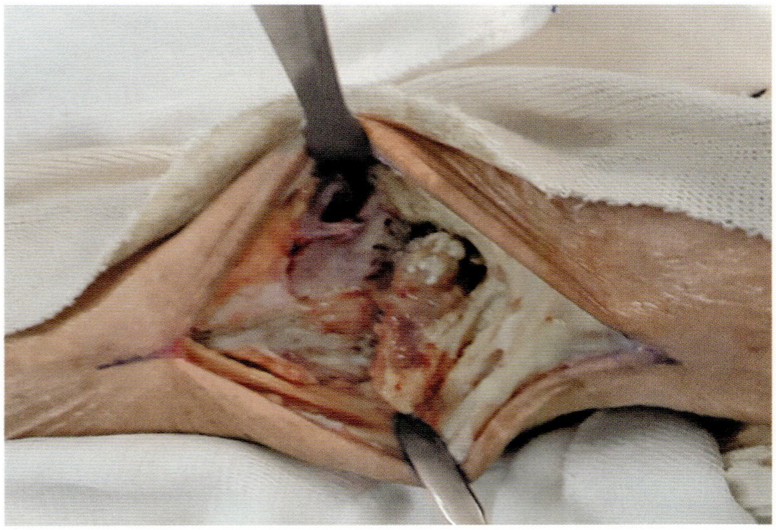

Fig. 11: Ankle joint is exposed.

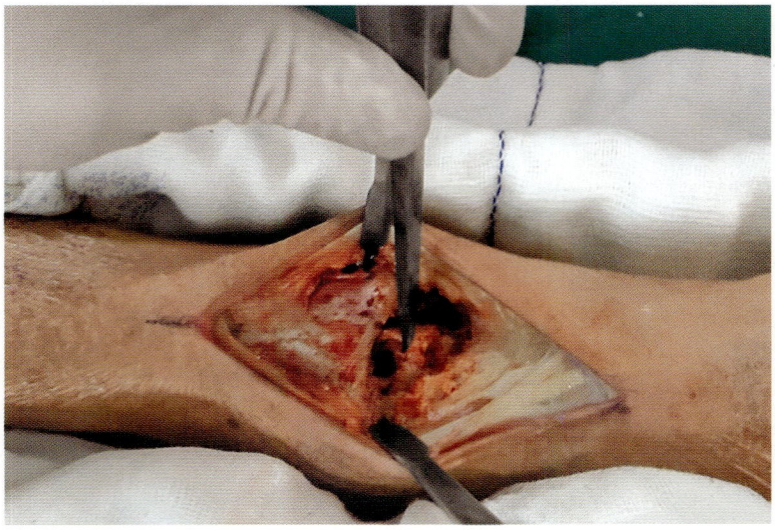

Fig. 12: Joint surfaces are prepared.

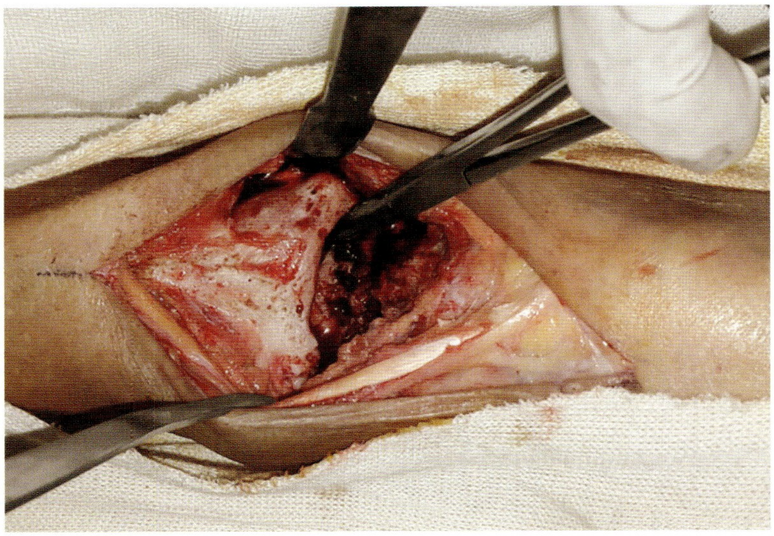

Fig. 13: Cartilage is removed from articular surface of tibia, lateral malleolus and talus.

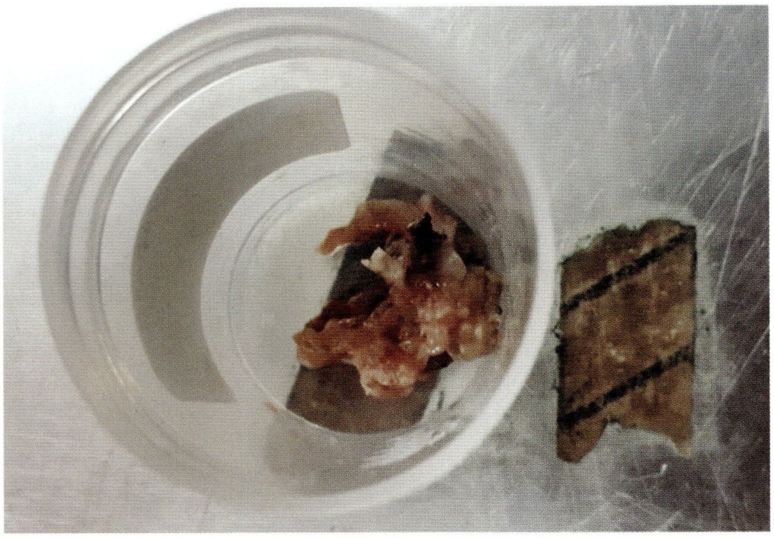

Fig. 14: Denuded cartilage.

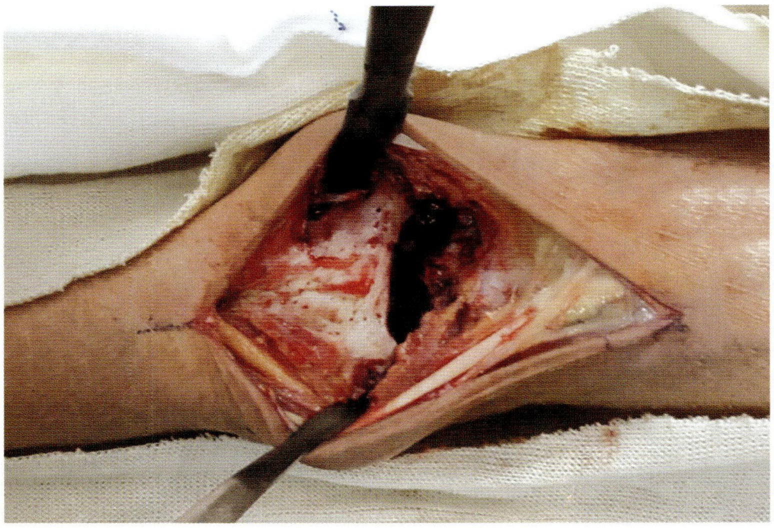

Fig. 15: Adjacent raw surfaces are ready for arthrodesis.

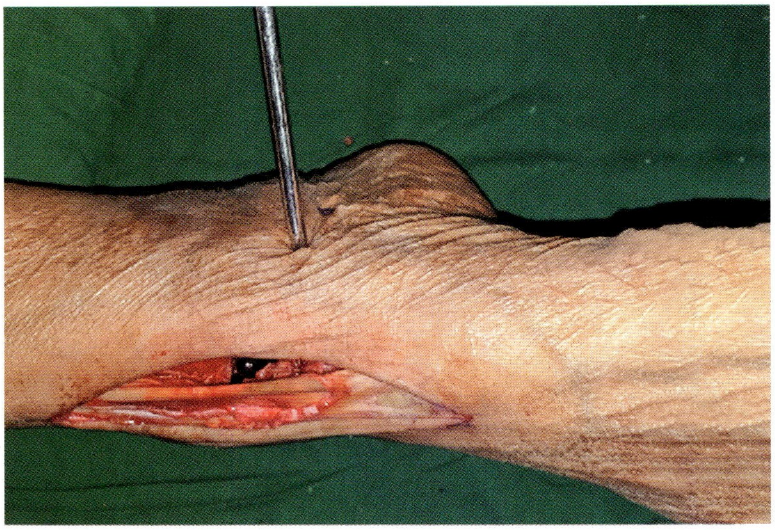

Fig. 16: Position of ankle is neutral for arthrodesis. Steinmann pin entry point for talus over medial aspect after taking stab incision and protecting neurovascular bundle.

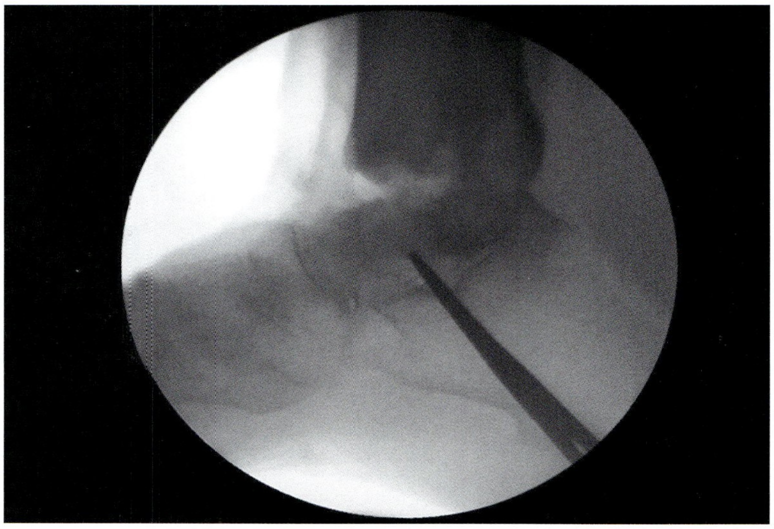

Fig. 17: Entry point confirmed on C-arm for talus.

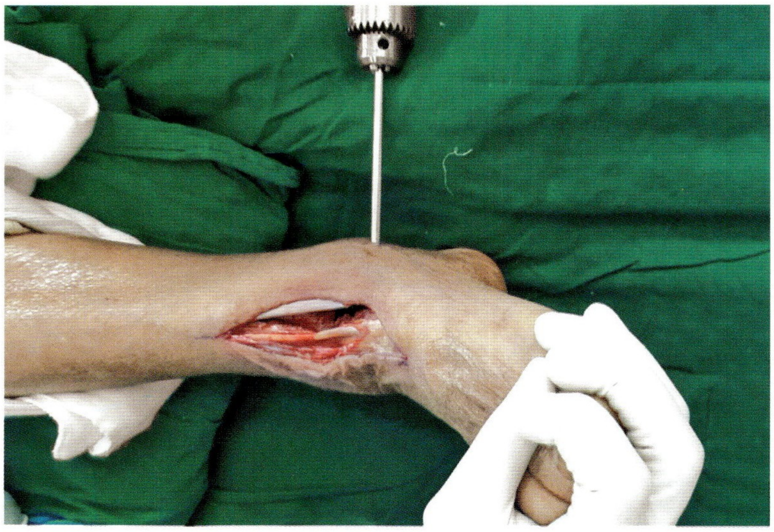

Fig. 18: Steinmann pin was passed through talus under C-arm control from medial to lateral direction so avoiding medial neurovascular bundle is ensured.

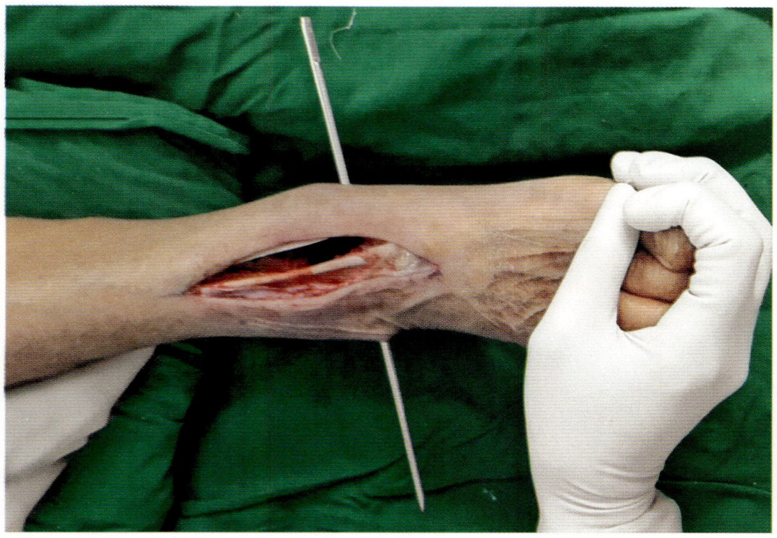

Fig. 19: Final position of talar Steinmann pin.

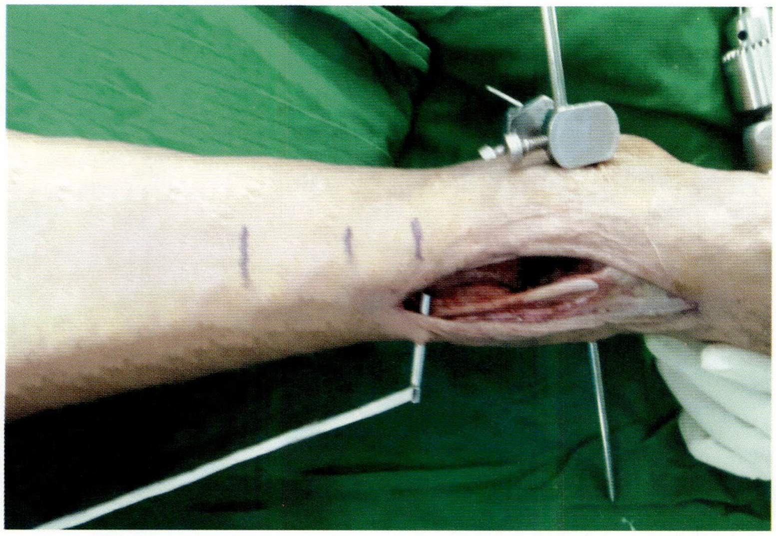

Fig. 20: Entry point for distal tibia Steinmann pin marked and drill sleeve inserted after stab incision over lateral aspect with protection of neurovascular bundle. Location of this pin should be such that sufficient compression can be applied using the compression device. Direct visualization and sleeve positioning through proximal corner of incision ensure avoiding neurovascular bundle.

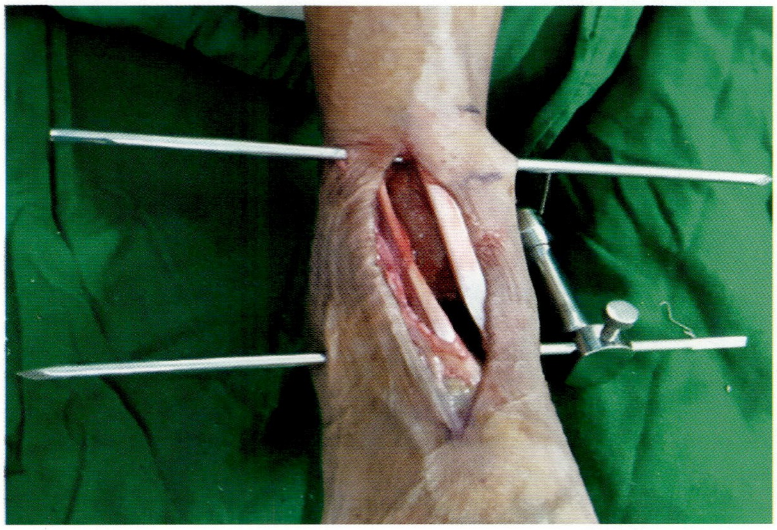

Fig. 21: Steinmann pin was passed through distal tibia under C-arm control from lateral to medial direction.

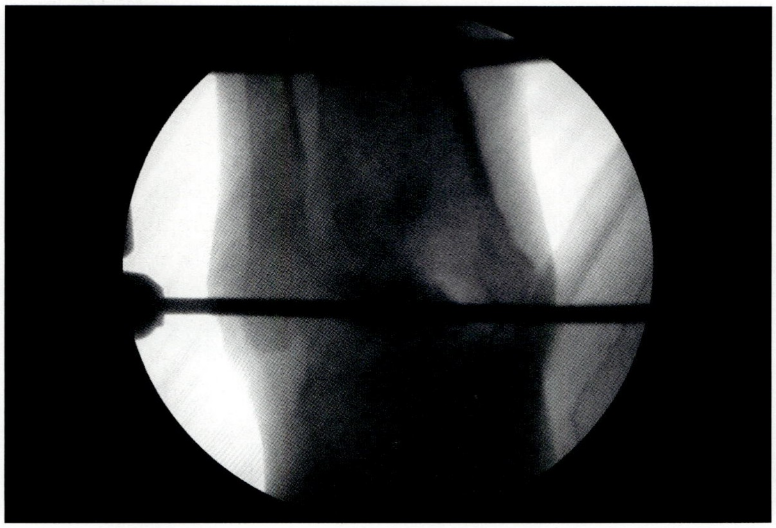

Fig. 22: Final pin position confirmed under C-arm.

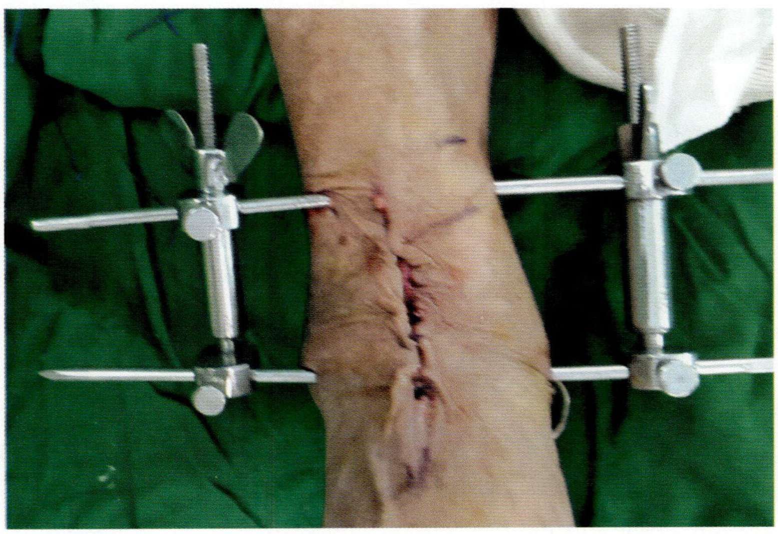

Fig. 23: Compression is achieved with Charnley compression device. Slight bending of pins indicates good compression effect.

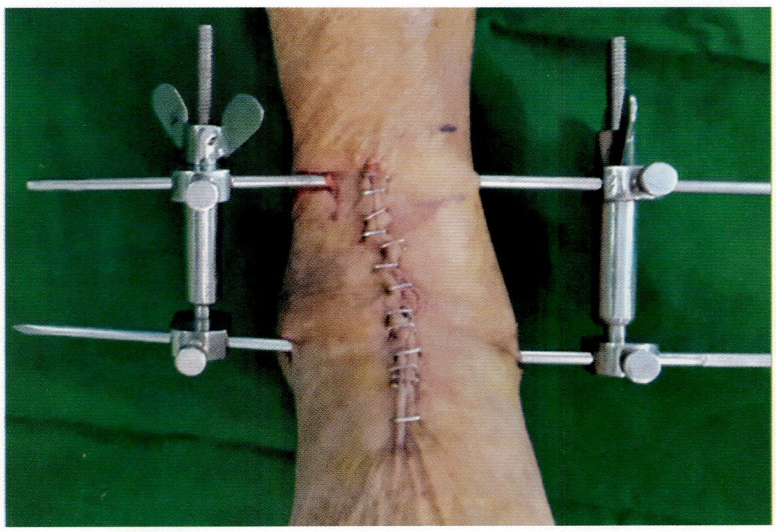

Fig. 24: Wound is closed in layers over drain and posterior slab support is applied.

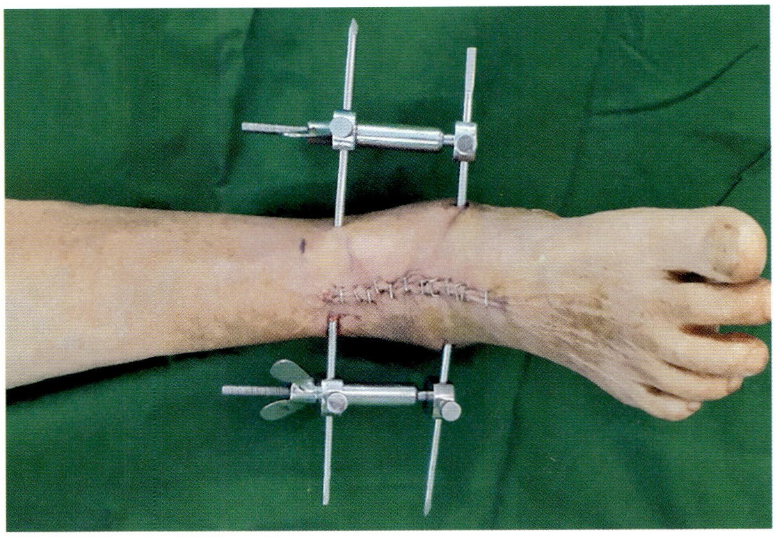

Fig. 25: Final picture of ankle arthrodesis.

COMPLICATIONS

Common complications after ankle fusion surgery are nonunion, delayed union, wound infection, intractable pain, tibial fracture, and unsightly scars.

OPERATIVE TECHNIQUES

- *Chevron ankle fusion*: This procedure allows excellent cosmetic result, high incidence of early fusion, and few complications. This approach involves bilateral (from both sides) exposure of the ankle joint, internal fixation, and medial tibial onlay bone graft.
- Charnley compression arthrodesis is indicated in sepsis when internal fixation and bone grafting are contraindicated.
- The white posterior fusion technique is used when posterior incision is desirable and physis is still open.

Ankle arthrodesis is used as a salvage procedure in aseptic necrosis of talus, chronic infections, failed previous fusions, and failed arthroplasties.

SUGGESTED READING

1. Charnley J. Compression arthrodesis of the ankle and shoulder. J Bone Joint Surg. 1951;33B(2):180-91.
2. Johnson EW Jr, Boseker EH. Arthrodesis of the Ankle. Arch Surg. 1968;97:766-73.
3. Mazur JM, Schwartze E, Simon SR. Ankle arthrodesis. Long-term follow-up with gait analysis. J Bone Joint Surg Am. 1979;61(7):964-75.
4. Randall EM, Kingsbury GH. Arthrodesis of the Ankle. In: Chapman MW (Ed). Operative Orthopedics, 2nd edition. Philadelphia: JB Lippincott Company; 1993.
5. White AA 3rd. A Precision posterior ankle fusion. Clin Orthop. 1974;(98):239-50.
6. Wilson HJ Jr. Arthrodesis of the ankle: a technique using bilateral hemimalleolar onlay grafts with screw fixation. J Bone Joint Surg. 1969;51(4):775-7.

SECTION 8

TRAUMATOLOGY

Section Editors: *Shrinivas S Shintre, Vijay M Panchanadikar*

CHAPTER 81

Fracture Clavicle: Plate Fixation Middle Third/Distal Third

Yash K Shah

INTRODUCTION

The clavicle is a S-shaped bone which looks like the musical symbol clavicula. It is broader at the medial and lateral ends and thin in the middle, hence it is vulnerable for fracture at this middle transition zone. Hence fractures are most common at this middle 1/3rd zone.

FRACTURE BIOMECHANICS

For Midshaft Clavicle

There are various forces acting on the clavicle. In case of a mid-shaft clavicle fracture here are the relevant forces (Fig. 1).

- The Sternocleidomastoid muscle pulls the medial segment superiorly.
- The sternoclavicular ligaments stabilize the medial segment medially.
- The pectoralis major pulls the lateral segment inferiorly and medially.
- Finally the weight of the arm pulls the lateral segment inferiorly via the coracoclavicular ligaments.

For Lateral End Clavicle

- In case of fractures of the lateral end of the clavicle, here are the relevant forces (Fig. 2).
- The medial segment is pulled superiorly by the sternocleidomastoid and the trapezius muscles.
- The distal segment is pulled medially by the pectoralis muscles and the latissimus dorsi muscle, and it is pulled inferiorly by the weight of the arm.

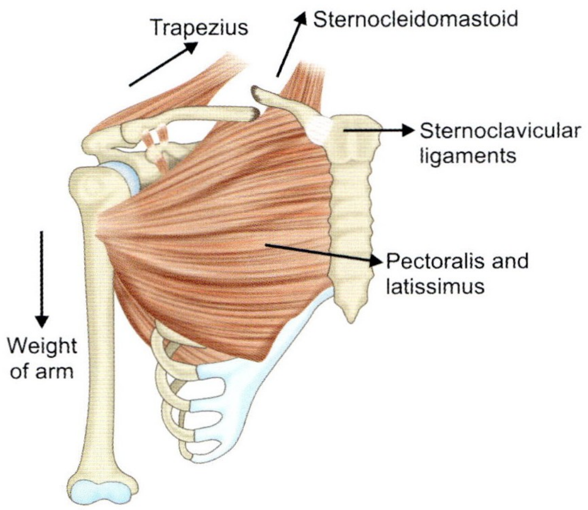

Fig. 1: Displacing forces for a midshaft fracture.

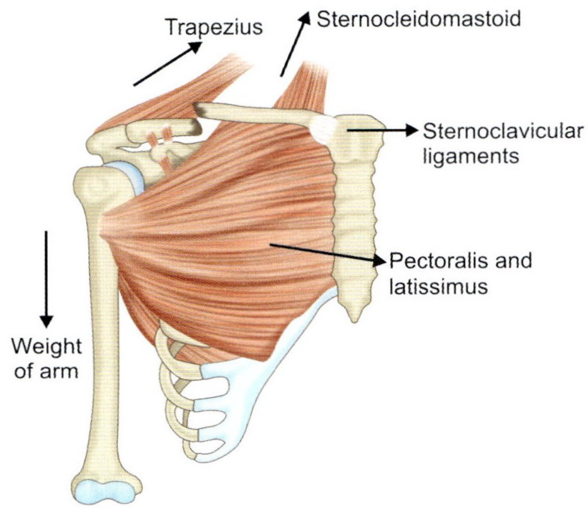

Fig. 2: Displacing forces for lateral fracture.

CLASSIFICATION

The classification of clavicle fractures was proposed by Craig for which the reader is suggested to refer the standard textbooks.

INDICATIONS FOR OPEN REDUCTION AND INTERNAL FIXATION OF DISPLACED MIDSHAFT FRACTURES (TABLE 1)

TABLE 1: Indications for open reduction and internal fixation of displaced midshaft fractures.

Absolute	*Relative*
• Shortening of more than 20 mm • Open wound • Neurovascular injuries • Scapulothoracic dissociation • Pathologic fracture • Trapezius paralysis	• Displacement of more than 20 mm • Head Injury • Seizures or any neurological disorder • Prolonged bed ridden condition • Floating shoulder • Bilateral fractures • Noncompliance with conservative treatment • Cosmetic reasons

INDICATIONS FOR DISTAL CLAVICLE FRACTURE

There is no clear consensus, but generally the coracoclavicular ligaments are disrupted in this type and hence these fractures must be operated upon.

OPERATIVE OPTIONS: MIDDLE THIRD CLAVICLE

- It is better to do a plate fixation than a nail fixation.
- Anatomical locked plates and reconstruction plates are commonly used.
- At least six to eight cortices hold seems sufficient for non-comminuted fractures.

OPERATIVE OPTIONS: DISTAL CLAVICLE

Kirschner Wire Fixation

K wires have a high failure rate and a migration rate of up to 50%. Hence, they have fallen out of favor.

CC Screw Fixation

Insertion is technically demanding, and the screws can limit shoulder motion.

Plate or Hook Plate Fixation

The distal fragment should be big enough for good fixation to allow a plate fixation.

Hook Plate Fixation

This plate can be hooked under the acromion and can be used when the distal fragment does not have sufficient hold.

Suture and Sling Technique

These techniques reconstruct the coraco-clavicular ligaments and are more anatomic.

TIMING OF SURGERY

A delayed surgery can cause more complication rate (7% to 36%). There is a more chance of intra-articular degeneration in case of lateral end clavicle fractures, in which case even an excision of the distal end of clavicle may be needed at times.

SURGICAL STEPS: FRACTURE MIDSHAFT CLAVICLE (FIGS. 1 TO 19)

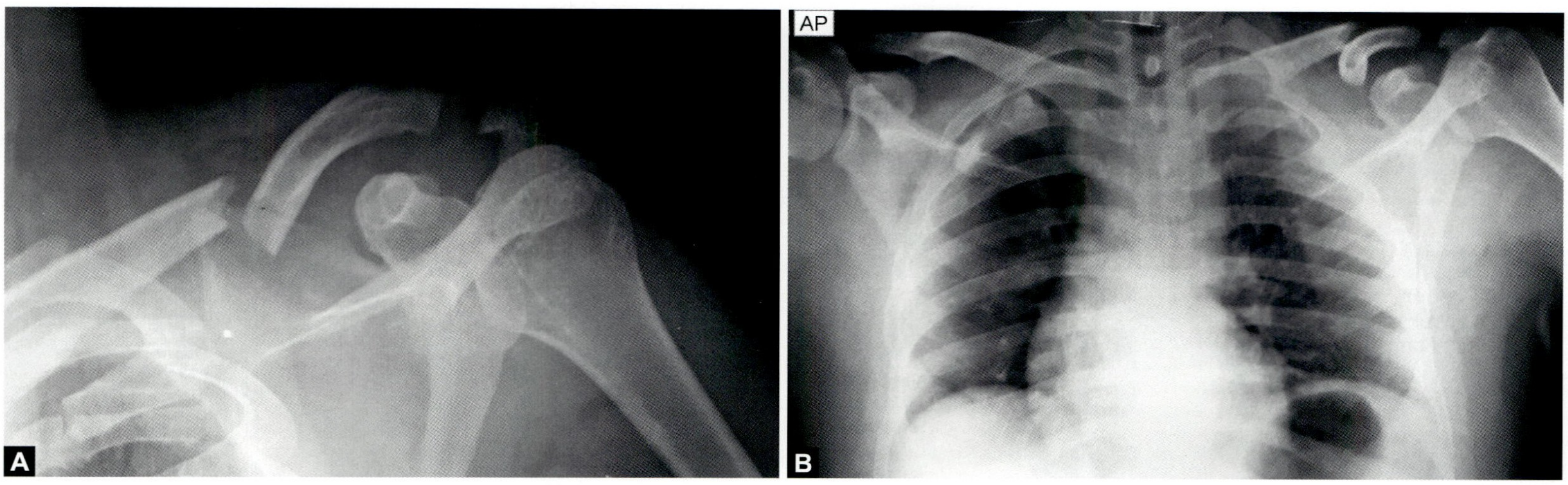

Figs. 3A and B: Preoperative X-ray of a patient with a left clavicle fracture. Always the X-ray of the chest is taken as well to rule out any other injuries.

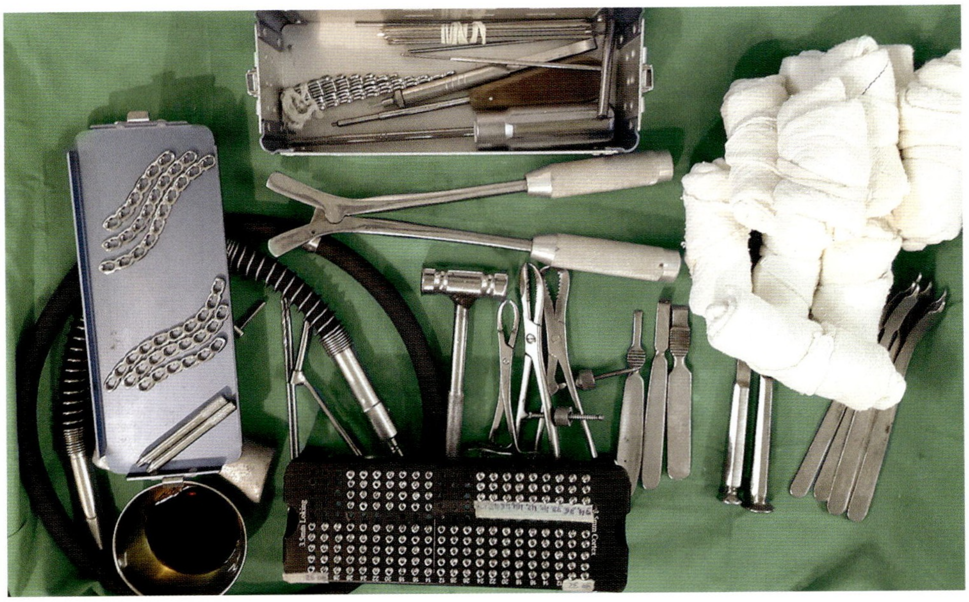

Fig. 4: Instrument trolley. Always keep various types and sizes of bone holders and spike retractors at disposal. Specially contoured locking plates are to be used.

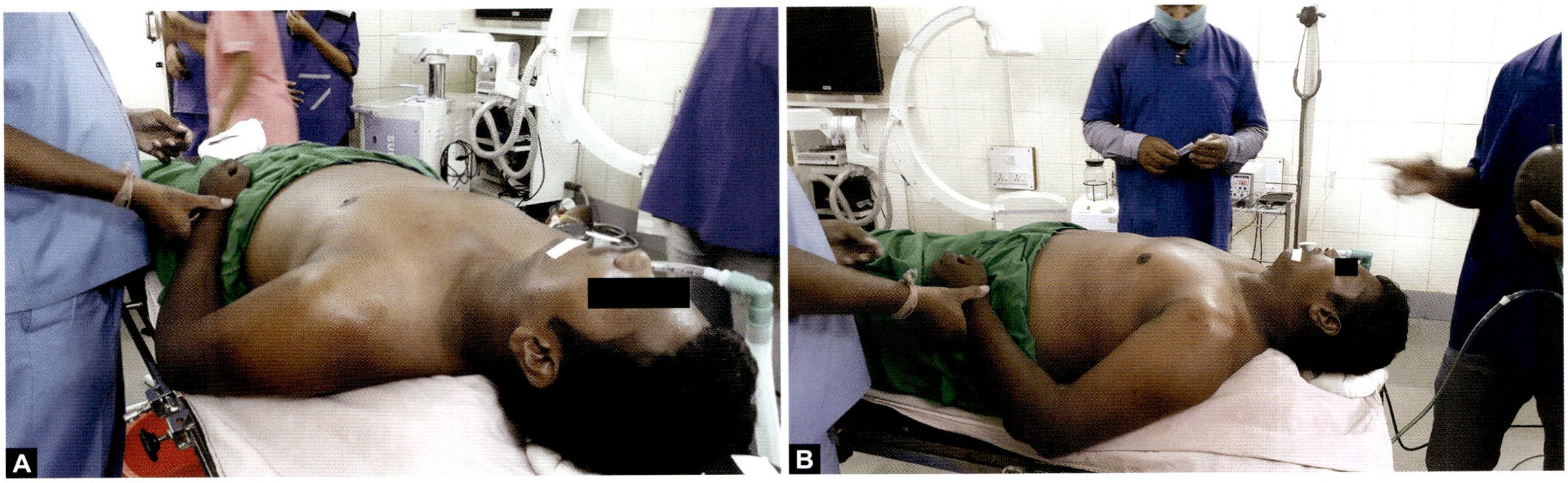

Figs. 5A and B: Position of the patient. Head end is slightly elevated.

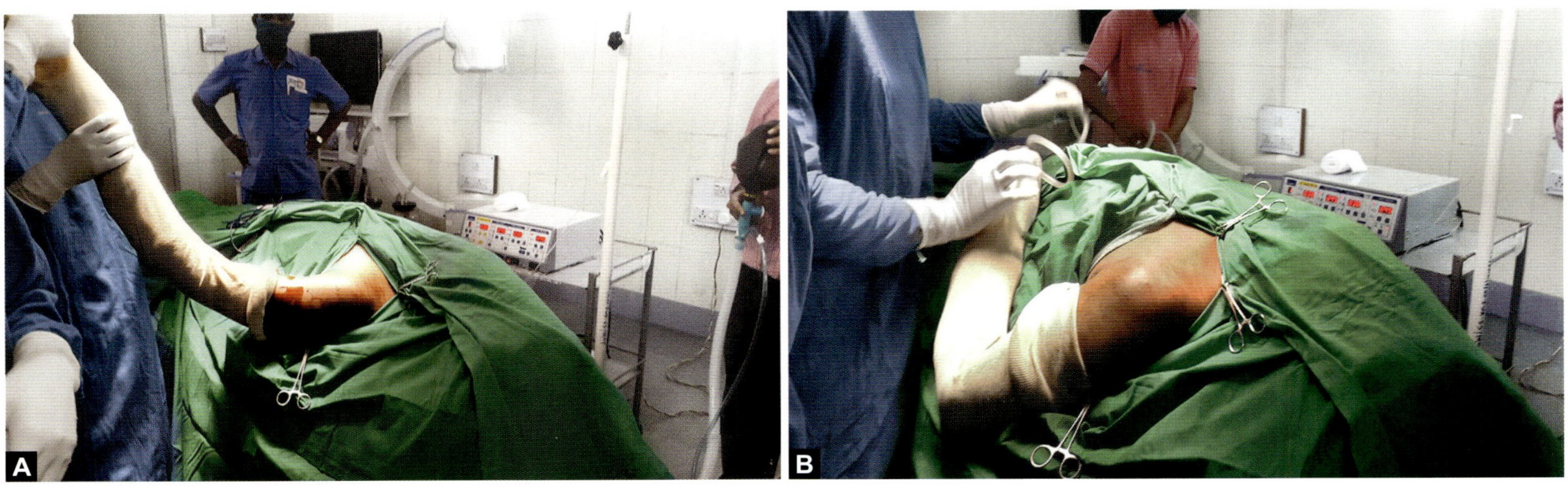

Figs. 6A and B: Draping of the patient should be such that the arm should be able to freely externally and internally rotate.

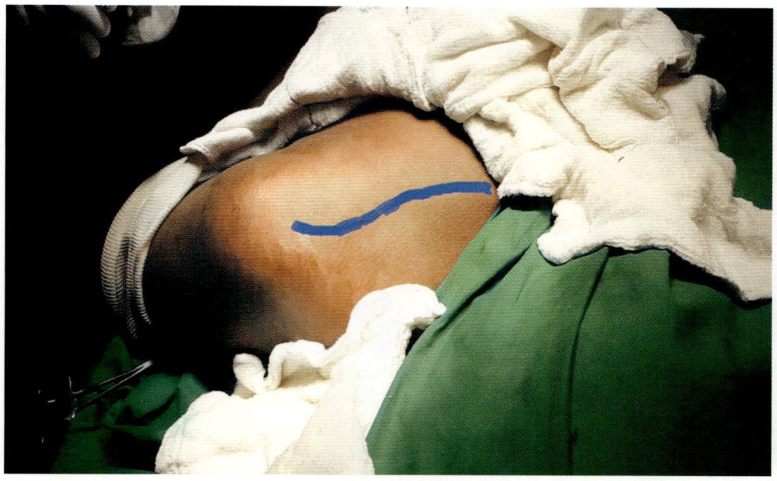

Fig. 7: Always better to mark your incision as many a times the patient is obese and it is easy to veer off into the wrong plane.

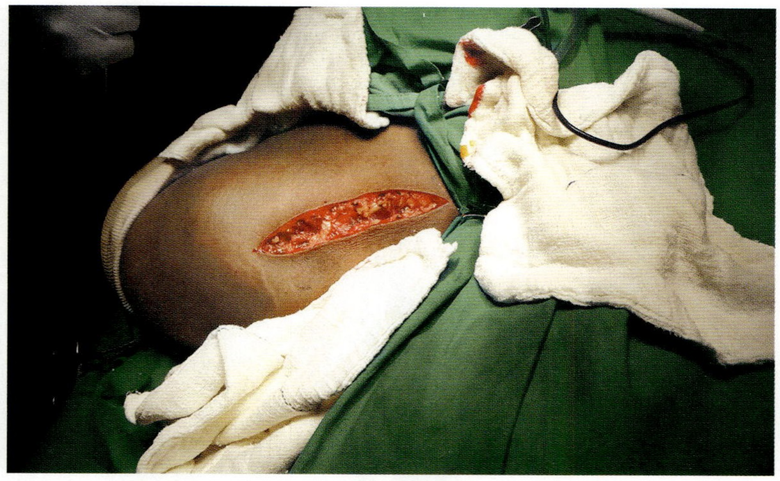

Fig. 8: A skin incision of about 8–10 cm is made.

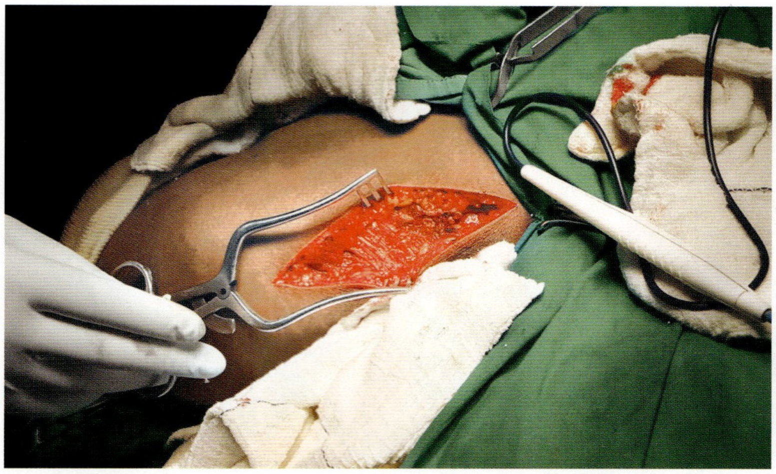

Fig. 9: A self-retaining retractor reduces the work of the assistant. Care should be taken to relieve the pressure off the skin in case the surgery is taking too much time.

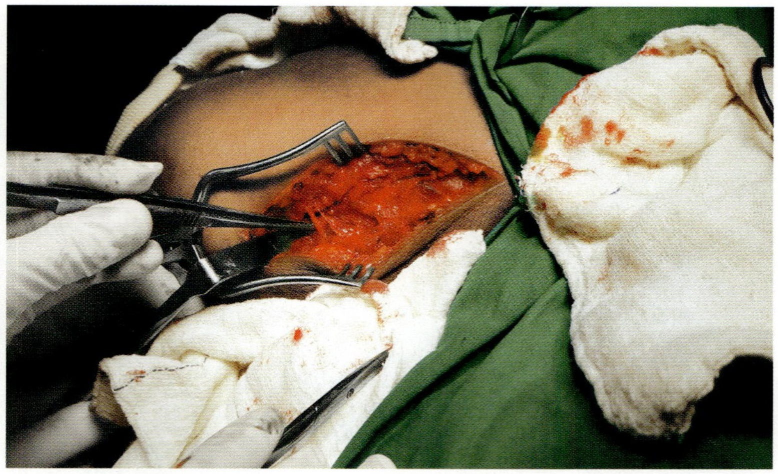

Fig. 10: Dissect out the supraclavicular nerves.

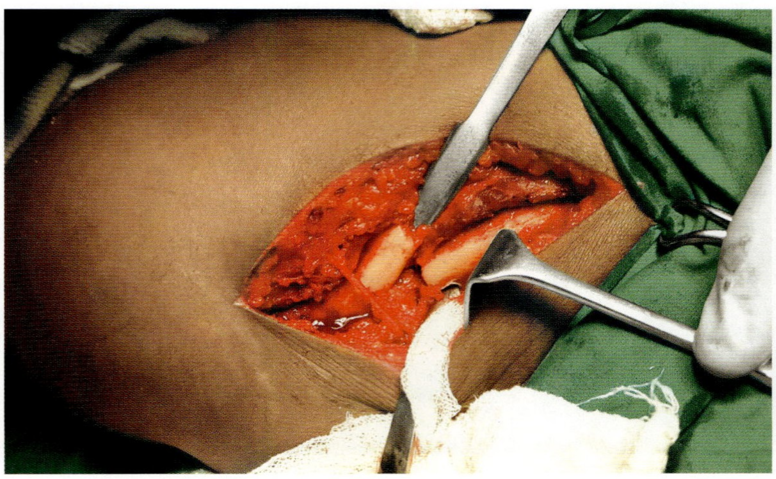

Fig. 11: Identify the fractured ends and freshen the edges.

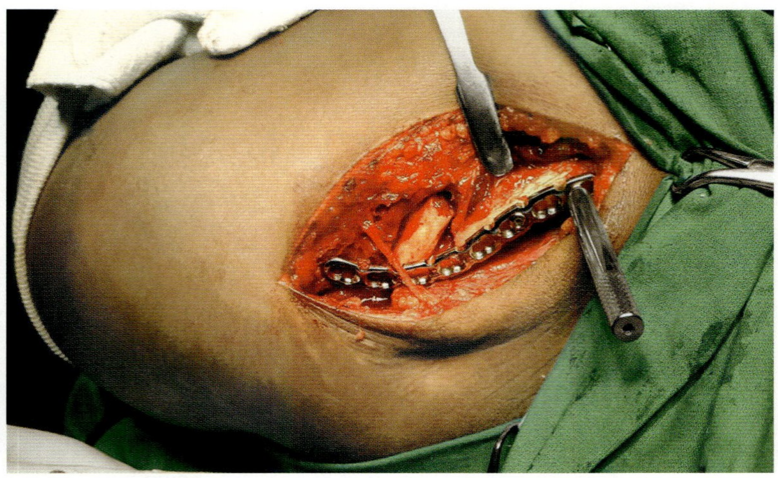

Fig. 12: Position the plate on the medial end of the clavicle using locking sleeve.

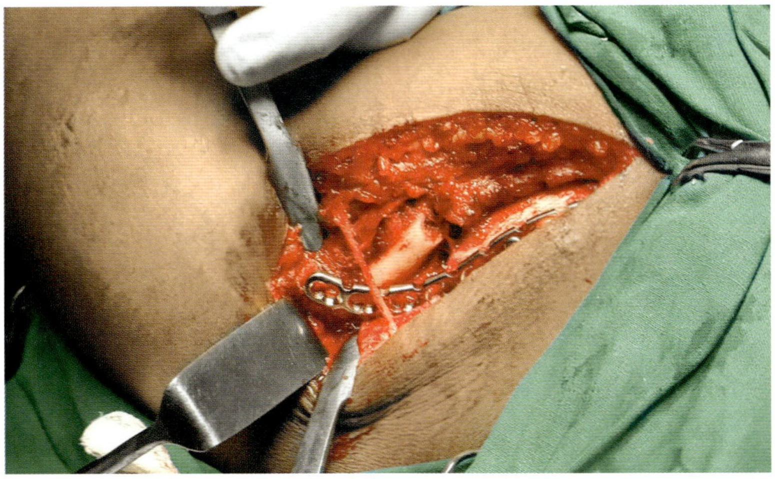

Fig. 13: Apply two screws, first being cortical to pull bone to plate on the medial fragment. Application of two screws on medial fragment ensures that all screws placement is in center of shaft. This is important for medial fragment as it is comparatively narrower.

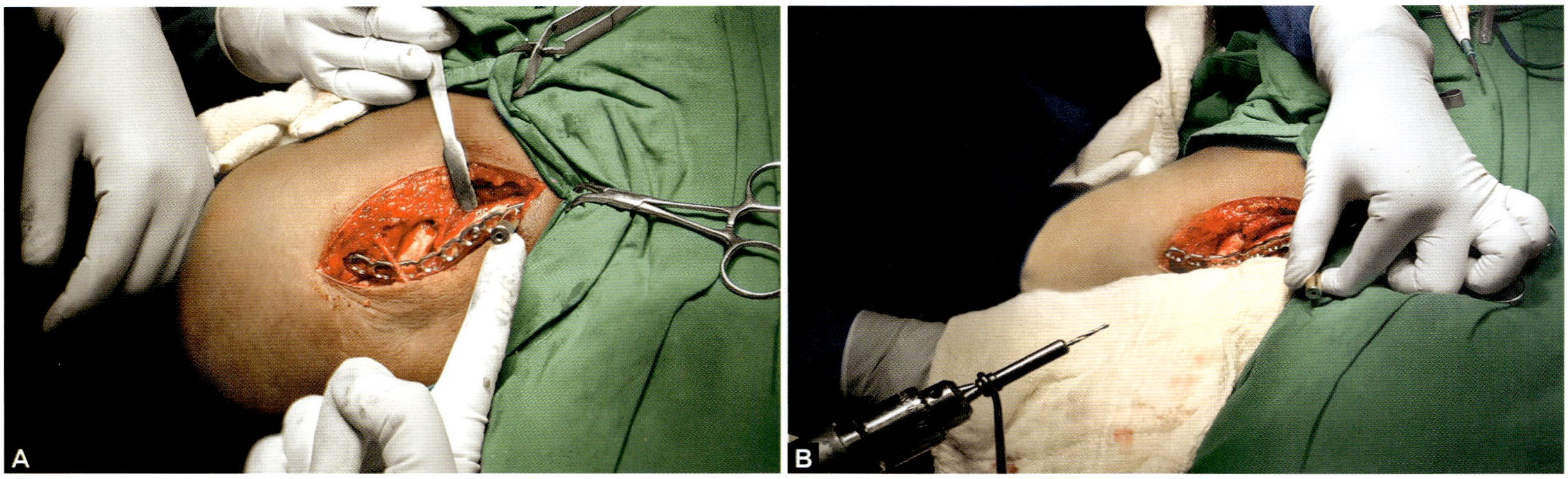

Figs. 14A and B: Patient's head comes in way of drill for more medial screws. The sleeve can be lifted up after application of first screw to create space for the drill. The drill bit length outside sleeve to be only slightly longer than bone width to prevent accidental plunge into adjacent vital structures.

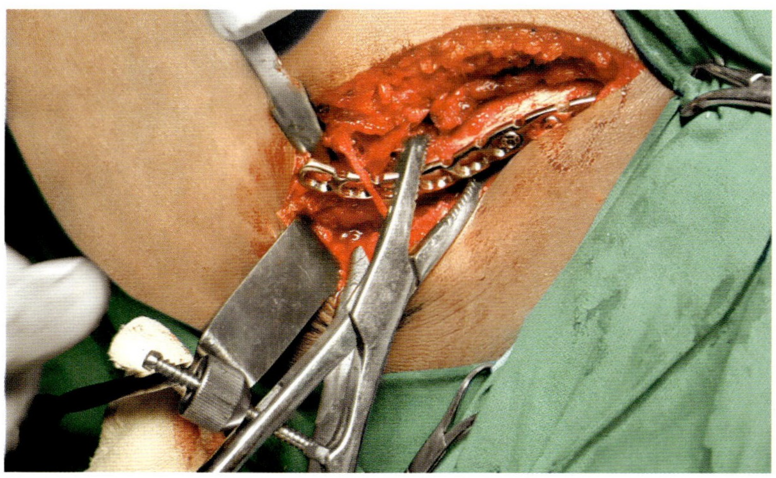

Fig. 15: Reduce the fracture with the help of a bone holding forceps.

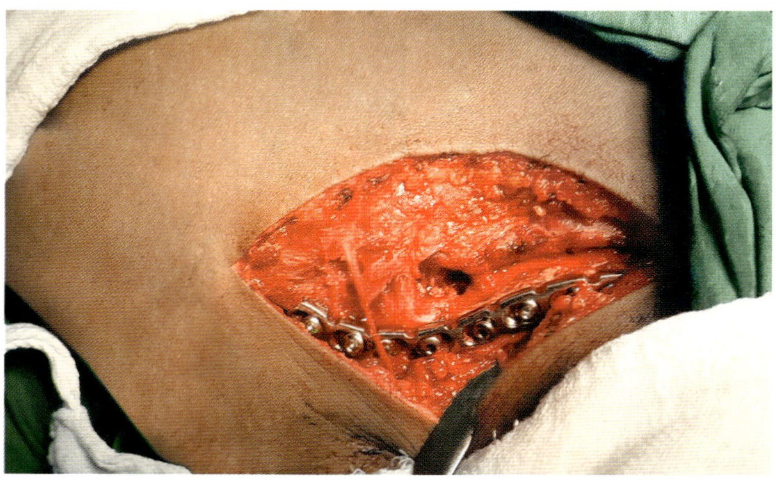

Fig. 16: Apply the remaining screws on the lateral end of the clavicle as well.

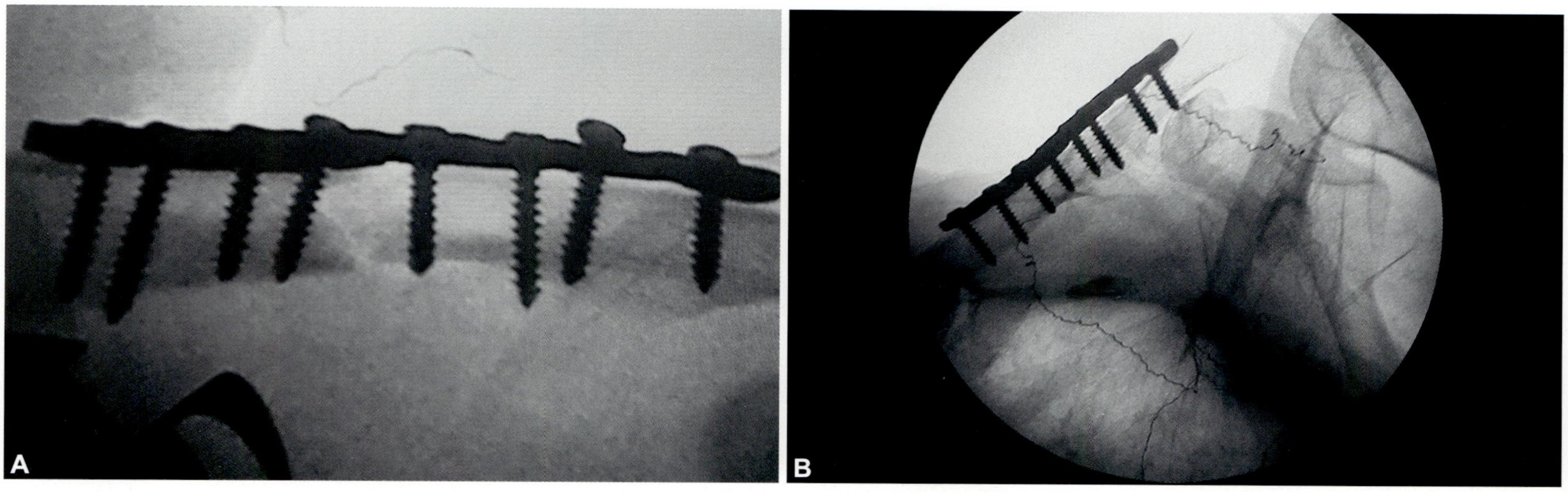

Figs. 17A and B: An intraoperative radiograph image is used to verify the correct length of the screws. Too long screws can damage the neurovascular structures underneath.

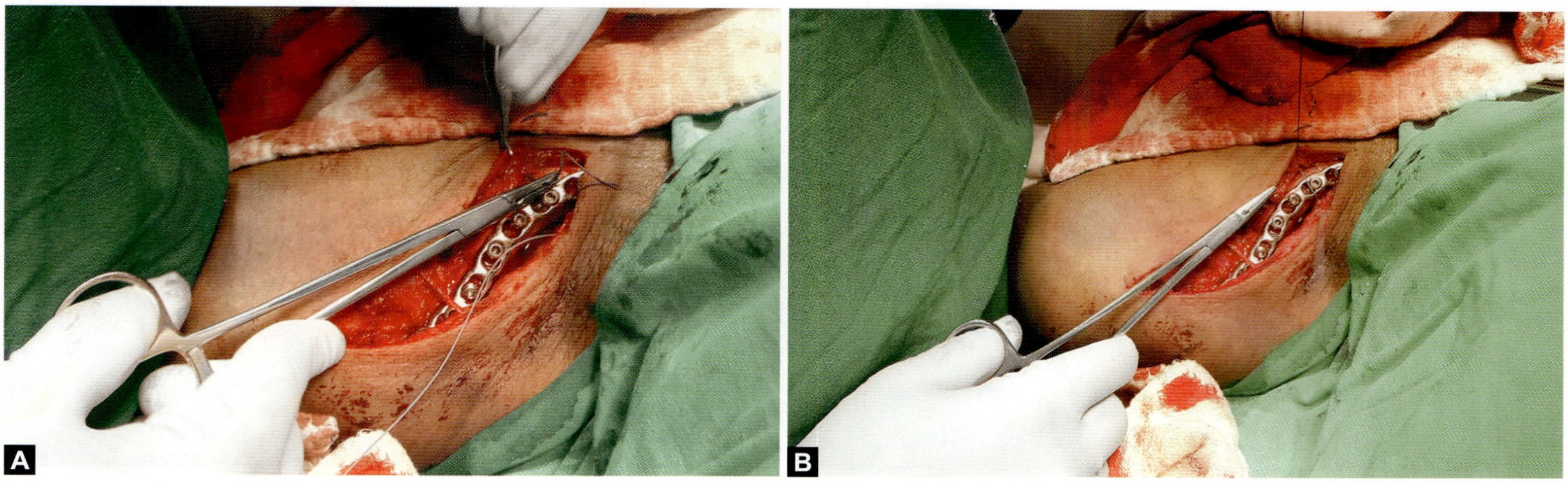

Figs. 18A and B: Sometimes, a butterfly fragment is attached to the plate by a sling suture of strong nonabsorbable material.

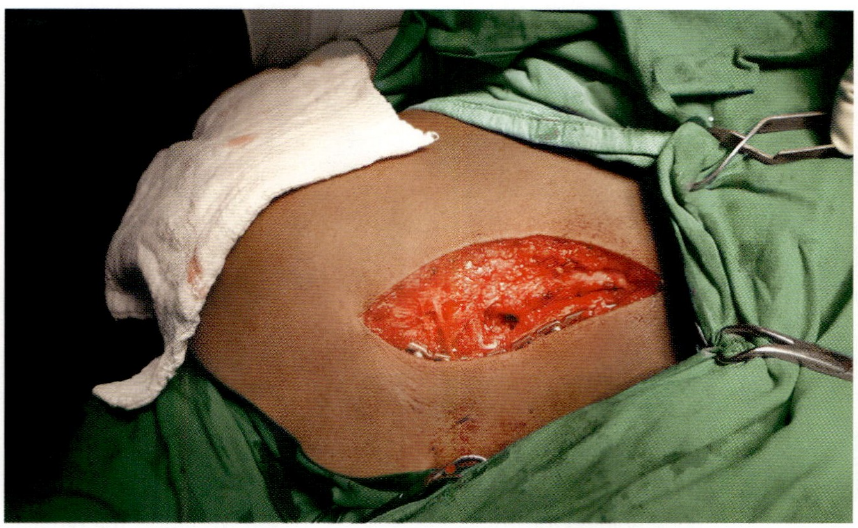

Fig. 19: Closure is performed in layers in a routine manner.

SURGICAL STEPS: FRACTURE OF DISTAL CLAVICLE (FIGS. 20 TO 33)

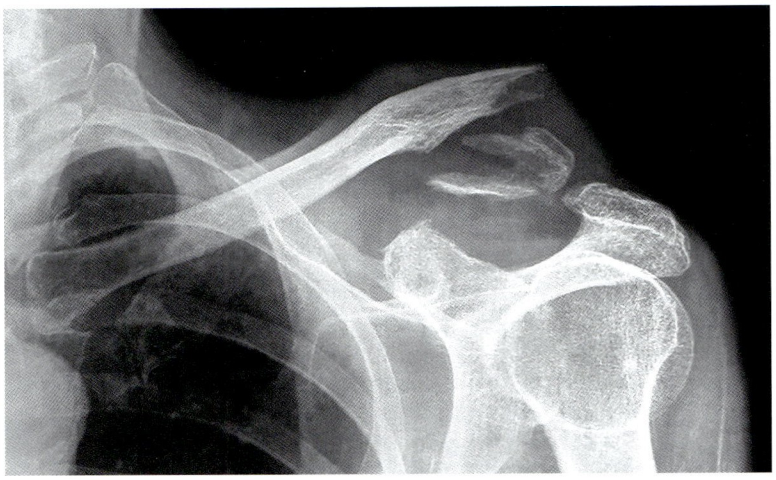

Fig. 20: Preoperative anteroposterior radiograph showing a fracture in the distal end of the clavicle.

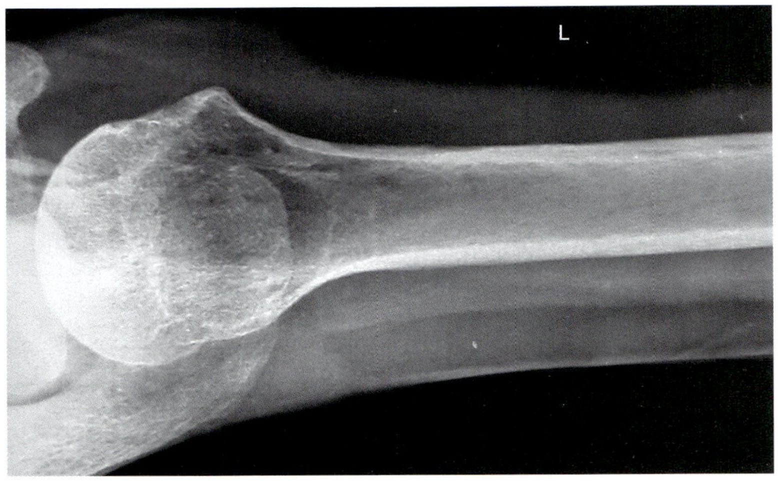

Fig. 21: Axillary view of the shoulder of the same patient.

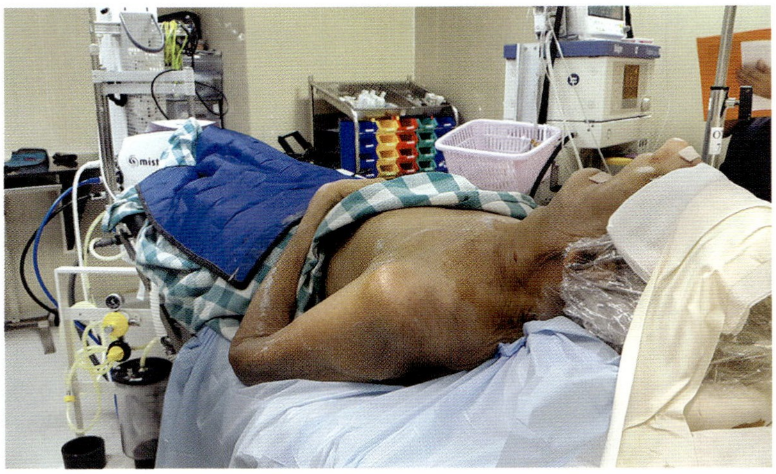

Fig. 22: Position of the patient. Anesthetist is at the foot end of the patient. The head end of the patient is raised by a pillow or the table is put in a beach chair position. The head of the patient is securely strapped to the table. Prior to painting and draping, a test shoot is taken to see if a proper view of the clavicle is obtained.

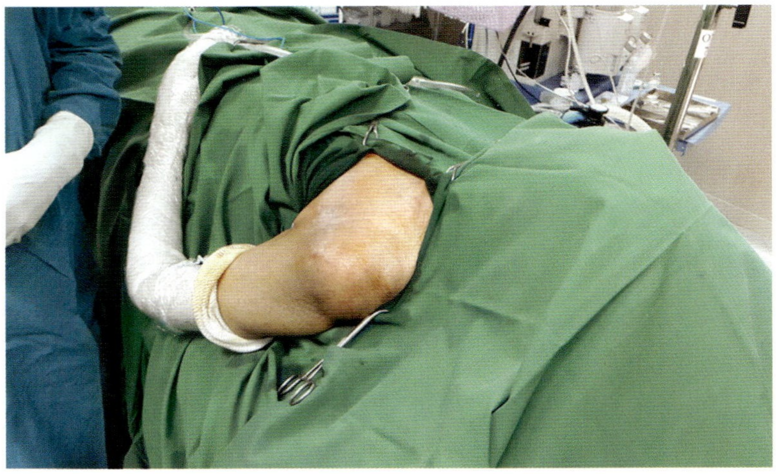

Fig. 23: Draping of the patient. The arm of the patient is draped in a sterile stockinette and a waterproof seal and a sticky drape is applied.

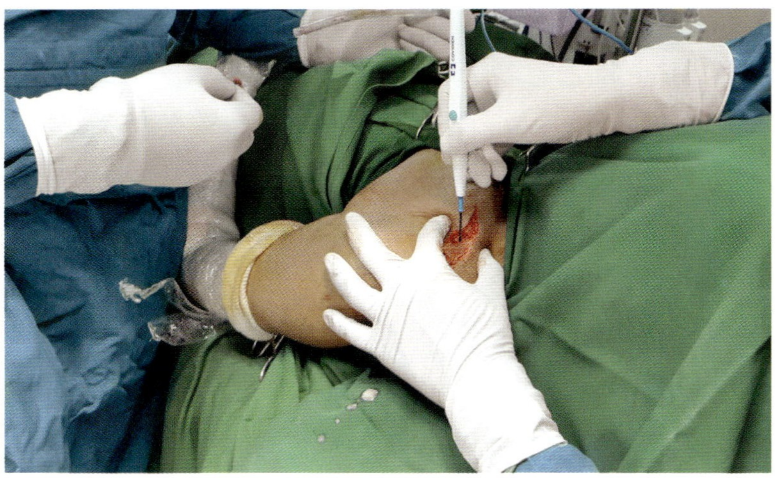

Fig. 24: An incision approximately 6–7 cm long is taken on the clavicle at the fracture site. A cautery is used to coagulate bleeders if any. Avoid injury to the supraclavicular nerve.

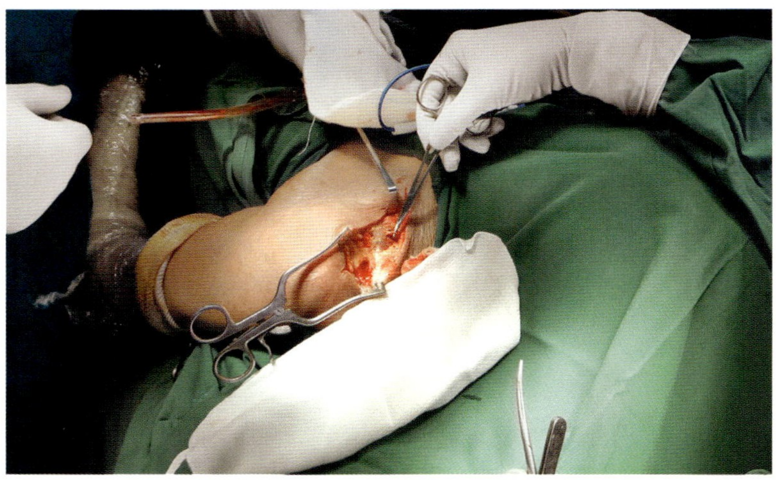

Fig. 25: Retraction is done by a mastoid/self-retaining retractor and the supraclavicular nerve is identified.

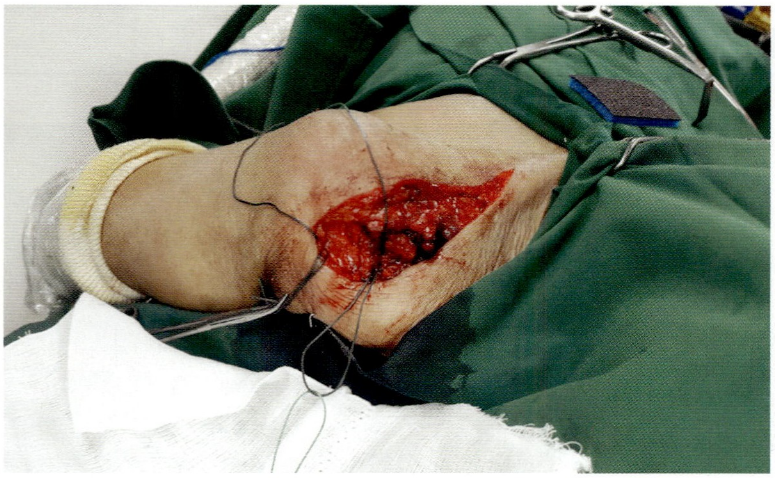

Fig. 26: Sometimes, reduction has to be done by using strong nonabsorbable sutures or similar to pull up the distal end of clavicle. This suture application has to be done at exposure prior to plate application as later on it is difficult.

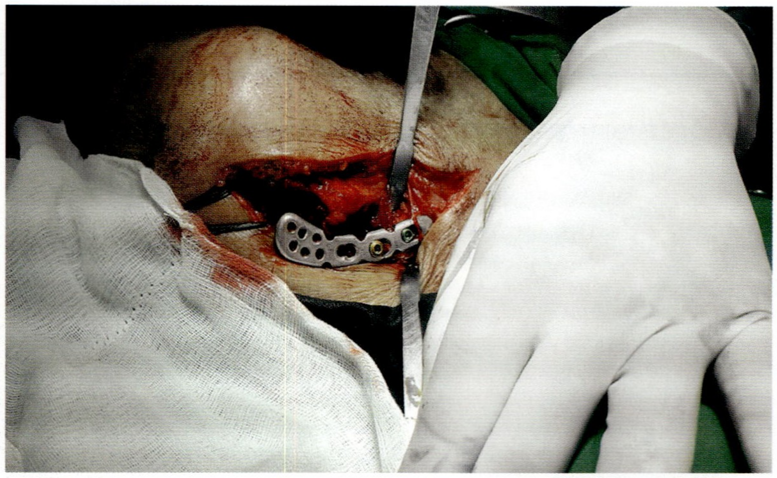

Fig. 27: A specially contoured anatomical locked plate is applied to the clavicle and screws are applied to the medial fragment.

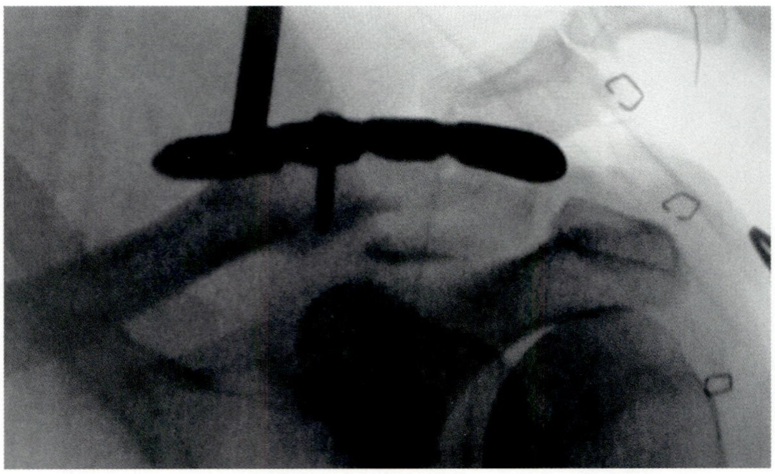

Fig. 28: Plate position is checked on C-arm image.

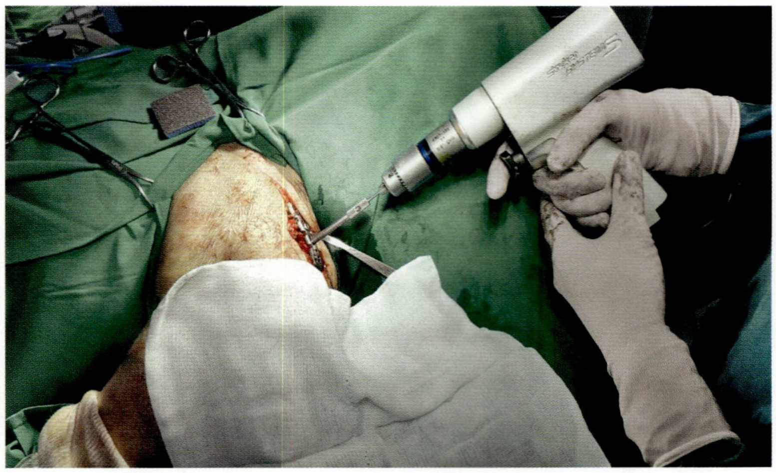

Fig. 29: After reduction is confirmed, the remaining screws are applied in the similar fashion.

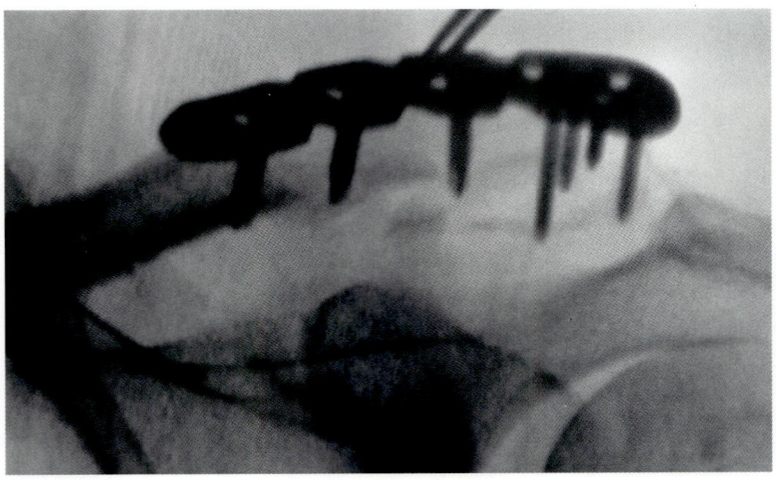

Fig. 30: After all screws are applied a final C-arm image is taken to confirm the placement and reduction. Lateral screws are carefully checked to ensure that they are not encroaching on joint.

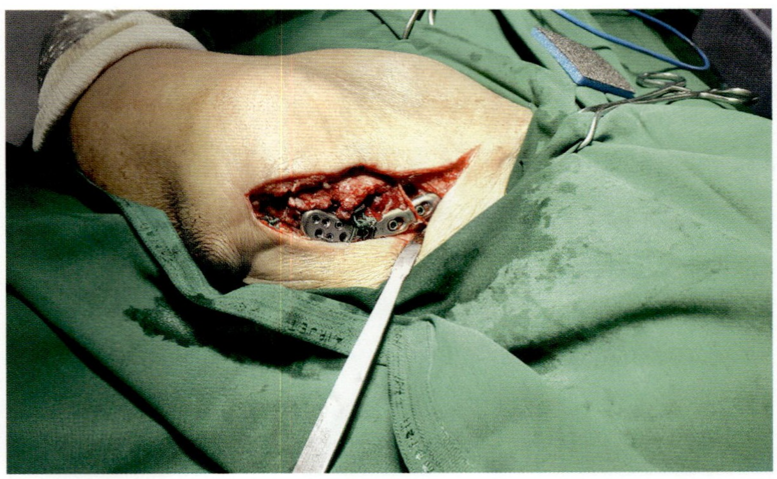

Fig. 31: The nonabsorbable sutures, which were passed under the distal fragment, are now tied securely over the plate. Care should be taken to cut them short after the knot else there will be irritation to the overlying skin.

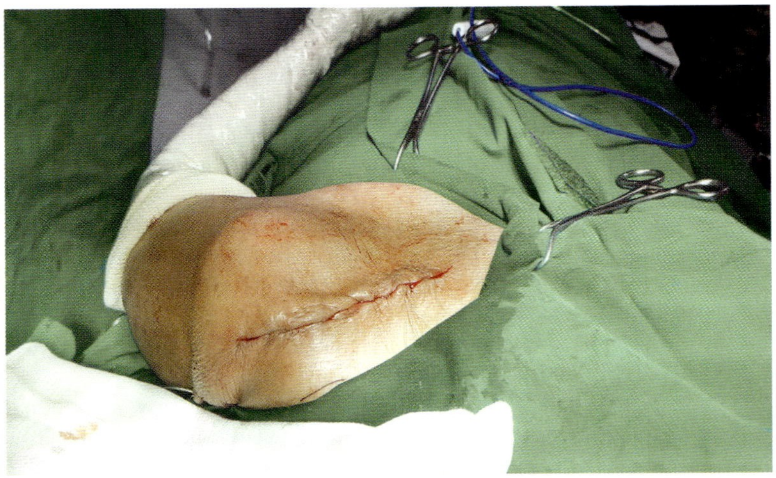

Fig. 32: Suturing is done in layers. Subcutaneous tissue is sutured with either 2-0 or 3-0 absorbable and skin is sutured with either 3-0 nylon or Staples.

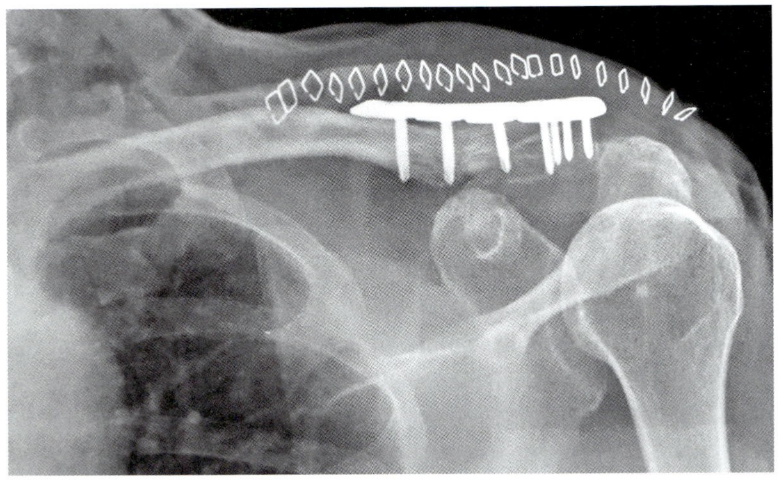

Fig. 33: A postoperative radiograph shows good placement of the plate and reduction.

COMPLICATIONS

Infection

Since the soft tissue coverage is not much, clavicle fractures are prone to infection (5%). However, they can be successfully managed with local wound care, antibiotics, and hardware removal after fracture union.

Malunion

Every clavicle fracture treated conservatively has some amount of malreduction, but some recent studies have shown a loss of function as well.

If the clavicle is shortened more than 15 mm, it can change the shoulder dynamics.

This malunion can cause pain, neurologic symptoms and even weakness.

Nonunion

All displaced fractures have a high rate of non union. It is 1–15% in mid shaft clavicle fractures and 11–40% in distal end clavicle fractures. Female sex, age, degree of displacement and comminution are risk factors for non union of the clavicle fracture.

Non union can cause pain, restriction of movement of the shoulder and neurovascular symptoms.

Plate fixation with or without bone grafting is the treatment for a symptomatic non union of fracture clavicle. In cases of nonunion of the distal end of the clavicle, excision of the distal end of the clavicle may be needed in case the fragment is small and the coracoclavicular ligaments are intact, and open reduction and internal fixation if the distal fragment is large enough.

Refracture

It is reported at rate of between 1% and 2%.

Hardware Prominence

In case the hardware is prominent, and causes irritation which is often seen with backpacks and similar straps it may need removal. The hardware reportedly needs to be removed in 8% of patients.

Pain

The other complications are:

- Restriction of shoulder movement, Weakness and neurovascular symptoms, Thoracic outlet syndrome and Subclavian vein compression.

SUGGESTED READING

1. Ballmer FT, Gerber C. Coracoclavicular screw fixation for unstable fractures of the distal clavicle. A report of five cases. J Bone Joint Surg Br. 1991;73:291-4.
2. Canadian Orthopaedic Trauma Society. Nonoperative treatment compared with plate fixation of displaced midshaft clavicular fractures. A multicenter randomized clinical trial. J Bone Joint Surg Am. 2007; 89(1):1-10.
3. Chan KY, Jupiter JB, Leffert RD, et al. Clavicle malunion. J Shoulder Elbow Surg. 1999;8(4):287-90.
4. Edwards DJ, Kavanagh TG, Flannery MC. Fractures of the distal clavicle: a case for fixation. Injury. 1992;23:44-6.
5. Eskola A, Vainionpaa S, Patiala H, et al. Outcome of operative treatment in fresh lateral clavicular fracture. Ann Chir Gynaecol. 1987;76:167-9.
6. Ghormley RK, Black JR, Cherry JH. Ununited fractures of the clavicle. Am J Surg. 1941;51:343-9.
7. Goldberg JA, Bruce WJ, Sonnabend DH, et al. Type 2 fractures of the distal clavicle: a new surgical technique. J Shoulder Elbow Surg. 1997;6:380-2.
8. Goldberg JA, Bruce WJ, Sonnabend DH, et al. Type 2 fractures of the distal clavicle: a new surgical technique. J Shoulder Elbow Surg. 1997;6(4): 380-2.
9. Harrington MA Jr, Keller TS, Seiler JGD, et al. Geometric properties and the predicted mechanical behavior of adult human clavicles. J Biomech. 1993;26:417-26.
10. Hessmann M, Kirchner R, Baumgaertel F, et al. Treatment of unstable distal clavicular fractures with and without lesions of the acromioclavicular joint. Injury. 1996;27(1):47-52.
11. Hill JM, McGuire MH, Crosby LA. Closed treatment of displaced middle-third fractures of the clavicle gives poor results. J Bone Joint Surg Br. 1997;79(4):537-9.
12. Jupiter JB, Leffert RD. Nonunion of the clavicle. Associated complications and surgical management. J Bone Joint Surg Am. 1987;69:753-60.
13. Katznelson A, Nerubay J, Oliver S. Dynamic fixation of the avulsed clavicle. J Trauma. 1976;16:841-4.
14. Khan LA, Bradnock TJ, Scott C, et al. Fractures of the clavicle. J Bone Joint Surg Am. 2009;91(2):447-60.

15. Klein SM, Badman BL, Keating CJ, et al. Results of surgical treatment for unstable distal clavicular fractures. J Shoulder Elbow Surg. 2010;19(7):1049-55.
16. Levy O. Simple, minimally invasive surgical technique for treatment of type 2 fractures of the distal clavicle. J Shoulder Elbow Surg. 2003;12(1):24-8.
17. McKee MD, Wild LM, Schemitsch EH. Midshaft malunions of the clavicle. Surgical technique. J Bone Joint Surg Am. 2004;86-A (Suppl 1):37-43.
18. Moseley HF. The clavicle: its anatomy and function. Clin Orthop Relat Res. 1968;58:17-27.
19. Neer CS. Fractures of the distal clavicle with detachment of the coracoclavicular ligaments in adults. J Trauma. 1963;3:99-110.
20. Neer CS. Fractures of the distal third of the clavicle. Clin Orthop. 1968;58:43-50.
21. Neviaser JS. The treatment of fractures of the clavicle. Surg Clin North Am. 1963;43:1555-63.
22. Neviaser RJ. Injuries to the clavicle and acromioclavicular joint. Orthop Clin North Am. 1987;18:433-8.
23. Robinson CM, Court-Brown CM, McQueen MM, et al. Estimating the risk of nonunion following nonoperative treatment of a clavicular fracture. J Bone Joint Surg Am. 2004;86-A(7):1359-65.
24. Rockwood CA. Chapter 32. Rockwood and Green's Fractures in Adults, 6th edition. Philadephia:Lippincott Williams & Wilkins; 2006. pp. 1236-49.
25. Webber MC, Haines JF. The treatment of lateral clavicle fractures. Injury. 2000;31(3):175-9.
26. Wood VE. The results of total claviculectomy. Clin Orthop Relat Res. 1986;(207):186-90.
27. Yamaguchi H, Arakawa H, Kobayashi M. Results of the Bosworth method for unstable fractures of the distal clavicle. Int Orthop. 1998;22(6):366-8.

CHAPTER 82

Fracture Greater Tuberosity Fixation with Nonabsorbable Suture

Ajay Chandanwale, Rajkumar Ekambaram, Rachit Vipul Shah

INTRODUCTION

Isolated undisplaced fracture of greater tuberosity is comparatively less common than proximal humerus involving the neck of humerus.

These types of fractures are generally classified under type 1 of Neer classification of proximal humerus fractures.

The mechanism of injury is impaction and avulsion injury of proximal humerus.

- The impaction type of injury is mostly due to forced hyperflexion and hyperabduction of the shoulder.
- The avulsion type of injuries is associated with glenohumeral dislocation of shoulder joint.

Lesser tuberosity fracture is also extremely rare and associated with posterior dislocation or comminuted proximal humerus fractures.

CLINICAL FEATURES

- Pain, swelling, and tenderness on palpation. Pain can be located mostly anterior to bicipital groove and increased on active overhead abduction.
- Pain on abduction of arm is characteristic.

INVESTIGATIONS

- Anteroposterior (AP) and lateral radiographs are useful.
- Magnetic resonance imaging (MRI) scan is used when there is any suspicion of recurrent dislocations and rotator cuff rupture.

TREATMENT

- Conservative management (for undisplaced fractures) includes initiation of passive range of motion 1 week postinjury and active range of motion 6 weeks postinjury.
- Open reduction and internal fixation are indicated in displaced fractures of greater tuberosity. (1) Screws, (2) Tension band, (3) Nonabsorbable suture.

SURGICAL STEPS (FIGS. 1 TO 6)

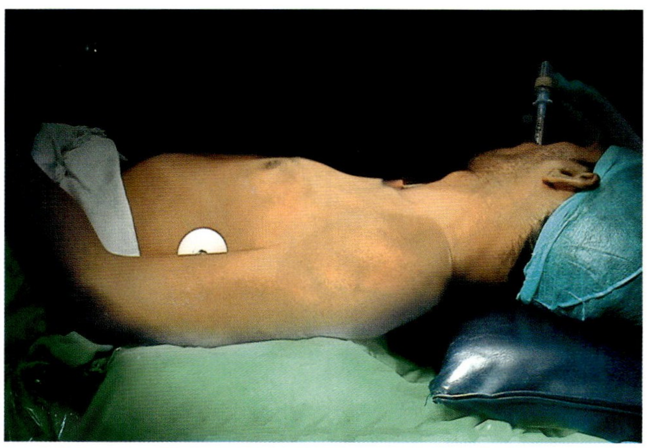

Fig. 1: *Position*: Supine position; Arm by the side of the body; Sandbag under the shoulder; Head up to reduce intraoperative hemorrhage.

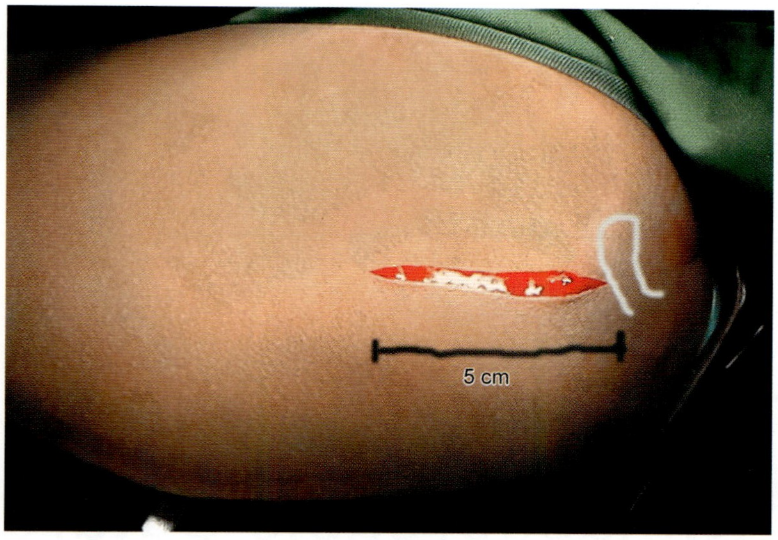

Fig. 2: *Approach and incision—Lateral approach*: Incision starting from the level of the tip of acromion descending distally up to 5 cm.

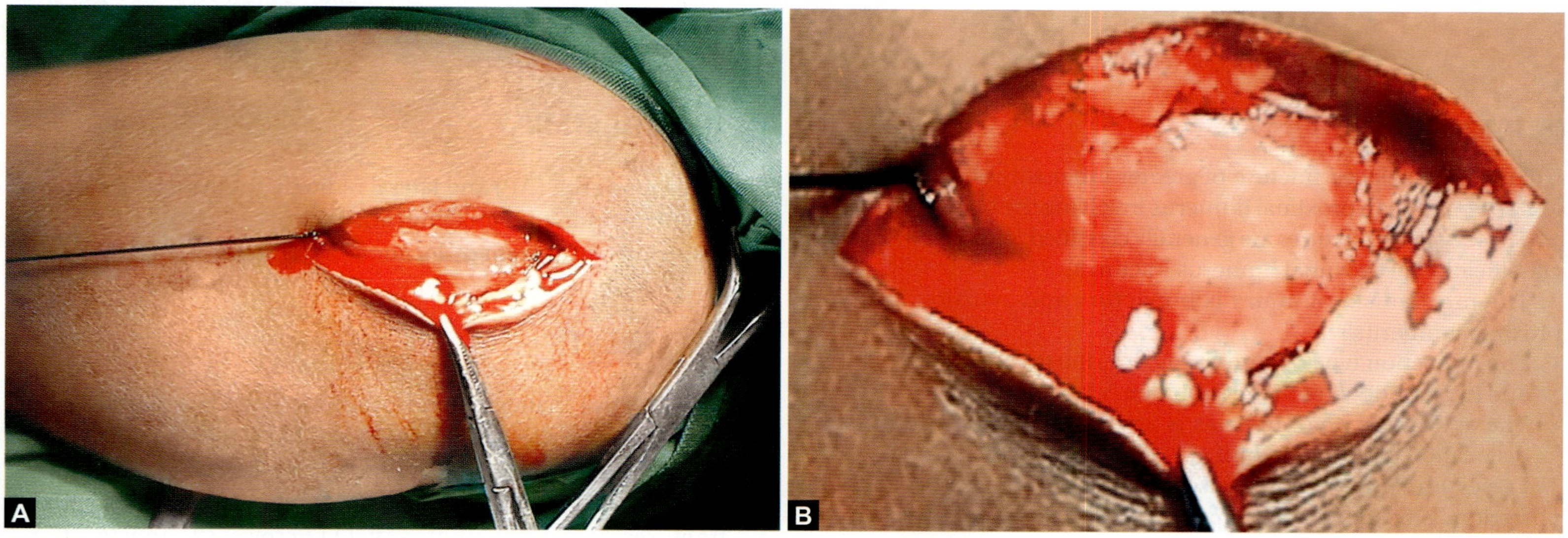

Figs. 3A and B: *Exposing the deltoid*: After exposing the deltoid (A), a stay suture is passed through the fibers of the muscle at the distal end of the incision; (B)—to limit the undesirable splitting of deltoid beyond the distal end of incision, which may endanger the axillary nerve.

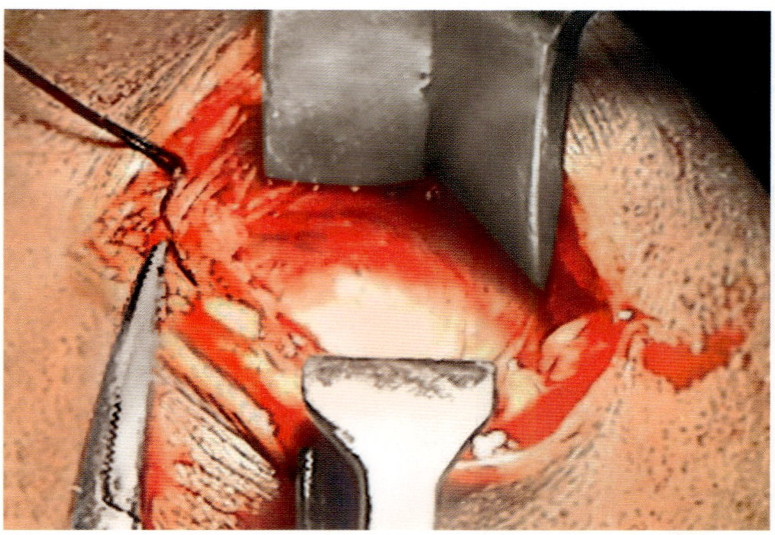

Fig. 4: *Identifying supraspinatus insertion*: Deltoid is split to expose rotator cuff and greater tuberosity.

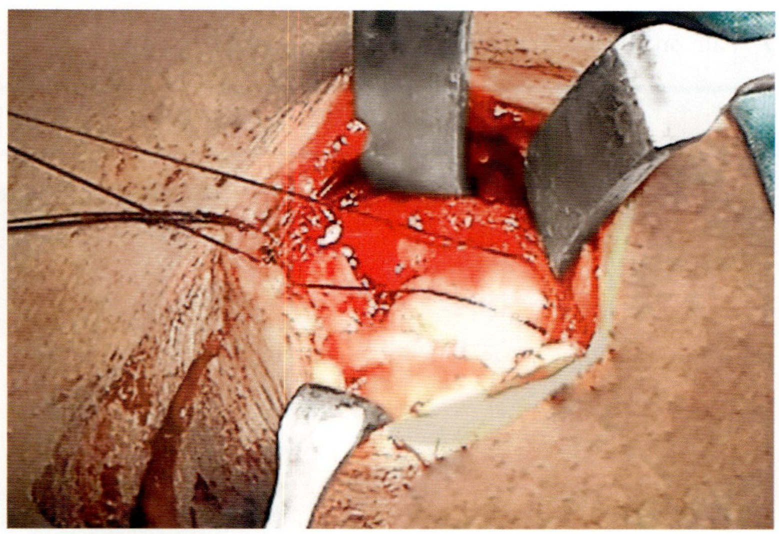

Fig. 5: *Passing nonabsorbable suture underneath supraspinatus insertion*: A thick nonabsorbable suture on reverse cutting needle (e.g. 3 number or 5 number polypropylene (nonabsorbable).

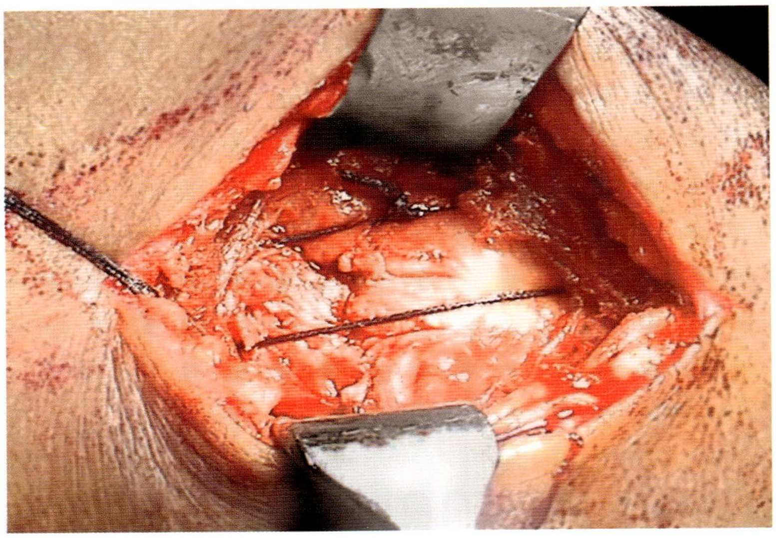

Fig. 6: *Passing suture through distal fragment and tying knot*: Make a drill hole through lateral cortex of upper part of distal fragment using drill bit or K-wire. Then, pass the suture using the needle. Then, the knot is tied after approximating the fracture site by abducting the shoulder.

SUGGESTED READING

1. Court-Brown CM, Garg A, McQueen MM. The epidemiology of proximal humeral fractures. Acta Orthop Scand. 2001;72(4):365-71.
2. Mattyasovszky SG, Burkhart KJ, Ahlers C, et al. Isolated fractures of the greater tuberosity of the proximal humerus: a long-term retrospective study of 30 patients. Acta Orthop. 2011;82(6):714-20.
3. Murray IR, Amin AK, White TO, et al. Proximal humeral fractures: current concepts in classification, treatment and outcomes. J Bone Joint Surg Br. 2011;93(1):1-11.
4. Park MC, Murthi AM, Roth NS, et al. Two-part and three-part fractures of the proximal humerus treated with suture fixation. J Orthop Trauma. 2003;17(5):319-25.

CHAPTER 83

Fracture Proximal Humerus Fixation

Shrinivas S Shintre, Vijay M Panchanadikar, Prateek Charuchandra Joshi, Chittanand Mendhe, Rajkumar Ekambaram

TWO PART FRACTURE PROXIMAL HUMERUS–PLATE FIXATION

Shrinivas S Shintre, Vijay M Panchanadikar

INTRODUCTION

Proximal humerus fractures are defined as the ones occurring at or proximal to the surgical neck of the humerus. It is the most common fracture affecting the shoulder girdle in adult population. Osteoporosis is one of the main contributory factors. Proximal humerus fractures have a unimodal distribution in the adult population and in patients above the age of 65 years, it accounts for more than 10% of upper extremity fractures.

The most common mechanism of injury is a fall from standing height. Other causes for fracture of proximal humerus include higher energy trauma such as fall from a height, motor vehicle accidents, sports injuries, and assaults. There are three main loading modes as a consequence of which proximal humerus can fracture: compressive loading of glenoid onto the humeral head, bending loads at the surgical neck and tension loads of the rotator cuff at the greater and lesser tuberosities.

INDICATIONS

Locked plate fixation is indicated for open reduction and internal fixation of fractures of proximal humerus, which include displaced and unstable fractures of either anatomical neck or surgical neck. Anterior deltopectoral approach is most commonly used for fractures of proximal humerus.

External fixator may be a method of definitive fixation in some carefully selected elderly morbid patients.

Other conditions, which may alter the management, include soft tissue or bony injuries of the shoulder and/or elbow joints, concomitant dislocation of the ipsilateral shoulder, floating elbow and less commonly injury to median and/or ulnar nerves.

POSTOPERATIVE PROTOCOL

Patients are kept on regular follow-up at 2 weeks, 6 weeks, and 3 months after surgery. Sling immobilization is done for 6 weeks after surgery and active range of motion exercises of the elbow, wrist, and hand are encouraged simultaneously. Passive range of motion exercises at shoulder are started between 2 weeks and 4 weeks after surgery depending on the fracture configuration and stability that was achieved along with forward elevation, external rotation, and pendulum exercises. Active assisted range of motion is started at 6 weeks if healing has progressed both clinically and radiographically. Suture removal is done 12–15 days after surgery.

POSSIBLE COMPLICATIONS

Apart from anesthetic complications, this surgery may be complicated by shoulder stiffness, screw back out, screw cut out, plate failure, malunion, and nonunion, primary screw perforation of the humeral head. Proper wound care must be taken to prevent postoperative surgical site infection and wound gaping. Other possible complications include malunion with varus angulation, superficial/deep wound infections, loss of fixation, subacromial impingement, vascular disruption of the proximal humerus, malreduction, glenoid erosion from screw perforation/penetration, and axillary nerve injury.

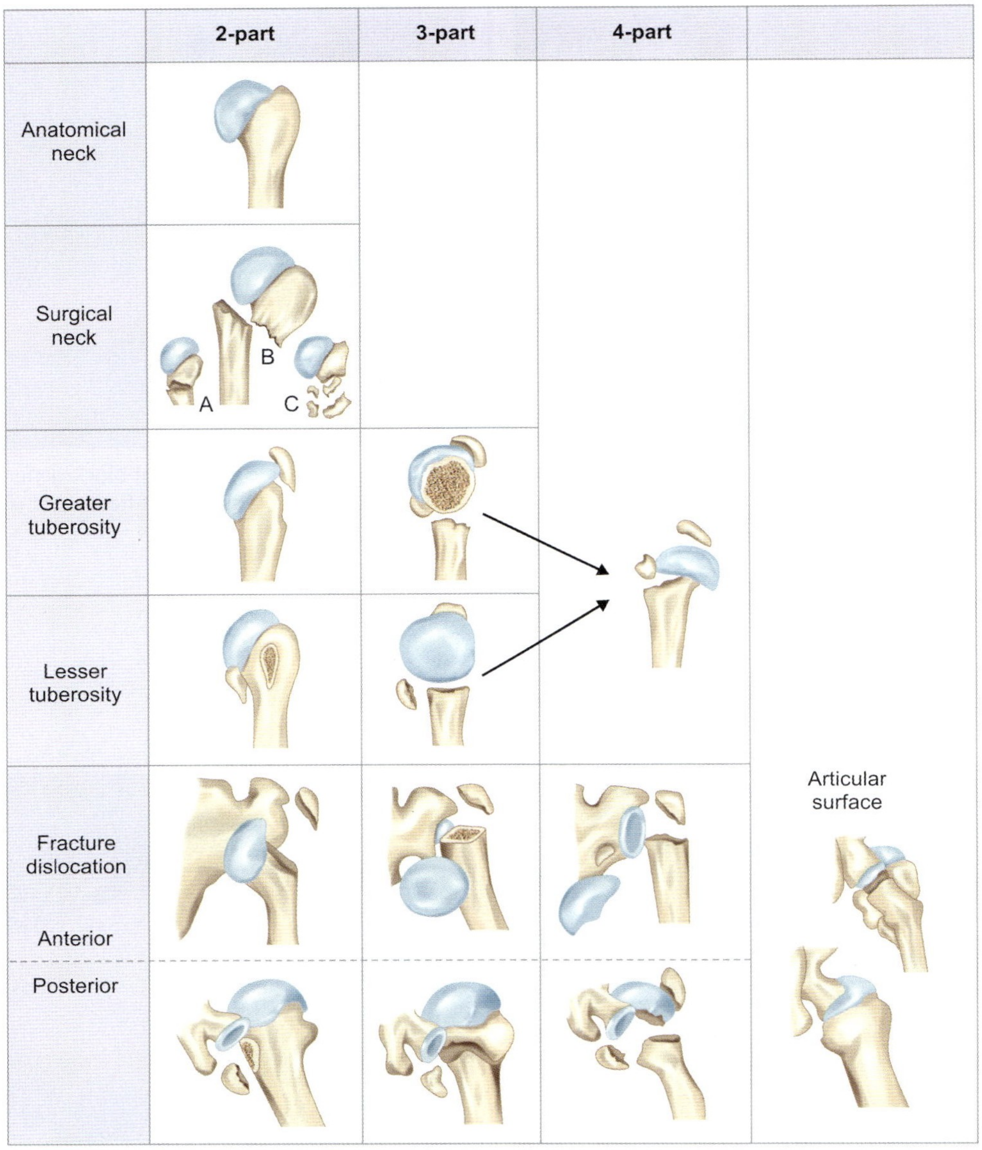

Fig. 1: Neer's classification.

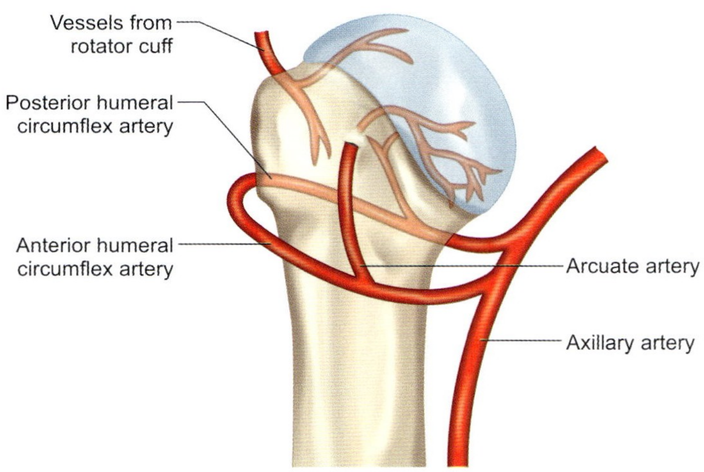

Fig. 2: Circulation around humeral head.

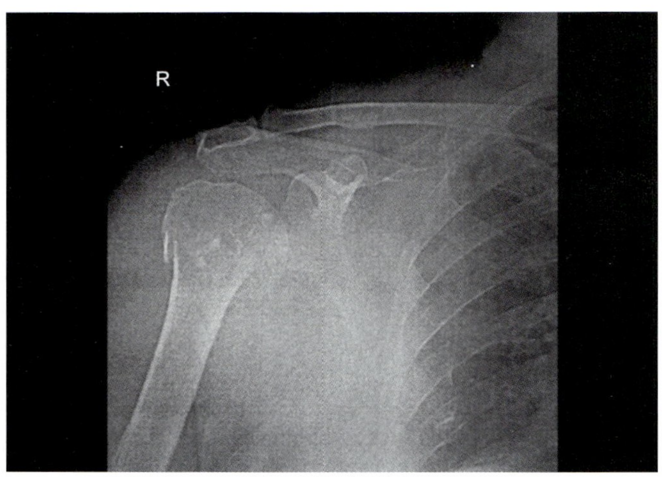

Fig. 3: X-ray—showing this to be two part fracture—however, both AP and lateral views necessary

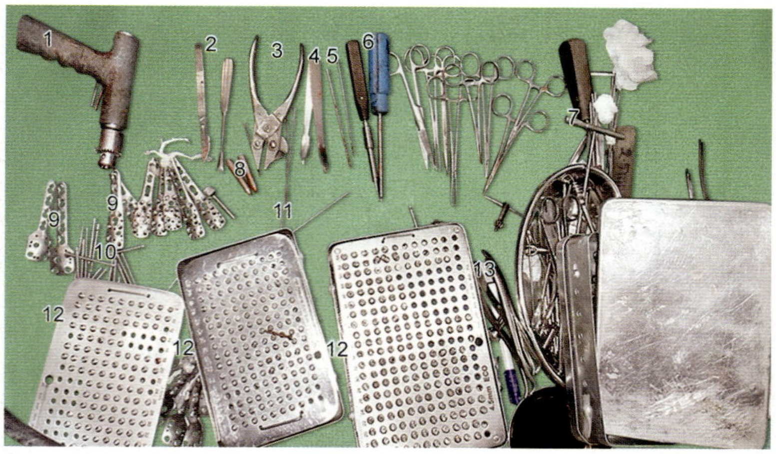

Fig. 4: Instruments—(1) Drill machine, (2) Periosteum elevator, (3) Plier with side cutter, (4) Bone levers (spikes), (5) Drill bits, (6) Screw drivers including torque limiting screw driver, (7) Tap, (8) Drill sleeves for locking screws, (9) Proximal humerus locking plates, (10) Locking screws, (11) K-wires, (12) Screw stands, (13) Bone holding clamps.

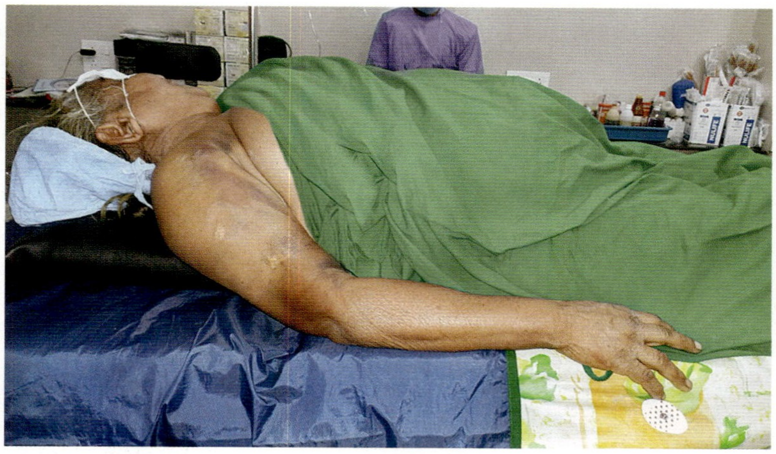

Fig. 5: Position—under regional block/general anesthesia, supine position on operating table, ensure that fracture is visualized in both C-arm views.

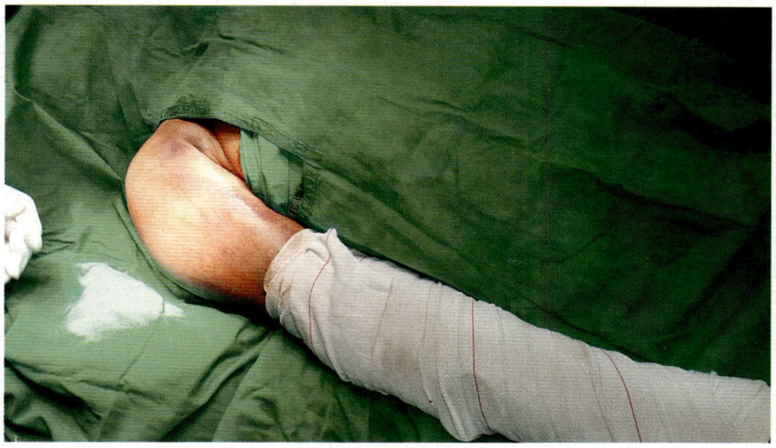

Fig. 6: Draping—upper limb draped separately for ease of manipulation.

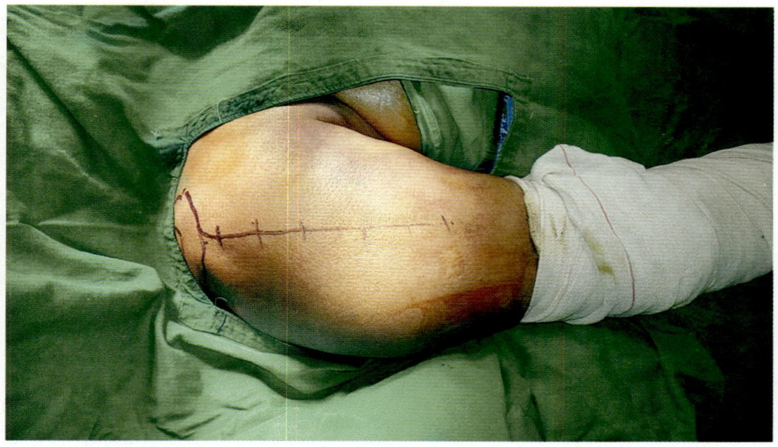

Fig. 7: Incision marking—starting from tip of acromion going distally—of length depending on length of plate to be fixed.

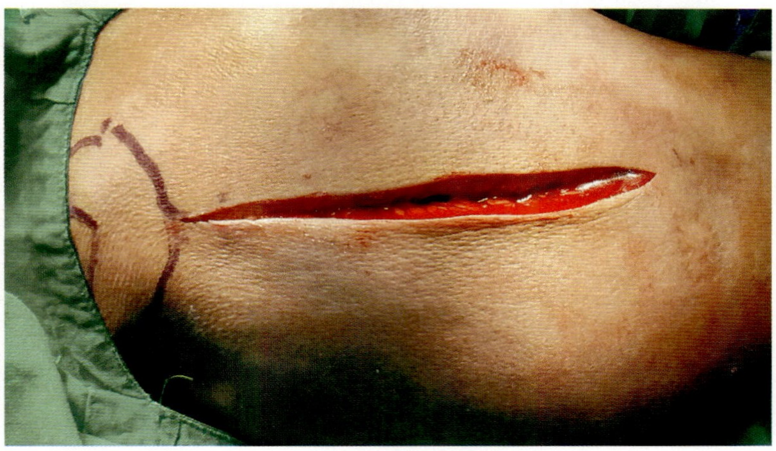

Fig. 8: Skin incision with 22 number blade.

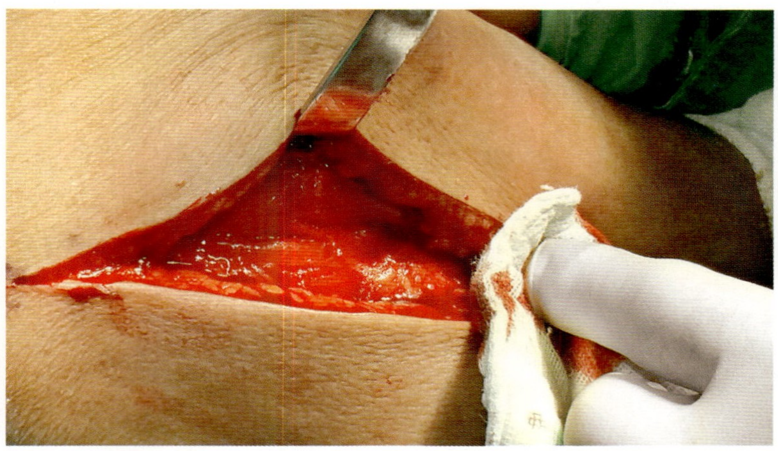

Fig. 9: Blunt sub cutaneous dissection using finger after cauterizing bleeders.

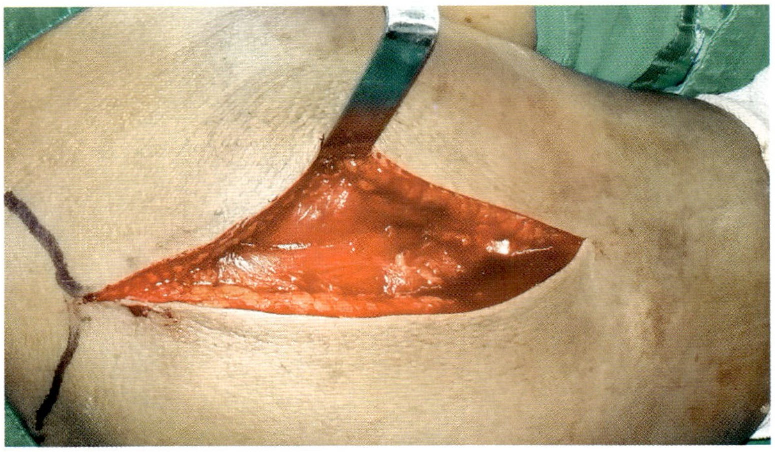

Fig. 10: Splitting deltoid muscle fibers with special care to protect axillary nerve at 5 cm distal to tip of acromion.

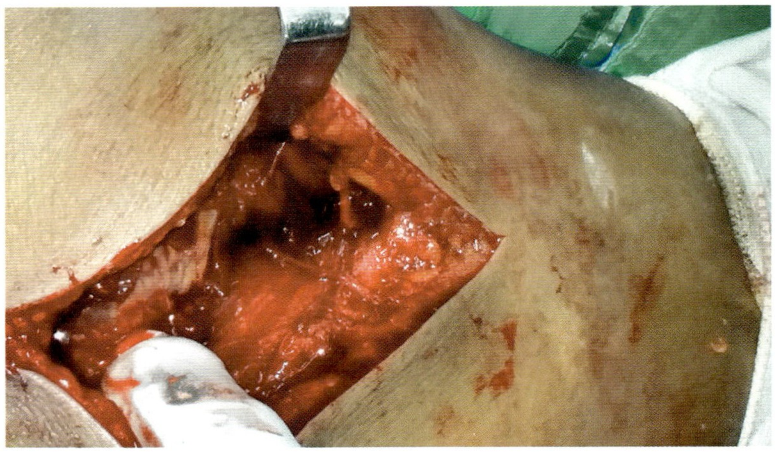

Fig. 11: Searching for axillary nerve—by blunt dissection with finger only.

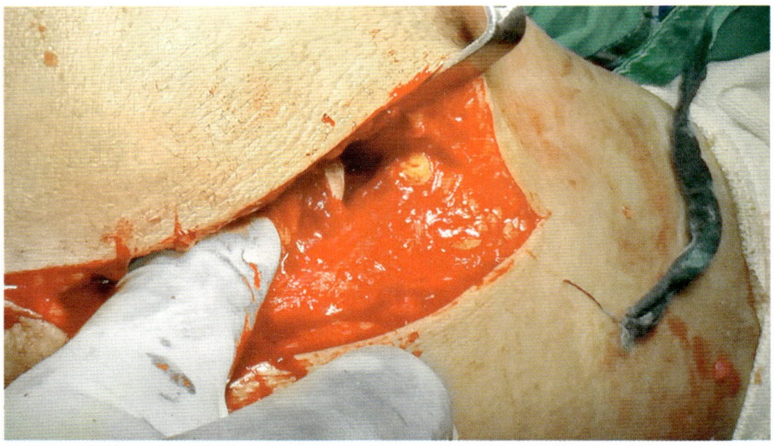

Fig. 12: Index finger is passed deeper to axillary nerve which is separated from surrounding soft tissue.

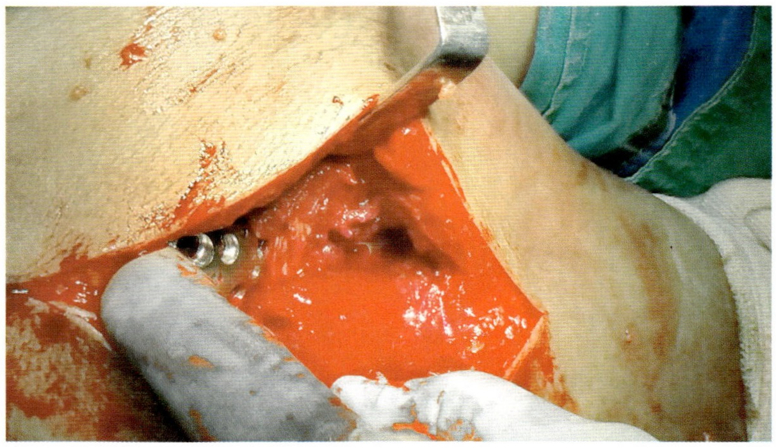

Fig. 13: Proximal humerus locking plate inserted protecting axillary nerve.

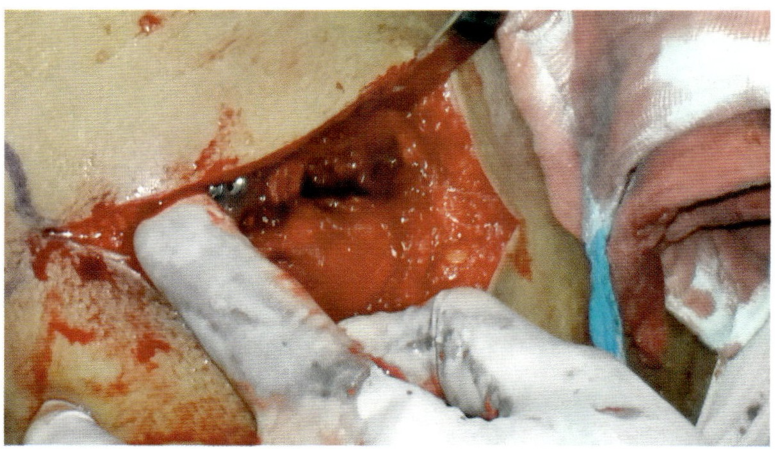

Fig. 14: Plate is pushed further.

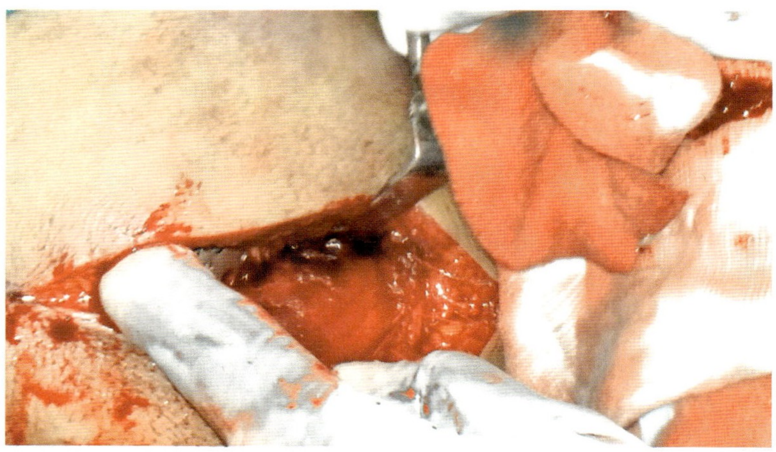

Fig. 15: Plate positioned finally so that its upper end is one finger breadth inferior to tip of greater tuberosity.

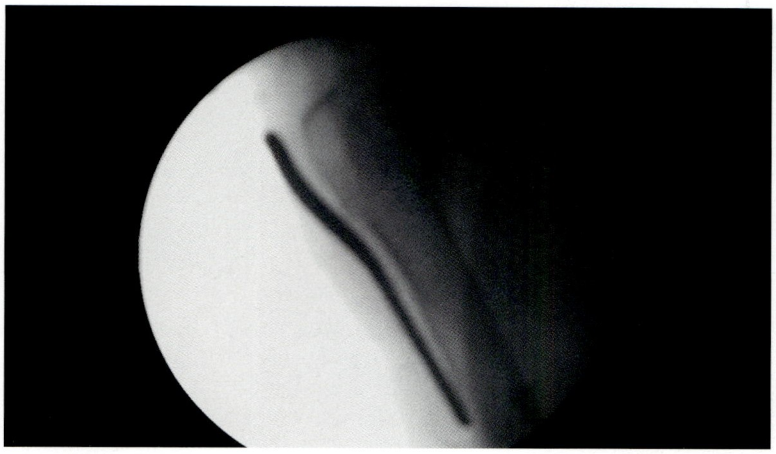

Fig. 16: Position confirmed under C-arm.

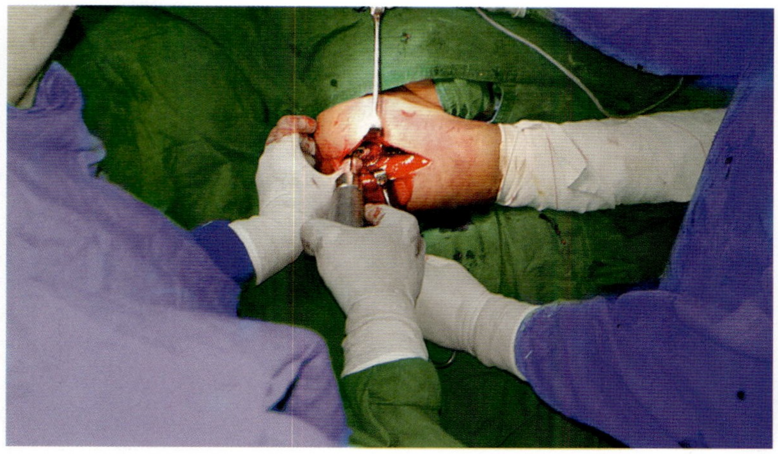

Fig. 17: Fixing locking plate provisionally with k-wire.

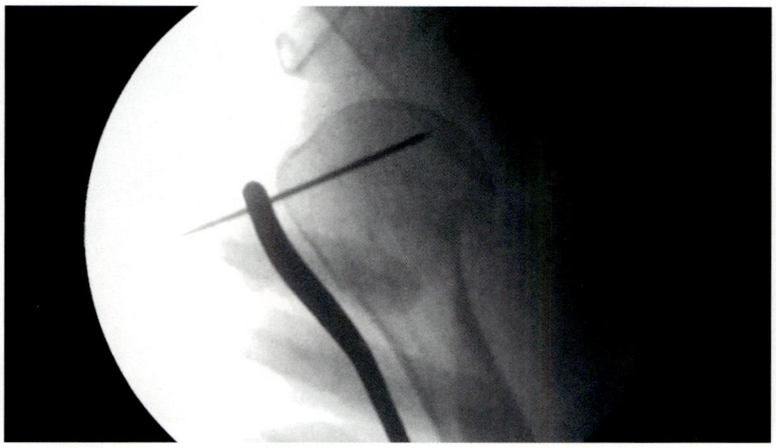

Fig. 18: C-arm image confirming length of wire inserted.

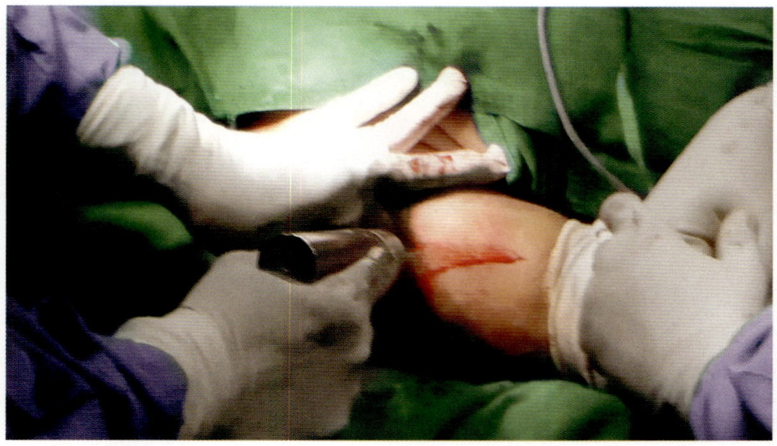

Fig. 19: Passing k-wire through other end of the plate.

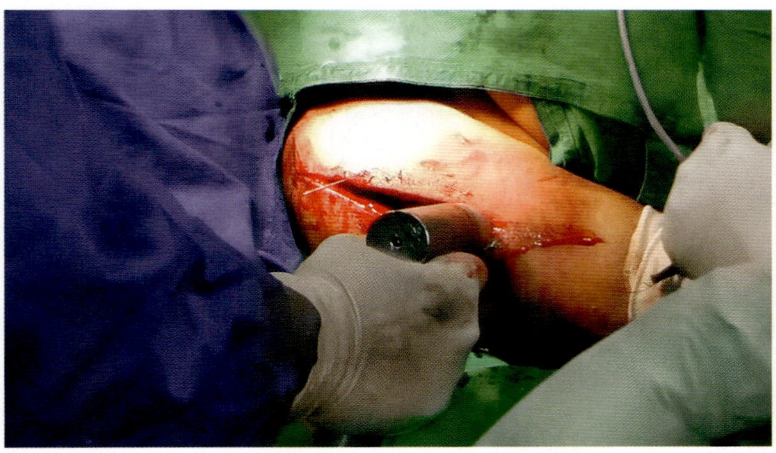

Fig. 20: Distal k-wire progressing further.

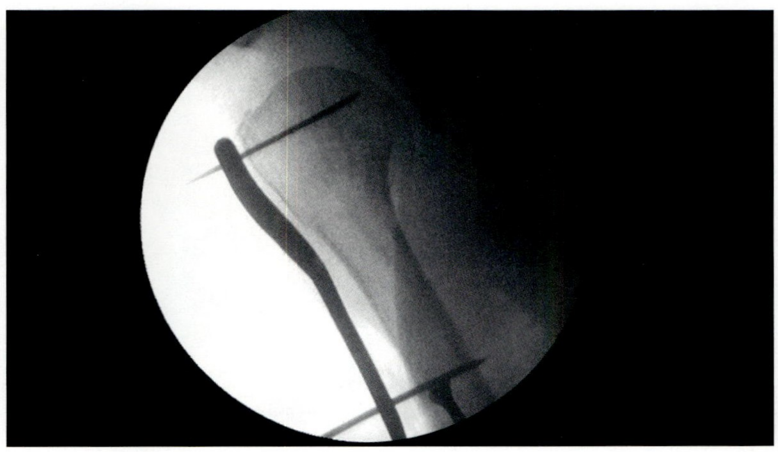

Fig. 21: C-arm imaging.

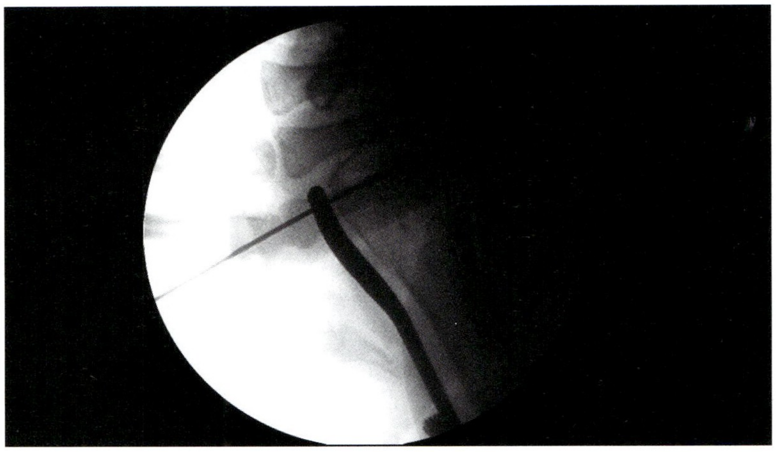

Fig. 22: C-arm visualization—pushing plate against bony surface.

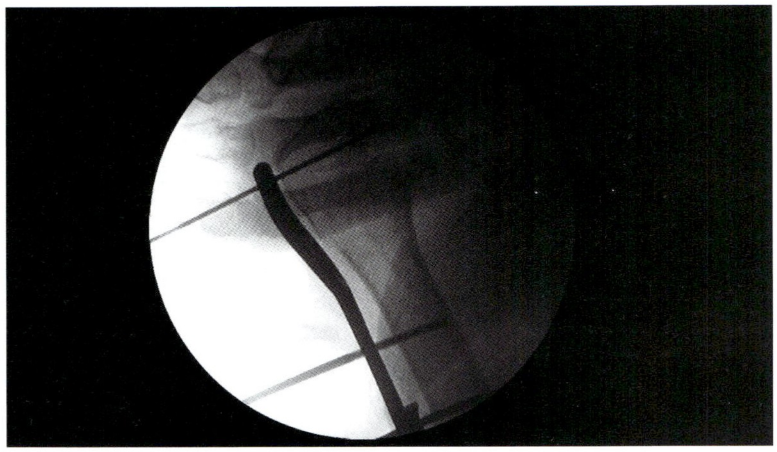

Fig. 23: C-arm image of passing drill bit through plate hole.

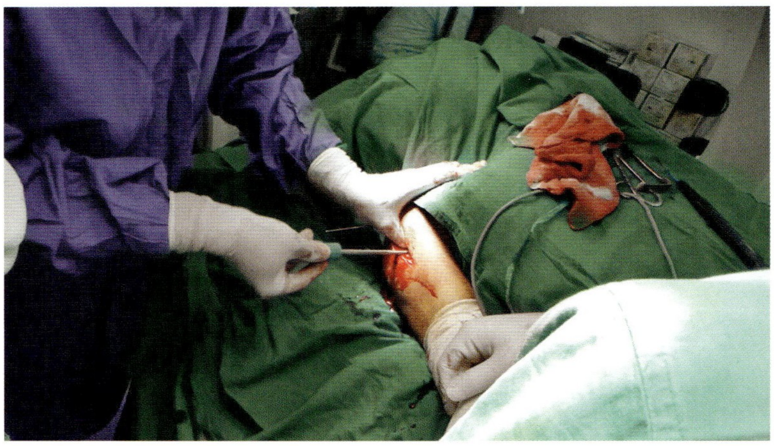

Fig. 24: Intraoperative photograph of passing of screw through plate.

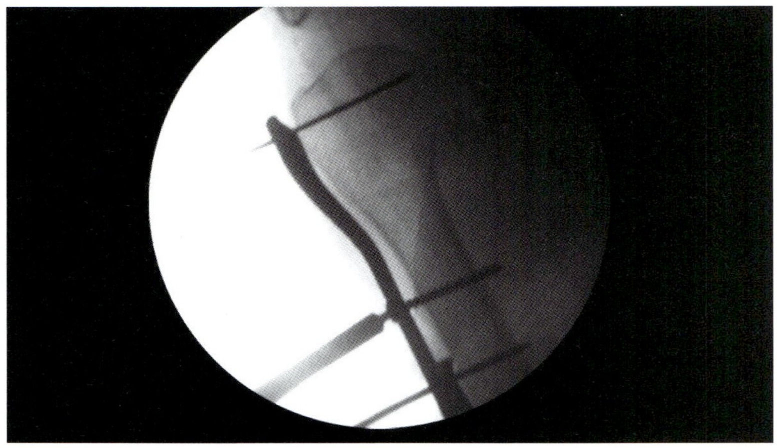

Fig. 25: C-arm image showing reducing gap between plate and bone by tightening the screw.

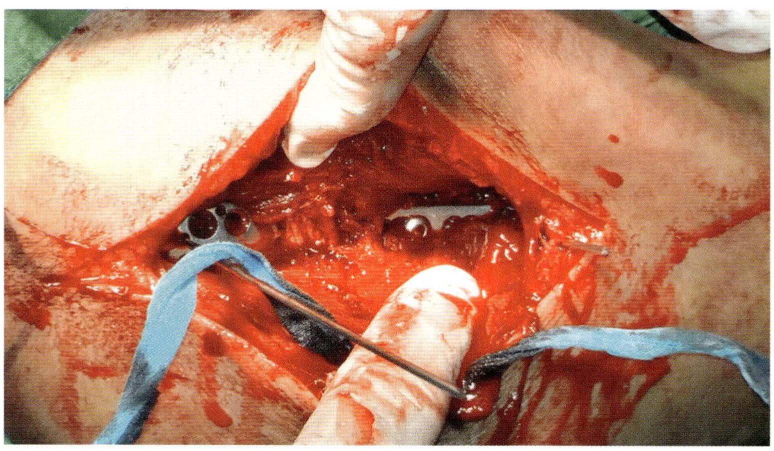

Fig. 26: Intraoperative photo showing screw and plate in proper position.

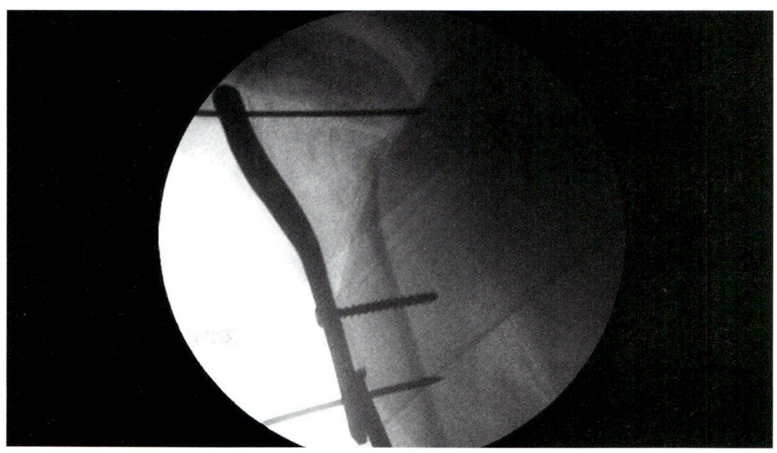

Fig. 27: C-arm image showing plate flush with the bone.

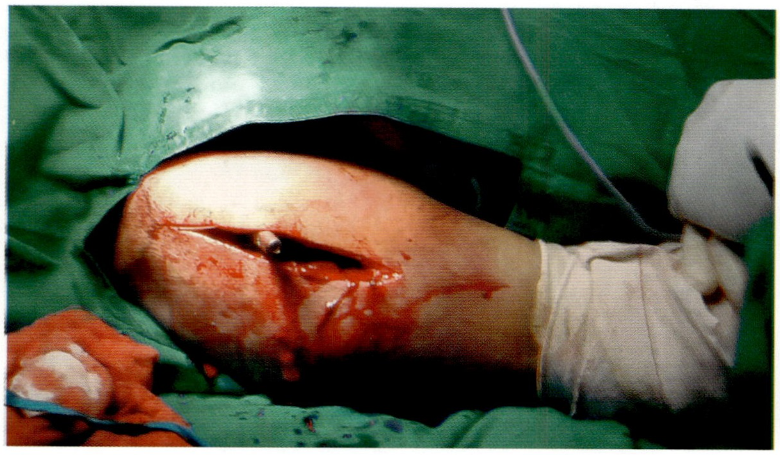

Fig. 28: Fixing drill sleeve for locking screw hole.

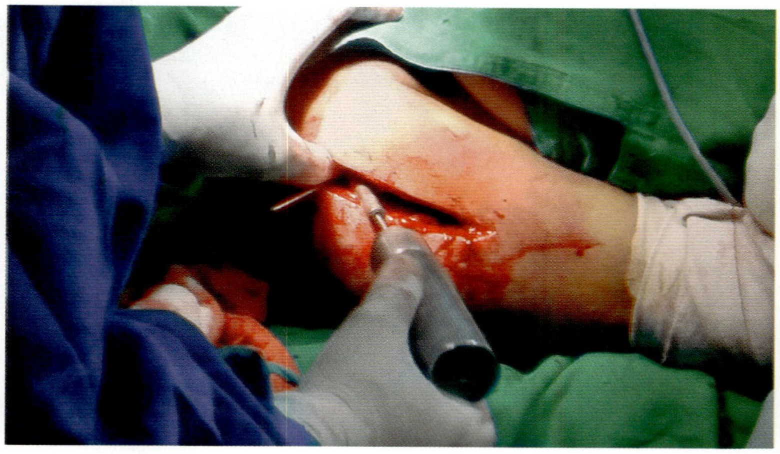

Fig. 29: Drilling for locking screw through sleeve.

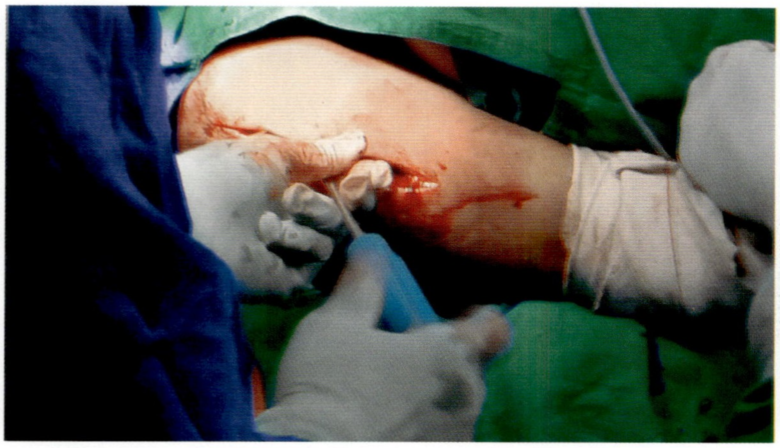

Fig. 30: Passing locking screw and tightening with torque limiting screw driver.

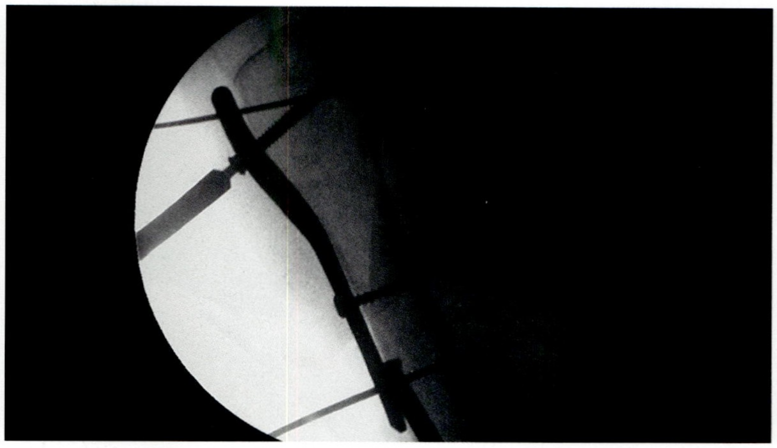

Fig. 31: C-arm image of locking screw position.

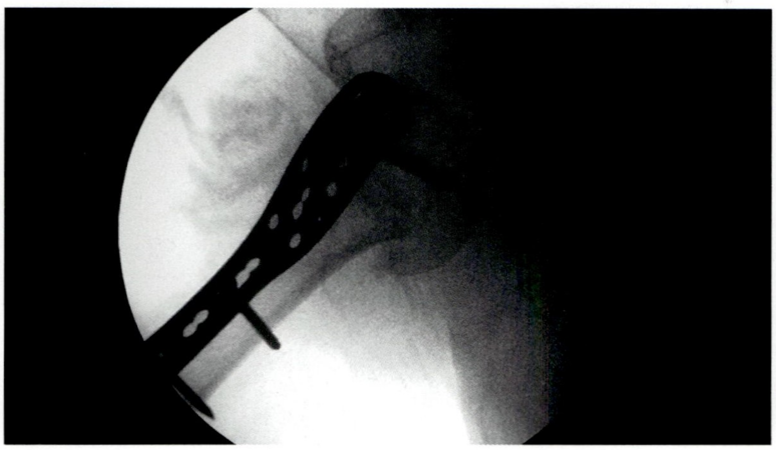

Fig. 32: Oblique projection of C-arm.

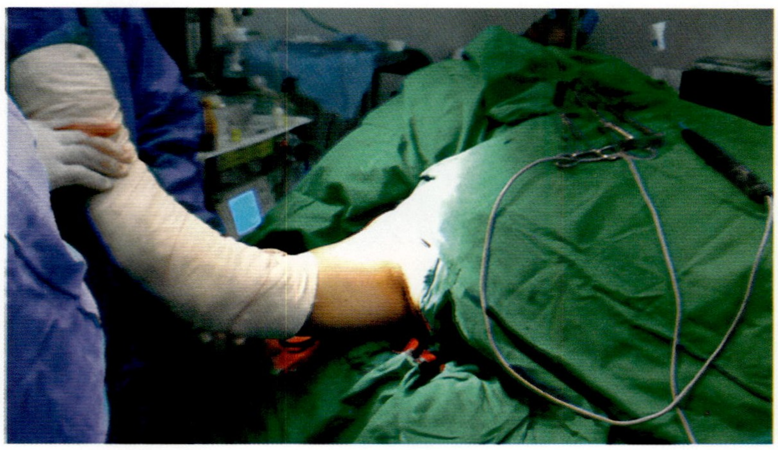

Fig. 33: Checking provisional stability of fracture fixation—position 1.

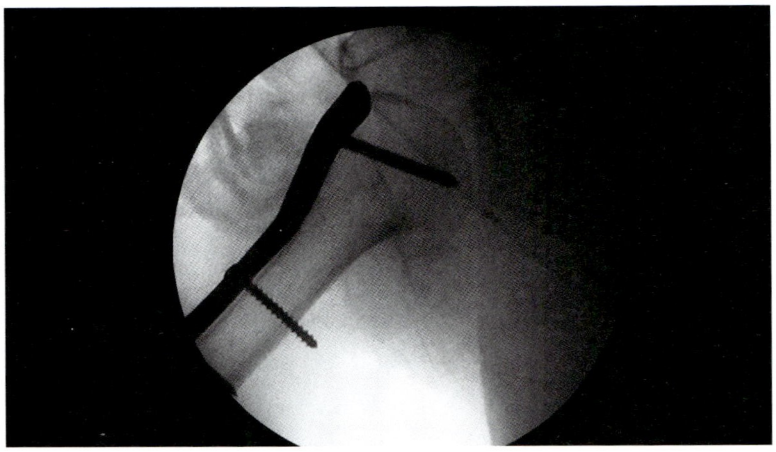

Fig. 34: C-arm image of position 1.

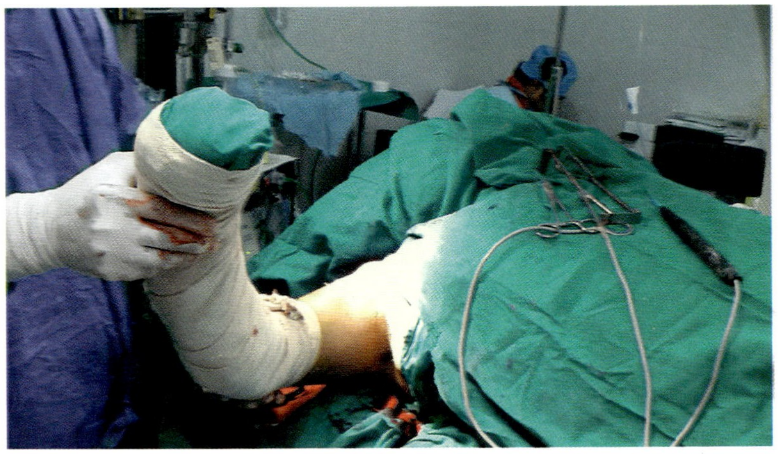

Fig. 35: Checking stability by internal rotation through shoulder position 2.

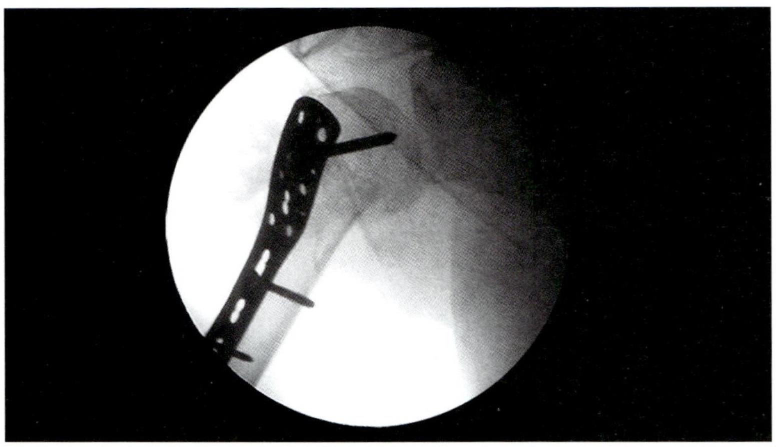

Fig. 36: C-arm image of position 2.

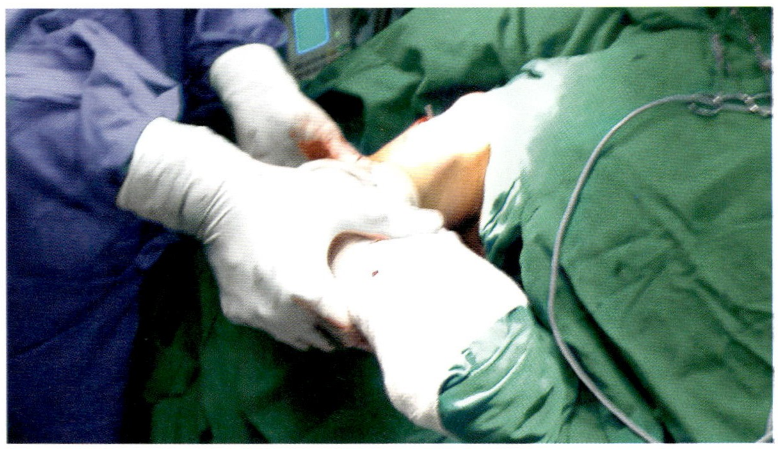

Fig. 37: Checking stability in full internal rotation position 3.

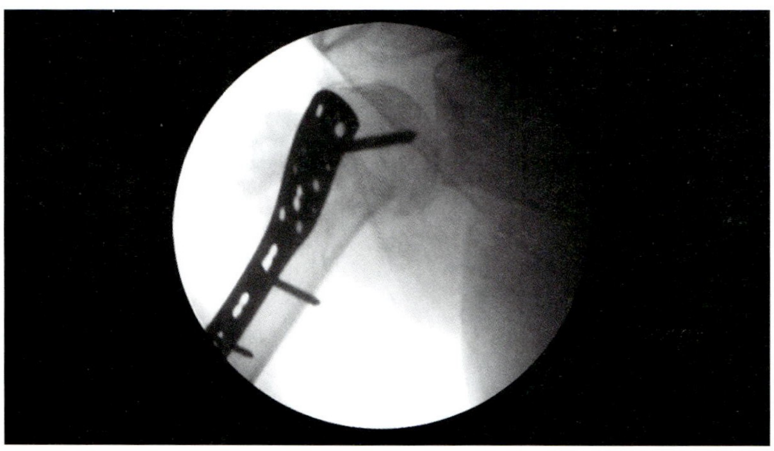

Fig. 38: C-arm image position 3.

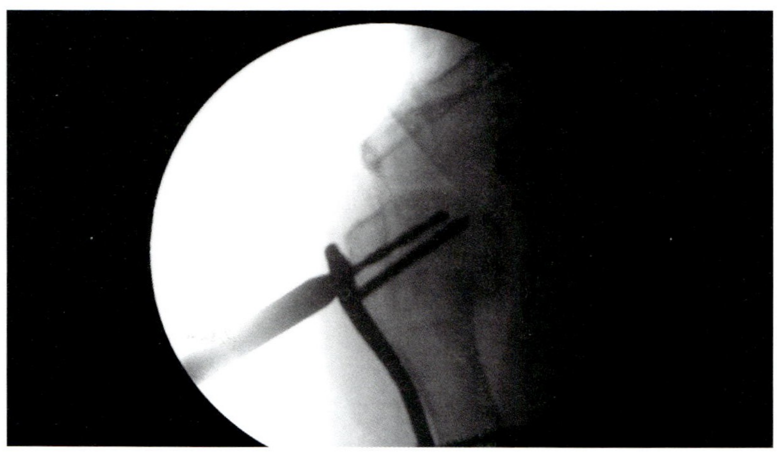

Fig. 39: C-arm image of passing additional locking screw for proximal fragment.

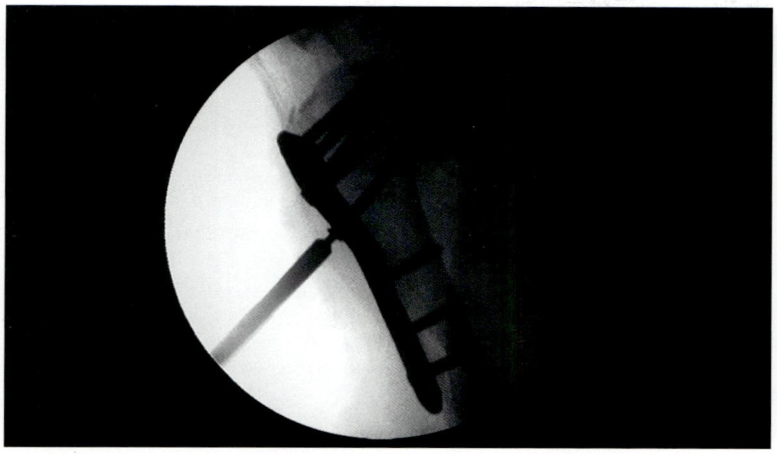

Fig. 40: C-arm image of insertion of last locking screw.

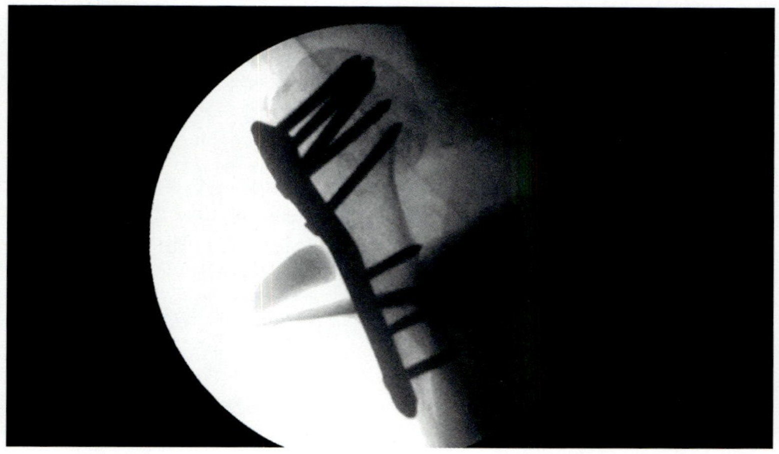

Fig. 41: Final C-arm image of fixation.

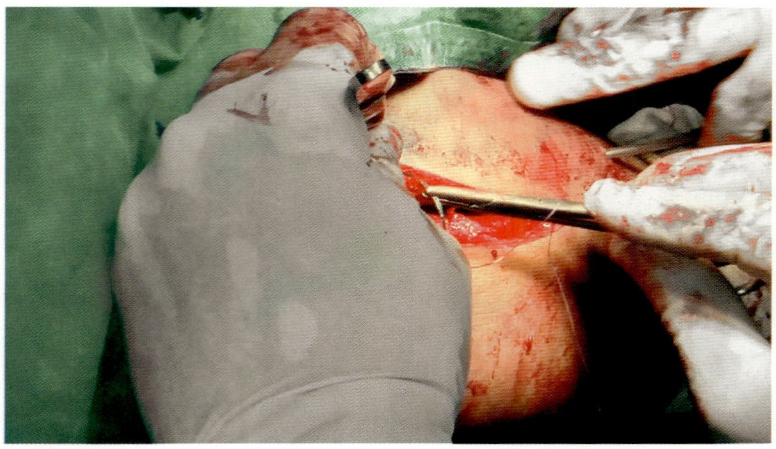

Fig. 42: Hemostasis, wash and suction drain followed by deltoid muscle sutured with 2-0 absorbable suture with interrupted sutures.

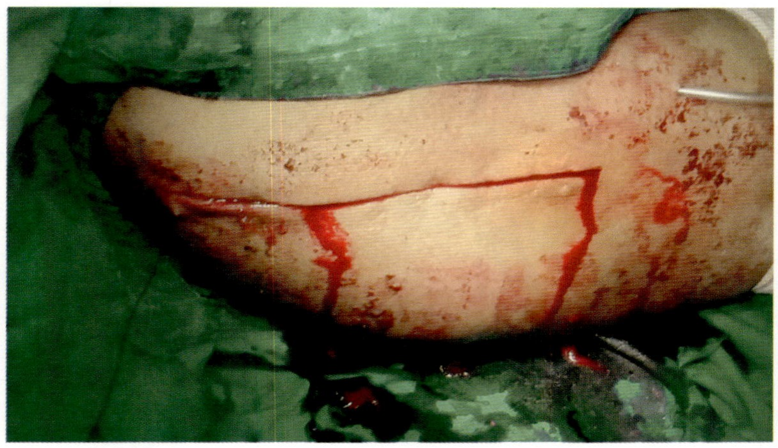

Fig. 43: Subcutaneous suturing done with inverted interrupted sutures using 3-0 absorbable suture.

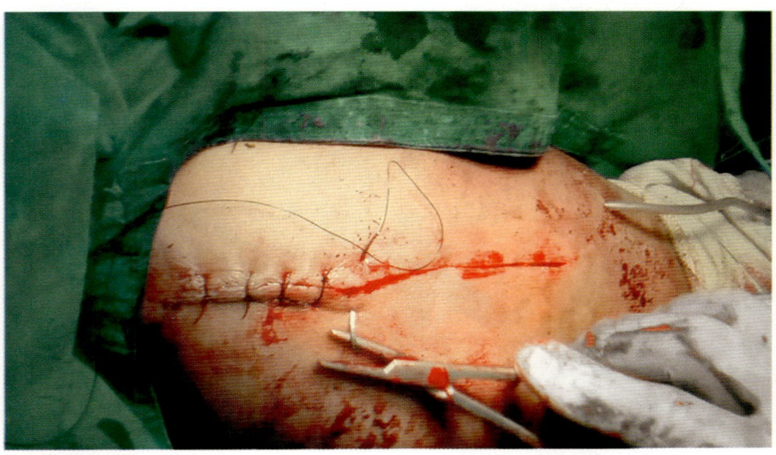

Fig. 44: Skin suturing using 3-0 nylon on reverse cutting curved needle.

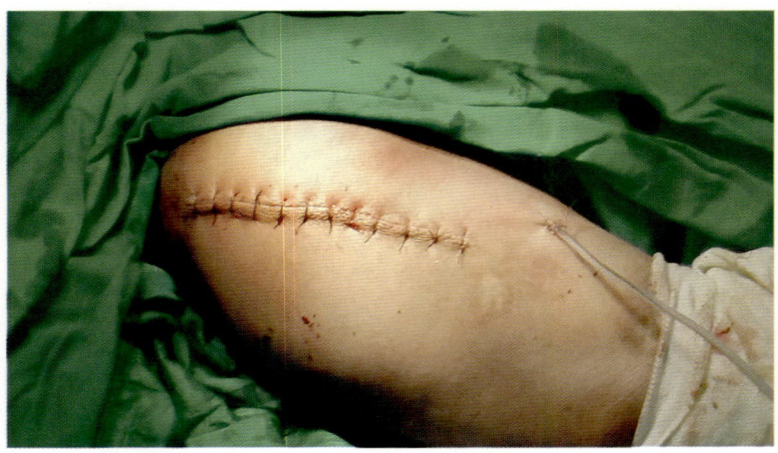

Fig. 45: Skin suturing completed.

SUMMARY

Many of proximal humerus fractures are treated nonoperatively. This is done mainly for all nondisplaced fractures and most of the valgus impacted fractures in patients with lower functional expectations. Patients with severely displaced and complex proximal humerus fractures are mostly candidates for operative intervention. In most cases requiring surgery, anatomical reduction and adequate fixation of the fracture is vital to reestablish the normal biomechanical relationship between the rotator cuff and the viable humeral head. All efforts should be made to reconstruct the proximal humerus and achieve anatomical reductions and stable fixation of the tuberosities. Shoulder arthroplasty should be considered in elderly patients with high chances of head nonviability such as in severely displaced fractures through anatomical neck, medial hinge disruption, and frank dislocation. Hemiarthroplasty is preferred for relatively younger patients and reverse shoulder arthroplasty is preferred for elderly patients. Currently, the preferred method of reconstruction of the proximal humerus is open reduction internal fixation (ORIF) with a locking screw construct via the deltopectoral approach in most cases.

Meticulous wound care when combined with patient-specific rehabilitation protocol minimizes postoperative complications.

SUGGESTED READING

1. Aggarwal S, Bali K, Dhillon MS, et al. Displaced proximal humeral fractures: An Indian experience with locking plates. J Orthop Surg Res. 2010;5:60.
2. Agudelo J, Schürmann M, Stahel P, et al. Analysis of efficacy and failure in proximal humeral fractures treated with locking plates. J Orthop Trauma. 2007;21(10):676-81.
3. Angibaud L, Zuckerman JD, Flurin PH, et al. Reconstructing proximal humeral fractures using the bicipital groove as a landmark. Clin Orthop Relat Res. 2007;458:168-74.
4. Badman B, Frankle M, Keating C, et al. Results of proximal humeral locked plating with supplemental suture fixation of rotator cuff. J Shoulder Elbow Surg. 2011;20(4):616-24.
5. Gardner MJ, Weil Y, Barker JU, et al. The importance of medial support in locked plating of proximal humeral fractures. J Orthop Trauma. 2007;21(3):185-91.

THREE/FOUR PART FRACTURE PROXIMAL HUMERUS–PLATE FIXATION

Prateek Charuchandra Joshi, Shrinivas S Shintre, Vijay M Panchanadikar

SURGICAL STEPS

For more complex fractures of the neck of humerus such as those with 3 or more fracture fragments, a different technique needs to be applied.

Step 1: The fracture fragments are identified after dissection and elevated using bone levers. The muscular and rotator cuff attachment of each piece is identified (Fig. 46).

Step 2: Stout suture tag is taken for subscapularis and Supraspinatus muscles attached to the upper fracture fragment (Fig. 47).

Step 3: Similar suture tag is taken for teres minor and Infraspinatus muscles on the lower fracture fragment. Overlying deltoid muscle is retracted using a posteriorly placed bone lever (Fig. 48).

Step 4: The fracture fragments are pulled together using the attached suture tags, and along with bone levers, fracture reduction is attempted. Also, applying an distal and lateral traction on the fracture fragments prevents the fracture from falling into varus (Fig. 49).

Step 5: In this case, one fragment which was depressed below the cortical surface, is levered upwards using the bone lever. This step may or may not be essential depending on the fracture pattern, and preoperative computed tomography (CT) scanning can help in predicting whether this maneuver will be necessary (Fig. 50).

Step 6: Holding the suture tags in traction to pull the fragments together and prevent varus position, the plate is applied and provisionally fixed with K-wires. Subsequently, definitive fixation with locking screws is done (Fig. 51).

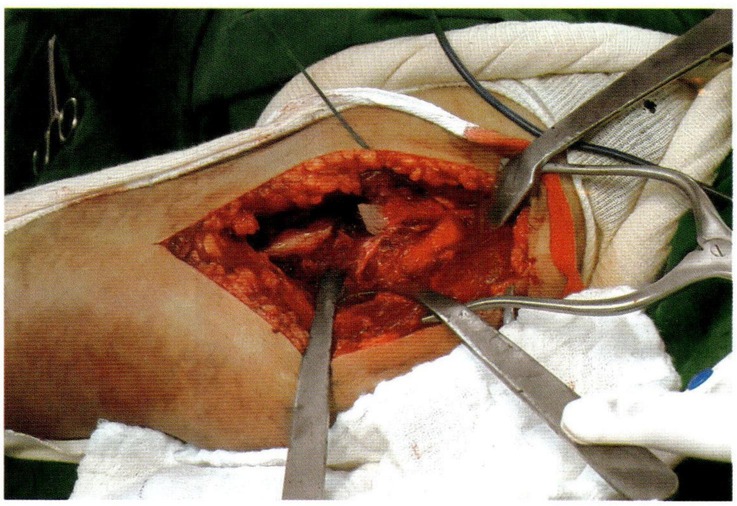

Fig. 46

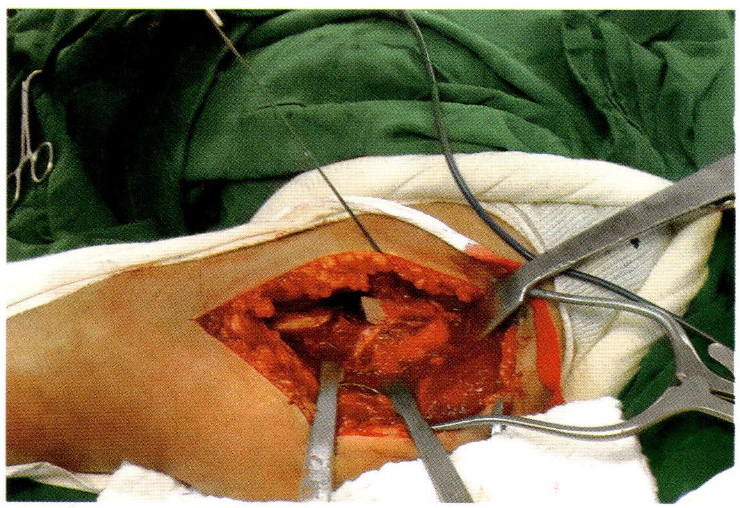

Fig. 47

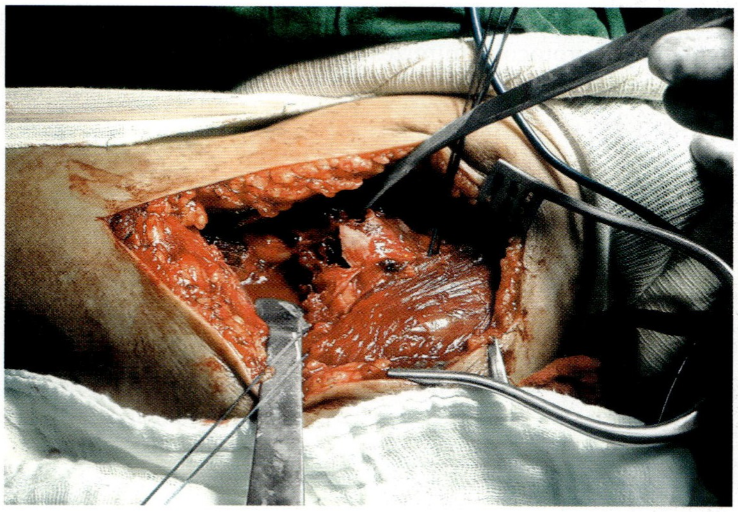

Fig. 48

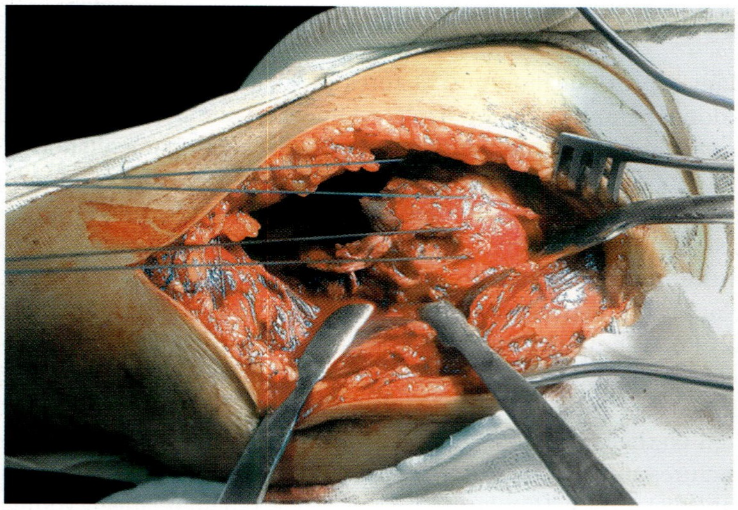

Fig. 49

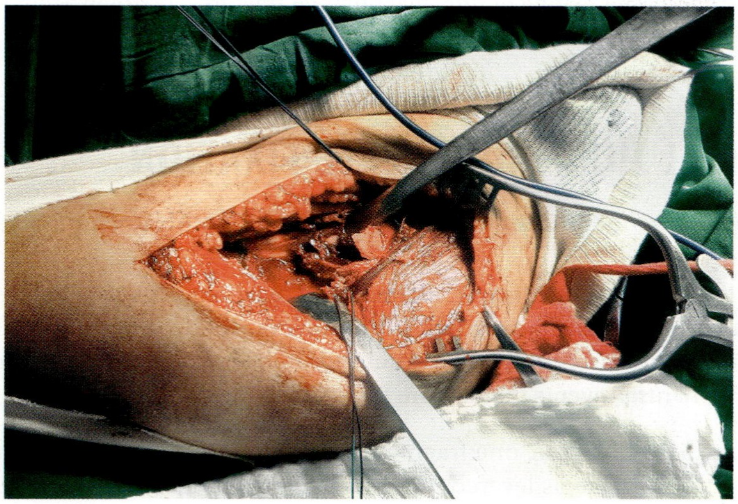

Fig. 50

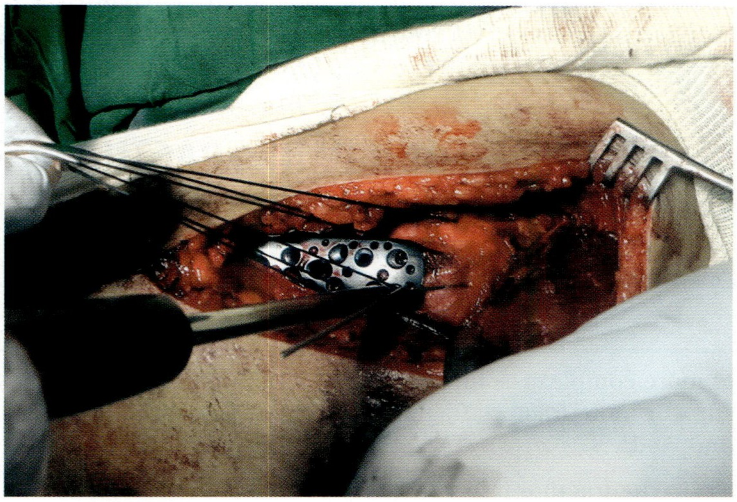

Fig. 51

K-WIRES AND EXTERNAL FIXATION (FIGS. 52 TO 62)

Shrinivas S Shintre, Vishal Patil, Chittanand Mendhe

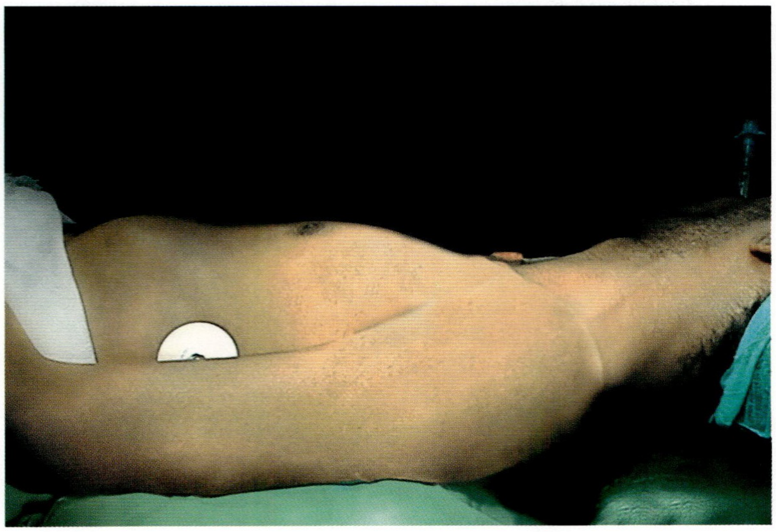

Fig. 52: Patient position.

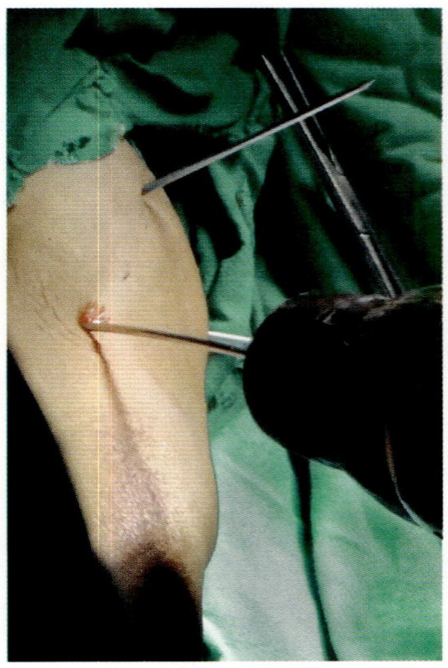

Fig. 53: Passing of 2 K-wires in proximal fragment.

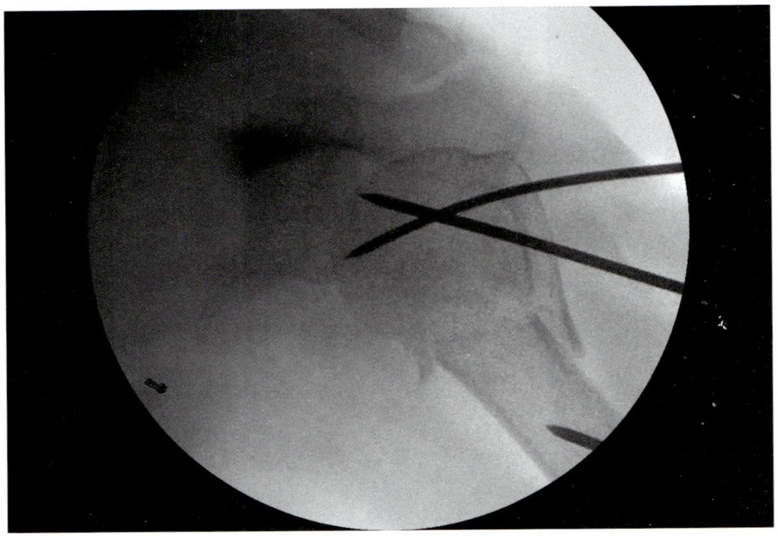

Fig. 54: Position confirmed with C-arm image.

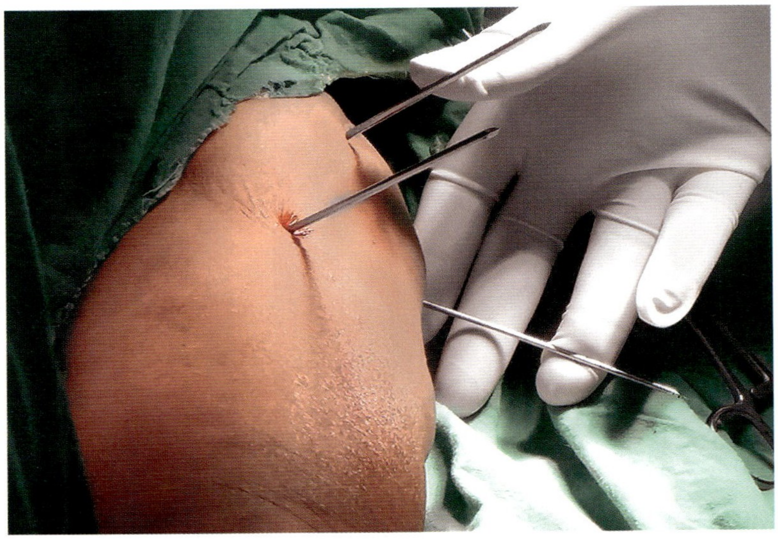

Fig. 55: Passing of K-wire in distal fragment.

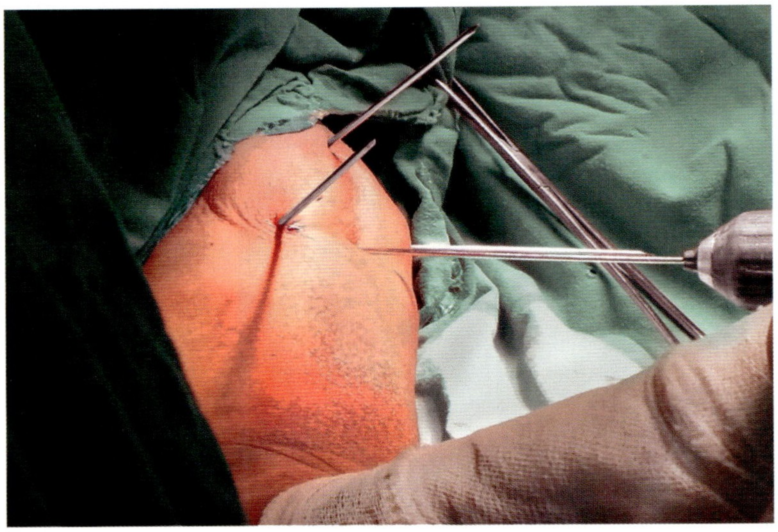

Fig. 56: Passing of 2 K-wires in distal fragment.

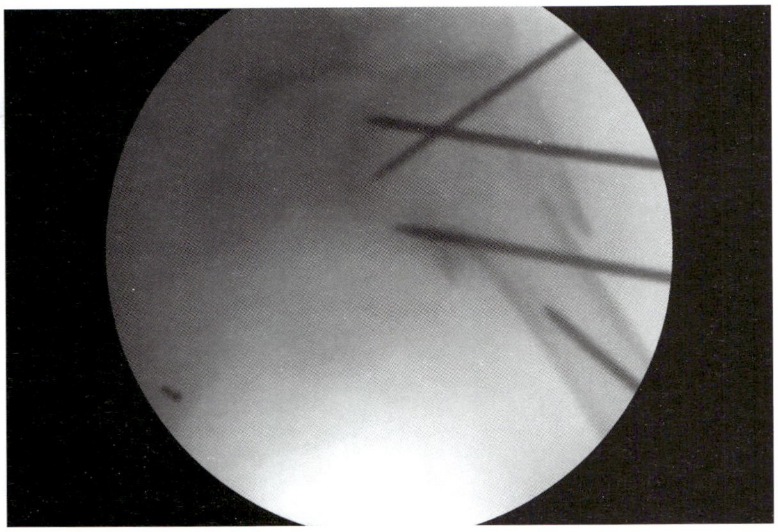

Fig. 57: Position confirmed with C-arm image.

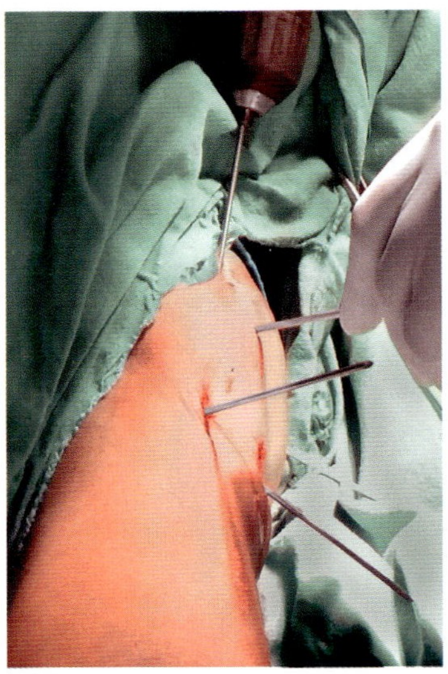

Fig. 58: Intraoperative photograph.

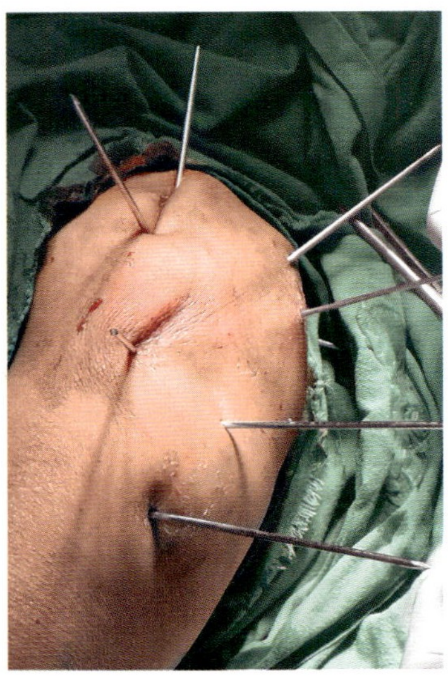

Fig. 59: Passing 2 additional K-wires.

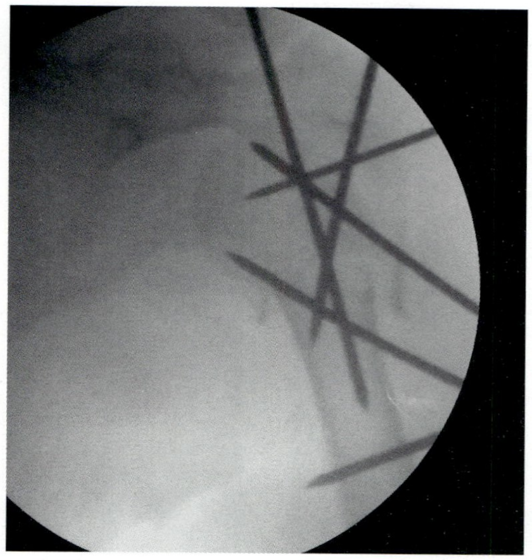

Fig. 60: Position confirmed with C-arm image.

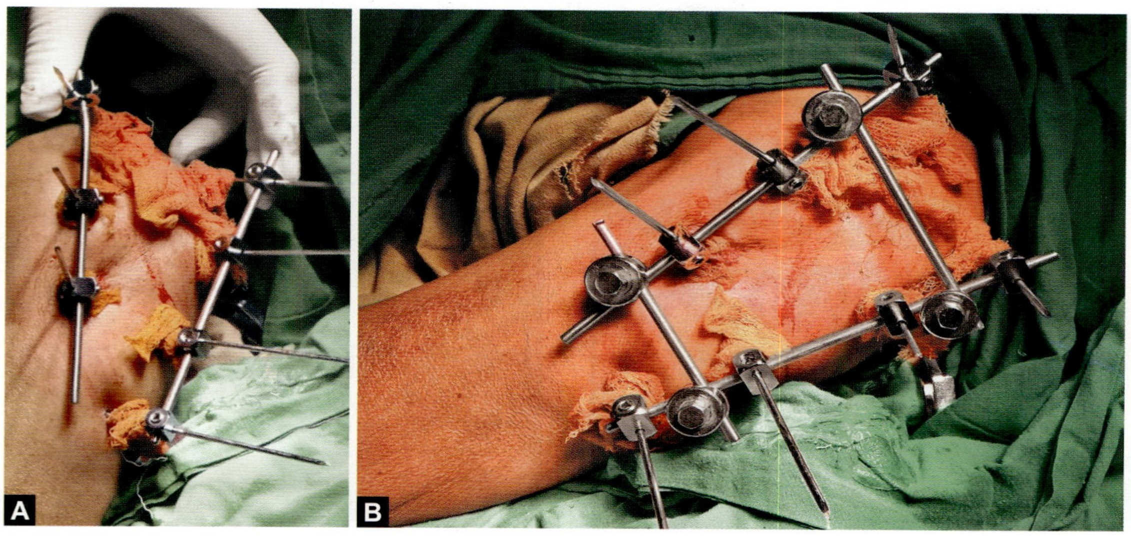

Fig. 61: External fixator applied.

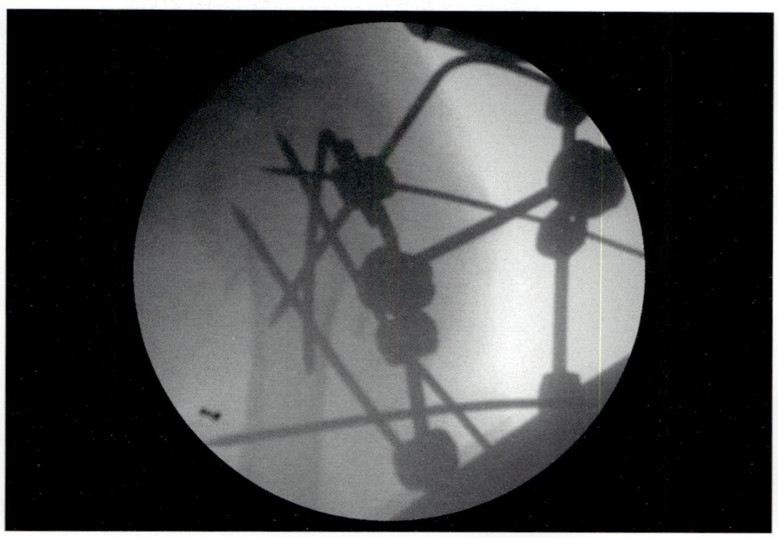

Fig. 62: Final position confirmed with C-arm image.

CHAPTER 84

Fracture Proximal Humerus: Hemireplacement

Umesh Jadhav, Aditya Upase

INTRODUCTION

Hemiarthroplasty is a surgical procedure that replaces one-half of the shoulder joint. The head of humerus is replaced with the stemmed humerus prosthesis. Glenoid is left intact.

INDICATIONS

Shoulder hemiarthroplasty should be considered the procedure of choice with following:

- Displaced Neer's type 4 fracture with or without dislocation in elderly patients
- Impression fractures involving greater than 40% of articular area
- Three-part fracture—dislocation in elderly with osteopenia
- Anatomical neck fractures not amenable to ORIF (open reduction and internal fixation)
- Fractures associated with comorbidities: Diabetes mellitus, smokers and steroids.

CONTRAINDICATIONS

- Infection
- Neuropathic joint
- Paralytic disorders
- Deficiency in shoulder cuff and deltoid muscle function
- Unmotivated patient.

IMAGING

X-rays

- True anteroposterior (AP) view of shoulder joint helps in determining extent of fracture pattern and degenerative joint disease.
- Axillary view of shoulder joint helps to identify fracture displacement and wear of glenoid.

Computed Tomography Scans

Computed tomography (CT) scan is useful to study the fracture patterns, to determine glenoid bone stock, and glenoid version.

Magnetic Resonance Imaging Scans

Magnetic resonance imaging (MRI) scan is useful for evaluation of rotator cuff status.

SHOULDER HEMIARTHROPLASTY: SURGICAL TECHNIQUE

Following is the step-by-step approach to shoulder hemiarthroplasty technique in case of proximal humerus Neer's four-part fracture and detailed surgical procedure.

SURGICAL STEPS (FIGS. 1 TO 28)

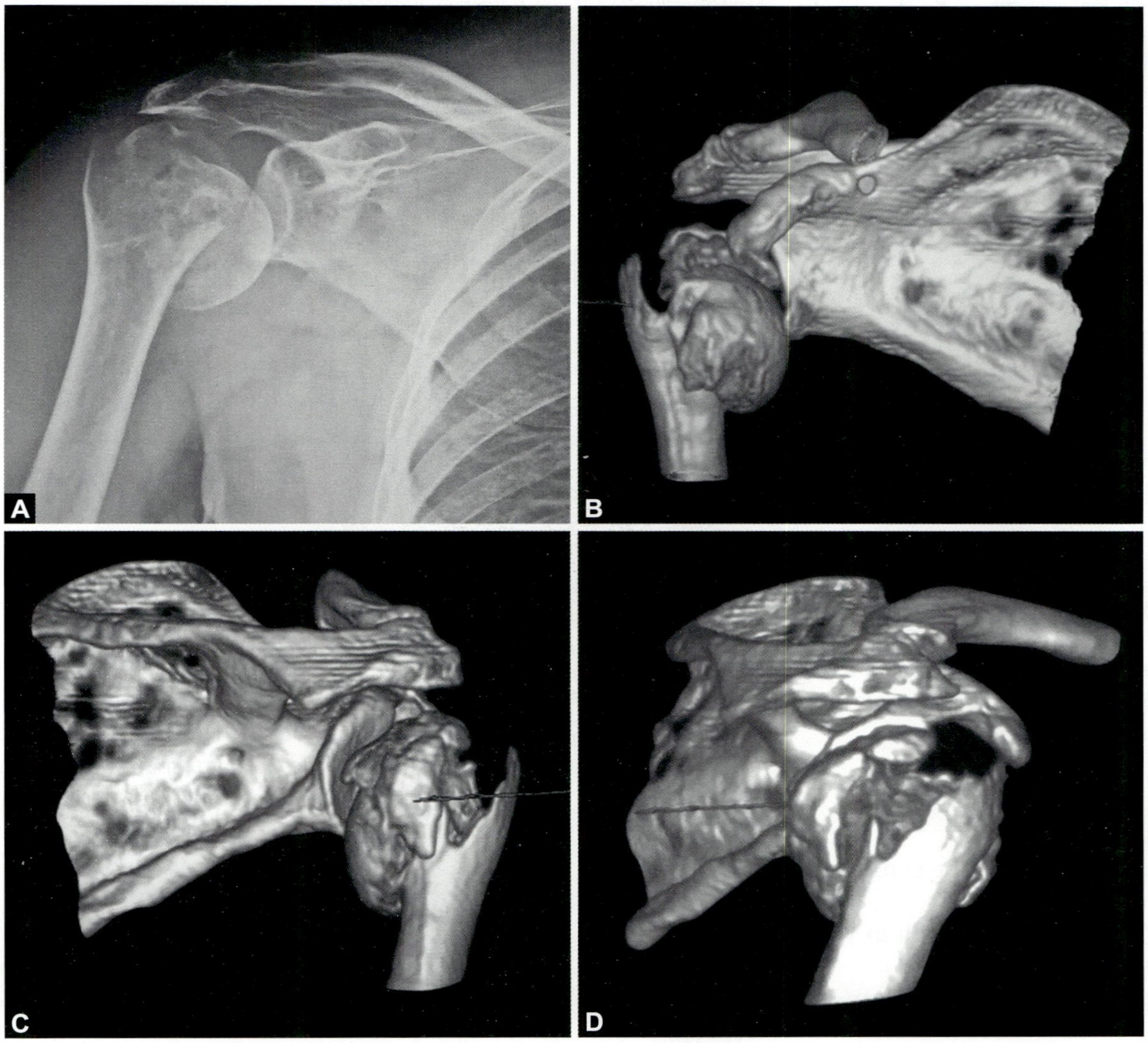

Figs. 1A to D: Neer's four-parts fracture proximal humerus in elderly lady. Above X-ray and 3D computed tomography (CT) scan confirm fracture pattern with osteoporosis.

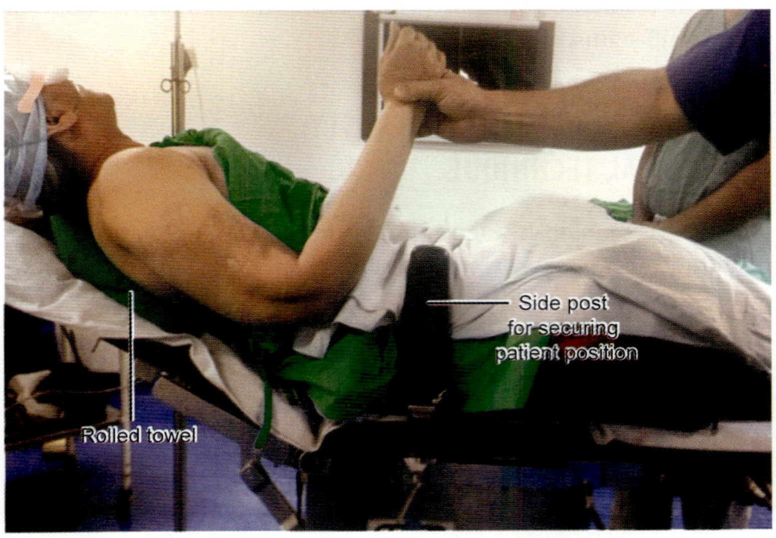

Fig. 2: Place the patient is beach chair position with rolled towel under scapula to correct the version of glenoid. Patient should be placed at the edge of the table to facilitate the extension for reaming of humeral canal. Secure patients position with leg holder and straps. Patient's head should be secured with straps.

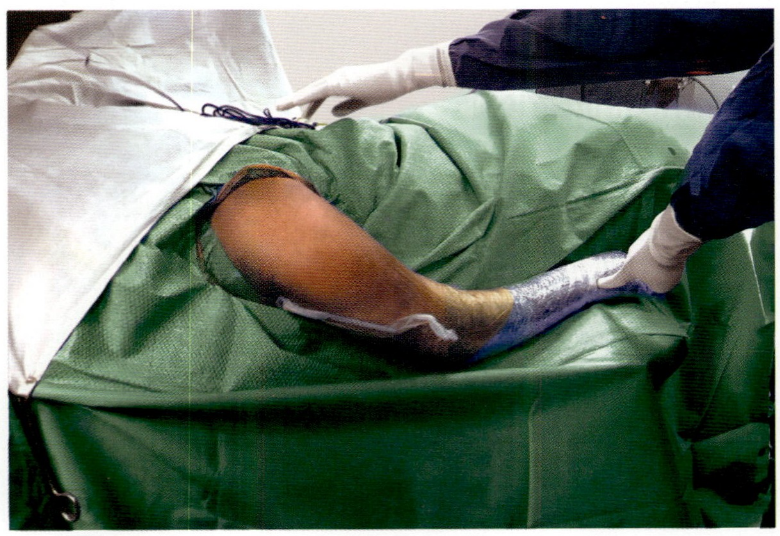

Fig. 3: Painting and draping should be done in standard fashion after primary scrubbing the parts.

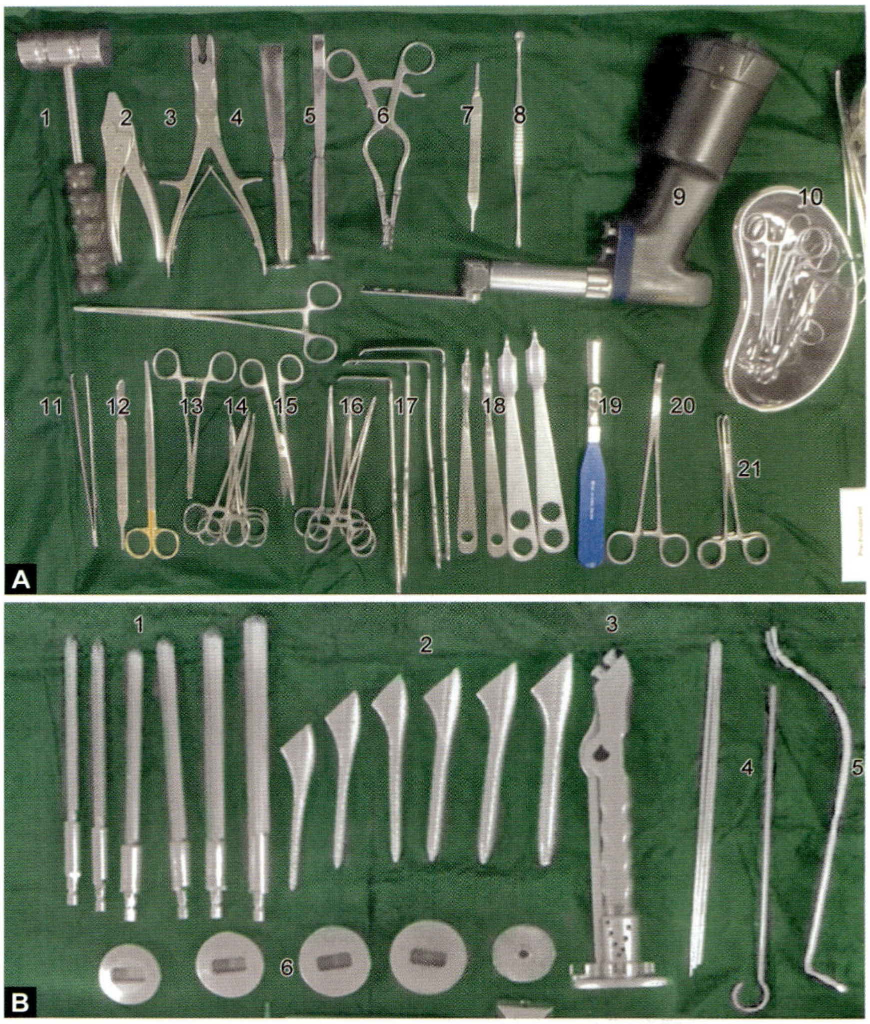

1. Mallet
2. Plier
3. Nibbler
4. Osteotome
5. Osteotome
6. Mastoid retractor
7. BP handle
8. Scoop
9. Drill saw
10. Kidney tray with towel clips
11. Tooth forceps
12. Knife and tissue dissecting scissor
13. Needle holder
14. Mosquito forceps
15. Scissor
16. Artery forceps
17. Retractors
18. Spikes
19. Periosteum elevator
20. Artery forceps
21. Allis forceps

1. Different sizes of reamers for humerus canal
2. Different sizes of humerus broaches and trial stems
3. Broach and trial stem holder
4. Guide pin
5. Retractor
6. Different sizes of trail head

Figs. 4A and B: General set of instruments with specific instruments (canal reamers, broaches, guide pins, trial prosthesis, etc.) required for hemiarthroplasty should be arranged and ready before start of the procedure.

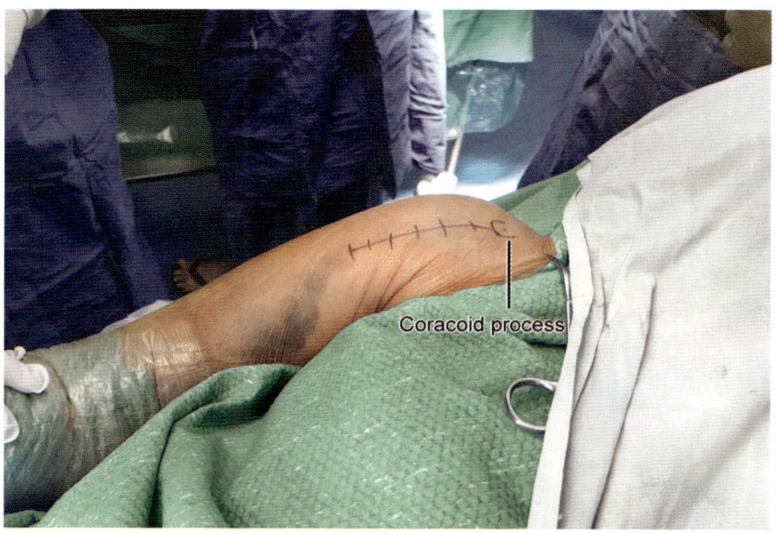

Fig. 5: Palpate clavicle, acromion, and coracoid process and identify deltopectoral interval. Mark the incision distally from coracoid process.

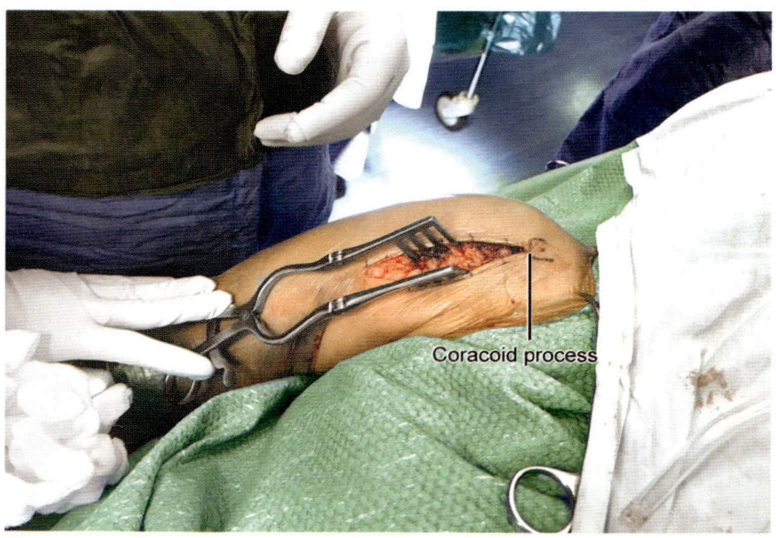

Fig. 6: Begin the procedure with skin incision and subcutaneous dissection.

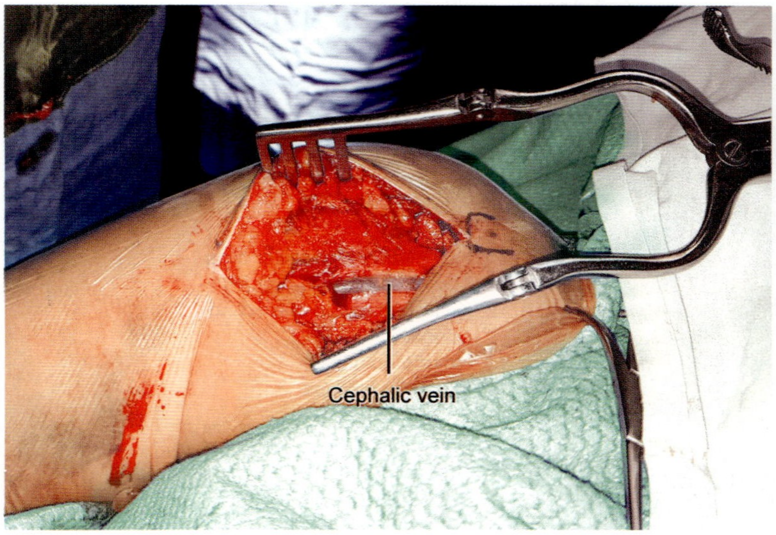

Fig. 7: Carry out dissection in deltopectoral interval to find cephalic vein. Allow the cephalic vein to fall medially and proceed further dissection.

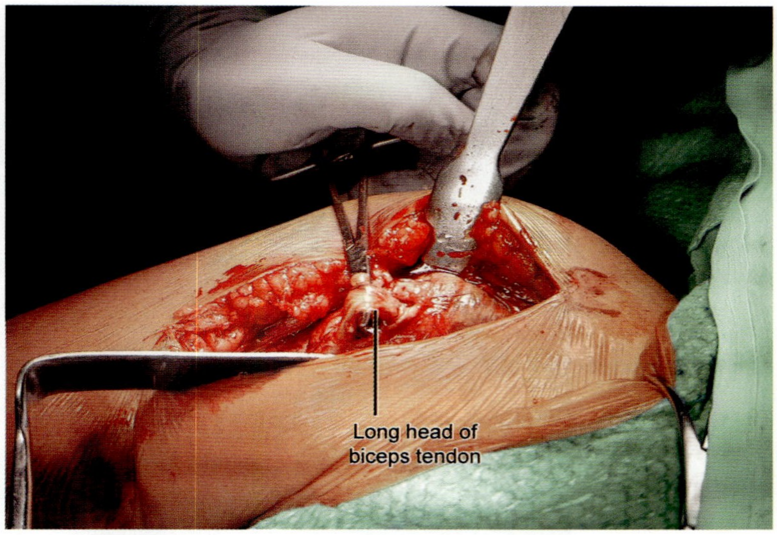

Fig. 8: Identify the bicipital groove and biceps tendon.

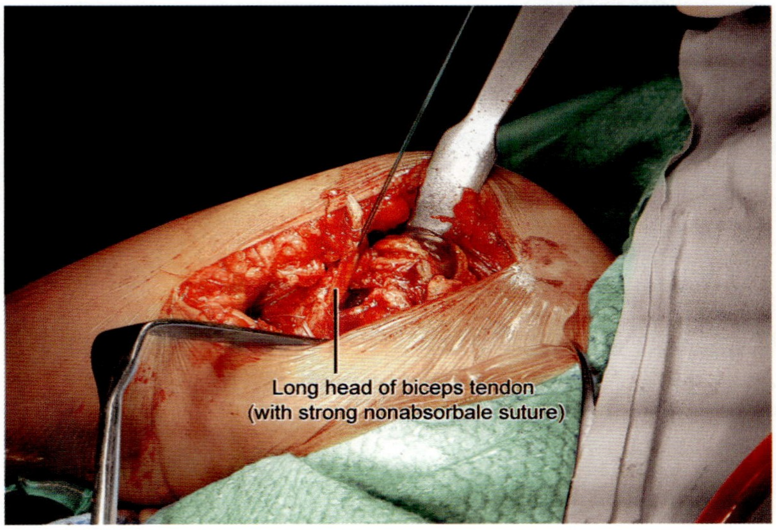

Fig. 9: Tie the long head of biceps tendon with strong nonabsorbable suture number 2. Perform the biceps tenotomy.

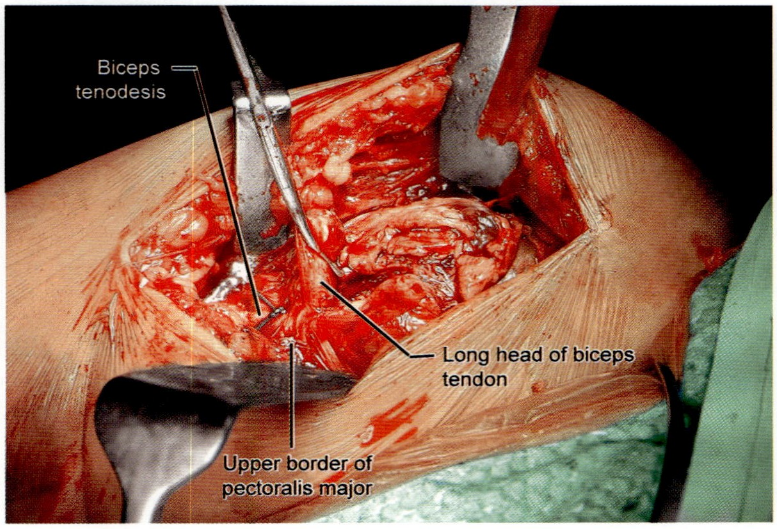

Fig. 10: Achieve the biceps tenodesis by suturing it at the level of upper border of pectoralis major.

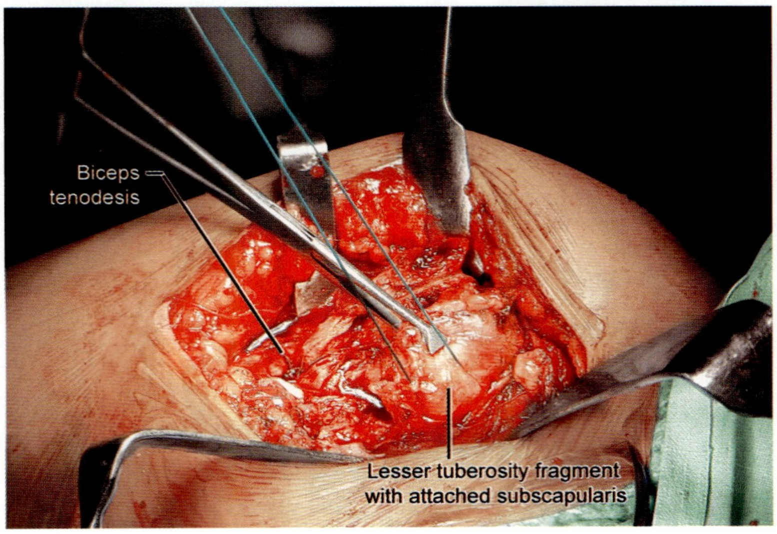

Fig. 11: Identify the fracture fragments. Tag the lesser tuberosity fragment with strong nonabsorbable suture number 2. Carry out dissection further into rotator interval to visualize head.

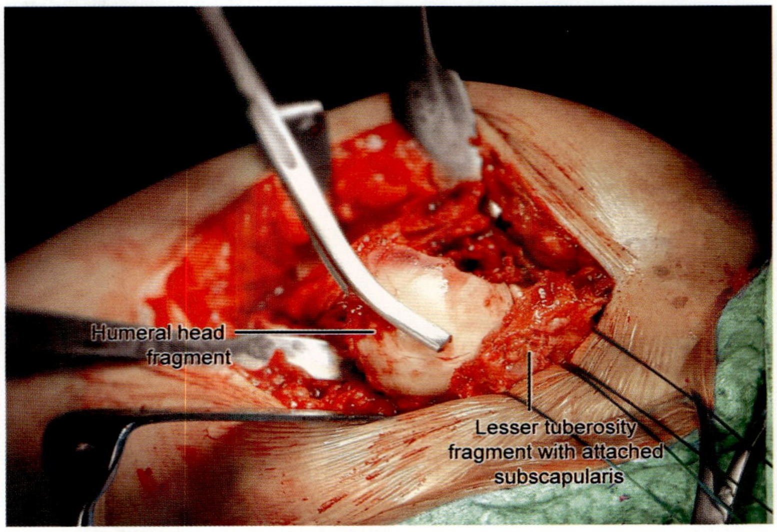

Fig. 12: Visualize the head and extract it out.

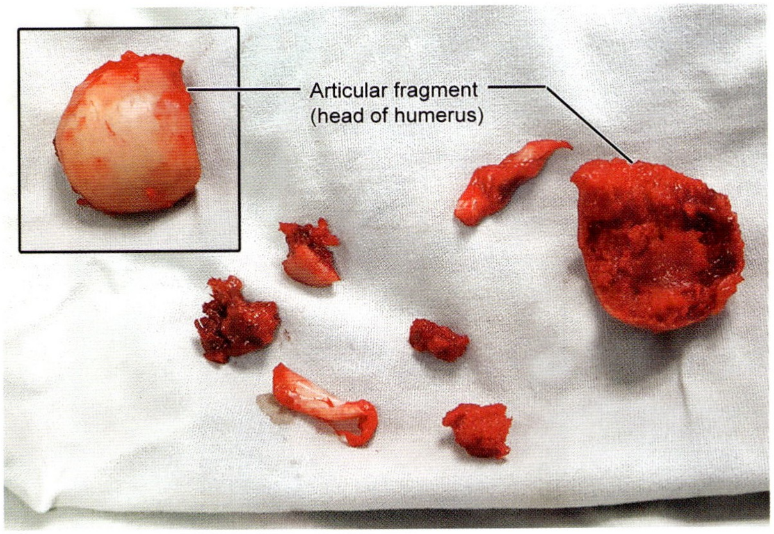

Fig. 13: Comminution of head fragment.

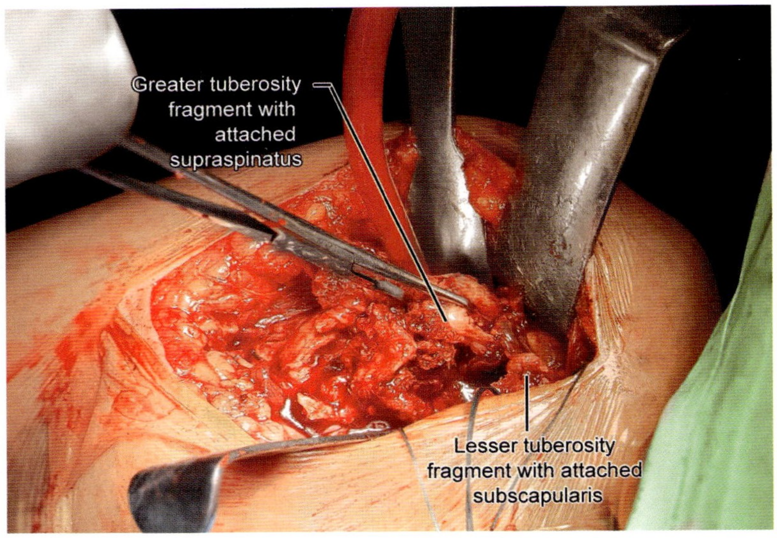

Fig. 14: Identify greater tuberosity fragments and tag them with strong nonabsorbable suture number 2.

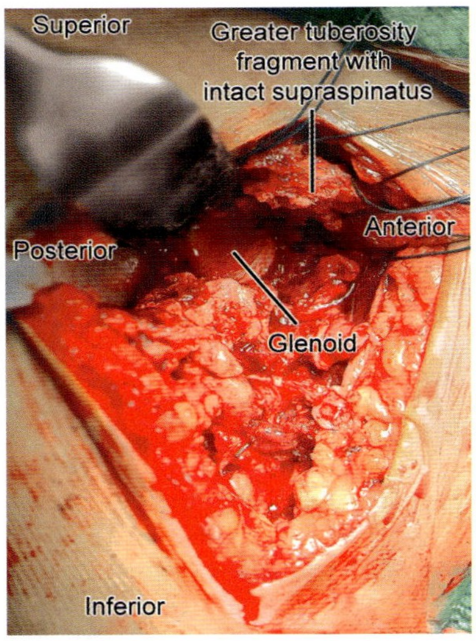

Fig. 15: Visualize the glenoid surface and check for any remaining small fragments inside joint.

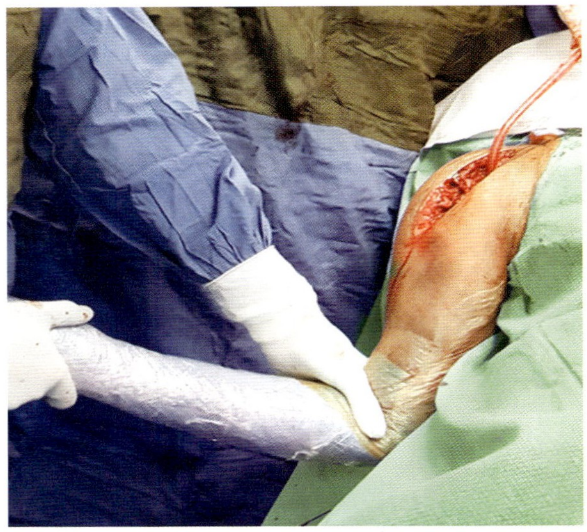

Fig. 16: Position the upper limb in extension and external rotation and elbow at 90° flexion so as to visualize humerus canal.

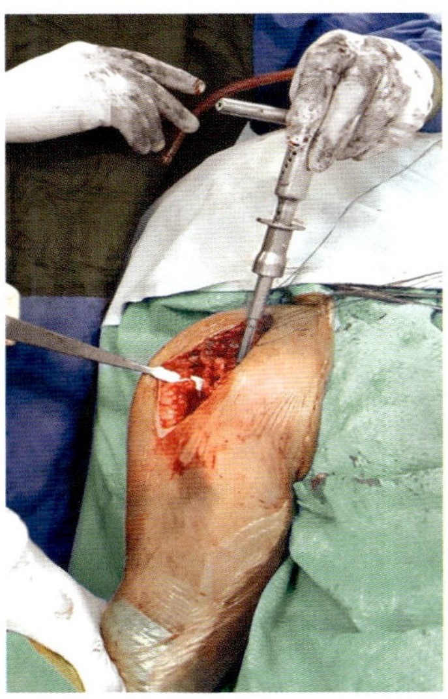

Fig. 17: Canal opening and reaming should be done keeping the upper limb in above mentioned position. Start with the smallest size reamer and advance further.

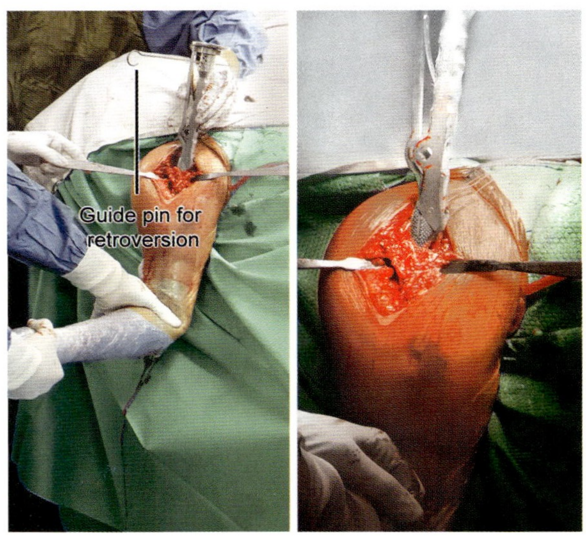

Fig. 18: Broaching should be done starting from small size broach stem and advancing further till broach gets snugly fit into the canal. Keep it in mind to maintain 20–30° of retroversion with the guide pin as shown in picture. Use forearm axis as reference for maintaining retroversion here.

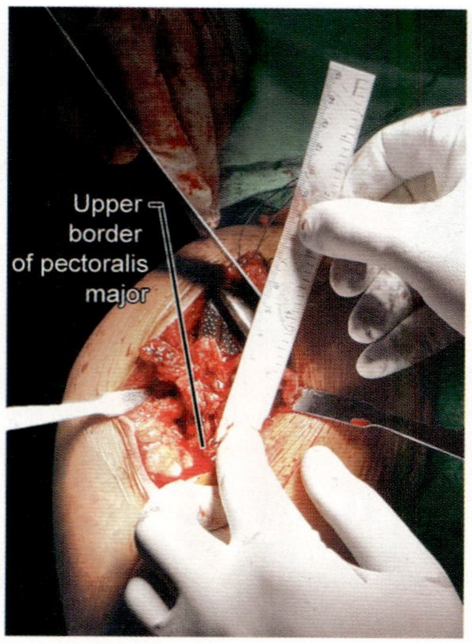

Fig. 19: Restoring the center of rotation for the humeral head in relation to the axis of the humeral diaphysis plays an important role. As a rule of thumb, the most superior aspect of the humeral head should be 1 cm superior to the greater tuberosity. Distance from top of prosthesis head to upper border of pectoralis major should be 50–56 mm.

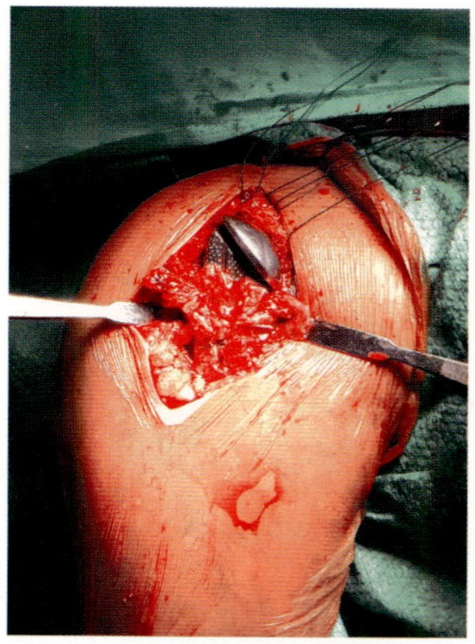

Fig. 20: Measure the extracted head size. Place the trial head on stem and reduce the glenohumeral joint with gentle traction and internal rotation. Check for stability and movements.

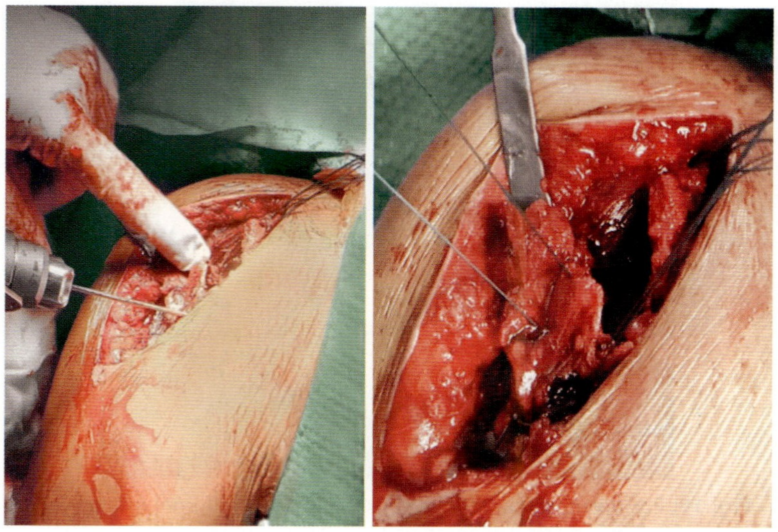

Fig. 21: Two holes should be drilled over shaft humerus and pass strong nonabsorbable suture threads through them in order to suture all tuberosity fragments together with the shaft after putting final prosthesis.

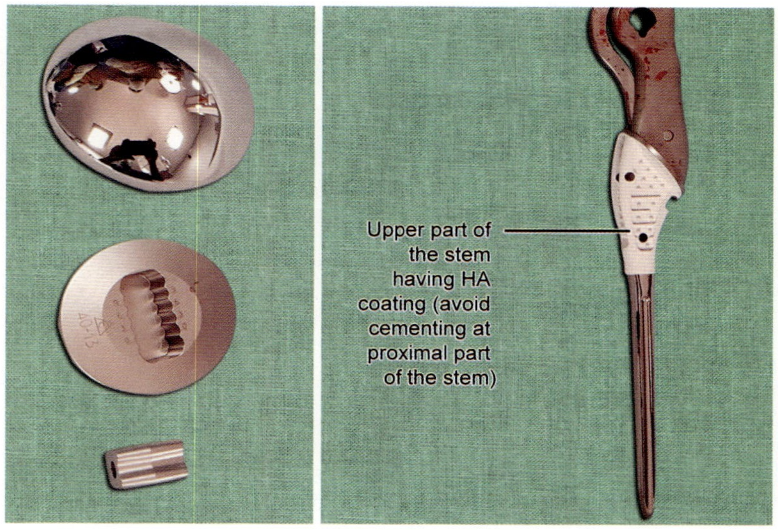

Fig. 22: After checking stability and movements with trial prosthesis insert final prosthesis of same size.

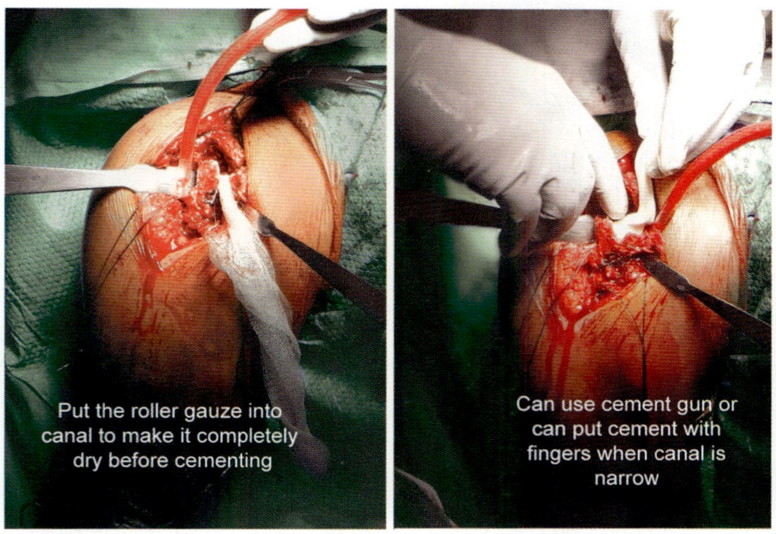

Fig. 23: After completing canal preparation, one may put bone plug or cement into the canal. Here, we are using cement because of osteoporotic bone.

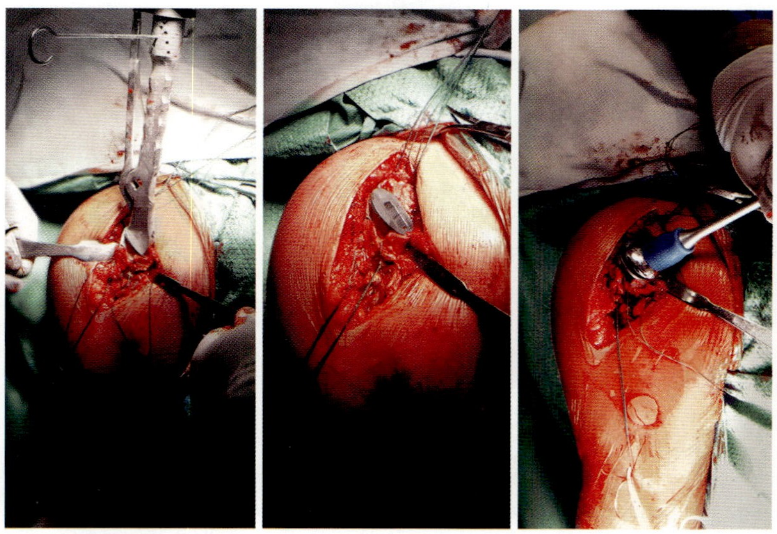

Fig. 24: After cementation of the canal, insert final humerus stem. Guide pin is used to maintain retroversion here. Place the head and reduce the glenohumeral joint.

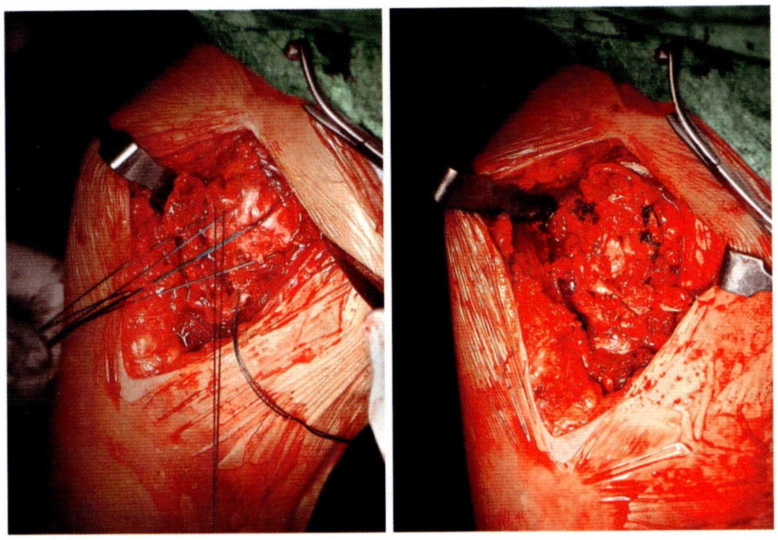

Fig. 25: Approximate greater tuberosity and lesser tuberosity fragments and suture it together and also to the shaft. One can use bone graft here to fill defect, if any.

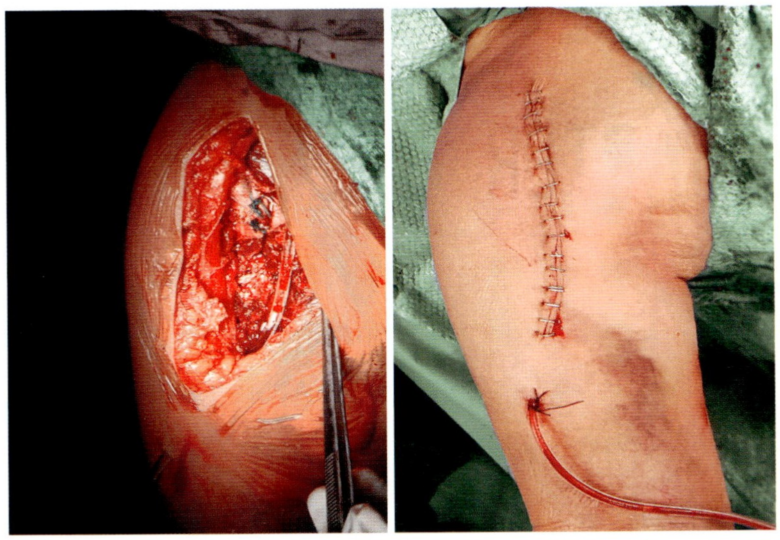

Fig. 26: Keep 12 number suction drain and perform tight closure of rotator interval. Perform deltopectoral interval and skin closure and dressing.

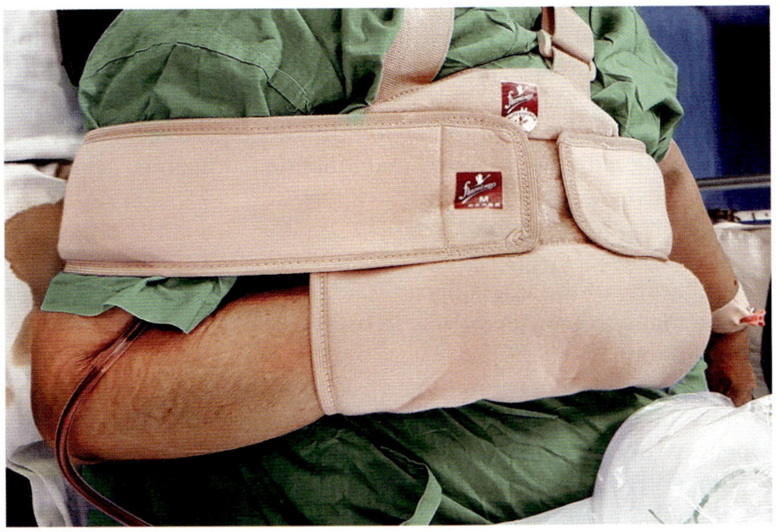

Fig. 27: Upper limb should be kept in shoulder immobilizer postoperatively.

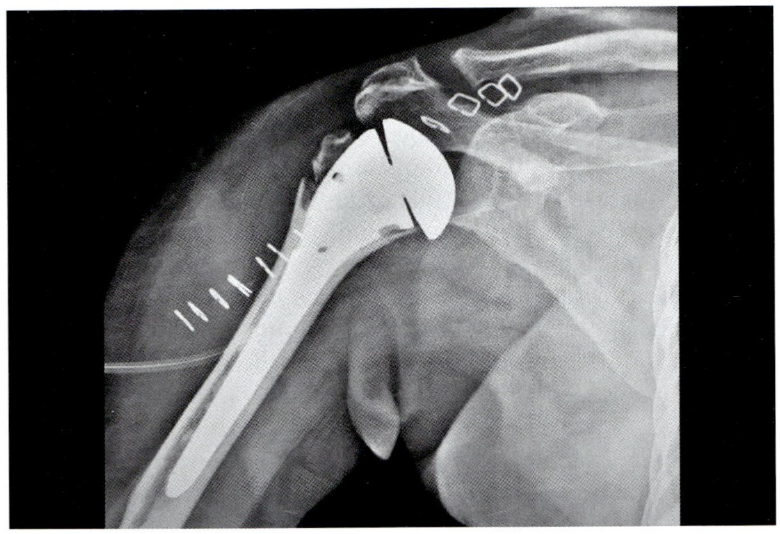

Fig. 28: Immediate postoperative X-ray shows perfect position of prosthesis with good approximation of greater tuberosity and lesser tuberosity fragments.

REHABILITATION

Upper limb is protected in shoulder immobilizer for 3 weeks with early start of elbow, wrist, and hand range of motion (ROM). After 3 weeks, passive range of motion is started till greater tuberosity fracture unites (fracture union usually takes 6–8 weeks). Strengthening exercises are started after full union of tuberosity fracture.

COMPLICATIONS

- Secondary osteoarthrosis of shoulder
- Tuberosity displacement/malunion (when used to treat fracture)
- Overstuffing of Joint (may cause stiffness of joint)
- Subluxation (anterosuperior) (in case of deficient coracoacromial arch and deficient rotator cuff).

SUGGESTED READING

1. Antuna SA, Sperling JW, Cofield RH. Shoulder hemiarthroplasty for acute fractures of the proximal humerus: a minimum five-year follow-up. J Shoulder Elbow Surg. 2008;17(2):202-9.
2. Godeneche A, Boileau P, Favard L, et al. Prosthetic replacement in the treatment of osteoarthritis of the shoulder: early results of 268 cases. J Shoulder Elbow Surg. 2002;11(1):11-8.
3. Neer CS 2nd. Displaced proximal humeral fractures. II. Treatment of three-part and four-part displacement. J Bone Joint Surg Am. 1970;52(6):1090-103.
4. Sanchez-Sotelo J, Cofield RH, Rowland CM. Shoulder hemiarthroplasty for glenohumeral arthritis associated with severe rotator cuff deficiency. J Bone Joint Surg Am. 2001;83-A(12):1814-22.
5. Sperling JW, Cofield RH, Rowland CM. Minimum fifteen-year follow-up of Neer hemiarthroplasty and total shoulder arthroplasty in patients aged fifty years or younger. J Shoulder Elbow Surg. 2004;13(6):604-13.

CHAPTER 85

Fracture Shaft Humerus: Interlocked Nailing

Mahesh Mone, Umesh Birole

INTRODUCTION

Humeral shaft fractures comprise small proportion of all adult fractures (3%) with annual incidence of 13 per 100,000.

With bimodal age distribution, domestic fall in elderly and high-velocity trauma in young population are the most common causes.

The association of radial nerve injury with diaphyseal humerus fracture is quite high (26.7%) and the most common location is middle-third fractures. The close anatomical relation and spiral course make radial nerve vulnerable to injury in humeral shaft fracture.

Traditionally, humerus diaphyseal fractures were treated nonoperatively using functional casts, brace, or coaptation splints. However, many treatment options are available nowadays like intramedullary nail. Open reduction internal fixation using plates and screws, and minimally invasive percutaneous plate osteosynthesis (MIPPO).

CLASSIFICATION

AO classification has given the most comprehensive description of fracture pattern:

- *Simple*: 12-A1 (spiral), 12-A2 (oblique > 30°), 12-A3 (oblique < 30°)
- *Wedge*: 12-B1 (spiral), 12-B2 (bending), 12-B3 (fragmented)
- *Complex*: 12-C1 (spiral), 12-C2 (segmental), 12-C3 (irregular).

CLINICAL FEATURES

Patient presents with swelling, tenderness, shortening of arm, and restricted movement at both shoulder and elbow.

It is important to check for radial nerve palsy by asking the patient to dorsiflex the wrist and digits, assessing sensations at dorsolateral hand and dorsum of thumb.

RADIOLOGICAL IMAGING

- Standard anteroposterior and lateral view of humerus with ipsilateral shoulder and elbow is the mainstay of imaging.
- Ultrasonography is used in localizing site of nerve injury and identifying cause of compression following trauma or after fracture stabilization.
- EMG NCV studies have limited role in assessing nerve recovery rate following radial nerve injury and functional outcome.

TREATMENT OPTIONS

Vast majority of the undisplaced fractures in low demand patients can be managed conservatively in brace, cast, or splint followed by physiotherapy.

Grossly displaced, comminuted fractures, multiple fractures often require internal fixation for stability and early range of motion (ROM). Operative options include:

- Closed reduction and internal fixation using intramedullary interlocking nail
- Open reduction and internal fixation using 4.5 mm dynamic compression plate (DCP)
- Open reduction and internal fixation using locking compression plate (LCP)
- Minimal invasive percutaneous plate osteosynthesis.

POTENTIAL COMPLICATIONS

Possible complications are mainly neurovascular injuries.

Intraoperative

- Radial nerve crushed between fracture ends during closed nailing
- Radial nerve entrapped underneath plate during ORIF/MIPPO
- Injury to brachial artery, while inserting the distal locking bolts of the interlocked nail
- Cuff tear during closed prograde nailing.

Postoperative

- Shoulder impingement, if nail protrudes more than 2 mm.
- Nonunion of the fracture
- Malunion.

SURGICAL PROCEDURE

Closed Intramedullary Interlocked Nailing of Fracture of Shaft Humerus

Indications:

- Inability to maintain acceptable reduction following conservative treatment
- Grossly displaced comminuted fracture
- Bilateral fracture
- Segmental fractures
- Pathological fracture.

Contraindications:

- Presence of radial nerve palsy.

Here, we describe the technique of closed intramedullary nailing of fracture shaft humerus.

Structures at risk:

- Supraspinatus insertion is at risk while making entry point.
- Axillary nerve injury during proximal locking as it winds around the neck of humerus approximately 5 cm distal to tip of acromion, from posterior to anterior
- Radial nerve entrapment during fracture manipulation and reduction
- Brachial artery is at risk during insertion of distal locking bolts.

STEPS OF SURGERY (FIGS. 1 TO 30)

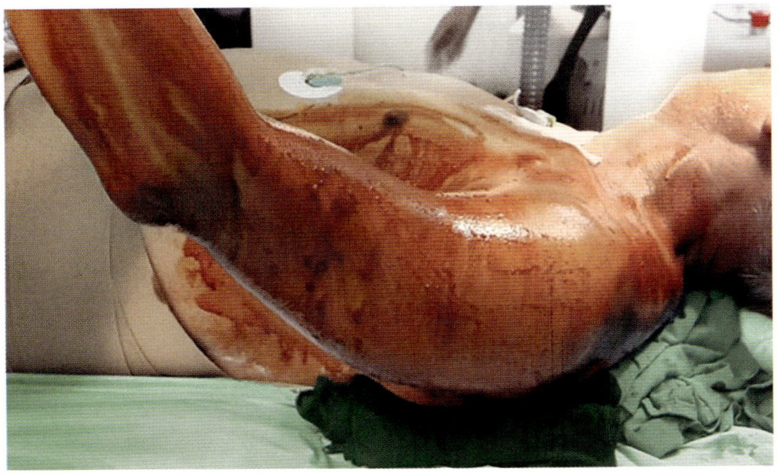

Fig. 1: Patient is positioned supine and parts painted and draped. Axilla is painted last to prevent operative site contamination.

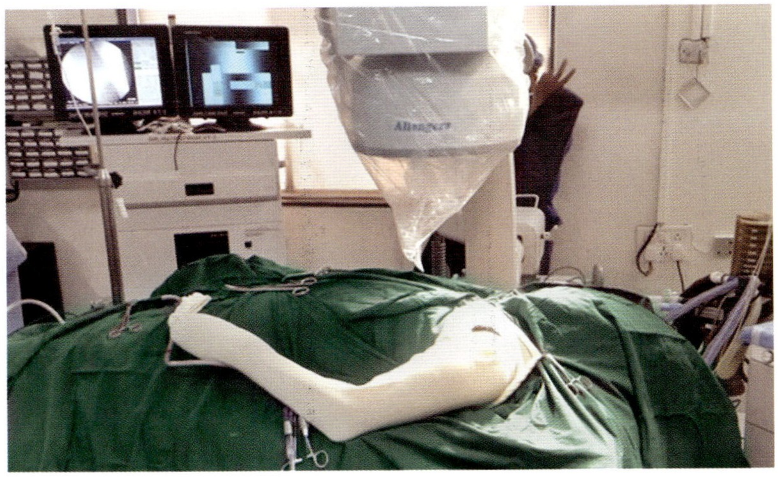

Fig. 2: C-arm should be positioned from opposite side. Stockinette is used to cover the entire limb.

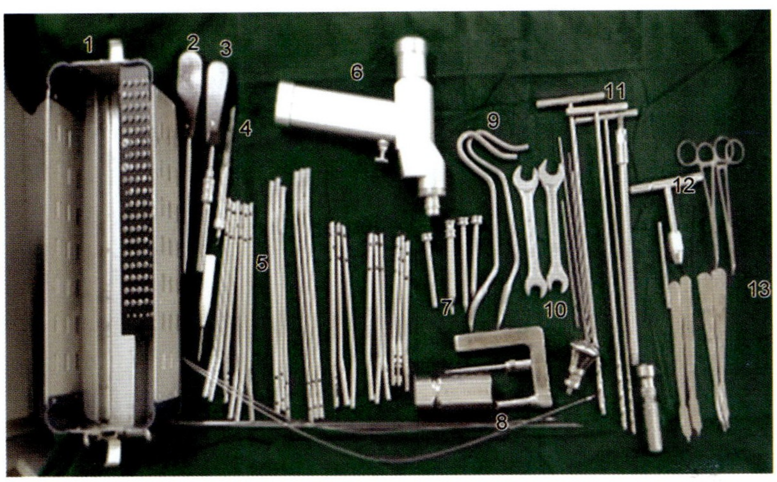

Fig. 3: Instruments on the trolley. (1) Implant set; (2) 4.5 mm screwdriver; (3) Entry reamer; (4) Depth gauge; (5) Nails of various sizes and lengths; (6) Cordless power drill; (7) Sleeves with trocar for proximal locking; (8) Jig along with guidewires and hammer assembly; (9) Pointed entry awl; (10) Spanners; (11) Canal reamers; (12) T-handle; (13) General orthopaedic instruments such as spike and artery forceps.

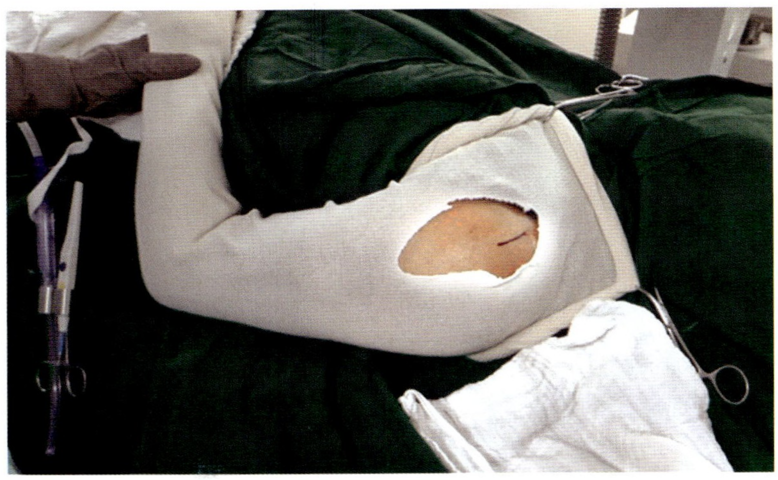

Fig. 4: Incision site is marked over superolateral aspect of shoulder. Arm to be extended, so greater tuberosity can be easily palpated and approached.

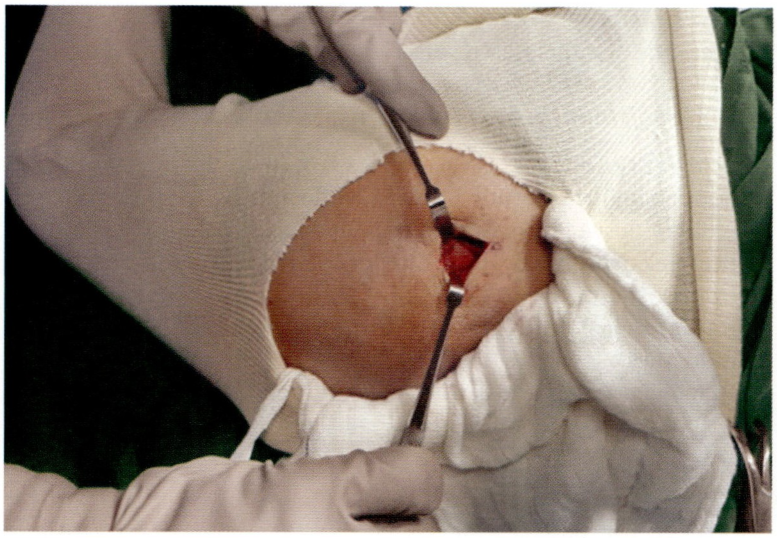

Fig. 5: Deltoid fibers separated and supraspinatus tendon is exposed.

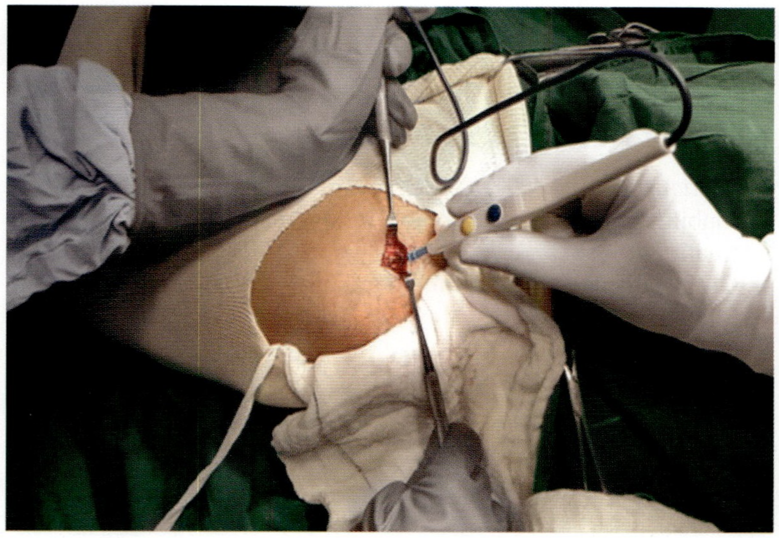

Fig. 6: Incision made in supraspinatus tendon longitudinally using electrical cautery. Entry is made just lateral to humeral articular cartilage.

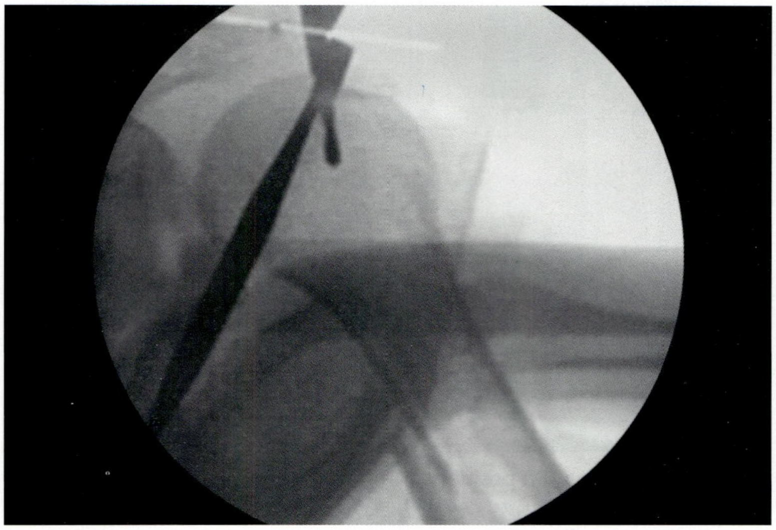

Fig. 7: Entry point is confirmed on C-arm. Entry is taken by drill bit.

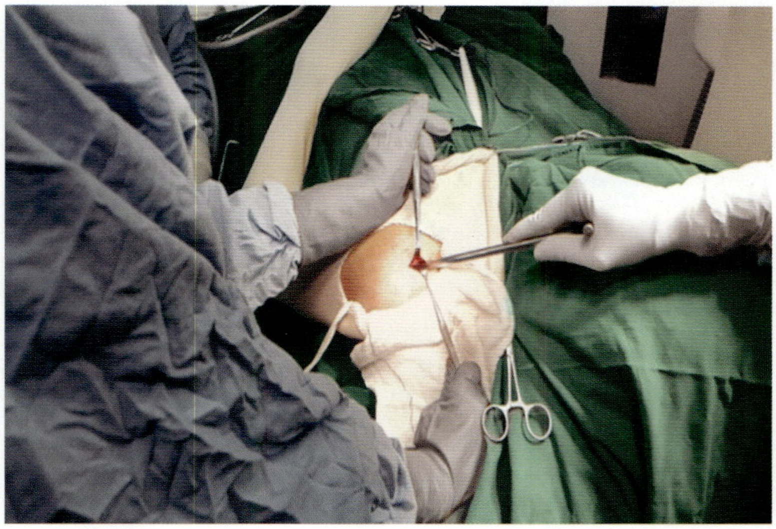

Fig. 8: Entry point enlarged by cannulated awl. Passage created in proximal humerus.

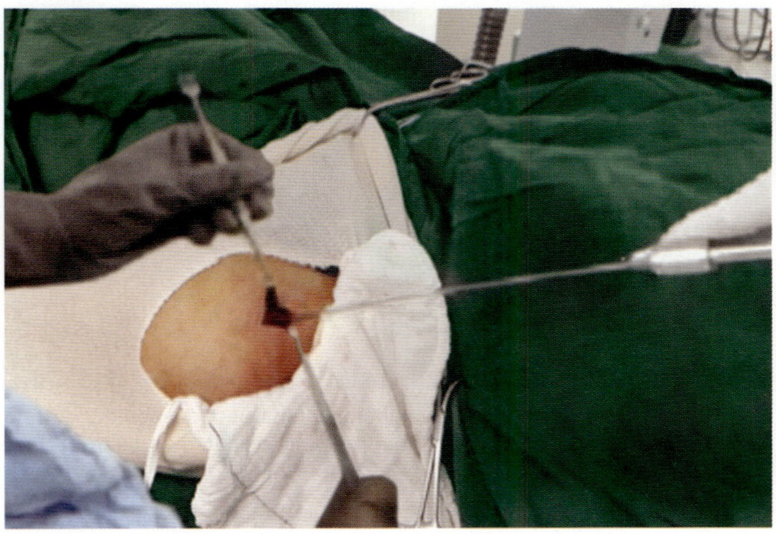

Fig. 9: Beaded guidewire is passed through the entry point of humerus.

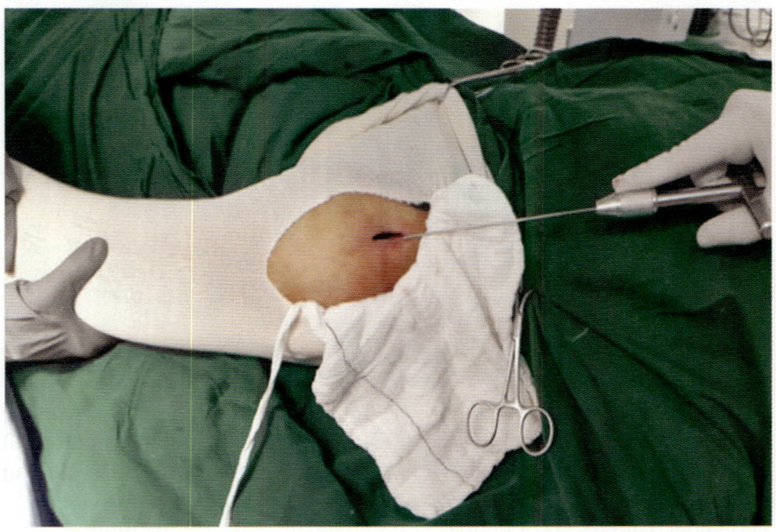

Fig. 10: Guidewire is advanced till fracture site.

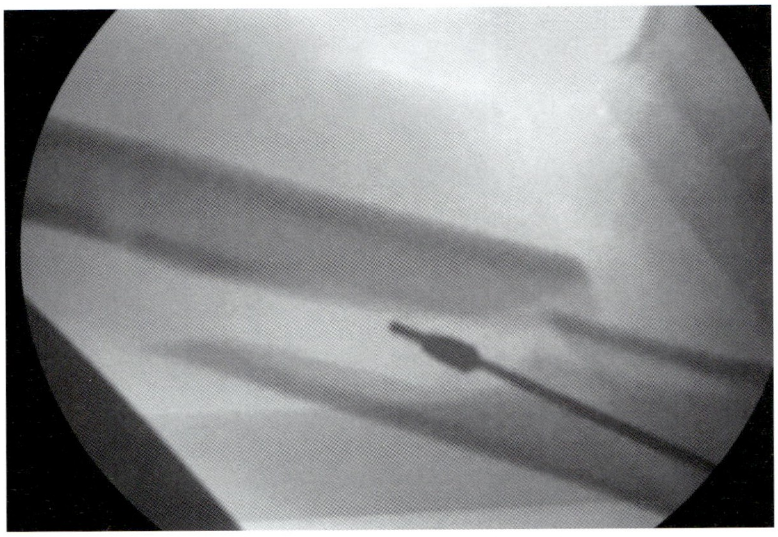

Fig. 11: Position of guidewire is confirmed in C-arm.

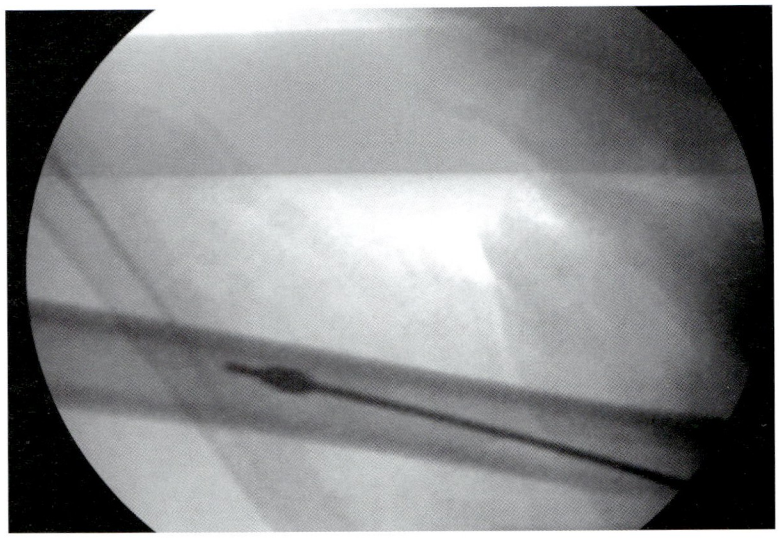

Fig. 12: Guidewire is further advanced, once it has negotiated the fracture site.

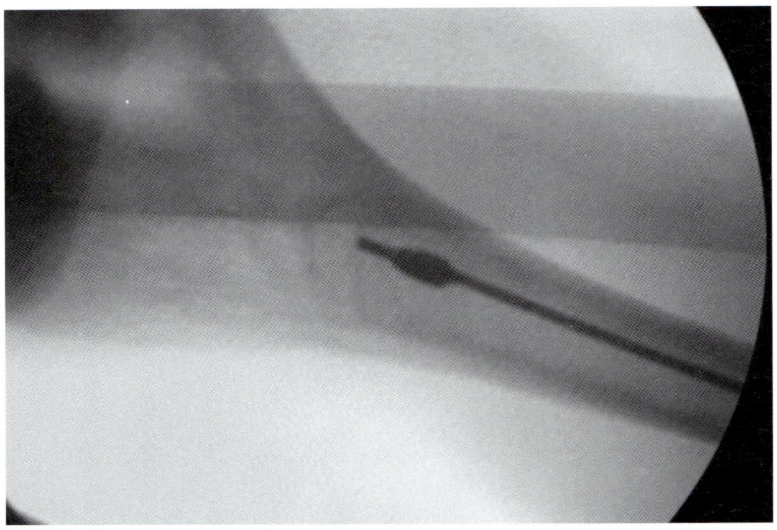

Fig. 13: Tip of guidewire should reach till the superior edge of olecranon fossa.

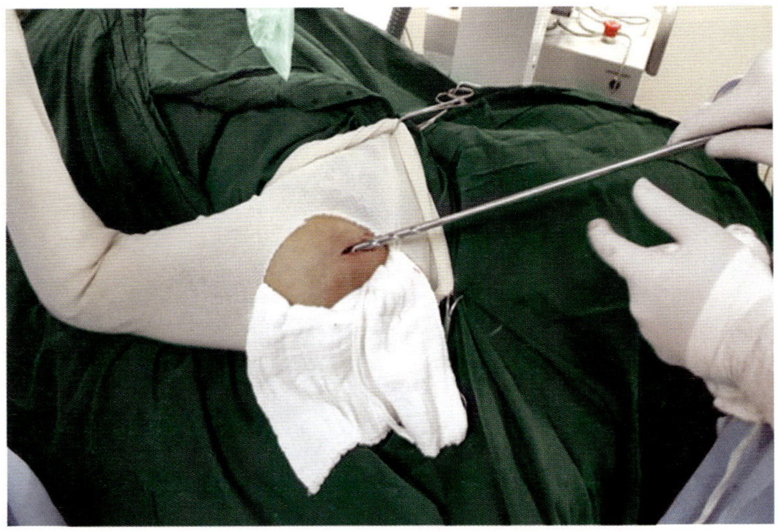

Fig. 14: Proximal humeral canal is reamed using hand reamer to accommodate broad proximal part of nail.

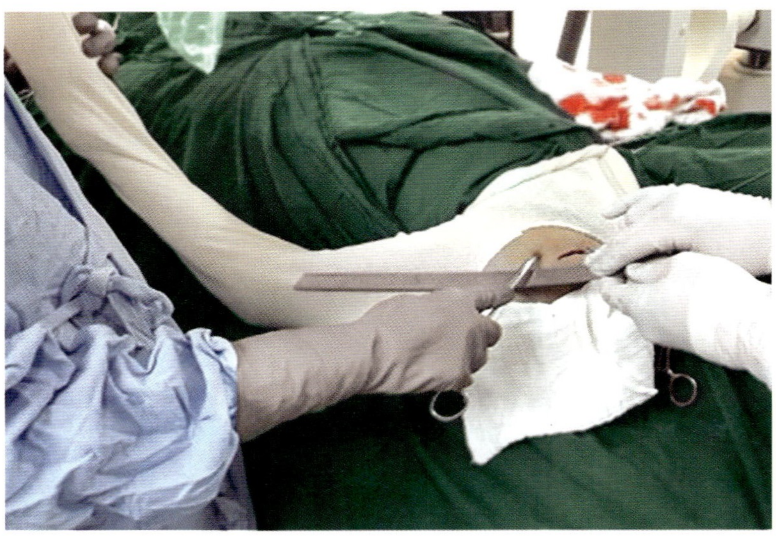

Fig. 15: Measure the length of nail required.

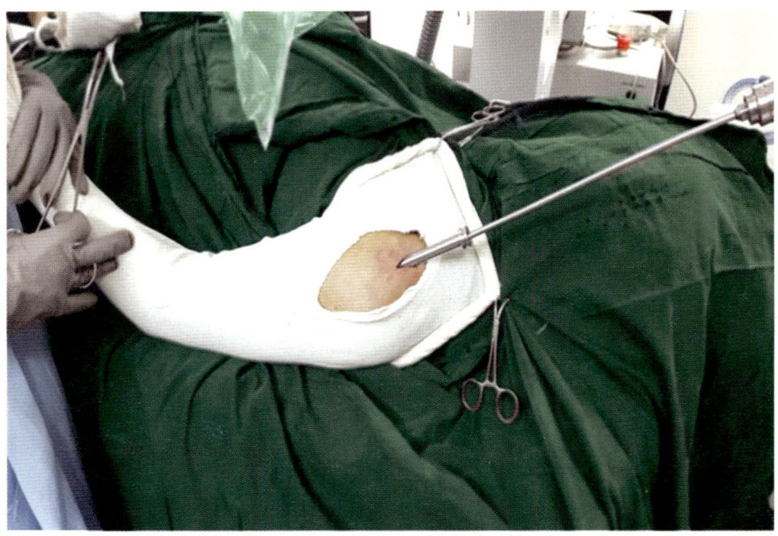

Fig. 16: Serial reaming using power drill, up to as distal as possible. Use of drill sleeve is recommended to prevent soft-tissue damage.

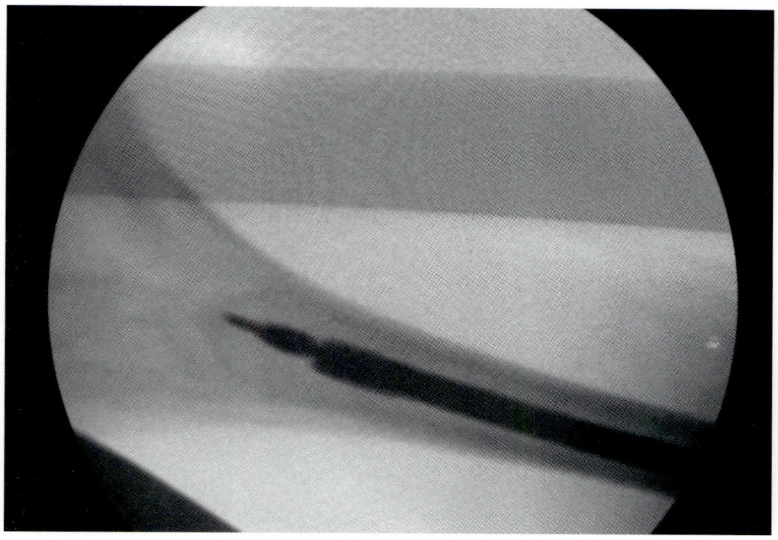

Fig. 17: Ball tipped guidewire limits the extent of reaming.

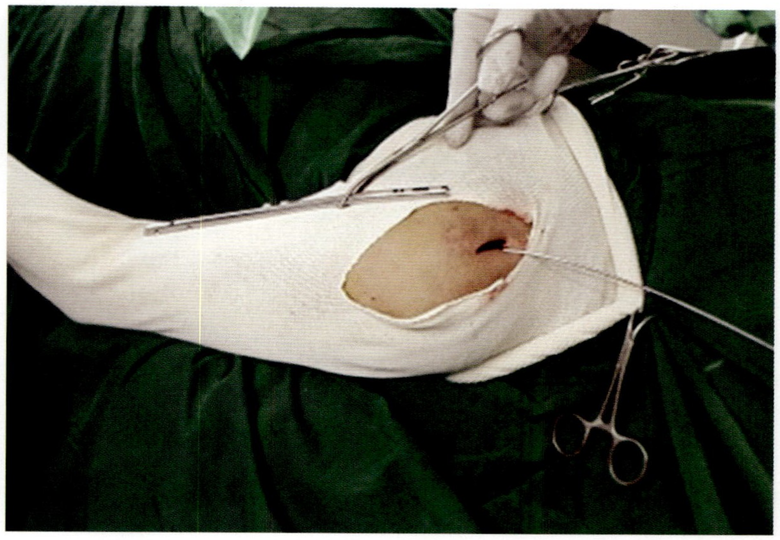

Fig. 18: Confirm the anticipated position of nail and confirm length before insertion.

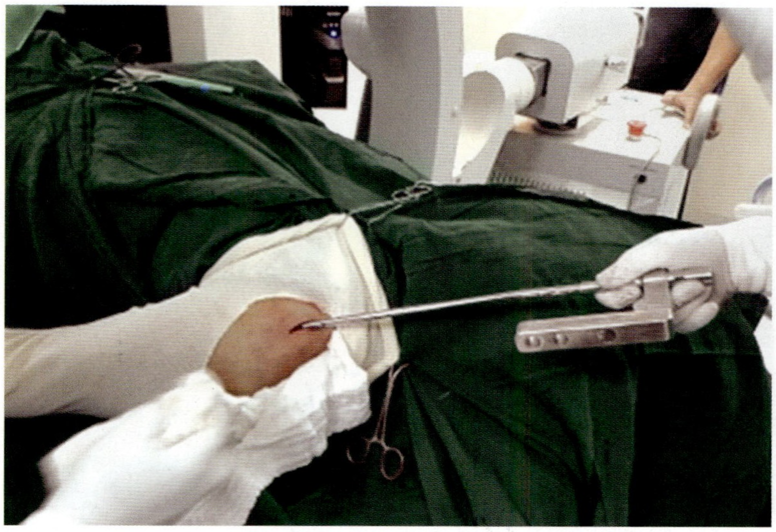

Fig. 19: Nail is assembled over jig and inserted through the entry point. Check size of nail, tighten all assembly bolts, and confirm easy passage of drill bit through jig and proximal nail holes beforehand.

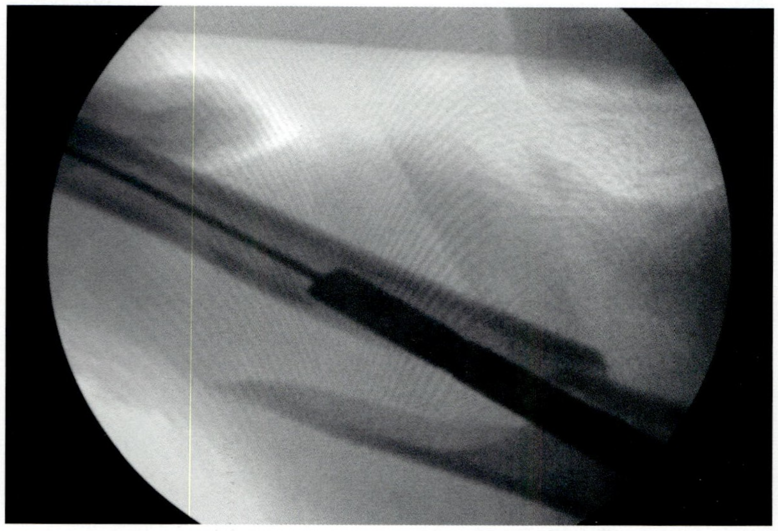

Fig. 20: Check and confirm the position of nail when negotiating the fracture site.

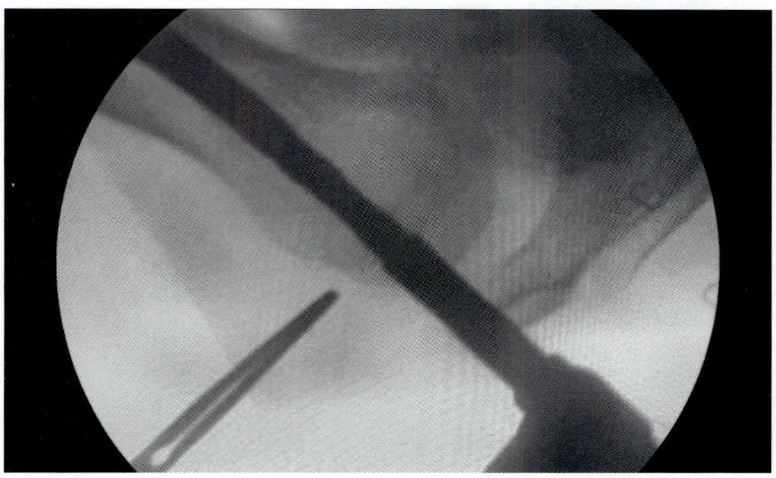

Fig. 21: Confirm that the proximal portion of the nail is sunk well below the bone surface. This will protect the supraspinatus tendon.

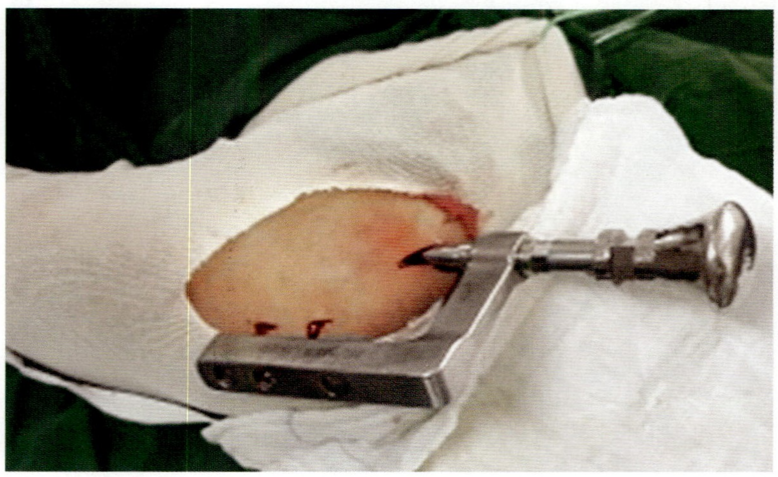

Fig. 22: Marking and incision for proximal locking.

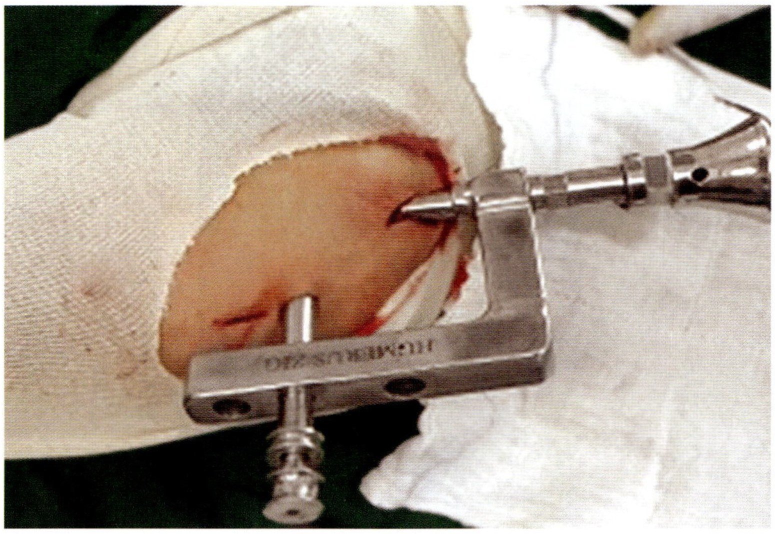

Fig. 23: Proximal locking may be done first as per surgeon preference. Through stab incisions sleeves are passed and drilling of bone performed. Ensure that drill bit does not plunge too much beyond. Bolts are passed.

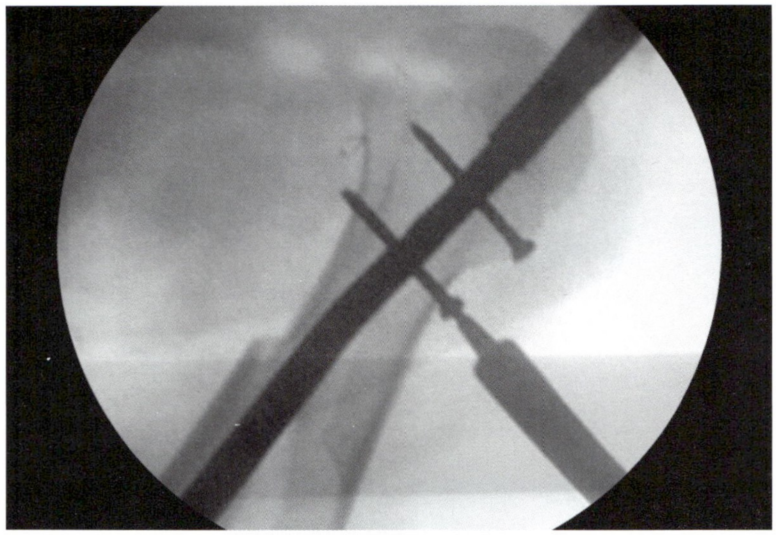

Fig. 24: Position of locking bolts confirmed in C-arm.

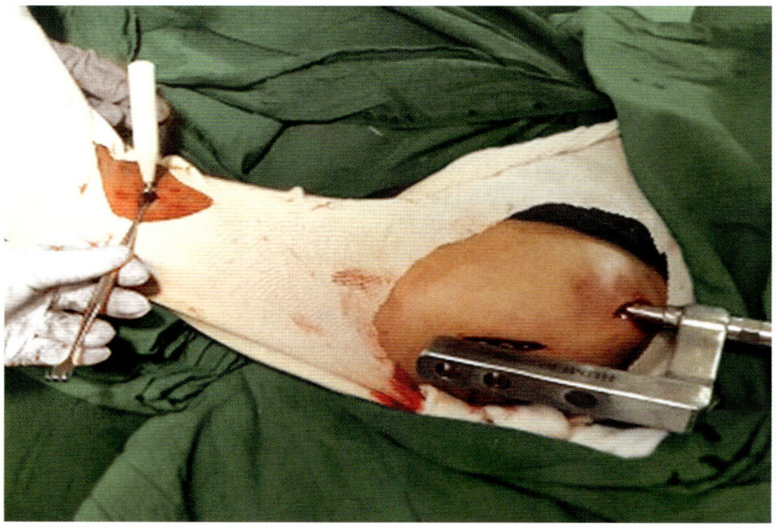

Fig. 25: Distal locking position is confirmed on C-arm, soft tissue is separated by blunt dissection. Take an incision large enough for the sleeves to pass. Drill only when on the anterior humeral cortex.

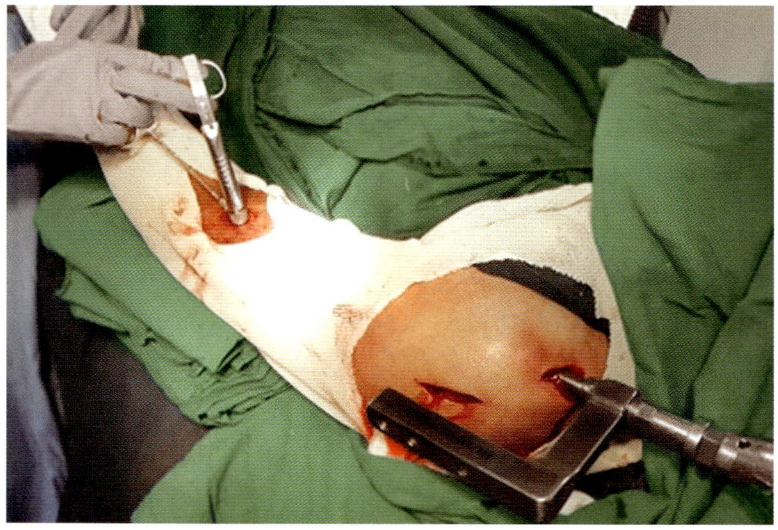

Fig. 26: Depth gauge is used to measure required length of distal bolt.

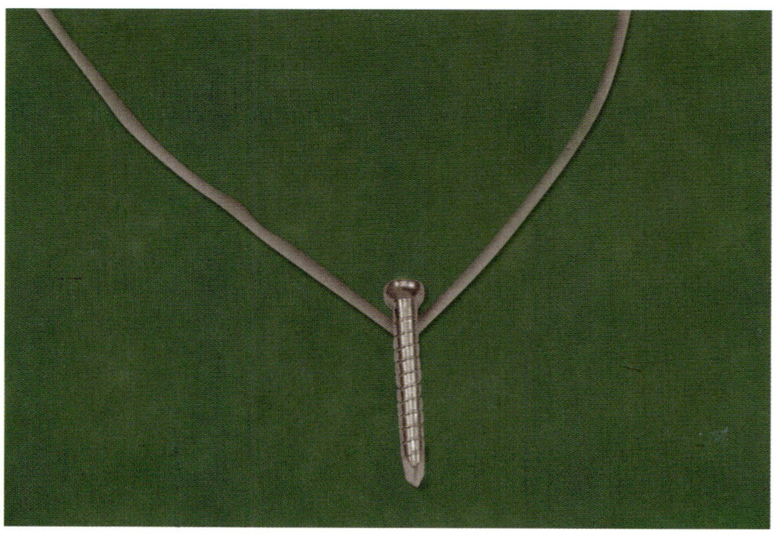

Fig. 27: Distal bolt may be tied with 2-0 absorbable suture. This helps in screw retrieval if it is malpositioned or exchange needed as it is often lost in surrounding soft tissue.

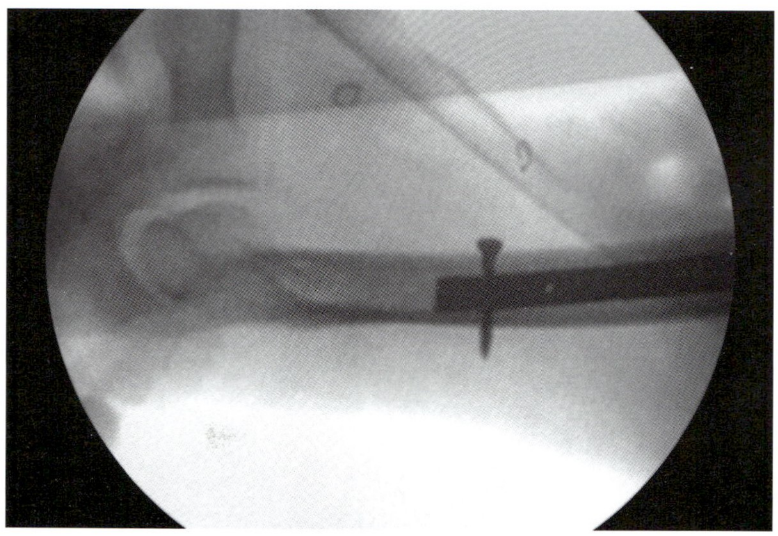

Fig. 28: Position of distal locking bolt and length confirmed on C-arm.

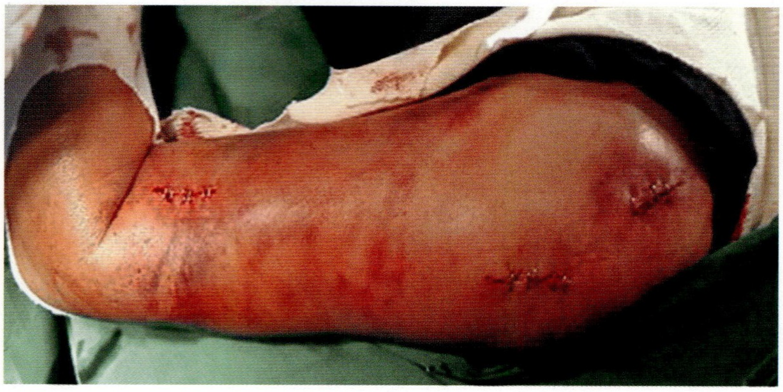

Fig. 29: Mini portals are closed in layers.

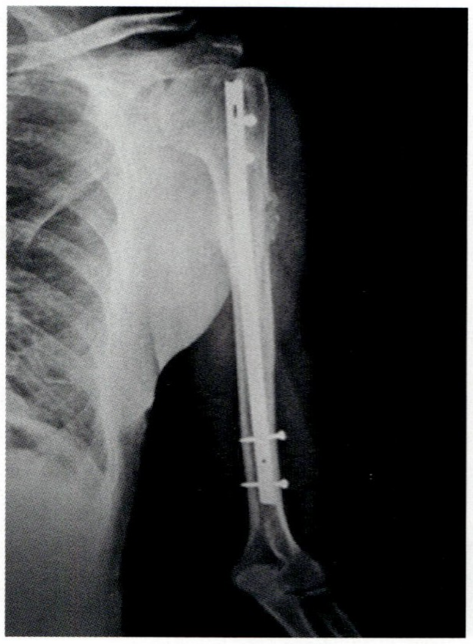

Fig. 30: X-ray at 3 months showing good position of implant and screws.

POSTOPERATIVE PROTOCOL

- Elbow range of motion exercises from day 3
- Shoulder pendulum exercises from day 7
- Stitch removal on day 14
- No driving for 6 weeks
- No swimming for 10 weeks.

SUGGESTED READING

1. Kim SH, Szabo RM, Marder RA. Epidemiology of humerus fractures in the United States: nationwide emergency department sample, 2008. Arthritis Care Res. 2012;64(3):407-14.
2. Kulkarni VS, Kulkarni MS, Kulkarni GS, et al. Comparison between antegrade intramedullary nailing (IMN), open reduction plate osteosynthesis (ORPO) and minimally invasive plate osteosynthesis (MIPO) in treatment of humerus diaphyseal fractures. Injury. 2017;48:S8-13.
3. Lawande AD, Warrier SS, Joshi MS. Role of ultrasound in evaluation of peripheral nerves. Indian J Radiol Imaging. 2014;24(3):254-8.
4. Ricci FP, Barbosa RI, Elui VM, et al. Radial nerve injury associated with humeral shaft fracture: a retrospective study. Acta Ortop Bras. 2015;23(1):19-21.
5. Schoch BS, Padegimas EM, Maltenfort M, et al. Humeral shaft fractures: national trends in management. J Orthop Traumatol. 2017;18(3):259-63.

CHAPTER 86

Fracture Shaft Humerus: Dynamic Compression Plate Anterolateral Approach

Sushrut Pulgaonkar, Prateek Charuchandra Joshi, Rajkumar Ekambaram

INTRODUCTION

Humerus shaft fractures are a relatively common occurrence in the adult population. Diaphyseal humeral fractures occur equally in males and females up to the age of 60 years. Incidence does not increase with advancing age.

The most common mechanism of injury is a fall in elderly osteoporotic patients, followed by motor vehicle accident in younger patients thus having a bimodal age distribution and accounting for 3–5% of all fractures. Other causes for fracture of humerus shaft include sporting activities, working accidents, falling from a height, violence and bone pathology. Approximately 7–8% are pathologic fractures and 3–5% are open fractures.

INDICATIONS

Associated conditions such as open wound, compound fracture, poor skin condition, and neurovascular injury may initially need to be stabilized with temporary external fixation before attempting a definitive fixation in order to fully optimize the patient for definitive surgery. This is called damage control orthopaedics.

If associated with radial nerve palsy, then nerve exploration should be carried out at the time of operative intervention as indicated for the fracture and in cases of open fractures.

SURGICAL STEPS (FIGS. 1 TO 16)

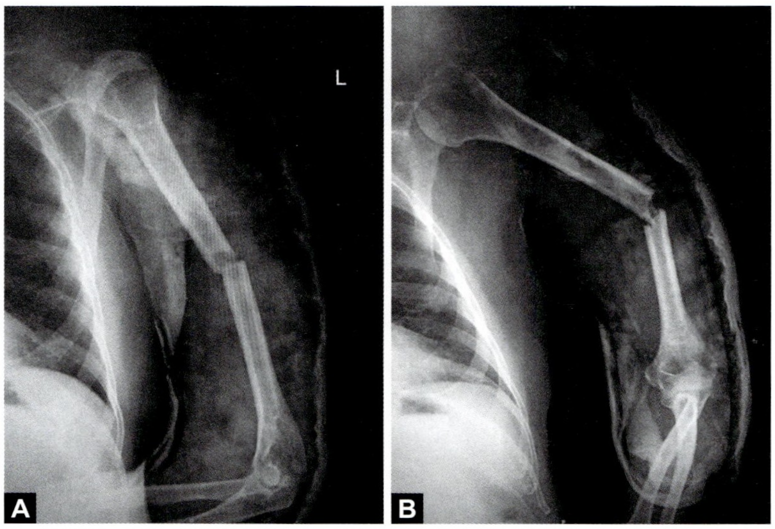

Figs. 1A and B: Preoperative radiograph of the patient with humerus shaft fracture. The fracture was closed without any neurovascular injury or associated infection.

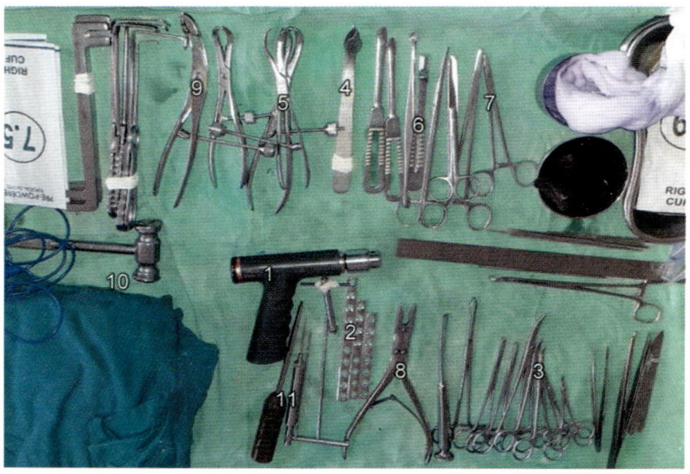

Fig. 2: Sterile instrument trolley as arranged for anterolateral plating for humerus. (1) Drill machine, (2) Humerus DCP plates, (3) Artery forceps, (4) Bone spike, (5) Bone holding forceps, (6) Perisoteum elevator and scoop, (7) Needle holder, (8) Bone nibbler, (9) Plate holding forceps, (10) Hammer, (11) Screw drivers and depth gauge.

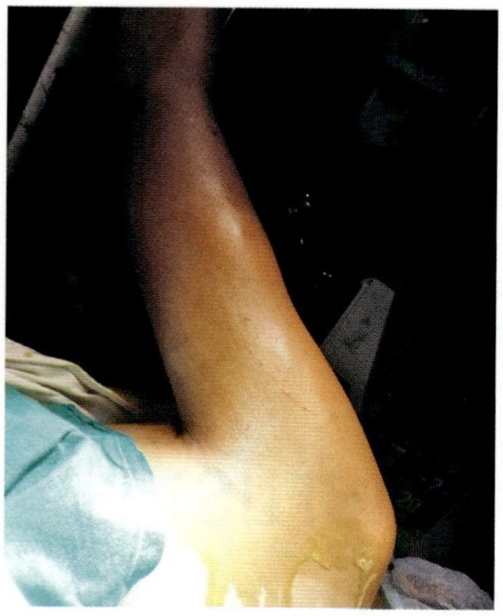

Fig. 3: The operative limb is cleaned with povidone iodine scrub and wiped down with surgical spirit.

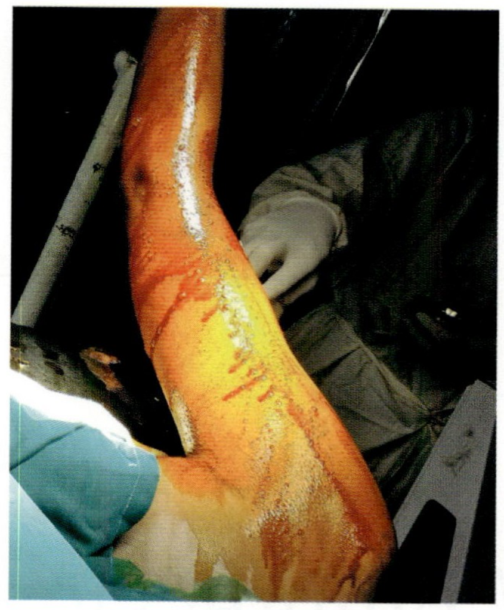

Fig. 4: After the limb is scrubbed, povidone-iodine painting is done.

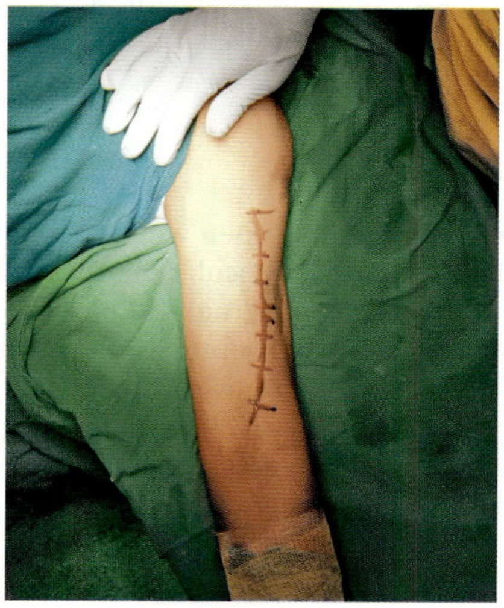

Fig. 5: Draping done. The limb ready for surgery. The incision site is marked on the skin using a sterile marker. Skin incision starts at the distal end of deltopectoral groove. From here, the incision continues distally following the lateral border of the biceps until about 5 cm proximal to the flexion crease of the elbow joint.

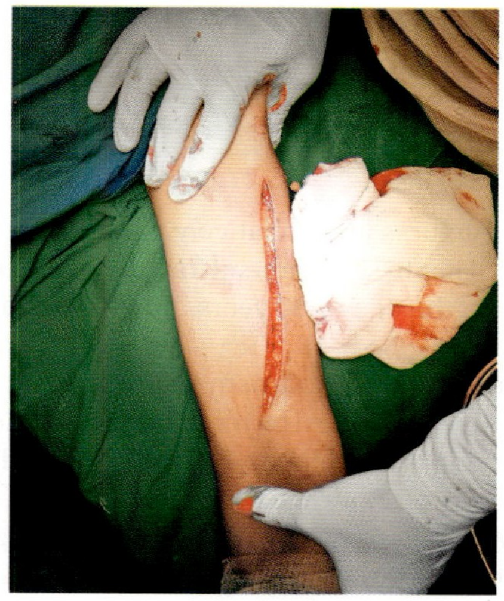

Fig. 6: Skin is incised along the marked incision line. Superficial and deep fascia is incised in line with the skin incision.

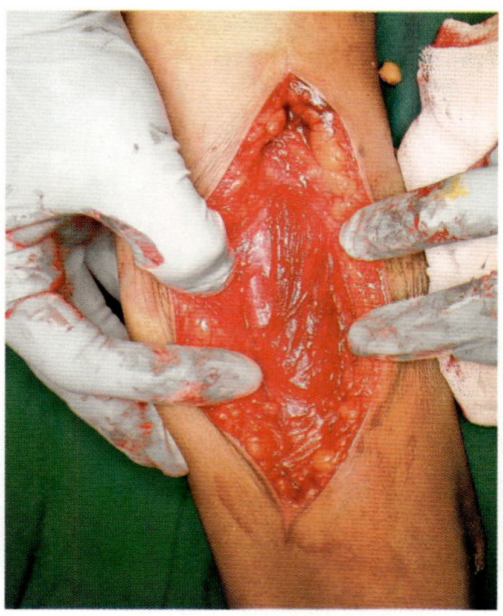

Fig. 7: The deep fascia is incised in line with the skin incision to identify the interval between the biceps brachii and the brachialis.

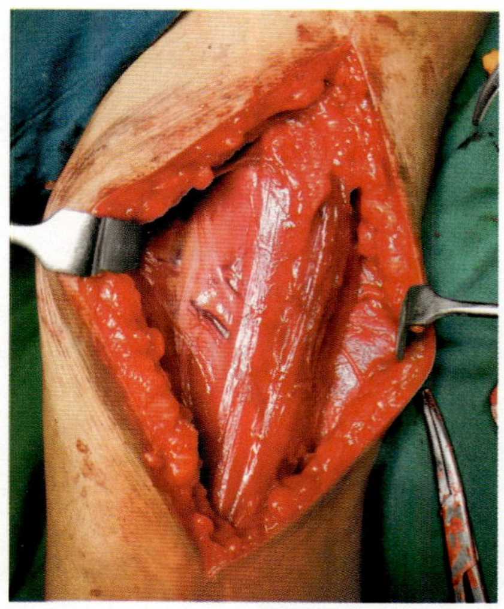

Fig. 8: Biceps is retracted medially, being careful to identify the musculocutaneous nerve. Proximally, the anterior circumflex humeral artery is identified as it crosses the field of dissection in a medial-to-lateral direction.

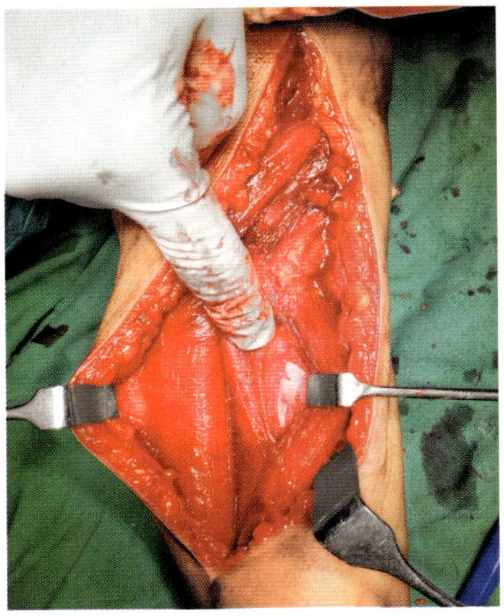

Fig 9: The fibers of the brachialis are split to expose the periosteum of the anterior humerus. The periosteum is incised and brachialis is stripped off the bone. Elbow is flexed to take tension off the brachialis, making the exposure easier.

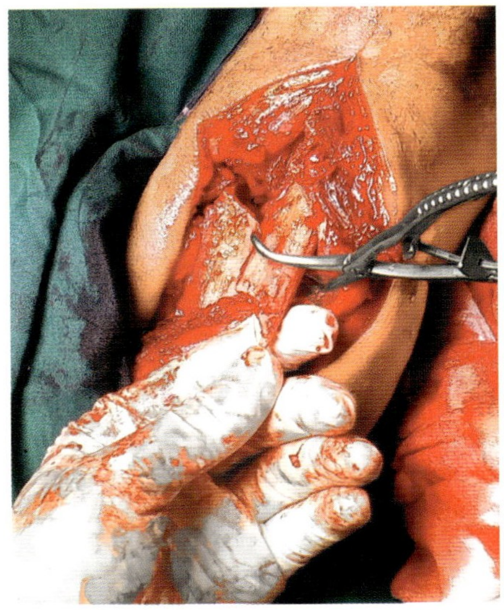

Fig 10: Bone fragments are held with bone holding forceps for exposing fracture site. Fracture edges are freshened by removing debris and soft tissue.

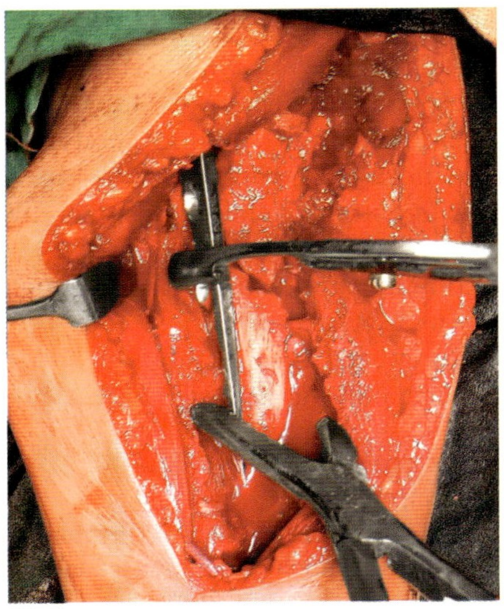

Fig 11: Reduction is achieved and plate is held over it by plate holding forceps.

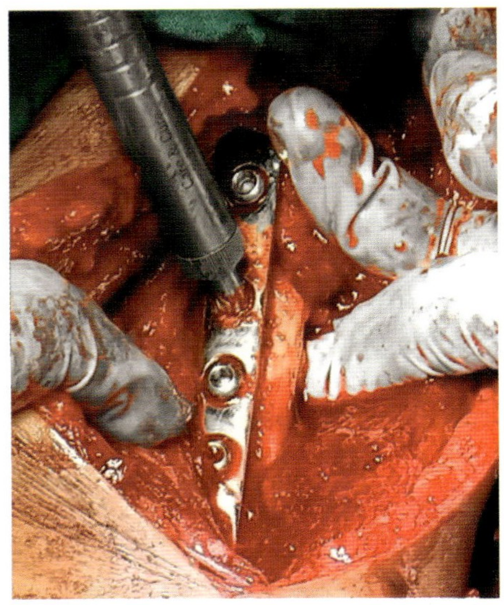

Fig 12: Once plate is held over the bone surface, holes are drilled through the bone and depth is measured with depth gauge for ideal screw length insertion.

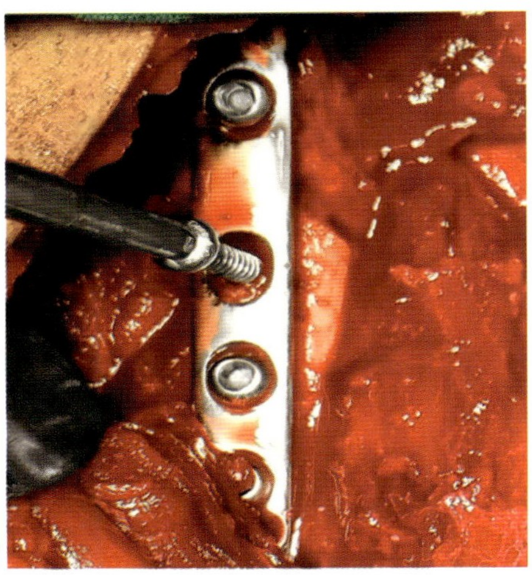

Fig 13: Screws of ideal length are introduced and tightened.

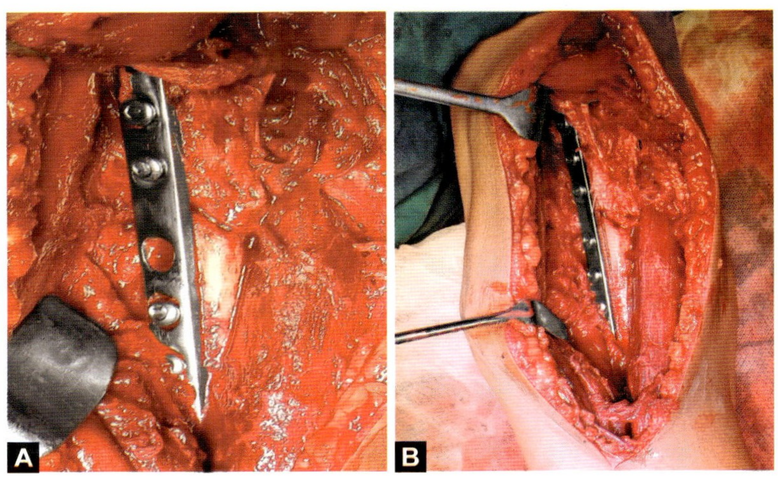

Figs. 14A and B: Images showing fixation of humerus fracture with DC plate with anatomical reduction.

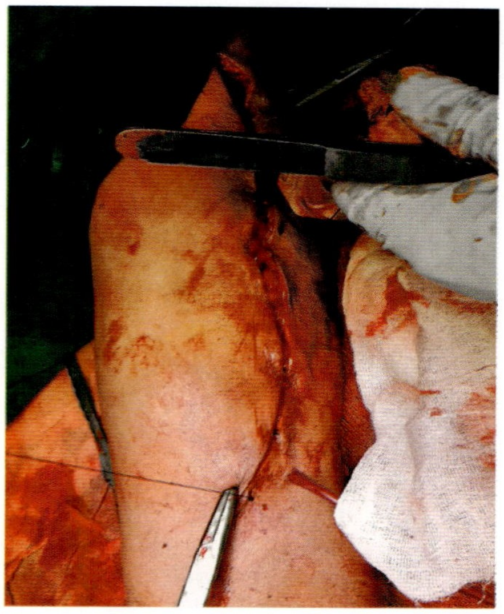

Fig. 15: Plate is covered with the muscles and fascia and then subcutaneous tissue is closed with absorbable suture over the suction drain.

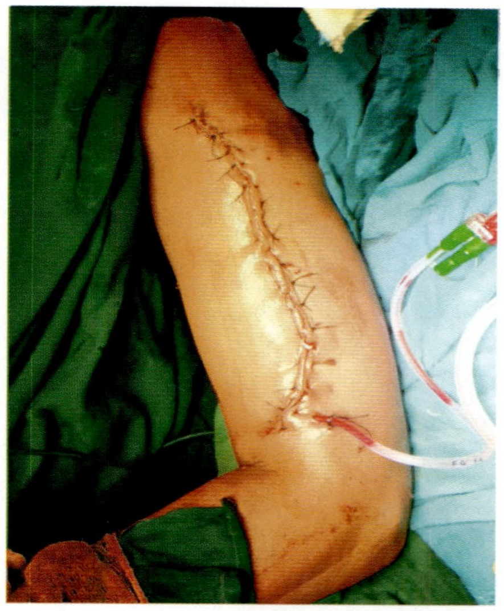

Fig 16: Skin closure is done with nonabsorbable suture and proper sterile dressing in done.

POSTOPERATIVE PROTOCOL

Goals of postoperative rehabilitation protocol after anterolateral plating of humerus include increasing the range of motion of shoulder and elbow joints while protecting the fracture site, controlling pain and swelling and preventing adhesion formation. Normally bony healing occurs after 12 to 14 weeks and limb returns to normal function 3–4 months after surgery.

Postsurgical protocol generally consists of early motion phase (0–5 weeks), active motion phase (5–12 weeks) and aggressive stretching and strengthening phase (after 12 weeks).

Suture removal is done 12–15 days after surgery.

POSSIBLE COMPLICATIONS

Apart from anesthetic complications, this surgery may be complicated by inadvertent injury to neurovascular structures during surgical dissection, if appropriate care is not taken. Injury can occur to the radial nerve (most commonly), axillary nerve and anterior circumflex humeral vessels. Proper wound care must be taken to prevent postoperative surgical site infection and wound gaping. Other possible complications include nonunion of fracture shaft humerus, malunion with varus angulation and superficial/deep wound infections.

SUMMARY

Fractures of shaft of humerus are commonly seen as an outcome of fall or motor vehicle accidents leading to blunt trauma to the arm.

Anterolateral plating appears to produce good results with high rate of fracture union in proximal and mid-third fractures of humerus shaft when combined with a strictly followed postoperative rehabilitation protocol.

Careful dissection and good surgical technique are essential to prevent iatrogenic neurovascular injury.

Meticulous wound care when combined with patient specific rehabilitation protocol minimizes postoperative complications.

SUGGESTED READING

1. Abalo A, Dosseh ED, Adabra K, et al. Open reduction and internal fixation of humeral non-unions: Radiological and functional results. Acta Orthop Belg. 2011;77(3):299-303.
2. Ajmal M, O'Sullivan M, McCabe J, et al. Antegrade locked intramedullary nailing in humeral shaft fractures. Injury. 2001;32(9):692-4.
3. Albritton MJ, Barnes CJ, Basamania CJ, et al. Relationship of the axillary nerve to the proximal screws of a flexible humeral nail system: an anatomic study. J Orthop Trauma. 2003;17(6):411-4.
4. Holstein A, Lewis GM. Fractures of the humerus with radial nerve paralysis. J Bone Joint Surg [Am]. 1963;45-A:1382-8.
5. Thompson JE. Anatomical methods of approach in operating on the long bones of the extremities. Ann Surg. 1918;68:309-29.

CHAPTER 87

Fracture Shaft Humerus: Dynamic Compression Plate by Posterior Approach

Shrinivas S Shintre, Prateek Charuchandra Joshi, Rajkumar Ekambaram

POSTERIOR APPROACH TO SHAFT HUMERUS: SURGICAL STEPS (FIGS. 1 TO 13)

Implant choice:

1. Patients having good bone quality dynamic compression plate (DCP). Limited contact dynamic compression plating (LC-DCP) plating can be done.
2. Patients with poor bone quality (osteoporotic) locking plate to be used.

How many cortices?

Screws must engage minimum of eight cortices in both the fragment.

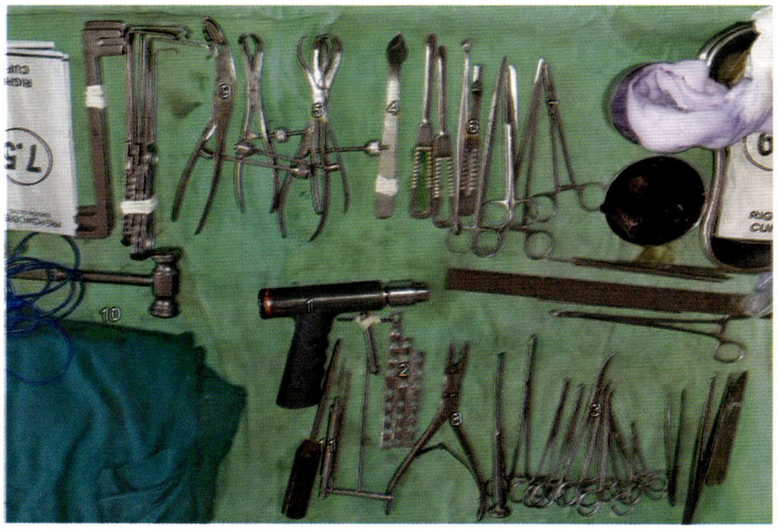

Fig. 1: Sterile instrument trolley as arranged for anterolateral plating for humerus. (1) Drill machine, (2) Humerus DCP plates, (3) Artery forceps, (4) Bone spike, (5) Bone holding forceps, (6) Perisoteum elevator and scoop, (7) Needle holder, (8) Bone nebbler, (9) Plate holding forceps, (10) Hammer, (11) Screw drivers and depth gauge.

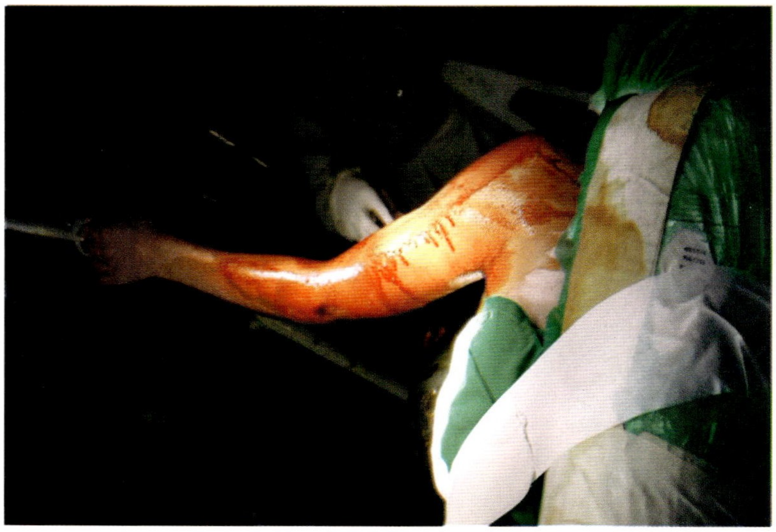

Fig. 2: Position of the patient: Lateral with arm over the top of the body elbow flexion 90°, with elbow at end of the lateral support). Painting and draping of the operative limb is done using povidone iodine.

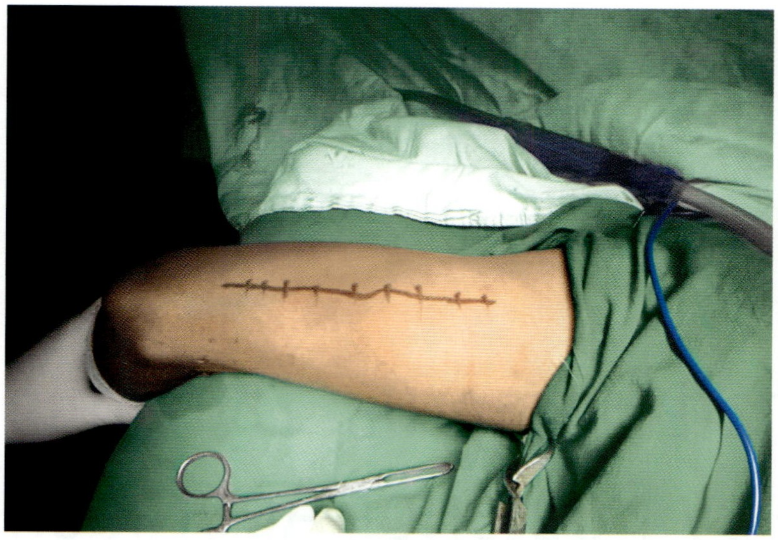

Fig. 3: Skin incision is marked with a sterile marker extending from 8 cm distal to the acromion to the olecranon fossa.

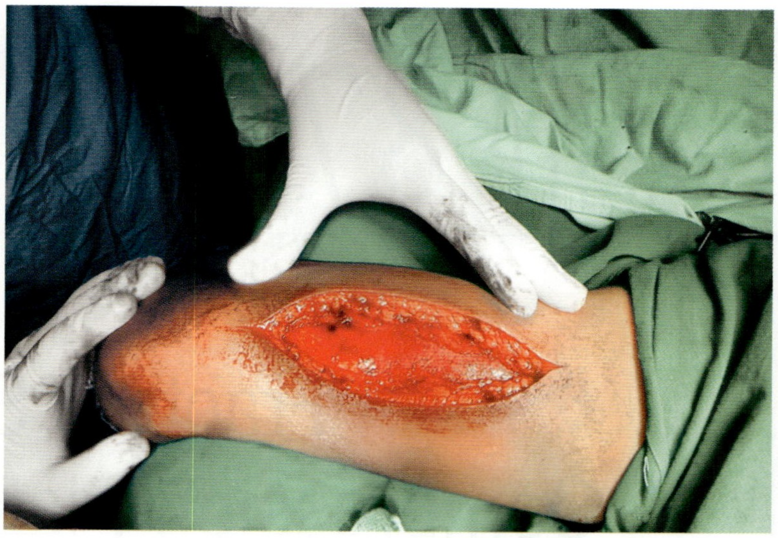

Fig 4: Skin and superficial fascia is incised along the marked line.

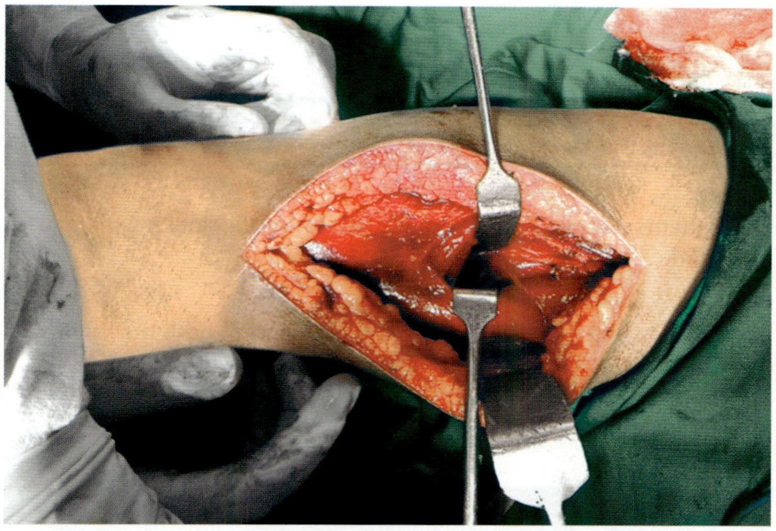

Fig. 5: Blunt dissection is done with a plane created between the long and lateral head of triceps.

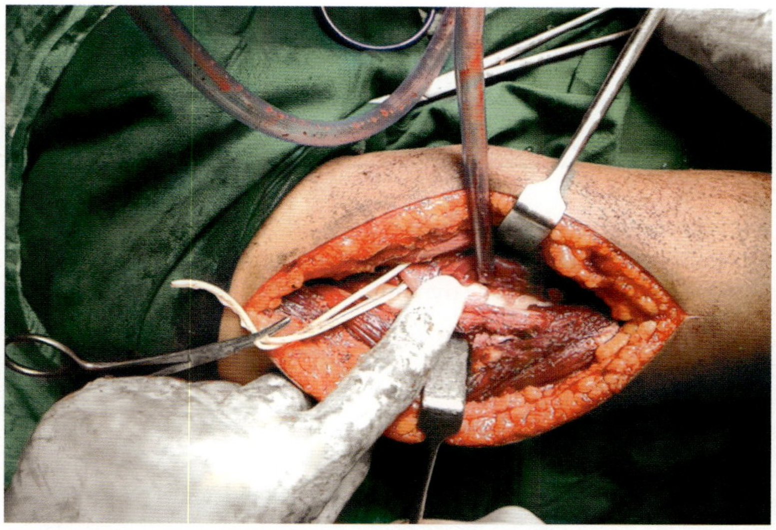

Fig. 6: Radial nerve is identified. It can be palpated over the spiral groove of humerus for ease of identification. Profunda brachii and venae comitantes run along the nerve and to be secured together. A stretchable strip of rubber glove is put under the nerve to aid for surgical dissection of the nerve (5 cm below the deltoid tuberosity) till it pierces the lateral intermuscular septum.

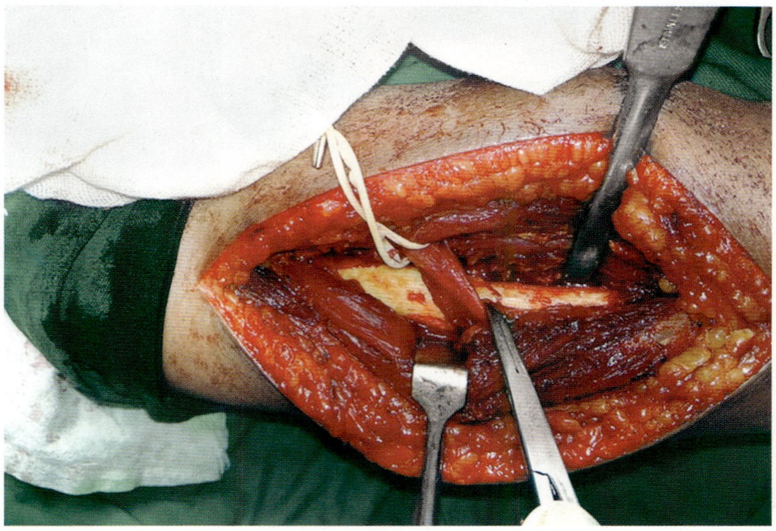

Fig 7: Intermuscular plane between the two heads of triceps is developed further till the bone is reached. Fracture site is visualized. Radial nerve along with the vessels needs to be secured.

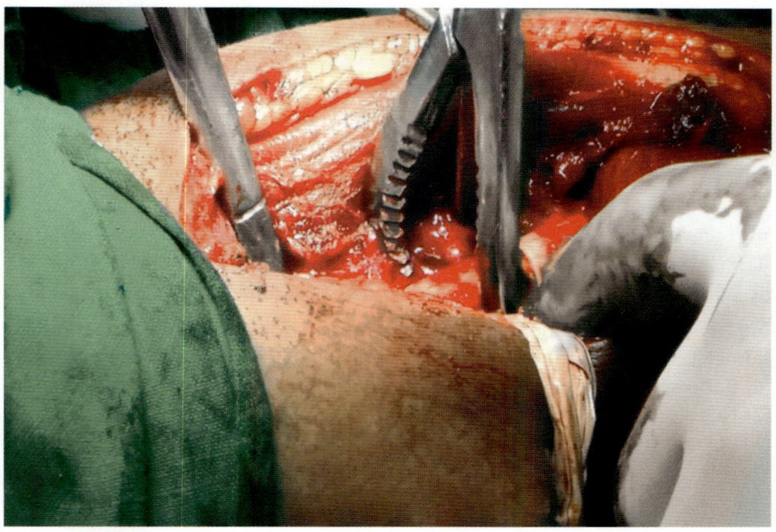

Fig. 8: Fracture site is exposed with aid of bone holding forceps and fracture edges freshened with curette.

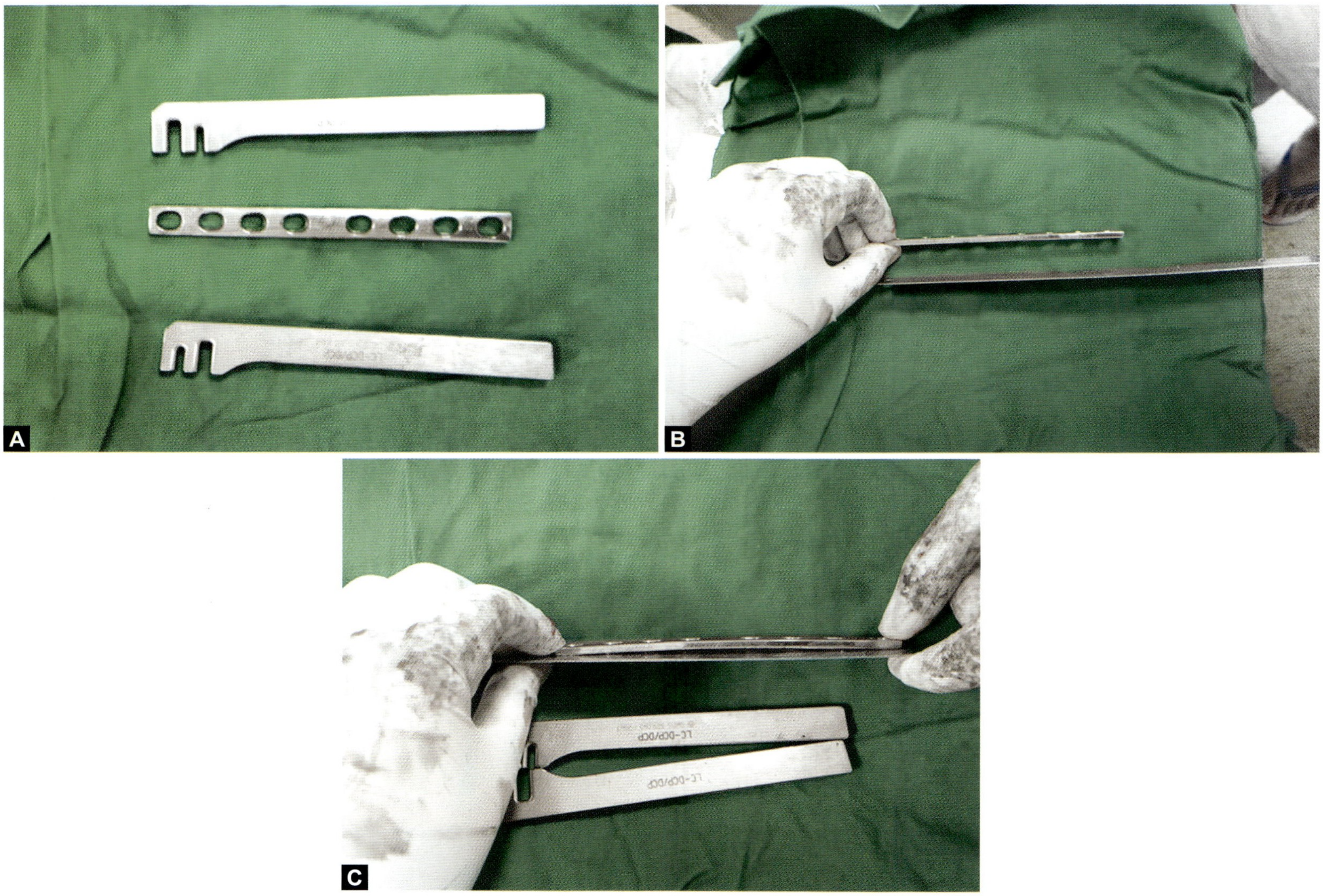

Figs. 9A to C: Prebending of the plate done over the fracture site (prevents opening up of the far cortex).

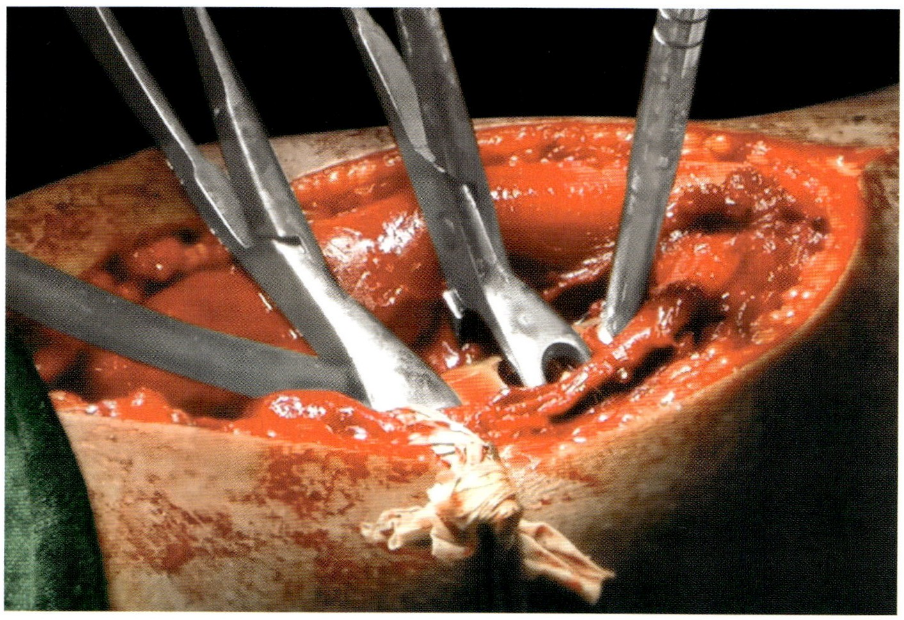

Fig. 10: 4.5 dynamic compression plate (DCP) is positioned over the shaft under the radial nerve and stabilized to the bone with plate holding forceps. Fracture reduction is maintained.

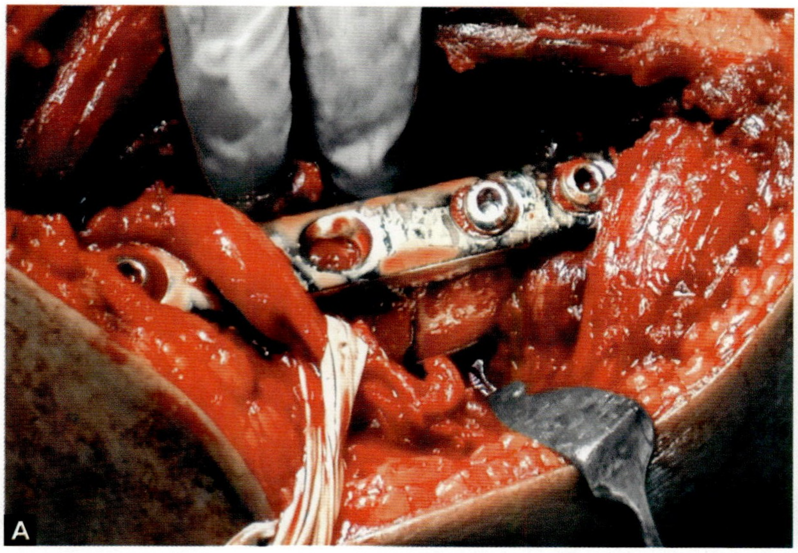

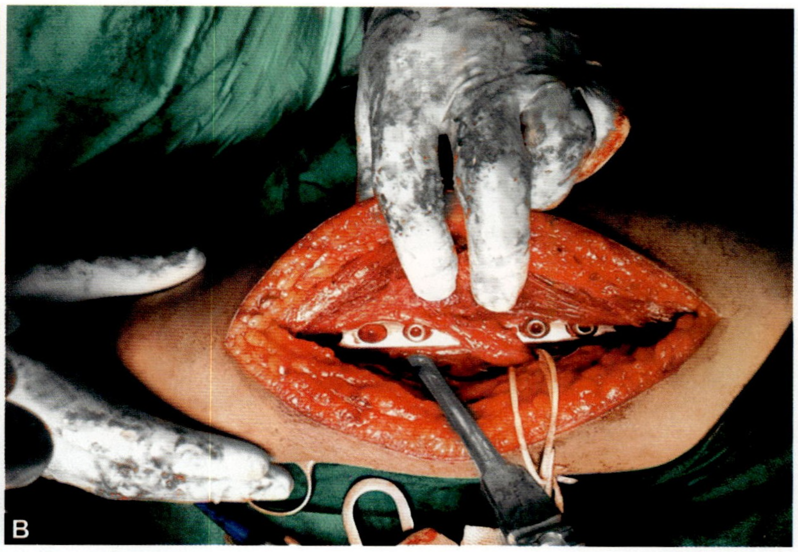

Figs. 11A and B: Open reduction and internal fixation with dynamic compression plate (DCP) (eight cortices purchase in both the proximal and distal fragment) done. Radial nerve and its relation with the plate and screws need to be mentioned. Usually, it lies over the 2nd–4th screw in the proximal fragment.

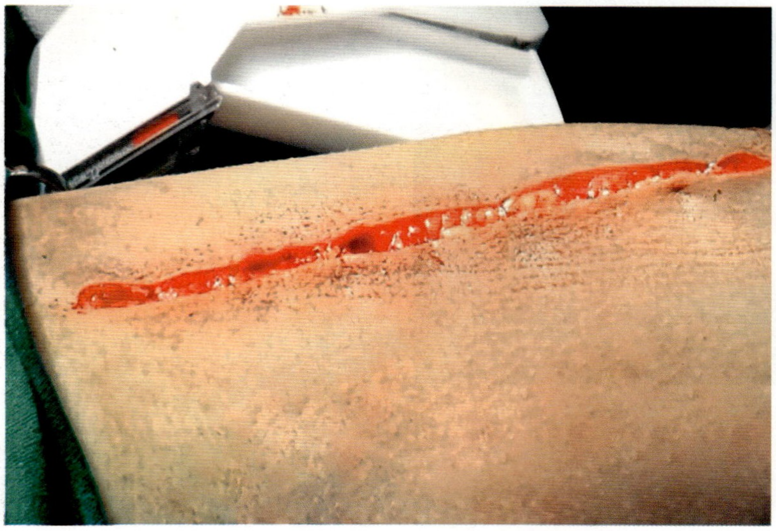

Fig. 12: Subcutaneous closure is done over the suction drain using nonabsorbable suture.

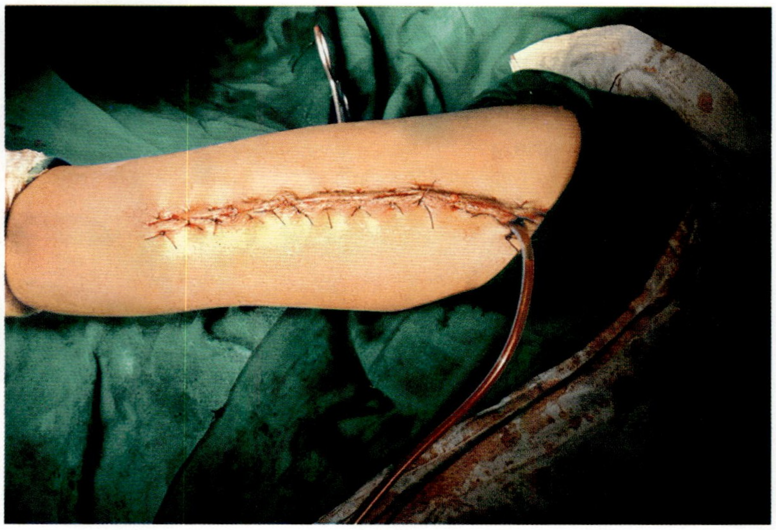

Fig. 13: Skin closure is done with nonabsorbable suture and proper sterile dressing is applied.

POSTOPERATIVE PROTOCOL

- Elbow range of motion exercises from day 3
- Shoulder pendulum exercises from day 7
- Stitch removal on day 14
- No driving for 6 weeks
- No swimming for 10 weeks.

SUGGESTED READING

1. Kim SH, Szabo RM, Marder RA. Epidemiology of humerus fractures in the United States: nationwide emergency department sample, 2008. Arthritis Care Res. 2012;64(3):407-14.
2. Kulkarni VS, Kulkarni MS, Kulkarni GS, et al. Comparison between antegrade intramedullary nailing (IMN), open reduction plate osteosynthesis (ORPO) and minimally invasive plate osteosynthesis (MIPO) in treatment of humerus diaphyseal fractures. Injury. 2017;48: S8-13.
3. Lawande AD, Warrier SS, Joshi MS. Role of ultrasound in evaluation of peripheral nerves. Indian J Radiol Imaging. 2014;24(3):254-8.
4. Ricci FP, Barbosa RI, Elui VM, et al. Radial nerve injury associated with humeral shaft fracture: a retrospective study. Acta Ortop Bras. 2015;23(1):19-21.
5. Schoch BS, Padegimas EM, Maltenfort M, et al. Humeral shaft fractures: national trends in management. J Orthop Traumatol. 2017;18(3): 259-63.

CHAPTER 88

Periprosthetic Fracture Fixation of Humerus by Dynamic Compression Plate

Shrinivas S Shintre, Chandan V Bhole, Jignesh Yeshwant Tandel

INTRODUCTION

Periprosthetic fractures of humerus arthroplasty are rare and relatively uncommon, with a prevalence of 1–2%. As a result of this, there is limited published literature on such cases, making the management of such cases difficult. However due to the rapidly increasing number of shoulder arthroplasties, periprosthetic fractures after shoulder arthroplasties, which were previously described as rare, might increase in the near future.

Techniques of fixation and management will be different as per patient profile and thus require improved understanding and innovation in their management.

RISK FACTORS AND PREDISPOSING FACTORS

- Nutritional status
- Bone quality
- Systemic diseases
- Steroid medications
- Occupational factors

Advancing age, female sex are some of the predictors of periprosthetic fracture.

CLASSIFICATION

There are quite a few classifications in the literature published about periprosthetic fractures after shoulder arthroplasty.

Wright and Cofield introduced the first classification system, which is discussed below.

The more widely accepted classification is given by Worland et al. in 1999, which accounts for implant stability and also gives treatment options according to the class.

Wright and Cofield Classification of Periprosthetic Fractures

Type	*Fracture location in relation to the stem of the prosthesis*
A	Fracture is centered at the tip of the prosthesis with an extension of more than one-third of the length of the stem
B	Fractures are centered at the tip but extension is less than one-third of the length of the stem
C	Fractures are distal to the tip of the prosthesis with extension in the distal humeral metaphysis

	Fracture angulation and displacement
None	No angulation
Mild	Less than 15° of angulation, or less than one-third displacement of the shaft diameter
Moderate	16–30° of angulation or 1/3–2/3 fracture displacement of the shaft diameter
Severe	More than 30° of angulation, and more than two-thirds displacement of the shaft diameter

Worland Classification of Implant Stability

Classification	*Description*	*Treatment*
Type A	Fracture about tuberosities	Conservative or ORIF
Type B	Fracture around the stem	
Type B1	Spiral fracture, stable stem	Conservative or ORIF
Type B2	Transverse or short oblique fracture, stable stem	Revision with long stem
Type B3	Unstable stem	Revision with long stem
Type C	Fracture well distal to the stem	Conservative or ORIF

CLINICAL EXAMINATION

A careful clinical examination is required to assess neurovascular status, swelling of soft tissue, skin condition at fracture site, mobility at fracture site.

There is high risk of radial nerve injury due to its course around the humerus, resulting in sensorimotor loss due to impingement or compression of the nerve.

Evaluation by radiographs by anteroposterior and lateral projection of humerus will be helpful for proper classification and treatment planning of the fracture.

CLINICAL FEATURES

The present patient is a case of 50-year-old diabetic and hypertensive lady, an operated case of hemiarthroplasty of right shoulder with Neer's prosthesis 2 years back. Now patient presented with a history of fall over the outstretched hand. She had complaints of pain and deformity in the right arm. On clinical examination, patient had weakness of wrist dorsiflexion and sensory loss in radial autonomous zone. Radiographic examination showed right humerus shaft fracture at the level of lower end of Neer's prosthesis (type B by Wright and Coffield classification and type B2 by Worland). Patient was immobilized in U-slab.

PREOPERATIVE PLANNING

Considering the age and activity of the patient before present trauma, it seems patient is a physically less active. Considering porosity of the bone, and level of fracture, fixation of the fracture with 4.5 narrow LC-DCP was planned.

SURGICAL STEPS (FIGS. 1 TO 8)

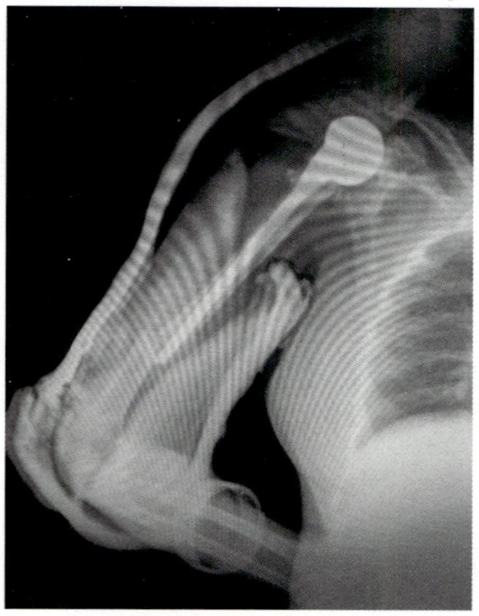

Fig. 1: Preoperative radiograph lateral view.

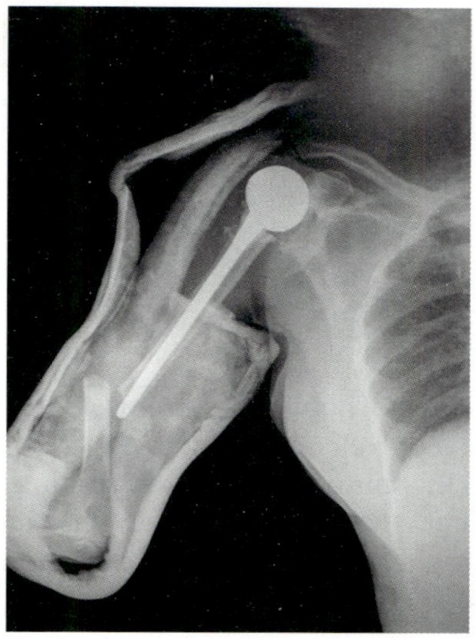

Fig. 2: Preoperative radiograph anteroposterior (AP) view.

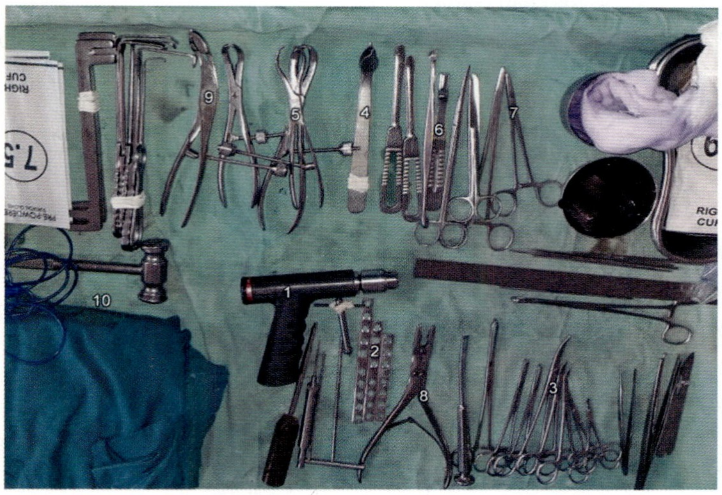

Fig. 3: Sterile instrument trolley as arranged for anterolateral plating for humerus. (1) Drill machine, (2) Humerus DCP plates, (3) Artery forceps, (4) Bone spike, (5) Bone holding forceps, (6) Perisoteum elevator and scoop, (7) Needle holder, (8) Bone nebbler, (9) Plate holding forceps, (10) Hammer, (11) Screw drivers and depth gauge.

Under brachial block, patient was given lateral position. Appropriate aseptic precautions were taken. Painting and draping of the operative area was done.

- Posterior midline skin incision taken after adrenaline infiltration.
- Subcutaneous soft tissue, superficial and deep fascia incised.
- Interval between long and medial head of triceps identified ion proximal part of the incision. Both the muscles were separated from above downward. Long head retracted laterally and medial head retracted medially.
- Short head of triceps visualized through the interval. Radial nerve was found to be tented and attenuated over sharp end of distal fragment. With blunt and gentle dissection, radial nerve isolated outside the operative area.

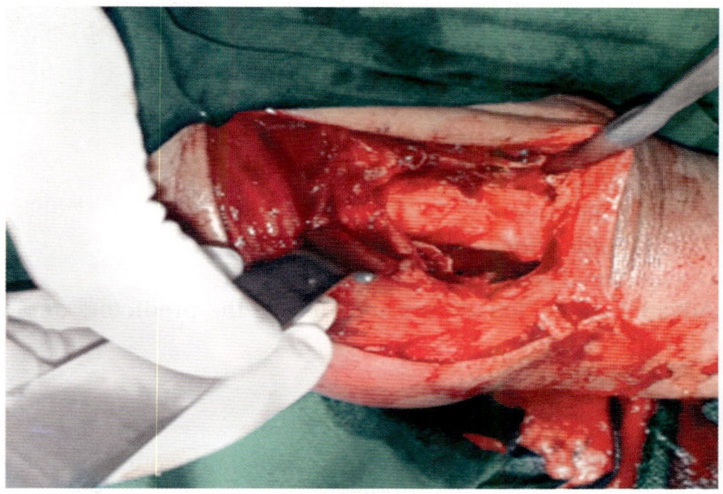

Fig. 4: Short head of triceps visualized.

- After subperiosteal elevation of short head, distal fragment was isolated and ends cleaned.
- Medullary canal of distal fragment was found to be obliterated by sclerotic bony reaction. Medullary canal created with a drill bit.
- Tip of the stem was seen protruding from the end of the proximal fragment. The stem was found to be well fixed.

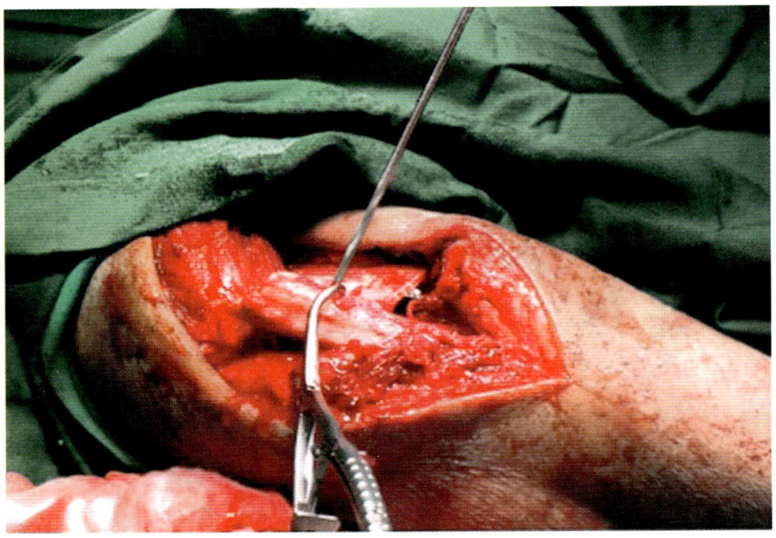

Fig. 5: Tip of the implant seen through the proximal fragment.
- Fracture reduced by holding fragments with bone-holding forceps.
- Prebent 9 hole 4.5 narrow locking DCP applied. Locking screws inserted in distal fragment and cortical screws inserted in proximal fragment, missing the stem of the Neer's prosthesis. Unicortical locking screw/circlage wire is an option for the proximal fragment in difficult situations.

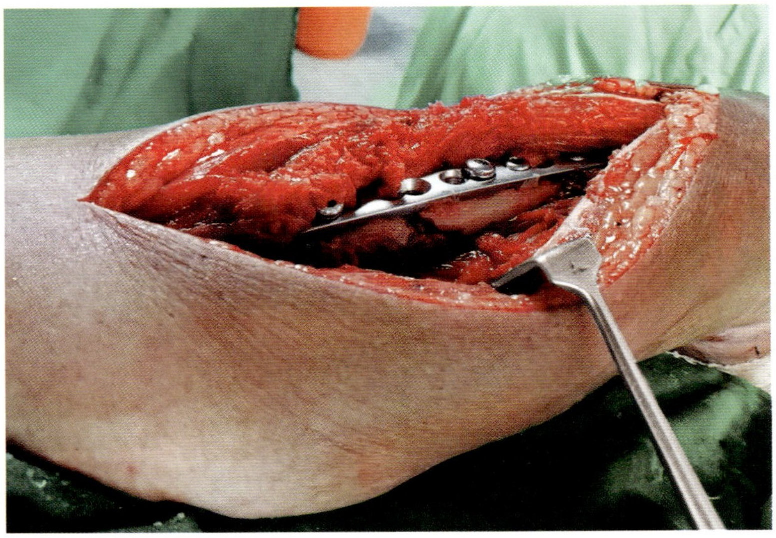

Fig. 6: Reduced fracture with plate in situ.

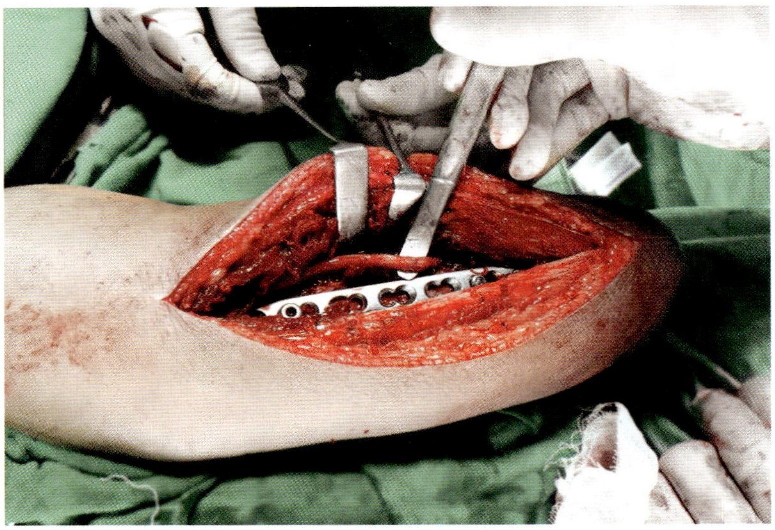

Fig. 7: Attenuated radial nerve freed and isolated away from the fracture.
- Copious wash given with betadine and normal saline.
- Wound closed in layers and sterile dressing done.

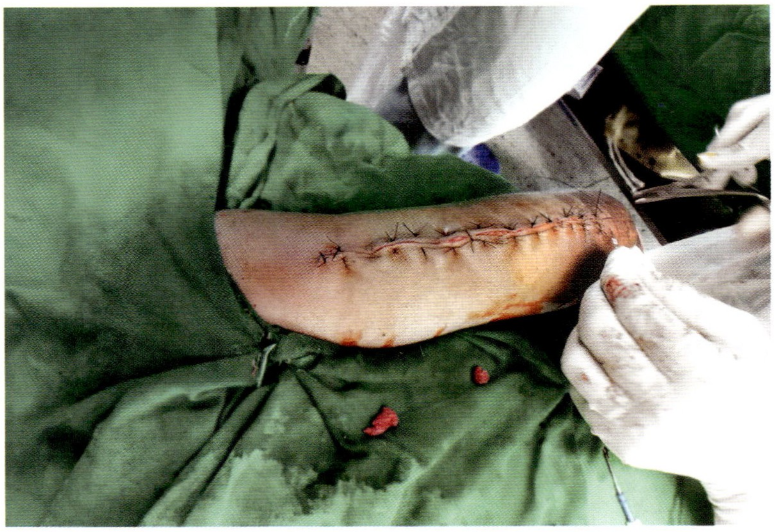

Fig. 8: Postoperative sutured incision.

POSTOPERATIVE MANAGEMENT (FIGS. 9 AND 10)

Postoperatively patient was immobilized in universal shoulder immobilizer. Cock up splint given for wrist drop. Usual postoperative intravenous antibiotics were given for 3 days. On fourth postoperative day, patient was discharged from hospital after wound found satisfactory.

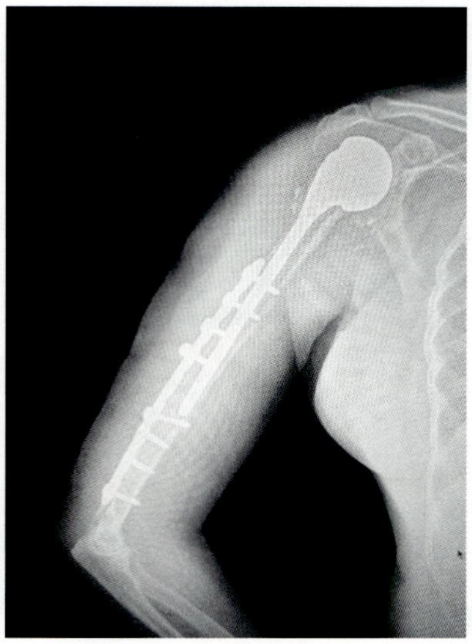

Fig. 9: Postoperative lateral radiograph.

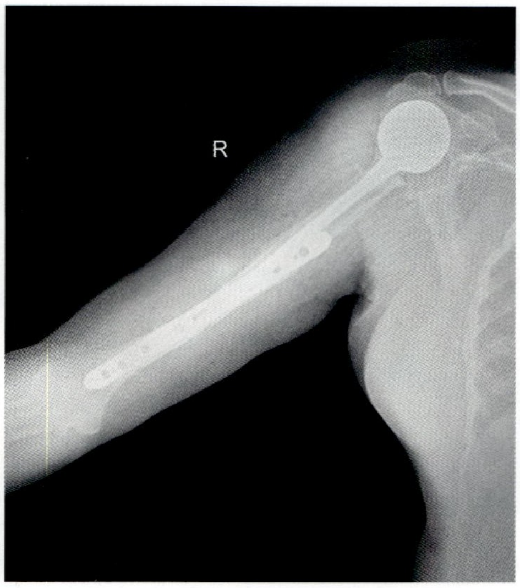

Fig. 10: Postoperative anteroposterior (AP) radiograph.

BIBLIOGRAPHY

1. Am J Orthop. (Belle Mead NJ). 2005;34(12):586-91.
2. Campbell JT,Moore RS, Iannotti JP, Norris TR, Williams GR, et al. J Shoulder Elbow Surg. 1998.
3. Andersen JR, et al. J Bone Joint Surg Am. 2013;95(1):9-18.

CHAPTER 89

Fracture Distal Humerus in Adults (Supracondylar-Intercondylar)

Vijay M Panchanadikar, Ajinkya Nitin Deshpande

INTRODUCTION

Distal humeral fractures in adults are technically challenging injuries to manage as most of them are complex. Nearly all of these cases require surgical intervention. Surgery is technically demanding due to inadequate exposure, comminuted fracture or osteoporotic bones. Incidence of these fractures in adults has shown an increasing trend in recent times. Incidence of these fractures in elderly is recently on the rise and these osteoporotic fractures should be fixed with locking plates. In addition to fracture fixation, management of osteoporosis plays a pivotal role for treating these injuries.

PATHOANATOMY AND CLASSIFICATION

The anatomy of the distal end of humerus is such that it consists of two columns viz medial and lateral column which together give support to the articular surface. Capitellum forms the distal end of lateral column which articulates with radial head and medial epicondyle forms distal end of medial column. Trochlea is situated between these two structures which articulates with the ulna. This articulating surface functions as the tie arch (Fig. 1). Distal humeral fractures involve the supracondylar region of the humerus and the articular surface of the distal part of the humerus.

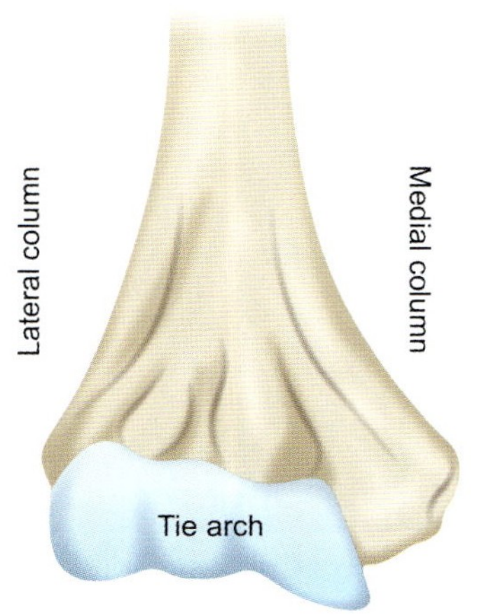

Fig. 1: Anatomy of distal humerus.

Distal humerus fractures are most commonly classified according to the Orthopaedic Trauma Association/Arbeitsgemeinschaft für Osteosynthesefragen (OTA/AO) classification system. Here "A" stands for an extra-articular fracture, "B" stands for a partial articular fracture, and "C" stands for complete articular fracture. These are further divided into 1, 2, and 3 to indicate the degrees of comminution (Fig. 2).

CLINICAL FEATURES

The patient presents with pain, swelling, contusion, tenderness, and limitation of elbow movements. One should actively look for brachial artery or nerve injury.

RADIOLOGICAL IMAGING

Standard anteroposterior and lateral views of the elbow joint are obtained in order to decide about further management. Computed tomography (CT) scan with 3D reconstruction of the elbow joint will greatly help in classifying the fracture and plan the surgical management accordingly.

TREATMENT OPTIONS

Conservative Option

The elbow joint is to be mobilized early on to avoid stiffening. However secondary displacement can occur if the joint is mobilized early because of the axial loads acting on the joint. So, conservative option in form of immobilization is advised only in undisplaced fractures or in elderly individuals not fit for surgery.

Surgical Option

Preferred modality of treatment in these fractures is surgical management is in the form of internal fixation. Arthroplasty may be performed

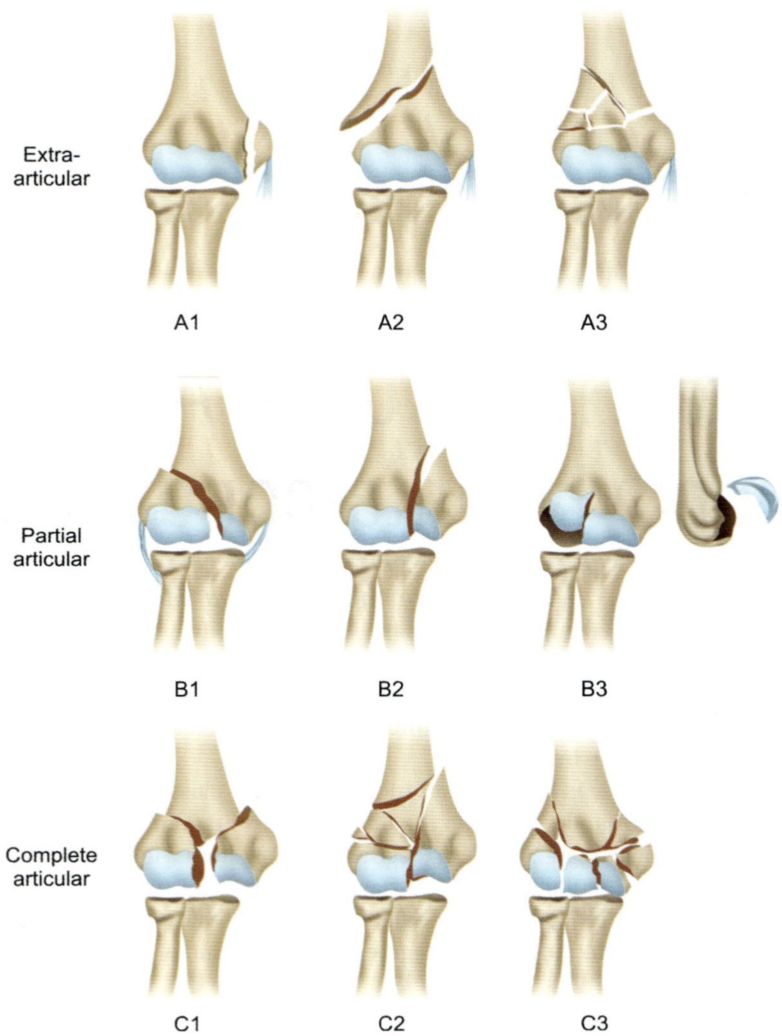

Fig. 2: Orthopaedic Trauma Association/Arbeitsgemeinschaft für Osteosynthesefragen (OTA/AO) classification of distal humerus fractures.

in select elderly with severely comminuted fractures. Main aim of internal fixation is to achieve stable accurate articular reduction to enable early postoperative mobilization of the elbow joint so as to prevent stiffening.

POTENTIAL COMPLICATIONS

The potential complications associated with these fractures include elbow stiffness, malunion, nonunion, heterotopic ossification, nerve palsies, and brachial artery injuries.

SURGICAL PROCEDURES

The most commonly used technique for internal fixation is the dual plate fixation. Anatomical articular surface reduction and rigid fixation is the basic principle that is to be followed while treating these fractures. Accurate articular reduction is the first important step that is to be achieved. One interfragmentary screw (CCS) is needed most often to stabilize the intra-articular component that creates a distal block. After achieving the articular reduction, the metaphyseal reduction should be achieved. For this plates are fixed on medial and lateral column in parallel or 90-90 configuration. Nowadays, distal humerus anatomical locking plates are available. Care should be taken to reconstruct the olecranon fossa adequately so as to avoid restriction of full extension postoperatively.

Various approaches for distal humerus are: paratricipital approach, triceps splitting approach, triceps reflecting (Bryan–Morrey), triceps reflecting anconeus pedicle (TRAP), olecranon osteotomy technique. Olecranon osteotomy approach provides better exposure and may be preferred in complex intra-articular fractures although it adds to the complexity of procedure.

Here, we are describing the triceps splitting approach. The structure which is at risk during this procedure is the ulnar nerve which is situated medially.

SURGICAL STEPS (FIGS. 3 TO 28)

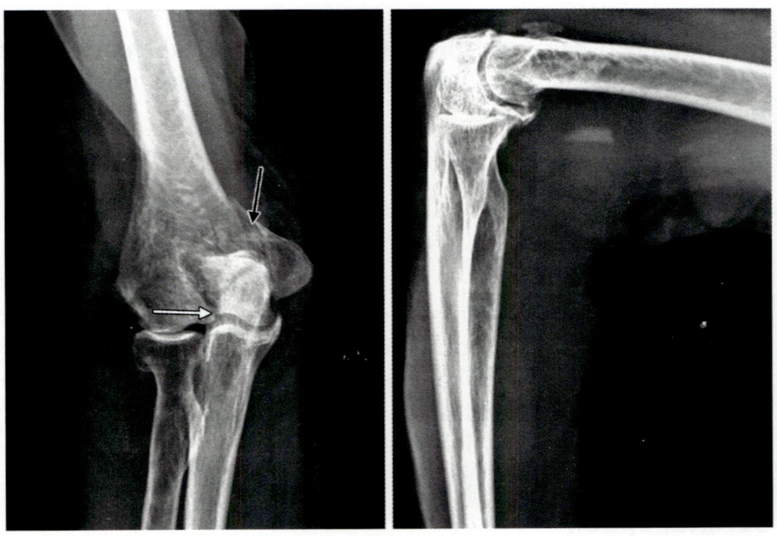

Fig 3: X-ray elbow AP and lateral views showing displaced medial condyle fracture of distal humerus (Black arrow) with intercondylar extension and articular step (White arrow).

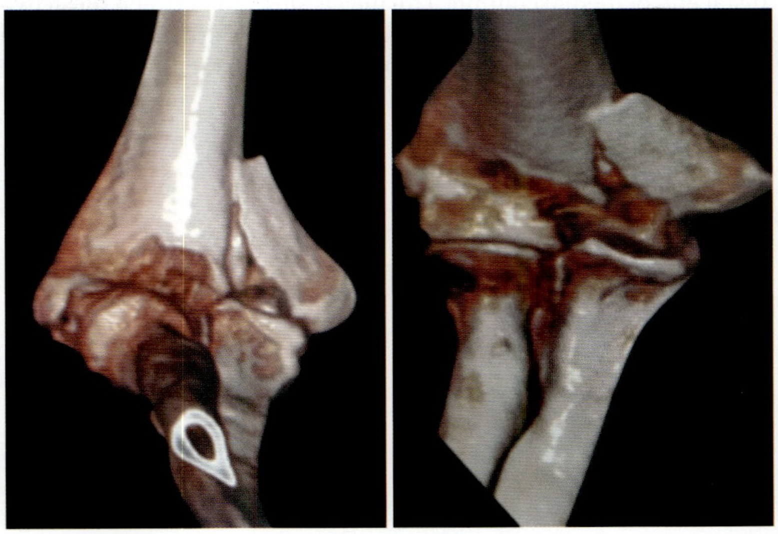

Fig. 4: 3D-CT reconstruction of elbow joint (preoperative) showing the exact fracture pattern. Fracture involves lateral pillar also.

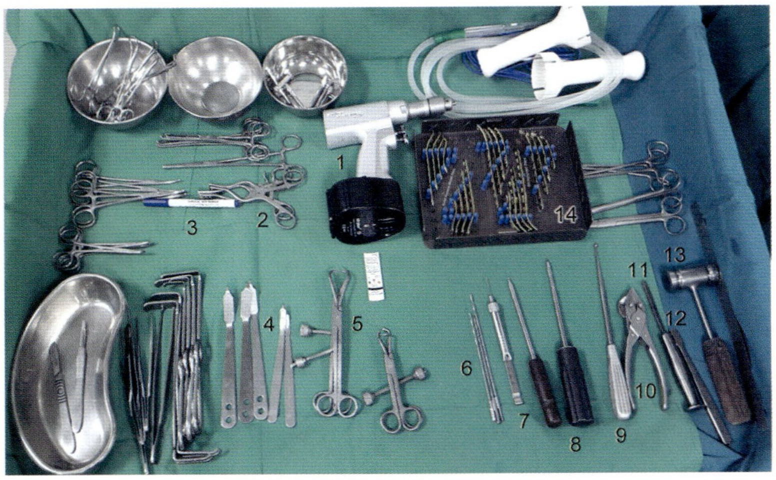

Fig. 5: Instruments. (1) Drill machine, (2) Self retaining retractors, (3) Surgical skin marker, (4) Bone levers(spikes), (5) Pointed reduction clamps, (6) Drill bits, (7) Depth gauge, (8) Screw drivers including torque limiting screw driver, (9) Bone curette, (10) Plier with side cutter, (11) Osteotome, (12) Bone punch, (13) Hammer, (14) Medial column and lateral column humerus locking plates.

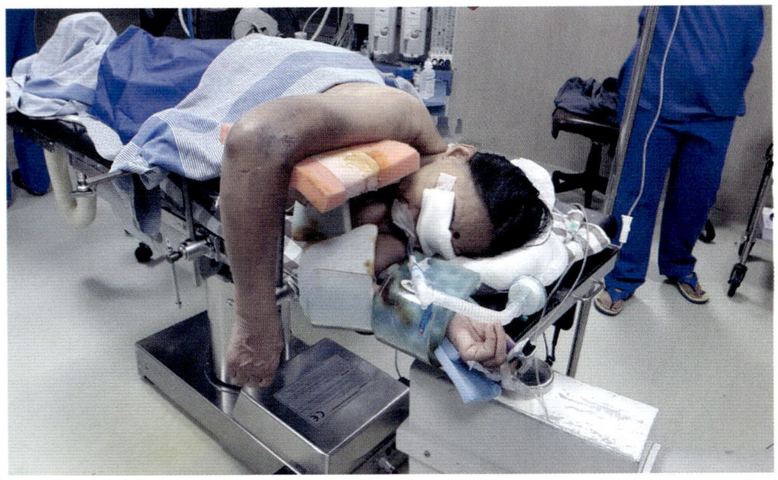

Fig 6: Position under regional block/general anesthesia, lateral decubitus position on operating table with arm on a radiolucent support with adequate padding.

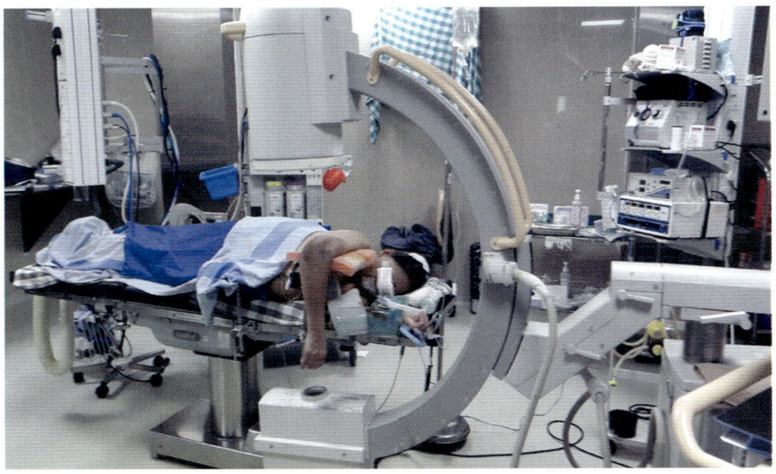

Fig 7: C-arm position: C-arm to be brought in from the head end of the table, ensuring that fracture is visualized in both C-arm views.

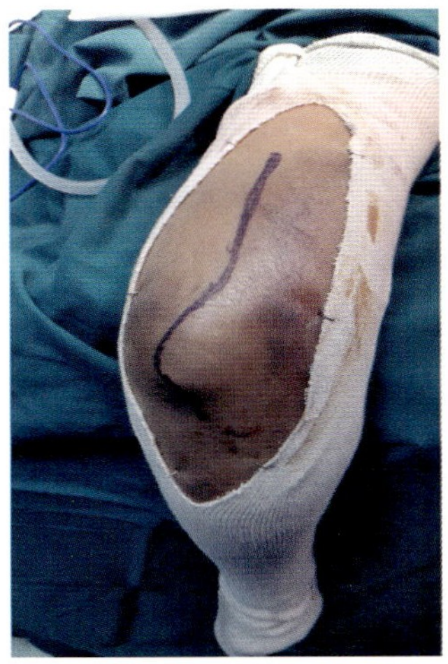

Fig. 8: Draping: Whole upper limb prepared and draped. Incision marked. Skin incision-straight incision beginning level with the junction of middle and distal third, centered on humeral shaft and curving around olecranon to ulnar side to end over the ulnar diaphysis.

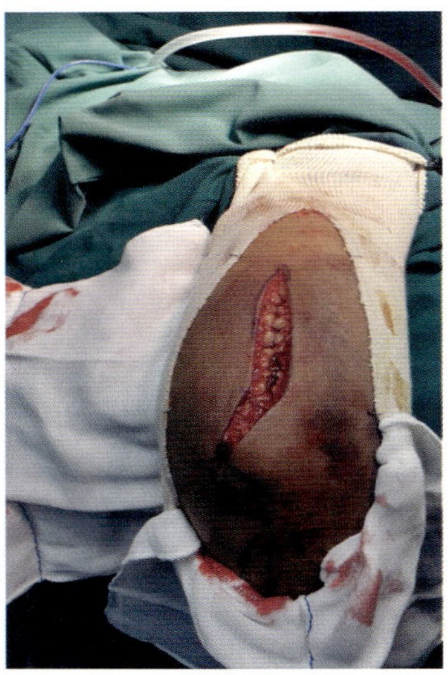

Fig 9: Skin incision with 22 number blade and subcutaneous dissection with 15 number blade.

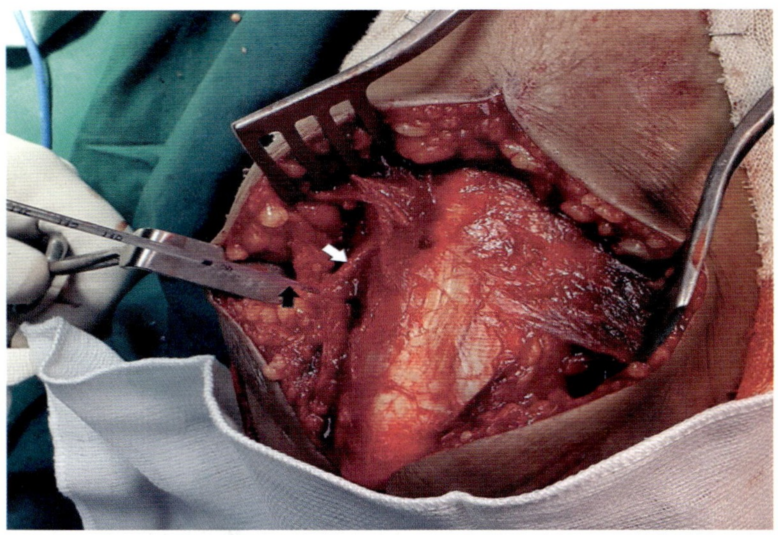

Fig. 10: Ulnar nerve dissection along the medial aspect of triceps. Ulnar nerve (White arrow). Infant feeding tube (Black arrow). Care to be taken to prevent accidental stretch to Infant feeding tube. May use soft rubber catheter. Ulnar nerve to be protected for all subsequent operative steps.

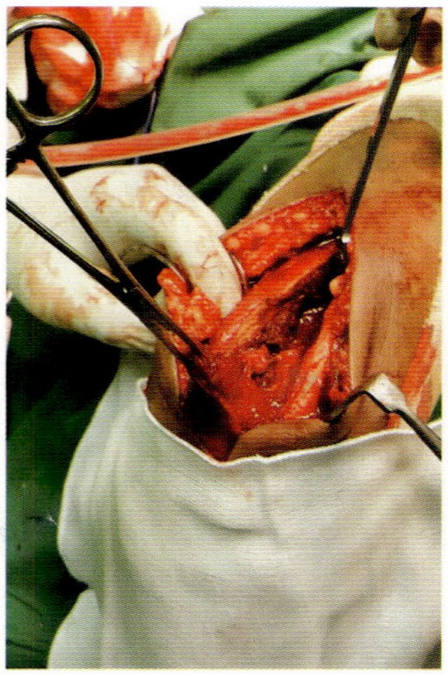

Fig 11: Triceps split (with distal V-Y) approach incision through the distal triceps muscle tendon junction in inverted V shape and split proximally in order to reach the distal humerus.

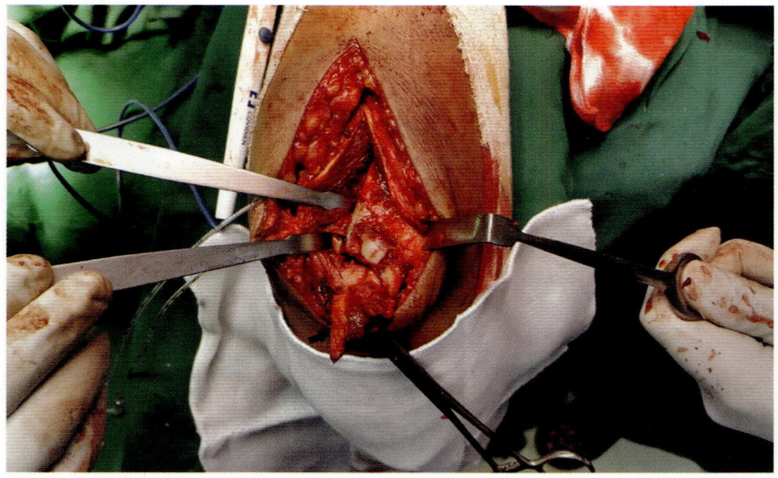

Fig 12: Exposed fracture site. The triceps insertion over olecranon kept intact.

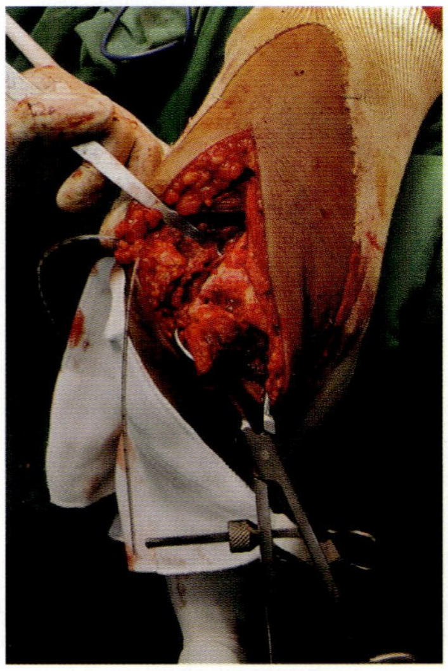

Fig. 13: The articular fragments reduced with the help of pointed reduction clamp. May perform "inside out technique of K-wire insertion" and "joystick maneuvre" instead.

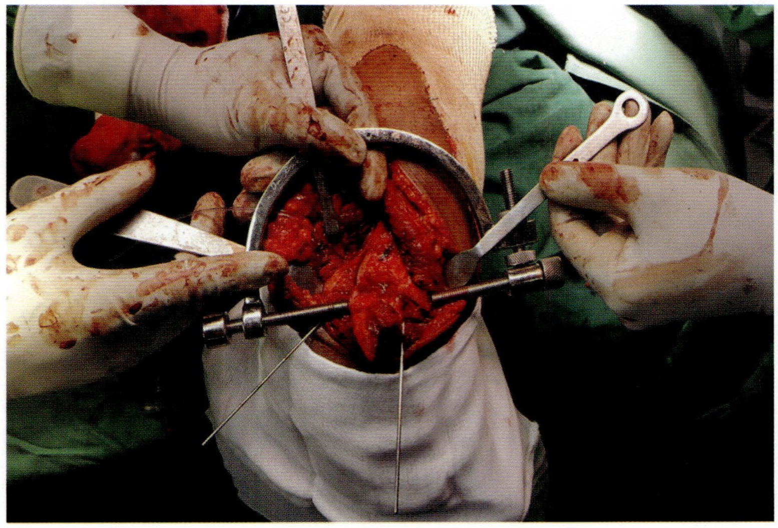

Fig 14: Reduced fracture fragments held in position with the help of K-wires.

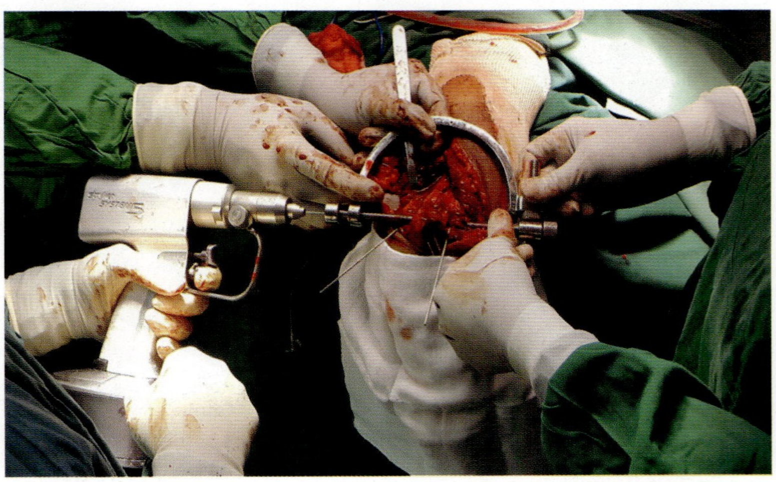

Fig. 15: Inserting the guidewire for cannulated intercondylar cancellous screw using the aiming device. Need to protect ulnar nerve.

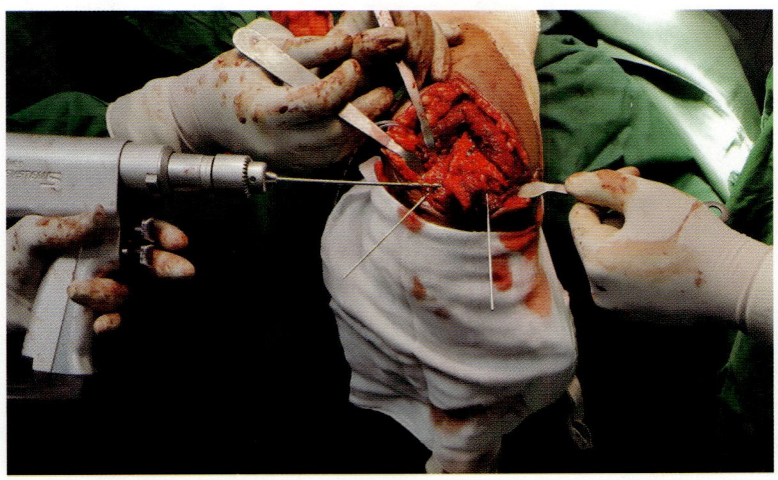

Fig 16: Drilling with cannulated drill bit over the guidewire.

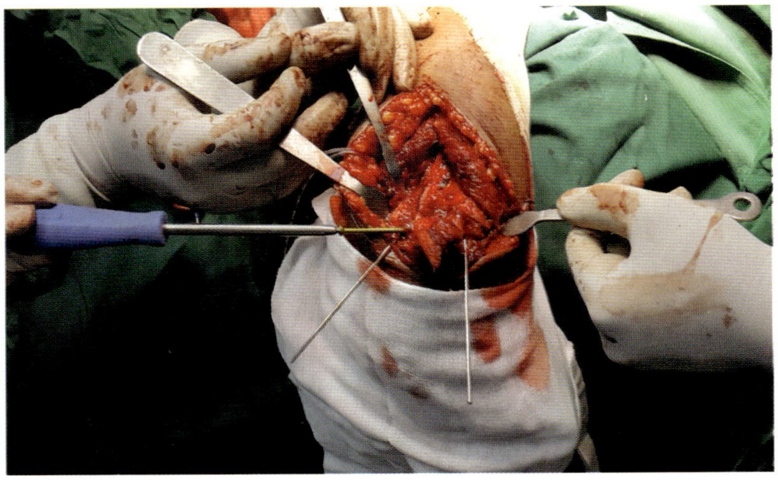

Fig 17: Partially threaded cannulated cancellous screw insertion over the guidewire to fix the articular fragments. Partially threaded screw used as an interfragmentary screw in order to achieve compression at the fracture site. Fully threaded preferred as position screw in case of comminution. Use the cannulated screwdriver.

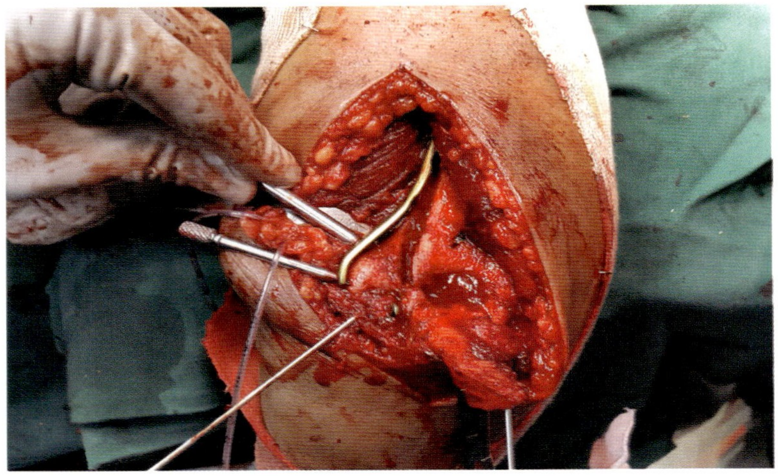

Fig. 18: Medial column distal humerus locking plate placed along the medial column and medial border with locking drill sleeves in place. Ensure that there is no gap between distal end of plate and bone.

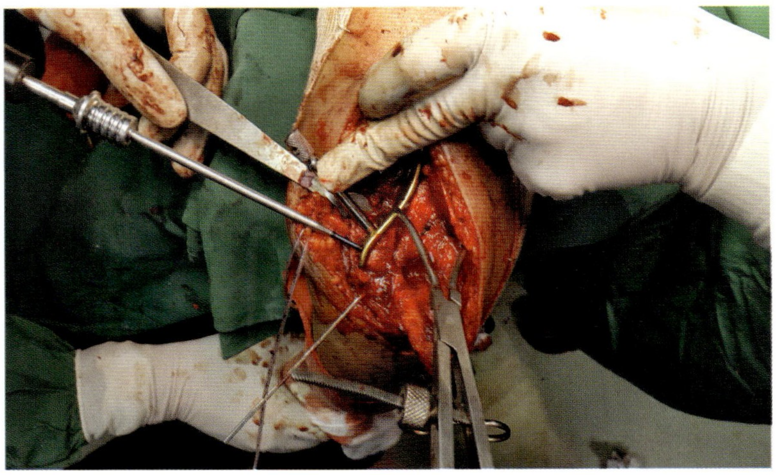

Fig. 19: Reduction of the medial column held in reduced position with help of pointed reduction clamp. Passing distal locking screw through the plate with help of torque limiting screwdriver. This step fixes the distal position of plate. Then first proximal screw is passed and tightened preferably cortex screw. This ensures that there is no gap between plate and bone and plate is not off bone proximally. Other locking screws are added.

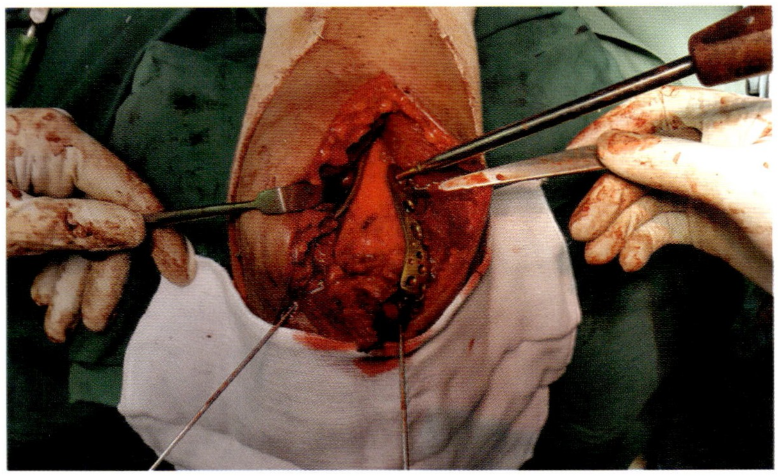

Fig. 20: Lateral column distal humerus locking plate placed over the dorsal surface of the lateral column in order to achieve the biplanar (orthogonal or 90-90) fixation. Spike retractors to be used gently at proximal corner to avoid radial nerve compression. Passing cortical screw with normal screwdriver. Parallel placement of plates is an option.

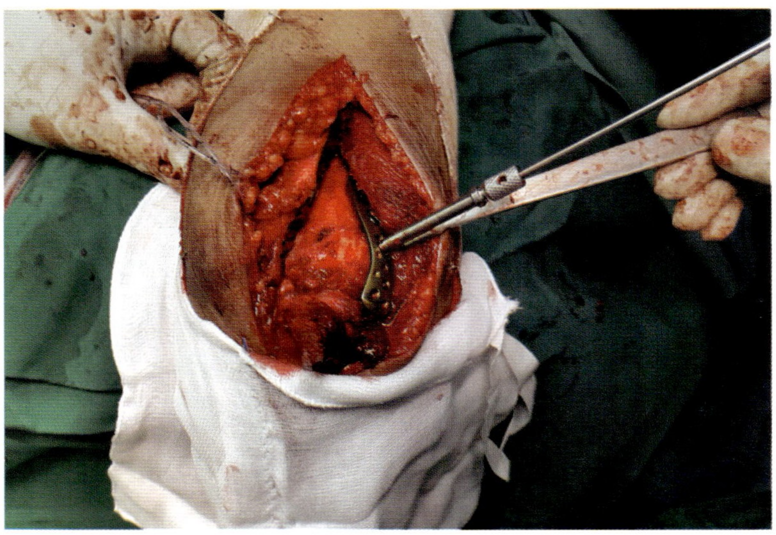

Fig. 21: Drilling for locking screw through the locking drill sleeve.

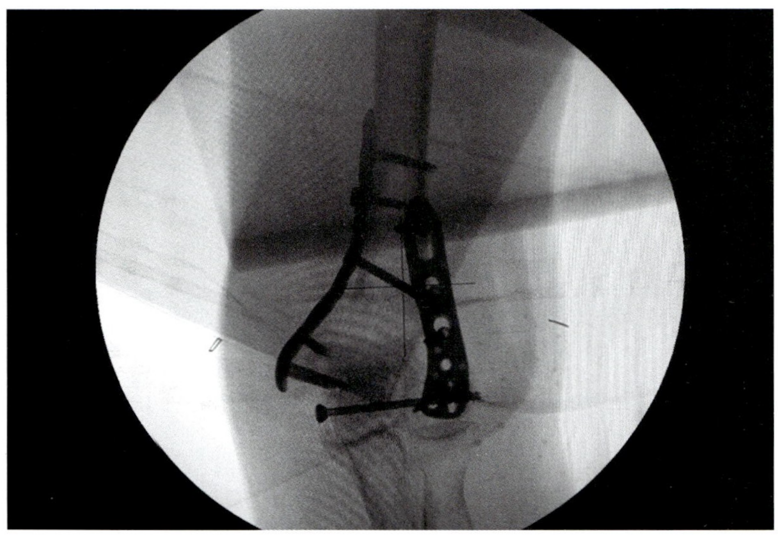

Fig. 22: Final C-arm image in AP view of biplanar fixation.

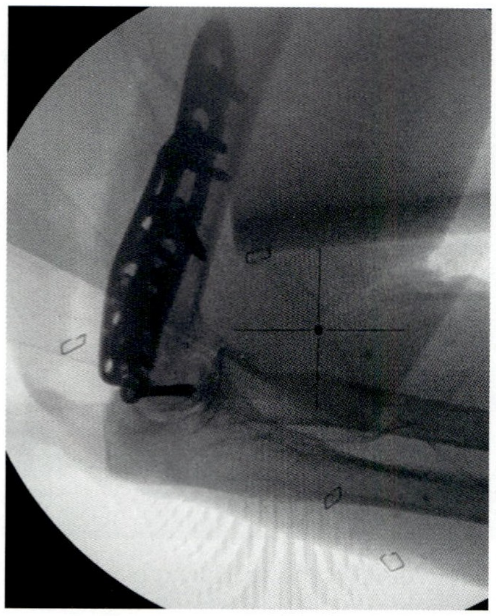

Fig 23: Final C-arm image in lateral view of biplanar fixation.

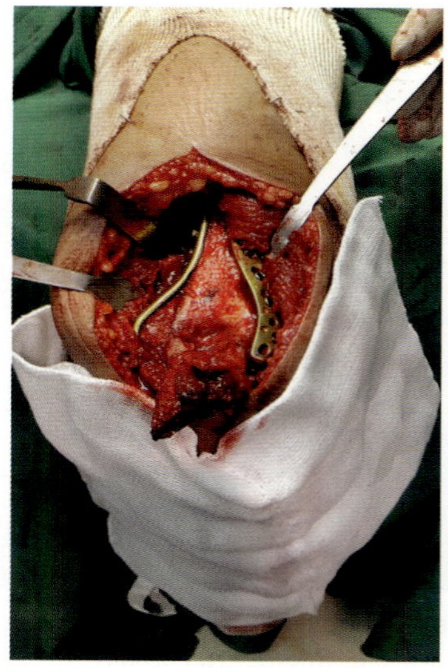

Fig 24: Final intraoperative image of biplanar fixation with reduced fracture fragments.

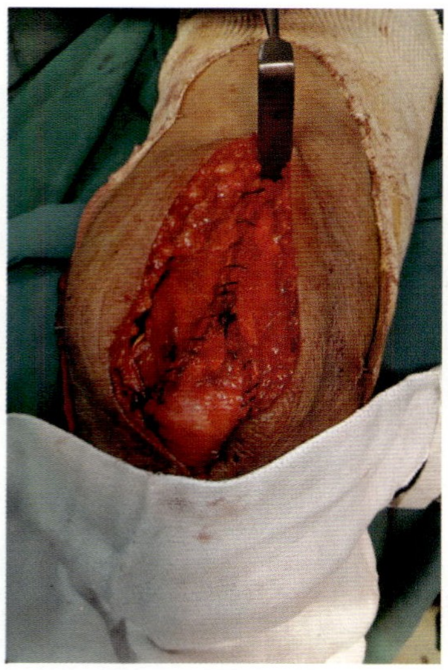

Fig 25: Hemostasis, wash and closure of the triceps.

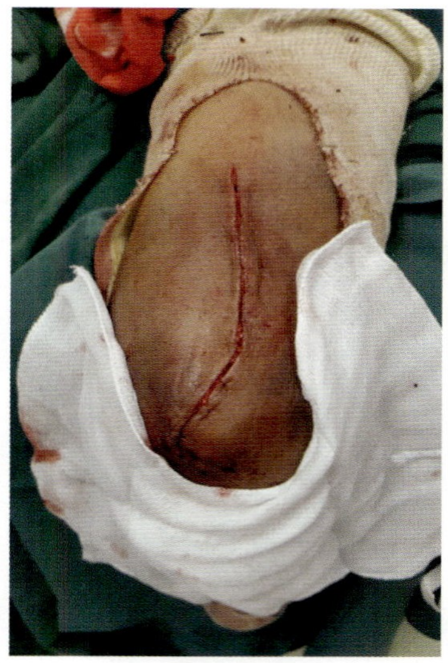

Fig 26: Subcutaneous layer closure with inverted interrupted sutures using 2-0 absorbable suture material.

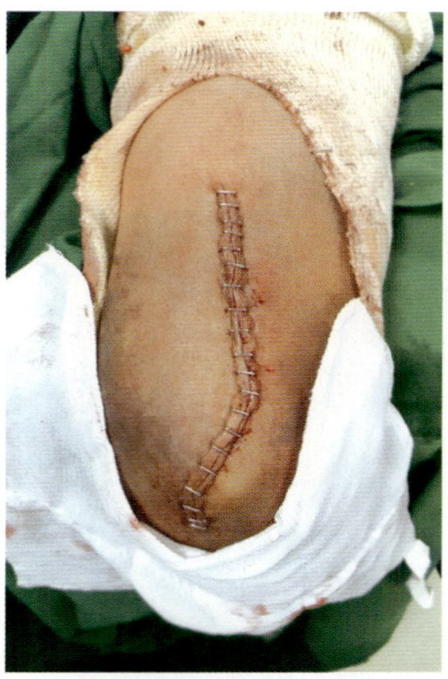

Fig 27: Skin closure with surgical staples.

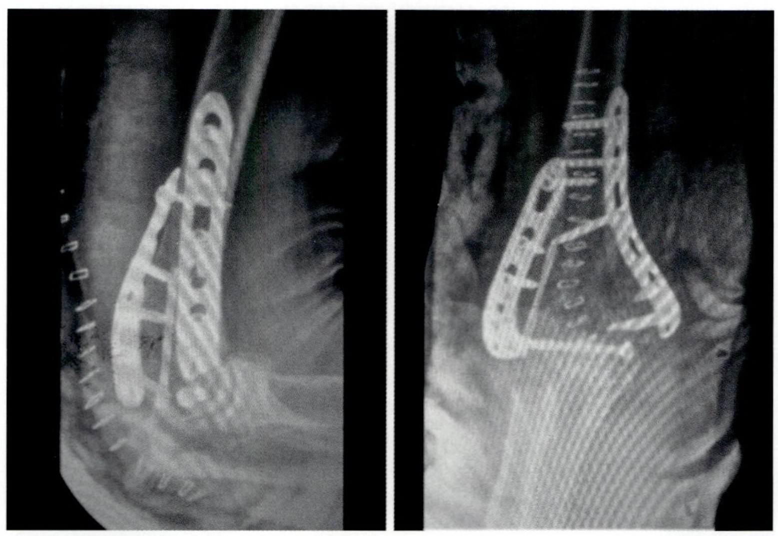

Fig. 28: Postoperative X-ray of elbow joint in AP and lateral views showing reduced fracture with biplanar fixation and articular surface fixation with interfragmentary screw.

SUGGESTED READING

1. Bégué T. Articular fractures of the distal humerus. Orthop Traumatol Surg Res. 2014;100(1):S55-63.
2. Nauth A, McKee MD, Ristevski B, et al. Distal humeral fractures in adults. JBJS. 2011;93(7):686-700.

CHAPTER 90

Fracture Neck Radius: Fixation with Mini-Fragment T-plate

Kartikeya Promod Joshi, Nishant Goyal, Ranjit Rajure

INTRODUCTION

Radial head and neck fractures account for 75% of the fractures of the forearm. Radial head fractures incidence is twice as common as compared to radial neck fractures. These fractures occur due to fall on the outstretched hand with elbow in pronation and partial flexion.

FRACTURES OF HEAD OF RADIUS

Radial head fractures account for one-third of all fractures of the elbow in adult population. According to gender distribution, there is no significant difference. The fracture incidence in men peaked at 3rd decade with high-energy traumas, whereas simple falls were dominant in women of postmenopausal age group.

The intricate anatomy of elbow joint is formed by humeroulnar, humeroradial, and proximal radioulnar joint (PRUJ). The stability of the elbow joint relies on both soft-tissue stabilizer (muscles and ligaments) and the bony articulations. Of the three separate articulations, the radial head influences all the biomechanics and contributes to elbow's functionality. The lateral aspect of the elbow joint is formed by radiocapitellar joint. The stability of radiocapillar joint is due to opposite congruity of the hemispherical shaped capitellum with the concave radial head. The lateral collateral ligament, prevents varus angulation and posterolateral rotatory instability. The radiocapitellar articulation is important to maintain both valgus and longitudinal stability of elbow and forearm. The radial head prevents the proximal progression of radius in axial loading of the forearm. At the elbow, approximately 60% of the mechanical load goes through the radial column. Loss of the radial head shifts 100% of the loading onto the ulnar column.

Mechanism of Injury

Three mechanisms leading to radial head fracture are:

1. A valgus force over extended elbow causing impaction of head with capitellum and which may be associated with injury to medial collateral ligament
2. Posterolateral rotatory force
3. Axial forearm loads may be associated with more complex Essex-Lopresti injury.

Signs and Symptoms

- Pain and swelling around the lateral side of the elbow
- Ecchymosis is a late feature
- Tenderness over radial head
- Pain is experienced more while forearm rotations and may be associated with the clicking sound
- Limitation of forearm rotations
- One must examine shoulder and wrist for associated injuries.

Classification of Radial Head Fracture

The original classification system described by Mason distinguished according to the displacement of radial head fracture.

Modified Mason classification:

- *Type 1*: Marginal undisplaced fracture
- *Type 2*: Marginal displaced fracture
- *Type 3*: Comminuted and displaced fracture with complete radial head involvement.

Broberg and Morrey attempted to quantify the extent of the radial head involvement and concomitant radial neck fracture.

Broberg and Morrey modification of Mason classification:

- *Type 1*: Undisplaced fracture or displacement less than 2 mm involving less than 30% for the head articulation
- *Type 2*: Displacement more than 2 mm with head greater than 30% head involvement
- *Type 3*: Comminuted fracture of radial head
- *Type 4*: Fracture of radial head associated with elbow dislocation.

Mason classification system modified by Johnston, which includes associated elbow dislocation with variety of complex fracture dislocation patterns about elbow and forearm.

Rineer classification (based on the detail whether there was cortical contact between the fragments, or not):

- *Cortical contact between fragments:* Stable
- *No cortical contact between fragments:* Unstable.

FRACTURE OF RADIUS NECK

Radial neck fractures are relatively uncommon in adults compared to children. In adults there is no separate classification system described, hence they are generally grouped along with radial head fractures. Radial neck fractures account for slightly more than 1% of all fractures in children and they represent about 5–10% of elbow injuries. The management of these type of fractures is a controversial topic which is generally guided by the degree of displacement and angulation. Undisplaced fractures can be managed by nonoperative treatment and displaced fractures need surgical fixation. There is no remodeling potential in adults as in pediatric population, hence significant displacement and angulation of radial neck fractures not acceptable. Open reduction internal fixation (ORIF) with plates and screws is advised for displaced fractures, but the procedure carries the risk of devascularization and avascular necrosis of the radial head.

Mechanism of Injury

- Fall on outstretched hand with elbow extended with valgus force.
- These fractures are also associated with elbow dislocation while injury can occur during the reduction of the dislocations. The direction of the angular deformity depends upon the position of the forearm rotation at the time of the injury.

Signs and Symptoms of the Radial Neck Fracture

- Pain over elbow may or may not be associated with the swelling
- Typical tenderness is over radial head
- Restricted forearm rotations mainly pronation, elbow flexion and extension are occasionally restricted
- Bruising is the late sign, seen over the lateral aspect of the elbow
- Referred pain over the wrist
- Posterior interosseous nerve (PIN) must be examined as it may be injured during radial neck fracture.

Classification

The Judet classification describes four types of fracture, depending on the displacement of the radial head.

Judet classification of the radial neck fracture:

1. *Type 1*: Undisplaced
2. *Type 2*: Angulation is less than 30°
3. *Type 3*: Angulation is between 30° and 60°
4. *Type 4*:
    - *Type 4a*: Angulation is between 60° and 80°
    - *Type 4b*: Angulation is more than 80°

Imaging for Radial Head and Neck Fractures

- Standard anteroposterior (AP) and lateral view of the elbow
- Anteroposterior and lateral view of the contralateral elbow for the comparison in pediatric age group
- An oblique view known as radiocapitellar view suggested by Greenspan and Hallcraig X-ray view, where the center of the X-ray beam is directed 45° to separate the proximal radius and the ulna.
- Magnetic resonance imaging (MRI), ultrasonography (USG), and arthrogram may be helpful in case of occult injuries.

TREATMENT GUIDELINES

Stable, Undisplaced Fractures and Isolated, Stable Partial Articular Fractures

The undisplaced and stable or minimally displaced partial articular fractures of the radial head are treated nonoperatively.

Unstable Partial Articular Fractures

These may be treated by ORIF or partial or complete excision of head. To restore the stability in case of ligamentous disruption, soft tissue repair is indicated along with ORIF.

Complete Articular Fracture (Mason Type 3)

Open reduction and internal fixation is indicated in a young patient with a complete multifragmentary articular injury. Every attempt should be made to salvage the native radial head, if a stable fixation can be achieved. In the case of a highly comminuted fracture in which stable fixation cannot be achieved, prosthetic replacement is preferred.

Acute radial head excision is not preferred for fear of aggravating an unrecognized elbow instability. Superior results are obtained by open reduction internal fixation as compared to radial head excision.

Radial Head and Neck Fractures associated with Complex Elbow and Forearm Injuries

Unstable, displaced Mason type 2 and 3 fractures of the radial head and neck are associated with complex fracture dislocation patterns about the elbow and forearm. These fracture patterns include spectrum of posterolateral instability, valgus injuries of elbow, posterior transolecranon fracture dislocation, Monteggia variant (Bado type 2), and Essex-Lopresti lesion. These are better managed by ORIF or radial head arthroplasty and soft tissue repairs. One has to be careful as there can be early or late failures seen after suboptimal fixation.

SURGICAL STEPS (FIGS. 1 TO 24)

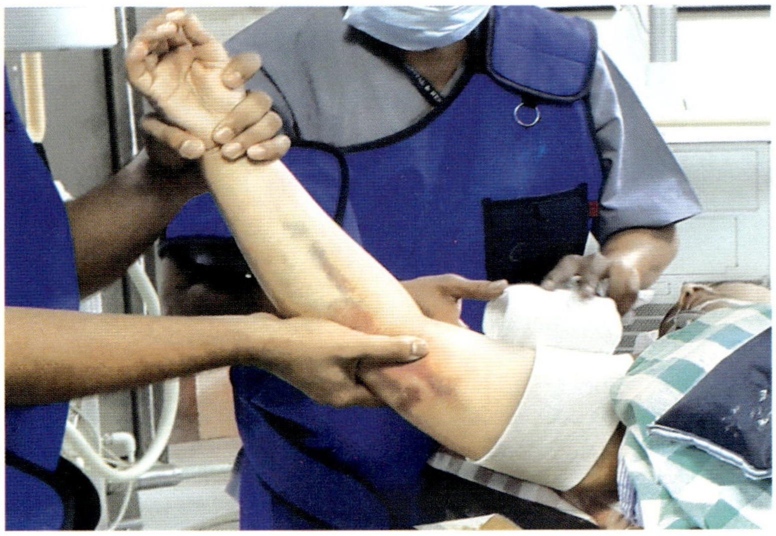

Fig. 1: Tourniquet application.

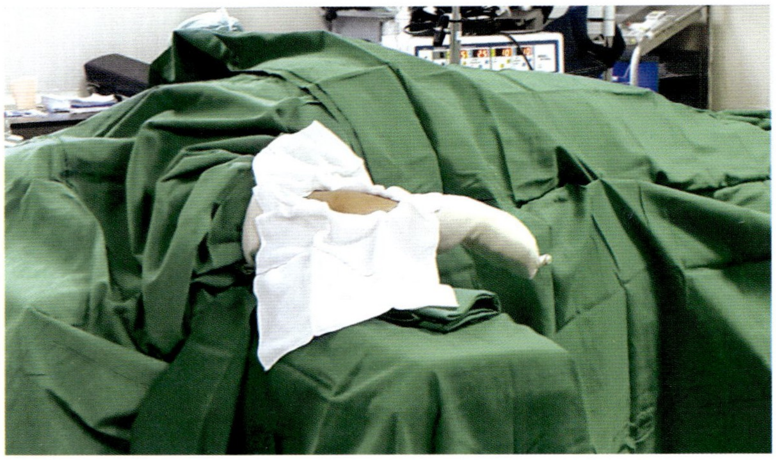

Fig. 2: *Positioning of the operative limb*: Supine position on a standard operating table with right upper limb supported on radiolucent hand table. C-arm perpendicular to the operating table in line with the affected extremity.

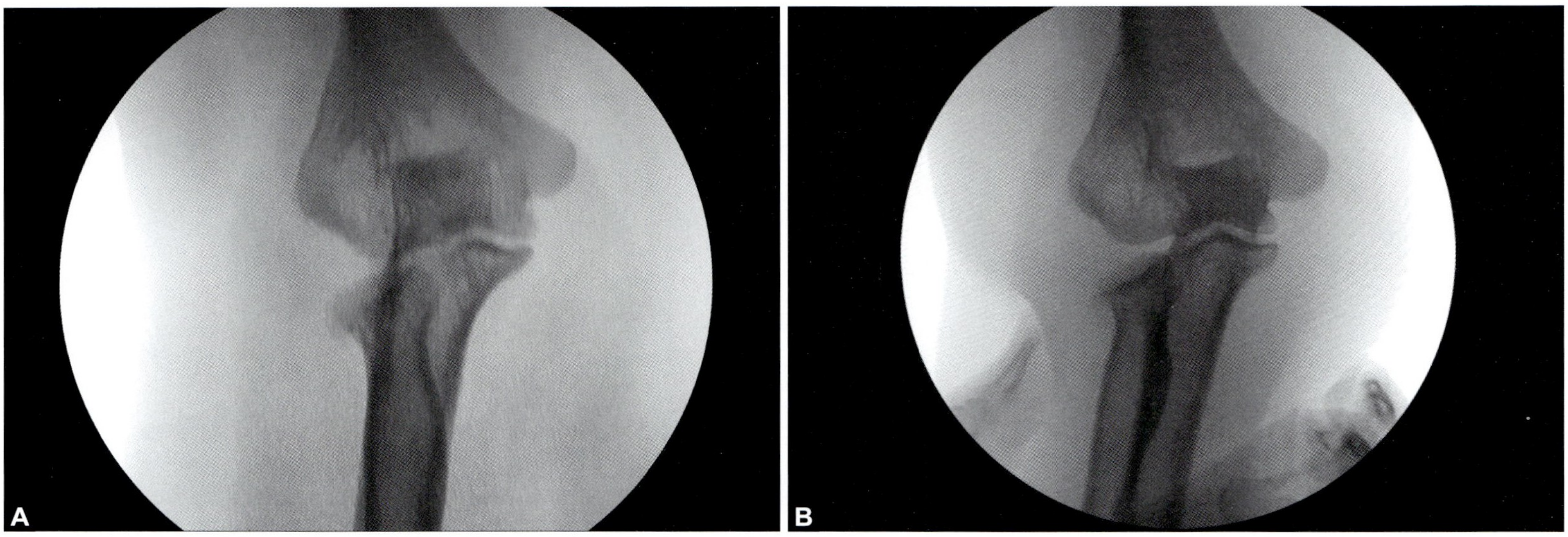

Figs. 3A and B: (A) Image intensifier television (IITV) images: (A) Radial fracture position in pronated position; (B) Valgus stress anteroposterior (AP) view.

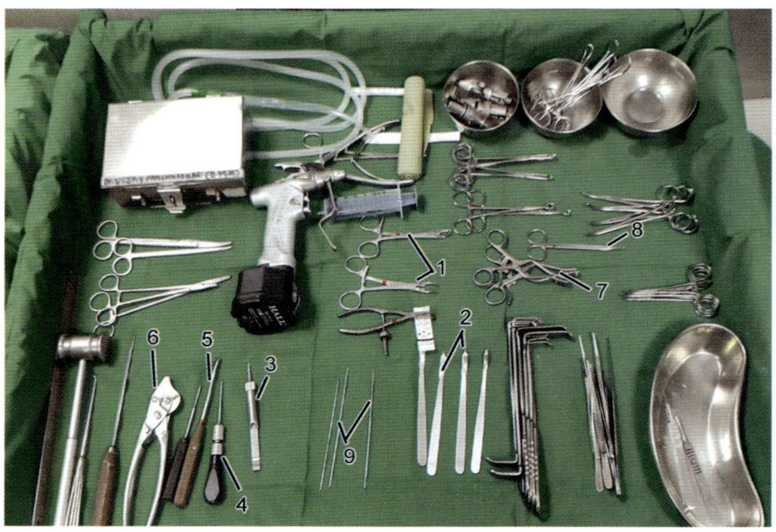

Fig. 4: Image showing required inventory. Mini-fragment plates (low profile) with 2–2.7 mm screws required. (1) Reduction forceps; (2) Small sized bone lever; (3) Depth gauge; (4) Hexagonal screwdriver; (5) Periosteal elevator; (6) Plier; (7) Mastoid retractor; (8) Dissecting scissor; (9) K-wires.

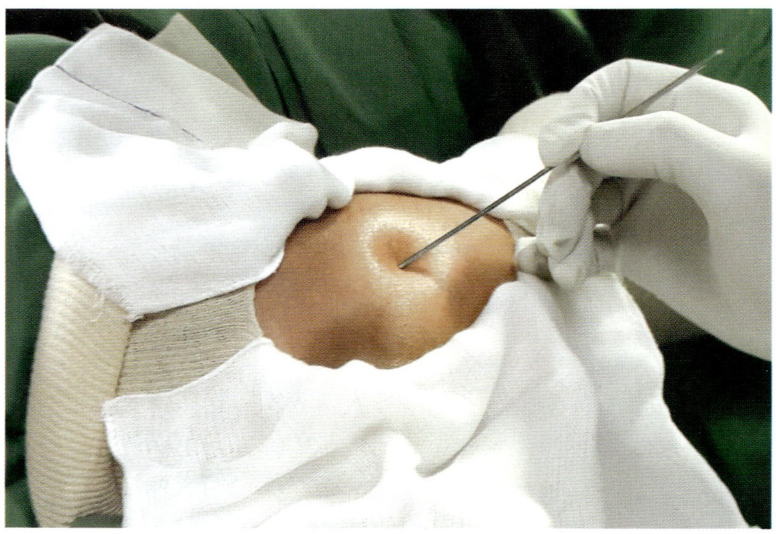

Fig. 5: Attempted closed reduction with K-wire.

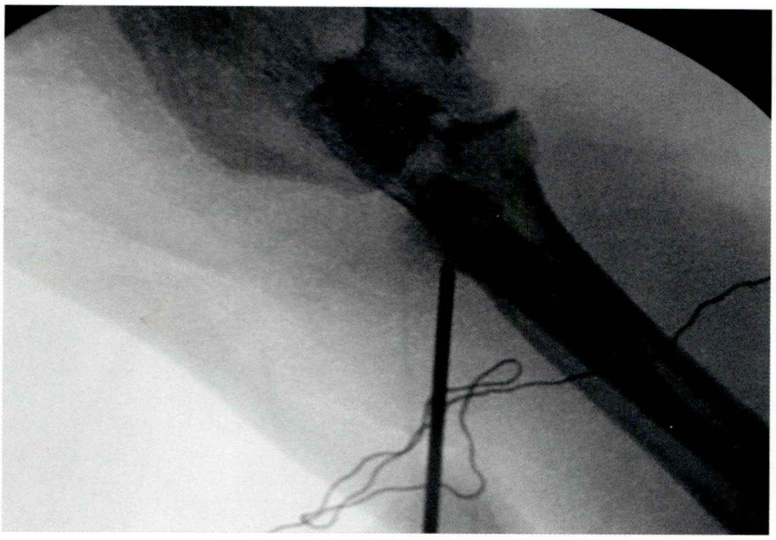

Fig. 6: Image intensifier television (IITV) confirmation of attempted closed reduction by disengaging the fracture site. Decision taken to proceed with open reduction and internal fixation. Head may have to be excised in cases of severe comminution, which cannot be reconstructed.

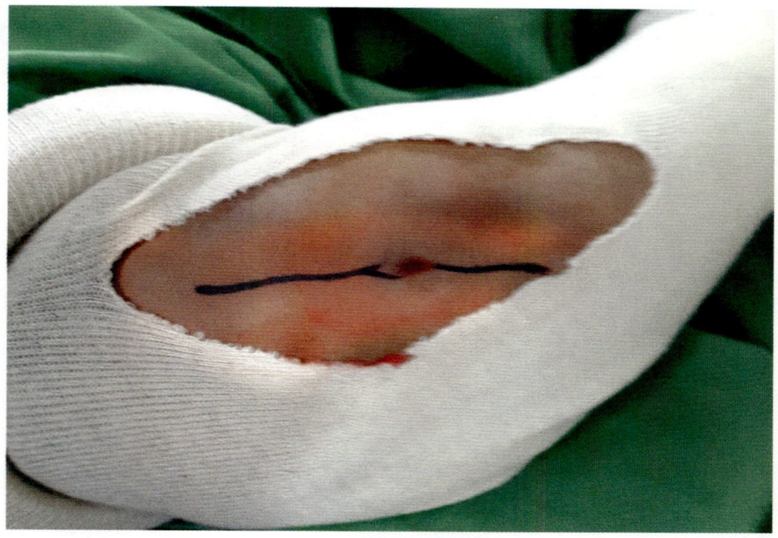

Fig. 7: Skin marking done for Kocher approach. Landmarks identified—lateral ridge of distal humerus, lateral epicondyle, and radial head (sometimes it is difficult to identify bony landmarks in cases of severe swelling).

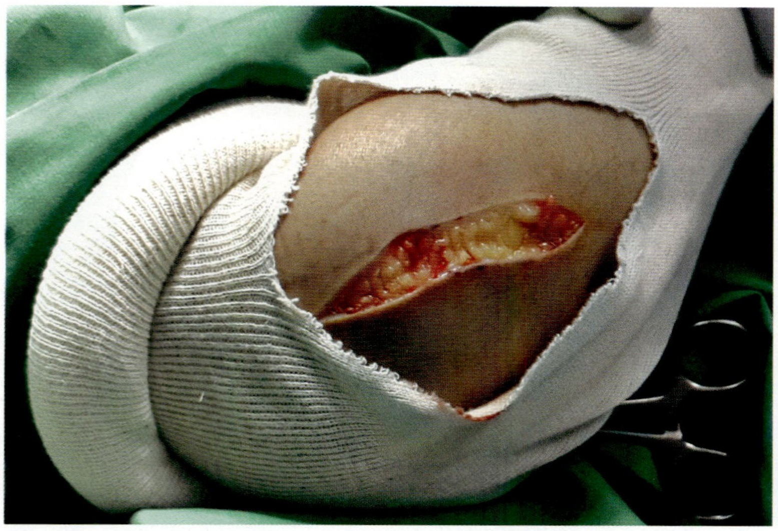

Fig. 8: Skin and subcutaneous tissue dissected.

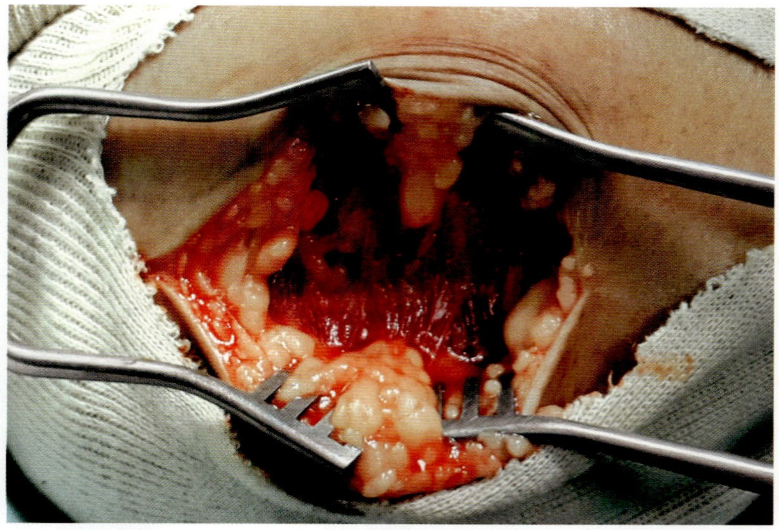

Fig. 9: Deep dissection done to identify interval between extensor carpi ulnaris (ECU) and anconeus.

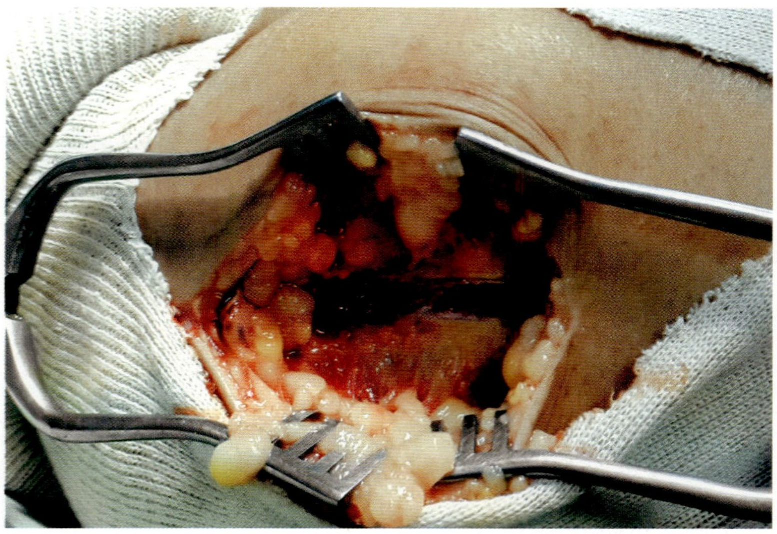

Fig. 10: Interval exposure done between extensor carpi ulnaris (ECU) and anconeus keeping the forearm pronated to avoid posterior interosseous nerve injury.

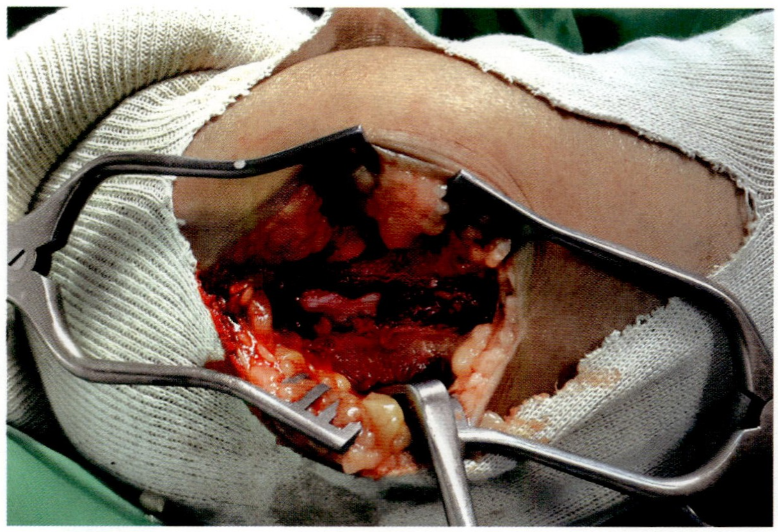

Fig. 11: Identification of proximal radius along with the impacted fracture and periosteum is elevated after incising the annular ligament for proper exposure. Lateral collateral ligament is protected during the deep dissection and its integrity is checked.

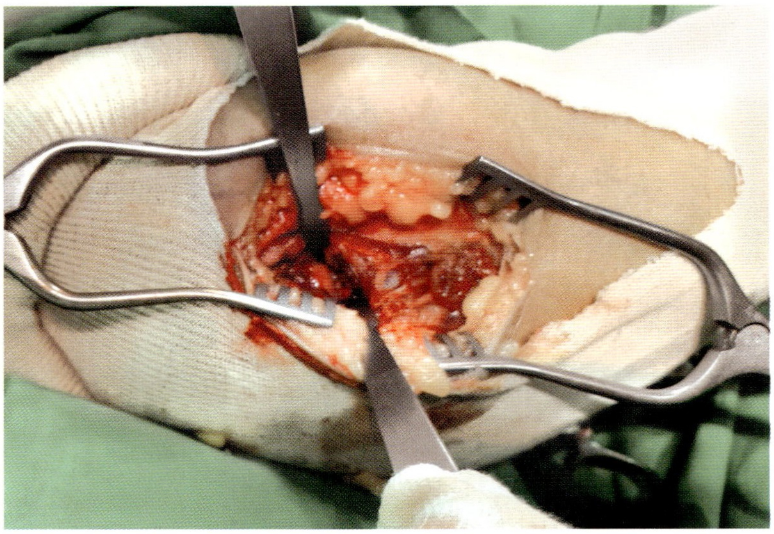

Fig. 12: Exposure of radial head using Homan spike. Excessive anterior retraction is avoided to avoid posterior interosseous nerve damage.

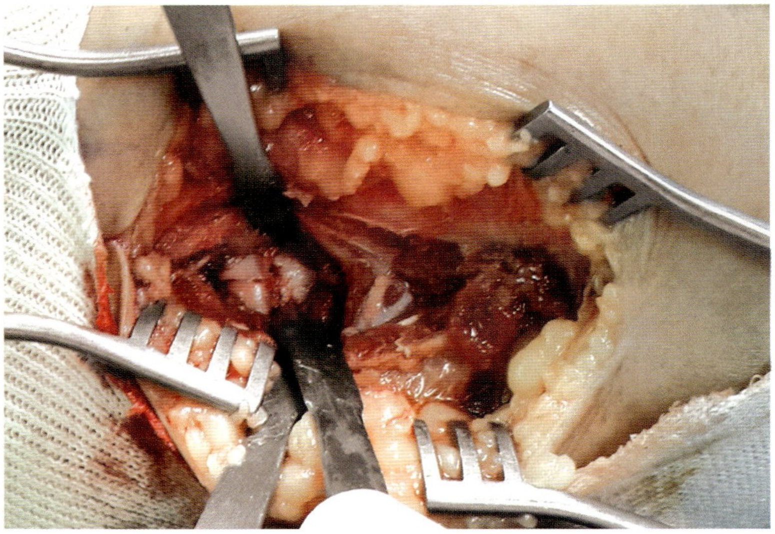

Fig. 13: Disimpaction of radial head and alignment with the shaft under direct vision.

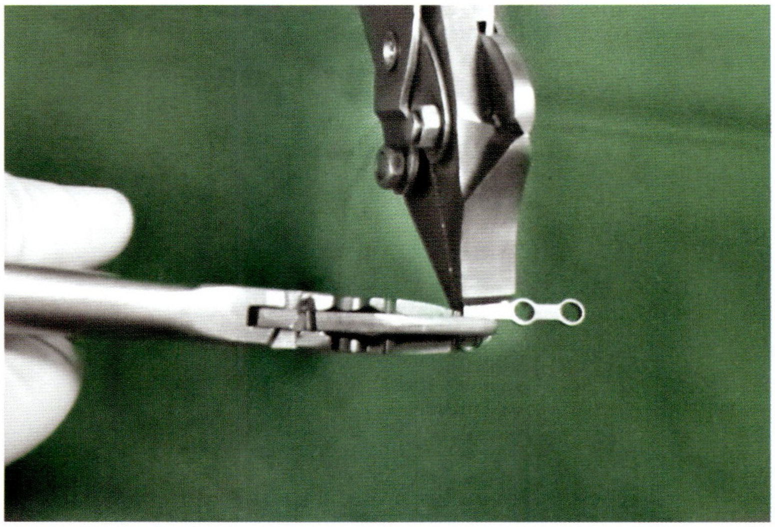

Fig. 14: Contouring of the low-profile minifragment T-plate using pliers before fixation.

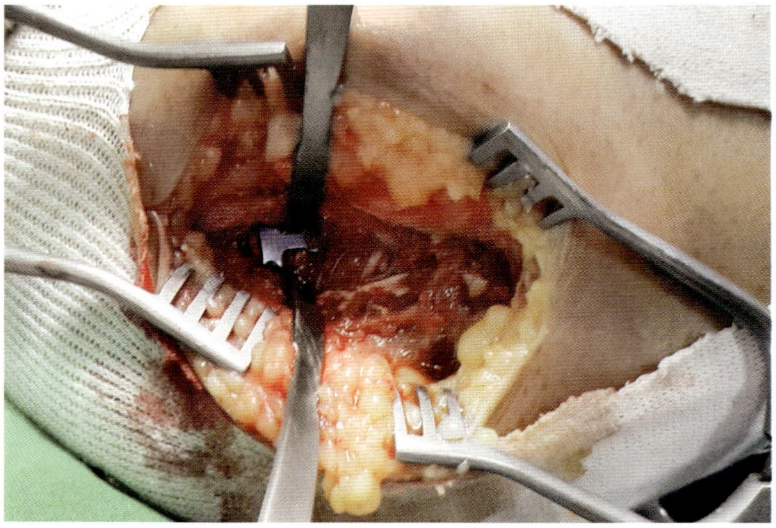

Fig. 15: Positioning of the plate in safe zone, which corresponds approximately to area between parallel lines passing through Lister's tubercle and radial styloid. First screw may be applied distally which temporarily buttresses head fragments. Head screws should be unicortical to avoid the impingement.

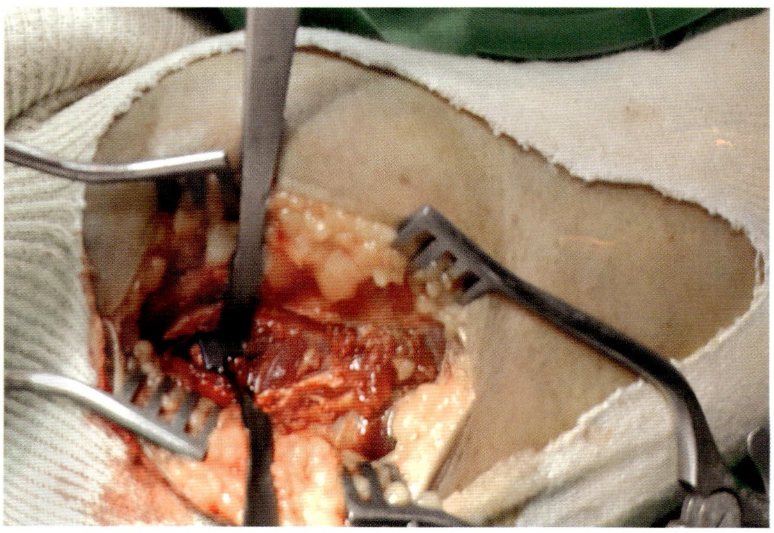

Fig. 16: Confirmation of the plate position in safe zone by pronosupination of the forearm.

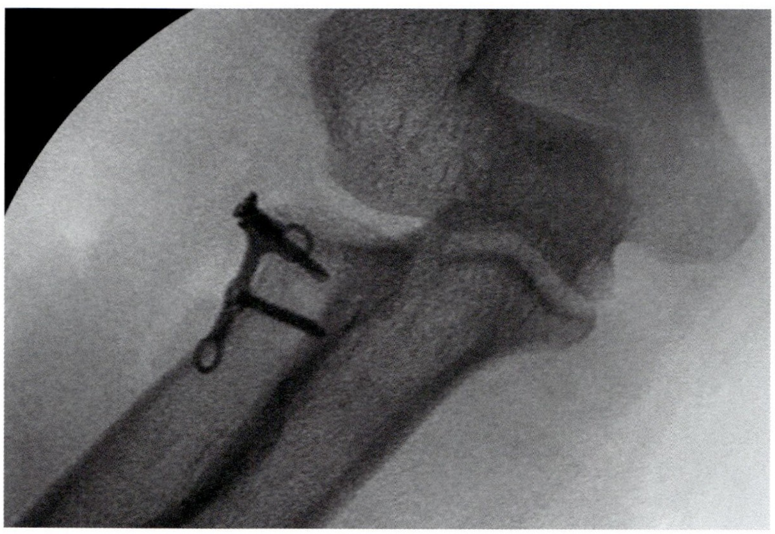

Fig. 17: Image intensifier television (IITV) image showing radial head in neutral position.

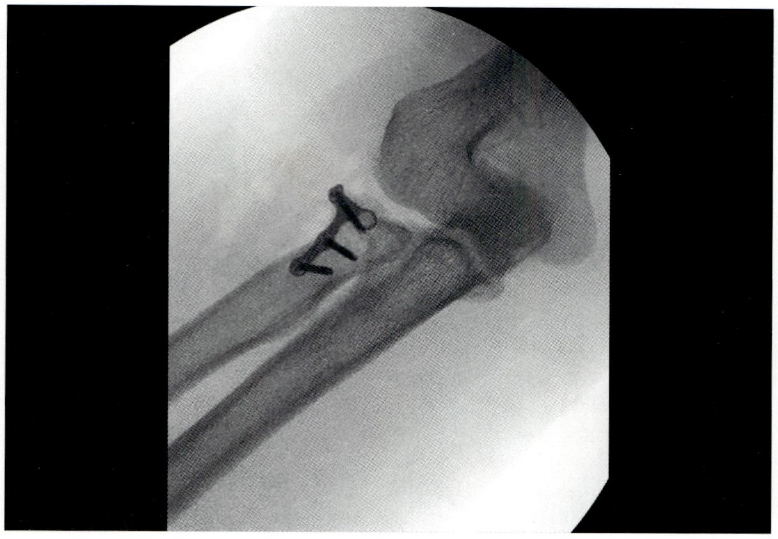

Fig. 18: Confirmation of plate position and stability of fixation in full supination.

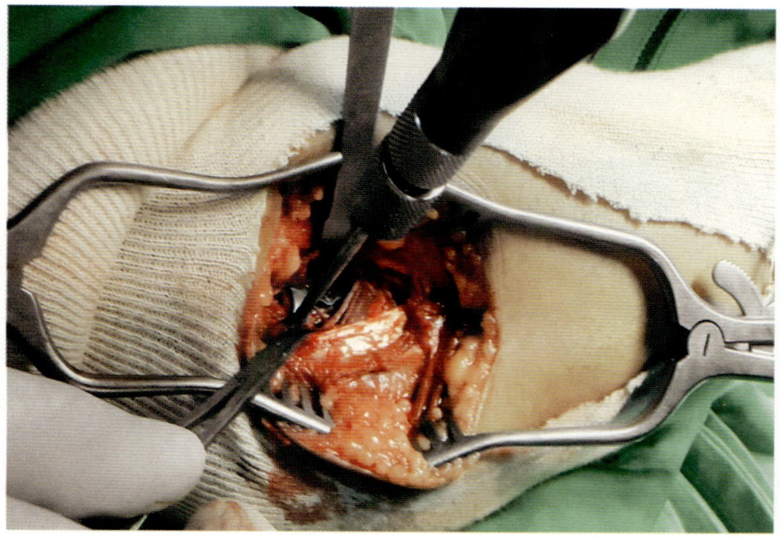

Fig. 19: Fixation of the remaining proximal screws.

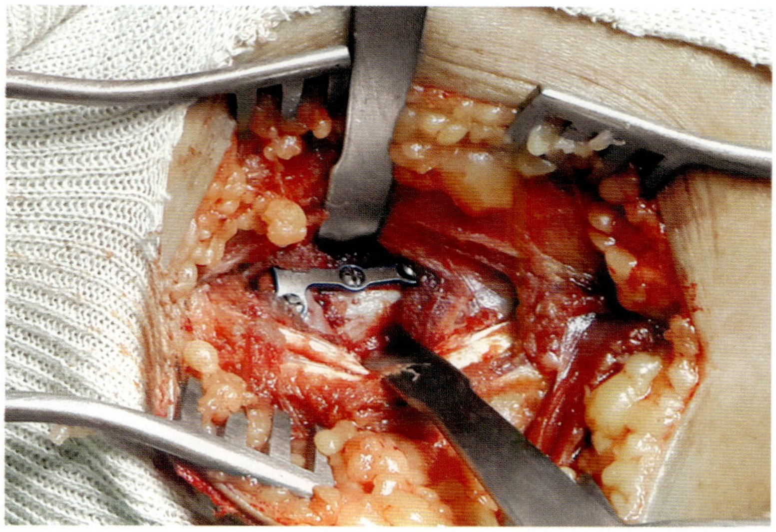

Fig. 20: Final plate position showing good reduction of fracture fragment.

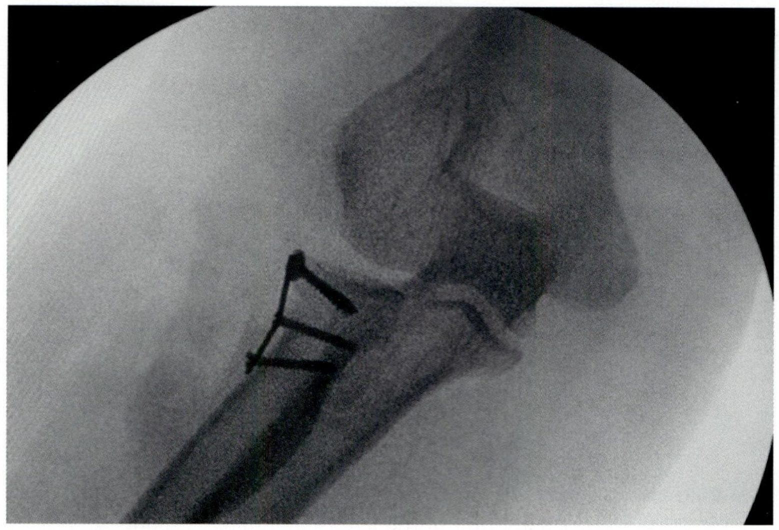

Fig. 21: Image intensifier television (IITV) anteroposterior (AP) image showing good reduction and stable fixation of the radial head fracture.

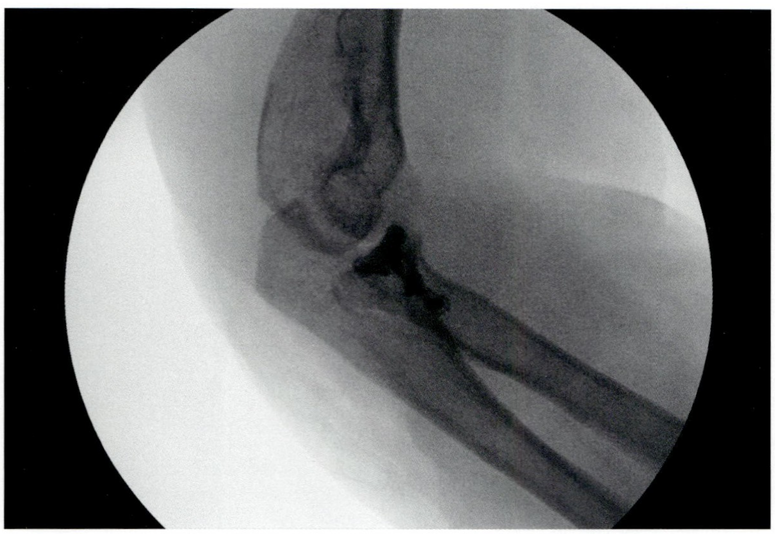

Fig. 22: Image intensifier television (IITV) image showing lateral image with stable fixation and proper alignment of radiocapitellar joint.

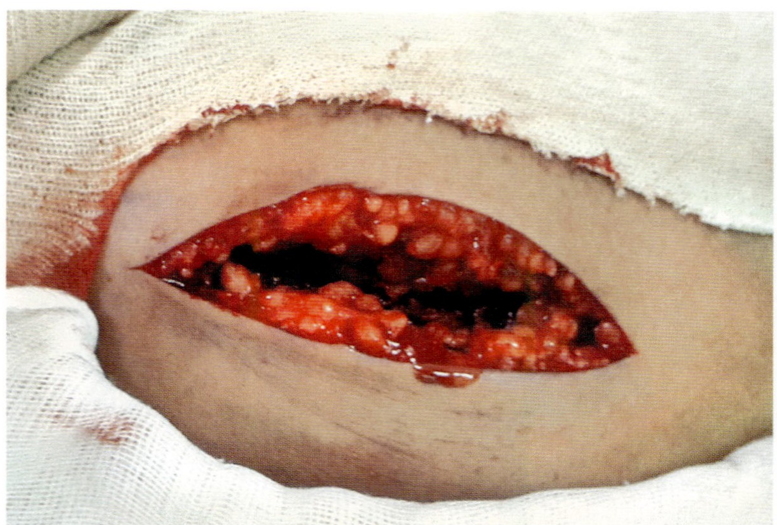

Fig. 23: Closure in layers. Annular ligament and any injured lateral collateral ligament are repaired before closure of the wound.

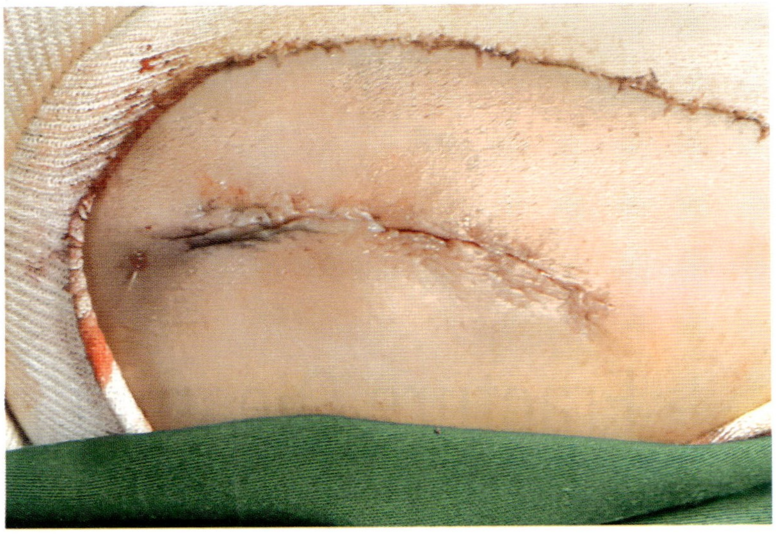

Fig. 24: Subcuticular closure of the wound.

POSTOPERATIVE PROTOCOL

- Posterior splint to be given for 15 days till soft-tissue healing occurs.
- Slab removal is done after 15 days and protected gradual range of motion exercises is started as tolerated.

COMPLICATIONS OF THE RADIAL HEAD AND NECK FRACTURE SURGERY

- Posterior interosseous nerve palsy
- Myositis ossification
- Osteonecrosis of radial head
- Cubitus valgus
- Loss of forearm rotations
- Nonunion though is the rare complication
- Cross-union.

SUGGESTED READING

1. Broberg MA, Morrey BF. Results of treatment of fracture-dislocations of the elbow. Clin Orthop Relat Res. 1987;(216):109-19.
2. Chapman CB, Su BW, Sinicropi SM, et al. Vitallium radial head prosthesis for acute and chronic elbow fractures and fracture dislocations involving the radial head. J Shoulder Elbow Surg. 2006;15(4):463-73.
3. Court-Brown CM, McQueen MM, Tornetta P. Proximal forearm fractures and elbow dislocations. In: Court-Brown C, McQueen MM, Tornetta P (Eds). Orthopaedic Surgery Essentials: Trauma, 1st edition. Philadelphia: Lippincott Williams & Wilkins; 2006. pp. 124-40.
4. de Haan J, Schep NW, Eygendaal D, et al. Stability of the elbow joint: relevant anatomy and clinical implications of in vitro biomechanical studies. Open Orthop J. 2011;5:168-76.
5. Dubberley JH, Faber KJ, Macdermid JC, et al. Outcome after open reduction and internal fixation of capitellar and trochlear fractures. J Bone Joint Surg Am. 2006;88(1):46-54.
6. Eilert RE, Erickson MA. Fractures of the proximal radius and ulna. In: Beaty JH, Kasser JR (Eds). Fractures in children. Philadelphia: Lippincott Williams and Wilkins; 2006. pp. 444-90.
7. Fuentes-Salguero L, Downey-Carmona FJ, Tatay-Diaz A, et al. Radial head and neck fractures in children. Rev Esp Cir Ortop Traumatol. 2012;56(4):300-5.
8. Ikeda M, Sugiyama K, Kang C, et al. Comminuted fractures of the radial head. Comparison of resection and internal fixation. J Bone Joint Surg Am. 2005;87(1):76-84.
9. Johnston GW. A follow-up of one hundred cases of fracture of the head of the radius with a review of the literature. Ulster Med J. 1962;31: 51-6.
10. Kaas L, van Riet RP, Vroemen JP, et al. The epidemiology of radial head fractures. J Shoulder Elbow Surg. 2010;19:520-3.
11. Lindenhovius AL, Felsch Q, Doornberg JN, et al. Open reduction and internal fixation compared with excision for unstable displaced fractures of the radial head. J Hand Surg Am. 2007;32(5):630-6.
12. Mason ML. Some observations on fractures of the head of the radius with a review of one hundred cases. Br J Surg. 1954;42(172):123-32.
13. Rineer CA, Guitton TG, Ring D. Radial head fractures: loss of cortical contact is associated with concomitant fracture or dislocation. J Shoulder Elbow Surg. 2010;19:21-5.
14. Ring D, Quintero J, Jupiter JB. Open reduction and internal fixation of fractures of the radial head. J Bone Joint Surg Am. 2002;84-A(10):1811-5.
15. Rosenblatt Y, Athwal GS, Faber KJ. Current recommendations for the treatment of radial head fractures. Orthop Clin North Am. 2008;39: 173-85.
16. Tejaswani NC, Mehta H. Fractures of the radial head and neck: current concepts in management. J Am Acad Orthop Surg. 2007;15:380-7.

CHAPTER 91

Fracture Olecranon Fixation by Olecranon Plate

Shrinivas S Shintre, Rahul Puranik, Rajkumar Ekambaram

INTRODUCTION

Olecranon fractures occur in 11.5 per lakh population in adults. This accounts for 8–10% of elbow fractures.

MECHANISM OF INJURY

Most commonly occurs due to fall on outstretched hand. Also occurs by direct trauma to elbow in which case fracture is usually comminuted and in some cases patient may have abrasions over elbow.

CLINICAL FINDINGS

Patient presents with pain and tenderness above elbow and swelling over the elbow with a typical deformity. Inability to extend the elbow; both active and passive elbow movements are restricted. In case of direct trauma to elbow patient may have abrasions over olecranon. Ulnar nerve injury can occur though less common but can be seen in case of comminuted fractures. One should look for any tingling or numbness in ring and little finger, decreased fine finger movements to rule out ulnar nerve damage.

INVESTIGATIONS

X-ray is the first investigation to be ordered and usually diagnosis suffices with X-ray. True anteroposterior (AP) and dead lateral X-rays are necessary. In case of elbow dislocations traction X-ray may be needed if elbow instability persists. CT scan can be helpful in case of comminuted fractures and to look for associated coronoid fractures and radial head dislocation.

MAYO CLASSIFICATION

Based on fracture displacement, comminution and ulnohumeral stability:
- Type I: Undisplaced
- Type II: Displaced, stable
- Type III: Unstable

Each type further divided into type A (noncomminuted) and type B (comminuted).

MANAGEMENT

It is based on the type of fracture, age of the patient and associated comorbidities. In case of undisplaced fracture conservative management is preferred. In case of displaced fractures operative management is to be done. Tension band wiring or plate fixation are among options. In case of comminuted fractures plating is the treatment of choice. In case of comminuted fractures when the comminution is too proximal, fragment excision and triceps repair has to been described. However, in elderly patient with comorbidities conservative management can be done even in comminuted fractures.

INDICATIONS OF OLECRANON PLATING

- Comminuted fractures (Mayo Types II and III)
- Fracture dislocation
- Monteggia fractures
- Pseudoarthroses of proximal ulna
- Olecranon repair after osteotomy in distal humerus surgery

SURGICAL STEPS (FIGS. 1 TO 14)

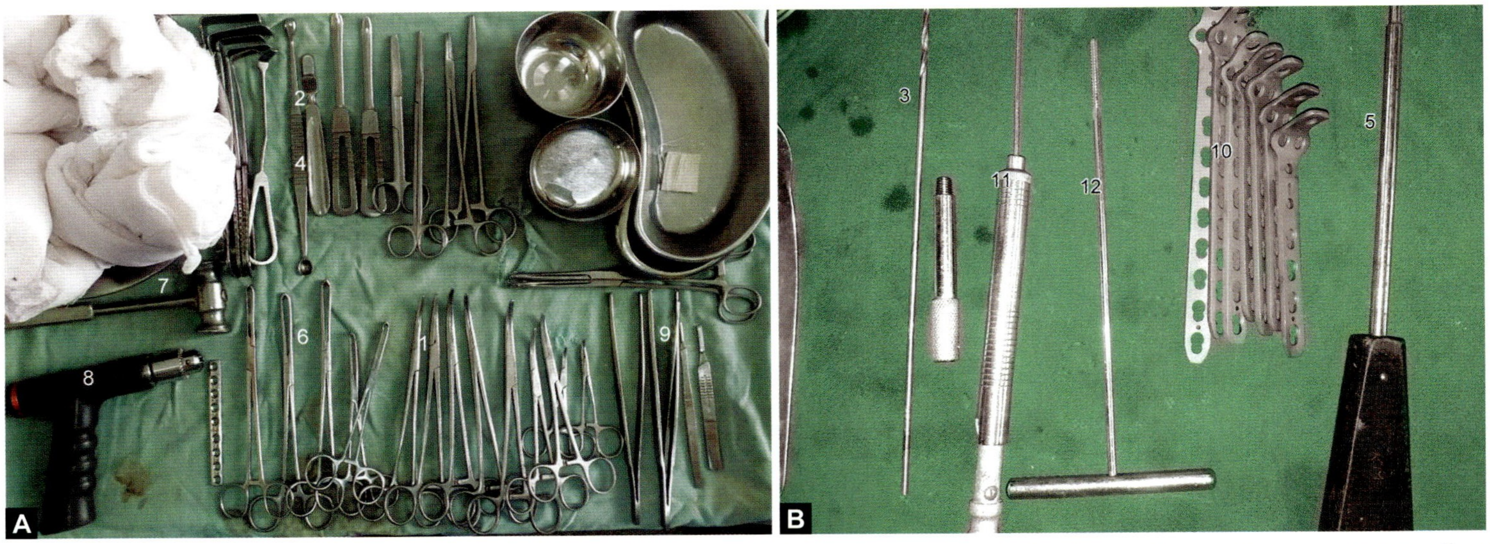

Figs. 1A and B: Instrument trolley needed for surgery. (1) Artery forceps, (2) Periosteum elevator, (3) Drill bits of 2.7 mm, (4) Scoop, (5) Screwdriver, (6) Allis forceps, (7) Mallet/Hammer (8) Drill machine, (9) Tissue holding forceps, (10) Olecranon hook plate, (11) Depth gauge, (12) Tap.

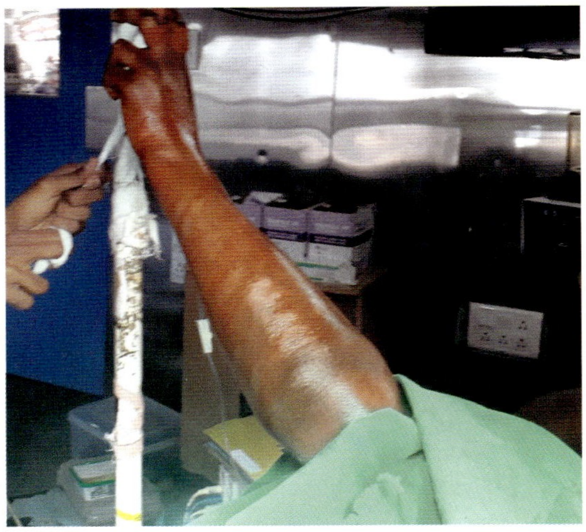

Fig. 2: After painting and draping of limb is done. Tourniquet is applied to prevent blood loss.

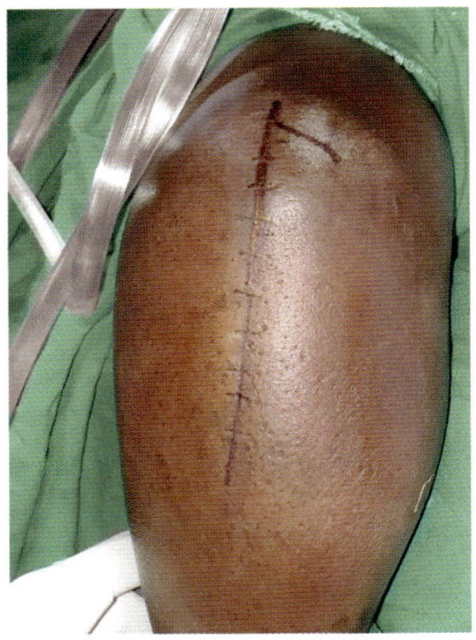

Fig. 3: Skin is marked for incision from tip of olecranon to 8–10 cm distally along the shaft of ulna.

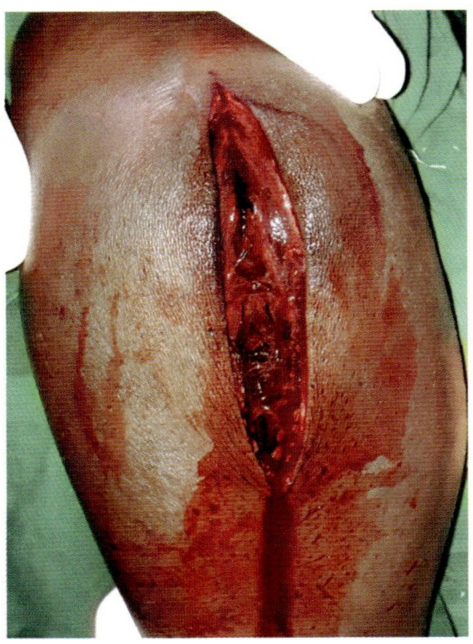

Fig. 4: Skin incision is done and soft tissues are separated.

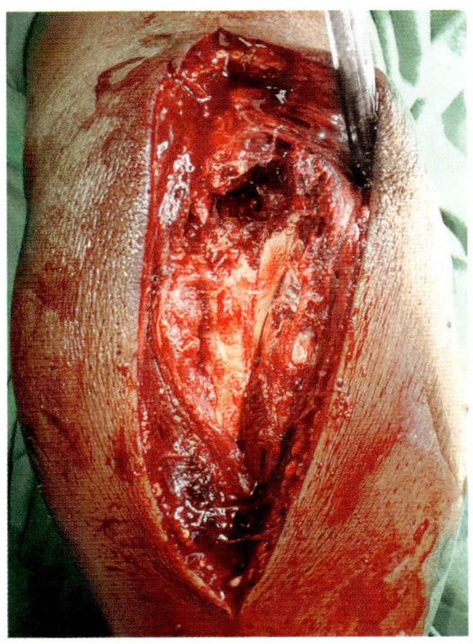

Fig. 5: Deep dissection is carried out and bone reached. Note the presence of comminuted fragments and fracture hematoma around the fracture site.

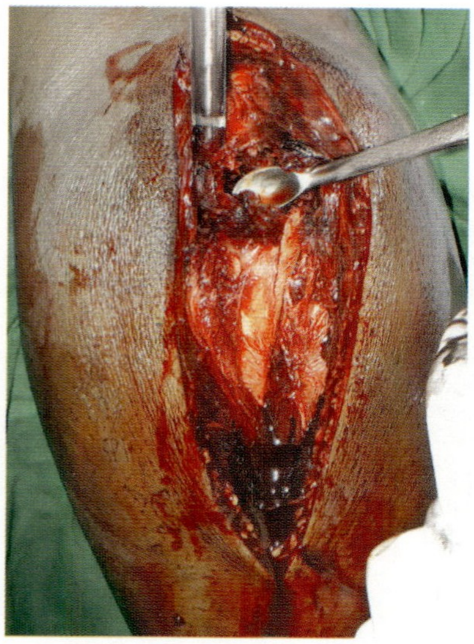

Fig. 6: Hematoma and soft tissue is removed and scooped out to ease the reduction and healing process.

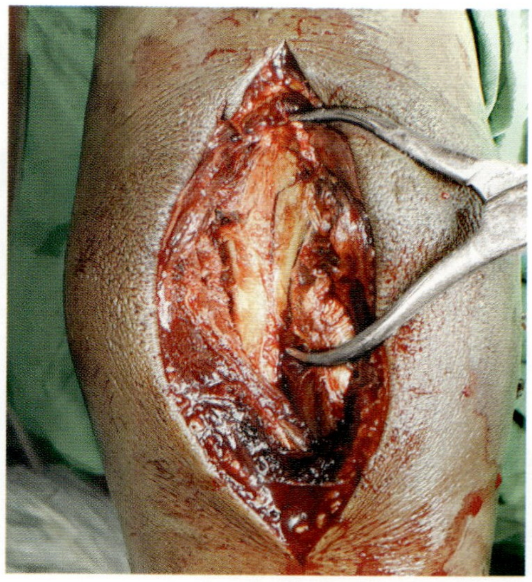

Fig. 7: Fracture fragments are held together using reduction forceps.

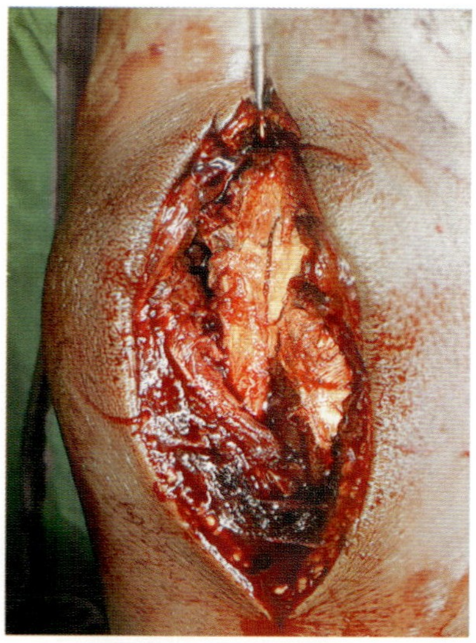

Fig. 8: K-wire is introduced from the tip of the olecranon and fixed to opposite cortex to hold the fragment in reduction.

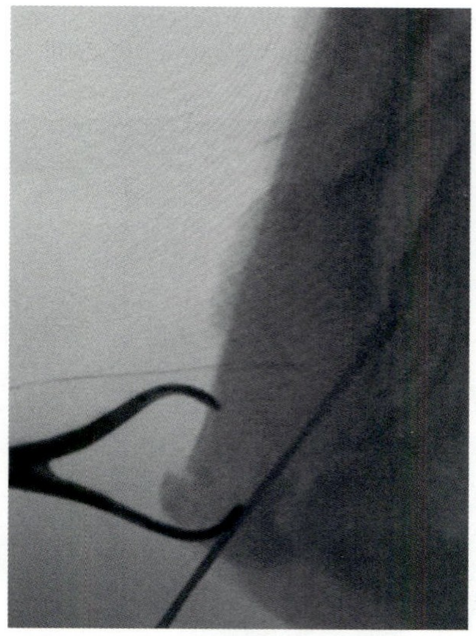

Fig. 9: K-wire visualized under C-arm.

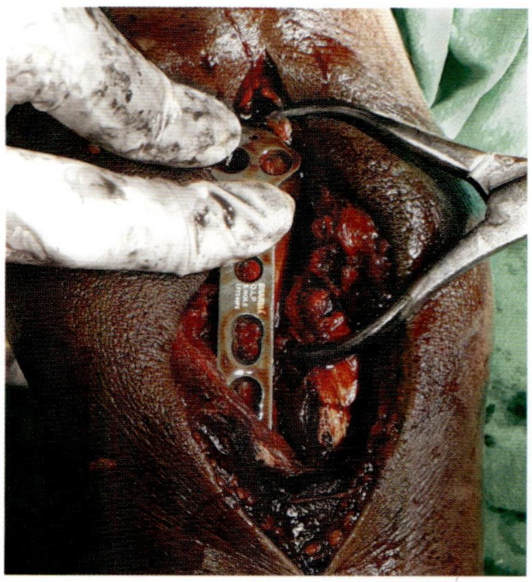

Fig. 10: Olecranon plate is introduced while reduction is maintained by reduction forceps and K-wire.

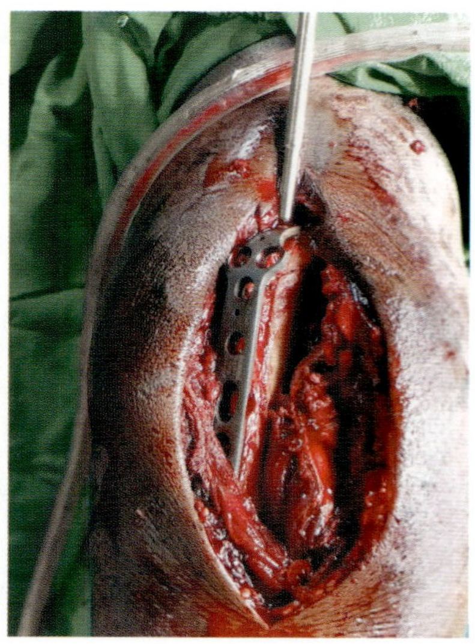

Fig. 11: Screw is introduced and tightened in the tip of olecranon.

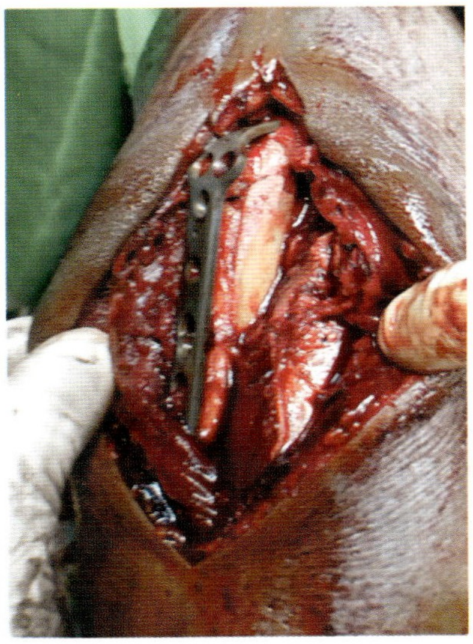

Fig. 12: Reduction is confirmed at this stage before fixing further.

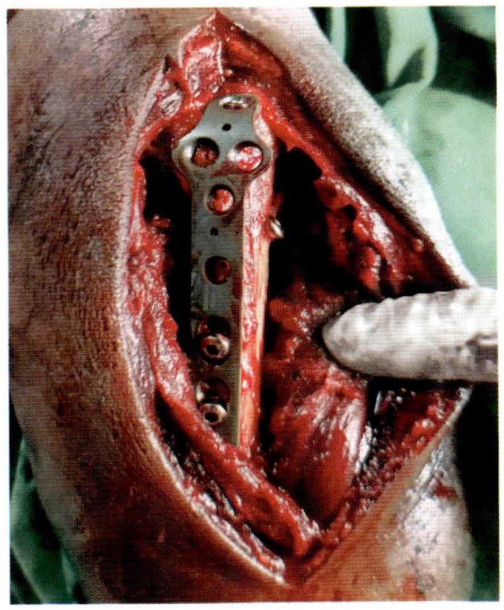

Fig. 13: Distal screws are fixed to the plate.

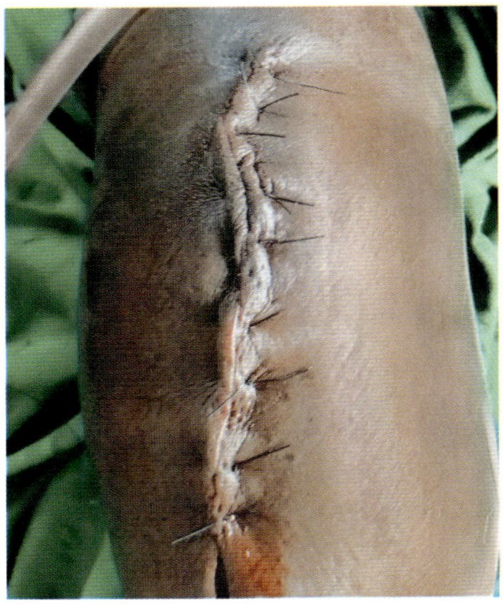

Fig. 14: After proper wash is given with povidone-iodine and normal saline. Subcutaneous tissue is closed with absorbable suture and skin is closed with nonabsorbable suture material 2-0.

COMPLICATIONS

- *Symptomatic (painful) implant*: Subcutaneous location of bone and faulty techniques predispose. Incidence can be reduced by proper surgical technique and using precontoured locking plates. Implant removal may be needed in 33% cases.
- *Heterotopic ossification*: Incidence is 2–13%. Patient presents with elbow stiffness. This can be reduced by good fixation and starting early range of motion exercises. Tablet indomethacin may be useful.
- *Infection*: At times due to improper wound care or uncontrolled BSL in diabetic patients. Patient presents with fever, discharge from wound site. Management includes antibiotics as per culture reports and wound wash under anesthesia. Sometimes implant removal may be needed.
- *Implant failure*: Proper preoperative planning, good fixation and addressing any associated injuries will help to prevent this issue.
- *Nonunion and malunion*: Occurs in about 5% cases. Proper fixation techniques help in minimizing this complication.

SUGGESTED READING

1. Azar FM, Terry Canale S, H. Beaty J. Campbell's Operative Orthopaedics, 13th edition. Netherlands: Elsevier; 2016.
2. Court-Brown C, Heckman JD, McKee M, et al. Rockwood and greens fracture in adults, 8th edition. Netherlands: Wolters Kluwer; 2014.
3. Egol K, Koval KJ, Zuckerman J. Handbook of fractures, 5th edition. Netherlands: Wolters Kluwer; 2014.
4. Hoppenfeld S, De Boer P, Buckley R. Surgical Exposure in Orthopaedics: The Anatomic Approach, 5th edition. Netherlands: Wolters Kluwer; 2016.
5. Thakur AJ. The elements of fracture fixation, 3rd edition. Netherlands: Elsevier; 2015.

CHAPTER 92

Monteggia Fracture Fixation with Dynamic Compression Plate

Ajay Chandanwale, Rahul Puranik, Rajkumar Ekambaram

INTRODUCTION

- Monteggia fractures are considered as fracture involving proximal shaft ulna with disruption of proximal radioulnar joint.
- Mechanism of injury is mostly through direct blow to the dorsum of upper forearm.

CLASSIFICATION

Bado Classification

- *Type 1:* Ulnar fracture with anterior angulation and anterior dislocation of radial head.
- *Type 2:* Ulnar fracture with posterior angulation and posterior dislocation of radial head.
- *Type 3:* Ulnar fracture with lateral dislocation of radial head.
- *Type 4:* Fracture of both proximal radius and ulna at same level with anterior dislocation of radial head.

CLINICAL FEATURES

- Pain, tenderness, and swelling of forearm. Deformity seen when there is obvious displacement of elbow joint.
- Neurovascular injury is always checked for as injury to median and posterior interosseous nerve can occur.

INVESTIGATION

- Anteroposterior (AP) and lateral radiograph of forearm with elbow and wrist joint. Computed tomography (CT) can be done, if needed.

TREATMENT

- Closed reduction and cast are done in pediatric population.
- Mostly open reduction with internal fixation using plate is required. Once ulna is reduced, radius is relocated most of the time with ease.

SURGICAL STEPS

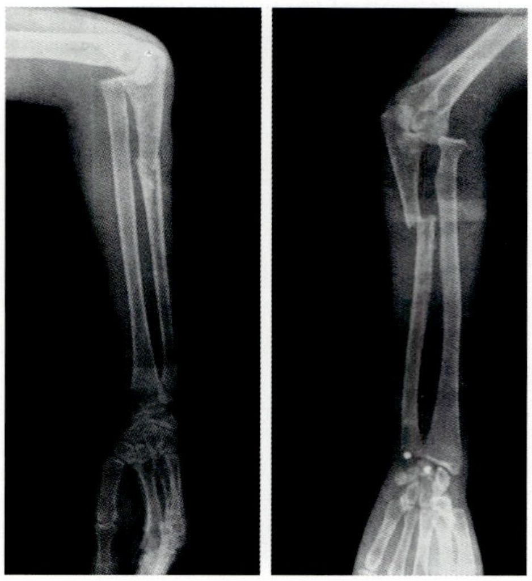

Fig. 1: Preoperative radiograph showing right Monteggia fracture.

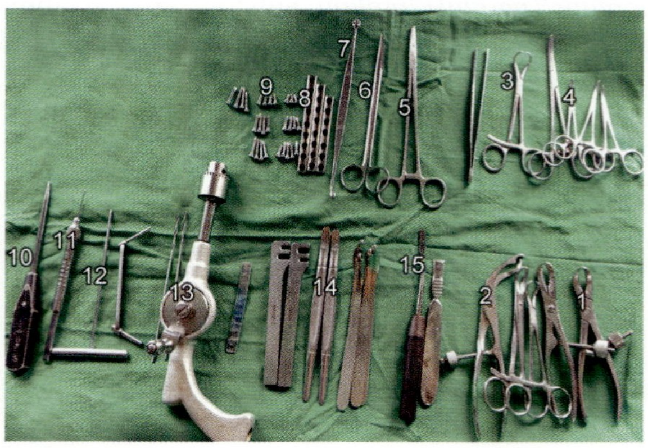

Fig. 2: Instrument trolley showing: (1) bone holding forceps, (2) plate holding forceps, (3) pointed reduction forceps, (4) artery forceps, (5) needle holder, (6) scissors, (7) scoop, (8) 3.5-mm dynamic compression plate, (9) screws, (10) screw driver, (11) depth gauge, (12) tap, (13) drill machine, (14) spikes, and (15) periosteal elevator.

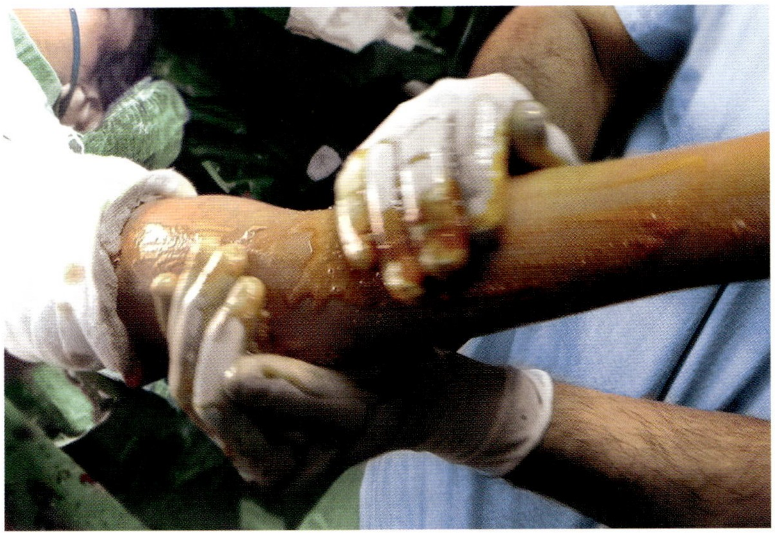

Fig. 3: Scrubbing of the limb with povidone–iodine scrub. Tourniquet applied to reduce blood loss. Painting and draping will be done later.

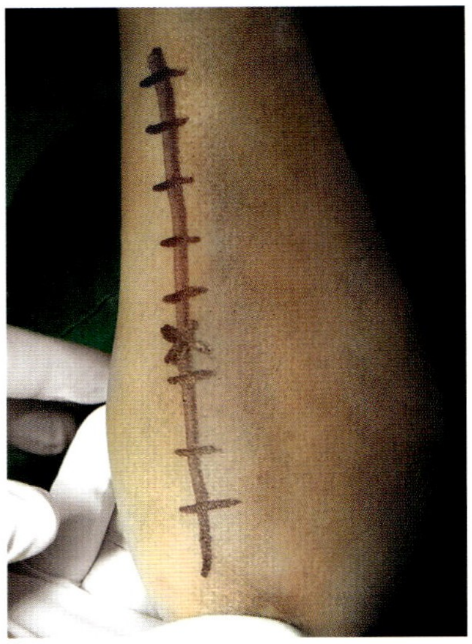

Fig. 4: Skin to be incised is marked with a marker along the subcutaneous border of the shaft of ulna.

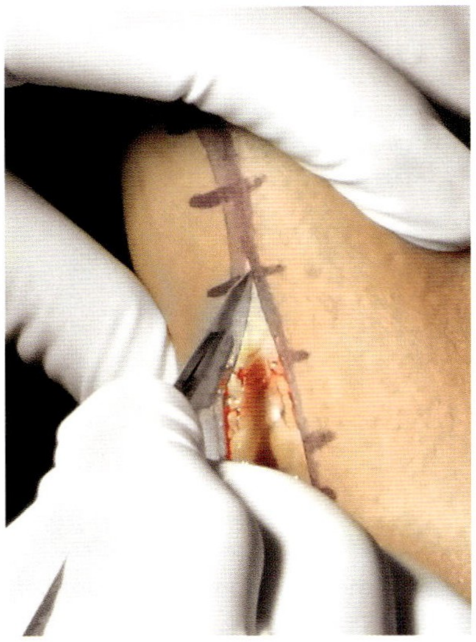

Fig. 5: Skin is incised with knife over the marked line.

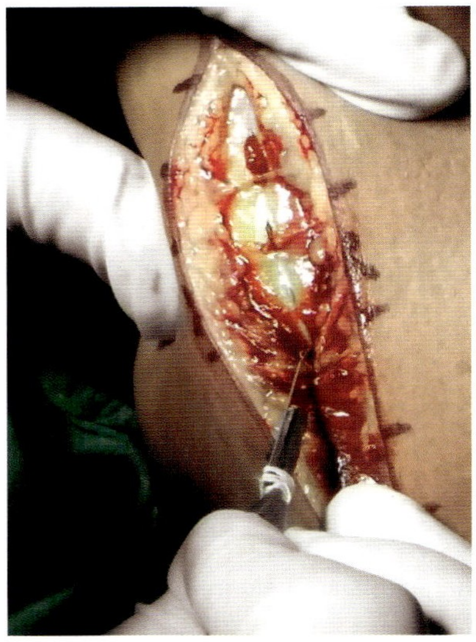

Fig. 6: Deep dissection is carried out through the fat and fascia.

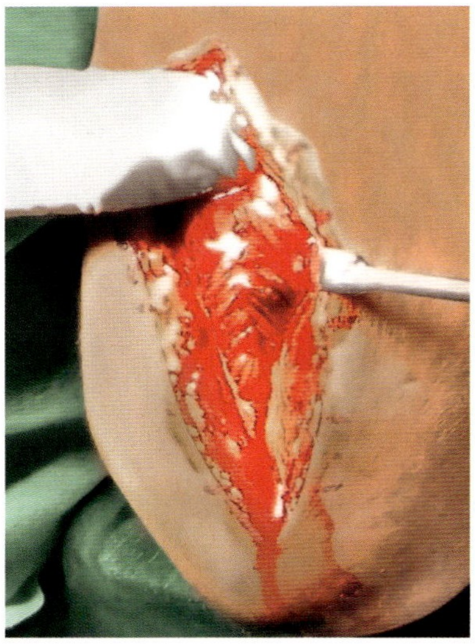

Fig. 7: On further dissection, an intermuscular plane is developed between extensor carpi ulnaris and flexor carpi ulnaris.

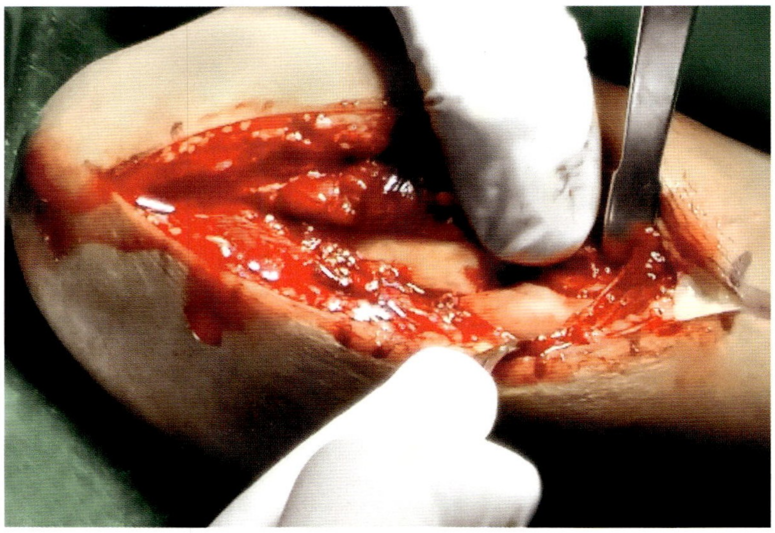

Fig. 8: Through the plane bone is reached out and fracture site visualized.

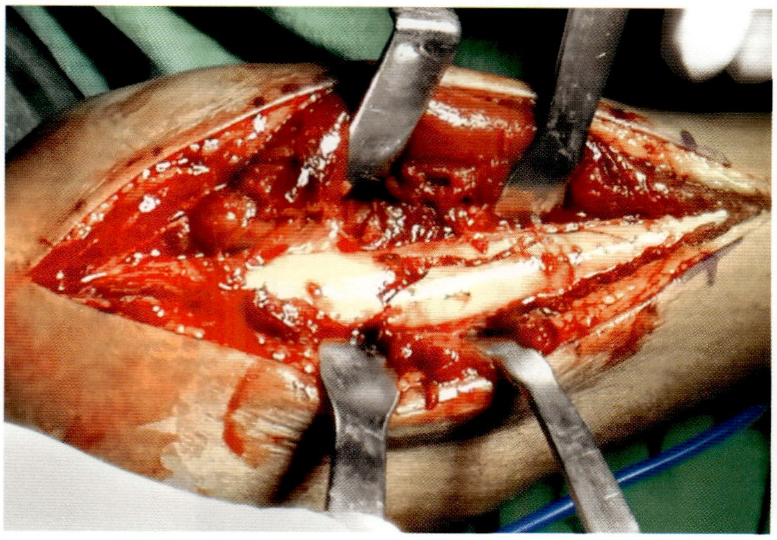

Fig. 9: After proper dissection, muscles are retracted to give a better view of fracture site.

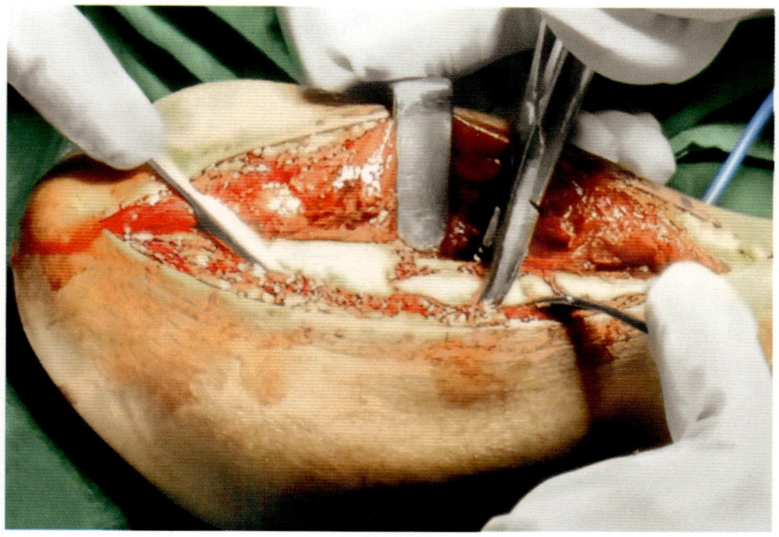

Fig. 10: Periosteum is elevated using periosteal elevator.

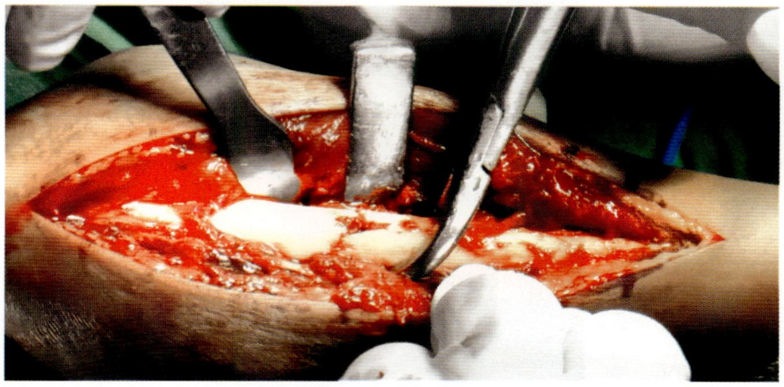

Fig. 11: Fracture fragments are held in position using reduction forceps.

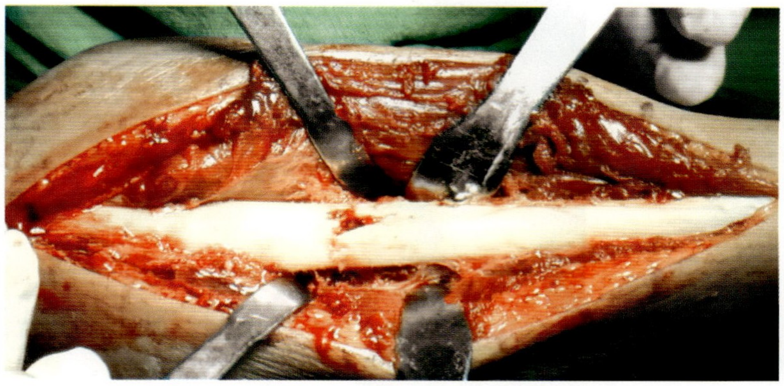

Fig. 12: After removal of the hematoma and loose soft tissue, fragments at fracture site is removed to get fresh healthy margins.

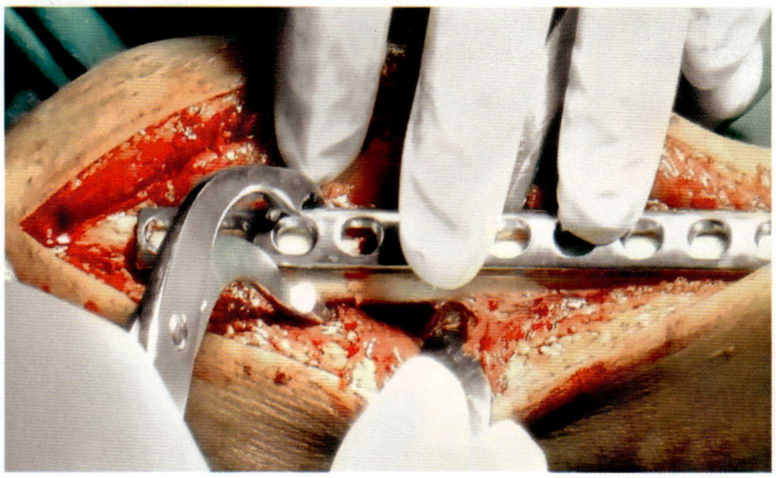

Fig. 13: Dynamic compression plate (DCP) is introduced and held with plate holding forceps.

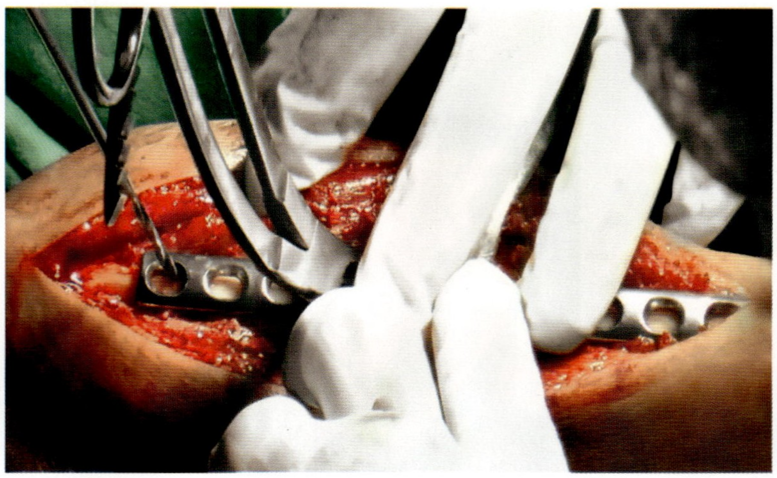

Fig. 14: Drilling of cortex is done using 2.7-mm drill bit in proximal fragment.

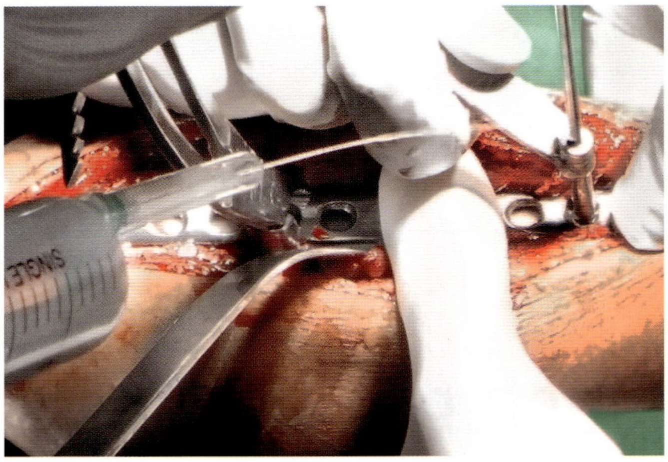

Fig. 15: Simultaneously drilling of cortex using 2.7-mm drill bit and sleeve is done in distal fragment. Syringing of normal saline is done to prevent heat necrosis of bone.

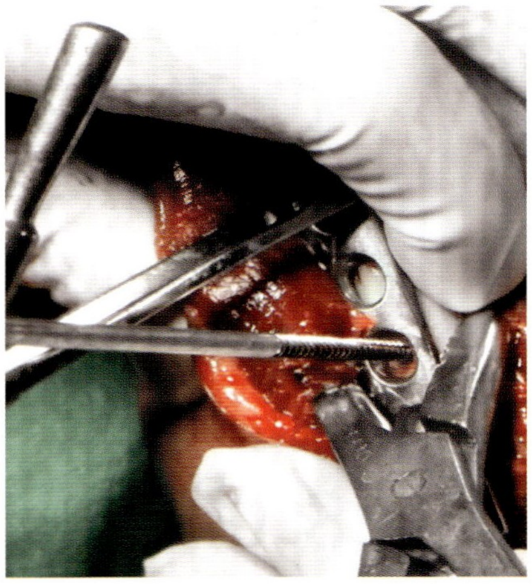

Fig. 16: Tapping of the cortex is done.

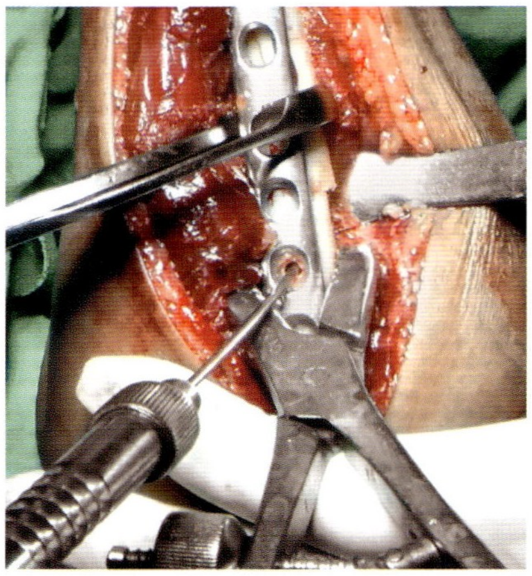

Fig. 17: Length of the screw is measured by the depth gauge introduced in the drill hole made.

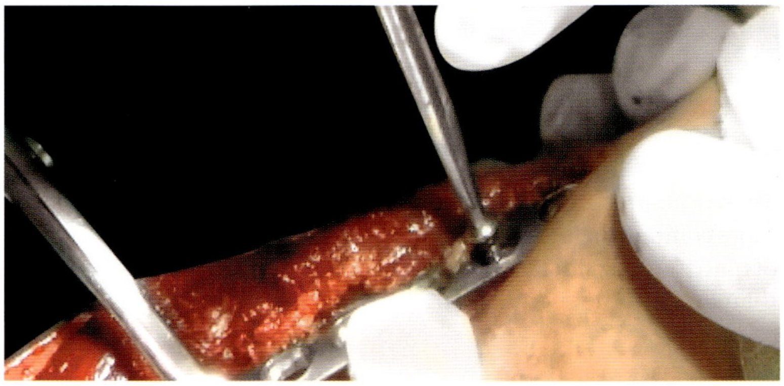

Fig. 18: Screw is tightened ensuring bicortical purchase of the bone. Similarly, other screws are introduced on both distal and proximal fragments ensuring the hold of minimum six cortices on either side. After provisional fixation, reduction of radial head reduction is confirmed by C-arm.

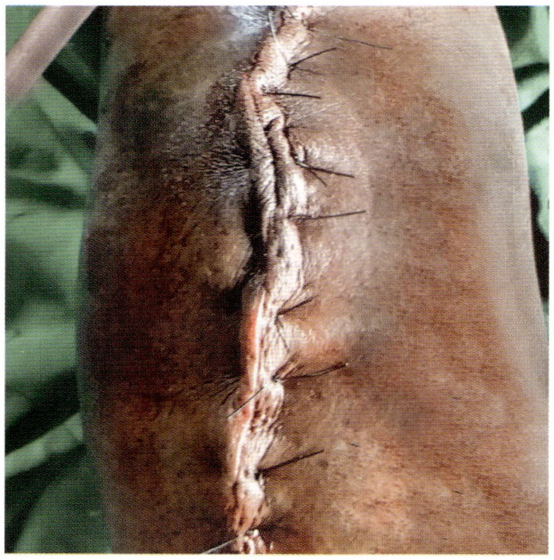

Fig. 19: After plate is fixed, wash is given with povidone–iodine and subcutaneous tissue is closed with absorbable suture and skin is closed with nonabsorbable suture 2-0.

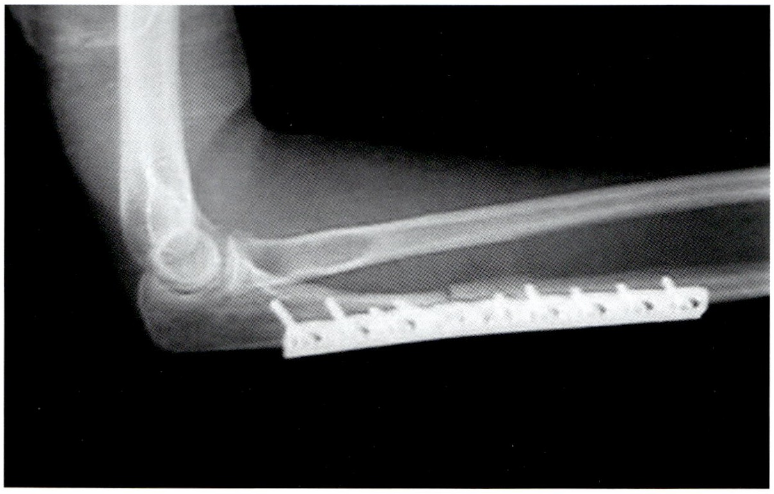

Fig. 20: Postoperative lateral radiograph showing superior radioulnar joint is in reduced position. Hence open reduction of superior radioulnar joint was not required.

COMPLICATIONS

- Nonunion
- Radial head instability rarely
- Elbow stiffness.

SUGGESTED READING

1. Ring D, Jupiter JB. Fracture dislocation of the elbow. J Bone Joint Surg Am. 1998;80(4):566-80.
2. Teasdall R, Savoie FH, Hughes JL. Comminuted fractures of the proximal radius and ulna. Clin Orthop Relat Res. 1993;(292):37-47.

CHAPTER 93

Radius Ulna Midshaft Fracture Fixation with Dynamic Compression Plate

Madan Hardikar, Hardik Shah, Ranjit Rajure

INTRODUCTION

These fractures are also known as, "both bone forearm fractures". It is more common in men than women, secondary to the higher incidence of road traffic accidents. The ratio of open to closed fractures is higher than for any other bone except tibia.

ANATOMY

Forearm is like a ring. The ulna is relatively straight bone which acts as an axis around which laterally bowed radius rotates in supination and pronation. Trauma leading to shortening of one bone has to cause fracture or dislocation of other forearm bone. The interosseous membrane is located in the space between the radius and ulna (Fig. 1).

Deforming forces:

- Radial fractures distal to the supinator insertion but proximal to pronator teres insertion—supination of proximal fragment.
- Radial fractures distal to supinator and pronator teres—neutral rotation alignment of the proximal fragment (Fig. 2).

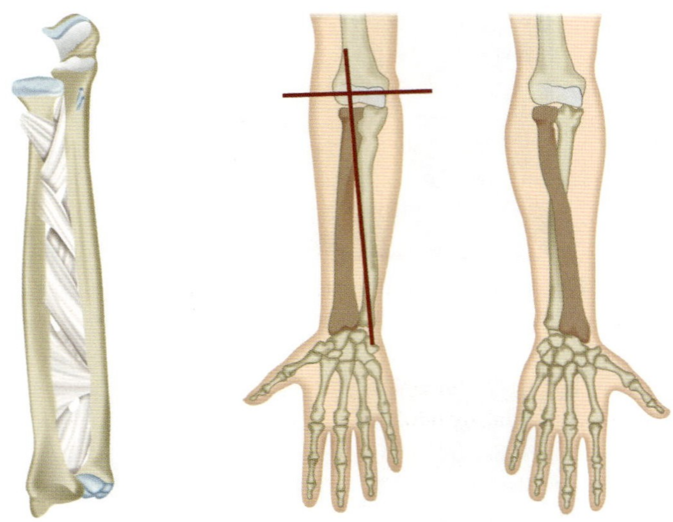

Fig. 1: Special anatomy—the two bones of the forearm function as a joint.

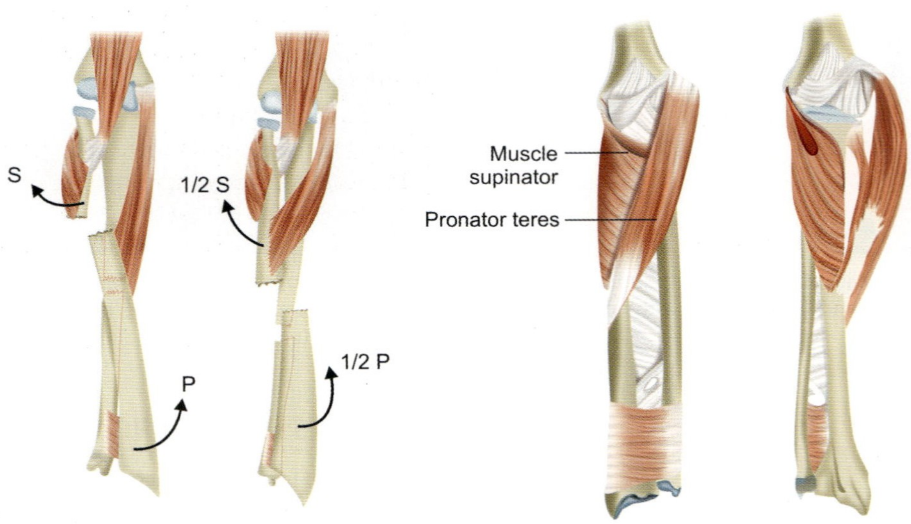

Fig. 2: Special anatomy—muscle forces tend to displace fractures.

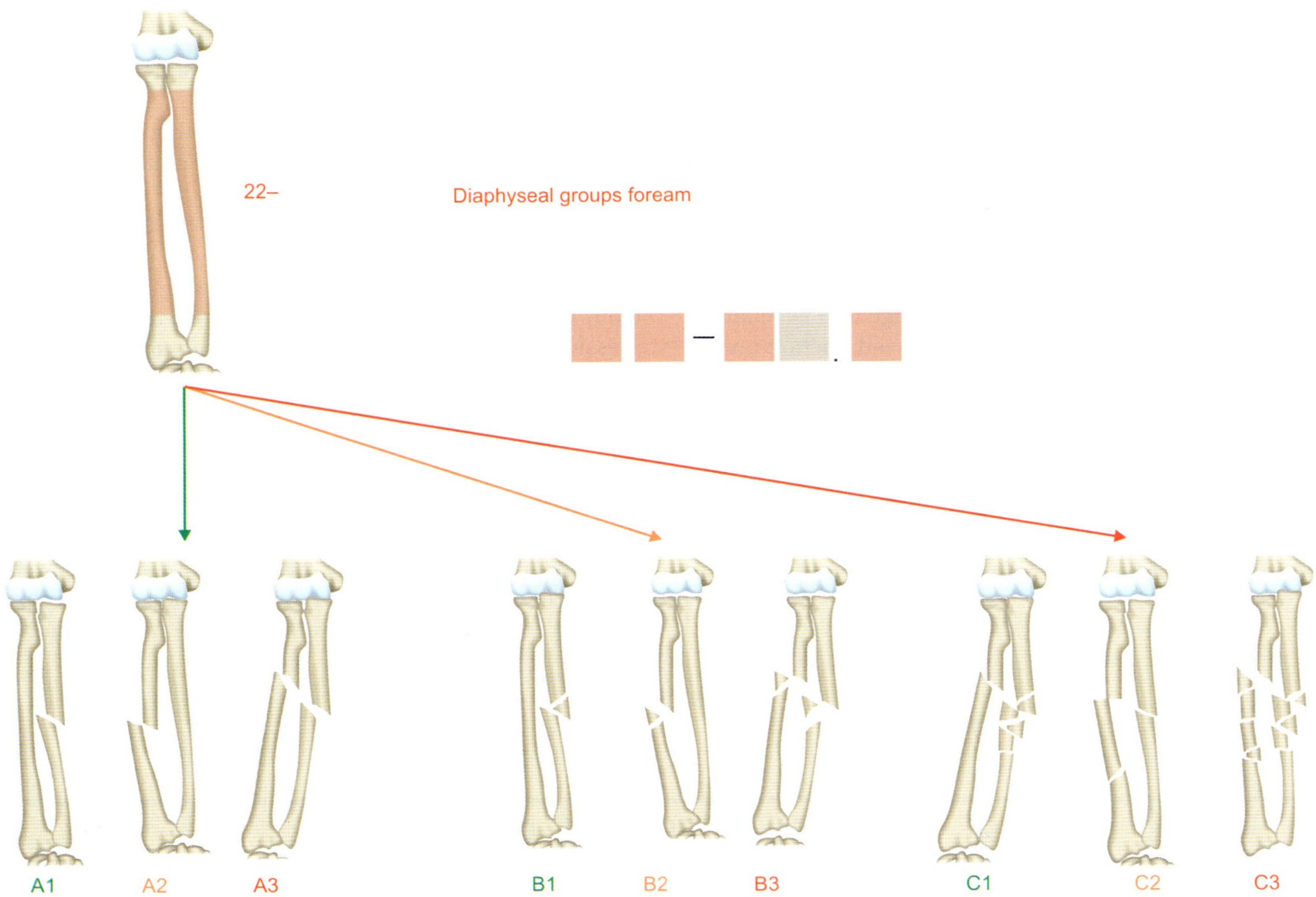

Fig. 3: AO/OTA classification.

MECHANISM OF INJURY

Mechanism of injury is either direct or indirect trauma.

Direct trauma mainly while protecting ones head. *Indirect trauma* may be in motor vehicle accidents, fall from height or athletic competition

CLASSIFICATION

- Descriptive
  - Closed versus open
  - Location
  - Comminuted, segmental, multifragmented
  - Displacement
  - Angulation
  - Rotational alignment
- Orthopaedic Trauma Association (OTA) classification:
  - Radial and ulna diaphyseal fractures (Type 2.2) (Fig. 3)
    - Type A
      Simple fracture of ulna (A1), radius (A2), or both bones (A3)
    - Type B
      Wedge fracture of ulna (B1), radius (B2), or both bones (B3)
    - Type C
      Complex fractures.

PRESENTATION

The patients usually presents with complaints of pain, swelling, loss of movements and gross deformity following traumatic episode.

One should actively look for open injuries, assess radial and ulnar pulses document median, radial, and ulnar nerve function. Pain with passive stretch, tense compartment may indicate impending compartment syndrome.

INVESTIGATIONS

For diagnosis, radiograph in two planes is mandatory and it should include elbow and wrist joints. CT scan is rarely indicated. MRI is useful for assessing damage to articular cartilage of distal radioulnar joint. Angiography is necessary in cases involving vascular trauma.

TREATMENT

Closed reduction and cast application may be indicated in younger age groups with minimal angulation and displacement. In adults patients, open reduction and internal fixation is the preferred modality of treatment.

Anatomical reduction is mandatory for these fractures because malunion of forearm affects range of supination and pronation.

Diaphyseal forearm fractures should be stabilized to maintain axial and rotational alignment. Open reduction and internal fixation with plate provides adequate reduction and high union rates.

However, periosteal stripping and excessive cortical contact may disrupt the blood supply.

To reduce the plate interference with cortical perfusion, thus reducing the cortical porosis. Limited contact dynamic compression plates was developed.

Subsequently, locking compression plate was developed which provides stronger biological fixation. However, plates still have some disadvantages such as causing soft-tissue damage and evacuation of the fracture hematoma that may result in delayed fracture union, nonunion and infection.

Intramedullary (IM) nailing can also be performed for the stabilization of fracture shaft radius and ulna. However, these methods of fixation have higher risk of decreased rotation motion of forearm due to lack of rotational and axial stability and under-reduction of radial bowing and have higher risk of nonunion.

AIMS

(1) Restore ulnar and radial length, (2) Restore rotational alignment, (3) Restore radial bow.

Radius fractures may be approached either by anterior (Henry) or posterior (Thompson) approach whereas ulna is always approached posteriorly.

Using two separate incisions decreases the incidence of radioulnar synostosis.

Implants that are commonly used are: (1) DCP 3.5 (dynamic compression plate); LC-DCP 3.5 (limited-contact dynamic compression plate), (3) LCP 3.5 (locking compression plate). At least three screws in each main fragment are mandatory. While using locking plates it is important to ensure that fracture is compressed prior to use of locked screws or else chances of nonunion are increased.

External fixator is indicated in case of open fractures.

Intramedullary nailing is indicated in following situations: (1) Segmental fractures, (2) Poor soft-tissue integrity, (3) Pathological fractures, and (4) Failed plate fixation.

It is not preferred routinely due to lack of rotational and axial stability and difficulty maintaining radial bow (higher nonunion rate).

SURGICAL STEPS (FIGS. 4 TO 35)

Here we are describing "Open reduction and internal fixation of radius ulna midshaft fracture with a dynamic compression plate (DCP) using a volar approach for radius and dorsal approach for ulna".

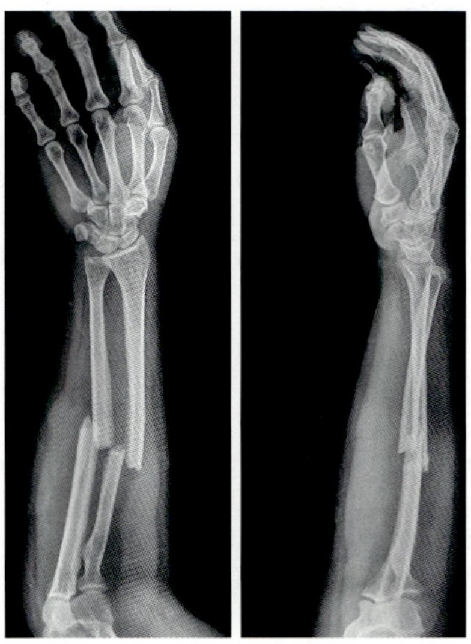

Fig. 4: Preoperative X-ray AP/lateral.

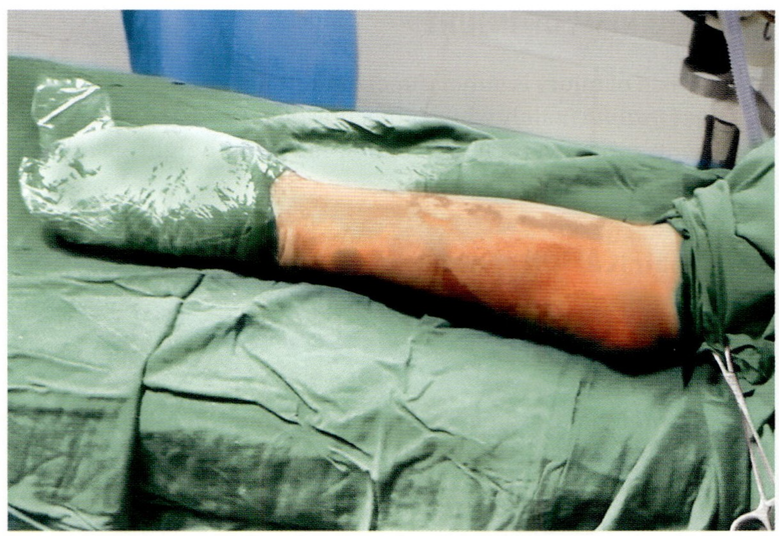

Fig. 5: Limb position with draping.

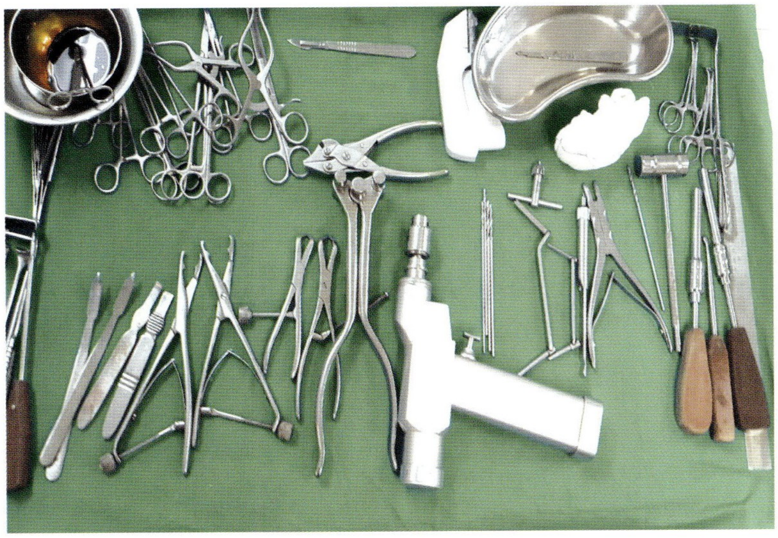

Fig. 6: Instrument trolly.

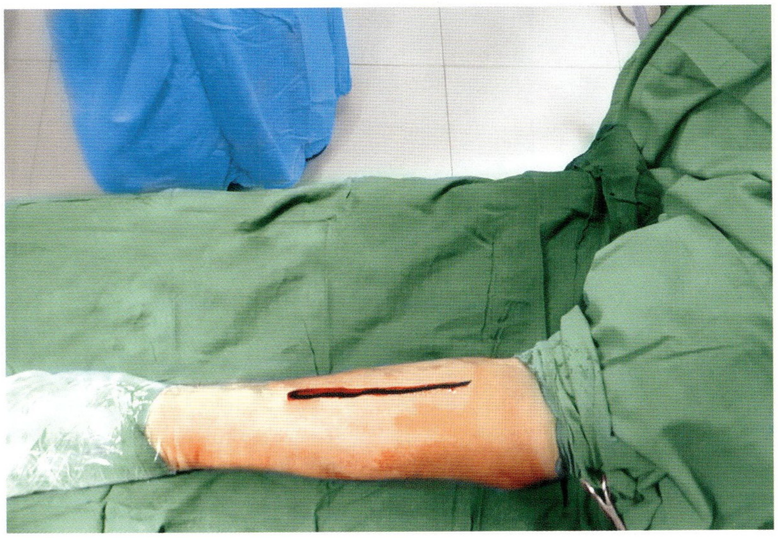

Fig. 7: Radial volar Henry approach incision.

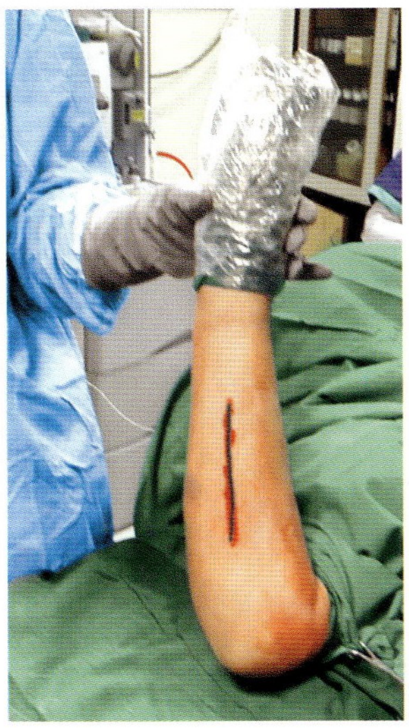

Fig. 8: Ulna dorsal approach incision.

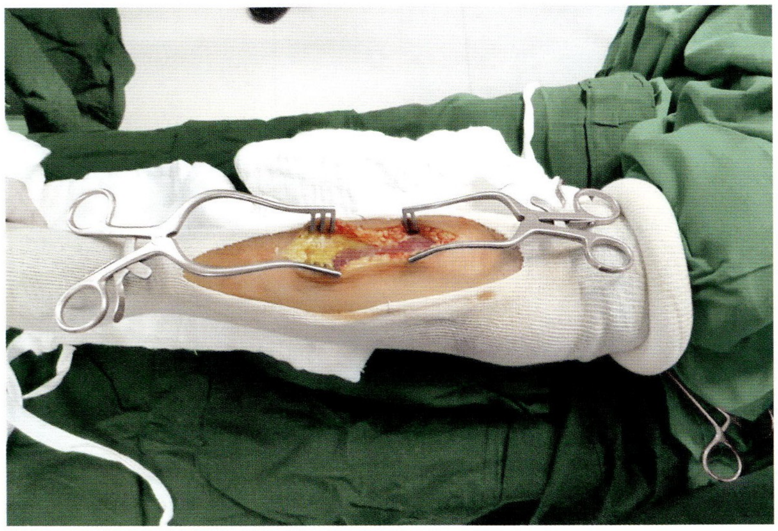

Fig. 9: Radial superficial dissection.

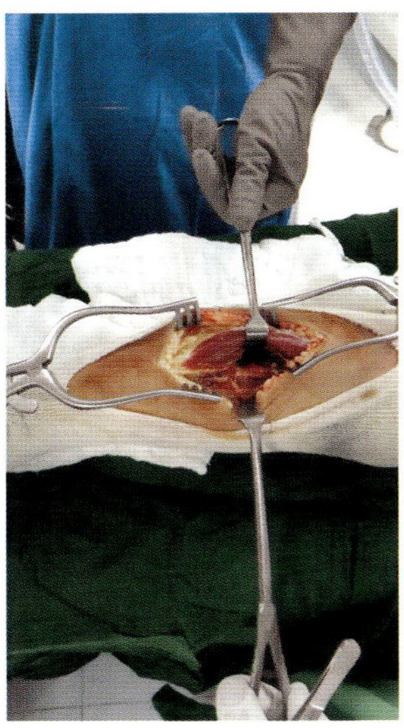

Fig. 10: Radial deep dissection—Interval between brachioradialis and flexor carpi radialis (Modified Henry's approach). Brachioradialis is a bulky muscle and occupies more than radial half of forearm in its proximal part. Radial artery is immediately deep to deep fascia hence opening of deep fascia needs to be done carefully.

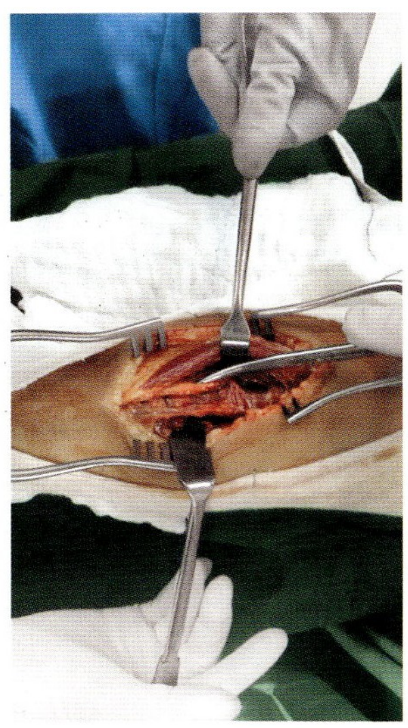

Fig. 11: Radial artery retracted medially along with flexor carpi radialis and superficial branch of radial nerve retracted laterally along with brachioradialis.

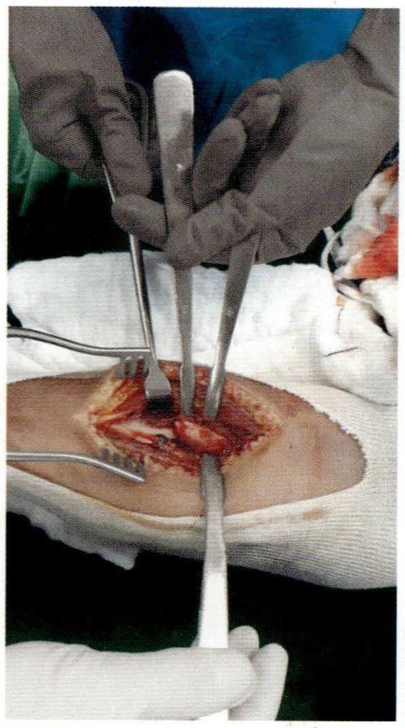

Fig. 12: Radius fracture exposed.

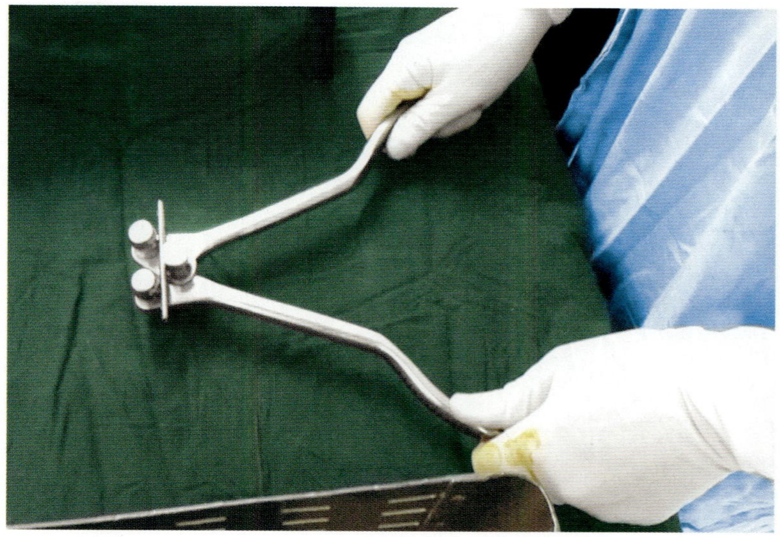

Fig.13: Contouring of dynamic compression plate (DCP) with plate bender is done to avoid opening of opposite cortex at fracture site in view of radial bow.

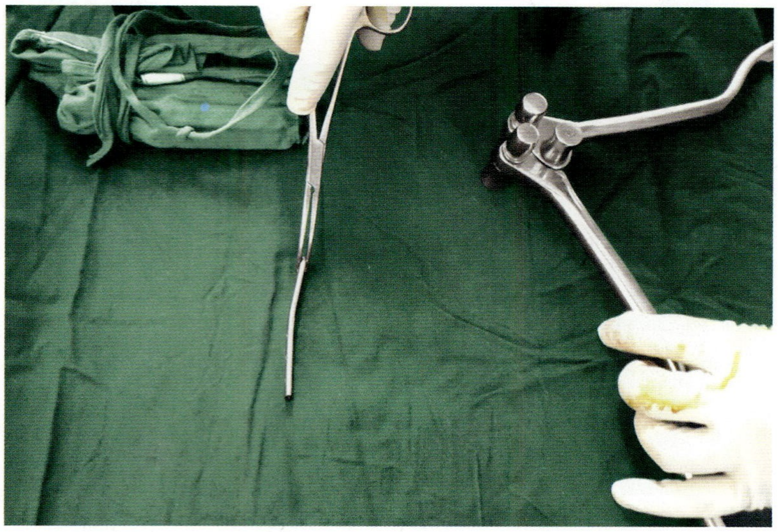

Fig. 14: Contoured plate [dynamic compression plate (DCP)].

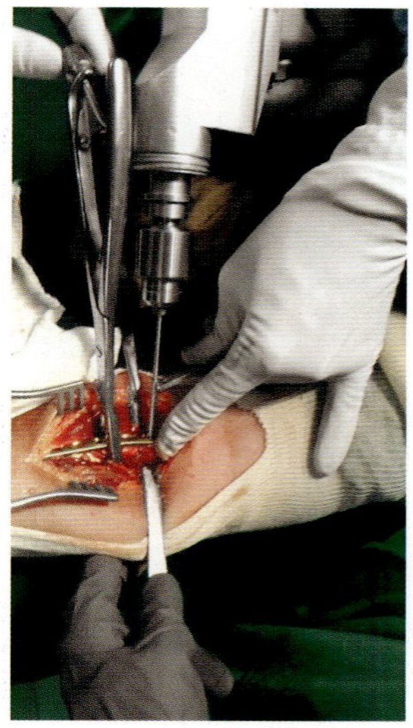

Fig. 15: Reduction done with forceps application and drilling of proximal cortical screw performed. Always drilling is performed first in the fragment which is having obtuse angle with the fracture line. Consider interfragmentary screw insertion in oblique fracture pattern to provide more stability.

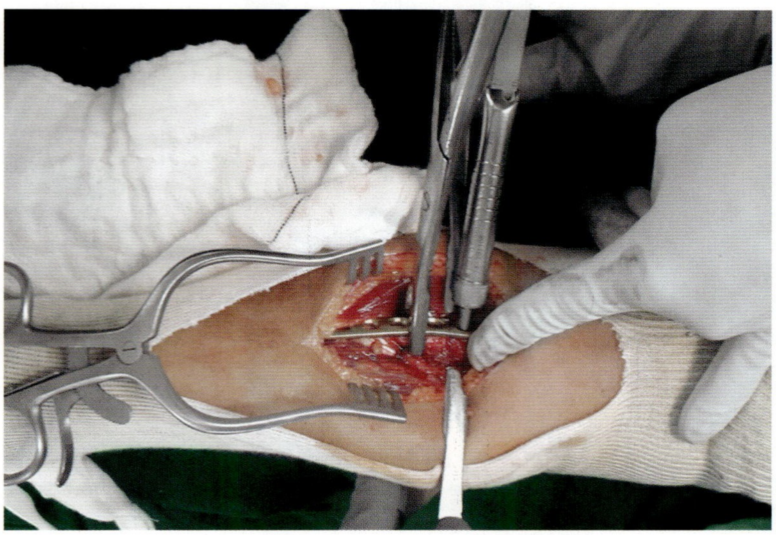

Fig. 16: Measuring proximal screw length.

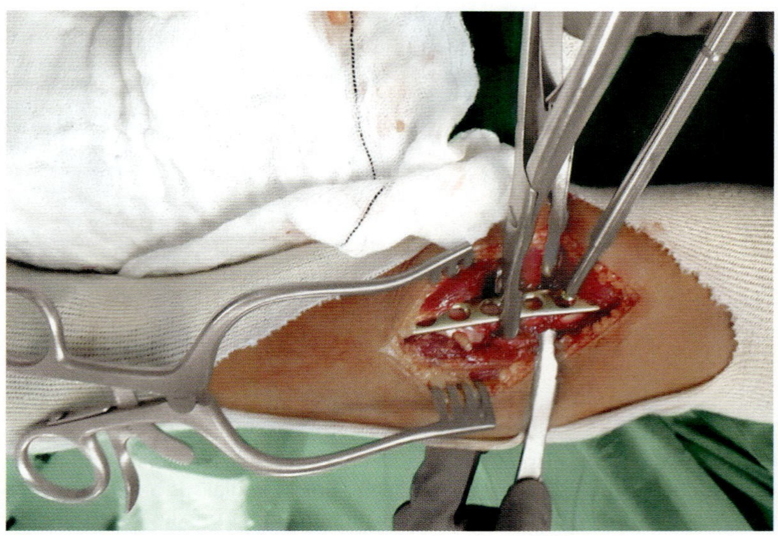

Fig. 17: Proximal cortical screw insertion (Do not tighten the screw completely).

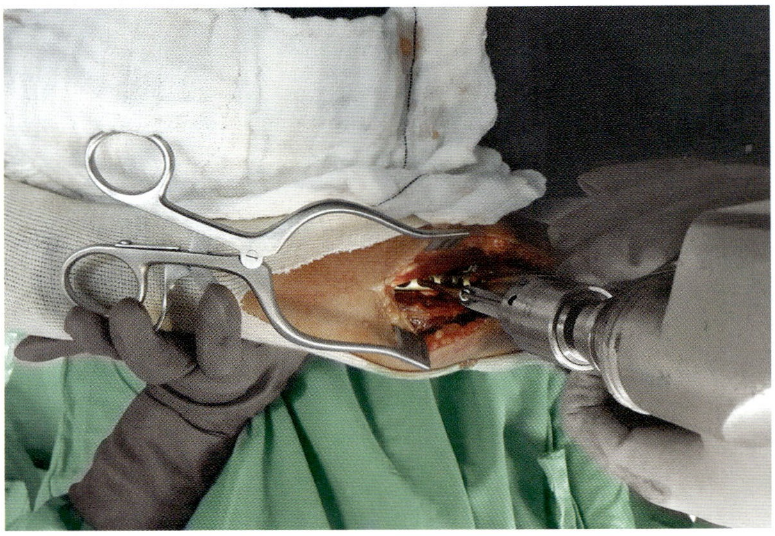

Fig. 18: Drilling of distal cortical screw. Eccentric drilling is an option in case of transverse fracture as it enables compression at fracture site. Care to be taken to ensure that end screws are not eccentrically located on shaft.

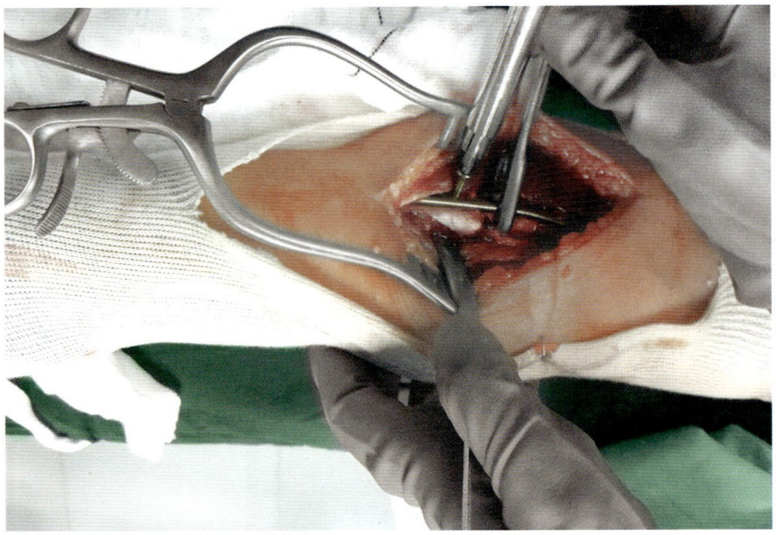

Fig. 19: Distal cortical screw insertion (both the screws are tightened alternatively while checking of compression at fracture site). In comminuted fracture compression is avoided.

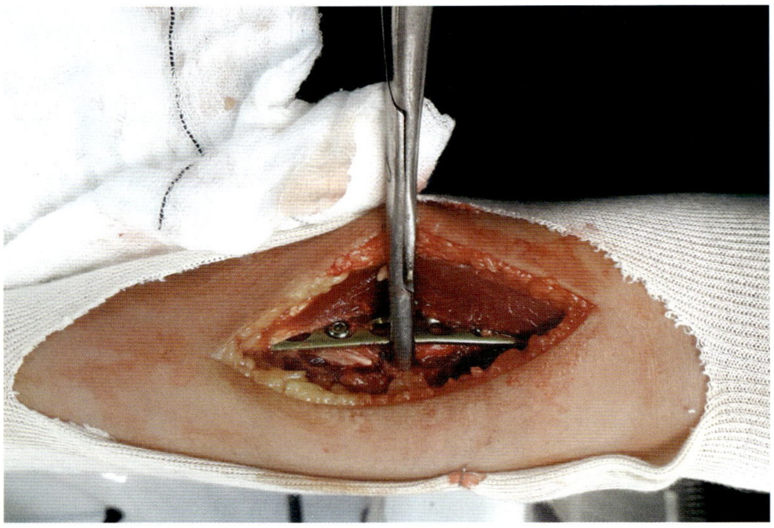

Fig. 20: Check the reduction of the fracture and then complete the rest of screws insertion.

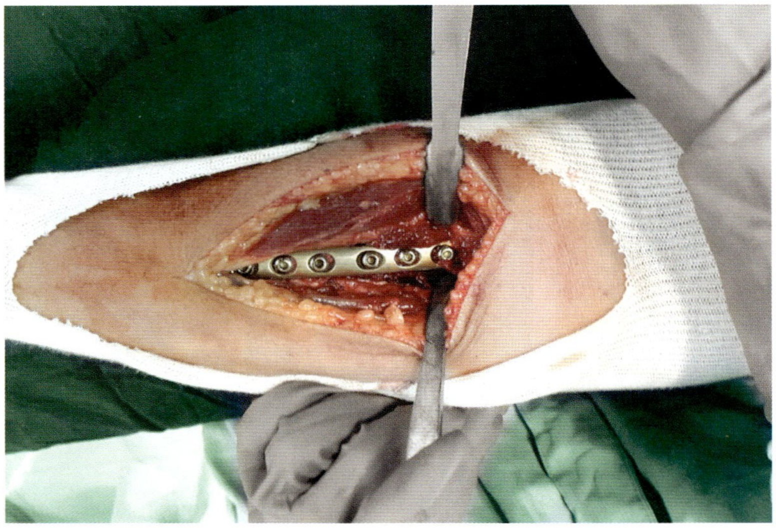

Fig. 21: Final radial [dynamic compression plate (DCP)] fixation.

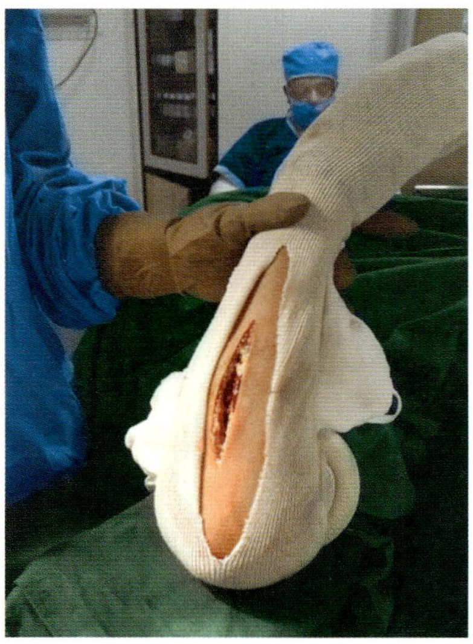

Fig. 22: Dorsal approach over subcutaneous border of ulna.

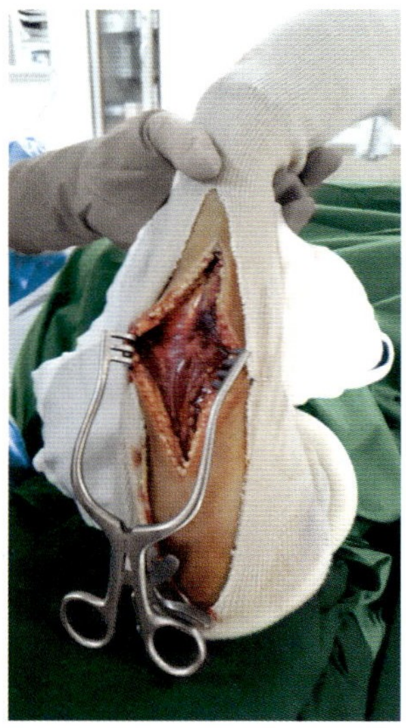

Fig. 23: Ulnar superficial dissection.

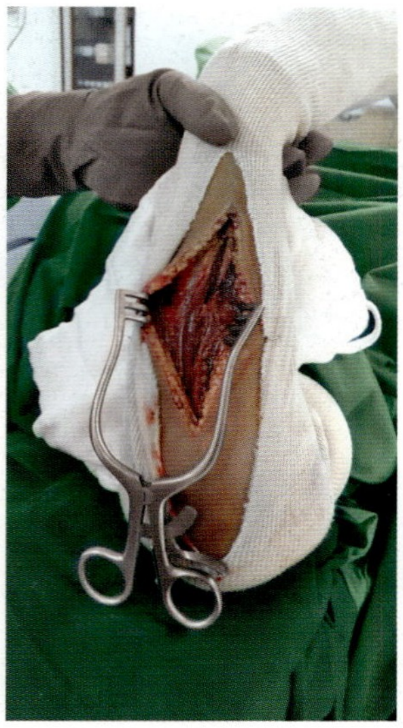

Fig. 24: Ulnar deep dissection between extensor carpi ulnaris and flexor carpi ulnaris.

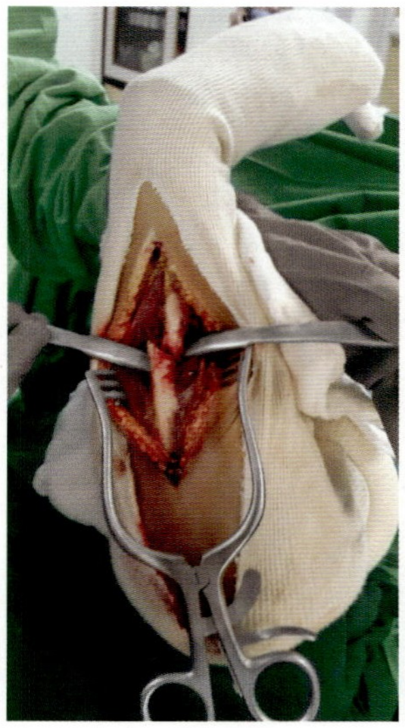

Fig. 25: Ulna fracture exposed.

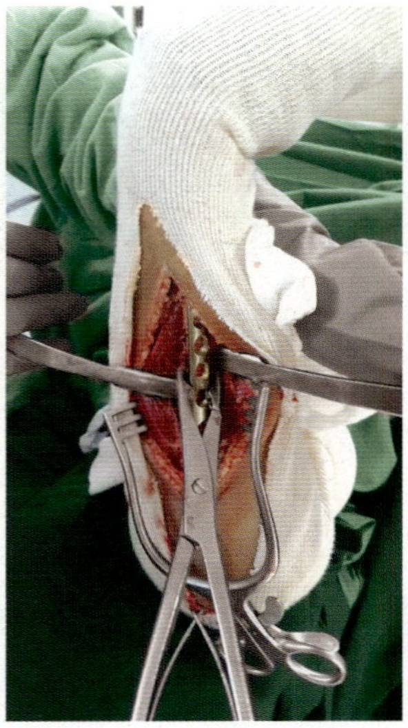

Fig. 26: Reduction forceps application over dynamic compression plate (DCP) over dorsal aspect of ulna.

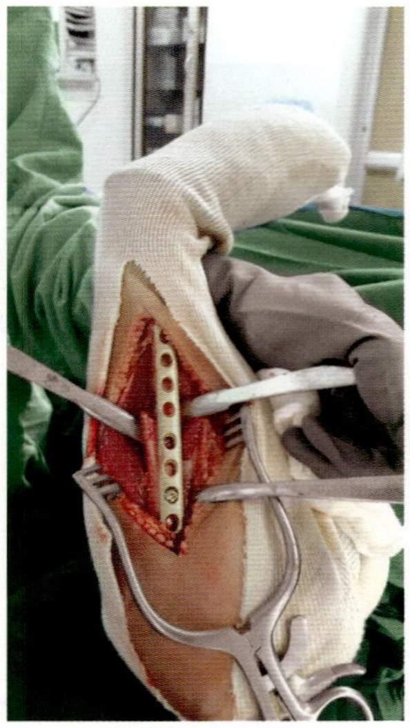

Fig. 27: Proximal cortical screw inserted.

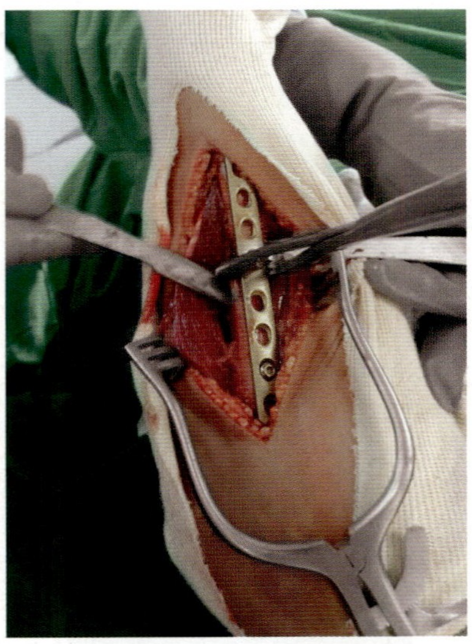

Fig. 28: Final reduction with reduction forceps achieved.

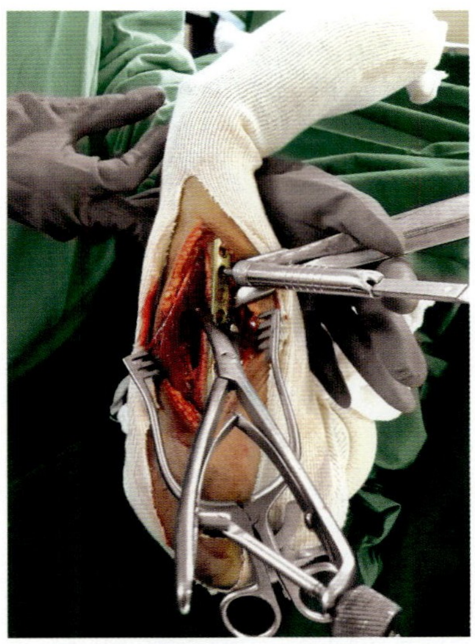

Fig. 29: Distal cortical screw length measurement and screw insertion. Care to be taken to ensure that end screws are not eccentrically located on shaft.

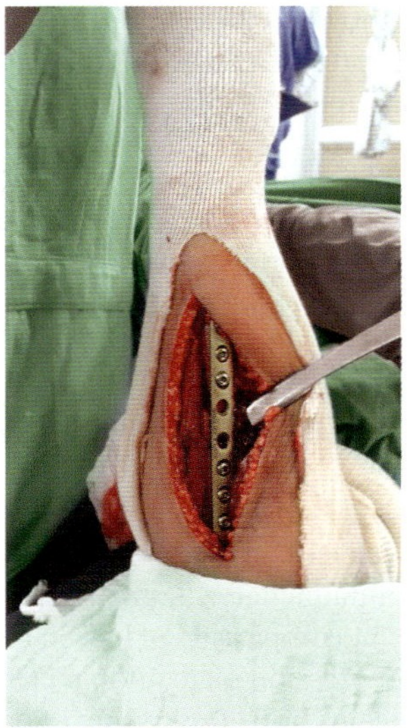

Fig. 30: Ulna final [dynamic compression plate (DCP)] fixation (Leaving two central holes overlying comminuted fragment).

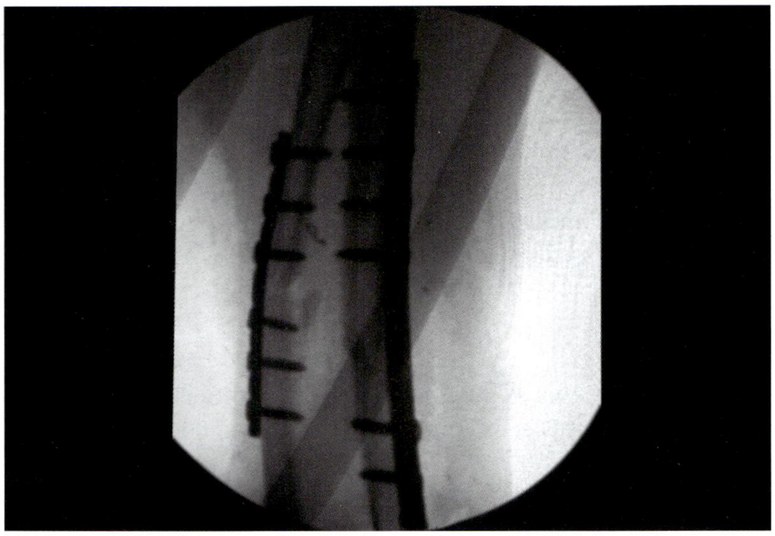

Fig. 31: Final C-arm image of radius-ulna [dynamic compression plate (DCP)] fixation.

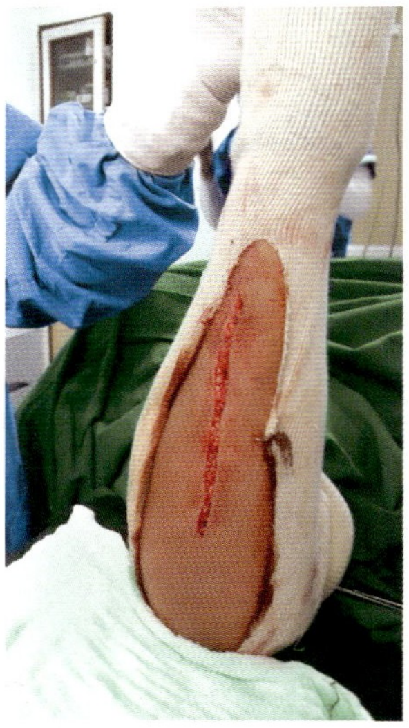

Fig. 32: Ulnar incision subcutaneous tissue closure.

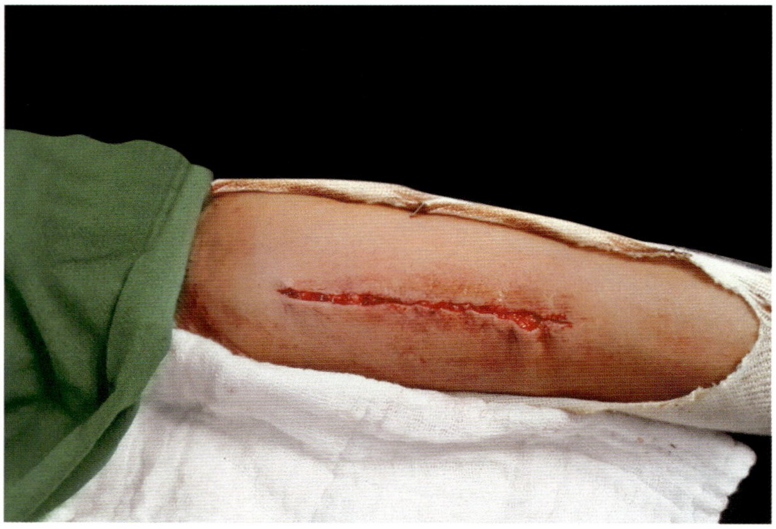

Fig. 33: Radial incision subcutaneous tissue closure.

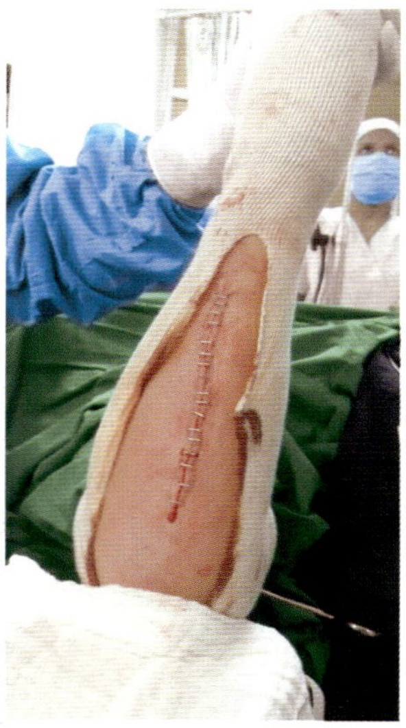

Fig. 34: Ulnar incision staples application.

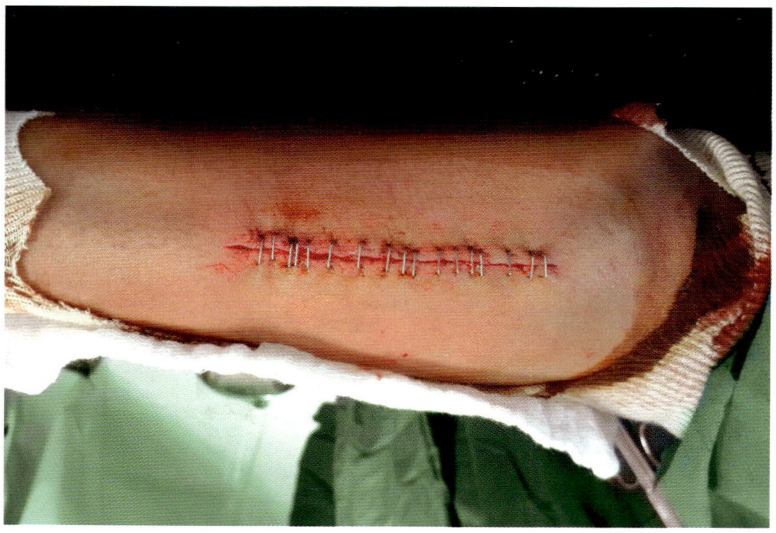

Fig. 35: Radial incision staples application.

COMPLICATIONS

- Nonunion and malunion
- Infection
- Neurovascular injury
- Compartment syndrome
- Volkmann contracture
- Posttraumatic radioulnar synostosis.

SUGGESTED READING

1. Anderson LD, Sisk D, Tooms RE, et al. Compression-plate fixation in acute diaphyseal fractures of the radius and ulna. J Bone Joint Surg Am. 1975;57:287-97.
2. Azboy I, Demirtas A, Uçar BY, et al. Effectiveness of locking versus dynamic compression plates for diaphyseal forearm fractures. Orthopedics. 2013;36:e917-22.
3. Frigg R. Locking Compression Plate (LCP). An osteosynthesis plate based on the Dynamic Compression Plate and the Point Contact Fixator (PC-Fix). Injury. 2001;32(Suppl 2):63-6.
4. Matthews LS, Kaufer H, Garver DF, et al. The effect on supination-pronation of angular malalignment of fractures of both bones of the forearm. J Bone Joint Surg Am. 1982;64(1):14-7.
5. Perren SM, Cordey J, Rahn BA, et al. Early temporary porosis of bone induced by internal fixation implants. A reaction to necrosis, not to stress protection? Clin Orthop Relat Res. 1988;232:139-51.
6. Perren SM, Klaue K, Pohler O, et al. The limited contact dynamic compression plate (LC-DCP). Arch Orthop Trauma Surg. 1990;109:304-10.
7. Sage FP, Smith H. Medullary fixation of forearm fractures. J Bone Joint Surg Am. 1957;39-A(1):91-8.
8. Saikia K, Bhuyan S, Bhattacharya T, et al. Internal fixation of fractures of both bones forearm: comparison of locked compression and limited contact dynamic compression plate. Indian J Orthop. 2011;45:417-21.
9. Wahsh AA. Exposure of both the radius and ulna through a single posterior incision: a technical note. SICOT J. 2015;1:21.

CHAPTER 94

Galeazzi Fracture Fixation with Dynamic Compression Plate

Mayur Purandare, Ranjit Rajure

INTRODUCTION

Galeazzi fracture is the fracture of radius at junction of middle-third and distal third with associated subluxation or dislocation of distal radioulnar joint (DRUJ). Galeazzi first described it in 1934.

CLASSIFICATION

Galeazzi fracture is seen among 3% of all forearm fractures and is more common in Males. Rettig et al. classified it into two types: *type 1*: Fracture lies in distal third radius (within 7.5 cm of distal radial articular surface) and *type 2*: Fracture lies in middle-third (more than 7.5 cm of articular surface). Type 2 fractures are more likely to have DRUJ instability.

CLINICAL FEATURES

Patients usually present with history of trauma, pain, swelling in forearm, deformity, and abnormal mobility. One should always do neurovascular evaluation and look for passive stretch pain as well.

RADIOLOGICAL EVALUATION

Anteroposterior and lateral radiographs usually provide sufficient information for further treatment.

TREATMENT

Galeazzi fracture dislocation is also called "the fracture of necessity". Open reduction and internal fixation of radial shaft with 3.5 dynamic compression plate (DCP) is treatment of choice in adults. Reduction and rigid anatomical fixation of radial shaft usually reduces the DRUJ dislocation.

SURGICAL STEPS

Full length radiographs anteroposterior (AP) and lateral view of forearm showing Galeazzi fracture dislocation (Figs. 1A and B).

Step 1: Instruments required. (1) Drill, (2) 3.5 dynamic compression plate (DCP) set, (3) reduction forceps, (4) retractors, and (5) periosteum elevator (Fig. 2).

Step 2: Position should be supine with arm on radiolucent side table. Use Tourniquet whenever feasible (Figs. 3A and B).

Step 3: Forearm in supination. Incision marked (Fig. 4).

Step 4: Skin incision centered on fracture. Henry's anterior approach is used to reach fracture site (Fig. 5). Internervous plane is between brachioradialis and flexor carpi radialis. Sensory branch of radial nerve lies below brachioradialis, identified and protected. Radial artery and flexor carpi radialis are mobilized and retracted medially. Pronator teres and flexor pollicis longus elevated subperiosteally to expose fracture site.

Step 5: Plate is contoured on table before fixation for better far cortex approximation (Fig. 6).

Step 6: Fracture is reduced anatomically. Plate is positioned (Fig. 7).

Step 7: Drilling with 2.7 mm drill bit. Eccentric drilling done for first screw to achieve compression at fracture site.

Step 8: Tapping done.

Step 9: Depth gauge used to estimate screw length (Fig. 8).

Step 10: Screw inserted with screw driver. Minimum six cortices hold in either side.

Step 11: Eccentric screw placement usually helps in achieving compression at fracture site (Fig. 9).

Step 12: Interfragmentary position screw after plate fixation is an option (at surgeon's discretion) (Fig. 10).

After anatomical and rigid fixation of radius (Fig. 11), stability of distal radioulnar joint (DRUJ) is assessed.

If DRUJ is still unstable, it can be transfixed with single Kirschner wire temporarily with forearm in supination.

Step 13: Closure is performed in a standard manner in layers. Absorbable for subcutaneous tissue and nonabsorbable for skin.

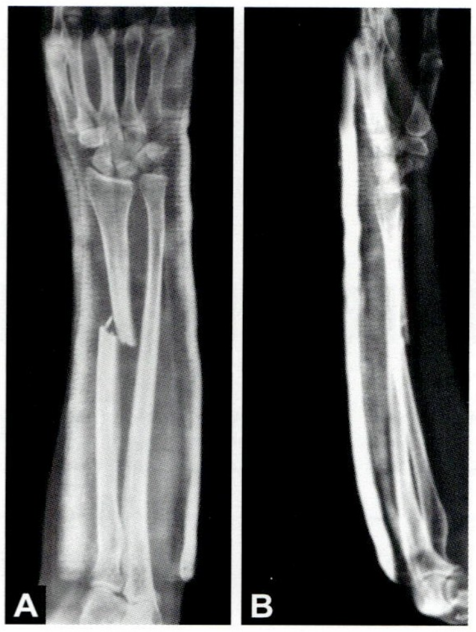

Figs. 1A and B: Anteroposterior and Lateral views of Forearm X-ray.

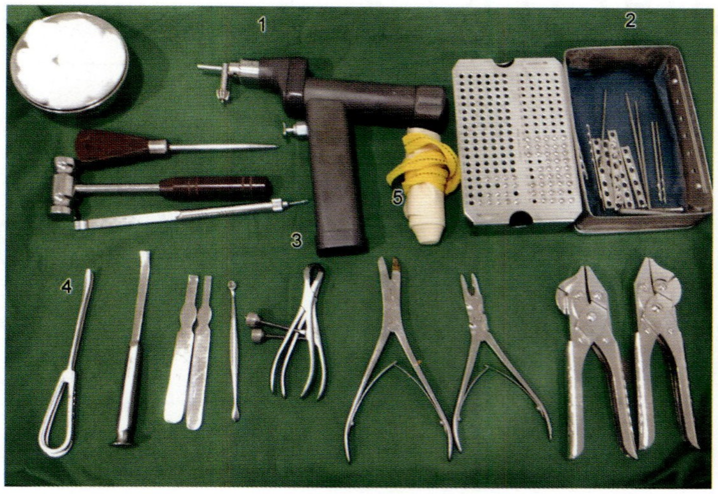

Fig. 2: Instruments required.

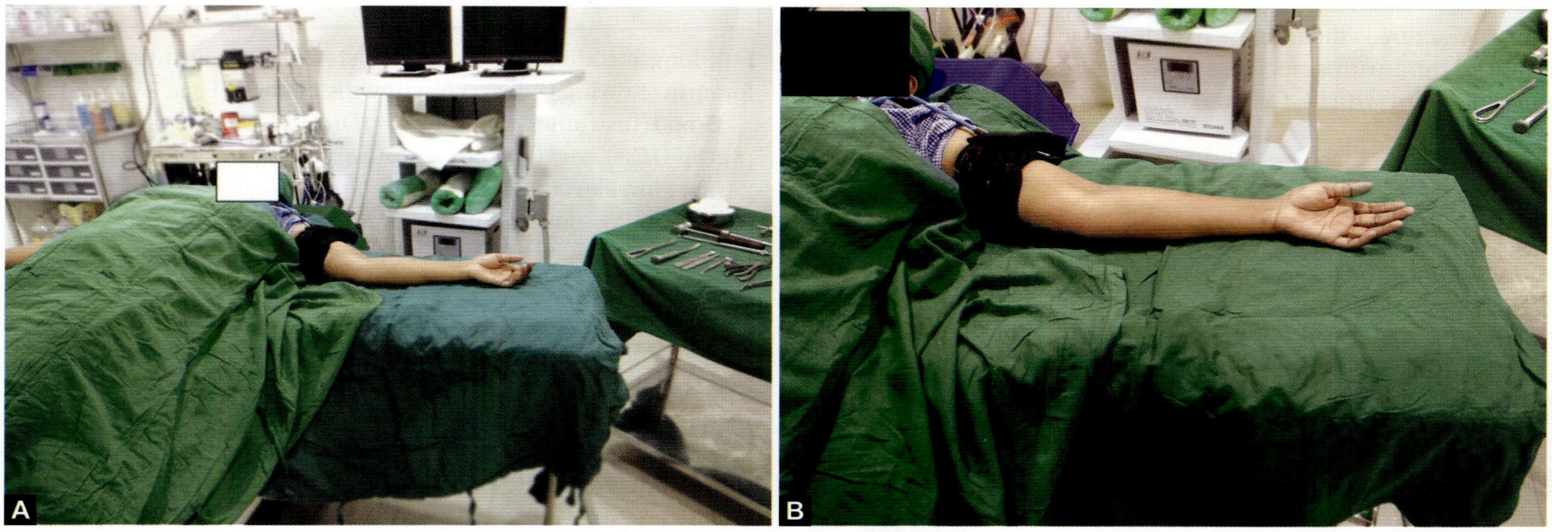

Figs. 3A and B: Position of Patient.

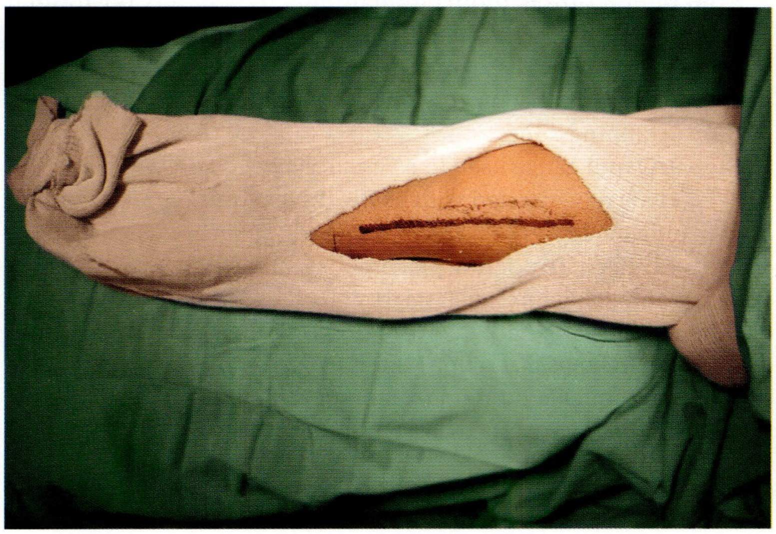

Fig. 4: Incision marked.

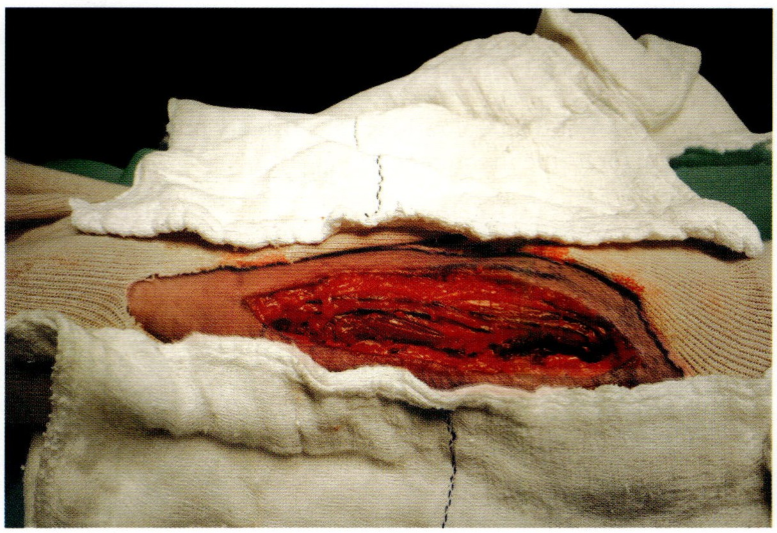

Fig. 5: Surgical exposure by Henry's anterior approach.

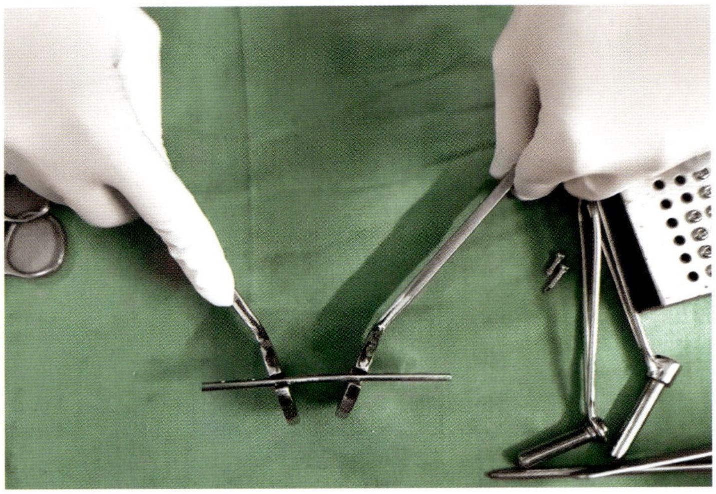

Fig. 6: Plate contoured.

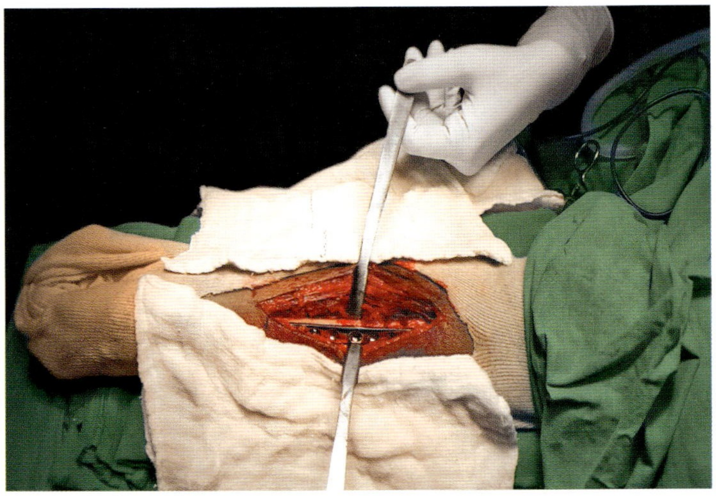

Fig. 7: Plate positioning.

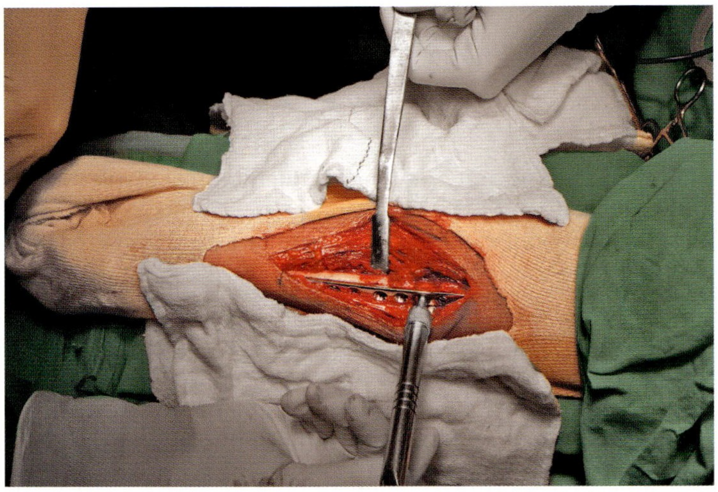

Fig. 8: Depth gauge used to measure screw length after drilling.

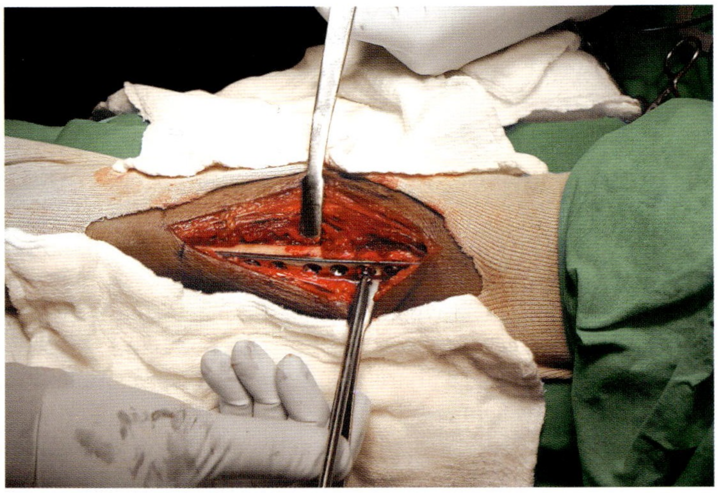

Fig. 9: Eccentric screw placement to achieve compression at fracture site.

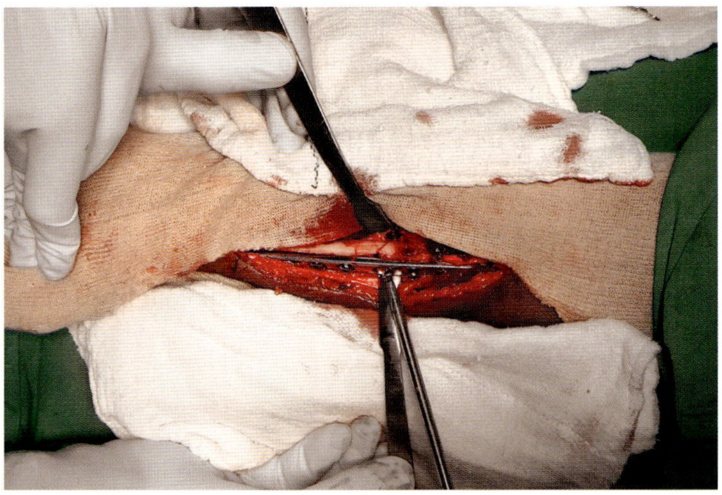

Fig. 10: Interfragmentary screw through plate can be placed.

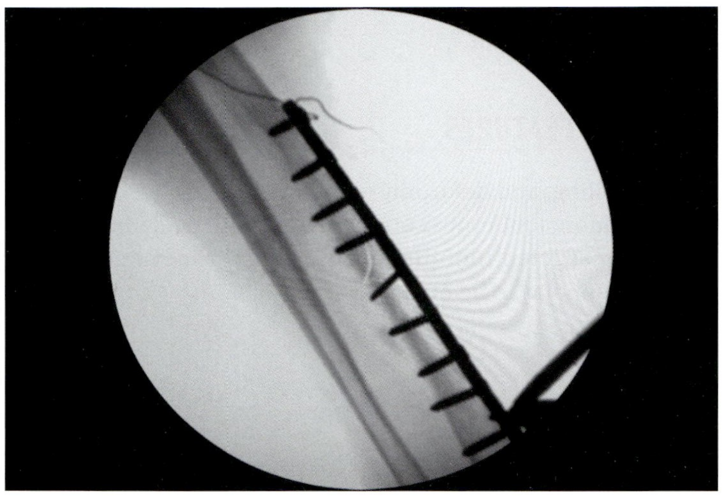

Fig. 11: Satisfactory reduction and implant placement/screw lengths noted. DRUJ stability assessed under image intensifier.

POSTOPERATIVE PROTOCOL

- Forearm may be immobilized in slab for 4 weeks after which range of motion active and passive is started.
- Postoperative X-ray immediately and then every month.

SUGGESTED READING

1. Galeazzi R. Ueber ein besonderes syndrom bei verletzungen im Bereich der unterarmknochen. Arch Orthop Unfallchir. 1934;35:557-62.
2. Mikic ZD. Galeazzi fracture dislocations. J Bone Joint Surgery Am. 1975;57(8):1071-80.
3. Rettig ME, Reskin KB. Galeazzi fracture dislocation: a new treatment oriented classification. J Hand Surg Am. 2001;26(2):228-35.

CHAPTER 95

Fracture Distal End Radius Fixation by External Fixator

Trimbak Dapkekar, Rajkumar Ekambaram, Prateek Charuchandra Joshi

INTRODUCTION

- Fracture distal end radius is one of the most common fractures of the upper extremities.
- Most commonly seen in elderly females due to osteoporosis.
- The mechanism of injury is fall on outstretched hand.
- Can also be associated with triangular fibrocartilage complex injury and interosseous ligament injuries.
- *Colle's fracture* is extra-articular fracture with dorsal displacement in corticocancellous junction.
- *Smith's* (reverse Colle's) fracture is extra-articular fracture with ventral displacement.
- *Barton's fracture is* intra-articular fracture with either dorsal or ventral displacement.

CLINICAL FEATURES

- Pain, swelling, and deformity of the wrist.
- On palpation, tenderness on the styloid with irregularity of radial border, restricted mobility is observed. Proper neurovascular examination has to be made.
- "Dinner fork deformity" is typical due to dorsal displacement of radius distally.
- The radial styloid can be at the same or higher level than ulnar styloid.

INVESTIGATIONS

- Anteroposterior (AP) and lateral radiographs of wrist are mandatory. Normal parameters in distal end radius radiographically are:
  - Radial inclination of 18–25°
  - Radial length with 8–18 mm range
  - Palmar tilt of 8–24°
  - Positive ulnar variance.
- Computed tomography (CT) scan is required to understand fracture type and for surgical planning.

TREATMENT

- Above elbow slab with proper limb elevation to reduce swelling followed by cast immobilization for 6 weeks.
- Open reduction internal fixation can be done for Barton's fractures.
- Distractor/ligamentotaxis should be done for comminuted intra-articular fractures or unstable Colle's fractures.

SURGICAL STEPS

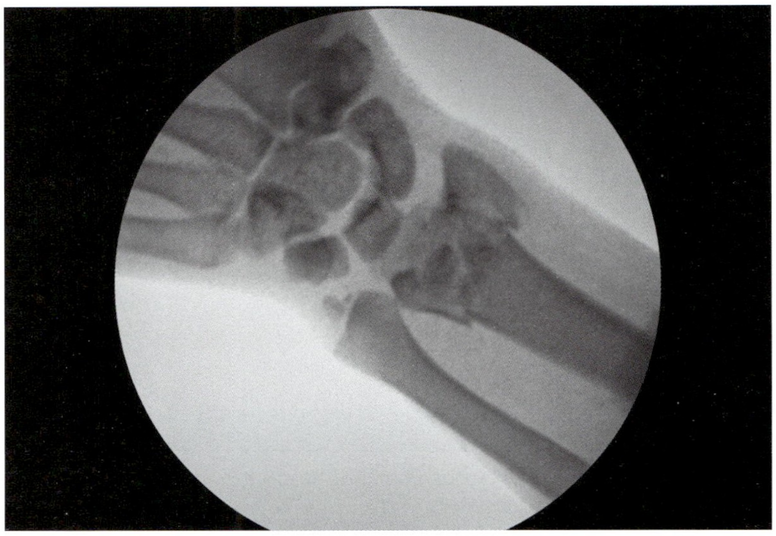

Fig. 1: Fluoroscopy showing fracture distal end radius with comminution.

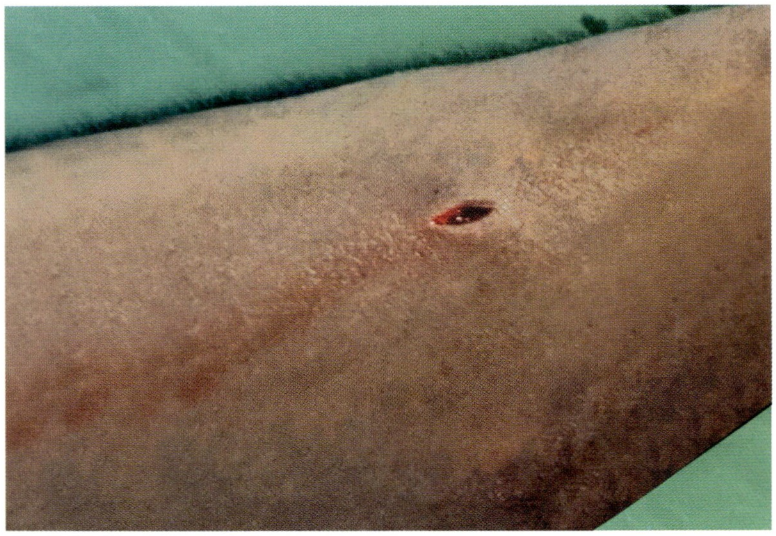

Fig. 2: Under proper sterile conditions painting and draping of the operative limb is done. Now a stab incision is taken about 5–6 cm proximal to distal end radius along the lateral border of radius.

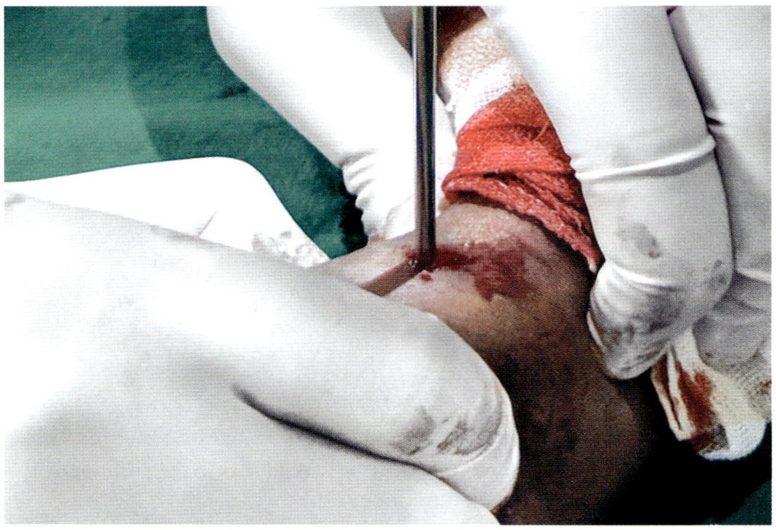

Fig. 3: Drill hole is made using 2.7-mm drill bit.

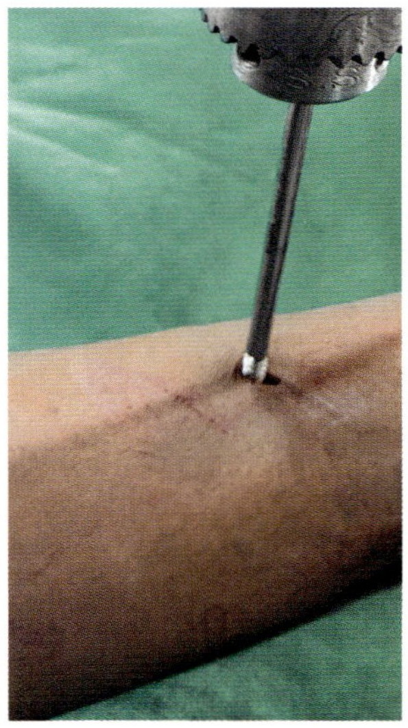

Fig. 4: Using T handle 3.2-mm Schanz pin is introduced such that there should be a bicortical purchase of radial shaft.

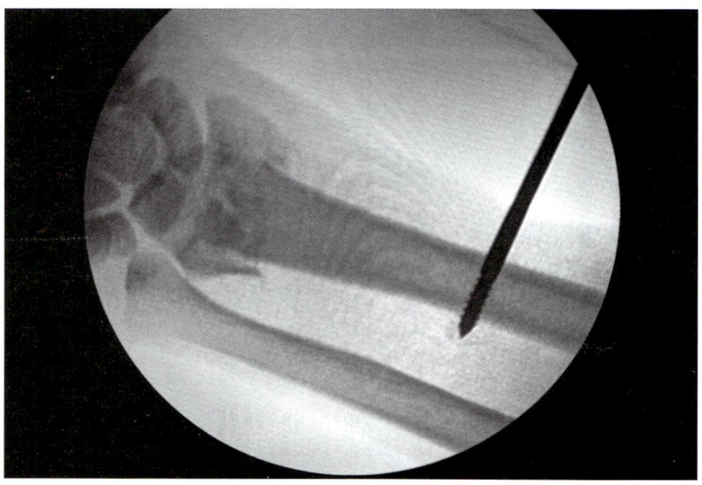

Fig. 5: Confirmation under C-arm.

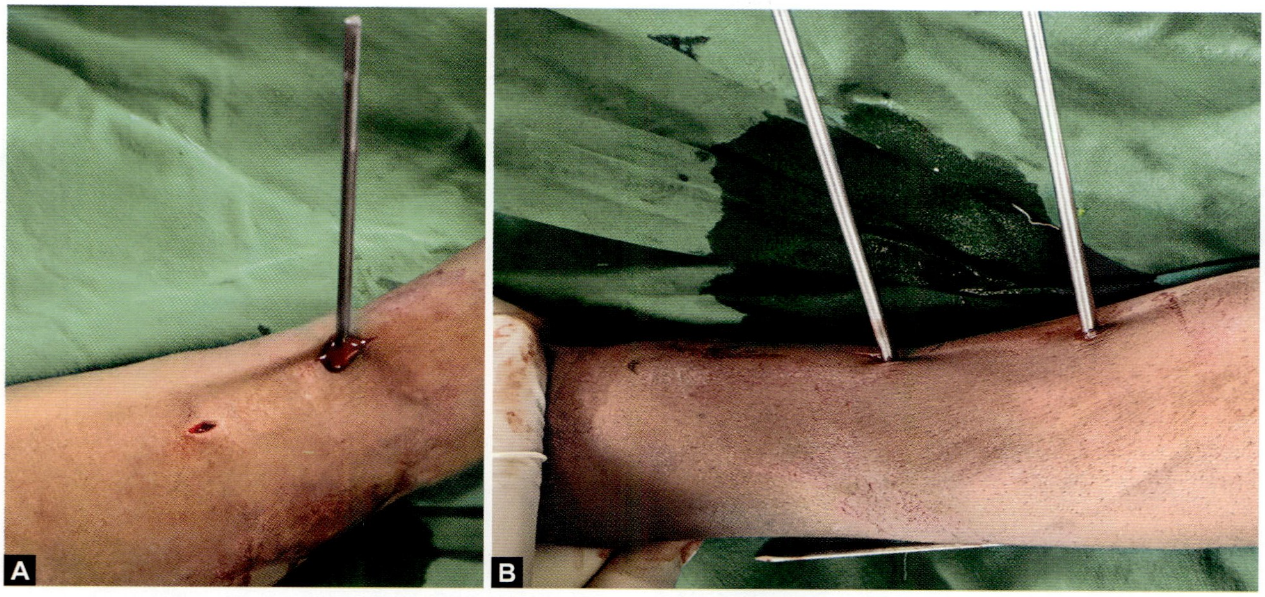

Figs. 6A and B: Another stab incision is taken three-finger proximal to the previous one and the same steps are repeated until another 3.2 mm pin is introduced.

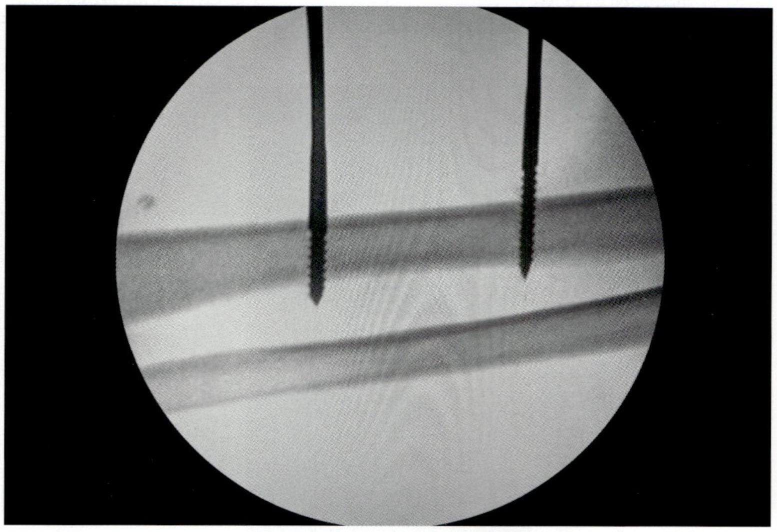

Fig. 7: Pins visualized under C-arm.

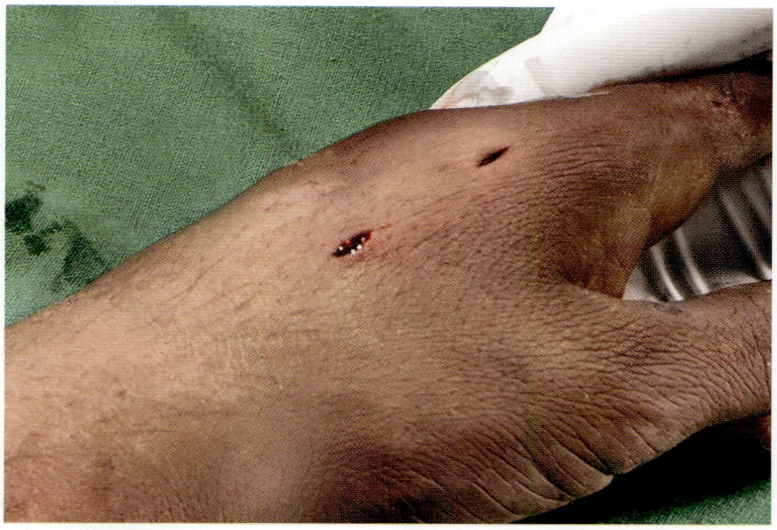

Fig. 8: Now two more stab incisions are made over base and neck of second metacarpal.

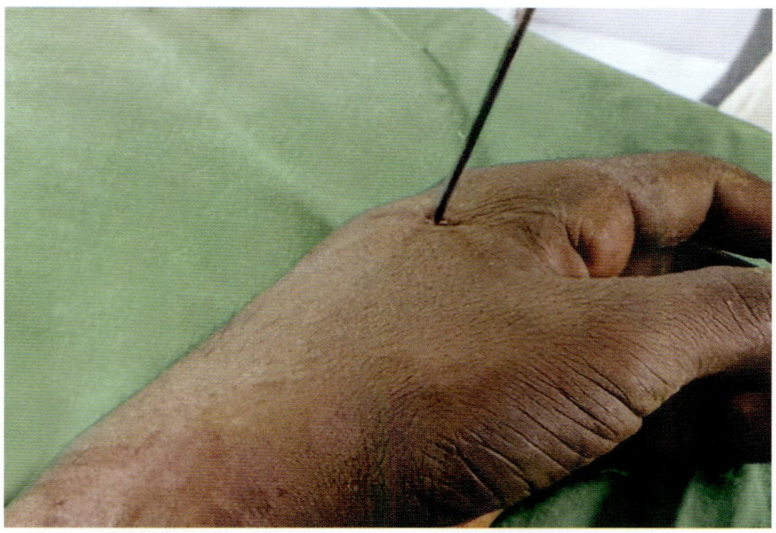

Fig. 9: Drill holes are made using 2 mm drill bit.

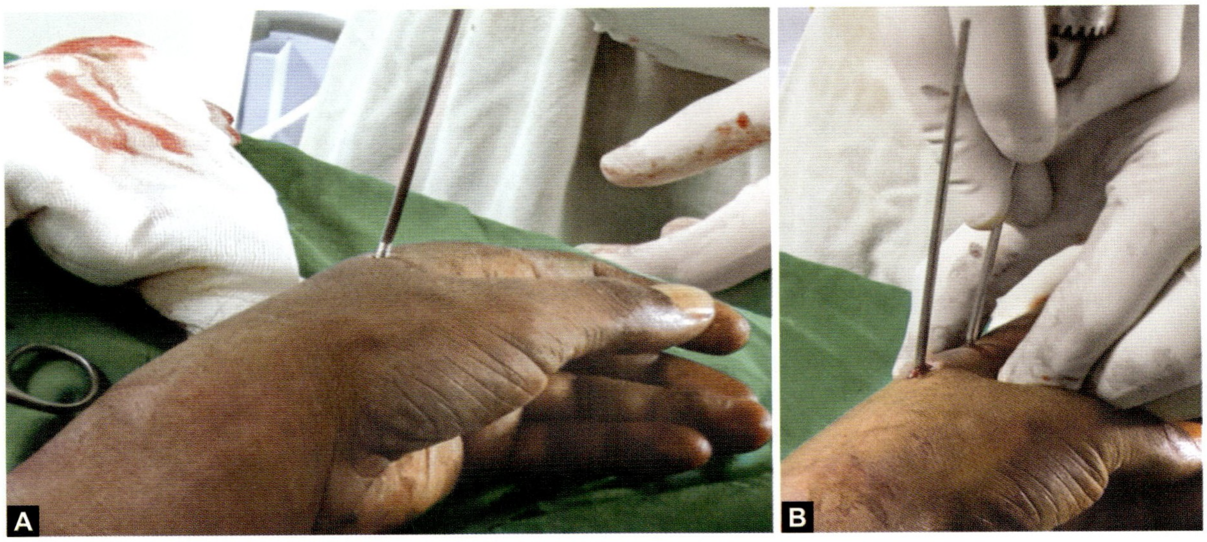

Figs. 10A and B: 2.7-mm metacarpal pins are introduced through T handle on both sites.

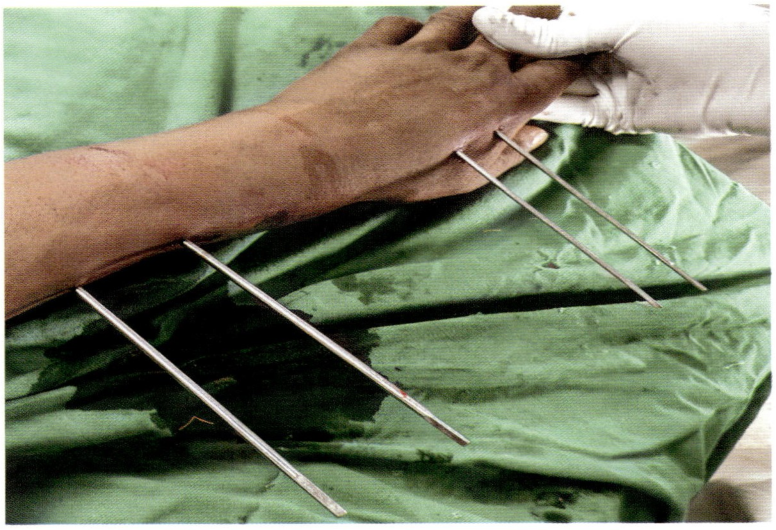

Fig. 11: Both distal pins are introduced.

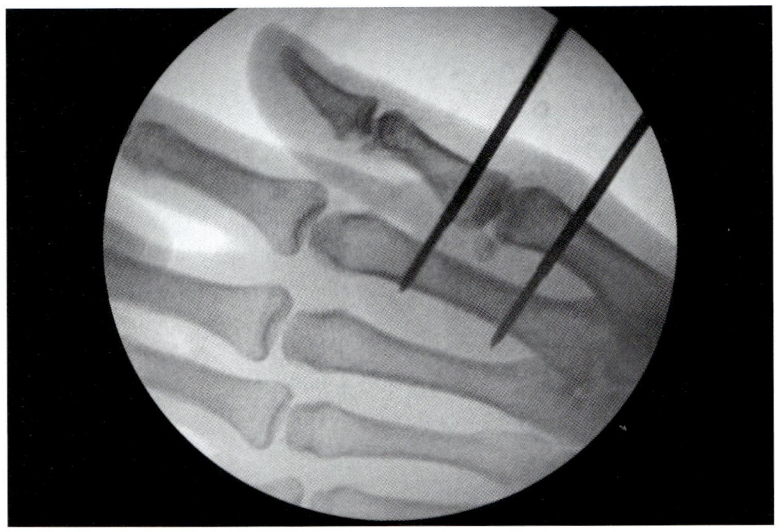

Fig. 12: C-arm confirmation of metacarpal pin insertion.

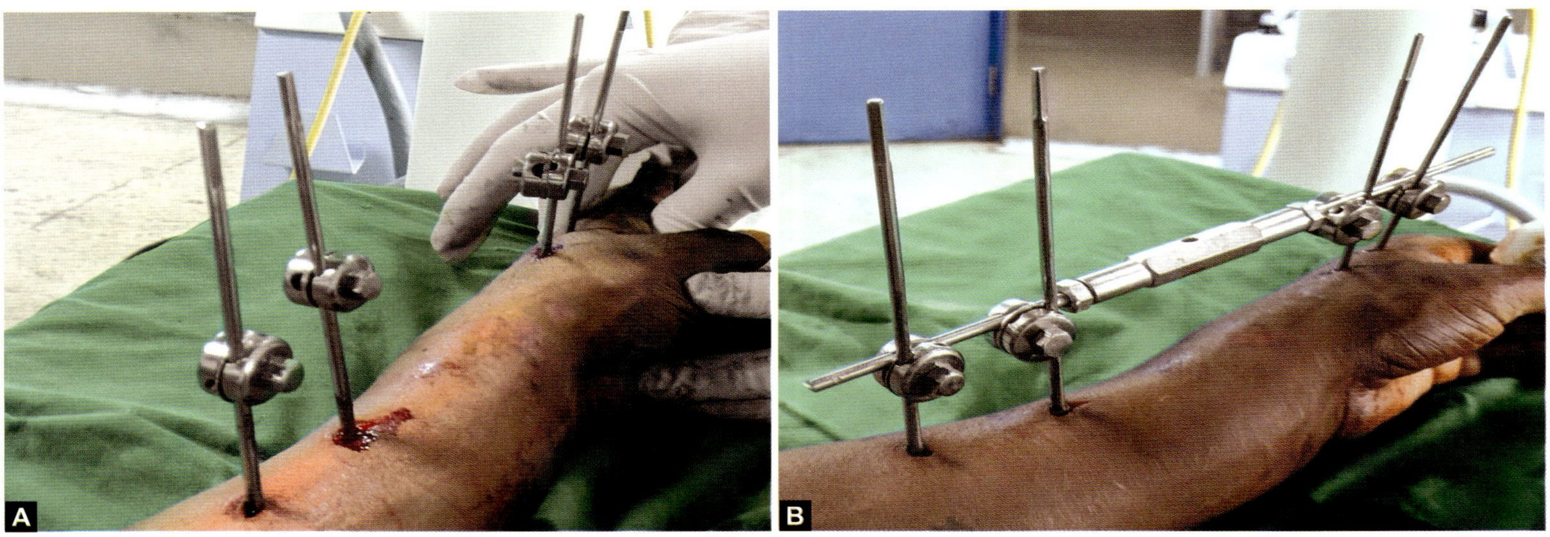

Fig. 13A and B: (A) Pins are connected to the clamps, tightened and to be checked for stability; (B) Radius distractor attached to the pins through the clamps.

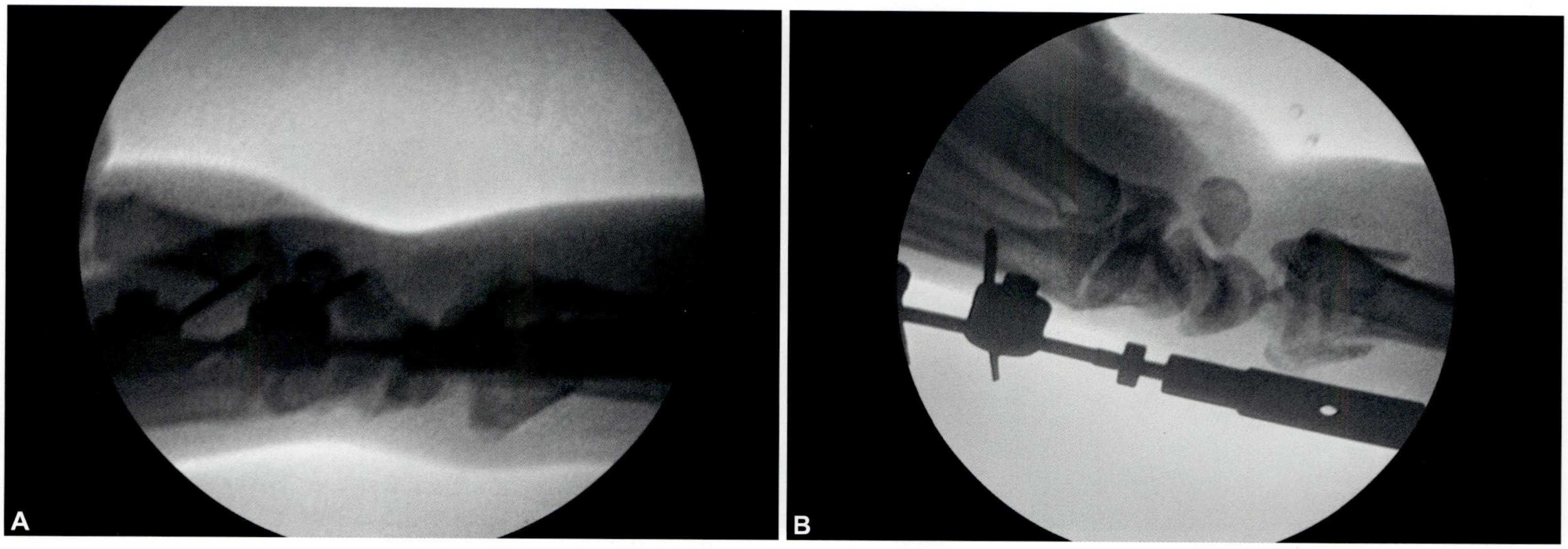

Figs. 14A and B: Visualized under C-arm after distraction.

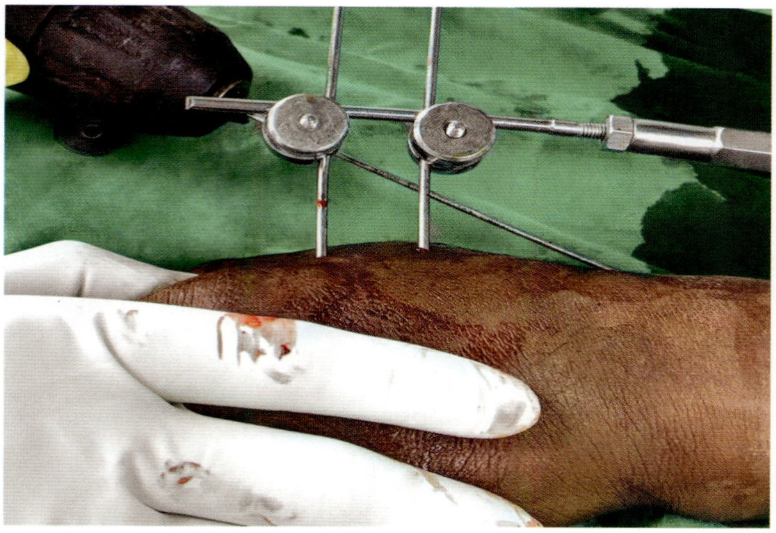

Fig. 15: After manipulation K-wire is introduced through styloid process and fixed to opposite cortex.

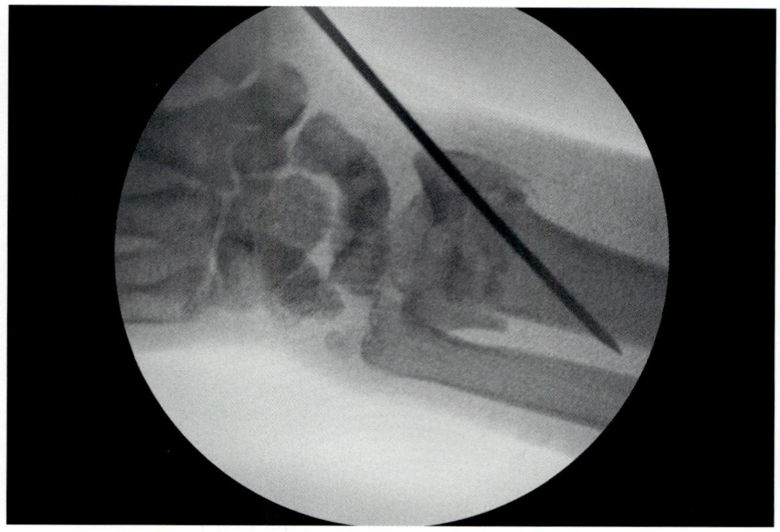

Fig. 16: K-wire seen under C-arm.

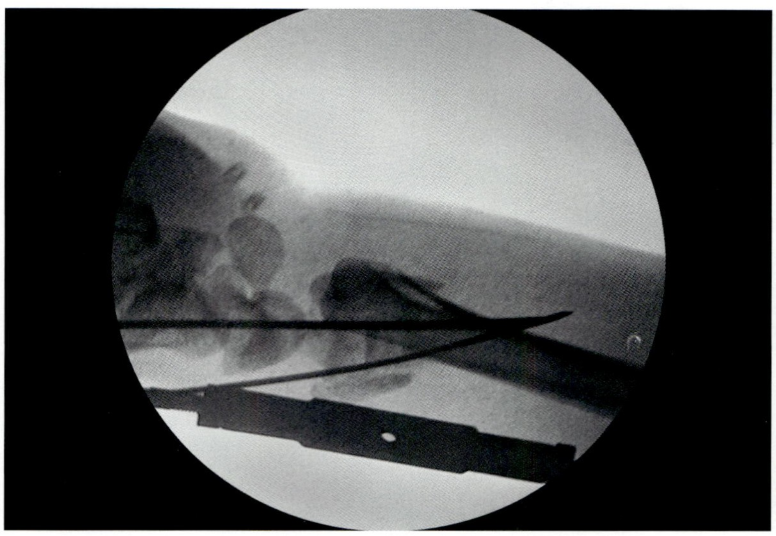

Fig. 17: Another K-wire is passed through the Lister's tubercle and fixed to opposite cortex, which is confirmed under C-arm.

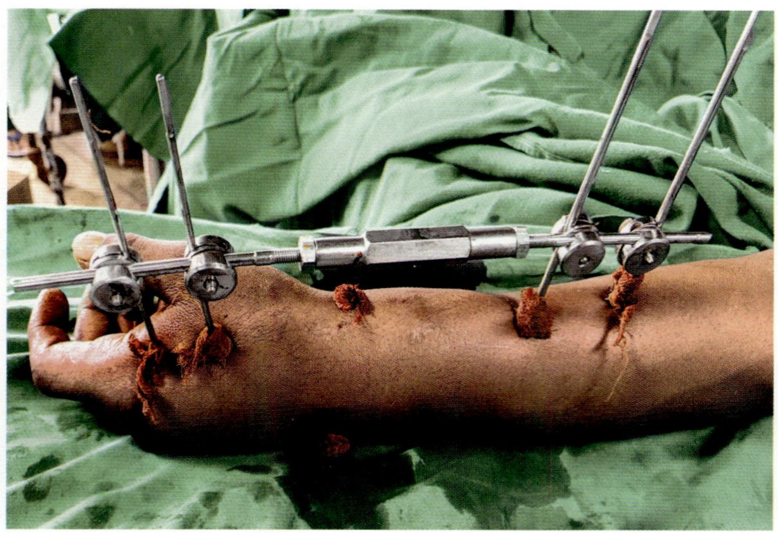

Fig. 18: Pin tract dressing done using povidone–iodine.

COMPLICATIONS

- Stiffness of wrist
- Malunion
- Inferior radioulnar joint subluxation
- Sudeck's osteodystrophy
- Rupture of extensor pollicis brevis tendon rarely.

SUGGESTED READING

1. Azar FM, Canale ST, Beaty JH. Campbell's operative orthopaedics, 13th edition. USA: Elsevier; 2017.
2. Blom A, Warwick D, Whitehouse M. Apley and Solomon's system of orthopaedics and trauma, 10th edition. Florida, USA: CRC Press; 2017.
3. Charles MC, James HD, Margaret MM, et al. Rockwood and Green's fractures in adults, 8th edition. Philadelphia: Lippincott Williams & Wilkins; 2014.
4. Miller M, Thompson S. Miller's Review of orthopaedics, 7th edition. USA: Elsevier; 2016.

CHAPTER 96

External Fixator Application for Pubic Diastasis

Nikhil Shah, Shrikant Sagane, Chittanand Mendhe

INTRODUCTION

Pubic symphysis plating is usually performed in cases of pubic diastasis. Separation of pubic symphysis without evidence of any fracture constitutes pelvic diastasis.

Separation of more than 10 mm is considered significant. One must always assess sacroiliac joint involvement in pubic diastasis.

Causes of pubic diastasis involve: pregnancy complications, trauma, sports injury, inflammatory arthritis following long-term corticosteroid intake.

INDICATIONS

Pubic symphysis plating is indicated for pubic diastasis with unstable pelvic ring injury. Symphyseal separation of more than 2.5 cm of diastasis is considered unstable and is usually treated using symphyseal plates.

Associated conditions such as wound infection, compound fracture, or neurovascular injury may necessitate temporary external fixation before the patient can be optimized for definitive fixation.

For the often-associated fracture or displacement of the posterior pelvic ring, fixation of the fracture should be done. If there is no vertical displacement (B-type injuries) then anterior reduction should usually be first.

If there is vertical displacement (C-type injuries) or if anterior reduction fails to achieve posterior reduction then posterior reduction should be performed first.

SURGICAL STEPS

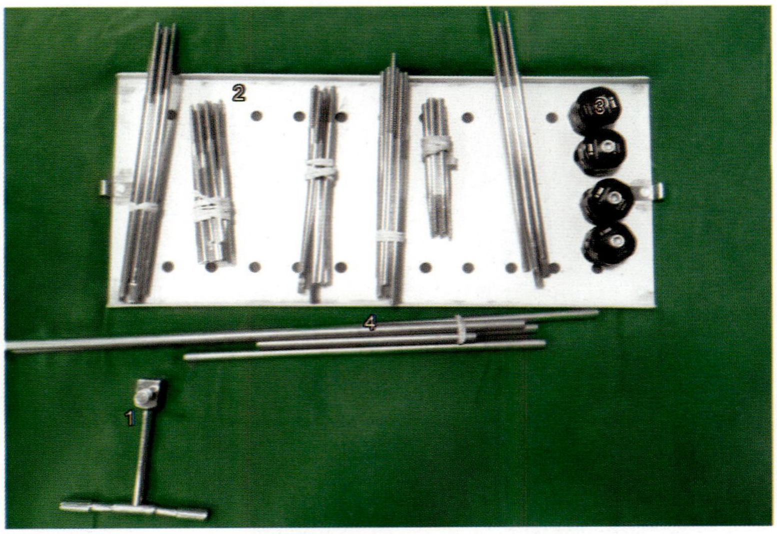

Fig. 1: External fixation requires following instruments (Fig. 1). (1) T handle or chuck, (2) Schanz pins mainly 6.5 mm of diameter, (3) Clamp(pin-to-rods and rod-to-rods variety), (4) Connecting rods of various lengths, (5) Drill bit of size 4.5 mm (not shown).

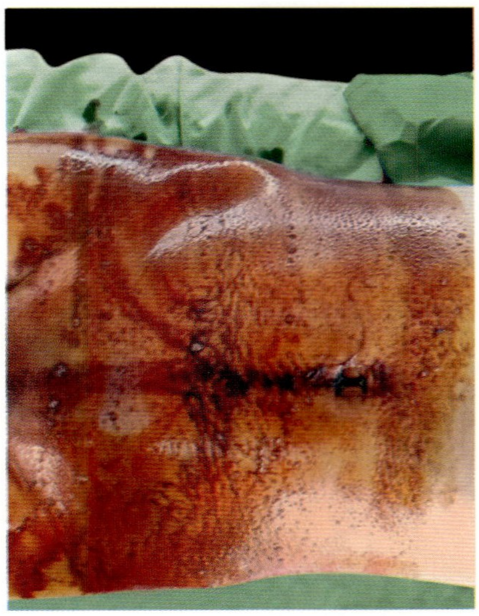

Fig. 2: Scrub and paint with povidone–iodine. The surgical site from costal margin to groin region covering both iliac borders and lateral aspect of pelvis.

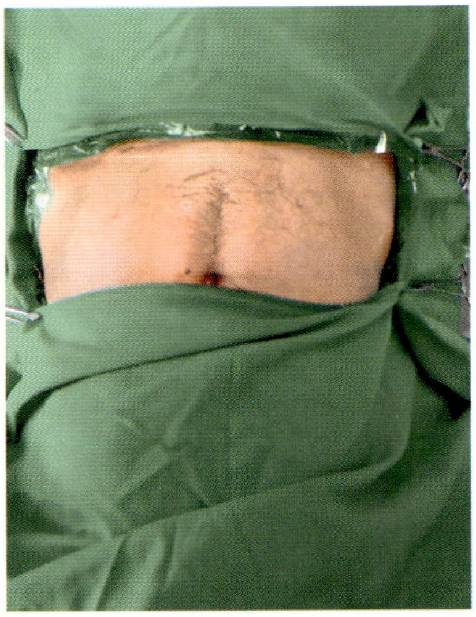

Fig. 3: Drape the surgical area with sterile drape so that anterior superior iliac spine (ASIS) and iliac crest should be visible.

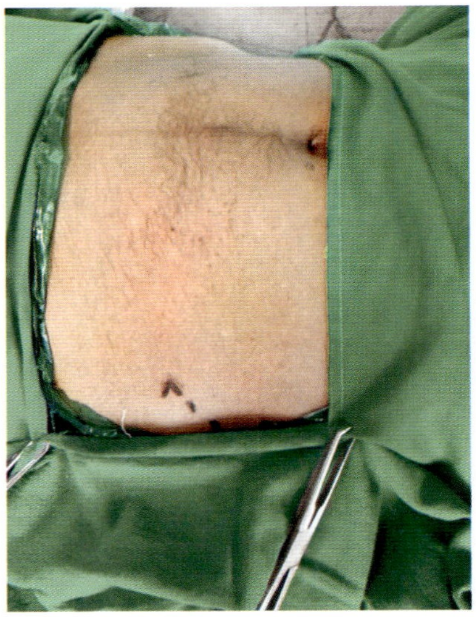

Fig. 4: Mark both anterior superior iliac spine (ASIS) with the skin marker as reference point for incision though which Schanz pin has to be inserted.

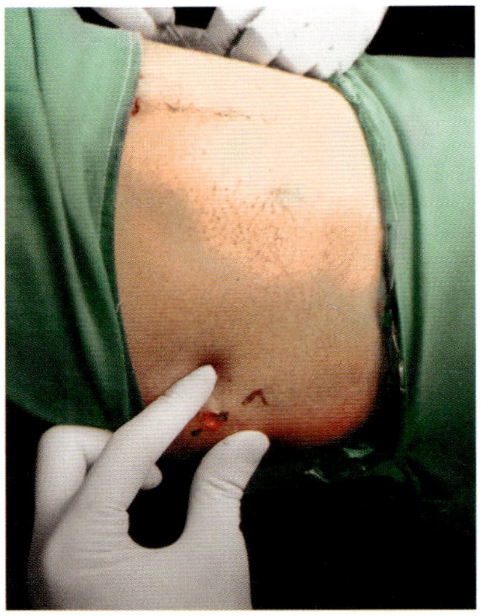

Fig. 5: Take first incision 1–2 cm posterior to anterior superior iliac spine (ASIS). Soft tissue separated with artery forceps till gritty sensation of bone is felt.

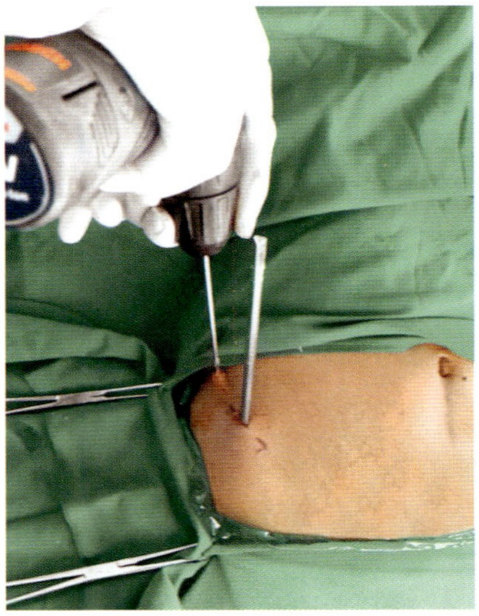

Fig. 6: Predrill with 4.5 mm drill bit with holding iliac blade between thumb and index fingure so that drill bit should not slip off from bone.

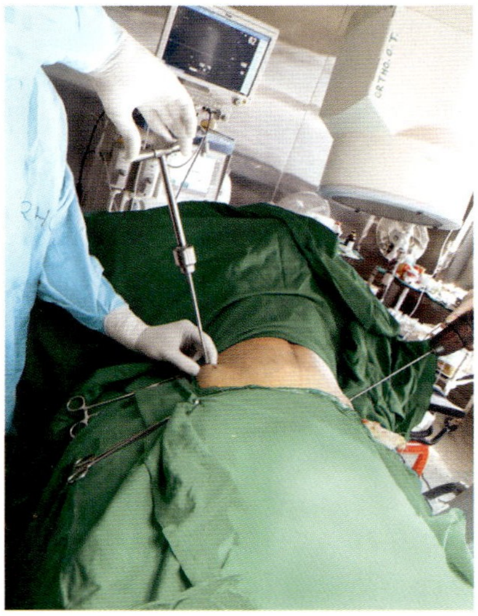

Fig. 7: Insert 6.5 mm Schanz pin with help of T handle. Bony resistance should be felt till the end during insertion to ensure positioning of the Schanz pin in bone.

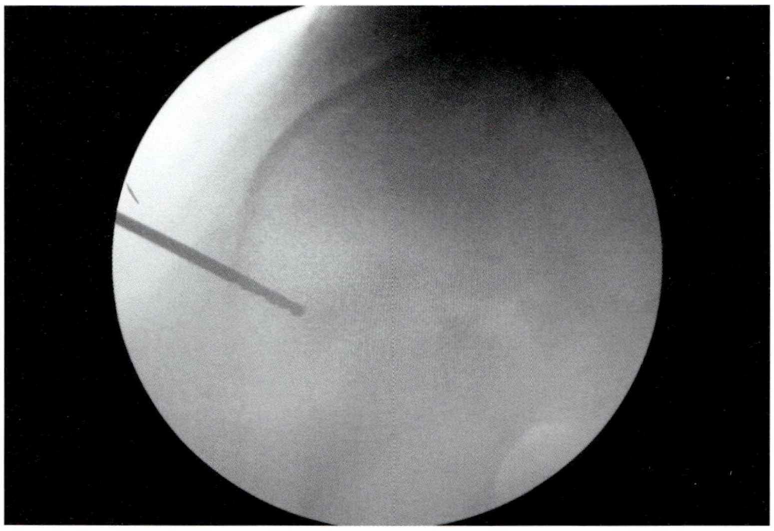

Fig. 8: Check the insertion in C-arm.

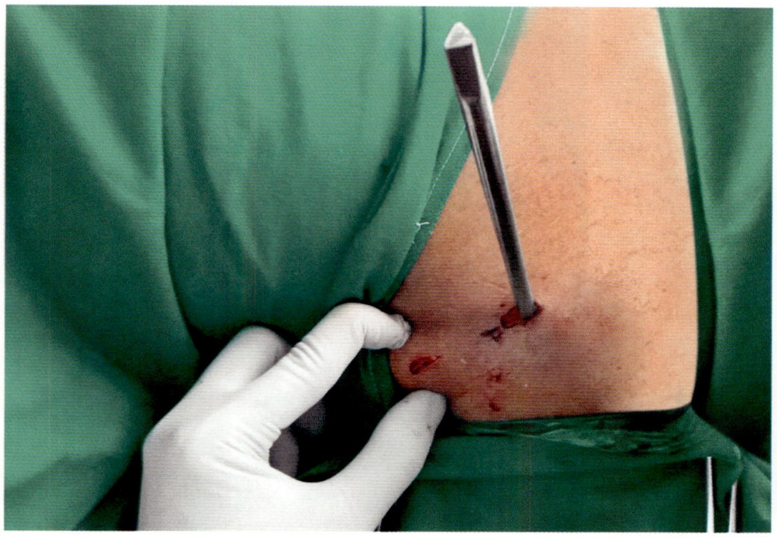

Fig. 9: Make second incision 2 cm posterior to the first one. Separate the soft tissue over the bone with forceps.

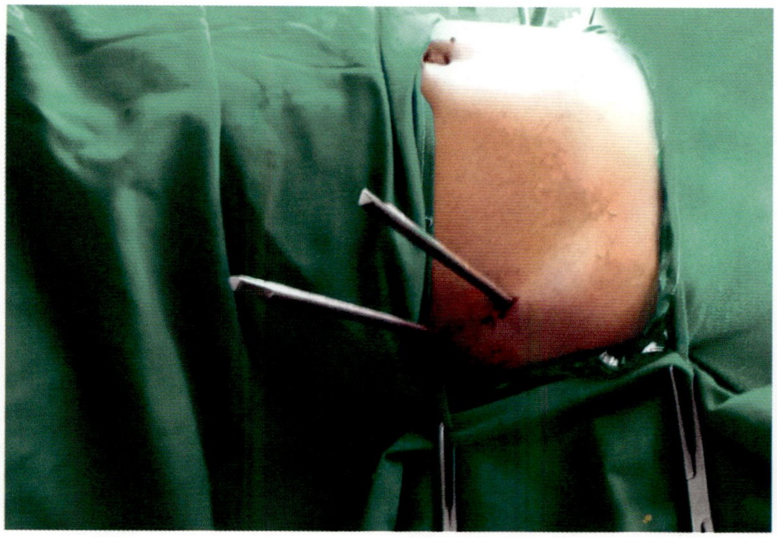

Fig. 10: Insert second Schanz pin after predrilling parallel to the first and confirm the screws are in bone.

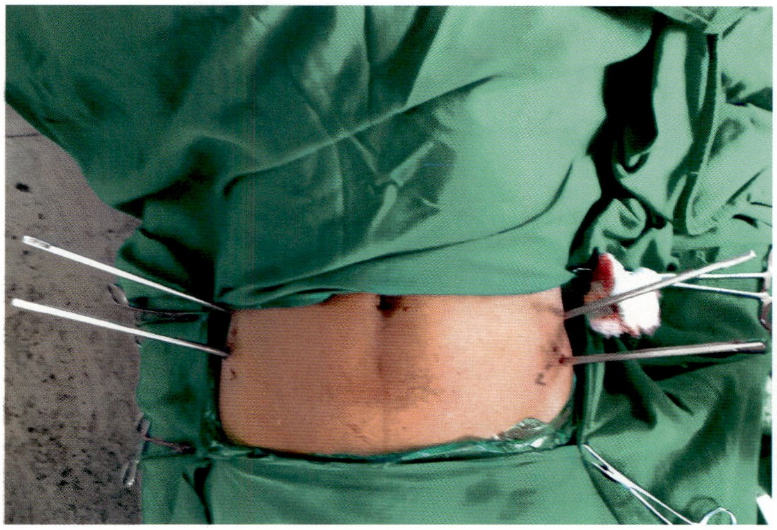

Fig. 11: Insert two Schanz screws on opposite side same as before.

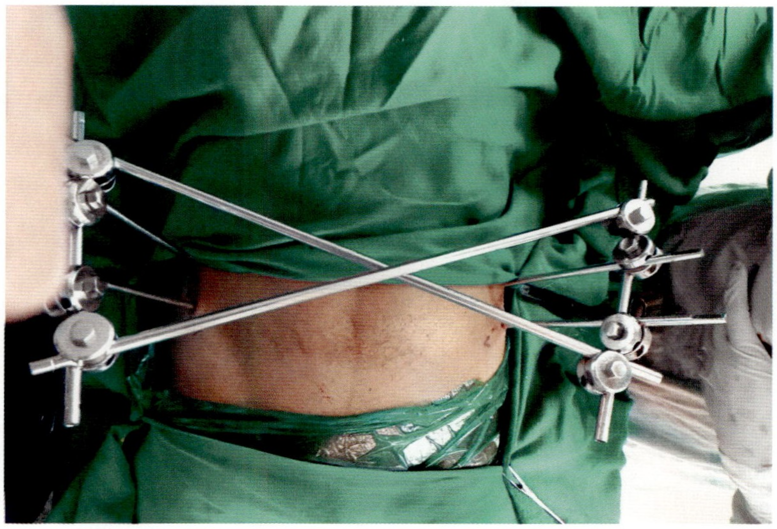

Fig. 12: Connect both side with long-connecting rods and check for stability.

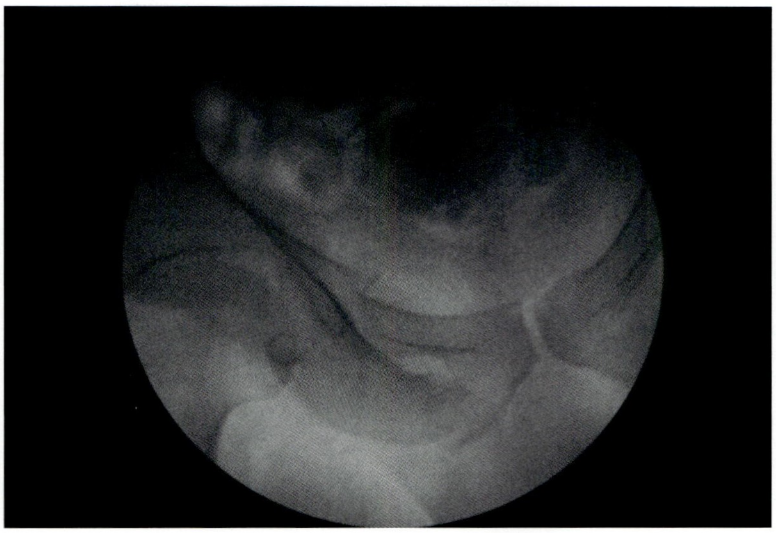

Fig. 13: Under C-arm guidance reduction achieved is confirmed.

POSTOPERATIVE PROTOCOL

- Postoperatively, weight bearing is restricted on the side of posterior ring injury for 3 months. Drain is removed after 2 days.
- After radiological evidence of fracture healing, the patient can be given trial of partial weight bearing.
- Regular wound dressing and cleaning should be done to minimize the chances of wound infection.
- Suture removal can be done after 12–15 days postoperatively.

POSSIBLE COMPLICATIONS

Apart from anesthetic complications, this surgery may be complicated by inadvertent injury to corona mortis with extensive lateral dissection.

Bladder injury is also common during drilling. A Foley's catheter should be used so as to decompress the bladder.

Postoperative surgical site infections and suture gaping can be prevented by proper wound care.

SUGGESTED READING

1. Azar FM, Canale ST, Beaty JH. Campbell's operative orthopaedics, 13th edition. USA: Elsevier; 2017.
2. Blom A, Warwick D, Whitehouse M. Apley and Solomon's system of orthopaedics and trauma, 10th edition. Florida, USA: CRC Press; 2017.
3. Charles MC, James HD, Margaret MM, et al. Rockwood and Green's fractures in adults, 8th edition. Philadelphia: Lippincott Williams & Wilkins; 2014.
4. Miller M, Thompson S. Miller's Review of Orthopaedics, 7th edition. USA: Elsevier; 2016.

CHAPTER 97

Pubic Symphysis Plate Fixation

Ambrish Mathesule, Nikhil Shah, Shrinivas S Shintre, Chittanand Mendhe

INTRODUCTION

Pubic symphysis plating is usually performed in cases of pubic diastasis. Separation of pubic symphysis without evidence of any fracture constitutes pelvic diastasis.

Separation of more than 10 mm is considered significant. One must always assess sacroiliac joint involvement in pubic diastasis.

Cause of pubic diastasis involves: pregnancy complications, trauma, sports injury, inflammatory arthritis following long-term corticosteroid intake.

INDICATIONS

Pubic symphysis plating is indicated for pubic diastasis with unstable pelvic ring injury. Symphyseal separation of more than 2.5 cm of diastasis is considered unstable and is usually treated using symphyseal plates.

Associated conditions such as wound infection, compound fracture, or neurovascular injury may necessitate temporary external fixation before the patient can be optimized for definitive fixation.

If there is associated posterior ring fracture with vertical displacement of hemipelvis (C-type injuries) or if anterior reduction fails to achieve posterior reduction then posterior reduction should be performed first.

SURGICAL STEPS

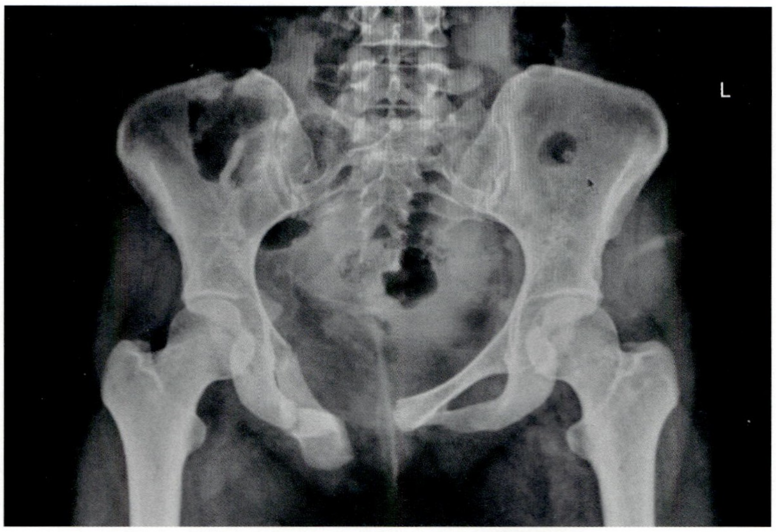

Fig. 1: Preoperative radiograph of the patient with pubic diastasis and pubic rami fracture with anterior displacement of the distal fragment. The fracture was closed without any neurovascular injury or associated infection.

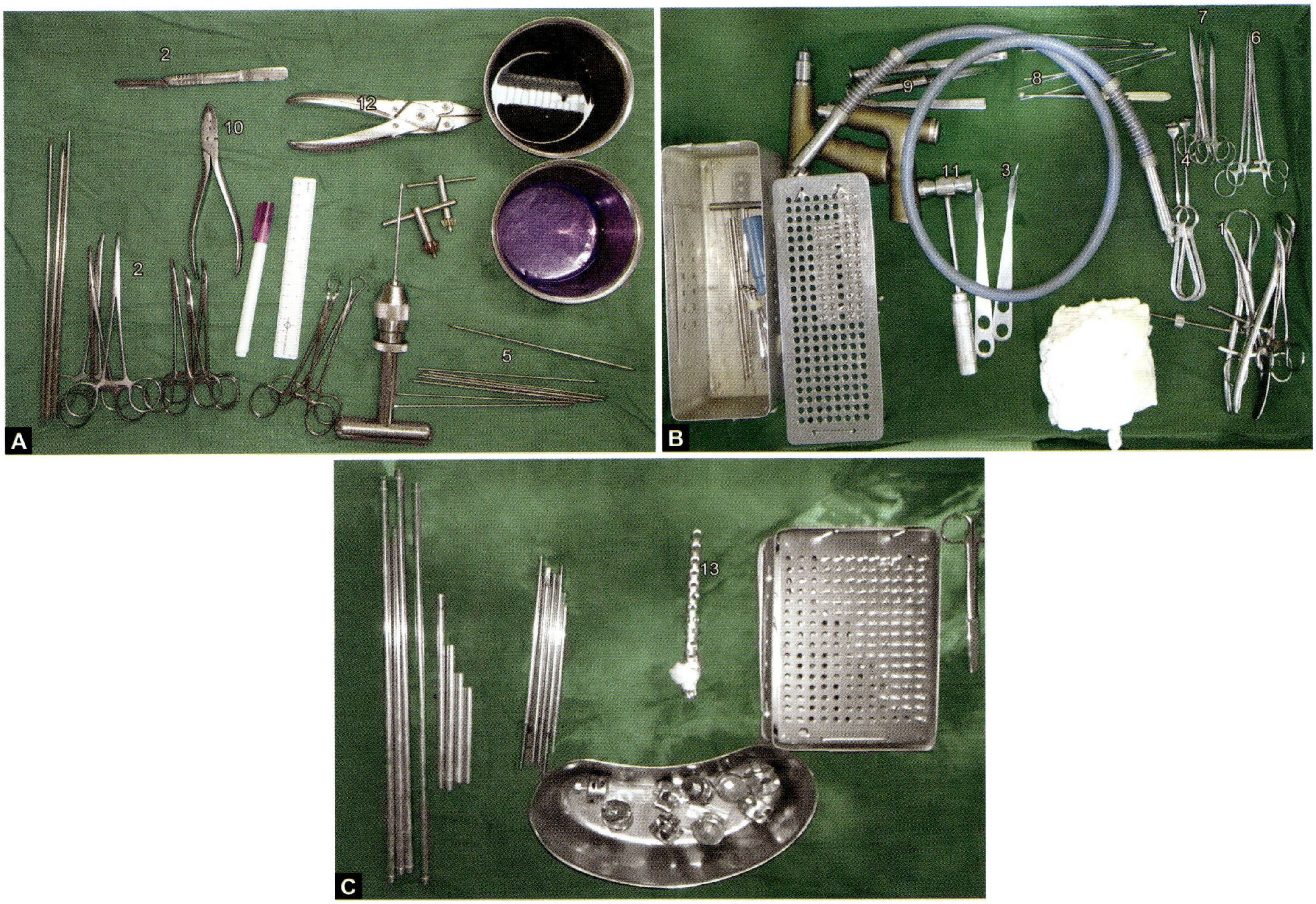

Figs. 2A to C: Sterile instrument trolley as arranged for open reduction and internal fixation for pubic diastasis. (1) Pointed bone reduction holder, (2) General surgical instruments including surgical blades, artery forceps, toothed and plain forceps, (3) Bone spikes, (4) Retractors, (5) Kirschner wires of varying thickness (0.5–3.0 mm), (6) Needle holders, (7) Dissecting scissors (stout and fine), (8) Scoop, (9) Osteotome, (10) Pointed plier, (11) Mallet, (12) Bone nibbler and stout plier. In addition, general orthopaedic instruments, sterile drapes and dressing and drill machine with 3.2 mm and 2.7 mm drill bits should be available, (13) Locking compression or combi plate.

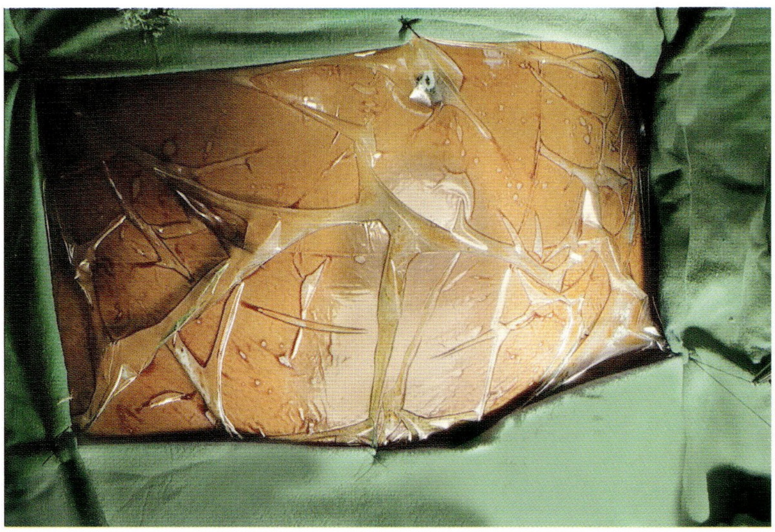

Fig. 3: The operative site is cleaned with povidone–iodine scrub and wiped down with surgical spirit.

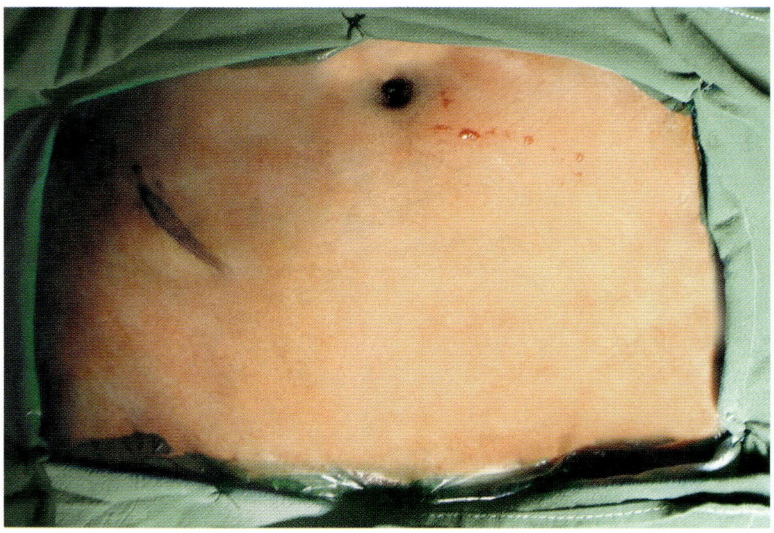

Fig. 4: Site is draped.

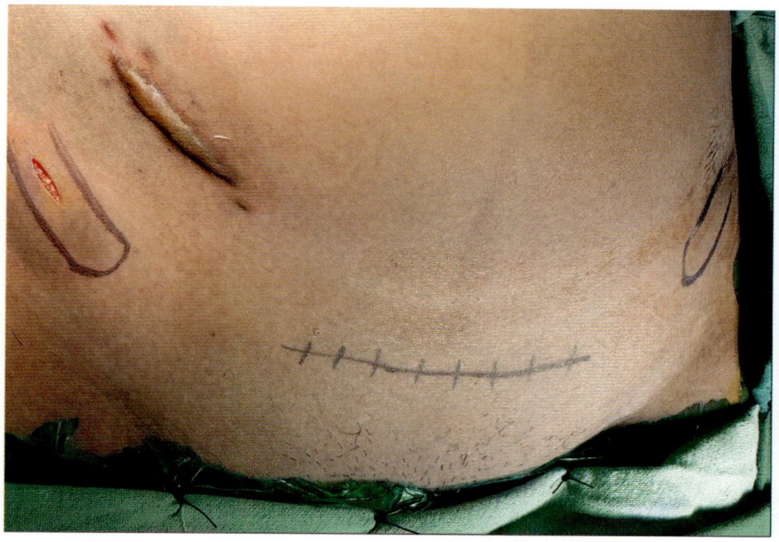

Fig. 5: The incision site is marked on the skin using a sterile marker. Pfannenstiel incision is taken about 1 cm proximal to pubic symphysis avoiding underlying neurovascular structures.

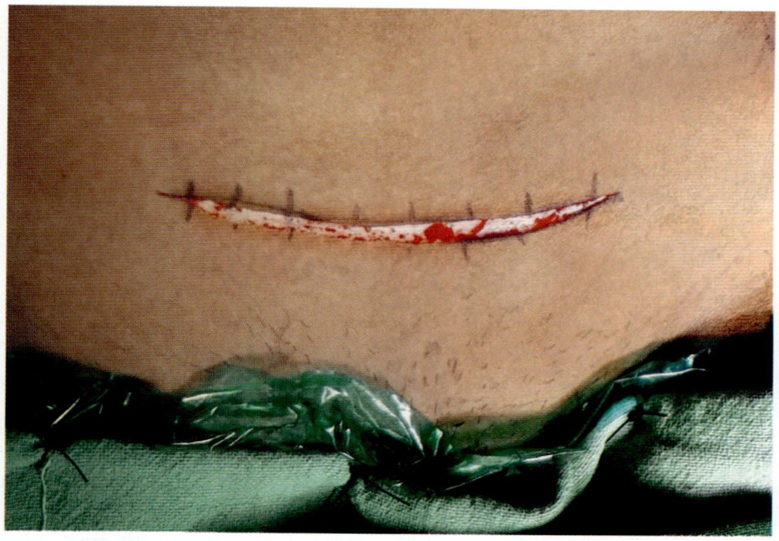

Fig. 6: Skin is incised along the marked incision line then superficial and deep fascia is incised in line with the skin incision.

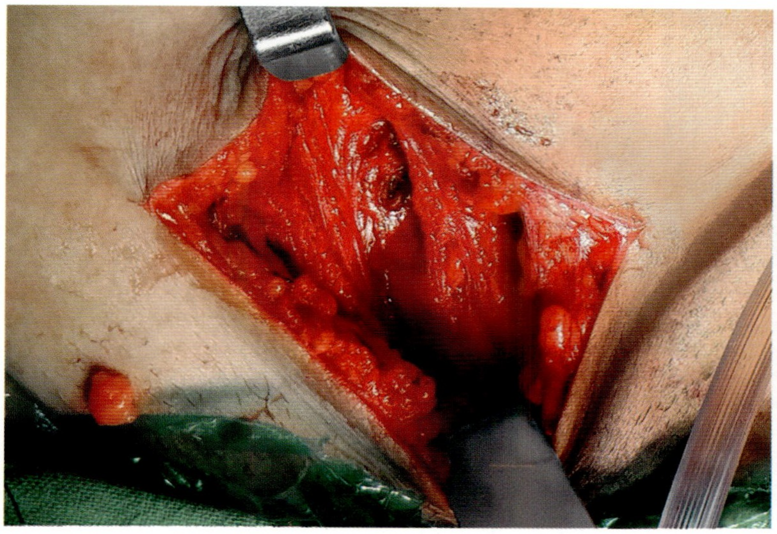

Fig. 7: Rectus abdominis is visible.

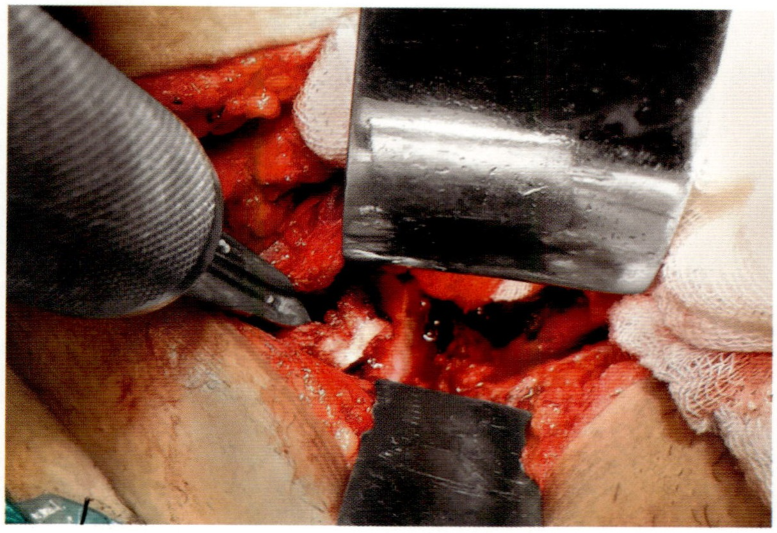

Fig. 8: Sharp dissection being employed to separate muscle attachment from symphysis pubis, to expose all fracture fragments with their overlying periosteal coverings. Bladder is separated from fracture fragment and symphisis pubis with the help of Deaver retractor and secured.

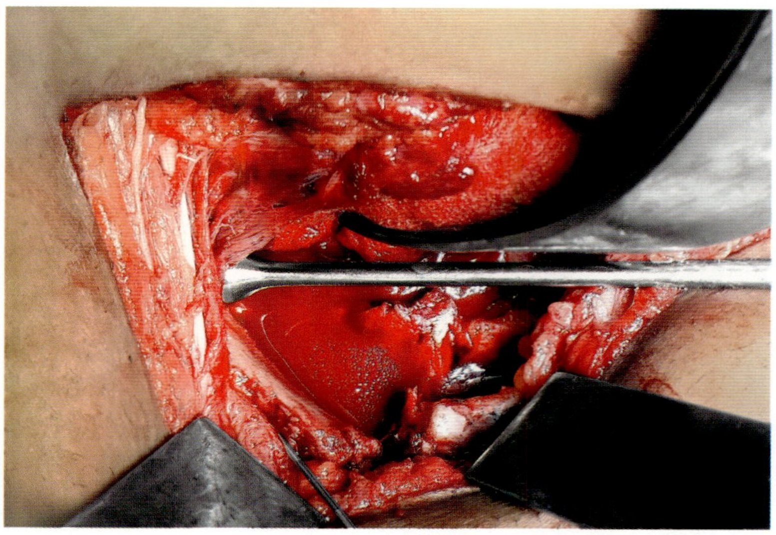

Fig. 9: The fracture site is cleaned and debris is removed using a sharp curette and artery forceps. Opposing edges of the bone at the fracture site are freshened.

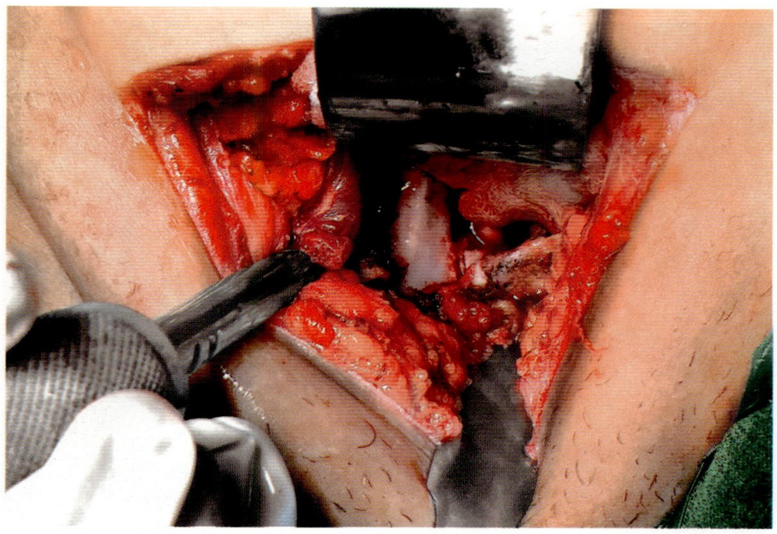

Fig. 10: The superior pubic ramus fragment is lying vertically because of displacement.

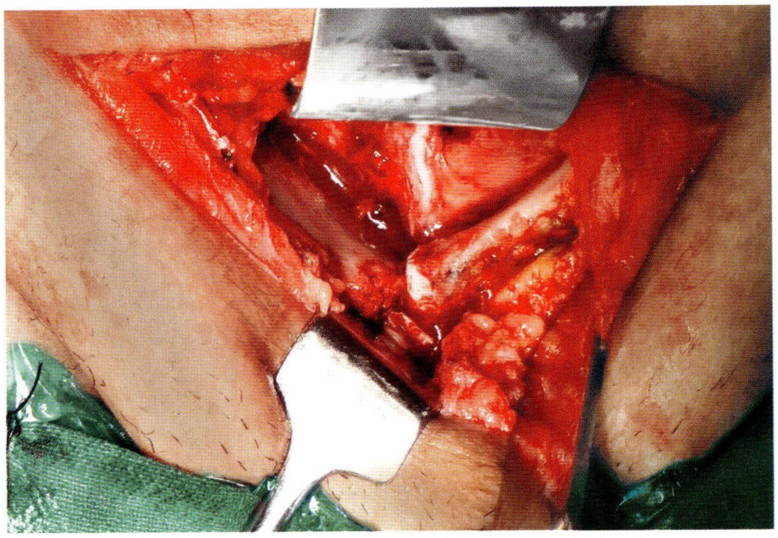

Fig. 11: After intervening soft tissue and bony debris is cleared from the fracture site, reduction is attempted. The figure above shows anatomical reduction with complete approximation of the fracture fragments.

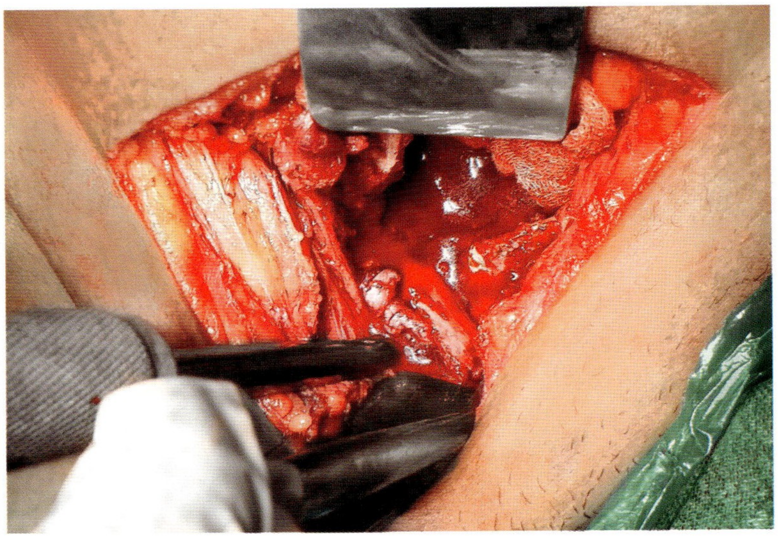

Fig. 12: The ramus being reduced and held in reduced position using a bony lever. Alternatively, spikes may also be used, however care should be taken to not traumatize the nearby vasculature (corona mortis).

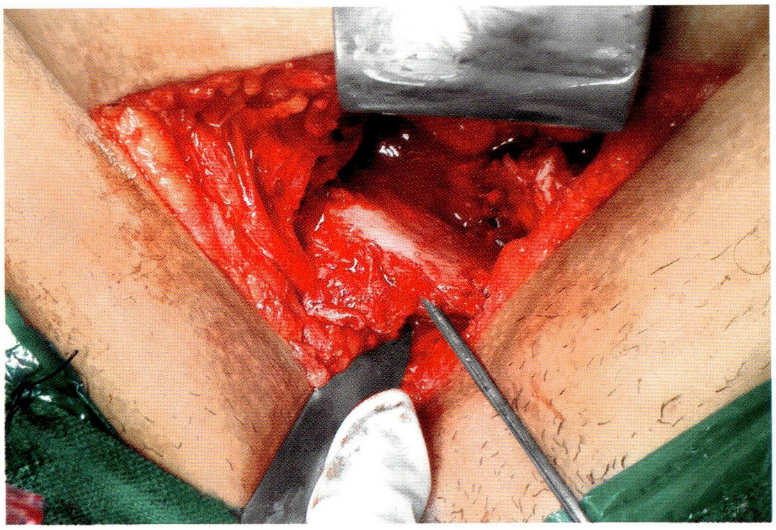

Fig. 13: A guidewire is inserted into the pubic rami, across the fracture site into the opposite cortex.

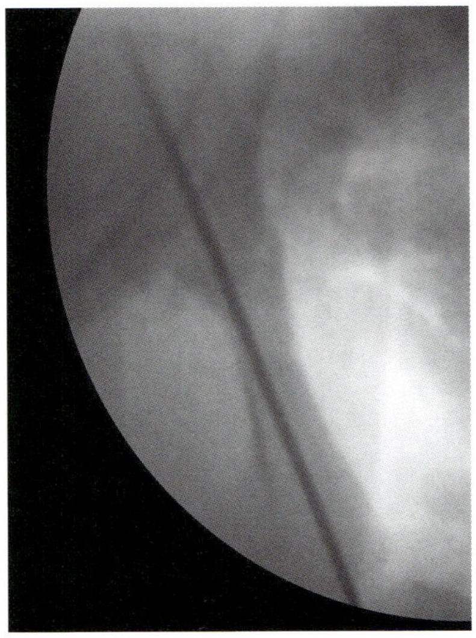

Fig. 14: Fluoroscopic view to confirm hold on the fracture fragment as well as bicortical purchase into the bone. C-arm shoot should be taken to prevent insertion of the wire in acetabulum.

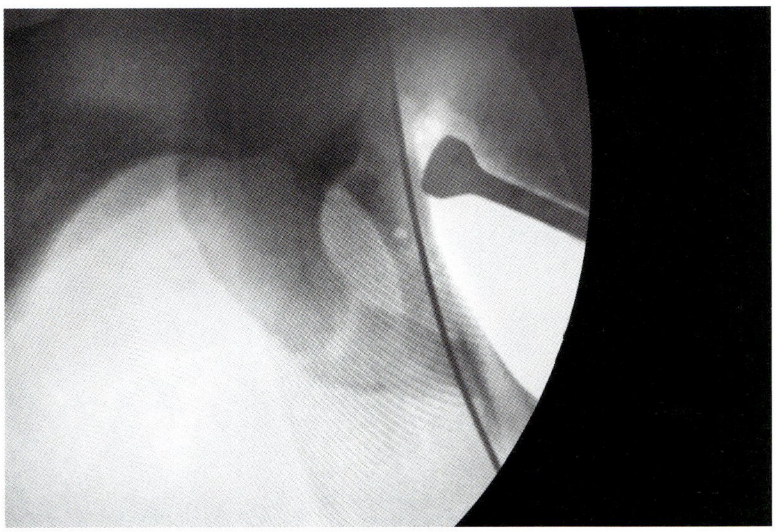

Fig. 15: The corresponding lateral view on intraoperative fluoroscopy.

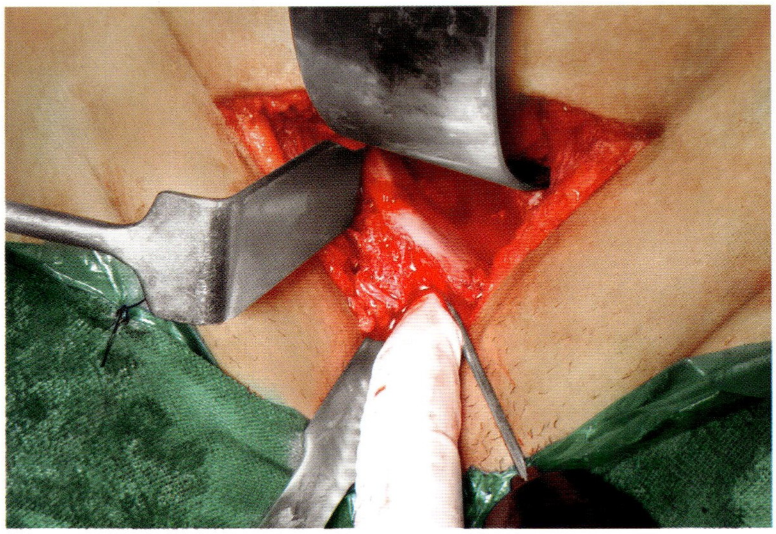

Fig. 16: Clinical photograph of the guidewire in situ. Fracture has been held in anatomic reduction.

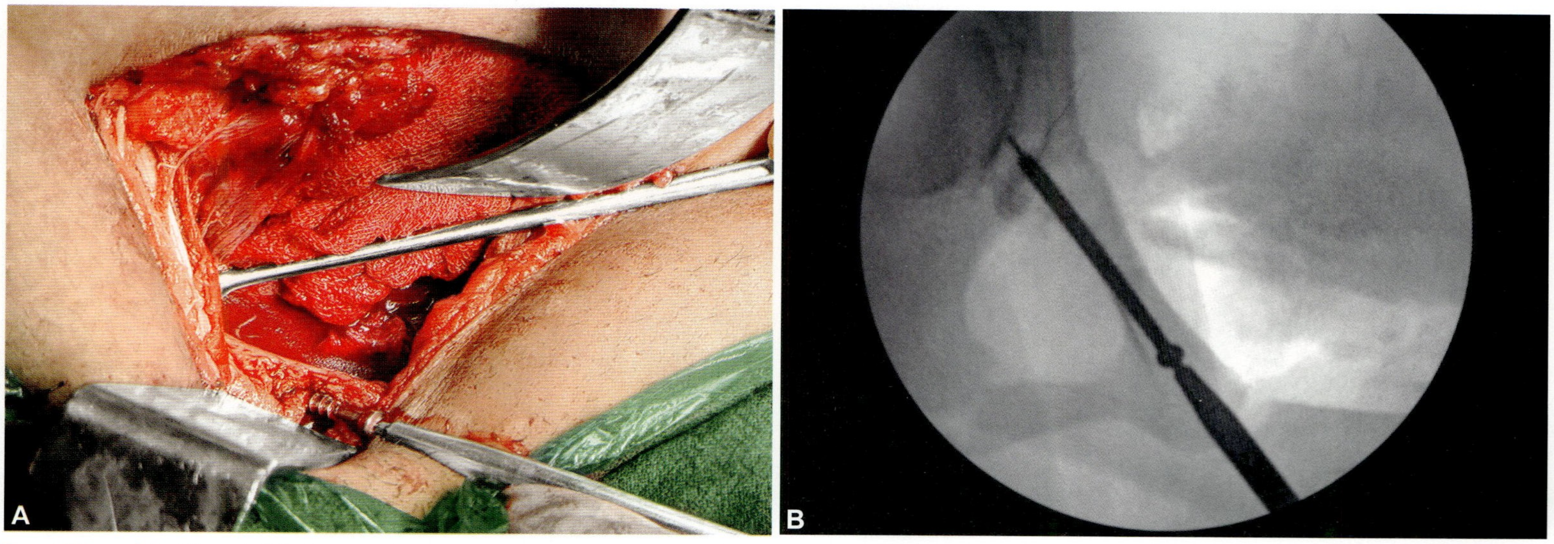

Figs. 17A and B: (A) A drill hole is made over the guidewire from the fracture site. The screw should be partially tightened and have bicortical purchase in the bone. (B) C-arm visualization of screw position over the guidewire.

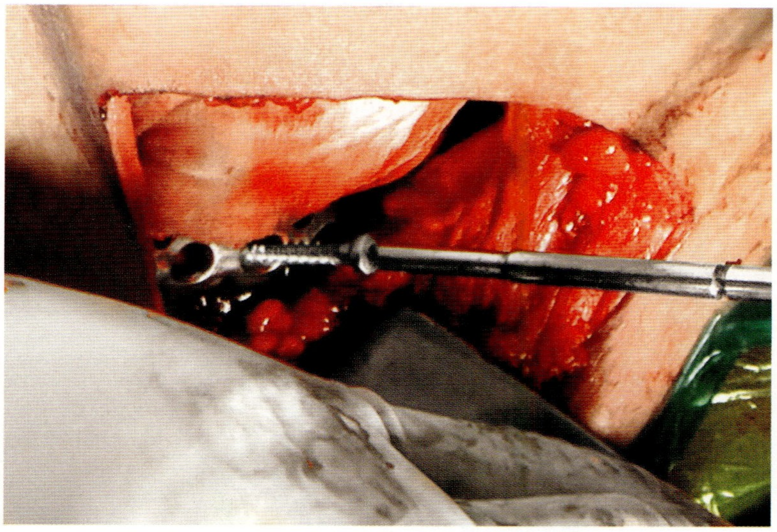

Fig. 18: A precontoured locking plate is held over the anterosuperior surface of the superior pubic rami, in such a way that symphysis pubis in the center of the plate. After drilling the cortical screws are inserted through medial plate holes.

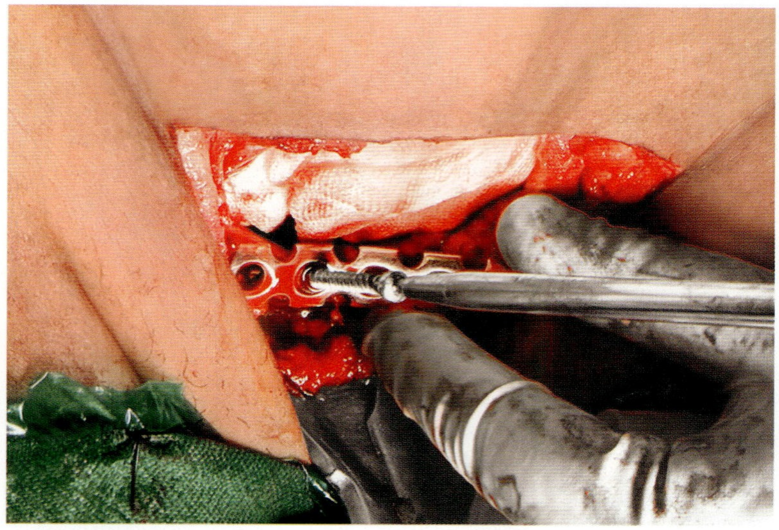

Fig. 19: After insertion of the medial screws, lateral locking screws are inserted in the locking plate.

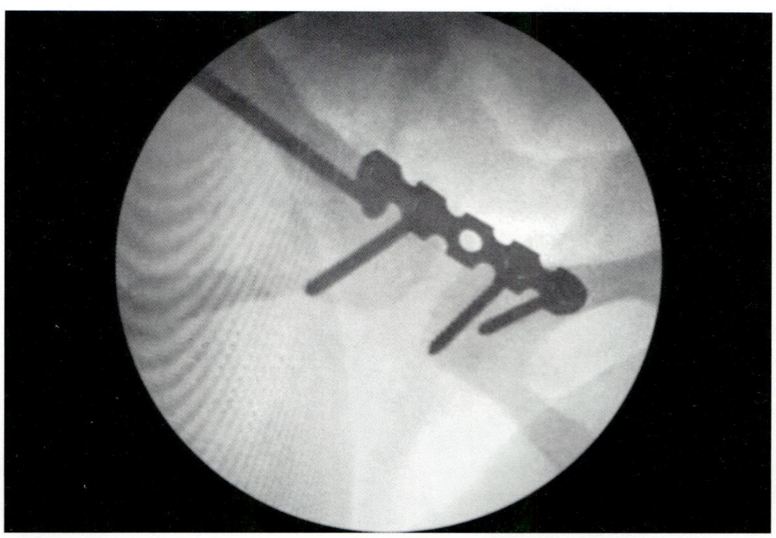

Fig. 20: After the construct has been fully tightened, confirm with fluoroscopic images.

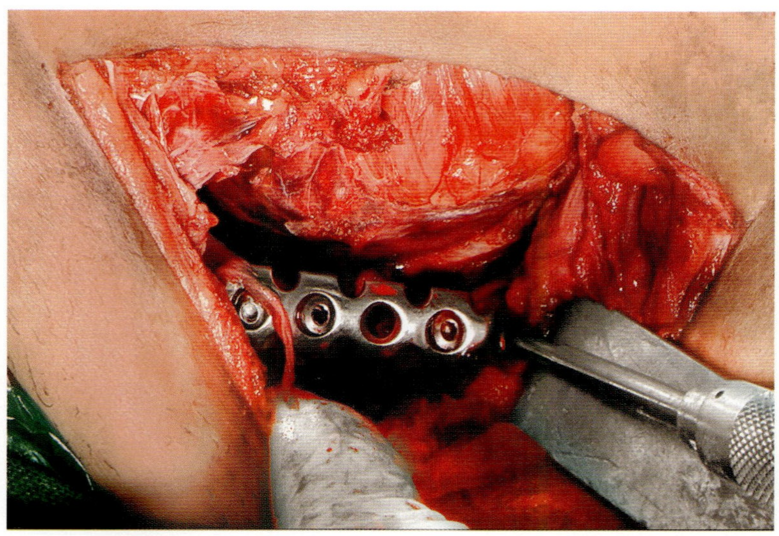

Fig. 21: The final construct before closure. Anatomic reduction at the fracture site with compression at the fracture site.

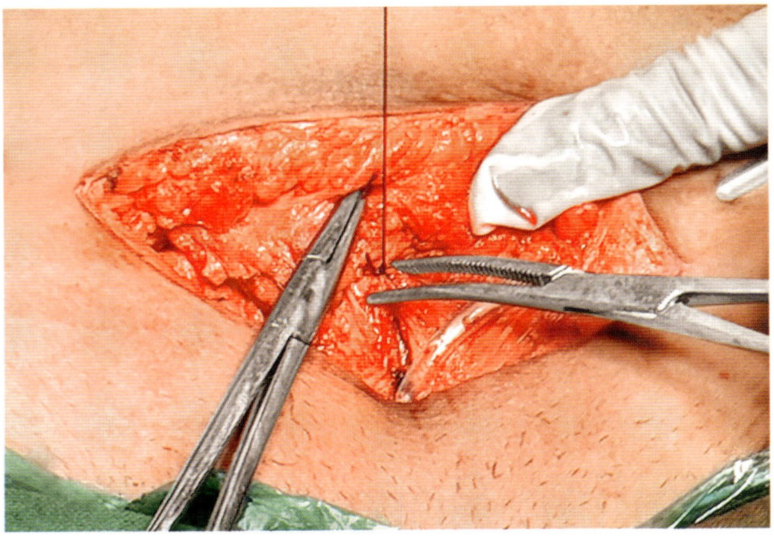

Fig. 22: Subcutaneous tissue is sutured using interrupted polyglactin sutures (2-0) later skin is closed using nonabsorbable nylon sutures taken in mattress fashion. Aseptic dressing is done.

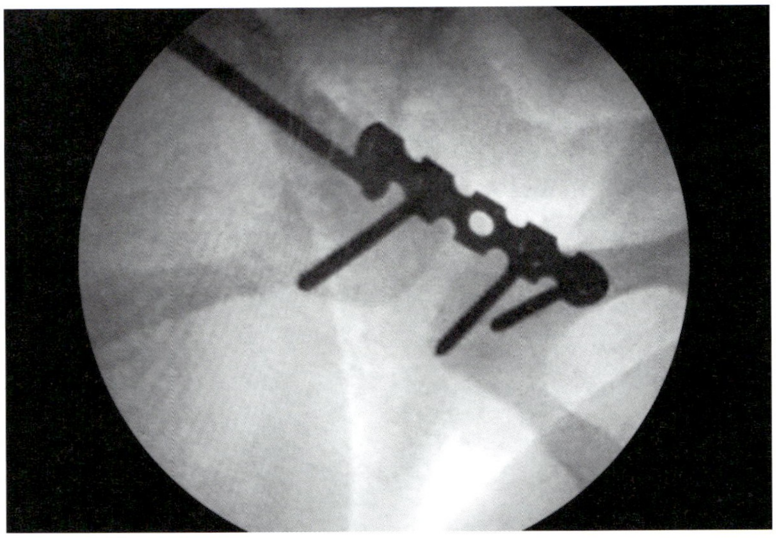

Fig. 23: Final postoperative fluoroscopy view.

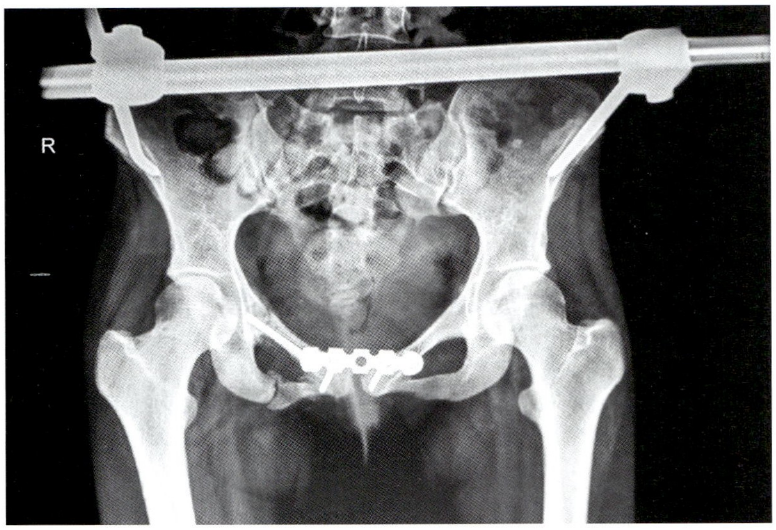

Fig. 24: Post operative radiograph.

POSTOPERATIVE PROTOCOL

- Postoperatively, weight bearing is restricted on the side of posterior ring injury for 3 months.
- Drain is removed after 2 days.
- In case of associated ramus fracture after radiological evidence of fracture healing, the patient can be given trial of partial weight bearing.
- Regular wound dressing and cleaning should be done to minimize the chances of wound infection.
- Suture removal can be done after 12–15 days postoperatively.

POSSIBLE COMPLICATIONS

Apart from anesthetic complications, this surgery may be complicated by inadvertent injury to corona mortis with extensive lateral dissection.

Bladder injury is also common during drilling. A Foleys catheter should be used so as to decompress the bladder.

Postoperative surgical site infections and suture gaping can be prevented by proper wound care.

SUGGESTED READING

1. Becker I, Woodley SJ, Stringer MD. The adult human pubic symphysis: a systematic review. J Anat. 2010;217(5):475-87.
2. Owens K, Pearson A, Mason G. Symphysis pubis dysfunction—a cause of significant obstetric morbidity. Eur J Obstet Gynecol Reprod Biol. 2002;105(2):143-6.
3. Parker JM, Bhattacharjee M. Images in clinical medicine. Peripartum diastasis of the symphysis pubis. N Engl J Med. 2009;361(19):1886.

CHAPTER 98

Sacroiliac Screw Fixation

Mahesh Kulkarni, Ranjit Mohan Modak

INTRODUCTION

Pelvic fractures are rare injuries with only 3 out of 100 of all bony injuries, with most being stable injuries. However instability is higher after posterior pelvic ring involvement; reaching 40% of total pelvic injuries.

Pelvic fractures are classified into high energy and low energy injuries.

High energy traumatic injuries are associated with major blood loss causing hypovolemic shock; such injuries usually involve posterior pelvic ring dysruptions including sacroiliac (SI) joint dislocations.

Such posterior pelvic ring injuries carry a higher mortality rate of around 20% compared to anterior ring injuries. This high mortality rate has not changed with advent of modern practices of resuscitation.

CLASSIFICATION

Classification of pelvic fractures into high- and a low-energy injury carries a good prognostic guideline for the management and prediction of the outcome. The pelvic injuries can involve any part of the pelvic ring including the hemipelvis, the sacrum, or acetabular fractures. Each injury can happen in isolation or in association with other injuries and each carries a different morbidity.

Sacroiliac joint disruption is commonly associated with high-energy pelvic ring fractures when a vertical shear force, the lateral compression or anteroposterior compression force were the mechanism of injury. Disruption of the SI joint could be associated with incomplete or complete posterior ligamentous disruption, the mechanism of injury and its severity decide whether the injury is rotationally unstable or rotationally and vertically unstable.

Technique of Iliosacral Screw Fixation: Surgical Steps

Iliosacral screw fixation has become a popular technique for treating unstable injuries of the pelvis that involve the posterior ring. In this procedure, one or two large screws (6.5–7.3 mm diameter) are inserted under fluoroscopic guidance through the ilium, across the sacroiliac (SI) articulation, and into the superior sacral vertebral bodies using percutaneous technique.

SURGICAL STEPS

Step 1: *Preparation and patient positioning*:

- *Anesthesia*: Spinal or general anesthesia with adequate muscle relaxant.
- *Antibiotics*: Third-generation cephalosporin.
- Shaving and preparation of private parts and thorough scrubbing with povidone–iodine 7.5%.
- *Position*: Preferred position is supine as simultaneous fixation of anterior pelvic ring fractures and use external fixator is feasible.

Prone position may complicate cases with chest injury, there is a problem of using external pelvic fixator and complicates fracture deformity.

Advantages of supine position include familiarity of positioning by anesthetist and nursing, ability of multiple teams working simultaneously and access to anterior pelvis, if additional reduction methods are required.

Two operating tables with opposite ends attached to each other are frequently used as they provide a large radiolucent area for better visualization with fluoroscopy. In some cases where this is not feasible, use of a radiolucent extension board may suffice (Figs. 1 to 3).

Step 2: *How to take intraoperative X-rays*?

After patient positioning before starting with the actual procedure, preliminary fluoroscopy images are obtained to confirm the fracture site, orientation of fracture fragments, and to assess reducibility of fracture.

Pelvic inlet and outlet views are obtained and a true lateral view is necessary for proper placement of screw.

For obtaining pelvic inlet view the head of C-arm is placed cephalad at 45° (Figs. 4 and 5).

For obtaining pelvic outlet view, the head of C-arm is placed caudal at 45° (Figs. 6 and 7).

A true lateral view is necessary to confirm screw position (Figs. 8 and 9).

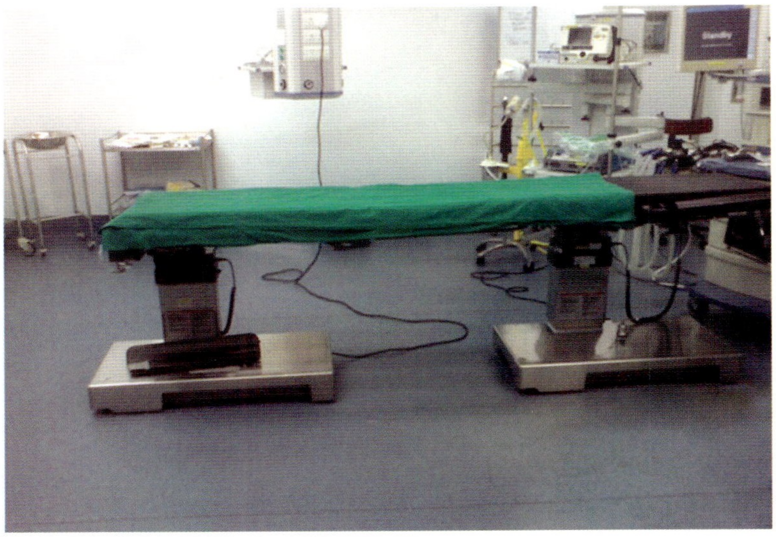
Fig. 1: Patient positioning with two operating tables joined end to end.

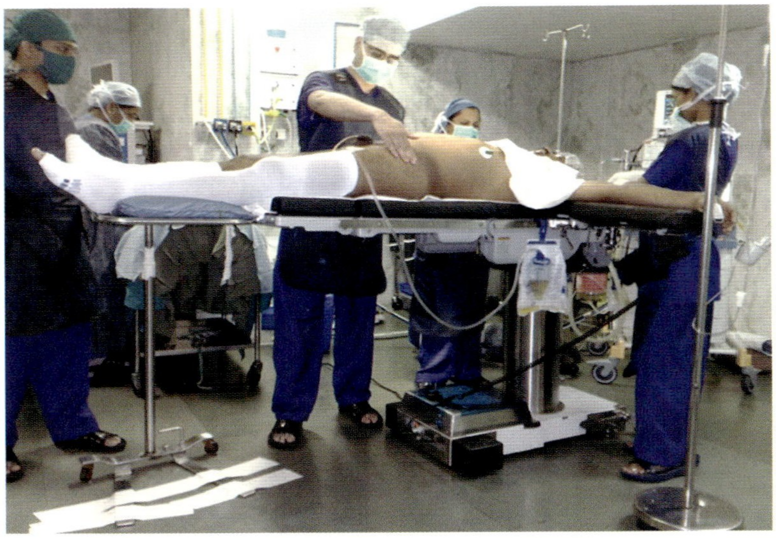
Fig. 2: Patient positioning with Mayo's trolley at leg end.

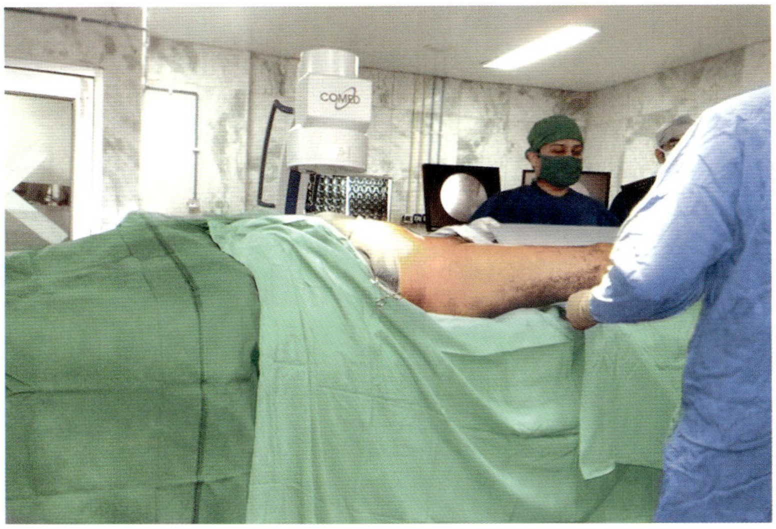
Fig. 3: Patient draping.

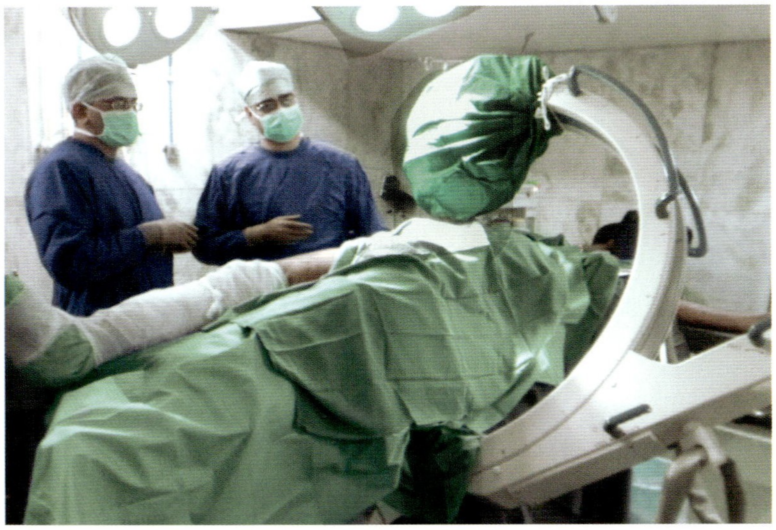
Fig. 4: Pelvic inlet view C-arm position.

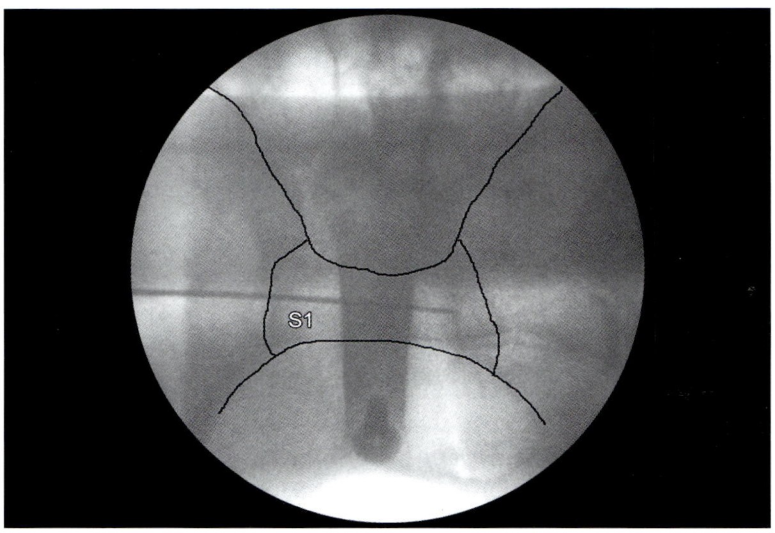

Fig. 5: Pelvic inlet view.

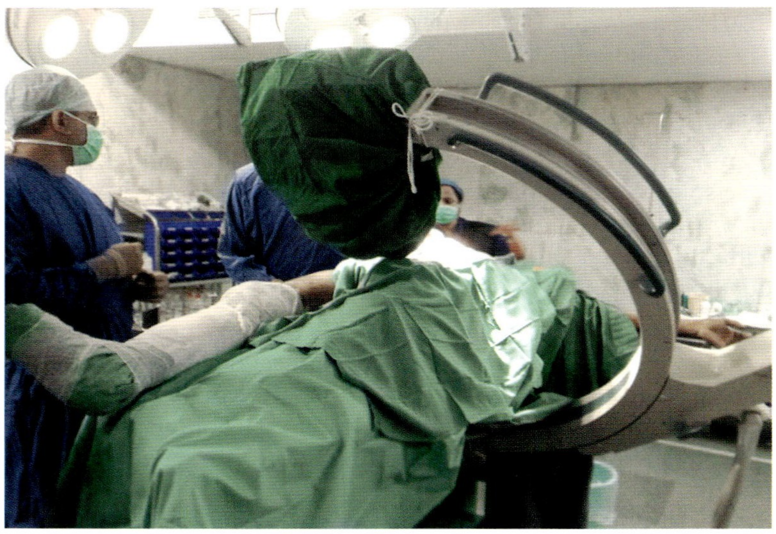
Fig. 6: Pelvic outlet view C-arm position.

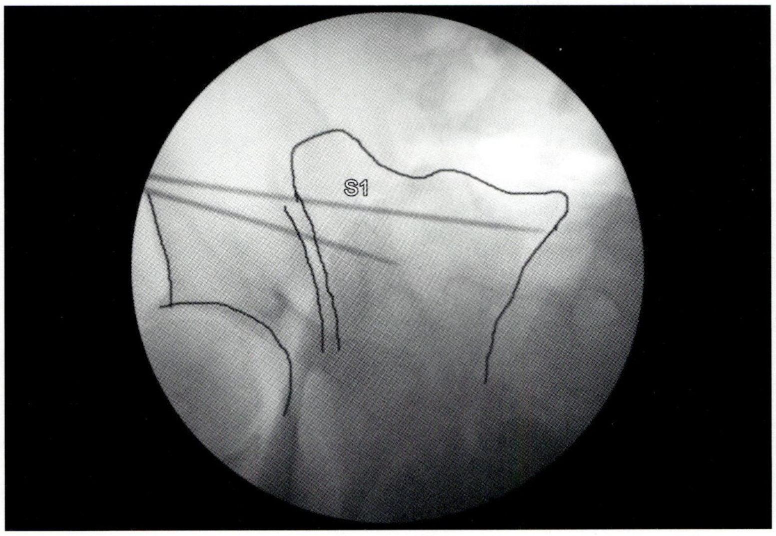

Fig. 7: Pelvic outlet view.

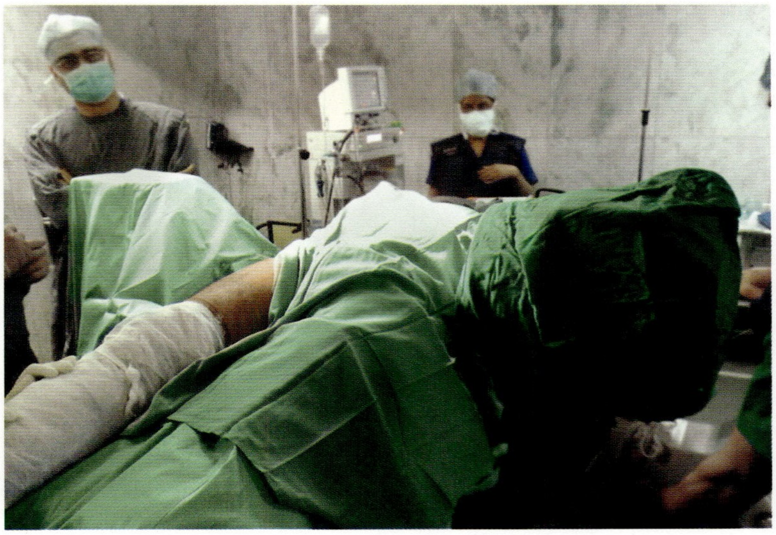

Fig. 8: Pelvis lateral view C-arm position.

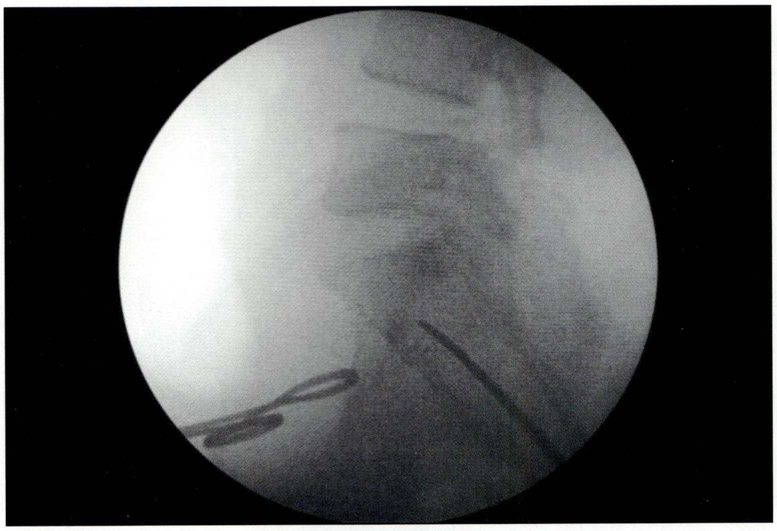

Fig. 9: Pelvic lateral view.

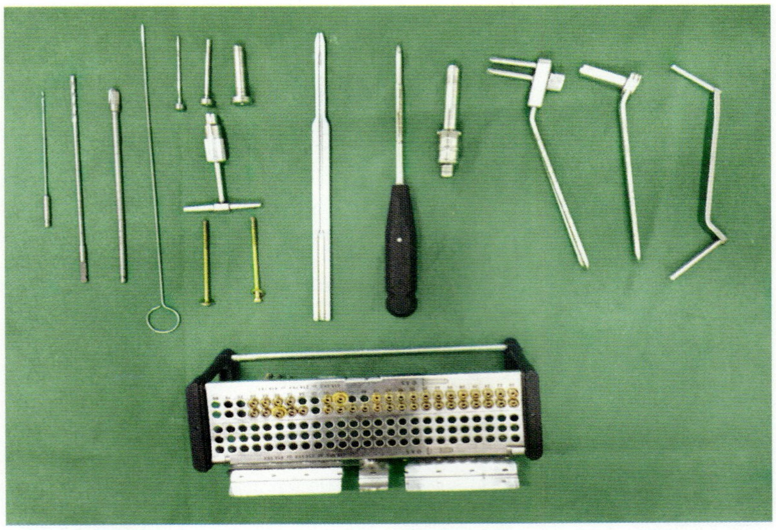

Fig. 10: Instrument set.

When indicated, an external fixator for pelvis is used for preliminary stabilization of the fracture and reduction of fracture/SI joint is achieved.

Step 3: *Instruments required and trolley set-up*: A set of specialized instruments is required for percutaneous iliosacral screw fixation. These include reduction clamps, ball tip spikes, and other instruments for screw insertion like long guidewires, drill bit, tap, and screw drivers (Figs. 10 and 11).

Step 4: *Surgical approach*: In the supine position, the anterior superior iliac spine (ASIS) is palpated and a line drawn from the ASIS and directed perpendicularly to the floor. A second line, drawn in line with the femoral shaft, intersects the first line and thus forms four quadrants (Fig. 12).

Step 5: *Location of screw entry point*: The entry point should be anterior in S1 and inferior to the iliac cortical density (ICD), which parallels the sacral alar slope, usually slightly caudal and posterior (Fig. 13). The ICD thus marks the anterosuperior boundary of the safe zone for an iliosacral screw, which may injure the L5 nerve root, if it penetrates this cortex.

An instrument handle can help to target the desired entry site for the guidewire.

A stab incision is made with a scalpel followed by insertion of a Kirschner wire (K-wire) through the incision until the outer table of the ilium is contacted. Instrumentation is directed toward the area of the bone between the anterior sacral ala and S1 neural foramina (Fig 14).

Step 6: *Fixation*: After closed reduction is confirmed, a smooth or drill bit tipped K-wire is inserted under triplanar (AP, both outlet views), fluoroscopic control through the stab incision and onto the lateral aspect of the ilium. Threaded wires are avoided as tactile feedback for detecting a bony tunnel breach is limited.

The starting point of wire at the entry to bone is tapped with light mallet and further insertion is with the help of drill. After appropriate starting point is confirmed, skin incision is elongated around the wire and blunt dissection is done.

The guidewire is now advanced further with a power drill though the lateral cortex of the ilium and under C-arm guidance to confirm its safe position (Fig. 15).

Step 7: *Position of the screws*: On the outlet view, the screw is angled approximately 20° cranially and on the inlet view, the screw is angled approximately 5° anteriorly. For cases of SI joint dislocation, the SI screw trajectory is posterior to anterior; while for sacral fractures, the screws are directed transversely. Care must be taken to avoid

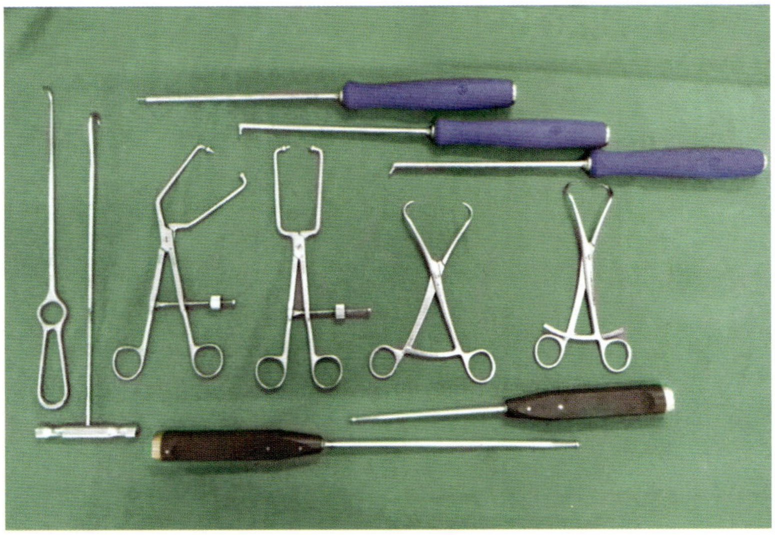

Fig. 11: Instrument set.

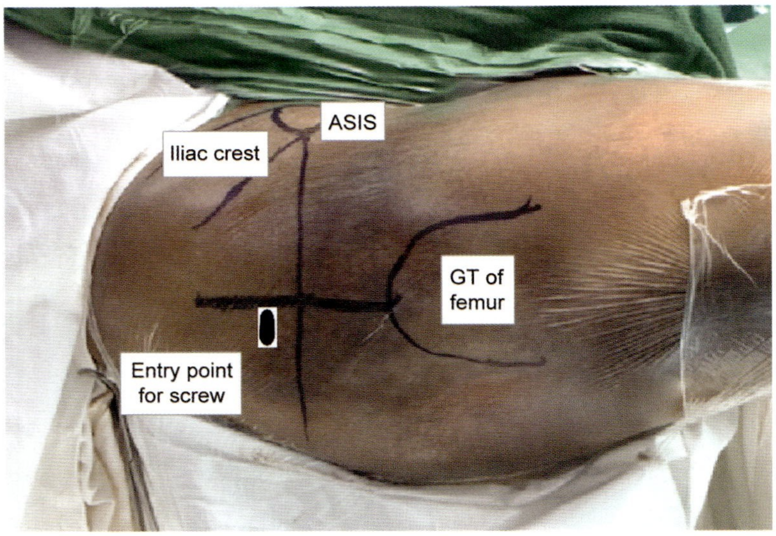

Fig. 12: Entry point location.

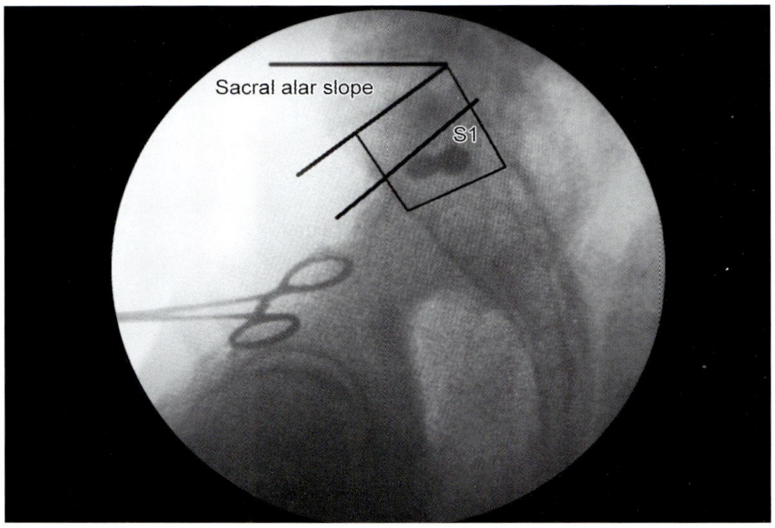

Fig. 13: Entry point location in accordance with Sacral ala.

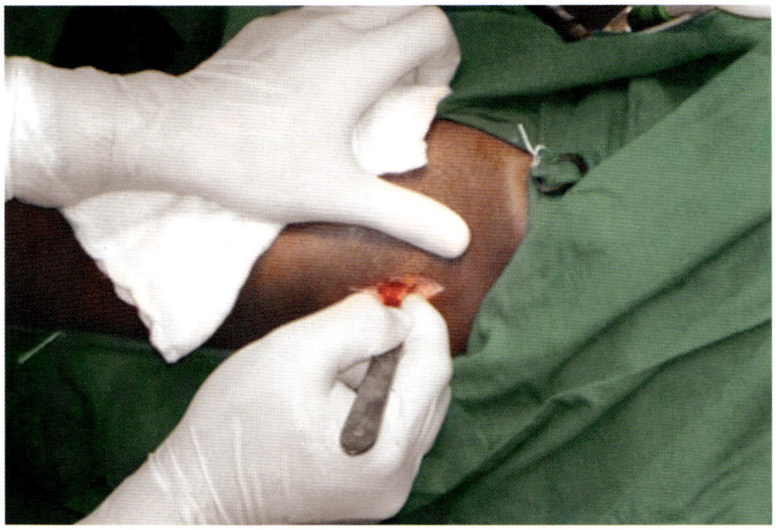

Fig. 14: Incision site.

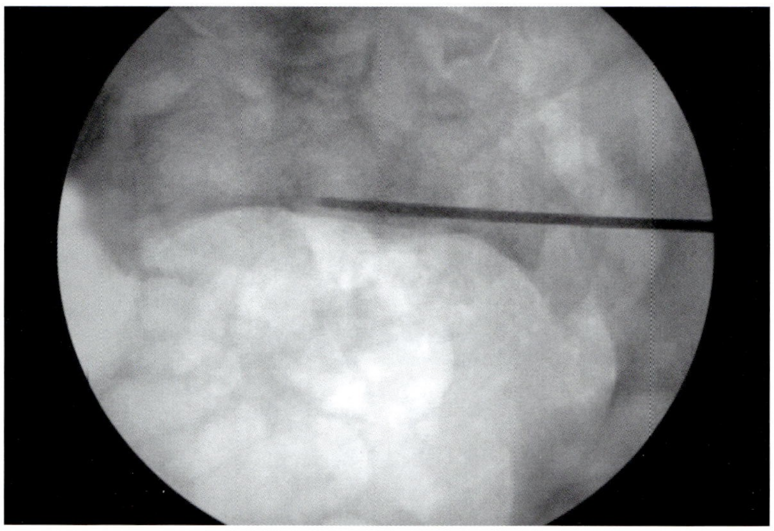

Fig. 15: Guidewire placement.

damage to nerve roots, which pass from posterior to anterior, midline to peripheral, and superior to inferior. Ideally, the screw should be positioned at the center of the S1 and S2 vertebral bodies, in order to avoid penetration of the recess of the sacral wing, foramina of the nerve roots, spinal canal, L5/S1 disc space and anterior cortex of the sacrum.

Safety of guidewire position is checked and it is further advanced till midline of the vertebral body avoiding passing through opposite ala.

Once position confirmed, depth is measured and cannulated drill bit of appropriate length is advanced over the guidewire (Fig. 16).

A cannulated tap is used over the guidewire (Fig. 17).

A 6.5 mm partially threaded cancellous screw is used when compression is desired. Screw is almost always used with washer to prevent further migration of screws in posterior direction. Full-threaded screws are used when compression is not desired (Fig. 18).

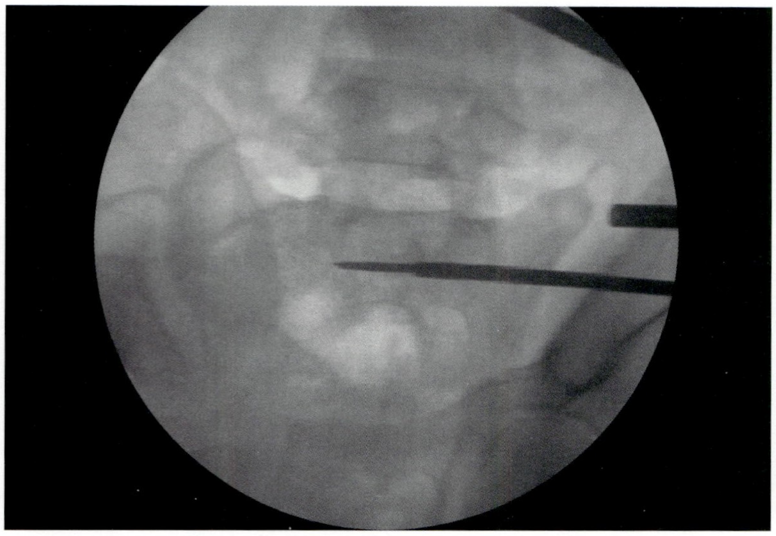

Fig. 16: Drilling over guidewire.

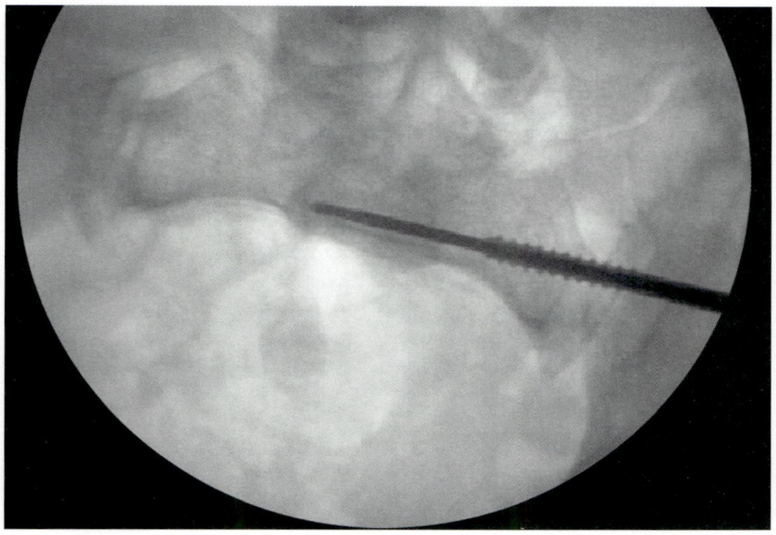

Fig. 17: Screw placement over guidewire.

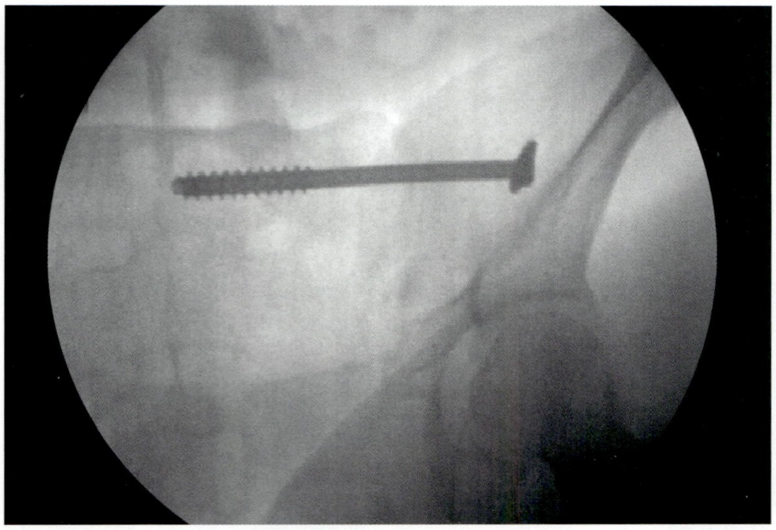

Fig. 18: Final screw position.

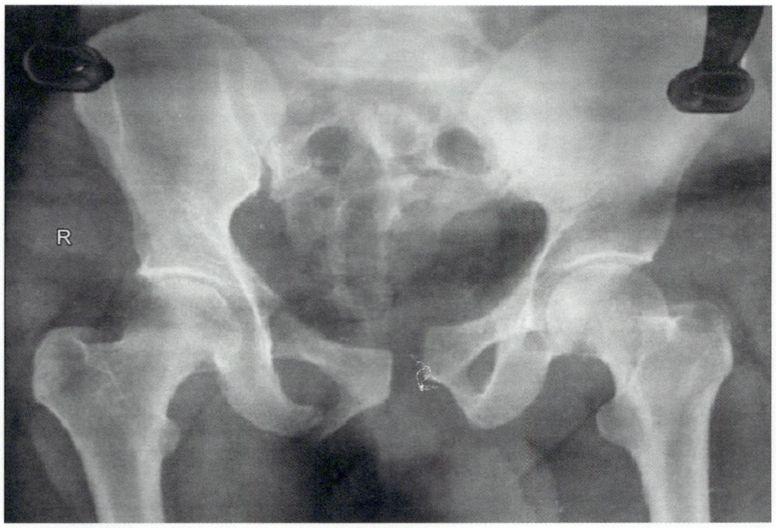

Fig. 19: Plain X-ray pelvis with both hips showing pubic symphysis diastasis with right sacroiliac joint disruption, and superior and inferior pubic ramus fracture.

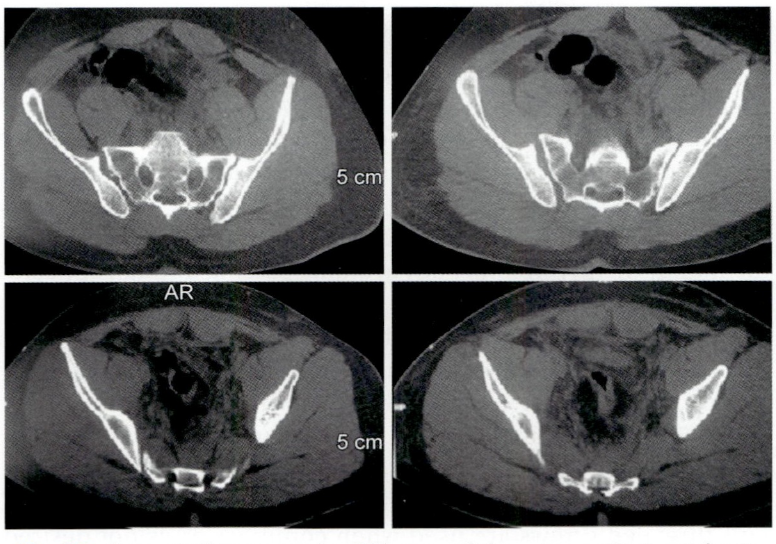

Fig. 20: Computed tomography (CT) scan of the same patient, axial cuts showing widening of sacroiliac joint.

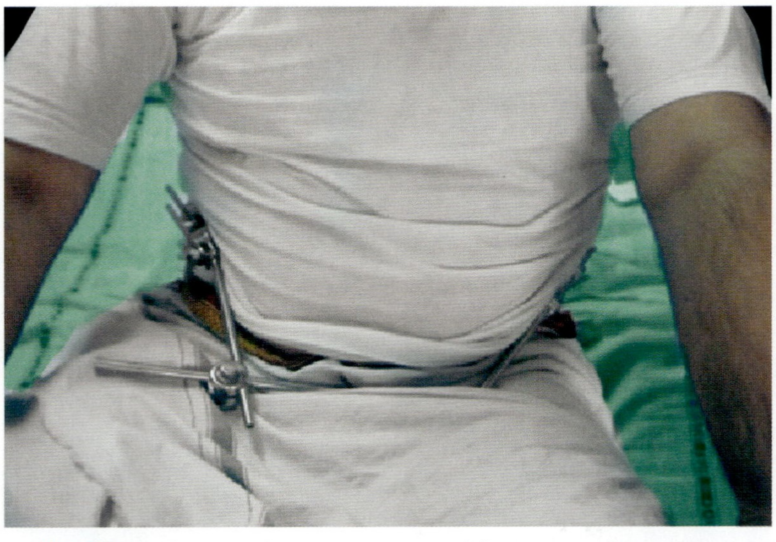

Fig. 21: Application of temporary external fixator in such a way that patients personal hygiene can be maintained.

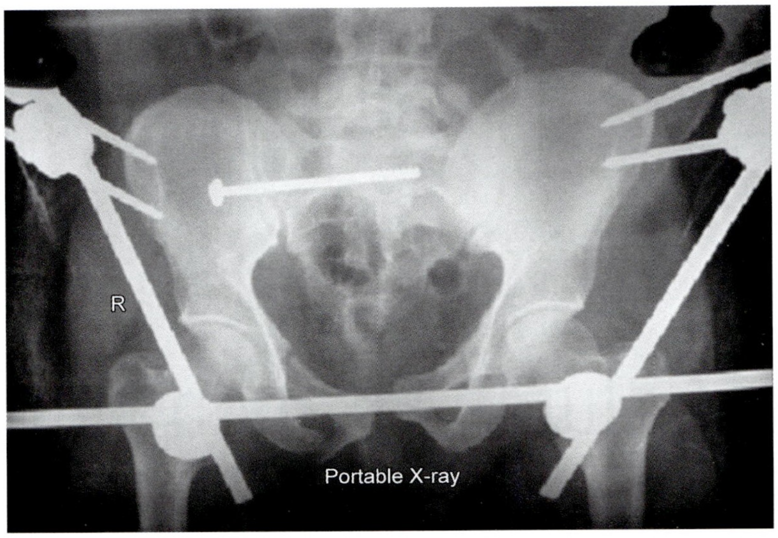

Fig. 22: Postoperative plain X-ray pelvic outlet view, showing well-reduced right sacroiliac (SI) joint by percutaneous SI screw fixation method with reduction of pubic diastasis within acceptable limits.

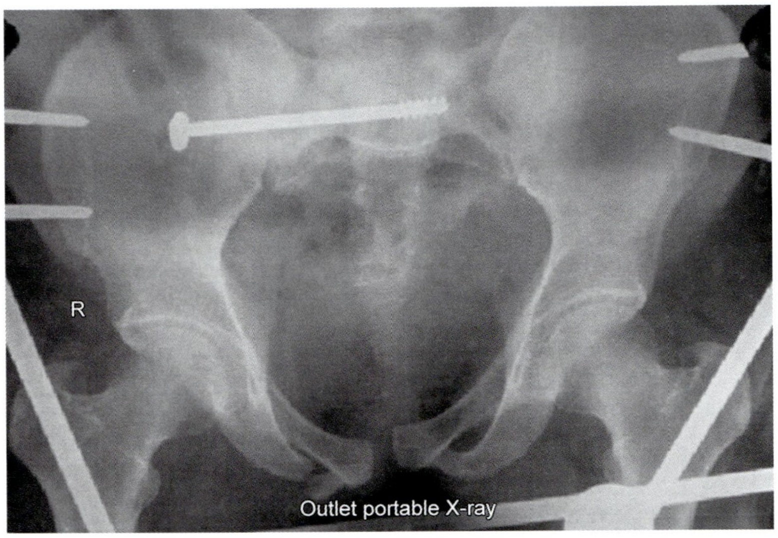

Fig. 23: Postoperative plain X-ray pelvic inlet view, showing well reduced right sacroiliac (SI) joint by percutaneous SI screw fixation method with reduction of pubic diastasis within acceptable limits.

Frequent fluoroscopic images are taken to confirm that the guidewire is not accidently advancing. Care is taken not to overtighten the screw and penetrate the lateral iliac cortex as it may cause change in screw position especially in osteoporotic bones in elderly.

The guidewire is then removed and stress views are taken to check stability of the construct.

After confirmation of stability, wound is closed and dressed under aseptic precautions.

Step 8: *Postoperative care*: The goals of postoperative management are to maximize the functional status of the patient, facilitate early return to function, and detect complications quickly and manage them appropriately.

SURGICAL FIXATION

Traditional method for treatment of SI joint injuries involved either conservative management or use of sacral bars or plates by openly reducing the fractures. This meant potential for long duration of the hospital stay, iatrogenic neurovascular injuries and more blood loss.

It is recommended to fix unstable types of pelvic fractures as this leads to better radiological outcome along with reduction of number of days spent in hospital, faster mobilization and better functional outcome with reduced morbidity and mortality rates.

TREATMENT

Routt popularized the technique of closed reduction and percutaneous sacroiliac screw fixation of the posterior pelvic ring injuries. This involves minimally invasive approach with reduced blood loss and less soft tissue handling leading to reduced postoperative infection rates.

The known complications of this percutaneous technique are improper reduction, implant failure and iatrogenic neurovascular injuries.

SUGGESTED READING

1. Burkhardt M, Nienaber U, Pizanis A, et al. Acute management and outcome of multiple trauma patients with pelvic disruptions. Crit Care. 2012;16(4):R163.
2. Canale T, James H, Beaty S. Campbell's Operative Orthopaedics, 11th edition. Amsterdam, Netherlands: Mosby Elsevier; 2007; pp. 2964-75.
3. Dalal SA, Burgess AR, Siegal JH. Pelvic fracture in multiple trauma: classification by mechanism is key to pattern of organ injury, resuscitative requirement, and outcome. J Trauma. 1989;29:981-1002.
4. Fallinger MS, McGanity PL. Unstable fractures of the pelvic ring. J Bone Joint Surg Am. 1992;74:781-91.
5. Gänsslen A, Hildebrand F, Pohlemann T. Management of hemodynamic unstable patients "in extremis" with pelvic ring fractures. Acta Chir Orthop Traumatol Cech. 2012;79(3):193-202.
6. Goris RJ, Gimbrere JS, van Niekirk JL, et al. Early osteosynthesis and prophylactic mechanical ventilation in the multi-trauma patient. J Trauma. 1982;22:895-903.
7. Langford JR, Burgess AR, Liporace Fa, et al. Pelvic fractures: part 2. Contemporary indications and techniques for definitive surgical management. J Am Acad Orhtop Surg. 2013;21:458-68.
8. Latenser BA, Gentilello LM, Tarver AA, et al. Improved outcome with early fixation of skeletally unstable pelvic fractures. J Trauma. 1991;31: 28-31.
9. Moed BR, Hartman MJ, Ahmad BK, et al. Evaluation of intraoperative nerve monitoring during insertion of an iliosacral implant in an animal model. J Bone Joint Surg Am. 1999;81(11):1529-37.
10. Moreno C, Moore EE, Rosenberger A, et al. Hemorrhage associated with major pelvic fracture: a multi-specialty challenge. J Trauma. 1986;26:987-94.
11. Nelson DW, Duwelis PJ. CT-guided fixation of sacral fractures and sacroiliac joint disruptions. Radiology. 1991;180:527-32.
12. Poole GV, Ward EF. Causes of mortality in patients with pelvic fractures. Orthopedics. 1994;17(8):691-6.
13. Riemer BL, Butterfield SL, Diamond DL, et al. Acute mortality associated with injuries to the pelvic ring: the role of early patient mobilization and external fixation. J Trauma. 1993;35:671-7.
14. Routt ML Jr, Kregor PJ, Simonian PT, et al. Early results of percutaneous sacroiliac screws placed with the patient in the supine position. J Orthop Trauma. 1995;9:207-14.
15. Schulman JE, O'Toole RV, Castillo RC, et al. Pelvic ring fractures are an independent risk factor for death after blunt trauma. J Trauma. 2010;68(4):930-4.
16. Wolinsky PR. Assessment and management of pelvic fracture in haemodynamically unstable patient. Orthop Clin North Am. 1997; 28:321-9.

CHAPTER 99

Anterior Column Fixation with Reconstruction Plate

Shrinivas S Shintre, Shrikant Sagane, Rajkumar Ekambaram

SURGICAL STEPS (FIGS. 1 TO 15)

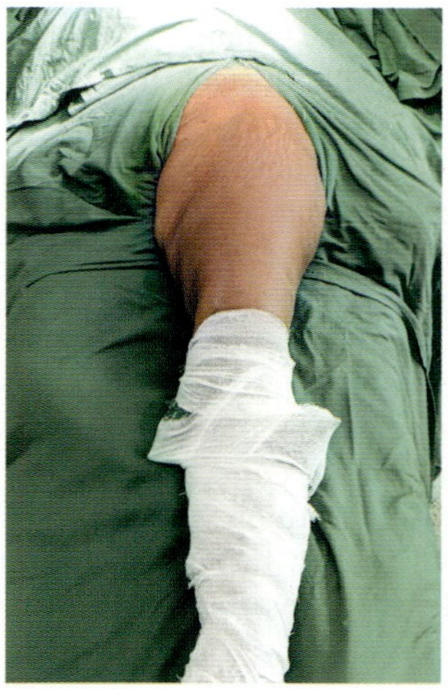

Fig. 1: Patient is positioned supine. Painting and draping of the operative site is done with povidone–iodine solution.

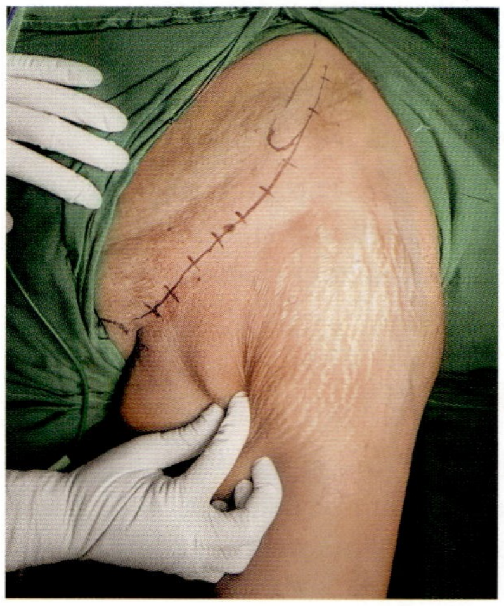

Fig. 2: Using sterile skin marker, marking is made with anterosuperior iliac spine and pubic symphysis as reference point and a line is drawn connecting both.

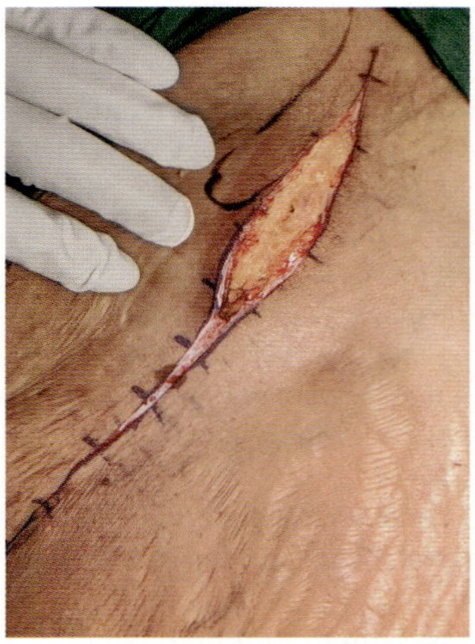

Fig. 3: Incision is made in layers over the line drawn from anterosuperior iliac spine to pubic symphysis.

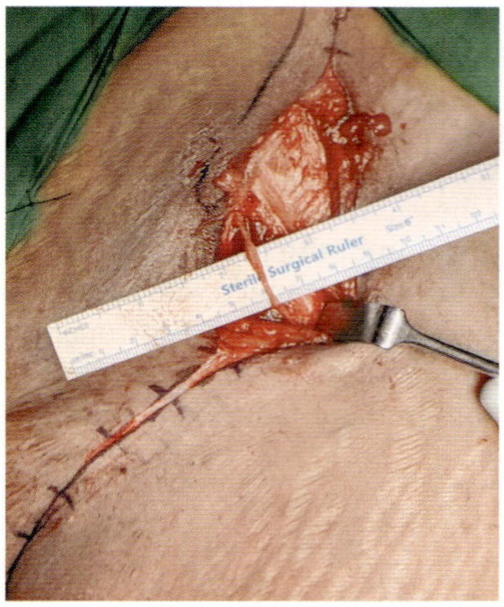

Fig. 4: After dissection, lateral femoral cutaneous nerve of thigh is identified and secured.

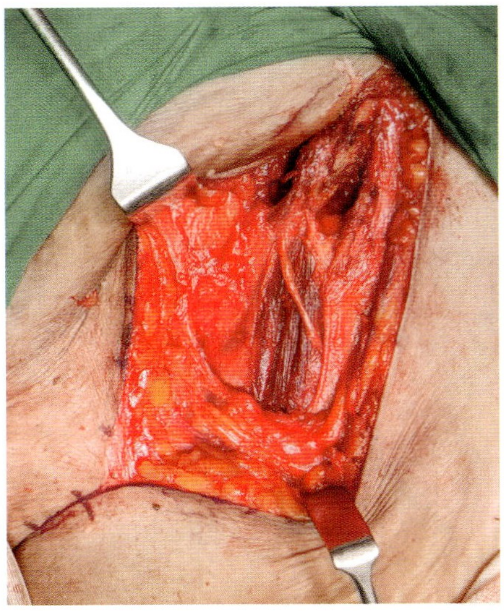

Fig. 5: Once the nerve is secured, further dissection is carried out.

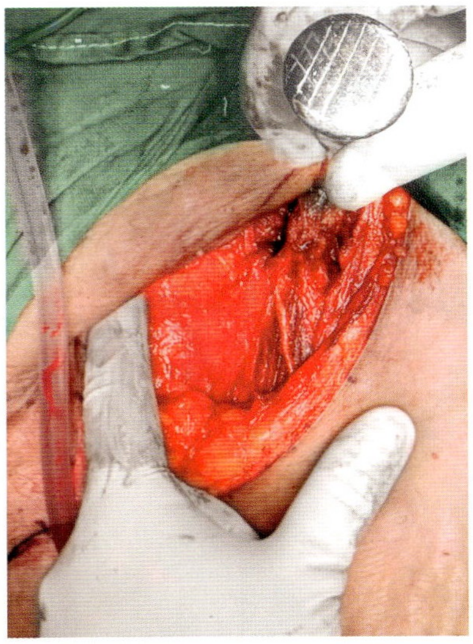

Fig. 6: After adequate dissection a lateral window for fracture fixation is made.

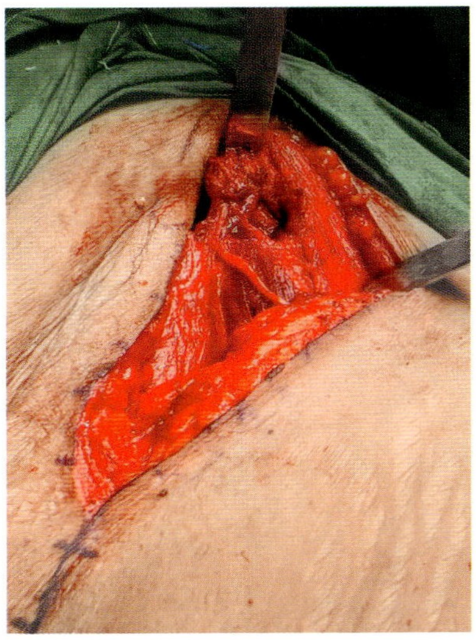

Fig. 7: Further deep dissection showing anterosuperior iliac spine.

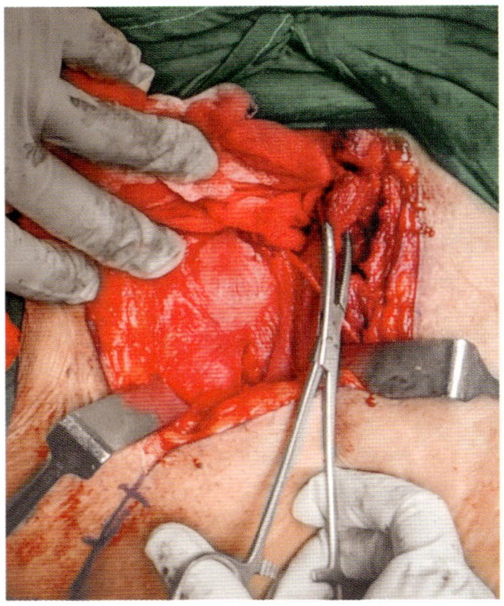

Fig. 8: Anterosuperior iliac spine is then osteotomized with osteotome.

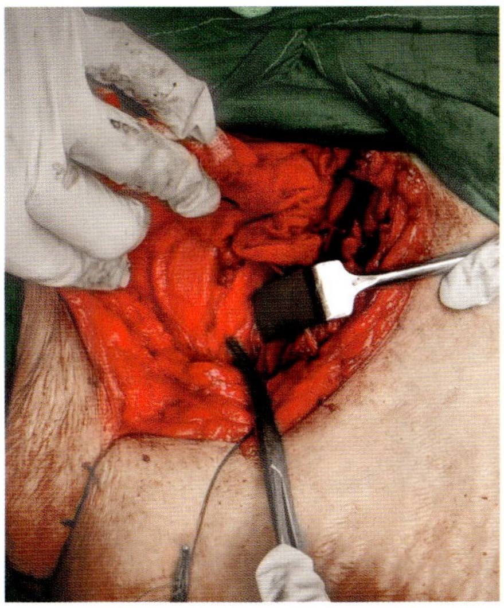

Fig. 9: Once lateral window is made, femoral vessels are identified and retracted medially.

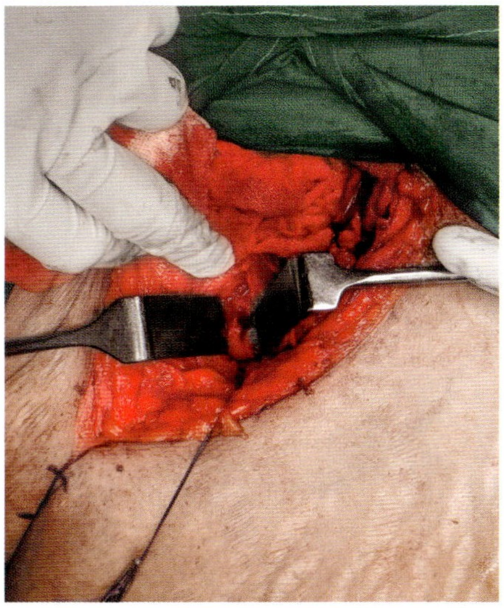

Fig. 10: The fractured anterior wall of acetabulum is exposed.

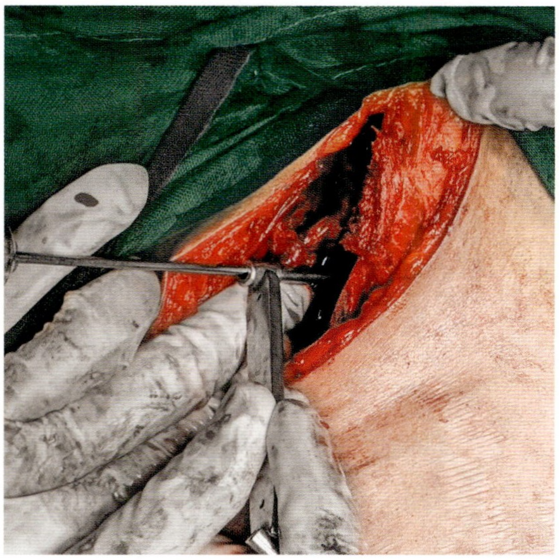

Fig. 11: Reduction of the fractured anterior wall is maintained with the help of a K-wire.

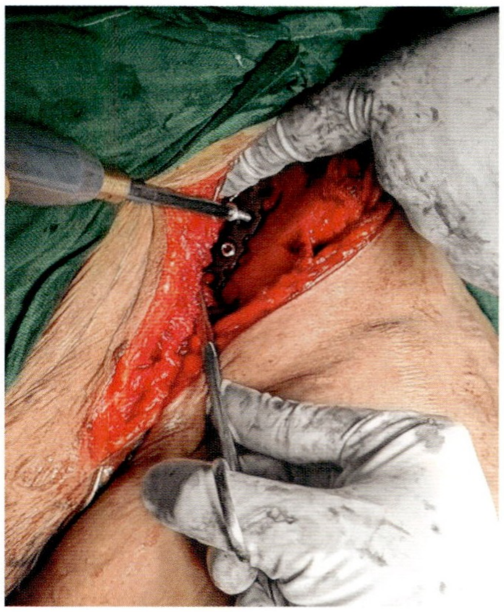

Fig. 12: A reconstruction plate is used for fixation of acetabular fractures and is positioned along iliac blade.

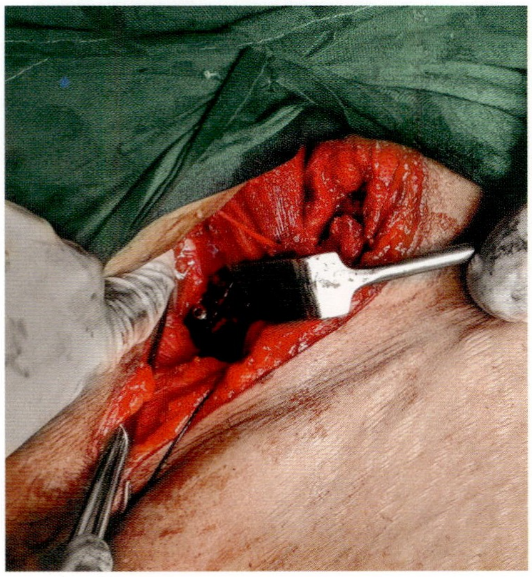

Fig. 13: Properly positioned reconstruction plate with screws tightened.

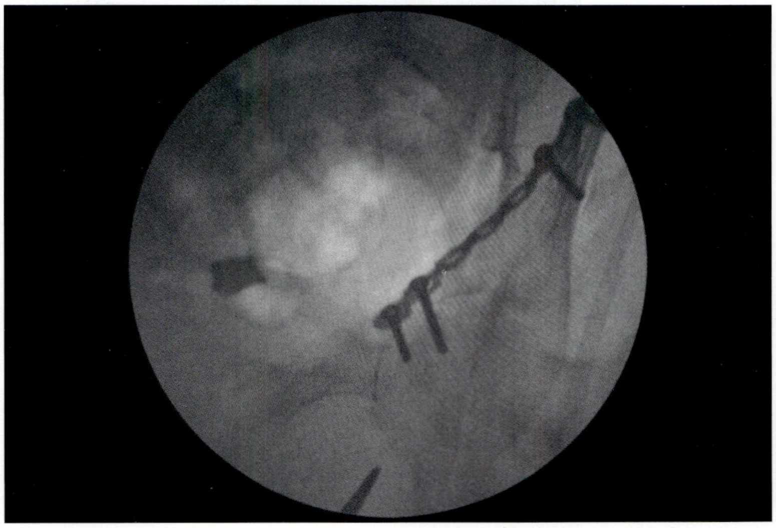

Fig. 14: Reduction is confirmed under C-arm.

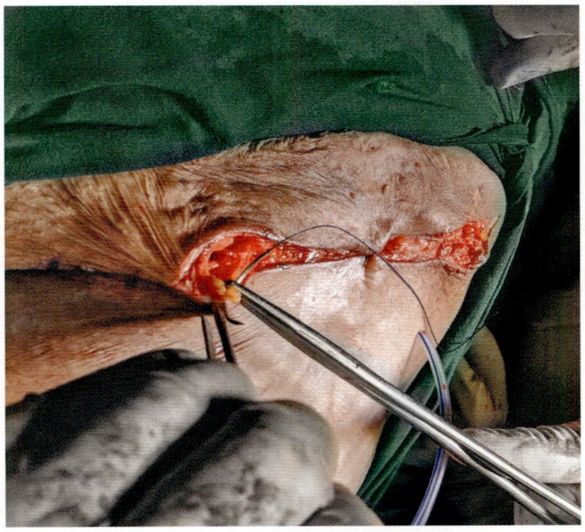

Fig. 15: Closure is done in layers of subcutaneous tissue by absorbable suture material followed by skin closure by nonabsorbable suture material along with a drain.

CHAPTER 100

Posterior Column Fixation with Reconstruction Plate

Ranjit Deshmukh, Rishikesh Ghalke, Anurag Daxini

INTRODUCTION

Acetabular fractures present with great treatment challenge to the orthopaedic surgeon primarily because of the complexity of the fracture, surgical decision making, and difficulty in gaining exposure of the fragments and reduction of the articular surface.

Acetabular fractures occur in a bimodal age distribution. In elderly, they occur with a low-energy trauma because of poor bone quality and in young population, they occur due to high velocity motor vehicle accidents.

Acetabulum fracture can occur in any one or more of the structures that make the acetabulum namely, the anterior wall, anterior column, posterior wall, posterior column, the roof, and quadrilateral plate.

The mainstay of treatment for displaced fractures is surgery, the goal being achieving an articular congruity and gaining stable fixation.

ANATOMY AND PATHOANATOMY OF ACETABULAR FRACTURES

Acetabulum is mainly made up of two columns—the anterior and posterior, which forms an inverted "Y". It is connected with the sacrum via the sciatic buttress. The anterior column is composed of the anterior ilium, anterior wall, iliopectineal eminence, and lateral superior pubic ramus. The posterior column is made up of the posterior wall, quadrilateral surface, ischial tuberosity, and the sciatic notch.

The acetabulum has an inclination of 40–45° and anteversion of 18–20°.

The mechanism of injury is usually a high-velocity injury and the pattern usually depends on the intensity and the vector of the force and the position of femoral head at the time of impact. In elderly individuals, the mechanism can be low-velocity injury in osteoporotic bones.

These fractures may be associated with other injuries in the lower limb, spine injuries, sciatic nerve injuries, abdominal and genitourinary tract injuries. It is therefore of importance to screen these patients where the mechanism of injury is a high-velocity trauma.

CLASSIFICATION (FIG. 1)

The Letournel and Judet classification is the most widely used classification system for acetabular fractures. It classifies the fractures as five elementary fractures and five associated fracture patterns.

CLINICAL FEATURES

Patient presents with pain, bruising, and inability to move the extremity. Sometimes, there might be associated lower limb fractures. One should always suspect abdominal or a genitourinary tract injury and look for signs like hematuria and hypotension.

RADIOLOGICAL IMAGING

Standard anteroposterior view of pelvis along with Judet, inlet and outlet views provide good information of the fracture anatomy. The obturator oblique and the iliac oblique Judet views provide a good view of the anterior column and posterior column, respectively.

Computed tomography (CT) scan with optional 3D reconstruction has an indispensable role for knowing the fracture anatomy.

TREATMENT OPTIONS

Nonoperative treatment in the form of protected weight bearing is indicated for patients who carry a high risk for surgery with highly morbid conditions and also who present late, i.e. more than 3 weeks after injury. Conservative management can also be considered for patients who have minimally displaced fractures, stable fractures, where articular congruity is maintained. Definitive indications for surgery include displaced fractures of the roof, unstable fracture pattern, marginal impaction, intra-articular loose bodies, and irreducible fracture dislocations.

Structures at Risk during Surgery

The sciatic nerve must be protected from traction injury by keeping the hip extended and knee flexed throughout the procedure. Care must be taken to isolate and protect the sciatic nerve and avoid unwanted retraction.

Medial femoral circumflex artery should be protected by avoiding excessive retraction and elevation of the quadratus femoris insertion.

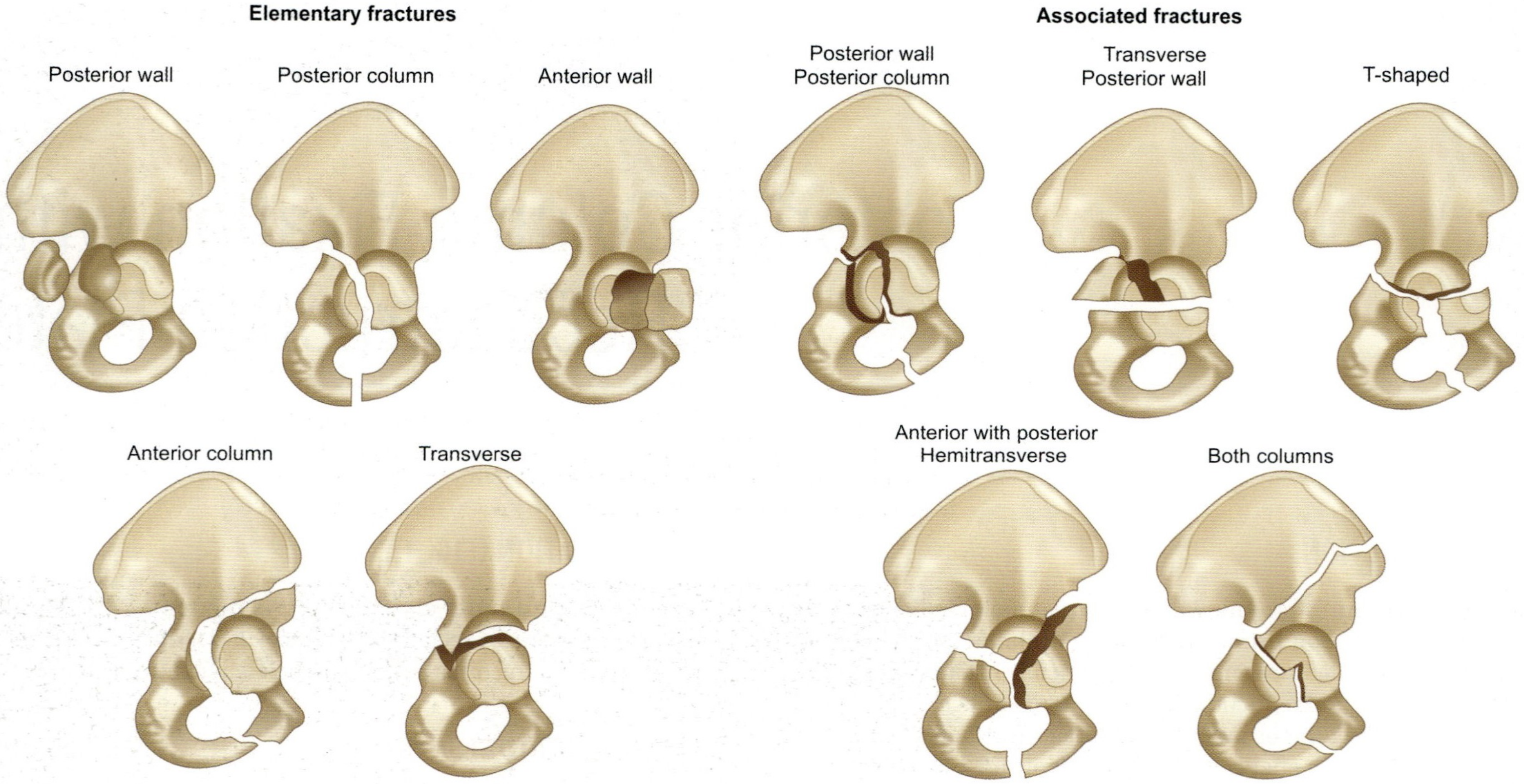

Fig. 1: Classification of acetabular fracture.

SURGICAL PROCEDURE

Here, we are describing open reduction and internal fixation of posterior column and wall fracture with a reconstruction plate using a Kocher–Langenbeck approach.

1. X-ray pelvis with both hips anteroposterior view showing posterior wall and posterior column fracture (Figs. 2A and B).
2. Computed tomography (CT) scan images axial sections (Fig. 3A) and CT scan images coronal sections (Fig. 3B).

Step 1: Patient positioning on operation table (Fig. 4).

Step 2: Position of C-arm (Fig. 5).

Step 3: Trolley with set of instruments (Fig. 6).

Step 4: Various plates used for fixation (Fig. 7).

Step 5: Painting and draping (Fig. 8).

Step 6: Kocher–Langenbeck skin incision mark (Fig. 9).

Step 7: Skin incision deepened (Fig. 10).

Step 8: Rotators tagged 1.5 cm away from insertion (Fig. 11).

Step 9: Capsule rent identified and extended, dislocated head visualized (Fig. 12).

Step 10: Wash given to the joint and loose fragments removed (Fig. 13).

Step 11: Impacted fragments elevated, fracture reduced and provisionally fixed with K-wire (Fig. 14).

Step 12: Postspring plate application (Fig. 15).

Step 13: Precontouring of plate with plate bender (Fig. 16).

Step 14: Plate fixation being done (Fig. 17).

Step 15: Cortex drilled with power drill (Fig. 18).

Step 16: Screw fixation requires special long screw driver with screw holder to help in the depth of working field. (Fig. 19).

Step 17: For superficial screw fixation normal long screw driver is useful (Fig. 20).

Step 18: C-arm image after provisional plate and screw application (Fig. 21).

Step 19: C-arm image after final screw application (Fig. 22).

Step 20: Final plate position after application (Fig. 23).

Step 21: Closure of rotators (Fig. 24).

Step 22: Closure of fascia (Fig. 25).

Step 23: Closure of deeper tissues (Fig. 26).

Step 24: Closure of subcutaneous tissue (Fig. 27).

Step 25: Skin closure (Fig. 28).

SURGICAL STEPS

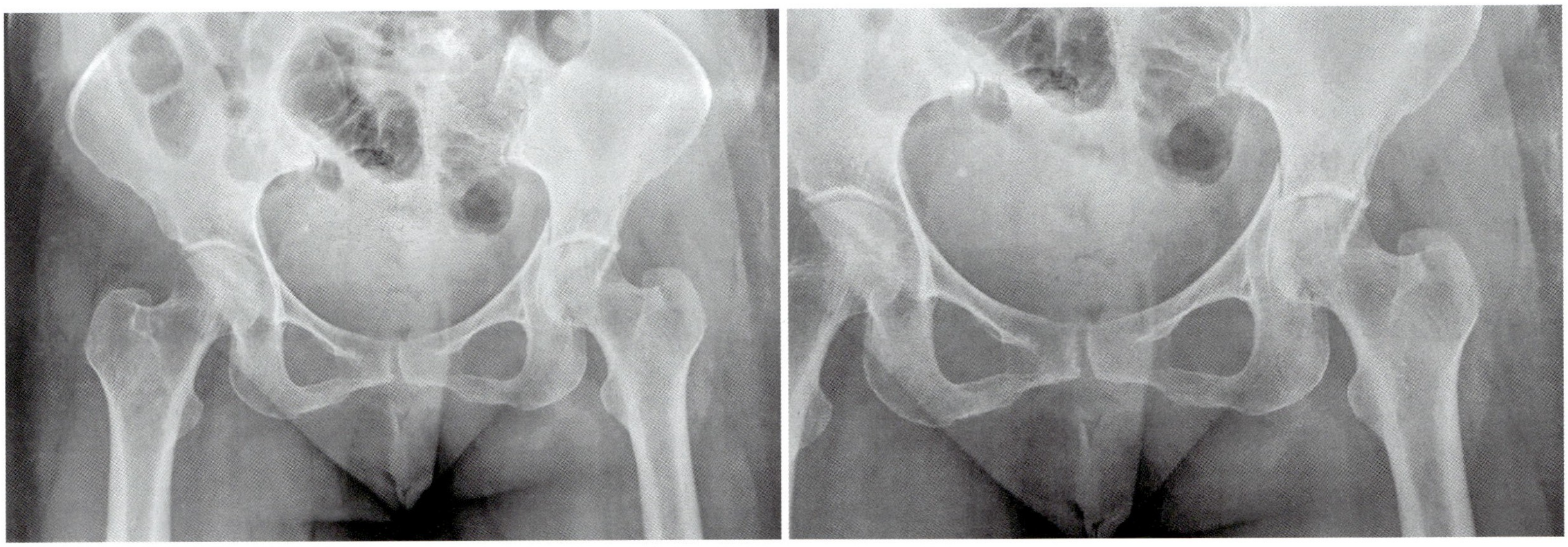

Figs. 2A and B: Preoperative X-rays showing posterior wall and column fracture.

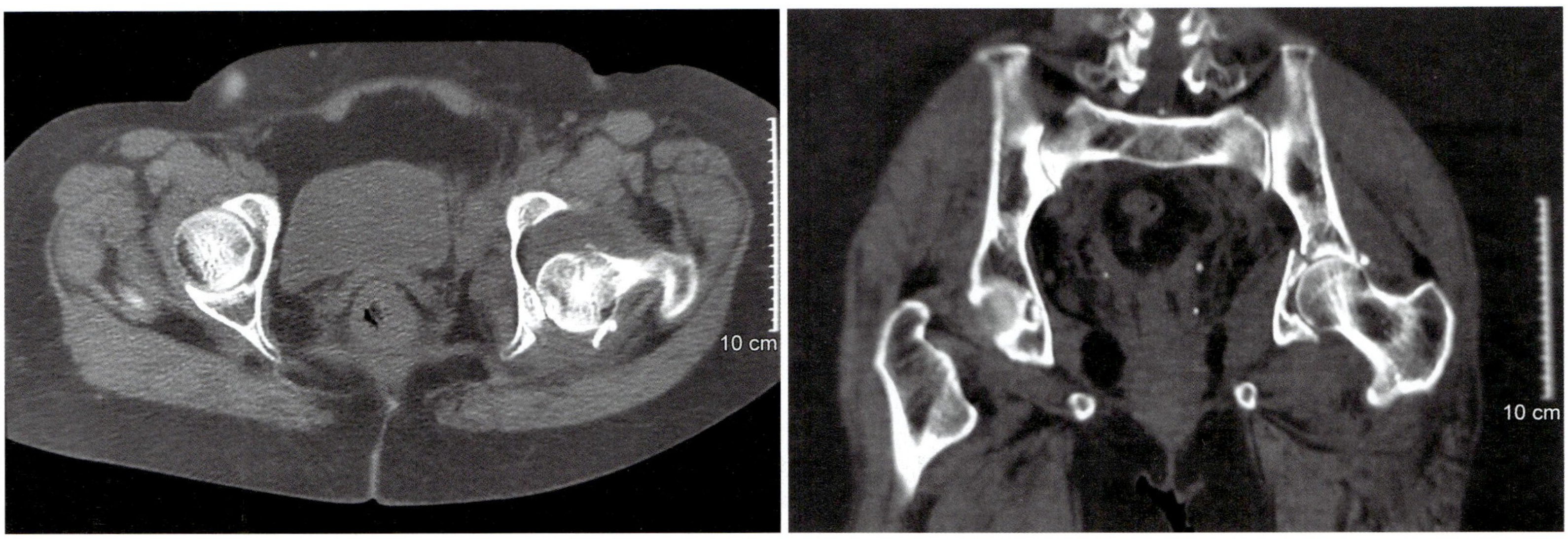

Figs. 3A and B: Preoperative CT scan images showing posterior subluxation of hip with posterior wall and column fracture.

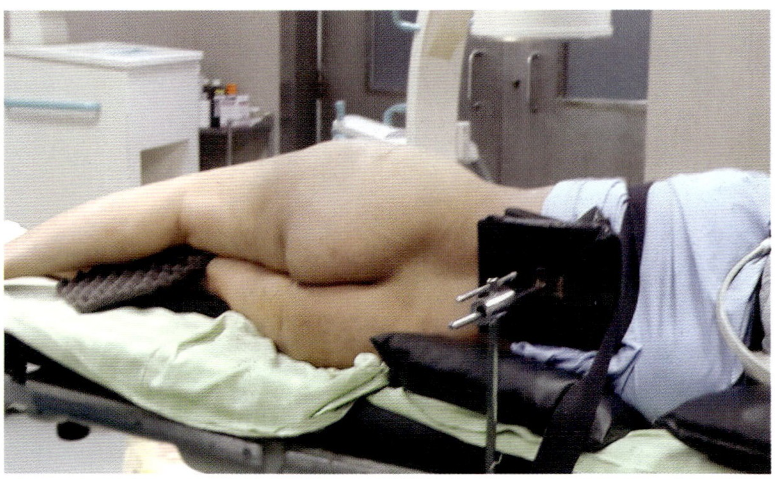

Fig. 4: Lateral position with supports.

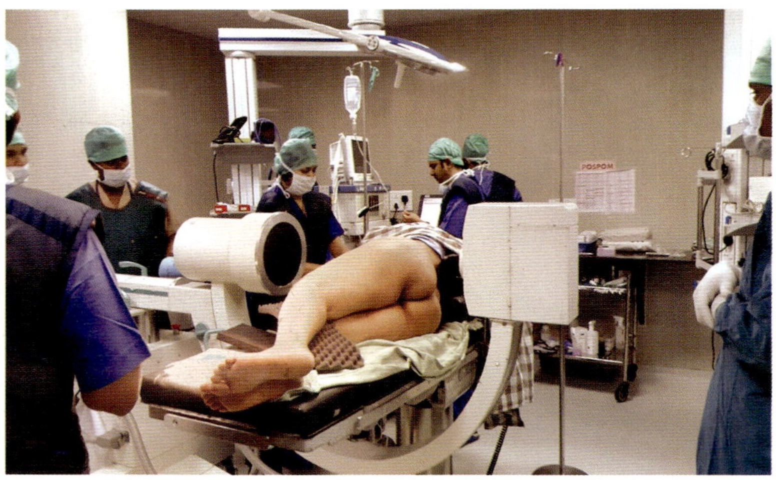

Fig. 5: Position of C-arm such that acetabulum is visible in all views of C-arm especially the Judet views.

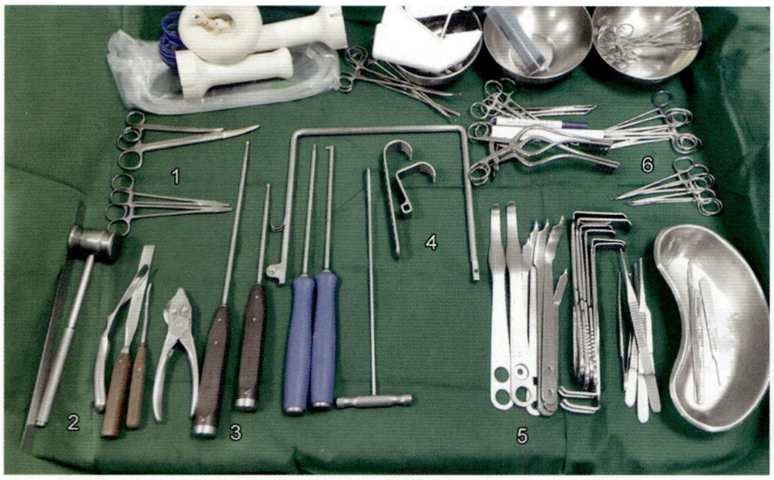

Fig. 6: Instrument set (1=Needle holder, 2=Osteotomes, chisel, periosteum elevator and hammer, 3=Ball spike with pointed ball tip (brown handle), in situ plate benders (blue handles), 4=Charnleys retractor, 5=Hohmann retractors blunt and pointed, 6=Artery forceps all sizes).

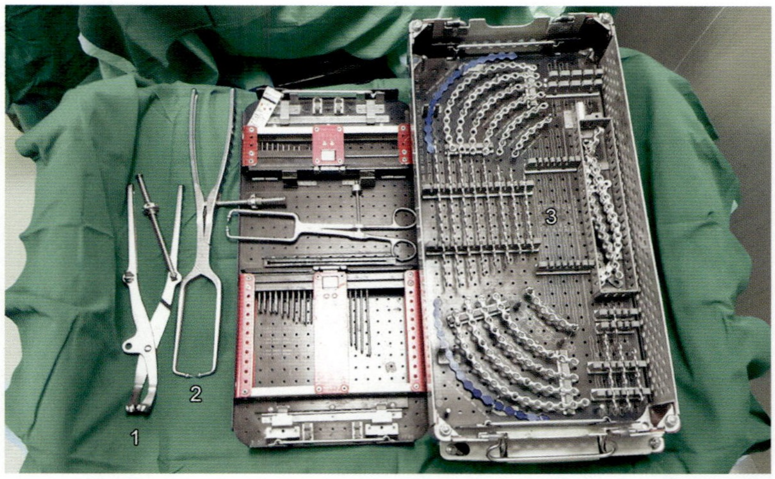

Fig. 7: Implant set (1=Pelvic reduction forceps using screws, 2=Reduction clamp, 3=Plates of all sizes).

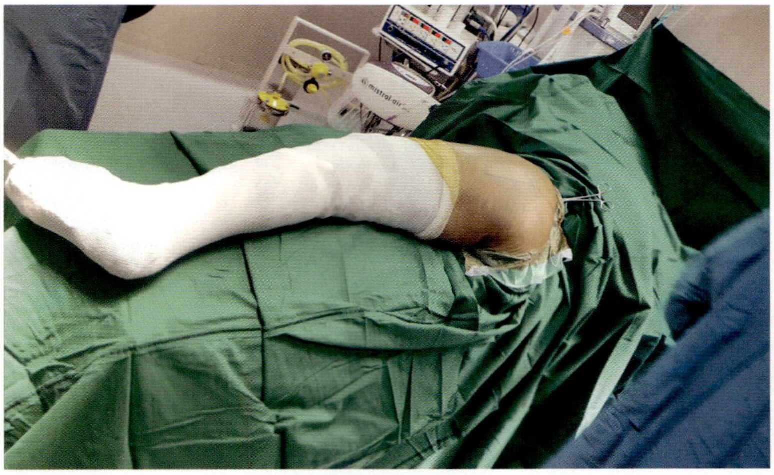

Fig. 8: Patient painting and draping.

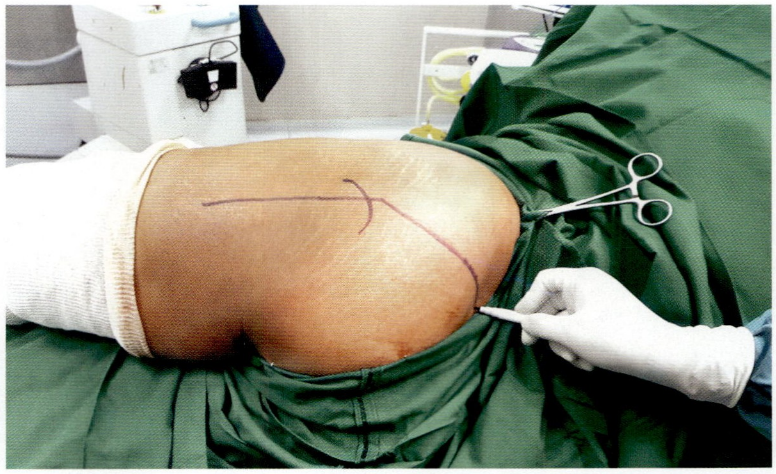

Fig. 9: Kocher Langenbeck incision marked.

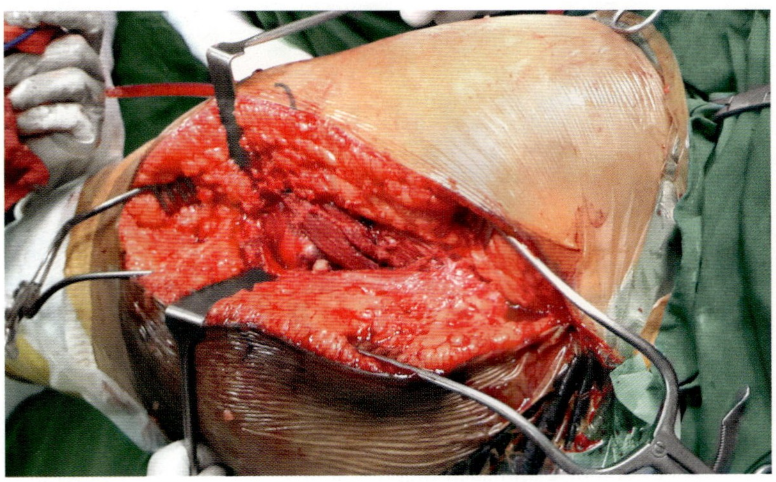

Fig. 10: Dissection deepened, Gluteus and rotators identified.

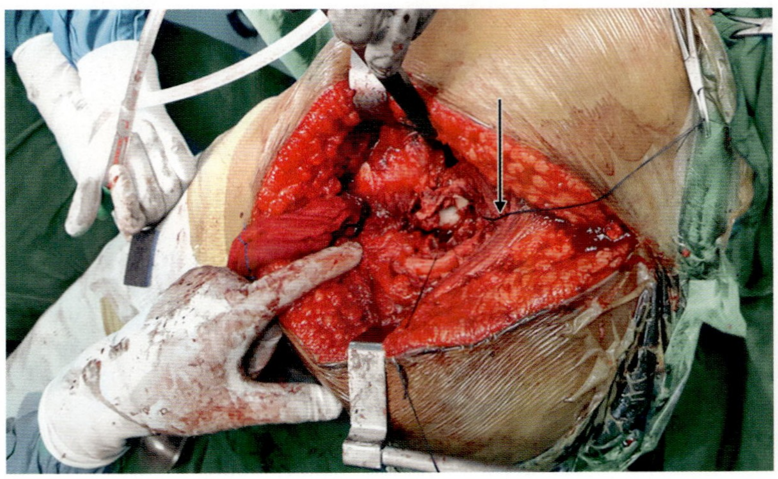

Fig. 11: Rotators tagged.

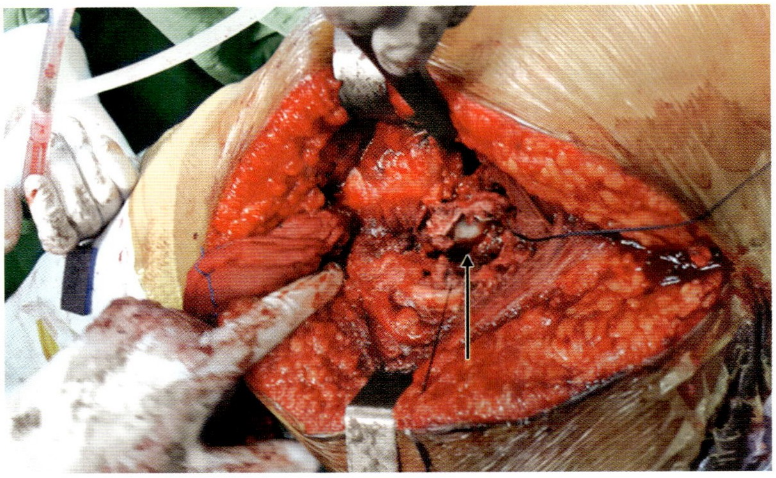

Fig. 12: Dislocated head identified.

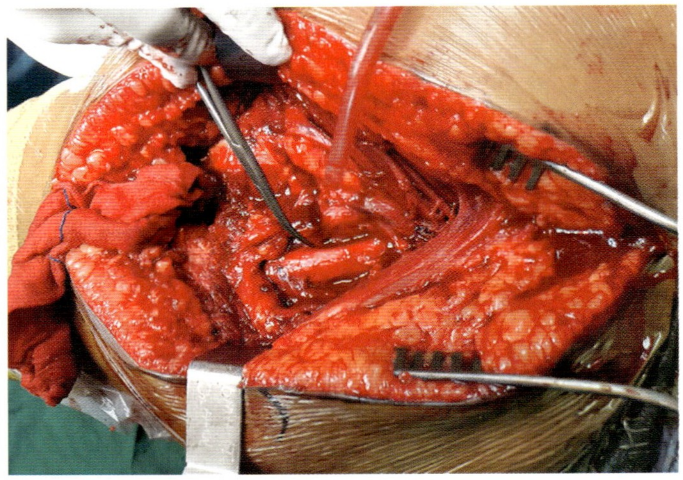

Fig. 13: Wash given and fragments from joint removed.

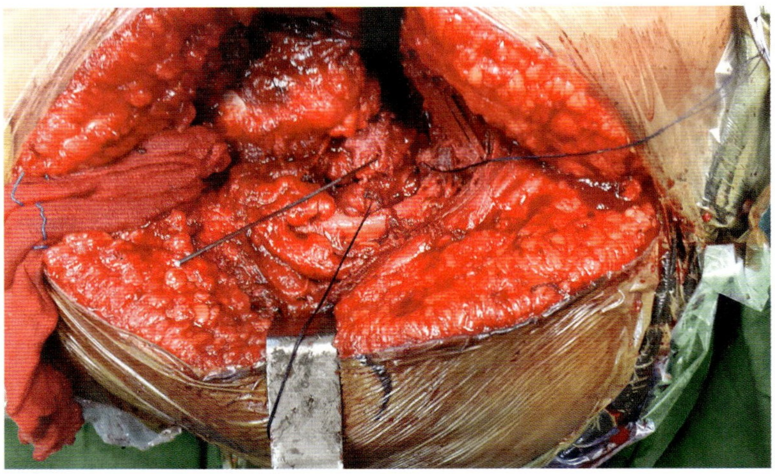

Fig. 14: Provisional fixation with K-wire.

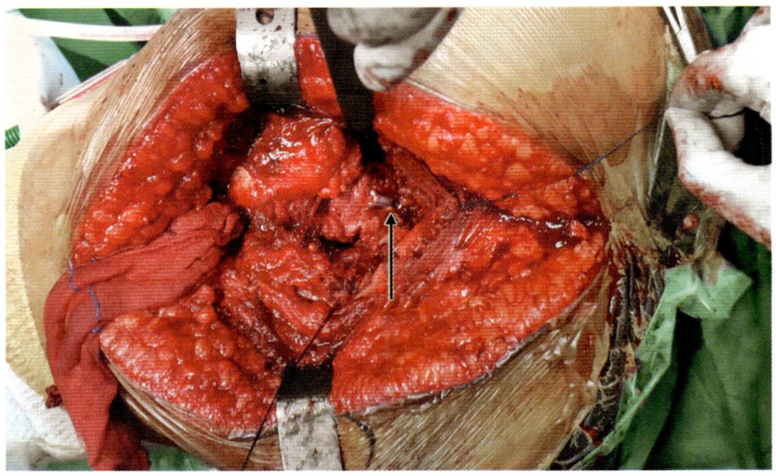

Fig. 15: Spring plate applied to support posterior wall fragment, since fragment is too small for interfragmentary screw.

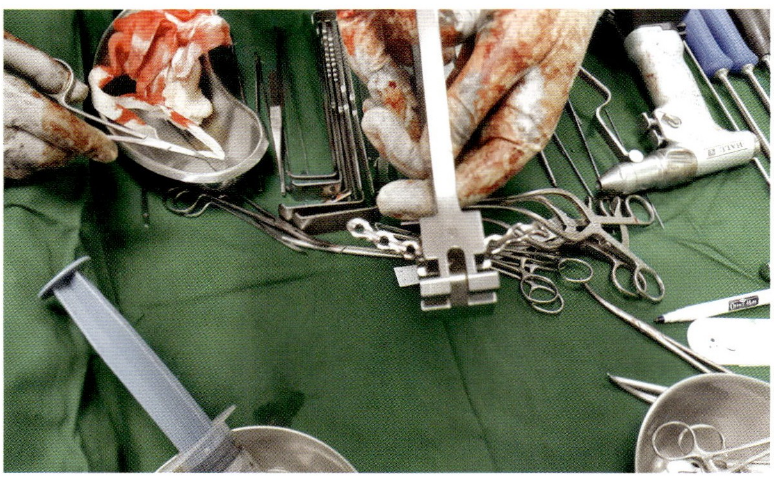

Fig. 16: Plate bender for contouring of plate.

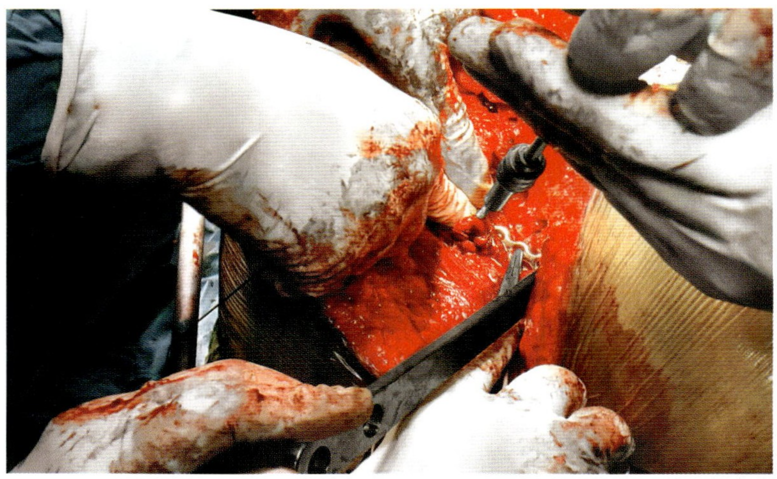

Fig. 17: Check the position and contouring of plate on patient.

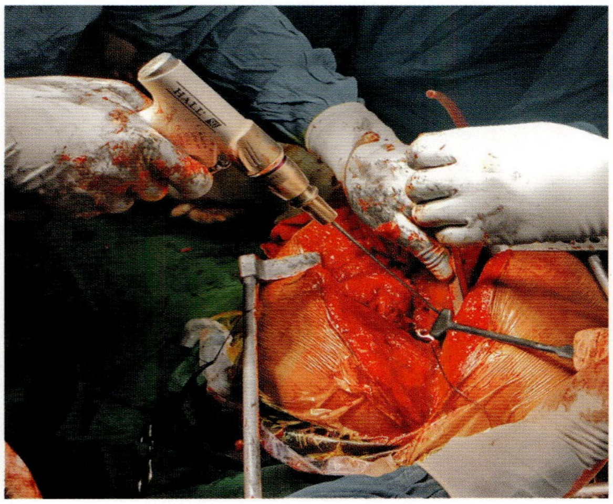

Fig. 18: Drilling of cortex.

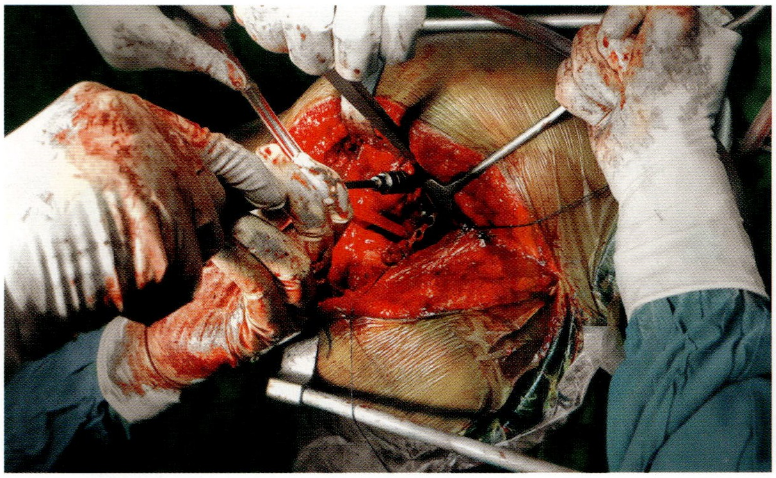

Fig. 19: Screw fixation in depth with long screw driver having screw holder.

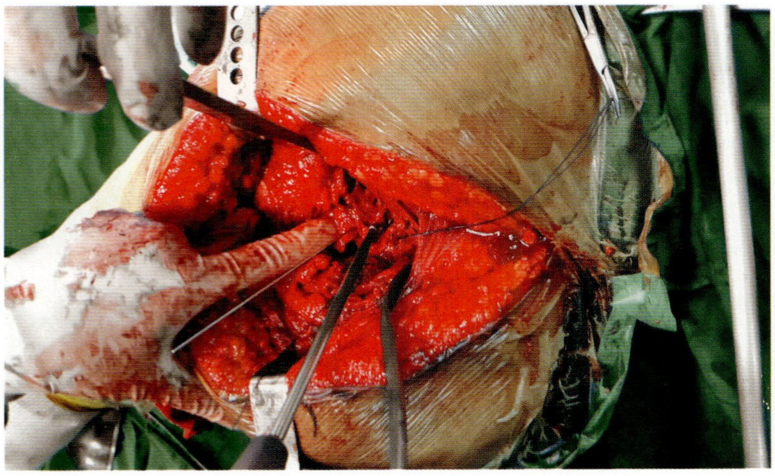

Fig. 20: Screw fixation with normal long screw driver.

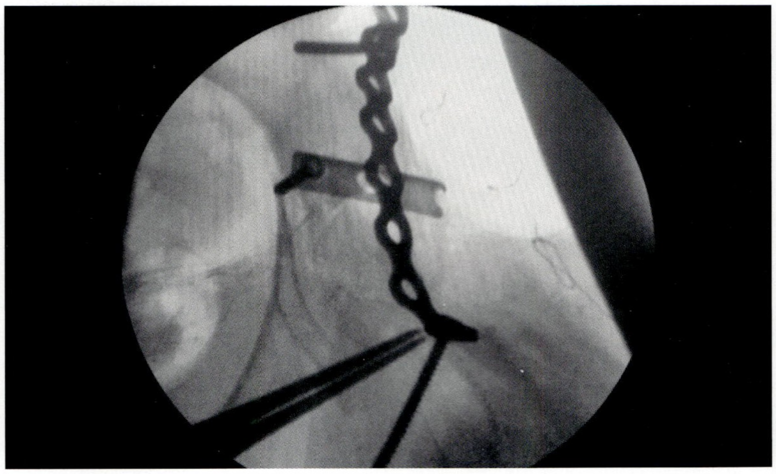

Fig. 21: C-arm image following provisional plate fixation.

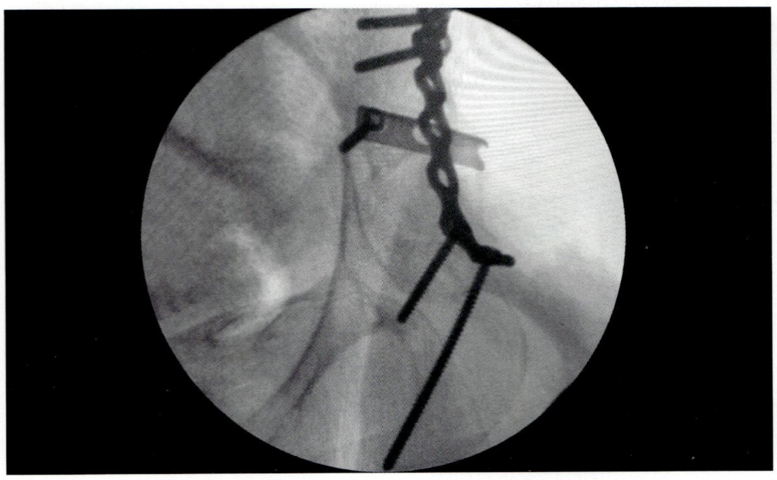

Fig. 22: Final C-arm image following plate fixation.

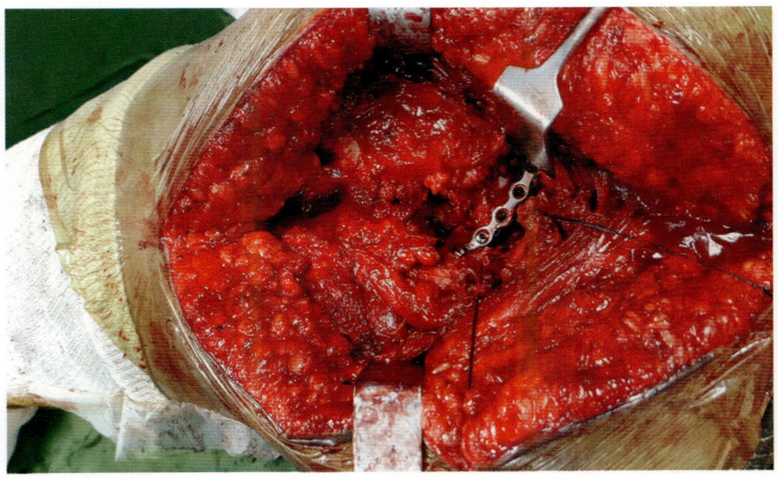

Fig. 23: Final plate position.

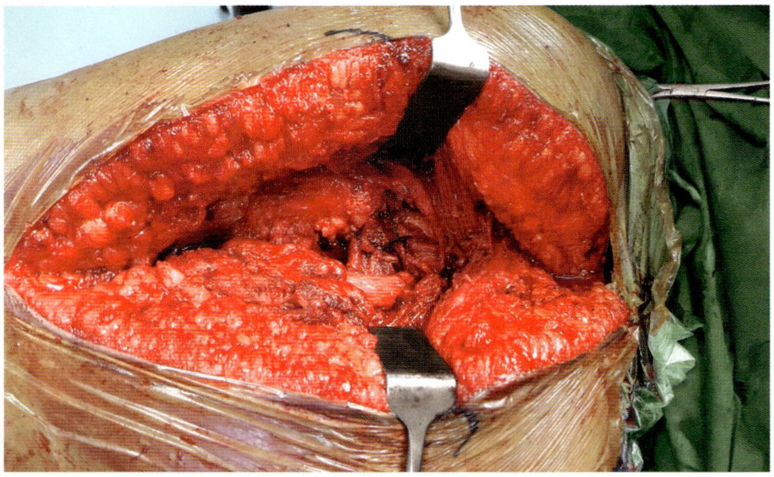

Fig. 24: Closure of rotators.

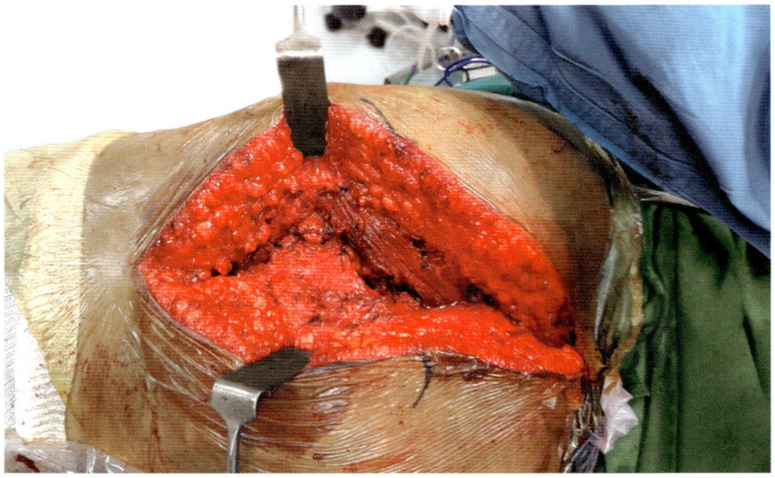

Fig. 25: Closure of fascia.

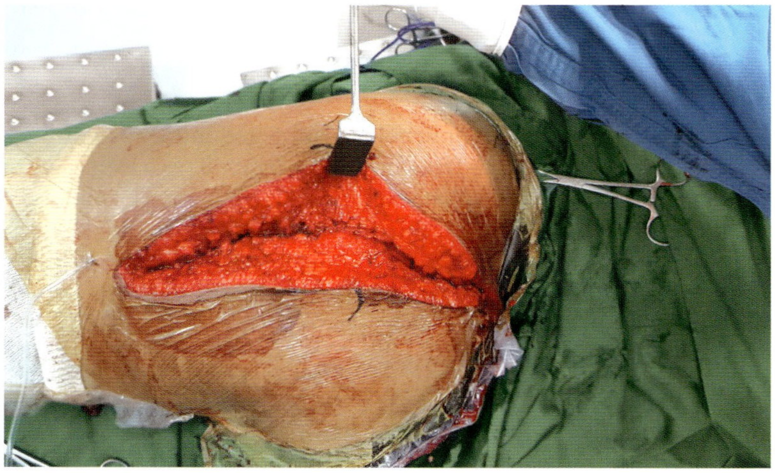

Fig. 26: Closure of deeper tissue.

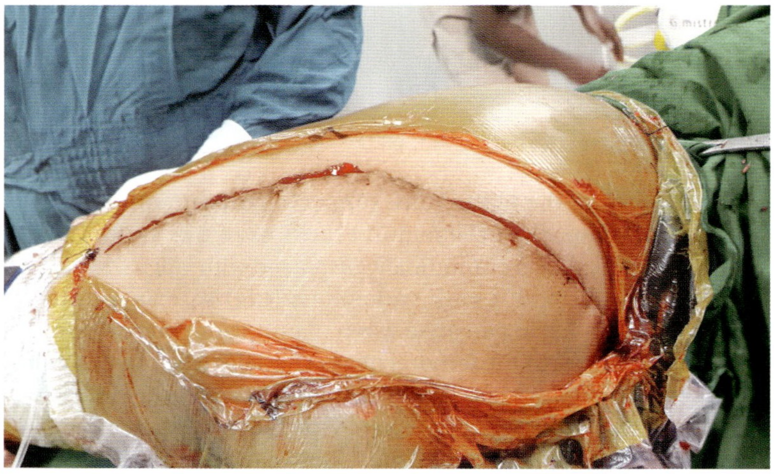

Fig. 27: Subcutaneous tissue closure.

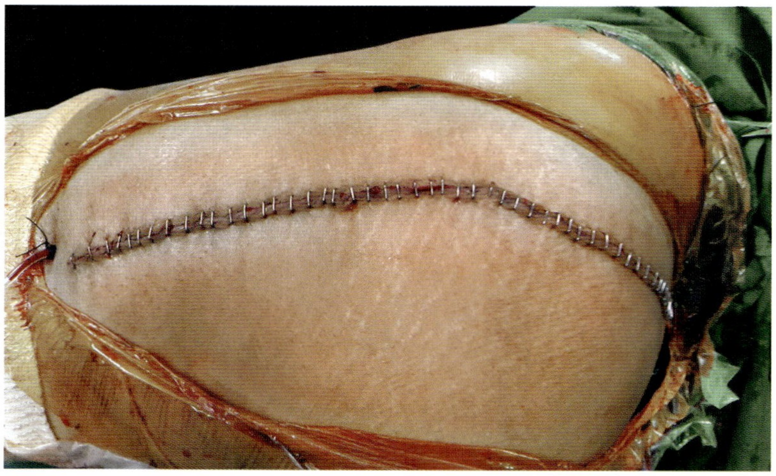

Fig. 28: Skin closure.

POSTOPERATIVE PROTOCOL

Following surgery, patient is advised nonweight-bearing mobilization till adequate union is seen on X-ray, following which patient is gradually shifted to partial weight-bearing ambulation and ultimately full weight-bearing ambulation with the help of walking stick. Gradually, the walking stick is taken off when fracture heals and patient is symptom free.

SUGGESTED READING

1. Letournel E. Fracture of the Cotyloid cavity, study of a series of 75 cases. J Chir(Paris). 1961;82:47-87.
2. Letournel E. Acetabulum fractures: classification and management. Clin Orthop Relat Res. 1980;(151):81-106.
3. Letournel E, Judet R. Fractures of the Acetabulum, 2nd edition. New York: Springer-Verlag; 1993.
4. Judet R, Judet J, Letournel E. Fractures of the acetabulum, Classification and surgical approaches for open reduction. J Bone Joint Surg Am. 1964;46A:1615-38.

CHAPTER 101

Fracture Neck of Femur Cannulated Cancellous Screw Fixation

Niranjan Chavan, Sharad M Hardikar

INTRODUCTION

Most fractures at the hip require surgical management, especially fractures of the neck of the femur. Fractures of the neck of femur which are undisplaced or minimally displaced with valgus impaction should be fixed in situ with cancellous (lag) screws. Choice of fixation and confusion can arise when planning the management of displaced fractures of the femoral neck. The selection of the surgical treatment for each patient has to be individualized on the basis of fracture pattern, time lapse since injury, patient acceptance, patient's physiological condition, age and most importantly, achieving fracture reduction. The surgeon has to be ready with all armamentarium with regards to options for surgical management of the fracture, and should be able to change his decision of surgical option, if needed.

Multiple cannulated cancellous screws act on the principle "lag screws", achieving compression at the well-reduced fracture site. Hence, this procedure is applicable to impacted intracapsular neck fractures as well as displaced fractures of the femoral neck especially in younger patients. However, "satisfactory" reduction must be obtained.

At the same time, caution must be exercised and other options such as hemireplacement should be considered, especially in elderly patients, if reduction cannot be achieved. In cases of fractures with intertrochanteric extension other implants such as dynamic hip screw are to be preferred.

PREOPERATIVE PREPARATION

Hip Radiographs

- Pelvis with both hips—anteroposterior view with 10° internal rotation (Fig. 1).
- Involved proximal femur—cross-table lateral view (Fig. 2).

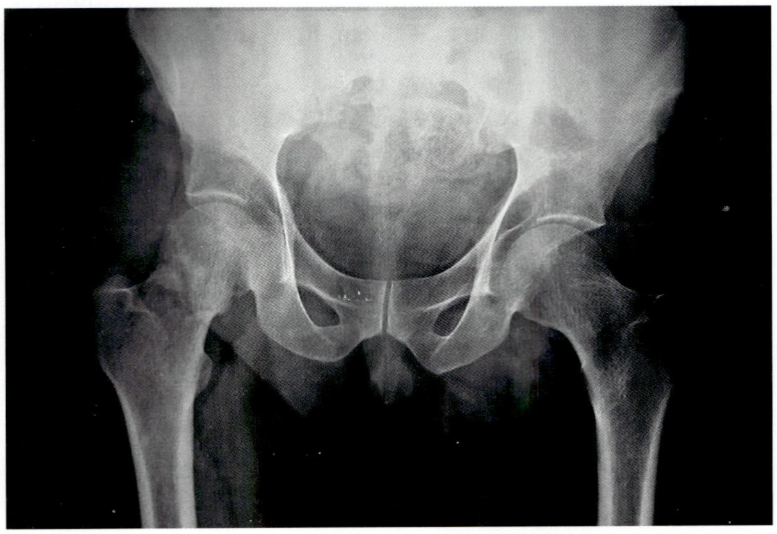

Fig. 1: Anteroposterior view with 10° internal rotation.

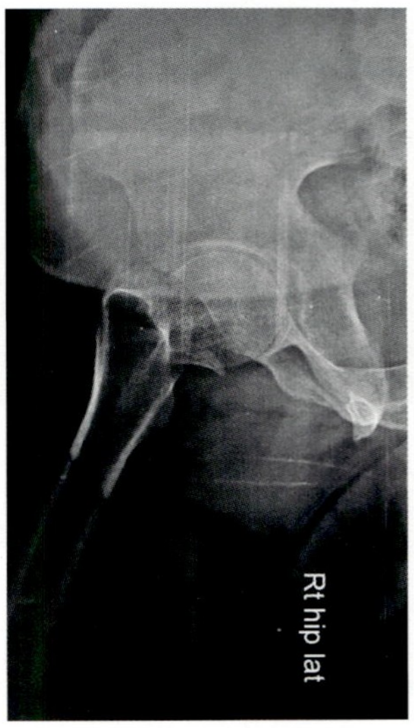

Fig. 2: Cross-table lateral view.

Good-quality radiographs are imperative for proper preoperative evaluation of the fracture pattern and for decision making. If missed or error in evaluation, C-arm evaluation after anesthetizing the patient can also be done without the fear of patient's discomfort due to pain.

Computed tomography (CT) scan has a role in cases of doubts of intertrochanteric of subtrochanteric extensions of the fracture pattern. Magnetic resonance imaging (MRI) has a role to confirm the viability of the femoral head in late presentations with displacement of fracture fragments, condition in which the vascular supply of the head may be compromised.

EXAMINATION AND DOCUMENTATION

Documenting status of preoperative neurovascular examination of the lower limbs to rule out sciatic injury, spinal injuries, or any other fragility fractures in elderly should be done to avoid any missed injuries.

SURGICAL STEPS

EQUIPMENT

- Radiolucent operating table with traction attachments (should be able to convert to flat table in case of change of operative plans, prosthetic replacement, etc.)
- C-arm image intensifier
- General instruments set (Fig. 3)
- Orthopaedic instruments set (drill, bone levers, mallet, screwdrivers, etc.) (Fig. 3)
- Cannulated screw instruments set (guidewires, angle guide, guidewires insertion device, depth gauge, cannulated reamer, cannulated screw driver, 6.5-mm cannulated cancellous partial threaded screws) (Figs. 4 and 5).

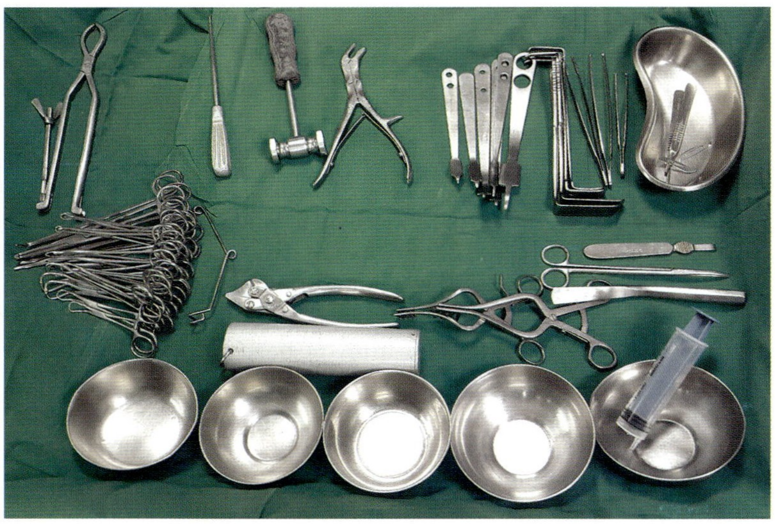

Fig. 3: General and general orthopaedic instruments.

ANESTHESIA, PATIENT POSITIONING, AND FRACTURE REDUCTION

Spinal or epidural anesthesia is the anesthesia of choice in almost all patients. Patients with concomitant upper limb injuries can be administered general anesthesia, subjective to physiological fitness.

Under anesthesia, the patient is placed supine on the fracture table with all pressure points well padded. Extra care should be taken to avoid incarceration of the genital area by the perineal post (Figs. 6 and 7).

Assessment of the adequacy of the fracture reduction is then done after positioning the patient on the fracture table. Fluoroscopy by C-arm is done in two or more planes to evaluate the reduction of the fracture fragments.

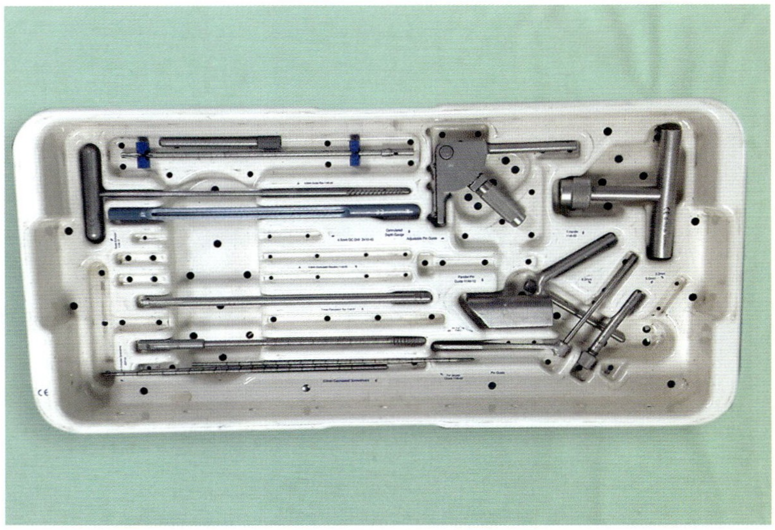

Fig. 4: Cannulated screw instruments set.

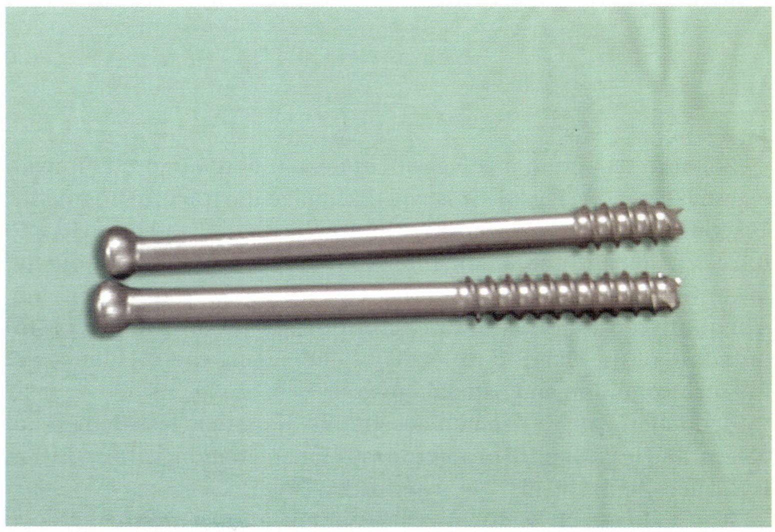

Fig. 5: 6.5-mm cannulated cancellous partial threaded screws.

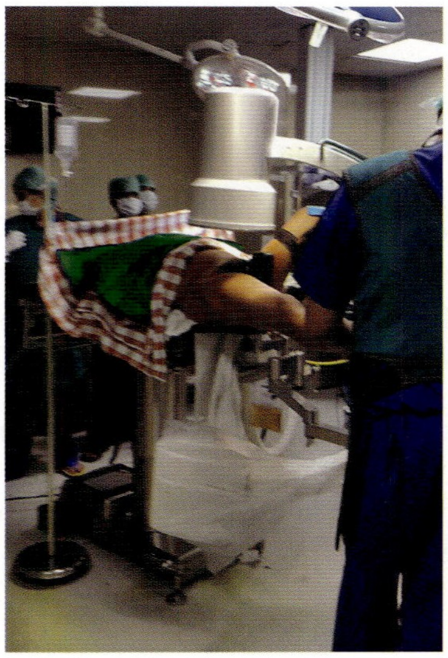

Fig. 6: C-arm position for anteroposterior (AP) view.

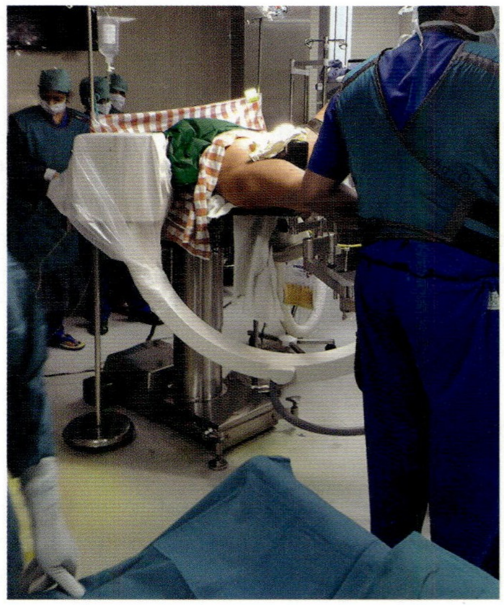

Fig. 7: C-arm position for lateral view.

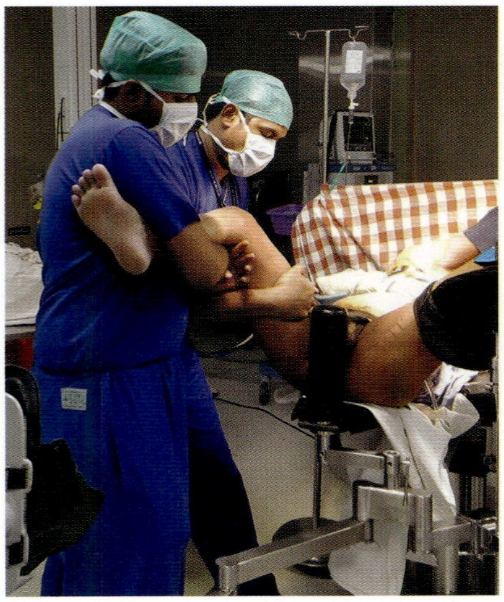

Fig. 8: Closed manipulation for fracture reduction.

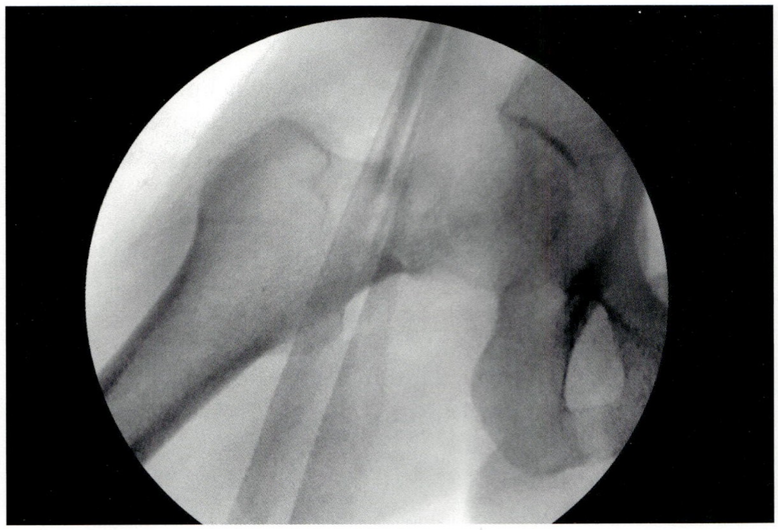

Fig. 9: Good reduction in AP view.

Fracture reduction involves 90° of flexion of the injured hip with external rotation (Fig. 8). This will disengage the fracture fragments. Traction is then given as the leg is internally rotated and brought into full extension and abduction. Internal rotation and length of both the lower limbs are then compared to confirm the fracture reduction. Adequate reduction is the most important factor for successful outcome of the fixation in terms of decreasing the incidences of fracture nonunion and osteonecrosis.

Reduction can be deemed acceptable, if there is less than 15° of valgus, and less than 10° of anteroposterior angulation. varus position is not acceptable at all (Figs. 9 and 10).

Post a successful reduction, the patient's limbs are then placed in the foot holders, positioning of the limbs are made as such that they do not interrupt the C of the image intensifier. Good aseptic scrubbing, painting, and draping should follow accepted positioning. A dose of intravenous antibiotic appropriate for the patient's infection prophylaxis is then administered prior to skin incision.

SURGICAL PROCEDURE

The screws can be inserted percutaneous, if the bony landmarks are well demarcated or in case of anticipated wound complications due to contusion or bruising at the trochanters and proximal lateral thigh. Routinely, limited open lateral approach is used for screw insertion. A straight lateral incision is made from the base of greater trochanter, extending 5–8 cm distally (Fig. 11).

After superficial dissection, the iliotibial band is then divided in line with the skin incision. Care should be taken to ensure that the deep dissection lies posterior to the tensor fascia lata proximally. The vastus lateralis fascia and muscle are then divided longitudinally, and two parts of muscle are retracted anteriorly and posteriorly. Alternatively, vastus lateralis fascia and muscle are elevated off the fascia posteriorly down to linea aspera then retracted anteriorly.

Soft tissues are retracted using a Hohmann bone lever placed just proximal to the insertion of gluteus maximus (Fig. 12). The lateral

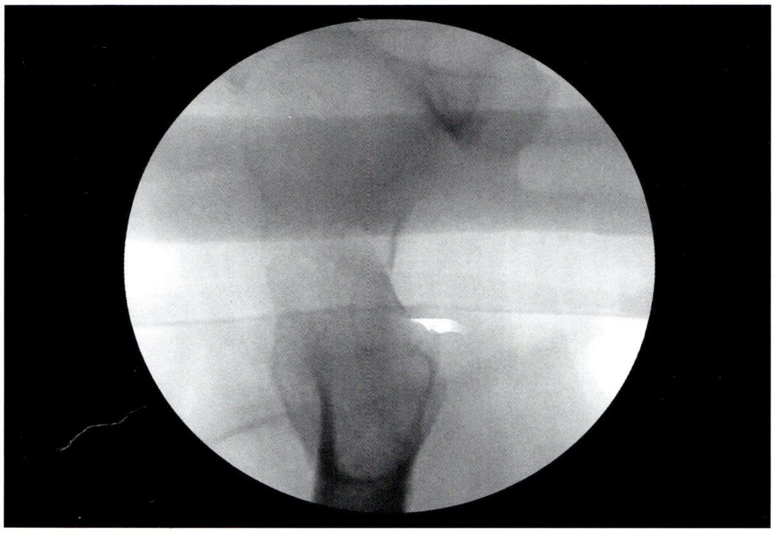

Fig. 10: Good reduction in lateral view.

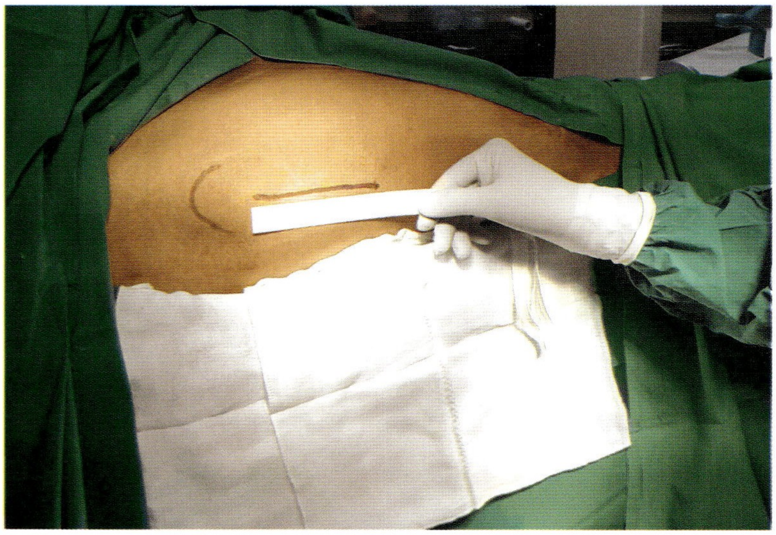

Fig. 11: Incision mark.

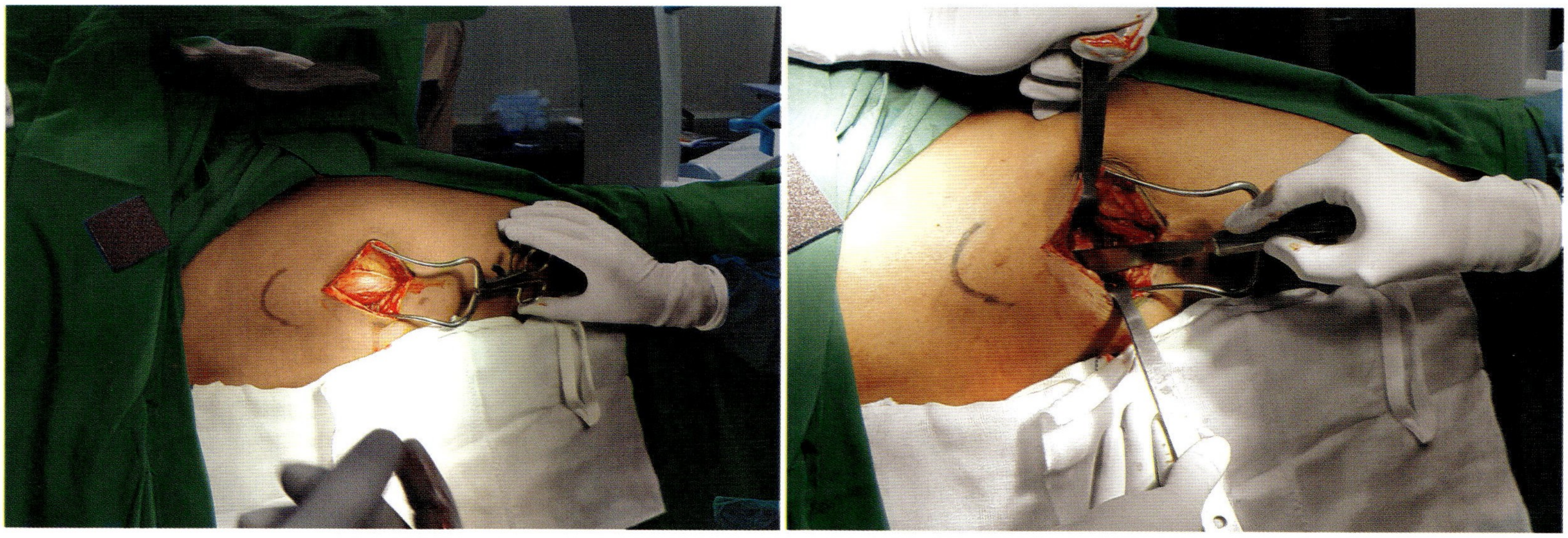

Fig. 12: Deeper dissection is done. A plane is created between the fibers of vastus lateralis.

cortex of the subtrochanteric area is then laid exposed for guidewires insertion.

Guidewires Insertion

Before starting insertion of the guidewires, a guidewire or blunt probe can be placed anterior to the femoral neck to estimate the femoral neck anteversion. A forceps or closed pair of scissors may also be used carefully. The same can be used to perform a closed capsulotomy at a later stage to drain off the fracture hematoma (Figs. 13 and 14). Drainage of hematoma eliminates tamponade effect and improves circulation to femoral head and may have a role in preventing avascular necrosis.

The guidepins are then inserted in an inverted triangular configuration. The apex pin of the triangle should be inserted first and it should be in the inferior and central or inferior and posterior aspect of the femoral neck. Care should be taken so as to avoid placing the inferior wire below the level of the lesser trochanter. Placing the inferior screw through the cortical subtrochanteric region may cause a stress riser effect, increasing the risk of a subsequent fracture. Biplanar fluoroscopy by C-arm is used to confirm wire placements in the anteroposterior and lateral planes through the neck. Two to three guidewires in parallel or divergent planes are inserted. The guidewires are inserted right up to a good hold by subchondral bone can be appreciated (Figs. 15 and 16). A cannulated depth gauge is then used to measure the length of the screws (Fig. 17A).

Fixation

Depending on the fracture pattern (subcapital vs transcervical vs basicervical), one-half threaded or one-fourth threaded screws are selected, making sure that the threaded portion should cross beyond the fracture site. Drilling with 4-mm drill bit (Fig. 17B) and

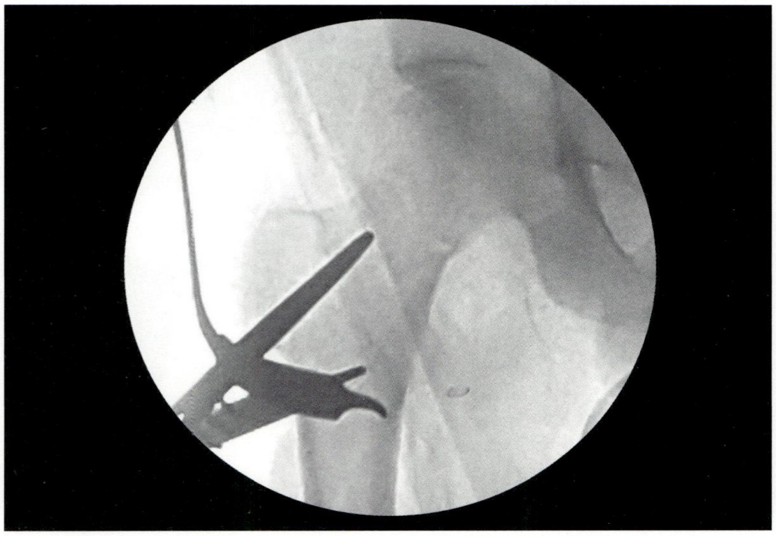

Fig. 13: Capsulotomy and drainage of fracture hematoma: C-arm guidance.

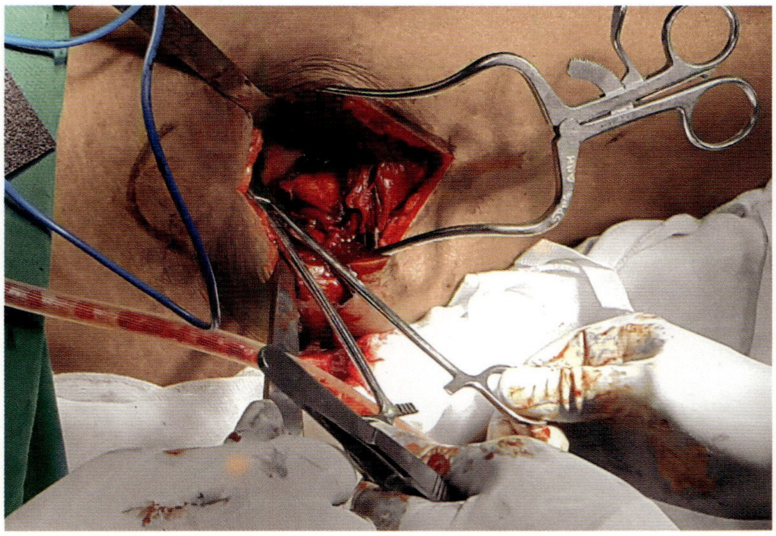

Fig. 14: Drainage of fracture hematoma.

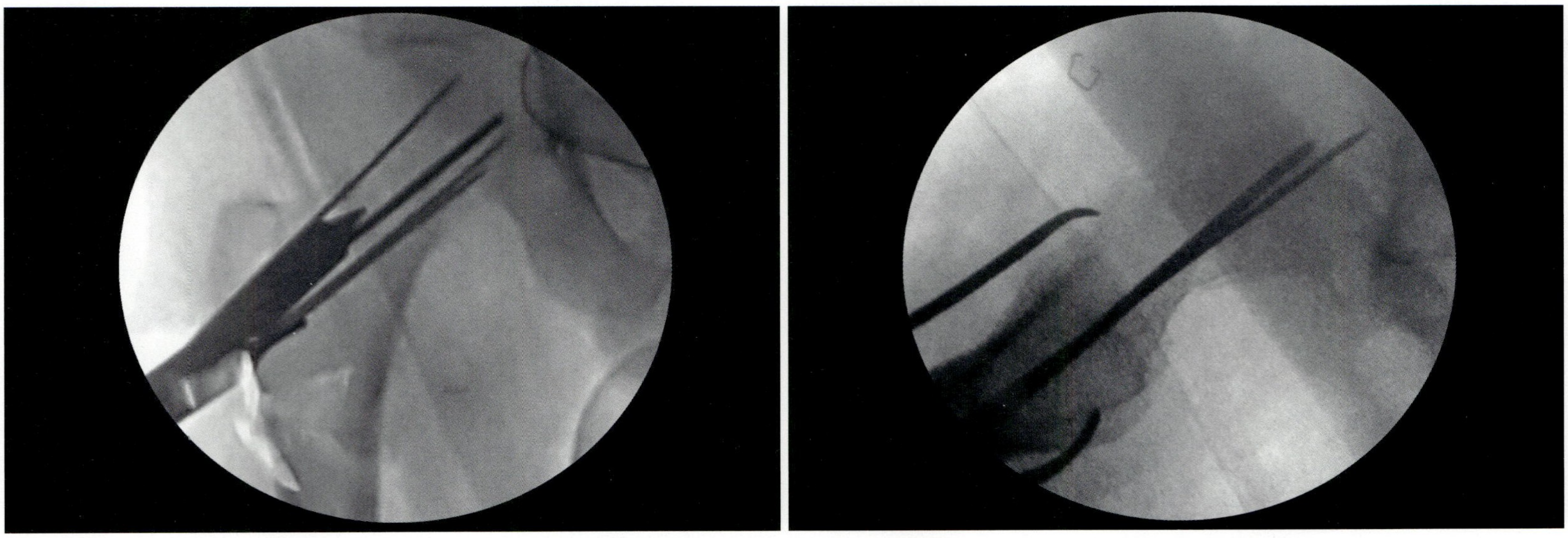

Fig. 15: The guidewires are inserted deep up to subchondral bone. Position checked in both AP and lateral C-arm views.

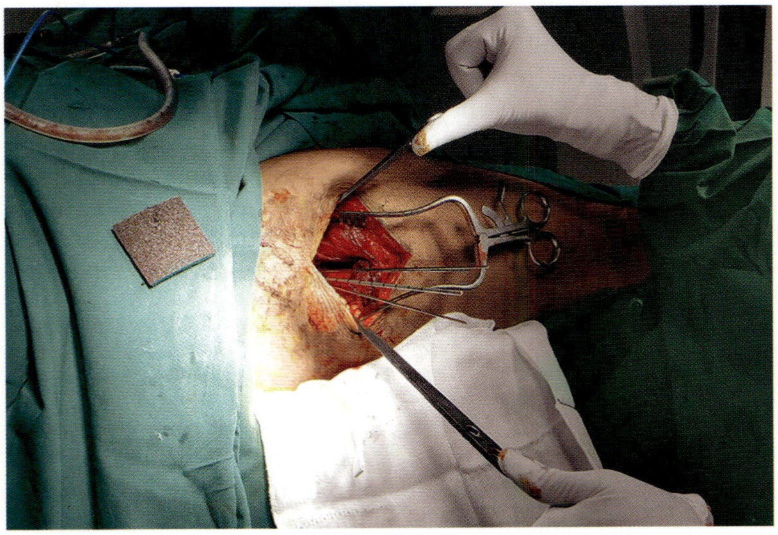

Fig. 16: Guidewires are inserted.

reaming/tapping is done along the intended path of the screws over the guidewires. Cannulated cancellous screws are then inserted with washers (Fig. 17C) to achieve compression at the fracture site. Position of the screws, length, and reduction is then confirmed by fluoroscopy (Figs. 18A and B).

A thorough sterile saline wash is given and closure of the surgical wound is achieved in layers. A thorough hemostasis should be achieved prior to closure of the wound. Placing of a vacuum drain is as per choice of the operating surgeon.

COMPLICATIONS

In spite of best efforts, a significant number of patients of this fracture develop complications:

- Avascular necrosis (23%)
- Nonunion (9%)
- Implant failure, cutout or backout.

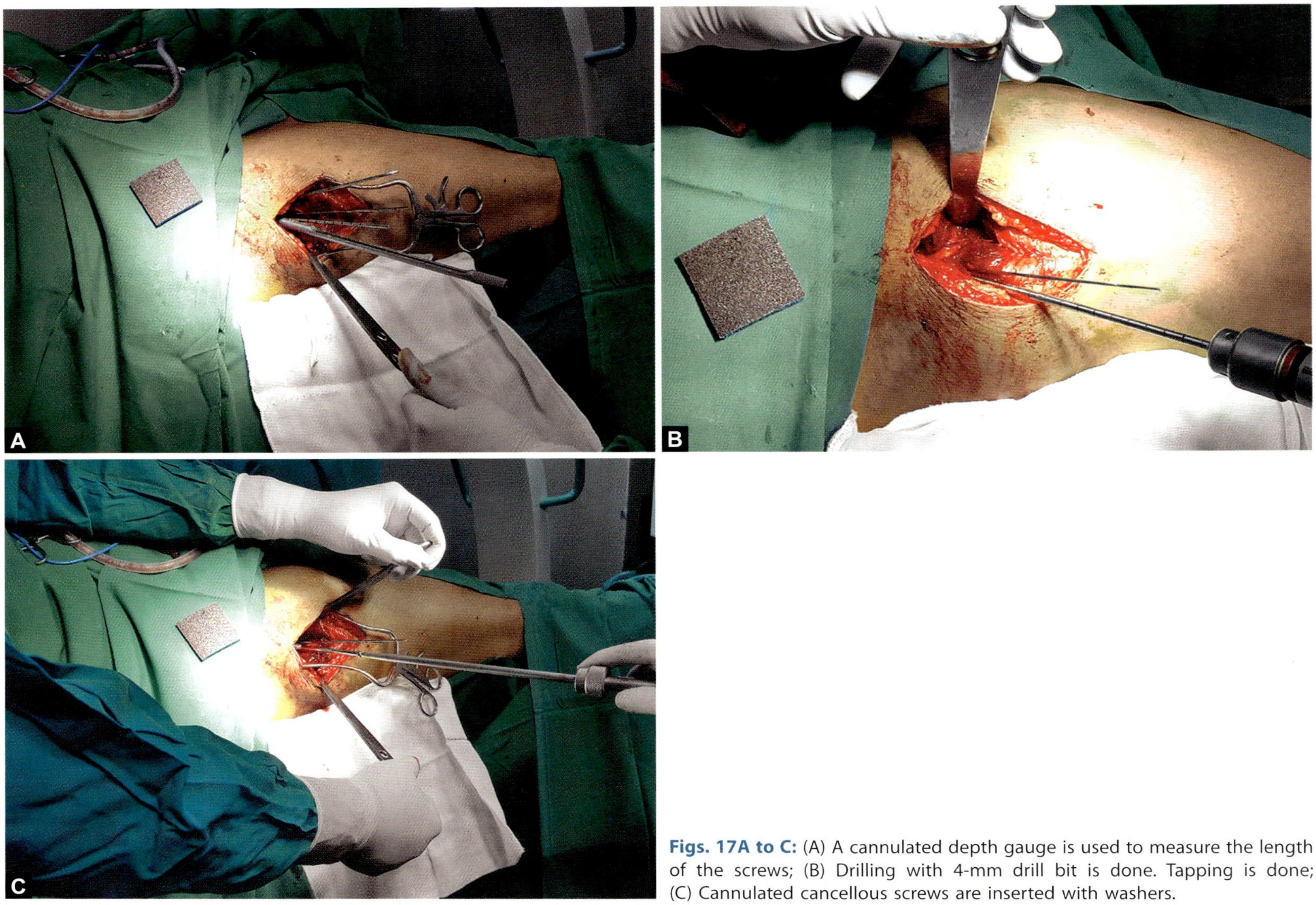

Figs. 17A to C: (A) A cannulated depth gauge is used to measure the length of the screws; (B) Drilling with 4-mm drill bit is done. Tapping is done; (C) Cannulated cancellous screws are inserted with washers.

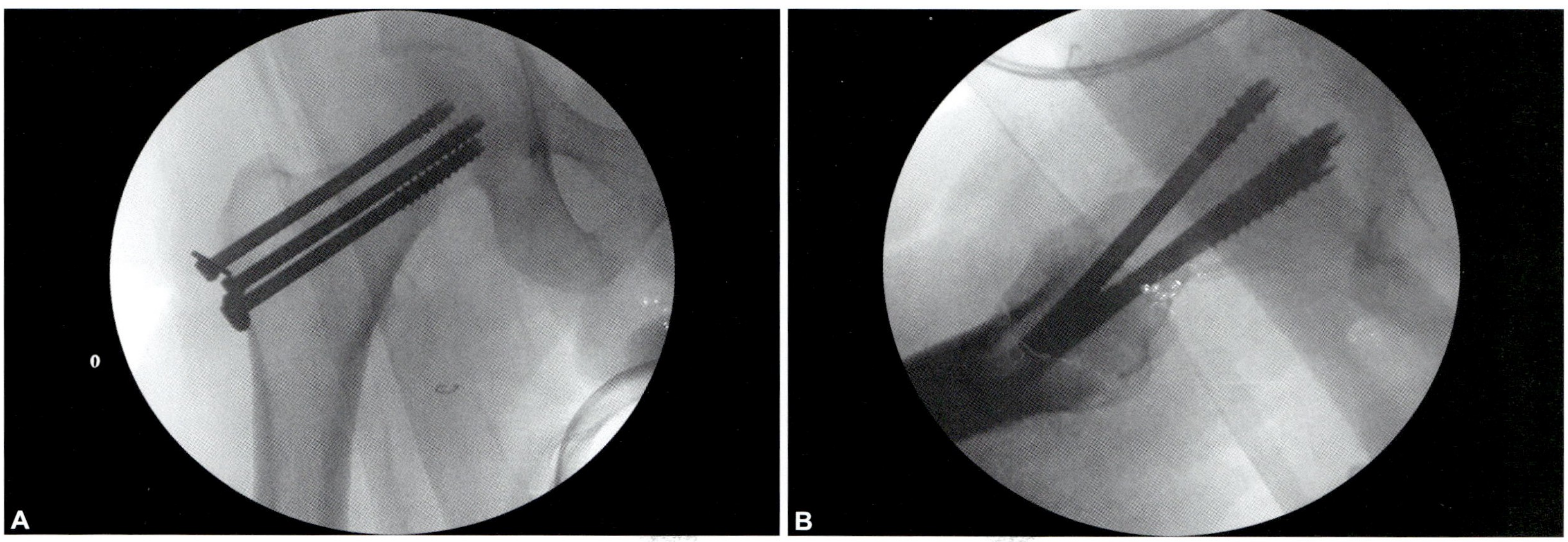

Figs. 18A and B

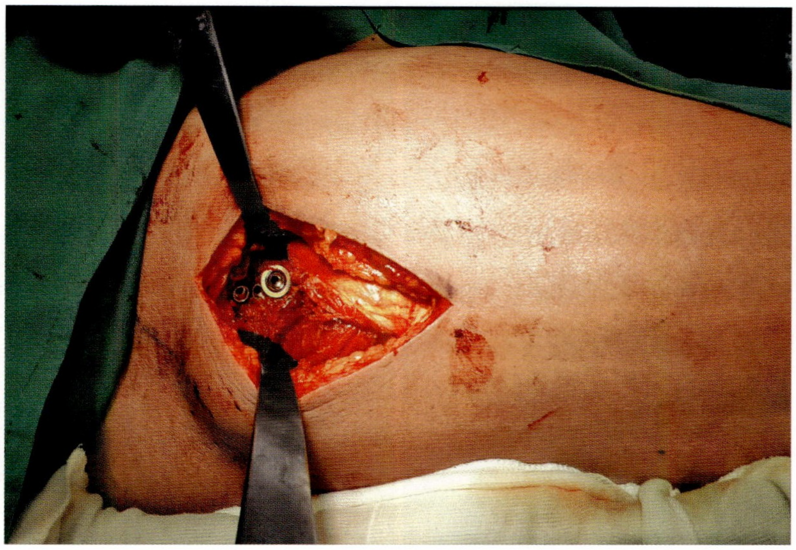

Fig. 18C

Figs. 18A to C: (A and B) Position of the screws, length, and reduction confirmed by fluoroscopy; (C) CC screws insertion completed and skin to be closed in layers.

POSTOPERATIVE CARE

The patient should be made to sit upright in bed and bedside legs dangling as early as possible subjective to patient's comfort and pain relief. If fracture is adequately reduced and fixed in a patient with good bone quality, ambulation can be initiated either with non-weight bearing (NWB), toe-touch weight bearing (TTWB), or weight bearing as tolerated (WBAT) with help of walking aids.

Postoperative neurovascular examination should be carried out and documented to rule out any iatrogenic injury pertaining to surgery or patient positioning. Prophylaxis for deep vein thrombosis in the form of low-molecular-weight heparin (LMWH), pneumatic compression devices, or compression stockings should be applied.

SUGGESTED READING

1. Angelini M, McKee MD, Waddell JP. Salvage of failed hip fracture fixation. J Orthop Trauma. 2009;23:472-8.
2. Bhandari M, Devereaux PJ, Swiontkowski MF. Internal fixation compared with arthroplasty for displaced fractures of the femoral neck. A meta-analysis. J Bone Joint Surg Am. 2003;85:1673-81.
3. Cserhati P, Kazar G, Manninger J. Non-operative or operative treatment for undisplaced femoral neck fractures: a comparative study of 122 non-operative and 125 operatively treated cases. Injury. 1996;27:583-8.
4. Haidukewych GJ, Rothwell WS, Jacofsky DJ. Operative treatment of femoral neck fractures in patients between the ages of fifteen and fifty years. J Bone Joint Surg Am. 2004;86:1711-6.
5. Rogmark C, Flensburg L, Fredin H. Undisplaced femoral neck fractures—no problems? A consecutive study of 224 patients treated with internal fixation. Injury. 2009;40:274-6.

CHAPTER 102

Fracture Neck of Femur Bipolar Hip Replacement

Dudani Baldev, Yash K Shah, Shrinivas S Shintre

BIPOLAR HIP REPLACEMENT (UNCEMENTED)

Dudani Baldev

INTRODUCTION

Austin-Moore and Thompson's prosthesis were introduced in 1950's as a primary prosthetic replacement for displaced femoral neck fractures. Since then hemi replacement has undergone a significant evolution in the indications as well as prosthetic design. The design of Austin-Moore prosthesis was such that it would be used without bone cement and was characterized by a fenestrated stem. The fenestrations were designed to enable bone ingrowth and thus allow "self-locking" of the prosthesis in the proximal femur. On the other hand, the Thompson prosthesis was inserted using bone cement. It had no fenestrations in stem. Many patients with these implants complained of thigh and groin pain. This was because of prosthesis loosening within the femoral canal (thigh pain)-as a result of cementless insertion in the case of Austin-Moore device and progressive acetabular erosion (groin pain). Protrusio acetabuli was quite common. Some factors could be correlated with the severity of acetabular erosion in patients with these devices, and these are patient activity level, duration of implantation, and fixation technique (cemented versus non-cemented).

To overcome these problems, the bipolar prosthetic design was introduced by James Bateman in 1974. In his design, an outer metal cup articulated with acetabular cartilage and enclosed an internal low-friction universal bearing. This bipolar bearing was expected to favor motion at the internal articulation and thereby to diminish cartilage wear. Since that time the bipolar prosthesis has undergone much refinement and is available today in both cemented and non-cemented options.

INDICATIONS

Bipolar prosthesis

- Displaced intracapsular fracture neck femur in elderly
- Pathological fracture neck femur
- Nonunion fracture neck femur
- Comminuted intertrochanteric fracture femur in elderly
- Avascular necrosis head femur.

FRACTURE NECK FEMUR

The most frequent indication for bipolar arthroplasty today is fresh fractures of neck of femur. This arthroplasty allows elderly patients to return to early weight bearing with shortened hospital stay, greater stability, more rapid rehabilitation and markedly decreased systemic complications with a reliable relief of pain.

SURGICAL TECHNIQUE

Preoperative Planning

It is important to plan the surgery properly, so that one can achieve good results. Proper history is of paramount importance. One should assess the present activity level of the patient. Elderly patients, who are active before the fall, usually do well after the surgery. One should also enquire whether the patient is suffering from diabetes mellitus, ischemic heart disease, hypertension or urinary tract infection, or any other medical illness or if the patient is on anti-platelet therapy (asprin) or on cortisones. Patients with cardiac, hepatic and renal disorders are more prone to complications related to bone cement. One has to be cautious in using cement in such cases, or else; press fit prosthesis can be chosen for proper fitting of prosthesis in the proximal femoral canal. Preoperative reading of X-ray is very important and if templates are available, one can make use of these, which will help in choosing the proper implant and whether bone cement to be used or not.

One can use monoblock or modular prosthesis (cemented or uncemented). We are describing here modular uncemented bipolar hip arthroplasty pictorially.

SURGICAL TECHNIQUE FOR MODULAR UNCEMENTED BIPOLAR ARTHROPLASTY (FIGS. 1 TO 27)

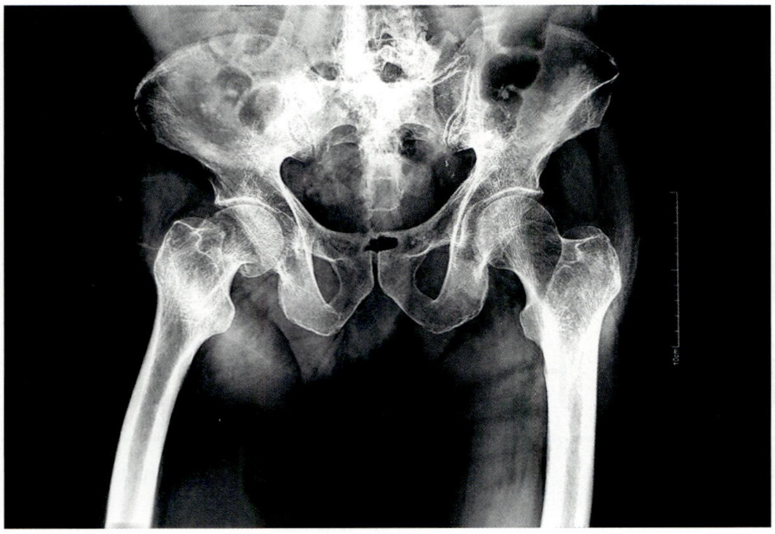

Fig. 1: Radiograph showing intracapsular fracture in elderly. Note gentle anterolateral bowing in this case.

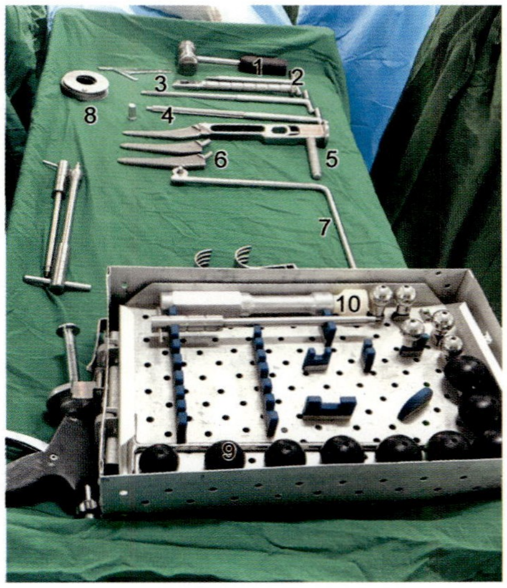

Fig. 2: Instruments on trolley: (1) Mallet, (2) Cork screw, (3) Box cutter, (4) Canal finding reamer, (5 and 6) Rasps of various sizes with handle, (7) Charnley self-retaining retractor, (8) Head sizer, (9) Different sizes of trial heads, (10) Head pusher.

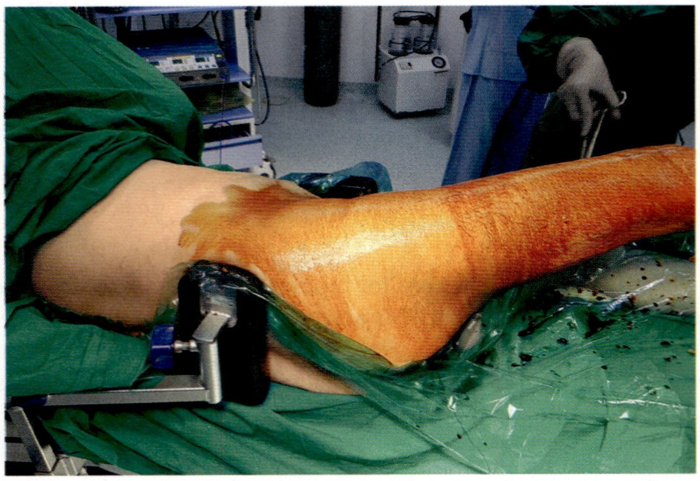

Fig. 3: Primary preparation of the surgical site with povidone–iodine in lateral position under spinal anesthesia.

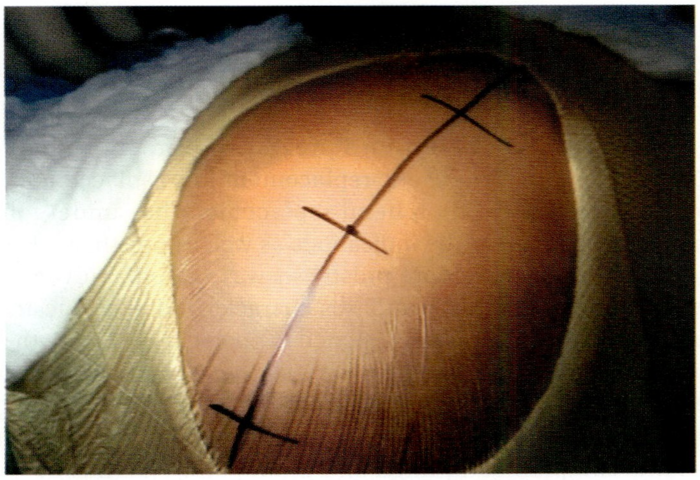

Fig. 4: Marking of incision centering on tip of greater trochanter, for posterolateral approach.

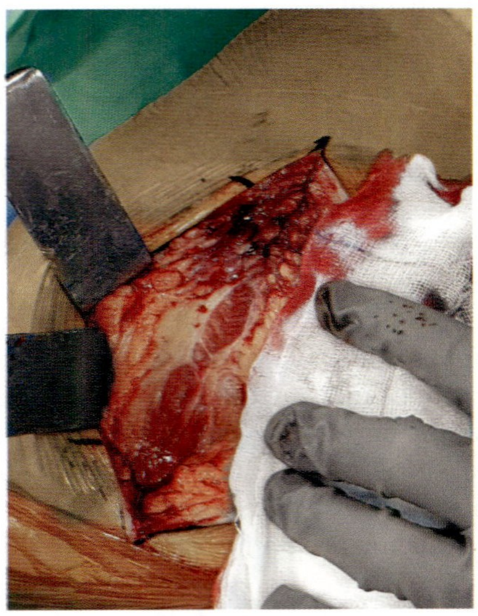

Fig. 5: Subcutaneous fat and fascia being cut in line with incision to expose the gluteus maximus fibers; after which splitting of gluteus maximus fibers is done.

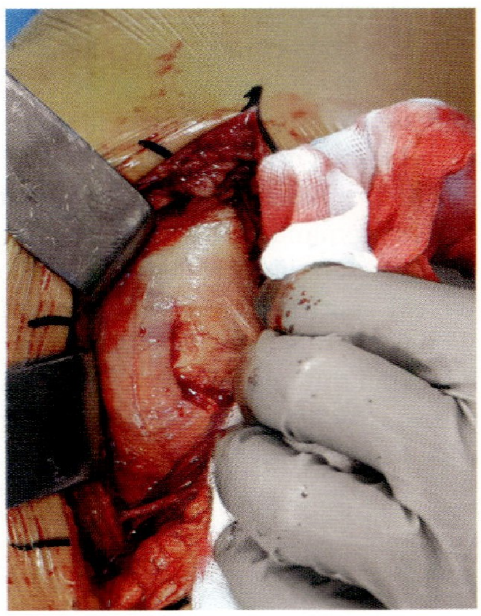

Fig. 6: Trochanteric bursa is being identified and cut.

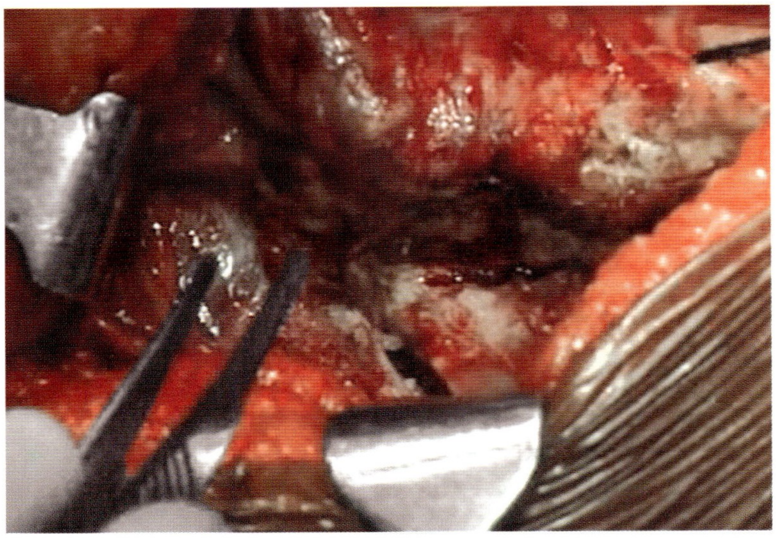

Fig. 7: Neck femur is being visualized after erasing short external rotators from the trochanteric crest.

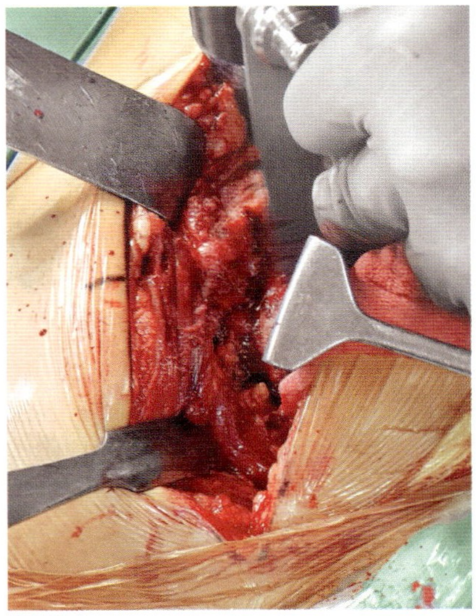

Fig. 8: Neck is being cut with the oscillating saw/osteotome, at 45° angle with longitudinal axis of femur, one finger breadth above the lesser trochanter with the leg in internal rotation at hip with knee flexed 90° till sole of foot is facing toward ceiling.

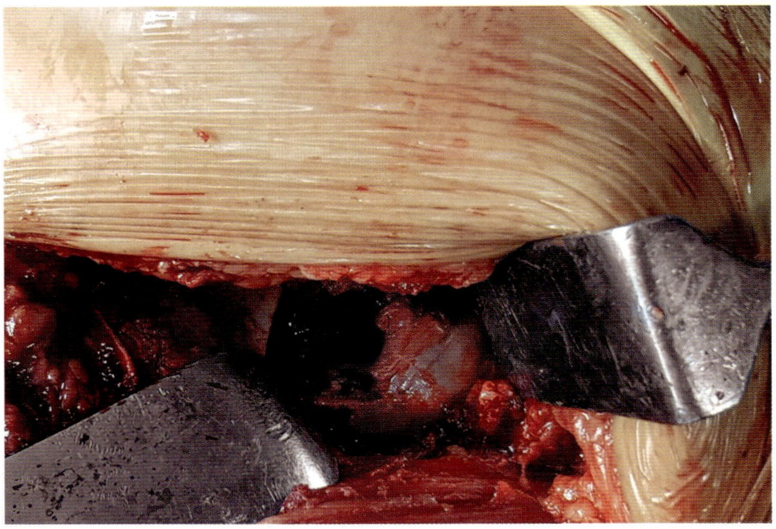

Fig. 9: Head of femur is visualized.

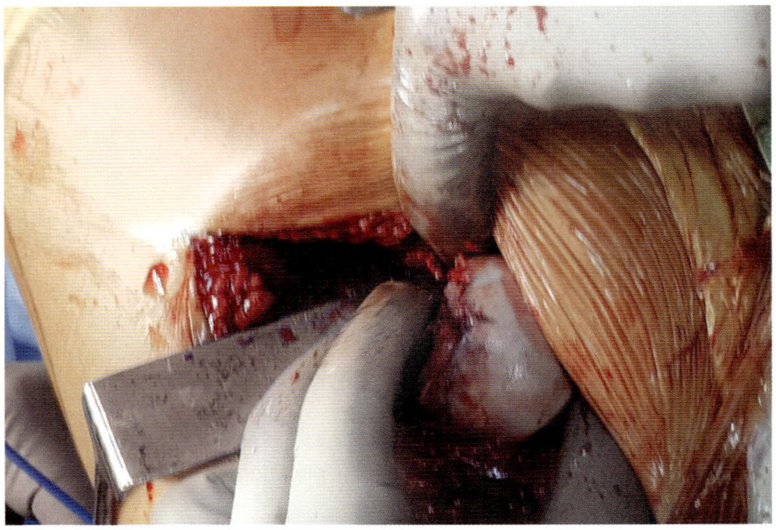

Fig. 10: Head is being extracted from the acetabulum after using cork screw and cutting ligamentum teres from acetabulum fovea to deliver head out.

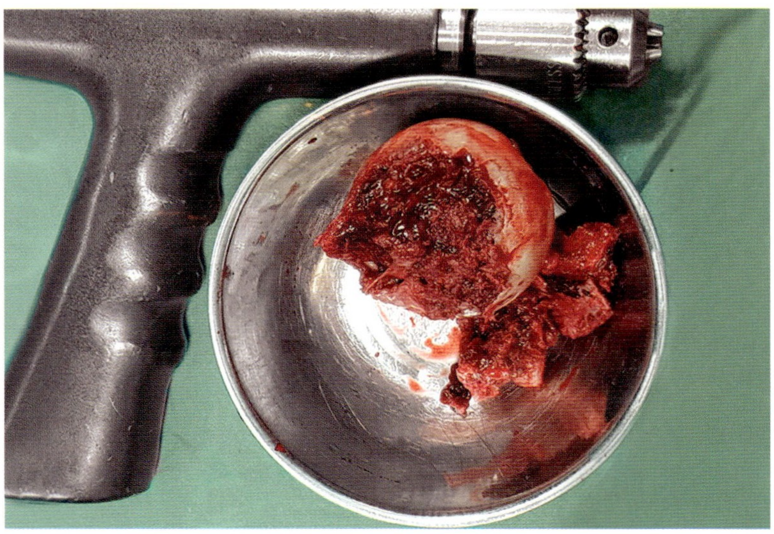

Fig. 11: Extracted head and loose pieces of bone.

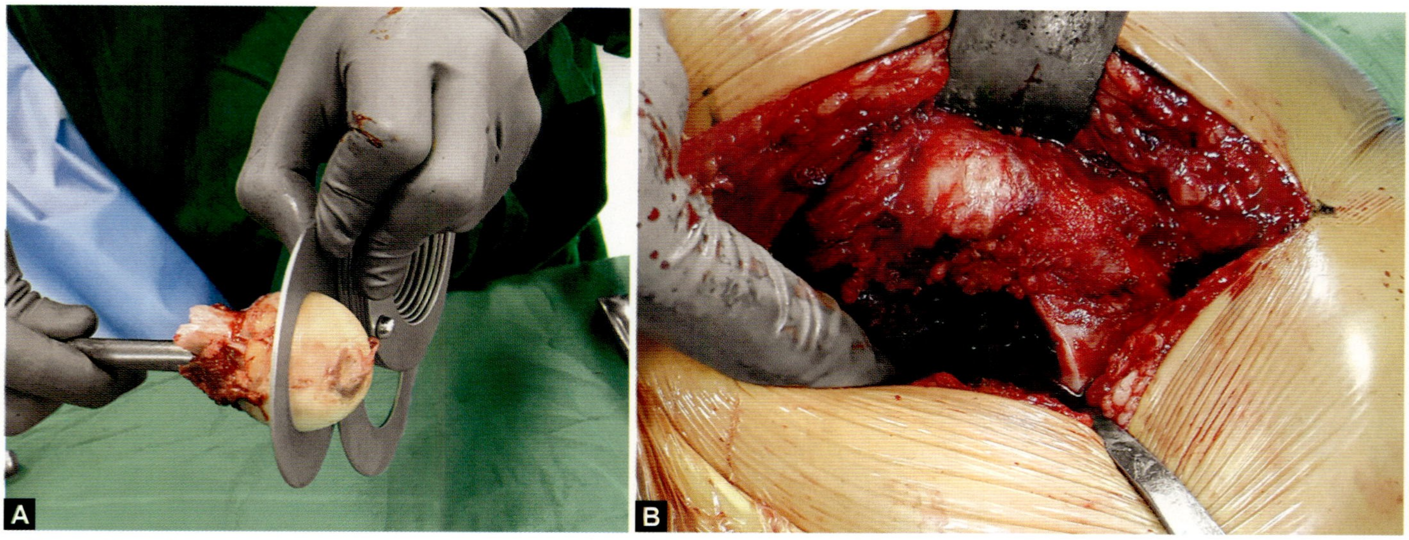

Figs. 12A and B: (A) Sizing of head is done and same size for final prosthesis is chosen; (B) The cut neck femur is properly exposed.

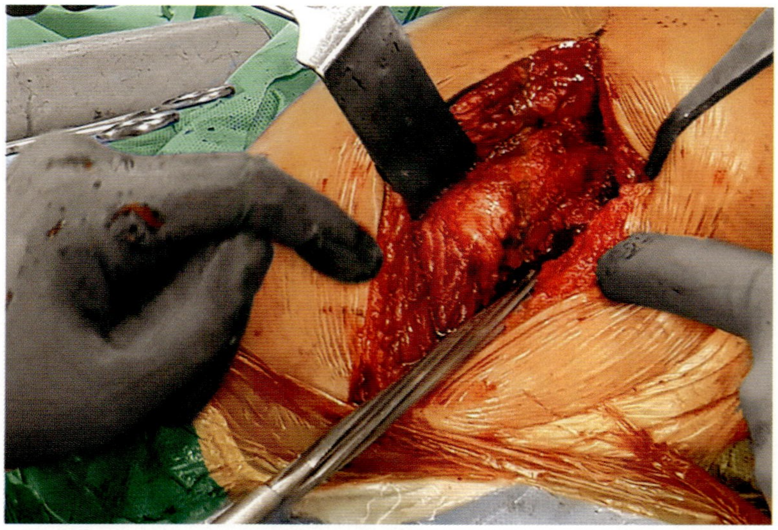

Fig. 13: Canal finder is used to assess direction of femoral canal.

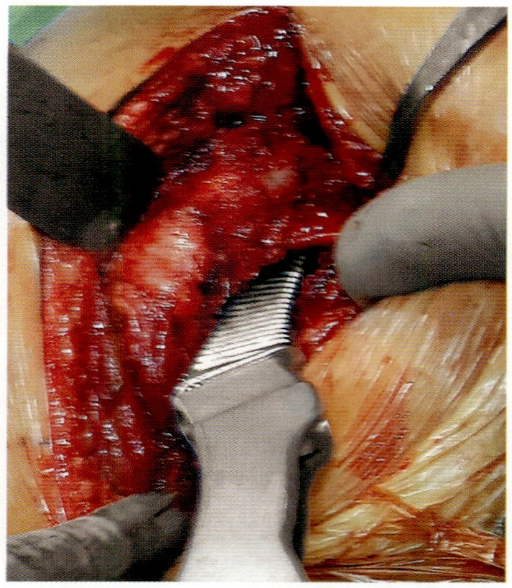

Fig. 14: Initial proximal rasping of canal is done with small size rasp starting from most lateral side.

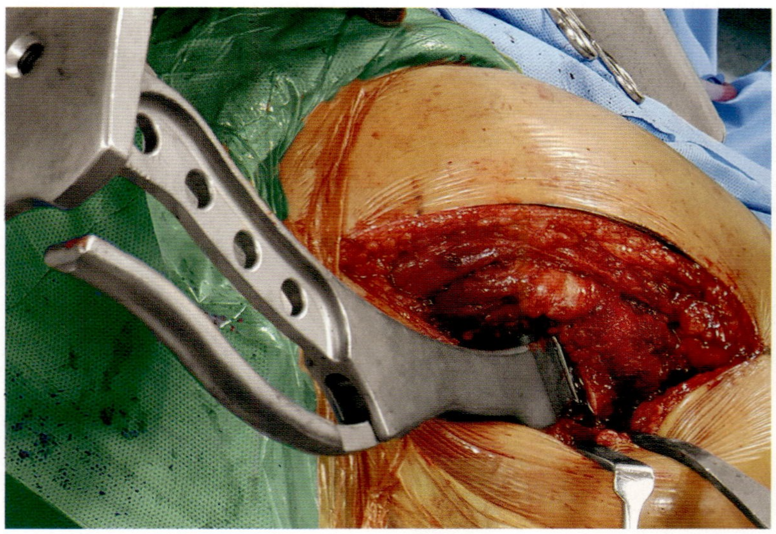

Fig. 15: Different sized rasps are used till one is chosen which fits snugly in canal. While rasping, care is taken to insert rasp in 10–15° of anteversion using either the position of the lesser trochanter as a reference; or sole of foot facing the ceiling as another.

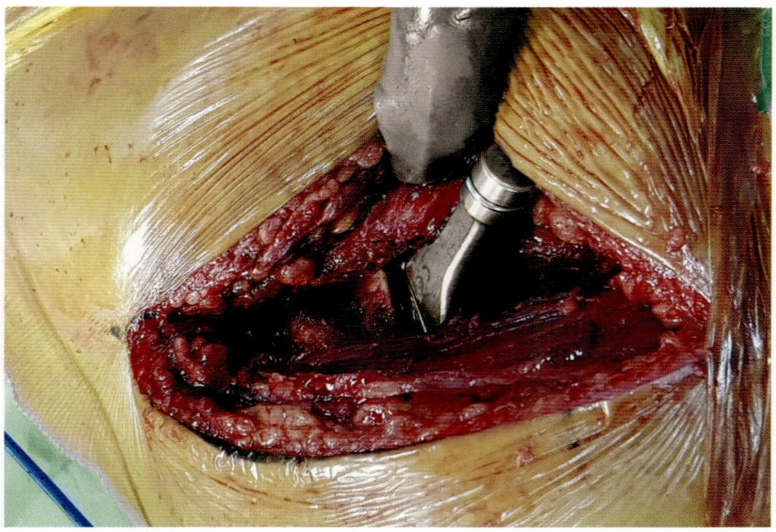

Fig. 16: Chosen trial prosthesis (femoral stem) is inserted.

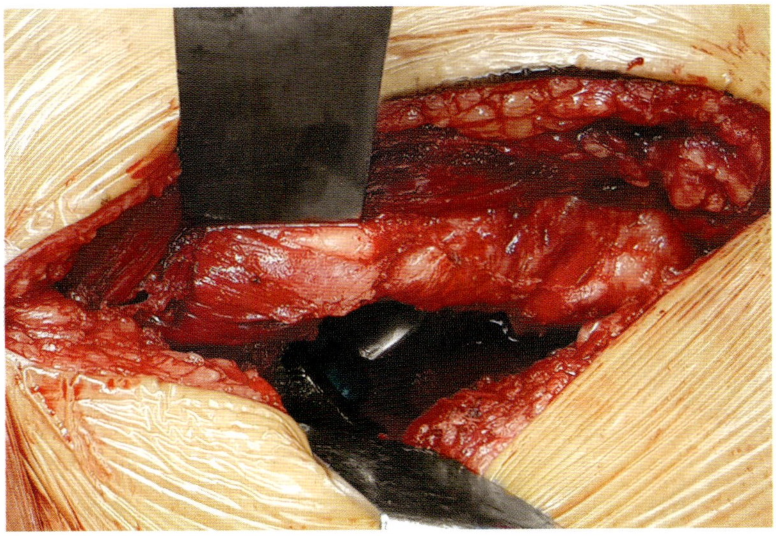

Fig. 17: Trial is done with chosen trial head and neck components and stability checked by flexing, adducting, and internally rotating hip 30°. Leg length is checked by comparing with knee and malleolar level of contralateral side.

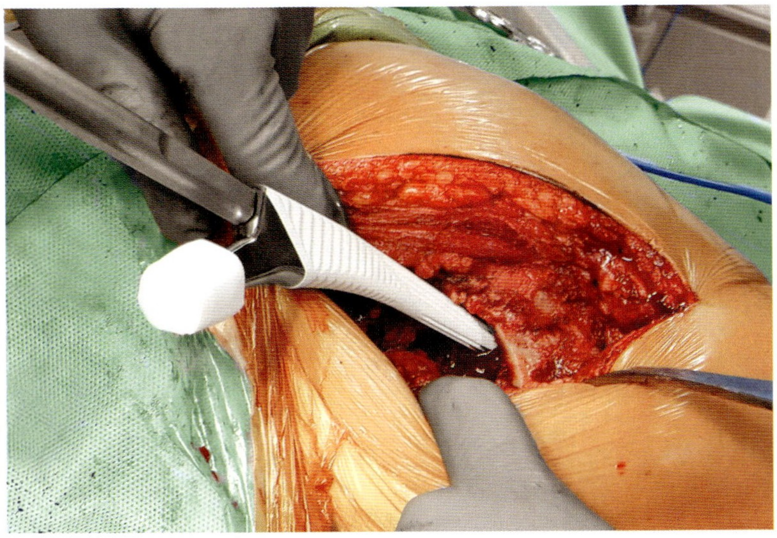

Fig. 18: Final prosthesis (Hydroxyapatite coated) is being pushed in the canal.

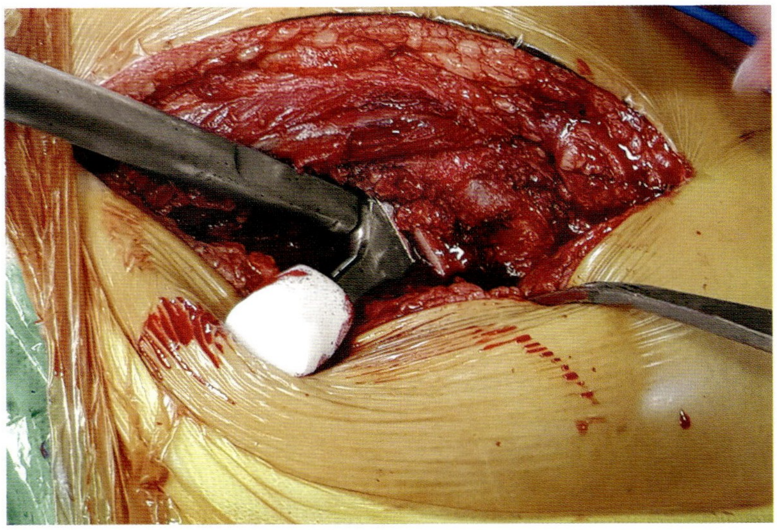

Fig. 19: Final hammering and seating of prosthesis in 10–15° anteversion.

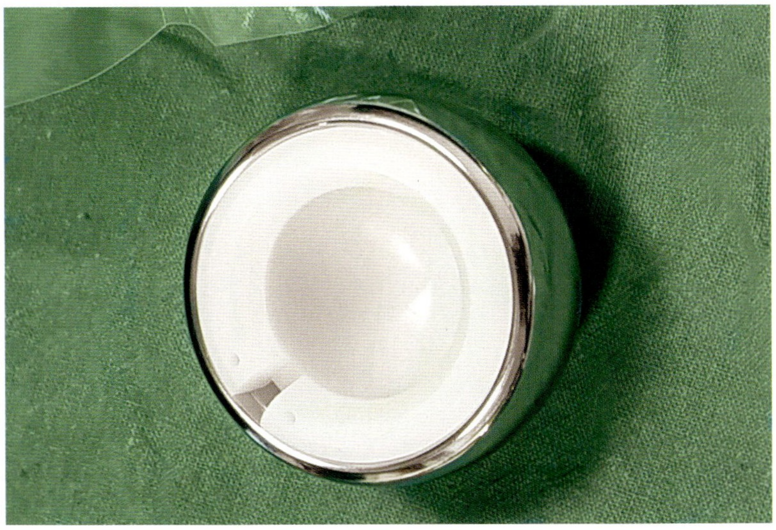

Fig. 20: Bipolar cup.

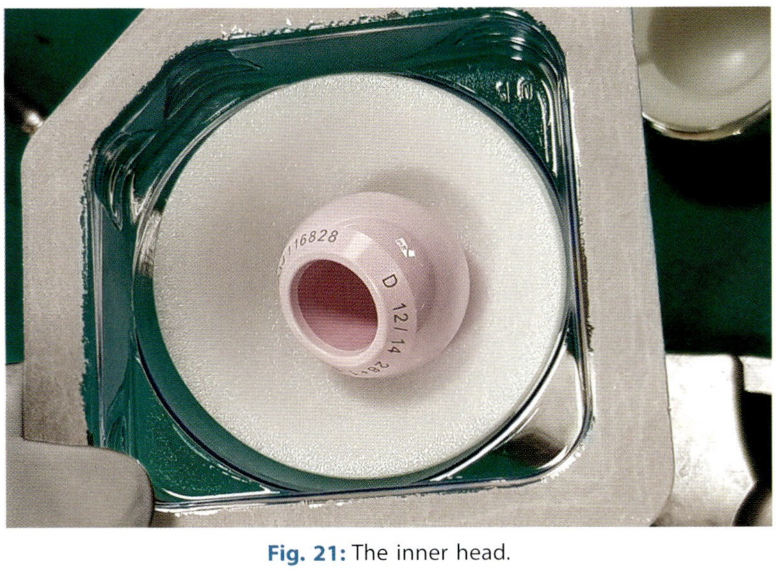

Fig. 21: The inner head.

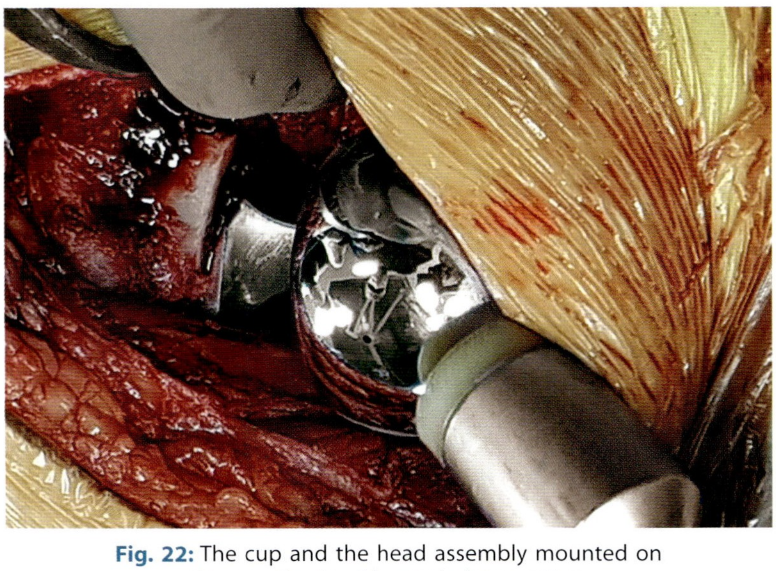

Fig. 22: The cup and the head assembly mounted on the prosthesis with gentle hammering.

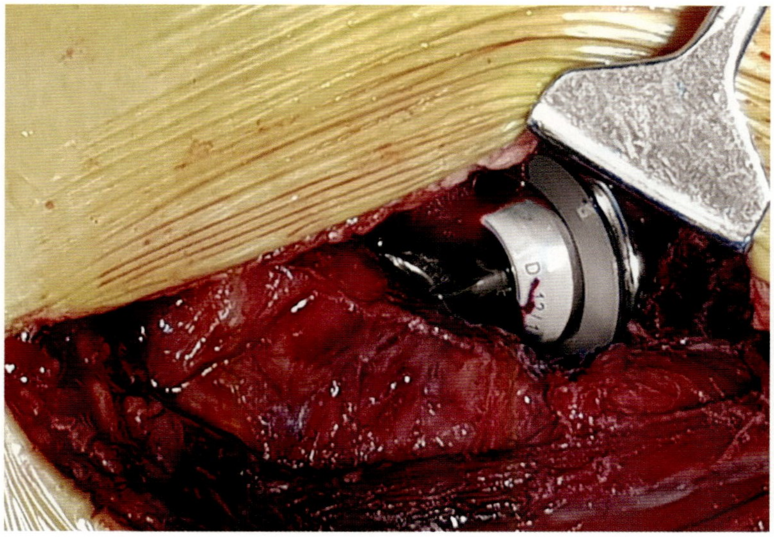

Fig. 23: Prosthesis is seated properly. Stability is again checked and shuck test is performed.

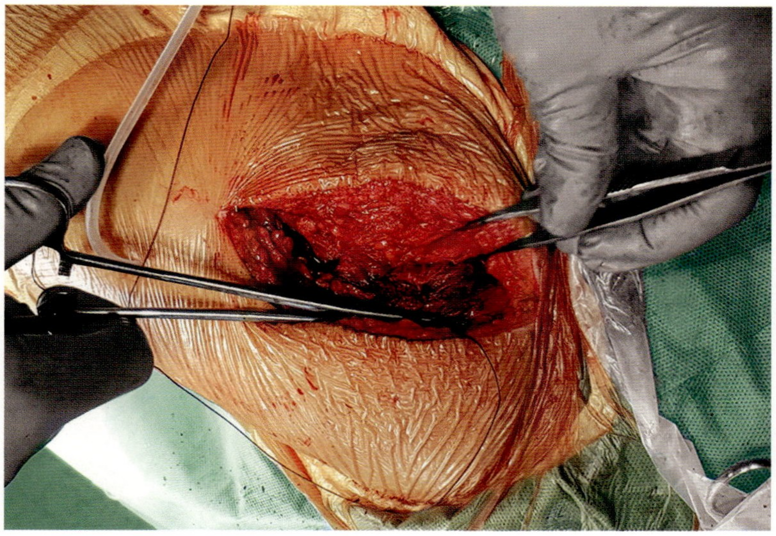

Fig. 24: The wound closure done in layers.

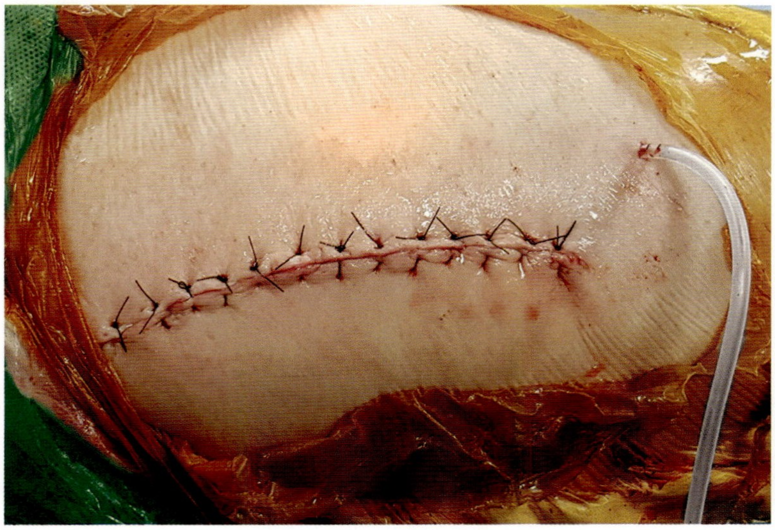

Fig. 25: Skin closure.

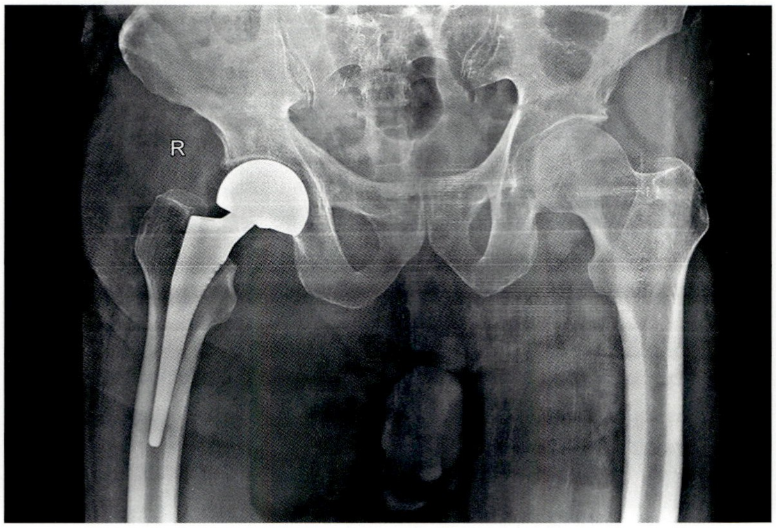

Fig. 26: Postoperative X-ray.

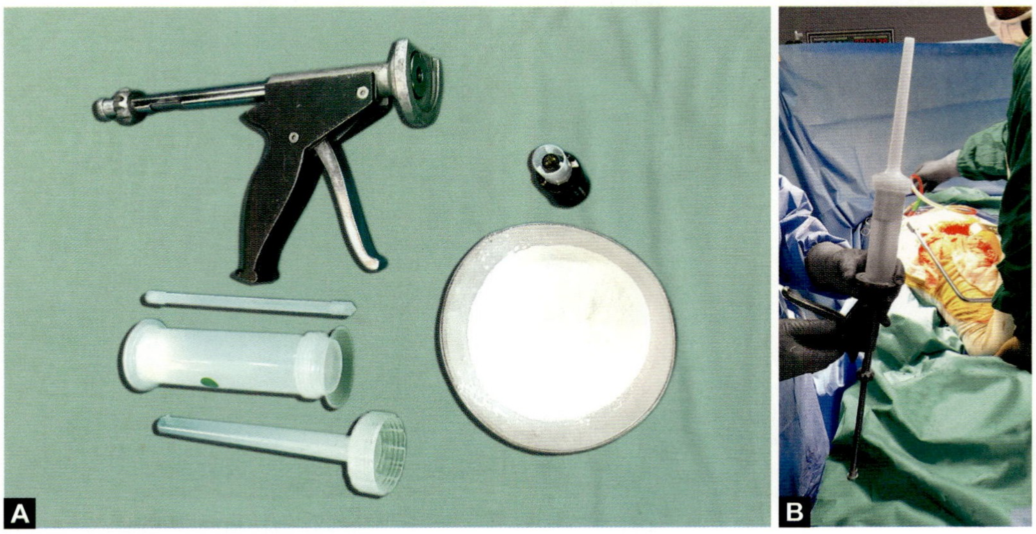

Figs. 27A and B: Bone cement and compatible prosthesis should be kept ready as a backup in case of problems encountered for uncemented prosthesis.

BIPOLAR HIP REPLACEMENT (CEMENTED)

Yash K Shah, Shrinivas S Shintre

CEMENTED BIPOLAR: SURGICAL STEPS (FIGS. 28 TO 57)

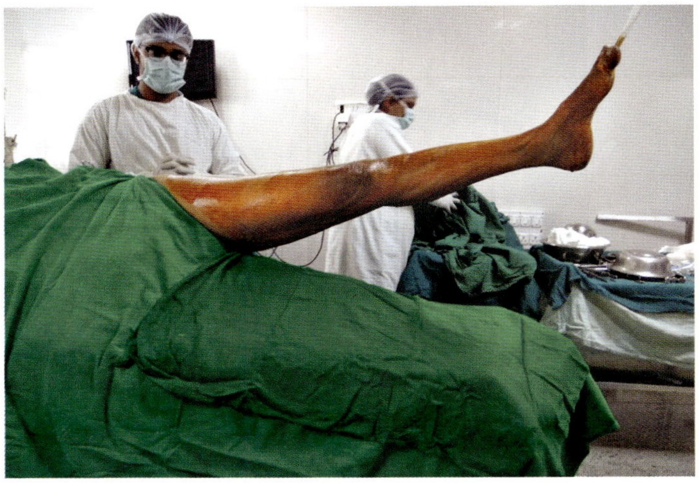

Fig. 28: In this case posterior approach is used. Lateral position is given and painting and draping are done. It is imperative to check the preoperative range of motion. If there is any restriction of abduction, due to adductor contracture, adductor tenotomy may be required either in beginning or at the end of the surgery after checking the range of motion.

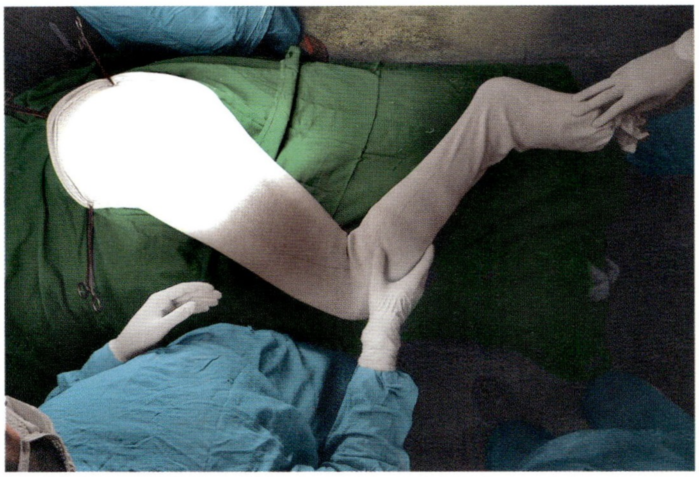

Fig. 29: Sterile stockinette is applied.

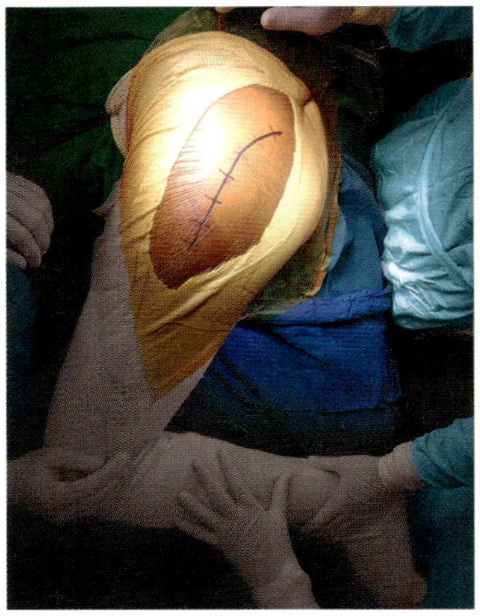

Fig. 30: Sterile povidone–iodine plastic sheet is applied and incision is marked.

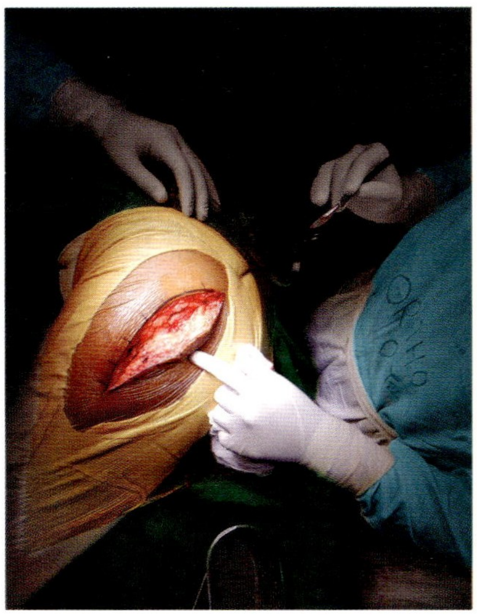

Fig. 31: Flex the hip at 90° and take straight incision starting from 6–8 cm proximal and posterior to greater trochanter (GT), it runs from this point to posterior border of GT continue distally over shaft about 5–7 cm from GT.

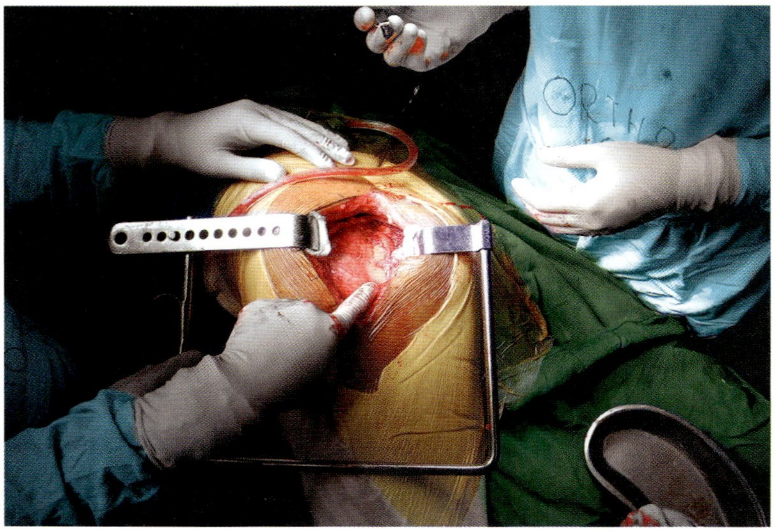

Fig. 32: Gentle retraction is done using a Charnley retractor.

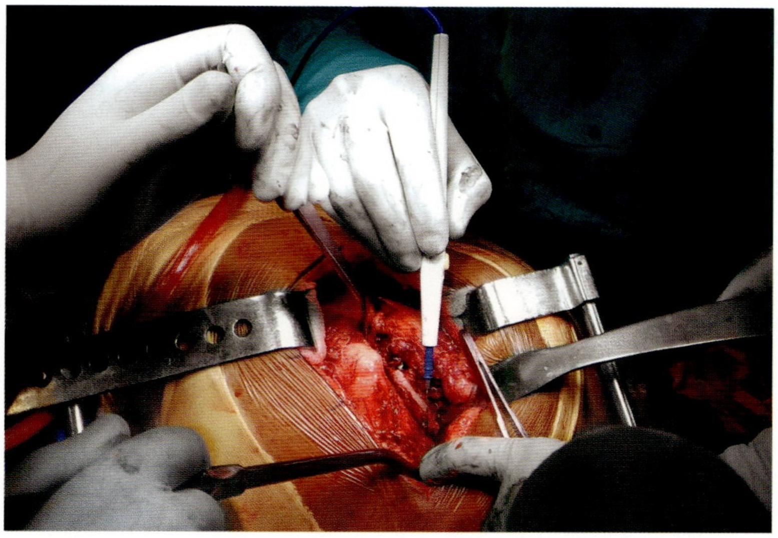

Fig. 33: Soft tissues are cut, viz. external rotators, trochanteric bursa. It is better to abduct the hip while cutting the fascia so that it gets relaxed and it cuts better better.

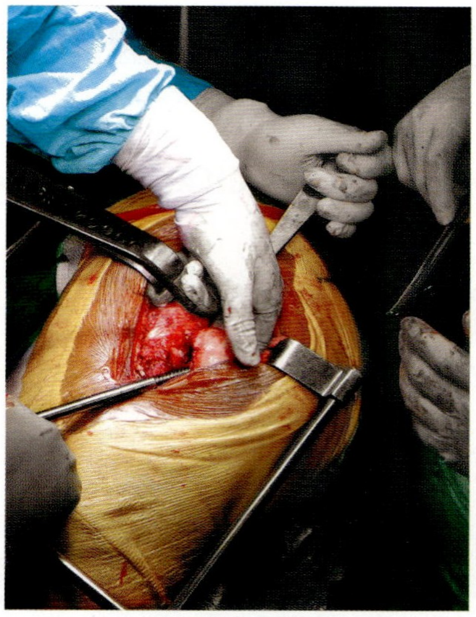

Fig. 34: Head is extracted using a cork screw extractor. Many a times, there is difficulty in extracting the head if there is an intact ligamentum teres. In those cases, it must be cut either with a cautery or a curved pair of scissors.

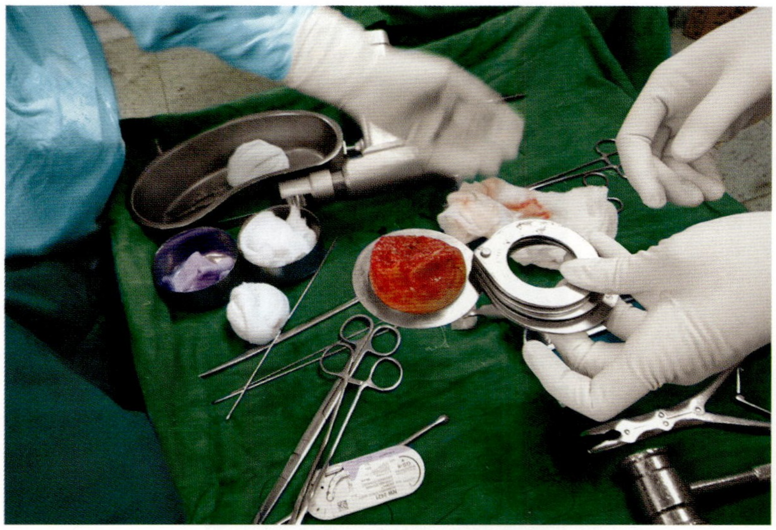

Fig. 35: Sizing of the extracted head is done using a template.

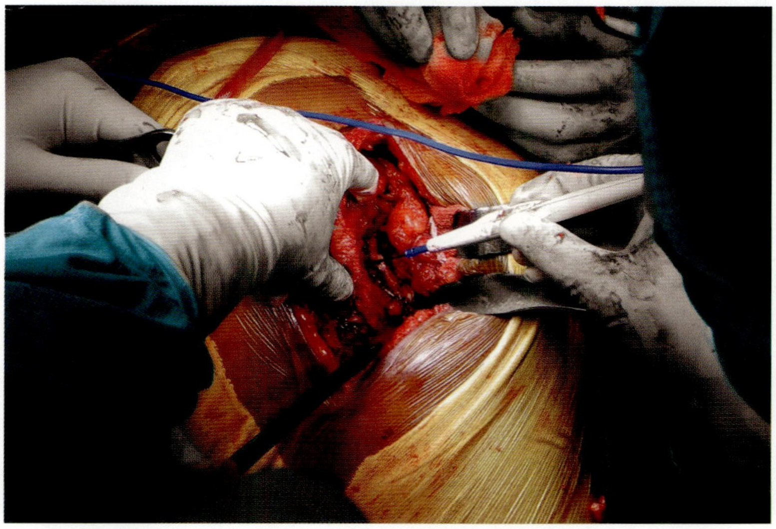

Fig. 36: Neck to be cut may be marked by a cautery pen. This avoids unnecessary errors while using the saw.

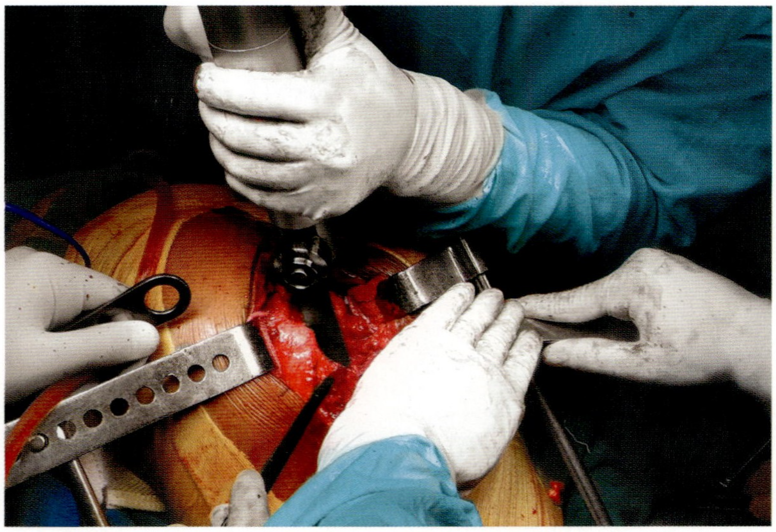

Fig. 37: Femoral neck is cut using a saw. Oscillating saw can be started before the saw blade touches the bone. This avoids slipping of the blade in the hands of a newcomer.

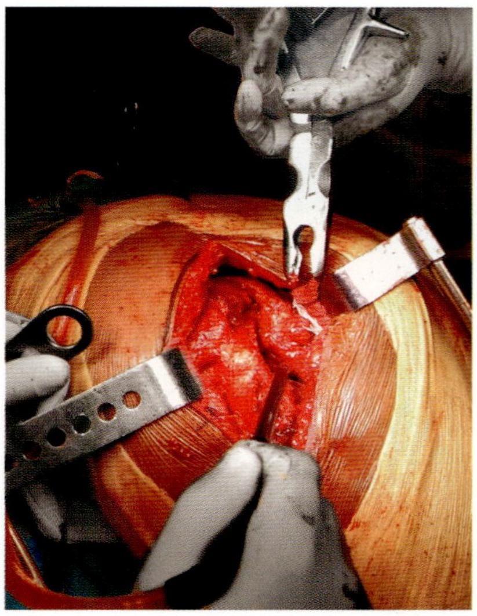

Fig. 38: Some bone near the piriform fossa is nibbled out. This helps in enabling as lateral access as possible in the piriform fossa.

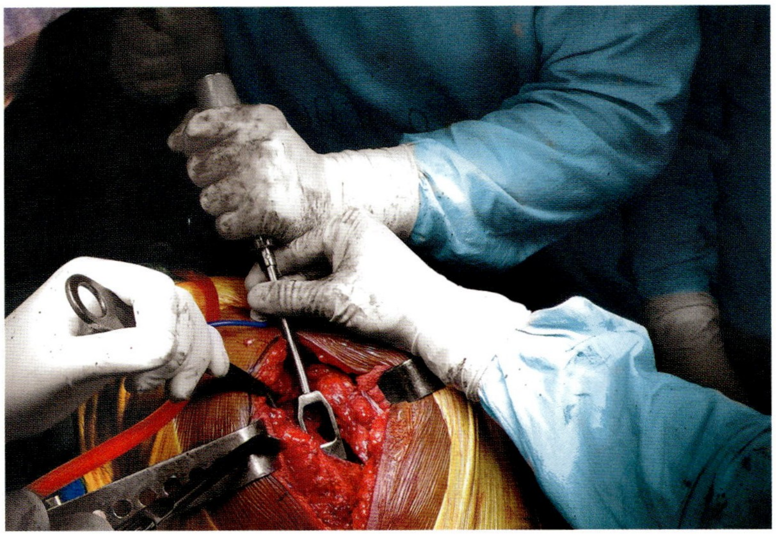

Fig. 39: A box cutting tool is used to make the initial box cut. Care must be taken to go as lateral as possible in the piriform fossa. This avoids a varus positioning of the stem. This is done in 15° anteversion. This can either be achieved by positioning the box chisel in 15° or positioning the box chisel in horizontal position and the assistant holding in limb in 15° internal rotation.

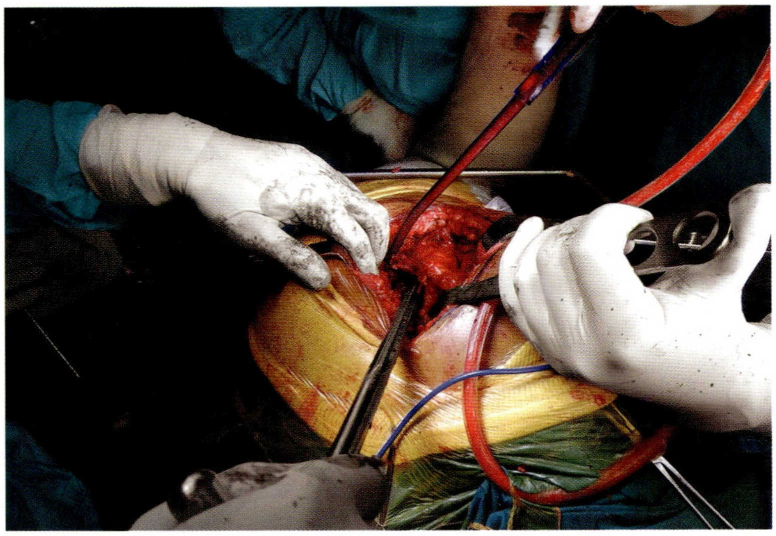

Fig. 40: A canal finder is used to judge the direction of the canal. This helps in wrong broaching and prevents disastrous penetration of the broach through the shaft.

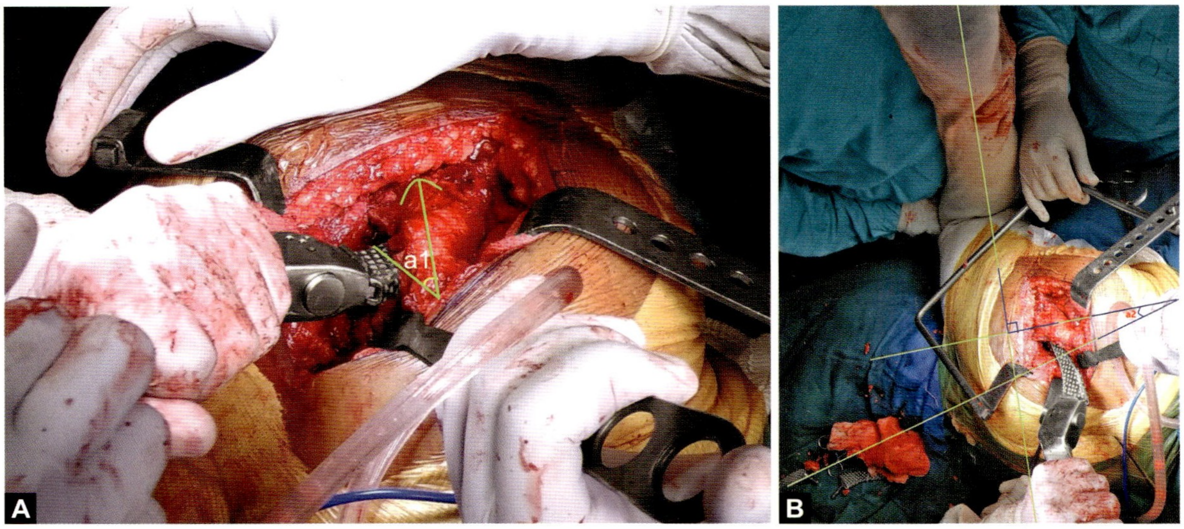

Figs. 41A and B: (A) In order to maintain anteversion, rasp is hammered such a way that superior edge of rasp is toward posterior cortex of neck and Inferior edge near anterior cortex. (a1) angle between the line tangential to posterior cortex of femur and another line tangential to posterior surface of broach; (B) The anteversion can also be judged by the angle between the line perpendicular to the long axis of leg and the other line tangential to the surface of broach (a2).

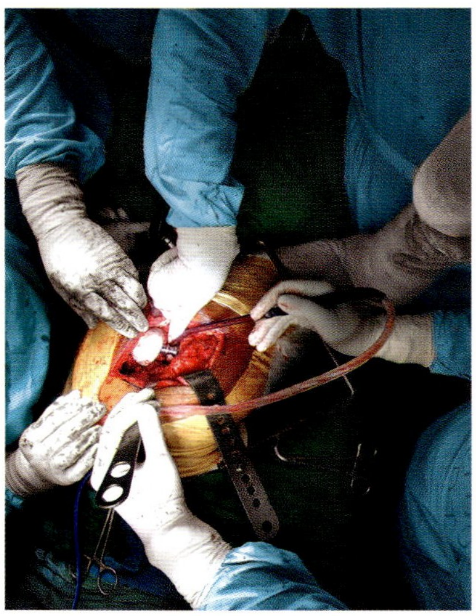

Fig. 42: Trial prosthesis is inserted. Length and version are checked.

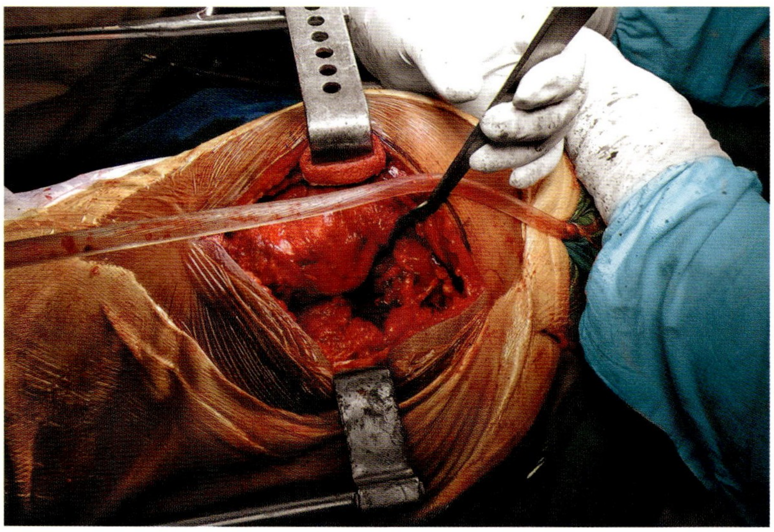

Fig. 43: Stability is checked. A shuck test is performed.

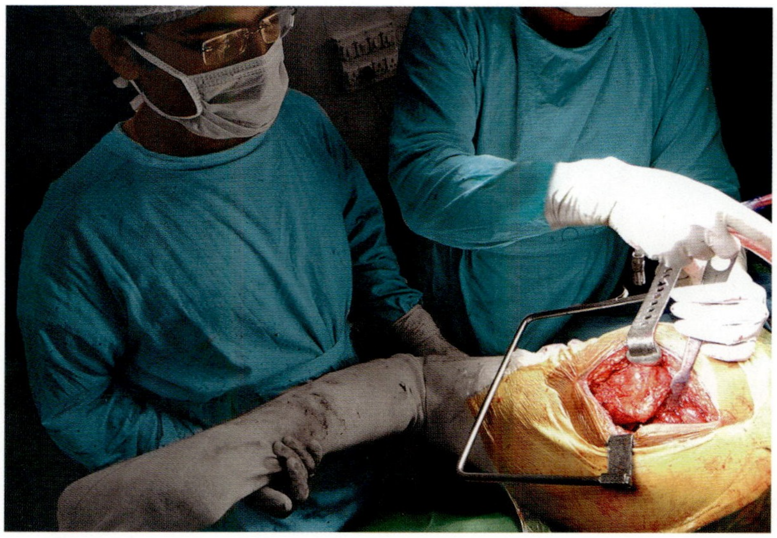

Fig. 44: An assistant is told to take the hip joint through all the normal ranges of motion to check the fit of the prosthesis.

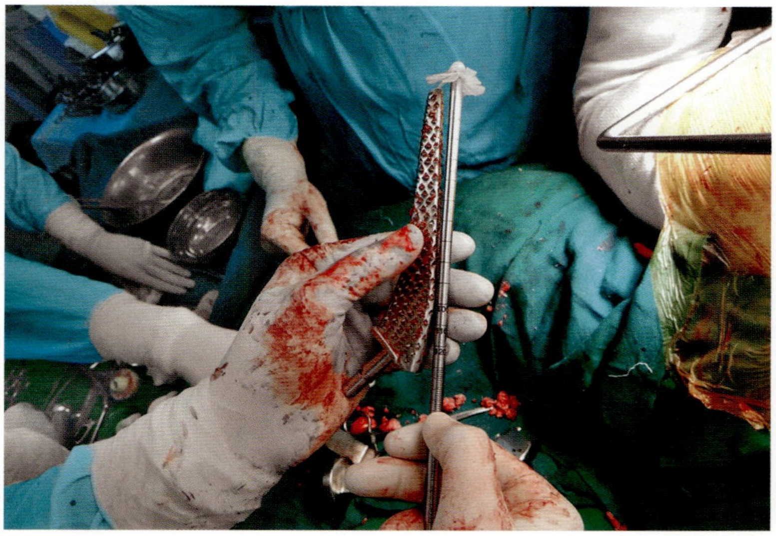

Fig. 45: The length as how deep to insert the cement restrictor is judged from either the trial stem/broach/actual prosthesis and the cement restrictor is inserted.

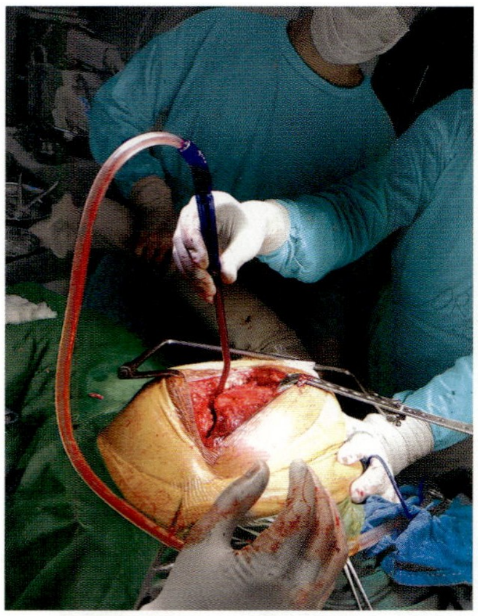

Fig. 46: The canal is cleared of all debris and blood by a suction. Any blood in-between the cement and bone is a cause of loosening.

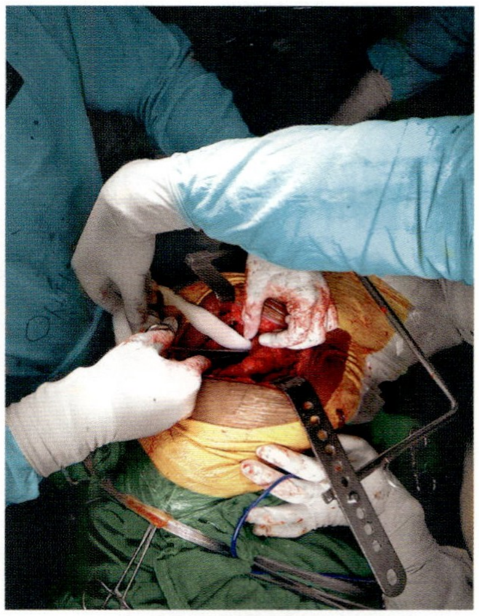

Fig. 47: Roller gauze/absorbent gauze is inserted in the femoral canal. This keeps the canal dry.

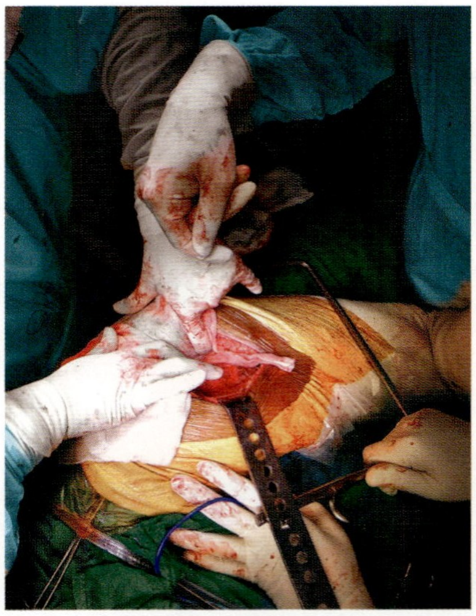

Fig. 48: Acetabulum pack is inserted. This prevents cement being impacted in the joint later on.

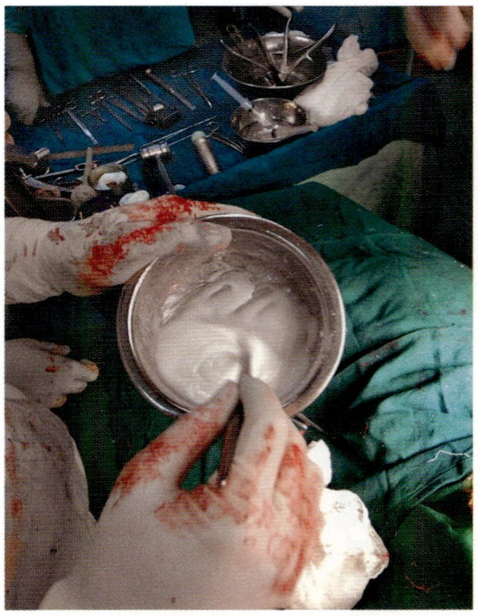

Fig. 49: Cement is mixed in a bowl. An assistant is told to keep track of the time and he/she is told to remind everyone of the time since mixing the cement till it hardens. Mixing can be done either with a spoon or a curette.

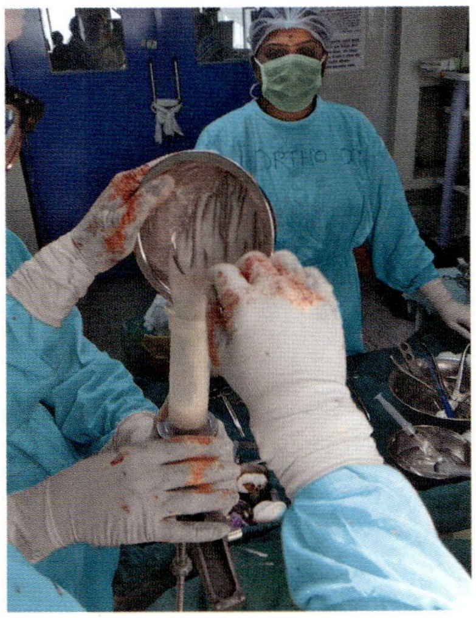

Fig. 50: After the cement turns into a semisolid state, it can be inserted in the cement syringe attached to cement gun.

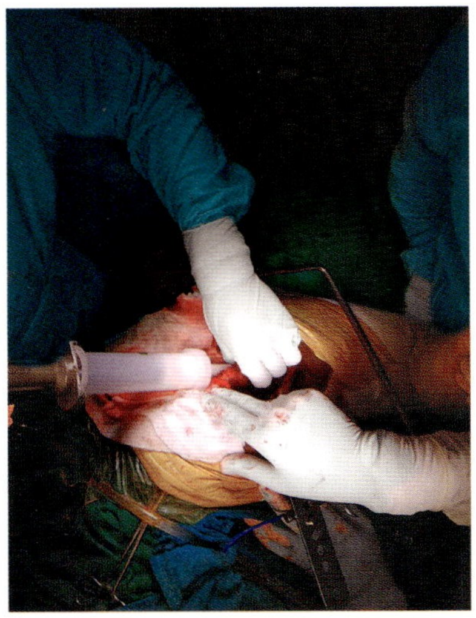

Fig. 51: The cement is then inserted into the femoral canal after removing the femoral pack while keeping the acetabulum pack. Any excess cement can be removed with an artery forceps after incising the excess with a scalpel/ with nibbler/osteotome, depending upon stage of hardening.

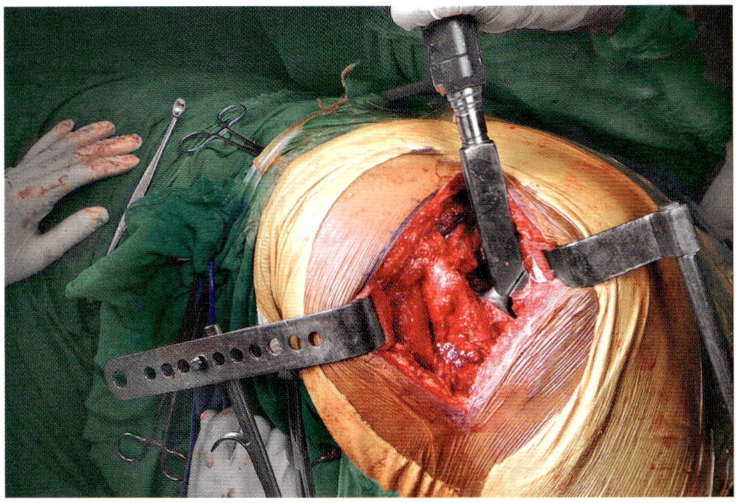

Fig. 52: The final prosthesis is inserted in around 15° of anteversion. After cleaning the trunnion selected modular head prosthesis is fitted over neck of stem. Then prosthesis is reduced in acetabulum by pushing with nylon punch.(Not shown here)

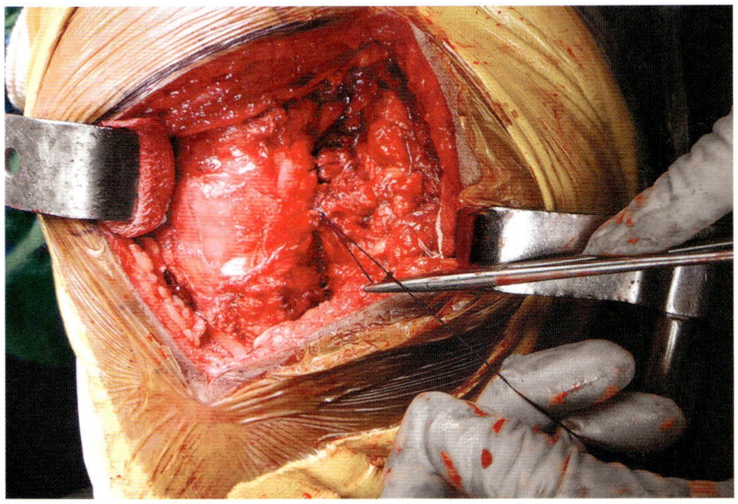

Fig. 53: Generally three sutures are taken on the short external rotator muscles of the hip. In any difficulty in passing the sutures directly through the bone, holes can be made in the bone either by a thick K-wire or drill so as to aid passage of the suture. 0 or 1 No. absorbable suture can be used here.

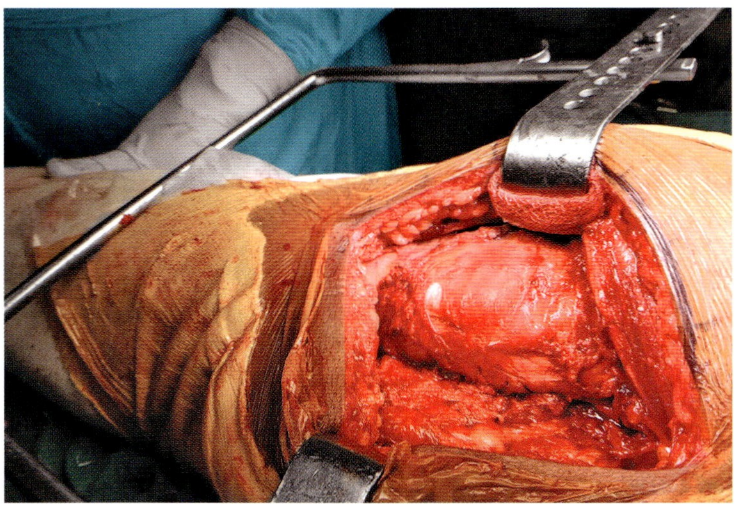

Fig. 54: The final picture after the suturing of these muscles to the trochanter.

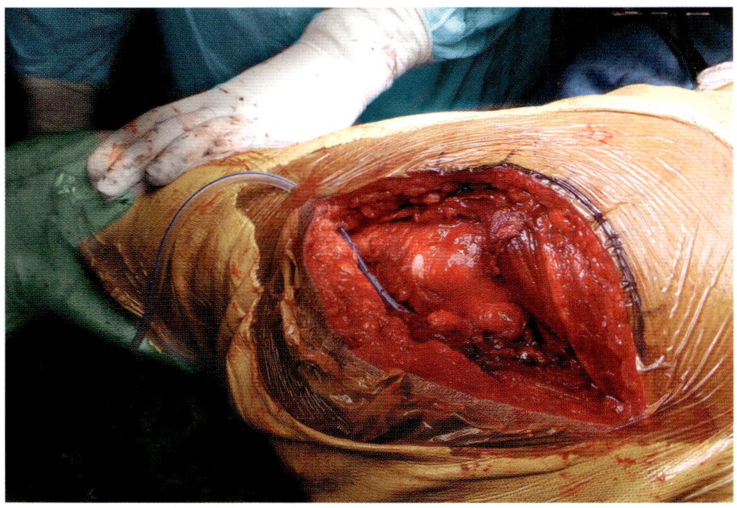

Fig. 55: Drain is inserted. It may be clamped for 2 hours and then opened. This causes a tamponade and reduces the postoperative blood loss.

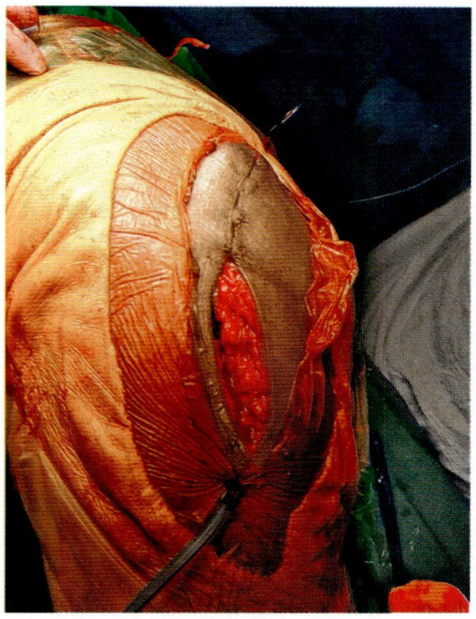

Fig. 56: Suturing is done in layers. 0 or 1 No. absorbable suture can be used for suturing gluteus maximus and No. 2-0 absorbable suture can be used for suturing fascia, and fat and subcutaneous layers. Skin can be closed with either staples or 2-0 or 3-0 nonabsorbable sutures.

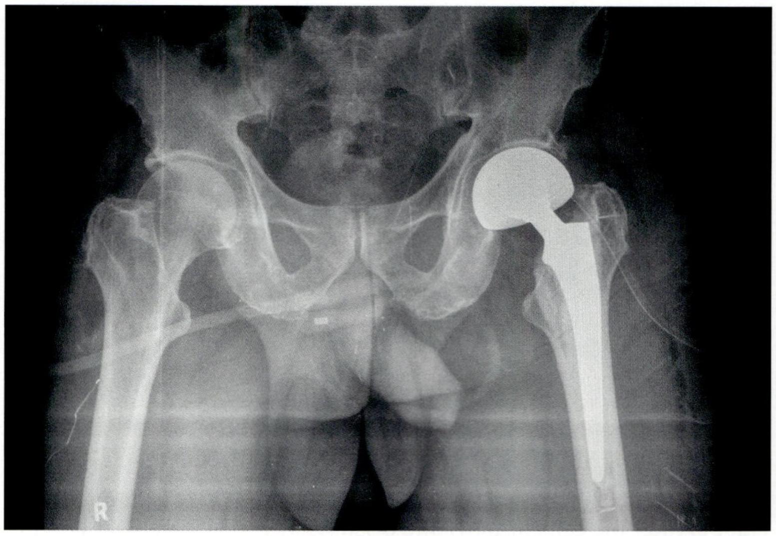

Fig. 57: Final postoperative radiograph. It shows a good cementing and a good placement of the stem.

POSTOPERATIVE MANAGEMENT

Post operatively patient is given long knee brace for few days which prevents patient from flexing knee and hip, and abduction pillow, hence preventing hip dislocation. Patient is made to walk full weight bearing with walker from 3rd day of surgery. Postoperative antibiotic is given for 3 to 5 days and patient is discharged from the hospital between 5 to 7 days.

SUGGESTED READING

1. Bateman JE. Single-assembly total hip: preliminary report. Orthop Digest. 1974;2:15-22.
2. Dudani BG, Azam SM, Madhukeshwar GV. Bipolar hemiarthroplasty for fractures of the neck of femur in the elderly. Ind J Orthop. 2004;38(1):12-5.
3. Giliberty RP. Bipolar endoprosthesis minimizes protrusio acetabuli, loose stems. Orthop Rev. 1985;14:27.
4. Vázquez-vela G, Vázquez-vela E. Acetabular reaction to the Bateman bipolar prosthesis. Clin Orthop. 1990;251:87-91.
5. West WF, Mann RA. Evaluation of the Bateman self articulating femoral prosthesis. Orthop Trans. 1979;3:17.

CHAPTER 103

Intertrochanteric Fracture Femur: Dynamic Hip Screw Barrel Plate Fixation

Vijay M Panchanadikar, Shrinivas S Shintre

INTRODUCTION AND CLASSIFICATION

Incidence of these fractures of the hip in elderly population is rising with increase in lifespan. Increasing number of motor vehicle accidents are contributing to the occurrence of these fractures in the younger populations. Various classifications are described. Boyd and Griffin described four types depending on level of fracture and comminution. Evans and Tronzo classified these fractures on basis of stability thus providing a guideline for fracture reduction and choice of implant (Fig. 1).

The Arbeitsgemeinschaft für Osteosynthesefragen (AO)/The Orthopaedic Trauma Association (OTA) classification is useful for communication and evaluation of results and allowing comparisons between studies. Untreated fractures are likely to go into malunion. These fractures tend to heal quickly and do not have complications like avascular necrosis of head of femur as compared to fractures of the neck (intracapsular).

CLINICAL FEATURES AND TREATMENT PLAN (FIGS. 2 TO 23)

Patients present with inability to bear weight following fall or accident and on examination have prominent external rotation deformity and shortening and severe painful restriction of hip movement. Treatment is surgical, so as to prevent serious and potentially fatal complications of prolonged immobilization and malunion. Choice of implant is dictated by fracture stability. Simple noncomminuted stable fractures are treated with hip screw and side plate device whereas those with medial or lateral wall comminution or having reverse oblique pattern or with subtrochanteric element are managed better with intramedullary fixation.

Dynamic hip screw and Barrel plate fixation continues to be the gold standard for a vast majority. As with all fracture surgery, principles of internal fixation are to be followed for a successful outcome. Good reduction either closed or open is mandatory. Ideal positioning of the hip screw in center of head or with slight inferior/posterior bias is important. Maintaining ideal tip apex distance will reduce chances of cutout. Barrel of plate is to be preferably long to reduce angular stress over screw as this may prevent free sliding inside barrel, but barrel should not cross fracture site. Otherwise controlled collapse at fracture is hampered. Four cortex screws in distal fragment to hold plate to shaft are adequate. Trochanteric support plate may be added to improve stability whenever needed.

Intramedullary fixations like proximal femur nail, trochanteric femoral nail, and variations of these are emerging as preferred fixation modalities in unstable fracture patterns. Intramedullary fixation has advantages of increased mechanical stability, minimal incisions, and lesser blood loss but suffers from drawback of being technically demanding with a learning curve. Good valgus reduction of fracture either closed or open is mandatory before nail insertion as nail will not ensure reduction. Entry point at tip of trochanter but with a medial bias is important so also is ideal positioning of hip screws. Good instrumentation is mandatory and one must be familiar with the set provided and instructions of individual manufacturer. Attention to all details will ensure good result or else complications will arise.

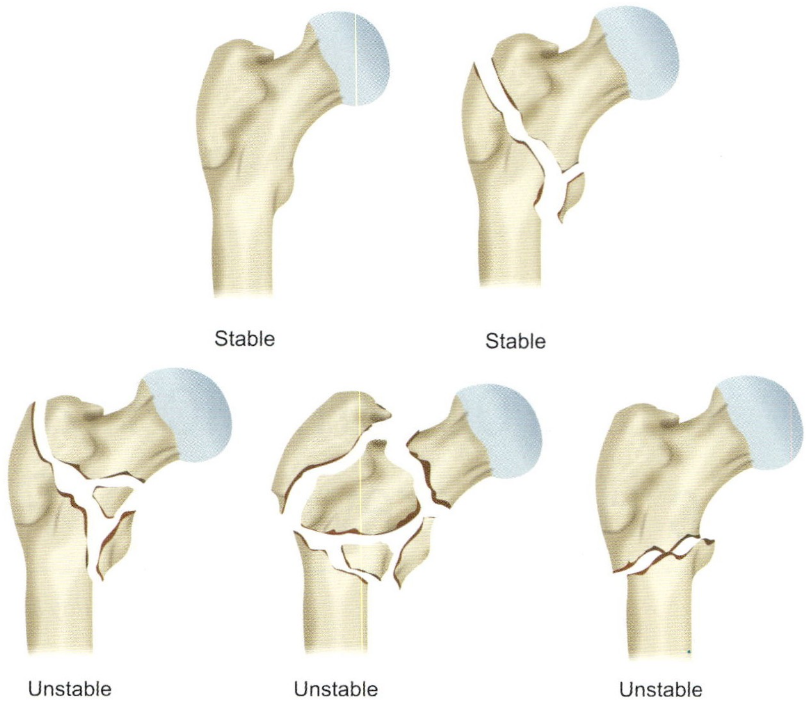

Fig. 1: Evans' classification.

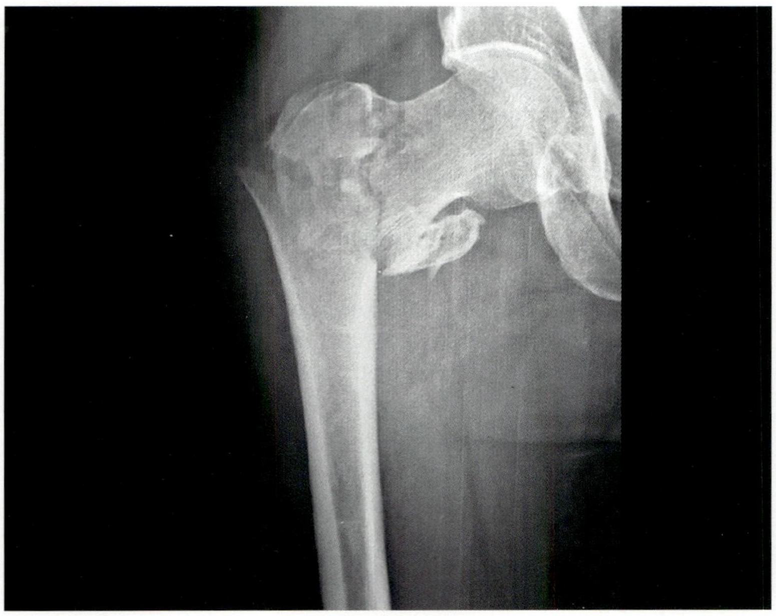

Fig. 2: Radiograph anteroposterior view.

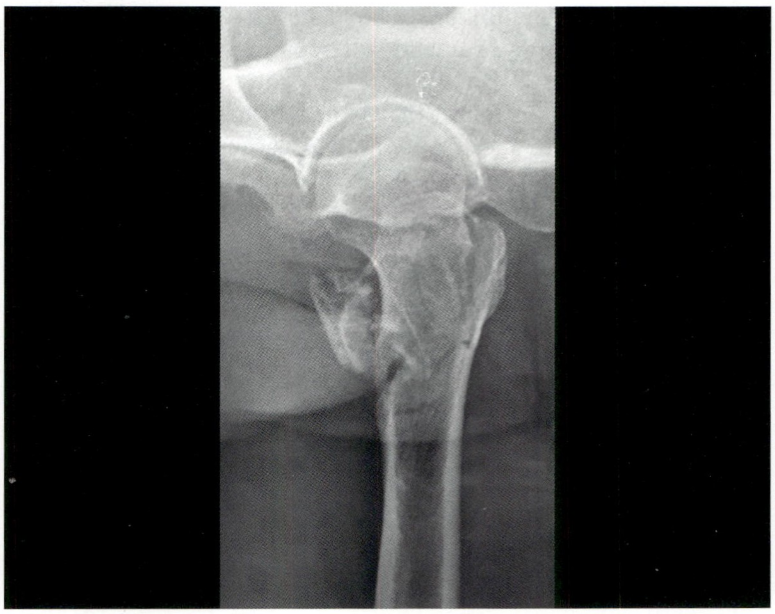

Fig. 3: Radiograph lateral view.

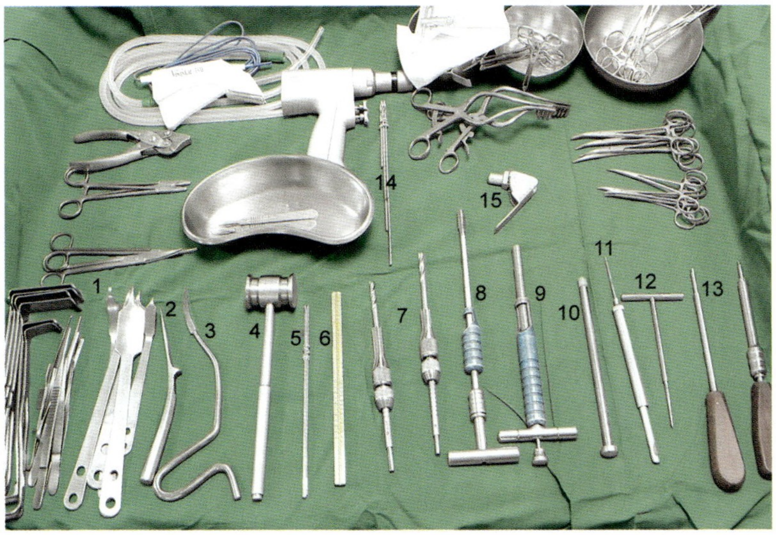

Fig. 4: Instruments trolley. Must have standard set. Key instruments are shown. (1) Spike retractors, (2) Periosteum elevator, (3) Diamond bone awl, (4) Hammer, (5) Guidewires, (6) Direct measure, (7) Triple reamer, (8) Tap for DHS, (9) T handle introducer/extractor for DHS, (10) Nylon punch, (11) Depth gauge, (12) Tap, (13) Screwdrivers, (14) Drills bits, (15) Angle guide.

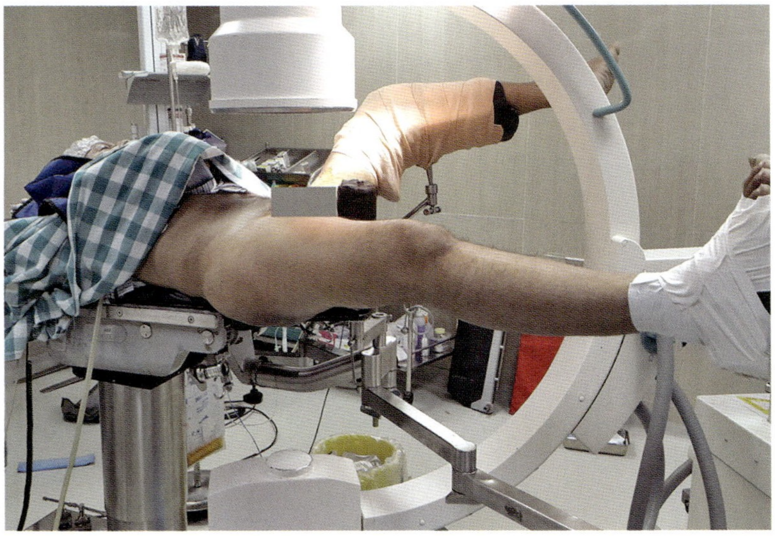

Fig. 5: C-arm position for anteroposterior view. Position of patient is secured after closed reduction. Reduction achieved by traction, abduction/adduction and appropriate rotation. Position of patella checked. Care taken not to position in excess internal/external rotation. Slight external rotation closes fracture gap posteriorly in case of posterior comminution (personal experience).

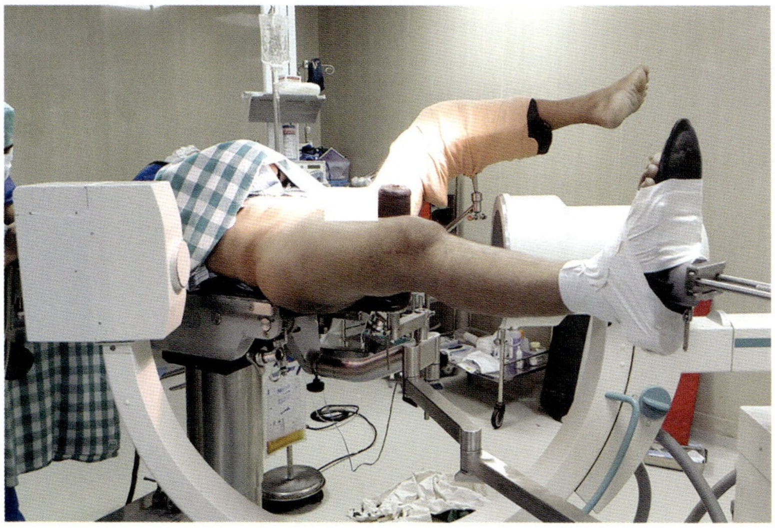

Fig. 6: C-arm position for lateral view.

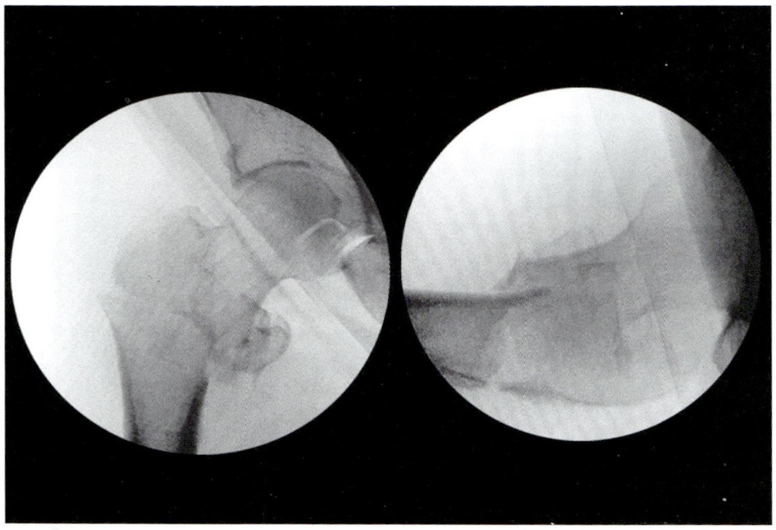

Fig. 7: C-arm image anteroposterior view and lateral view.

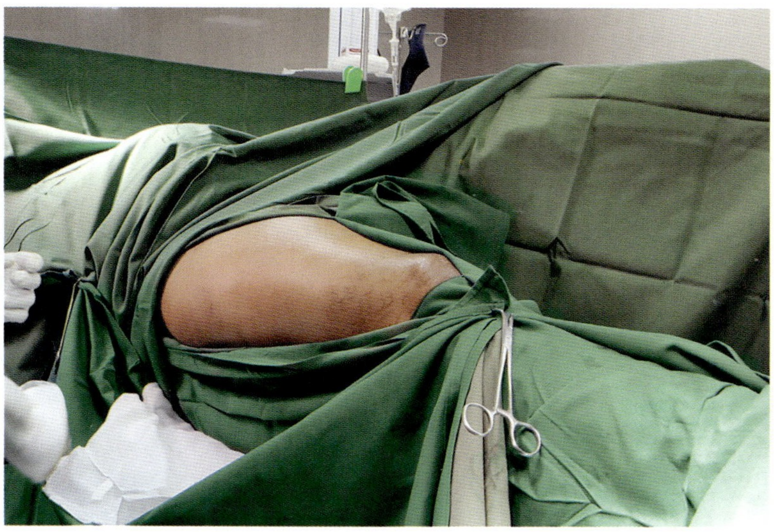

Fig. 8: Draping.

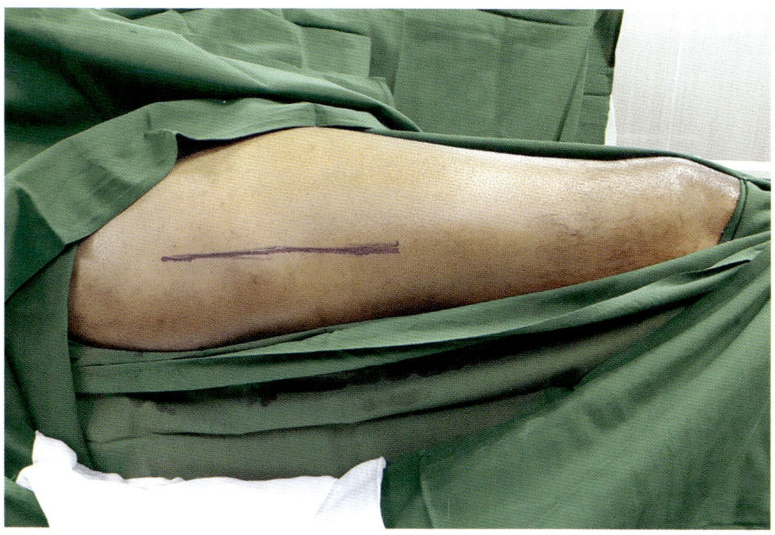

Fig. 9: Incision marked. Incision is located on lateral aspect of proximal thigh.

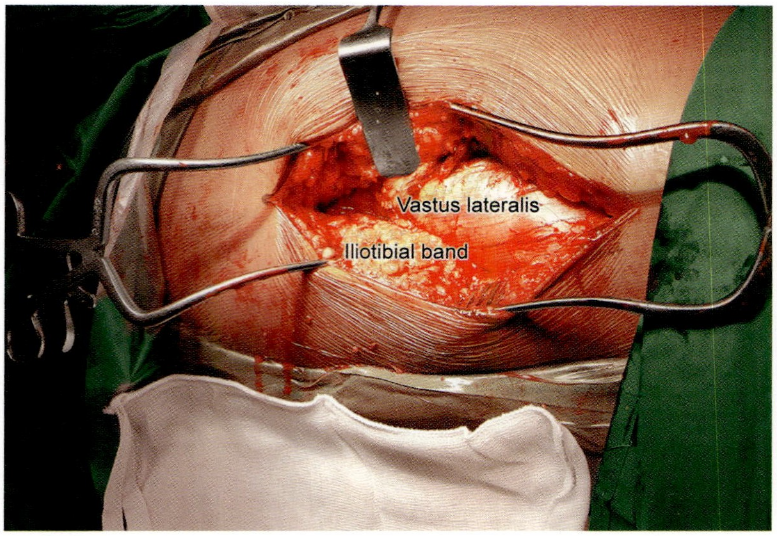

Fig. 10: Skin is incised about 5 inches in length extending distally from just proximal to tip of greater trochanter. Incision deepened through superficial fascia, fascia lata and iliotibial band.

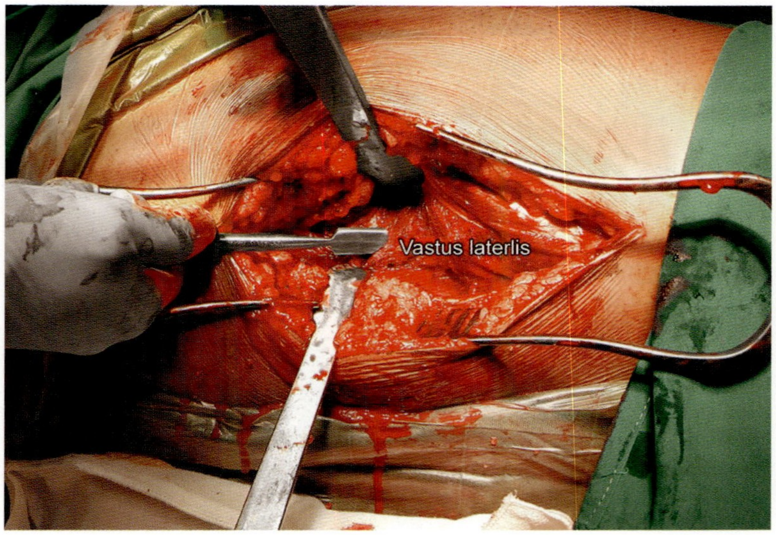

Fig. 11: Vastus lateralis is split nearer posterior border and erased subperiosteally from vastus ridge and shaft for required length. Trochanteric flare is exposed. If fracture reduction is not achieved earlier by closed technique, it is now performed under direct vision. Carefully inserted spike retractor on anterior part of neck helps, so also appropriately placed reduction clamps.

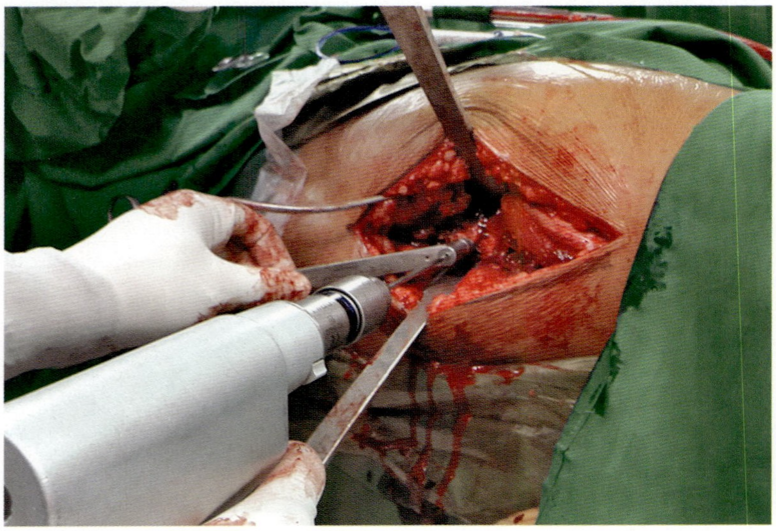

Fig. 12A: Entry point to be ¾ inch distal to vastus ridge and midway between anterior and posterior borders.

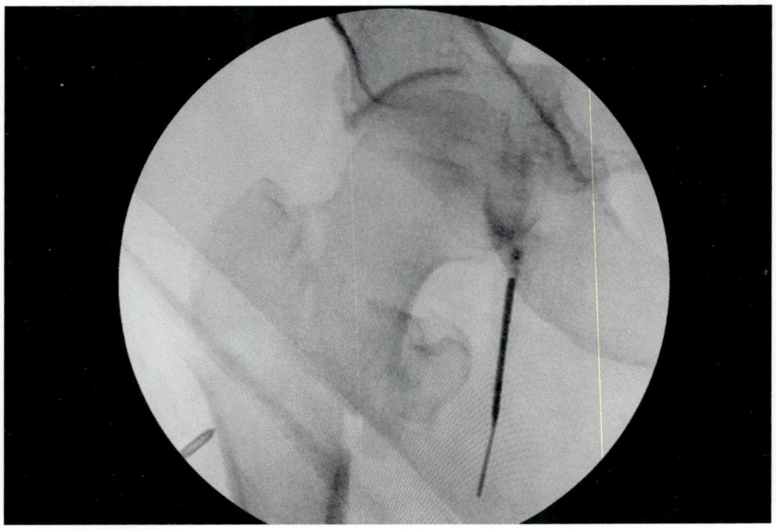

Fig. 12B: Accurate entry point is located by placing drill on bone surface while viewing anteroposterior C-arm image.

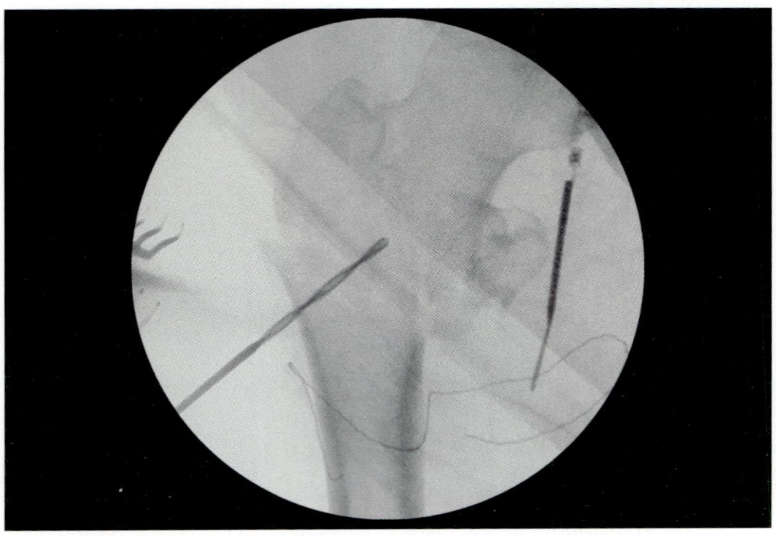

Fig. 12C: Drill advanced partly into neck.

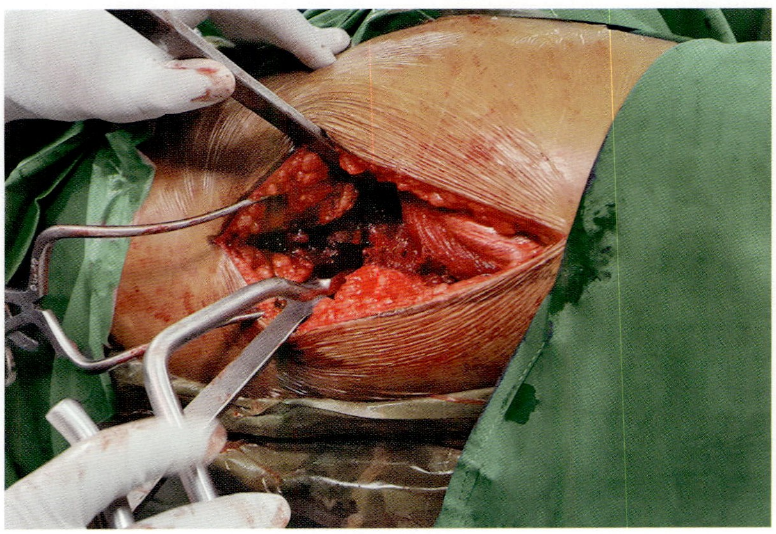

Fig. 13A: Entry enlarged with awl.

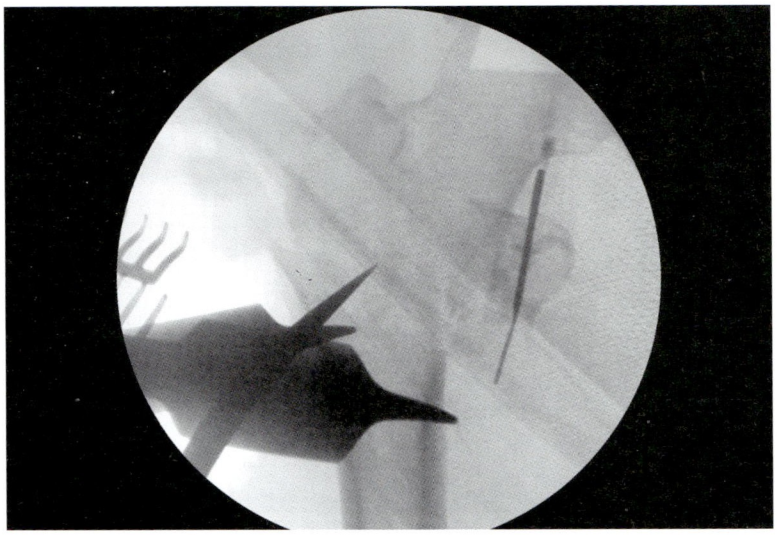

Fig. 13B: This enlarged entry point enables easy change of direction of guidewire as otherwise cortex firmly grips the guidewire, C-arm image.

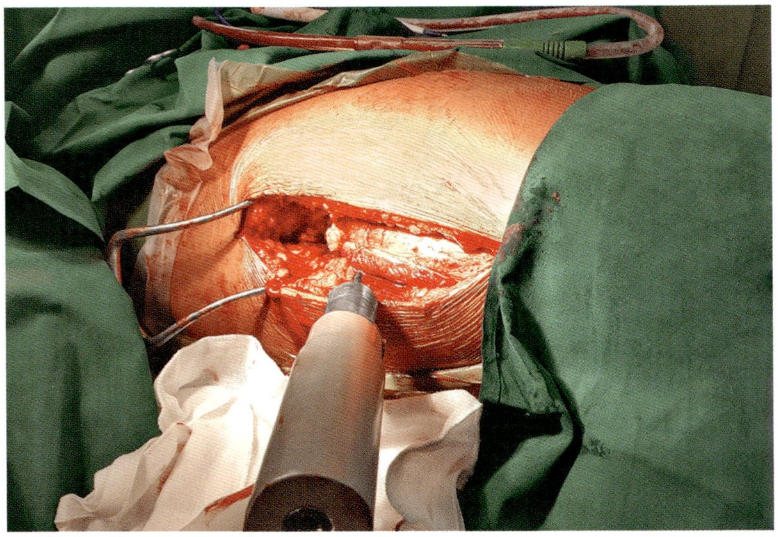

Fig. 14A: At first guidewire may be inserted on front of neck close to bone to judge version prior to introduction of definitive guidewire (not shown here). Guidewire is driven in deep up to subchondral cortex but never into or beyond joint, because accidental breakage of penetrating guidewire can be a major complication.

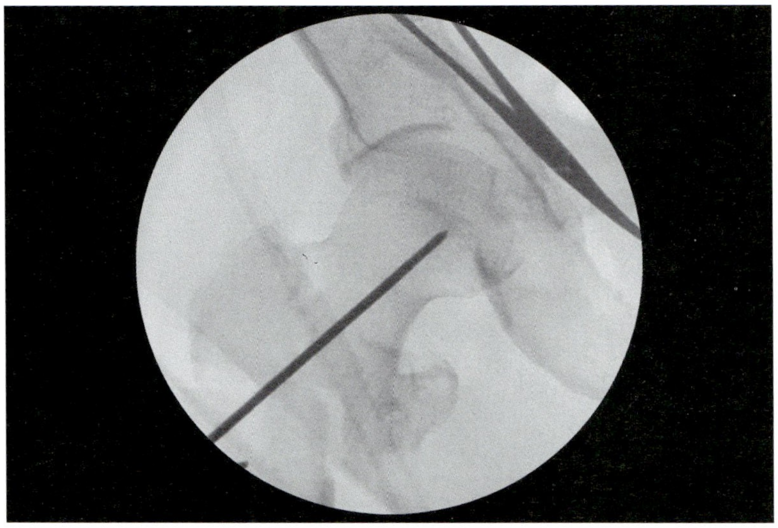

Fig. 14B: Guidewire position is checked in both C-arm views. It should be in center of head or slight inferior position in AP view.

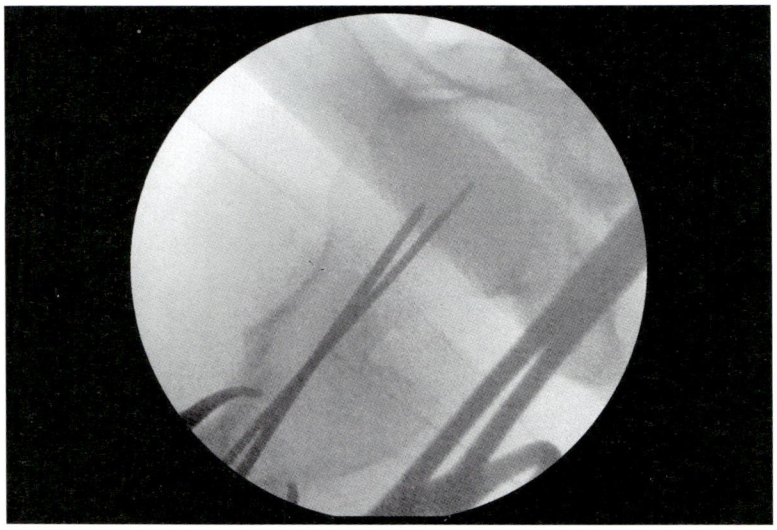

Fig. 14C: In lateral view it should be in center of head or slightly posterior.

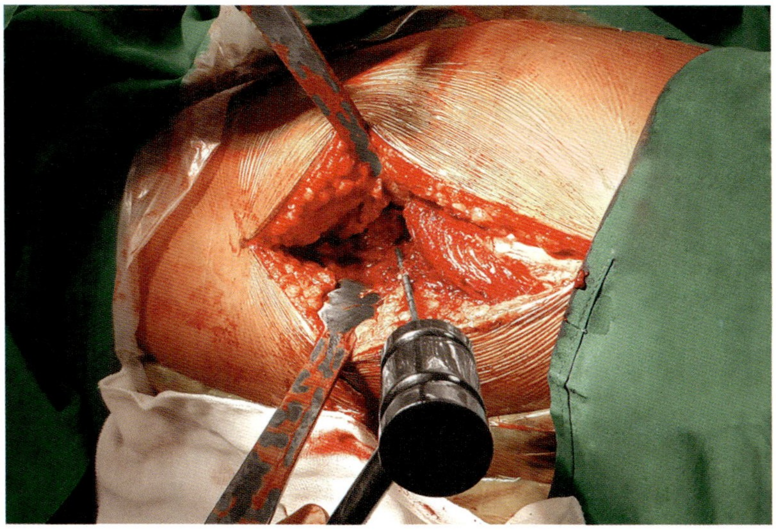

Fig. 14D: Guidewire is then gently tapped into firm position.

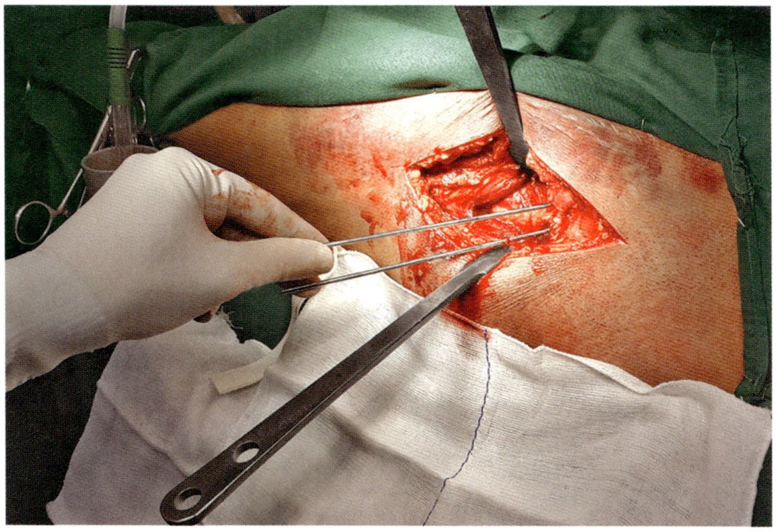

Fig. 14E: Another guidewire may be added to prevent rotation of head and neck during subsequent steps. Length of dynamic hip screw is estimated by direct measure. Angle for barrel plate is measured using angle guide.

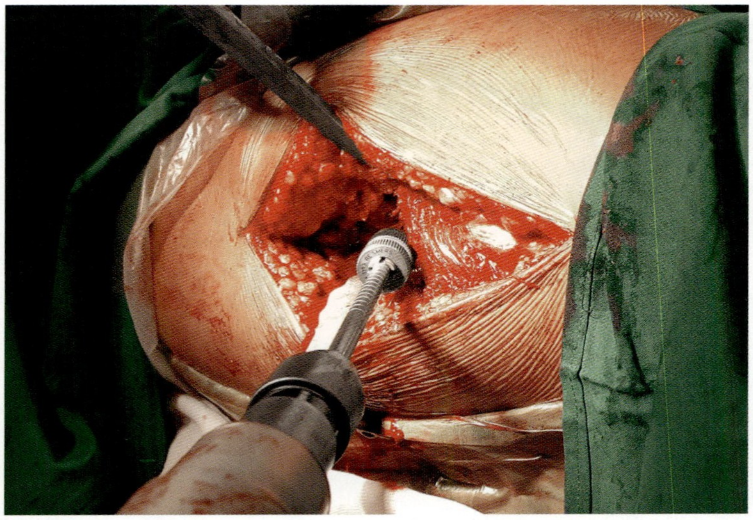

Fig. 15A: Reaming is done over the guidewire using special triple reamer (adjusted for correct length) and up to subchondral bone keeping in mind the requirements of tip apex distance. Power reamer may be preferred to prevent comminution of outer cortex and in hard bone.

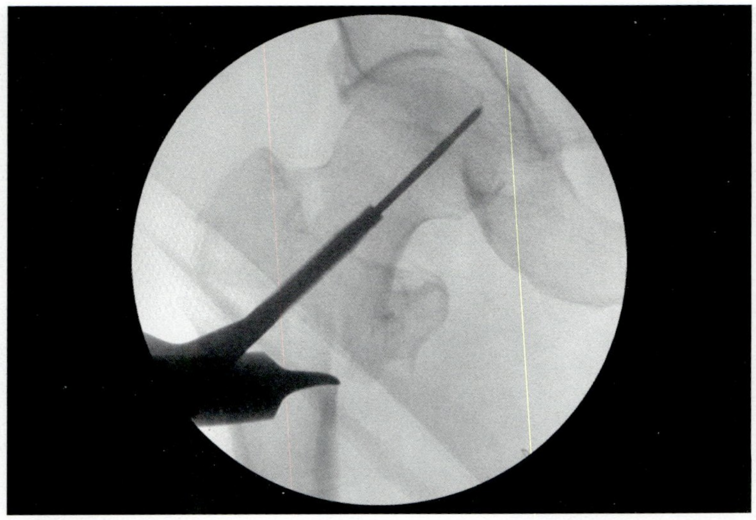

Fig. 15B: Care is taken not to drive guidewire into pelvis inadvertently by frequent monitoring of anteroposterior C-arm image. This can happen if guidewire is stuck inside reamer. Barrel of plate is inserted inside the enlarged entry point to test adequacy of reaming and removed. At times the guidewire comes out inadvertently while taking out the triple reamer. It can be accurately repositioned centrally in reamed hole by keeping the hip screw in reverse in reamed hole then reintroducing the wire in cannulated part.

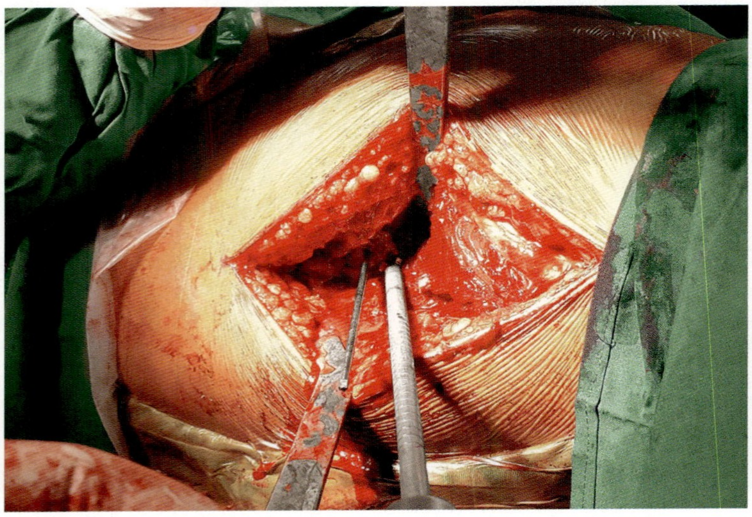

Fig.16A: Tapping is performed by cannulated tap over the guidewire to the desired depth gently but firmly while avoiding "tripping"..

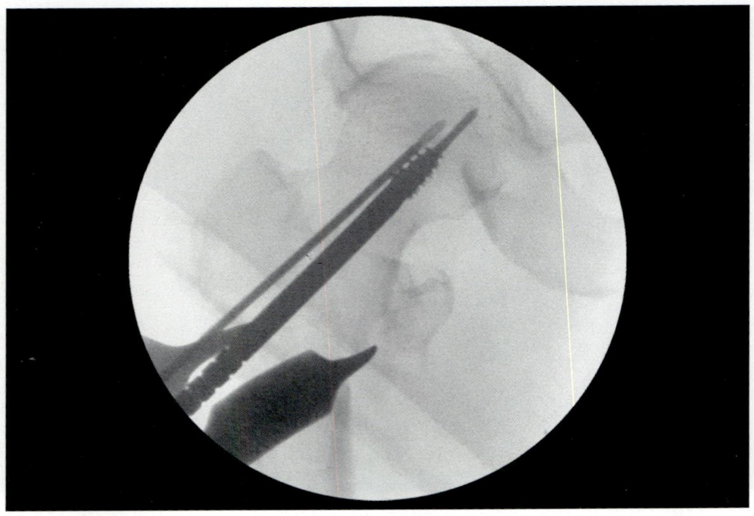

Fig. 16B: Tapping. C-arm image.

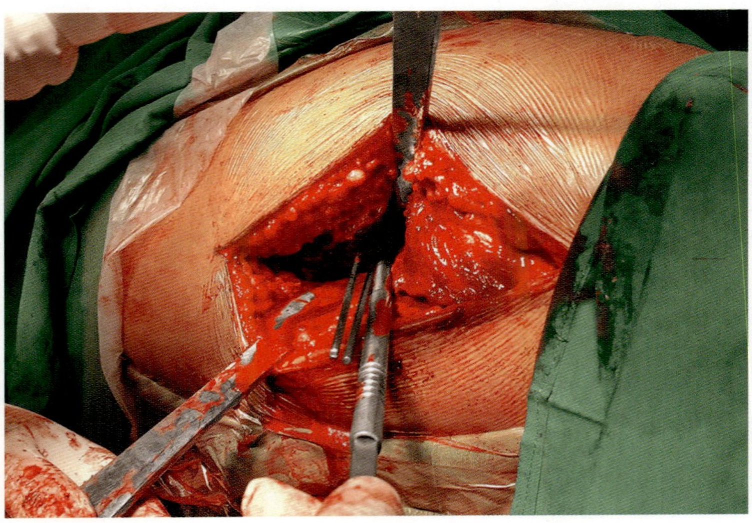

Fig. 17A: Length of dynamic hip screw is estimated by depth measure. (Practical tip)

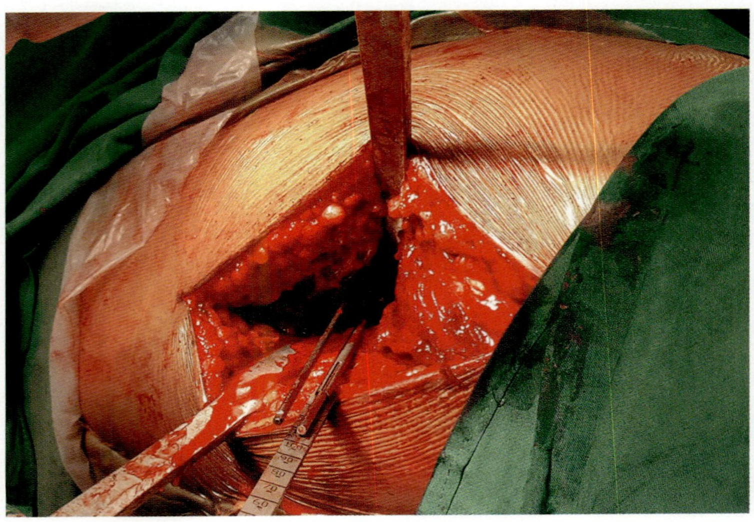

Fig. 17B: Length of dynamic hip screw is estimated more commonly by direct measure. Selected dynamic hip screw and barrel plate is checked priorly for compatibility. Four holed plate suffices in noncomminuted fractures. Long barrel is chosen for dynamic hip screw of more than 85 mms.

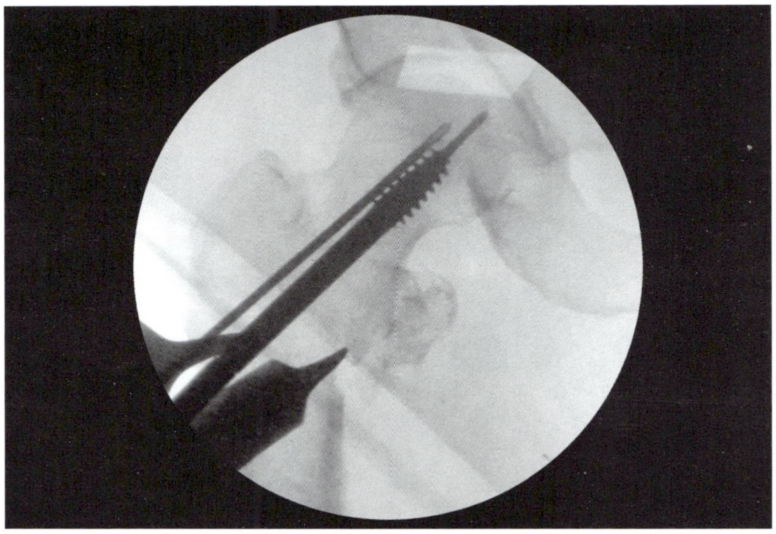

Fig. 18: Dynamic hip screw is inserted to appropriate depth over guidewire. Ensuring correct orientation helps subsequent easy insertion of barrel plate. Outer end of hip screw positioned slightly inside the outer cortex allows intraoperative compression by top nut.

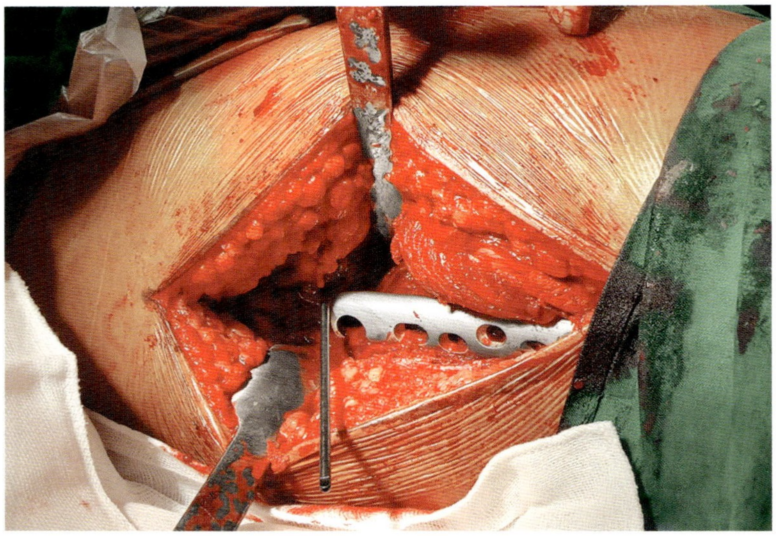

Fig. 19A: Barrel plate is inserted.

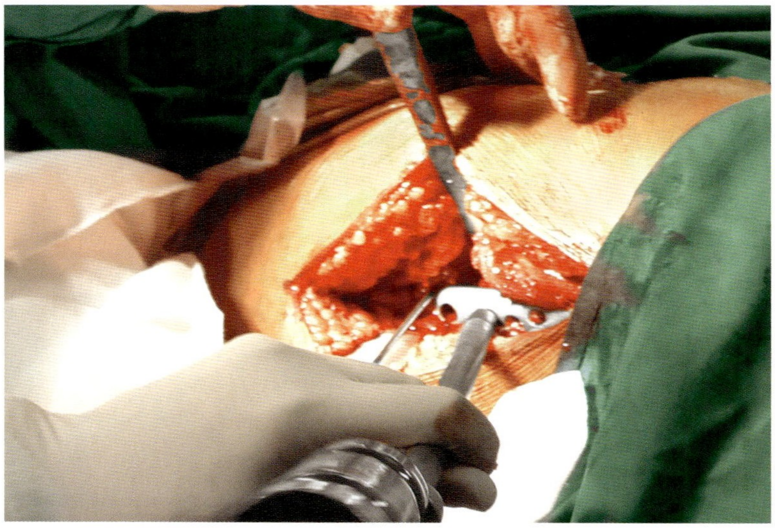

Fig. 19B: Barrel plate is lightly tapped into position by nylon punch.

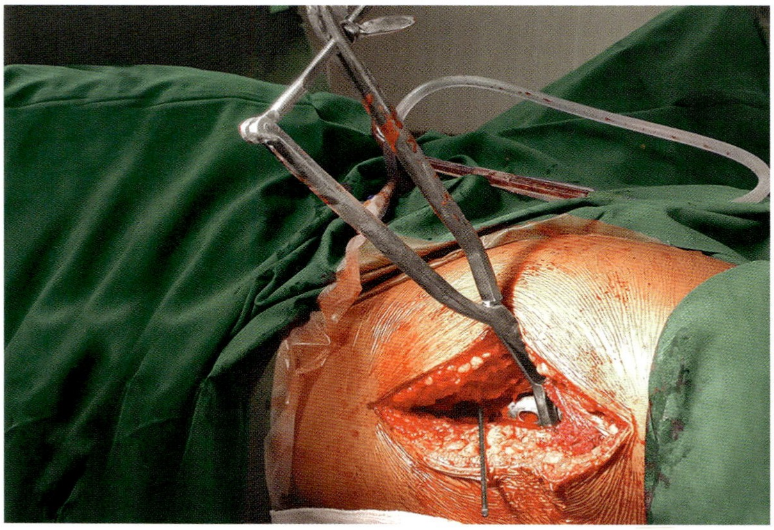

Fig. 19C: Barrel plate is held firmly to shaft by large bone holding forceps. Care is taken to ensure positioning of most distal cortex screw hole centralized on shaft.

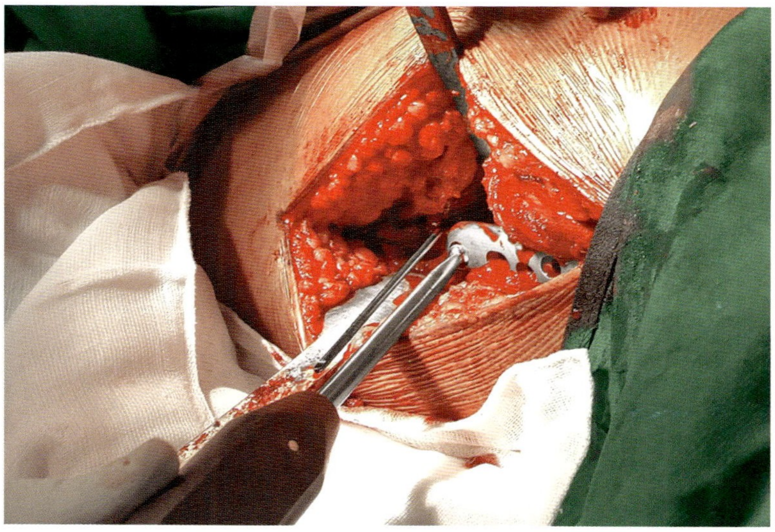

Fig. 19D: Top nut is applied but not tightened.

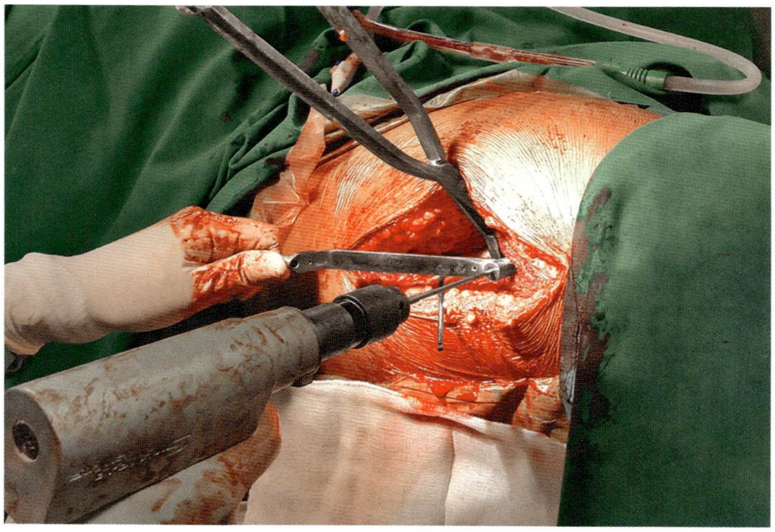

Fig. 20A: Cortex is drilled in distal screw hole of barrel plate. Position of distal most screw hole is rechecked to prevent eccentric positioning of distal end of plate over lateral surface.

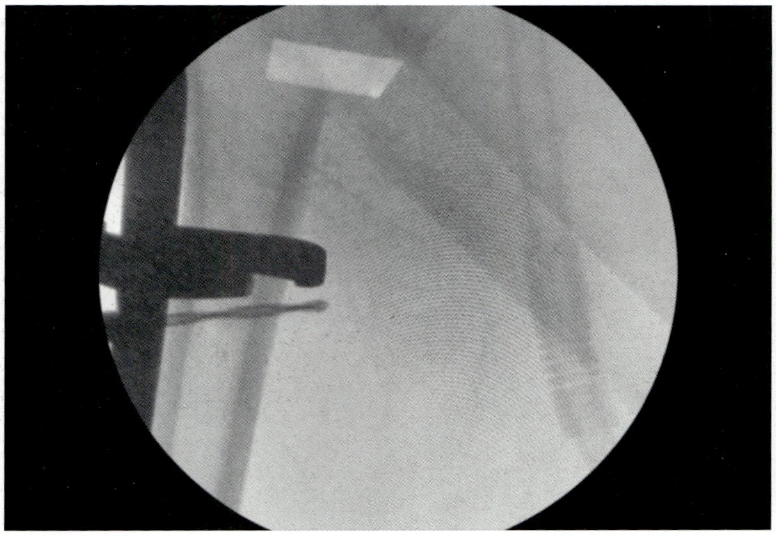

Fig. 20B: C-arm image of drilling.

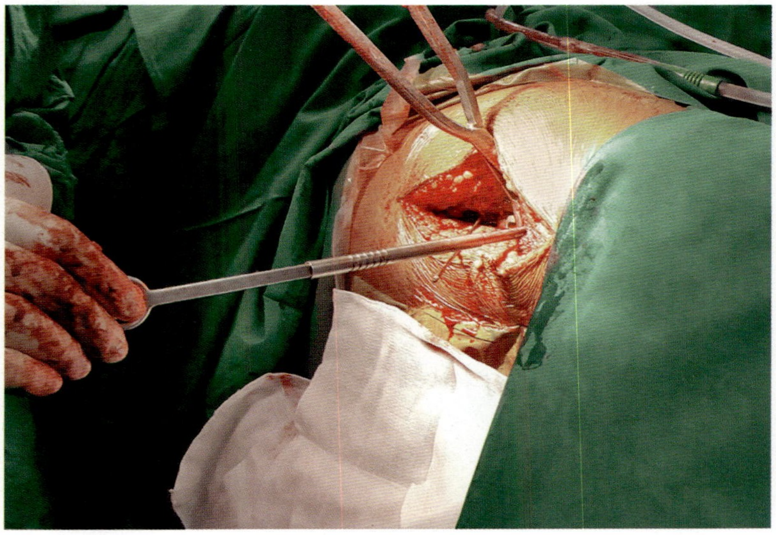

Fig. 20C: Use of depth measure to estimate screw length.

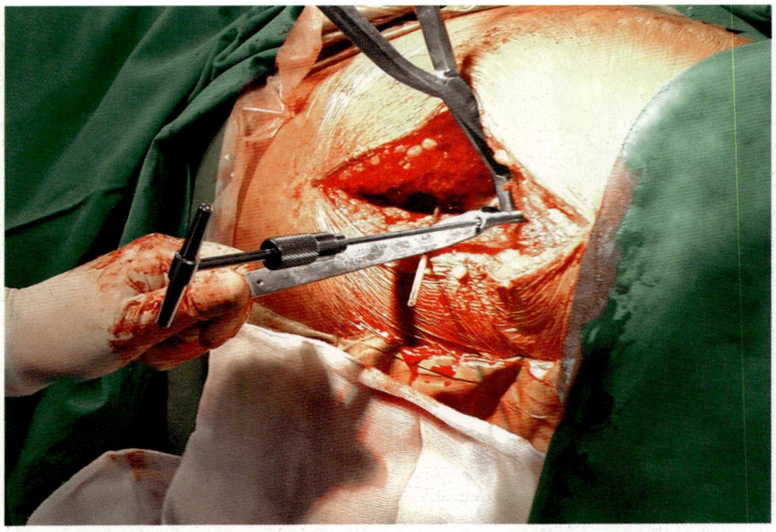

Fig. 20D: Tapping done to appropriate depth.

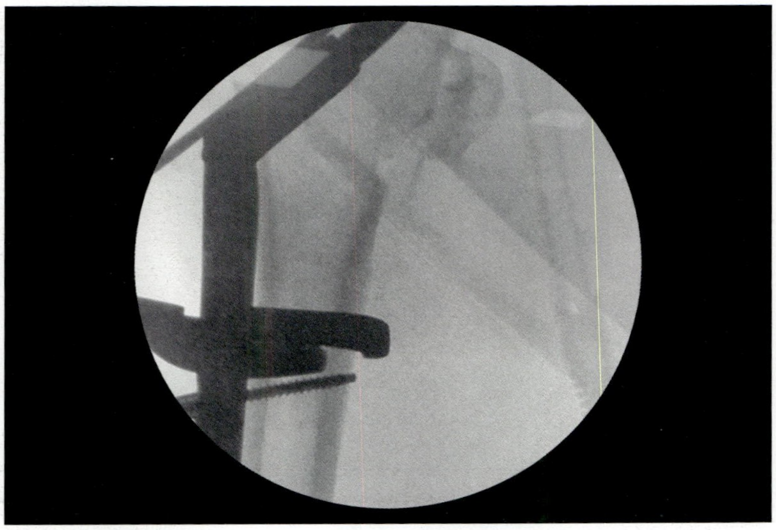

Fig. 20E: C-arm image of tapping.

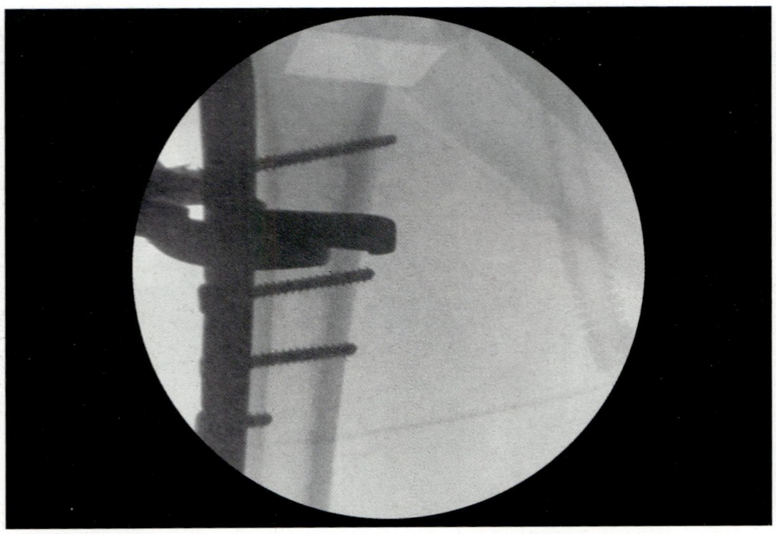

Fig. 21A: After tapping corresponding screw is inserted. Rest of the cortical screws are inserted in similar fashion.

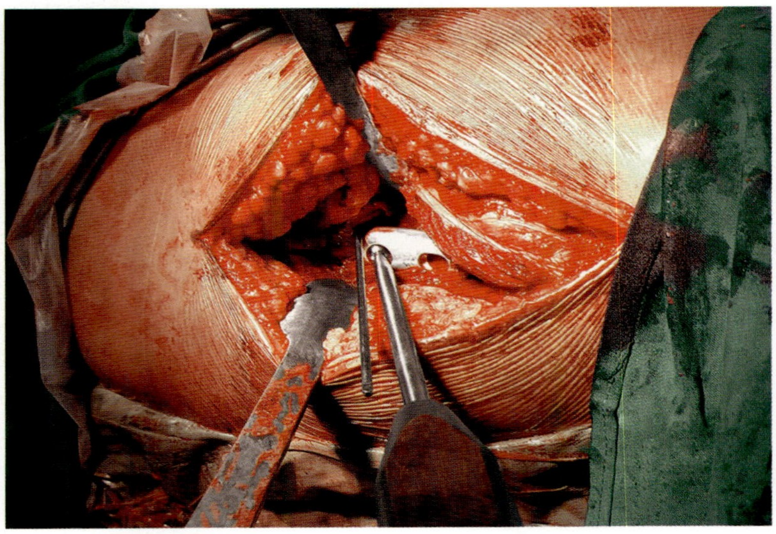

Fig. 21B: Compression given by tightening of top nut.

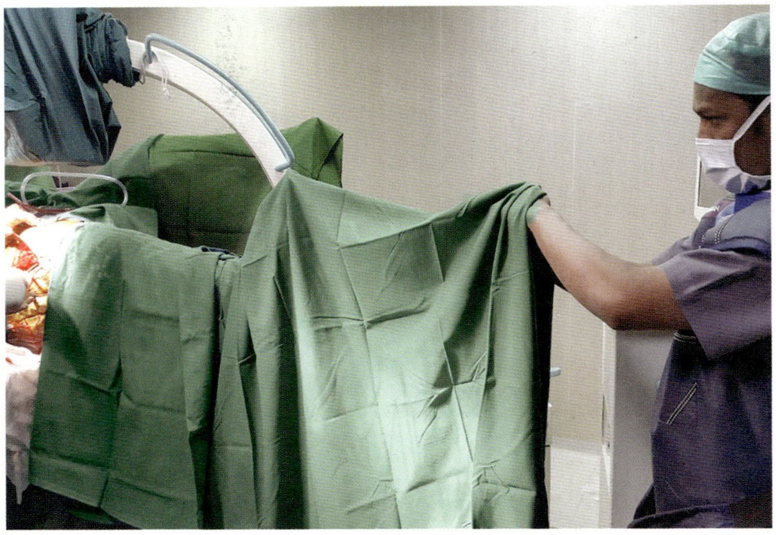

Fig. 21C: Traction released at fracture table prior to top nut tightening.

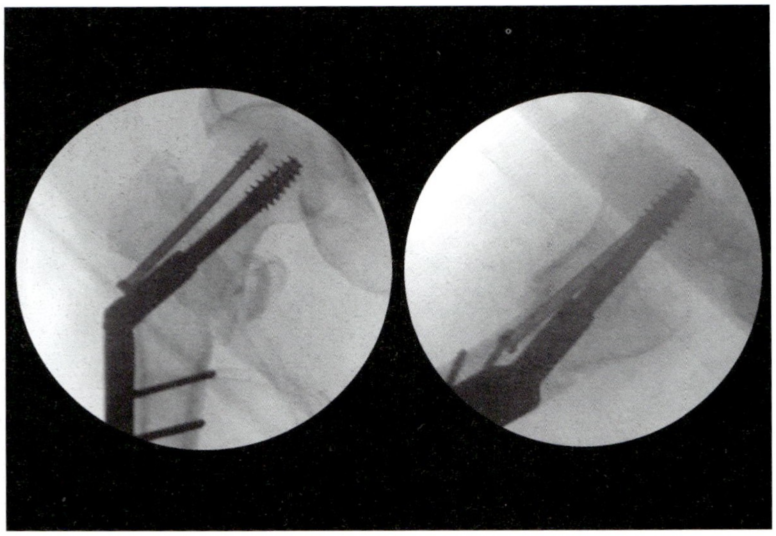

Fig. 22: Additional cancellous screw proximally is an option depending on stability. Position is checked in both C-arm views.

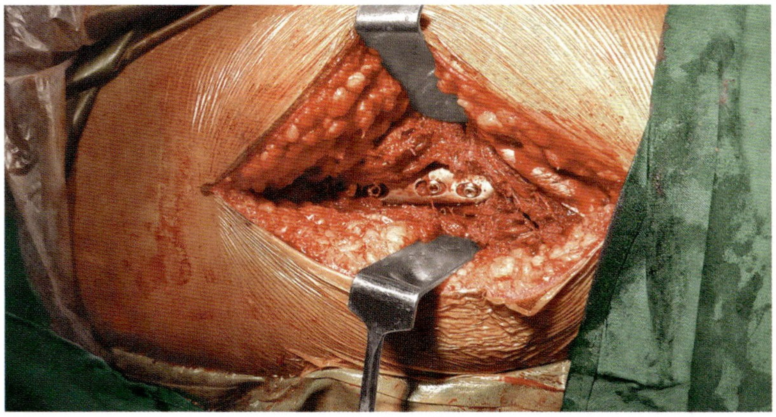

Fig. 23A: Hemostasis achieved.

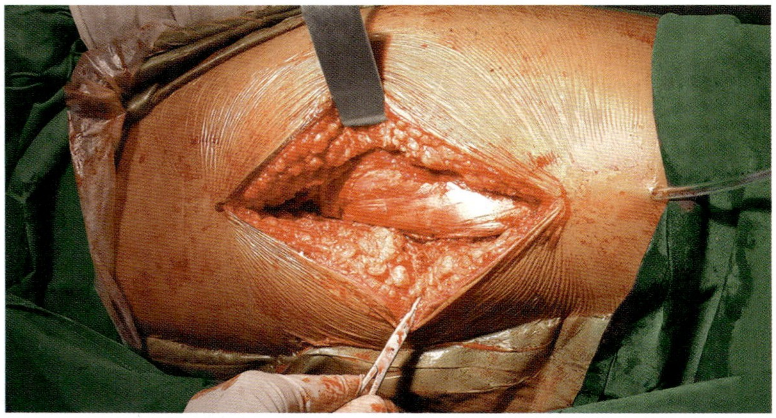

Fig. 23B: Vastus lateralis and tensor fascia lata sutured in layers over drains.

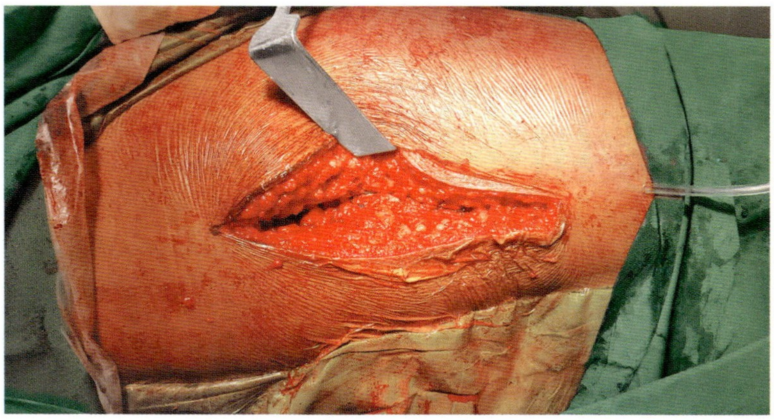

Fig. 23C: Subcutaneous tissues closed.

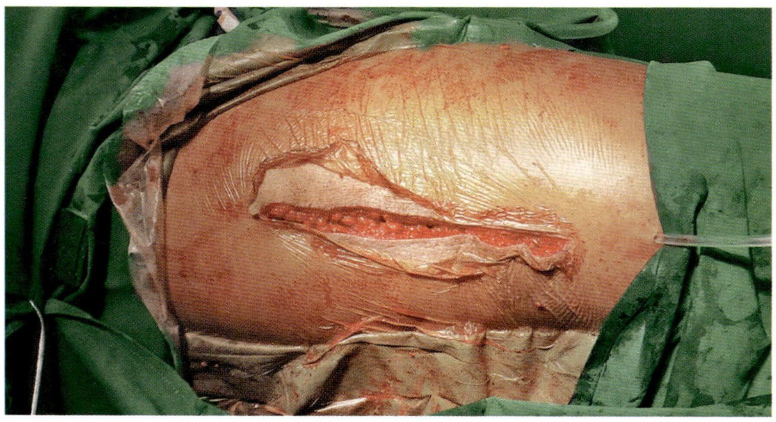

Fig. 23D: Further subcutaneous closure with absorbable sutures.

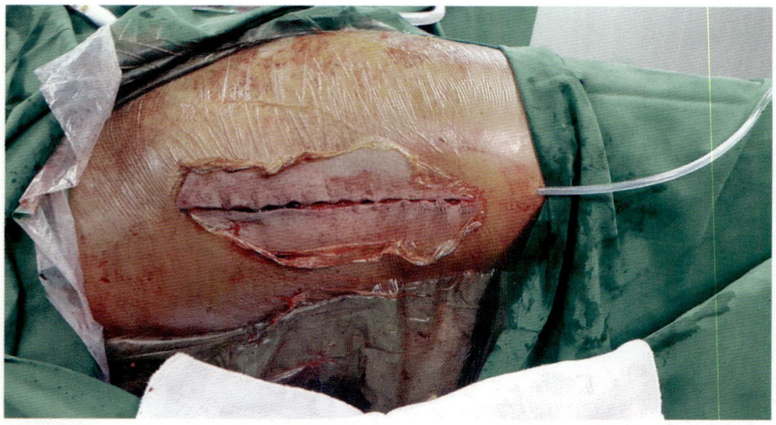

Fig. 23E: Adequate appoximation achieved.

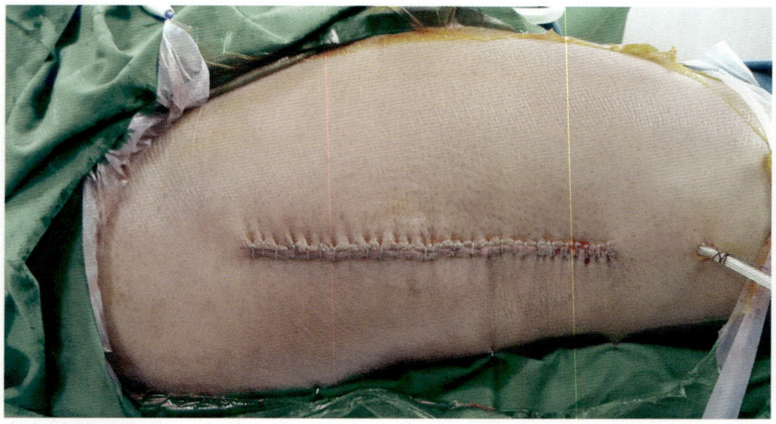

Fig. 23F: Skin closure.

POSTOPERATIVE PROTOCOL FOR DHS BARREL PLATE AND PROXIMAL FEMUR NAIL

- Bedside sitting encouraged on second postoperative day.
- Standing and partial weight-bearing walker walking as tolerated from second week onwards.
- Full weight-bearing after 3 months if follow-up radiographs are satisfactory.

COMPLICATIONS

Possible complications of surgery include implant failure and cut out especially in osteoporotic bones and these may require revision surgery. Other complications include shortening and malunion.

SUGGESTED READING

1. Baumgaertner MR, Curtin SL, Lindskog DM, et al. The value of the tip-apex distance in predicting failure of fixation of peritrochanteric fractures of the hip. J Bone Joint Surg. 1995;77A:1058.
2. Baumgaertner MR, Curtin SL, Lindskog DM. Intramedullary versus extramedullary fixation for the treatment of intertrochanteric hip fractures. Clin Orthop. 1998;348:87.
3. De Ridder VA, de Lange S. Use of an intramedullary hip screw compared with a compression hip screw with a plate for intertrochanteric femoral fractures: a prospective, randomized study of one hundred patients. J Bone Joint Surg. 1999;81A:1502.
4. Domingo LJ, Cecilia D, Herrera A, et al. Trochanteric fractures treated with a proximal femoral nail. Int Orthop. 2001;25:298-301.
5. O'Brien PJ, Meek RN, Blachut PA, et al. Fixation of intertrochanteric hip fractures: gamma nail versus dynamic hip screw—a randomized, prospective study. Can J Surg. 1995;38:516.

CHAPTER 104

Intertrochanteric Fracture Femur: Proximal Femur Nail Fixation

Vijay M Panchanadikar, Shrinivas S Shintre

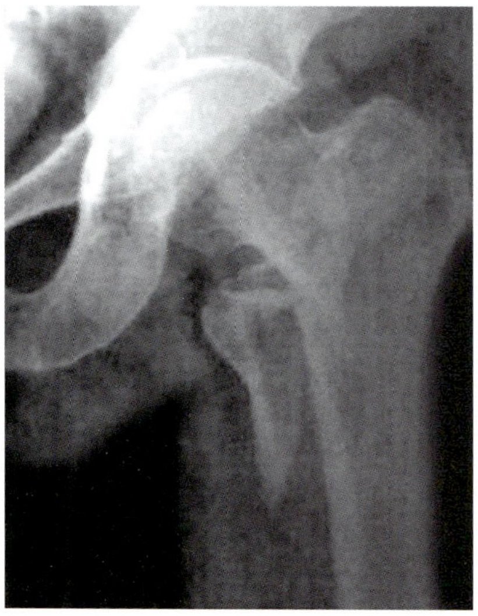

Fig. 1: X-ray—anteroposterior view.

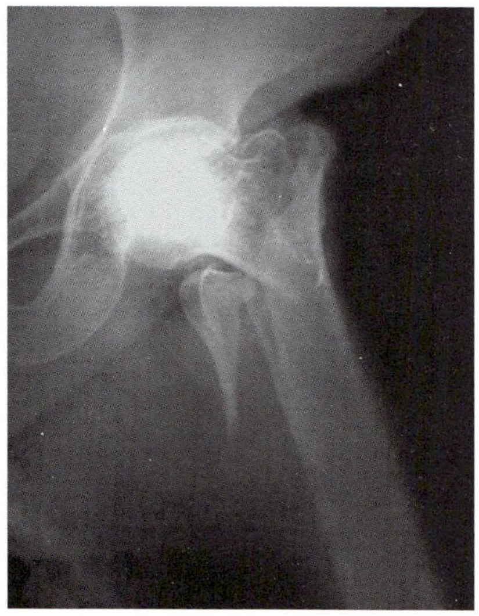

Fig. 2: X-ray—lateral view.

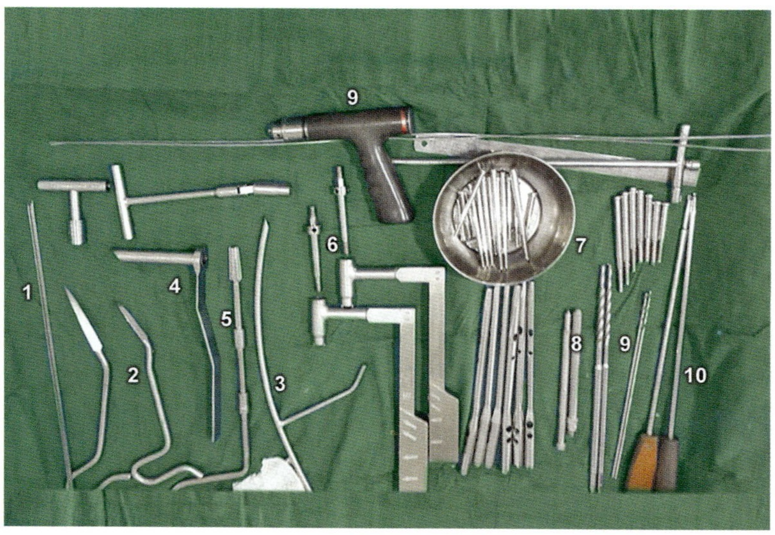

Fig. 3: Instruments trolley. Must have standard set. Key instruments are shown. 1—Guidewires, 2—diamond awl noncannulated/cannulated, 3—fossa finder device, 4—large sleeve, 5—proximal reamer, 6— jigs, nail bolts and socket wrench assembly, 7—nails, compression screw/hip pin, 8—sleeves, 9—power drill and drill bits, 10—screwdrivers.

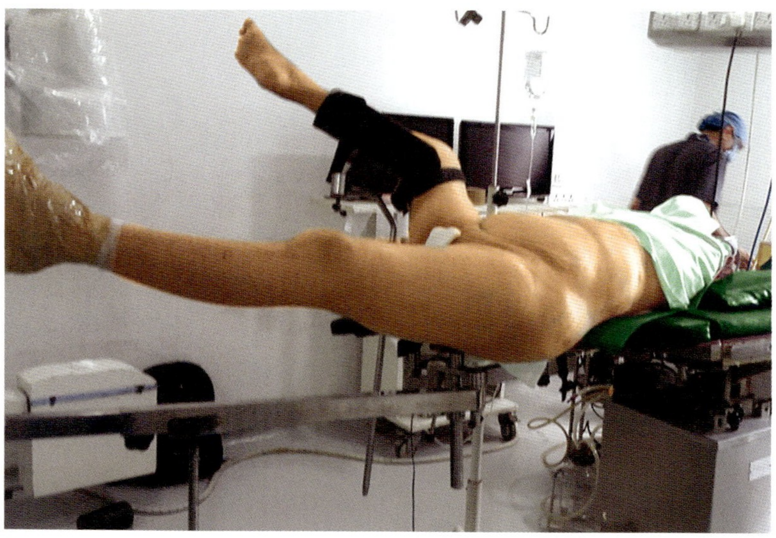

Fig. 4: Closed reduction is done by traction and rotation. C position of patient is secured with adducted thigh. If reduction is not adequate, open reduction is subsequently performed. Care is taken not to position limb in excess internal/external rotation.

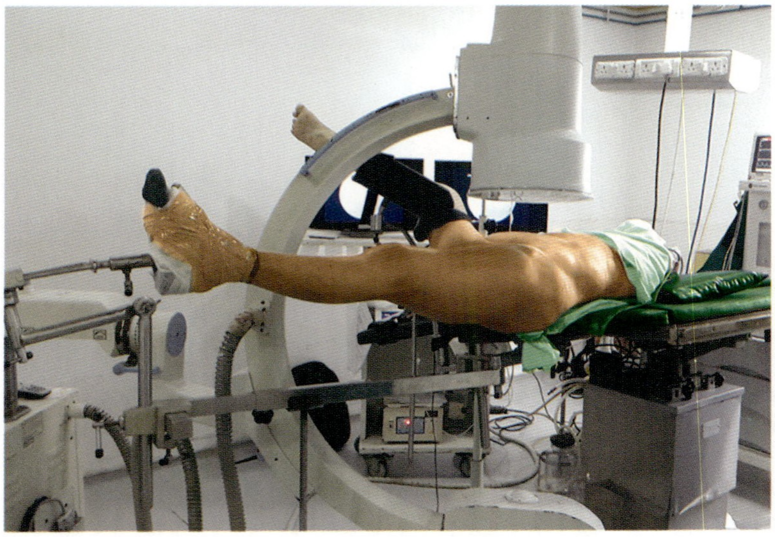

Fig. 5: C-arm position for anteroposterior view.

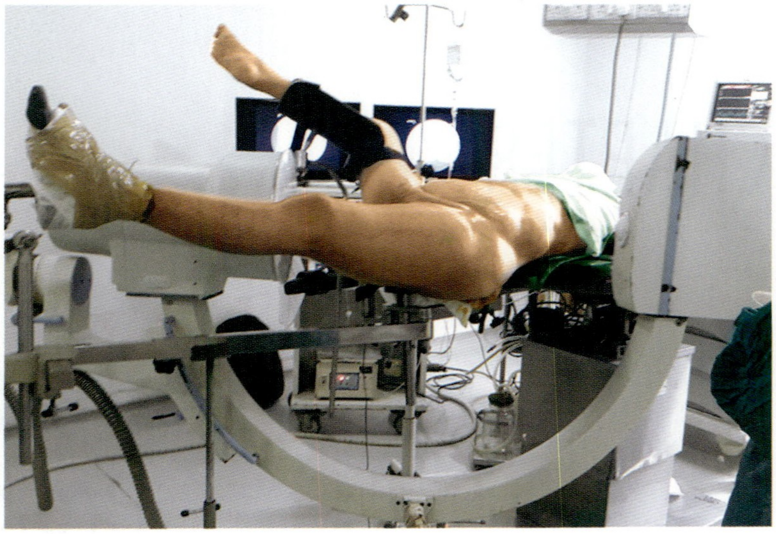

Fig. 6: C-arm position for lateral view.

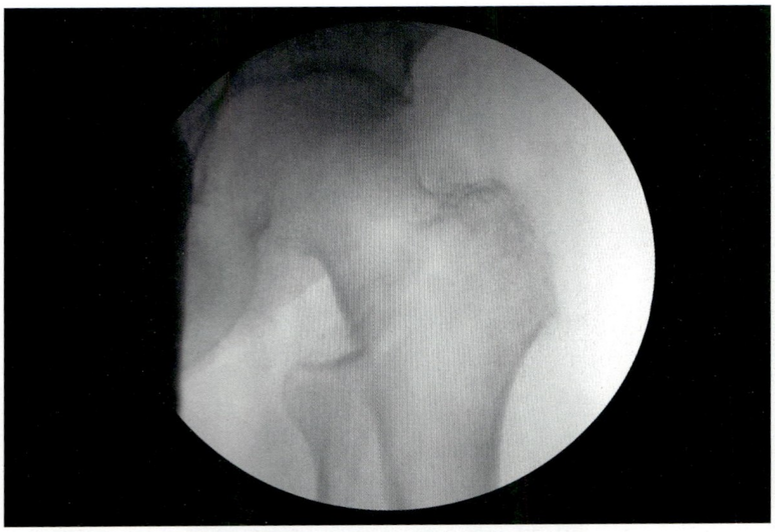

Fig. 7: C-arm image anteroposterior view.

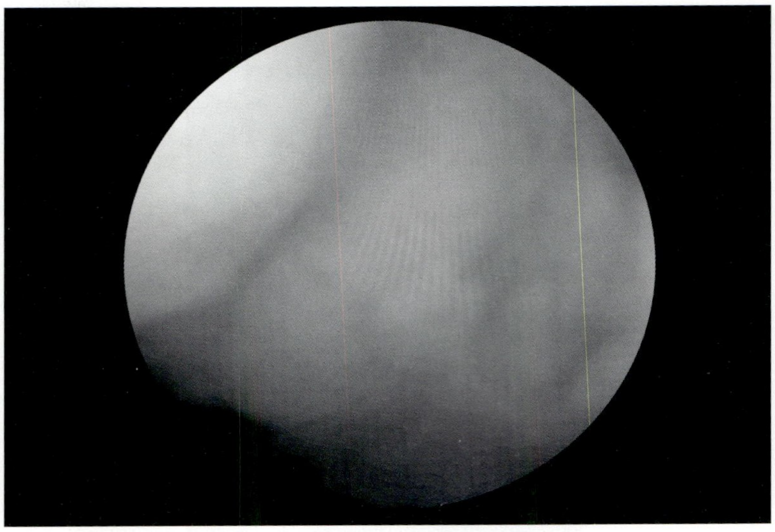

Fig. 8: C-arm image lateral view.

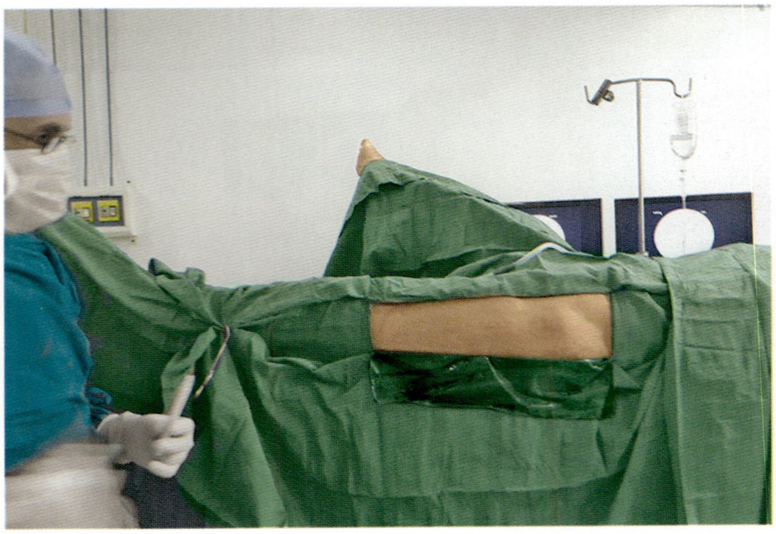

Fig. 9: Draping.

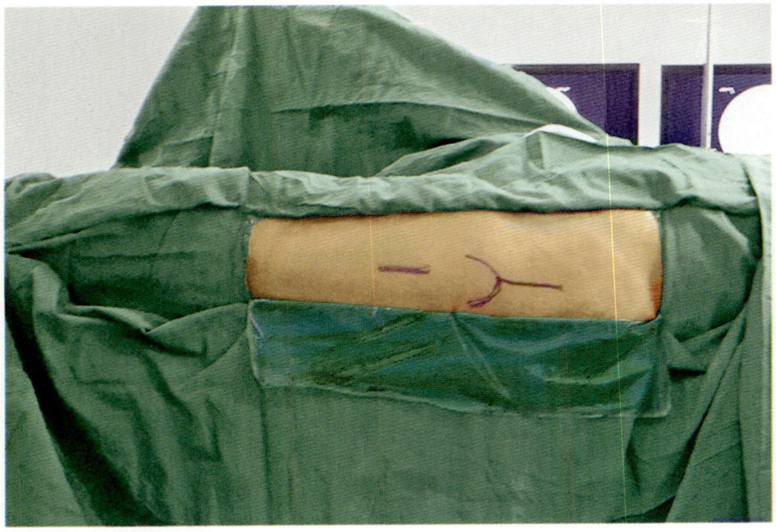

Fig. 10: Incisions. Proximal for nail entry and distal for compression screw (inferior lag screw)/hip pin entry are marked.

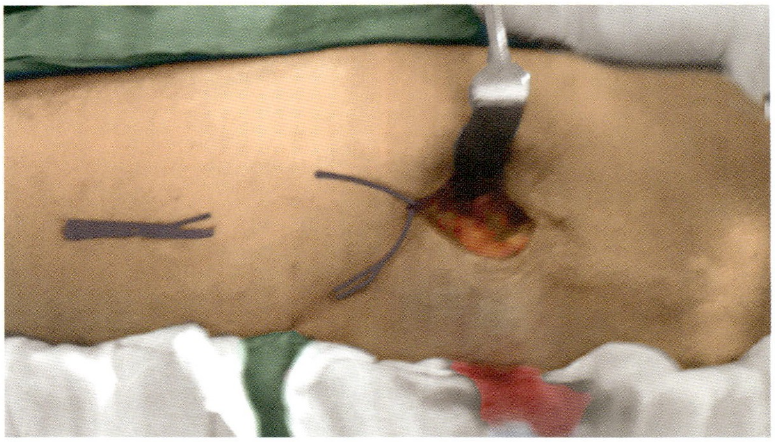

Fig. 11: Proximal incision is taken about 2 inches in length extending proximally starting at tip of greater trochanter. Incision is deepened through fascia and insertion of gluteus medius. Tip of trochanter is palpated.

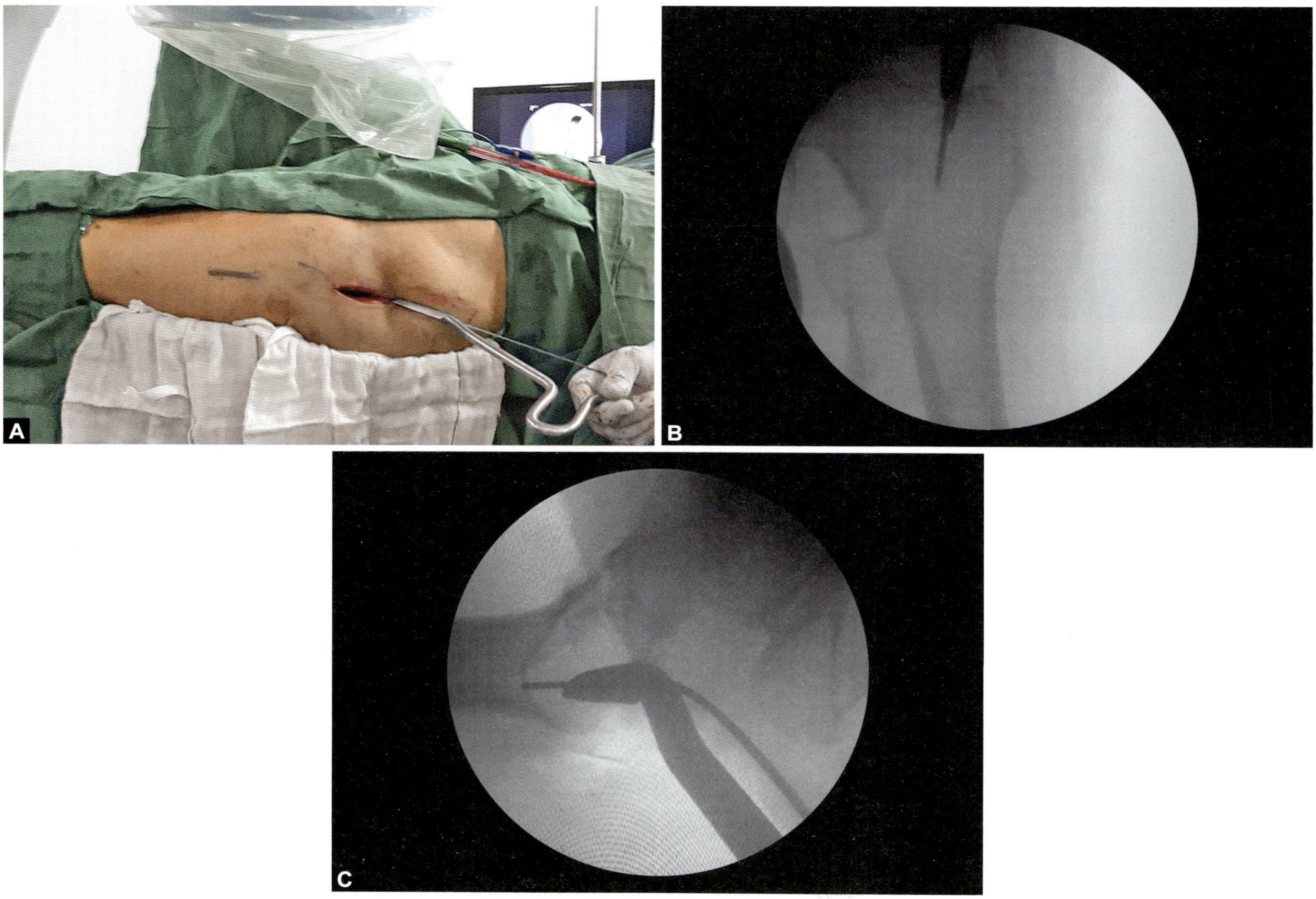

Figs. 12A to C: Cannulated awl is used to locate accurate entry point just medial to the tip of trochanter (A) in C-arm anteroposterior view (B), and middle of trochanter in line with femoral shaft in lateral view (C).

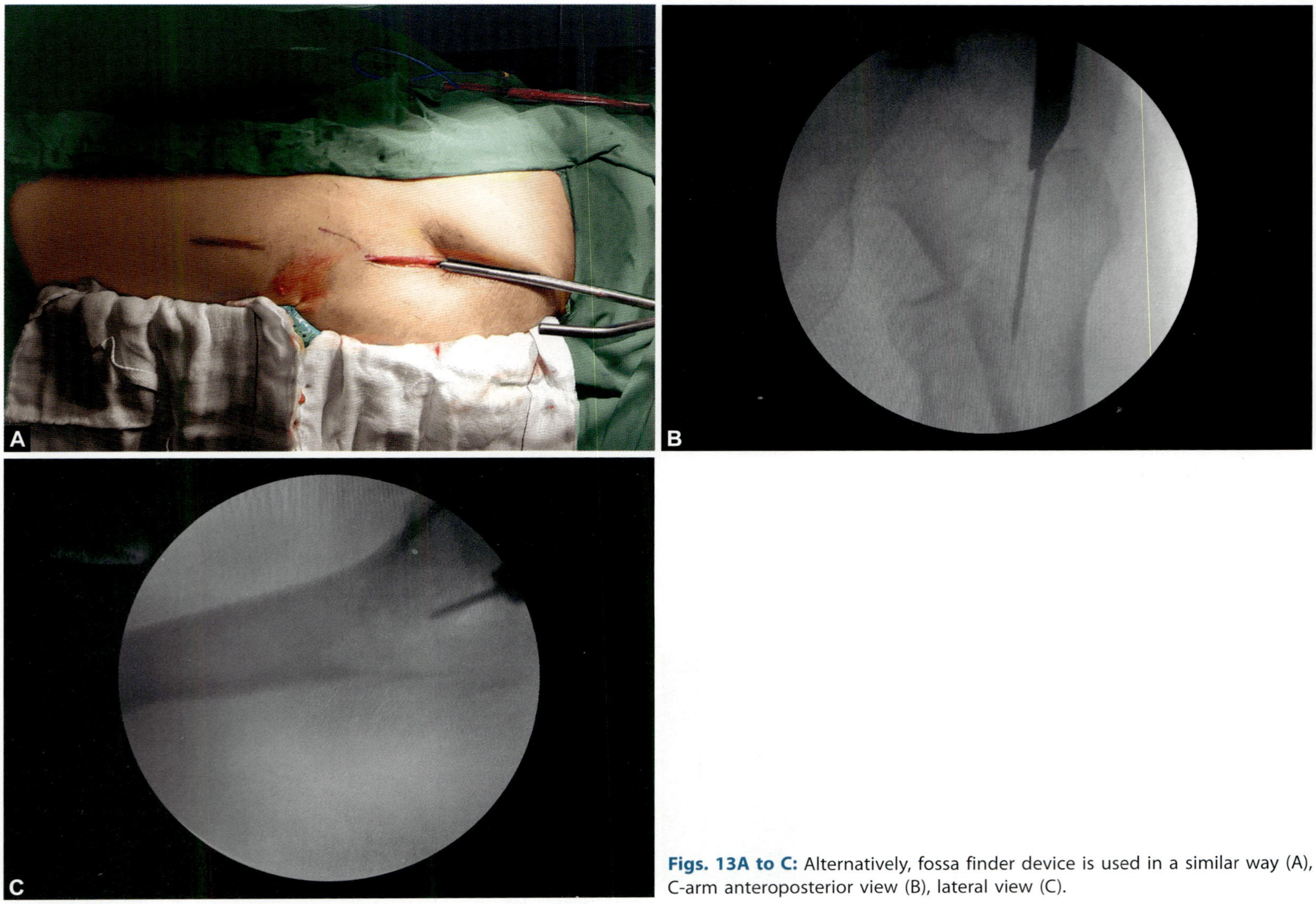

Figs. 13A to C: Alternatively, fossa finder device is used in a similar way (A), C-arm anteroposterior view (B), lateral view (C).

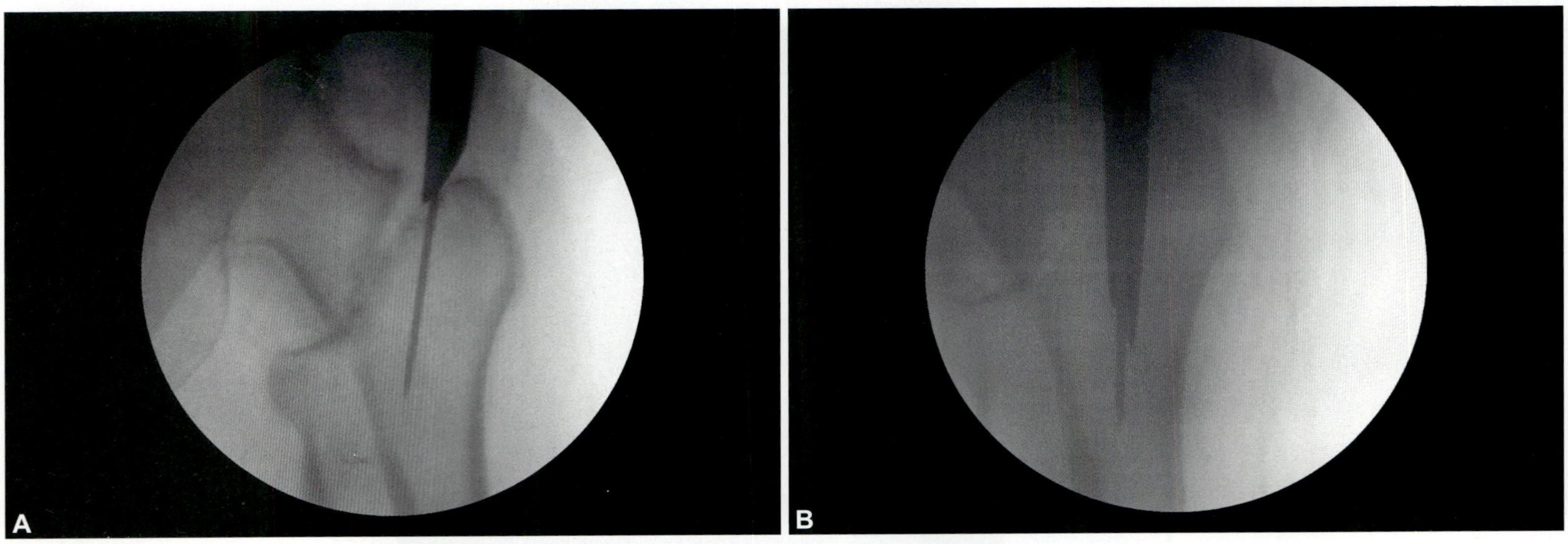

Figs. 14A and B: Guidewire tends to hit medial, anterior, or posterior cortex (A). It is redirected appropriately into the canal by use of cannulated awl or fossa finder device (B). Extreme care is taken to ensure that guidewire does not come out medially through fracture area and injure medial neurovascular structures.

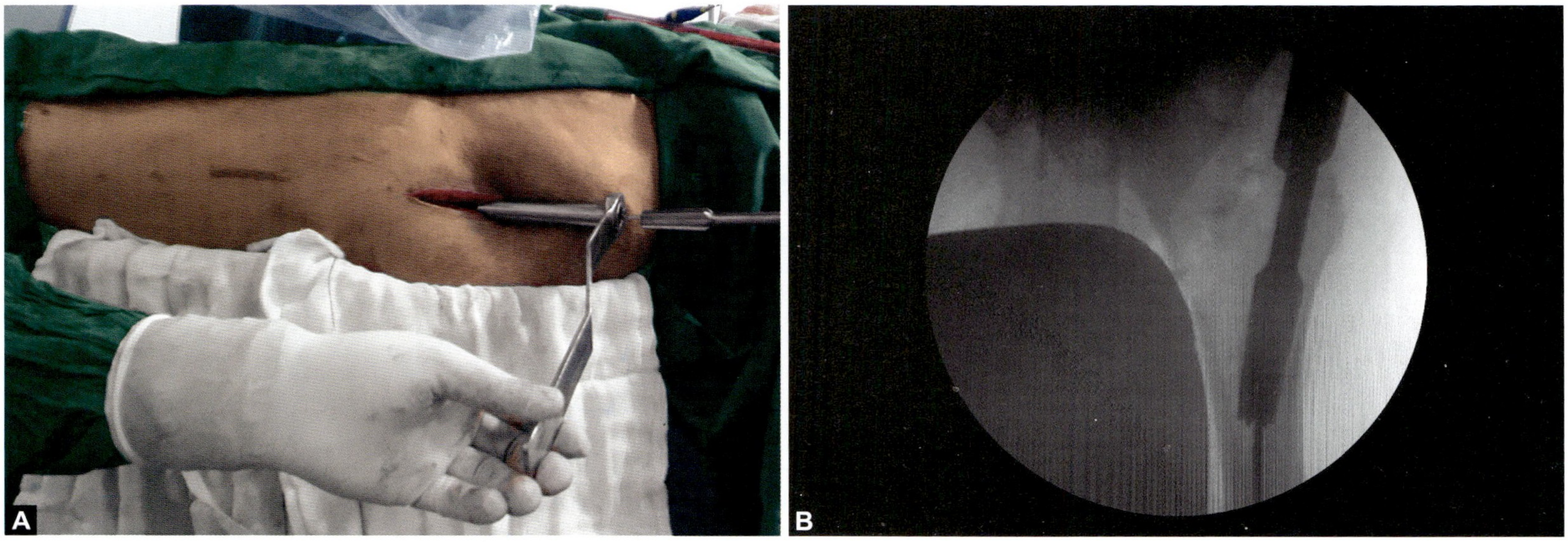

Figs. 15A and B: Reaming is done over the guidewire using special proximal reamer keeping it parallel to lateral cortex and up to recommended depth to accommodate broad proximal part of nail (A), C-arm image (B). Care is taken to keep reamer medially positioned at entry point to prevent lateralization of entry point.

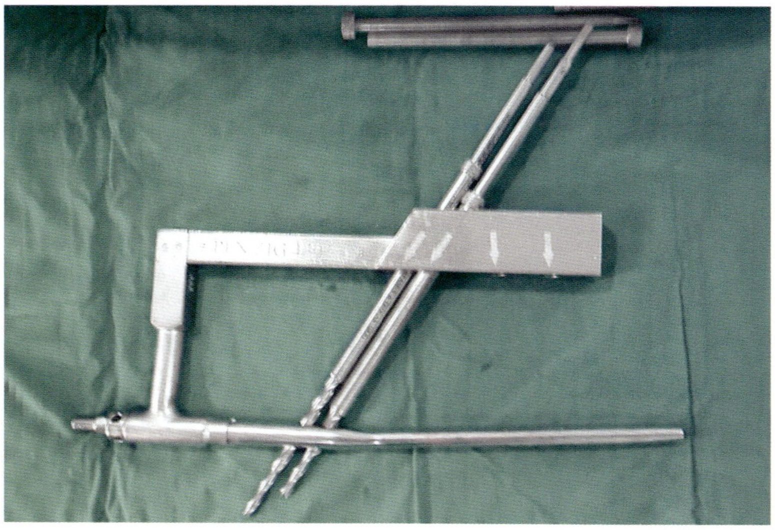

Fig. 16: Nail of appropriate length, angle and diameter is assembled over jig in correct orientation. Assembly checked carefully by surgeon himself for nail length, angle, diameter and orientation, all bolts are appropriately tightened and passage of sleeves through jig, and drills through screw hole of nail checked.

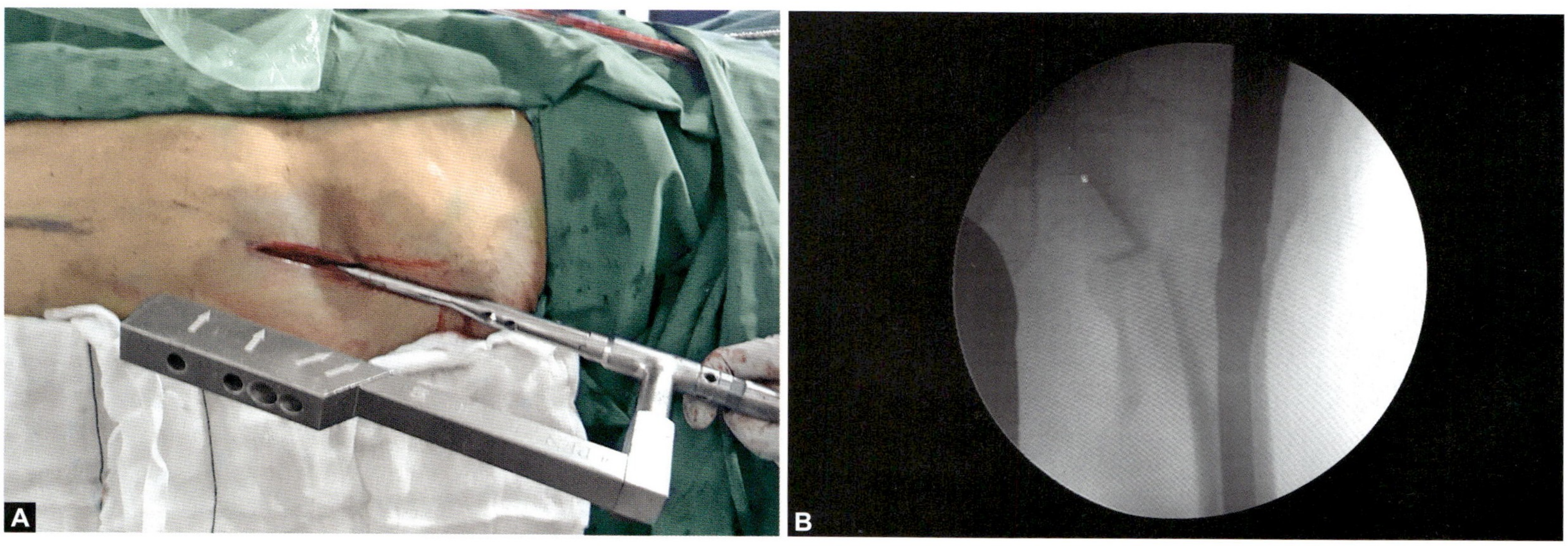

Figs. 17A and B: Nail is inserted to appropriate depth (A), C-arm image (B).

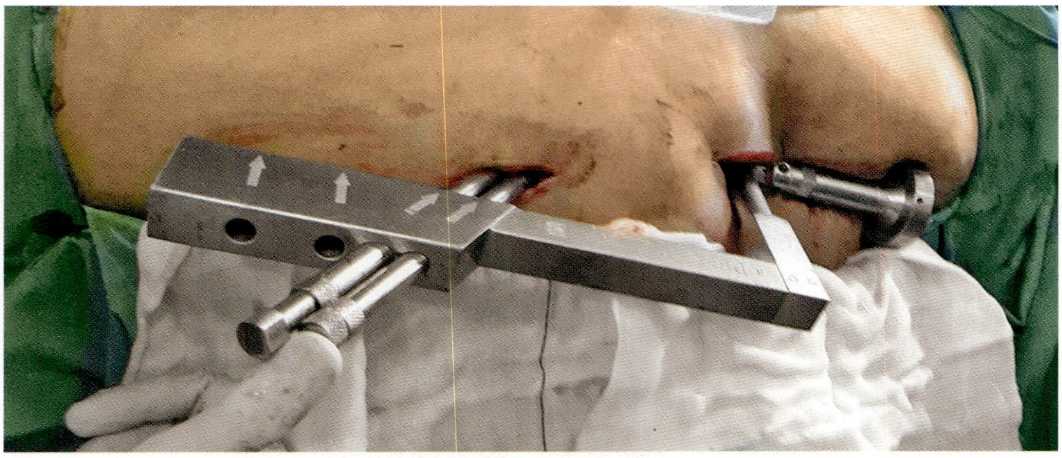

Fig. 18: Incision for inferior lag screw and superior hip pin taken, deepened through fascia lata, passage created up to bone by artery forceps. Sleeves passed, tapped into position touching bone surface.

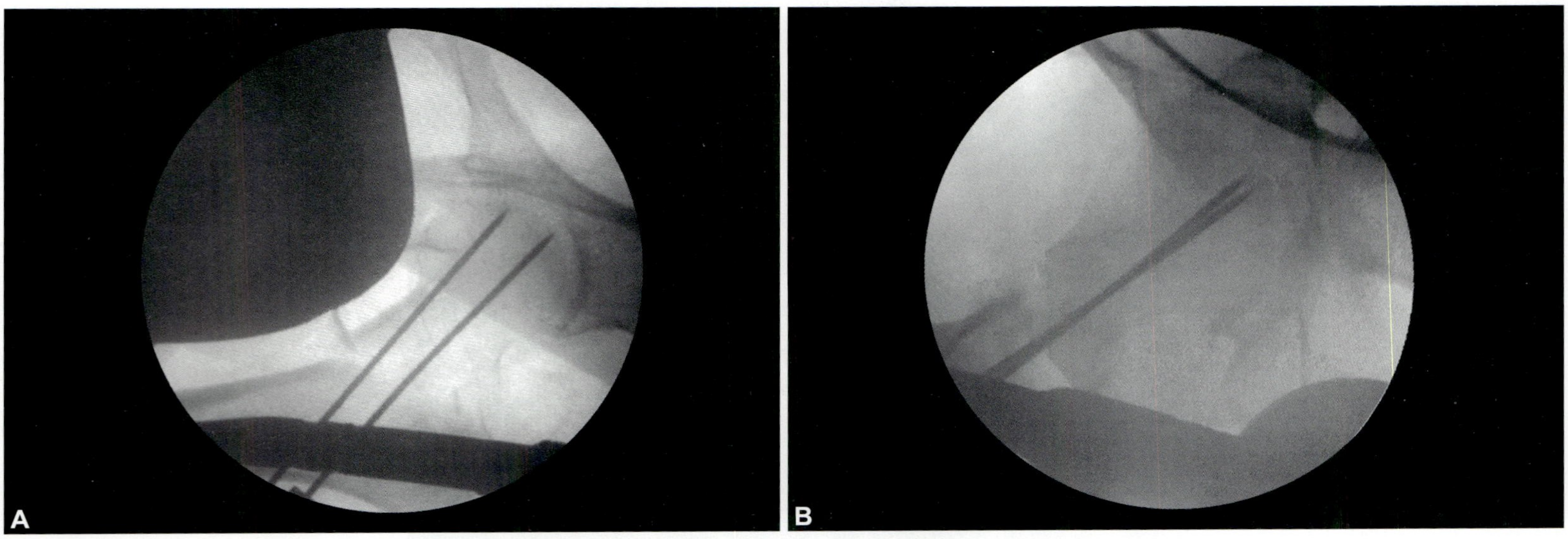

Figs. 19A and B: Outer cortex drilling is done. Guidewires passed into position through sleeves by trial error while checking in both C-arm views antero-posterior (A), lateral (B). Guidewires passed deep up to subchondral cortex but never into or beyond joint. For inferior lag screw guidewire, ideal position is center center or slight posteroinferior.

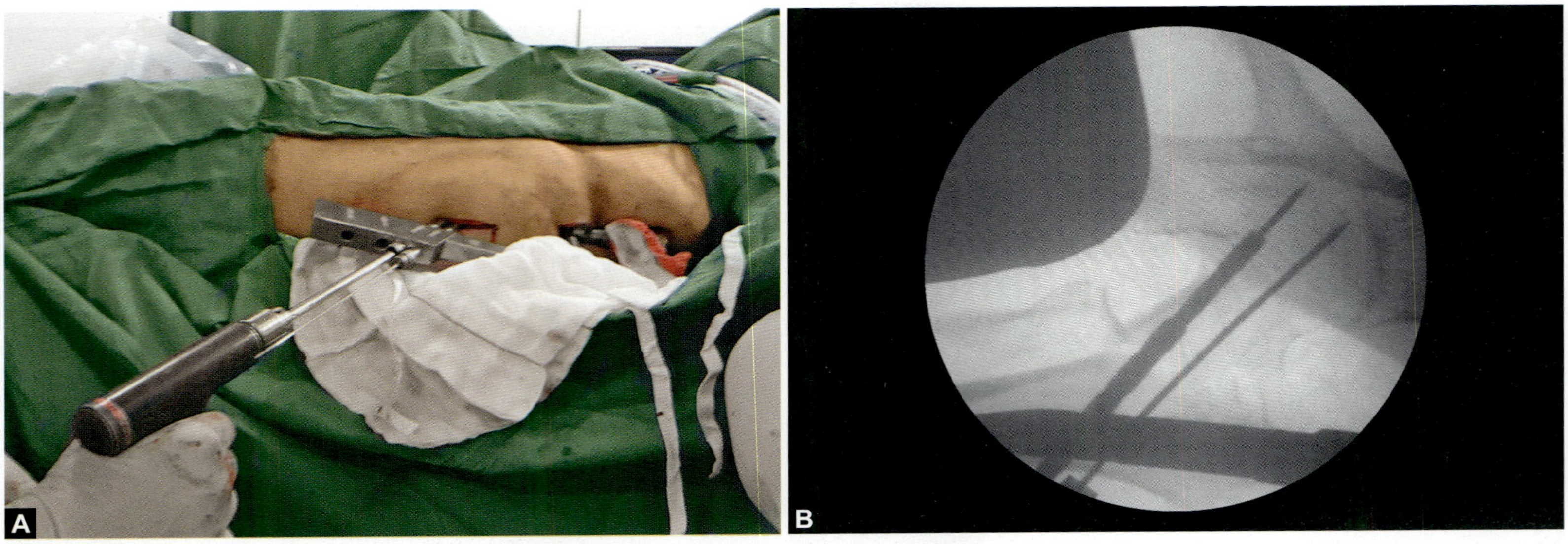

Figs. 20A and B

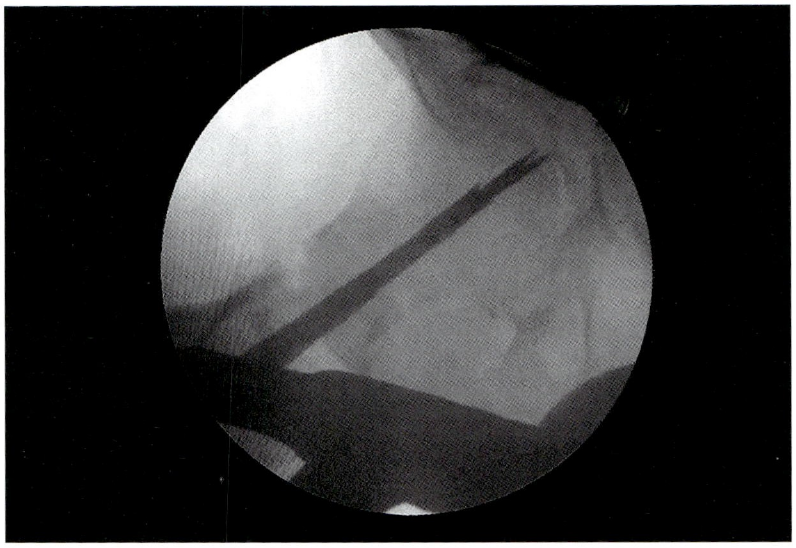

Fig. 20C

Figs. 20A to C: Drilling is done over guidewires to appropriate depth (A), C-arm image anteroposterior (B), lateral (C). At times, drill hits nail and does not progress. In that case, smaller diameter drill is used or in osteoporotic bone screws are passed directly.

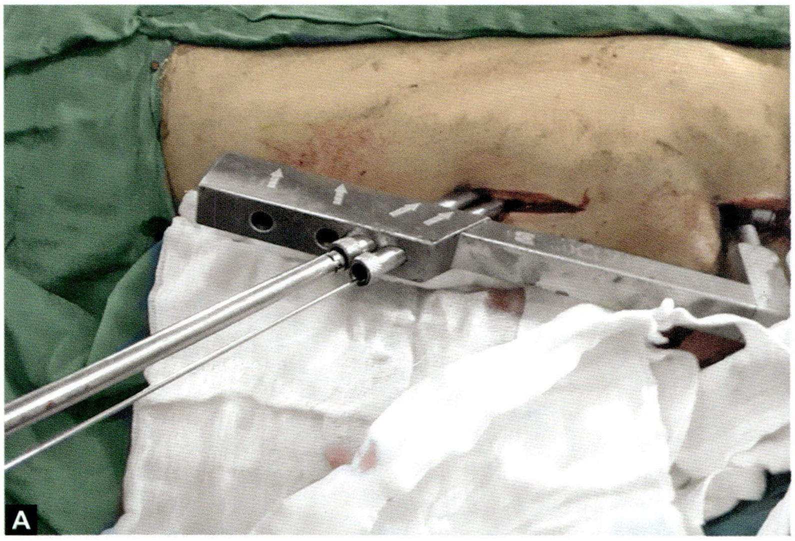

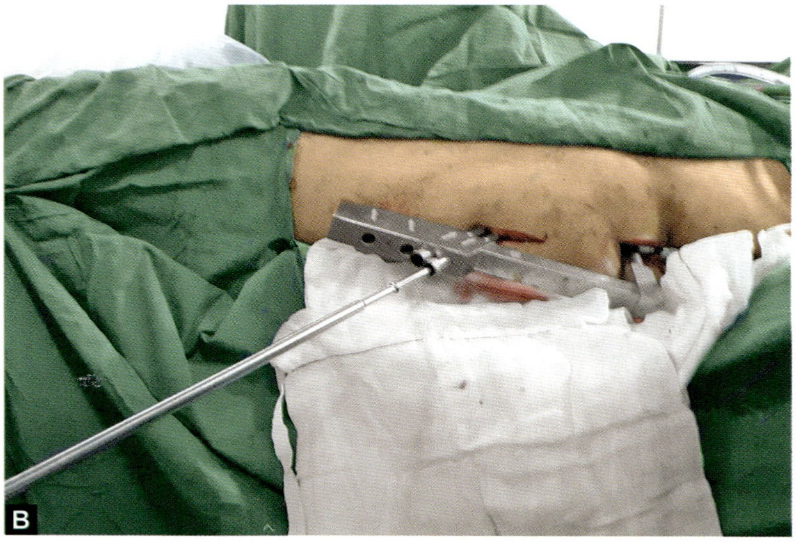

Figs. 21A and B: At times guidewire bends nearer tip while the cannulated screw is being inserted. In such situations, it is advisable to remove the guidewire and pass the screw. Inferior lag screw is passed first (A), and then superior hip pin (B). Superior hip pin is to be 15 mm shorter than the inferior lag screw.

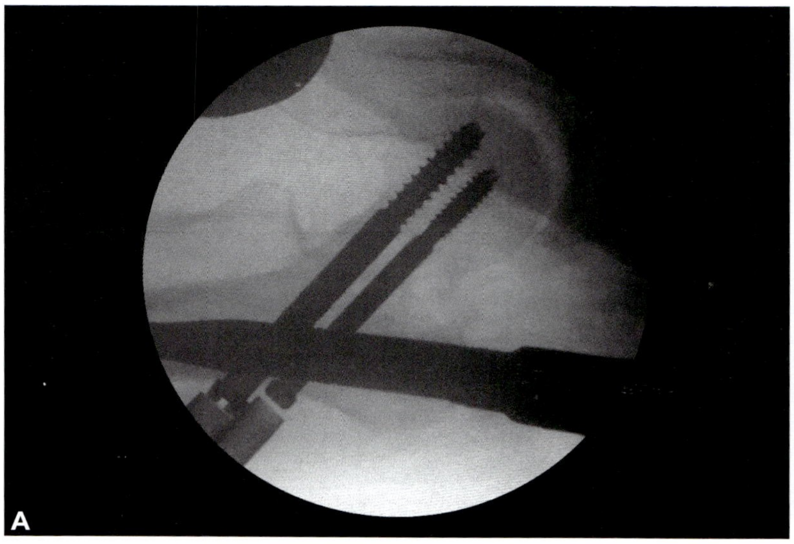

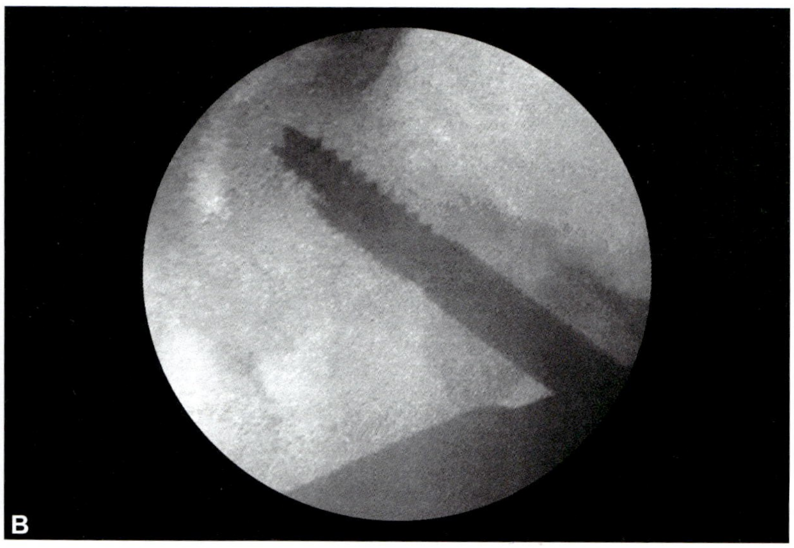

Figs. 22A and B: Position is checked in both C-arm views. C-arm image anteroposterior (A), lateral (B).

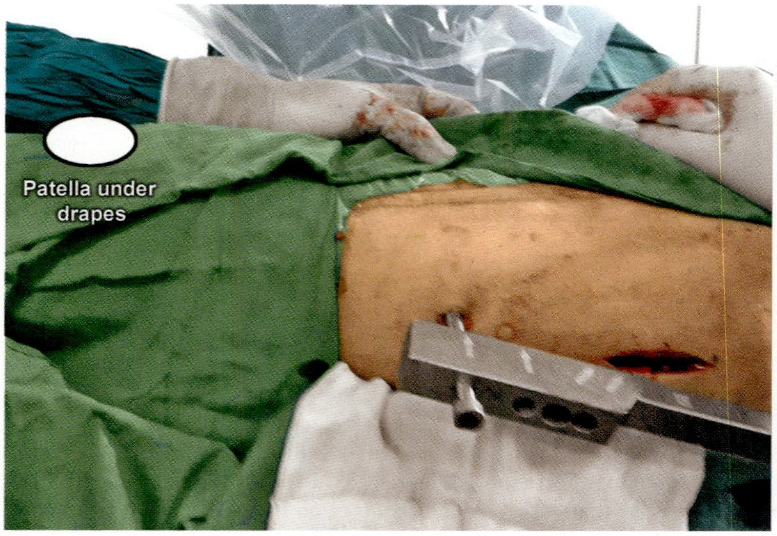

Fig. 23: Position of patella checked again under drapes to ensure appropriate rotation. Distal incision for entry of sleeve of distal bolt is taken and deepened. Sleeve tapped into position touching bone surface.

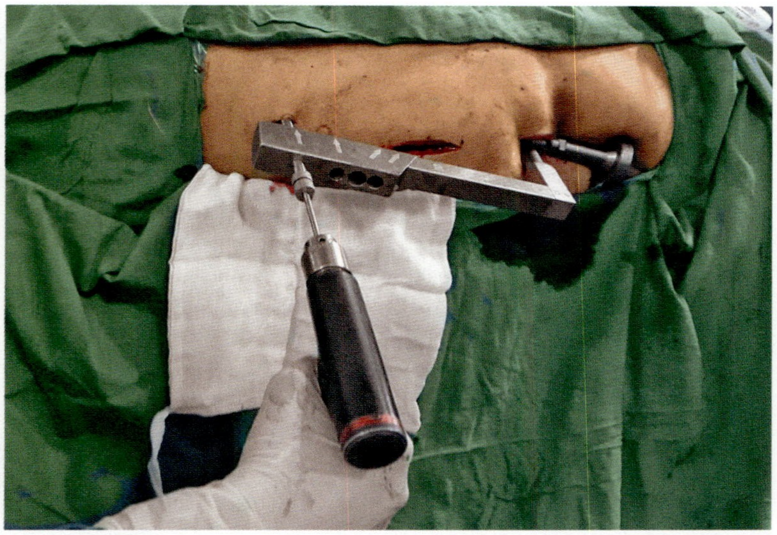

Fig. 24: Drilling is done with sharp and appropriate size drill bit. Far cortex drilling is done adequately and carefully to prevent drill plunge. Inadequate drilling of far cortex prevents easy passage of bolt.

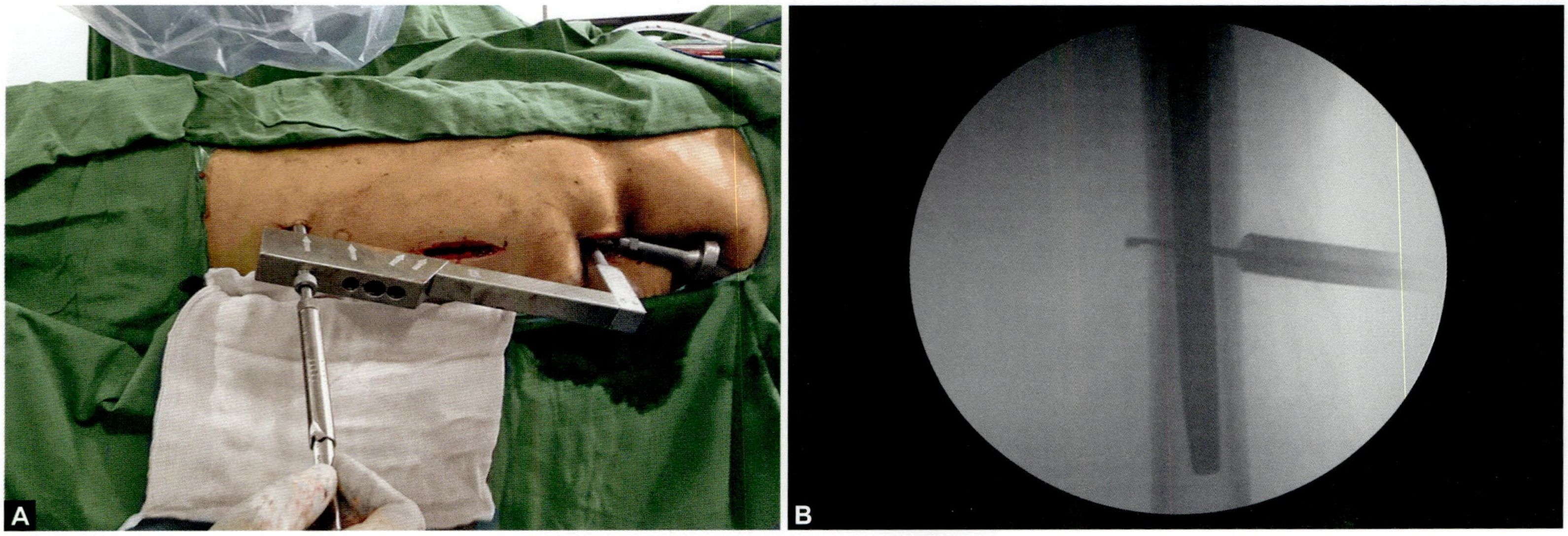

Figs. 25A and B: Length of bolts measured by depth gauge (A). C-arm image (B)

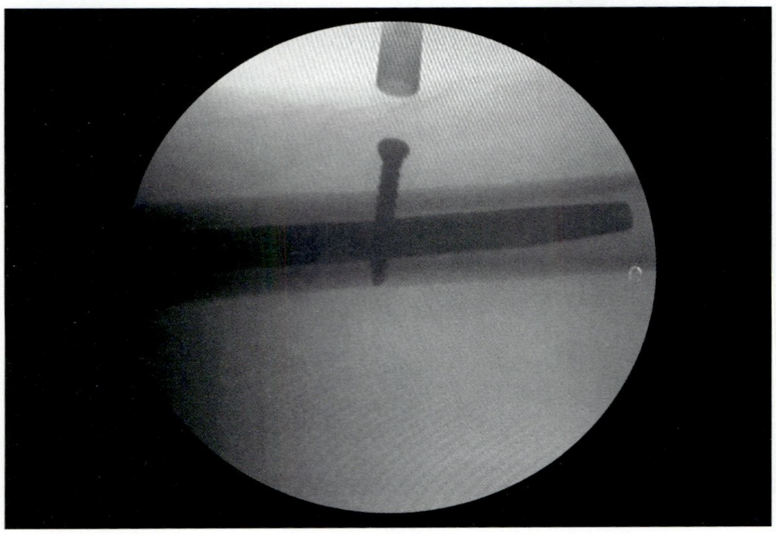

Fig. 26: Appropriate size static and/or dynamic bolts are inserted. C-arm monitoring for size while bolt is half way through allows easy change of bolt. Fully seated bolt is difficult to find and remove.

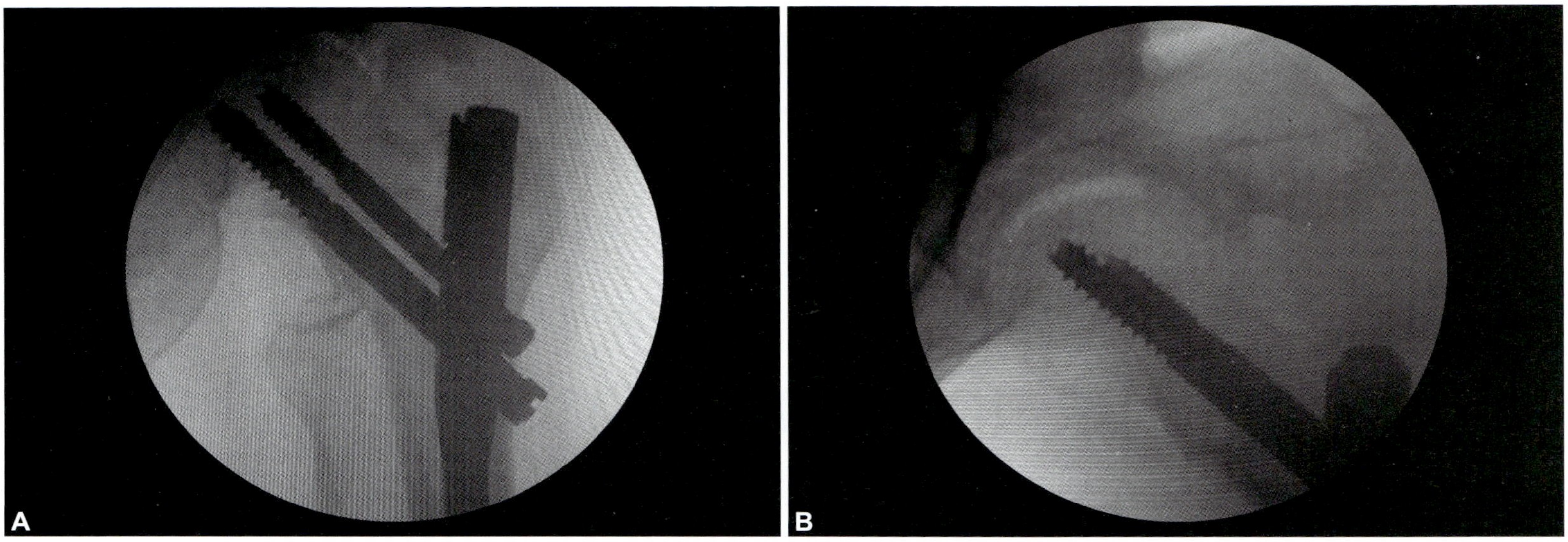

Figs. 27A and B: Final position of implant is checked in both C-arm views.

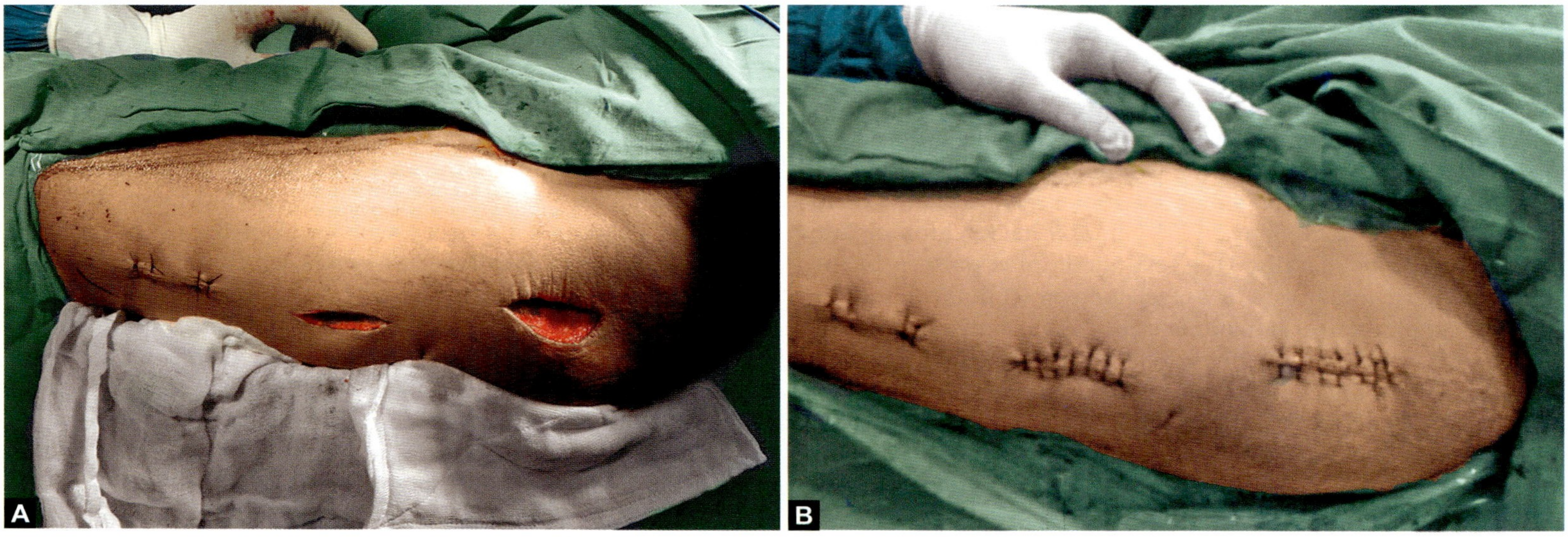

Figs. 28A and B: Wounds are closed in layers.

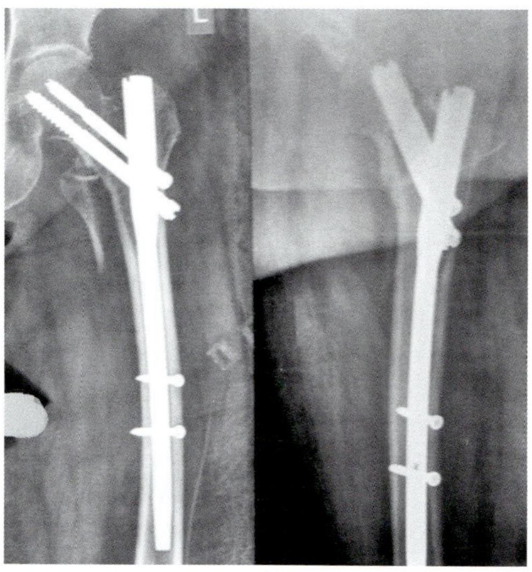

Fig. 29: Postoperative X-ray shows satisfactory position in both views.

CHAPTER 105

Subtrochanteric Fracture Femur: Proximal Femur Nail Fixation

Milind Modak, Neelkamal Sourav

INTRODUCTION

Fractures in the subtrochanteric region of femur are usually very difficult to manage. On the femur the region 3 inches below the lesser trochanter and towards the isthmus is the subtrochanteric region. The fracture line in subtrochanteric fractures may extend proximally into the trochanteric or femoral neck region or into the femoral shaft distally. Due to the complex pattern in the subtrochanteric fractures, it is associated with complications like nonunion, malunion, or implant failure. It is challenging to decide upon a single method of treatment to all patterns of subtrochanteric fractures. Due to the complex pattern of subtrochanteric fracture, it can be associated with various injuries like ipsilateral fractures of the femoral neck, ipsilateral distal femoral, supracondylar or condylar fractures, ipsilateral tibial fractures (floating knee) and ligament and meniscal injuries of the knee and polytrauma. Subtrochanteric fractures are associated with systemic complications and also nonunion, malunion, implant failure, and infections.

Bisphosphonates associated subtrochanteric fractures are increasingly encountered and they have unique pathophysiology. Pathological fractures due to metastasis are also increasing due to increase in life expectancy.

Management of subtrochanteric fractures have improved over time due to the development of new techniques and implants.

EPIDEMIOLOGY

Out of the entire hip fractures less than one-third of all the hip fractures are subtrochanteric. It has a trimodal age presentation with a relatively low peak among children, a high peak of young adults due to high-energy trauma and increasing peak in the elderly population above 65 years of age. The elderly group is affected due to osteoporosis, bisphosphonates-induced fractures, periprosthetic fractures, metastasis and increased activity level. The subtrochanteric fractures are associated with high mortality rate of 20%.

CLASSIFICATION

There are various classifications done in past to describe the fracture geometry and guide in fracture management.

Fielding gave the anatomical classification. Russell–Taylor classification was based on the piriformis involvement. Although this classification is not used anymore since the introduction of trochanteric entry cephalomedullary nail, which stabilizes fractures with or without piriformis extension.

Seinsheimer gave the most useful and practical classification based on the number of fracture fragment with or without the involvement of lateral or medial cortex. Loizou et al. classified the subtrochanteric fracture based on the degree of comminution but this classification did not gain popularity. The AO classification was recommended by OTA as they found it more convenient for communication. But, it classified fractures with different biological and mechanical fractures as diaphyseal fractures which was considered a disadvantage.

The ideal classification is yet to be described to guide in the management of such fractures with a good interobserver reproducibility.

MANAGEMENT OF SUBTROCHANTERIC FRACTURE

With current surgical advancement the nonsurgical management is an exception only in cases of severe comorbid conditions who cannot withstand anesthesia or surgical procedure.

Surgical management is advisable in most patients of the subtrochanteric fractures who are hemodynamically stable. The stabilization of the fracture done within first 48 hours reduces the associated complications and the mortality. The surgical method of fixation includes plates or intramedullary nails.

A retrospective study comparing extramedullary versus intramedullary fixation demonstrated that less bleeding with less operative time with intramedullary fixation though the complications were similar. Although after assessing the fracture geometry, the most familiar method of fixation should be done achieve an optimal functional outcome with low complication rates. Intramedullary fixation is biomechanically stronger and also causes lesser soft tissue trauma.

IMPLANT SELECTION

The nails have a biomechanical advantage over the plates due to their intramedullary placement. The intramedullary implants decreases bending stresses, decreases varus angulation and prevents shaft medialization. In spite of these advantages, technical difficulties can give rise to problems.

Proximal reaming done to accommodate the enlarged proximal nail, which incorporates the head screws results in the removal of substantial bone. In addition, injury to the abductor mechanism leads to gait disturbances with a lurch, persistence of pain in spite of a well-placed implant and difficulties can be faced, if revision is required. Sometimes, at the entry portal, an extension of fracture may occur while reaming or insertion of the nail causing fracture displacement or varus malalignment.

Although IIA and IIB are technically demanding for the use of the nail, augmenting cerclage wiring can be done prior to insertion of a nail. This, however, is not without difficulties and complications. IIB fractures are the best indications for plating. The implants could be 95° blade plate, a dynamic condylar screw (DCS) or a recent proximal femoral plate.

The Russell–Taylor classification helps in implant selection (Fig. 1).

The Russell-Taylor classification helps in implant selection. Type I versus Type II shows the involvement of piriformis fossa where a nail may propagate or deform fracture. Type A versus Type B shows the involvement of lesser trochanter and posteromedial buttress.

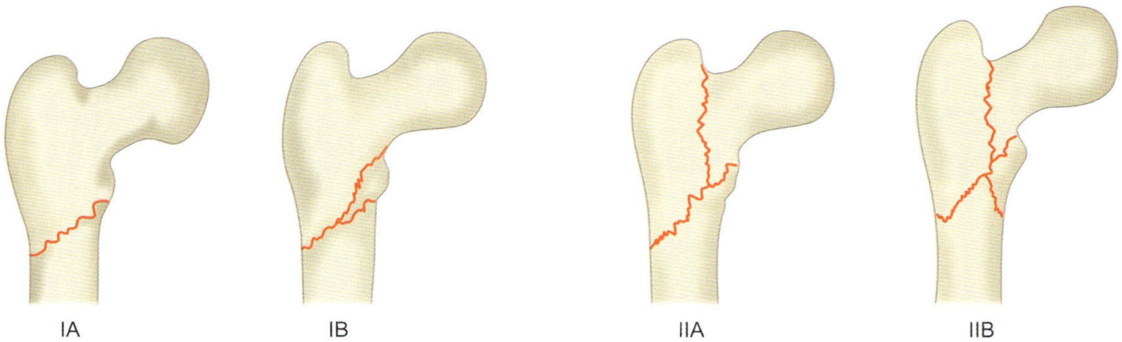

Fig. 1: Russell–Taylor classification.

SURGICAL STEPS (FIGS. 2 TO 68)

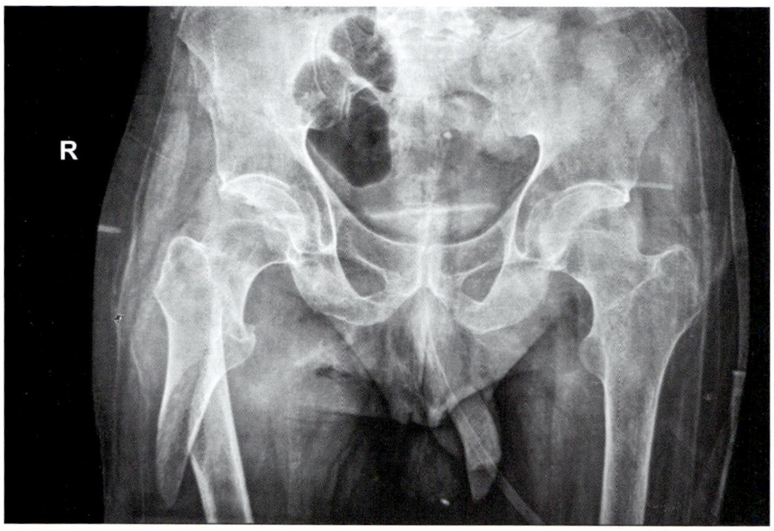

Fig. 2: Radiograph of the pelvis with both hips anteroposterior (AP) view showing subtrochanteric fracture right hip.

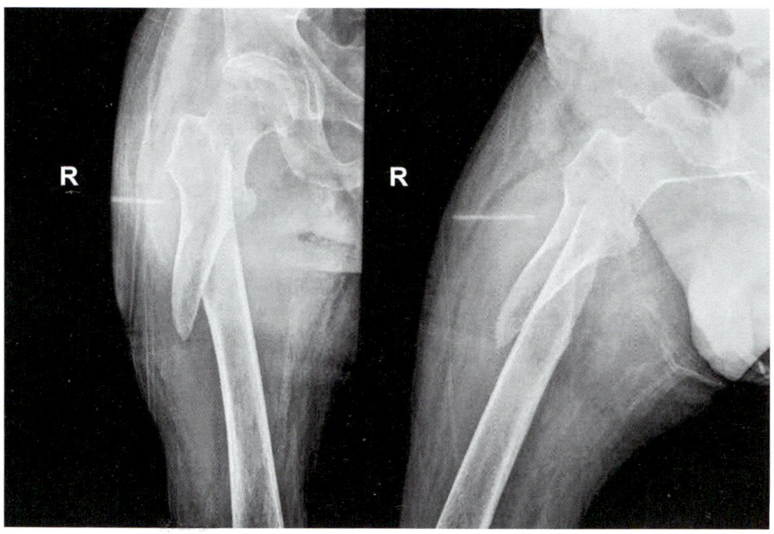

Fig. 3: Radiograph of right hip with shaft of the femur anteroposterior (AP) and a lateral view showing a subtrochanteric fracture.

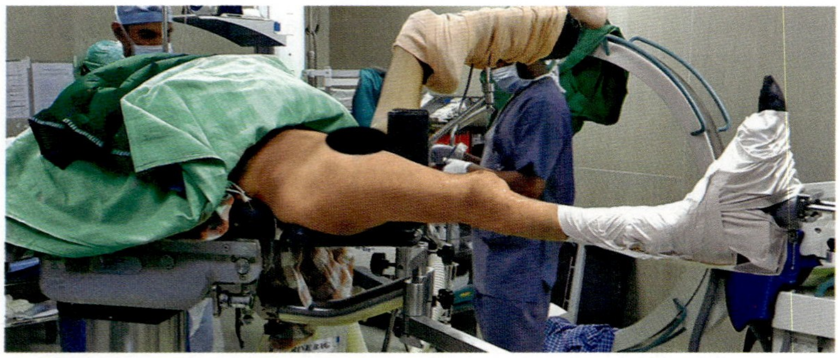

Fig. 4: Patient positioned supine, on the fracture table. The opposite limb supported in a lithotomy position. Closed reduction is done to align the fracture fragments.

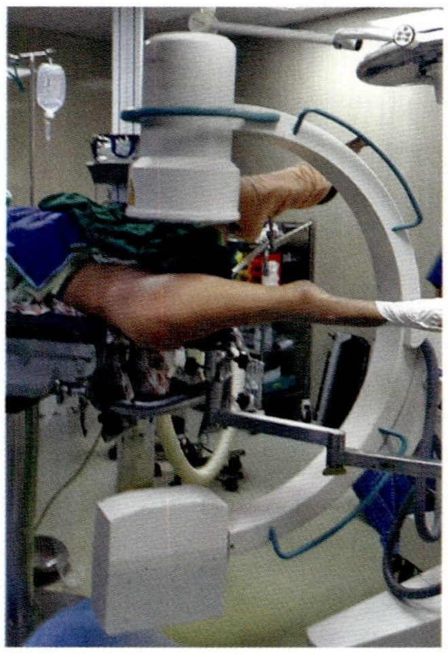

Fig. 5: "C" positioning of the patient on fracture table with image intensifier showing anteroposterior (AP) view. The operative side is kept in supine position on a fracture table under traction. The acceptable reduction is achieved under C-arm guidance.

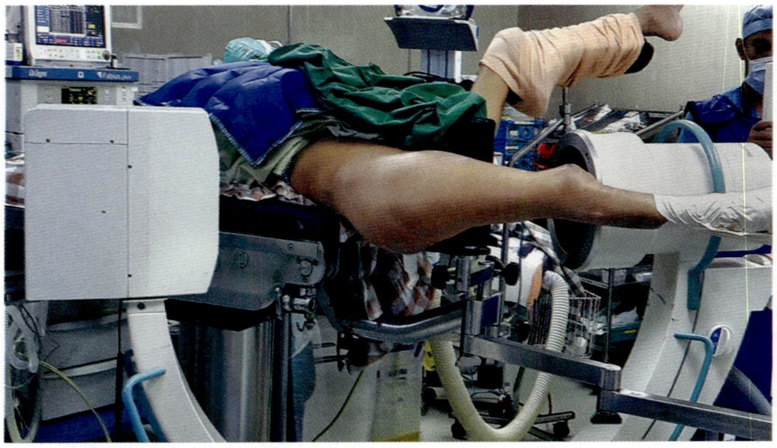

Fig. 6: Intraoperative positioning with image intensifier showing lateral view. After satisfactory reduction painting and draping done. Open reduction is considered if satisfactory close reduction is not achieved.

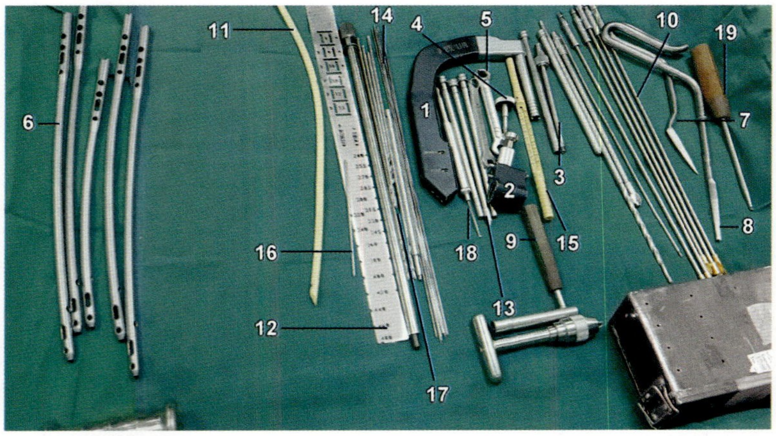

Fig. 7: Complete set of armamentarium for intramedullary nailing of subtrochanteric fracture, (1) Insertion handle with a jig, (2) Proximal sleeve insertion Jig, (3) Threaded conical bolt, (4) Driving head, (5) Combination wrench, (6) Long antegrade femoral nails of various diameters and lengths, (7) Curved awl, (8) Cannulated awl, (9) Protection sleeve, (10) Cannulated flexible reamers with increasing diameters, (11) Exchange tube, (12) Measuring device, (13) 6.5-mm and 8.0-mm proximal tissue protection sleeves (inner, outer) and a trocar, (14) Guidewires (2.8-mm diameter, length 350 mm) for proximal sleeve, (15) Depth gauge, (16) Thick K-wire, (17) Drill bits, (180) Depth gauge for locking bolts, (19) Hexagonal screw driver. Additional instrumentation for fracture manipulation and guidewire positioning used as required.

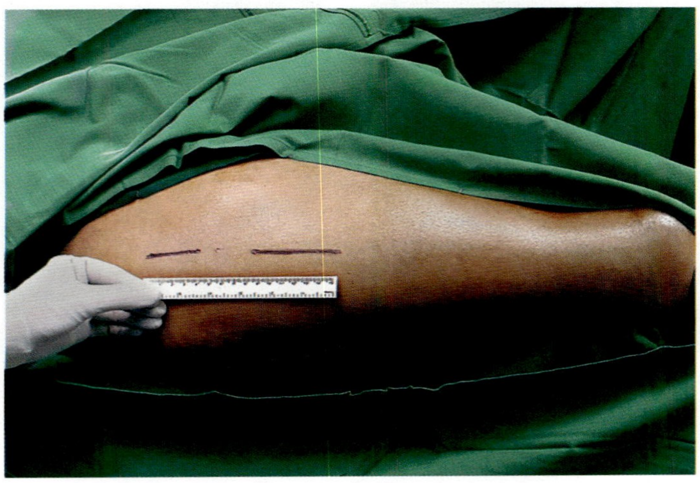

Fig. 8: Incision site marked on the patient.

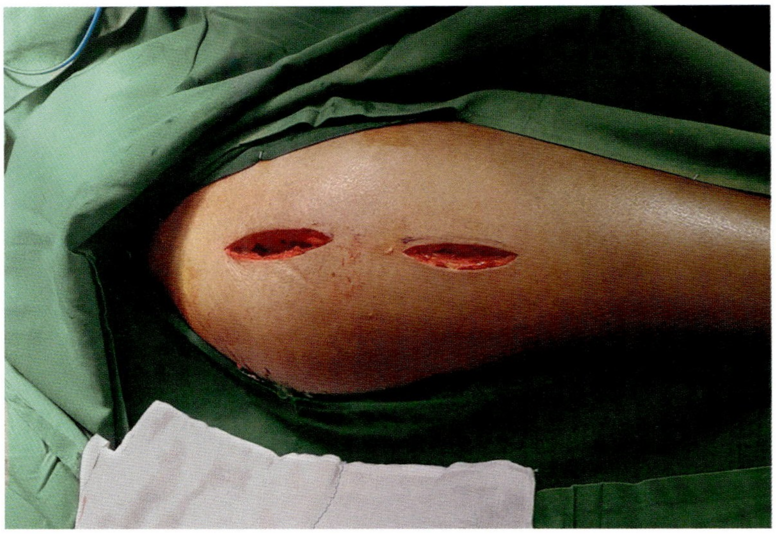

Fig. 9: Skin incision is taken. The proximal incision for the entry of nail is taken approximately 5 cm proximal to the tip of greater trochanter in the line of the shaft of the femur for open reduction. Subsequently, the second incision is taken at in the line of the shaft of femur for open reduction.

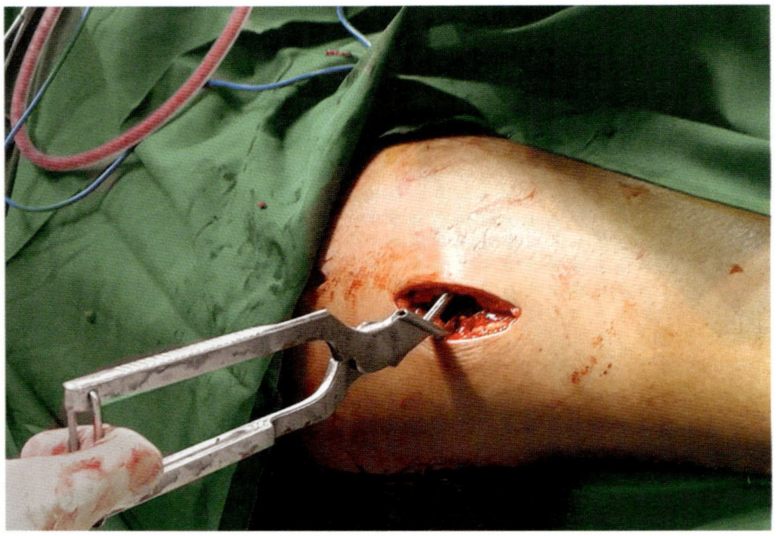

Fig. 10: Use of wire passer after open reduction of fracture fragments.

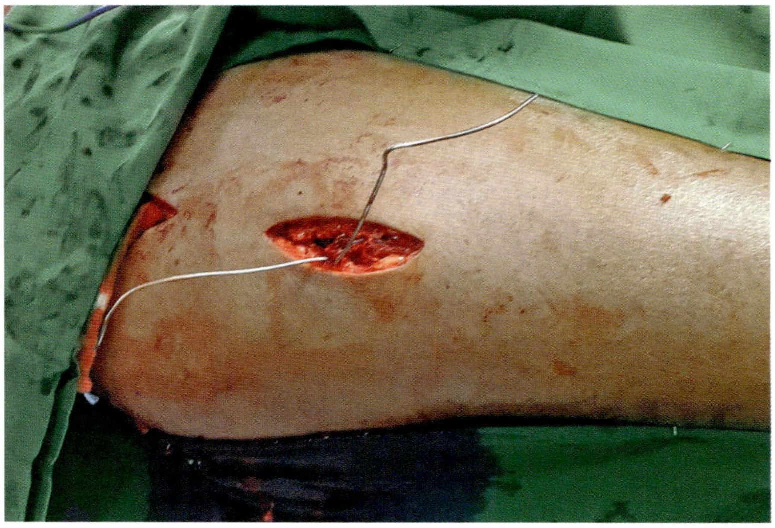

Fig. 11: Encerclage done using stainless steel wire.

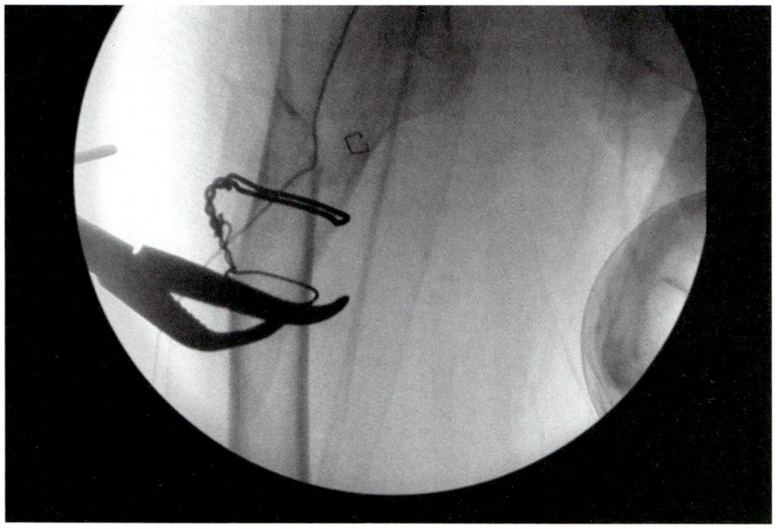

Fig. 12: Reduction of fracture attempted under image intensifier guidance with cerclage wire in situ.

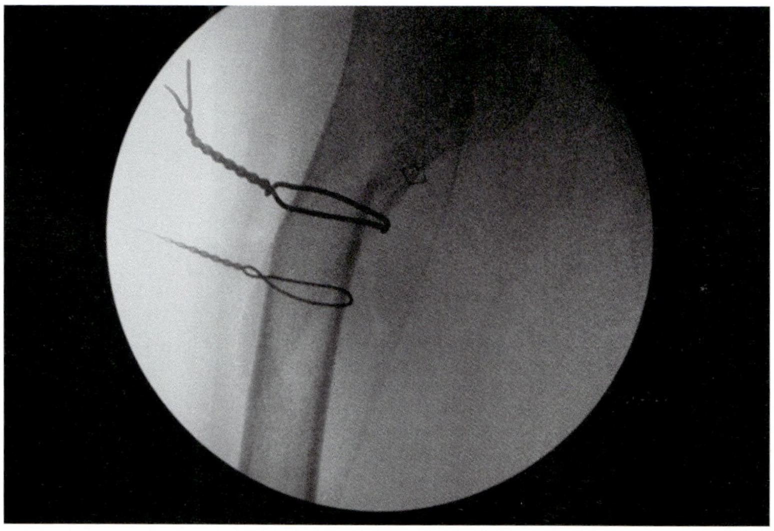

Fig. 13: Image intensifier showing reduction with cerclage wire in situ.

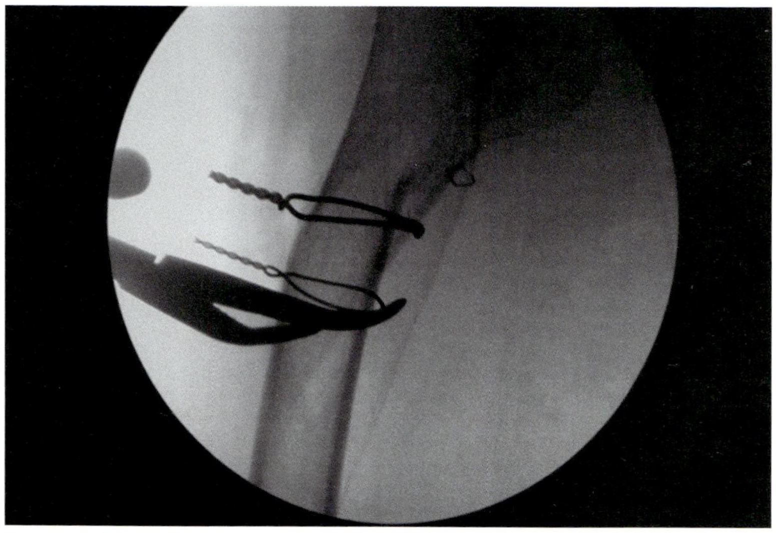

Fig. 14: Image intensifier showing fracture held with reduction clamp and cerclage wire.

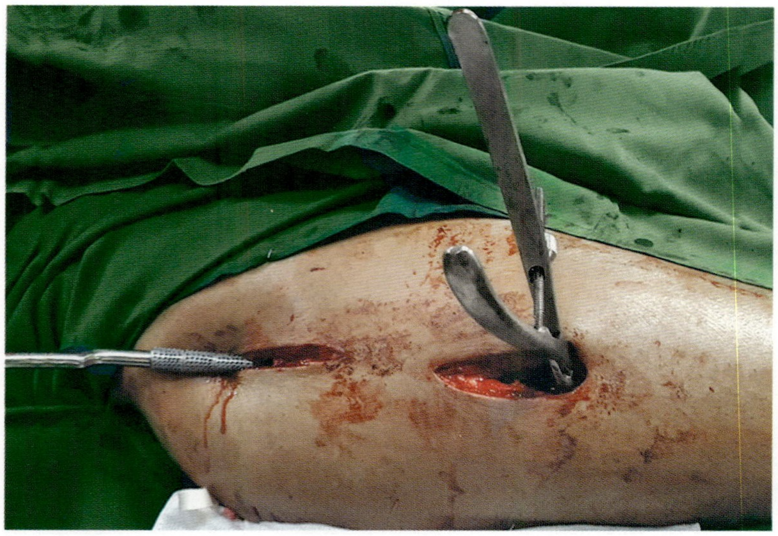

Fig. 15: Intraoperative image showing proximal entry done using guidewire followed by the awl and a simultaneous reduction of fracture fragments.

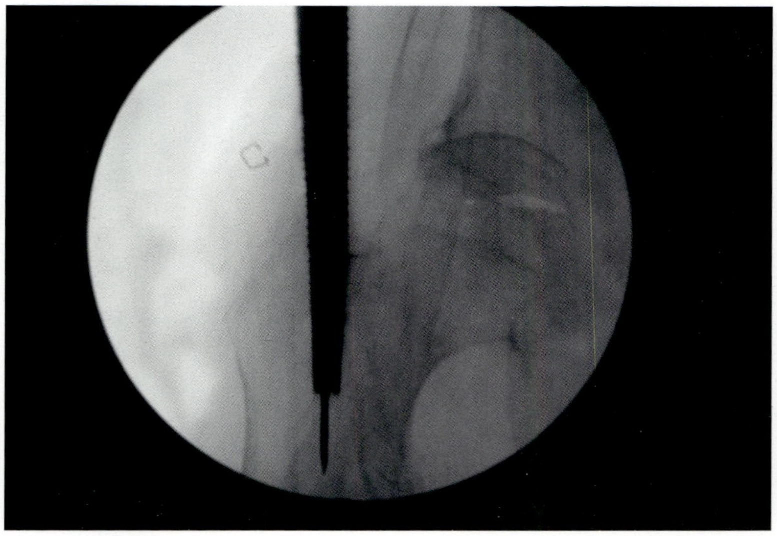

Fig. 16: Confirmation of the correct entry point showing cannulated angled awl with the guide pin in situ [image intensifier television (IITV) image anteroposterior (AP) view].

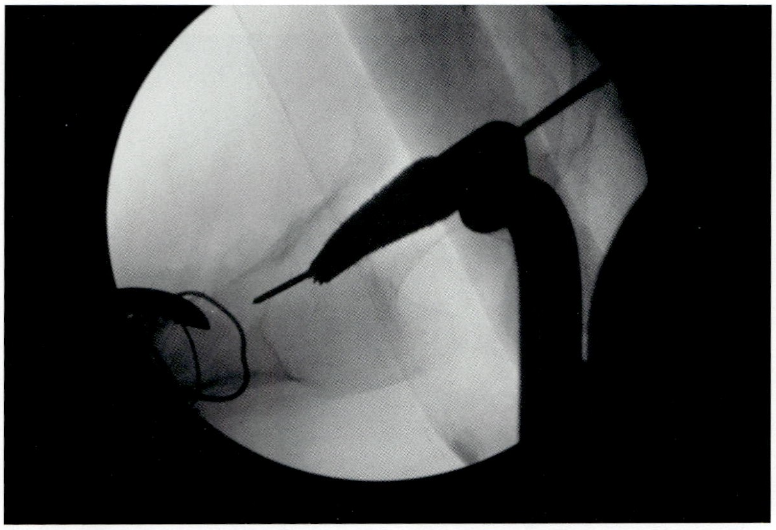

Fig. 17: Confirmation of the correct entry point showing cannulated angled awl with the guide pin in situ [image intensifier television (IITV) lateral view].

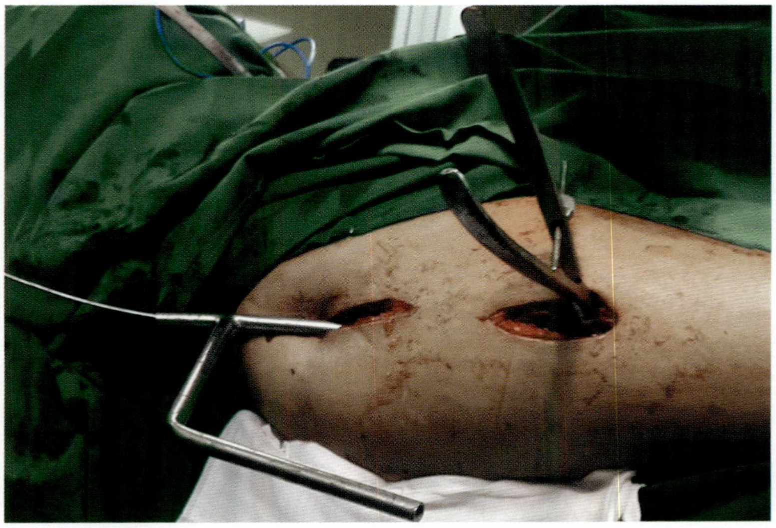

Fig. 18: Guide pin inserted further with simultaneous manipulation using fossa finder device.

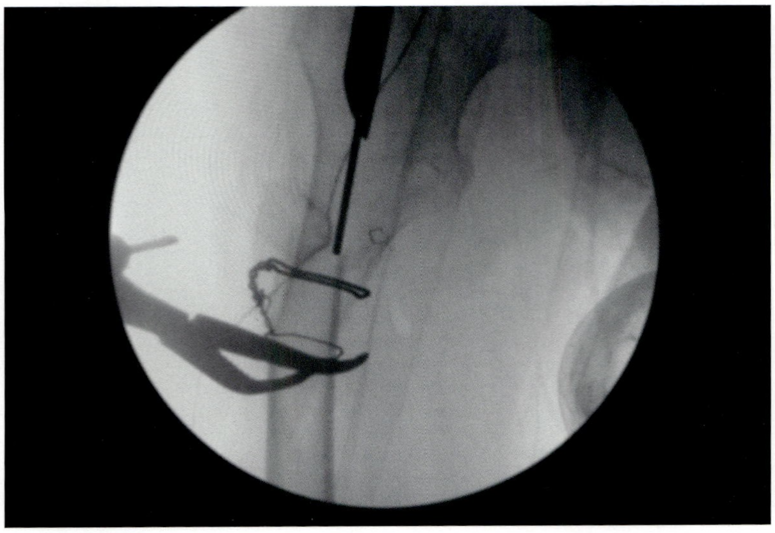

Fig. 19: Tip of the manipulating device in the proximal fragment [image intensifier television (IITV) image anteroposterior (AP) view].

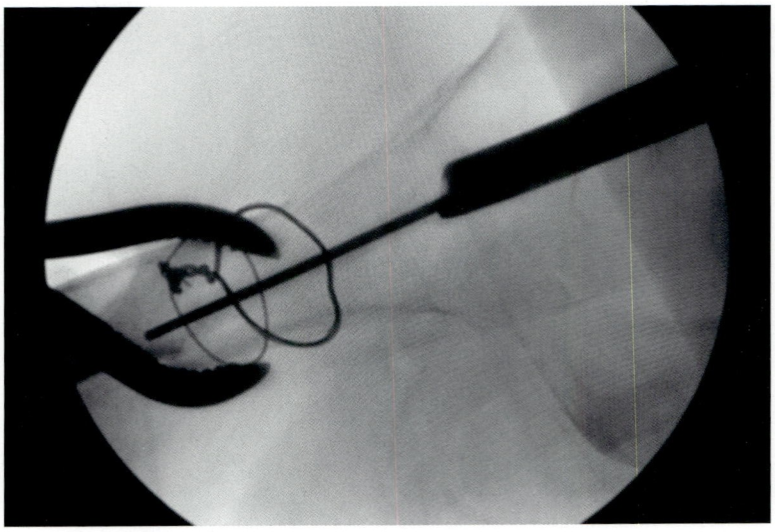

Fig. 20: Tip of the manipulating device in the proximal fragment [image intensifier television (IITV) image lateral view].

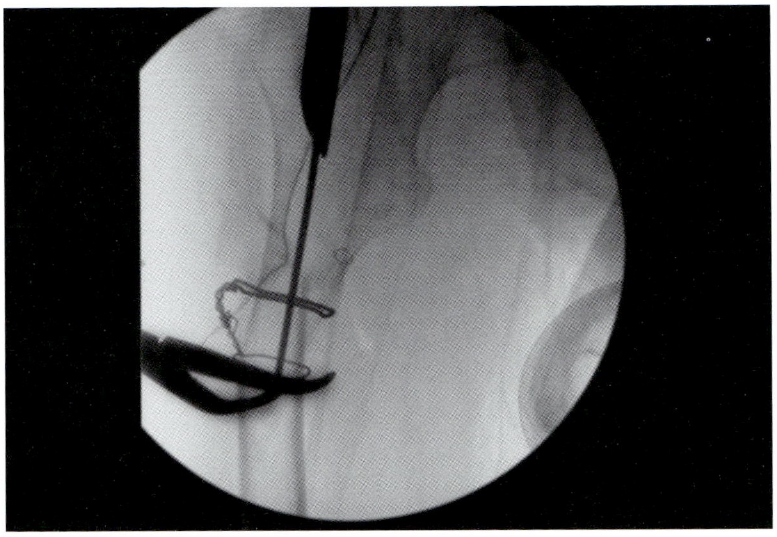

Fig. 21: Guidewire advanced further across the fracture site under the guidance of image intensifier television (IITV).

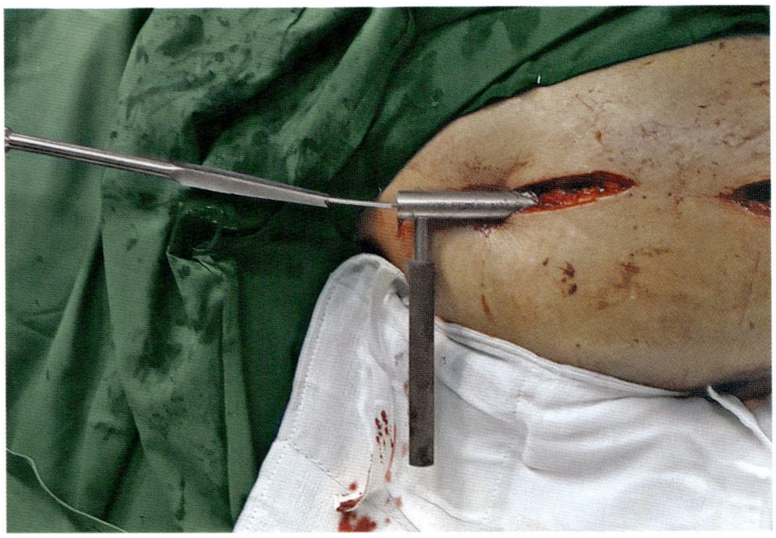

Fig. 22: Proximal reaming done. Proximal reamer advanced parallel to lateral cortex of proximal femur up to the level of the lesser trochanter. Use of proximal soft tissue protection sleeve is seen in this image.

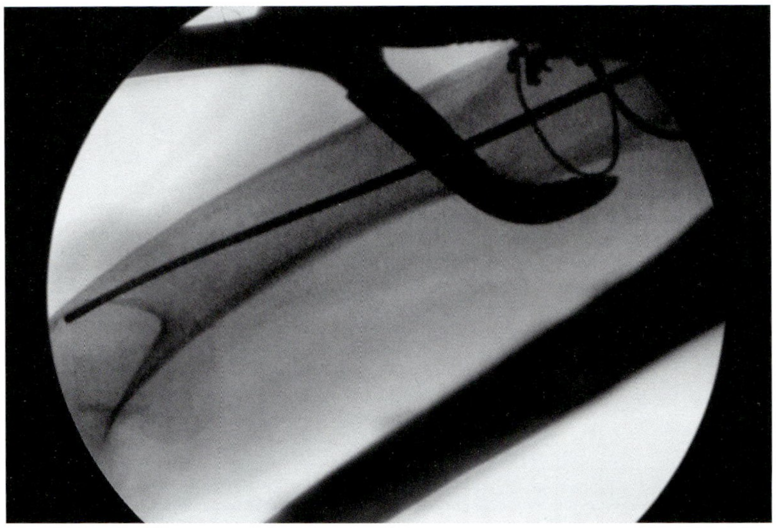

Fig. 23: Image intensifier television (IITV) image confirming intramedullary placement of guidewire on the lateral view.

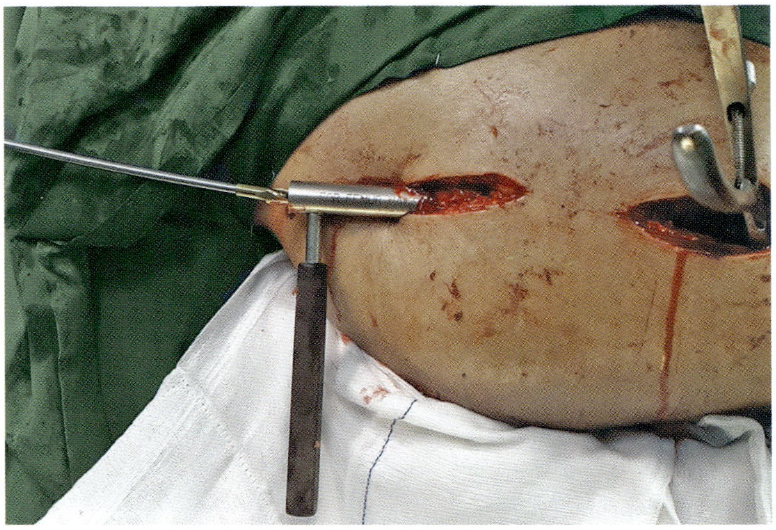

Fig. 24: Proximal protection sleeve positioned over the guidewire with 8 mm size flexible reamer in situ (intraoperative image).

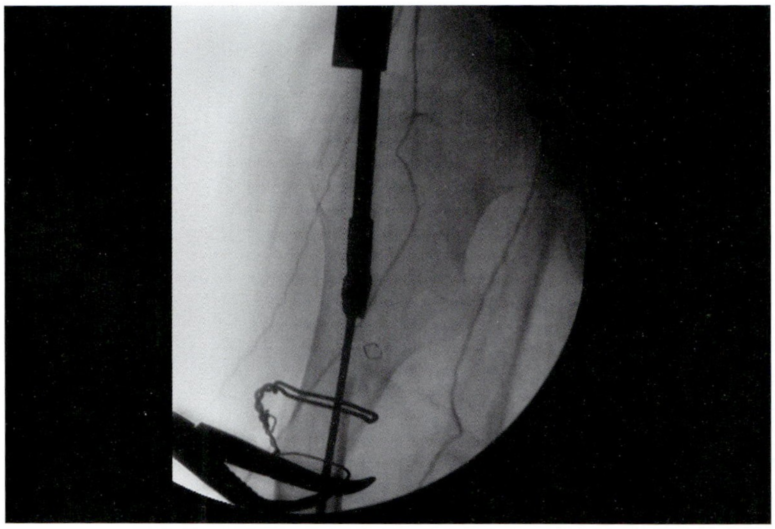

Fig. 25: Image intensifier television (IITV) image showing reaming over the guidewire.

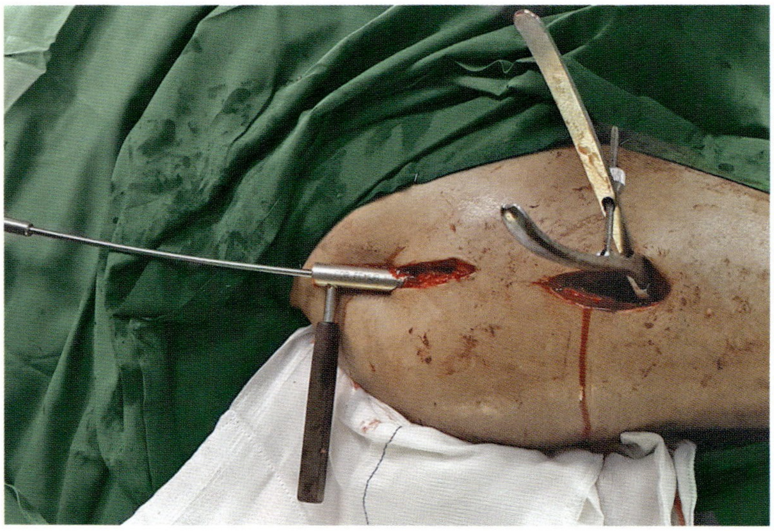

Fig. 26: Sequential reaming done over the guidewire with 0.5 mm increment. Final reaming done nail diameter selected 2 mm less than the final reamer diameter (intraoperative image).

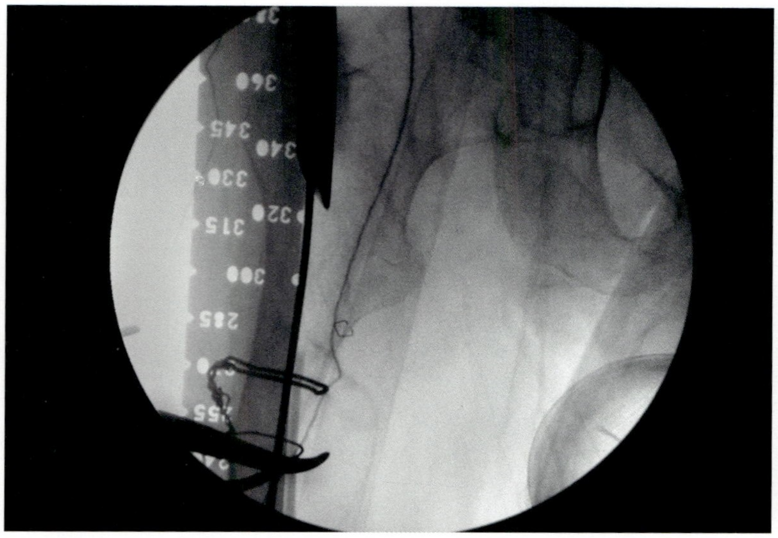

Fig. 27: Confirmation of nail length proximally [image intensifier television (IITV) image].

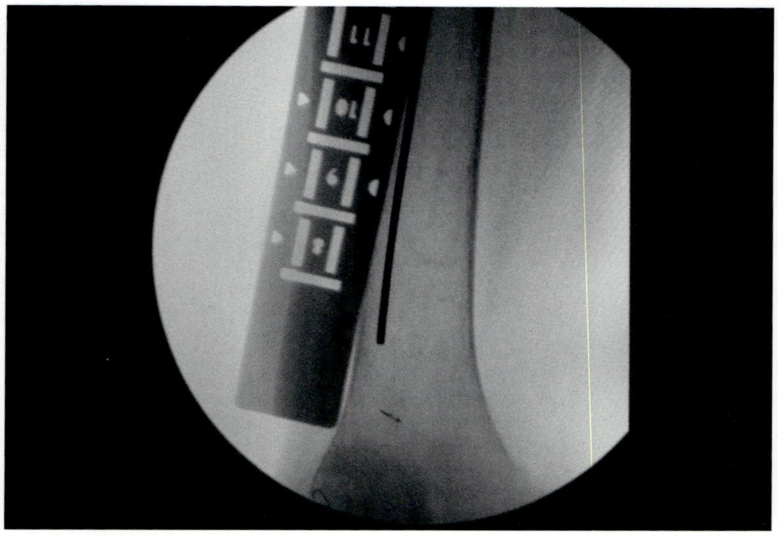

Fig. 28: Confirmation of nail length distally [image intensifier television (IITV) image].

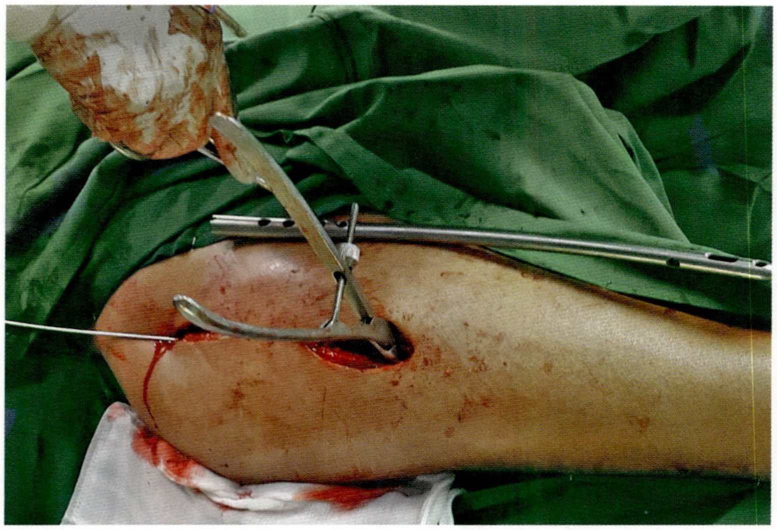

Fig. 29: Additional confirmation of nail length using another nail of the same length.

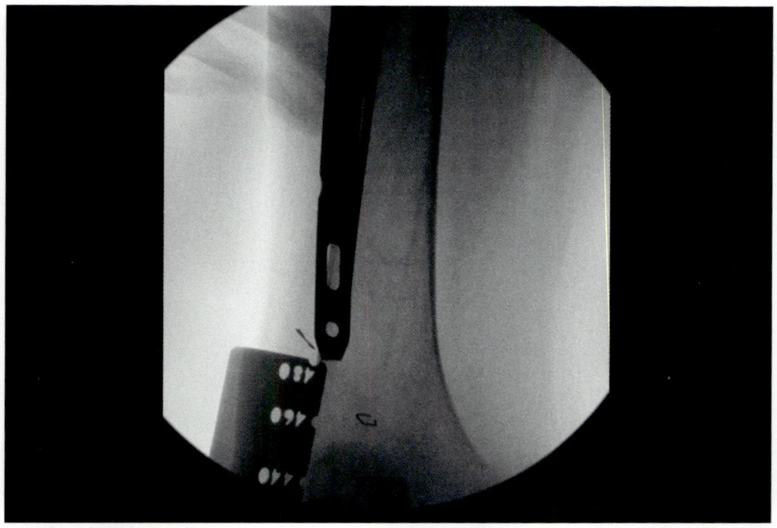

Fig. 30: Image intensifier television (IITV) image showing confirmation of nail length using another nail of the same length.

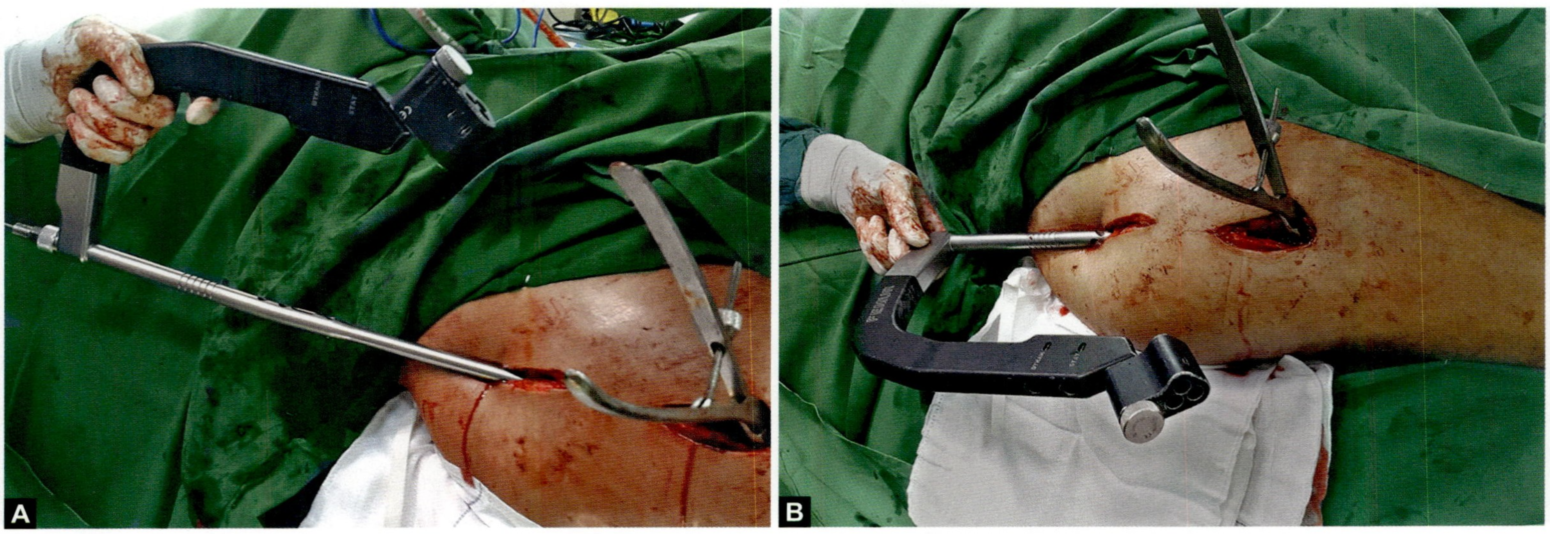

Figs. 31A and B: Insertion of the definitive nail. The size and side of the nail is confirmed and nail is secured to the jig keeping the correct right-left orientation in mind. The sleeves are positioned in the jig and the accurate passage of drill bit through the nail is confirmed. The jig is kept anteriorly/internally rotated on purpose initially to facilitate easy passage of the nail in the proximal canal, which is subsequently rotated laterally.

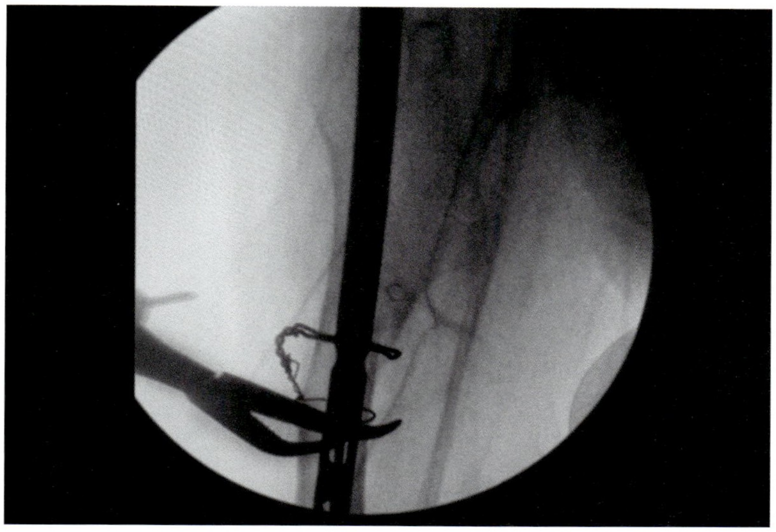

Fig. 32: Image intensifier television (IITV) image showing insertion of the nail across the fracture site.

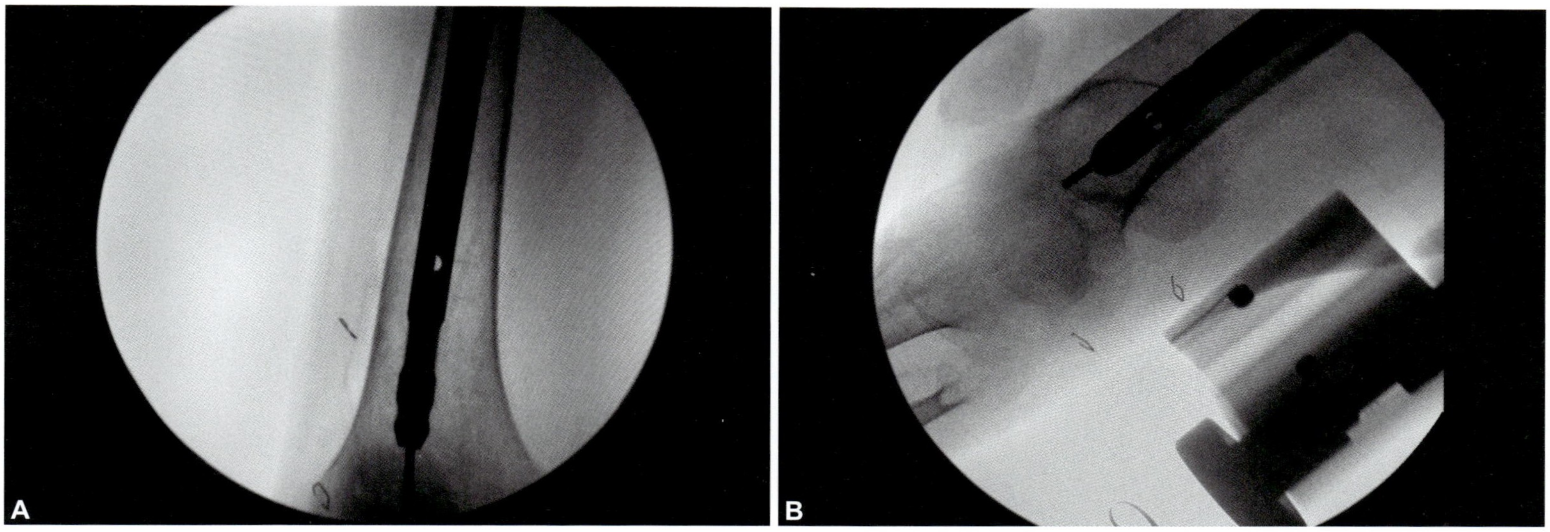

Figs. 33A and B: Confirmation of nail tip, which should be at the level of superior pole of the patella [image intensifier anteroposterior (AP) and lateral views].

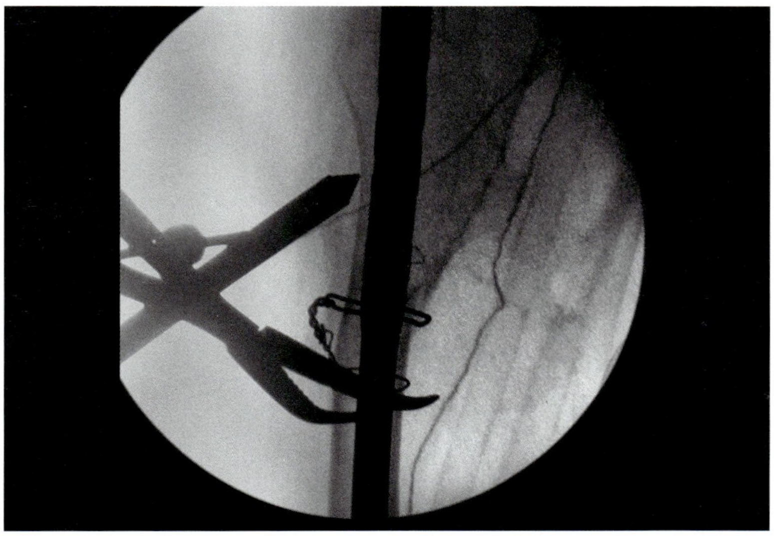

Fig. 34: Insertion of 8 mm outer sleeve with confirmation of complete seating of with inner sleeve on lateral cortex [image intensifier television (IITV) image].

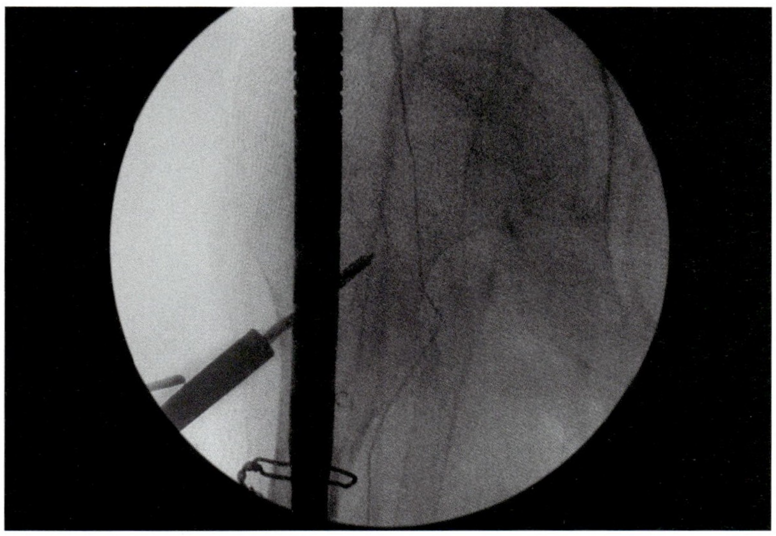

Fig. 35: Perforation of the outer cortex done using 3.5 mm drill bit [image intensifier television (IITV)].

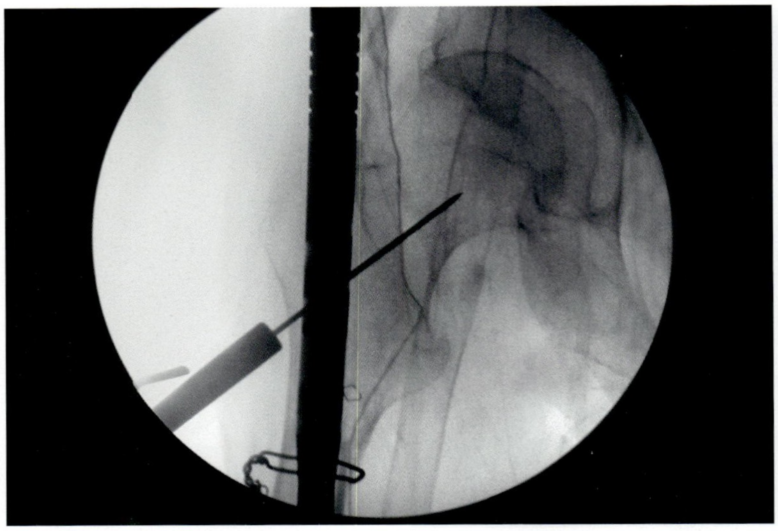

Fig. 36: Guidewire positioned near calcar [image intensifier television (IITV) image]

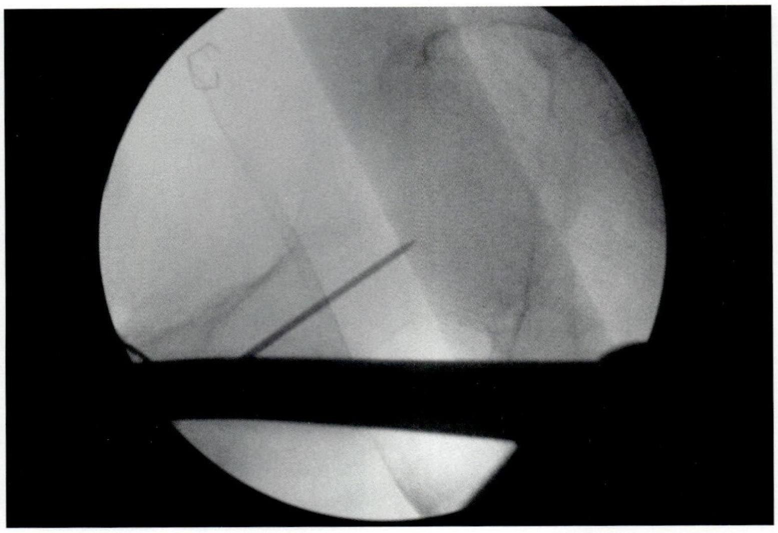

Fig. 37: Image intensifier television (IITV) confirmation of guidewire position on lateral view.

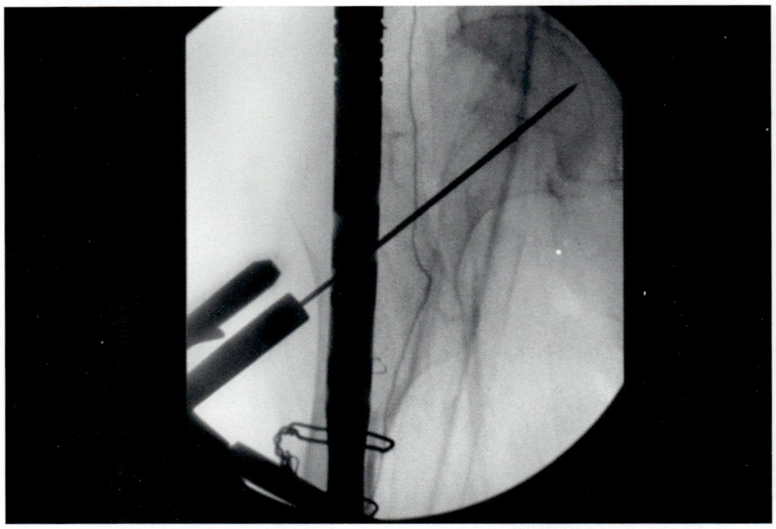

Fig. 38: Guidewire advanced and proximal 6.5 mm sleeve positioned [image intensifier television (IITV) image].

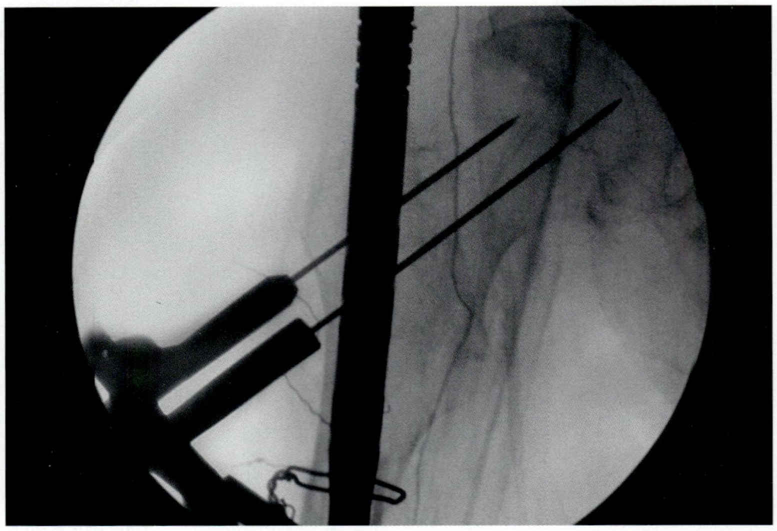

Fig. 39: Insertion of proximal guidewire and confirmation of the position of both the guidewires on anteroposterior (AP) view.

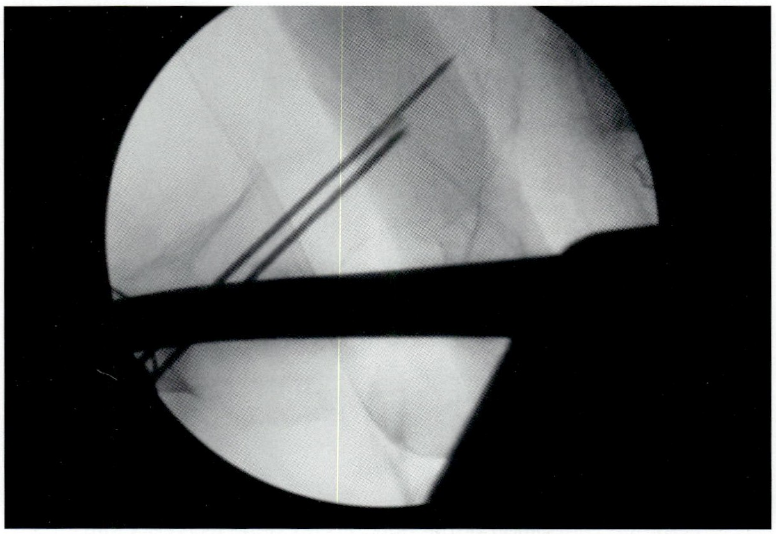

Fig. 40: Insertion of proximal guidewire and confirmation of the position of both the guidewires on the lateral view.

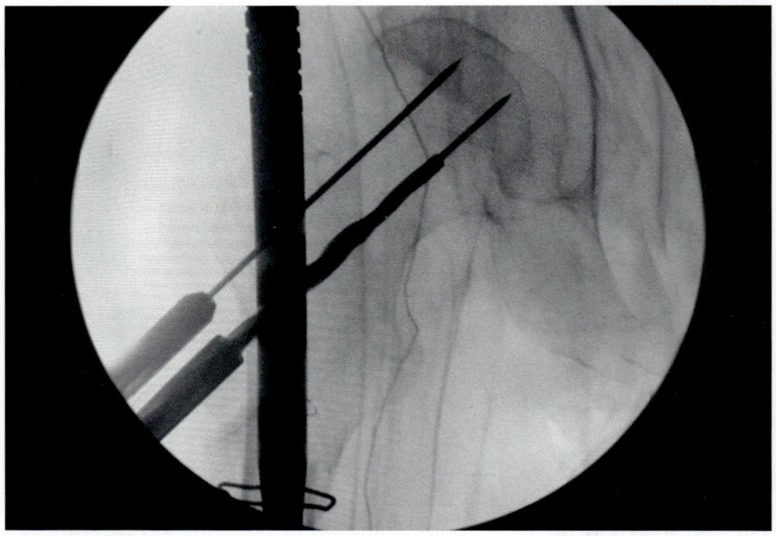

Fig. 41: Drilling with a 6.5 mm cannulated drill bit for calcar screw [image intensifier television (IITV) image].

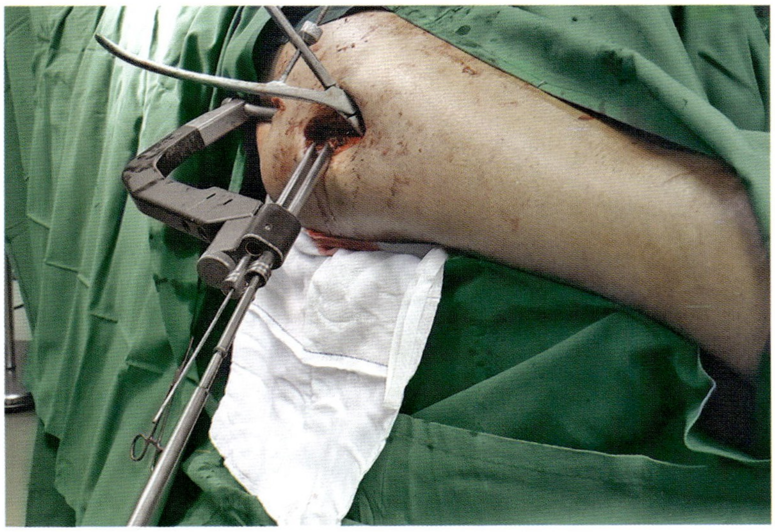

Fig. 42: Insertion of inferior (calcar) screw.

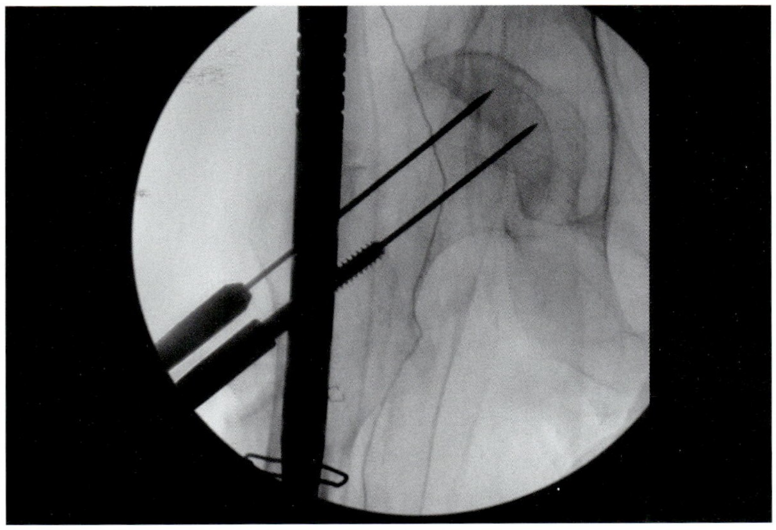

Fig. 43: Insertion of calcar screw on anteroposterior (AP) view [image intensifier television (IITV) image].

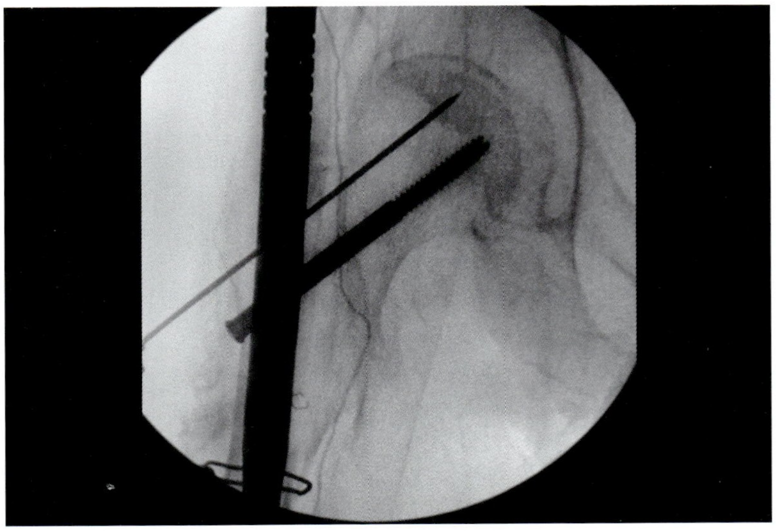

Fig. 44: Confirmation of complete seating of calcar screw on anteroposterior (AP) view Image intensifier image.

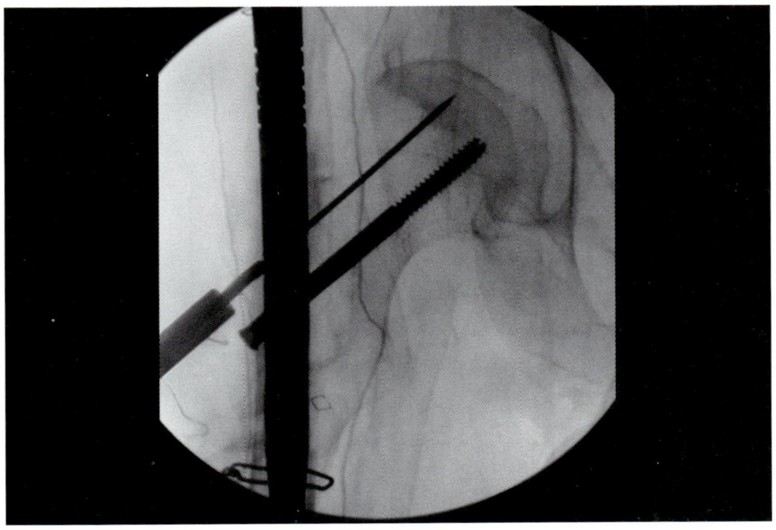

Fig. 45: Drilling with a 6.5 mm cannulated drill bit for the proximal screw [image intensifier television (IITV) image].

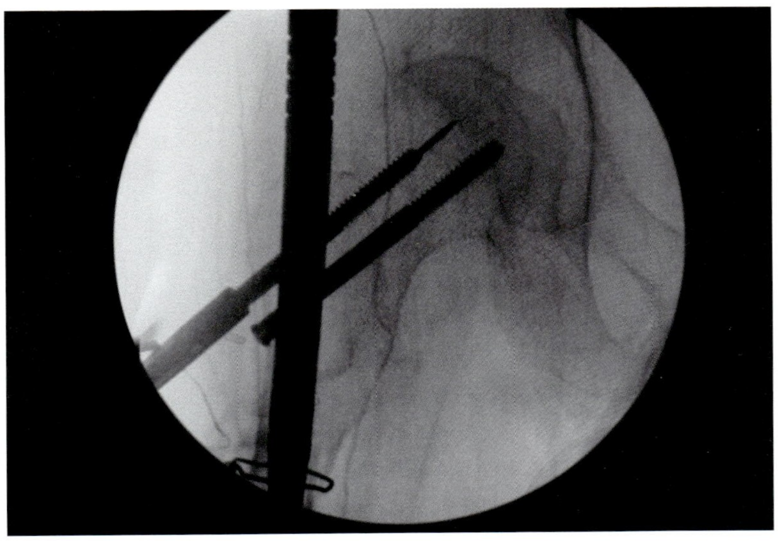

Fig. 46: Insertion of the proximal screw after drilling with 6.5 mm cannulated drill bit [image intensifier television (IITV) image].

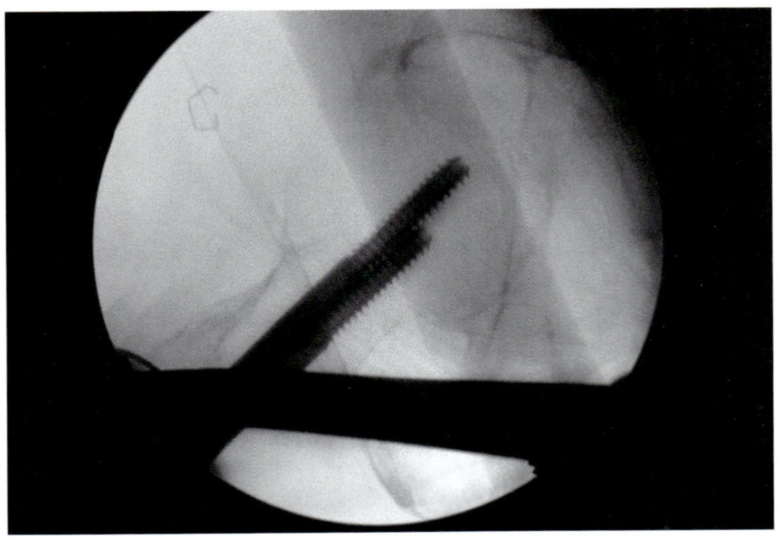

Fig. 47: Confirmation of both the screw position on the lateral view.

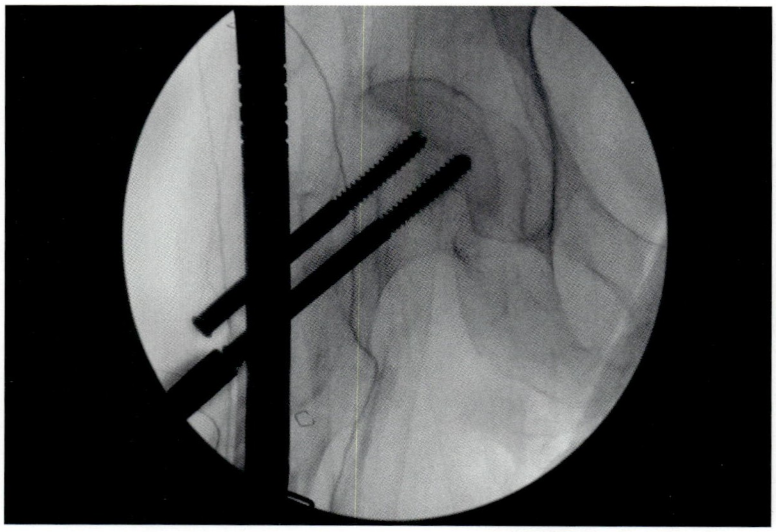

Fig. 48: Confirmation of screw position on anteroposterior (AP) view with final tightening of each screw [image intensifier television (IITV)].

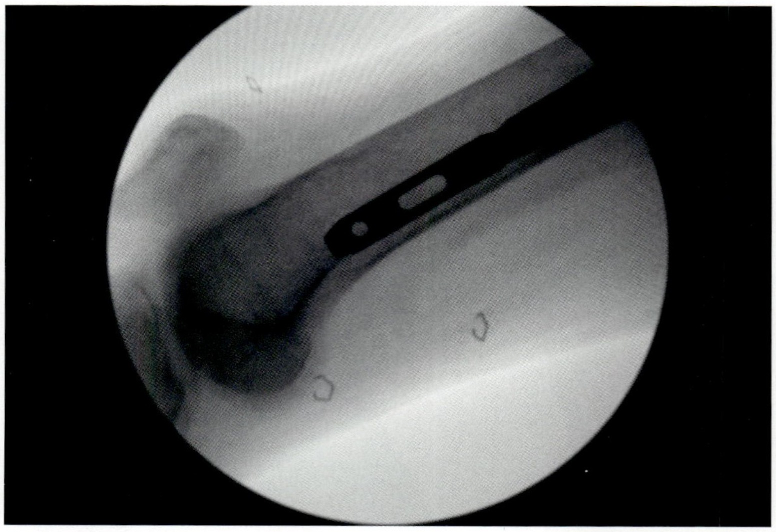

Fig. 49: Viewing of the distal holes in perfect alignment before drilling under image intensifier television (IITV) guidance.

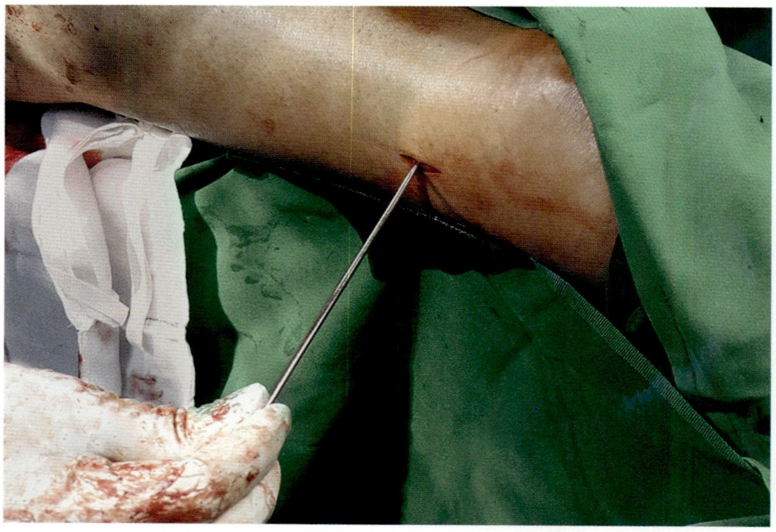

Fig. 50: Positioning of thick K-wire into the dynamic hole before entering the near cortex. Change over to drill is easy if the sleeve is firmly positioned (not seen in this figure).

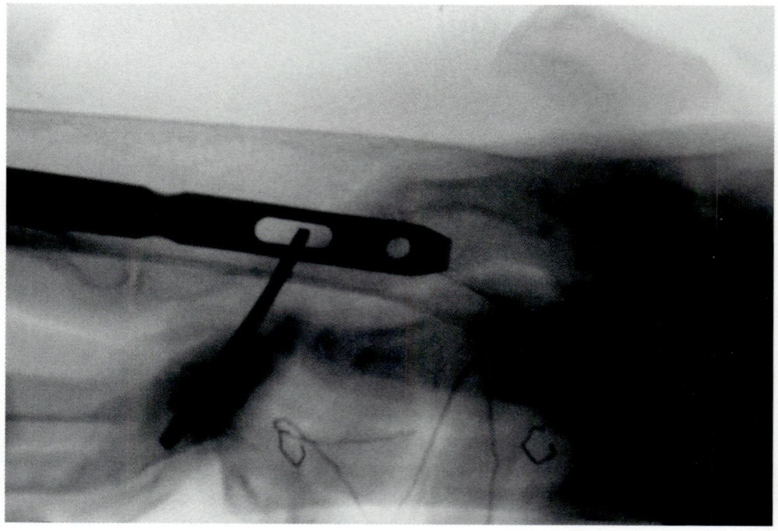

Fig. 51: Image intensifier television (IITV) confirmation of the position of K-wire onto the dynamic hole.

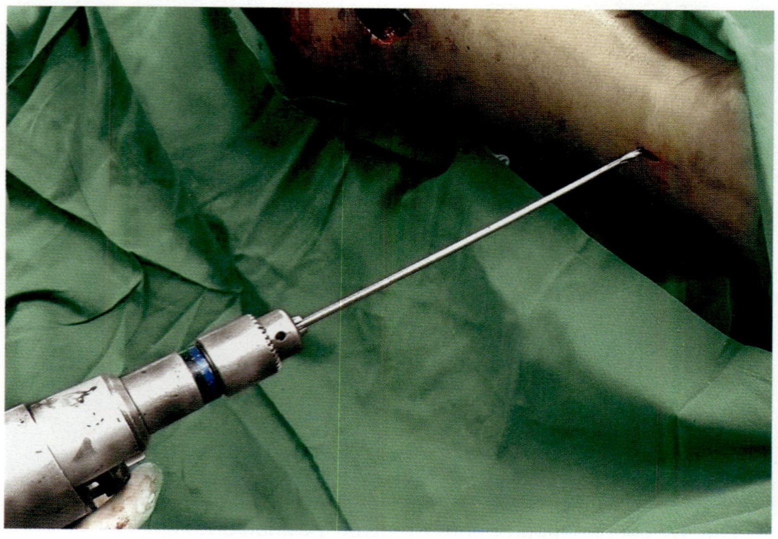

Fig. 52: Free hand drilling of the dynamic hole.

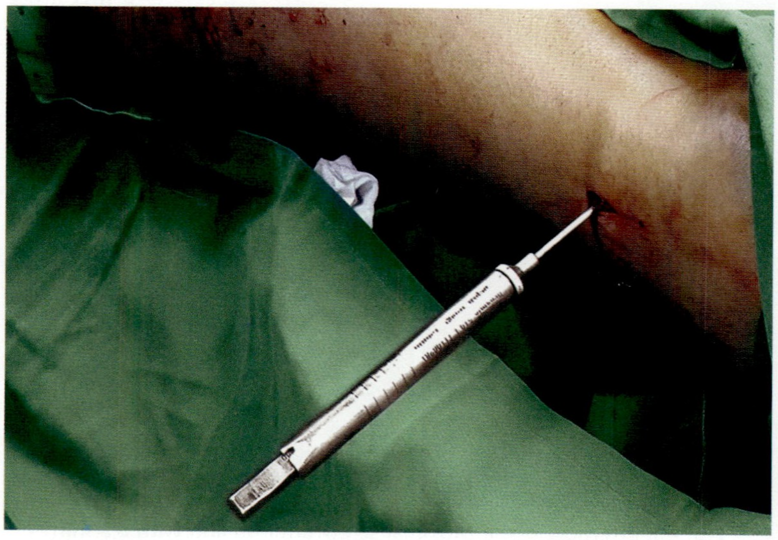

Fig. 53: Measurement of the length using depth gauge.

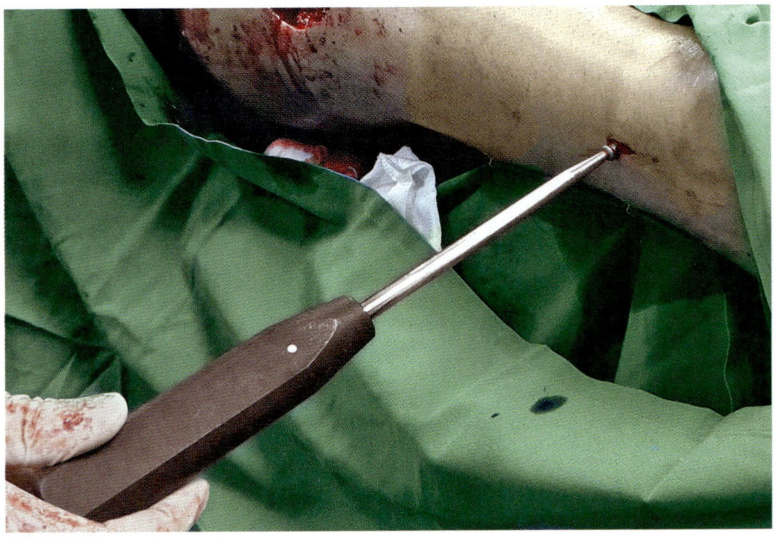

Fig. 54: Insertion of the screw in the dynamic hole.

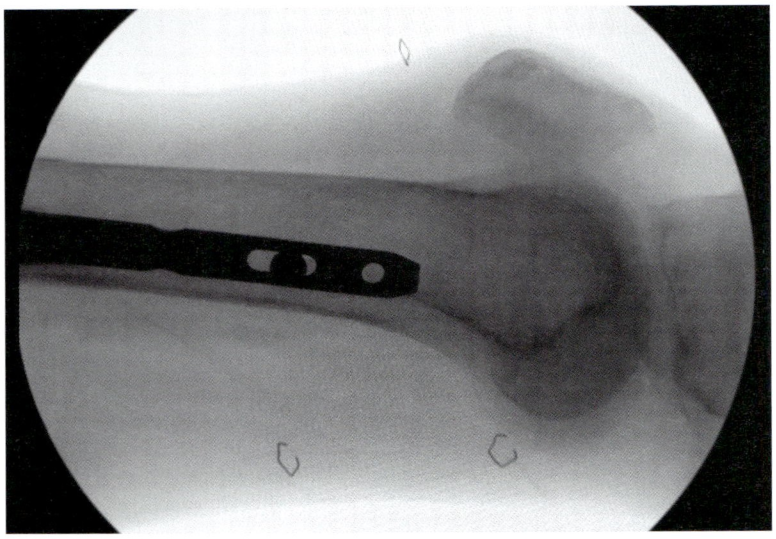

Fig. 55: Confirmation of screw position on lateral view [image intensifier television (IITV) image].

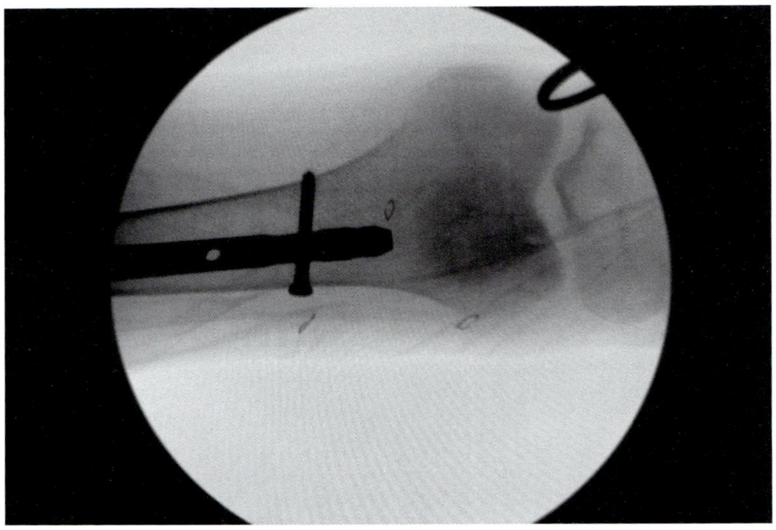

Fig. 56: Confirmation of screw position on anteroposterior (AP) view [image intensifier television (IITV) image].

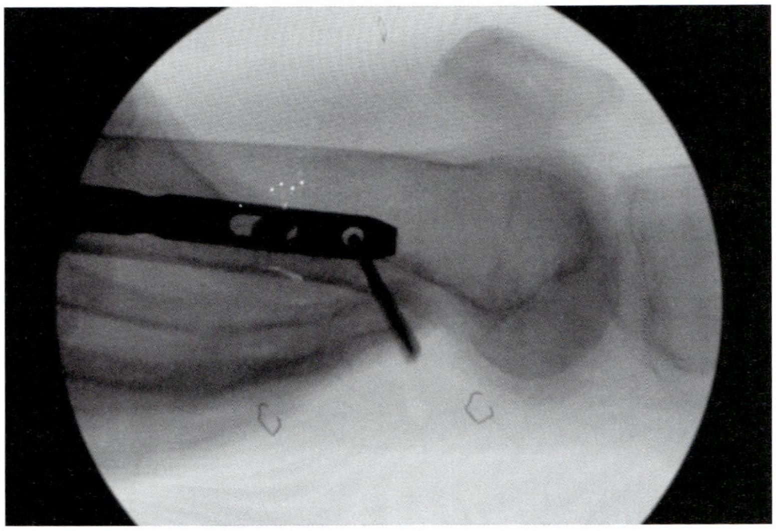

Fig. 57: Free hand technique for insertion of a distal bolt in the dynamic hole using a thick K-wire [image intensifier television (IITV) image].

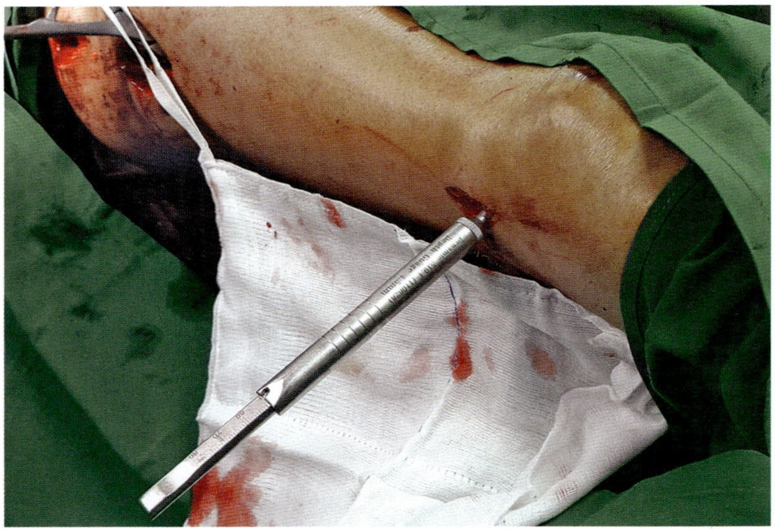

Fig. 58: Measurement of the static hole screw length using depth gauge.

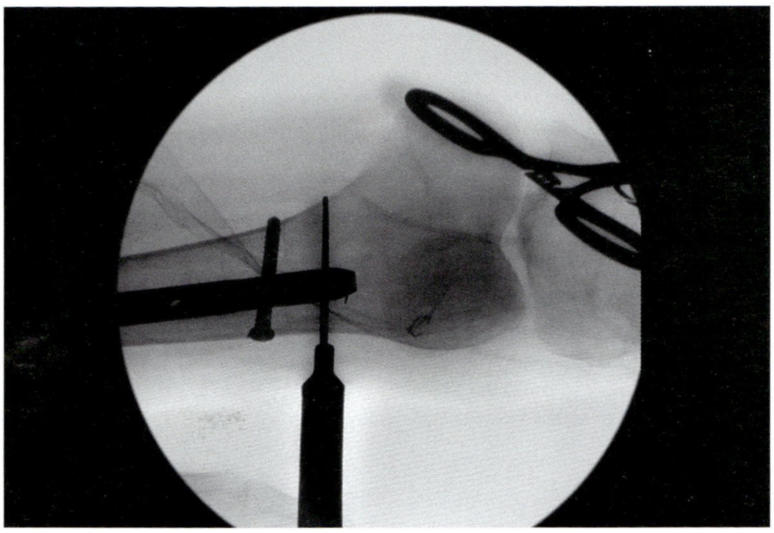

Fig. 59: Image intensifier television (IITV) confirmation of length on anteroposterior (AP) view.

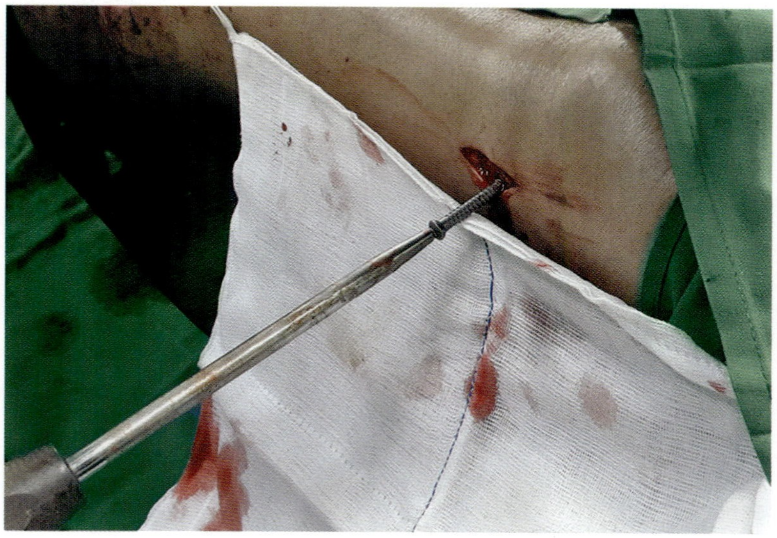

Fig. 60: Insertion of a screw in the static hole.

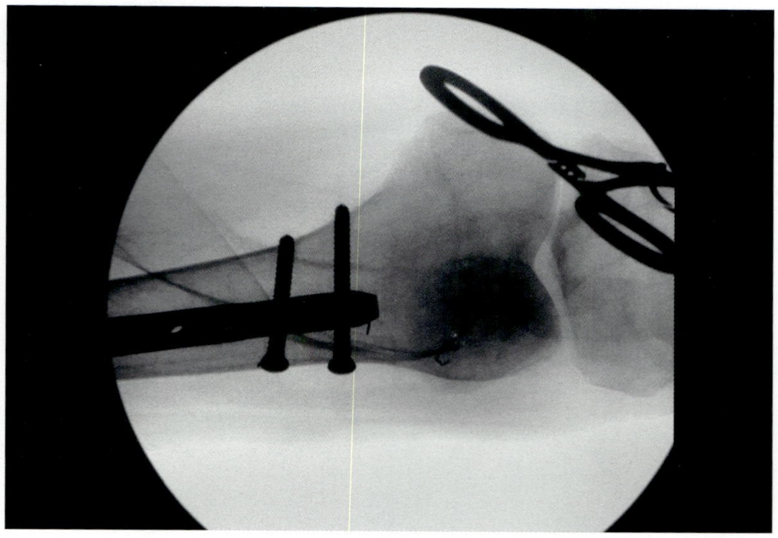

Fig. 61: Confirmation of both the bolts position on anteroposterior (AP) view [image intensifier television (IITV) image].

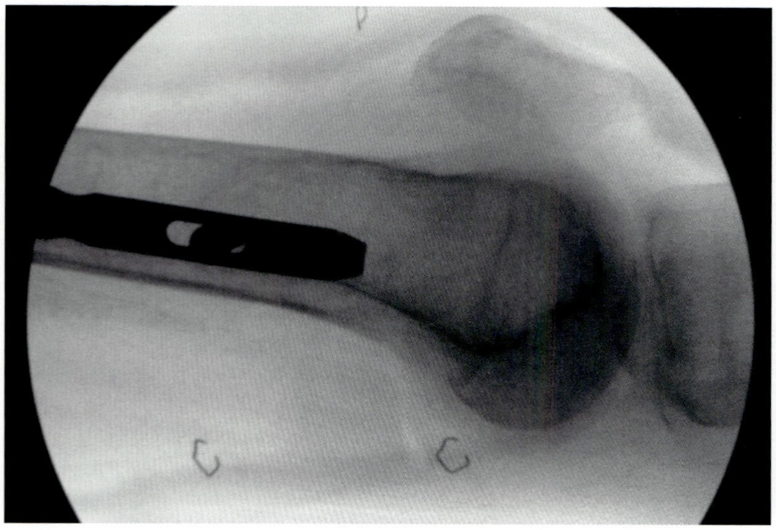

Fig. 62: Confirmation of both the bolts position on lateral view [image intensifier television (IITV) image].

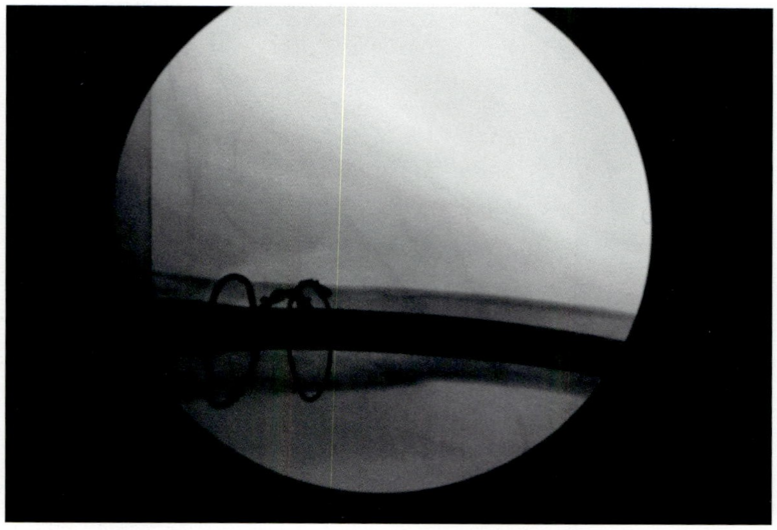

Fig. 63: Lateral image showing the final reduction of fracture with a nail in situ.

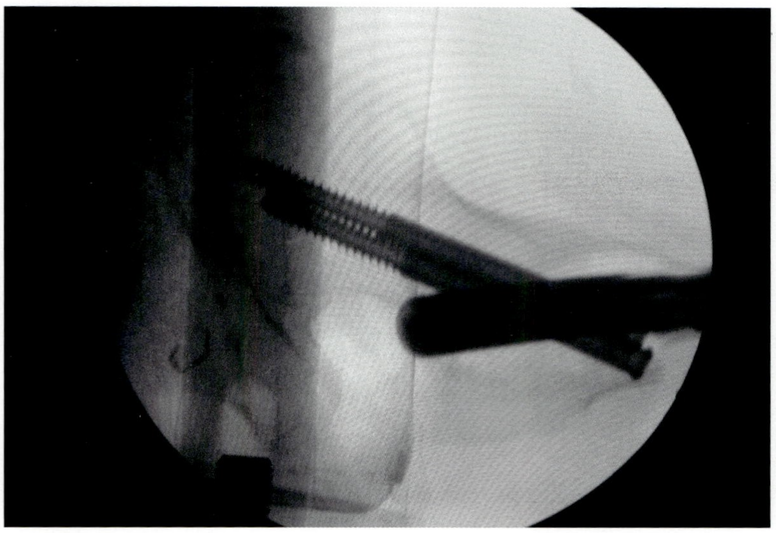

Fig. 64: Image intensifier television (IITV) image showing final screw position on the lateral view.

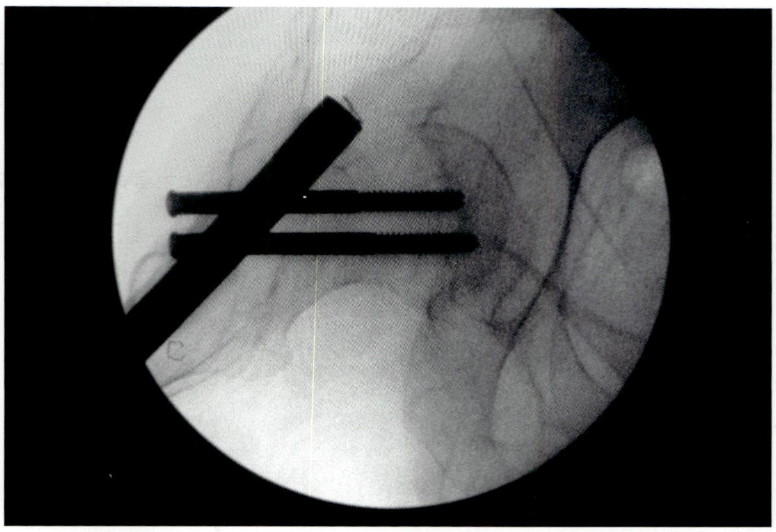

Fig. 65: Image intensifier showing final screw position on anteroposterior (AP) view.

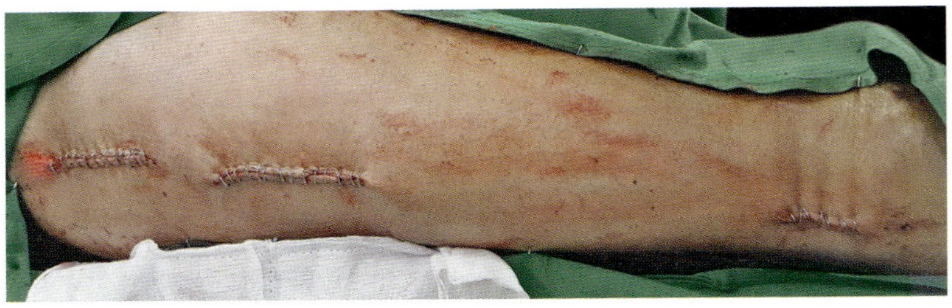

Fig. 66: Image showing suture line after the final implantation of an intramedullary nail.

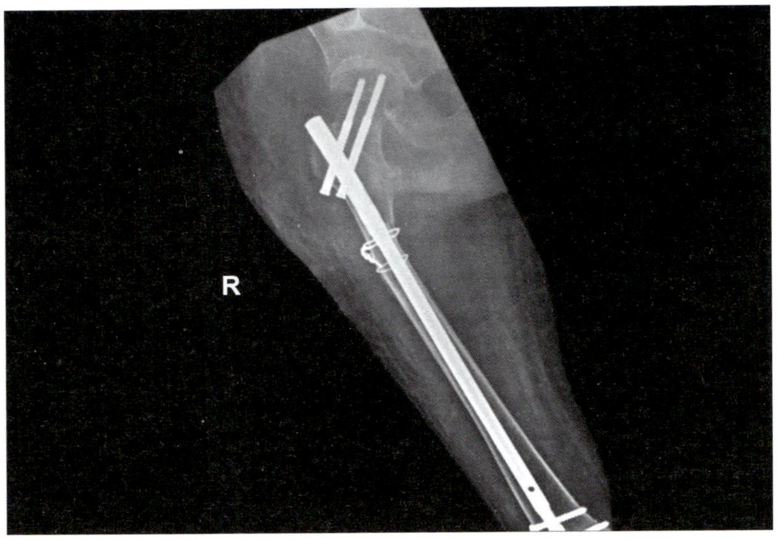

Fig. 67: Anteroposterior (AP) radiograph showing the final image after fixation.

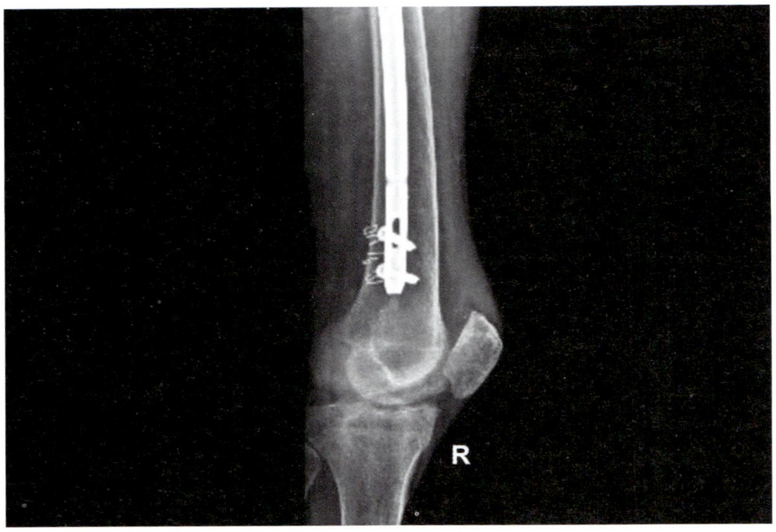

Fig. 68: Lateral radiograph showing the final image after fixation.

COMPLICATIONS

Even with the advent of new implants and technique, the complication rate with subtrochanteric fracture management still remains high (around 21%). The most frequent complications seen are loss of the reduction, pseudarthrosis, and infection.

SUGGESTED READING

1. Fielding JW. Subtrochanteric fractures. Clin Orthop Relat Res. 1973;(92):86-99.
2. Guyver PM, McCarthy MJ, Jain NP, et al. Is there any purpose in classifying subtrochanteric fractures? The reproducibility of four classification systems. Eur J Orthop Surg Traumatol. 2014;24(4):513-8.
3. Herscovici D Jr, Pistel WL, Sanders RW. Evaluation and treatment of high subtrochanteric femur fractures. Am J Orthop (Belle Mead NJ). 2000; 29(9 Suppl.):27-33.
4. Joglekar SB, Lindvall EM, Martirosian A. Contemporary management of subtrochanteric fractures. Orthop Clin North Am. 2015;46(1):21-35.
5. Khan SK, Kalra S, Khanna A, et al. Timing of surgery for hip fractures: a systematic review of 52 published studies involving 291,413 patients. Injury. 2009;40(7):692-7.
6. Kuzyk PR, Bhandari M, McKee MD, et al. Intramedullary versus extramedullary fixation for subtrochanteric femur fractures. J Orthop Trauma.2009;23(6):465-70.
7. Loizou CL, McNamara I, Ahmed K, et al. Classification of subtrochanteric femoral fractures. Injury. 2010;41(7):739-45.
8. Miedel R, Törnkvist H, Ponzer S, et al. Musculoskeletal function and quality of life in elderly patients after a subtrochanteric femoral fracture treated with a cephalomedullary nail. J Orthop Trauma. 2011;25(4): 208-13.
9. Mirbolook A, Siavashi B, Jafarinezhad AE, et al. Subtrochanteric fractures: comparison of proximal femur locking plate and intramedullary locking nail fixation outcome. Indian J Surg. 2015;77:795-8.
10. Murray RC, Frew JFM. Trochanteric fractures of the femur: a plea for conservative treatment. J Bone Joint Surg Br. 1949;31:204-19.

CHAPTER 106

Subtrochanteric Fracture Femur: Proximal Femur Plate Fixation

Milind Modak, Neelkamal Sourav

INTRODUCTION

Proximal femoral fracture poses a great challenge for management, especially if complicated by comminution and poor bone quality. The goal of surgery in such situation would be to restore length, restore alignment and rotation. Though intamedullary nailing is commonly used for management of pertrochaneric and subtrochanteric fractures, there is a definite rationale for the use of plating of the proximal femur to achieve good quality reduction and a stable fixation.

The challenges in proximal third femur fracture management are many, rotational instability, which is pronounced, if there is comminution with high-velocity polytrauma on the rise, one is faced with varied fracture patterns. Complex deforming forces cause displacement of the fragments. Severe osteoporosis is a challenge to achieve a stable construct and implants can back out and fail. Structural bowing in the femur due to age and arthritis makes implant selection and application a great challenge. Proximal femoral plate (PFP) can be used to meet the challenge.

INDICATIONS AND CONTRAINDICATIONS

The PFP is indicated in osteoporotic fracture of the proximal femur stable or even unstable fracture, especially if nail introduction is a cause of concern for increasing the comminution during the introduction of the nail. Open reduction and PFP would be indicated in the following situations:

- Presence of distal implant, e.g. knee prosthesis
- A pre-existing implant, which has to be removed through an open approach
- Lateral wall comminution or fracture extending into lateral cortex or piriformis fossa. This would not allow the use of an intramedullary nail
- Internal fixation for malunion, nonunion, revision of fixation, or corrective osteotomies of the proximal femur.

The advantage of plating over nailing is that, it reduces the risk of injury to the hip abductors and short-external rotators and also minimizes the incidence of heterotrophic ossification.

The 4.5 mm proximal femoral locking plate is indicated in a variety of situation like fracture of trochanteric regions: simple intertrochanteric fractures, reverse oblique trochanteric fractures, transverse trochanteric fractures, complex multifragmentary fracture with medial cortex instability.

Proximal femoral plate well addresses proximal femoral fracture with ipsilateral shaft femur fractures.

Proximal femoral plate is also useful in stabilizing proximal femoral osteotomy. The locking system stabilizes the construct even in severely osteoporotic fractures. It is also used in subtrochanteric femur fracture.

The ideal indication of PFP would be fracture with a large posteromedial fragment, a fracture with a reverse oblique pattern, a shattered lateral wall with a detached greater trochanter. On attempted nailing, if a satisfactory alignment is not achieved, the PFP would be useful, and can be kept as a standby implant.

IMPLANT SELECTION

The PFP would be the ideal implant for Russell–Taylor type IIA and type IIB fracture.

The PFP is an anatomically contoured locking plate. A stable construct is created with option out of six fixed angle screws occupying the head and neck. PFP is a more biological construct due to its minimally invasive submuscular placement with the help of jig.

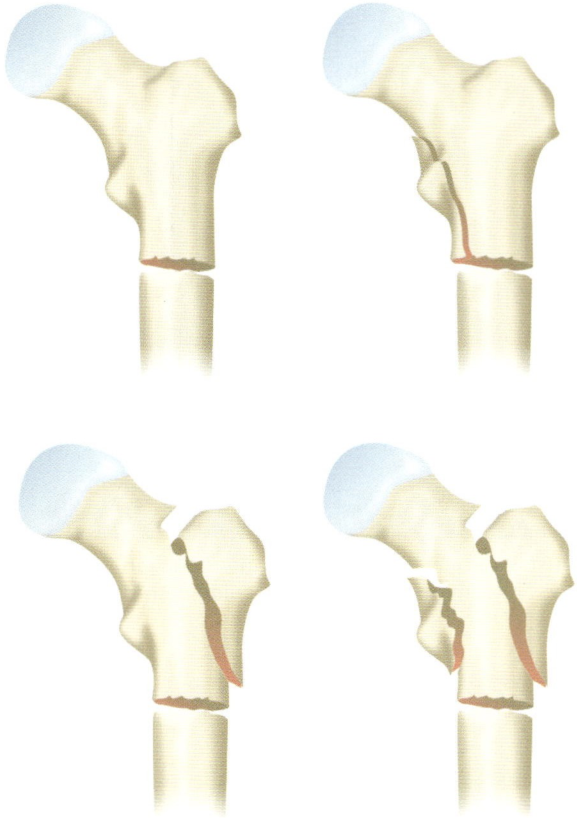

Fig. 1: Russell-Taylor classification.

SURGICAL STEPS (FIGS. 2 TO 11)

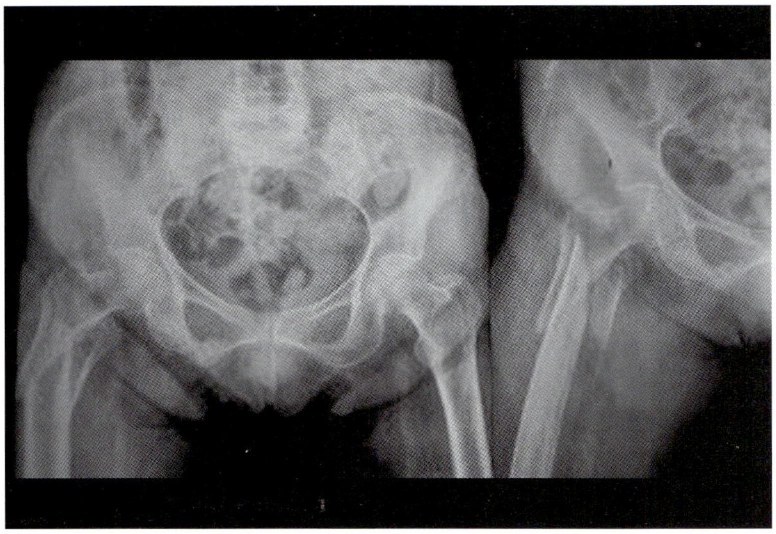

Fig. 2: Preoperative X-ray. These include the pelvis with both hips anteroposterior (AP) view and the fractured hip with shaft AP view. Lateral view and ipsilateral knee X-ray is also done.

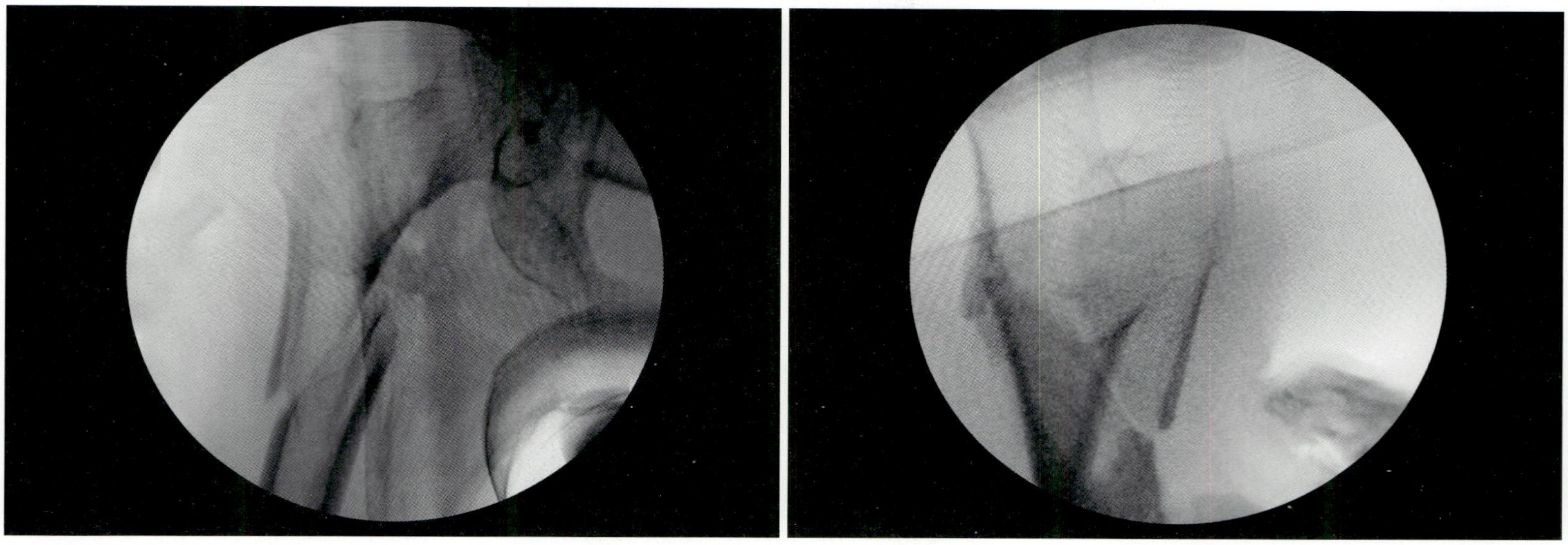

Fig. 3: C-arm image. The patient positioned on standard fracture table and the reduction is assessed on the C-arm. Adequate C-arm mobility and visualization are confirmed before proceeding with painting and draping.

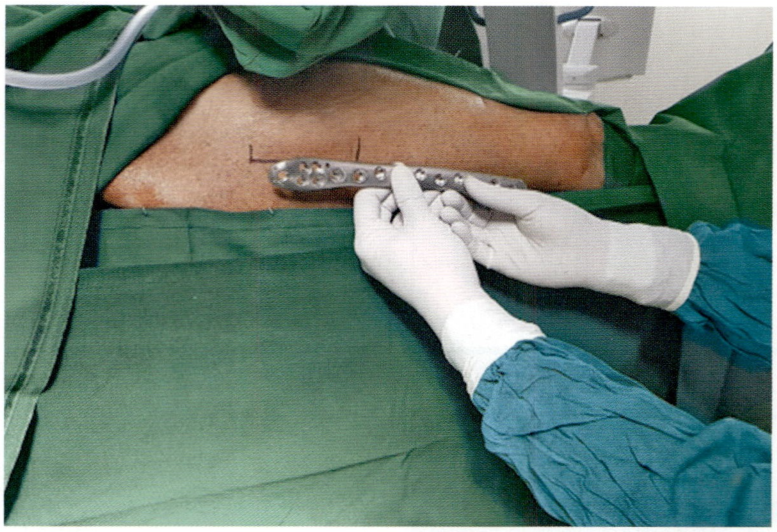

Fig. 4: Skin incision marked. The appropriate length of the proximal femoral plate is selected and the incision is marked by visualizing under the C-arm. Care taken that the plate does not touch the skin.

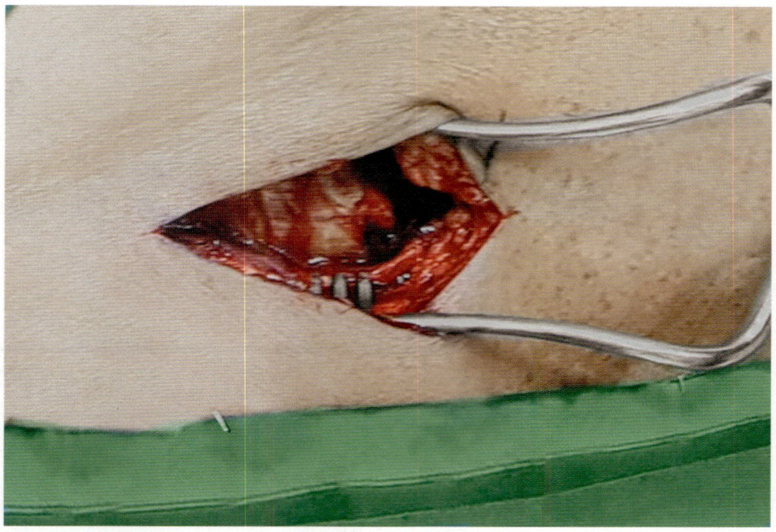

Fig. 5: Incision. Direct lateral approach to the proximal femur. Hemostasis achieved as one proceeds deeper.

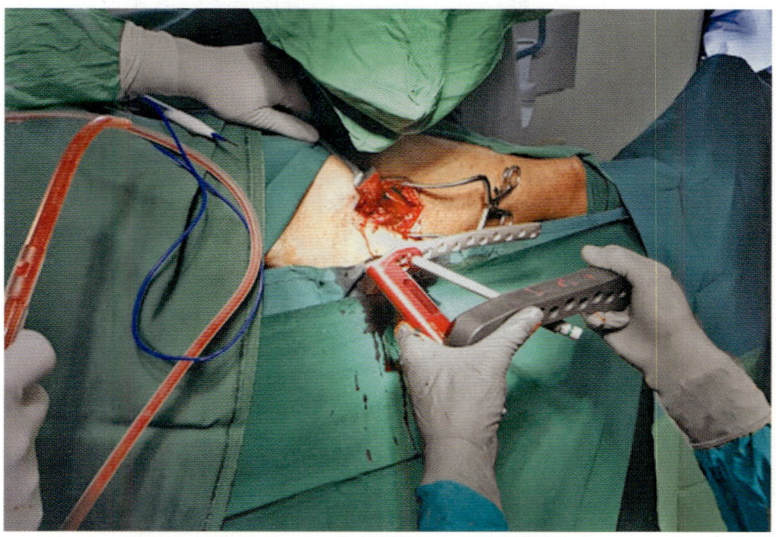

Fig. 6: Incision and implant. The proximal femur is exposed by cutting tensor fascia lata and splitting vastus lateralis muscle. Trochanteric flare and shaft of femur exposed. The implant along with the jig is aligned on the C-arm and plate length decided and confirmed.

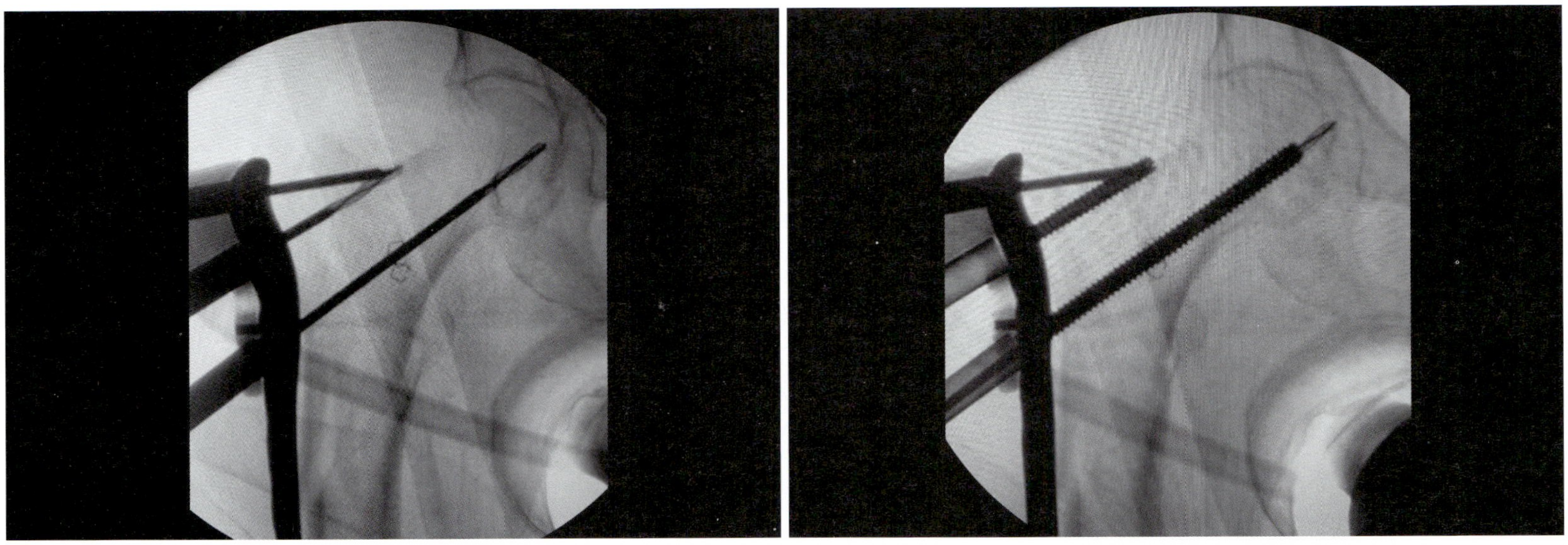

Fig. 7: C-arm image of alpha screw drill guide in anteroposterior (AP) and lateral view. The plate is slid by a minimally invasive technique in the submuscular plane. The position of the anatomically contoured proximal femoral plate (PFP) is adjusted on the C-arm. The 3.2 mm alpha screw drill guide is inserted under C-arm visualization. The drill guide is placed so as to lie above the femoral calcar in AP view and central position in the lateral view—in line with femoral neck axis. The drill guide is positioned so as not to penetrate the subchondral bone.

- *Proximal alpha and beta drill tip guidepin and guidepin*: The fixation steps proceed with the beta drill guide and subsequent progression of screw fixation
- *Alpha and beta screw*: The alpha screw of appropriate length with measurement taken off the drill tip guide pin. The various options of screw, which can fill any screw hole are 4.5 mm cortex screw, 4.5 mm locking screw, 5.7 mm cannulated locking screw, 6.5 mm cancellous, 6.5 mm cannulated conical, 6.5 mm cannulated locking screw.

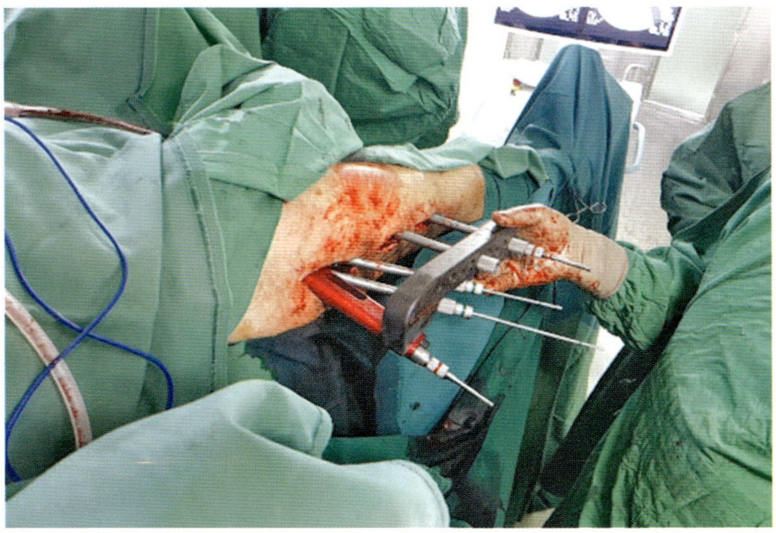

Fig. 8: Jig and plate in position. Once the alpha screw is placed in the desired position, the construct is stabilized by passing the superior 3.2 mm drill tip guide pin. The plate positioned so as to align with the shaft and the distal most locking screw hole is occupied by passing the distal 3.2 mm drill tip guide pin. The reduction and position of the plate are confirmed on the C-arm. The fracture reduction is facilitated by traction, ball spike pusher, reduction forceps, or cerclage wire, as required.

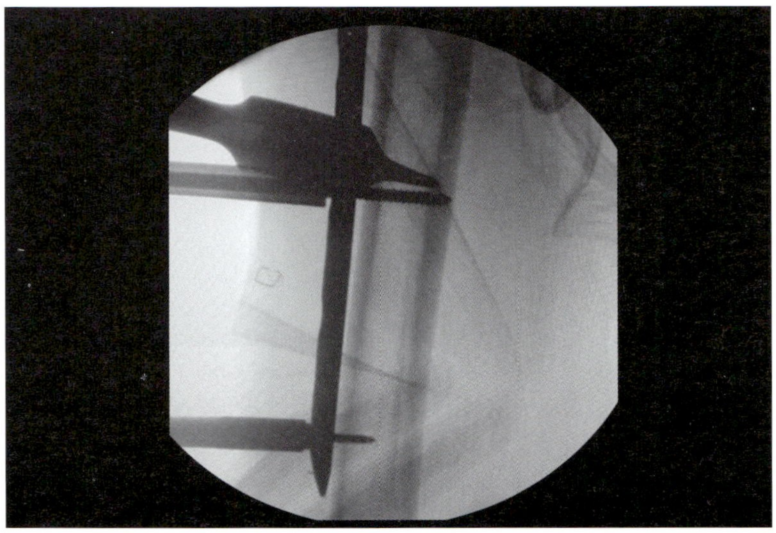

Fig. 9: Distal drill tip guide pin—in position. The distal drill tip guide pin position is confirmed and fixed after assessing the appropriate position of the plate on the shaft of femur.

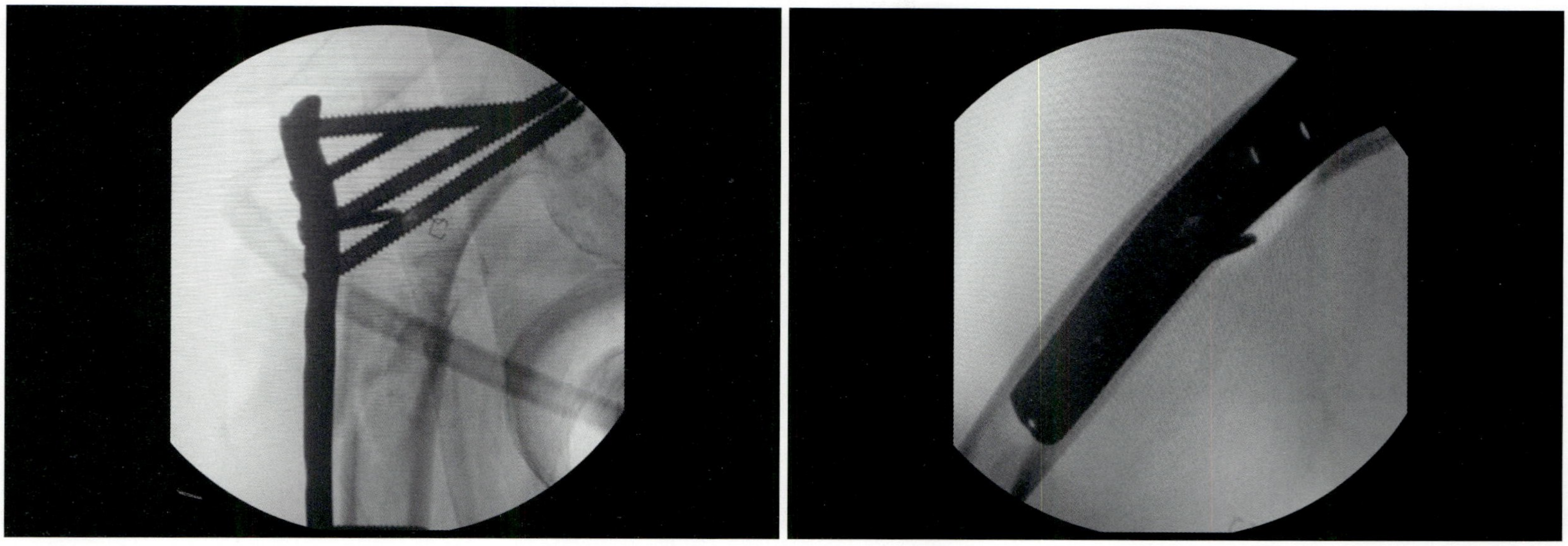

Fig. 10: Final C-arm image anteroposterior (AP) and lateral view. The proximal screws are fixed out of option of six screws. The alpha screw is mandatory followed by the other screws. All screw may not be filled. The plate is stabilized along the shaft of the femur. A 4.5 mm cortical nonlocking screw just distal to the fracture can be used to approximate the plate to the shaft. Subsequently, 4.5 mm locking screws are used to complete the construct.

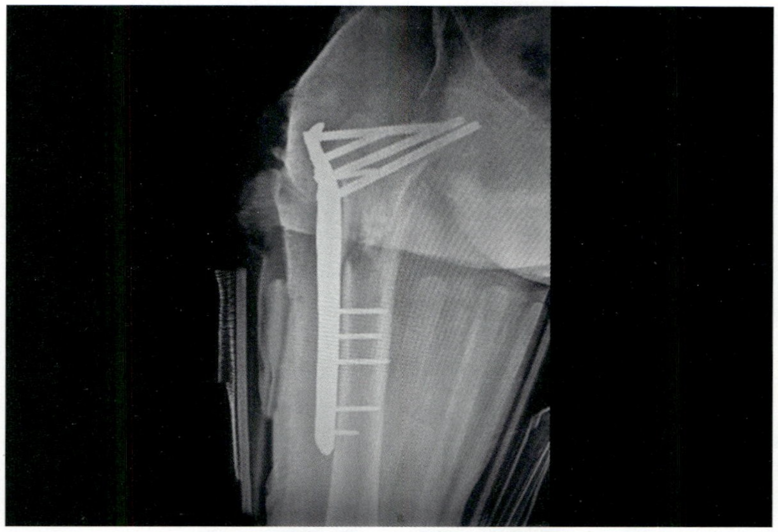

Fig. 11: Postoperative X-ray. Postoperative X-ray shows a good alignment with a stable construct. Five screws out of six options in the head neck have been used.

POSSIBLE COMPLICATIONS

The complications, which arise following the use of the proximal femoral plate, are due to technical errors. Various angular and rotational malalignment can be prevented by good preoperative planning and achieving a good reduction on table prior to fixation. Screw penetration into the hip can be very painful. This should be prevented by good C-arm imaging during surgery and screws not perforating into subchondral bone. Inadequate reduction and shortening should be prevented by meticulous reduction techniques on table. Improper implant selection should be avoided, short plate should be avoided. Torsional and axial failure should be prevented by fixation of at least eight cortices distally in the subtrochanteric fracture fixation.

SUGGESTED READING

1. Bergman GD, Winquist RA, Mayo KA, Hansen ST. Subtrochanteric fracture of the femur. Fixation using the Zickel nail. J Bone Jt Surg - Ser A. 1987;69(7):1032-40.
2. Article O, Asif N, Ahmad S, Qureshi OA, Jilani LZ, Hamesh T, et al. Unstable intertrochanteric fracture fixation – is proximal femoral locked compression plate better than dynamic hip screw. J Clin Diagn Res. 2016;9-13.
3. Kumar A, Jain A, Agrawal A. Outcome of proximal femur fracture treated with long proximal femoral nail and dynamic hip screw. International Journal of Orthopedics Sciences. 2017;3(3):600-6.
4. Mm H, Qs A, Fh Q, Mti N. Evaluation of the outcome of proximal femoral locking compression plate for the treatment of comminuted trochanteric and subtrochanteric femoral fractures in lateral decubitus approach without peroperative image intensifier; 2008.
5. Govindasamy R, Gnanasundaram R, Kasirajan S, Meleppuram JJ, Archit K, et al. Proximal femur locking compression plate in complex proximal femoral fractures: a retrospective analysis. Int J Res Orthop. 2016;2(3):104-8.

CHAPTER 107

Fracture Shaft Femur: Interlocking Nail Fixation

Prasad Joshi

INTRODUCTION

Fractures of the shaft of femur are very common in all strata of society. Fractures in young patients are generally secondary to high-energy trauma such as road traffic accidents and falls from height.

In elderly osteoporotic patients, the fractures may result from low energy trauma such as fall from standing height or domestic accidents.

The patient presents with a history of trauma, associated with pain and swelling of the thigh and inability to stand. Abnormal movement at the fracture site is a pathognomonic sign.

Fracture shaft femur results in blood loss into the hematoma of thigh roughly 1.5–2 liters, and hence a patient of fracture shaft femur may present with hypovolemic shock and hemodynamic stabilization with fluids and blood transfusion is necessary. The fractured limb should be temporarily stabilized using a Thomas splint with or without traction. Skeletal traction may be applied to maintain the alignment of the fractured fragments.

In fractures complicated by infection, gross contamination, distal neurovascular compromise (DNVC), open fractures, in hemodynamically unstable patients or in those with polytrauma, external fixation may be considered as a means of providing temporary stabilization of the fracture, after which definitive fixation can be undertaken later.

Depending on the type of fracture (transverse, oblique, or spiral) and the degree of comminution, the fracture is classified into various types. AO has also given a classification for fractures of shaft of femur.

Fractures of shaft of femur may be associated with dislocation of the hip or knee, fractures of ipsilateral tibia (floating knee), neurovascular injury, and fat embolism syndrome. Open fractures of the femur may also present with an associated neurovascular deficit.

In this chapter, we are describing the procedure of intramedullary interlocking nailing, which is the treatment of choice for all closed and Gustilo Anderson Grade 1 open fractures of femoral diaphysis.

OPERATIVE TECHNIQUE

STEPS OF OPERATION

Step 1: Patient position: On fracture table with traction (Fig. 1A) and other limb in lithotomy position, under C-arm control. Sterile draping is done (Figs. 1B and C).

Step 2: Fracture reduction checked under C-arm. Antroposterior (AP) (Fig. 2A) and lateral view (Fig. 2B).

Step 3:
Incision: 2–3 cm from tip of greater trochanter. Over the line drawn perpendicular to the line from anterior superior iliac spine tip downwards (Fig. 3A). Incision is taken (Fig. 3B).

Step 4: Entry point taken through the medial aspect of tip of the greater trochanter with the help of 4-mm Steinmann pin [C-arm view (Fig. 4A) and clinical photograph (Fig. 4B)]. Steinmann pin slightly advanced (Fig. 4C). Entry should be in the center of the neck in lateral view (Fig. 4D). Guidewire passed after removal of Steinmann pin through the same hole. AP view (Fig. 4E) and lateral view (Fig. 4F).

Step 5: Proximal reaming done over the guidewire from 8 mm to 13 mm. C-arm images (Figs. 5A and 5B); clinical picture (Fig. 5C).

Passing of beaded guidewire through the proximal fragment and across the fracture into the distal fragment after achieving closed reduction in both AP and lateral C-arm view (Figs. 5D to G). Guidewire is advanced till it reaches superior pole of the patella (Figs. 5H and I).

Step 6: Reaming of entire length of the canal over the beaded guidewire from 8 mm in 0.5 mm increments till 1.5 mm larger than the measured size (Figs. 6A to D).

Step 7: Exchange of the beaded guidewire with nonbeaded guidewire with help of exchange tube (Fig. 7A). Non-beaded guidewire in situ (Fig. 7B).

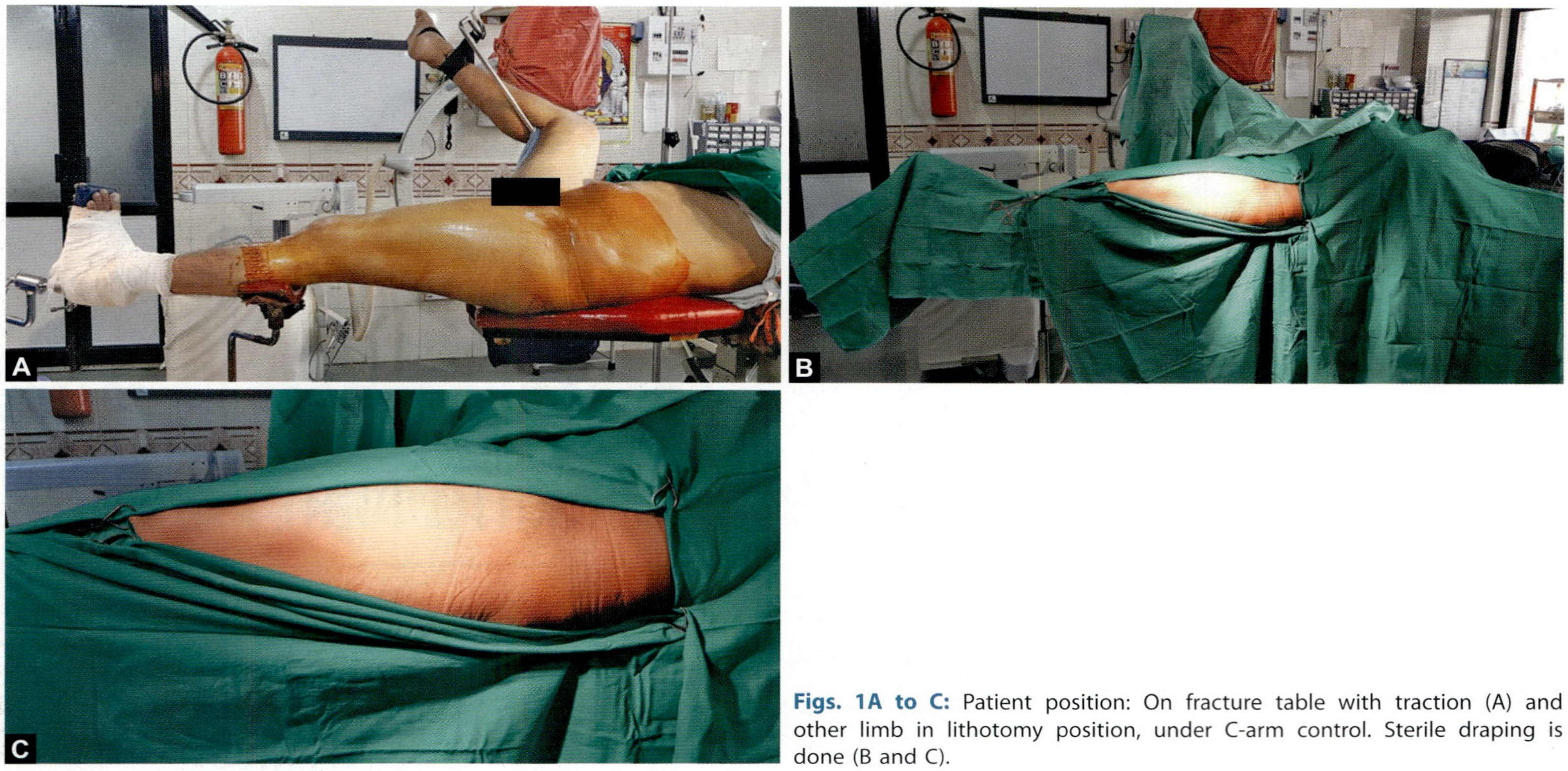

Figs. 1A to C: Patient position: On fracture table with traction (A) and other limb in lithotomy position, under C-arm control. Sterile draping is done (B and C).

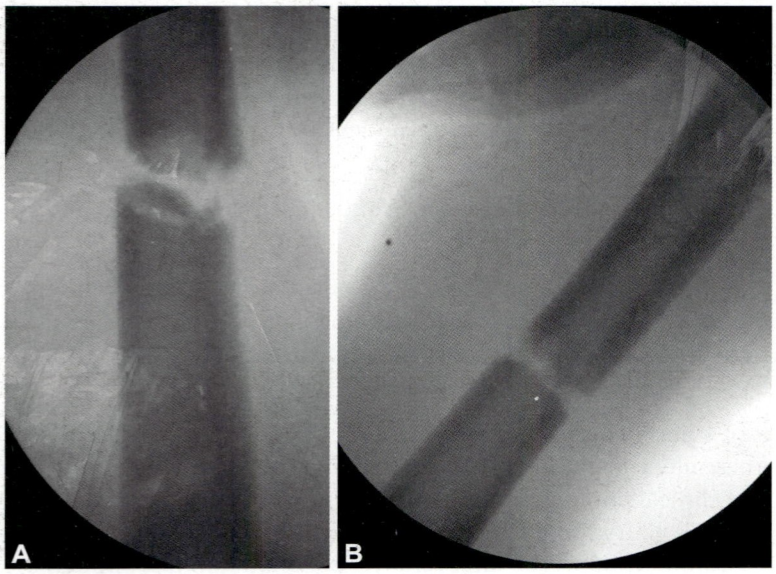

Figs. 2A and B: Fracture reduction. C-arm anteroposterior (AP) (A) and lateral view (B).

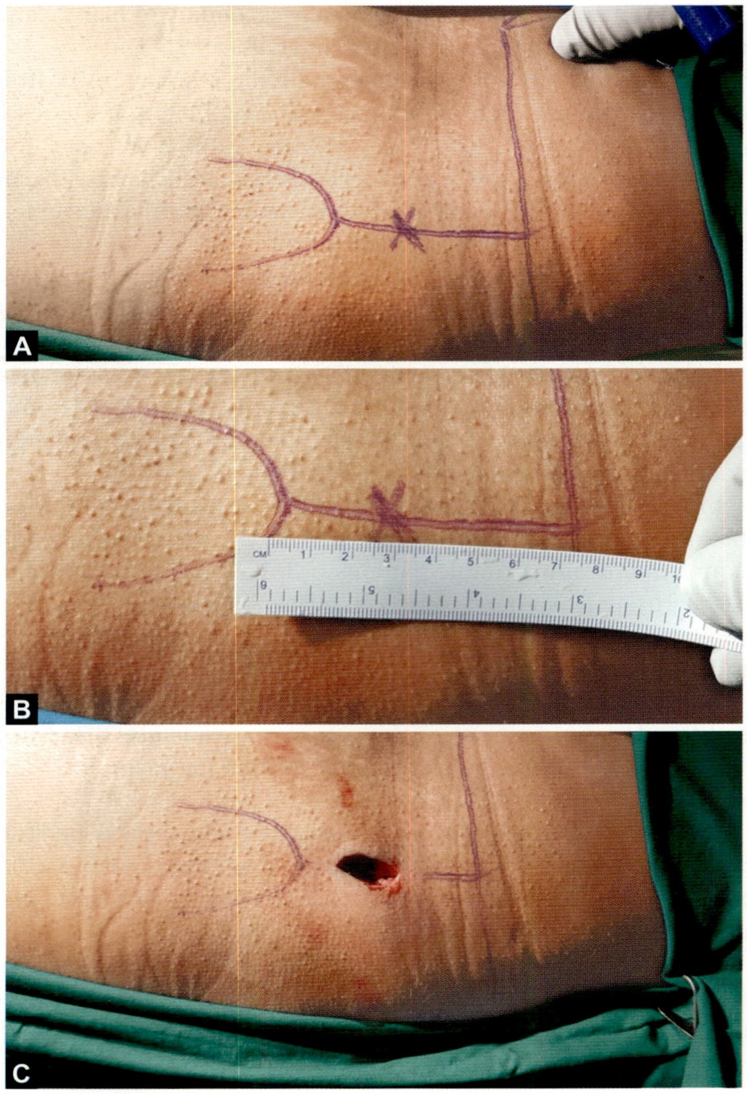

Figs. 3A to C: Incision

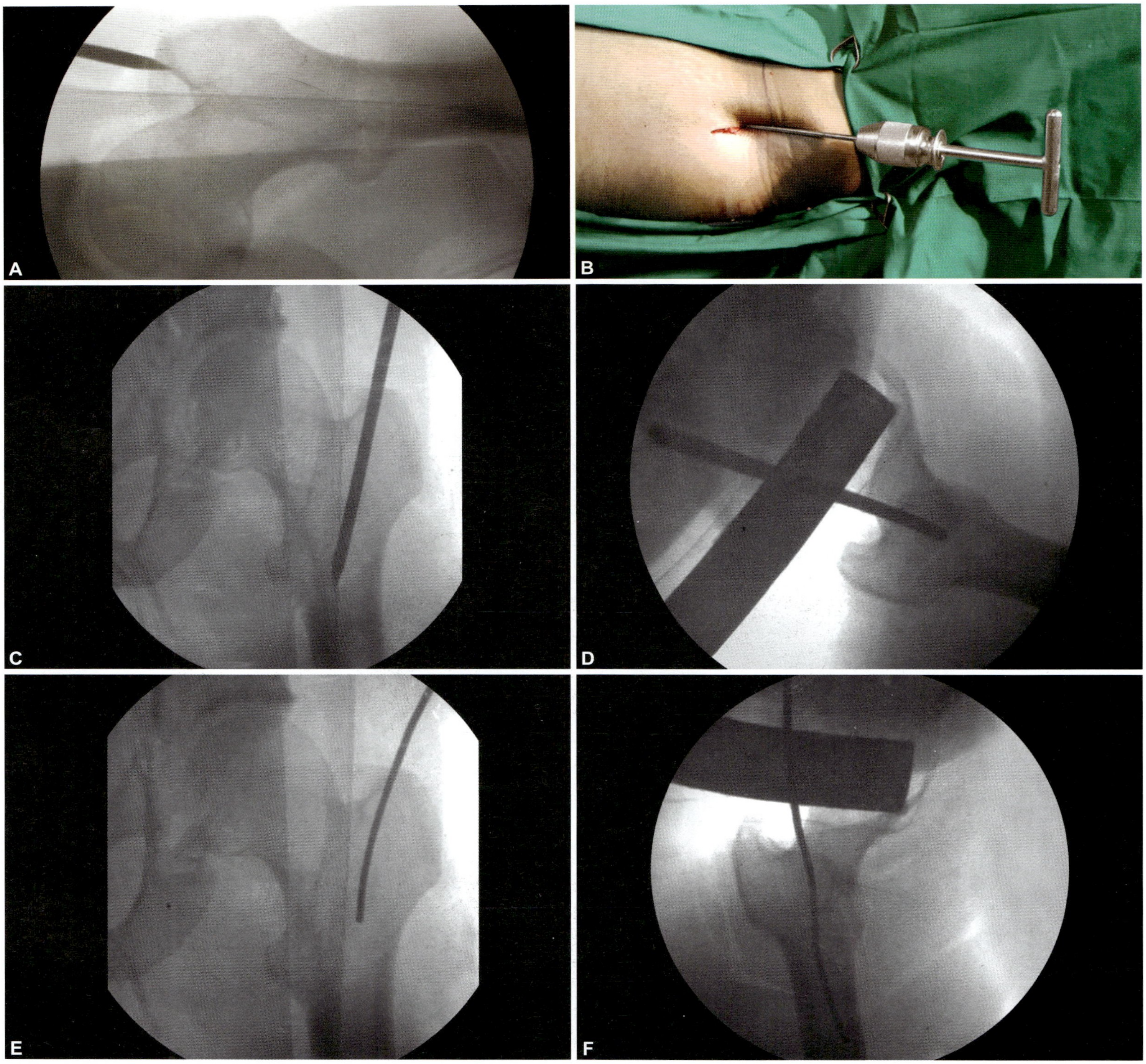

Figs. 4A to F: Entry point taken through the medial aspect of tip of the greater trochanter with the help of 4-mm Steinmann pin [C-arm view (A) and clinical photograph (B)]. Steinmann pin slightly advanced (C). Entry should be in the center of the neck in lateral view (D). Guidewire passed after removal of Steinmann pin through the same hole. AP view (E) and lateral view (F).

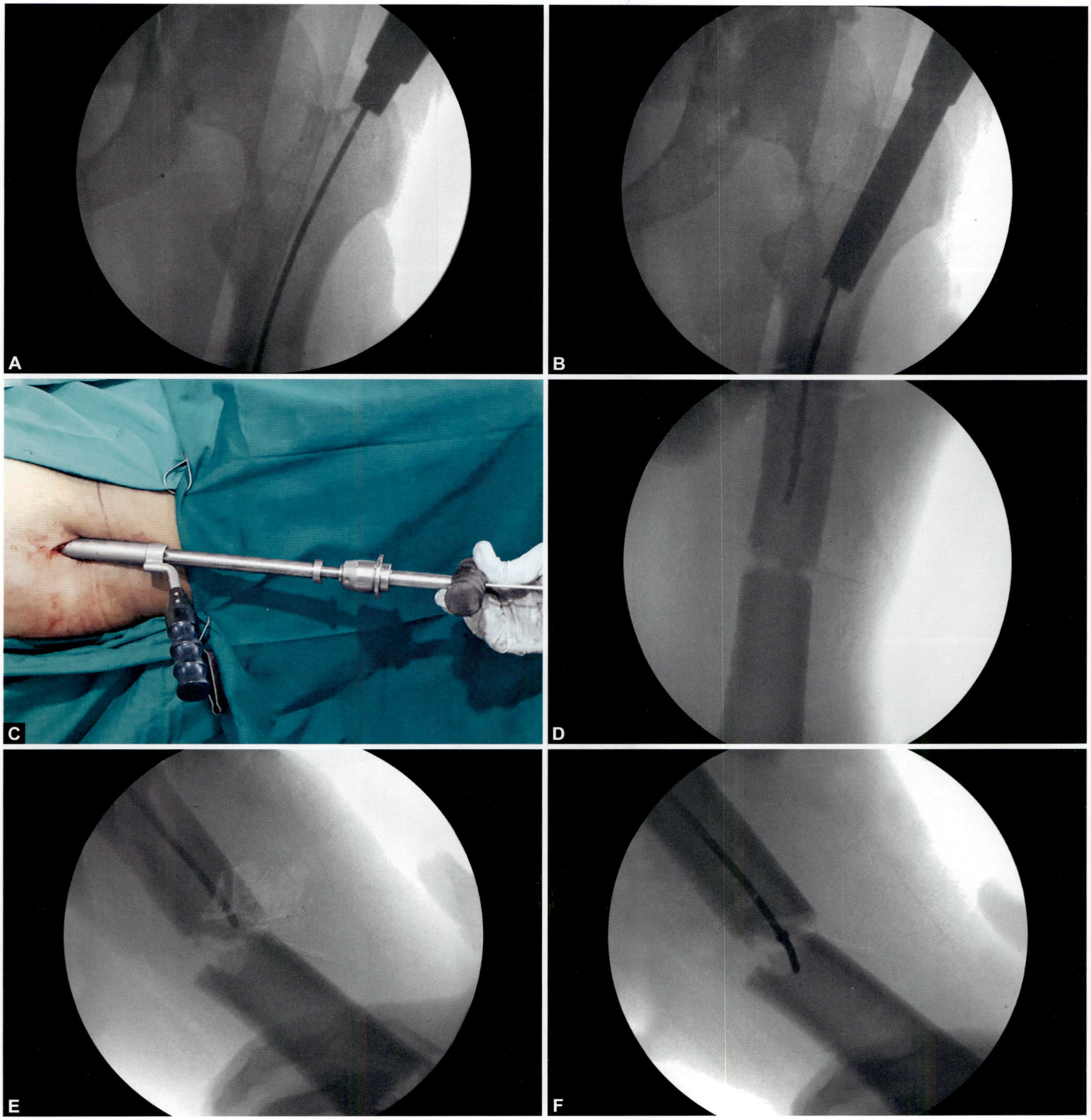

Figs. 5A to F: Reaming and passing of beaded guidewire.

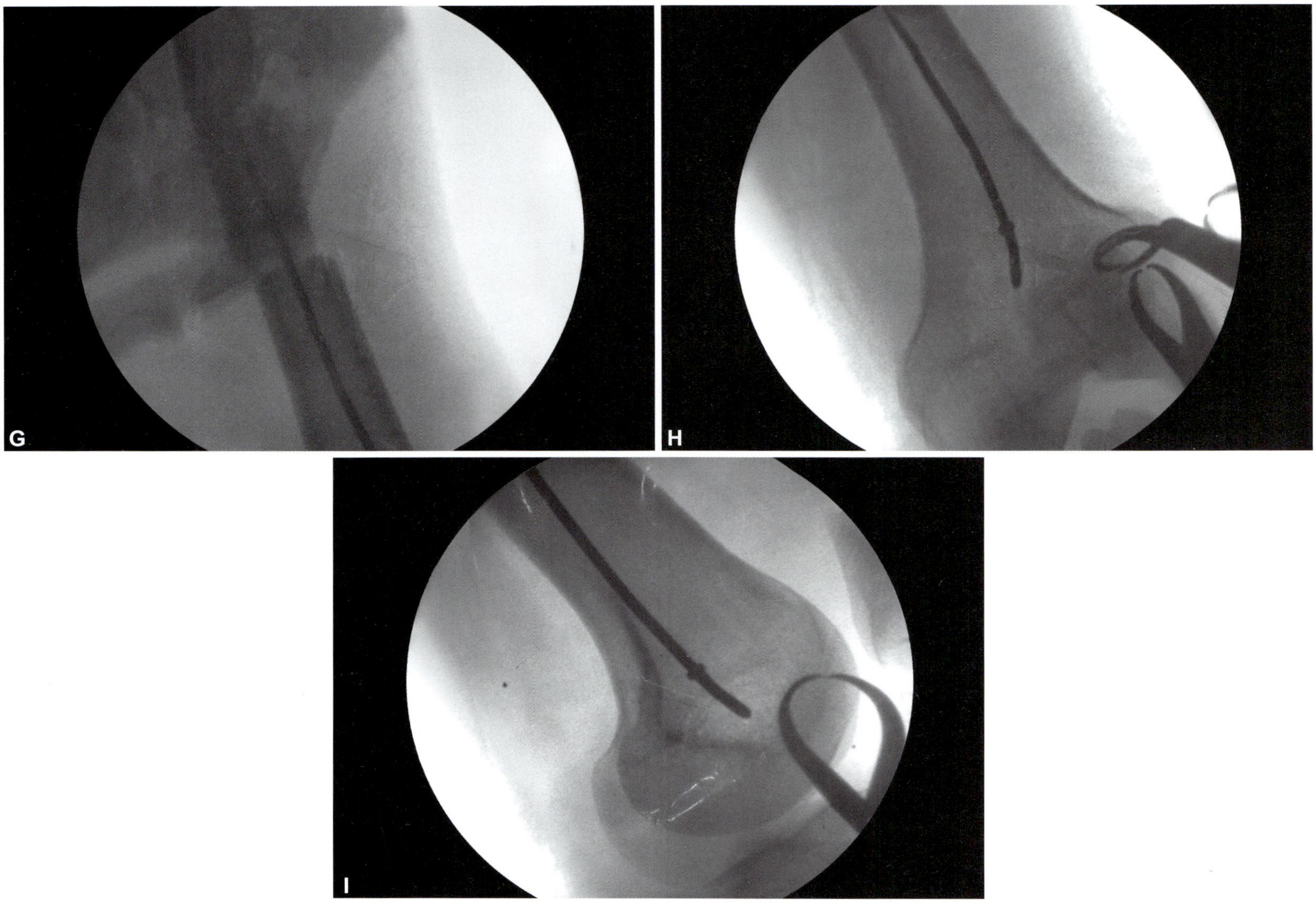

Figs. 5G to I: Guidewire passed at least till superior pole of patella.

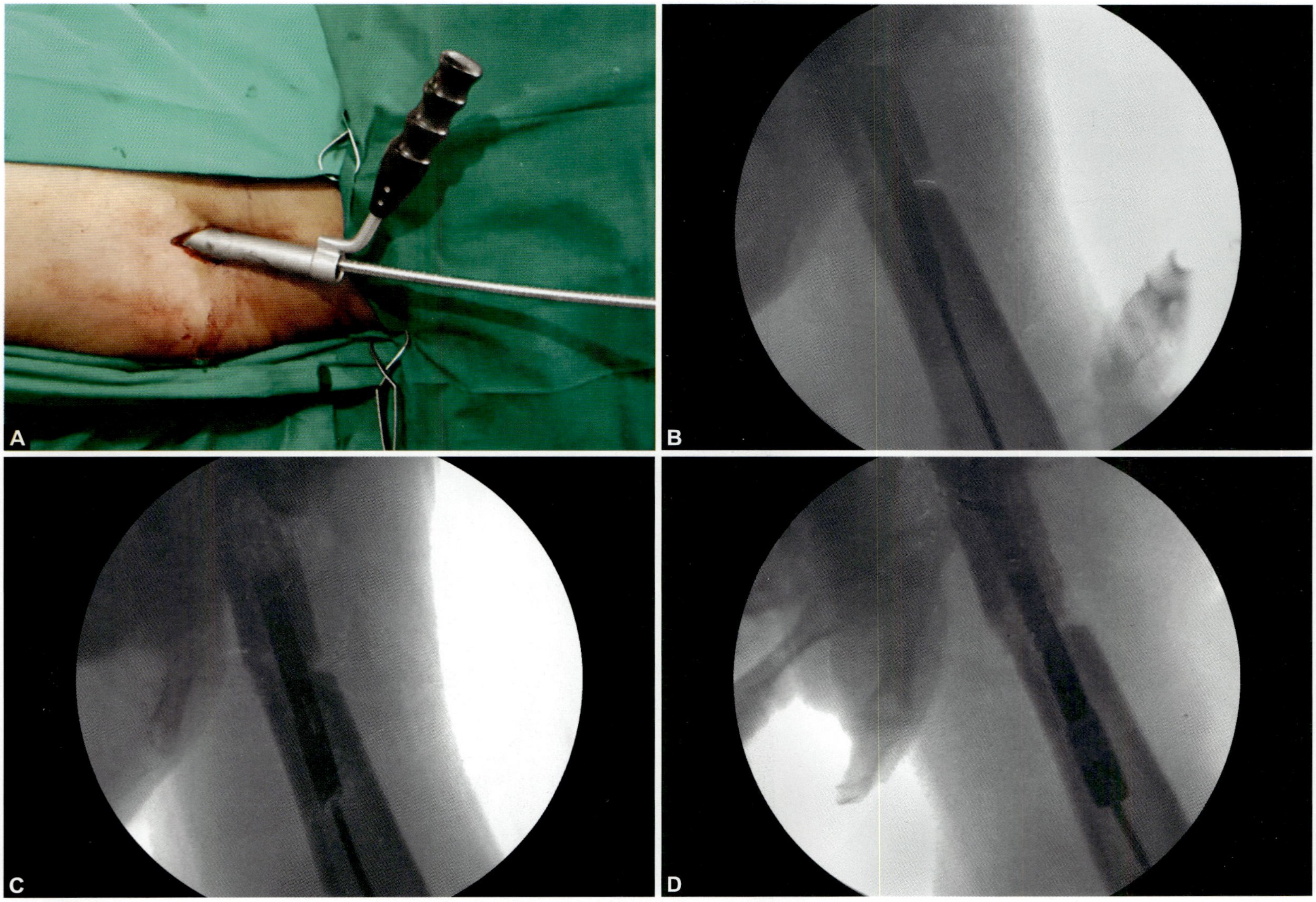

Figs. 6A to D: Reaming with flexible reamers over beaded guidewire.

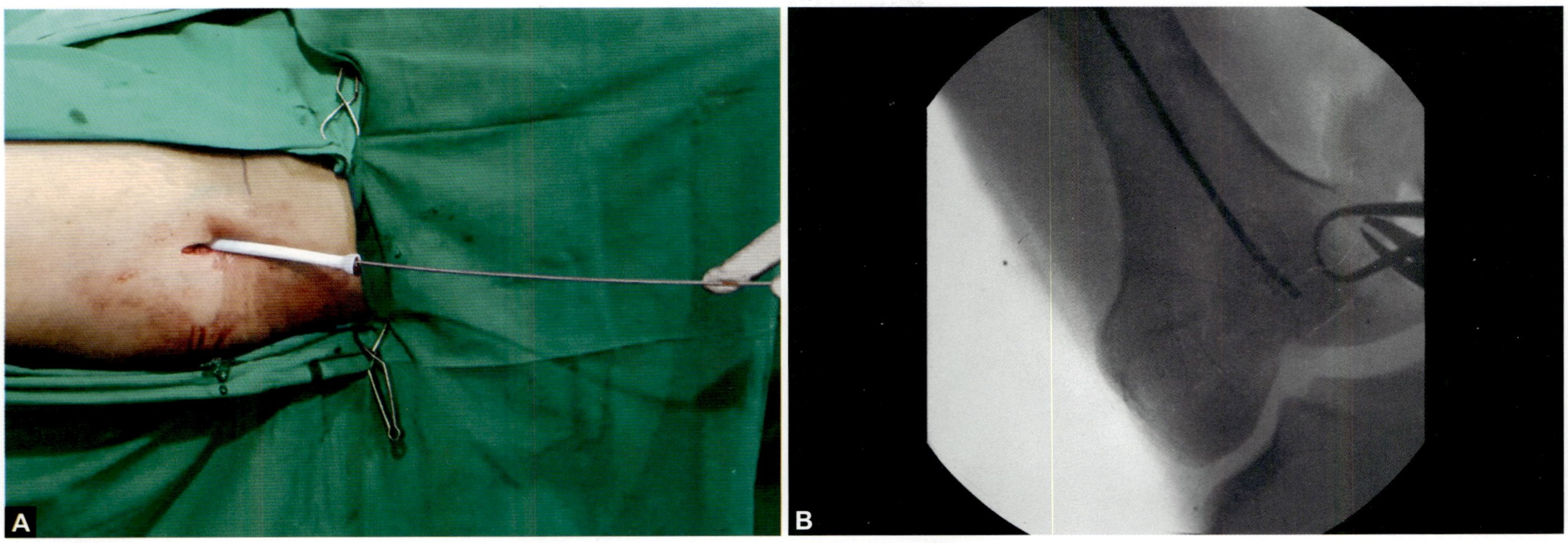

Figs. 7A and B: Through exchange tube guidewire changed to non beaded one.

Step 8: Measurement of nail length with measuring scale (Fig. 8A). Chosen nail is gently advanced over the guidewire, across the fracture site into the distal fragment under C-arm guidance (Figs. 8B to G).

Guidewire removed and distal end of the nail is visualized to confirm its level (Figs. 8H to J).

Similarly, the position of the proximal end of the nail is confirmed (Fig. 8K).

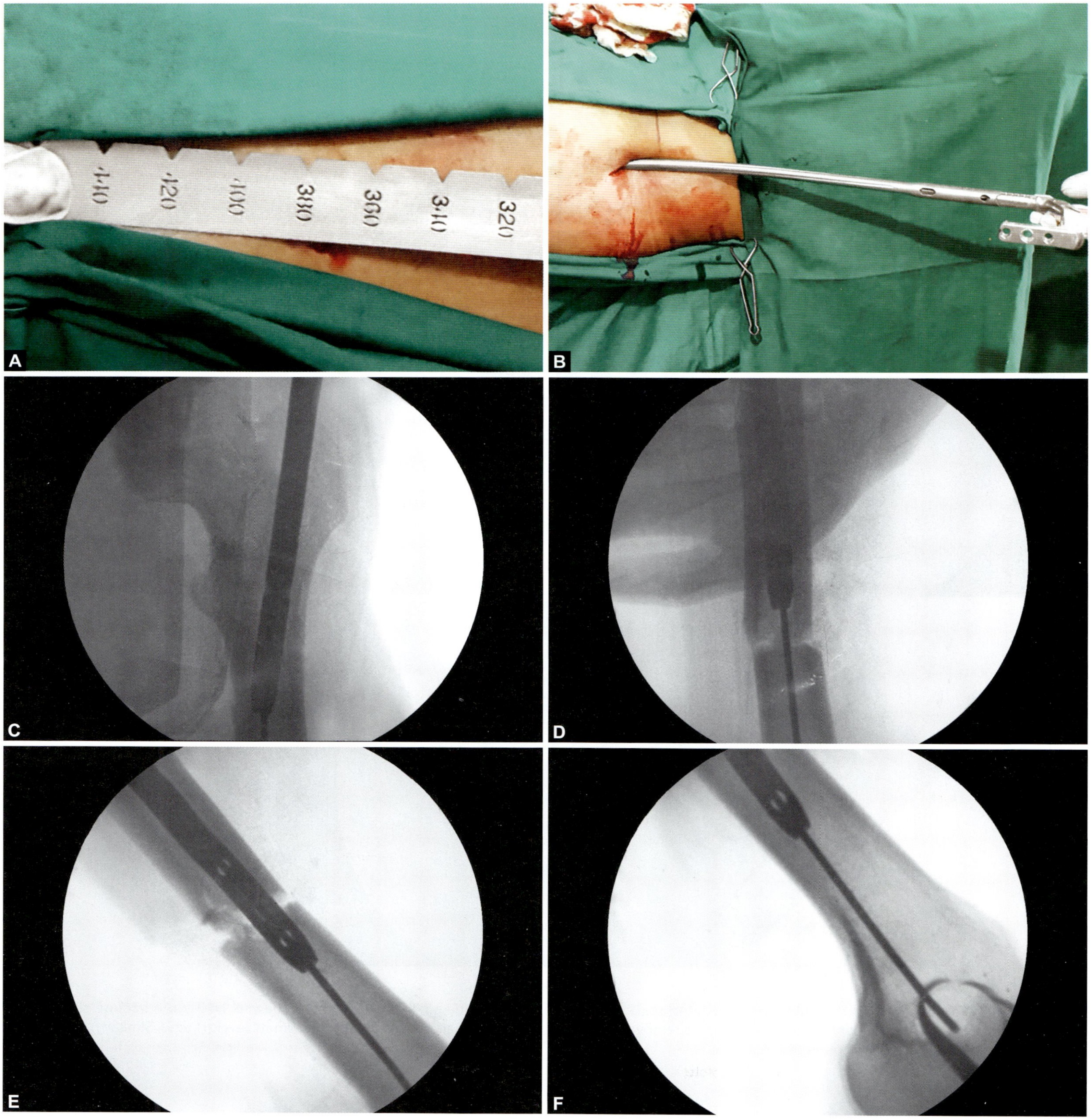

Figs. 8A to F

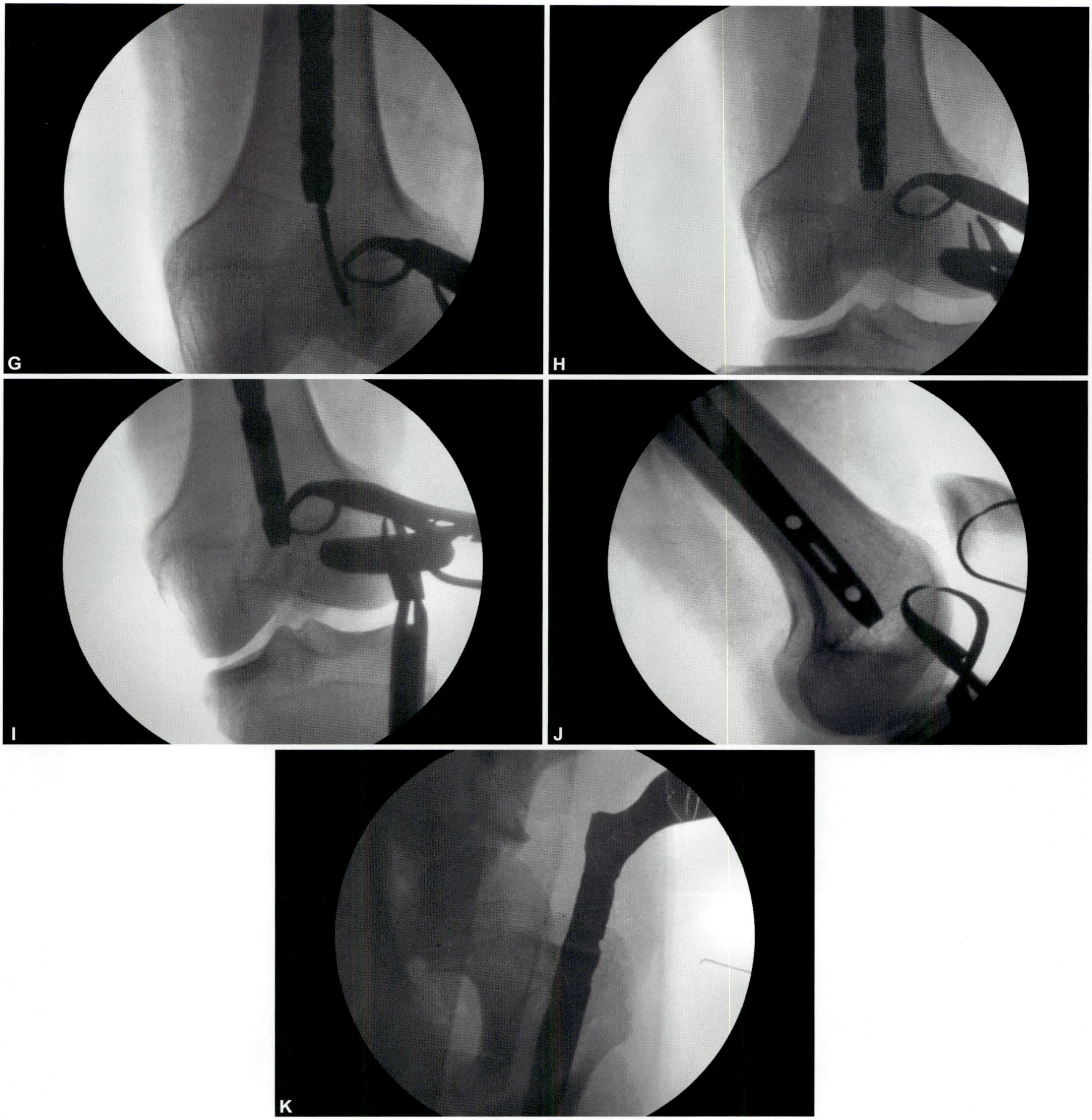

Figs. 8G to K

Figs. 8A to K: Measurement of nail length with measuring scale (A). Chosen nail is gently advanced over the guidewire, across the fracture site into the distal fragment under C-arm guidance (B to G). Guidewire removed and distal end of the nail is visualized to confirm its level (H to J). Similarly, the position of the proximal end of the nail is confirmed (K).

Step 9: Release of traction (in case of transverse fractures) to achieve intraoperative collapse (Fig. 9A), which is confirmed under C-arm (Fig. 9B).

Step 10: C-arm positioned to lateral view for distal locking (Fig. 10A). Lateral view should show distal lock holes as perfect circles (Fig. 10B).

Locating the hole with knife (Figs. 10C and D) and stab incision is taken (Fig. 10E).

Step 11: Drilling through both the cortices with the K-wire (Fig. 11A), checking on C-arm (Figs. 11B and C) and final drilling with 3.5-mm drill (Fig. 11D). Depth gauge being used to estimate the length of the bolt to be inserted (Fig. 11E). Bolt being inserted under C-arm guidance. Lateral view (Fig. 11F) and AP view (Fig. 11G).

The other distal locking bolt is put in a similar fashion (Figs. 11H to K).

Step 12: Reduction checked in AP (Fig. 12A) and lateral (Fig. 12B) before proximal locking. Impaction done in cases of transverse fractures.

Step 13: Proximal locking is done through dynamic hole with 4.9 mm bolt under C-arm guidance (Figs. 13A to F). Proximal locking may be done first as per surgeon's preference.

Step 14: Wound sutured in layers with 1-0 absorbable suture for fascia and subcutaneous tissue and 2-0 nonabsorbable nylon suture for skin closure (Figs. 14A and B).

Step 15: Postoperative X-ray AP view (Fig. 15A) and lateral view (Fig. 15B).

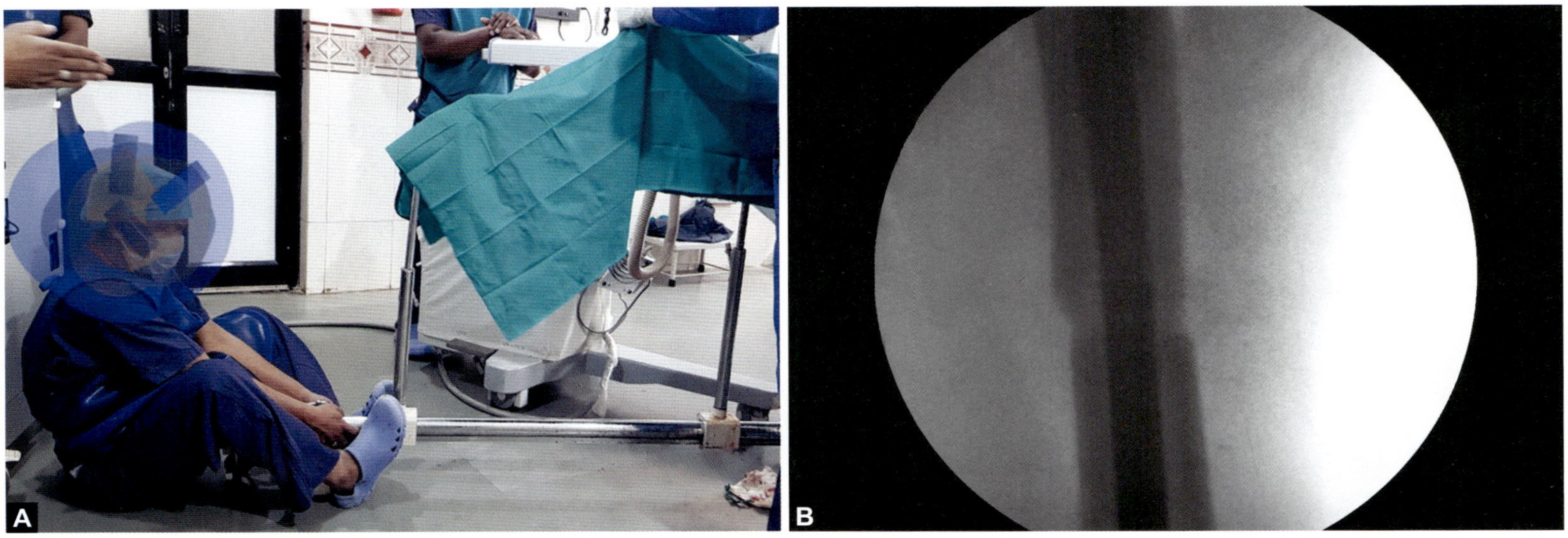

Figs. 9A and B: Release of traction and C-arm confirmation of collapse at fracture site.

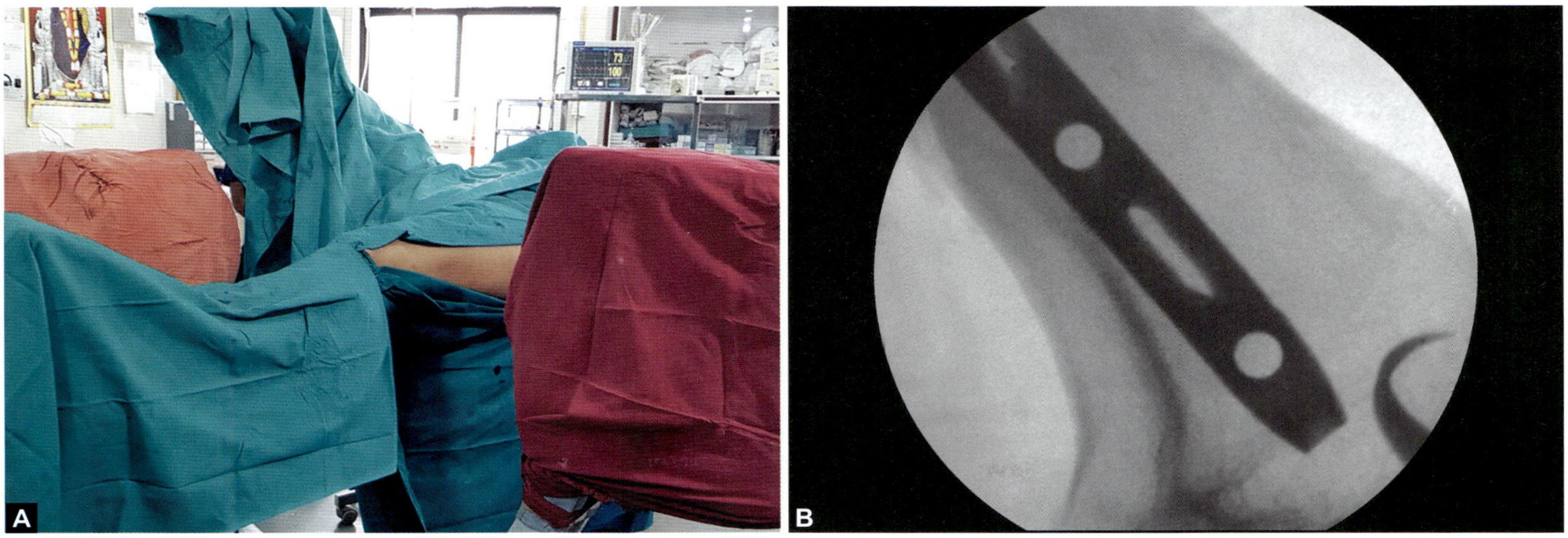

Figs. 10A and B: C-arm positioned to lateral view for distal locking (A). Lateral view should show distal lock holes as perfect circles (B).

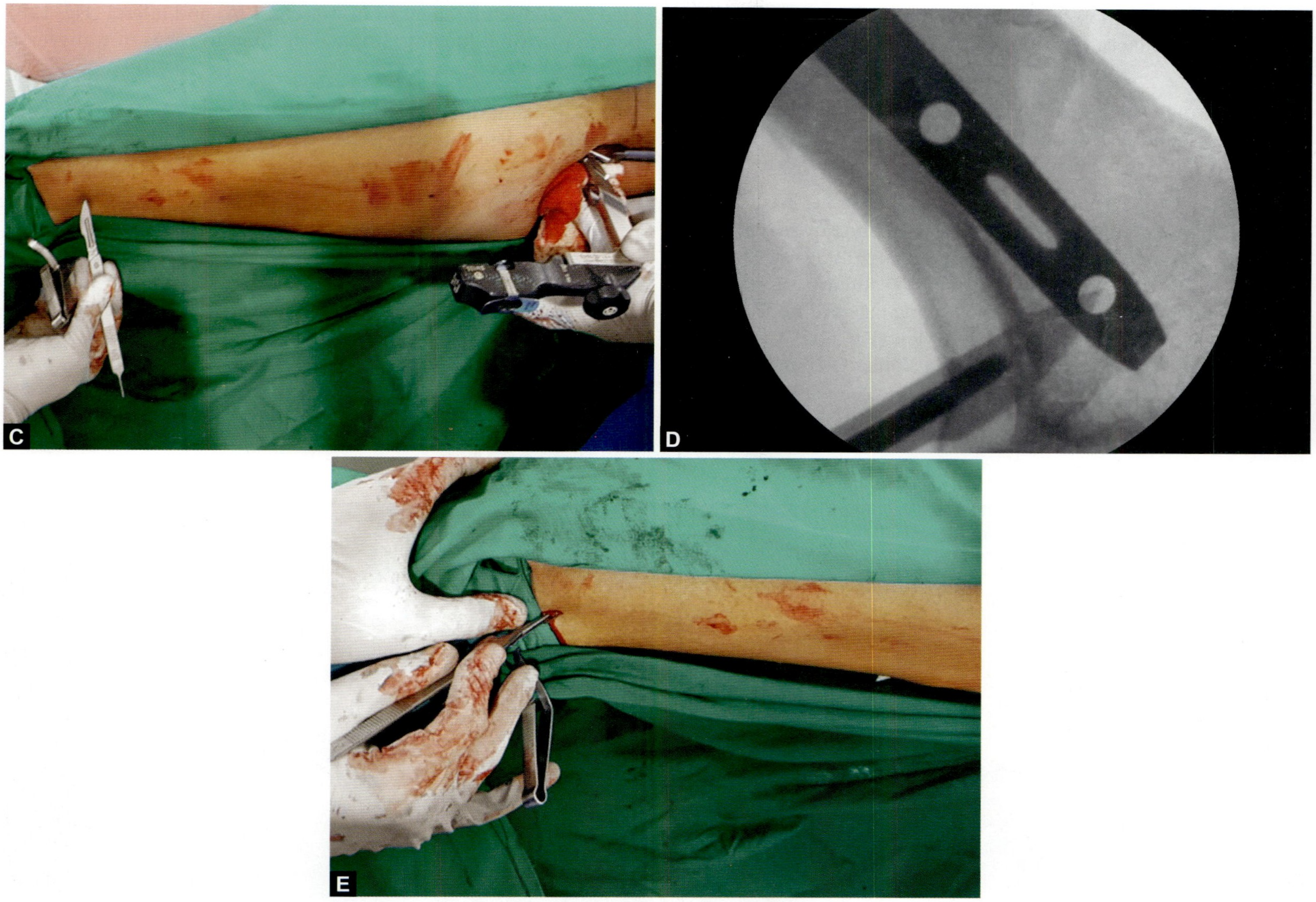

Figs. 10C to E: Locating the hole with knife (C and D) and stab incision is taken (E).

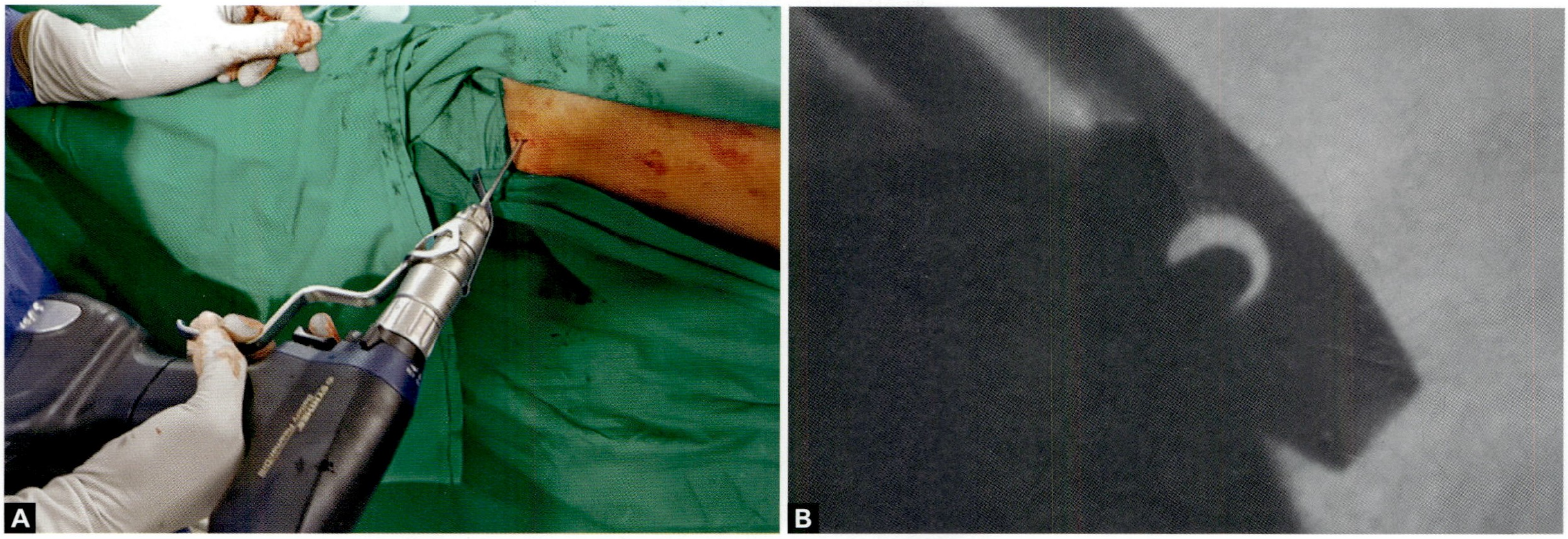

Figs. 11A and B: Drilling with K-wire.

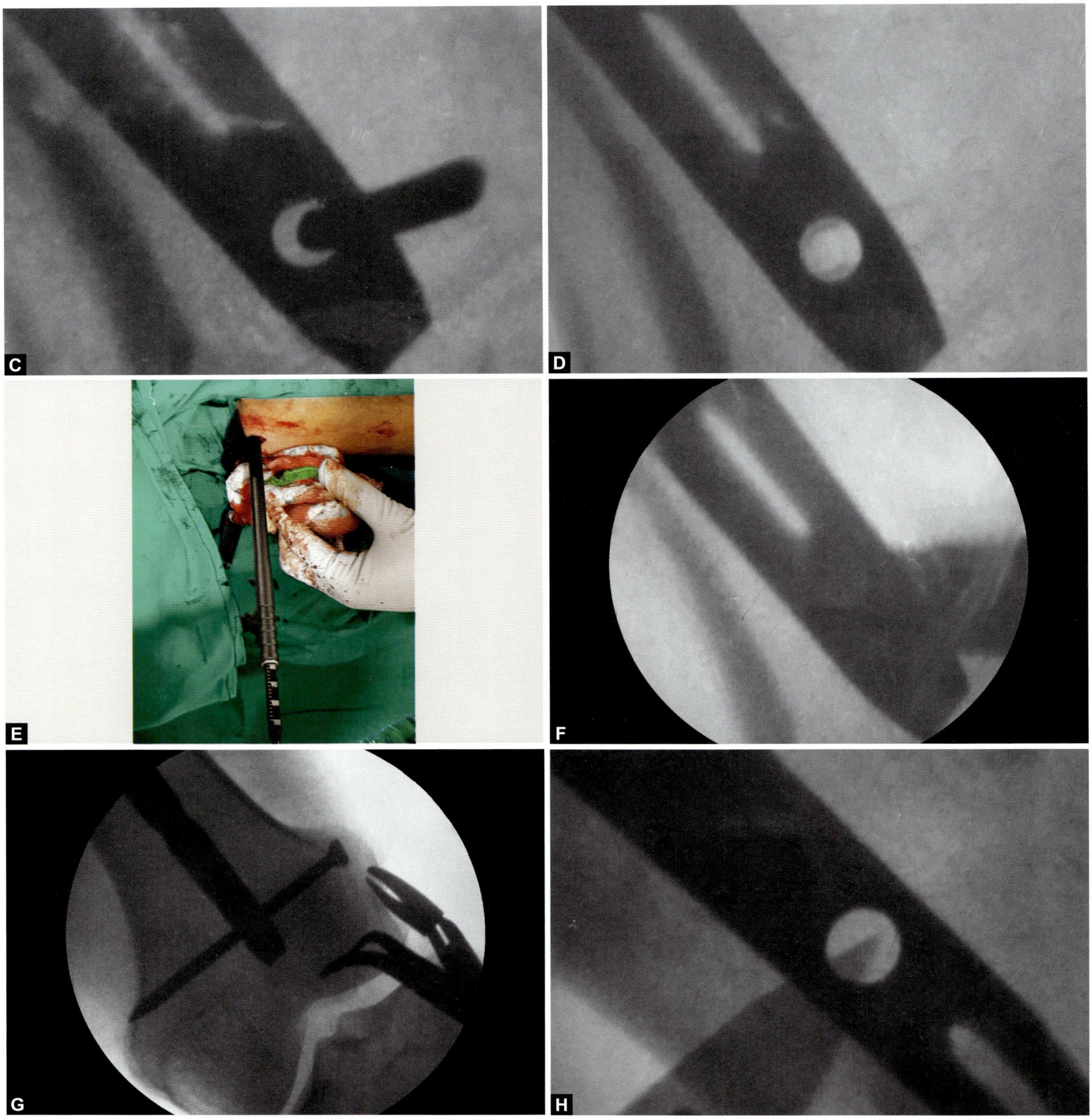

Figs. 11C to H: Bolt insertion after measuring depth.

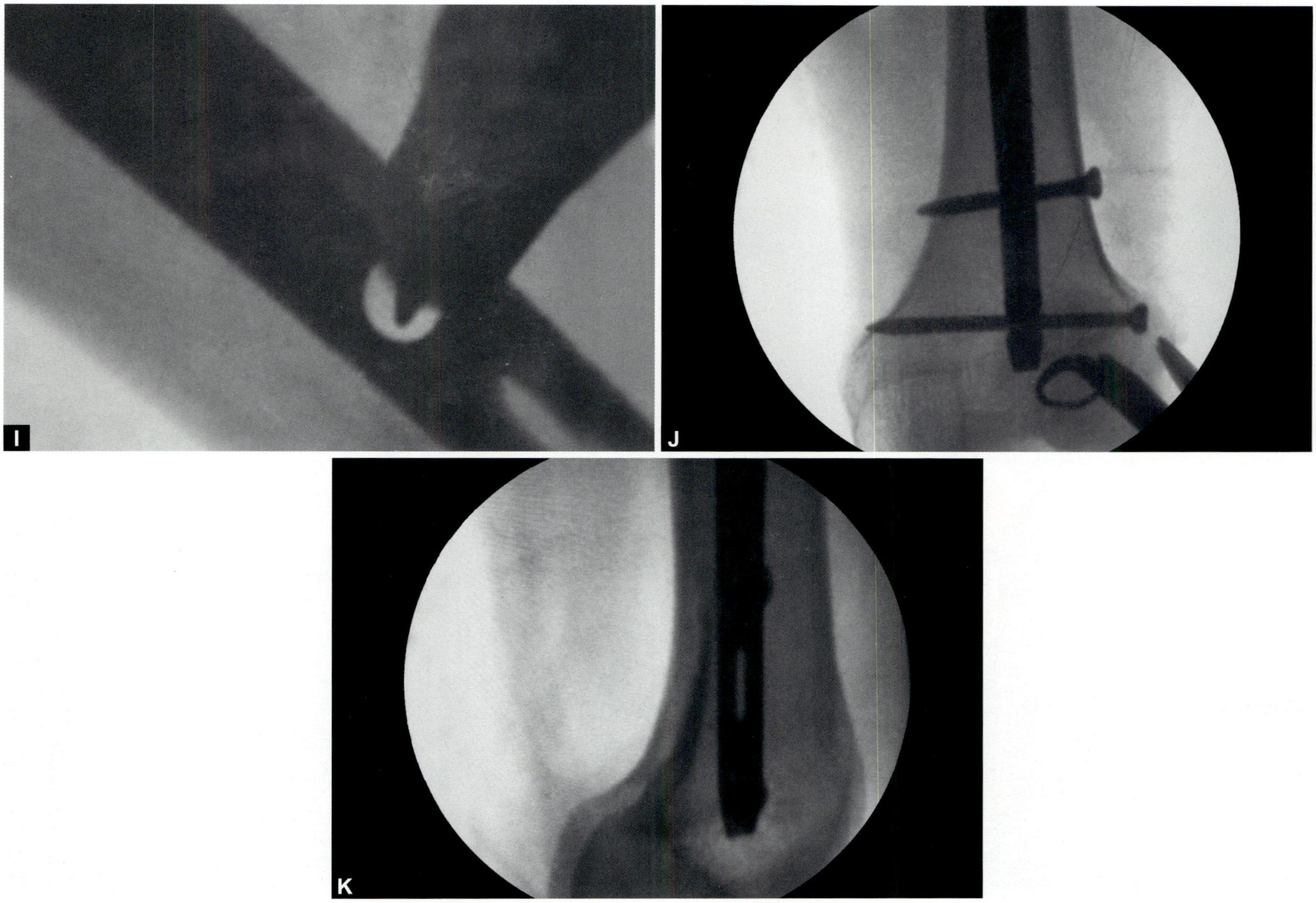

Figs. 11I to K: The other distal locking bolt is inserted in a similar fashion.

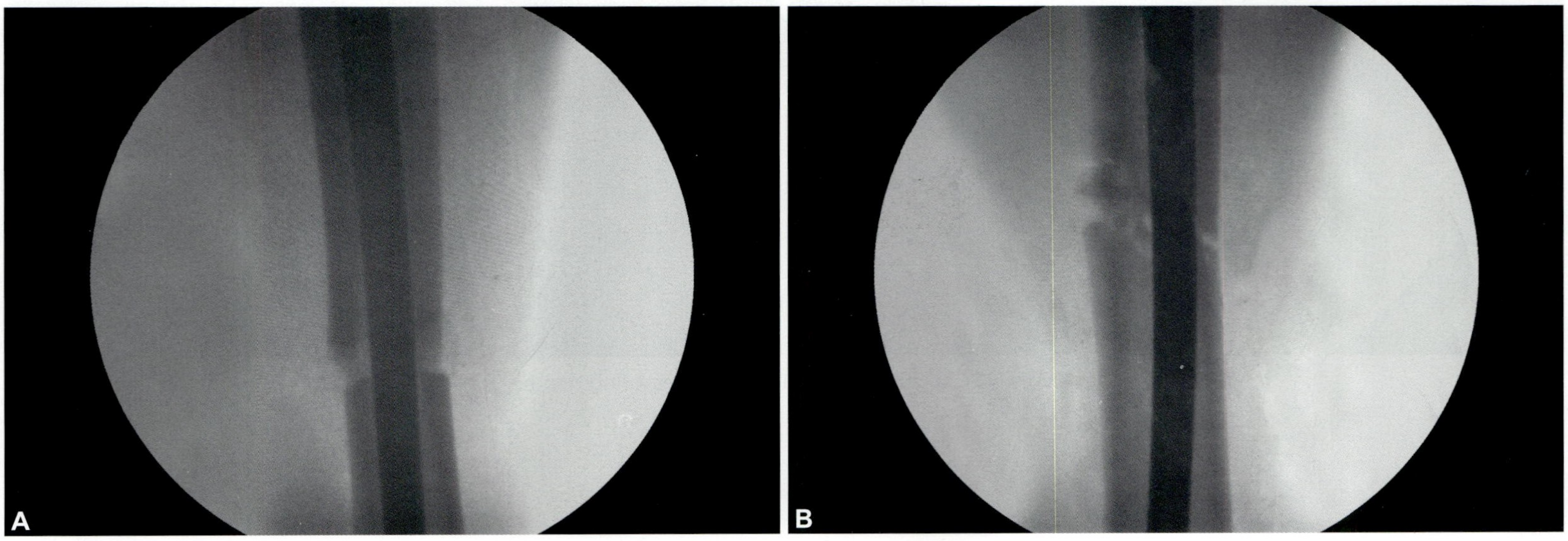

Figs. 12A and B: Reduction checked in AP (A) and lateral (B) before proximal locking. Impaction done in cases of transverse fractures.

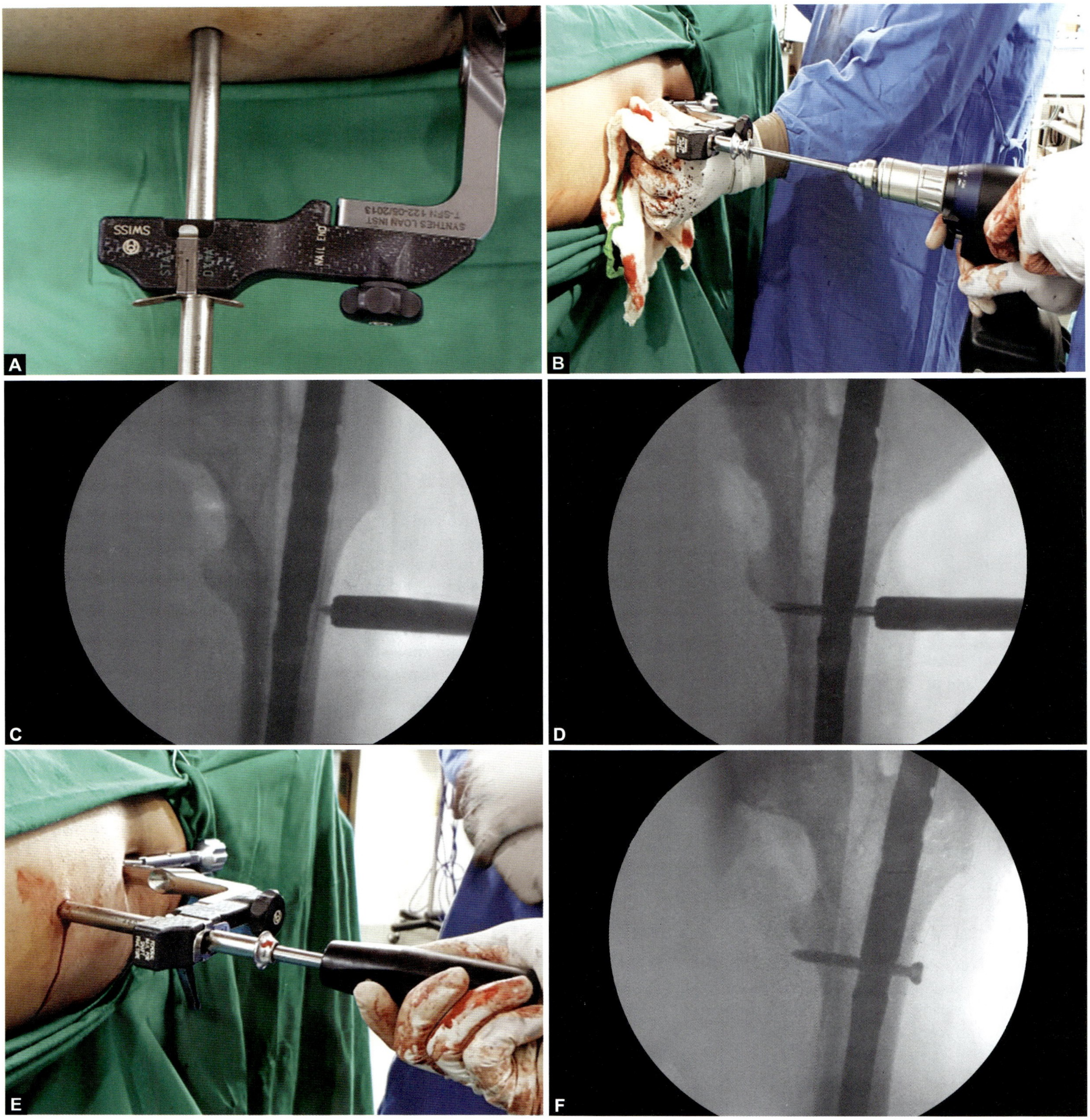

Figs. 13A to F: Proximal locking is performed.

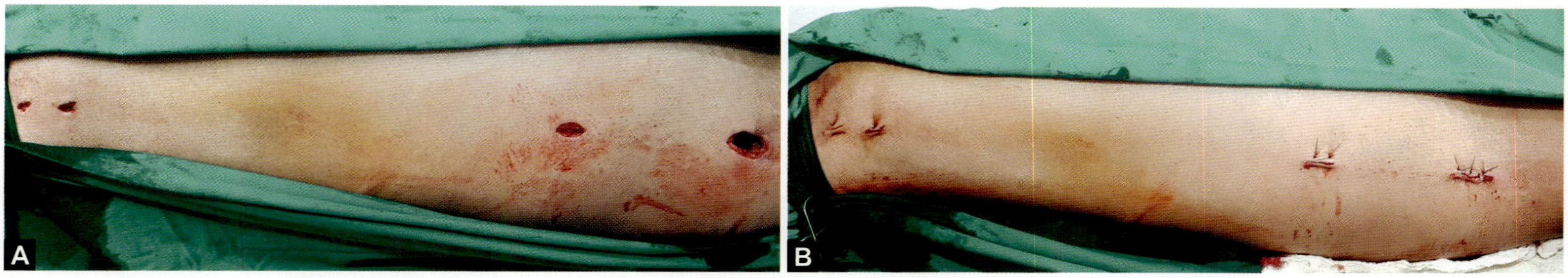

Figs. 14A and B: Closure in layers.

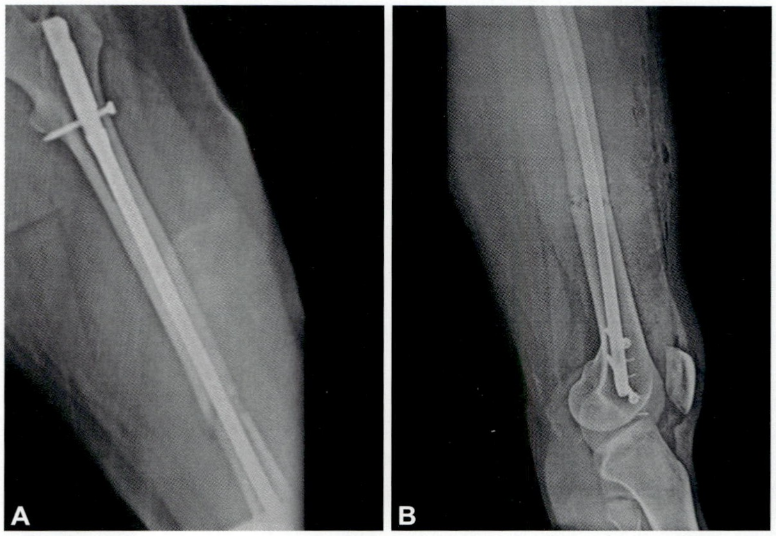

Figs. 15A and B: Postoperative radiograph showing satisfactory position of fracture and implant.

SUMMARY

Closed reduction and interlocking nailing is a very effective and less traumatic technique for any fracture shaft femur with very good results.

POSTOPERATIVE PROTOCOL

- Range of motion exercises for knee and hip joint without weight bearing may be started on the 1st postoperative day.
- Nonweight-bearing mobilization using crutches or walker can be started within a few days postoperatively. Partial weight bearing may be commenced depending on stability of fixation and degree of comminution and bone loss at the fracture site.
- Surgical dressings to be changed on 5th postoperative day.
- In case of immobilized patient (e.g. due to contralateral injuries or pelvic or spinal trauma) thromboembolism prophylaxis should be considered.

POSSIBLE COMPLICATIONS

- Hypovolemic shock, which may be fatal if not compensated in a timely manner
- Neurovascular injury
- Iatrogenic perforation to anterior or posterior cortex of femoral shaft due to misdirected reamer or entry awl
- Infection and implant failure
- Malunion/nonunion
- Fat embolism syndrome.

SUGGESTED READING

1. Bhandari M, Guyatt G, Khera V, et al. Operative management of lower extremity fractures in patients with head injuries. Clin Orthop. 2003;407:187-98.
2. Henry S, Seligson D. Ipsilateral femoral neck-shaft fractures: a comparison of therapeutic devices. Orthop Trans. 1990;14:269.
3. Nowotarski PJ, Turen CH, Brumback RJ, et al. Conversion of external fixation to intramedullary nailing for fractures of the shaft of the femur in multiply injured patients. J Bone Joint Surg Am. 2000;82:781-8.
4. Perren S, Claes L. Biology and biomechanics in fracture management. AO principles of fracture management. New York: Thieme; 2000. pp. 7-30.
5. Russell TA. Intramedullary nailing: evolutions of femoral intramedullary nailing: first to fourth generations. J Orthop Trauma. 2011;25(Suppl 3): S135-8.

CHAPTER 108

Supracondylar Fracture Femur: Locked Plate Fixation

Sarang Kasture, Vijay M Panchanadikar, Shrinivas S Shintre

INTRODUCTION

Bimodal distribution is seen in distal femur fractures. These occur in young adults after high-energy trauma and in elderly osteoporotic individuals after low-energy trauma. With increase in number of joint replacements periprosthetic distal femur fractures have become increasingly common.

SURGICAL ANATOMY

Distal femur is peculiar in terms of its trapezoidal shape in cross-section. Medial condyle extends more distal compared to lateral condyle and anatomical axis is 6–7° valgus. Gastrocnemius pull causes apex posterior deformity, extensors and hamstrings cause shortening while adductors cause varus deformity in supracondylar fractures.

PRESENTATION

These fractures present as pain swelling and deformity in the distal thigh region. One has to assess the distal perfusion and pulse as there is possibility of injury to popliteal vessels in severely displaced fractures.

IMAGING

Standard anteroposterior (AP) and lateral radiographs are mandatory. Traction views could be obtained to better assess the fracture pattern but are difficult to obtain because of pain. Computed tomography (CT) scan is indicated to assess intra-articular extension, establish osteochondral fragments, and identify coronal plane fracture (Hoffa fracture). Angiography is indicated, if popliteal vessel injury is suspected.

CLASSIFICATION

Descriptive classification includes supracondylar and intercondylar variants. OTA classifies distal femur fracture as 33 A, B, and C (extra-articular, partial articular, and complete articular, respectively).

TREATMENT

Undisplaced fractures can be treated nonoperatively in a cast or knee brace with immediate mobilization. Operative treatment is invariably preferred method in displaced fractures. Knee spanning external fixator can be used as a damage control tool in unstable or polytrauma patient. Displaced fractures with intra-articular extension are treated with open reduction and internal fixation with plate screw assembly, while extra-articular fractures in an osteoporotic bone could be treated with distal femur intramedullary nail.

OPERATIVE STEPS (FIGS. 1 TO 25)

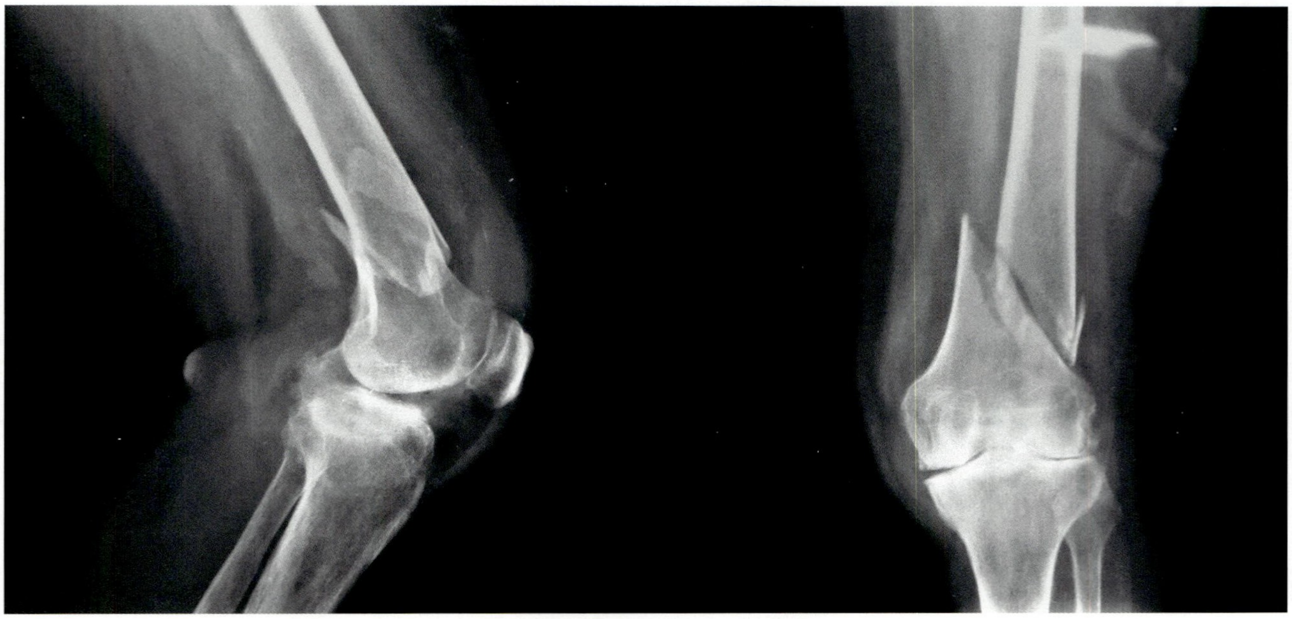

Fig. 1: Preoperative radiograph. AO A3 fracture (extra-articular with comminution).

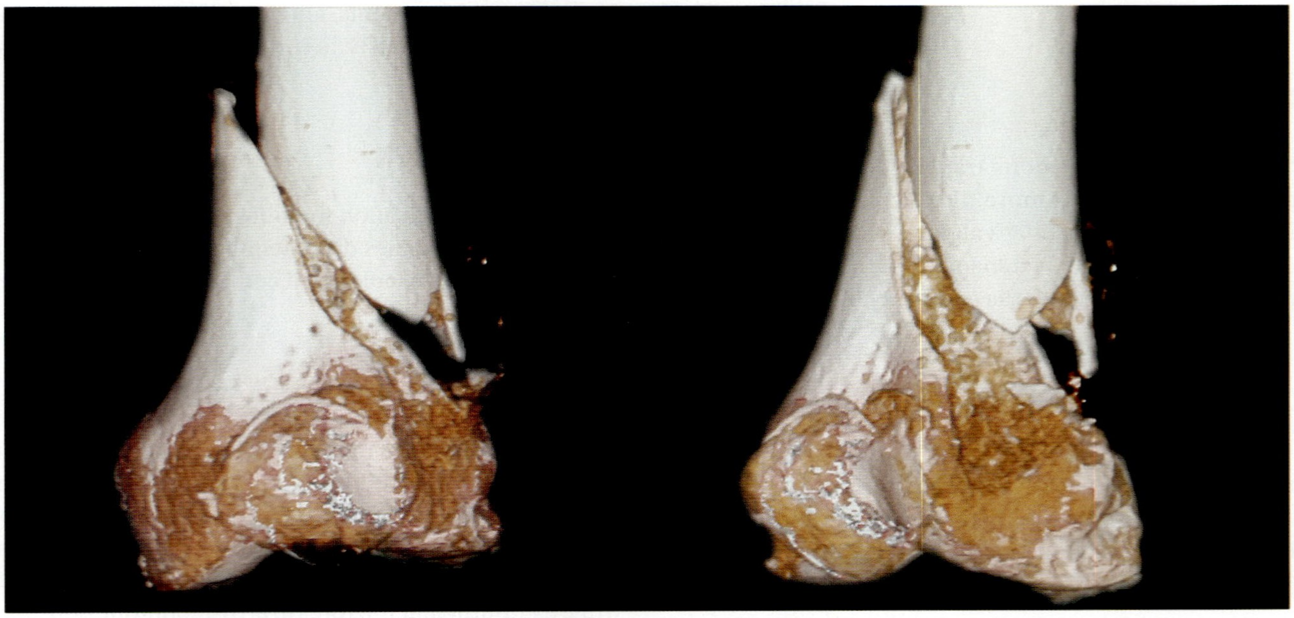

Fig. 2: Three dimensional (3D) reconstruction computed tomography (CT) images.

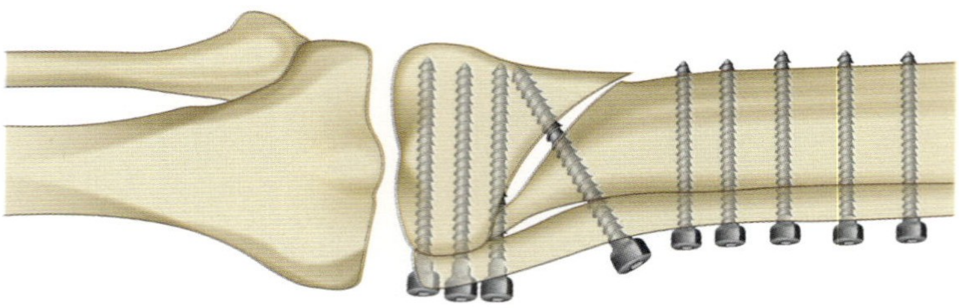

Fig. 3: Schematic representation of the plan of fixation. Interfragmentary screw with a neutralization locking plate to provide a rigid fixation.

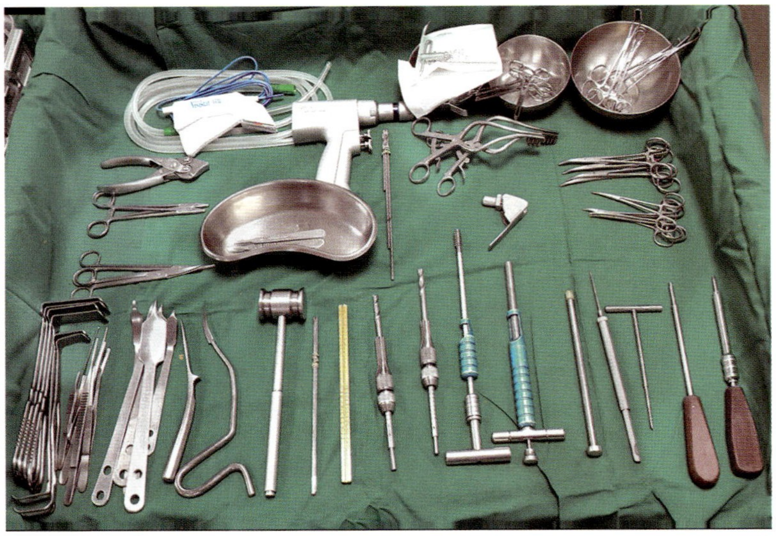

Fig. 4: Instrumentation.

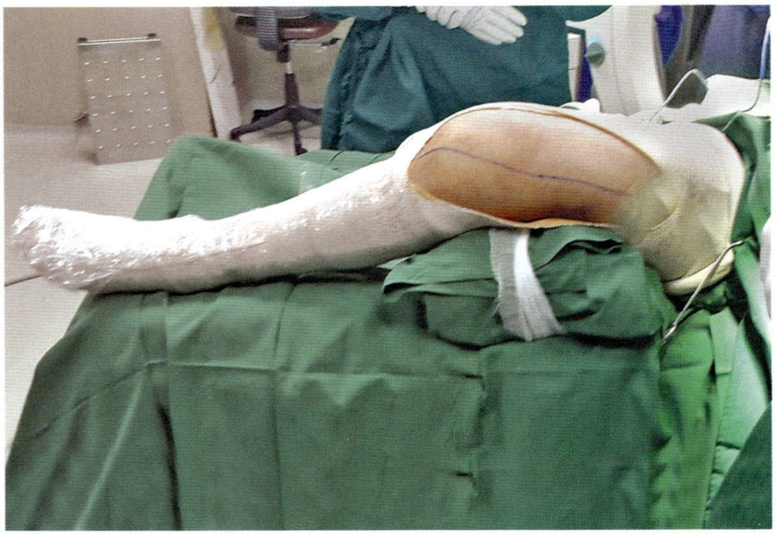

Fig. 5: Patient position. Flexion at the knee with a bolster to facilitate maneuvering reduction as well as relax the posterior neurovascular structures.

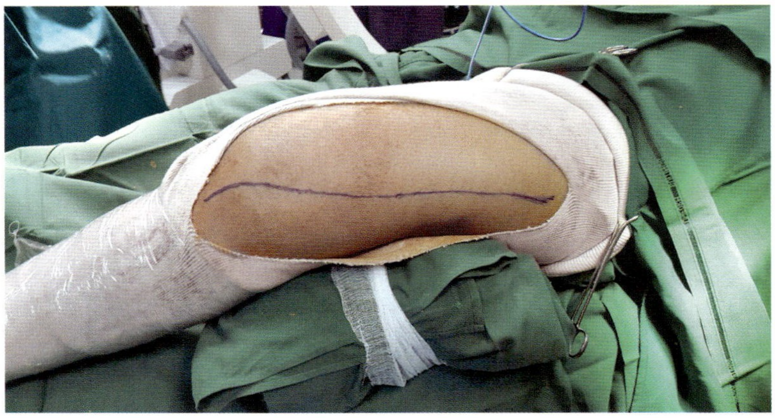

Fig. 6: Planned incision. Anterolateral approach. Skin incision starts proximally depending on the most proximal extent of the fracture in mid-lateral line of the femoral shaft. It curves anteriorly over the lateral femoral condyle, toward the tibial tubercle, if arthrotomy is required.

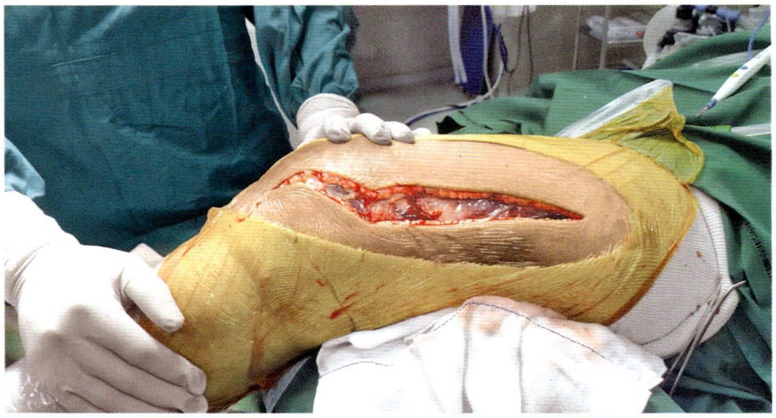

Fig. 7: Skin incision.

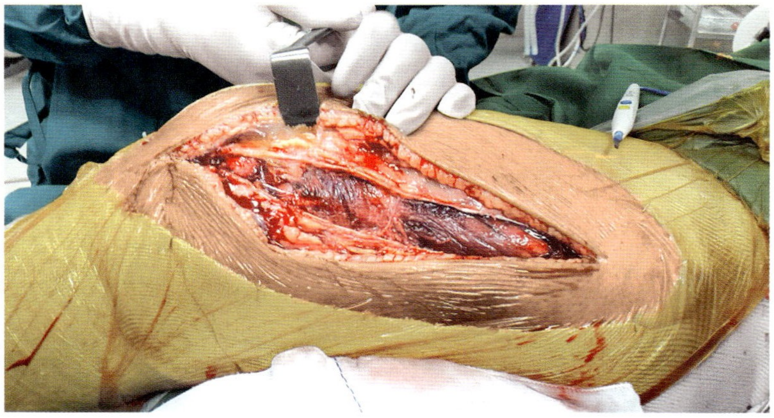

Fig. 8: Division of the iliotibial band in line with the skin incision.

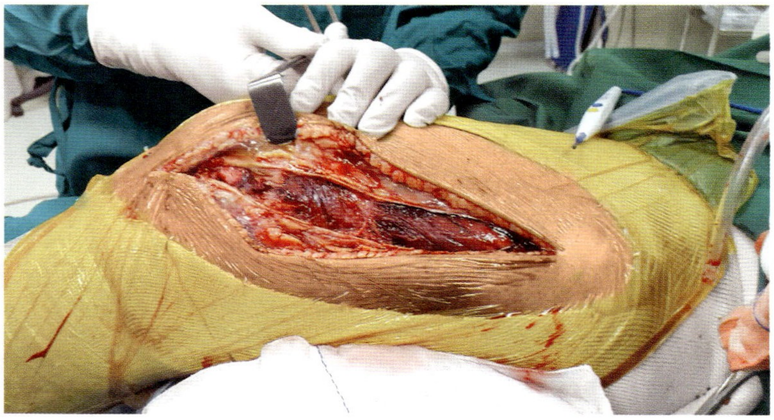

Fig. 9: Vastus lateralis exposed which needs anteromedial elevation to expose the fracture site. Several perforates may be encountered, which need ligating to avoid excessive bleeding.

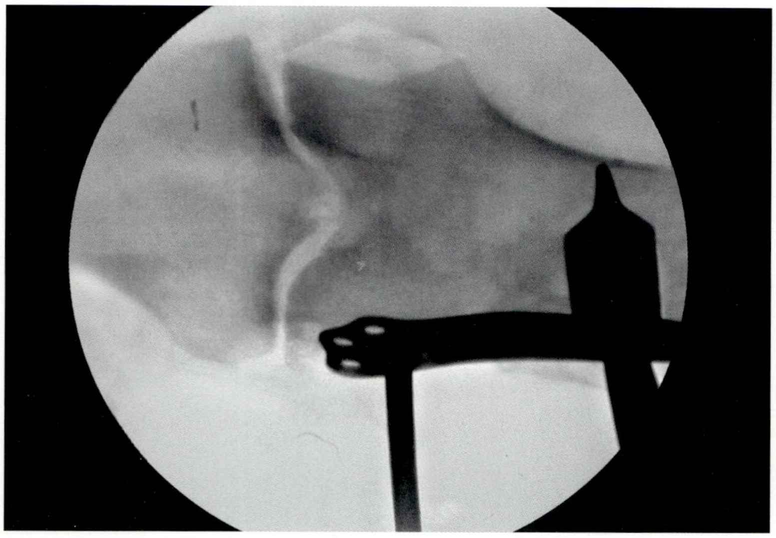

Fig. 10: Reduction achieved by traction and manipulation and broad Hohmann retractor to reduce the medial spike of the fracture.

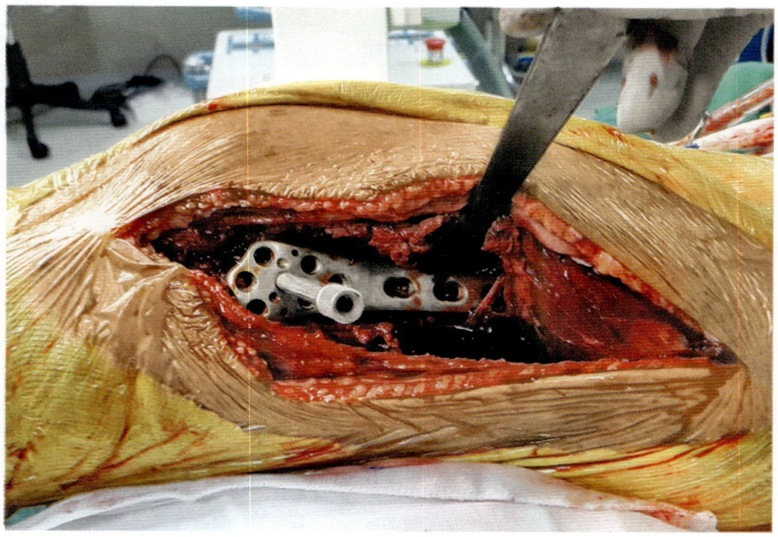

Fig. 11: Distal femur locking compression plate (LCP) plate is used for fixation. The locking guide can be used to hold and position the plate.

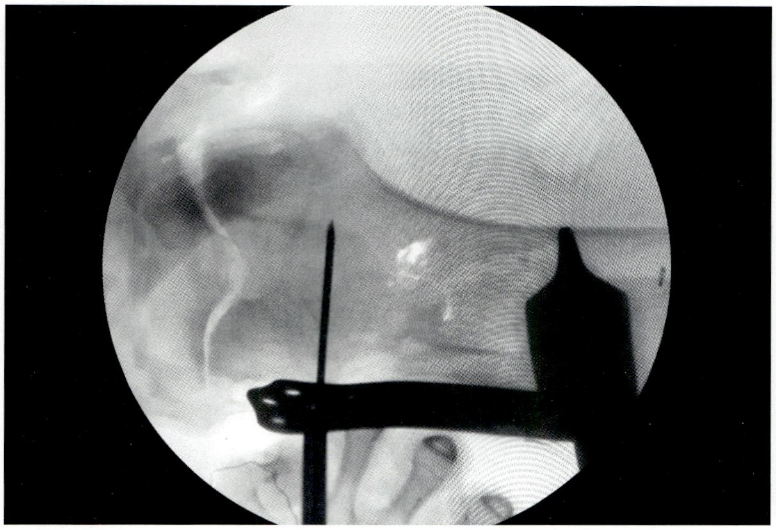

Fig. 12: Place a temporary K-wire to position the plate. This should be parallel to the articular surface in coronal and axial planes. Another K-wire could also be placed as a guide in the anterior aspect parallel to the trochlear surface of the patellofemoral joint.

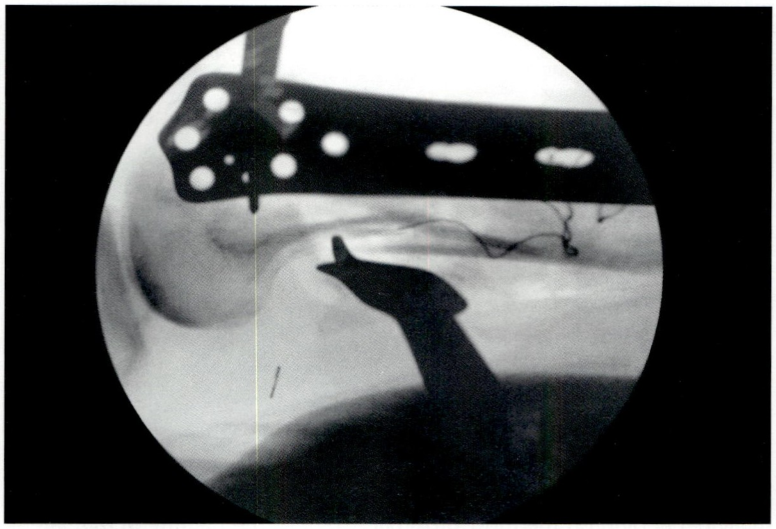

Fig. 13: Ensure proper and central placement of the plate over the condyle by taking anteroposterior (AP) and lateral views. Here, the reduction is secured by Hohmann retractor placed posteriorly (to reduce the flexed distal fragment) and anteromedially to reduce the medial spike of the distal fragment.

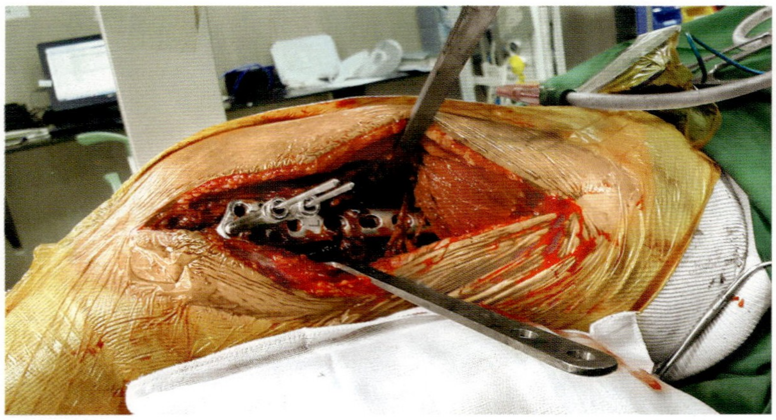

Fig. 14: Guidewires/K-wires placed in the two distal holes of the plate.

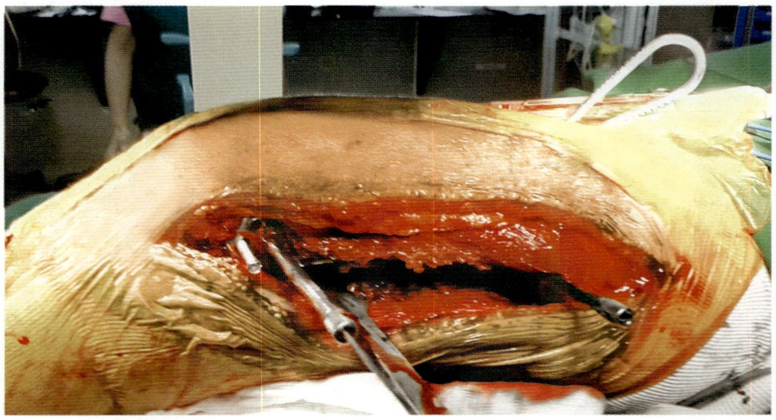

Fig. 15: Two distal locking screws placed. Ensure reduction is maintained. Also ensure proper placement of the plate over the proximal fragment. Locking sleeve inserted in the proximal locking hole is used to maneuver the plate.

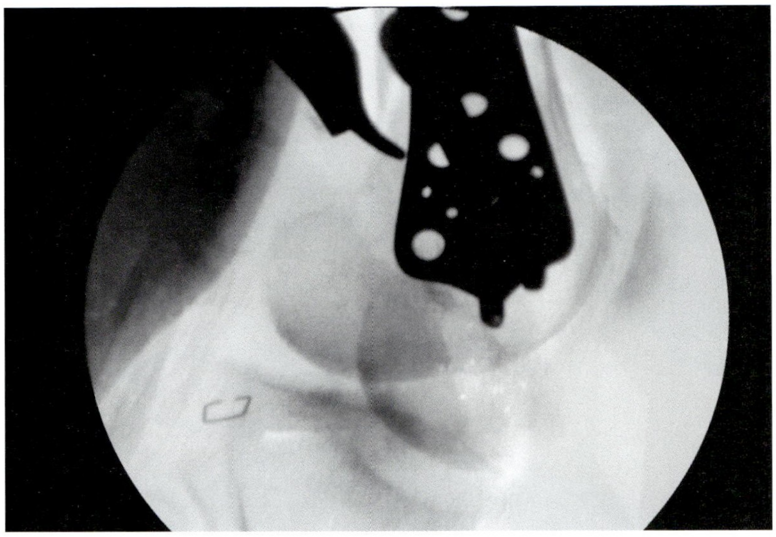

Fig. 16: Proper placement of the plate with two locking screws. Ensure reduction is maintained.

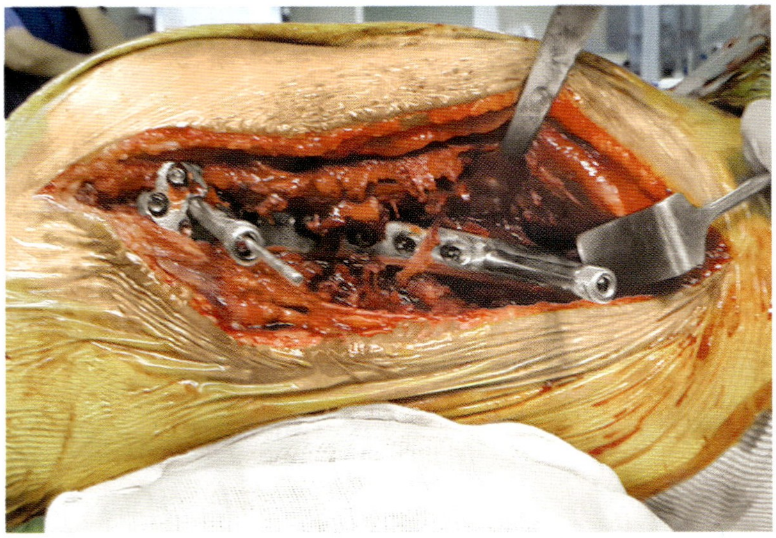

Fig. 17: Third distal locking screw applied.

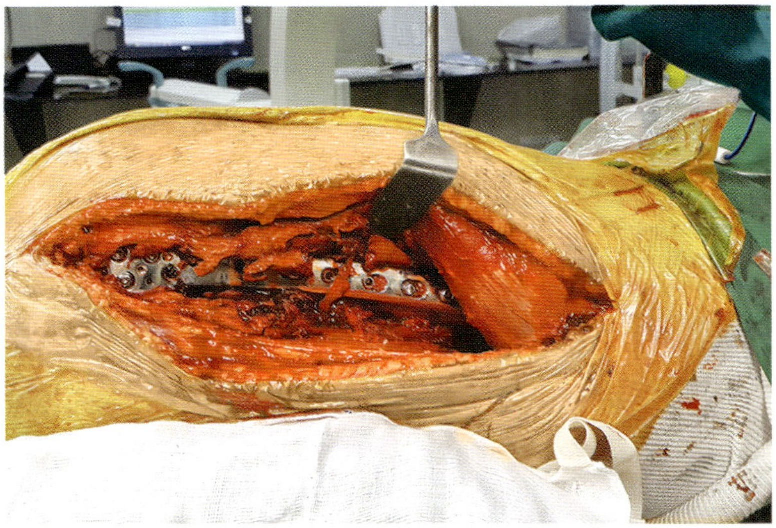

Fig. 18: Condyles then reduced to the shaft and proximal screws applied with an interfragmentary screw through the plate. First proximal screw may be cortex screw to pull bone to plate. Lateral C-arm view is now taken after this provisional fixation to note and correct sagittal malalignment, if any. Some earlier applied screws may have to be loosened for this step. Remaining locking screws are applied.

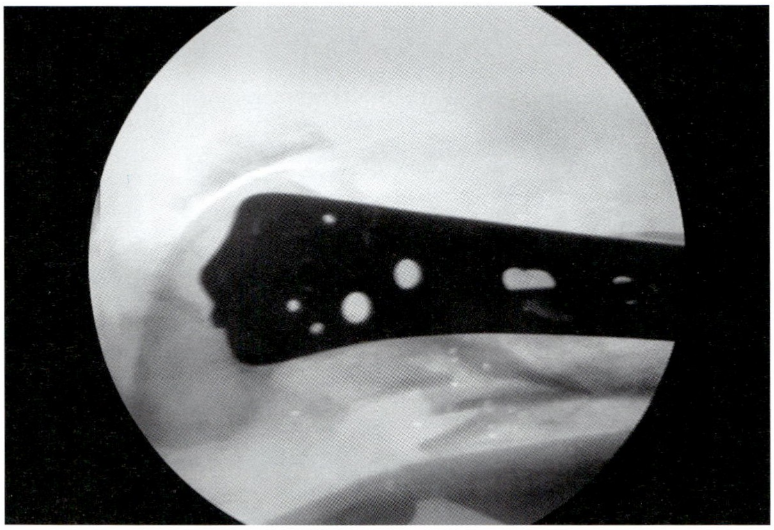

Fig. 19: Lateral view after fixation.

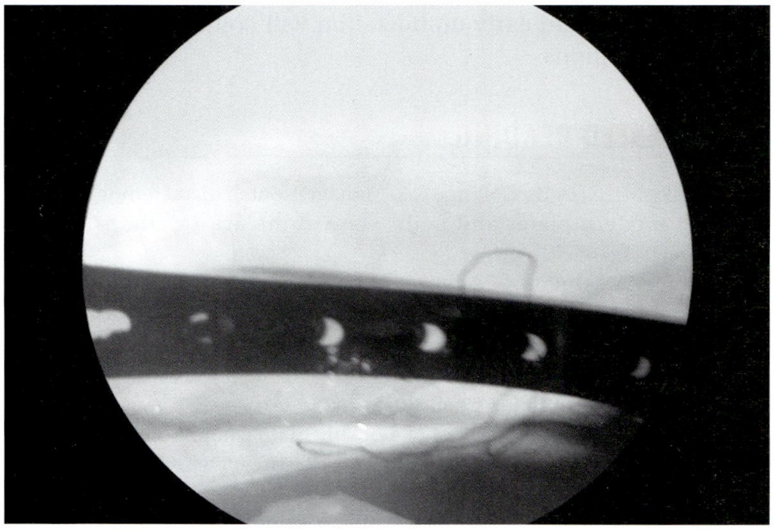

Fig. 20: Lateral view of the proximal fragment.

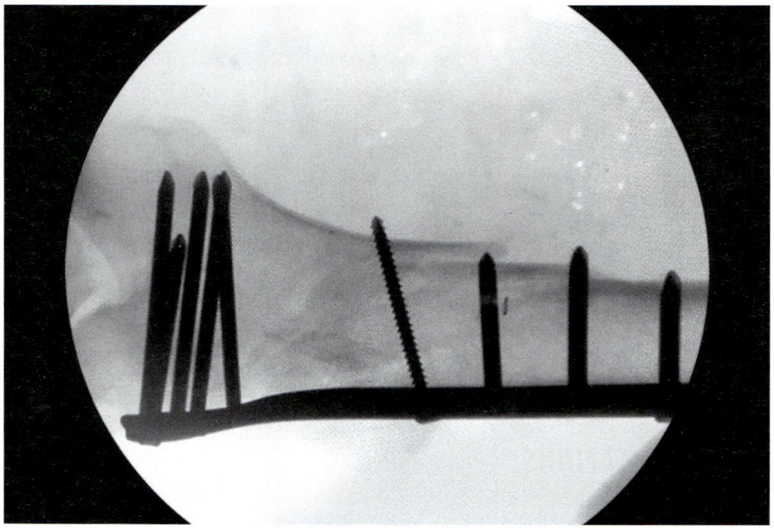

Fig. 21: Anteroposterior (AP) view of the fracture after fixation.

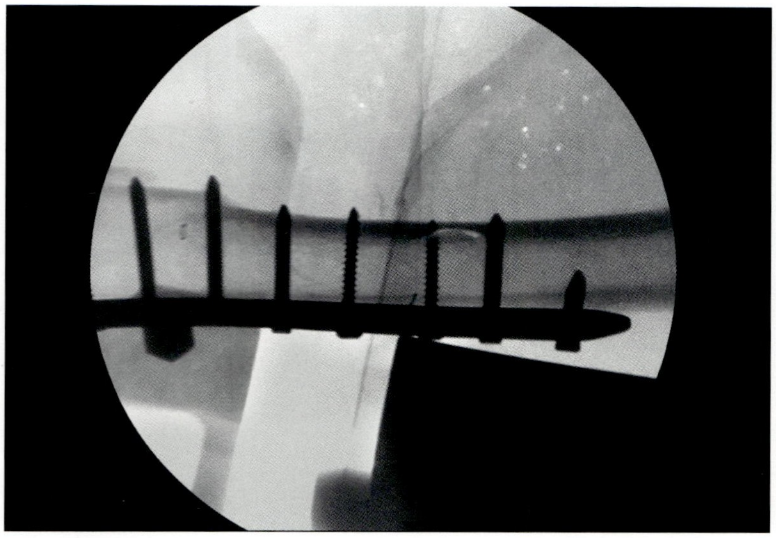

Fig. 22: Anteroposterior (AP) view of the proximal fragment. Note use of unicortical proximal locking screw to prevent stress riser at the proximal end of the plate. Some screw holes are better left unfilled.

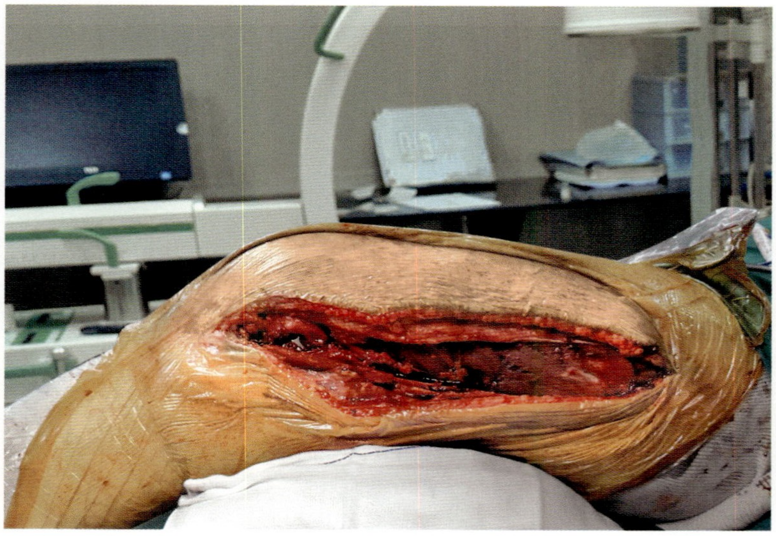

Fig. 23: Vastus lateralis covers the plate.

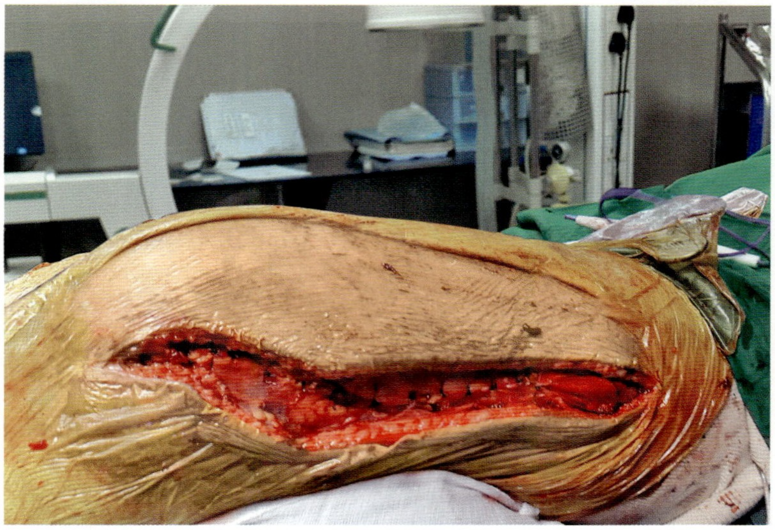

Fig. 24: Closure of iliotibial band.

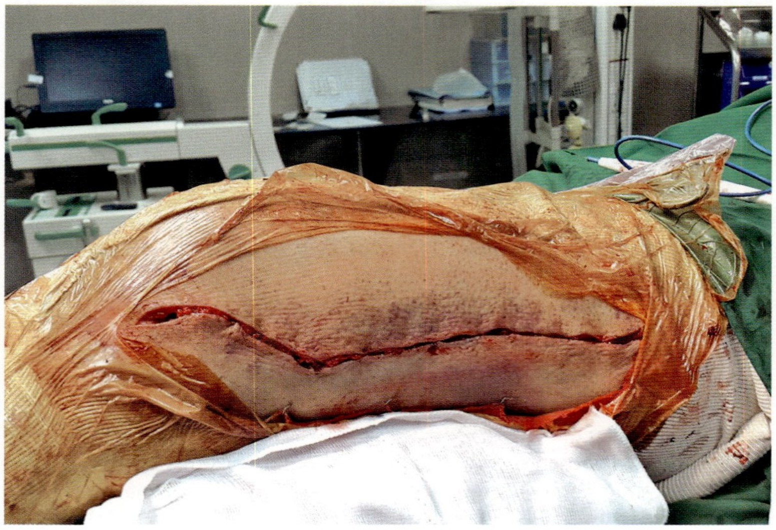

Fig. 25: Subcutaneous closure.

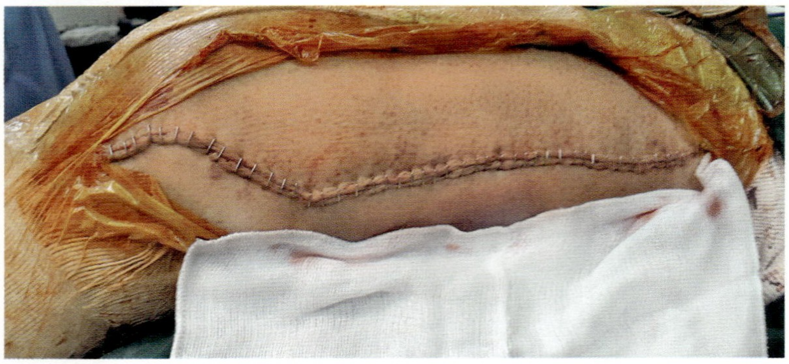

Fig. 26: Clips to the skin.

COMPLICATIONS

Possible complications include knee stiffness and malunion with later osteoarthritis of knee joint. Optimum joint surface restoration, strong fixation, and early mobilization will contribute to prevent these complications.

SUGGESTED READING

1. Beltran MJ, Gary JL, Collinge CA. Management of distal femur fractures with modern plates and nails: state of the art. J Orthop Trauma. 2015;29(4):165-72.
2. Ehlinger M, Ducrot G, Adam P, et al. Distal femur fractures. Surgical techniques and a review of the literature. Orthop Traumatol Surg Res. 2013;99(3):353-60.
3. Link BC, Babst R. Current concepts in fractures of the distal femur. Acta Chir Orthop Traumatol Cech. 2012;79(1):11-20.
4. Toro G, Calabrò G, Toro A, et al. Locking plate fixation of distal femoral fractures is a challenging technique: a retrospective review. Clin Cases Miner Bone Metab. 2015;12(Suppl 1):55-8.
5. Von Keudell A, Shoji K, Nasr M, et al. Treatment options for distal femur fractures. J Orthop Trauma. 2016;30 Suppl 2:S25-7.

CHAPTER 109

Hoffa Fracture: Buttress Plate Fixation

Vijay M Panchanadikar, Shrinivas S Shintre, Chandrashekhar Sathaye

INTRODUCTION

These are essentially coronal plane fractures of medial or lateral femoral condyle and may occur as either isolated or as a part of comminuted distal femoral fracture.

These fractures are at times difficult to diagnose on standard X-rays, hence computed tomography (CT) scan assessment is essential.

Treatment of these fractures is invariably surgical, in order to restore knee anatomy and function and to prevent future instability and osteoarthritis.

With minimally invasive technique, one may not be able to achieve a perfect anatomical reduction, so open reduction under direct vision is recommended.

Most of the times, these fractures are approached by lateral or medial parapatellar approach except posterior marginal fractures, which need to be approached posteriorly.

Fixation is by minimum two lag (cancellous) screws of 6.5-, 3.5-, or 4-mm diameter supplemented often by headless screws/small buttress plates (Fig. 1).

CLASSIFICATION (AO/OTA)

- *33-B3.1*: Flake lateral/anterior
- *33-B3.2*: Unicondylar posterior
- *33-B3.3*: Bicondylar posterior (Fig. 2).

DIFFICULTIES DURING SURGERY

- These are difficult fractures to expose and reduce.
- Ideal screw position may be difficult to achieve.

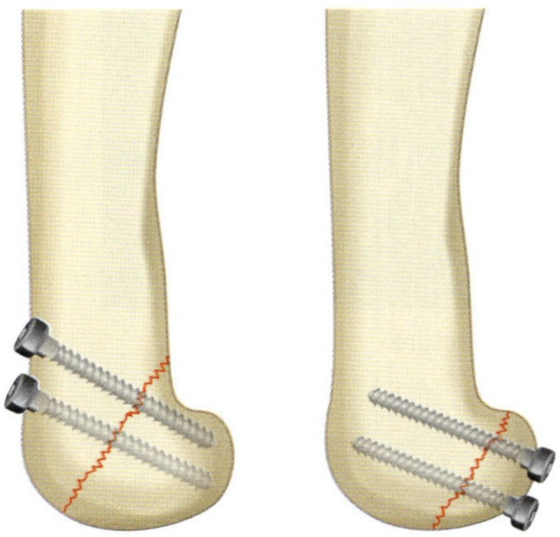

Fig. 1: Fixation plan: minimum two lag screws of 6.5, 3.5 or 4 mm diameter.

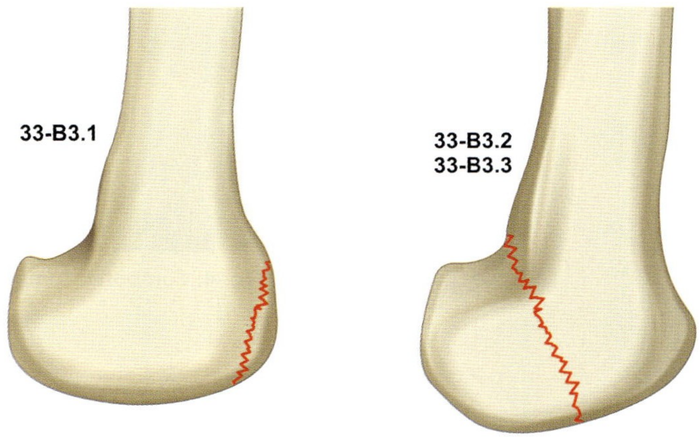

Fig. 2: AO/OTA classification.

SURGICAL STEPS (FIGS. 3 TO 21)

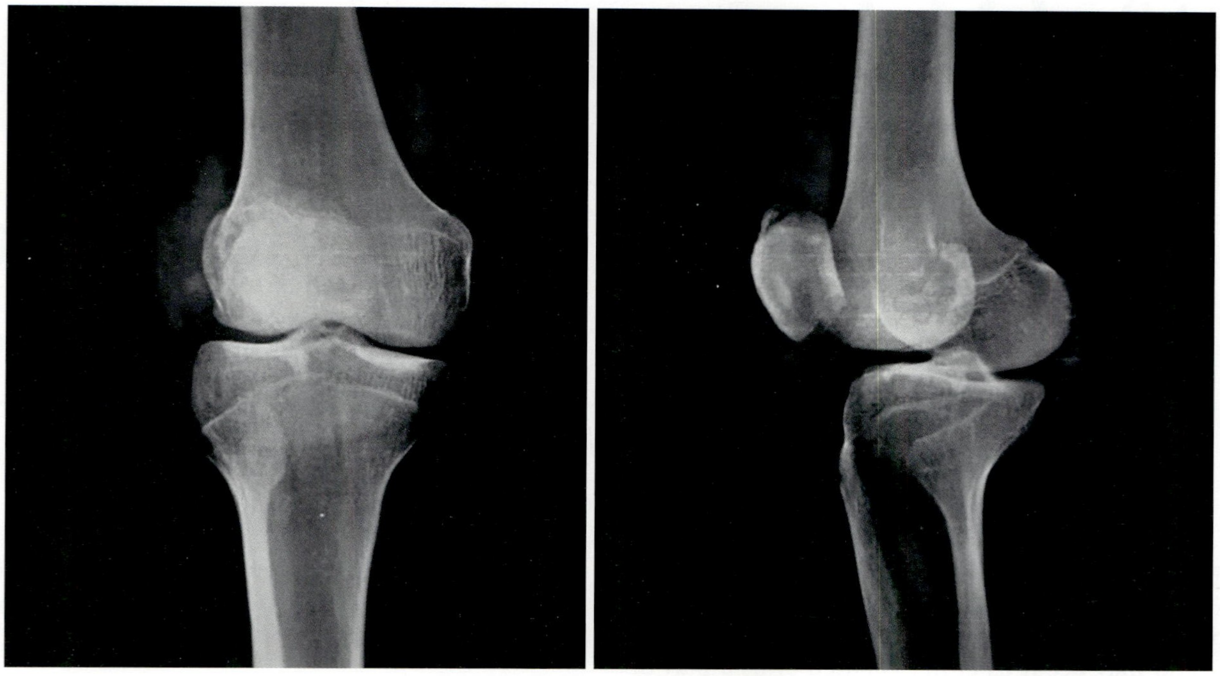

Fig. 3: X-rays: Fracture is barely seen.

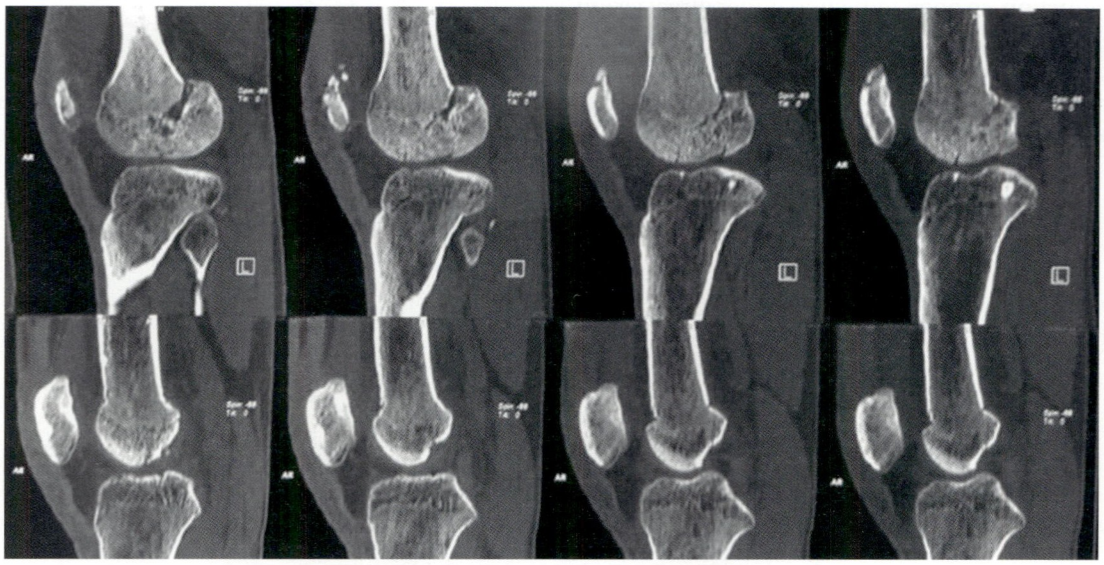

Fig. 4: Computed tomography (CT) scan clearly shows fracture.

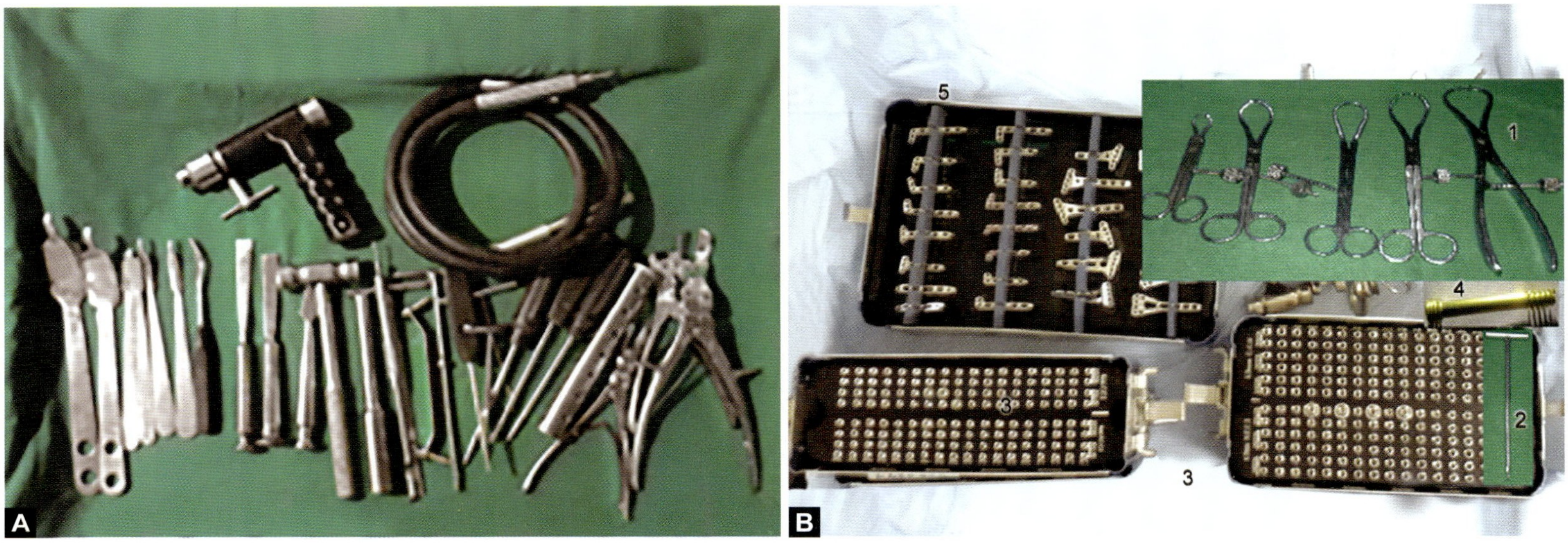

Figs. 5A and B: General/special instruments. (1) Reduction clamps, (2) Countersink, (3) Screw set CCS 4 and 6.5 mm 16, 32 mm thread length, (4) Headless screw, (5) Small plates.

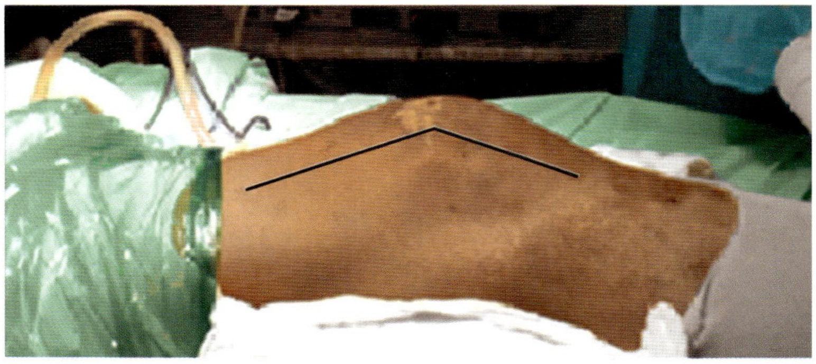

Fig. 6: Supine position and incision mark.

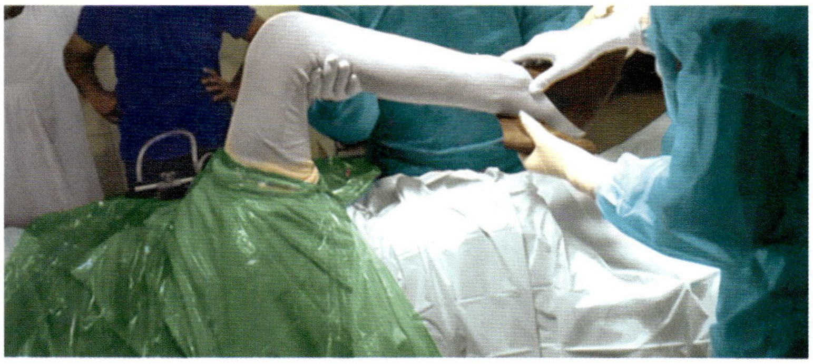

Fig. 7: Tourniquet is applied in flexion to gain length of quadriceps, which facilitates retraction.

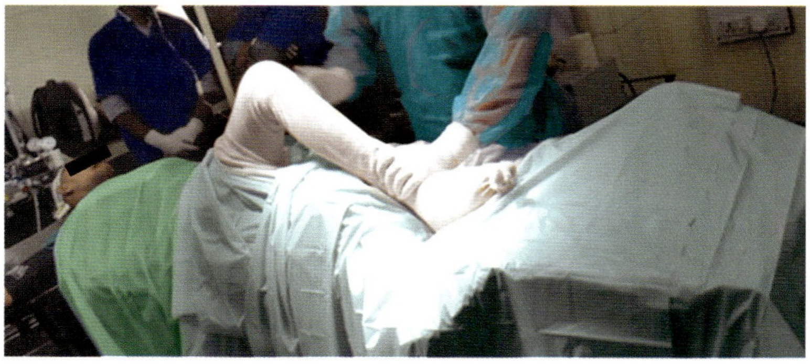

Fig. 8: Sandbag at foot end to maintain flexion of knee.

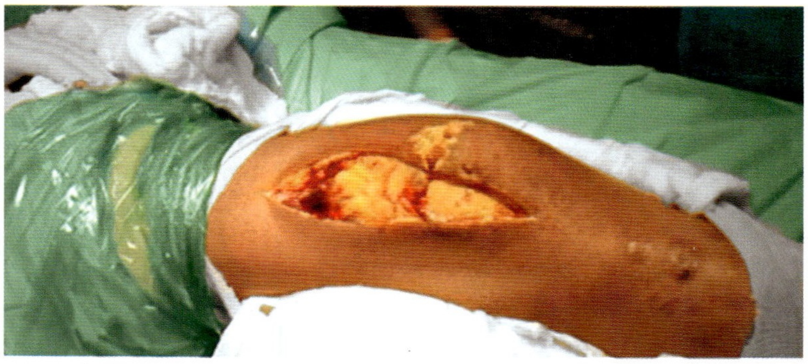

Fig. 9: Exposure. Fracture is exposed by lateral parapatellar approach. Medial parapatellar approach may be needed for medial Hoffa.

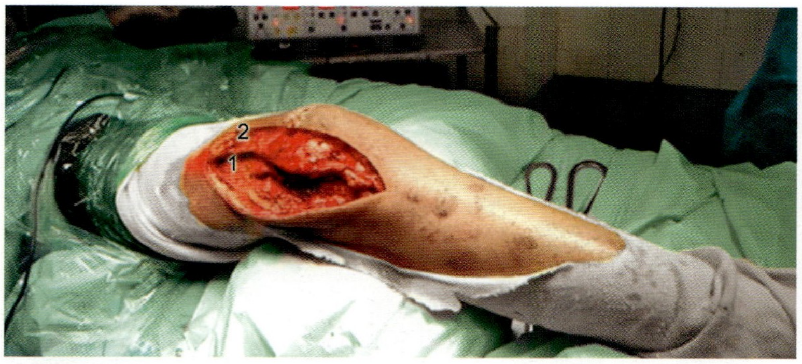

Fig. 10: Exposure is deepened between: (1) Vastus lateralis and (2) Vastus intermedius/rectus.

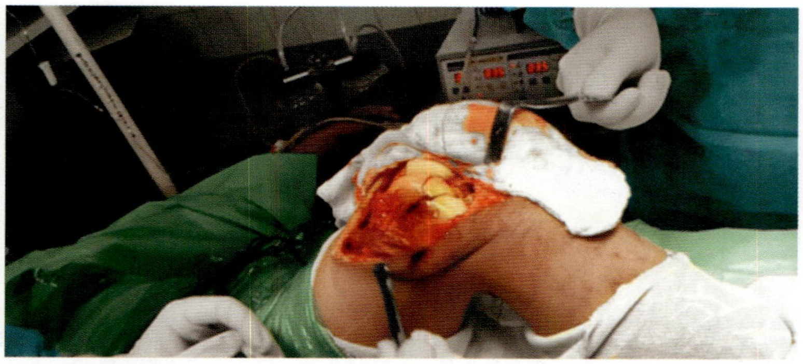

Fig. 11: Medial patellar dislocation is done. For this proximal release should be 4 inches proximal to proximal pole of patella and distal up to patellar tendon. Release of fat pad is needed but, meniscus is carefully preserved.

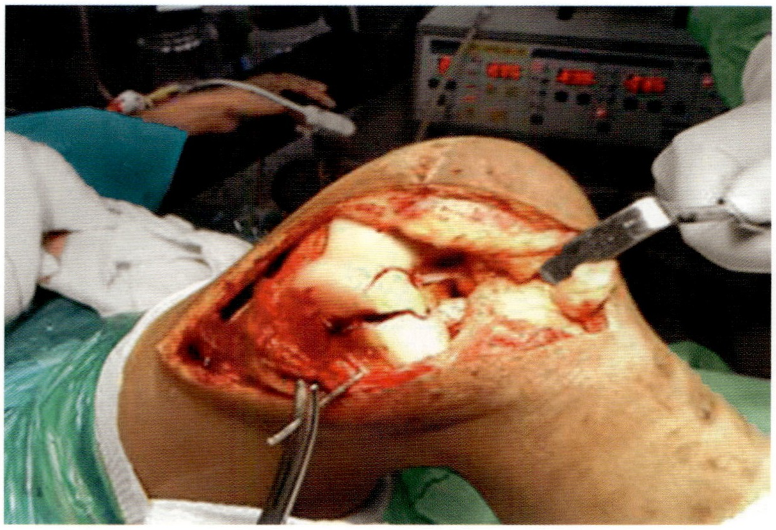

Fig. 12: K-wires are used like joystick. Reduction achieved and held by reduction clamps. Reduction clamp gripping around joystick will compress fracture. Knee is maintained in flexion.

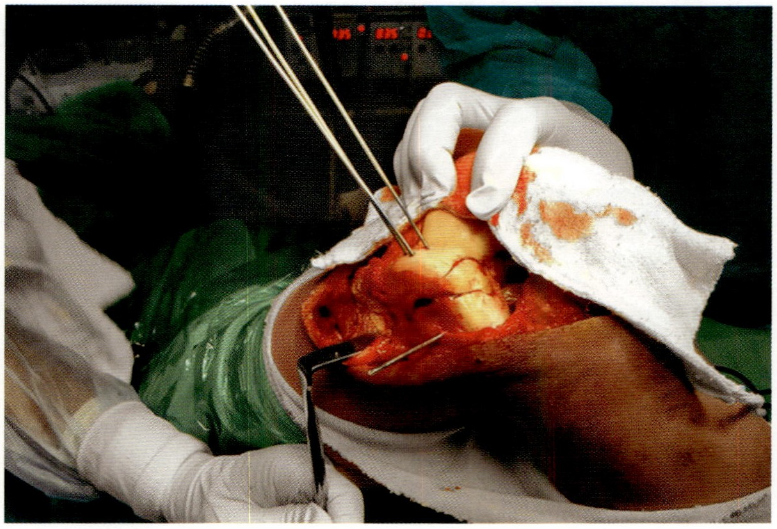

Fig. 13: Multiple guidewires are passed after reduction in an anteroposterior direction and as near right angles to fracture plane as possible.

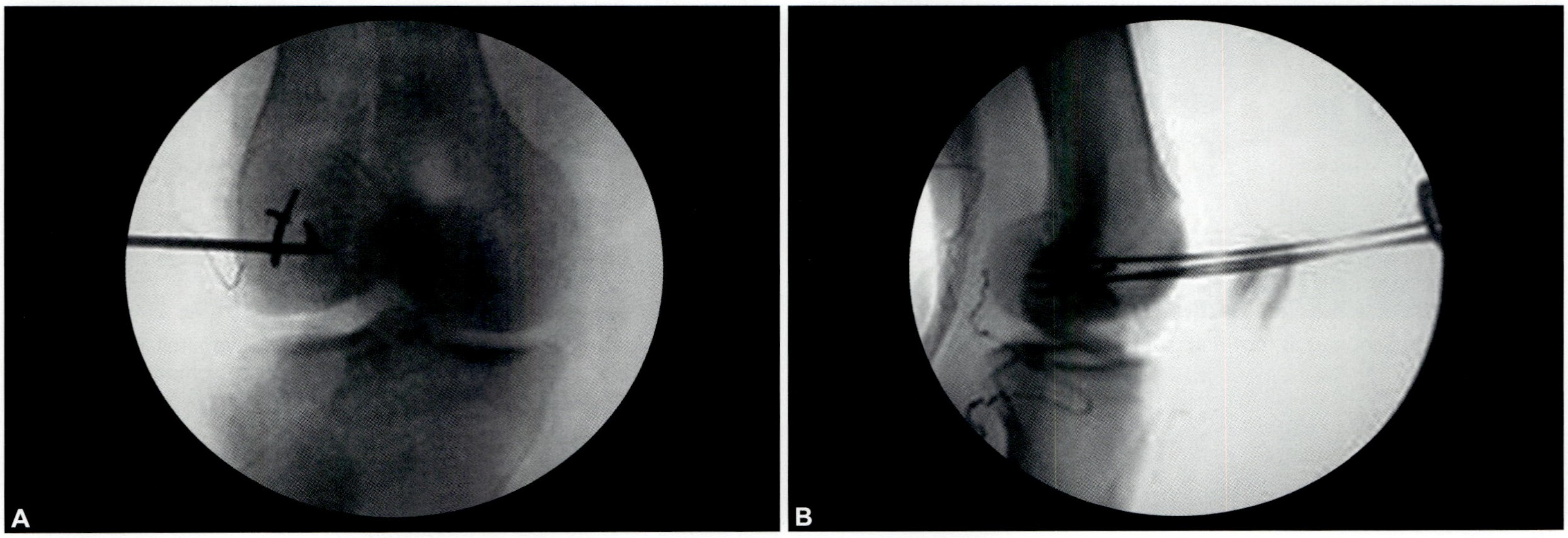

Figs. 14A and B: Care is taken so that guidewire does not pass beyond the posterior cortex.

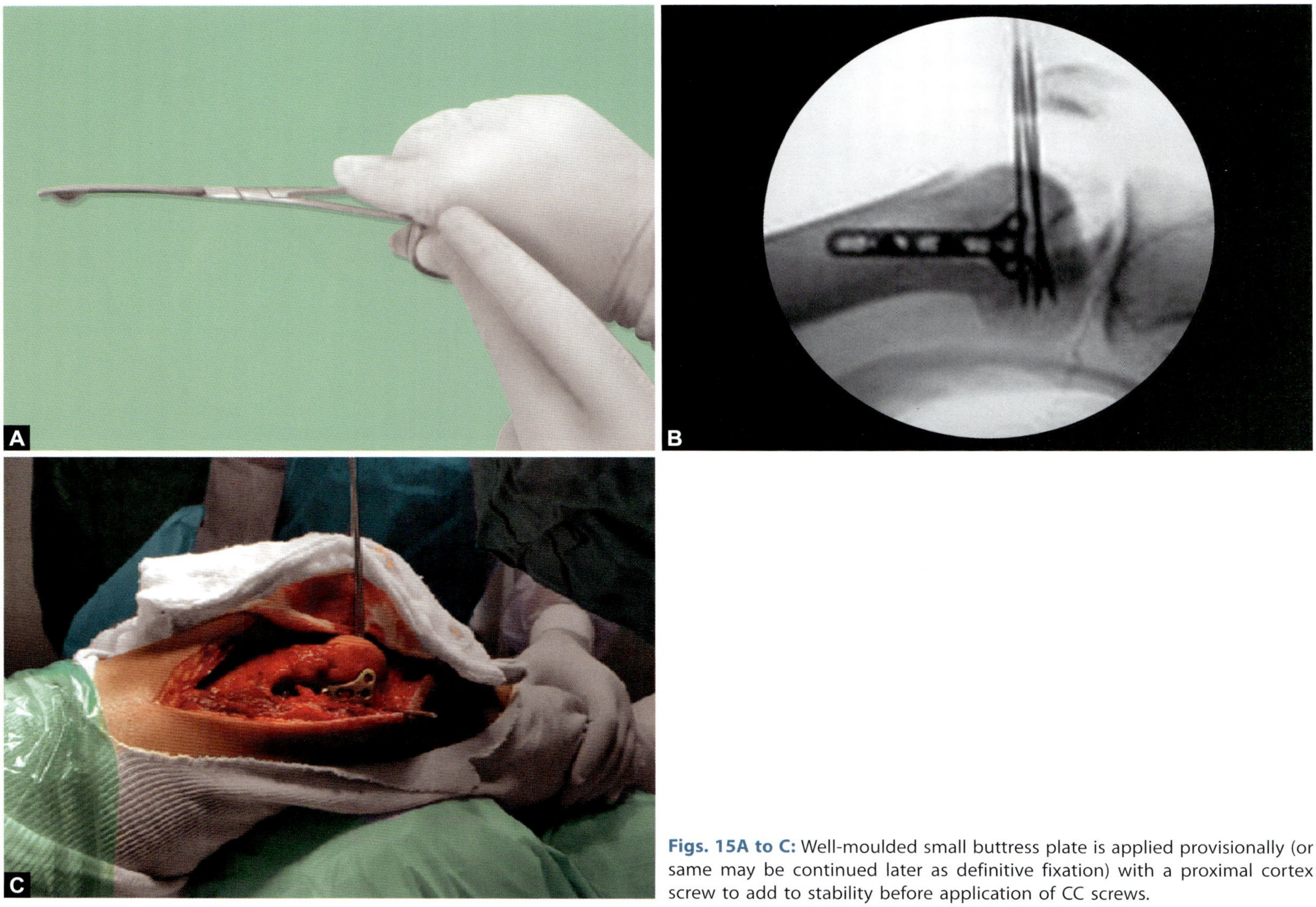

Figs. 15A to C: Well-moulded small buttress plate is applied provisionally (or same may be continued later as definitive fixation) with a proximal cortex screw to add to stability before application of CC screws.

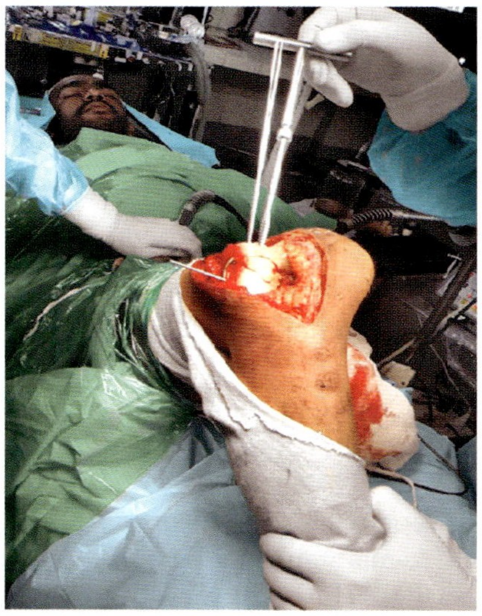

Fig. 16: Drilling and tapping are done over guidewire.

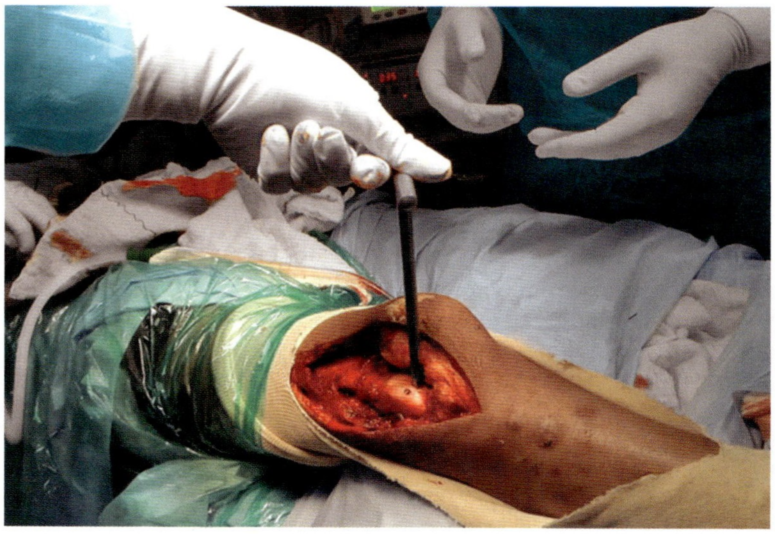

Fig. 17: Countersink is used to create space for head of screw so it can be buried deep underneath articular cartilage. Countersinks are often noncannulated adding difficulty to this step.

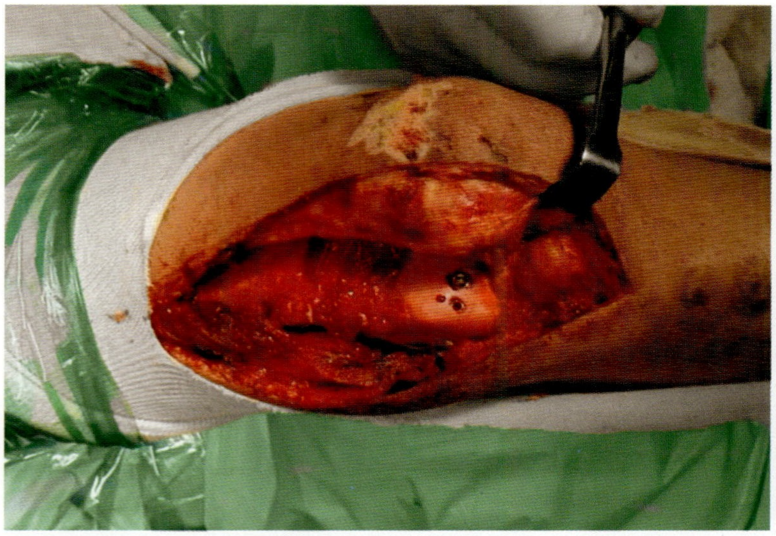

Fig. 18: CC screws are inserted and sunk below surface.

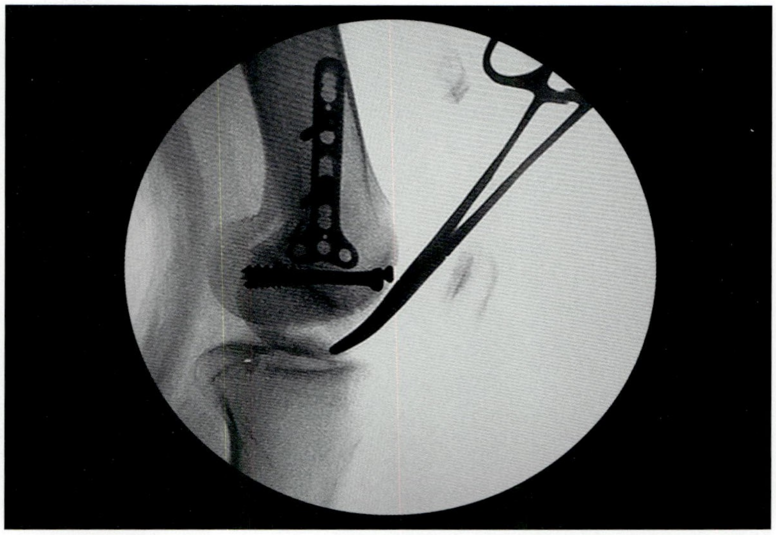

Fig. 19: Identify the correct condyle in lateral C-arm image. This prevents inadvertent crossing of posterior margin of condyle by screw threads.

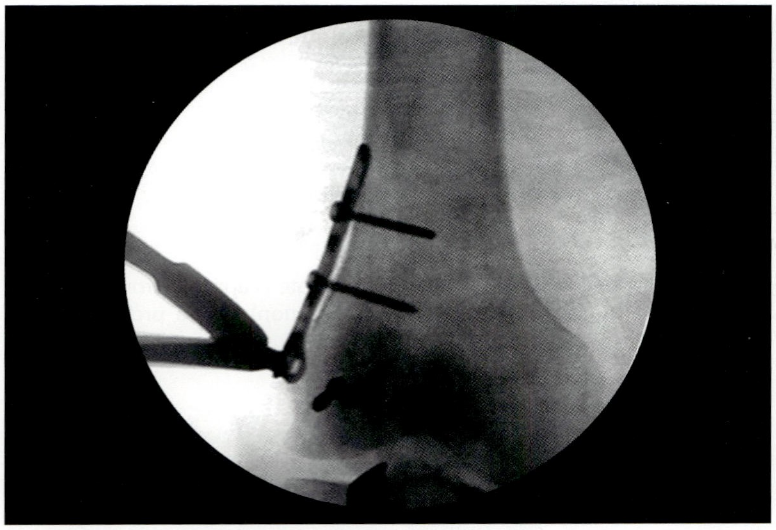

Fig. 20: Buttress plate fixation is completed.

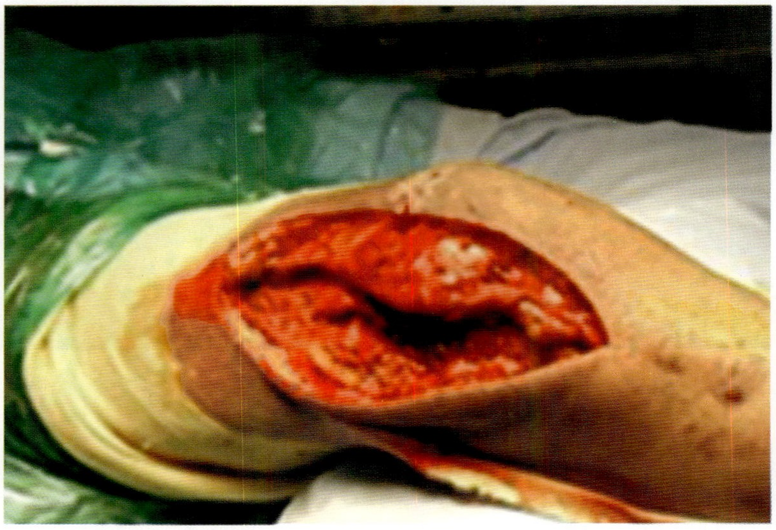

Fig. 21: Routine closure is performed. Drain may be used. Muscle, fascia sutured with strong absorbable and skin with nonabsorbable sutures.

STANDARD POSTOPERATIVE PROTOCOL

- *Mobilization*: Immediate postoperative active and passive range of motion exercises as tolerated by the patient.
- *Walking with brace*: Nonweight bearing for 6 weeks.
- Walking partial weight bearing for further period of 6 weeks.
- *Radiological evaluation*—every month.

COMPLICATIONS

- *Immediate*:
  - Loss of reduction producing deformity and instability.
  - Knee stiffness.
- *Late*: Osteoarthritis.

SUMMARY

- *X-ray is not enough:* At slightest suspicion scans should be ordered.
- *Key instruments:* Screw set CCS 4 and 6.5 mm 16, 32 mm thread length headless screws, reduction clamps, countersink, distal radius plates.
- *Tourniquet* to be applied in knee flexion.
- *Sandbag* is used to maintain knee flexion.
- *Exposure:* At least 4 inches proximal-to-proximal pole of patella. Distal up to patellar tendon insertion. Release of fat pad, spare meniscus.
- *K-wire as Joystick:* Are to be used for reduction.
- *Knee flexion:* Maintain knee in flexion for better exposure.

- *Reduction clamp* gripping around joystick is important for compressing fracture.
- *Multiple guidewires:* Guidewires should not cross posterior cortex of condyle.
- *Buttress plate has to be moulded well:* May be applied prior to CC screws.
- *Countersinking* of screws is important.
- *Screws should not cross posterior cortex.* Identify correct condyle on lateral C-arm image.
- *Immediate mobilization* will prevent stiffness.

SUGGESTED READING

1. Letenneur J, Labour PE, Rogez JM, et al. Fractures de Hoffa: a propos de 20 observations. Ann Chir. 1978;32:213-9.
2. Starr AJ, Jones AL, Reinert CM. The "swashbuckler": a modified anterior approach for fractures of the distal femur. J Orthop Trauma. 1999;13:138-40.
3. York SE, Segina DN, Aflatoon K, et al. The association between supracondylar-intercondylar distal femoral fractures and coronal plane fractures. JBJS. 2005;87-A(3):564-9.

CHAPTER 110

Fracture Patella Fixation by Tension Band Wiring

Amit R Kale, Vijay Kakatkar, Madan Hardikar, Chittanand Mendhe

INTRODUCTION

- Patella is the largest sesamoid bone in the human body located in quadriceps muscle.
- Power of quadriceps muscle is increased by about 30% because patella positions the quadriceps mechanism away from axis of rotation of knee thus increasing lever arm.

ETIOLOGY

- Indirect force from violent quadriceps contraction (hyperflexion of knee)
- Direct blow to patella (e.g. fall over front of knee, dashboard injury).

Rarely other causes like:

- After resurfacing patella in total knee arthroplasty (fatigue fracture)
- After anterior cruciate ligament (ACL) reconstruction using bone-tendon–bone graft (faulty technique)
- After medial patellofemoral ligament (MPFL) reinsertion surgeries (exact mechanism not known).

CLASSIFICATION (FIG. 1)

According to displacement of fracture fragments:

- Nondisplaced
- Displaced.

According to morphology:

- Transverse
- Longitudinal
- Comminuted.

TREATMENT GOALS

- To restore alignment
- Repair of the retinaculum
- To ensure stability.

All this can be achieved by restoring bony congruity with hardware to rigidly fix fracture.

Methods of Treatments

Cylindrical Cast or Knee Brace

- *Biomechanics*: Stress-sharing device
- *Mode of bone healing*: Secondary
- *Indications*: Used for nondisplaced fractures and longitudinal fractures
- Cylinder cast allows full range of motion (ROM) at ankle.

Open Reduction and Internal Fixation

- *Biomechanics*: Stress-shielding and sharing
- *Modes of fixation*: Tension band wiring, cerclage wiring ± lag screw fixation
- *Mode of bone healing*: Primary, unless solid fixation is not achieved, then also secondary
- *Indications*: Used for comminuted and displaced transverse fractures
- Open reduction is performed to align articular surface. Retinacular disruption is repaired.

Partial or Total Patellectomy

Used when grossly comminuted fracture cannot be repaired.

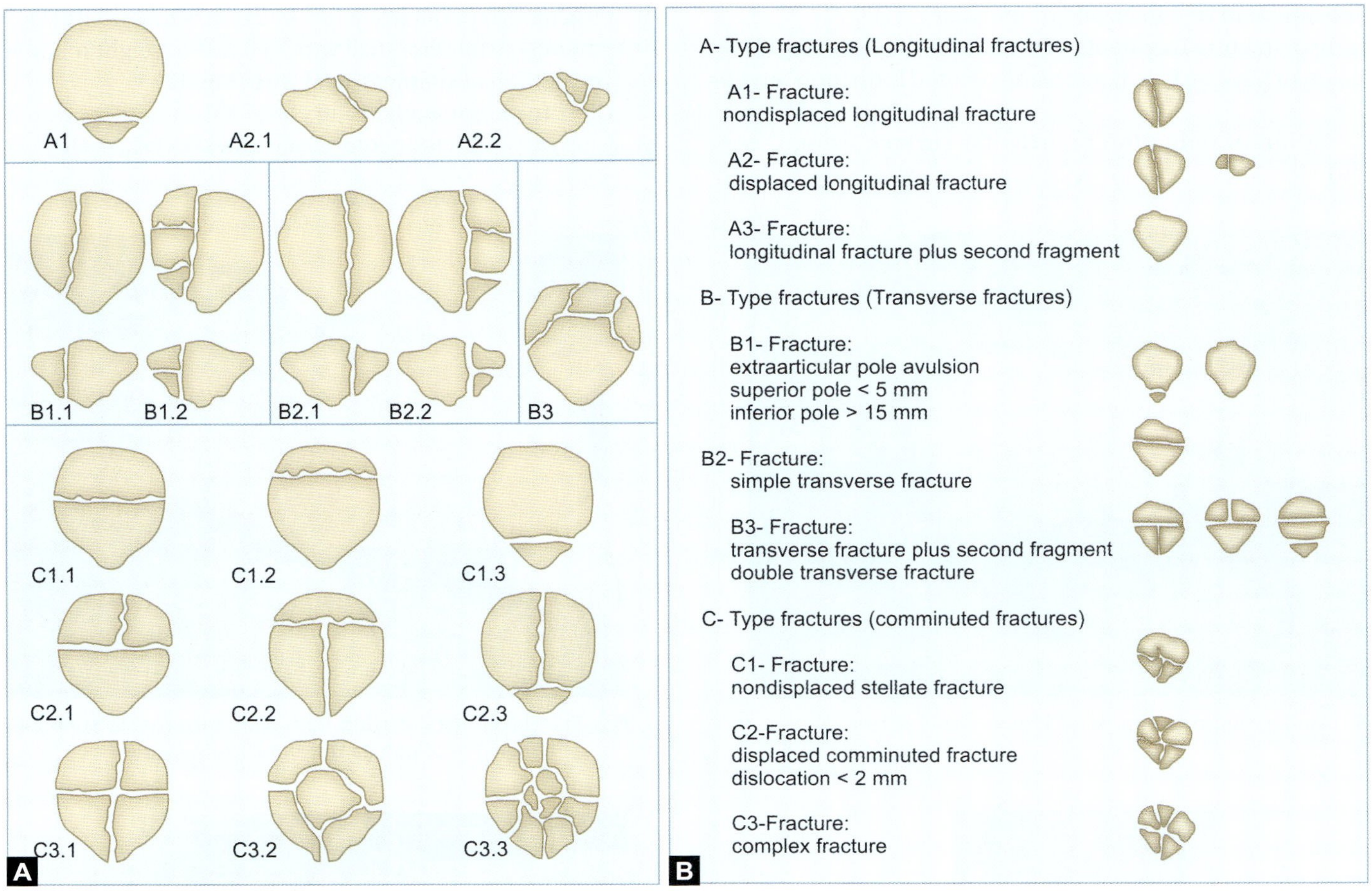

Fig. 1: Classification of fracture patella.

SURGICAL STEPS

PROCEDURE

1. Supine position with tourniquet and C-arm as shown in Figure 3
2. Painting and draping using water impermissible drapes (Fig. 4)
3. Palpation of bony landmarks like fracture fragments, tibial tuberosity (Fig. 5)
4. Vertical incision over knee 2.5 cm above patella to tibial tuberosity (Fig. 6)

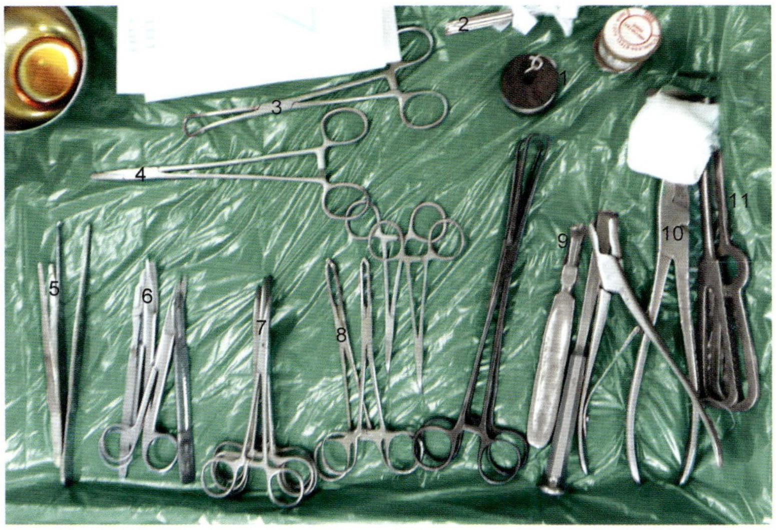

Fig. 2: Instrument trolley for surgery. (1) tension band wire, (2) K-wires, (3) reduction forceps, (4) needle holder, (5) tissue forceps, (6) scalpal blades, (7) artery forceps, (8) Allis forceps, (9) periosteum elevator, (10) plier, (11) tissue retractors.

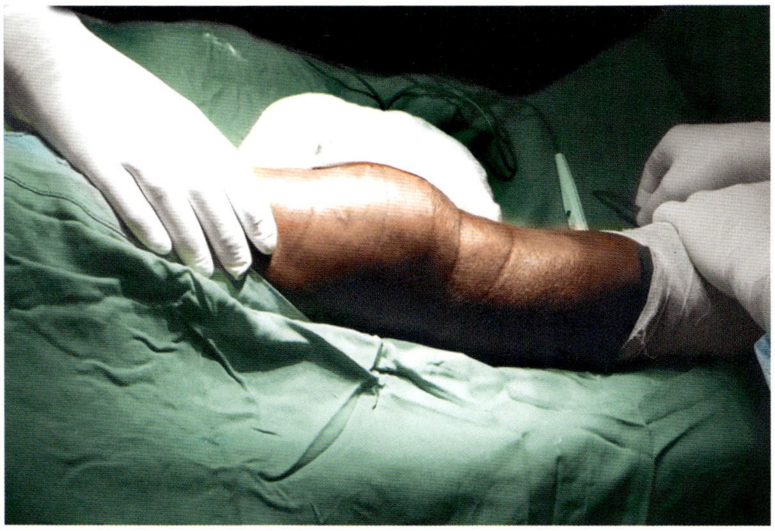

Fig. 3: Supine position and tourniquet applied, knee frame is preferable.

5. Demonstration of rent in extensor retinaculum (Fig. 7)
6. Exposure of fracture fragments and cleaning of edges (Fig. 8)
7. Reduction of fracture fragments using pointed reduction forceps (Fig. 9)
8. Confirmation of reduction of articular surface using C-arm (Fig. 10)
9. Passing two parallel K-wires in fracture fragments (Fig. 11)
10. Passing of stainless steel wire in figure-of-eight manner
11. Tensioning of stainless steel wire (Fig. 12)
12. Closure of retinacular injury (Fig. 13)
13. Closure of subcutaneous tissue and skin (Fig. 14).

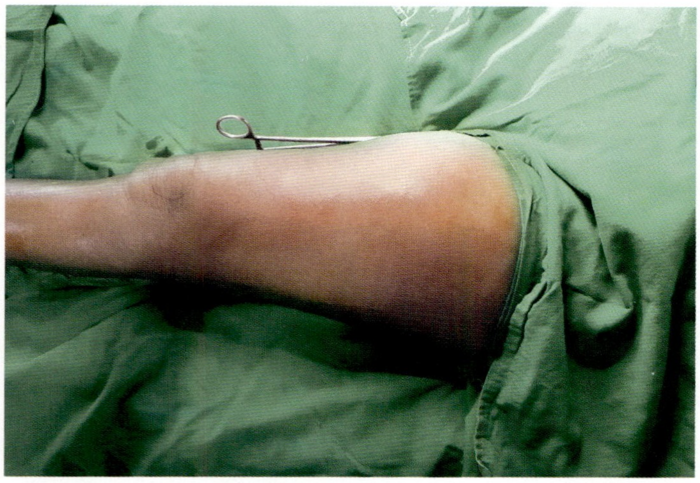

Fig. 4: Painting and draping use of impermeable plastic drapes.

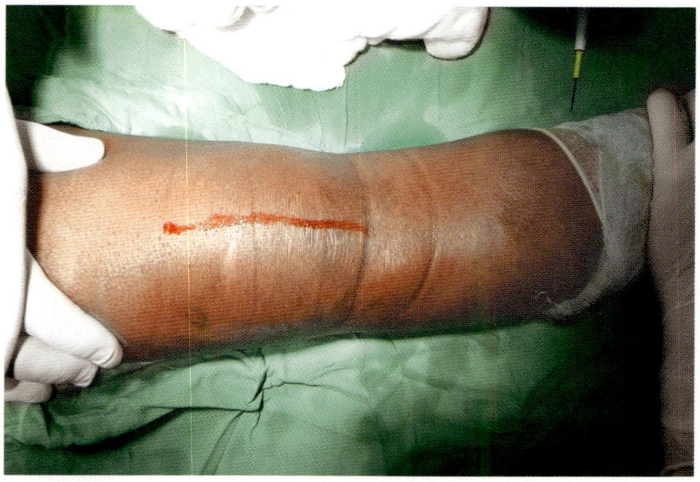

Fig. 5: Incision mark starting from 2 cm proximal to superior border of patella upto tibial tuberosity.

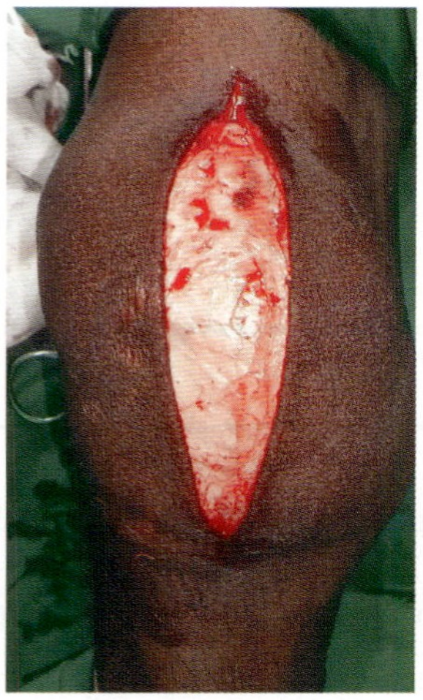

Fig. 6: Vertical incision slightly on lateral side of patella.

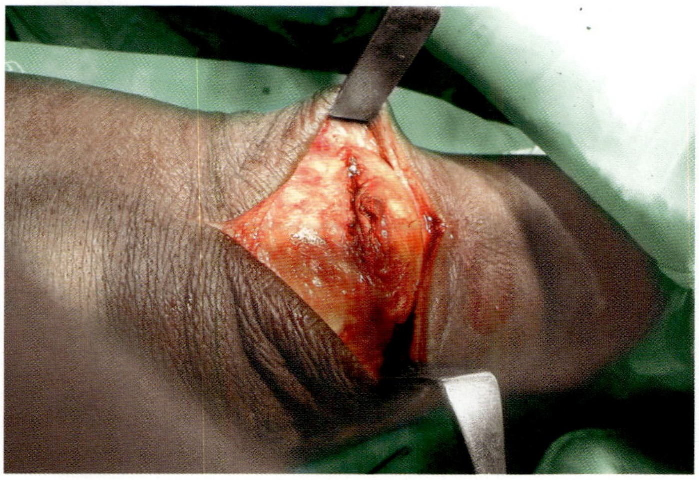

Fig. 7: Rent in extensor retinaculum.

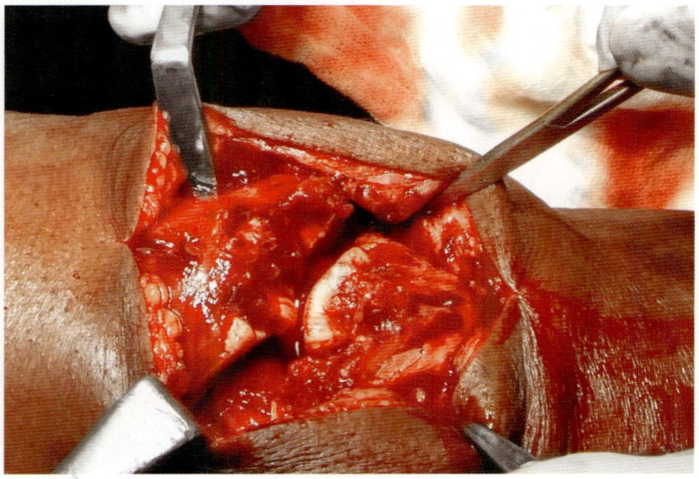

Fig. 8: Fracture fragments exposed and edges cleaned with scoop.

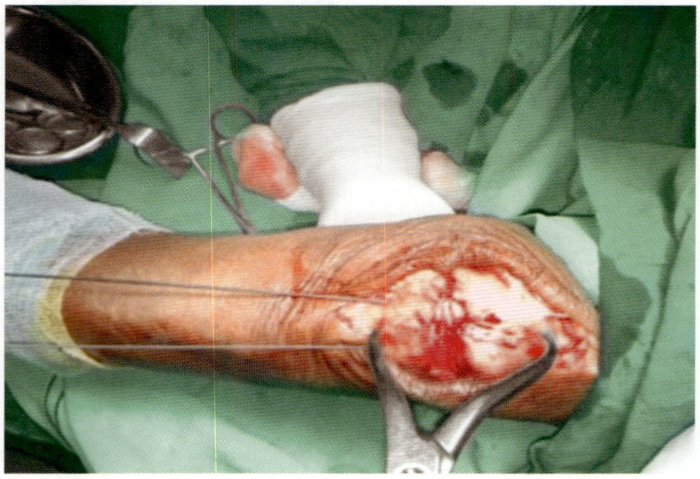

Fig. 9: Fracture reduced and held with pointed reduction forceps. In case of additional sagittal plane fracture, transverse K-wire is used to fix it. This converts three part fracture to two part fracture.

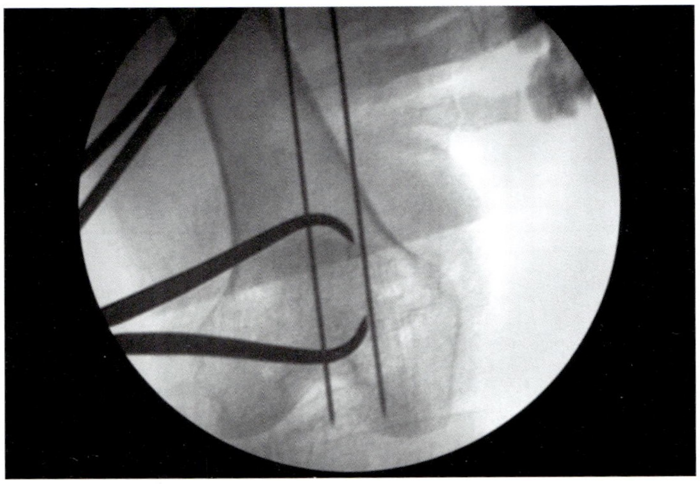

Fig. 10: Two parallel K-wires anteroposterior (AP) view.

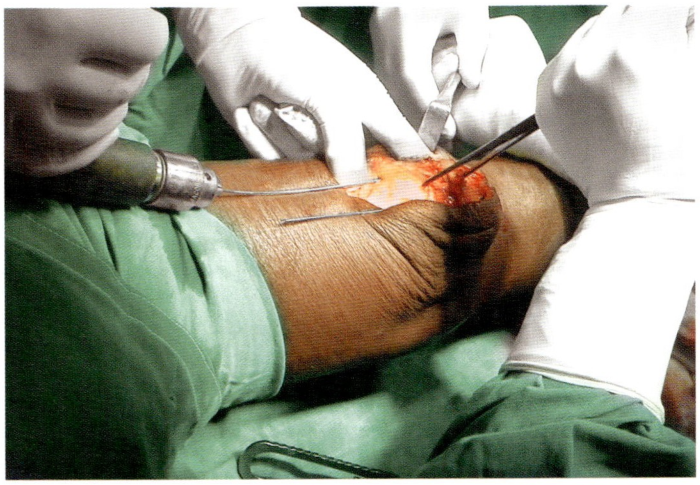

Fig. 11: Passing of two parallel K-wires holding fracture fragments.

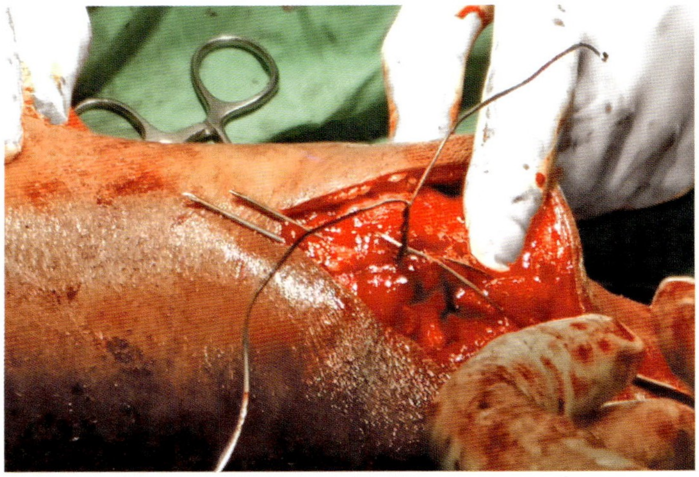

Fig. 12: Twist the both end of SS Wire. However repair the retinaculum tears before final tightening of SS wire.

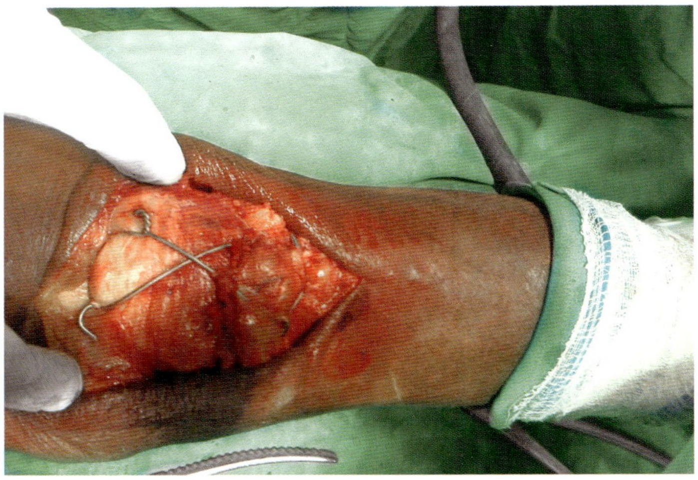

Fig. 13: Cut the proximal ends of both K wire and bend them.

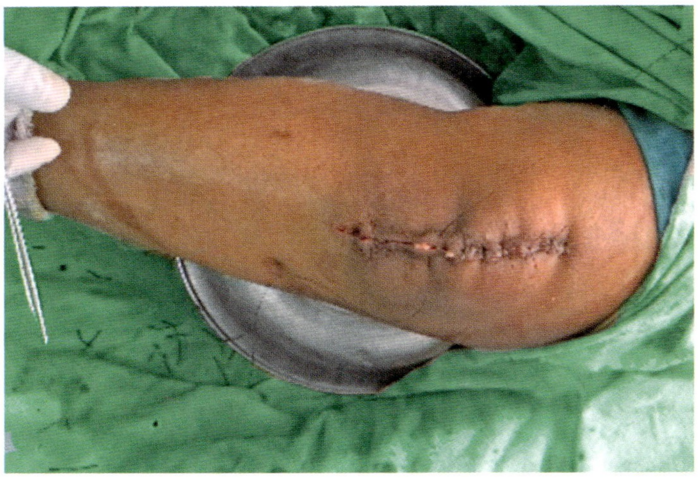

Fig. 14: Final skin closure in flexion of knee.

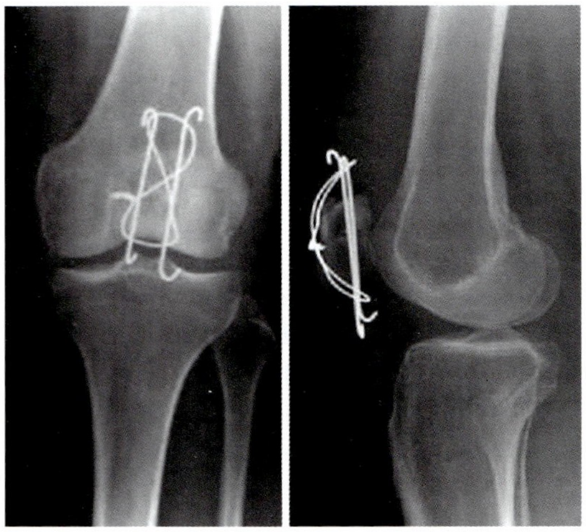

Fig. 15: Postoperative radiograph.

POSTOPERATIVE CARE

- Extremity immobilized in full extension for 4 weeks to allow tendon-to-bone healing
- Full active ROM begins after with gradual increasing flexion.

SUGGESTED READING

1. Smith ST, Cramer KE, Karges DE, et al. Early complications in the operative treatment of patella fractures. J Orthop Trauma. 1997;11(3): 183-7.
2. Weber MJ, Janecki CJ, Mcleod P, et al. Efficacy of various forms of fixation of transverse fractures of the patella. J Bone Joint Surg Am. 1980;62(2):215-20.

CHAPTER 111

Fracture Proximal Tibia Fixation

Onkar Lande, Nitish Agrawal, Hitesh J Mangukiya, Jignesh Yeshwant Tandel, Chittanand Mendhe, Madhav Khadilkar, Shrinivas S Shintre, Rachit Vipul Shah

BICONDYLAR FRACTURE TIBIA CANNULATED CANCELLOUS SCREW FIXATION

Onkar Lande, Nitish Agrawal

INTRODUCTION

Fractures of the tibial plateau are fracture involving the articular surface of proximal tibia and account for 1% of all fractures in adults. Of these nearly, two-thirds involve the lateral plateau only, one-fifth involve the medial plateau only, and the remaining involve both. This is because the medial articular surface and medial condyle are stronger than lateral articular surface and lateral condyle respectively. Correspondingly, medial plateau fractures are usually caused by high-energy injuries and most of the times it is associated with soft tissue injury presenting in form of skin blisters, disruption of lateral collateral ligament (LCL) complex, peroneal nerve lesions, and vascular damage.

MECHANISM OF INJURY

In young adults, tibial plateau fractures are usually due to high-energy trauma such as falls from height, road traffic accidents, etc. whereas in the elderly with osteopenic bone, even a simple fall on the knee can result in tibial plateau fractures.

CLINICAL PRESENTATION

As with most other fractures, initial presenting complaint of the patient is pain, swelling, and inability to move the affected limb. Careful evaluation of the patient is a must to rule out neurovascular compromise. At the same time, evaluation of ligament and soft tissue injury should be carried out.

INVESTIGATIONS

For delineating the fracture anatomy and pattern, standard anteroposterior and lateral radiographs should be obtained with additional oblique views if required. Evaluation with CT scan including 3D reconstruction should be done as it helps surgical planning. Soft tissue and/or ligament injury may be evaluated with MRI. Arterial color Doppler may be obtained if vascular compromise is suspected.

CLASSIFICATION OF TIBIAL PLATEAU FRACTURES (FIG. 1)

Schatzker Classification

- *Type I*: Lateral split fracture
- *Type II*: Split-depressed fracture
- *Type III*: Pure depressed fracture
- *Type IV*: Medial plateau fracture
- *Type V*: Bicondylar fracture

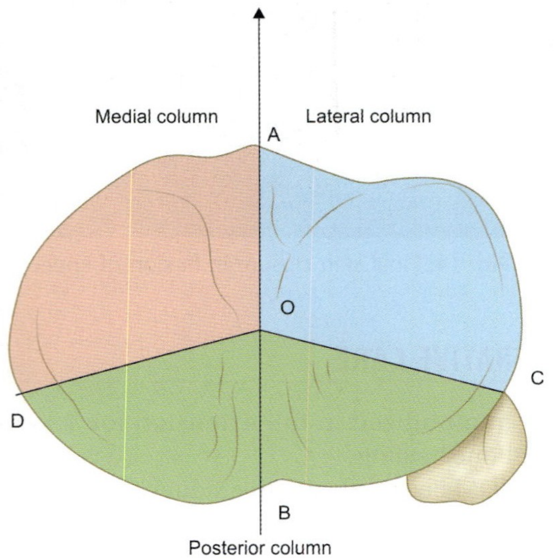

Fig. 1: Three-column concept for fixation of tibia plateau fractures.

- *Type VI*: Metaphyseal-diaphyseal dissociation
  - Types I–III are due to low-energy trauma
  - Types IV–VI are due to high-energy trauma
  - Type I usually occurs in younger individuals and is associated with medial collateral ligament injuries
  - Type III is usually extremely rare.

TREATMENT

Nonoperative

- Nondisplaced or minimally displaced may be treated nonoperatively
- Protected weight bearing is done in a hinged brace and early range of knee motion started.
- Isometric quadriceps exercises like progressive passive, active assisted, and active controlled range-of-knee motion exercises are started.
- Partial weight bearing with support of walking aid for 2–3 months is allowed, with progression to full weight bearing.

Operative Treatment

- *Indications*:
  - Articular depression more than 2 mm to 1 cm
  - Instability more than 10°.
- *Open fractures*:
  - Associated compartment syndrome
  - Associated vascular injury.
- *Operative treatment principles*: Tibial articular surface reconstruction and re-establishment of tibial alignment is the main goal.
  - Reduction and fixation of intra-articular fractures and buttressing of elevated articular segments with bone graft or bone substitute to maintain normal plateau
  - Plates and screws, screws only or external fixator devices may be used for definitive fixation depending on soft tissue and skin condition
  - Choice of implant depends on fracture patterns, degree of displacement and familiarity of the surgeon to the procedure
  - Adequate soft tissue repair/reconstruction, preservation and/or repair of the meniscus as well as intra-articular and extra-articular ligamentous structures are done.
- Spanning external fixator may be required in higher energy open injuries.
- Schatzker types I–IV fractures can be fixed with percutaneous screws or a laterally placed buttress plate. If satisfactory closed reduction (<1-mm articular step-off) cannot be achieved with closed techniques, open reduction and internal fixation are indicated.
- Depressed fragments are to be elevated from below en masse by using a bone tamp working through the split component or a cortical window. The metaphyseal defect may be filled with some type of osteoconductive material.
- Types V and VI fractures can be managed using plate and screws, ring fixator, or a hybrid fixator.
- Minimally invasive percutaneous plate osteosynthesis (MIPPO) is a valuable technique being used more often in recent times in properly selected cases.
- Fractures of the posterior medical plateau may require a posteromedial incision for fracture reduction and plate stabilization.
- *Postoperative care*: Nonweight bearing
- Weight bearing is allowed at 8–12 weeks.

COMPLICATIONS

- Arthrofibrosis
- Infection
- Compartment syndrome
- Malunion or nonunion
- Posttraumatic osteoarthritis
- Peroneal nerve injury
- Popliteal artery injury.

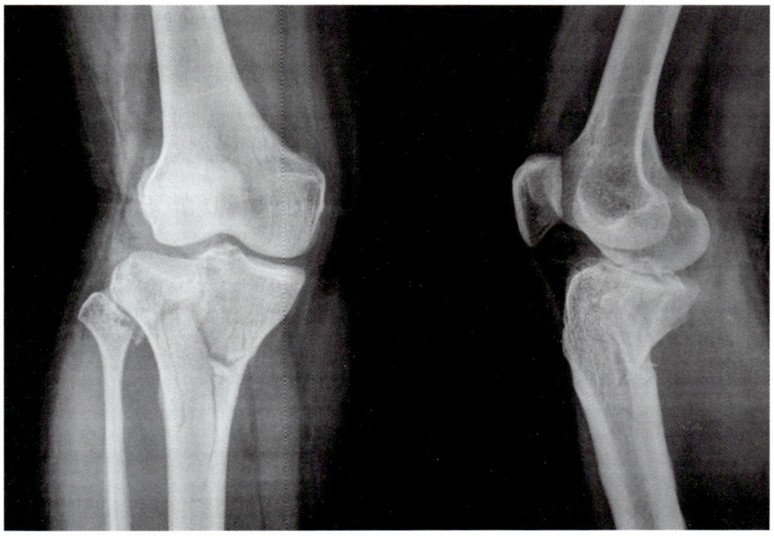

Fig. 2: X-ray of knee joint with proximal tibia and distal femur anteroposterior view and lateral view showing bicondylar fracture of proximal tibia with involvement of articular surface.

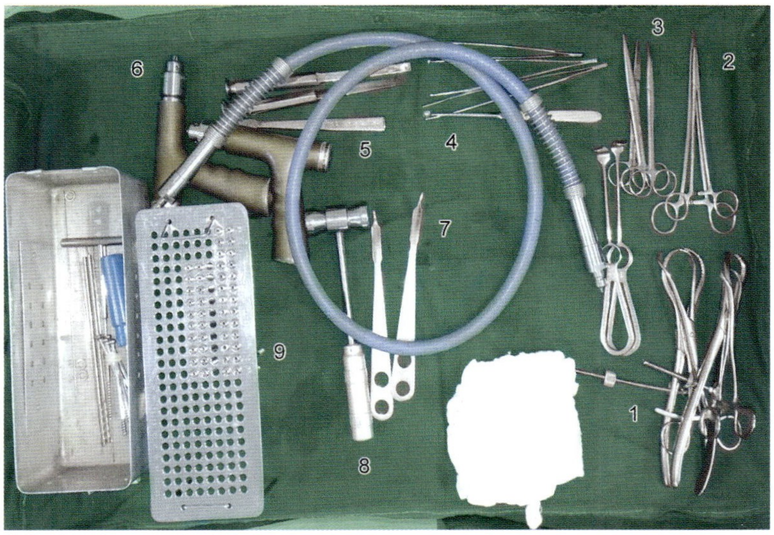

Fig. 3: (1) Bone holding reduction forceps; (2) Artery forceps; (3) Mosquito forceps; (4) Curette; (5) Osteotome; (6) Drill; (7) Hohmann bone lever; (8) Hammer; (9) Cannulated cancellous screw.

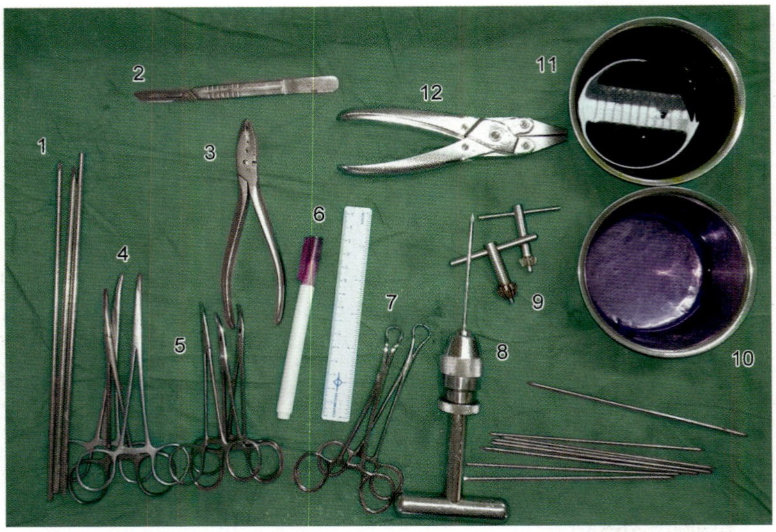

Fig. 4: (1) Steinmann pin; (2) Knife; (3) Wire cutter; (4) Artery forceps; (5) Mosquito forceps; (6) Measuring scale; (7) Towel clip; (8) T-handle with Steinmann pin; (9) Chuck key; (10) Spirit; (11) Povidone iodine solution; (12) Pliers.

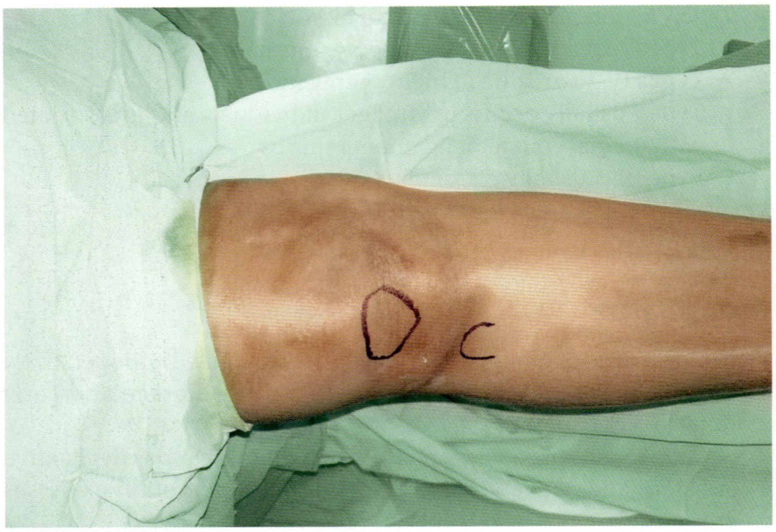

Fig. 5: Supine position given on traction table. Patella and tibial tuberosity marked.

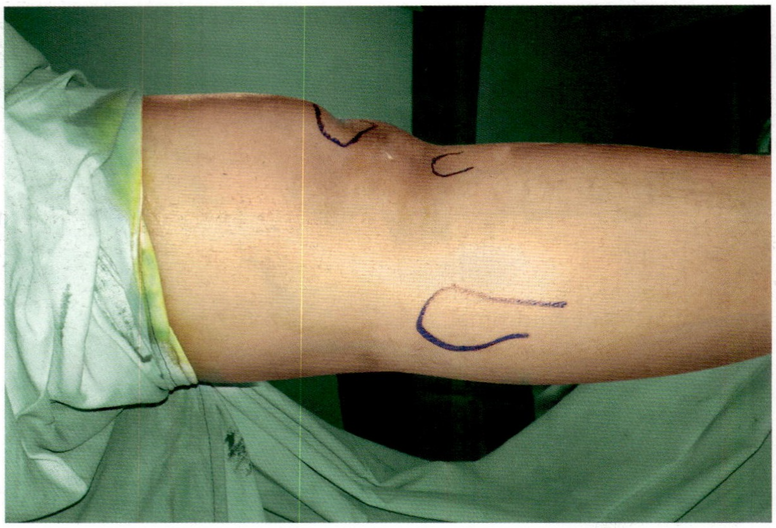

Fig. 6: Fibula head and neck marked with marker pen.

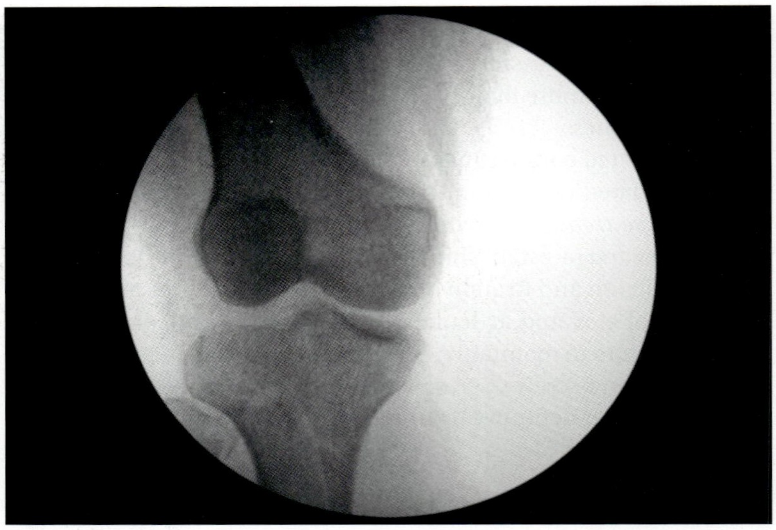

Fig. 7: Anteroposterior view over C-arm image intensifier showing depressed bicondylar fracture.

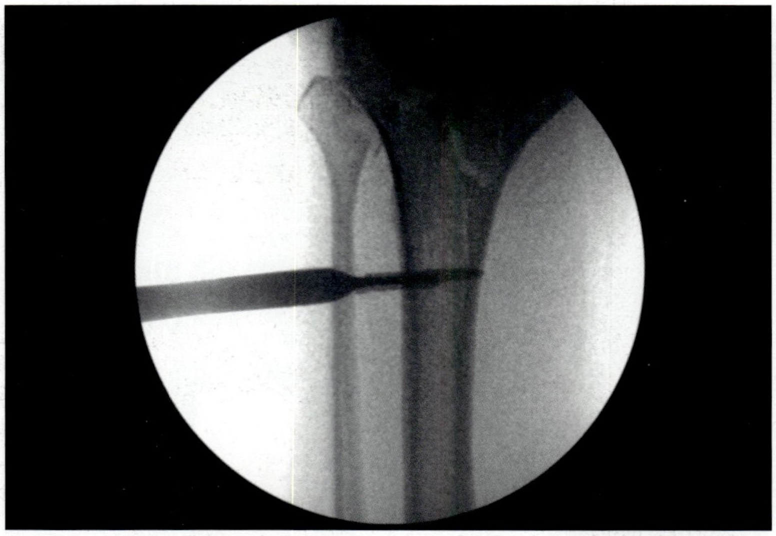

Fig. 8: Entry site for Steinmann pin identified over C-arm by placing knife.

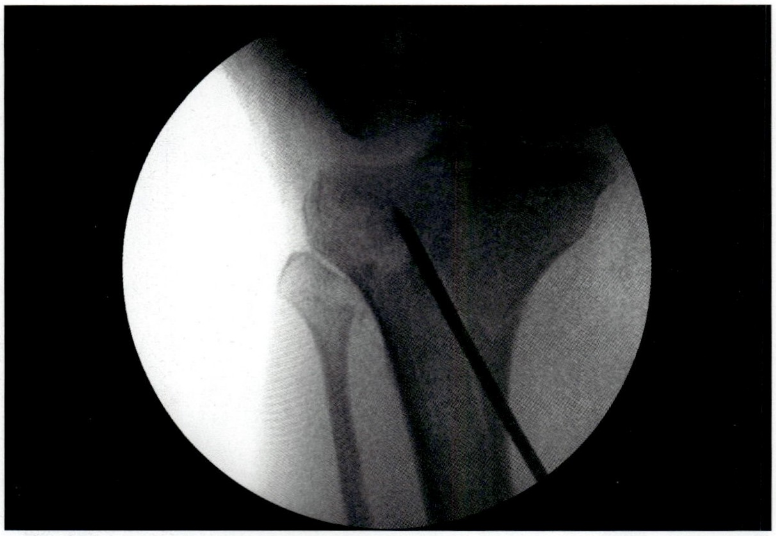

Fig. 9: Stab incision taken over medial side and Steinmann pin inserted from medial cortex towards lateral condyle. Position of Steinmann pin confirmed over C-arm anteroposterior view. Various bone punches or blunt periosteum elevators may also be used for this step but a larger cortical window is required.

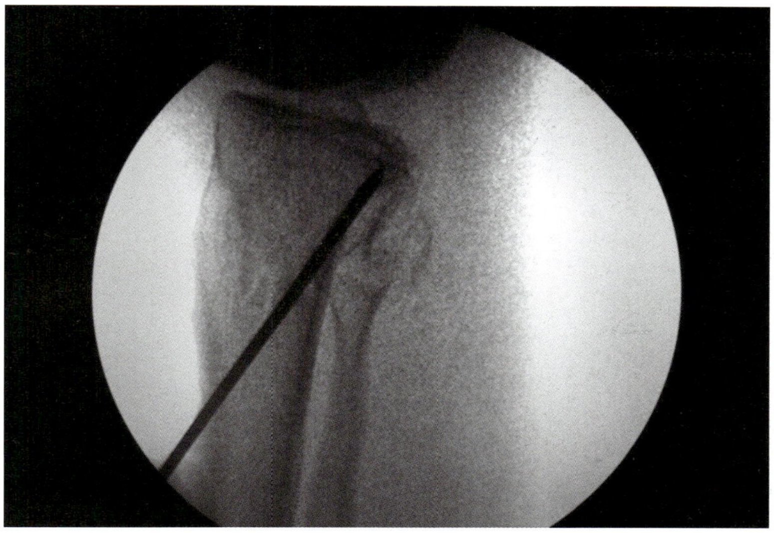

Fig. 10: Position of pin confirmed over C-arm lateral view.

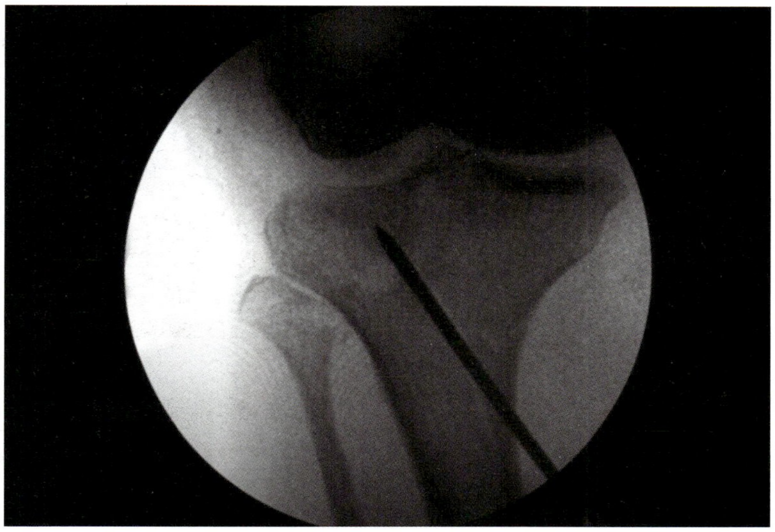

Fig. 11: Depressed lateral condyle elevated with Steinmann pin under C-arm guidance on anteroposterior view.

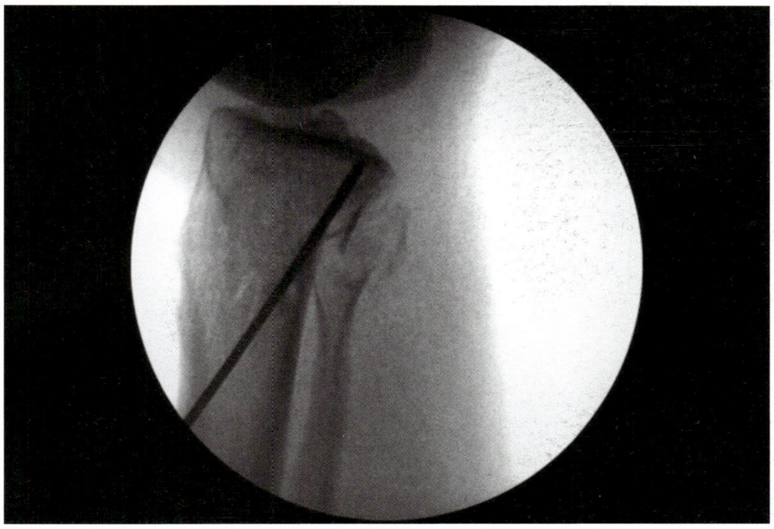

Fig. 12: Depressed posterior articular surface elevated with Steinmann pin under C-arm lateral view.

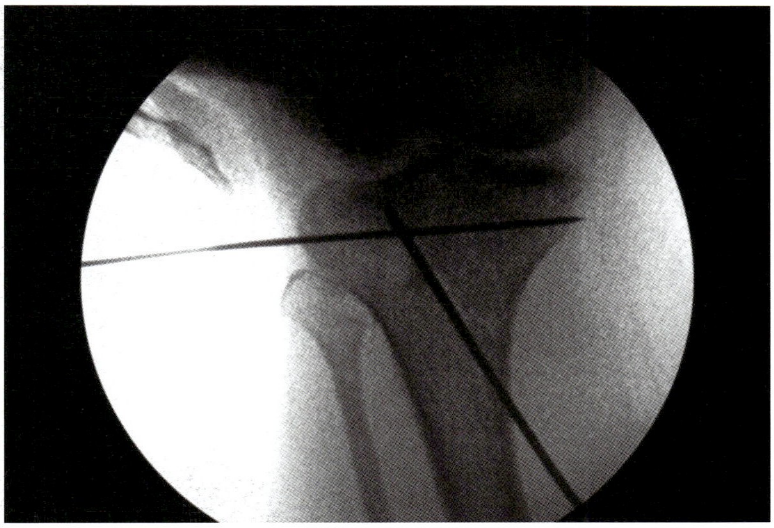

Fig. 13: A guidewire is inserted from lateral condyle to medial condyle under C-arm anteroposterior view to hold depressed condyle.

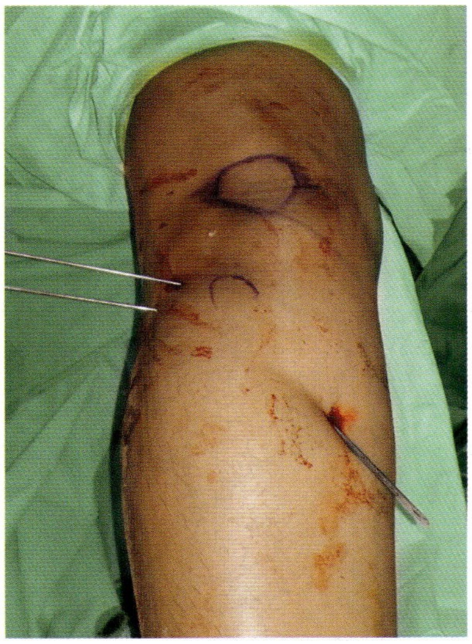

Fig. 14: A 2nd guidewire inserted from lateral cortex to hold depressed condyle.

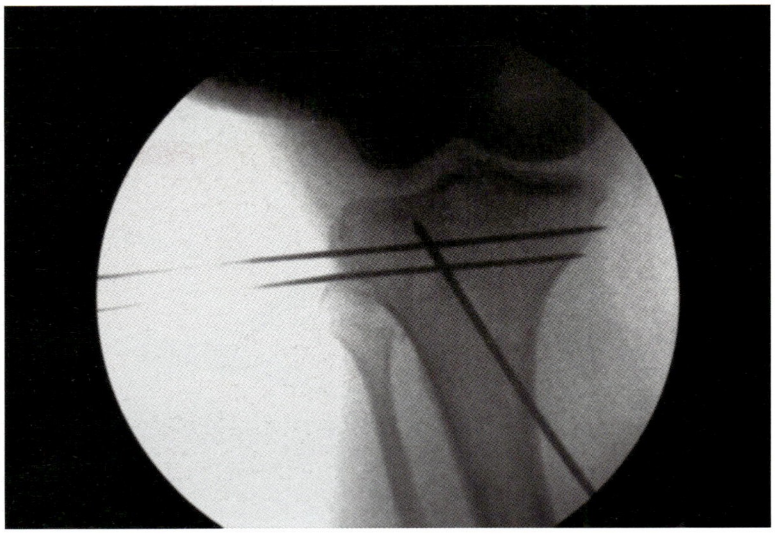

Fig. 15: Position of both guidewire confirmed over C-arm anteroposterior view.

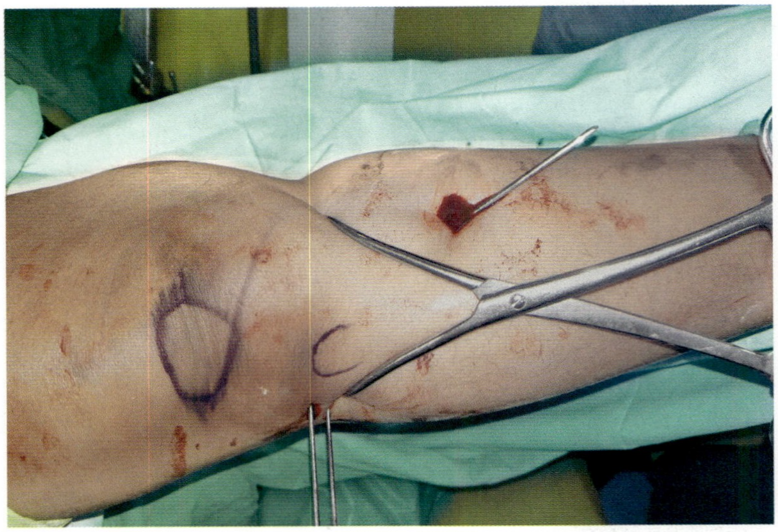

Fig. 16: Bone holding reduction forceps is used to compress both condyles together.

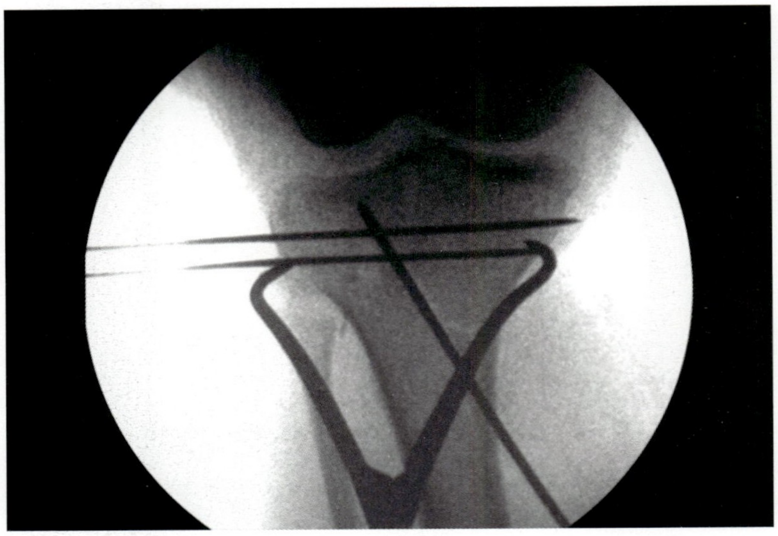

Fig. 17: Reduction confirmed over C-arm anteroposterior view.

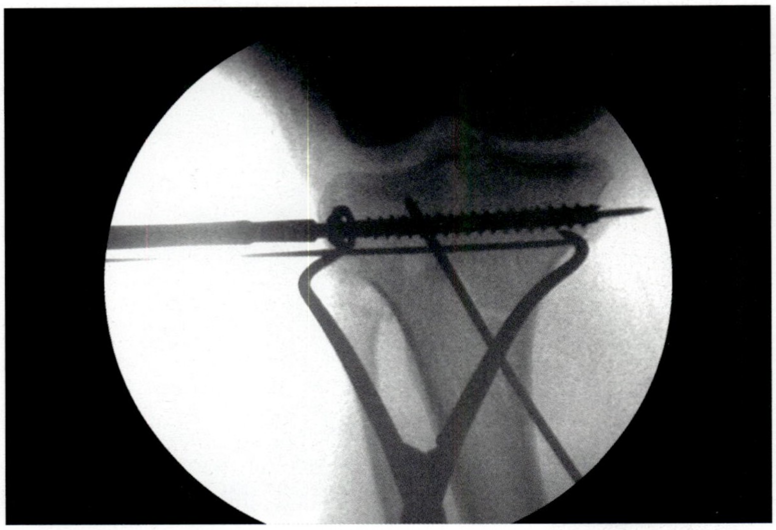

Fig. 18: Stab incision taken and 6.5 mm CC screw with washer inserted from lateral condyle to medial condyle over guide wire to hold anterior part of articular surface.

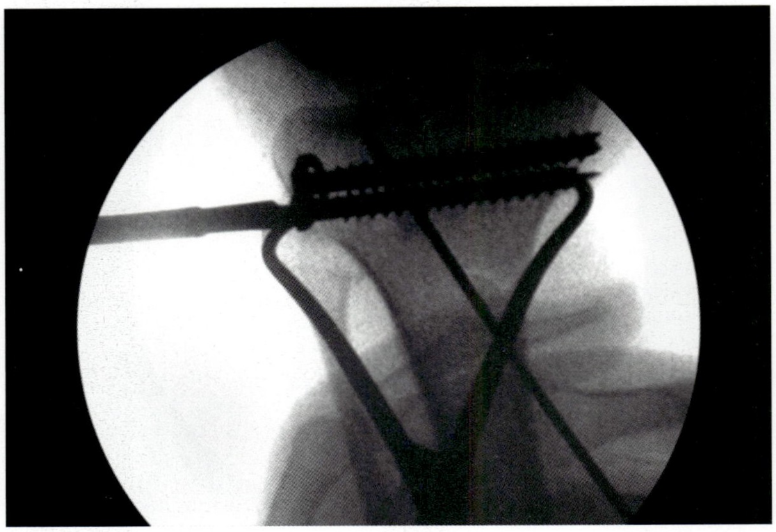

Fig. 19: Stab incision taken and 6.5 mm CC screw inserted over guide wire to hold posterior part of articular surface and fixation confirmed over C-arm anteroposterior view.

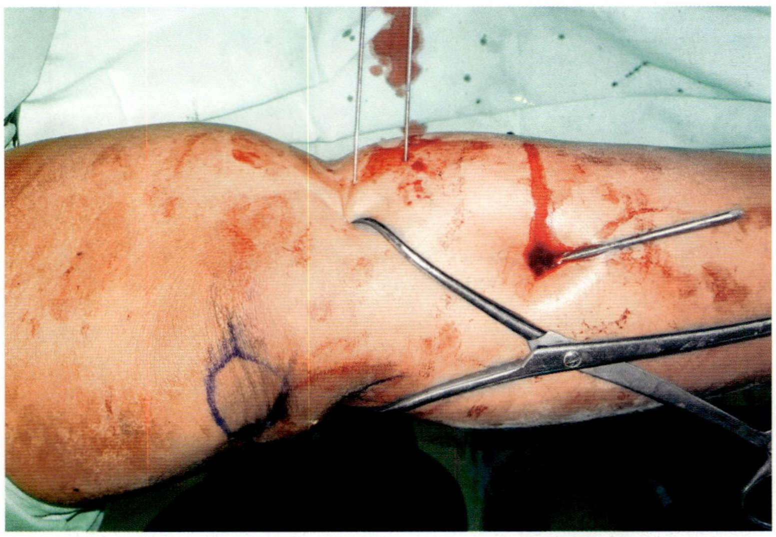

Fig. 20: 2 more guidewires inserted from medial side to lateral side under C-arm anteroposterior view.

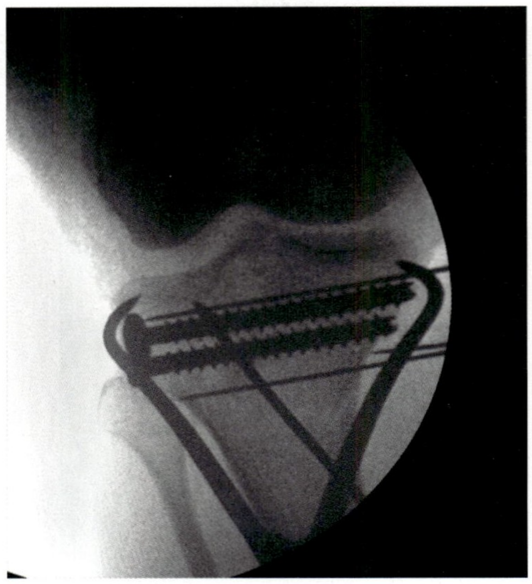

Fig. 21: Position of both guidewire confirmed over C-arm anteroposterior view.

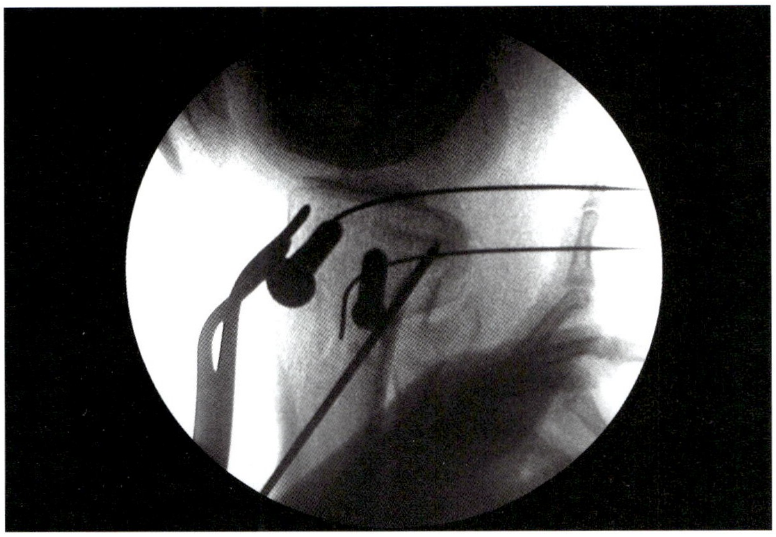

Fig. 22: C-arm lateral view showing position of both guide wires. Stab incision taken and two 4 mm CC screws are inserted on both guide wires from medial to lateral direction.

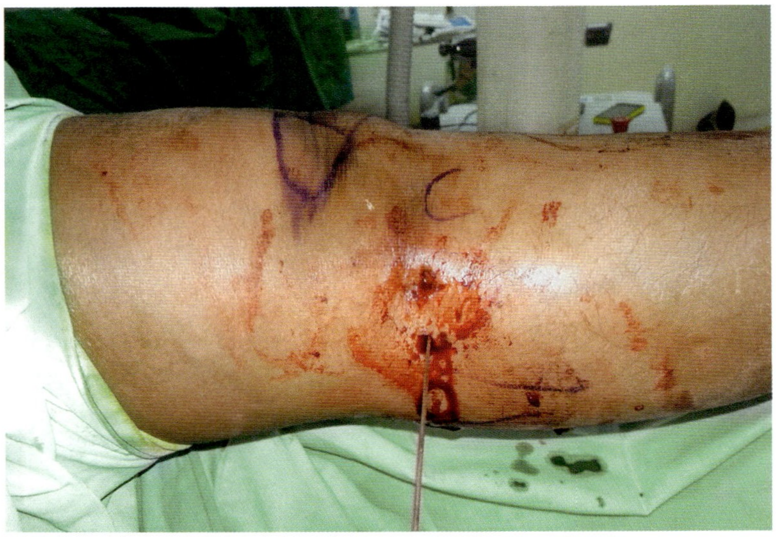

Fig. 23: An additional 5th guide wire inserted from lateral condyle to medial condyle to hold posterior part of articular surface.

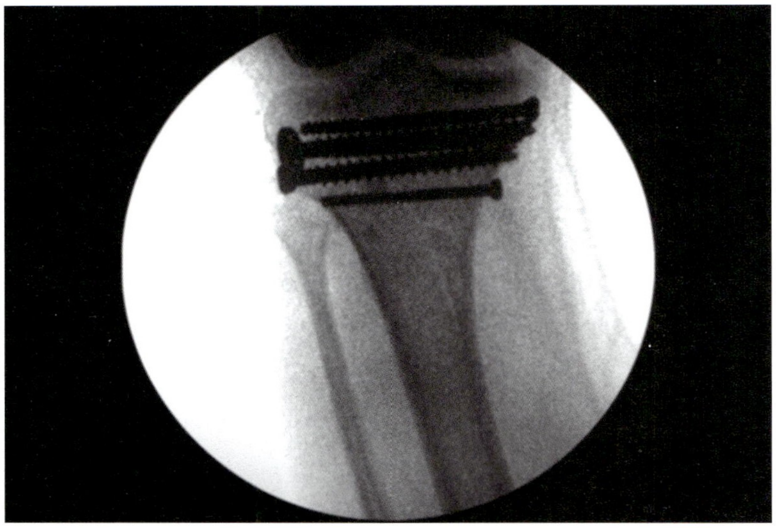

Fig. 24: Stab incision taken and 4 mm CC screw fixed over guide wire to hold posterior part of articular surface. Final fixation confirmed over C-arm anteroposterior view.

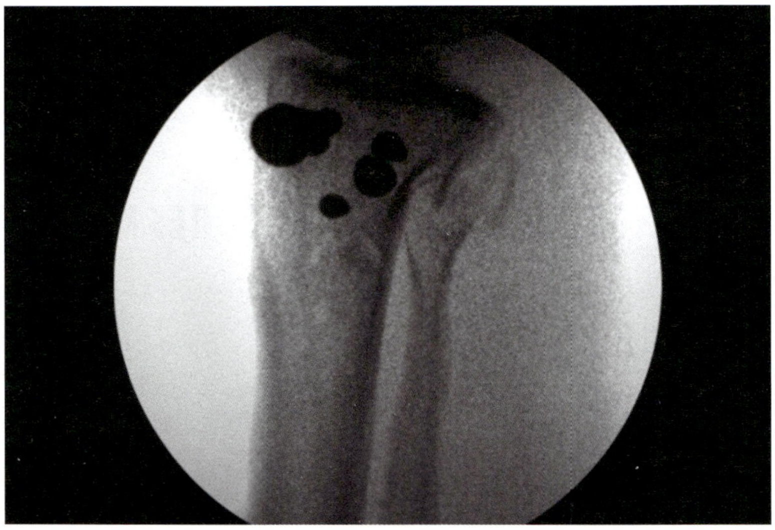

Fig. 25: Final fixation confirmed over C-arm lateral view.

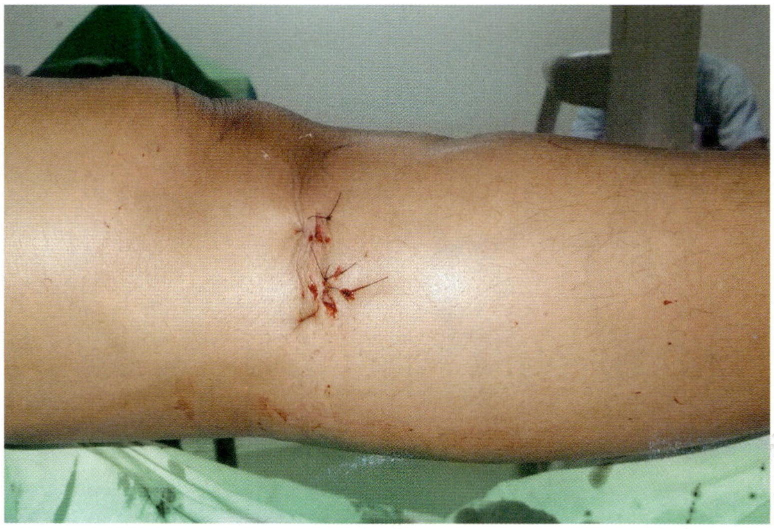

Fig. 26: Stab incisions are cleaned with povidone-iodine solution and skin suture taken with nonabsorbable suture material on lateral side. Total 3 screws are fixed from lateral to medial side.

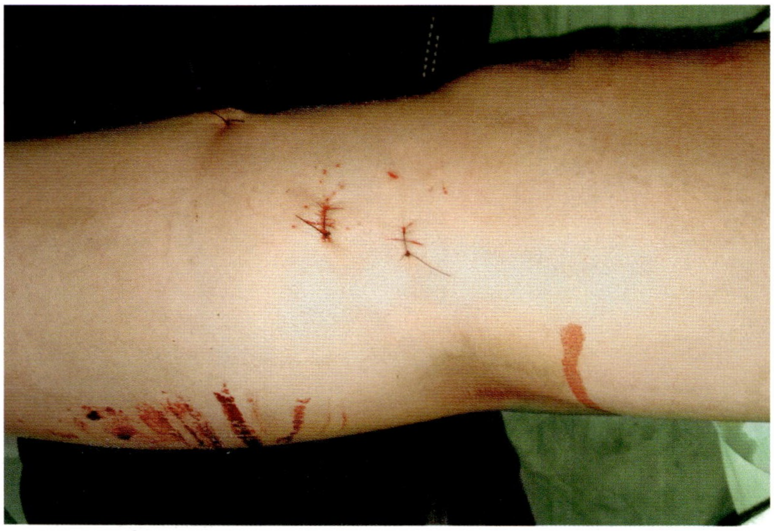

Fig. 27: Suturing done with nonabsorbable suture material on medial side. Total 2 screws are fixed from medial to lateral side.

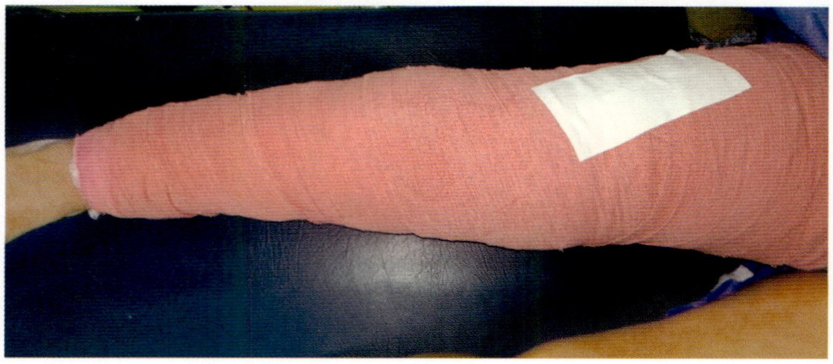

Fig. 28: A cylindrical slab given with knee in 15° flexion. Compression bandage applied.

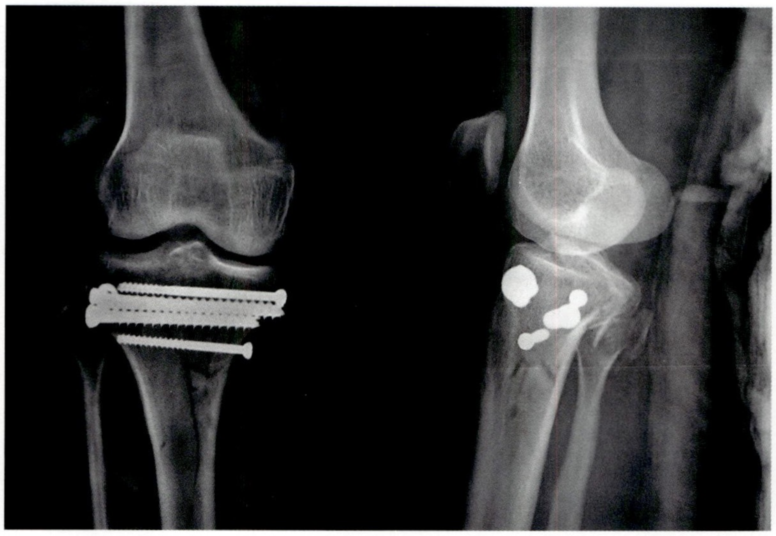

Fig. 29: Postoperative X-ray showing: Fracture Bicondylar proximal tibia fixed with CC screws fixation.

SUGGESTED READING

1. Berkson EM, Virkus WW. High-energy tibial plateau fractures. J Am Acad Orthop Surg. 2006;14(1):20-31.
2. Coleman M, Wright A, Gruen G. Prolonged operative time increases infection rate in tibial plateau fractures. Injury. 2013;44(2):249-52.
3. Zeng ZM, Luo CF, Putnis S, et al. Biomechanical analysis of posteromedial tibial plateau split fracture fixation. Knee. 2011;18(1):51-4.

PROXIMAL TIBIA FRACTURE: MINIMALLY INVASIVE PLATE OSTEOSYNTHESIS

Hitesh J Mangukiya, Jignesh Yeshwant Tandel, Chittanand Mendhe

INTRODUCTION

Minimally invasive plate osteosynthesis (MIPO) is indicated in Schatzker—Type 5 and 6 fractures especially in cases of long segment metaphyseo at diaphyseal comminution.

SURGICAL STEPS

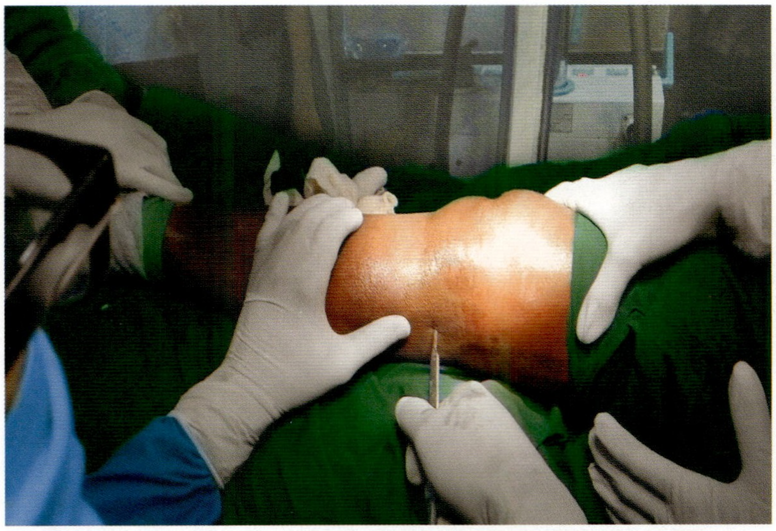

Fig. 30: Patient positioning (supine) with operative extremity kept in 20–30° flexion at hip and knee.

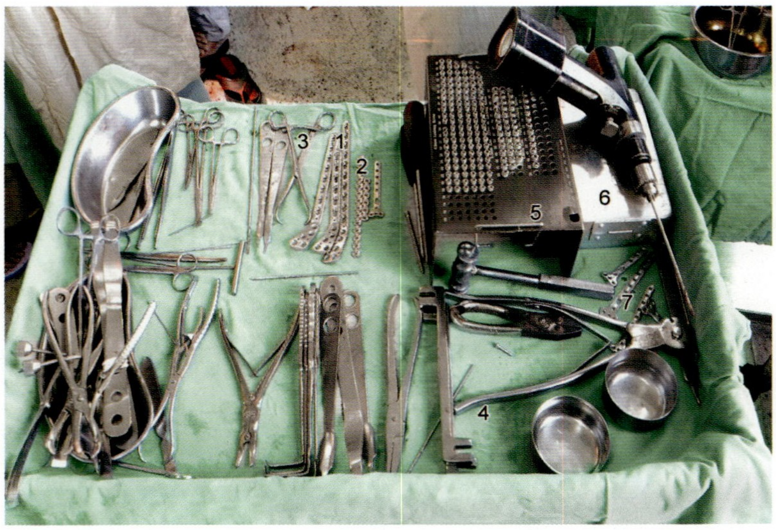

Fig. 31: Necessary implants and instruments for the procedure. (1) Hockey locking plate; (2) Reconstruction plate; (3) Pointed reduction forceps; (4) Plate benders; (5) Locking and nonlocking screws of 3.5 mm and 4.5 mm; and (6) Drill machine and other general instruments.

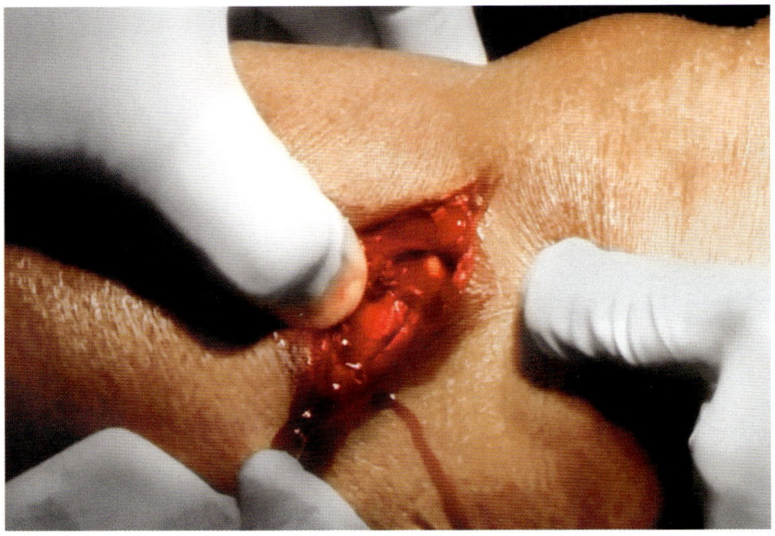

Fig. 32: Straight or oblique skin incision of 5 cm length is taken posterior to Gerdy's tubercle, running distally and posteriorly. Alternatively, the incision can begin at Gerdy's tubercle and continue distally and anteriorly.

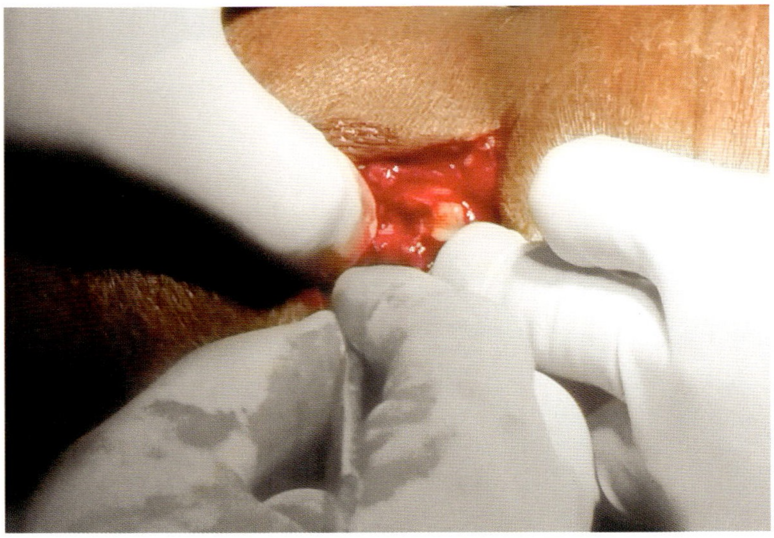

Fig. 33: Superficial sharp dissection done by opening the deep fascia and releasing the anterior attachment of tibialis anterior muscle.

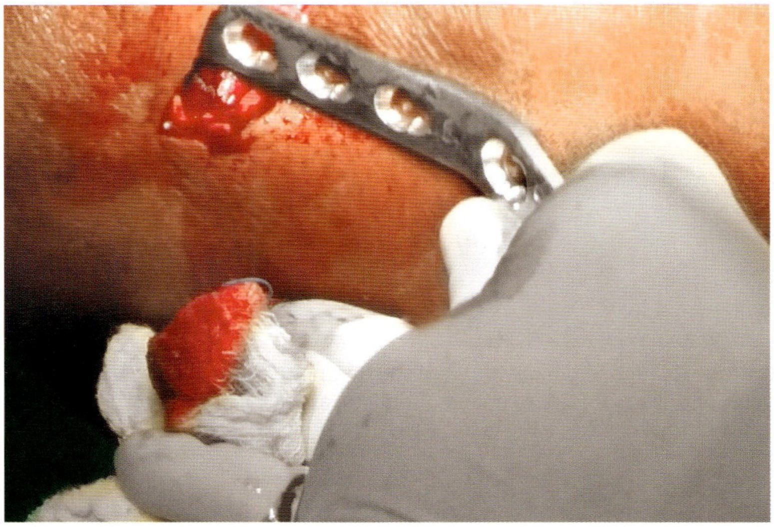

Fig. 34: Precontoured anatomical locking plate is passed in submuscular plane on anterolateral aspect of proximal tibia.

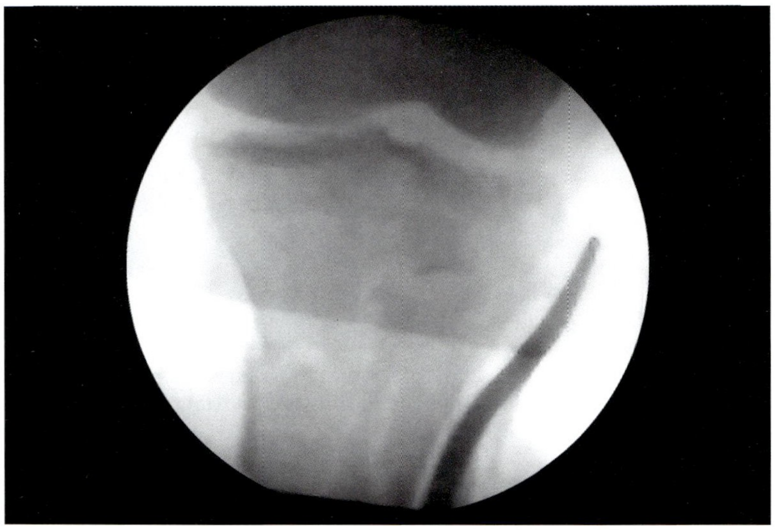

Fig. 35: Plate positioning is checked under C-arm image.

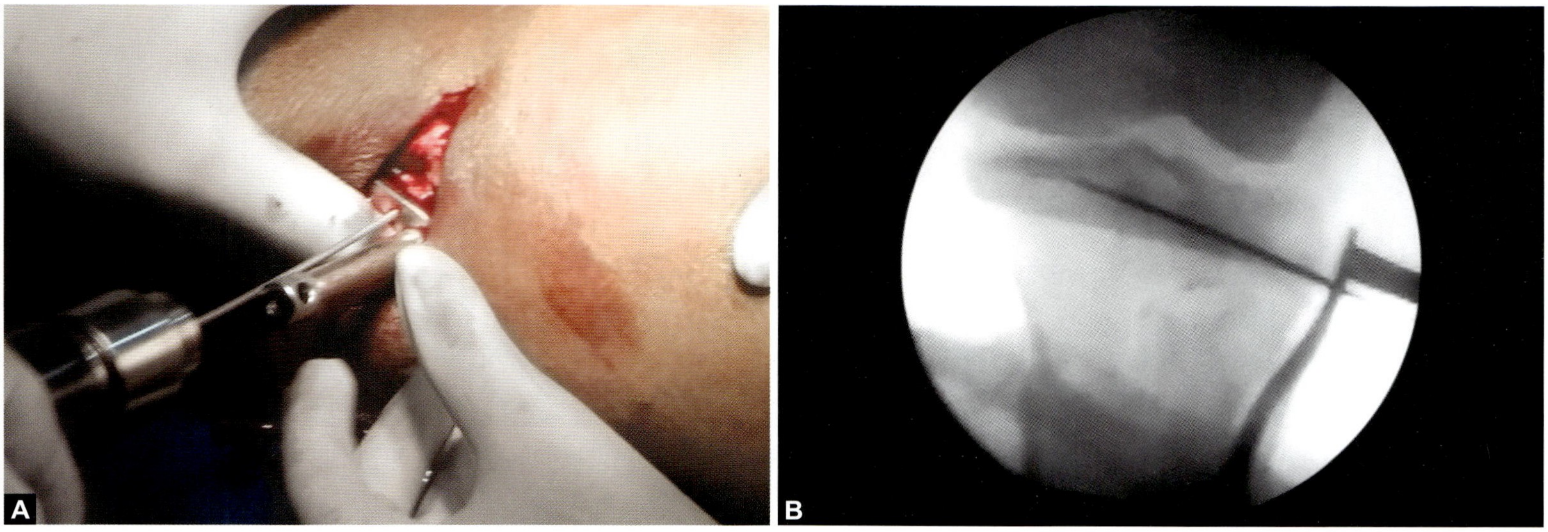

Figs. 36A and B: Preliminary K-wire fixation is done to secure plate positioning. (A) Clinical photo; and (B) C-arm image.

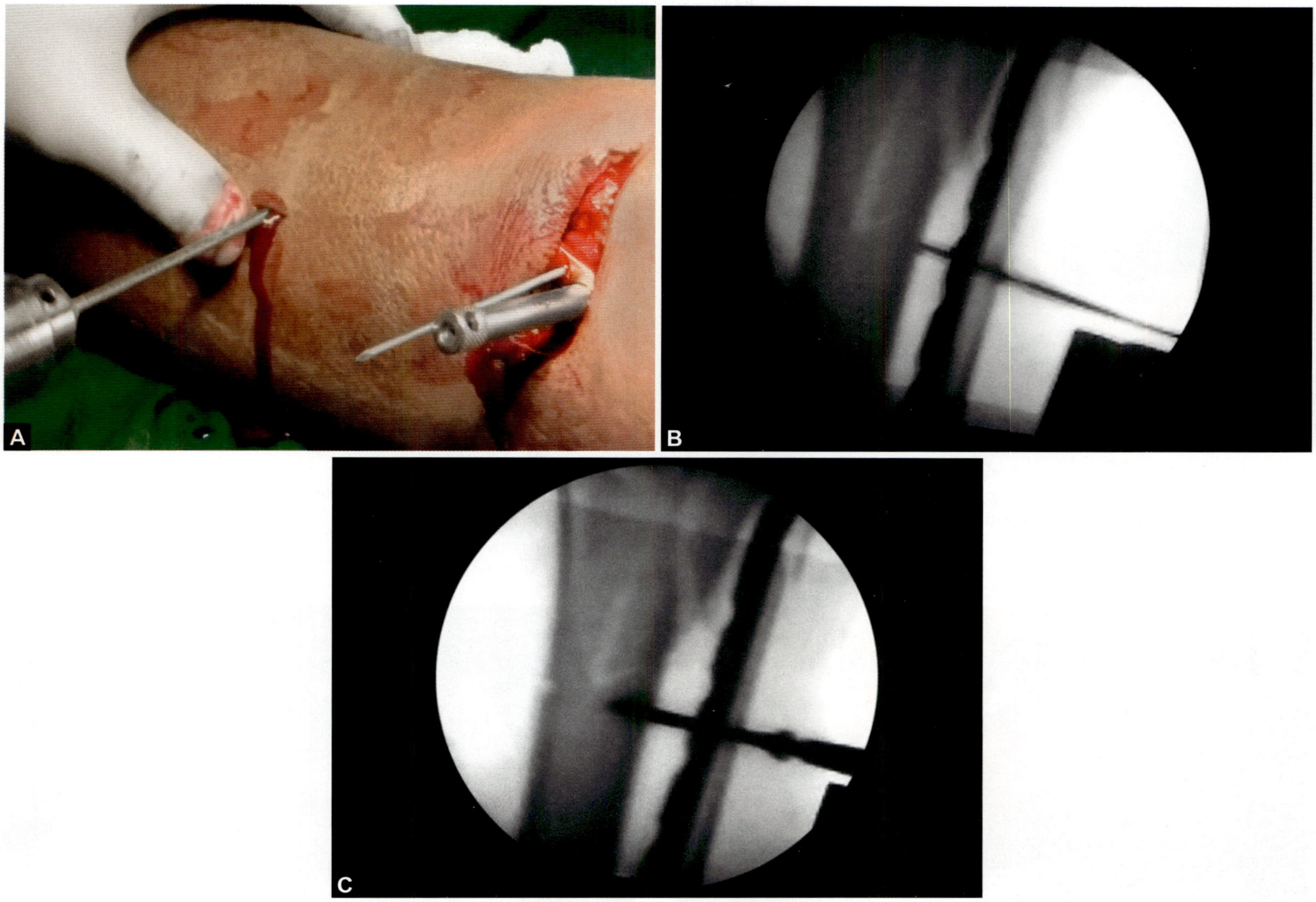

Figs. 37A to C: Indirect reduction of fracture fragments is carried out by manual traction. Plate is aligned with the distal fragment; a cortical screw is inserted just distal to extension of fracture line for provisional fixation. (A) Clinical photograph of drilling; (B) C-arm image of drilling; and (C) Screw insertion at C-arm image. Care is taken to ensure that the distal most screws are centrally located on the tibial cortex.

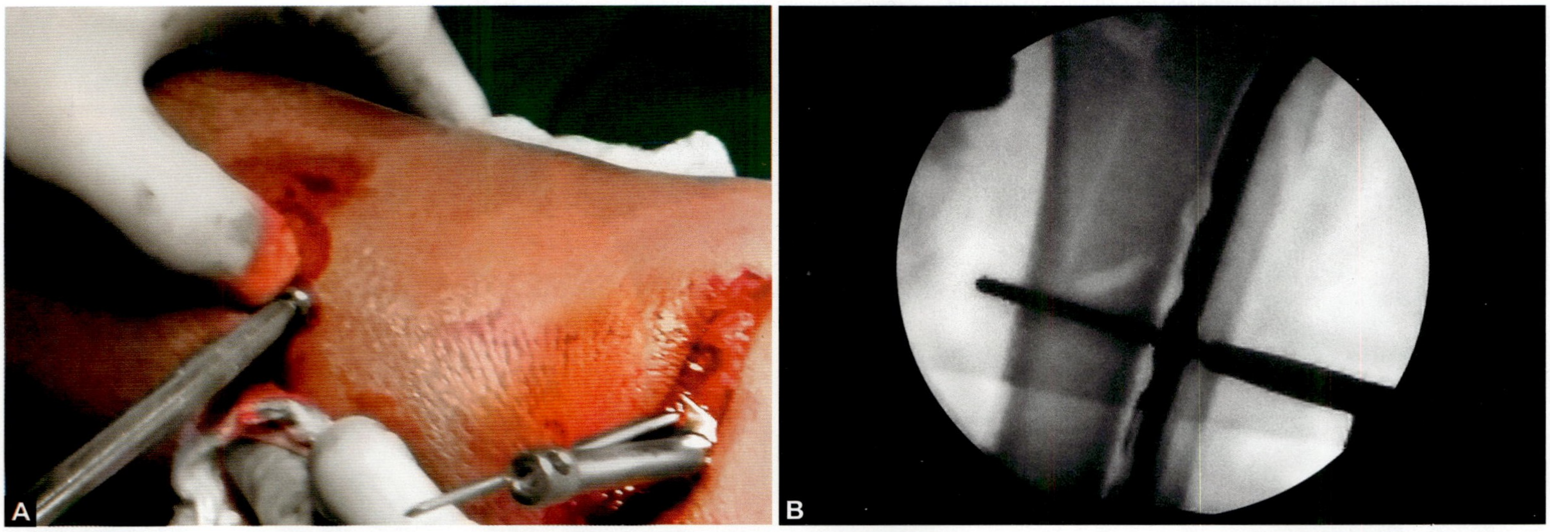

Figs. 38A and B: On final tightening of cortical screw, plate becomes flush with the bone. (A) Clinical photograph; and (B) C-arm image.

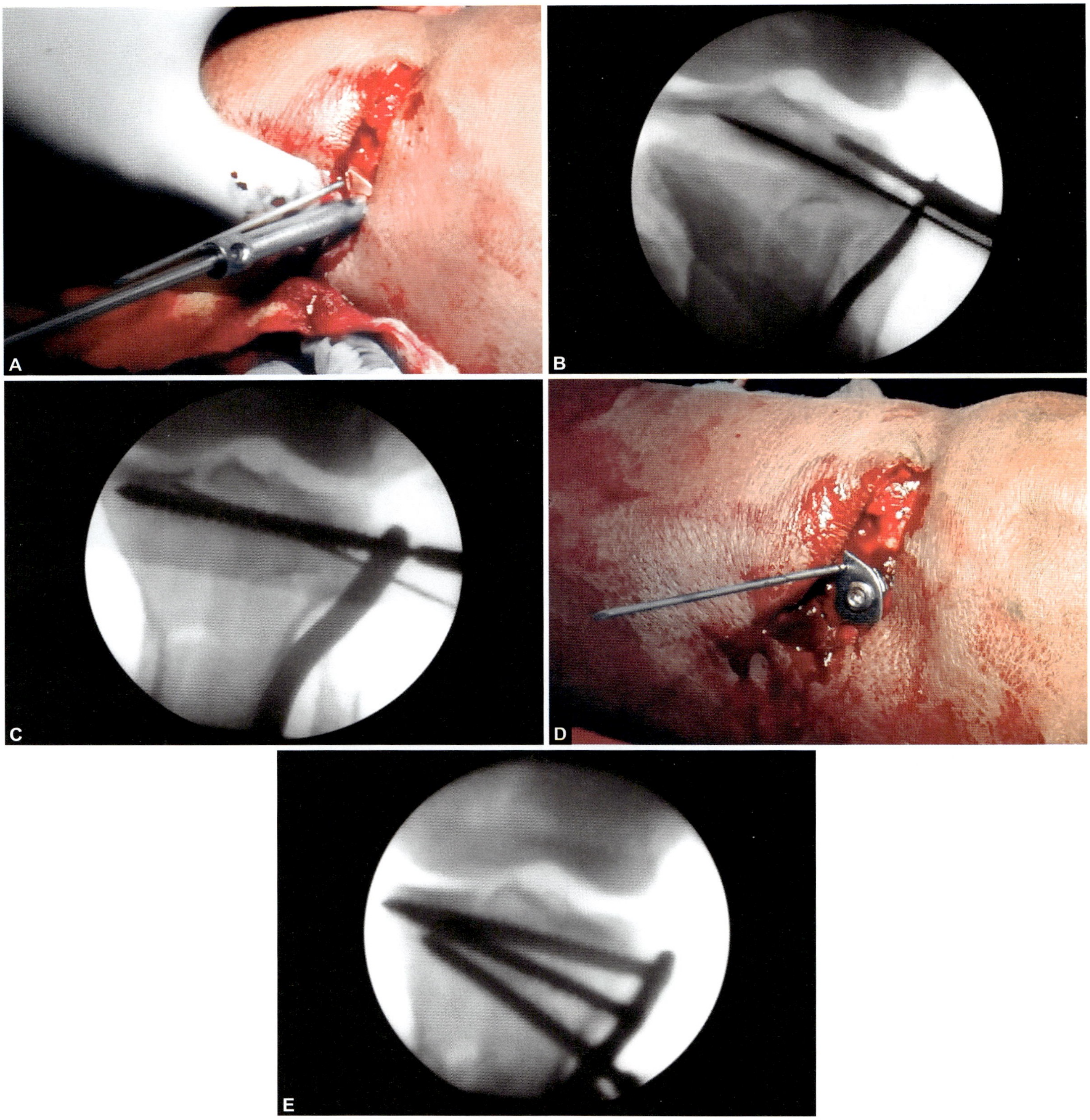

Figs. 39A to E: Proximal locking screw fixation is carried out under C-arm guidance to prevent intra-articular penetration. (A) Clinical photograph of drilling; (B) C-arm image of drilling; (C) C-arm image of screw insertion; (D) Final screw insertion clinical photograph; and (E) Remaining screws are inserted.

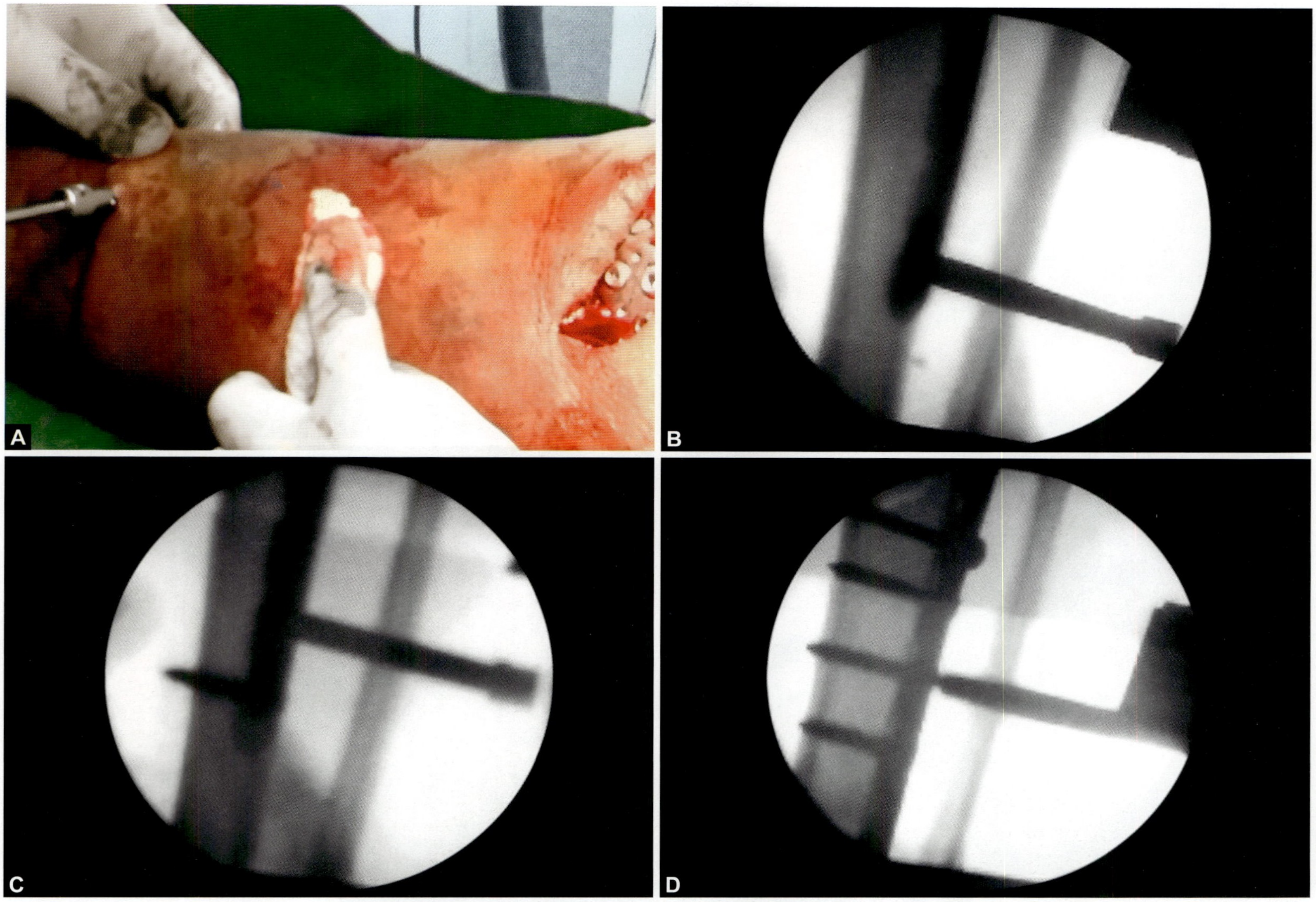

Figs. 40A to D: Distal locking screw fixation is done using stab incision placed directly overlying the plate holes under C-arm guidance. (A) Clinical photograph of drilling through sleeve; (B) C-arm image of drilling through sleeve; (C) C-arm image of screw inserted; and (D) C-arm image showing the remaining screws inserted.

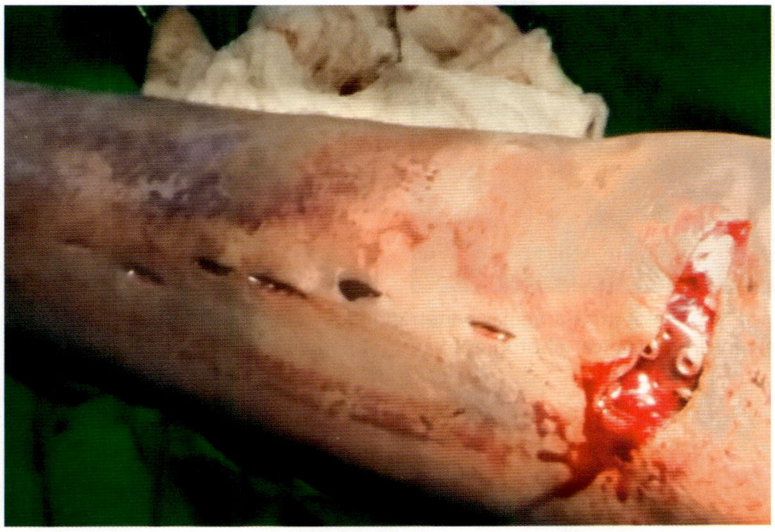

Fig. 41: Final implant placement showing minimal incision. Fascia and skin are closed in layers. Sterile dressing is applied.

POSTOPERATIVE MANAGEMENT

Static quadriceps exercise and ankle mobilization are started as soon as patients' pain is tolerated. Non-weight-bearing walking is initiated immedietely with passive movements at the knee joint. Active knee and ankle exercises and straight leg raising exercises are added gradually. At four to six weeks post operative partial weight bearing with crutches is started. Full weight bearing is allowed around three months provided follow up X-ray shows satisfactory healing.

POSSIBLE COMPLICATIONS

- Soft tissue disruption over the incision
- Malalignment of fracture as the surgery is performed closed; and the full length of the limb cannot be visualized on C-arm, which will lead to later malunion
- Iatrogenic injury to neurovascular structures
- Rarely nonunion.

SUGGESTED READING

1. Baumgaertel F, Buhl M, Rahn BA. Fracture healing in biological plate osteosynthesis. Injury. 1998;29 Suppl 3:C3-6.
2. Krettek C, Schandelmaier P, Miclau T, et al. Minimally invasive percutaneous plate osteosynthesis (MIPPO) using the DCS in proximal and distal femoral fractures. Injury. 1997;28 Suppl 1:A20-30.
3. Phisitkul P, McKinley TO, Nepola JV, et al. Complications of locking plate fixation in complex proximal tibia injuries. J Orthop Trauma. 2007;21:83-91.
4. Rhinelander FW. The normal microcirculation of diaphyseal cortex and its response to fracture. J Bone Joint Surg. 1968;50(4):784-800.
5. Sidhu AS, Brar BS, Mann HS, et al. Minimally invasive plate osteosynthesis for proximal and distal tibial fractures. Pb J Orthop. 2010;12(2):14-7.

BICONDYLAR FRACTURE TIBIA PLATE FIXATION

Madhav Khadilkar, Shrinivas S Shintre, Rachit Vipul Shah, Chittanand Mendhe

BICONDYLAR PLATING INDICATIONS ALL SCHATZKER 5 AND 6 PATTERNS.

Patient is laid supine on an operating table under spinal anesthesia with the hip buttressed with a small bolster to keep the limb in neutral rotation. Tourniquet is applied and under sterile precautions, the limb is scrubbed followed by painting and draping.

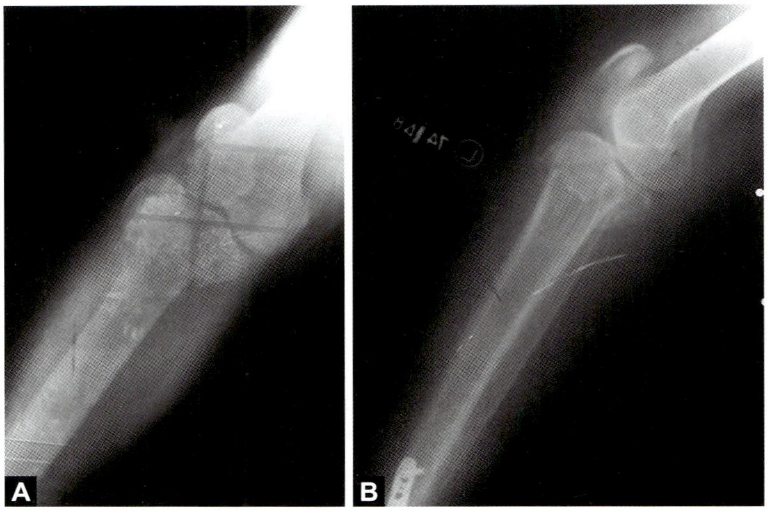

Figs. 42A and B: Preoperative anteroposterior and lateral radiographs.

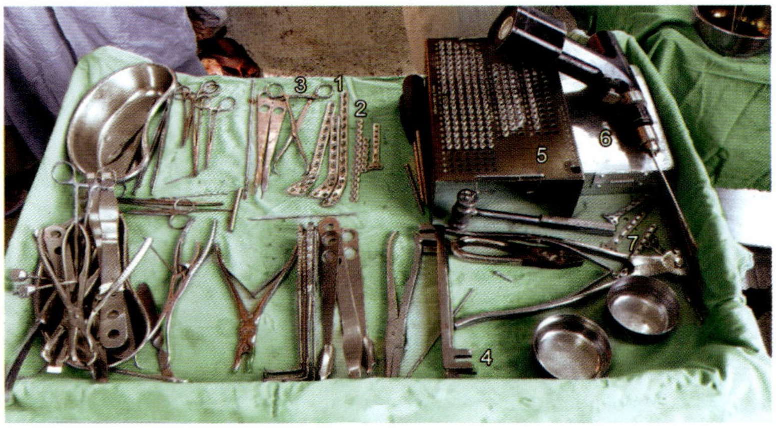

Fig. 43: Instrument trolley showing medial and lateral condylar plates along with instrument assembly. (1) Lateral condylar plate; (2) Reconstruction plate; (3) Pointed reduction forceps; (4) Plate benders; (5) Screw box; (6) Drill; and (7) Medial condylar plate.

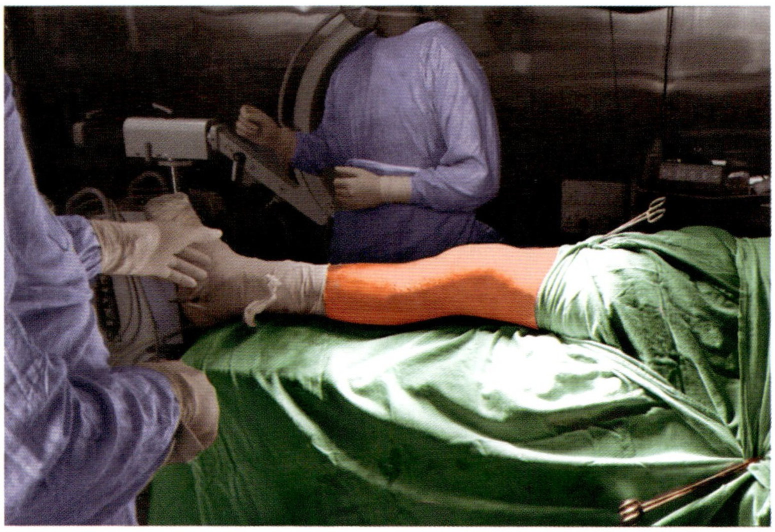

Fig. 44: Supine position of the patient for bicondylar plating of proximal tibia—painting and draping are done.

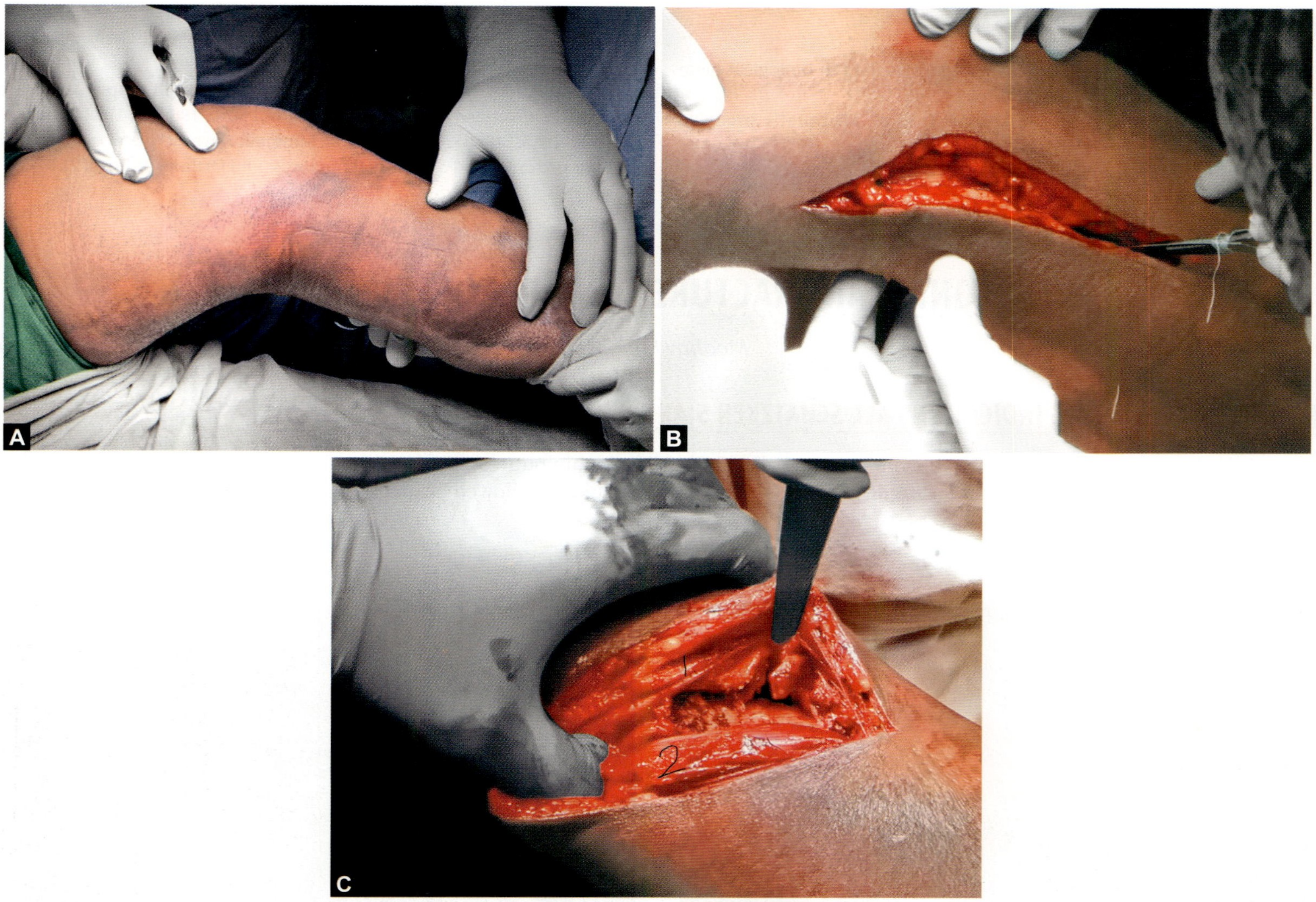

Figs. 45A to C: Incision for the posteromedial approach between the posterior pes (A) and the medial gastrocnemius muscle (B) is made; and (C) The medial head of the gastrocnemius is retracted to protect the structures in the popliteal fossa and visualize the medial tibial plateau.

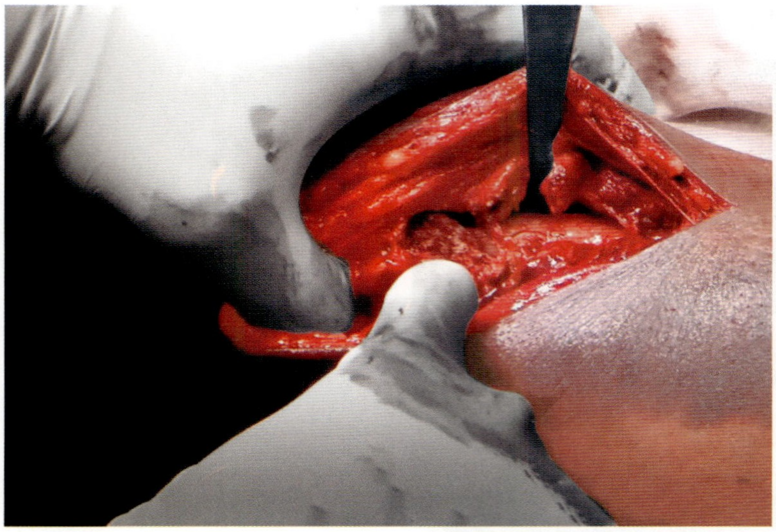

Fig. 46: With the help of blunt and sharp dissection using periosteum elevator, cautery or knife, the attached muscles are dissected away from the fracture to expose the fracture fragments.

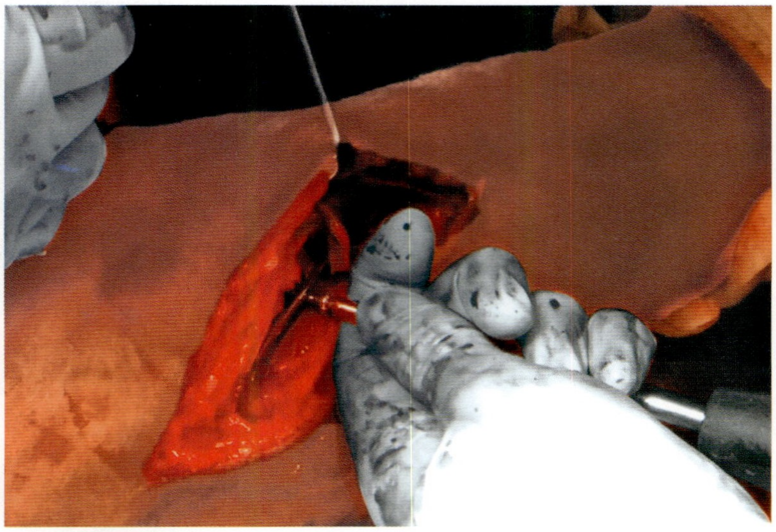

Fig. 47: Medial condylar plate is slid into the submuscular plane with the help of sleeve attached in one of the proximal screw holes.

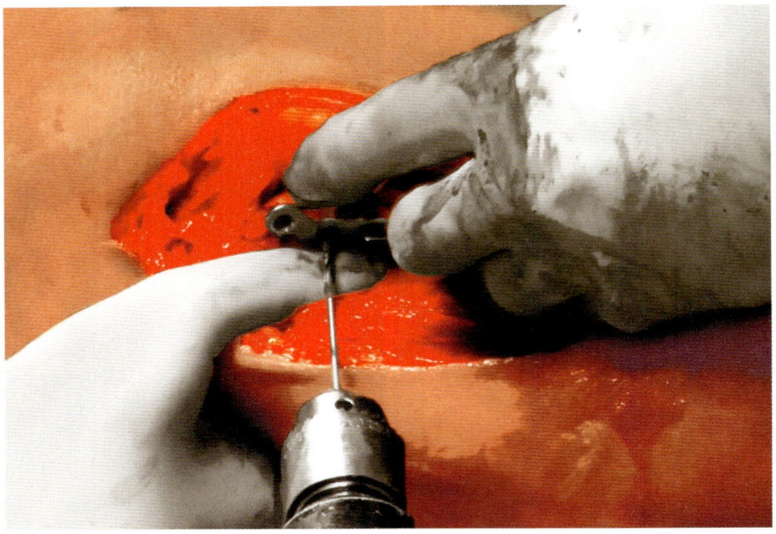

Fig. 48: Under fluoroscopic guidance, first cortical screw is passed through central hole of the plate to secure plate against surface of the bone.

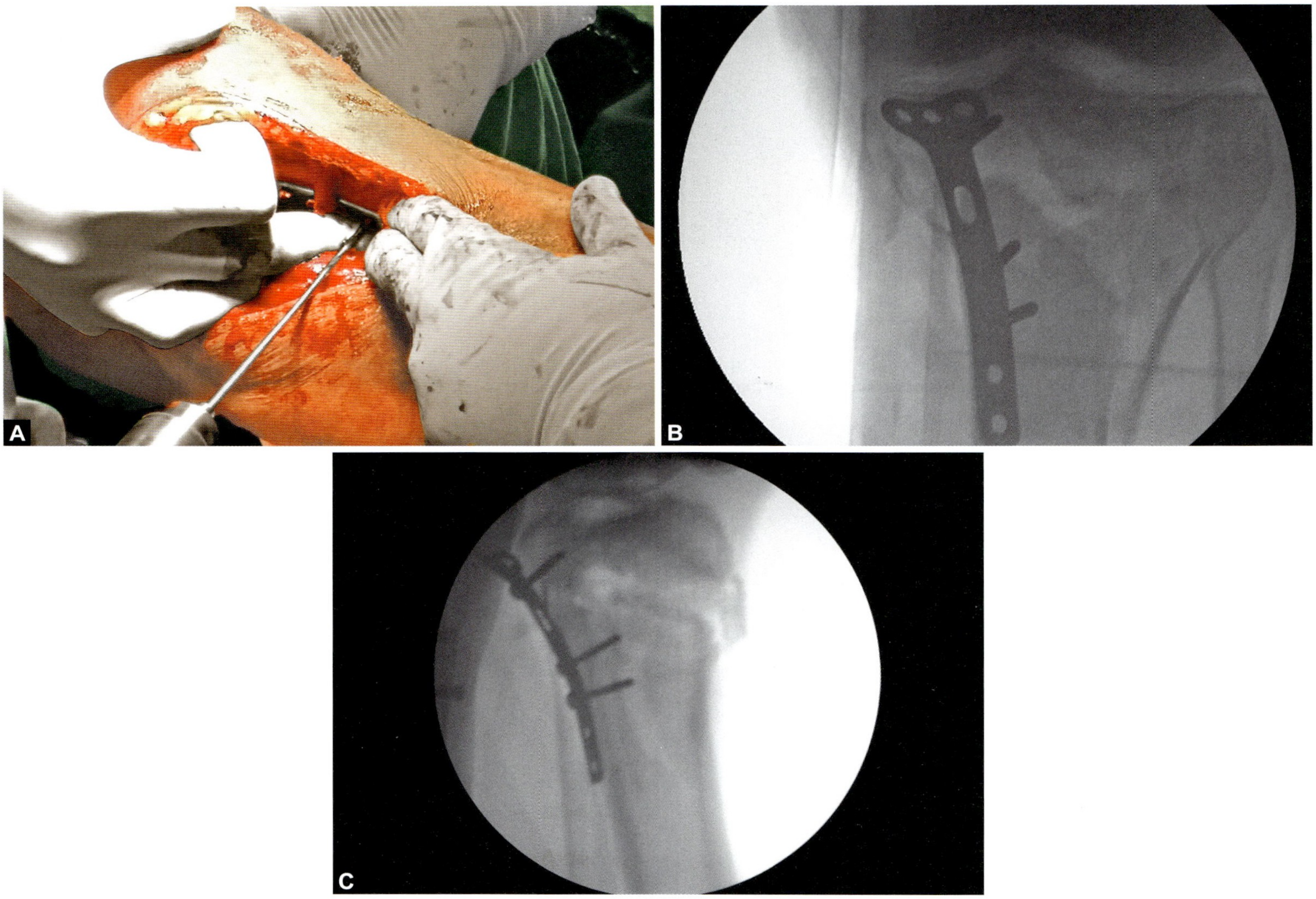

Figs. 49A to C: Additional screws are fixed to achieve buttressing of fracture fragments under the plate.

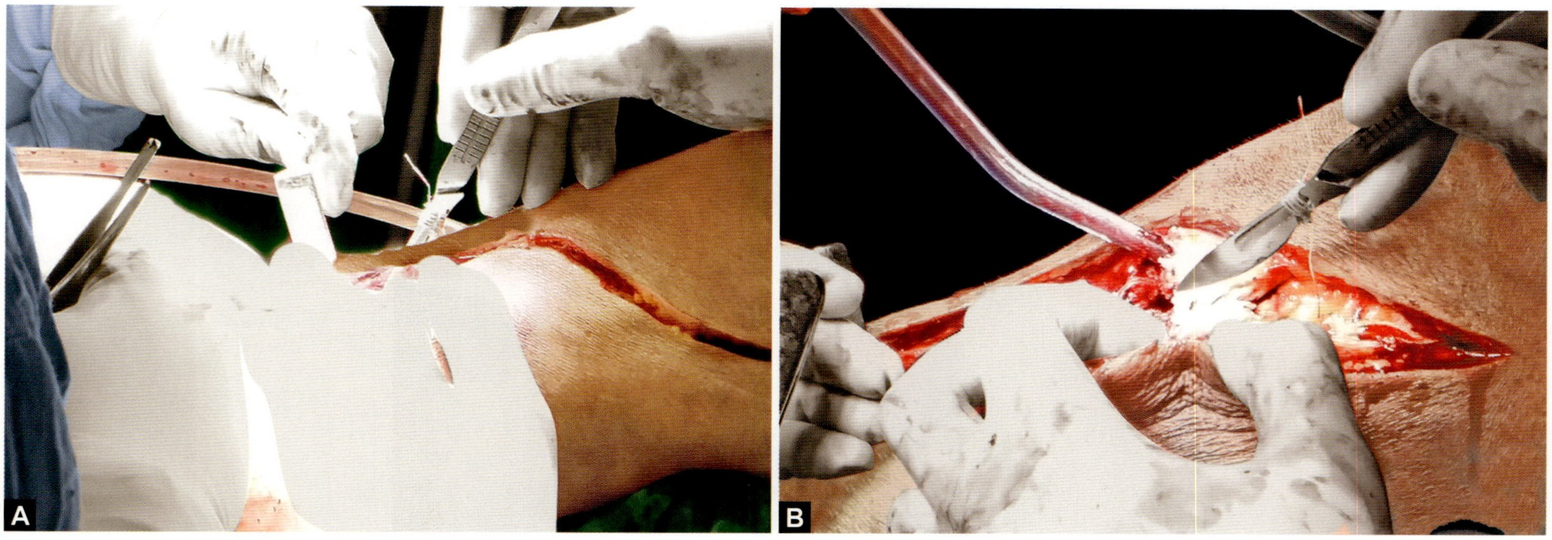

Figs. 50A and B: A curved incision based on the Gerdy's tubercle is made and extended distally over the anterior compartment. The anterior compartment muscles are incised continuously with the iliotibial band to provide adequate access to the anterolateral surface of proximal tibia.

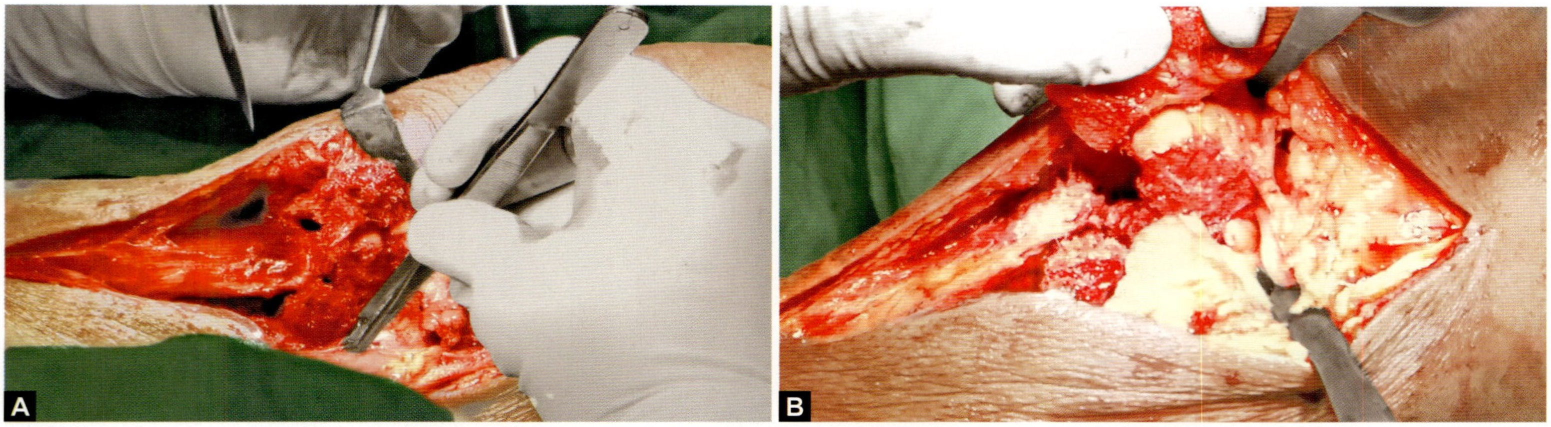

Figs. 51A and B: Under fluoroscopic guidance, the depressed fracture fragments are elevated through the window that is available throughout the split fracture.

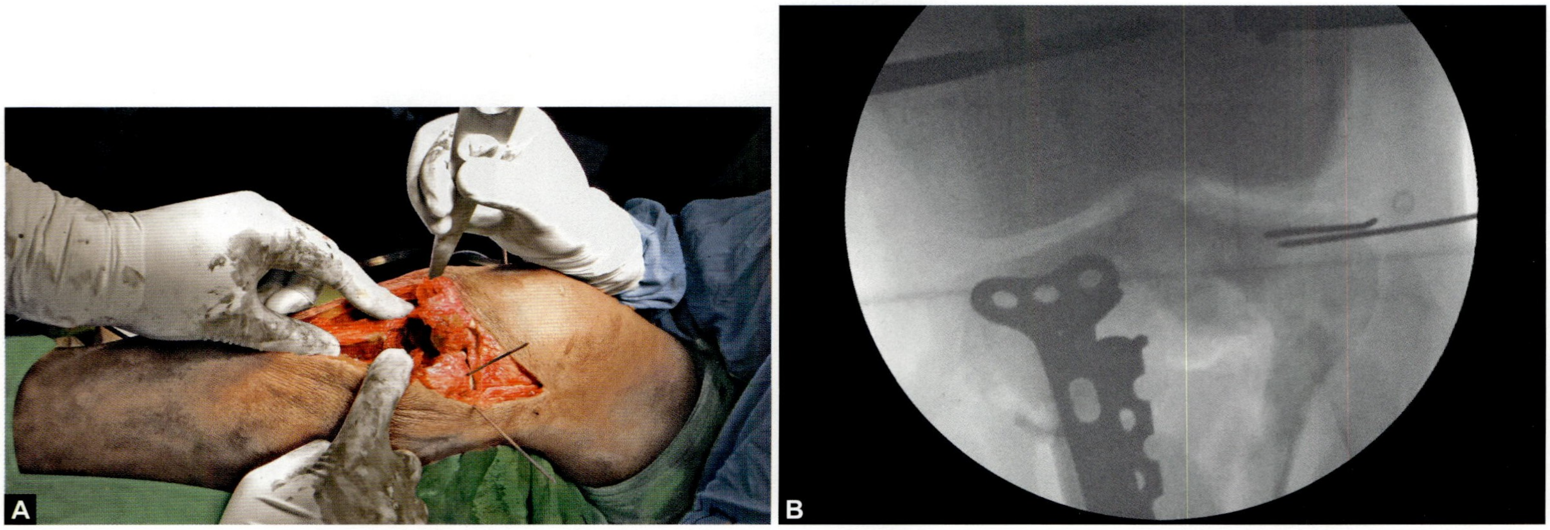

Figs. 52A and B: After adequate reduction of the articular surface, the surface is temporarily held in reduction with the help of a fluoroscopically-guided K-wire passed subarticularly.

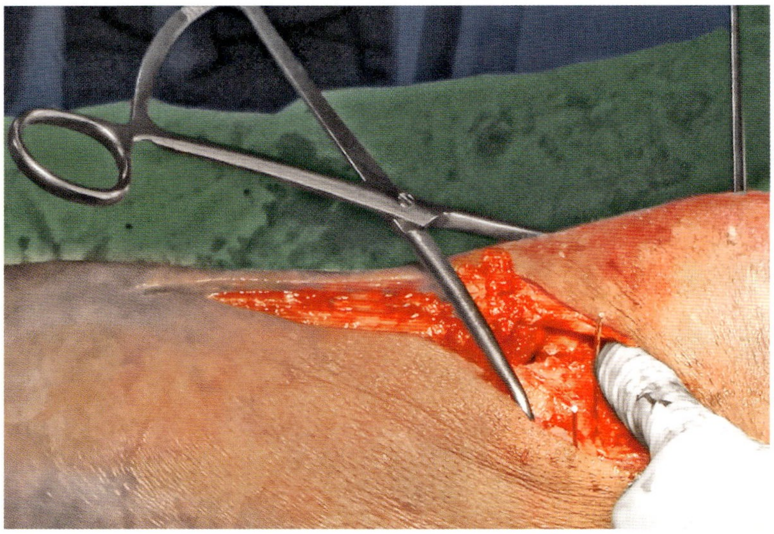

Fig. 53: Further reduction of the fracture surface and reduction of the bicondylar width are achieved with the help of pointed bone holding forceps and confirmed by fluoroscopy.

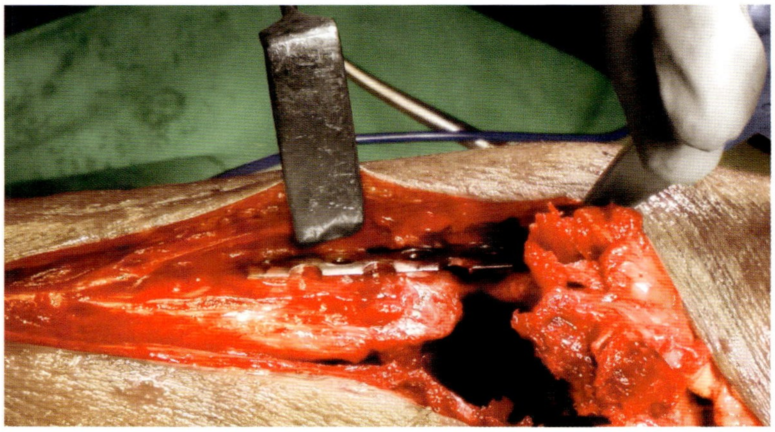

Fig. 54: A 3.5-mm reconstruction plate is introduced from the anterolateral incision and is used to buttress the anterior fragment.

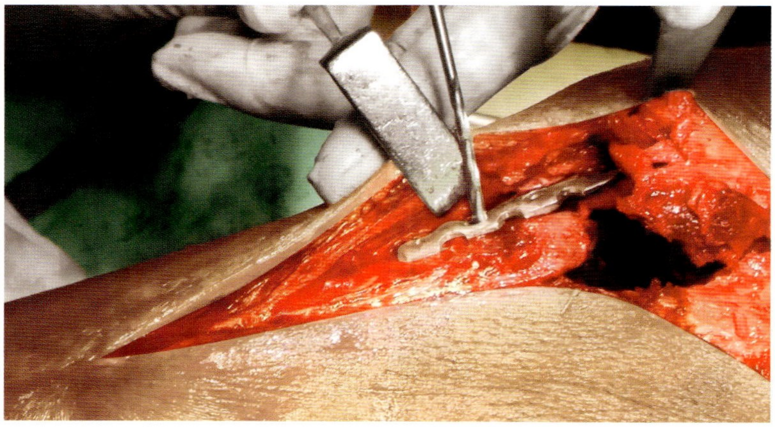

Fig. 55: The 3.5 mm reconstruction plate is fixed with help of cortical screws.

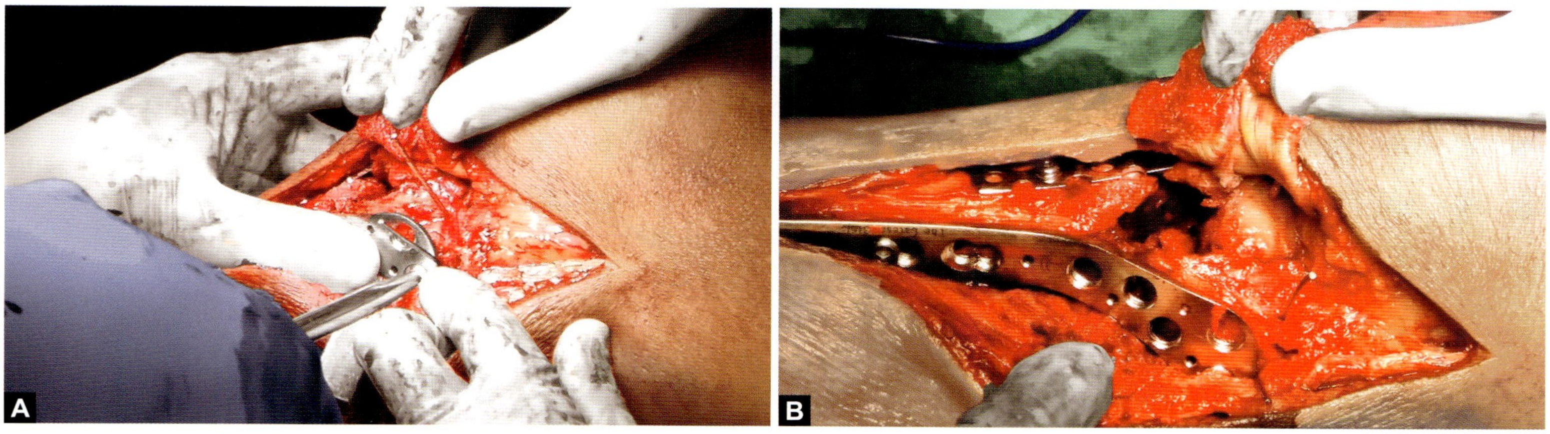

Figs. 56A and B: Lateral condylar plate for proximal tibia is introduced submuscularly with the help of sleeve.

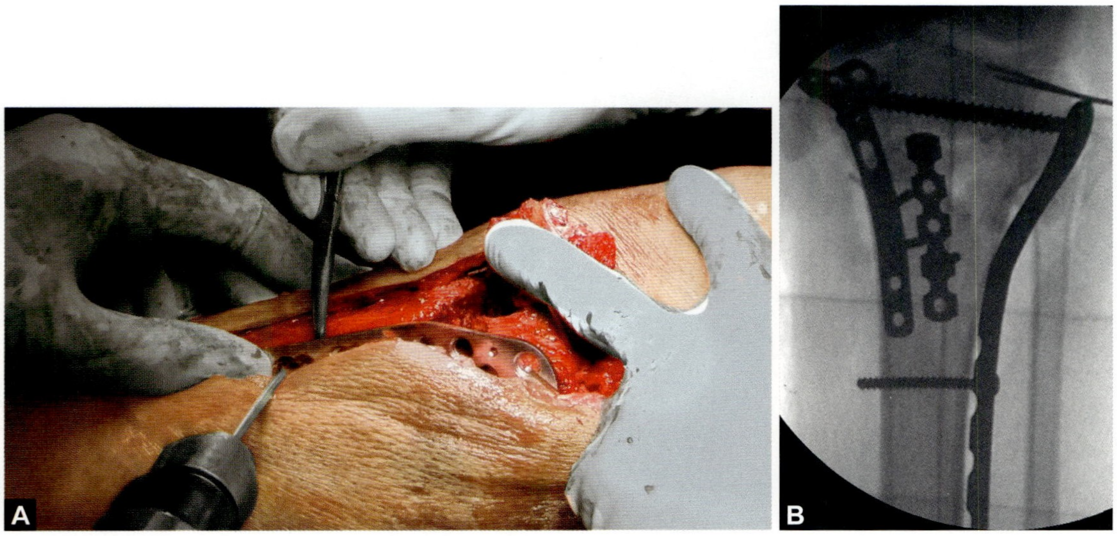

Figs. 57A and B: Plate is buttressed onto fracture anterolateral surface of the tibia with the help of cortical screws.

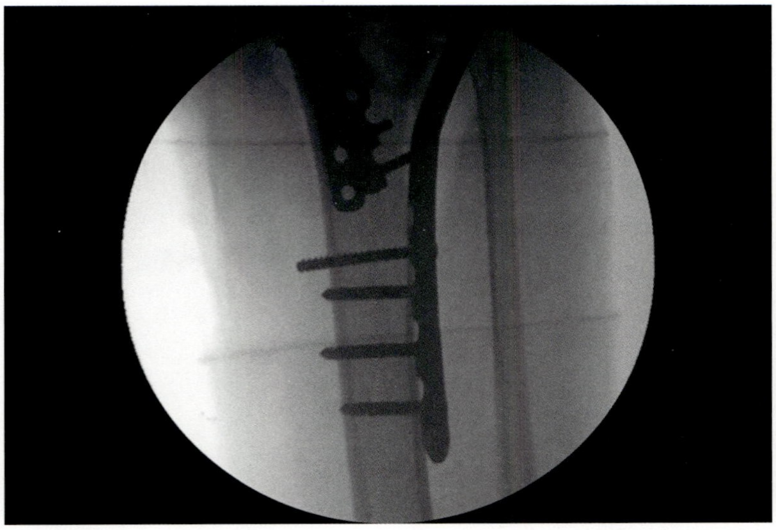

Fig. 58: Plate is fixed with locking and cortical screws and reduction is confirmed under fluoroscopy.

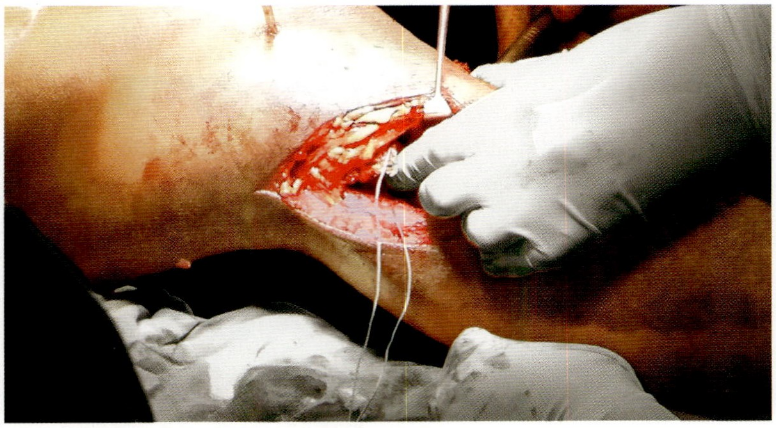

Fig. 59: Posteromedial incision is sutured first.

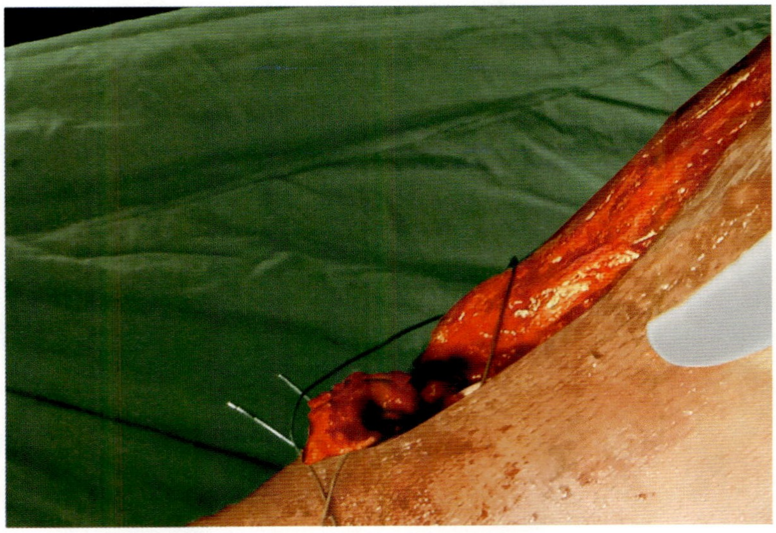

Fig. 60: Anterolateral incision is closed in layers.

CHAPTER 112

Fracture Shaft Tibia Interlocking Nail Fixation

Prateek Charuchandra Joshi, Rajendra Latkar, Shrinivas S Shintre, Rajkumar Ekambaram

INTRODUCTION

Fracture tibia is the most common long bone fracture. Almost 70–80% of tibial shaft fractures are associated with fibular fractures. The mechanism of injury is high-energy trauma in young age group and low energy trauma in older age group. It is more common in men than in women. Due to its subcutaneous location of bone, it often presents as open fracture and in that situation it is usually treated with external fixation. Neurovascular bundle injury should be looked for. Common peroneal nerve palsy must be ruled out in associated high fibula fractures.

CLINICAL FEATURES

Pain, restriction of motion, tenderness on palpation, and swelling are clinical features. Open fractures of tibial shaft can result in bleeding due to damage to tibial vessels. Open fractures may get infected hence all possible care has to be taken.

Foot drop can result from associated common peroneal nerve injury in neck of fibula fractures.

INVESTIGATIONS

Anteroposterior and lateral radiographs of the entire tibia with knee and ankle have to be done as diaphyseal fractures can be associated with knee and ankle injuries.

TREATMENT

- Good quality above knee slab.
- Proper hydration with intravenous fluids and diet.
- Patient is advised limb elevation and ice fomentation to reduce swelling. Once swelling subsides, slab can be converted to cast.
- Intramedullary interlocking nailing provides both translational and rotational stability.
- External fixator is an option reserved for open fractures with or without neurovascular complications.

INDICATIONS

Intramedullary interlocked nailing is employed for the vast majority of tibial shaft fractures. Acute stabilization of closed fractures as well as open fractures with minimal contamination can be performed with intramedullary nailing. Intramedullary nailing is unadvisable in grossly contaminated fractures, open tibial fractures of Gustilo Anderson grade III B or III C, or those associated with extensive soft tissue damage. Patients with medical comorbidities unfit for anesthesia, or those at a high risk of cardiopulmonary complications such as pulmonary thromboembolism or fat embolism may need stabilization with external fixation systems before definitive fixation can be undertaken. Proximal and distal shaft fractures with extensive comminution may benefit from plate fixation.

PREOPERATIVE RADIOGRAPH

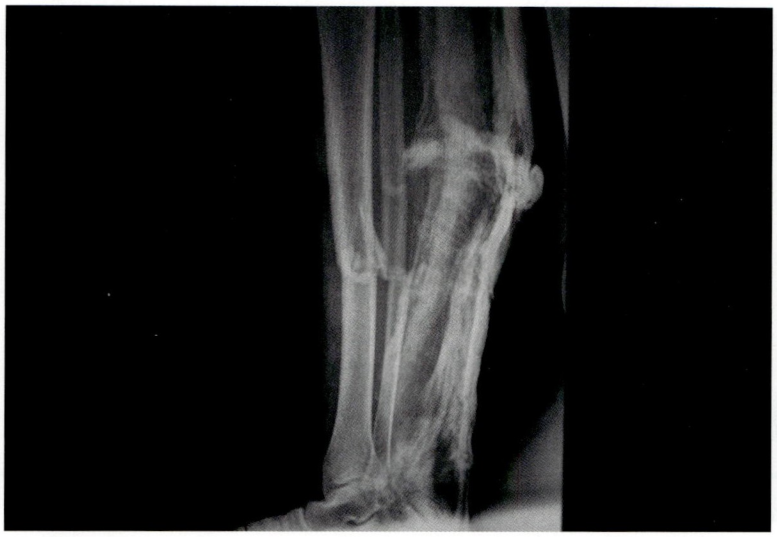

Fig. 1: Preoperative lateral radiograph of mid-shaft fracture of tibia, amenable to intramedullary nailing.

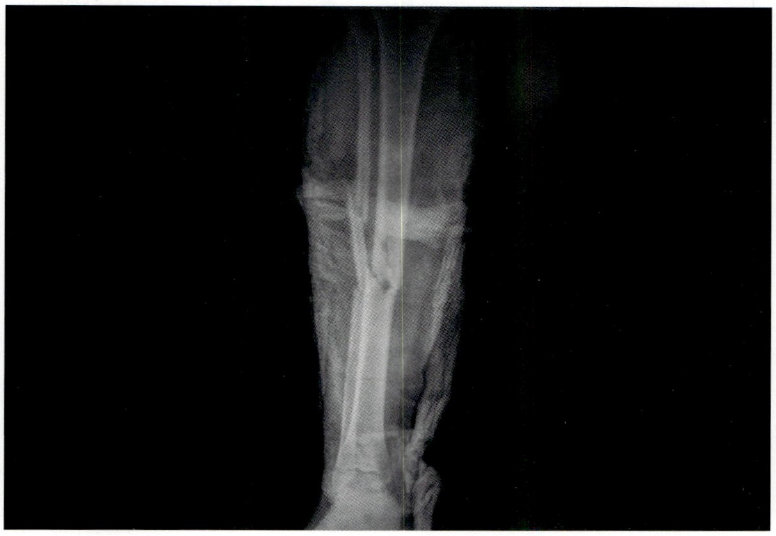

Fig. 2: Anteroposterior radiograph.

SURGICAL PROCEDURE

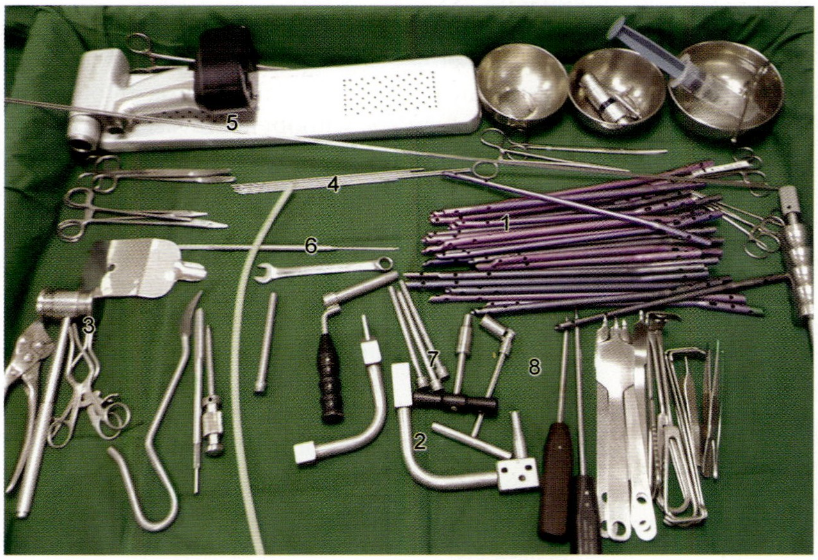

Fig. 3: Surgical instruments necessary for intramedullary nailing of the tibia. (1) Implant: Intramedullary nails in a range of lengths and diameters, (2) Tibia intramedullary interlocking nailing jig to direct the nails and locking screws, (3) Hammer, (4) Drill bits, (5) Guidewires, (6) Depth gauge, (7) T-handle, (8) Screw driver of 4.5 mm.

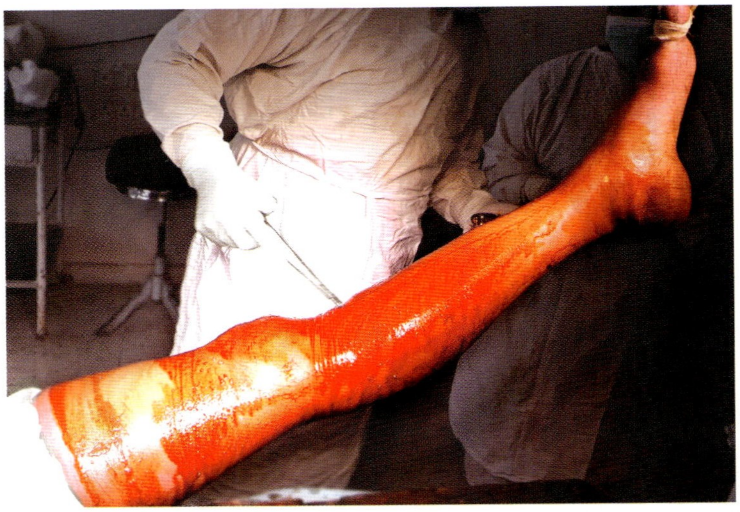

Fig. 4: The limb is scrubbed and povidone iodine painting is done. Optionally, a tourniquet may be applied in unsterile manner prior to painting and draping.

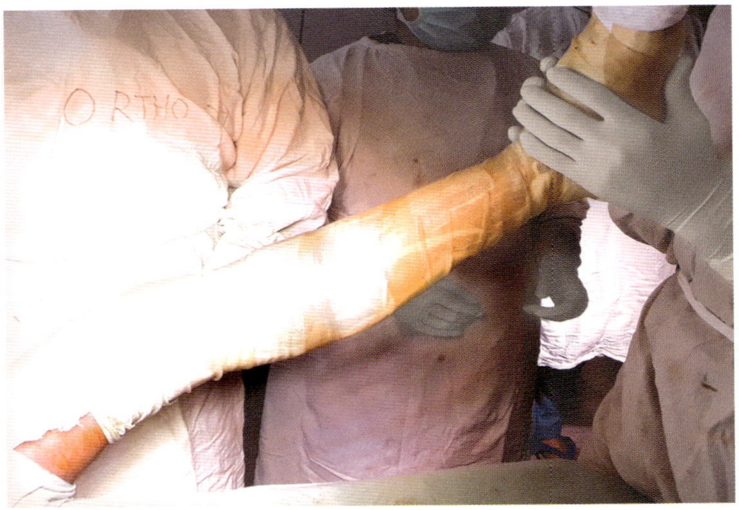

Fig. 5: Under all aseptic measures, painting and draping is done followed by elevation of the limb and exsanguination.

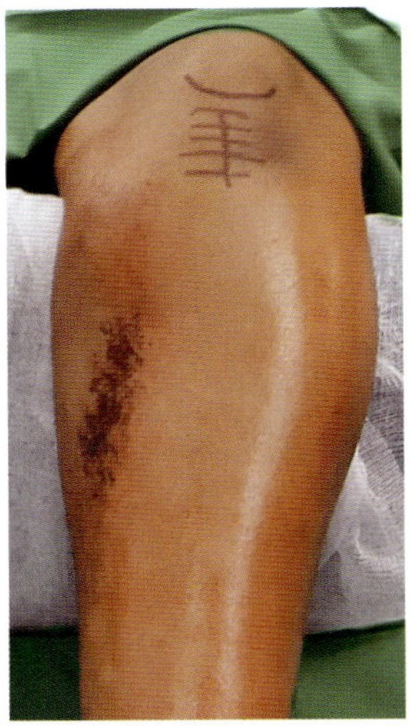

Fig. 6: The limb is placed in flexion at the knee joint on a radiolucent knee frame. The required incision line is marked on the skin surface with a sterile marker. Incision is a 5-cm midline incision on the anterior surface of the knee joint from lower pole of the patella to the upper part of tibial tuberosity.

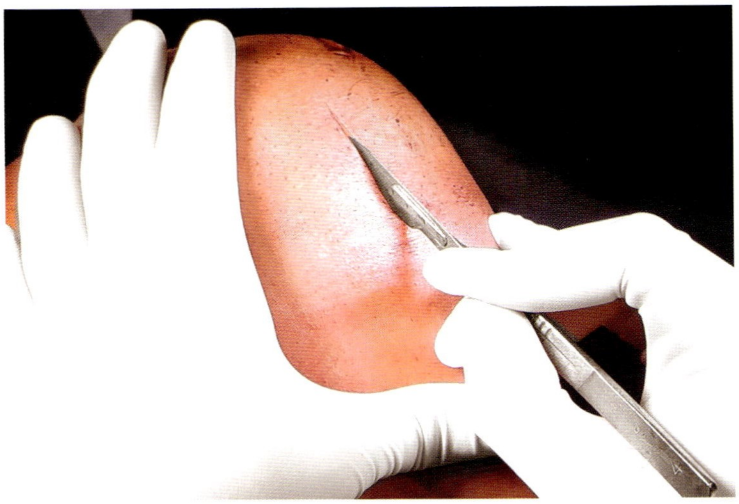

Fig. 7: The marked incision being made.

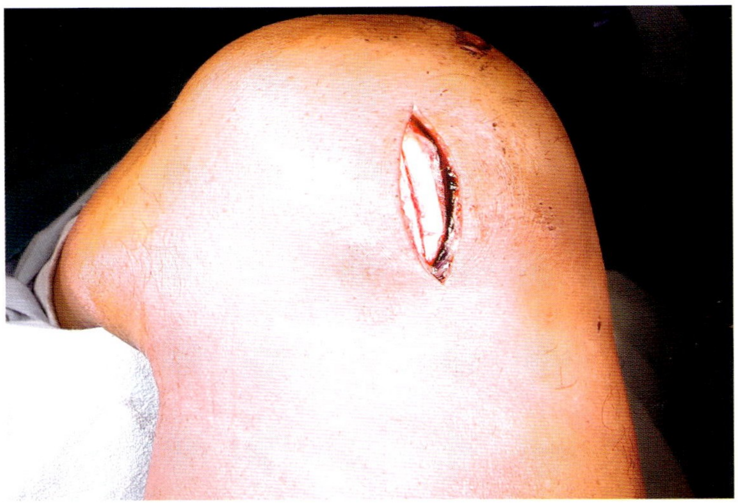

Fig. 8: Soft tissue is dissected and retracted to expose the underlying patellar tendon.

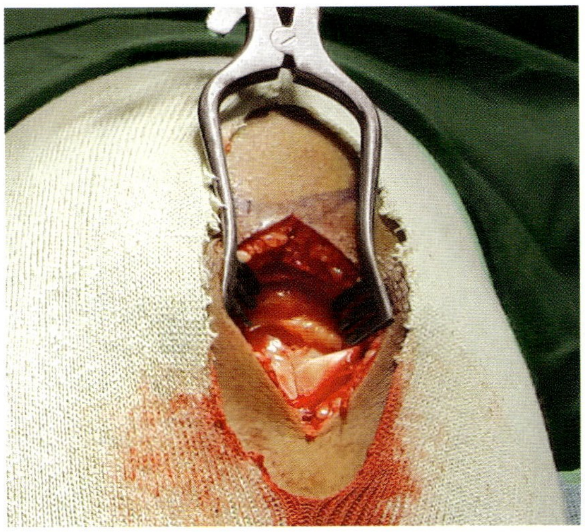

Fig. 9: Patellar tendon is split atraumatically and retracted with right-angled or Mollison retractors and underlying soft tissues are dissected to approach the nail entry site.

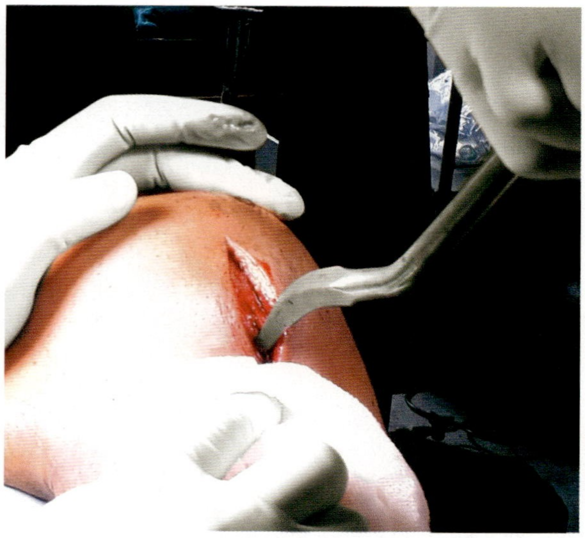

Fig. 10: Using the entry awl, the entry is taken on the anterosuperior facet of the tibial tuberosity in the midline. The awl is then used to create a path into the medullary canal of the tibia.

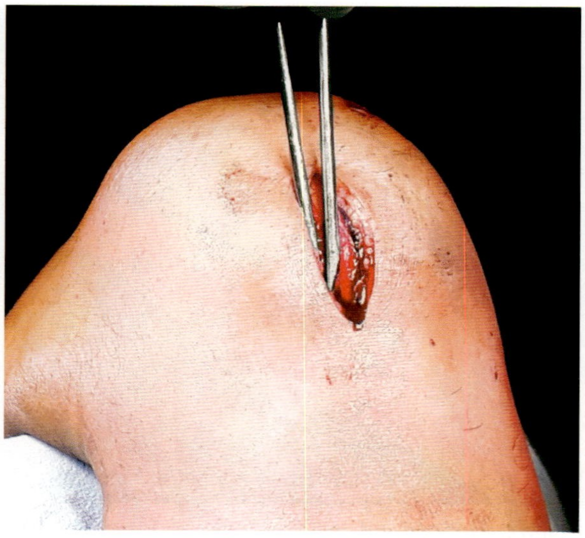

Fig. 11A: The tract created by the entry awl is cleaned and intervening soft tissue separated using the artery forceps. The artery forceps also help to confirm the continuity of the entry tract with the medullary canal of the tibia.

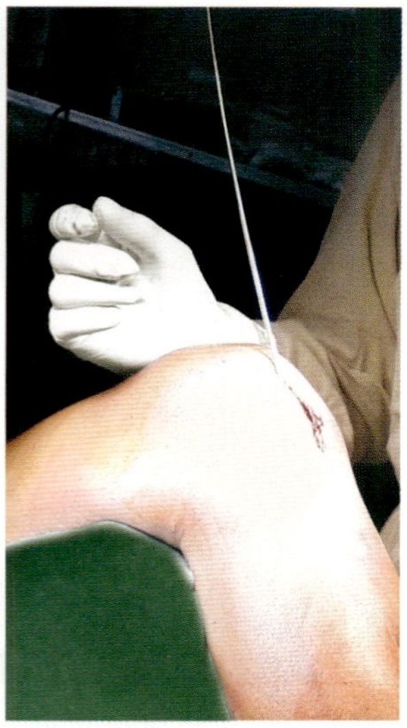

Fig. 11B: Closed reduction of the fracture is performed and the guidewire is passed from the proximal fragment through the fracture site into the distal fragment.

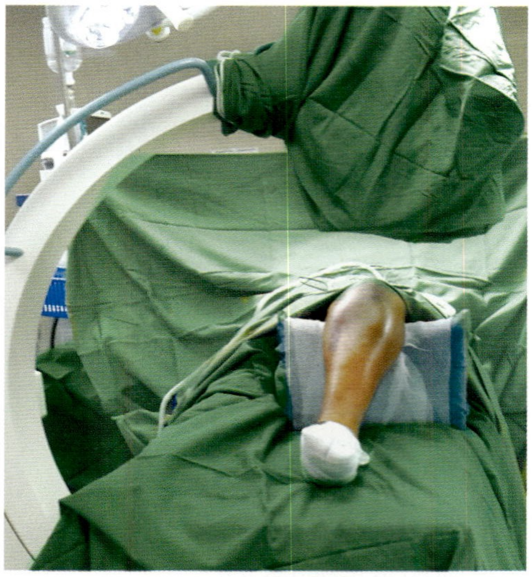

Fig. 12: C-arm positioning for intraoperative fluoroscopy. Views are taken in anteroposterior as well as lateral plane.

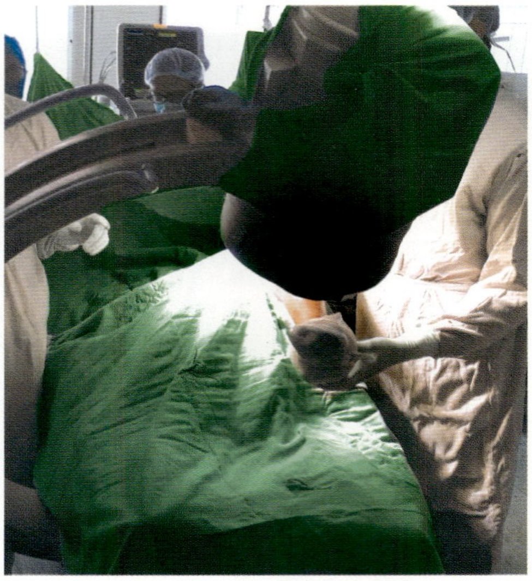

Fig. 13: The C-arm positioned in oblique with reference to the patient, provides an anteroposterior view of the tibia placed in flexion on the knee frame.

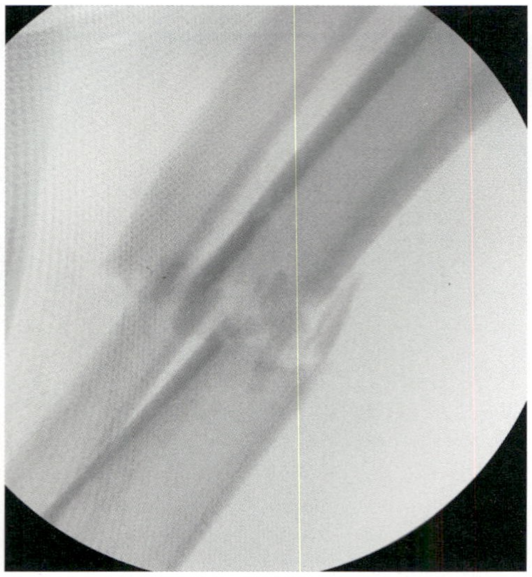

Fig. 14: The fracture site is visualized under fluoroscopy and reduction is attempted. Attempt is made to bring about cortical contact between the proximal and distal fracture fragments.

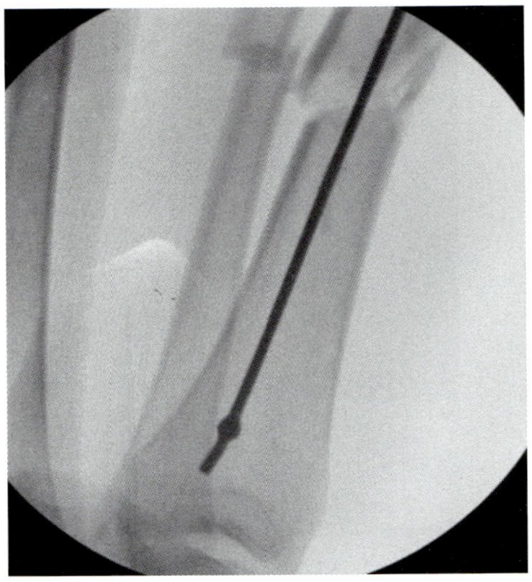

Fig. 15: Passage of the guidewire into the distal fragment is confirmed under intraoperative fluoroscopy. The guidewire should be centro-central in anteroposterior as well as lateral views.

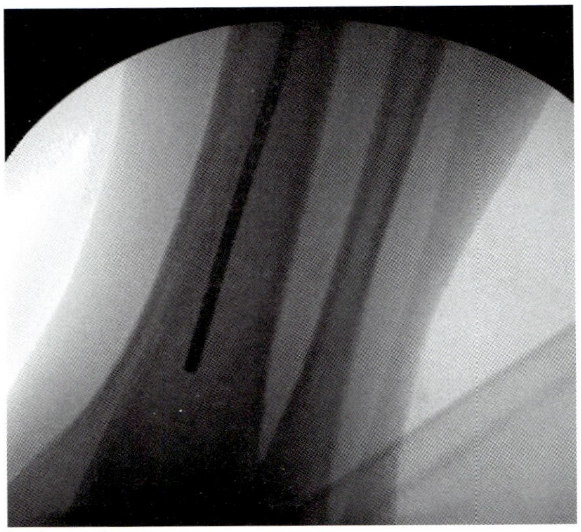

Fig. 16: The fracture reduction and position of the guidewire is confirmed under fluoroscopy. Fracture reduction should be anatomical and the guidewire should be centro-central in anteroposterior as well as lateral views.

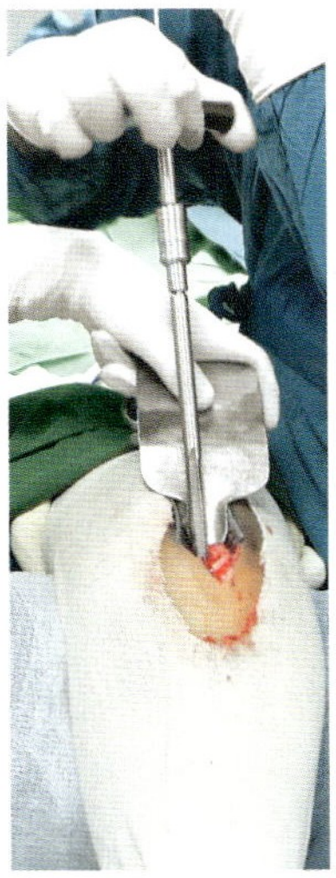

Fig. 17: Reaming of the medullary canal is performed using cannulated reamers passed over the guidewire starting with proximal hand reamer. Gentle reaming must be done in osteoporotic or elderly patients and those with comminuted fractures in order to prevent iatrogenic fractures or displacement of the comminuted fragments respectively.

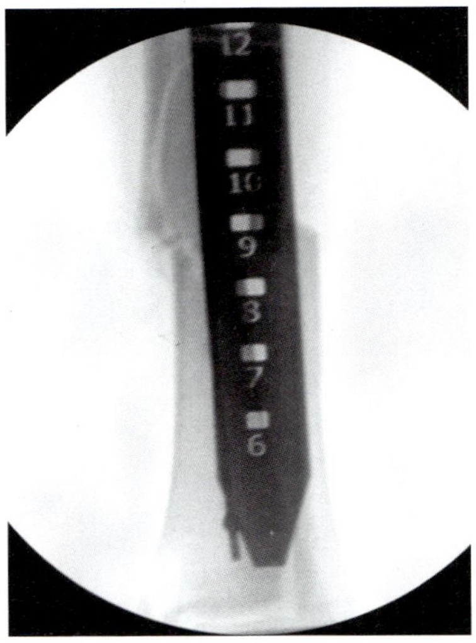

Fig. 18: A radiopaque scale placed over the bone is used to calculate the maximum diameter of nail to be inserted. Reaming is done up to 1.5 mm more than the projected nail size.

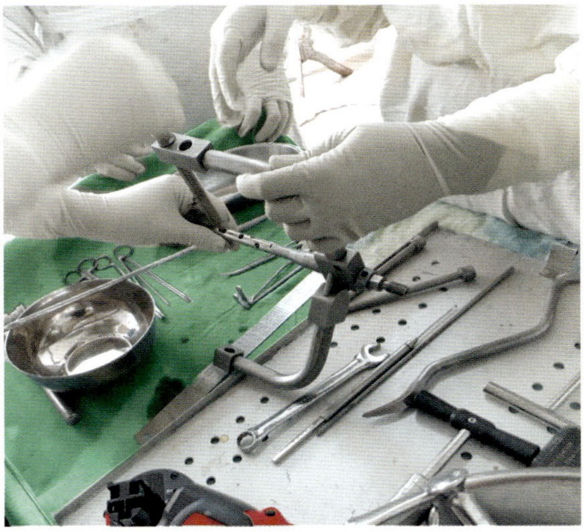

Fig. 19: After the canal has been prepared with adequate reaming, the nail of adequate length is loaded onto the jig. The jig should be medial and the concavity of the nail should face anteriorly. It is prudent to confirm the patency of the jig and the sleeve by passing a drill bit through it; this will detect mismatch of the nail and the jig.

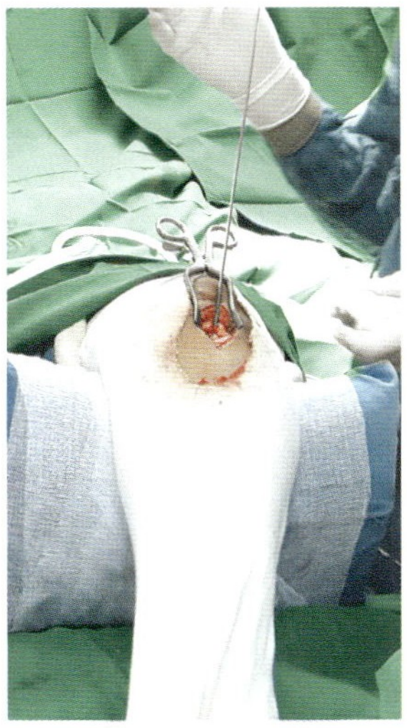

Fig. 20A: Just prior to nail insertion. The canal has been adequately reamed and the guidewire is in situ. If earlier for reaming a beaded guidewire was used, it is now exchanged using an exchange tube to a nonbeaded one. The nail is ready to be inserted.

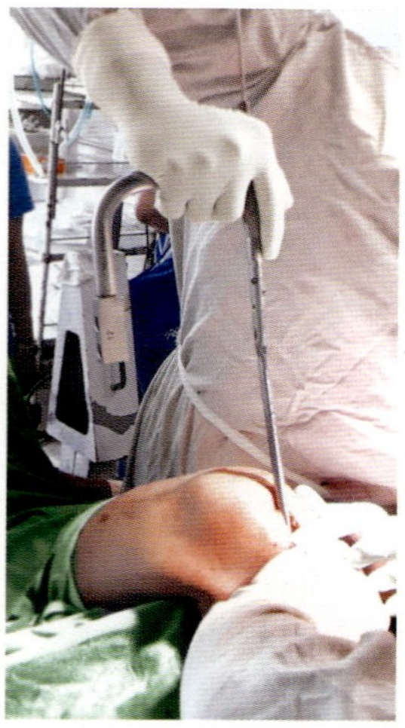

Fig. 20B: The surgeon passes the cannulated nail through the guidewire and into the entry site. The assistant provides a counterforce to stabilize the proximal fragment with one hand; with the other hand, the assistant provides traction to the distal fragment to maintain reduction at the fracture site. The nail should be pushed into the tibia using only the hand push. Sometimes light tapping may be required but it should never be hammered into the canal.

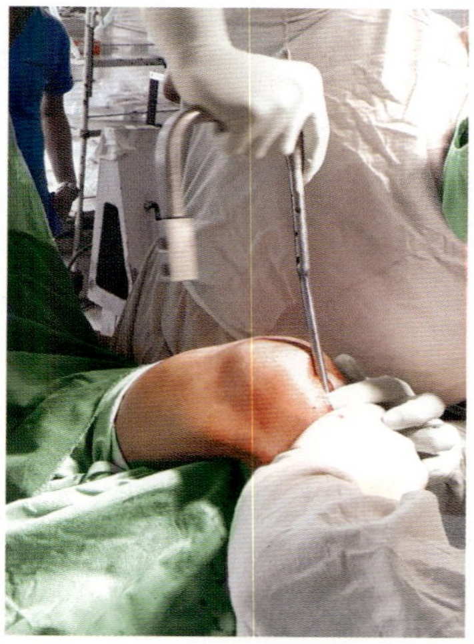

Fig. 21: The nail is advanced into the tibia. The assistant provides traction and maintains reduction throughout.

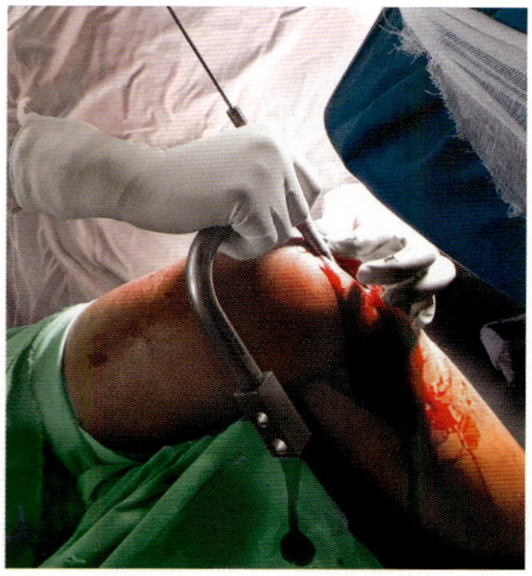

Fig. 22: The nail is advanced into the tibia to its full extent. Reduction must be maintained throughout the procedure.

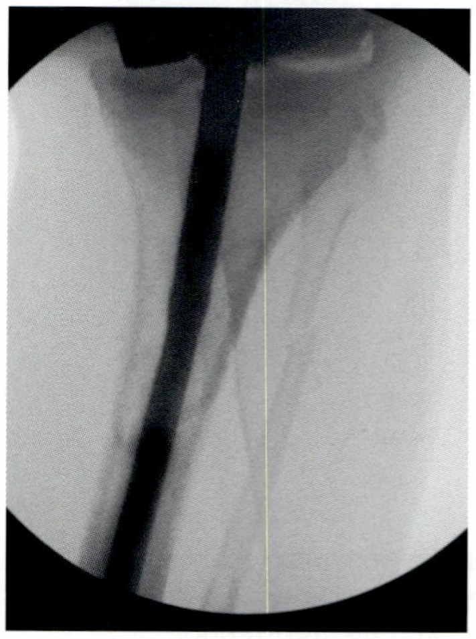

Fig. 23: Intraoperative fluoroscopy is used to confirm the position of the nail in the medullary canal. Fluoroscopic views should also be obtained at the knee and ankle joints to ensure that the nail is not proximally proud nor penetrating the subchondral zone of the distal tibial articular surface.

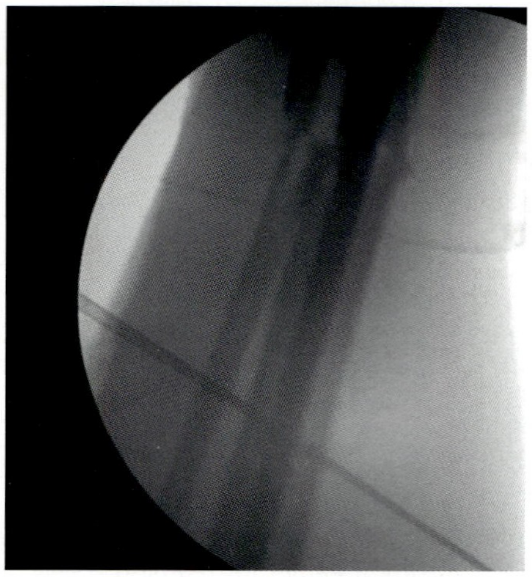

Fig. 24: Fluoroscopic views at the fracture site reveal anatomical reduction.

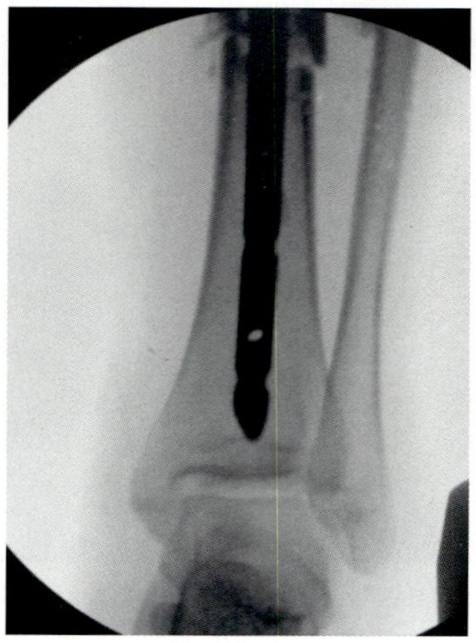

Fig. 25: Fluoroscopic image of the distal end of the tibia confirming fracture reduction as well as proper placement of the nail. The tip of the nail should stop just short of the periarticular subchondral zone.

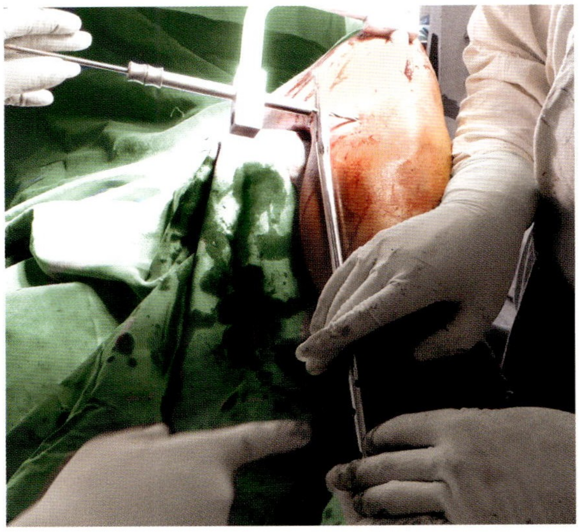

Fig. 26: A nail of the same length as the one inserted into the tibia is applied on the jig and placed parallel to the intramedullary nail. The screw holes for the distal lock screws on the outer nail are used to mark the incision sites for distal locking. Careful dissection should be undertaken in this area to avoid traumatizing the underlying neurovascular structures.

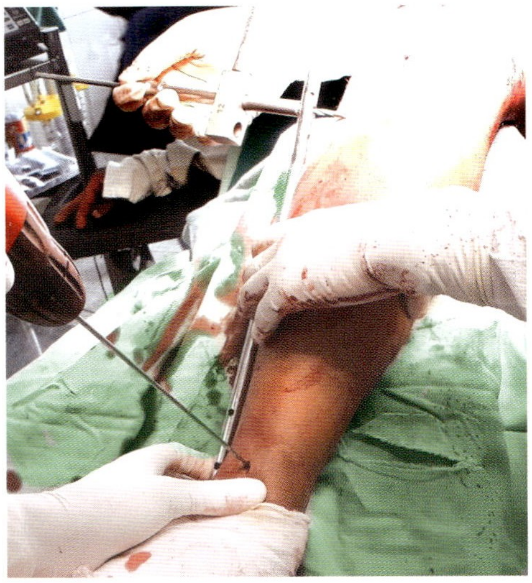

Fig. 27: Drill hole is made in the tibia at the site marked for distal lock after fluoroscopy confirmation. Drilling is done through the nail and both cortices of the tibia.

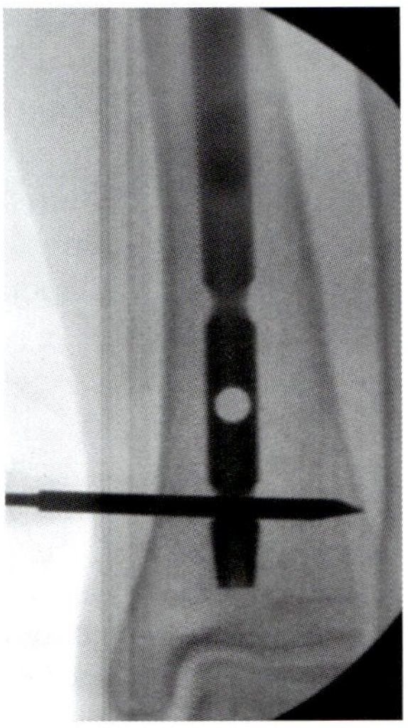

Fig. 28: Passing of drill/K-wire is confirmed on fluoroscopy.

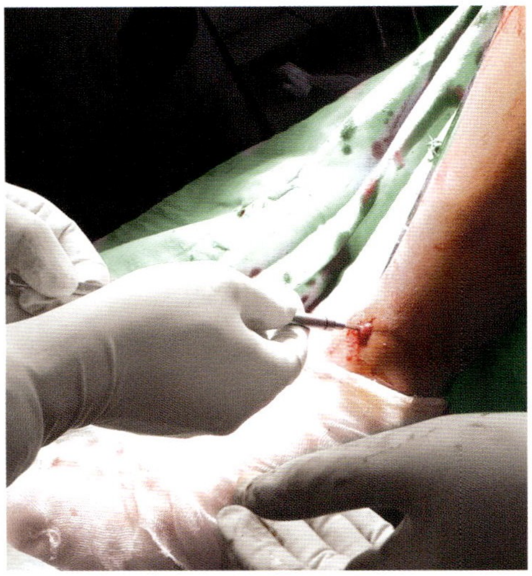

Fig. 29: The depth gauge being used to determine the length of the screw to be inserted.

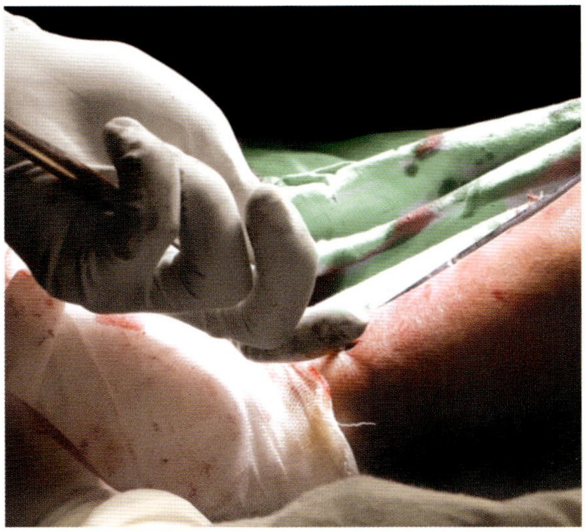

Fig. 30: 4.5-mm bolt of the obtained length is driven into the tibia, through the nail into the opposite cortex. Similarly, the other distal locking screw is also inserted. Screw position and bicortical purchase is confirmed on intraoperative fluoroscopy.

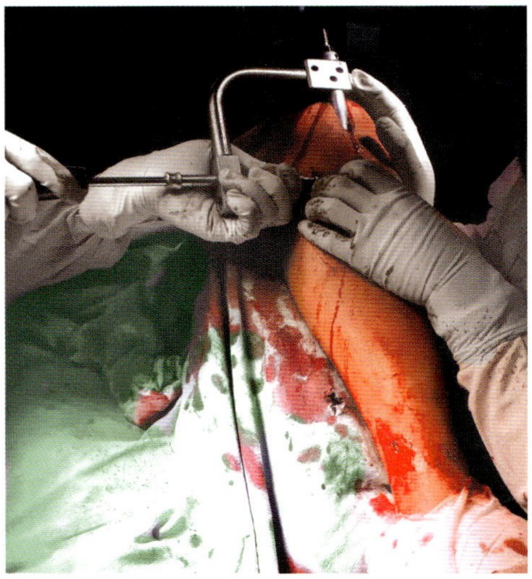

Fig. 31: Proximal interlocking of the nail is performed by drilling through the jig and percutaneously inserting screws of appropriate length. Screw position and bicortical purchase is confirmed on intraoperative fluoroscopy. The jig is then removed, the incisions washed and layer wise closure done.

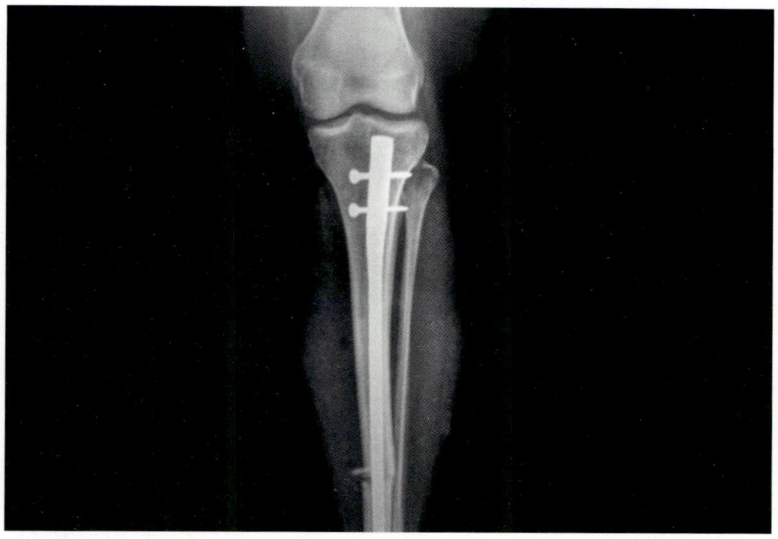

Fig. 32: Postoperative radiograph showing proximal tibia with bolts.

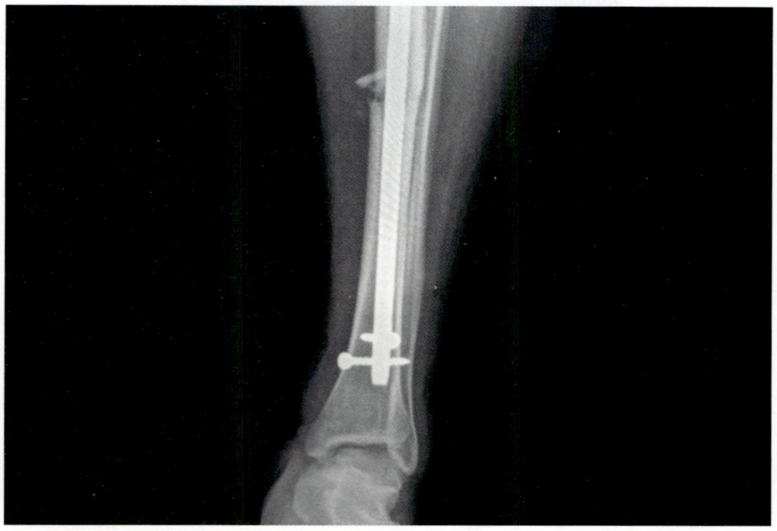

Fig. 33: Postoperative radiograph showing distal tibia with bolts in the nail.

POSTOPERATIVE PROTOCOL

The patient is provided strict limb elevation, ice fomentation and non-weight bearing. Range-of-motion for the knee and ankle joints can be started provided there is no injury. Meticulous wound care and regular dressing should be done to prevent surgical site infections.

POSSIBLE COMPLICATIONS

Intramedullary interlocking nailing of the tibia may be complicated by the following:

- Soft tissue trauma and injury to neurovascular structures
- Surgical site infections and osteomyelitis
- Fat embolism, especially in patients with underlying cardio-pulmonary comorbidities.
- Venous thromboembolic phenomena as a result of prolonged immobilization.
- Malunion or nonunion of fracture.

SUMMARY

Intramedullary interlocking nailing is the procedure of choice for closed fractures of shaft of tibia. It provides stable fixation of shaft fractures via a minimally invasive approach. Fracture reduction, guidewire placement, nail position and interlock screw placement should be confirmed under fluoroscopy intraoperatively. The procedure may be complicated by infections, fat embolism due to reaming of medullary canal and post-operative thromboembolic phenomenon due to prolonged immobilization. Osteomyelitis may present as a late complication.

SUGGESTED READING

1. Azar FM, Canale ST, Beaty JH. Campbell's Operative Orthopaedics, 13th edition. Philadelphia, PA: Elsevier; 2016.
2. Blom A, Warwick D, Whitehouse M. Apley and Solomon's System of Orthopaedics and Trauma, 10th edition. Boca Raton: CRC Press; 2017.
3. Court-Brown C, Heckman JD, McKee M, et al. Rockwood and Green's Fractures in Adults, 8th edition. Philadelphia: Wolters Kluwer Health; 2014.
4. Miller MD. Miller's Review of Orthopaedics, 7th edition. Philadelphia, PA: Elsevier; 2015.

CHAPTER 113

External Fixator Application for Open Tibia Fractures

Ajay Chandanwale, Prateek Charuchandra Joshi, Shrinivas S Shintre

INTRODUCTION

External fixation is one of the most commonly employed surgical techniques in the management of polytrauma. It employs the application of a rigid external construct made of pins and rods to stabilize the fracture until definitive fixation can be achieved.

INDICATIONS

In contemporary orthopaedics, external fixation is most often applied as a means of provisional fixation in order to maintain reduction or acceptable alignment of the fracture fragments until either definitive fixation can be achieved, or until any associated life- or limb-threatening conditions have been resolved. The common indications for external fixation are as follows:

- Compound (or open) fractures.
- Fractures associated with vascular injury, where bony stabilization is necessary before vascular repair can be undertaken.
- Fractures associated with compartment syndrome necessitating fasciotomy or compartment release.
- Gross infection in a compound fracture, wherein external fixation may be combined with the insertion of antibiotic impregnated cement beads or a cement spacer.
- As a means of rapid stabilization of fractures associated with polytrauma such as head, chest or abdomen injury in an unstable patient.
- Rarely, external fixation may be used as a definitive means of fixation in a patient with gross medical comorbidities who may be unfit for any other regional or general anesthesia.

In this chapter, external fixation of the lower limb will be discussed.

PREOPERATIVE RADIOGRAPHS (FIG. 1)

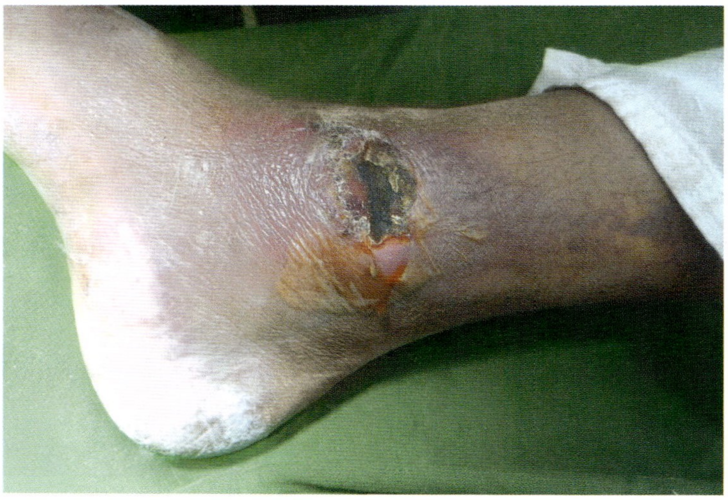

Fig. 1: A compound fracture of distal tibia and fibula (bimalleolar) with ankle dislocation Gustilo Andersen Grade II. (an indication for external fixation).

SURGICAL STEPS (FIGS. 2 TO 14)

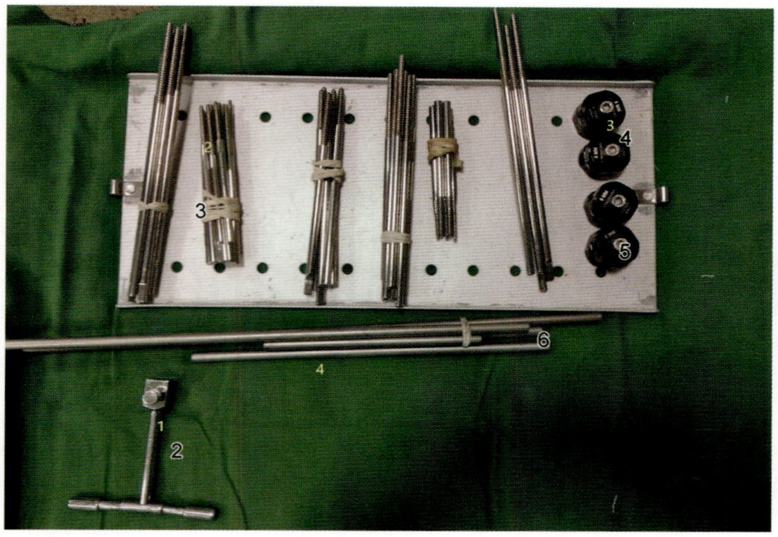

Fig. 2: Surgical instruments necessary for external fixation. External fixation requires the following instruments: (1) T-handle or chuck to drive the Schantz pins, (2) Schanz pins of various lengths and diameters, (3) Clamps (pin-rod as well as rod-rod variety), (4) Connecting rods of various lengths. In addition, a drill machine with 2.7 mm, 3.2 mm and 4.0 mm drill bits, sterile drapes, gauze swabs, and general orthopaedic and surgical instrumentation must be available.

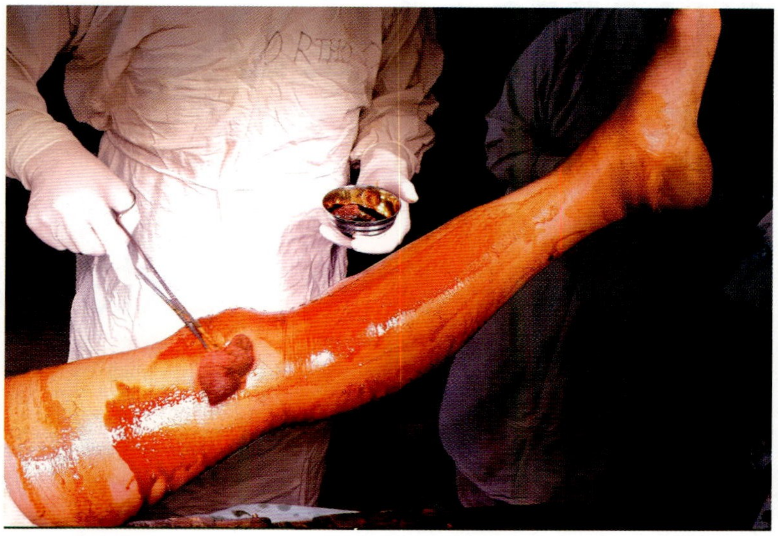

Fig. 3: The limb is scrubbed and povidone iodine painting is done. Optionally, a tourniquet may be applied as per the surgeon's preference.

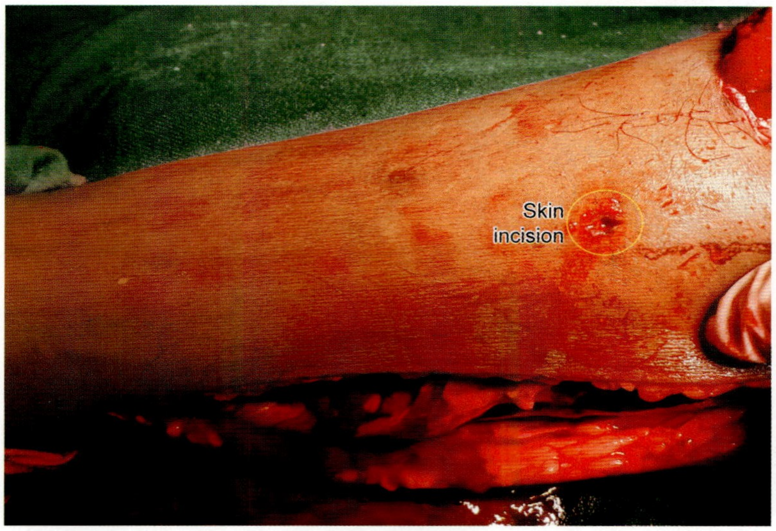

Fig. 4: Using a small size blade (no. 15 or 11), 5–7 mm stab incisions are made on the skin at three finger-breadth intervals. These serve as entry points for drill holes in the shaft of tibia.

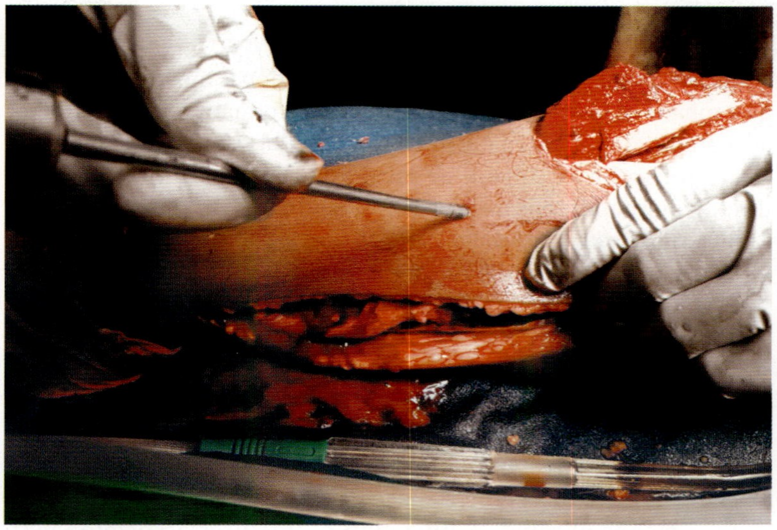

Fig. 5: A 3.2 mm drill bit is used to make drill holes on the shaft of the bone. Meticulous drilling should be undertaken given the close proximity of neurovascular structures to the posterior and posteromedial aspects of the tibia. Normal saline or distilled water should be irrigated using disposable syringe along the tract of the drill hole in order to prevent heat necrosis of the bone.

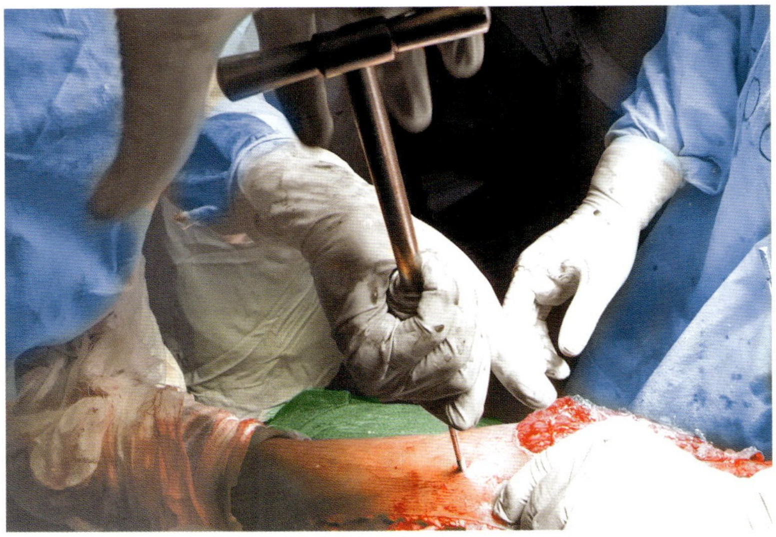

Fig. 6: Using a T-handle or chuck, Schanz pins are driven into the shaft of the tibia through the drill holes made previously. The pins should be perpendicular to the cortical surface of the bone and each pin should have bi-cortical purchase in the bone.

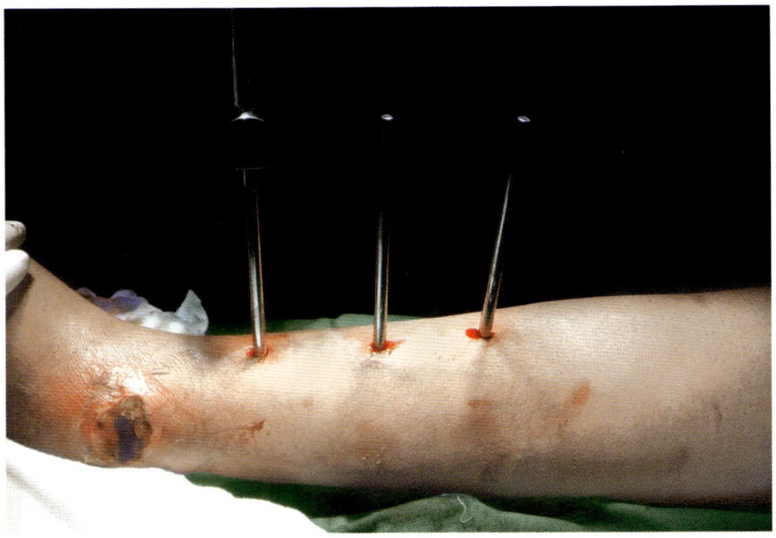

Fig. 7: Schanz pins being inserted into the tibia. A minimum of four to six cortices must be engaged on either side of the fracture. The fracture is reduced and the pins are fixed with connecting rods. The assembly is complete.

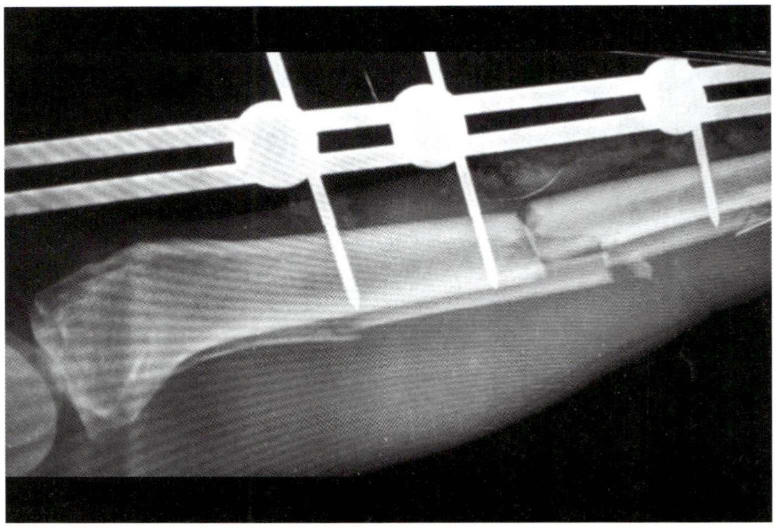

Fig. 8: Postoperative radiograph of the patient in Figure 2 showing fracture shaft tibia with external fixator in situ. Simple external fixation is generally sufficient for mid-shaft fractures. In case of distal or articular fractures, the involved joint may need to be spanned, as below.

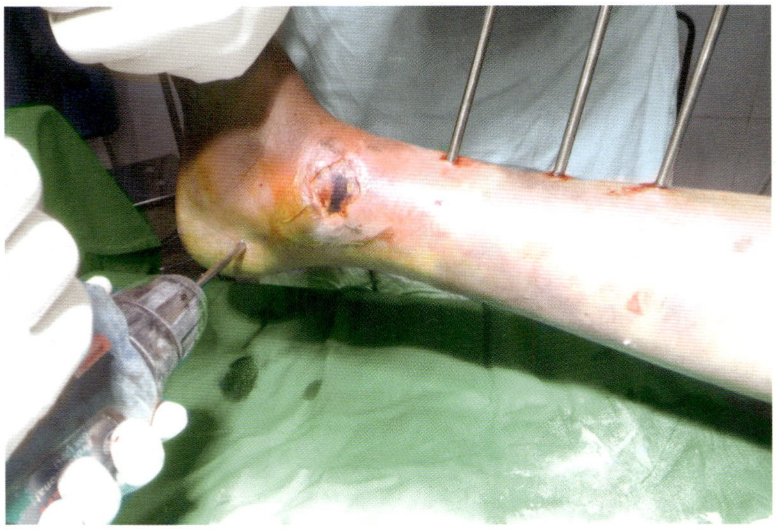

Fig. 9: Spanning of the ankle joint may be necessary in cases of distal tibiofibular fractures and/or those with disruption of the ankle mortise. A Steinman or Denham pin is passed percutaneously through the body of the calcaneum, forming the base of the "foot frame".

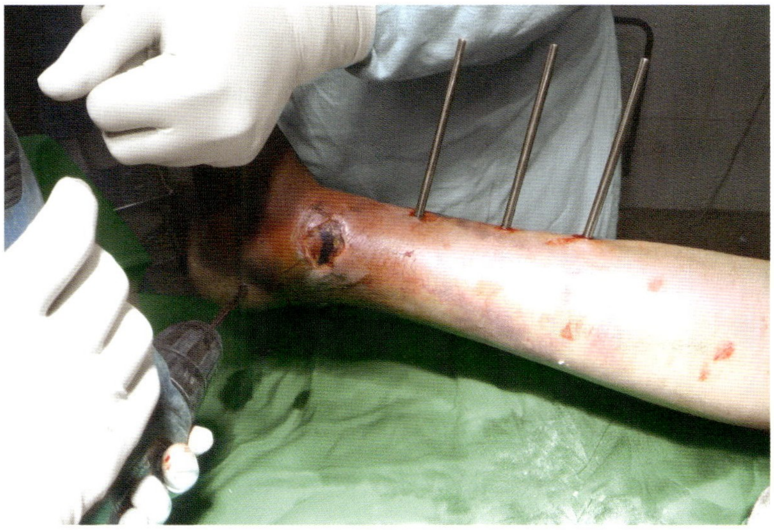

Fig. 10: Drill holes using a smaller (2.7 mm) drill bit are made in the shaft of the first and fifth metatarsals through stab incisions 1cm proximal to the metatarsal head. Small (3.5 mm) Schanz pins are driven into the metatarsal shaft on either side, with preferably a three- to four-cortex purchase on each side.

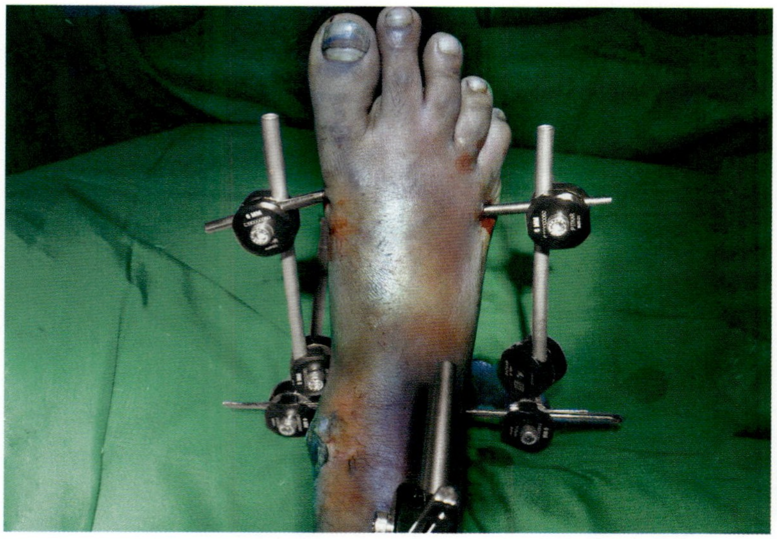

Fig. 11: Appropriate sized connecting rods are applied to the pins and fixed in place using clamps, hence completing the square "foot frame".

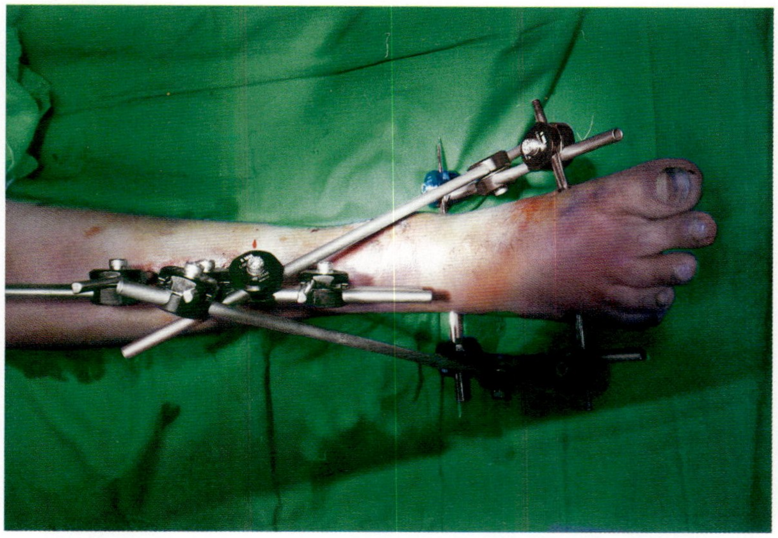

Fig. 12: The tibial pins are connected to each other using parallel connecting rods, and to the foot frame using obliquely applied rods. The proximal clamps of the oblique rods are fixed to the tibial assembly and tightened.

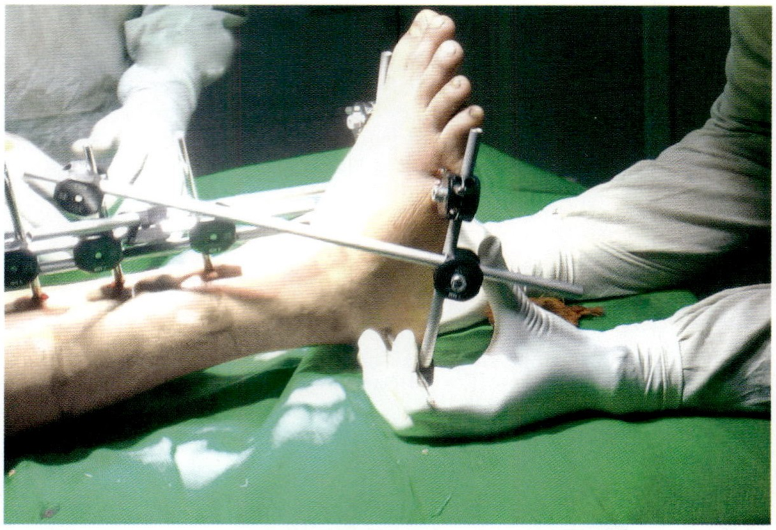

Fig. 13: Traction is applied to the ankle joint using a longitudinal pull applied to the foot frame. Care is taken to restore neutral rotation of the ankle and to prevent equinus positioning of the foot.

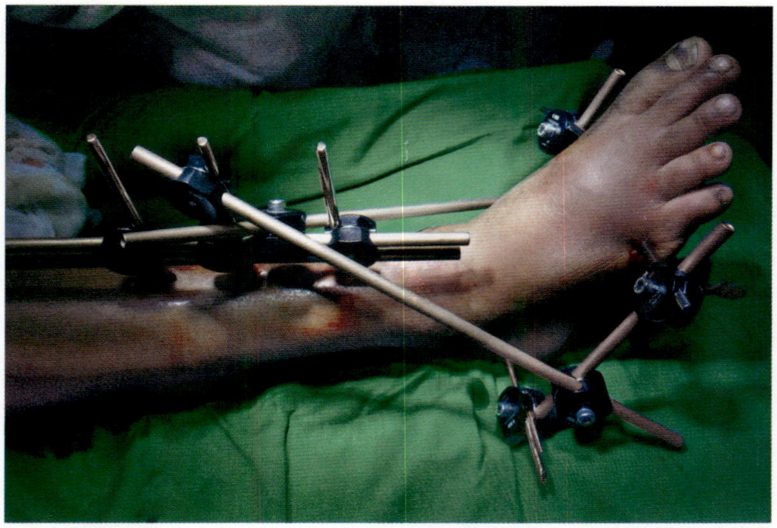

Fig. 14: The final external fixator assembly. Three 4.5 mm Schanz pins connected to two parallel rods stabilize the tibial shaft proximal to the fracture. One calcaneal Steinman or Denham pin and two 3.5 mm Schanz pins form the foot frame. The oblique rods connect the two assemblies and "span" the ankle joint. Pin tract cleaning is done and wounds if any are debrided. Sterile dressing is done. The patient is provided with limb elevation, ice fomentation and analgesics post operatively.

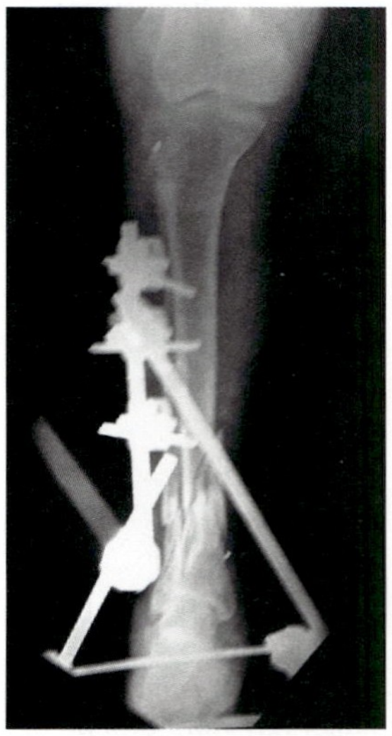

Fig. 15: Postoperative radiograph of the same patient confirming pin positioning, fracture reduction and stability of the ankle mortise. In this patient, the fibula fracture has been stabilized by an intramedullary Kirschner wire.

POSTOPERATIVE PROTOCOL

- Patient is advised not to bear weight on the operated limb and strict limb elevation.
- Range-of-motion for the joints proximal and distal to the fixator assembly can be started in the absence of injury to the joints concerned.
- Pin tract cleaning and wound care with reconstructive procedures such as skin grafting or flap application, if necessary, should be performed.

COMPLICATIONS

- Soft tissue trauma and injury to neurovascular structures
- Pin tract infections

- Wound-related complications such as secondary infections
- Plastic or reconstructive surgery related complications such as graft rejection, flap necrosis or infection of the flap with gaping of the wound
- Malunion or nonunion of fracture
- Osteomyelitis.

SUMMARY

External fixation is one of the commonly performed surgeries in orthopaedic practice. Compound fractures, vascular injuries, and gross infection are the common indications for external fixation. It may be used as a provisional or rarely a definitive fixation method. It may be complicated by neurovascular or soft tissue trauma, pin tract infections or wound complications.

SUGGESTED READING

1. Apley and Solomon's system of orthopaedics and trauma 10th edition.
2. Campbell's operative orthopaedics 13th edition.
3. Miller's Review of orthopaedics 7th edition.
4. Rockwood and Green's fractures in adults 8th edition.

CHAPTER 114

Fracture Distal Tibia: Minimally Invasive Plate Osteosynthesis

Onkar Lande, Madan Hardikar, Nitish Agrawal

INTRODUCTION

Fracture of the tibia and fibula shaft is most common fracture amongst all long bone fractures. Diaphyseal tibia fracture has the highest rate of nonunion amongst all long bones fractures.

MECHANISM OF INJURY

Direct

- High energy bending due to road traffic accident causes transverse, oblique, displaced types of fracture pattern.
- Penetrating gunshot injury usually causes comminuted fractures.
- Low energy bending injury causes short oblique fracture or transverse fracture pattern.
- Fibular shaft fracture occurs due to direct trauma to lateral aspect of leg.

Indirect

- In torsional mechanisms like twisting with foot fixed and fall from moderate height causes nondisplaced or displaced spiral fracture pattern with minimal comminution.
- Stress fracture is common in military recruits at metaphyseal-diaphyseal junction.
- In ballet dancers, stress fracture occurs in middle third tibia.

CLINICAL EXAMINATION

In neurovascular status of limb assessment, dorsalis pedis artery and posterior tibial artery pulsations are checked. Examination for tibial and common peroneal nerve are done.

- Assess soft tissue injury to the limb.
- Pain out of proportion to the injury is most reliable sign of compartment syndrome.
- Knee ligament injuries at times are associated with tibial fractures.

RADIOLOGICAL EVALUATION

Anteroposterior and lateral view of entire tibia fibula is taken. Additional oblique view is used to characterize the fracture pattern.

Presence of comminution in X-ray indicate high-energy injury. In missing bone or open wounds, osseous defect is seen on X-ray. Air in soft tissue on X-ray may indicate gas gangrene or other anaerobic infection.

Other modalities commonly used is computed tomography scan in case of metaphyseal fracture with articular extension, magnetic resonance imaging (for ligament injury) and technetium 99 bone scanning (for stress fracture) and angiography (arterial injury).

TREATMENT

Nonoperative

Long leg cast with knee in 0–5° flexion is given for undisplaced fractures. Average time for union is 16+–4 weeks.

Acceptable fracture position for nonoperative treatment is:

- Less than 5° of varus or valgus is acceptable.
- Less than 10° of anterior or posterior angulation is recommended.
- Less than 10° of rotational deformity.
- Less than 1 cm of shortening.
- More than 50% cortical contact is advised.

Tibial stress fracture is managed in short leg cast with partial weight-bearing mobilization till symptoms subside.

Operative

Intramedullary Nailing

- Locked nail is ideal for all fractures including comminuted fractures and it effectively prevents shortening.
- Nonlocked nail allows impaction at the fracture site with weight bearing but it is difficult to control rotation.

- Reamed nail enhances periosteal blood flow so indicated for most closed and open fractures.
- Unreamed nail preserves intramedullary blood supply but reserved for open fractures.

Flexible Nail

Only recommended in children or adolescents with open physes.

External Fixation

Indication: Primarily used to treat severe open fractures and in closed fractures which are complicated by compartment syndrome, in damage control orthopaedics and concomitant head injury or burn.

Plate and Screws

- Indicated for metaphyseal or epiphyseal fracture extension.
- Percutaneously inserted plate fixation done in proximal and distal tibia fractures by minimally invasive plate osteosynthesis (MIPO) technique.
- Minimally invasive plate osteosynthesis technique is most suitable in patients with multifragmentary or comminuted fracture, segmental fractures, narrow medullary canals, fractures extending up to the articular surfaces.
- In MIPO a plate is passed across a fracture using mini skin incisions on each end of the bone. It avoids prolonged surgery and large incisions associated with traditional plate fixation.
- Minimally invasive plate osteosynthesis is biological plating technique and benefits of MIPO are blood supply is maximally preserved at fracture site and fracture hematoma minimally disturbed.
- Contraindications of MIPO technique are:
  - Severe soft tissue loss with no coverage of exposed bone
  - Pathological fracture
  - Associated vascular injuries
  - Active local infection
  - Compartment syndrome.

In compartment syndrome emergency fasciotomy of all four-muscle compartments with multiple incision technique is necessary.

SURGICAL STEPS (FIGS. 1 TO 20)

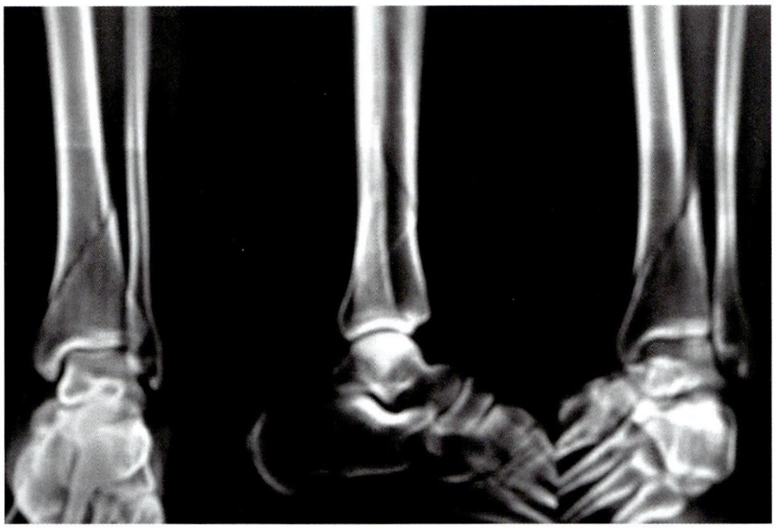

Fig. 1: Anteroposterior, lateral and oblique view of X-ray showing spiral fracture of distal third of tibia. 36-year-old patient presented with closed fracture tibia.

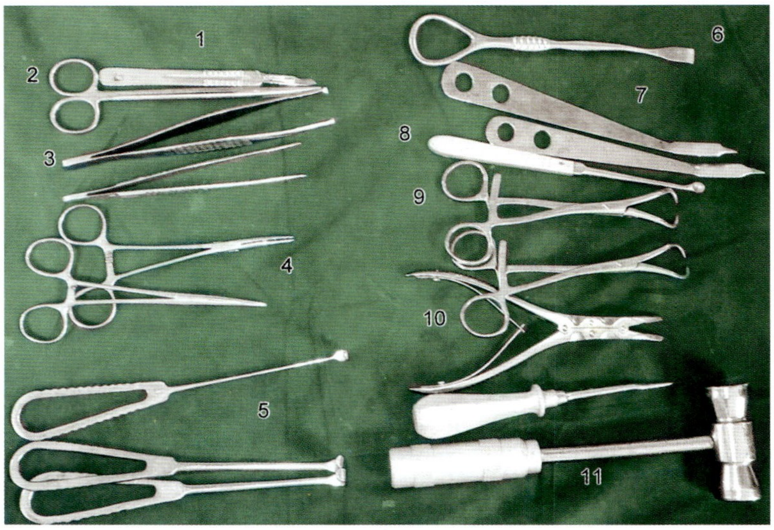

Fig. 2: Instruments used: (1) Knife blade, (2) Dissecting scissors, (3) Forceps, (4) Artery forceps, (5) Right angle retractors, (6) Periosteum elevator, (7) Bone lever, (8) Curette, (9) Bone holding reduction clamps, (10) Bone nibbler, (11) Hammer.

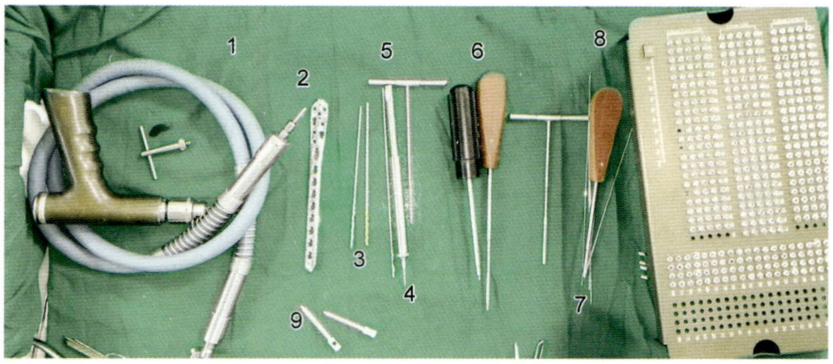

Fig. 3: (1) Drill with chuck key, (2) 9-hole locking plate for distal third tibia, (3) Drill bits 2.5 mm, (4) Depth gauge, (5) Tap, (6) Screwdriver for locking and nonlocking screws, (7) K-wire, (8) Screws (3.5 mm)—locking cancellous, nonlocking cancellous, locking cortical, and nonlocking cortical, (9) Locking sleeves.

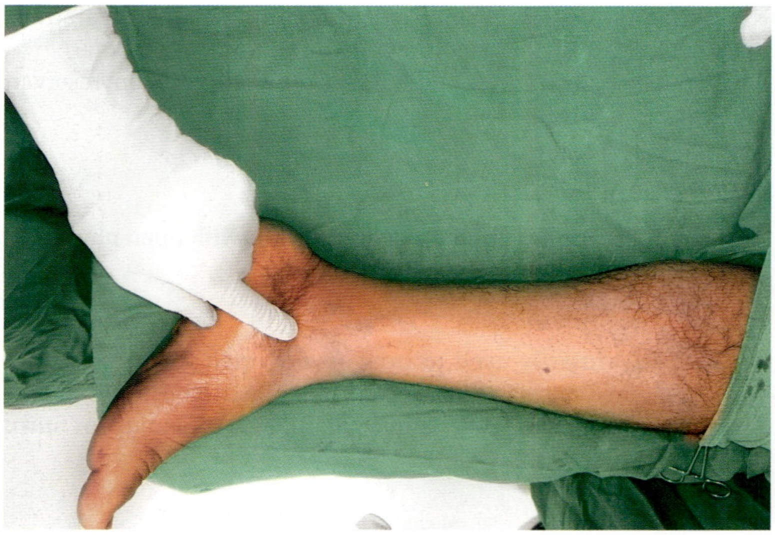

Fig. 4: Lateral position given with exposure of medial side of leg and medial malleolus palpated.

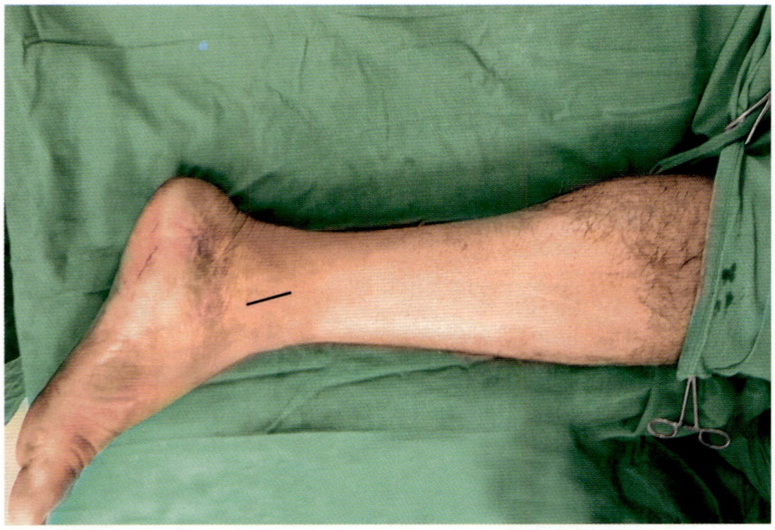

Fig. 5: Marking of incision slightly anterior to medial malleolus.

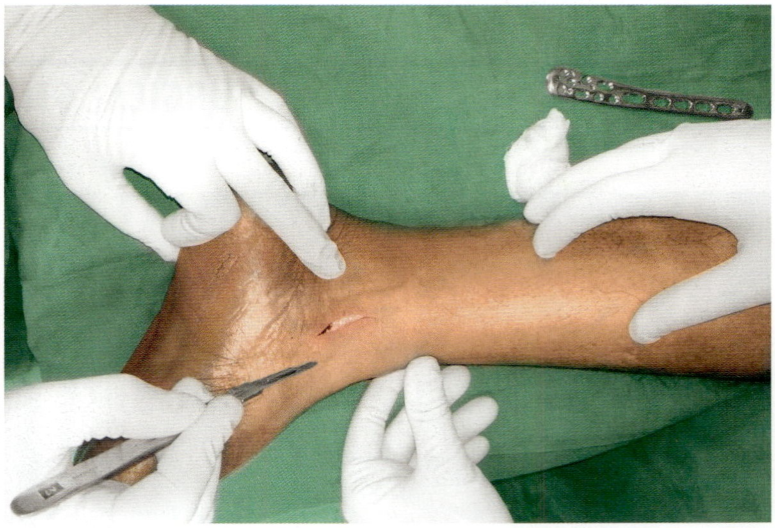

Fig. 6: Skin incision taken with skin knife and further dissection of soft tissue and fascia done.

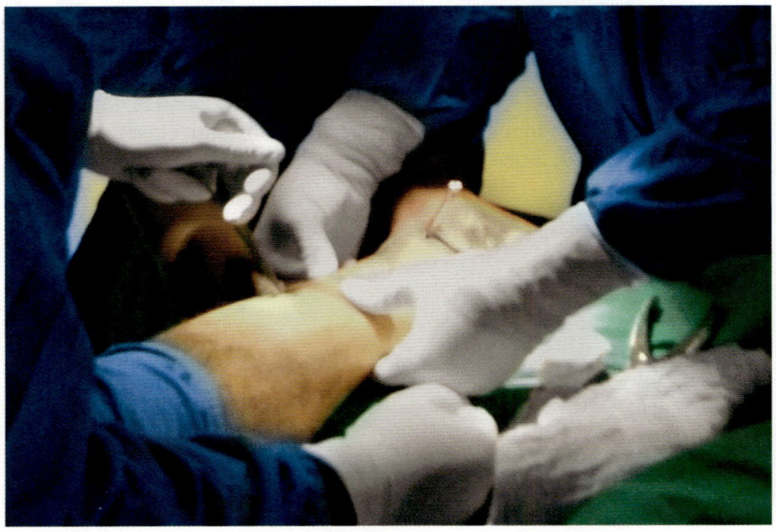

Fig. 7: 9-hole locking plate is inserted and slid proximally from incision site percutaneously crossing fracture side.

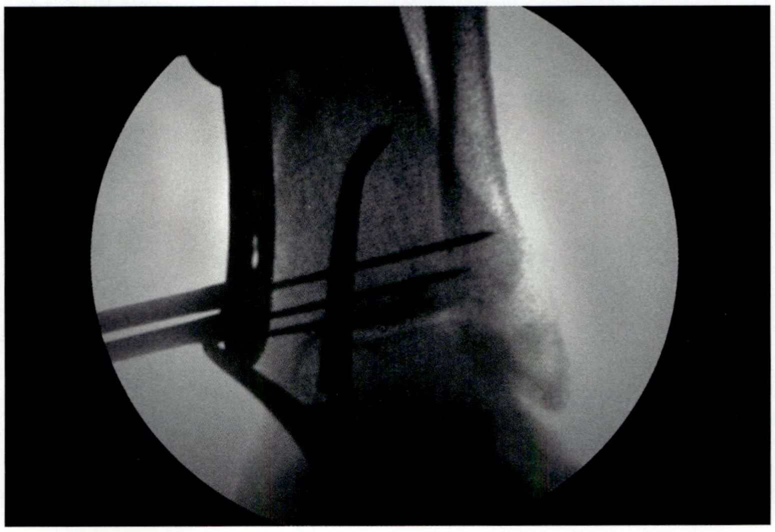

Fig. 8: Distal end of plate is temporarily fixed with K-wires through locking sleeves and confirmed over C-arm image intensifier anteroposterior view.

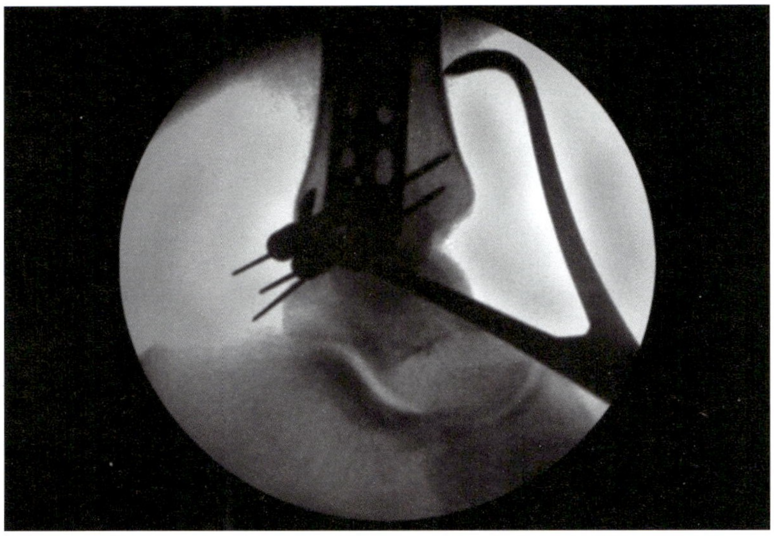

Fig. 9: Distal K-wire temporary fixation confirmed over C-arm lateral view.

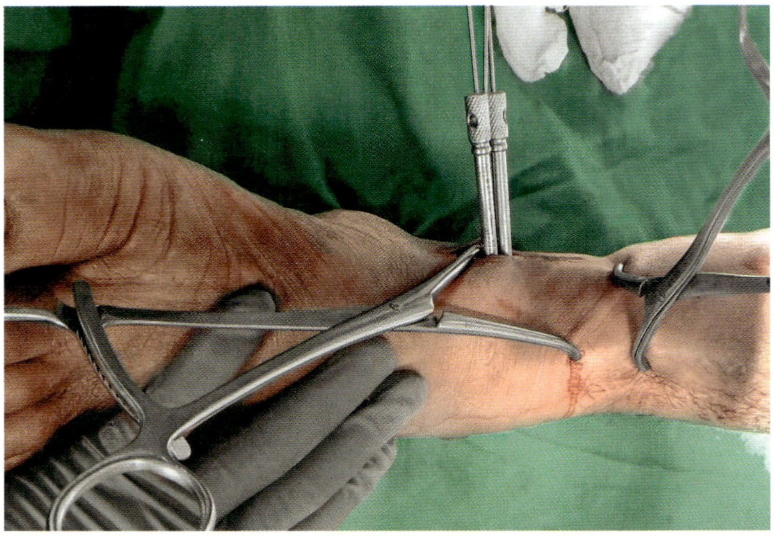

Fig 10: Fracture reduction done with bone holding reduction clamps.

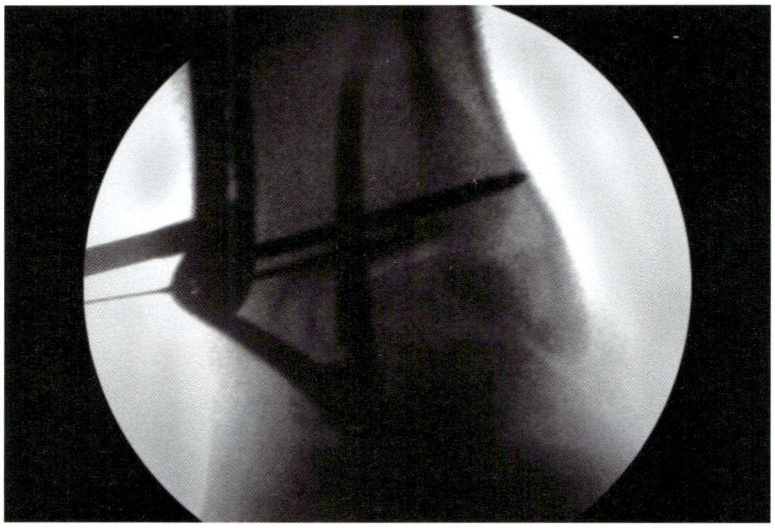

Fig. 11: Drilling done through sleeve and distal cancellous locking screw fixation done and confirmed by C-arm.

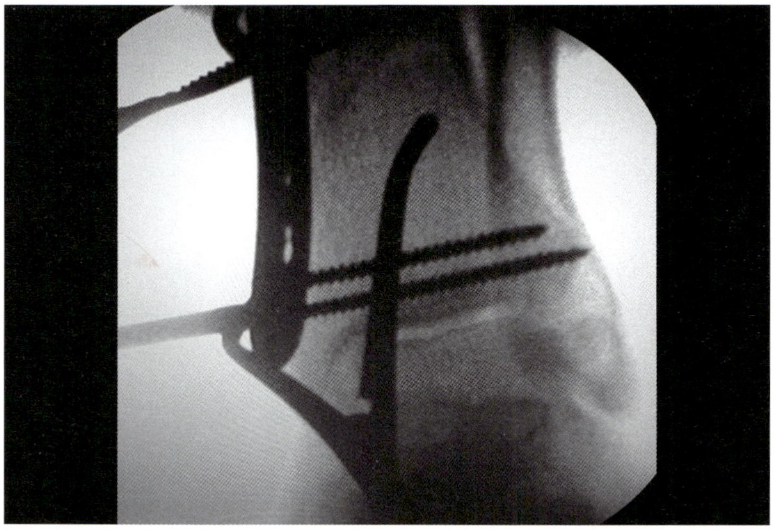

Fig. 12: Distally second cancellous locking screw fixation done under C-arm.

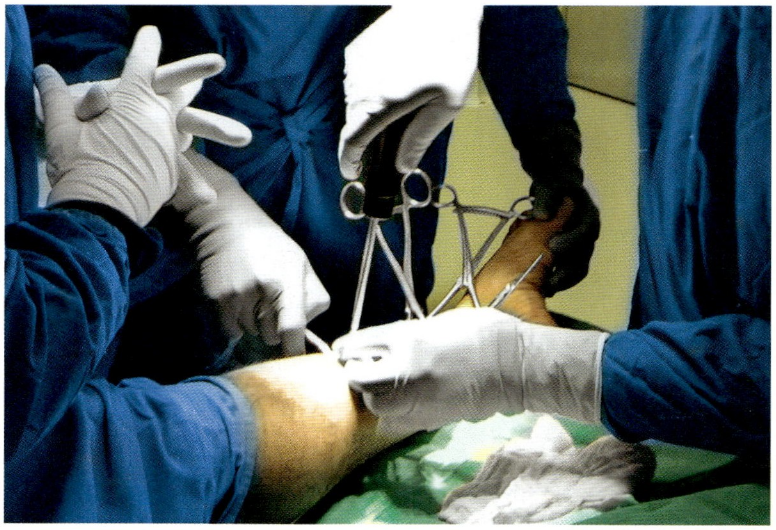

Fig. 13: Proximally cortical locking screw fixation done by using sleeve and drill. First screw may be nonlocked cortical so as to pull the plate to the bone.

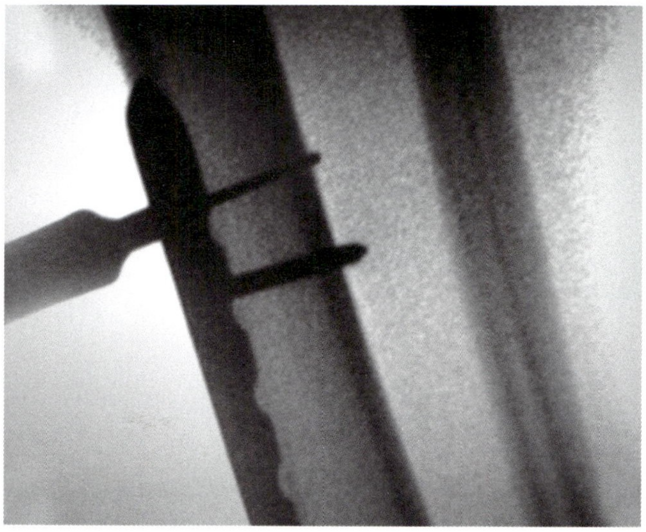

Fig. 14: Proximally cortical locking screw fixation confirmed under C-arm.

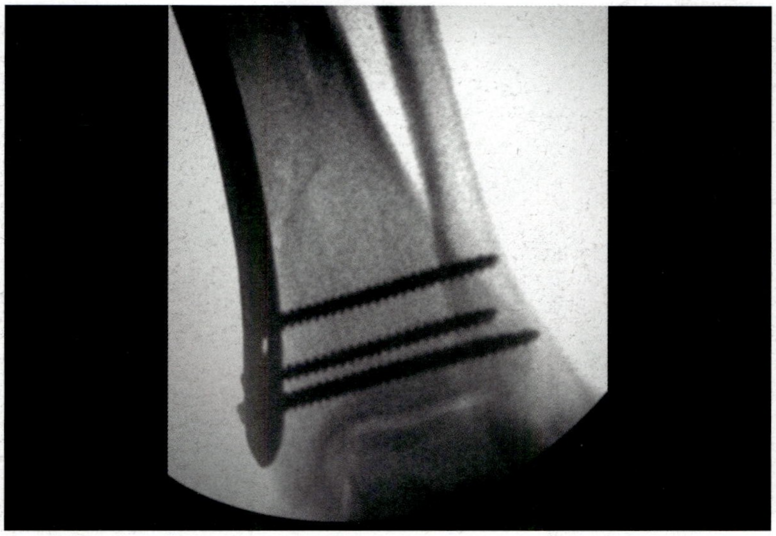

Fig. 15: Distally third cancellous locking screw fixation done under C-arm.

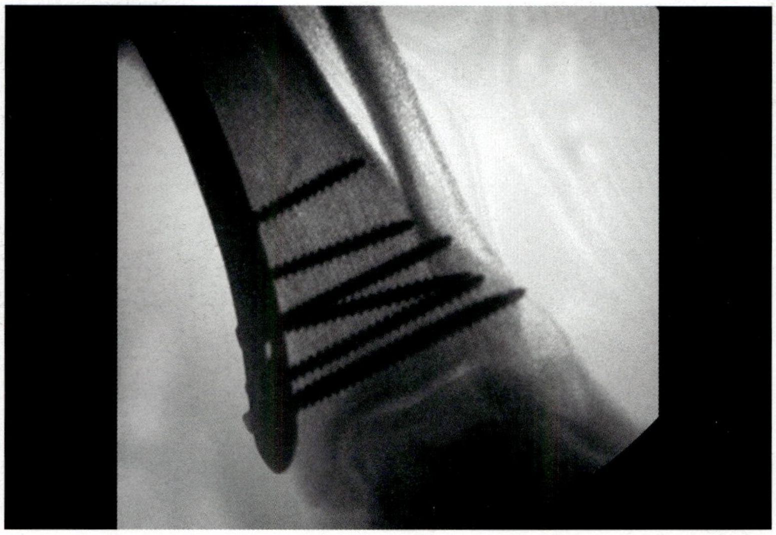

Fig. 16: Distally total seven cancellous locking screw fixation done under C-arm.

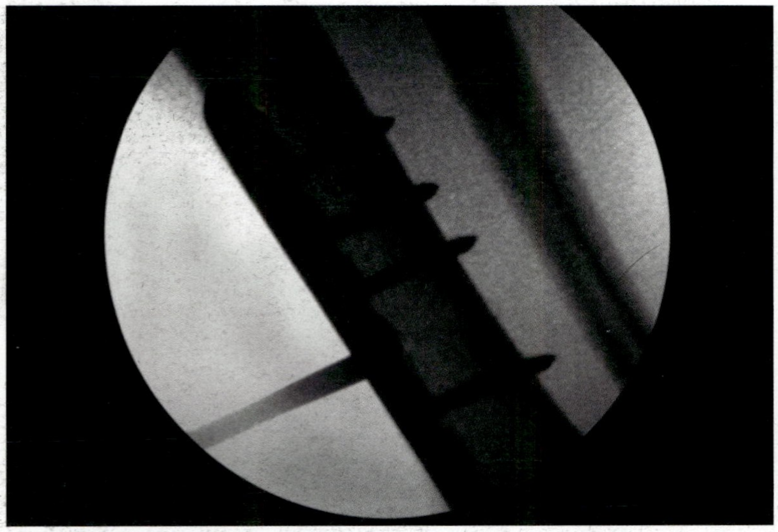

Fig. 17: Proximally total five bicortex locking screw fixation done under C-arm.

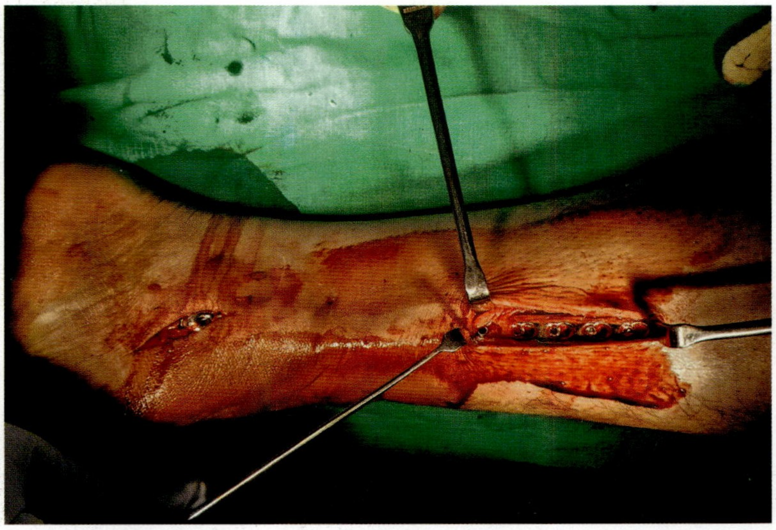

Fig. 18: Final fixation seen. Wash given with normal saline and povidone iodine.

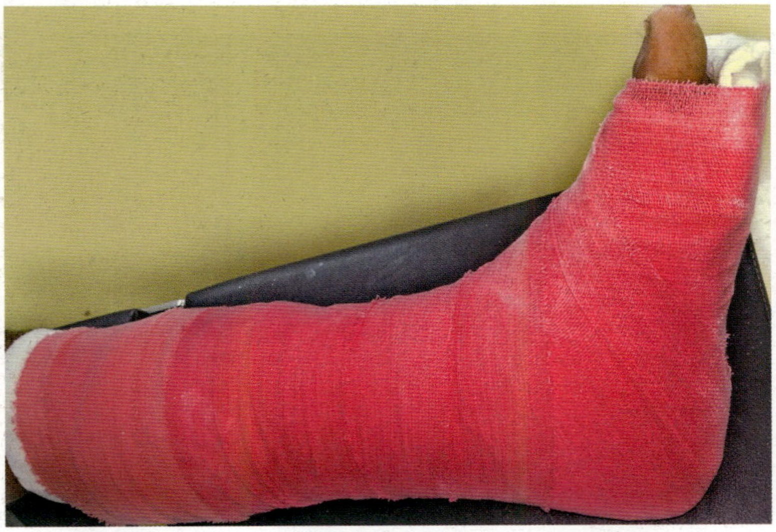

Fig. 19: After suturing skin with nonabsorbable suture material below knee slab given with ankle in neutral position. Compression bandage applied.

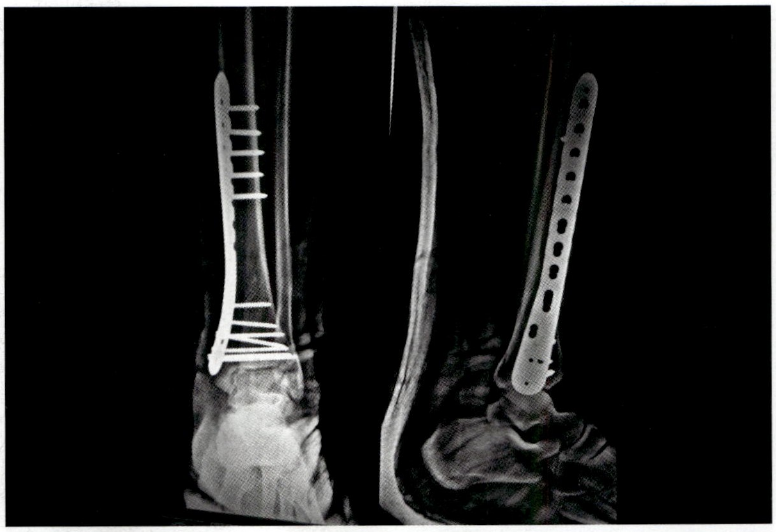

Fig. 20: Postoperative X-ray showing fixation of # distal third tibia with 9-hole locking plate and 12 screws by using minimal invasive percutaneous plate osteosynthesis technique.

POSTOPERATIVE MANAGEMENT

- Active toe movements initiated from day of surgery.
- Ankle dorsiflexion and plantar flexion exercises started from first day.
- Hamstring strengthening exercises and static quadriceps exercise started from first day.
- Non-weight-bearing mobilization with walker support started from second day.
- Suture removal done on day 15.
- Partial weight-bearing mobilization with walker support started after 6 weeks.
- Full weight-bearing mobilization with walker support started after 12 weeks if X-ray shows satisfactory healing.

COMPLICATIONS

- Malunion: Associated with nonoperative management and metaphyseal fracture
- Nonunion: Associated with high velocity injuries, open fractures, infection, inadequate fixation, and initial fracture displacement
- Soft tissue loss mostly in open fractures
- Stiffness at knee or ankle joint associated with nonoperative treatment
- Knee pain due to intramedullary nailing
- Implant breakage
- Reflex sympathetic dystrophy
- Compartment syndrome: Anterior compartment involvement is most common
- Fat embolism
- Claw toe deformity
- Neurovascular injury: Most common in high velocity trauma cases with compromise in anterior tibial artery.

SUGGESTED READING

1. Archdeacon MT, Wyrick JD. Reduction plating for provisional fracture fixation. J Orthop Trauma. 2006;20(3):206-11.
2. Cannada LK, Jones AL. Demographic, social and economic variables that effect lower extremity injury outcomes. Injury. 2006;37(12): 1109-16.
3. Lack WD, Starman JS, Seymour R, et al. Any cortical bridging predicts healing of tibial shaft fractures. J Bone Joints Surg. 2014;96(13): 1066-72.
4. Stuermer EK, Stuermer KM. Tibial shaft fracture and ankle joint injury. J Orthop Trauma. 2008;22(2):107-12.
5. Vallier HA, Cureton BA, Patterson BM. Randomised prospective comparison of plate versus intra medullary nail fixation for distal tibia shaft fracture. J Orthop Trauma. 2011;25(12):736-41.

SECTION 9

BONE TUMORS

Section Editor: *Arun Salunkhe*

CHAPTER 115

Exostosis Excision

Raghav Barve, Snehal Dantkale

INTRODUCTION

Osteochondromas constitute a vast majority of benign bone tumors. These tumors grow as cartilage-capped bony projections on the surface of bones (exostoses). Such tumors can occur in any bone undergoing endochondral ossification. Long bones in the leg, pelvis and scapula are the most common site of exostoses. Development of osteochondromas occurs generally during growth spurts around the ages of 13 and 15 and stops when the physis fuses at puberty. Incidence of these tumors is found up to 30 years of age mainly affecting children and adolescents. Mainly these tumors are solitary nonhereditary lesions and rarely (around 10–15%) some osteochondromas occur as a part of hereditary multiple osteochondromas (HMOs). Osteochondromas are nontraumatic and idiopathic in nature. The treatment of choice for osteochondroma is surgical excision of solitary lesion (excisional biopsy), when symptoms cause restriction of movements or nerve and blood vessel compression.

SYMPTOMS

The majority of exostoses present without any complaints and are found incidentally. Some of the most common symptoms are a hard immobile painless palpable mass and ache in surrounding muscles after excessive activity. Symptoms aggravate when complications like pathological fractures, deformity, or mechanical obstruction in joint movement occur. If the osteochondroma is in close proximity of neurovascular bundle, patient can have numbness, weakness, and rarely symptoms of venous engorgement or ischemic changes. 20% of patients who experience nerve compression also have problems of vascular compromise, arterial thrombosis, aneurysm, and pseudoaneurysm. Claudication, severe pain, acute ischemia, and symptoms of phlebitis are an indication of formation of pseudoaneurysm and venous thrombosis. If the tumor is found under a tendon, pain occurs during movement and thus results in restriction of joint motion. Pain can also be a result inflammation of overlying bursa, fracture at the base of the tumor stalk. Malignant transformation of osteochondroma can be suspected if patient experiences severe pain, swelling in surrounding soft tissues and rapidly enlarging mass.

DIAGNOSIS AND INVESTIGATIONS

Osteochondromas are generally asymptomatic and is very unlikely to cause any discomfort. They are often incidentally found when a radiograph is done for an unrelated cause.

- X-rays are the fundamental investigation done to evaluate the lesion. They also indicate bone growth related to osteochondroma. Serial radiographs help in assessing the rate of growth of the tumor.
- Computed tomography (CT) scan can show detailed bony anatomy of the tumor and detect the presence of calcification.
- Magnetic resonance imaging (MRI) is the most accurate method to get a clear picture of the exact morphology of the tumor, compression on surrounding soft tissue, grading, vascularity, and for differentiation from other lesions.
- Ultrasound is done when there are suspicion aneurysms or pseudoaneurysms and venous or arterial thrombosis.
- A biopsy of the tumor can also be done to find out if there is malignant transformation.

TREATMENT AND PROGNOSIS

Osteochondromas have a very low malignancy rate (<1%) and resection of the tumor is required only if symptoms such as pain, restriction of movements, or impingement on nerves or vessels occur. Treatment is not necessary for solitary osteochondromas, which are asymptomatic. While doing surgical resection, the entire lesion along with the cartilaginous cap should be excised to reduce any chances of reoccurrences. Surgical management is the treatment of choice, if complications such as fractures, paresthesias, paraparesis, neuropathy, and vascular compromise take place. A prophylactic excision can be done, if the lesion is in close proximity of a neurovascular bundle. Complete excision of osteochondroma is curative. Incomplete excision of tumor results in local recurrence. If multiple reoccurrences occur in a well-excised lesion, it may indicate malignant nature of tumor. Detailed investigation is required in case of symptoms suggestive of malignancy. Treatment for solitary osteochondroma is careful observation with periodic follow-ups. Regular X-rays help us to monitor and detect any changes in the tumor morphology.

SURGICAL STEPS (FIGS 1 TO 18)

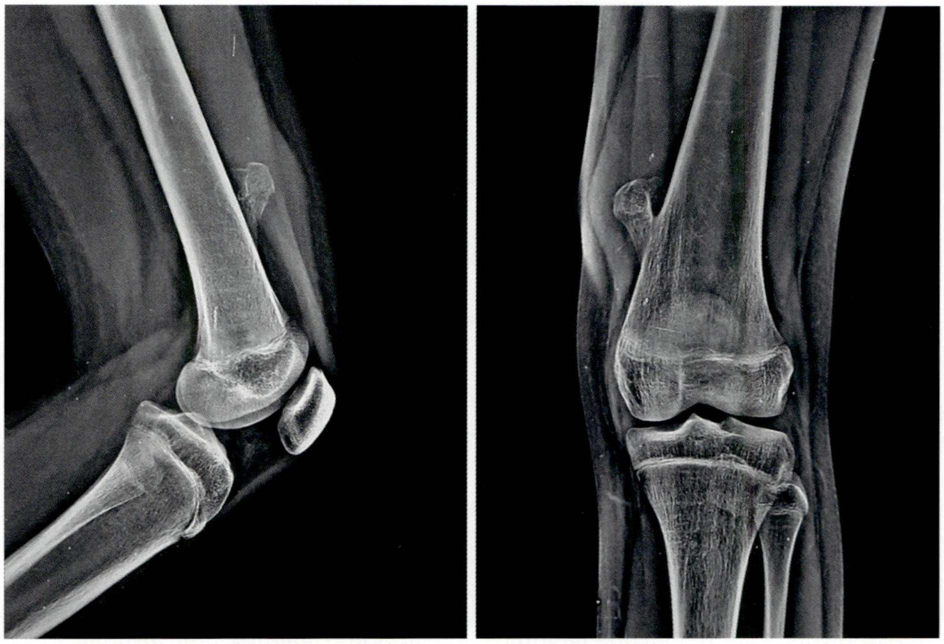

Fig. 1: Radiograph anteroposterior and lateral view showing osteochondroma.

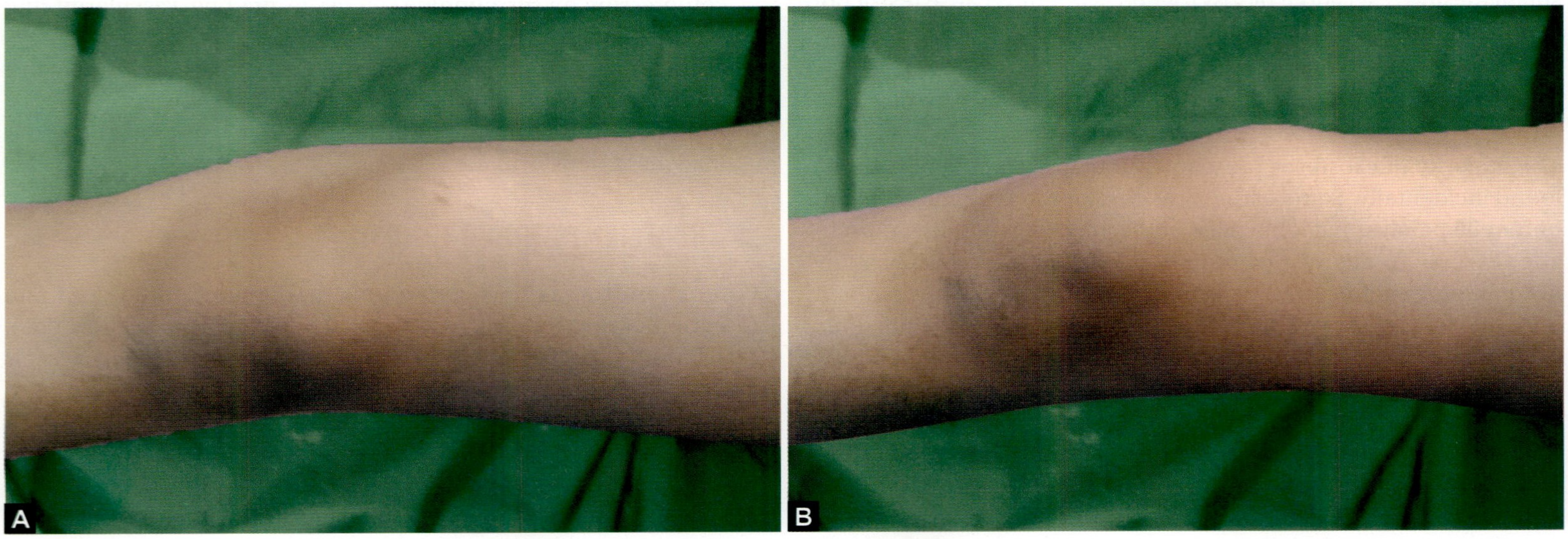

Figs. 2A and B: Clinical photograph of osteochondroma.

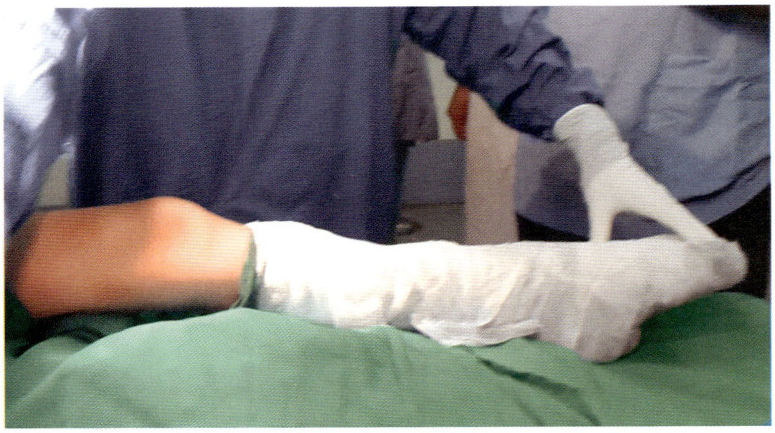

Fig. 3: Patient position.

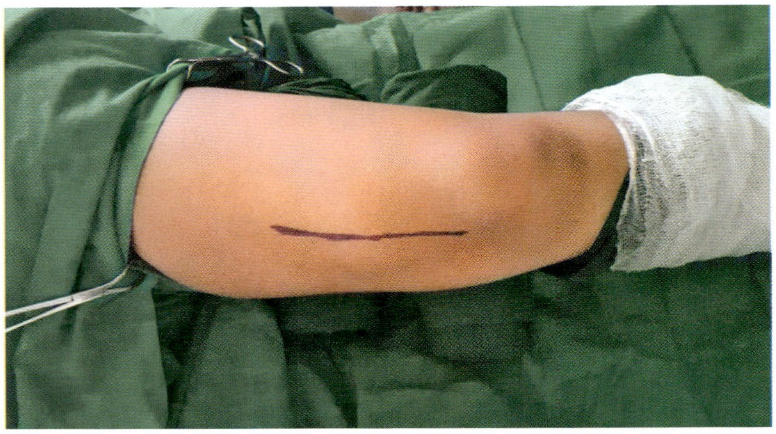

Fig. 4: Incision marked.

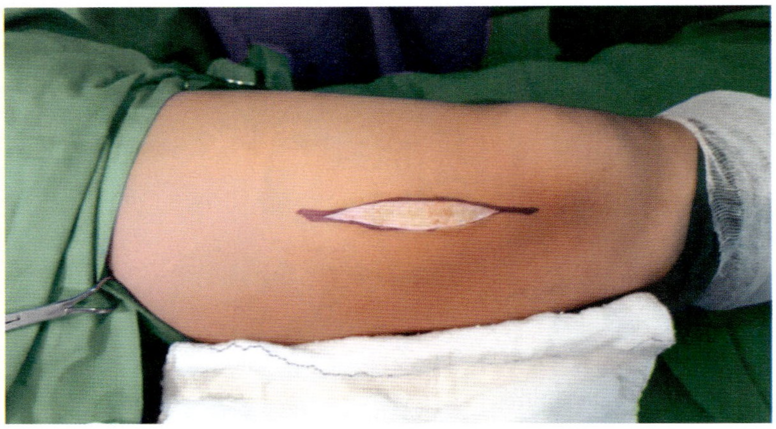

Fig. 5: Incision deepened through skin and fascia.

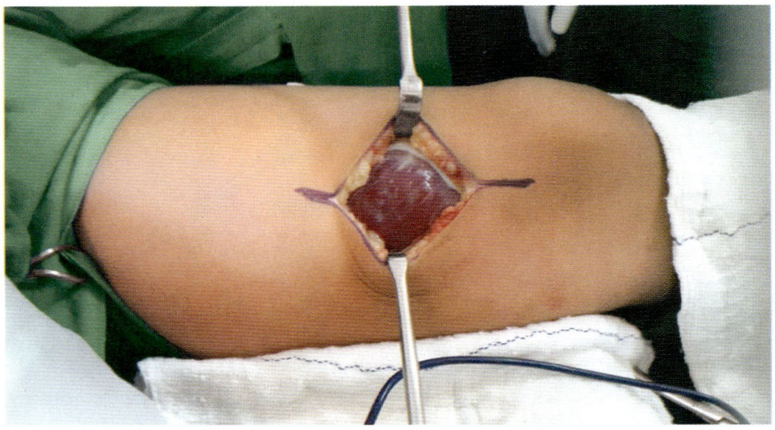

Fig. 6: Overlying muscle (vastus medialis) seen.

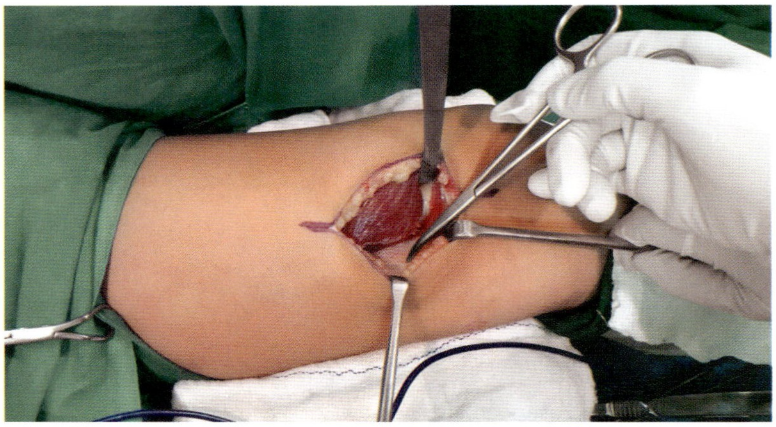

Fig. 7: Muscle fibers separated bluntly.

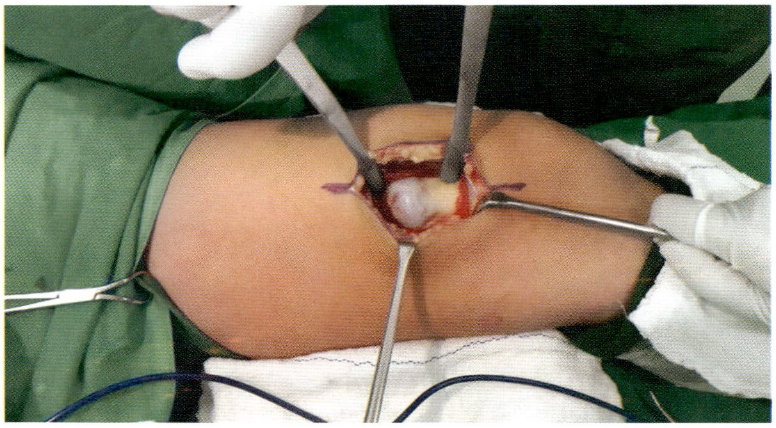

Fig. 8: Muscle fibers retracted.

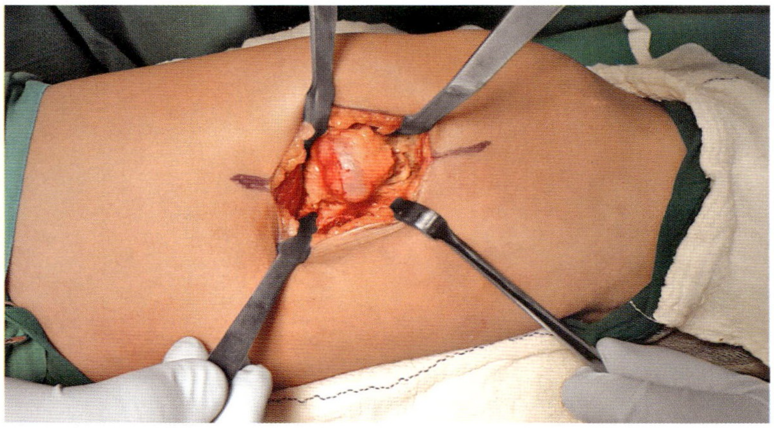

Fig. 9: Osteochondroma with intact cartilage cap seen. Care taken not to damage the cartilage cap.

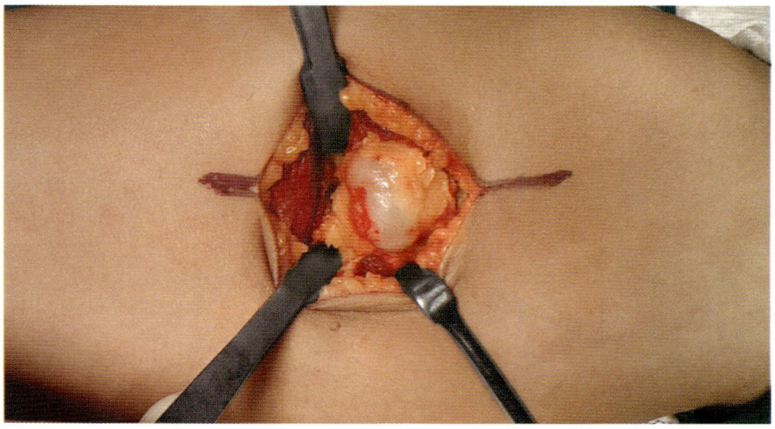

Fig. 10: Base of osteochondroma exposed from all sides.

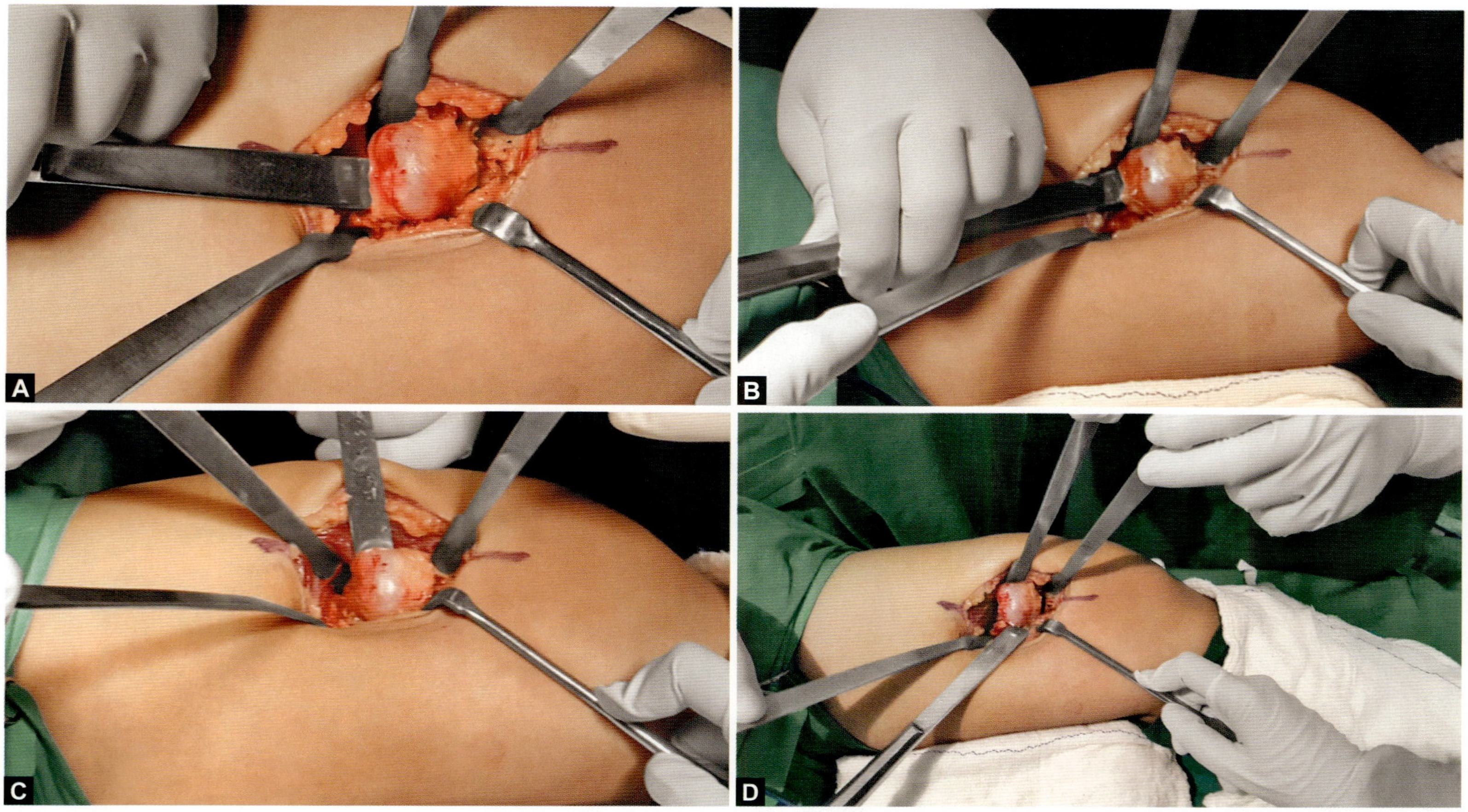

Figs. 11A to D: Osteotomy done at the base from all sides.

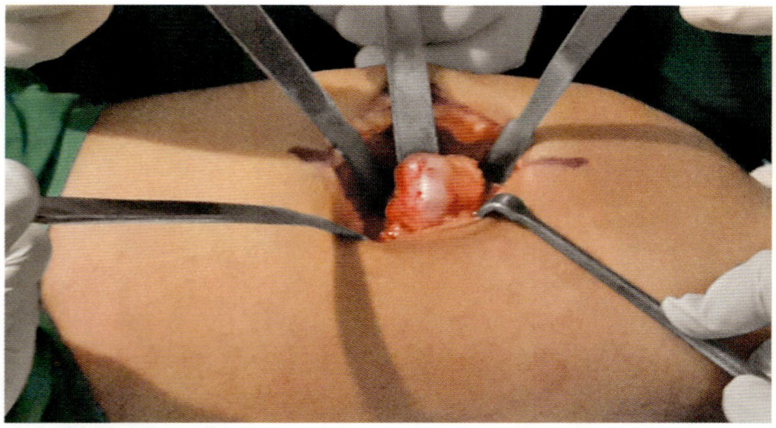

Fig. 12: Osteochondroma elevated.

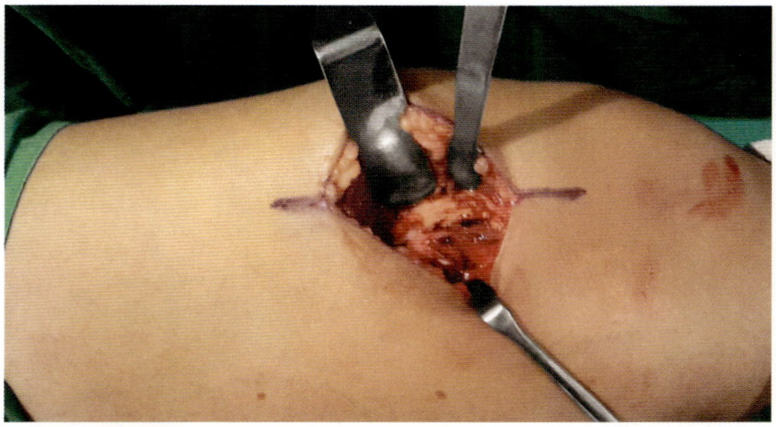

Fig. 13: Base seen after removal of osteochondroma.

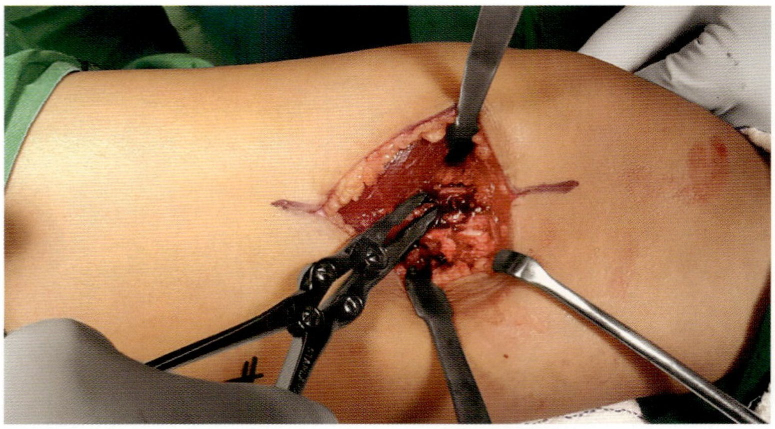

Fig. 14: Edges smoothened with nibbler.

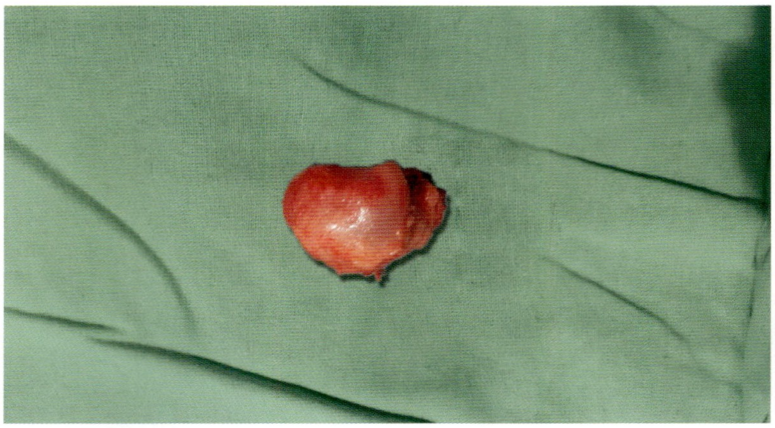

Fig. 15: Excised specimen.

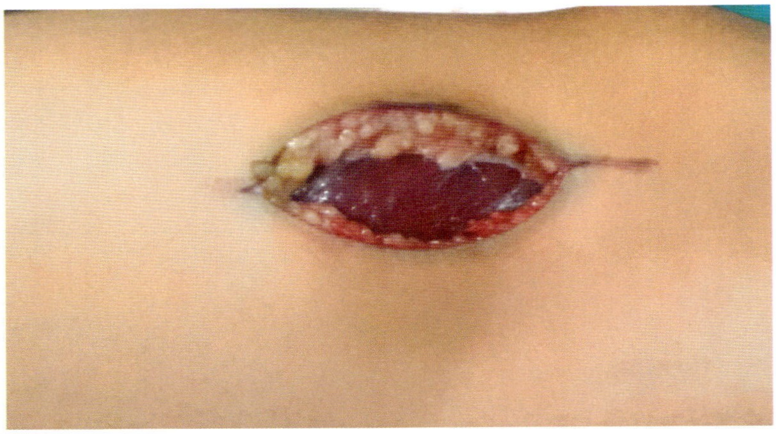

Fig. 16: Muscle repositioned.

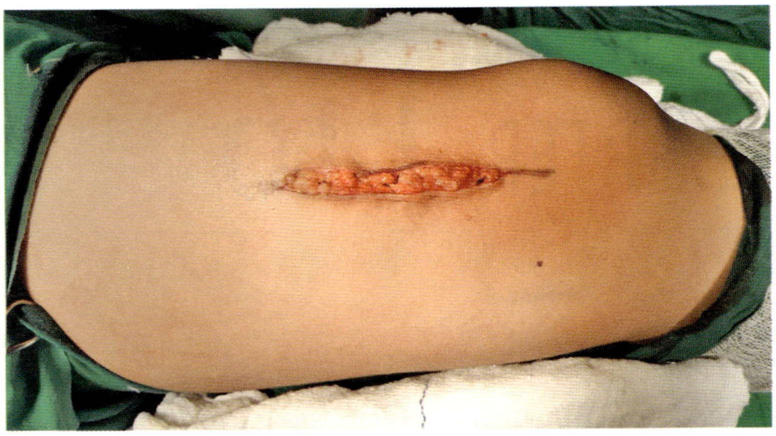

Fig. 17: Subcutaneous closure by absorbable 2-0.

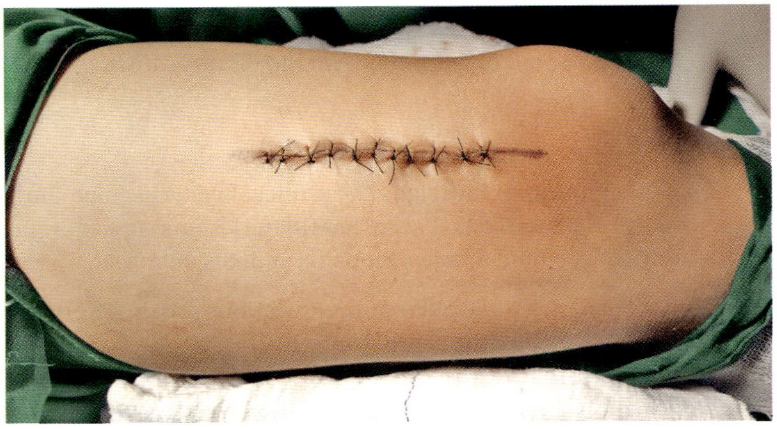

Fig. 18: Skin closure by nonabsorbable suture 3-0.

SUGGESTED READING

1. Bone Tumor.org. Osteochondroma. [online] Available from: http://www.bonetumor.org/tumors/pages/page31.html. [Accessed October, 2018].
2. Bovée JVMG. Multiple osteochondromas. Orphanet J Rare Dis. 2008;3(1):3.
3. Christianne R, Hameetman L, Bovée JVMG. Bone: Osteochondroma. Atlas Genet Cytogenet Oncol Haematol. 2009;13(9):678-80.
4. Kitsoulis P, Galani V, Stefanaki K, et al. Osteochondromas: Review of the Clinical, Radiological and Pathological Features. In Vivo. 2008;22(5):633-46.

CHAPTER 116

Excision of Soft-tissue Tumors

Sachin Nagapurkar, Harshal Saogi, Nitish Agrawal

HEMANGIOMA

Theory: Hemangioma is common benign bone lesion. Asymptomatic lesions of the vertebral bodies are present in 10% of the population. Soft tissue hemangiomas constitute of about 7% of all soft tissue tumors. These lesions are commonly encountered in skull and hemangioma of long bones of the extremities are rare. Spinal lesion are rarely symptomatic unless there is vertebral collapse or, rarely present with soft-tissue extension, nerve root or cord compression.

Histology of these lesions show blood filled spaces of cavernous type. Some may be of mixed variety involving cavernous and capillary type.

Radiographic appearance of spine is characteristic; with thickened, vertically oriented trabeculae pattern showing the classic "jailhouse" appearance or corduroy cloth sign. These thickened trabeculae show up as "polka dot" pattern on CT scan. In MRI the lesions appear bright on T1- and T2- weighted images. Biopsy is at times required.

Treatment: There are multiple treatment options for symptomatic lesions. Surgical resection is adequate for almost all soft tissue hemangiomas. Most lesions of the long bones can be treated adequately with extended curettage. Preoperative embolization can help minimize the massive intraoperative blood loss. Selective arterial embolization also can be used as definitive treatment for symptomatic lesions in surgically inaccessible location. Rare cases of vertebral collapse with neurologic compromise may require surgery of nerve root or cord decompression. Low-dose radiation is used in inoperable lesions but it carries the risk of malignant degeneration.

SURGICAL STEPS (FIGS. 1 TO 13)

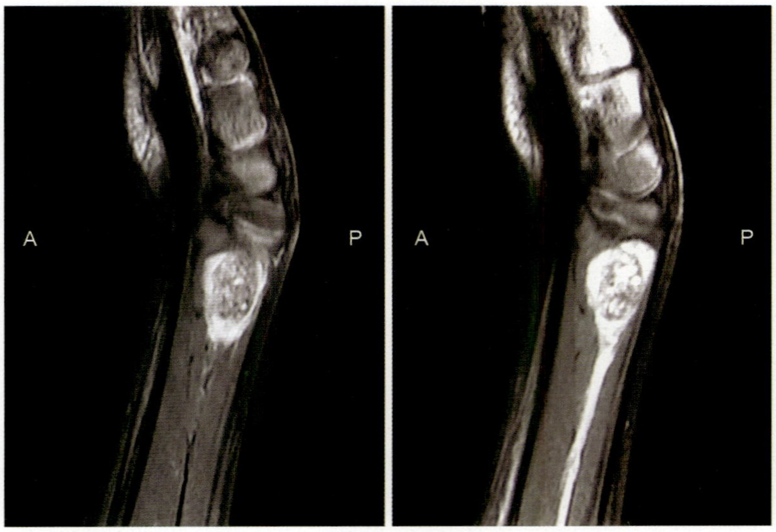

Fig. 1: Proton density weighted (PD) fat sagittal.

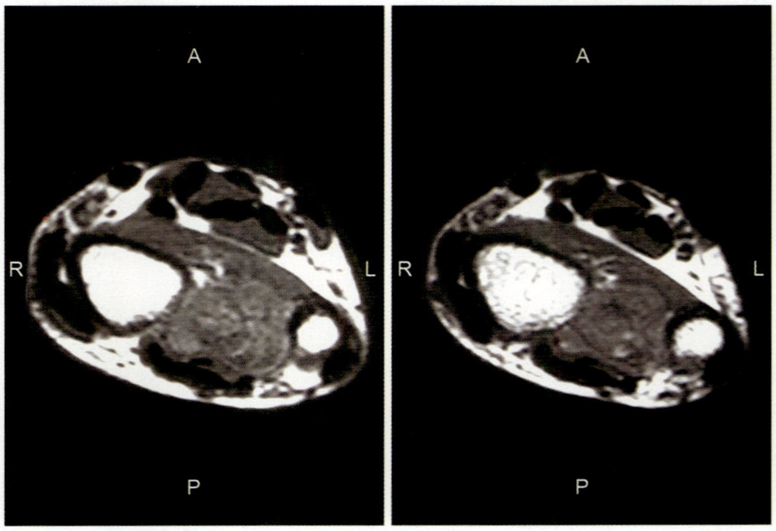

Fig. 2: T1 axial.

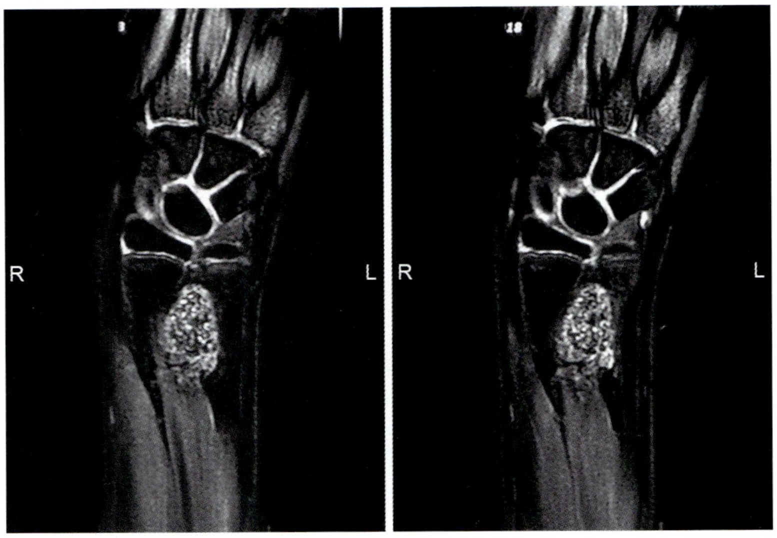

Fig. 3: Three dimensional (3D) WATSF.

A 13-year-old boy with pain in lower third forearm on dorsal aspect. Magnetic resonance imaging (MRI) left wrist and forearm showing 2.5 × 1.5 cm sized fusiform mass lesion along the ventral aspect of distal third of wrist with thickened posterior interosseous nerve leading to it. The lesion appears heterogeneously hyperintense on T2/PD (proton density) images and hypointense on T1-weighted images.

No evidence of any intramuscular extension of lesion is noted. Above features are suggestive of posterior interosseous nerve Schwannoma.

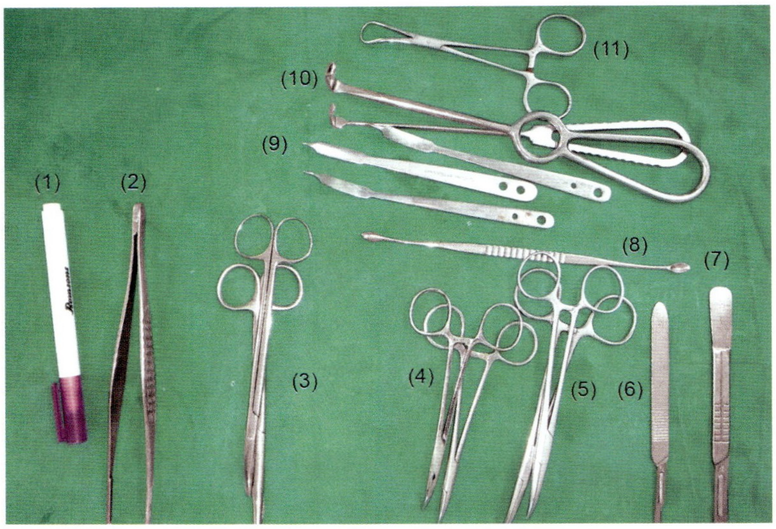

Fig. 4: Instruments: (1) Marker pen, (2) Tissue forceps, (3) Dissecting scissors, (4) Mosquito forceps, (5) Artery forceps, (6) Stab knife, (7) Skin knife, (8) Bone curette, (9) Hohmann bone lever, (10) Right angle retractor, (11) Towel clip.

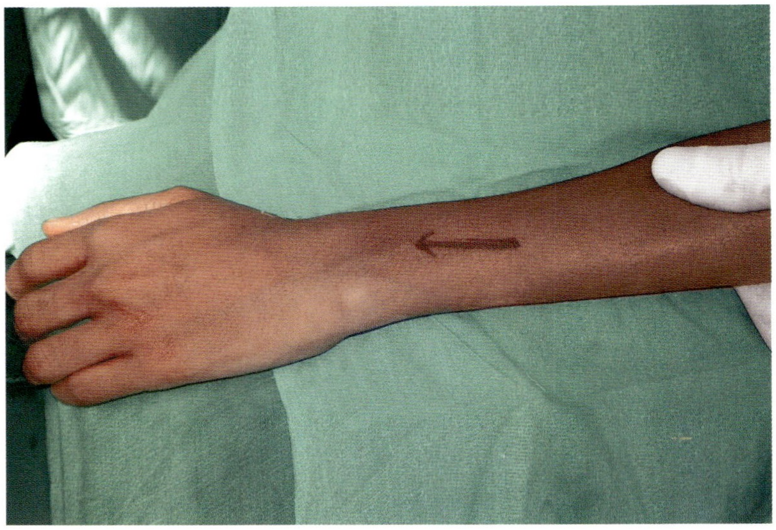

Fig. 5: Patient is positioned supine on operating table. Left hand is kept on hand rest support on side of operating table. Painting and draping are done in standard manner. Incision site is marked over abnormal mass lesion on dorsal aspect of lower third of forearm.

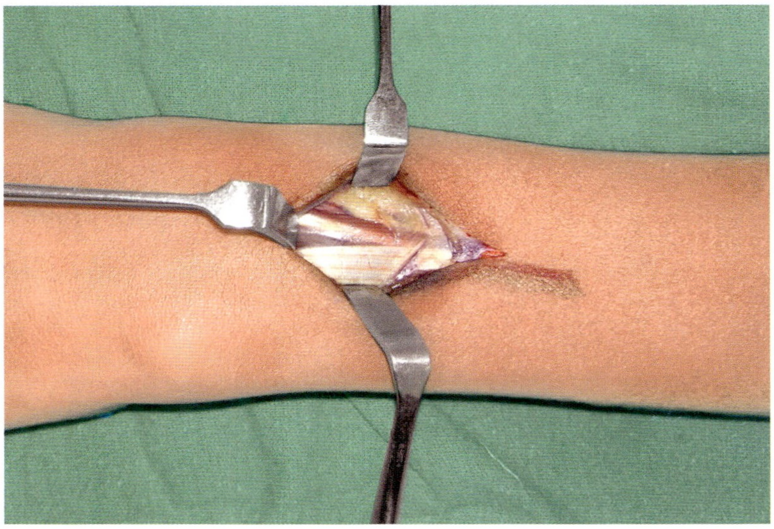

Fig. 6: Skin incision taken with knife and further soft tissue and fascia. Dissection done with stab knife.

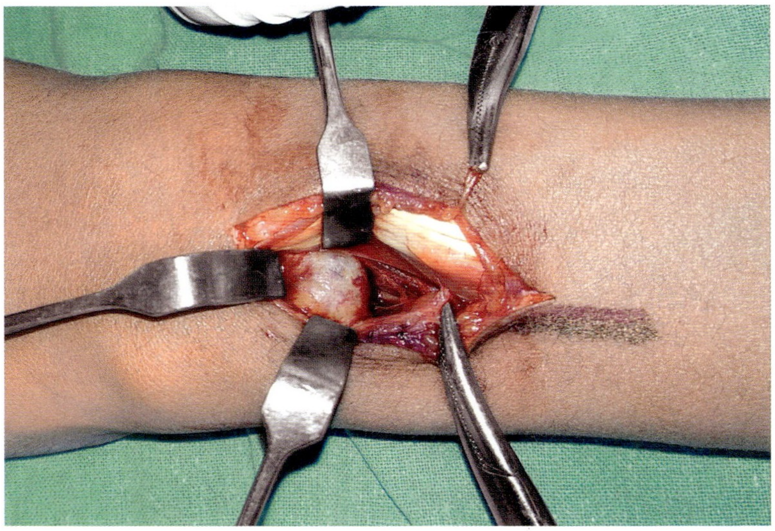

Fig. 7: Tendon and muscle sheath is separated with dissecting scissors. Small tributaries and capillaries clamped with mosquito forceps, muscle and tendon retracted with right angle retractor exposing the abnormal mass.

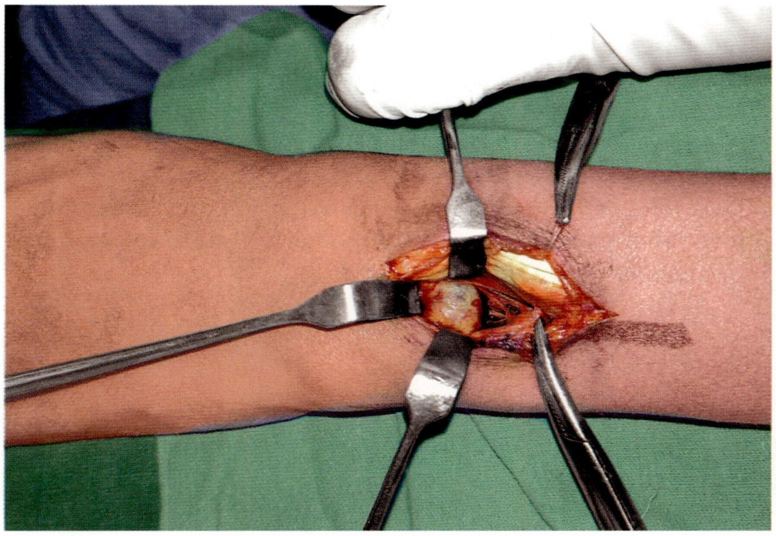

Fig. 8: Abnormal mass separated from surrounding soft tissue by blunt dissection with dissecting scissor and mosquito forceps.

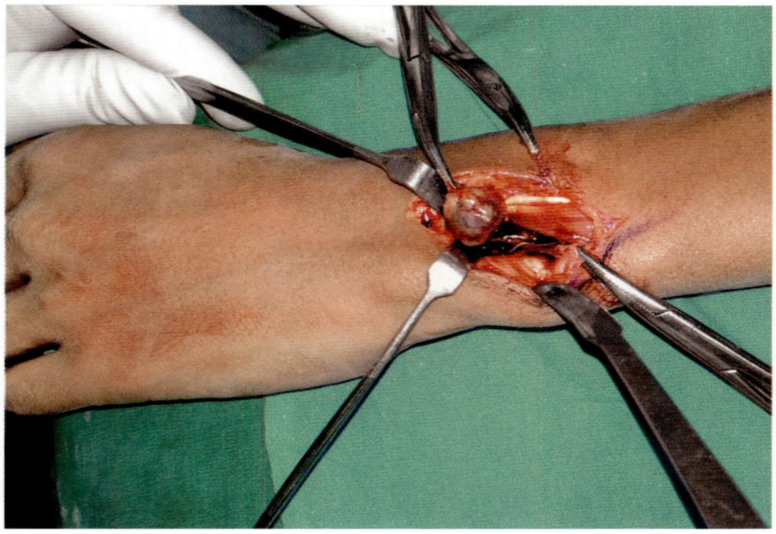

Fig. 9: Abnormal mass lifted with artery forceps.

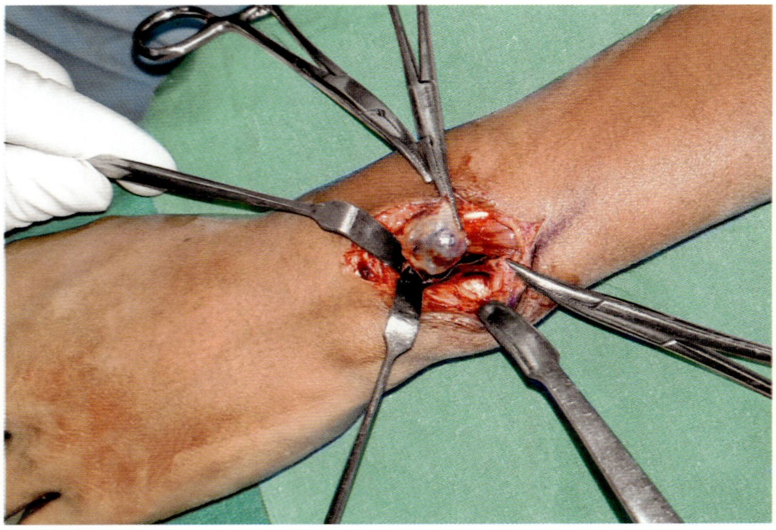

Fig. 10: Connection of abnormal mass with feeding vessels clamped with artery forceps and ligated with linen thread. Abnormal mass dissected from surrounding tissue with dissecting scissor and excised.

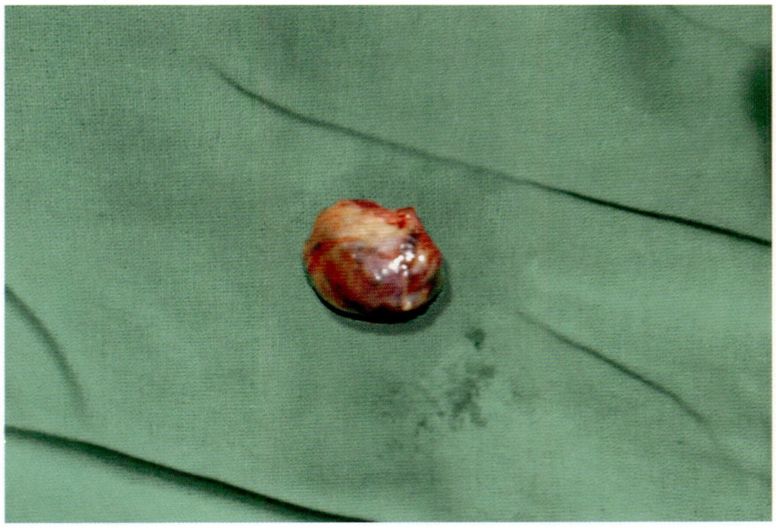

Fig. 11: Excised abnormal mass most likely filled with blood with dark brown hemorrhagic (approximately 2.5 × 1.5 cm) appearance most likely hemangioma. Excised mass sent for histopathological examination.

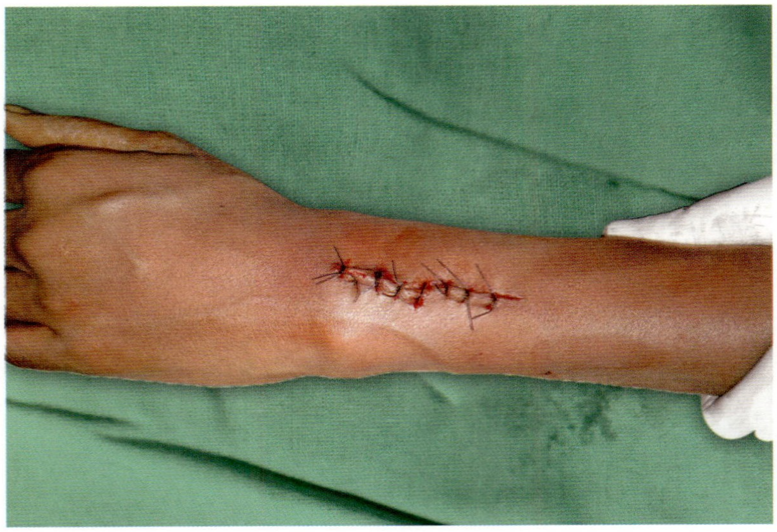

Fig. 12: Wash given with normal saline. Direct skin suturing done with nonabsorbable suture material.

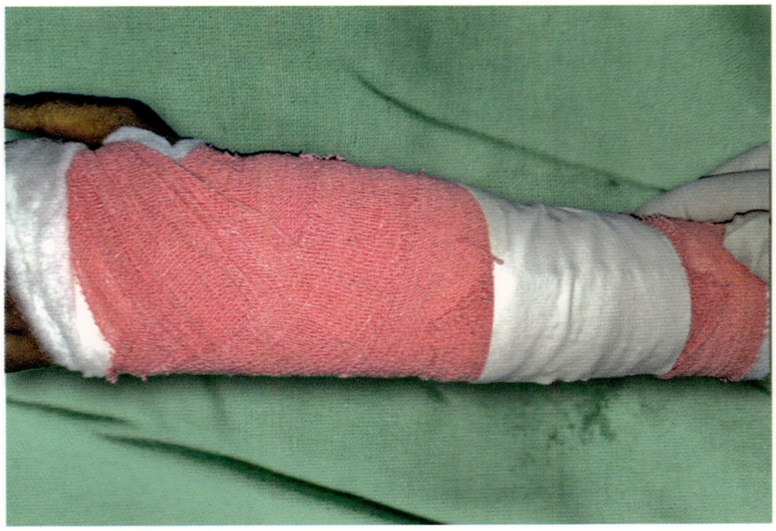

Fig. 13: Compression bandage given after dressing.

POSTOPERATIVE MANAGEMENT

- Active finger movements started from day 1.
- Active wrist, elbow, and shoulder range of motion started from day 1.
- Suture removal done on 14th day.
- Histopathology report showing well circumscribed masses composed of large cavernous spaces filled with blood. The intervening areas show proliferation of pericytes. Also seen few capillary sized vascular spaces few congested blood vessels seen.
- No evidence of atypia or malignancy.
- *Impression*: Hemangioma.

REFERENCES

1. Aich RK, Deb AR, Banerjee A, et al. Symptomatic vertebral hemangioma: treatment with radiotherapy. J cancer Res ther. 2010;6:199.
2. Alexander J, Meir A, Vrodos N, Yau YH. Vertebral hemangioma: an important differential in the evaluation of locally aggressive spinel lesion. Spine. 2010;35:E917.
3. Maverogenis AF, Rossi G, Calabro T, et Al. The role of embolization for hemoangioms. Musculoskeletal Surg. 2012;96:125.
4. Miszczyak SF. Tukiendrof A. Radiotherapy of painful vertebral hemoangioms: the single center retrospective analysis of 137 cases. Int J Radiat Oncol Biol Phys. 2012;82:e173.
5. Urruita J, Postigo R, Larrondo R, Martin AS. Clinical and imagine findings in patient with aggressive spinal hemoangioms requiring surgical treatment. J Clin Neurosci. 2011;18:209.

CHAPTER 117

Bone Cyst of Neck Femur: Curettage and Fixation

Arun Salunkhe, S Prakash, Sachin Nagapurkar, Nitish Agrawal

UNICAMERAL BONE CYST

- Unicameral bone cysts commonly affect children. These are more of a developmental or reactive lesion than a true tumor. In the first 2 decades male and female ratio is 2:1. These are found most commonly in proximal humerus and femur although any bone of the extremities can be affected. In adults, ilium and calcaneum are most common location. The lesions are highly active during skeletal growth period. Usually there is spontaneous healing at maturity. Cysts are usually asymptomatic unless pathological fracture occurs.
- Plain radiographs are typically diagnostic for unicameral bone cysts with a centrally positioned, purely lytic lesion and a well-marginated define. It by no means penetrates the cortex. No periosteal response is present except when there is a fracture. A thinned cortical fragment at times fractures and falls into the base of the lesion thus confirming its empty cystic nature. "Fallen fragment" sign is pathognomonic of a unicameral bone cyst with a fracture. Unicameral bone cysts grow as metaphyseal lesions abutting the physis in growing kids. With time, they appear to move into the diaphysis because the physis grows far away from the cyst, categorized active when they are within 1 cm of the physis latent while they are toward the diaphysis.
- Focal disorder in metaphyseal reworking blocks interstitial fluid drainage. Multiplied strain, which leads to focal bone necrosis and accumulation of fluid. This is most accepted theory for pathogenesis.
- Cyst fluid consists of prostaglandins, interleukins, oxygen-free radicals, metalloproteinases, cytokines, lead to bone resorption. It is packed with a clean yellow, serous fluid. Fibrous membrane, less than 1-mm thick, strains the cyst wall. Lining of fibroblasts takes place in place of endothelial cells. Deep to this membrane lining, the cyst wall includes fibrovascular tissue with fragments of immature, mesenchymal cells, osteoclast-like giant cells, and occasional lymphocytes.
- Monitoring by serial plain radiographs is all that required to treat small and asymptomatic lesions in the upper extremities. Symptomatic or large lesions are treated with curettage (with or without bone grafting or internal fixation) aspiration and injection (usually the usage of corticosteroids, bone marrow aspirate, demineralized bone matrix, or different substances). Pathologic fractures of upper limb can be treated conservatively, as fracture can also provoke cyst "healing". Fractures via proximal femur, curettage, bone grafting, and internal fixation.
- *Corticosteroid injection:* 80–200 mg of methylprednisolone is used, depending on the size, age of the affected person along with size of the lesion.
- Autogenous bone marrow mixed with allograft demineralized bone matrix, calcium sulfate, high-porosity hydroxyapatite, calcium phosphate bone graft substitutes cancellous allograft.
- Curettage, bone grafting, and internal fixation should be done for large painful lesions, the proximal femur that are at high risk for fracture.

ANEURYSMAL BONE CYST

Aneurysmal bone cysts (ABCs) are locally destructive, blood-stuffed reactive lesions of bone. These are not considered to be genuine neoplasms. It can affect any bone, but the maximum usual places include the proximal humerus, distal femur, proximal tibia, and spine.

Commonly affects 10–20-year-old patients. Can arise in any decade of adult life, however almost 80% affects within the 2nd decade. Can be primary or secondary (arising in other tumors).

Primary ABC can be neoplastic. Spontaneous regression may be visible in few active primary ABCs, however it is quite rare in aggressive or secondary lesion. ABCs can be of hydraulic strain foundation, secondary to be hemorrhage and may be traumatically caused. In the spine, 66% of ABCs will stand up from posterior elements and 33% will arise from the vertebral body. These progress as aggressive osteolytic lesions with extensive permeative cortical destruction. In humerus and femur pathological fracture is a common complication.

Campanacci Classification of Aneurysmal Bone Cysts

- Aggressive cysts show signs of reparative osteogenesis, ill-defined margins and no periosteal shell.
- Active cyst reveal an incomplete periosteal shell with a defined margin between the lesion and the host bone.
- Inactive cyst has a complete periosteal shell with sclerotic margin present between the cyst and the metaphysis.

Histology

Aneurysmal bone cysts are composed of blood-crammed space with intervening fibrous septae. True endothelial cells are not found generally. The tissue consists of sponge-like with cavernous spaces and filled with blood. Cavities are surrounded by means of grey or brownish tissue and have an osseous component. At the outer edge of the lesion an egg shell like layer of periosteal bone present around the lesion.

Radiographs screen an expansile lytic lesion elevating the periosteum but remains contained with the aid of a thin shell of cortical bone. An ABC may have properly-described margins or a permeative appearance that closely resembles a malignancy. It is far most usually eccentrically placed in metaphysis.

Computed tomography (CT) scan is beneficial to evaluate lesion of the pelvis or vertebral column greater exactly than radiography. It helps to assess cautiously the presence of periosteal rim of the bone around a lesion. Magnetic resonance imaging (MRI) shows the multiloculated cavities and fluid levels. When differentiating among a unicameral and ABC by the use of MRI, the presence of a double-density fluid and intralesional septations typically indicates an ABC.

An ABC can originate primarily, however legions much like an ABC are observed in numerous different lesions, consisting of giant cell tumors, chondroblastomas, osteoblastomas fibrous dysplasia, nonossifying fibromas, and chondromyxoid fibromas. Even though the pathogenesis is unsure, it is likely probable that ABC consequences from nearby circulatory disturbance leading to multiplied venous pressure and manufacturing of local hemorrhage.

Treatment of most of the ABCs are extended curettage and grafting with a bone graft substitute. During surgery tourniquet use is advised as there is a possibility of heavy bleeding. Marginal resection now and again is advised for lesions in expendable bones. Lesions in the spine or pelvis can be dealt with preoperative embolization to limit surgical loss. Arterial embolization has been used as definitive remedy of ABC in place where curettage could be extraordinarily tough. Low-dose radiation has been suggested to be an powerful approach of remedy, frequently associated with rapid ossification; but, because of the potential for malignant transformation it is not used routinely.

In patients treated with curettage a recurrence rate of 10–20% is expected. Recurrence is commonly asociated with age less than 15 years, centrally located cystic cavity contents. Recurrent cyst can be dealt with with the same technique as the primary lesion.

SURGICAL STEPS

A 12-year-male child came with complaint of pain in left hip.

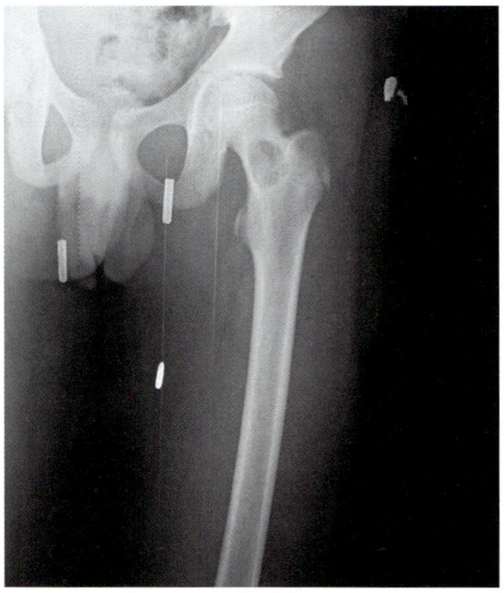

Fig. 1: X-ray left hip shows lytic lesion on inferocentral aspect of femoral neck. Cortex of neck intact.

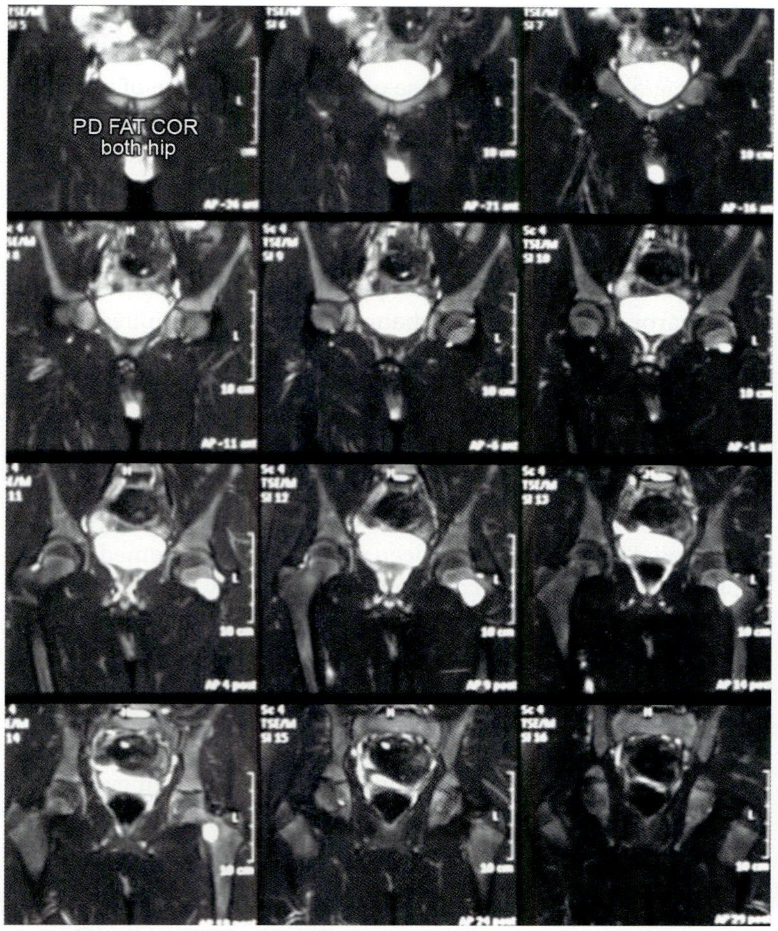

Fig. 2: Magnetic resonance imaging (MRI) proton density (PD) fat coronal view both hips showing intramedullary, eccentric, well-defined T1 hypointensed.

- MRI both hips T2, STIR (short inversion time inversion recovery) hyperintense lesion with lobulated margin measuring 31.0 × 28.1 × 19.3 mm in the neck of the left femur
- Endosteal scalloping of the neck of left femur is noted.
- No obvious adjacent bony/cortical destruction. No bone marrow edema adjacent to lesion
- No obvious extension of lesion into adjacent epiphysis/soft tissue
- Perifemoral muscles/soft tissue is normal
- Findings are suggestive of simple bone cyst.

DIFFERENTIAL DIAGNOSIS

- Enchondroma
- Brown tumor of the hyperparathyroidism.

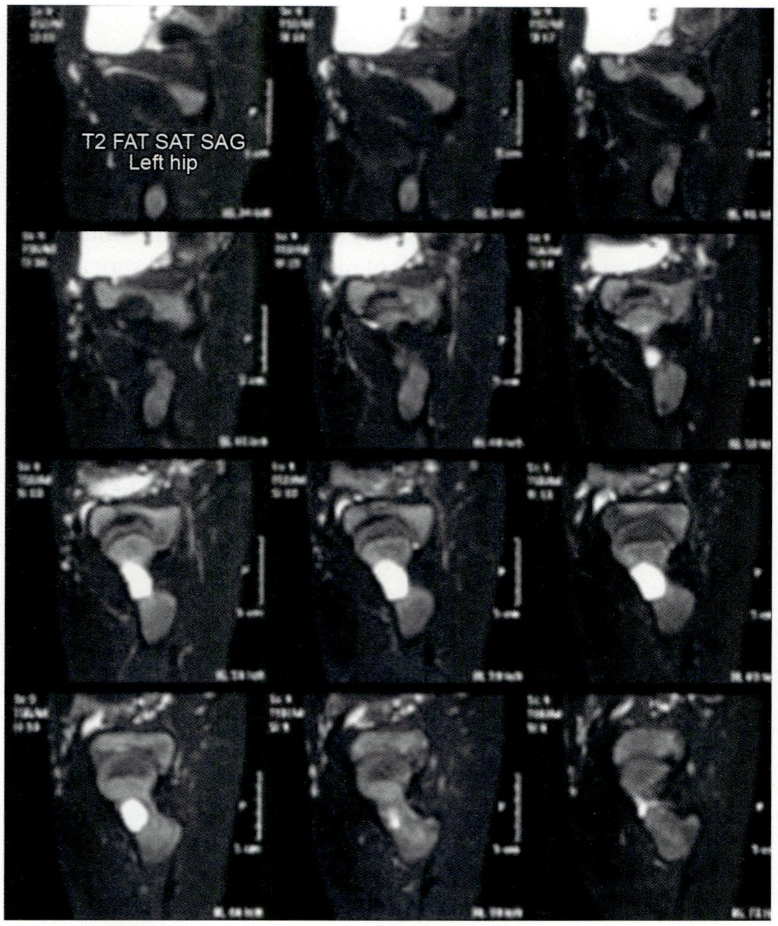

Fig. 3: Magnetic resonance imaging (MRI) T2 fat saturation sagittal view of left hip.

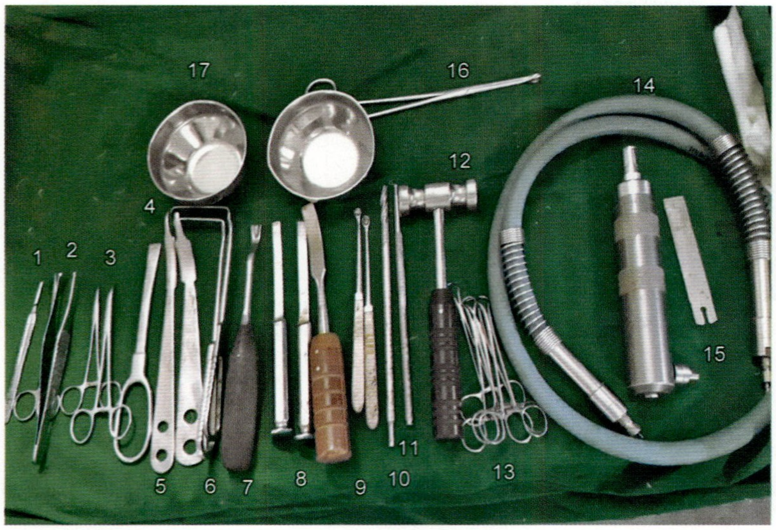

Fig. 4: Instruments: (1) Bard–Parker handle knife, (2) Tooth forceps, (3) Artery and mosquito forceps, (4) Periosteum elevator, (5) Hohmann bone lever, (6) Right angle refractor, (7) Curved chisel, (8) Osteotome, (9) Curette, (10) 6.5-mm reamer, (11) Bone punch, (12) Hammer, (13) Towel clip, (14) Drill, (15) Saw blade, (16) Sponge holding forceps, (17) Sterile container.

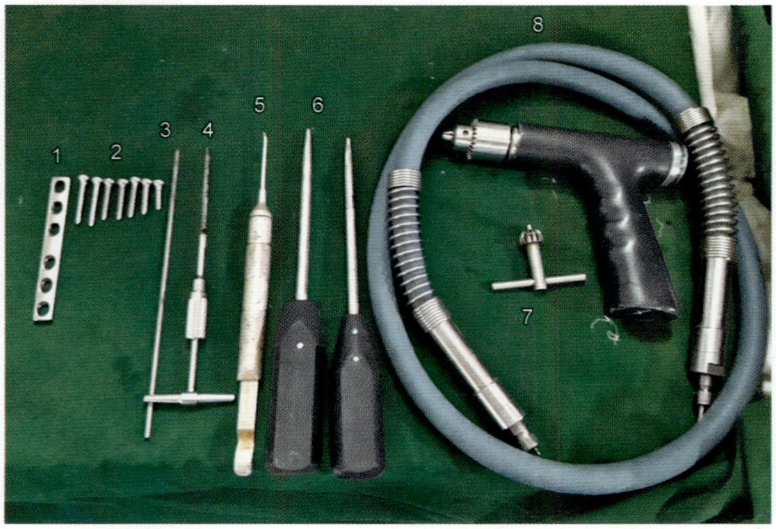

Fig. 5: (1) Six hole plate, (2) Cortical screws, (3) Drill bit, (4) Tap, (5) Depth gauge, (6) Screw driver, (7) Chuck key, (8) Power drill.

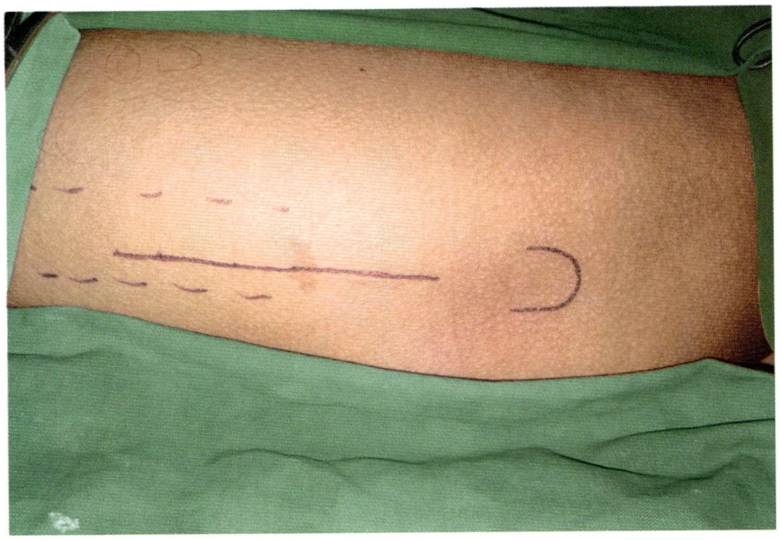

Fig. 6: Patient positioned supine on traction table. Scrubbing, painting, and draping of iliac crest and left hip operative site done in standard manner.

Cortical and cancellous bone graft harvested from left iliac crest. Greater trochanter, shaft of femur, and incision site marked on left side lateral side.

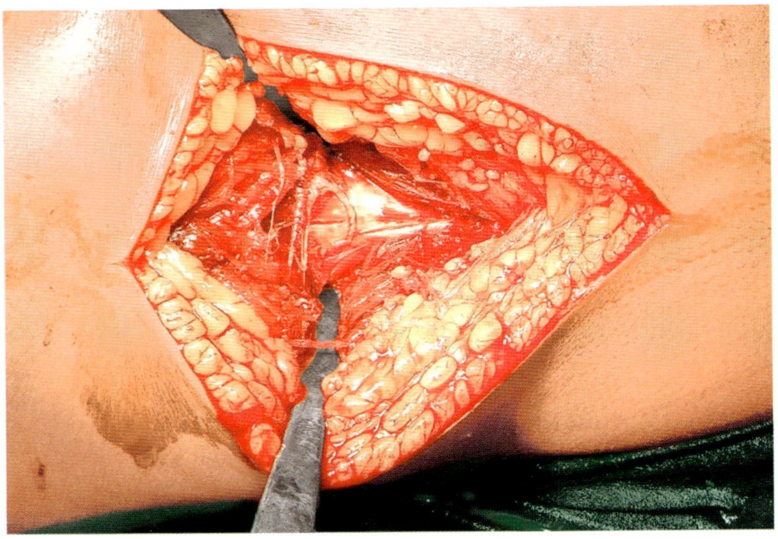

Fig. 7: Incision taken with knife blade No. 21. Soft tissue, subcutaneous fat, and fascia dissection done with stab knife blade No. 15. Further vastus lateralis separated along its fibers and retracted with Hohmann bone lever.

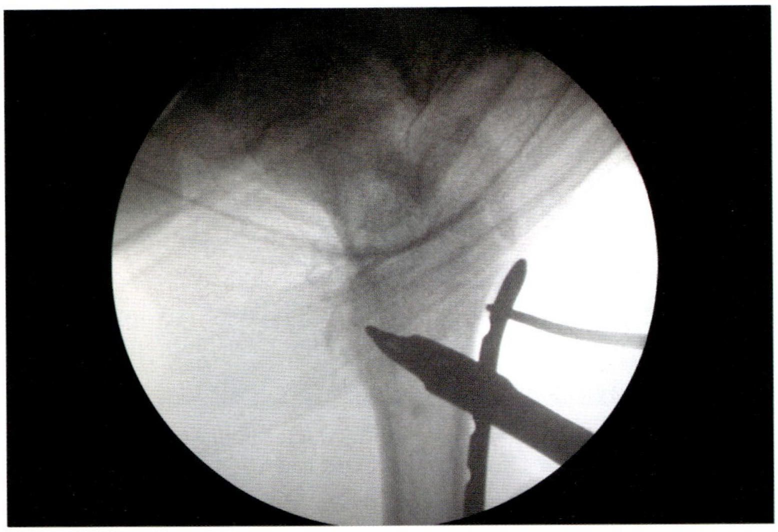

Fig. 8: Entry point for curettage and plate position confirmed on C-arm image intensifier on anteroposterior view.

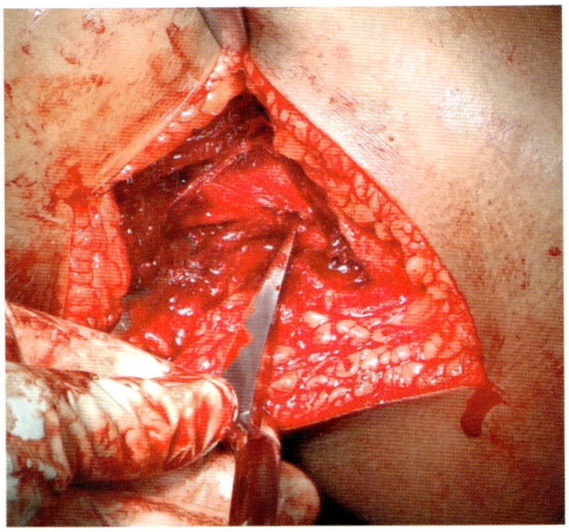

Fig. 9: Small impression made by awl for entry of guidewire on lateral cortex.

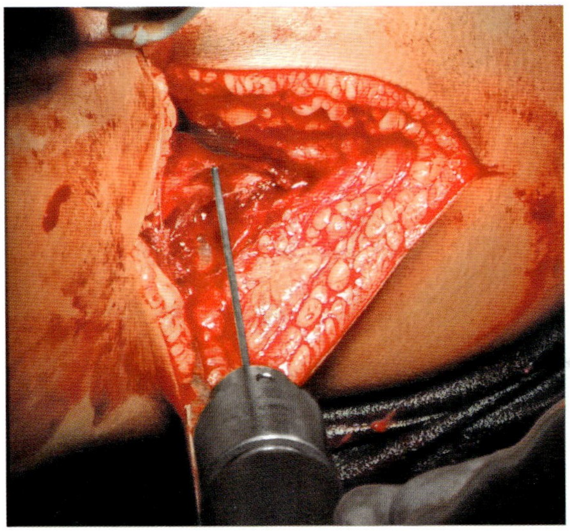

Fig. 10: Guidewire is inserted from lateral cortex on previous impression with the help of drill.

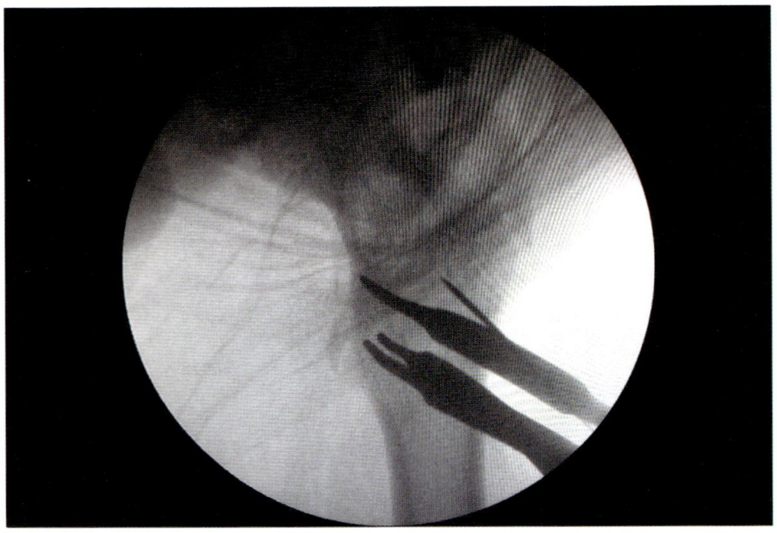

Fig. 11: Guidewire entry checked on C-arm anteroposterior (AP) view.

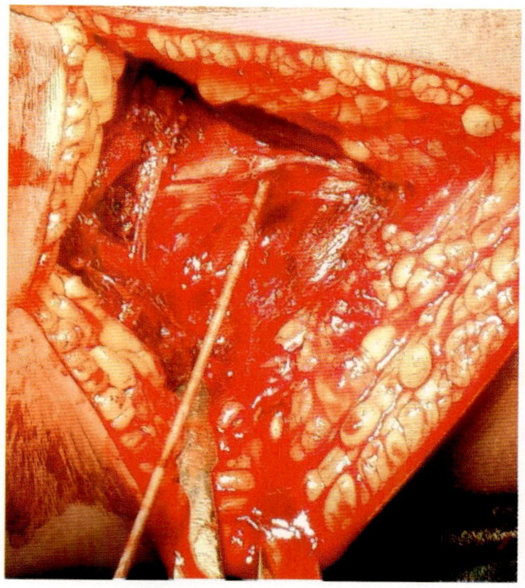

Fig. 12: Guidewire is inserted up to the cyst cavity.

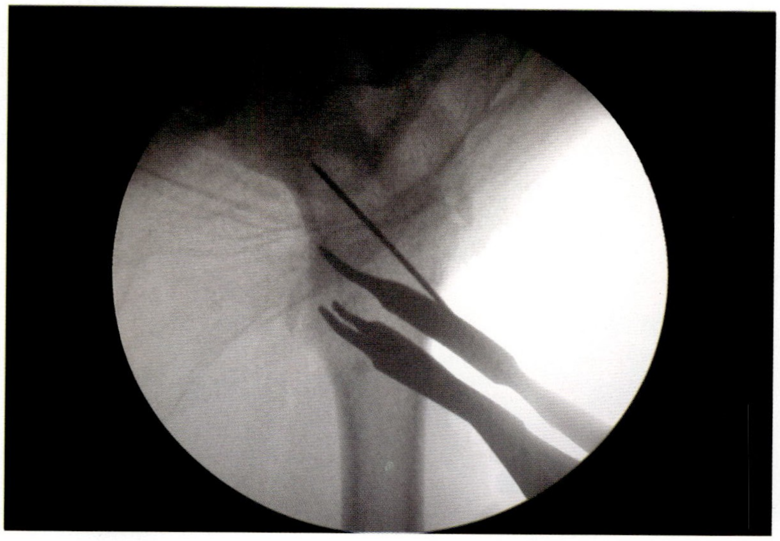

Fig. 13: Guidewire position into cyst cavity confirmed under C-arm guidance on anteroposterior (AP) view.

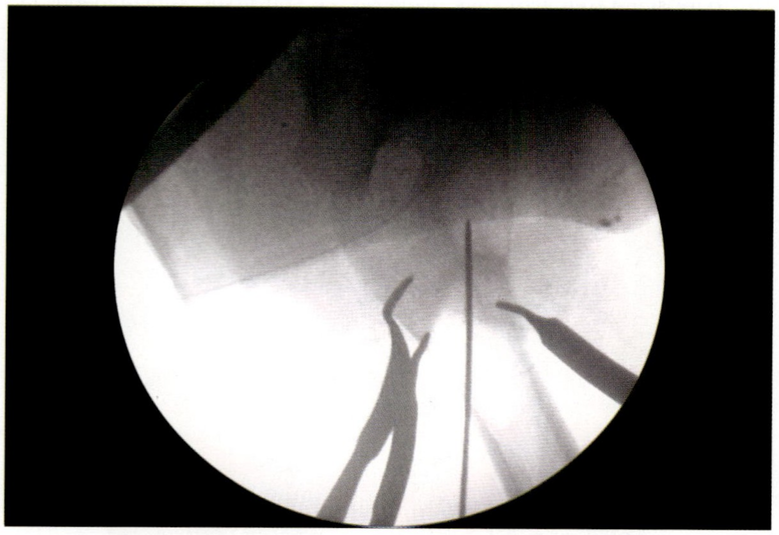

Fig. 14: Guidewire position into cyst cavity confirmed under C-arm lateral view. Care should be taken that entry is made with guidewire proximal to the level of lesser trochanter to prevent subtrochanteric fractures.

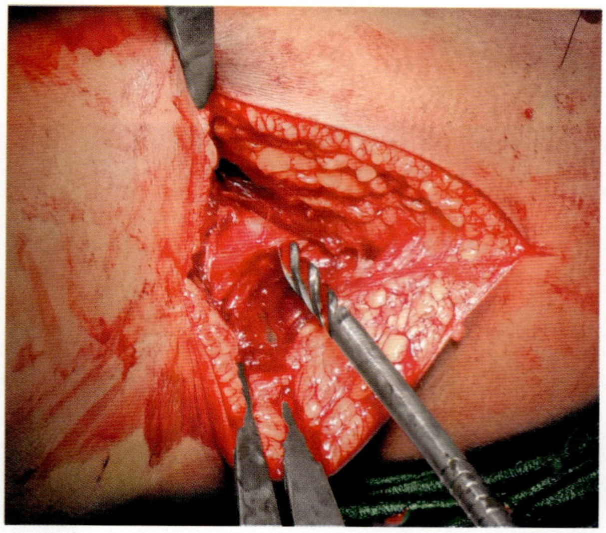

Fig. 15: 6.5-mm reamer inserted over the guidewire up to the cyst cavity for curettage of cyst cavity.

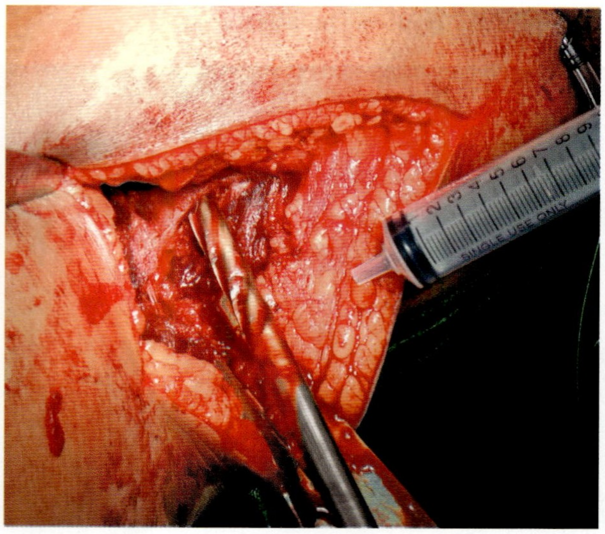

Fig. 16: Cyst cavity fluid is collected in sterile syringe.

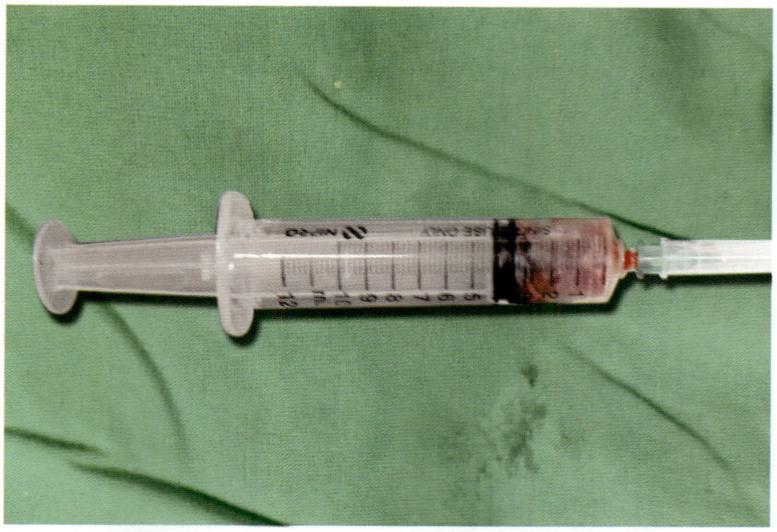

Fig. 17: 1–1.5 cc fluid is collected in 10 cc sterile syringe. Fluid is hemorrhagic/serous in nature. Fluid is send for further culture and sensitivity, (to check presence of any organism/bacteria) gram staining and ZN staining.

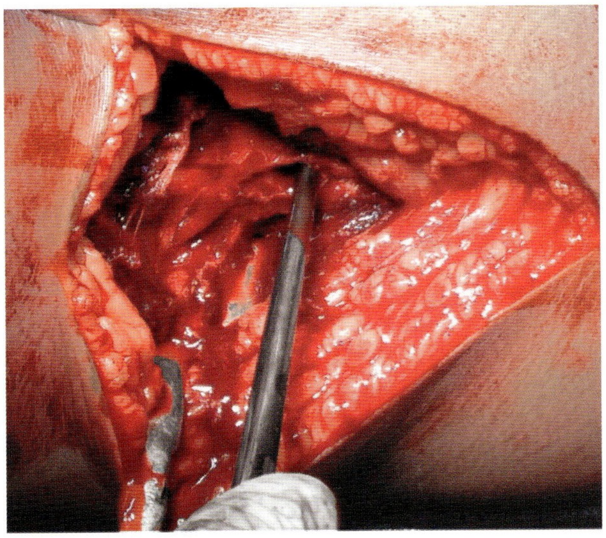

Fig. 18: Burns bone curette is used for curettage cyst cavity.

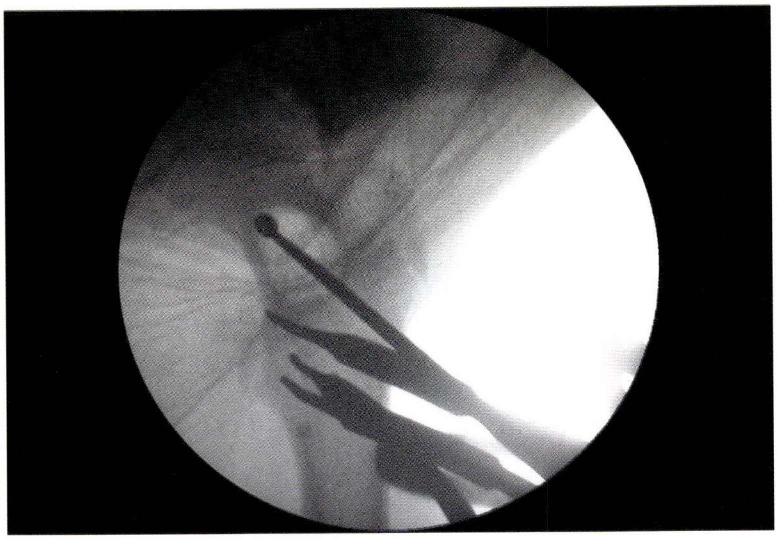

Fig. 19: Curettage of cyst cavity checked under C-arm.

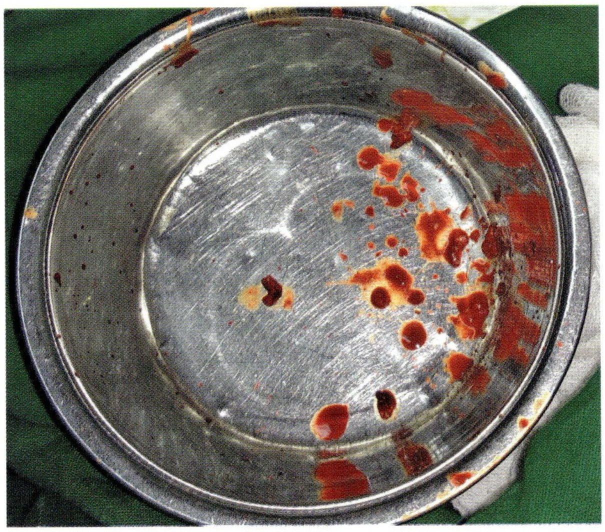

Fig. 20: Tissue from curettage of cyst cavity is collected in sterile container and send for histopathological examination.

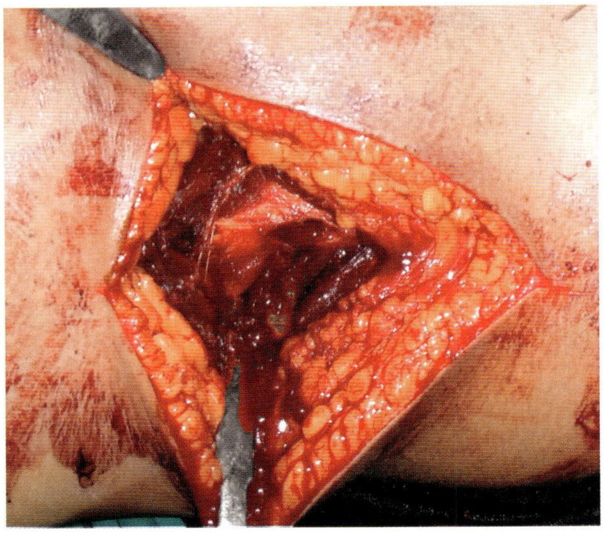

Fig. 21: Curettage of cyst cavity completed.

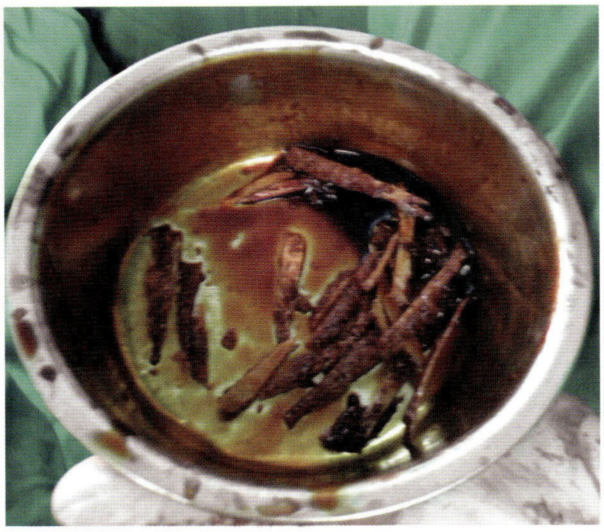

Fig. 22: Cancellous and cortical bone graft harvested from left iliac crest prepared in sterile container for bone grafting.

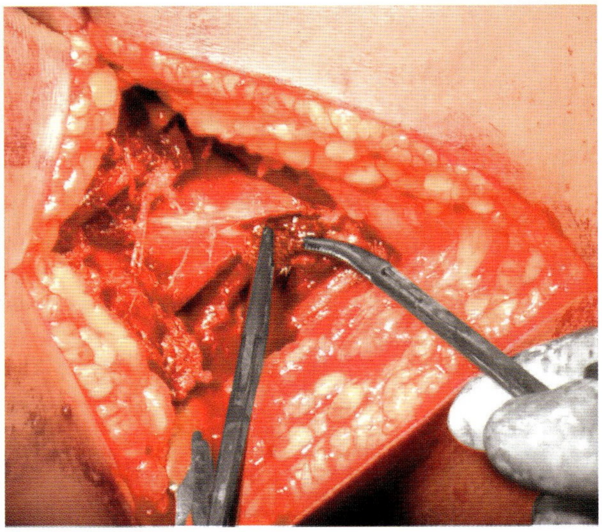

Fig. 23: Cancellous bone graft inserted into cavity.

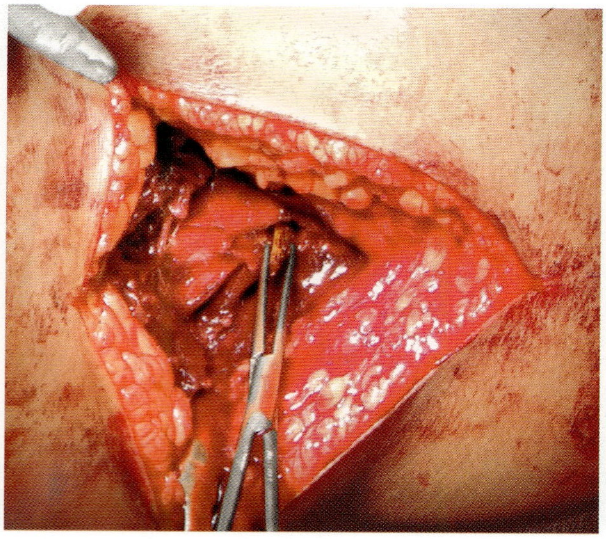

Fig. 24: Cortical bone graft inserted into cavity.

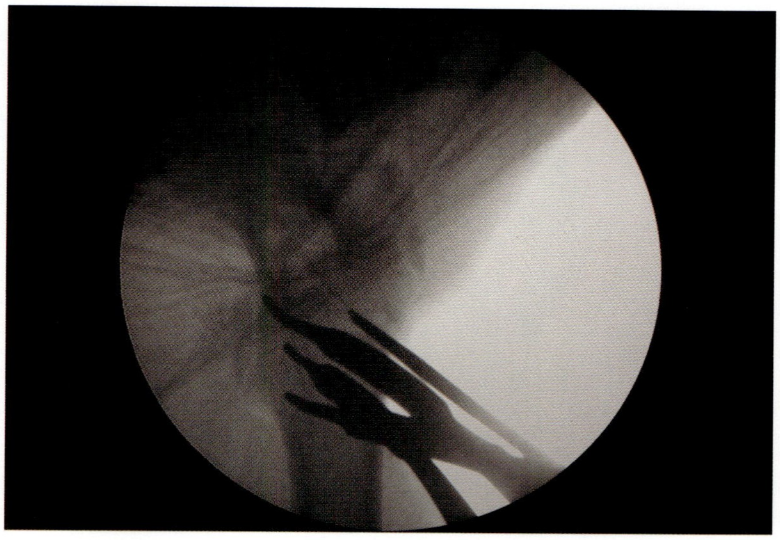

Fig. 25: Insertion of bone graft done under C-arm anteroposterior (AP) view.

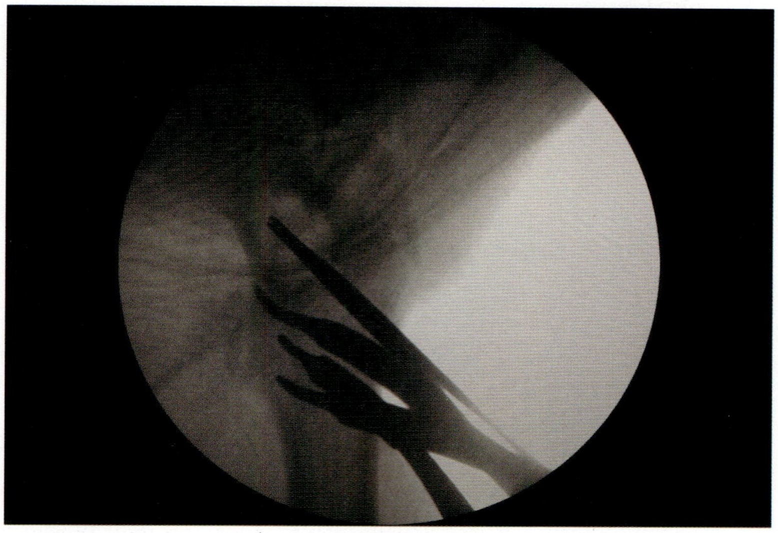

Fig. 26: Proper placement of bone graft into cyst cavity confirmed over C-arm anteroposterior (AP) view.

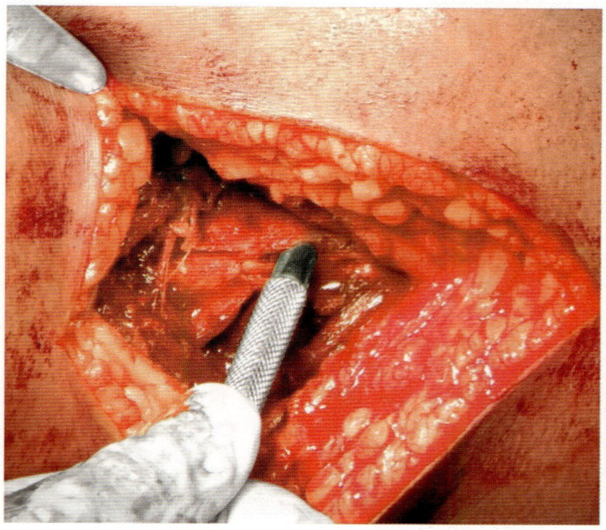

Fig. 27: Bone punch is used to punch bone graft into cavity.

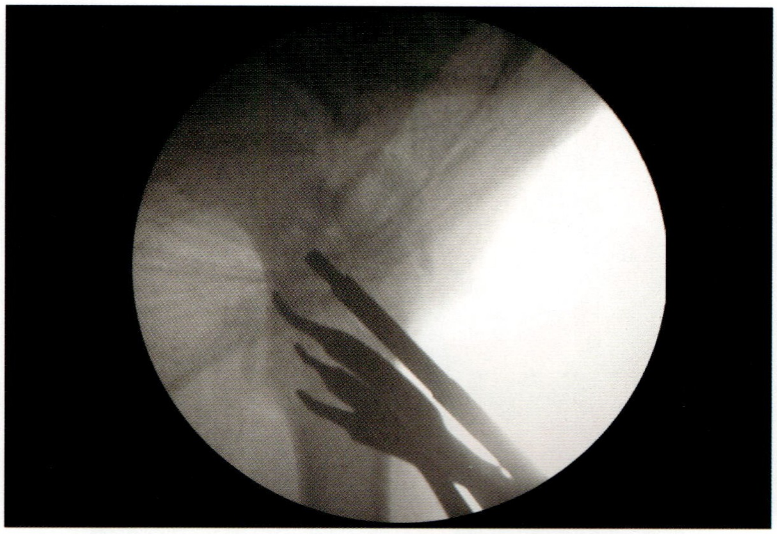

Fig. 28: Punch checked under C-arm anteroposterior (AP) view.

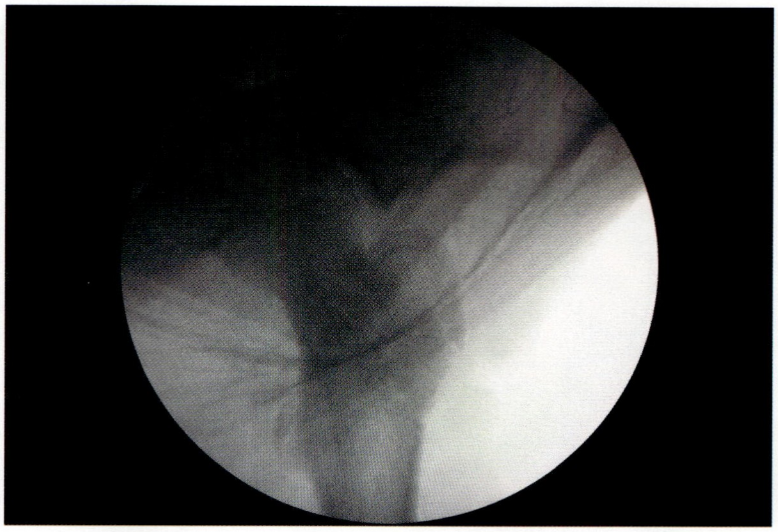

Fig. 29: Bone grafting completed with cancellous and cortical bone graft and confirmed over C-arm anteroposterior (AP) view.

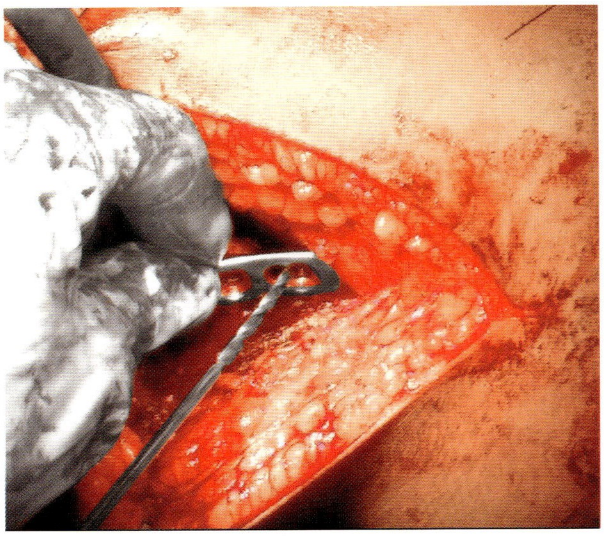

Fig. 30: Six-hole limited contact dynamic compression plate (LC-DCP) plate and drill used for internal fixation.

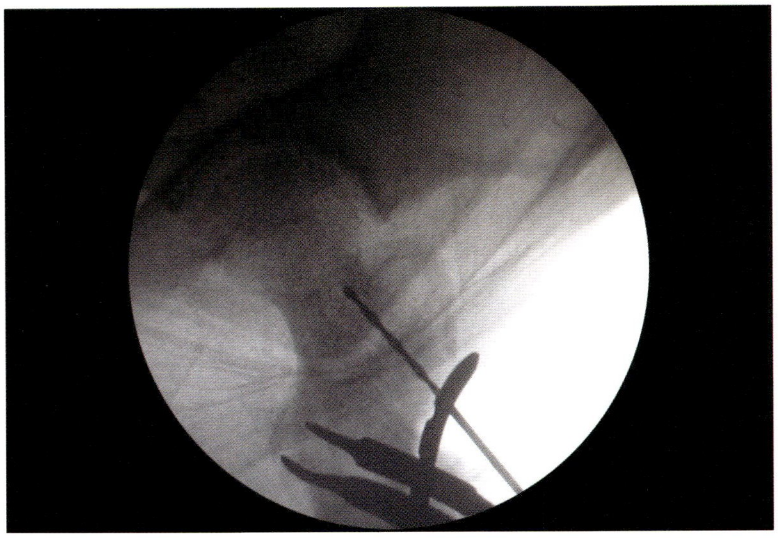

Fig. 31: Drilling for proximal screw fixation is done under C-arm on anteroposterior (AP) X-ray.

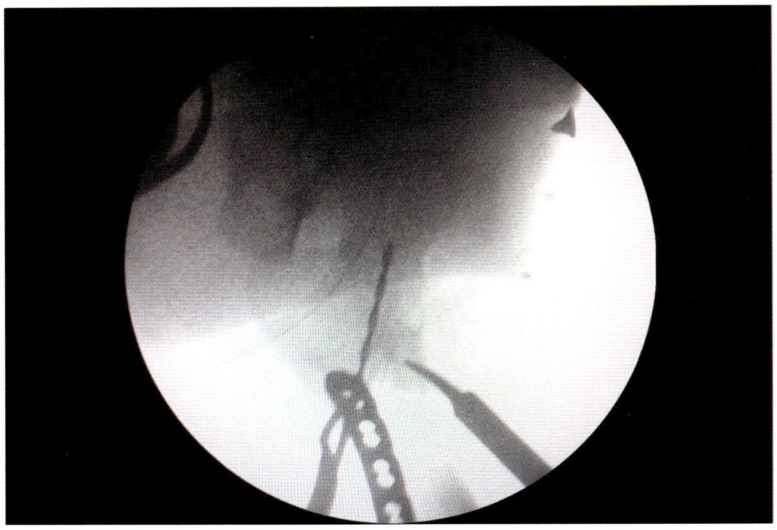

Fig. 32: Position of drill bit confirmed on C-arm lateral view.

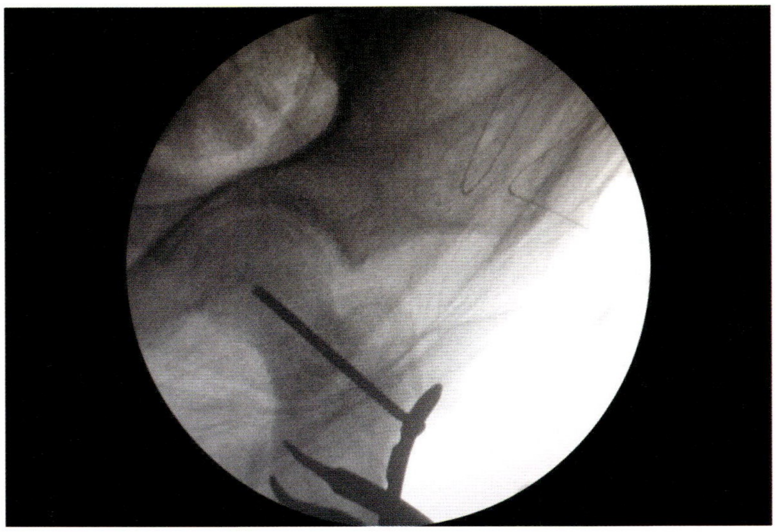

Fig. 33: Screw length is measured with depth gauge and most proximal screw is fixed in metaphyseal area. Care should be taken not to penetrate physis as bone is growing.

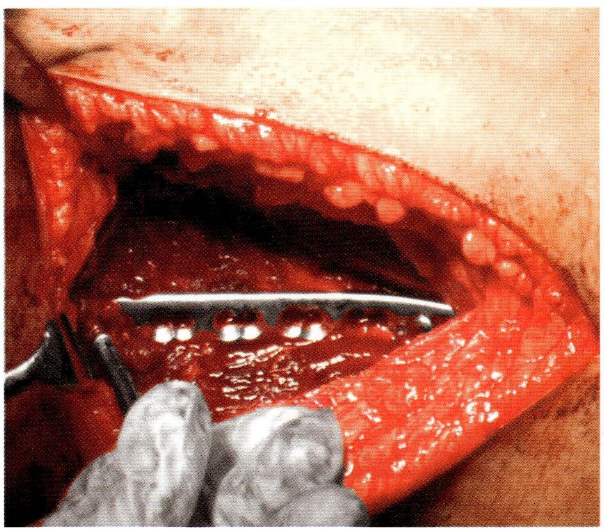

Fig. 34: Most distal screw fixation into femoral shaft done in similar manner.

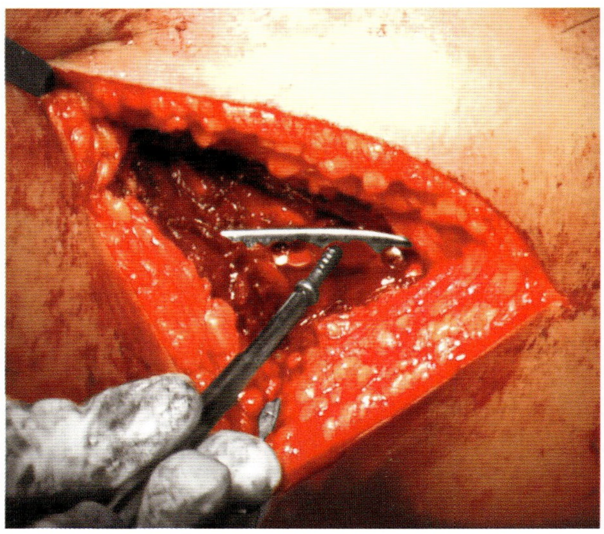

Fig. 35: Proximal 2nd screw fixation into metaphyseal area done in similar manner.

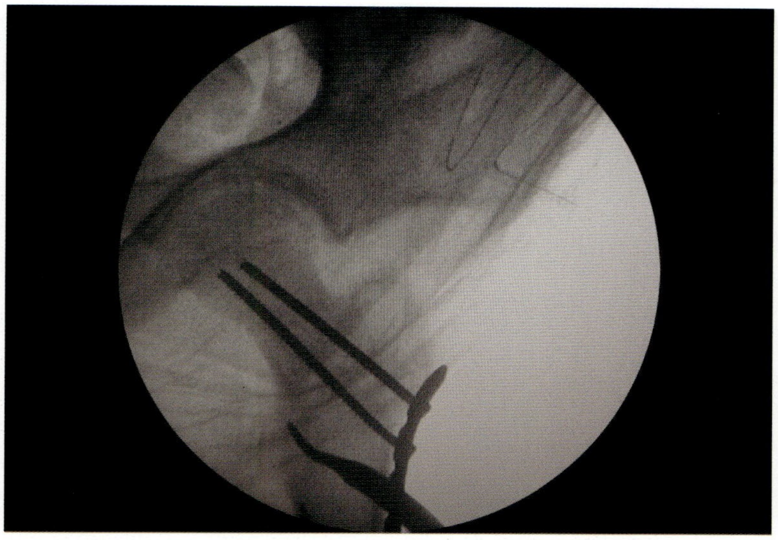
Fig. 36: Proximal 2nd screw fixation confirmed over C-arm anteroposterior (AP) view.

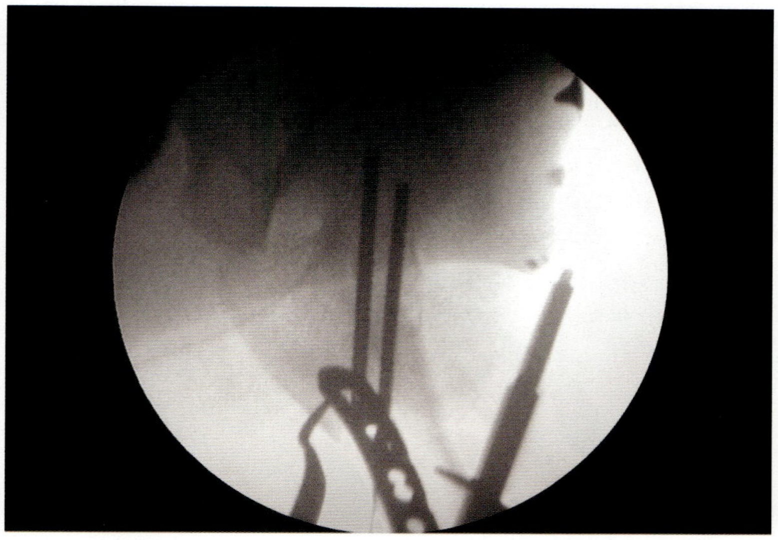
Fig. 37: Proximal two screw fixation confirmed over C-arm lateral view. Care should be taken not be break anterior or posterior cortex of neck.

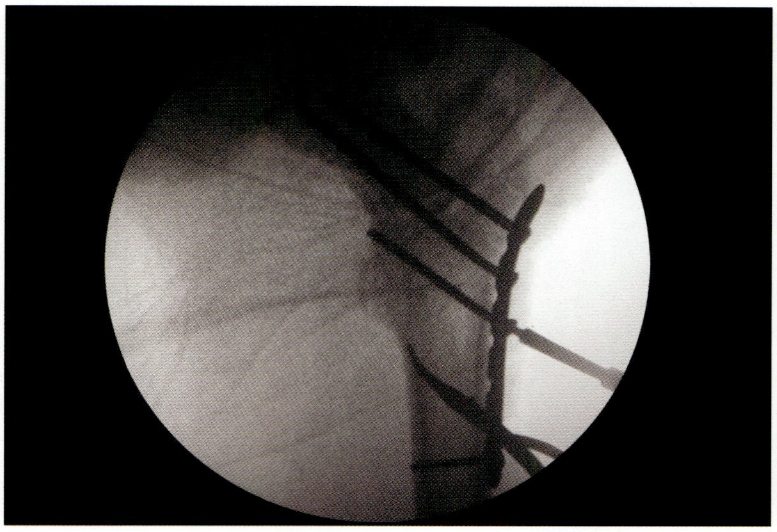
Fig. 38: Proximally 3rd screw fixation done under C-arm in similar manner.

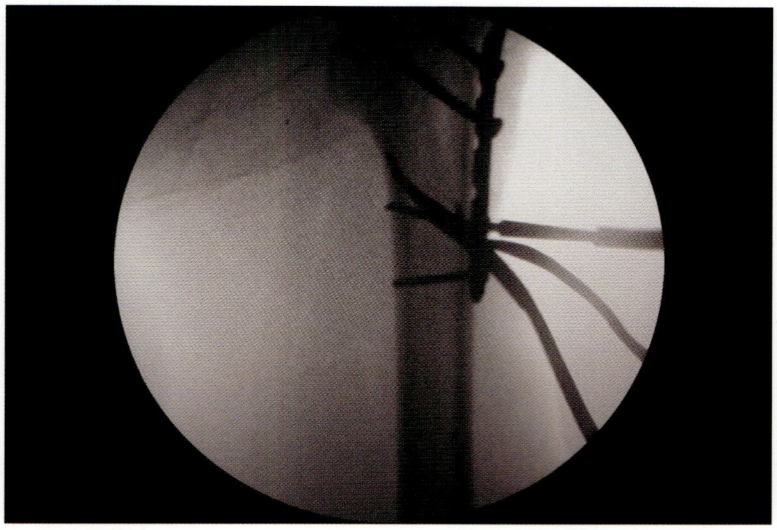
Fig. 39: Remaining two distal screws fixation into femoral shaft done under C-arm in similar manner.

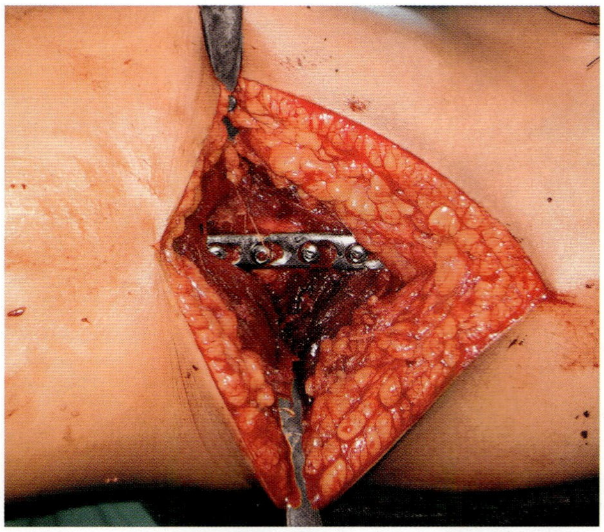
Fig. 40: Internal fixation is completed with six-hole limited contact dynamic compression plate (LC-DCP) and six screws.

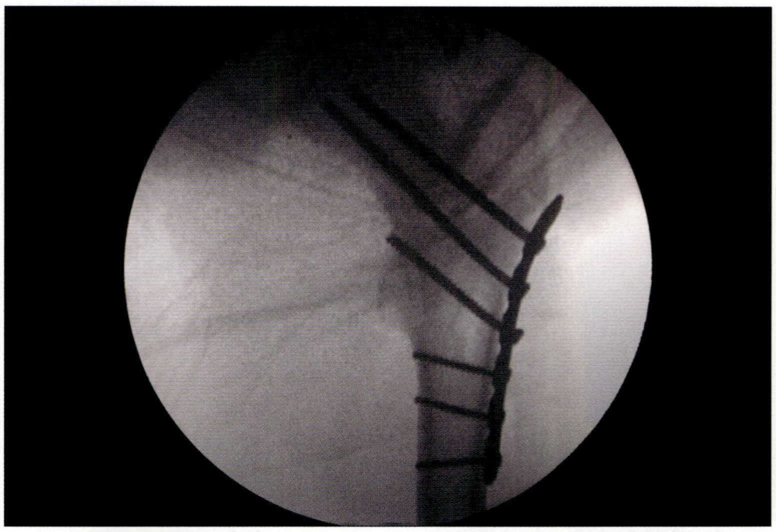
Fig. 41: Final fixation confirmed over C-arm anteroposterior (AP) view. Wash given with normal saline and povidone-iodine. Fascia is closed tightly over suction drain with absorbable suture material. Skin closure is done with nonabsorbable suture material. Drain fixed with nonabsorbable suture material. Dressing done.

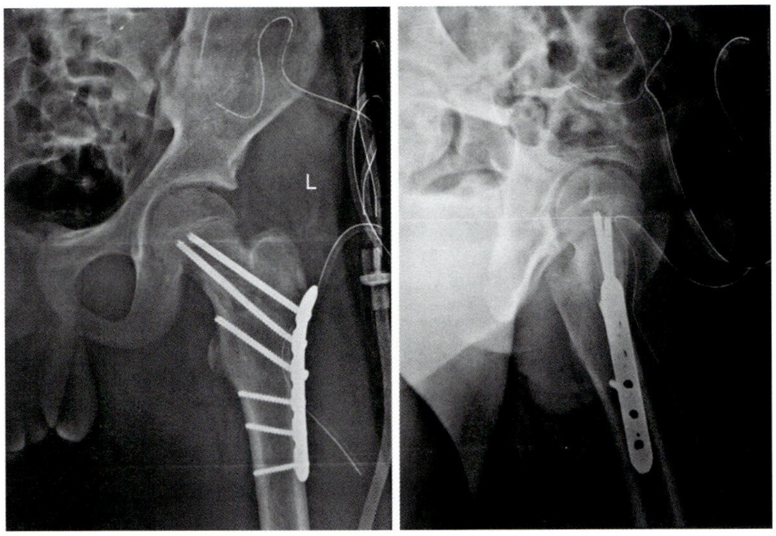

Fig. 42: Postoperative X-rays.

POSTOPERATIVE MANAGEMENT

- Active toe movements initiated from day of surgery.
- Ankle dorsiflexion and planter fixation exercises started from day 1.
- Hamstring strengthening exercises and static quadriceps exercise started from day 1.
- Non-weight-bearing mobilization with walker support started from day 2.
- Suture removal done on day 15.
- Postoperative patient is kept non-weight bearing for 3–4 weeks.
- Partial weight bearing mobilization with walker support started after 3–4 weeks.
- Full weight bearing with walker support started after 6 weeks.
- Culture and sensitivity report of fluid shows no growth.
- Gram stain report shows pus cell but no organism seen.
- Ziehl-Neelsen (ZN) stain of fluid no acid fast bacilli seen.
- Histopathology report of tissue taken from bone cyst cavity shows bone tissue with no evidence of any specific pathology.

SUGGESTED READING

1. Hou HY, Wu K, Wang CT, et al. Treatment of unicameral bone cyst a comparative study of selected techniques. J Bone Joint Surg. 2010;92A:855.
2. Pretell-Mazzini J, Murphy RF, Kushare I, et al. Unicameral bone cyst: general characteristics and management controversies. J Am Acad Orthop Surg. 2014;22:295.
3. Ramierz A, Abril JC, Touza A. Unicameral bone cyst, radiologist assessment of venous outflow by cystography as a prognostic index. J Pediatr Orthop. 2012;B21:233.
4. Sung AD, Anderson ME, Zurakowski D, et al. Unicameral bone cyst: a retrospective study of three surgical treatment. Clin Orthop Relat Res. 2008;466:2519.
5. Thawarani D, Thai CC, Welch RD, et al. Successful treatment of unicameral bone cyst by single percutaneous injection of alpha-BSM. J Pediatr Orthop. 2009;29:511.

CHAPTER 118

Aneurysmal Bone Cyst

Shrinivas S Shintre, Rajkumar Ekambaram, Chittanand Mendhe

INTRODUCTION AND CLINICAL FEATURES

- Aneurysmal bone cyst is a bone lesion-as the name suggests is eccentric in location, multiloculated and filled with blood
- Mostly presents in 2nd decade of life.
- Common site of involvement is metaphysis of long bones, posterior elements of vertebrae.

INVESTIGATIONS

- Anteroposterior (AP) and lateral radiographs showing radiolucent lesion situated mostly at metaphysis and extending outwards eccentrically with it's longitudinal diameter is more than transverse-a differentiating feature from Giant cell tumour
- Magnetic resonance imaging (MRI) is advised to know exact location and content of the lesion (with visible multiple fluid levels) with more precision.

HISTOPATHOLOGY

- Aneurysmal bone cysts are cavernous blood or serum-filled spaces devoid of a specific endothelial lining.
- It has thin strands of bone present in fibrous septa.

TREATMENT

- Curettage of the lesion and bone grafting.
- Amputation in extreme cases.
- Recently injection of sclerosant such as Polidocanol into the cyst is practised.

SURGICAL STEPS (FIGS. 1 TO 5)

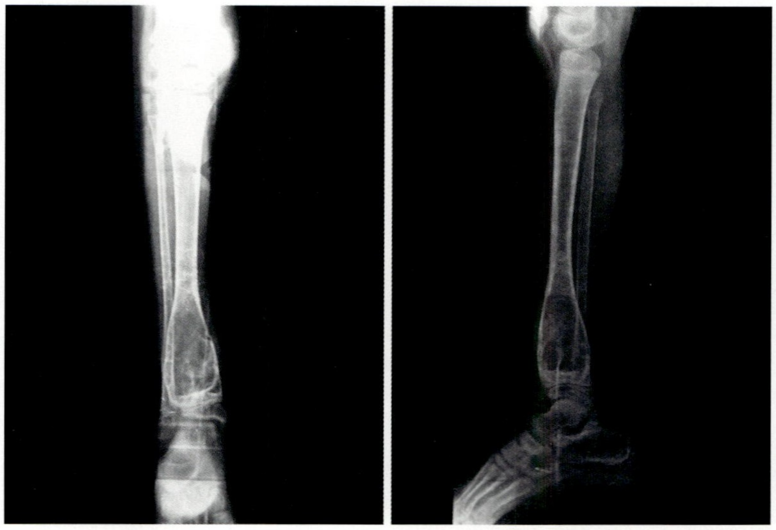

Fig. 1: Preopeartive X-ray showing lesion in right distal tibia.

- Patient is positioned supine and scrubbing done with povidone scrub.
- Painting and draping of the limb.
- Skin incision of 7–10 cm is taken over the bone where the lesion is noted.
- Then after removing the bone window, the cavity is curetted.
- After sealing with bone cement, closure of subcutaneous tissue is done by absorbable suture and skin closure done with non-absorbable suture 2-0.

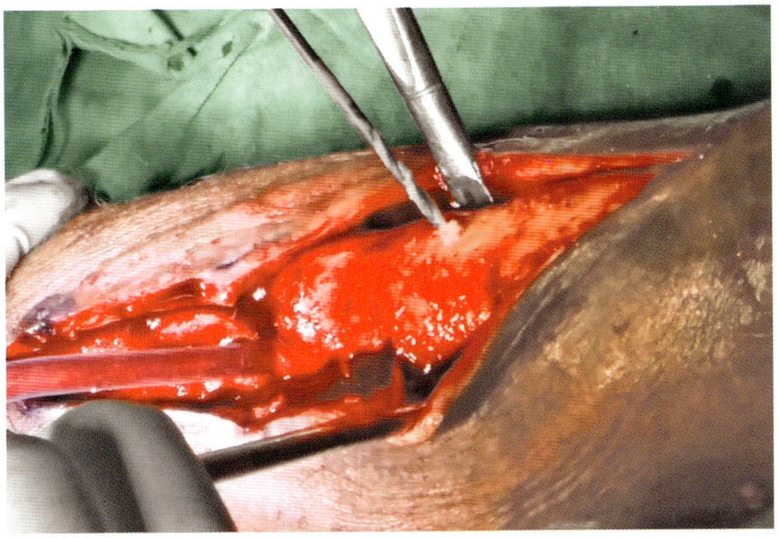

Fig. 2: Bone reached, skin is retracted using retractor and drill holes are made using 3.7 drill bit.

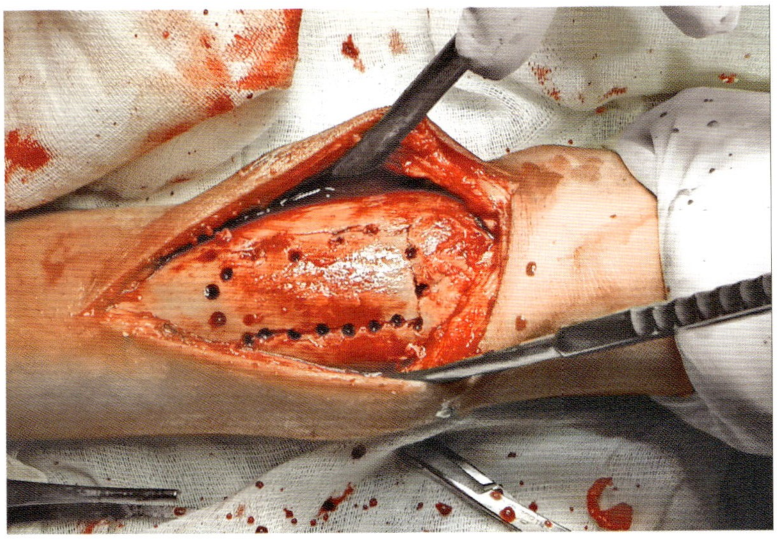

Fig. 3: The proposed bony window is marked with multiple drill holes and adjacent holes are joined to each other serially to cut the bone window using osteotome.

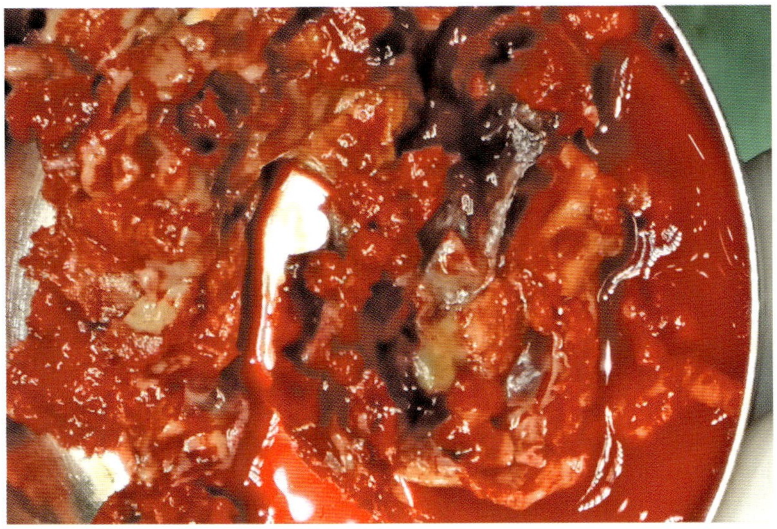

Fig. 4: The specimen obtained from curettage is sent for histopathological examination for confirmation.

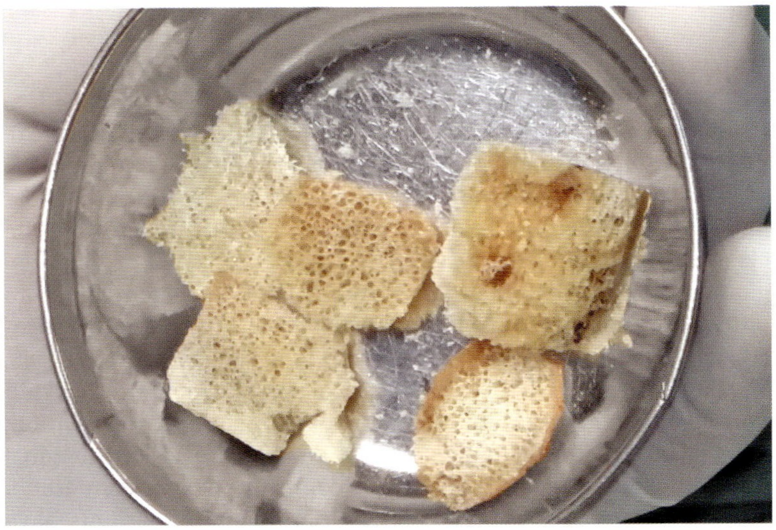

Fig. 5: Bone allograft, which is to be introduced to cover the bone defect in distal tibia.

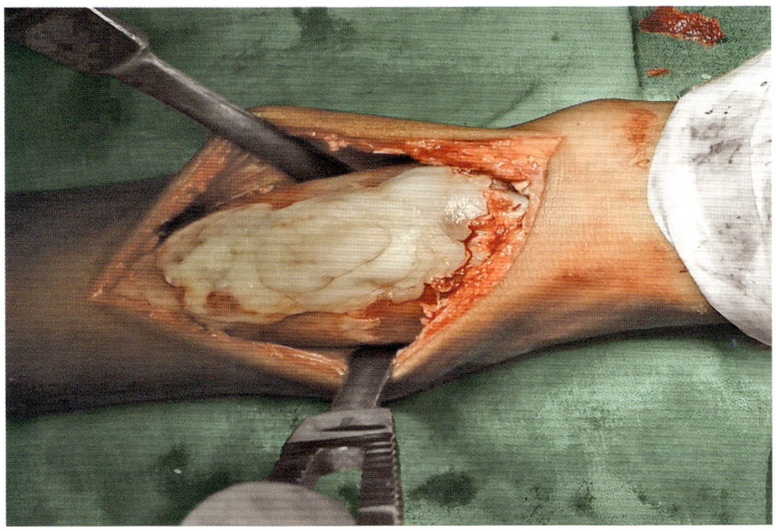

Fig. 6: Since the flap of the window is thinned out, bone defect is sealed with bone cement made of poly(methyl methacrylate) or PMMA.

COMPLICATIONS

- Pathological fractures
- Growth disturbances.

SUGGESTED READING

1. Mankin HJ, Hornicek FJ, Ortiz-Cruz E, et al. Aneurysmal bone cyst: a review of 150 patients. J Clin Oncol. 2005;23(27):6756-62.
2. Park HY, Yang SK, Sheppard WL, et al. Bernthal current management of aneurysmal bone cysts. Curr Rev Musculoskelet Med. 2016;9(4): 435-44.

CHAPTER 119

Excision of Recurrent Pigmented Villonodular Synovitis

Santosh Jeevannavar, Keshav Shenoy S, Prasanna Baindoor

INTRODUCTION

Pigmented villonodular synovitis (PVNS) is a progressive disease of the synovium. Commonly presents as either a localized (nodular) or diffuse type. Significant morbidity and joint destruction are present in advanced cases. Tenosynovial giant cell tumors (TGCTs) can be classified based on their location and growth patterns as localized giant cell tumor of the tendon sheath (TGCT, localized type) and diffuse giant cell tumor of tendon sheath (TGCT, diffuse type, or extra-articular PVNS) with those involving the joint space known as PVNS.

Like most benign lesions with clinical symptoms interfering with normal function, treatment of choice would be surgical intervention. Surgical intervention usually involves wide surgical excision/marginal excision, which may be done arthroscopically or by open method. The recurrence rate for PVNS is high and usually patients have undergone multiple procedures. Wide surgical excision combined with radiotherapy has given encouraging results, especially in recurrence.

CLINICAL PRESENTATION AND SYMPTOMS

Common age of presentation is between the ages of 30 and 50 with a higher incidence in females. The knee is the most common affected joint 75%. Recurrent episodes of pain, swelling, and stiffness associated with hemarthrosis are the common clinical presentation. The clinical course is insidious with recurrent episodes of joint swelling and discomfort, which may be confused with meniscal pathology.

INVESTIGATIONS

Plain radiographs in the initial stage are essentially normal apart from soft tissue swelling. In late stages of PVNS, secondary features of advanced stage disease like joint space narrowing, osteophytes, and erosion are seen. So, plain radiographs are not useful as a diagnostic tool.

Magnetic resonance imaging (MRI) is considered to be the gold standard in imaging PVNS. MRI findings in different sequences have been well described. The synovial proliferation pattern and hemosiderin deposits are characteristic of PVNS.

TREATMENT OPTIONS

Surgical resection through complete synovectomy is the mainstay of the treatment. Arthroscopic resection is adequate for localized or nodular form of PVNS; however in advanced cases or those with diffuse form of PVNS, open surgical synovectomy is the gold standard. Joint replacement surgery is also indicated if during open synovectomy joint erosion or cartilage destruction is severe. The recurrence rates after surgical intervention range from 20% to 30% and vary depending upon the management strategy. Adjuvant treatment modalities have been developed to decrease the recurrence rates, and also for resistant cases. Adjunct modalities include intra-articular radioisotopes and external beam radiotherapy.

SURGICAL PROCEDURES

Here, we are describing open surgical resection and synovectomy combined with postoperative external beam radiotherapy for recurrent PVNS.

CASE HISTORY

A 32-year-old man presented with recurrent episodes of pain and swelling of left knee for which he had undergone two previous surgical procedures: (1) arthroscopic procedure and (2) open synovectomy.

Knee pain, effusion, and limitation of knee movements are still persisting even after the second procedure. Fresh investigations revealed extensive PVNS involving the left knee joint.

Step 1 (Fig. 1)

Preoperative clinical photograph demonstrating:

1. Previous operative scar
2. Knee effusion.

Step 2 (Fig. 2)

Preoperative X-rays demonstrating knee effusion with maintained articular surfaces.

Step 3 (Fig. 3)

Preoperative MRI. Sagittal cuts showing extensive synovial thickening and hypertrophy in posterior medial and lateral compartment suggestive of recurrent PVNS. Periarticular erosions are also seen.

Step 4 (Fig. 4)

Preoperative MRI. Coronal cuts showing extensive synovial hypertrophy.

Step 5 (Fig. 5)

Preoperative MRI coronal cuts showing extensive synovial hypertrophy including patellofemoral joint.

Step 6 (Fig. 6)

Preoperative MRI axial cuts showing diffuse synovial hypertrophy involving the whole of the knee joint including posterior compartment.

Step 7 (Fig. 7)

Arthroscopy images confirming PVNS just before open synovectomy.

Step 8 (Fig. 8)

- Supine position with knee flexed, sterile tourniquet inflated.
- Standard anterior approach to knee
- Incision deepened and medial parapatellar arthrotomy done
- Figure 8 demonstrates the superior part of arthrotomy with synovial hypertrophy.

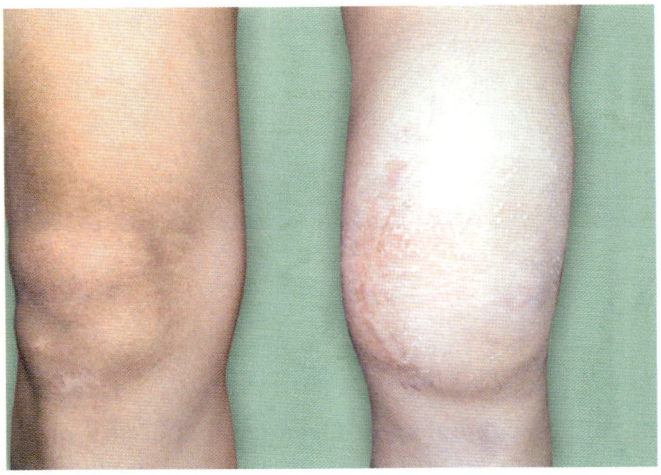

Fig. 1

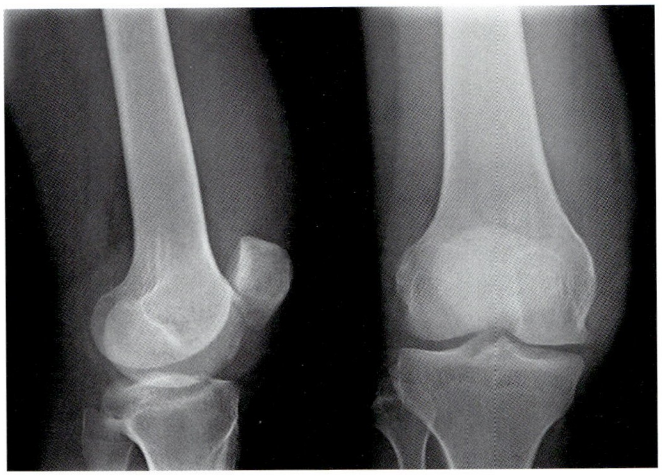

Fig. 2

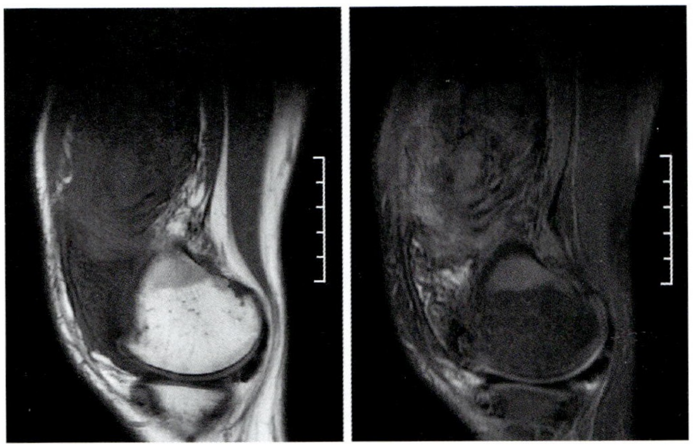

Fig. 3

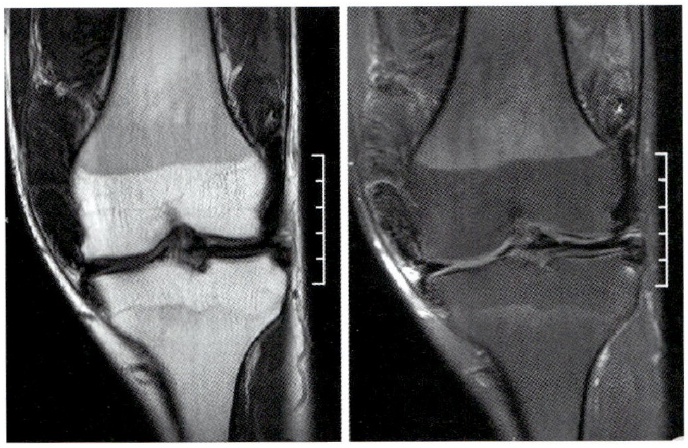

Fig. 4

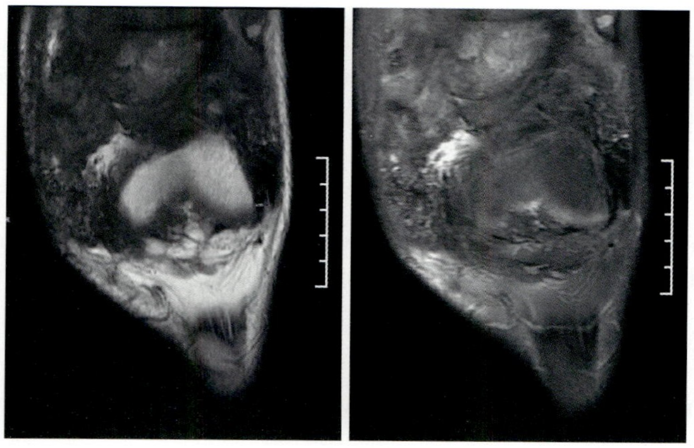

Fig. 5

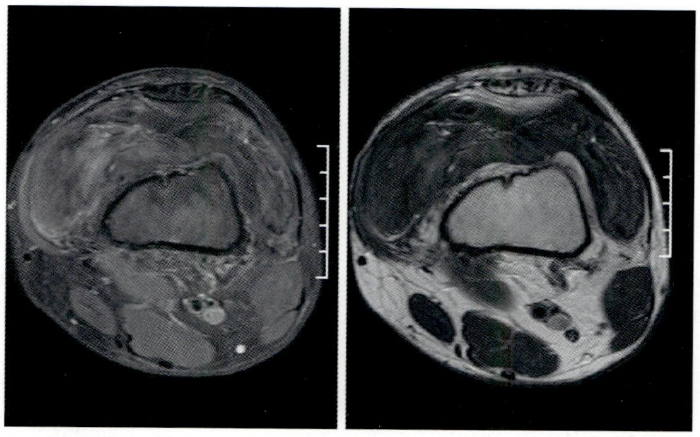

Fig. 6

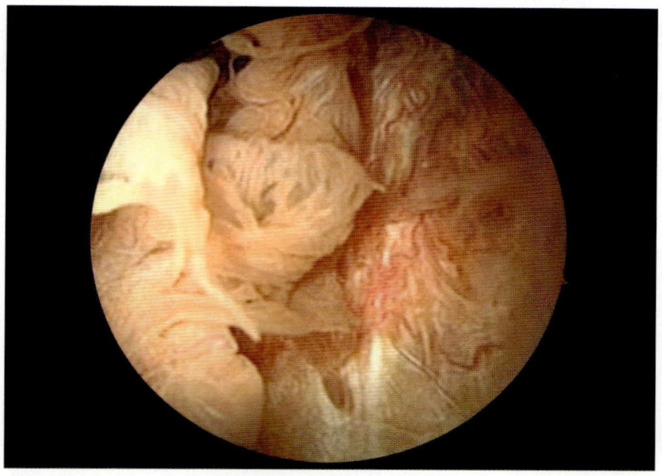

Fig. 7

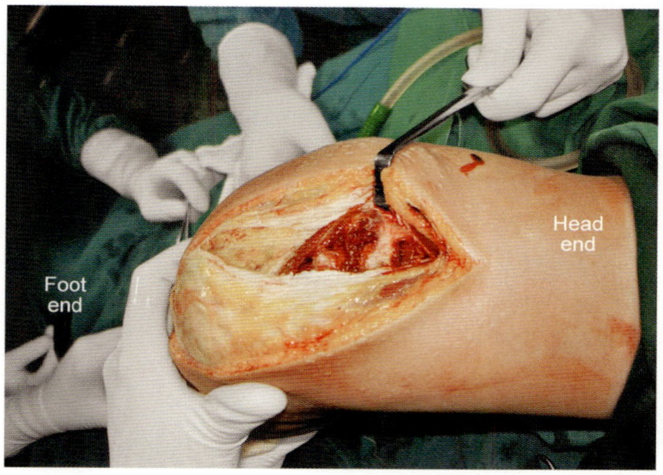

Fig. 8

Step 9 (Fig. 9)

Arthrotomy extended distally ending just medial to tibial tuberosity. Patellar retinaculum held and retracted laterally with alleys forceps and retractors on the medial side as the joint is further exposed. The typical synovial appearance of PVNS can be seen in the superior and inferior part of the wound.

Step 10 (Fig. 10)

Patella everted laterally as the knee is gently flexed to complete the arthrotomy. The diffuse involvement is seen in suprapatellar, parapatellar, and infrapatellar region. In recurrent cases and those patients with diffuse involvement, it is essential to get a wide exposure to see the extent of involvement.

Step 11 (Fig. 11)

Knee arthrotomy completed and the knee completely exposed with patellar everted. Joint retractors held by the assistant will expose the different joint areas so as to assess the extent of involvement. The complete exposure as in this case will help in assessing the cartilage status and also the joint destruction. In advanced cases of joint destruction and cartilage erosion, accessory procedures along with synovectomy and excision can be planned.

Step 12 (Fig. 12)

Suprapatellar synovium is excised completely till bone. The hypertrophied synovium is held with sponge-holding forceps and gently separated as a single layer starting from one corner of the joint and finishing at the other corner. Note the minimal degeneration seen at the trochlear groove.

Step 13 (Fig. 13)

The visible suprapatellar, intercondylar, and parapatellar synovium has been excised. The knee is gently brought forward by giving an anterior thrust and flexing the knee. This brings the posterior structure into greater visibility and helps in removing most of the posterior synovium. Frequent change of retractors by the assistant will aid in reaching posterior most structures.

Step 14 (Fig. 14)

Synovial excision is complete and we can see almost all the compartments of the knee cleared of disease tissue. The cartilage is clearly seen and shows minimal degeneration. The meniscus and the ligaments are also cleared of diseased tissue. Tissue samples for histopathological studies are obtained from three compartments and sent.

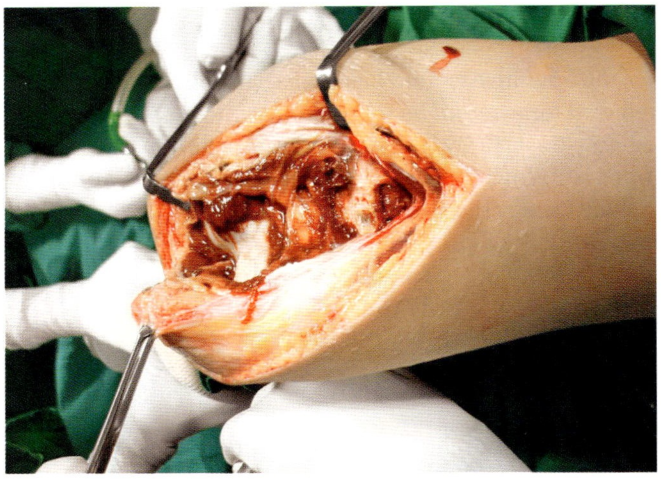

Fig. 9

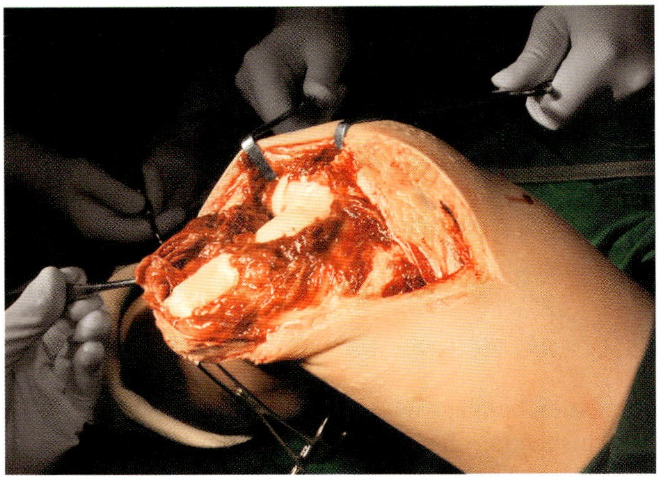

Fig. 10

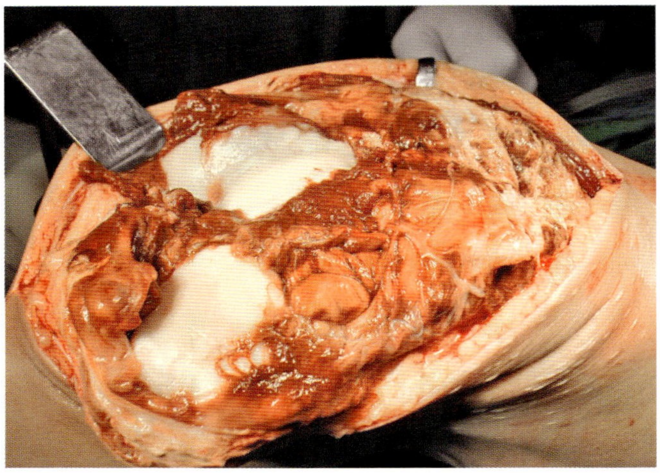

Fig. 11

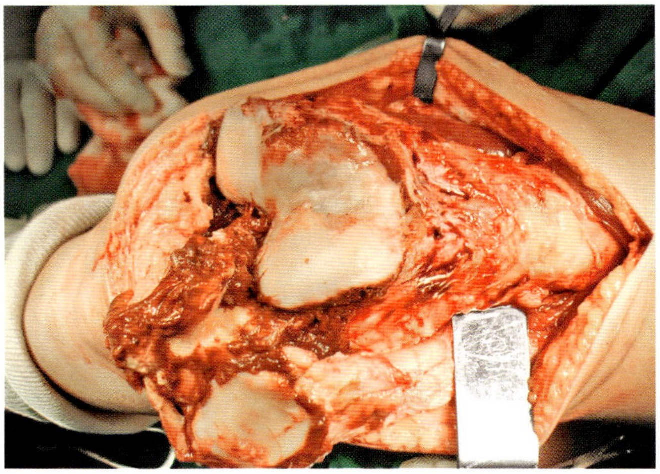

Fig. 12

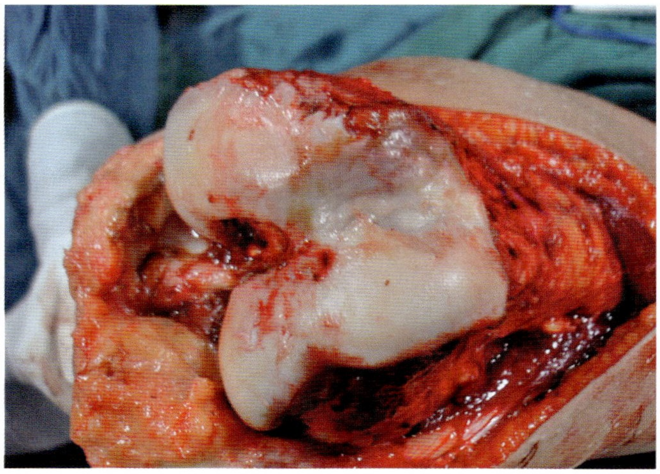

Fig. 13

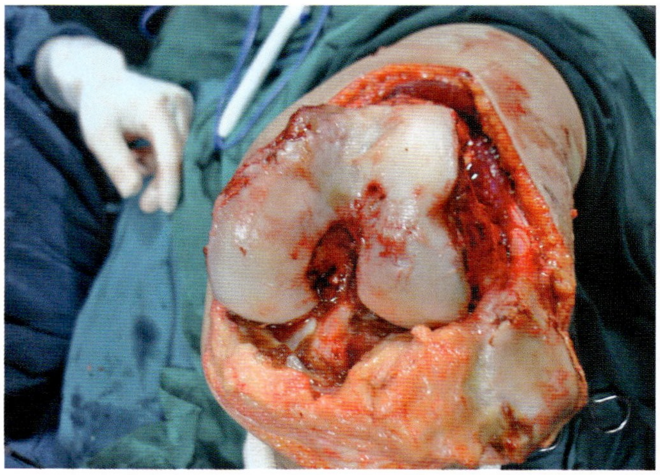

Fig. 14

Step 15 (Fig. 15)

The excised synovium with the diseased tissue can be seen here removed in one layer.

Step 16 (Fig. 16)

The wound closure is done in layers over suction drains after tourniquet release.

POSTOPERATIVE PROTOCOL

- Compression bandage with long leg knee brace
- Wound inspection after 48 hours and drain removal
- Nonweight-bearing mobilization and knee movements started as per patient comfort
- Suture removal at 14 days and full weight-bearing mobilization.

RADIOTHERAPY AUGMENTATION

- Once the operative wound has healed (usually at 3 months) patient is referred for *external beam radiotherapy*
- Moderate dose 30 Gy is used as per the radiotherapist protocol
- Patient is followed up at 3, 6, 9, and 12 months and examined clinically for any recurrence
- Repeat MRI done at 1 year.

Repeat MRI at 1 year showing no recurrence and complete remission of PVNS (Figs. 17 to 20).

SURGICAL TIPS AND TRICKS

- Thorough and complete preclinical workup is essential
- MRI is a must to map the disease and plan the surgery in detail and also rules out other pathology
- MRI will also assess the cartilage status

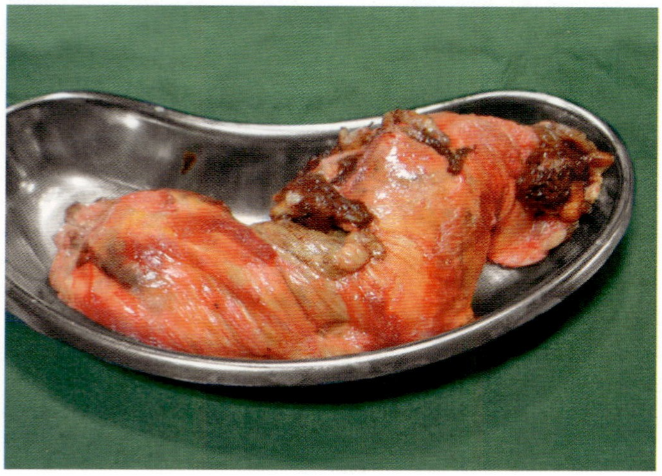

Fig. 15

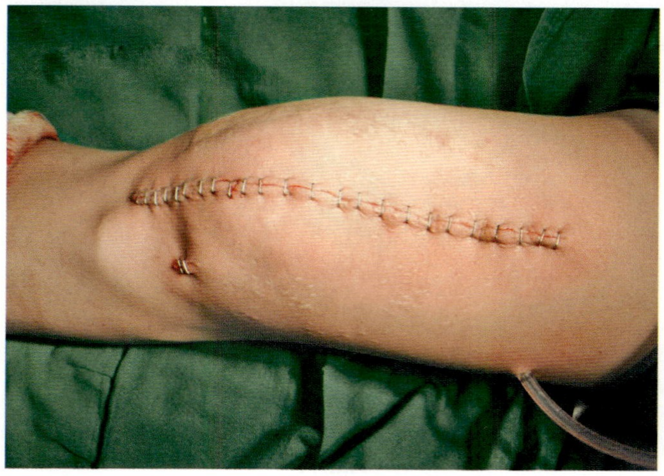

Fig. 16

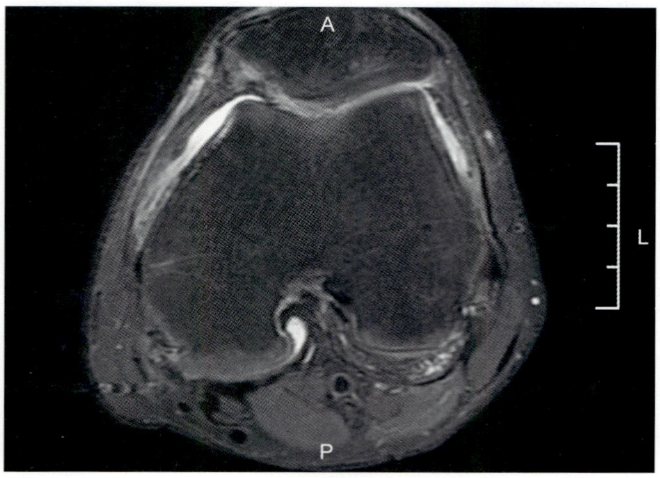

Fig. 17

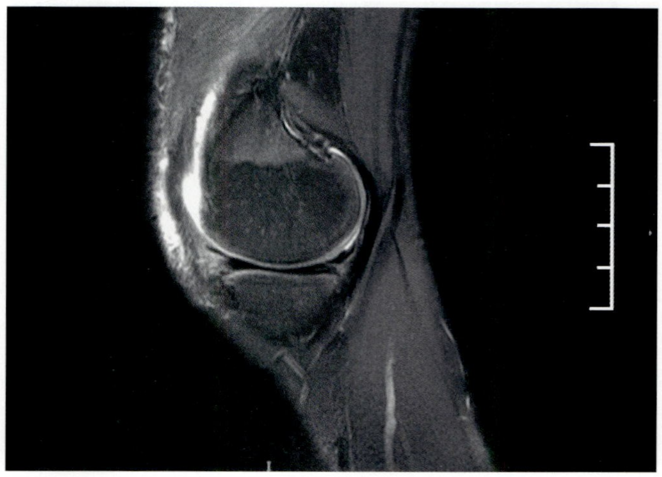

Fig. 18

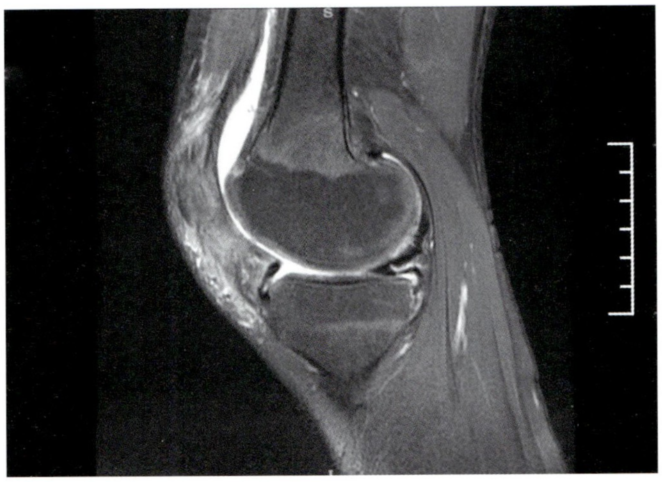

Fig. 19

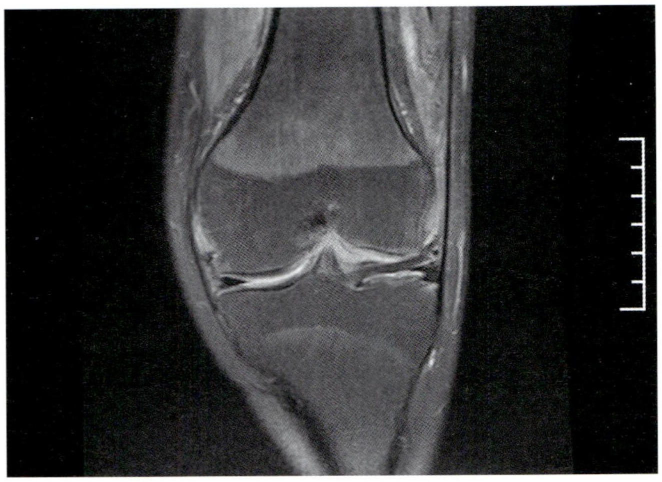

Fig. 20

- Arthroscopy is a good diagnostic tool and also can be used to excise localized form of PVNS
- Complete joint exposure with generous arthrotomy helps to assess the disease involvement and also in surgical excision
- Adjuvant radiotherapy is essential to decrease the recurrence rate.

SUGGESTED READING

1. Biermann JS. Orthopaedic Knowledge Update: Musculoskeletal Tumors 3. USA: American Academy of Orthopaedic Surgeons; 2014. pp. 282-5.
2. Cannada LK. Orthopaedic Knowledge Update 11. USA: American Academy of Orthopaedic Surgeons. 2014.
3. Horoschak M, Tran PT, Bachireddy P, et al. External beam radiation therapy enhances local control in pigmented villonodular synovitis. Int J Radiat Oncol Biol Phys. 2009;75(1):183-7.
4. Jaffe HL, Lichtenstein L, Sutro CJ. Pigmented villonodular synovitis, bursitis and tenosynovitis. Arch Pathol. 1941;21:731-65.
5. Mankin H, Trahan C, Hornicek F. Pigmented villonodular synovitis of joints. Surg Oneal. 2011;103(5):386-9.
6. Ottaviani S, Ayral X, Dougados M, et al. Pigmented villonodular synovitis: A retrospective single-center study of 122 cases and review of the literature. Semin Arthritis Rheum. 2011;40(6):539-46.
7. Park G, Kim YS, Kim IH, et al. Low-dose external beam radiotherapy as a postoperative treatment for patients with diffuse pigmented villonodular synovitis of the knee: 4 recurrences in 23 patients followed for mean 9 years. Acta Orthop. 2012;83(3):256-60.
8. Ravi V, Wang WL, Lewis YO. Treatment of tenosynovial giant cell tumor and pigmented villonodular synovitis. Curr Opin Oncol. 2011;23(4): 361-6.
9. Zook IE, Wurtz DL, Cummings IE, et al. Intra-articular chromic phosphate (32p) in the treatment of diffuse pigmented villonodular synovitis. Brachytherapy. 2011;10(3):190-4.

SECTION 10

PLASTIC SURGERY

Section Editor: *Pushkar Deshpande*

CHAPTER 120

Split Thickness Skin Graft

Parag Sahasrabudhe, Vijay M Panchanadikar, Snehal Dantkale, Anurag Daxini

INTRODUCTION

Skin grafting is most commonly performed procedure in plastic surgery. Depending upon the thickness of the skin harvested, skin grafting can be split-thickness skin grafting (Thiersch), or full thickness skin grafting (Wolff). In India, skin grafting rotation flap was performed around 600 BC for reconstruction of nose. In more recent times, Ollier used the split thickness grafting technique in 1872 and Thiersch later perfected it. Today, split-thickness graft is popularly known as Thiersch graft.

INDICATIONS

Skin loss due to any cause, e.g. trauma, surgery, burns, etc. having a healthy vascular bed.

- *Donor site*: Common sites include upper anterior and lateral thigh, upper inner arm, buttocks, thenar eminence (for finger grafts small areas).
- *Contraindications*: The harvested skin should not be directly placed over area where there is no vascular bed, e.g. directly over tendon or bone.

ADVANTAGES

- Large raw area can be covered
- Less donor site morbidity
- As the thickness is less, there is more chance of graft survival.

DISADVANTAGES

- Less resistance to trauma
- Poor cosmetic appearance, poor texture, and match
- Greater chance of graft contraction.

PROCEDURE

Though Humby knife use is ideal and common nowadays, in its absence, small graft can be harvested by meticulous use of 15 number blade. It is important to have thinner graft, which has better chances of survival. The graft size can be increased by dermatome, or by perforations with a knife. Saline storage after harvesting is important to prevent devitalization. While applying harvested skin, it should be spread evenly across the wound and sutured at the edges. At the conclusion of procedure, compression dressing is to be applied while taking care to cover the pits well with gauze to ensure uniform pressure. While changing dressing of the wound, the gauze is to be soaked well in normal saline and dressing is carefully peeled off (like a banana). This prevents accidental loss of graft. Nonsticky dressing is an option though not compulsory. Dressing is not to be disturbed for initial 5 days, though superficial layers may be changed. Excess graft can be saline stored in refrigerator and utilized later on for about 4 weeks though the exact duration of viability is unknown. (on same patient).

SURGICAL STEPS (FIGS. 1 TO 15)

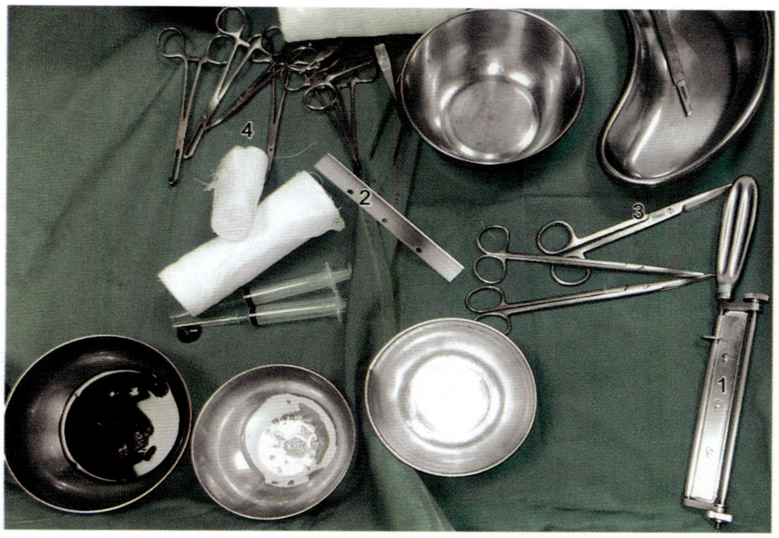

Fig. 1: Instrument trolley: (1) Humby knife, (2) Knife blade, (3) Scissors, (4) General instruments. Two sterile wooden boards are required to stretch the skin.

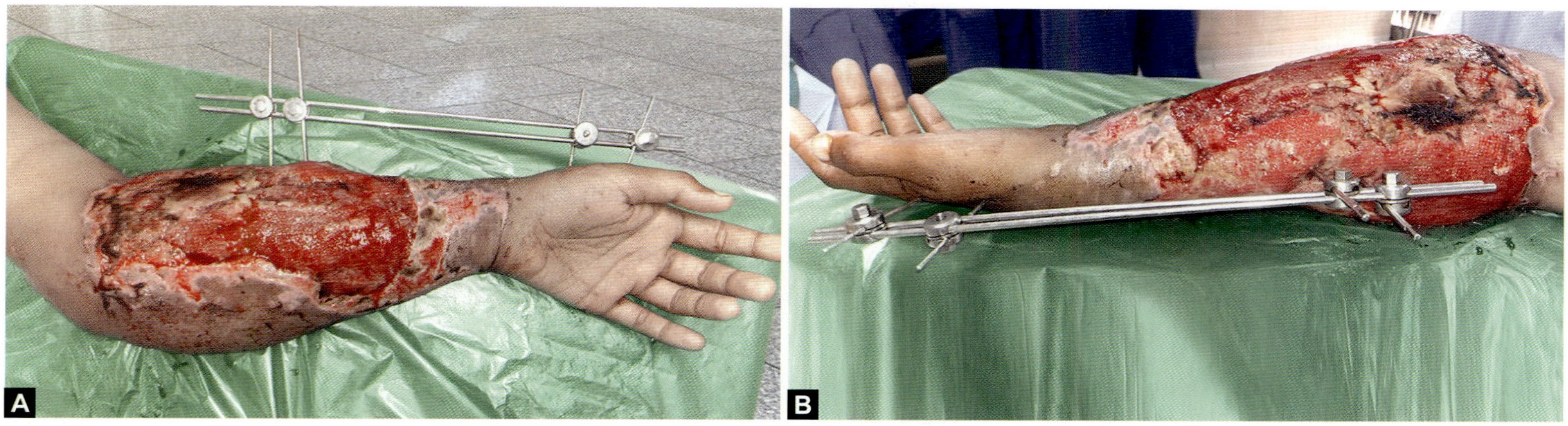

Figs. 2A and B: Raw area over forearm.

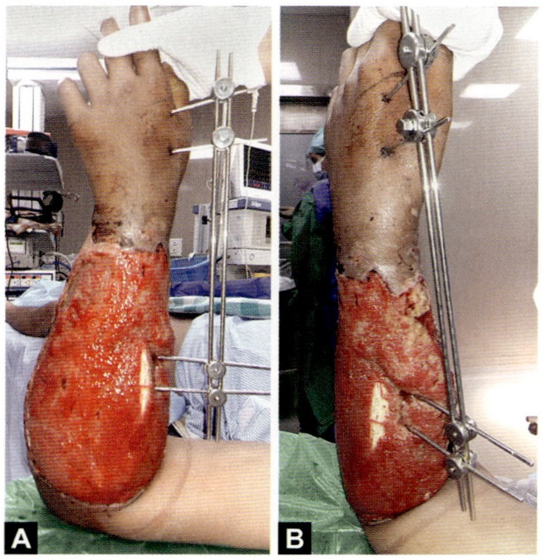

Figs. 3A and B: Raw area after wound debridement.

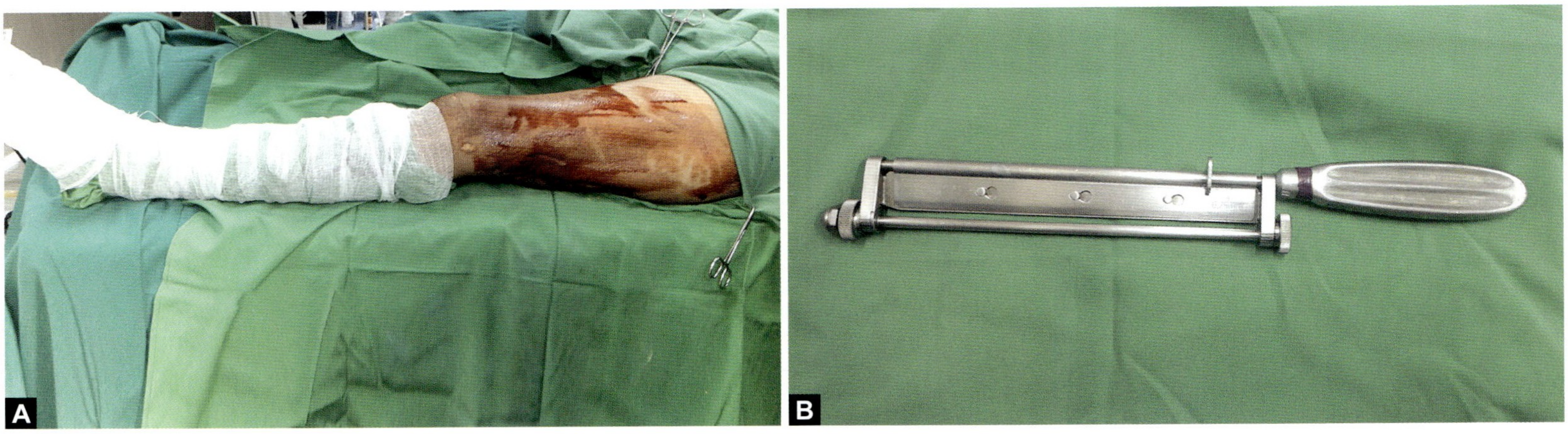

Figs. 4A and B: (A) Donor site is prepared; (B) Humby knife is adjusted to the medium thickness in most cases.

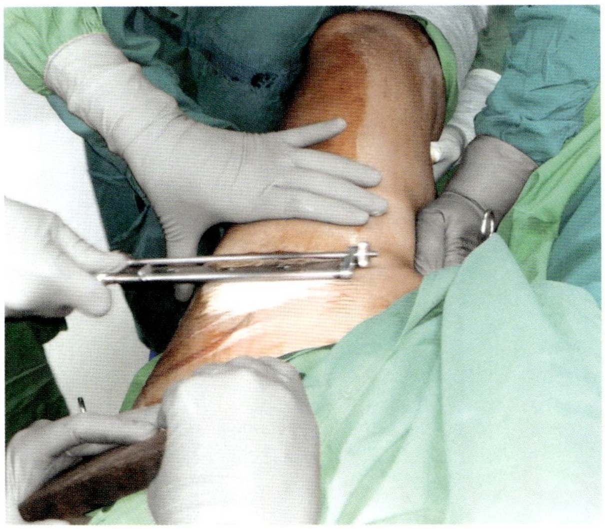

Fig. 5: Harvesting skin from donor site is done from anterior thigh.
- Liquid paraffin is applied for lubrication. Skin is stretched by hand or preferably by two wooden boards.
- Skin graft is harvested by slowly progressive to and fro movement of the knife.

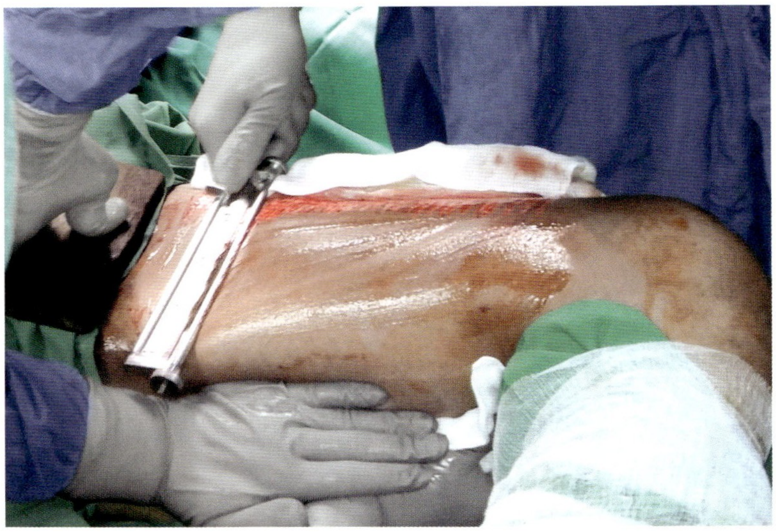

Fig. 6: Additional graft is harvested from medial side of thigh.

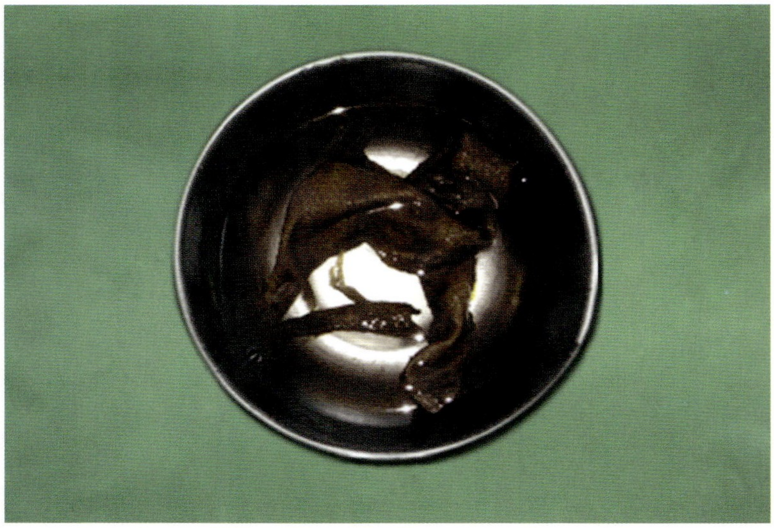

Fig. 7: Graft harvested and stored in saline.

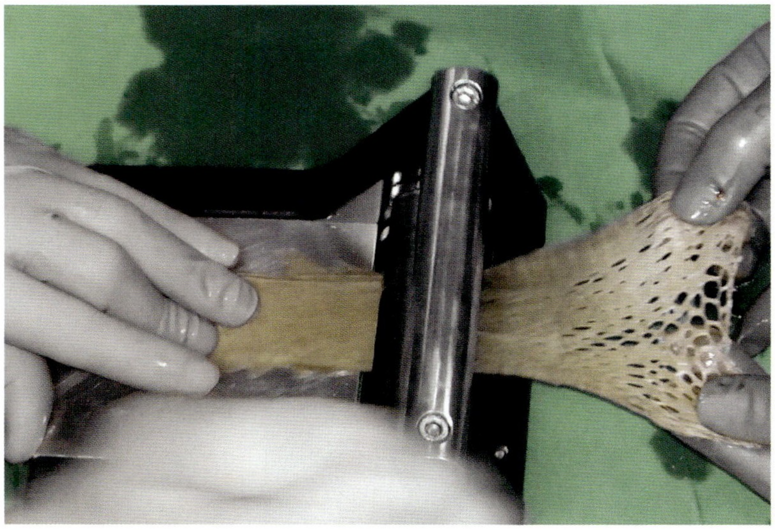

Fig. 8: Skin meshing is done using dermatome. Alternatively it can also be done by 15 number blade after placing the graft on wooden board.

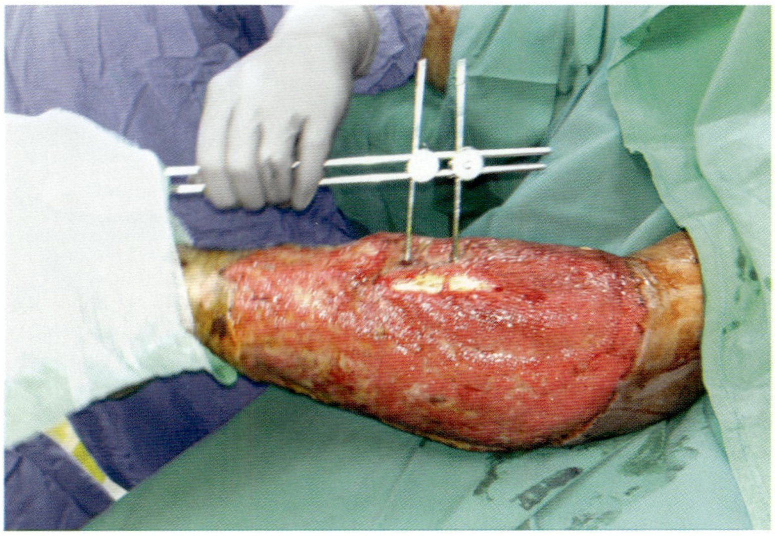

Fig. 9: Area to be grafted is cleaned with normal saline.

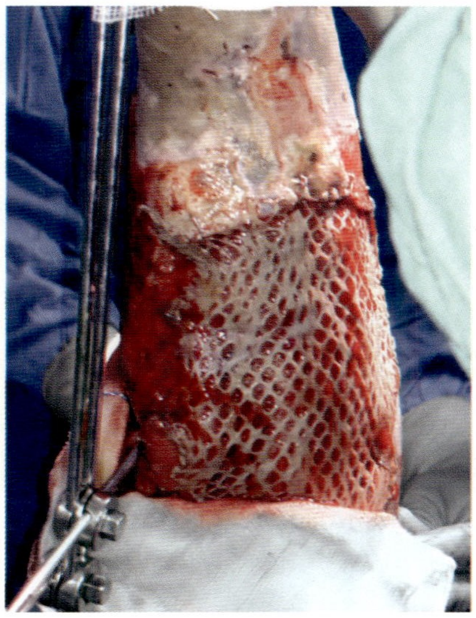

Fig. 10: Harvested graft is spread evenly over the prepared area.

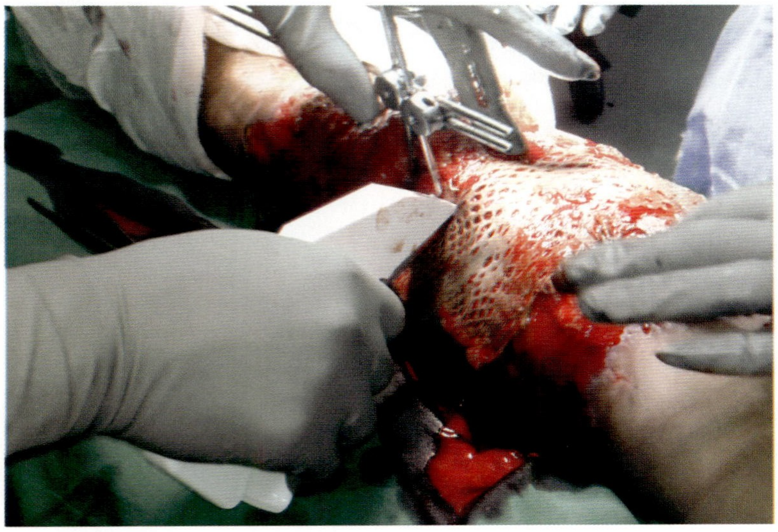

Fig. 11: Graft is sutured to the raw area at edges using stapler.

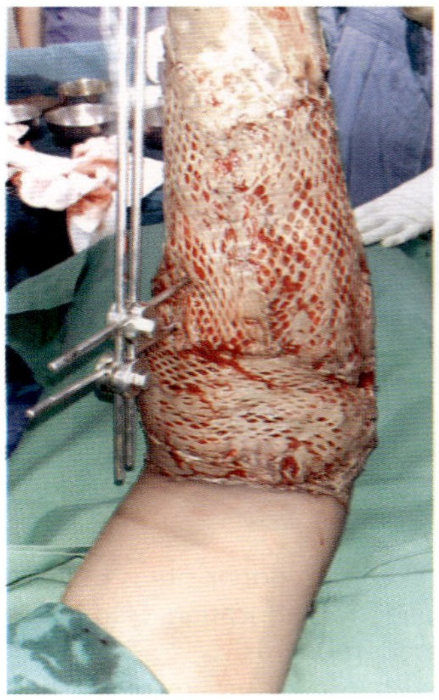

Fig. 12: Completed skin grafting.

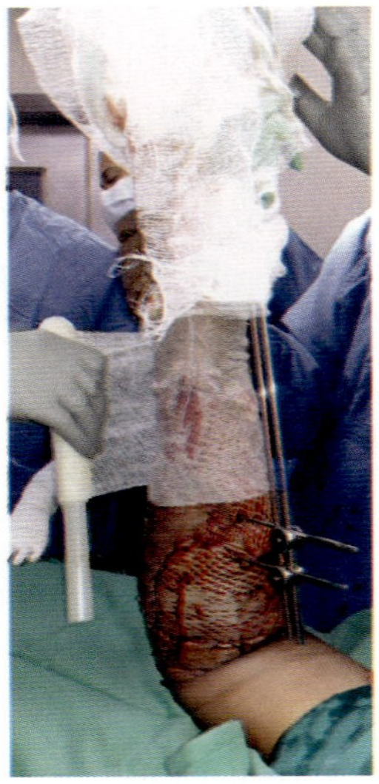

Fig. 13: Dressing of the grafted area using nonsticky dressing.

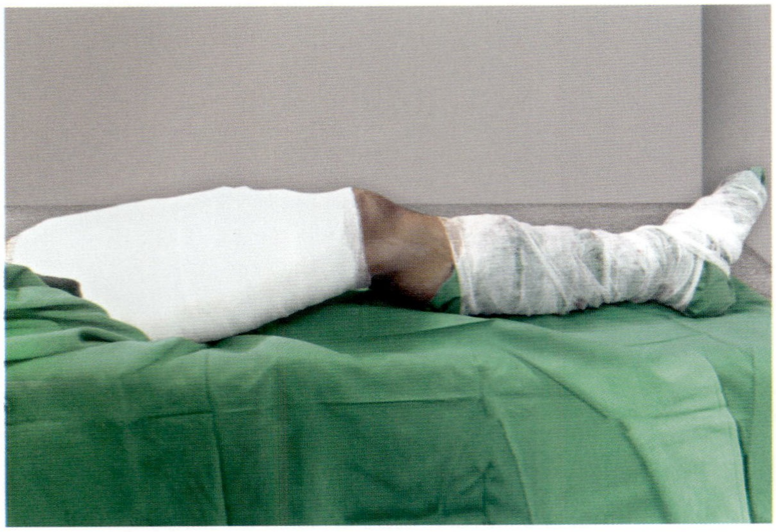

Fig. 14: Final dressing of donor area.

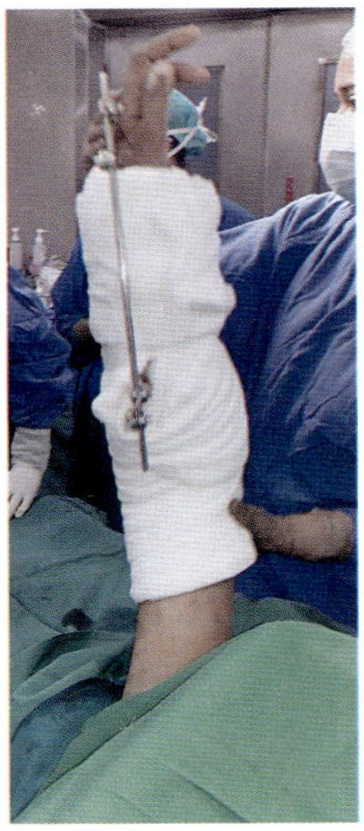

Fig. 15: Final dressing of grafted area.

COMPLICATION

Infection leading to loss of skin graft.

SUGGESTED READING

1. Ratner D. Skin grafting: from here to there. Dermatol Clin. 1998;16(1): 75-90.
2. Shimizu R, Kishi K. Skin graft. Plast Surg Int. 2012;2012:563493.
3. White N, Hettiaratchy S, Papini RP. The choice of split-thickness skin graft donor site: patients' and surgeons' preferences. Plast Reconstr Surg. 2003;112(3):933-4.

CHAPTER 121

Cross-finger Flap

Pushkar Deshpande

INTRODUCTION

Finger tip amputation carries significant importance among all severe hand injuries. The main aim of the treatment of these injuries is to restore the sensation and painless finger function. Cross finger flap (CFF) is versatile tool for these kind of injuries. Cronin described cross finger flap in 1951. It is a two stage reconstruction procedure. The donor site is dorsal surface of middle phalynx of the adjacent finger. The flap is raised in rectangular shape with base intact, after planning in reverse done.

INDICATIONS

Cross finger flap is generally indicated for covering volar soft tissue defects over middle and distal phalynx. It can be used primarily to replace an avulsed finger pad. It can be used secondarily to release a scar due to burn injury on volar aspect of middle and distal phalynx.

SURGICAL STEPS (FIGS. 1 TO 13)

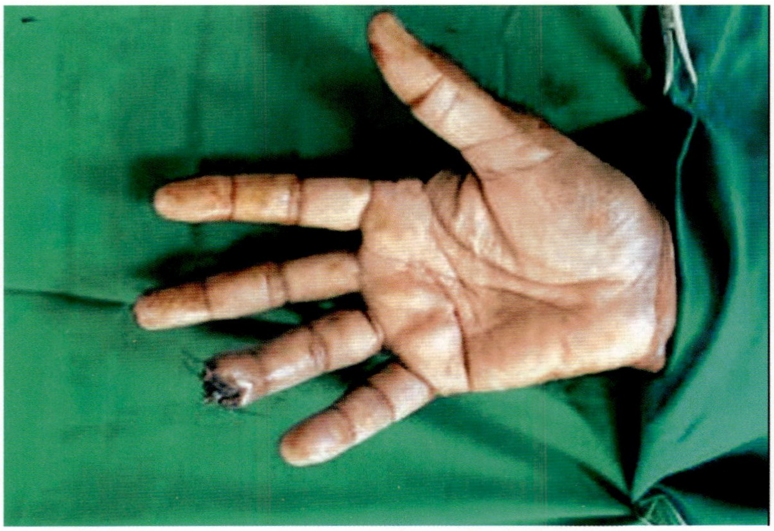

Fig. 1: Distal tip necrosis of right ring finger [anteroposterior (AP) view] post primary suturing 8 days before.

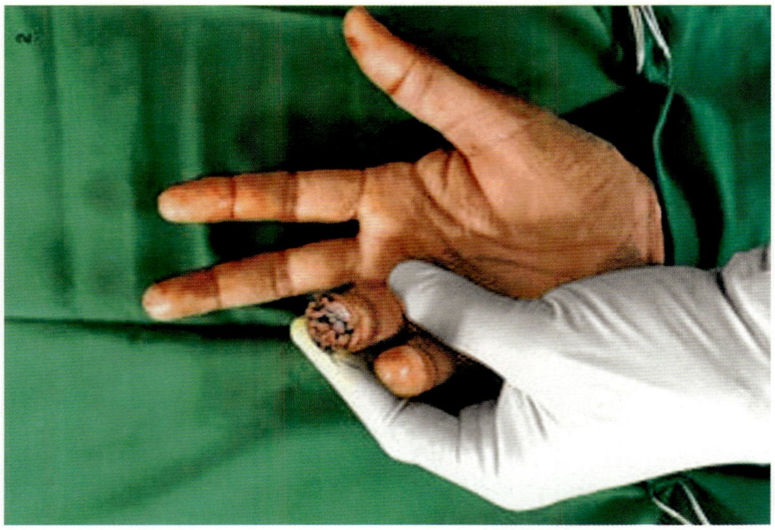

Fig. 2: Bird's eye view.

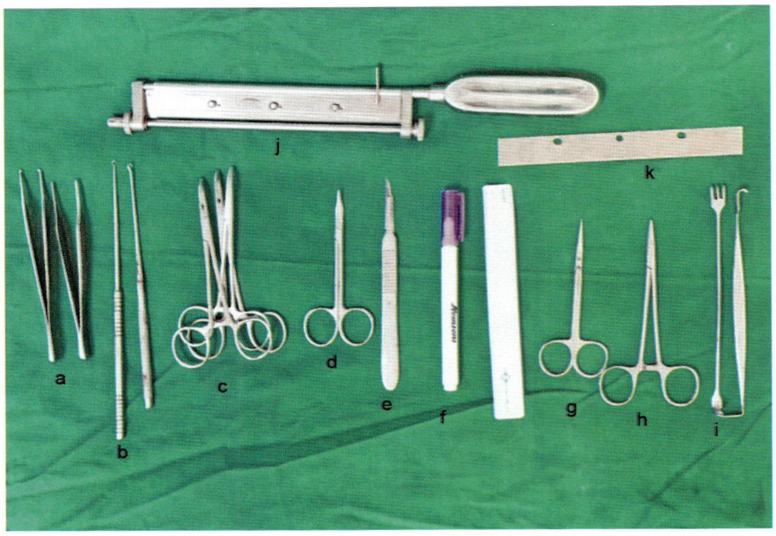

Figs. 3A to K: Instrumentation. (A) Pair of Adson's forceps, (B) Skin hooks, (C) Artery forceps, (D) Scissors, (E) BP handle with 15 number blade, (F) Marker pen with measuring scale, (G) Suture cutting scissors, (H) Needle holder, (I) Cat's paw retractor, (J) Humby's skin graft knife, (K) Skin graft blade.

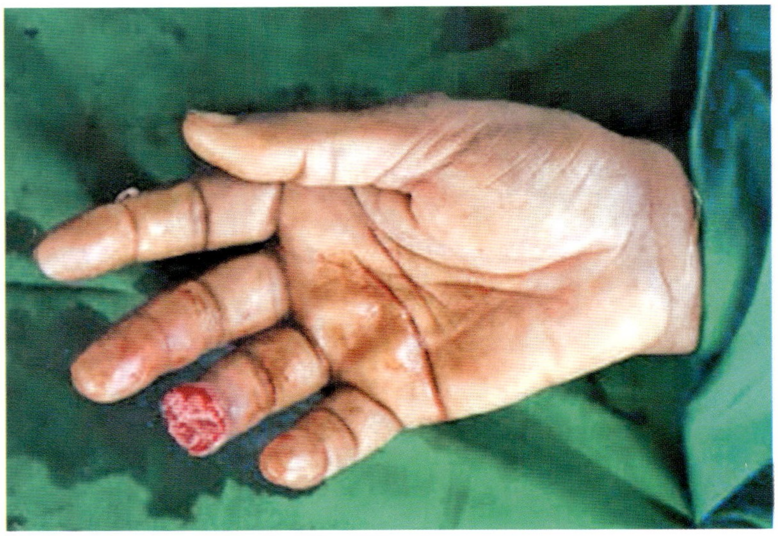

Fig. 4: Postdebridement defect of fingertip.

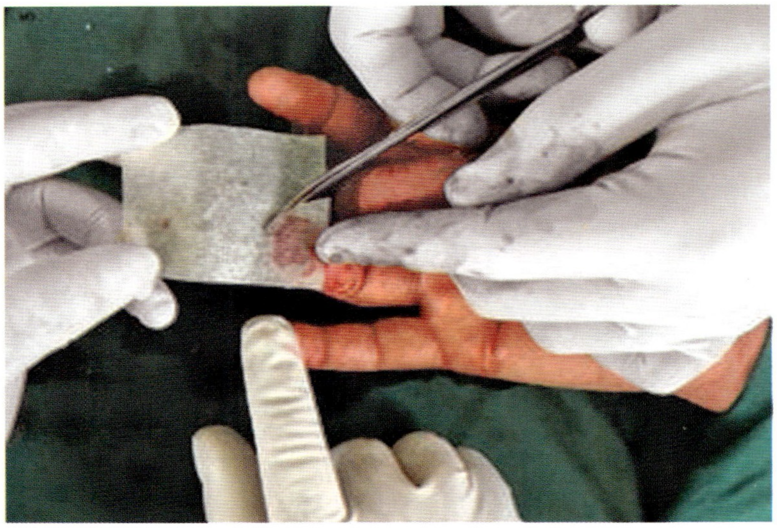

Fig. 5: Blood print taken.

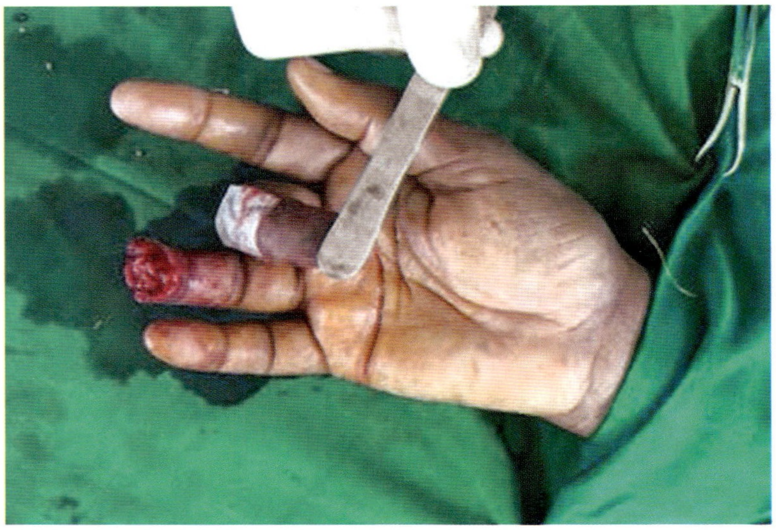

Fig. 6: Planning in reverse is done after transferring blood print to donor site.

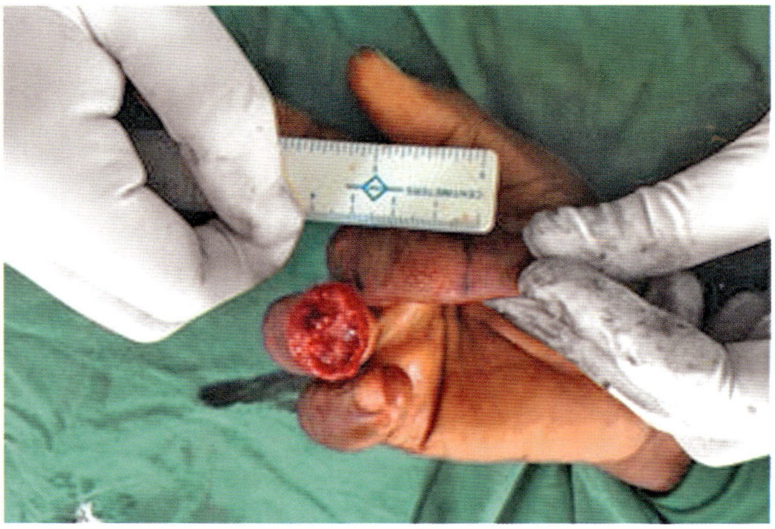

Fig. 7: Flap marked on the middle phalanx of dorsal aspect of middle finger.

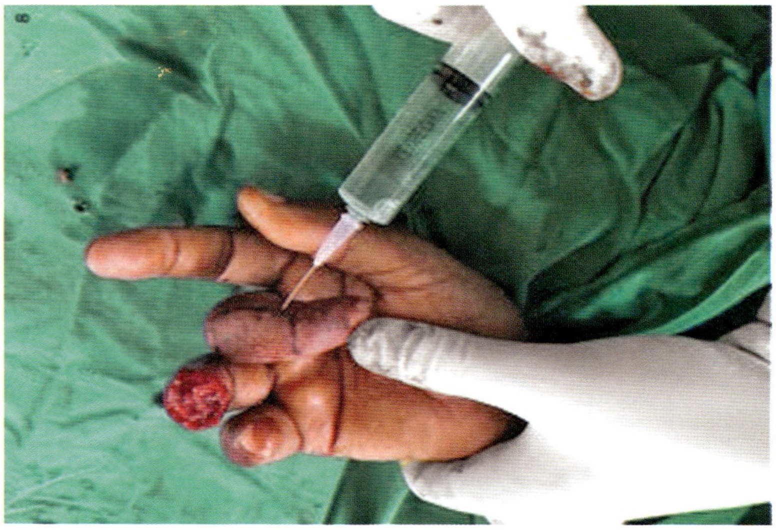

Fig. 8: Hydrodissection done with 2% diluted xylocaine.

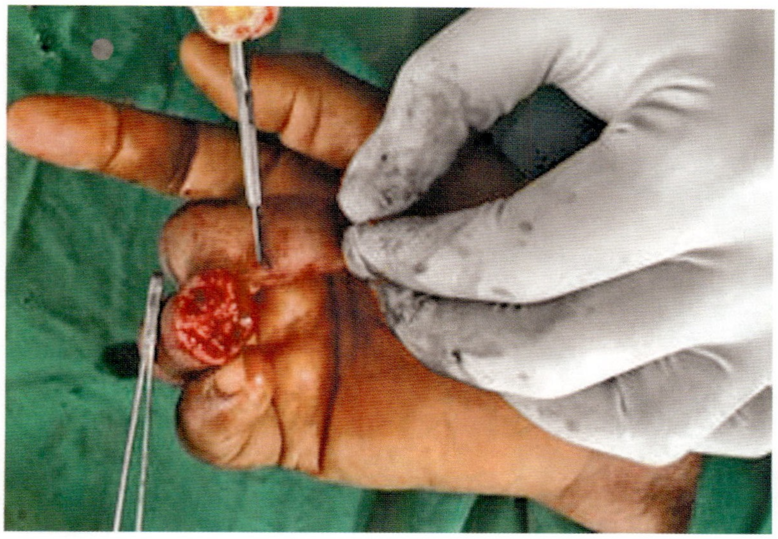
Fig. 9: Flap incision taken.

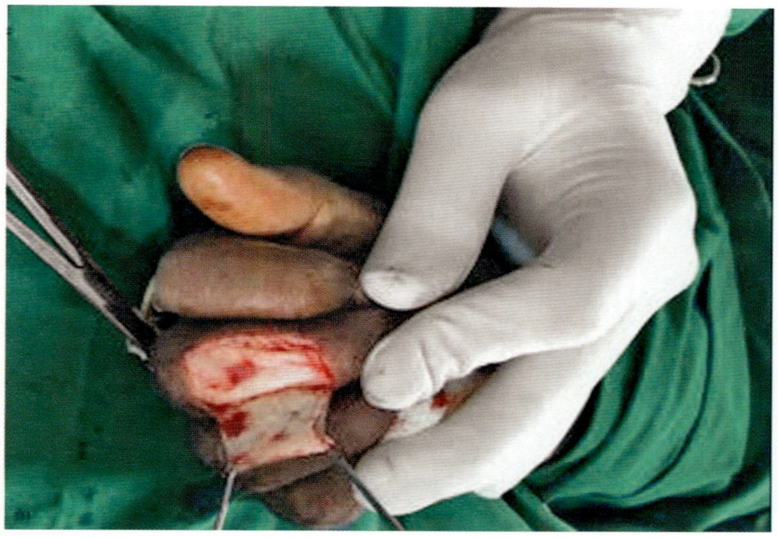
Fig. 10: Flap elevation with intact peritenon.

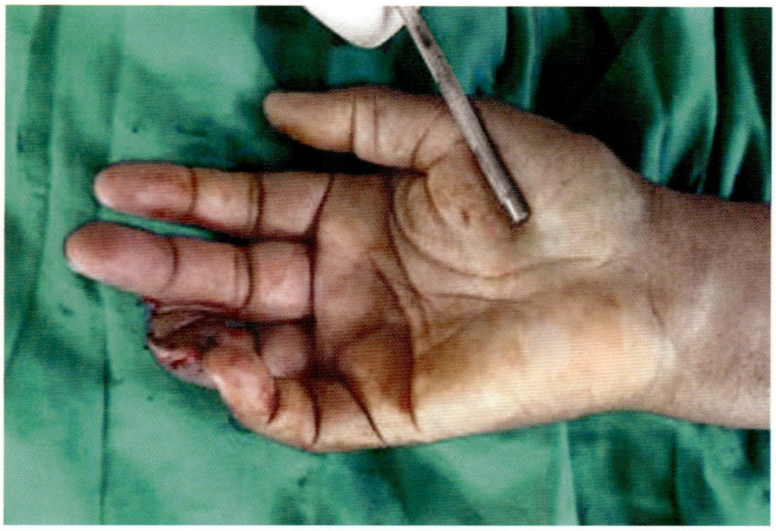
Fig. 11: Flap inset given.

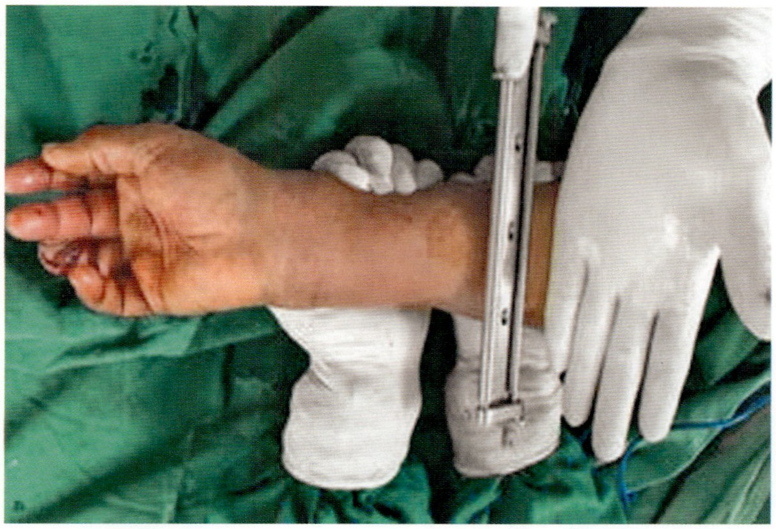
Fig. 12: Split skin graft (SSG) harvested from right forearm.

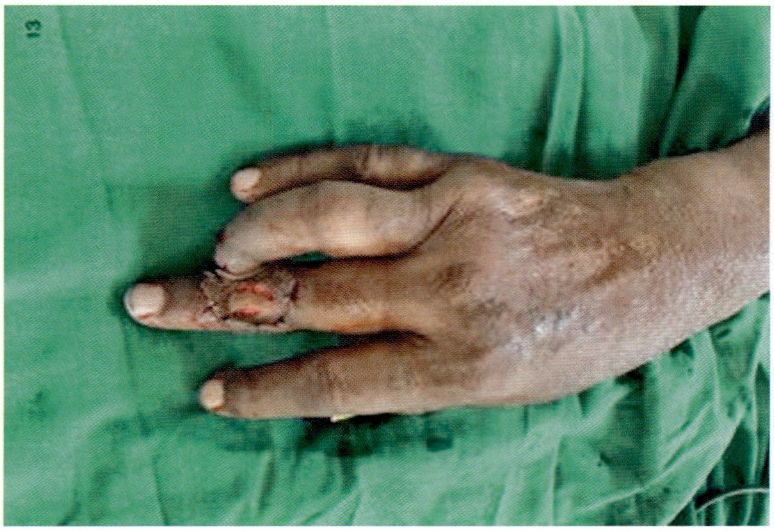
Fig. 13: Donor site coverage done with SSG.

COMPLICATIONS

Cross-finger flap dehiscence is very rare complication in children. Partial or complete skin graft loss at donor site is another complication noted in various studies. Mild stiffness is noted if joint movement is not started early in postoperative period.

SUGGESTED READING

1. Al-Qattan MM. De-epithelialized cross-finger flaps versus adipofascial turn over flaps for the reconstruction of small complex dorsal digital defects: a comparative analysis. J Hand Surg Am. 2005;30:549-57.
2. Cronin T. The cross finger flap: a new method of repair. Am Surg. 1951;17:419-25.
3. Curtis RM. Cross-finger pedicle flap in hand surgery. Ann Surg. 1957;145:650-5.
4. Johnson RK, Iverson RE. Cross-finger pedicle flaps in the hand. J Bone Joint Surg. 1971;53A:913-9.
5. Kappel DA, Burech JG. The cross-finger flap: an established reconstructive procedure. Hand Clin. 1985;1:677-83.
6. Kleinert HE, McAlister CG, MacDonald CJ, et al. A critical evaluation of cross finger flaps. J Trauma. 1974;14:756.

CHAPTER 122

Lower Extremity Reconstruction: A Holistic, Joint Approach

Ameya Bindu

INTRODUCTION

Complex polytrauma requiring stabilization of the patient before definitive limb fixation can be undertaken, is a common occurence in contemporary orthopaedics. In such cases, the patient has to be resuscitated and hemodynamically stabilized; planning for future definitive fracture fixation can start concurrently but is executed after stabilization.

Multidisciplinary approach is required for management of these polytrauma patients. Early involvement of plastic surgeons in the holistic approach, as per Levine's orthoplastic approach, is an integral part of patient management. It will emphasise selection of the most appropriate technique likely to achieve stable and reliable wound closure with minimal donor site morbidity.

PREOPERATIVE ASSESSMENT

Detailed and accurate preoperative survey of the patient with a lower extremity wound is of utmost importance in developing a successful treatment. Any execution of a reconstructive procedure is undertaken assuming the patient is vitally and physiologically stable and that life threatening and limb-threatening vascular injuries are adequately treated. Wound healing may be delayed in presence of comorbidities like diabetes. One should actively search for injury to neurovascular structures and joints in order to take care of them during soft tissue repair. Relevant investigations such as X-rays and vascular Doppler should also be done in view of possible complications of polytrauma.

DEBRIDEMENT

A complex lower extremity trauma defect should undergo thorough irrigation of compound fractures and debridement of necrotic tissues. A thoroughly performed, meticulous surgical debridement is the basic prerequisite to any form of further treatment strategy either in the form of fracture stabilization or wound coverage the cutting instrument must remain within the obviously dead tissue and progress is then made toward what is certainly normal and then stopped when there is evidence of some bleeding. Serial debridement can be preferred in majority of cases to avoid any excess and also because, as the wound evolves, more dead tissue becomes apparent.

There are certain basic principles that need to be followed for a good surgical debridement:

- Should be performed under tourniquet with adequate lighting and magnification.
- All the tissues that appear obviously dead and necrotic have to be radically excised. (Clues to devitalized tissues include: pale discolored tissues, thrombosed vessels, lack of blanching even after tourniquet application, and absence of pinpoint bleeding).
- Should be done from center to periphery, layer-by-layer.
- The longitudinal and vital structures that should be preserved are arteries, nerves and major tendons.
- Bone debridement should be conservative and the vascularity should be reconfirmed after releasing the tourniquet.
- A reconstructive surgeon should be preferably involved in the debridement process.
- A thorough wound wash or lavage is mandatory to remove all dirt and contamination prior to final defect assessment.

SKELETAL STABILIZATION

At this stage, fracture fixation should be considered in consultation with orthopaedic as well as plastic surgeons. Earlier, external fixation was the mainstay of treatment in such cases. However, in recent times, intramedullary nails or even plates have been used albeit in select cases.

TIMING OF RECONSTRUCTION

The factors which dictate the timing of definitive wound management in the injured extremity are the general condition of the patient as well as the condition of the wound like bacterial status, type of fracture, tissues involved in the injury, and the exposed vital structures. In a stable patient, after precise wound assessment, treatment of any limb-threatening vascular injury, removal of all devitalized tissue, control of infection, and fixation of fractures, definitive wound closure is performed. Optimum preparation of the patient as well as the wound is a prerequisite to definitive wound coverage.

RECONSTRUCTIVE OPTIONS

In majority of cases, the simplest and safest as well as least technically demanding method should be chosen. For smaller wounds with no exposure of vital structures (such as neurovasculature, bones, joints and tendons), healing by secondary intention can be opted for. A wound which is deemed unlikely to heal by secondary intention in about 3 weeks should be covered with a skin graft after confirming that the bed is well vascularized.

Full thickness flaps are undertaken as soon as wound condition permits, when there is exposure of vital structures.When local flaps are not practical or in the event of their failure, vascularized myocutaneous flaps are indicated. Good clinical judgment is essential in order to choose the most appropriate option.

There are multiple choices of local and regional flaps available according to the location and dimensions of the defect, including muscle flaps, musculocutaneous flaps, islanded perforator based propeller flaps, and axial flaps, but in this chapter, we will primarily be discussing local fasciocutaneous flaps (perforator plus peninsular flaps/ Ponten flaps) for small to moderate defects and a representative case record of a microvascular free tissue reconstruction for a foot defect.

LOCAL FASCIOCUTANEOUS FLAPS

Local fasciocutaneous flaps have now become a standard practice and a major tool for the reconstructive surgeon dealing with wounds in the leg. The majority of leg defects extending from knee to sole can be covered by these procedures.

Surface anatomy of the three major vessels of the leg in reference to fixed bony points can be marked preoperatively as per standard guidelines (Figs. 1A to C).

Indications

Small-to-moderate sized defects with locally available healthy tissues.

Contraindications

High-velocity injury with major degloving and extensive zone of trauma, with mutilated donor tissues.

Advantages

- Safe and robust vascularity
- Simple, easy, and rapid procedure
- Provides stable and pliable tissues
- Easy to re-explore for secondary bony/tendon procedures
- Does not require any special setup or training
- Can be used in presence of external fixators.

Disadvantages

- A skin graft is almost always necessary for donor site closure
- Large flaps used may lead to lymph edema and stasis in the long-term period
- Some contour deformity.
- May require two stages in some cases of inferiorly based flaps.

Planning of Flap

The nature of transfer of these flaps is transposition and rotation; the distal most incisions are taken first and the elevation proceeds proximally towards the base. Exposed vital structures mandate use of a flap but sometimes in a perticular wound, part of it can be managed by a skin graft and rest might require a flap cover.

Raising the Flap

The incision and dissection proceeds from the distal most margin of the flap from the base cited and the flap is raised in the subfascial

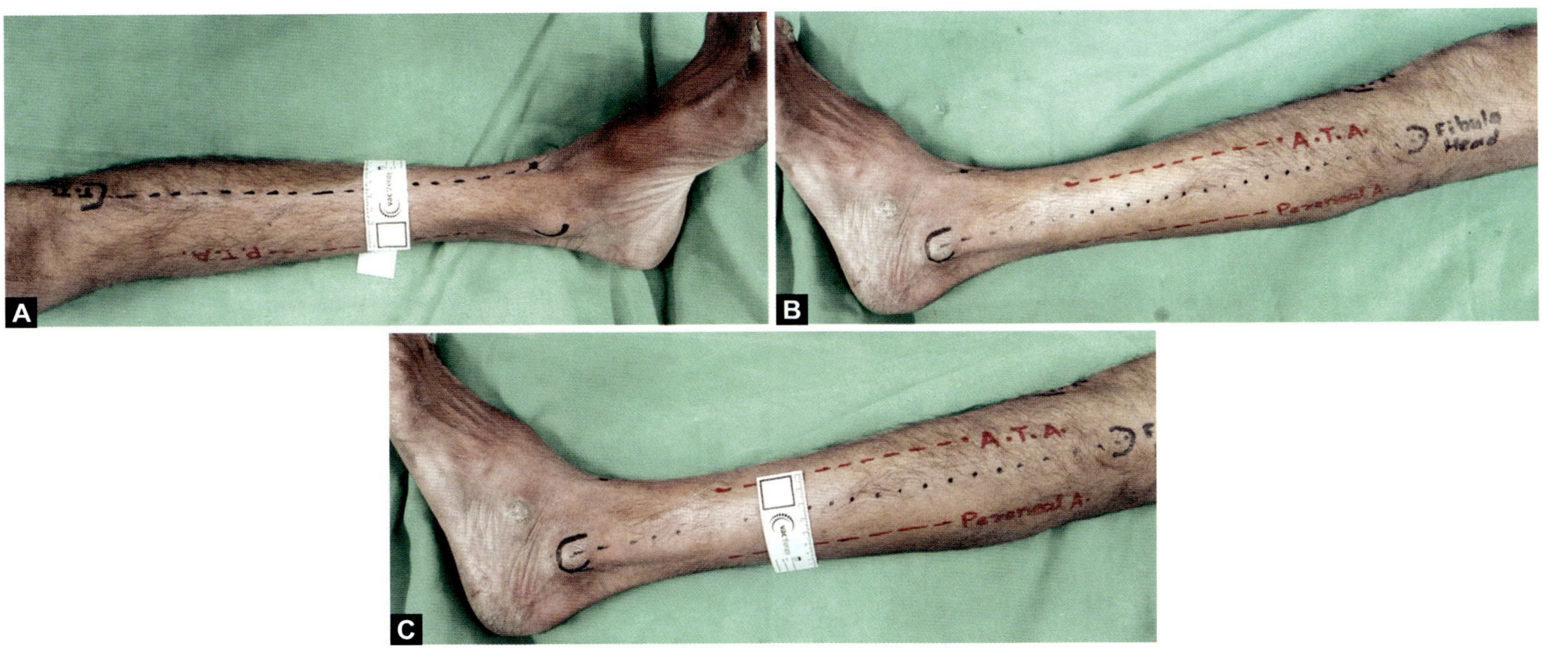

Figs. 1A to C: Markings of vascular axes of the three major vessels of the leg—posterior tibial, anterior tibial, and peroneal. Black dotted lines are the reference lines and the red ones are the vascular axes.

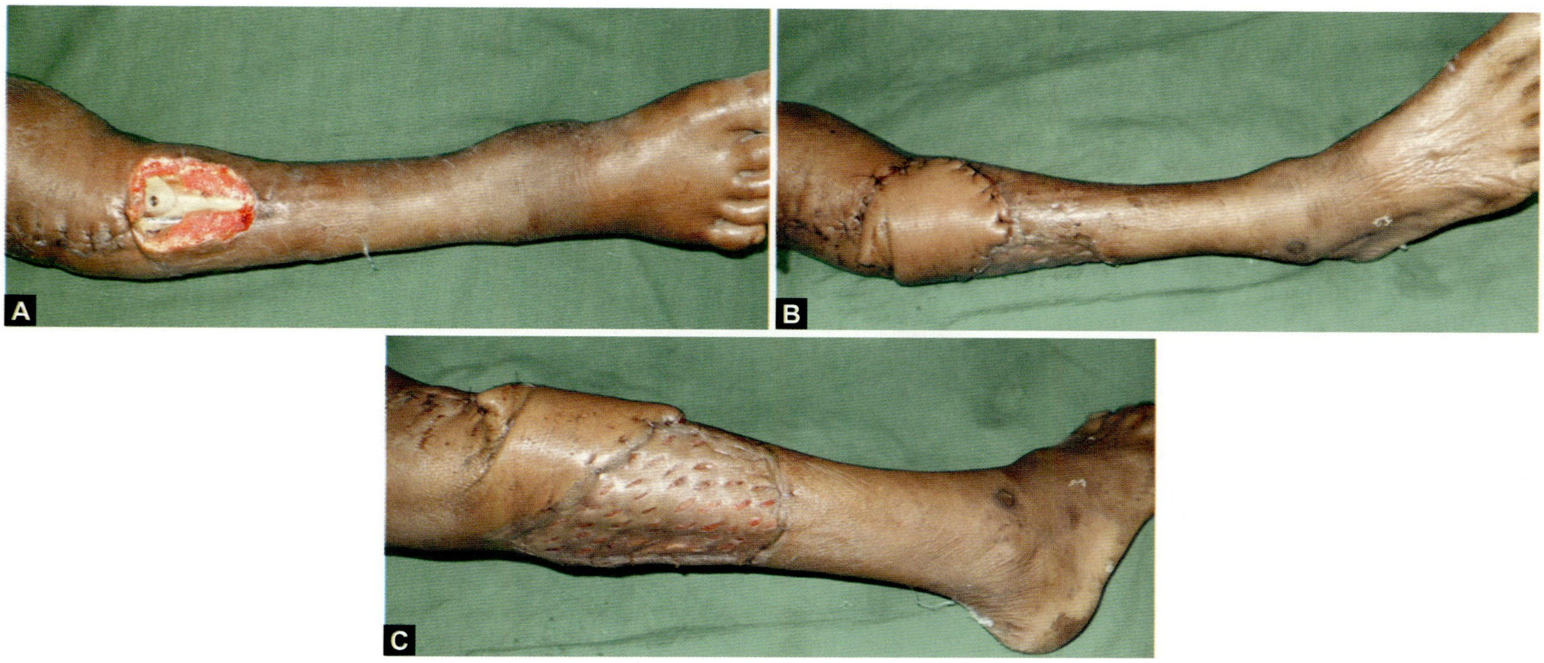

Figs. 2A to C: Proximal and middle one-third leg defect with exposed tibia. A superiorly based fasciocutaneous flap executed based on the perforators on peroneal vessel axis. Donor area is skin grafted.

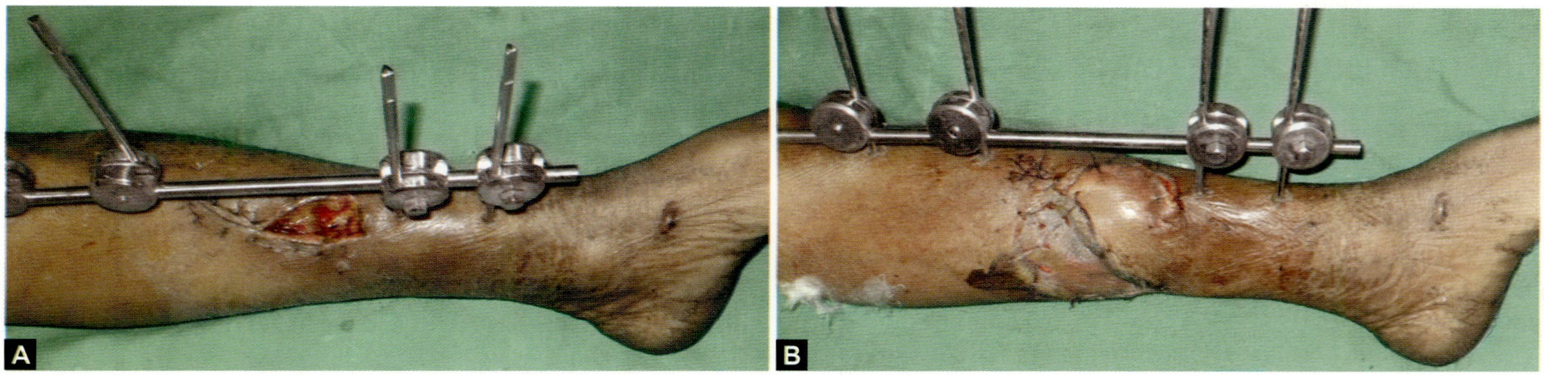

Figs. 3A and B: A middle and lower one-third junction leg defect with exposed bone. An inferiorly based fasciocutaneous flap planned on the posterior tibial artery (PTA) axis perforators.

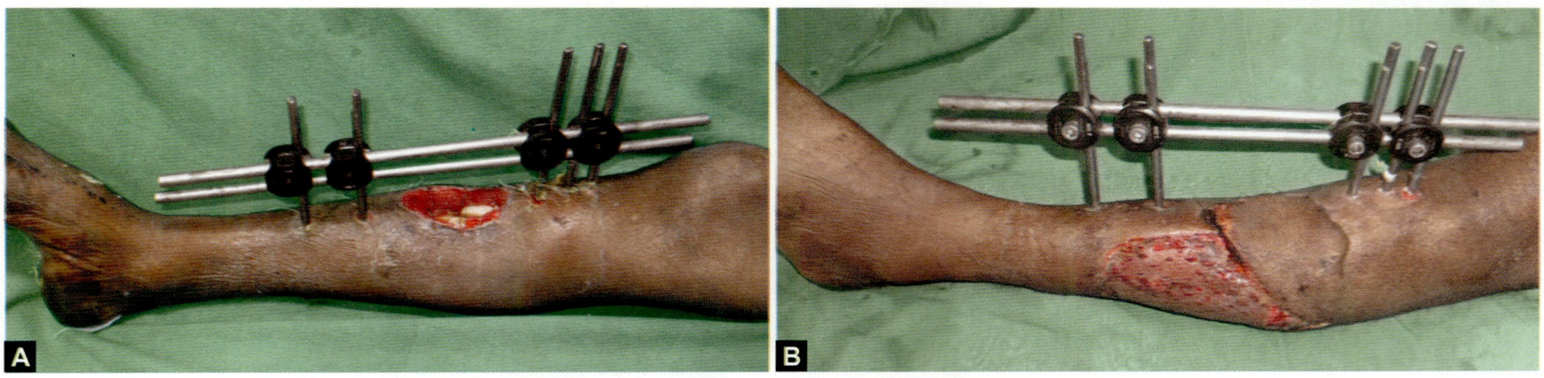

Figs. 4A and B: Proximal and middle one-third leg defect with exposed tibia. A superiorly based fasciocutaneous flap executed based on the perforators on peroneal vessel axis. Donor area is skin grafted.

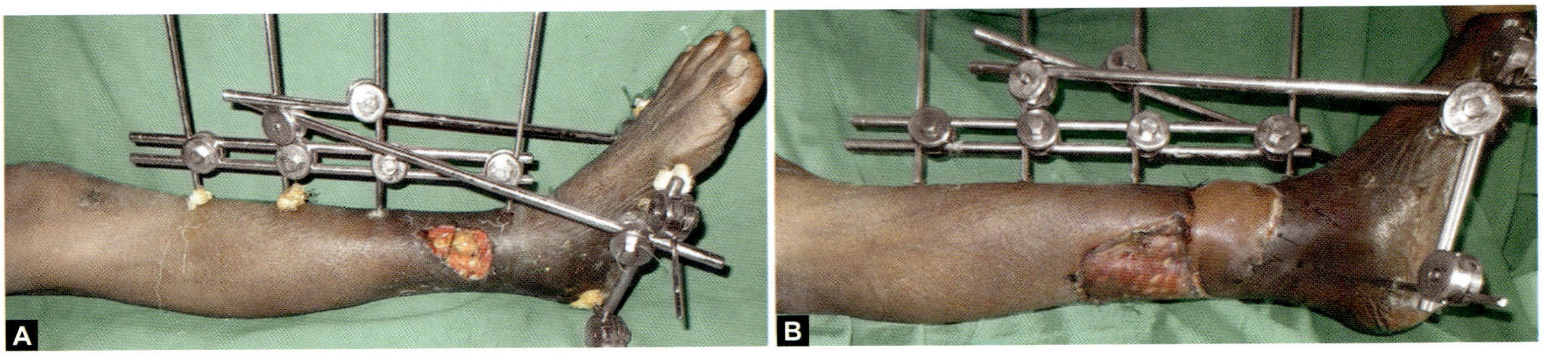

Figs. 5A and B: A middle and lower one-third junction leg defect with exposed bone. An inferiorly based fasciocutaneous flap planned on the posterior tibial artery (PTA) axis perforators. Donor area is grafted.

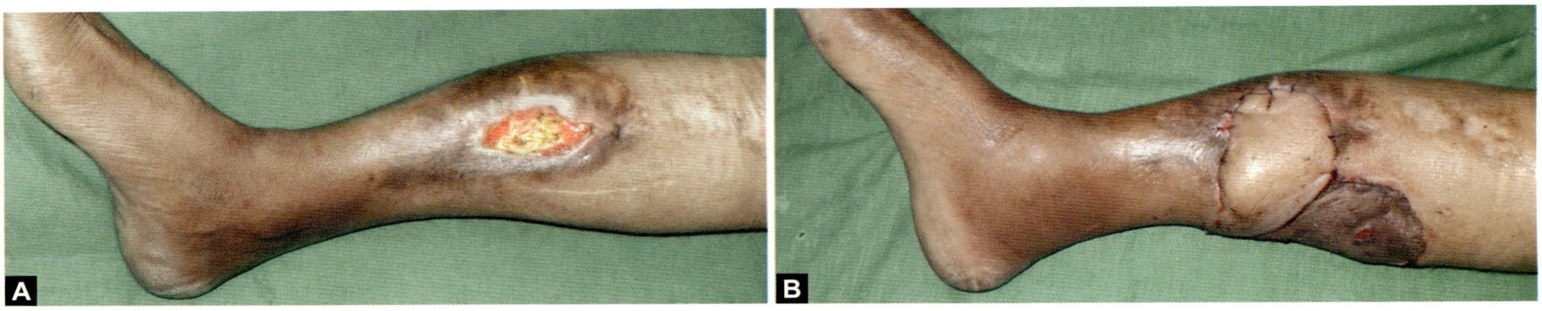

Figs. 6A and B: A middle one-third leg defect with exposed tibia. An inferiorly based fasciocutaneous flap executed based on the perforators on posterior tibial artery axis. Donor area is skin grafted.

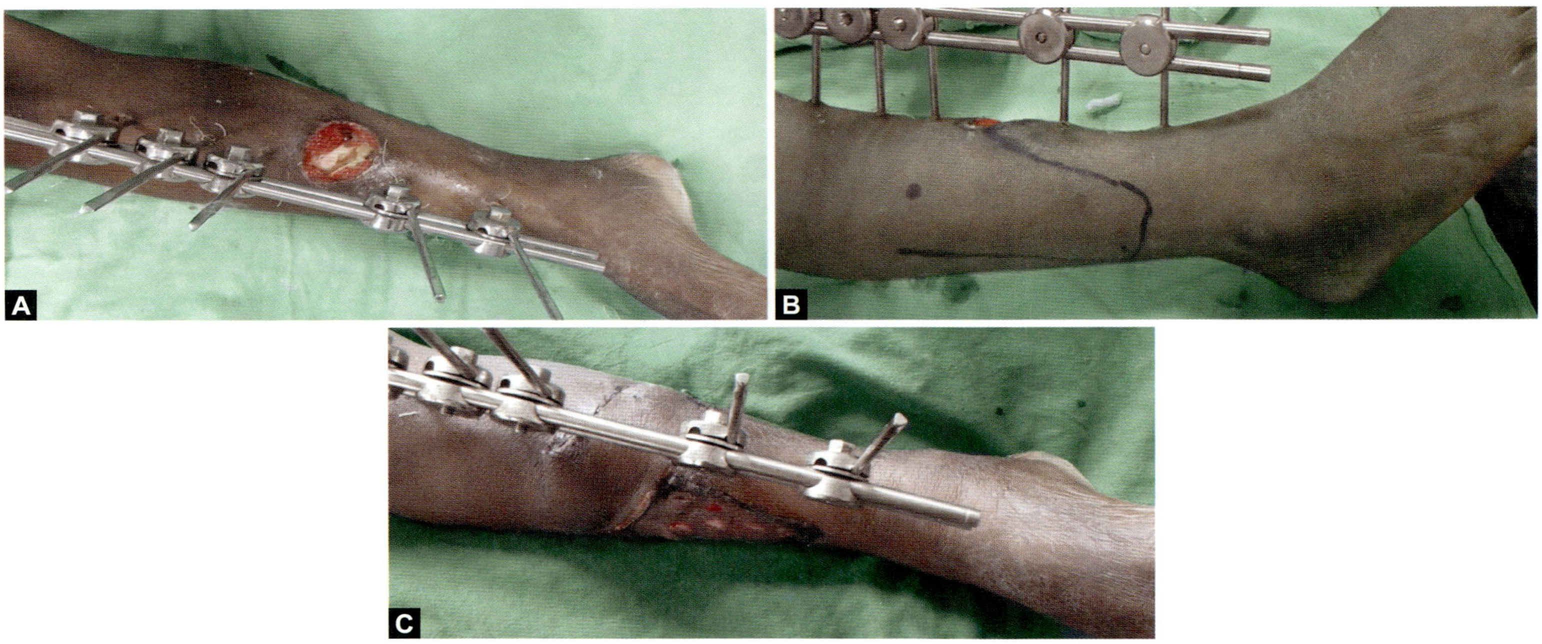

Figs. 7A to C: Middle and lower one-third junction leg defect with exposed tibia. A superiorly based fasciocutaneous flap executed based on the perforators on anterior tibial artery axis. The blue dot represents the perforator marked with a hand-held Doppler. Shin of tibia.

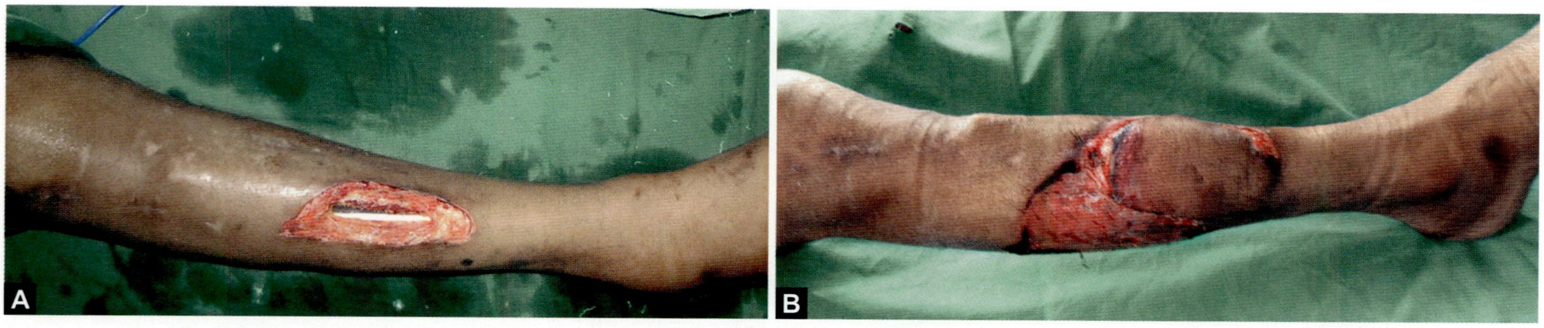

Figs. 8A and B: Middle one-third leg defect with exposed tibia and implant. An inferiorly based fasciocutaneous flap executed based on the perforators on anterior tibial artery axis. Donor area is skin grafted.

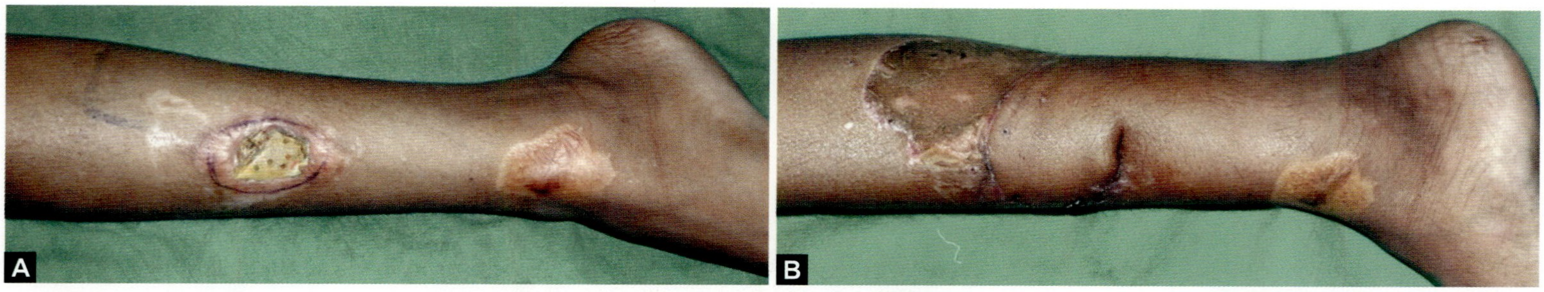

Figs. 9A and B: A middle one-third leg defect with exposed bone and surrounding scarring. An inferiorly based fasciocutaneous flap planned on the posterior tibial artery (PTA) axis perforators after excising the scarred and necrotic tissues and removing the dead outer cortex.

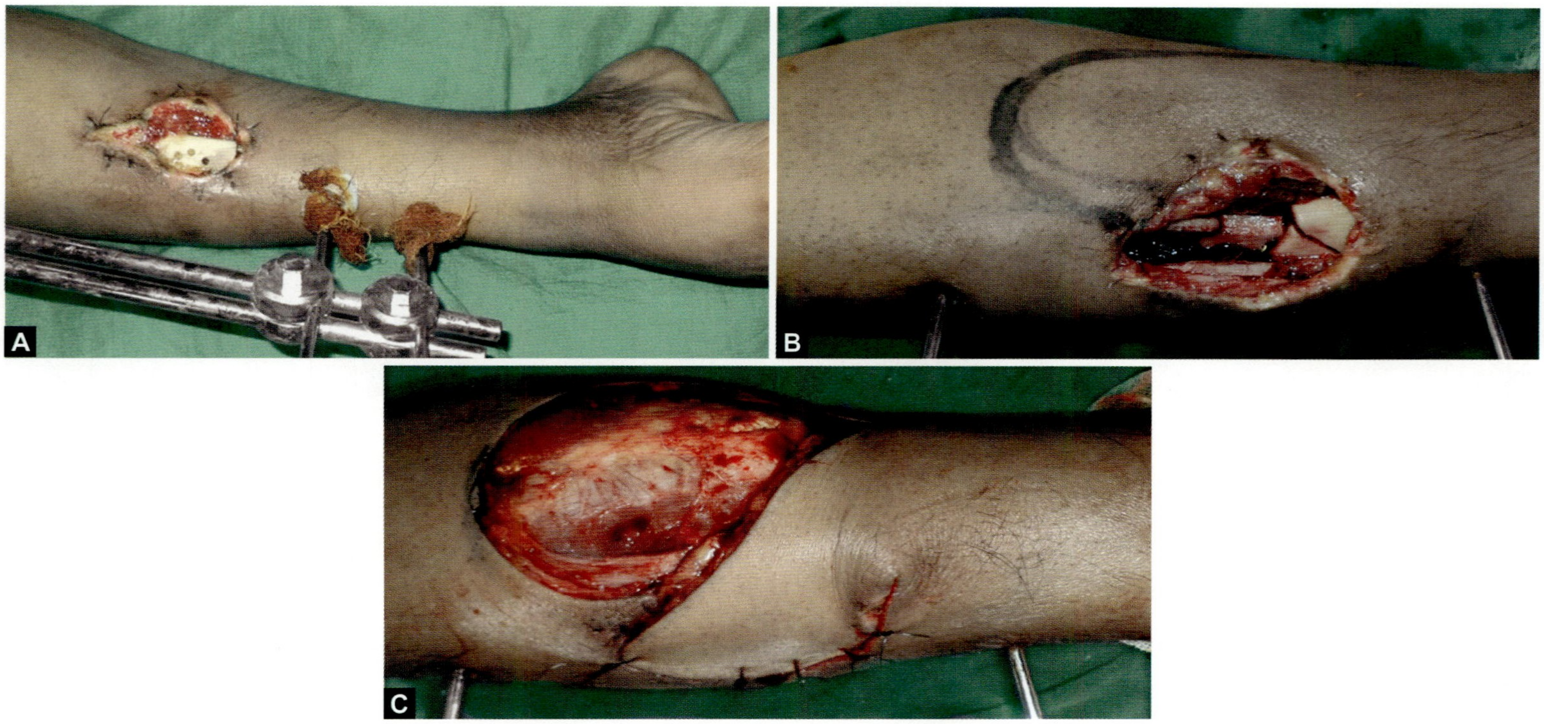

Figs. 10A to C: A middle one-third leg defect with exposed bone and fracture site involving tibia. An inferiorly based fasciocutaneous flap planned on the posterior tibial artery (PTA) axis perforators.

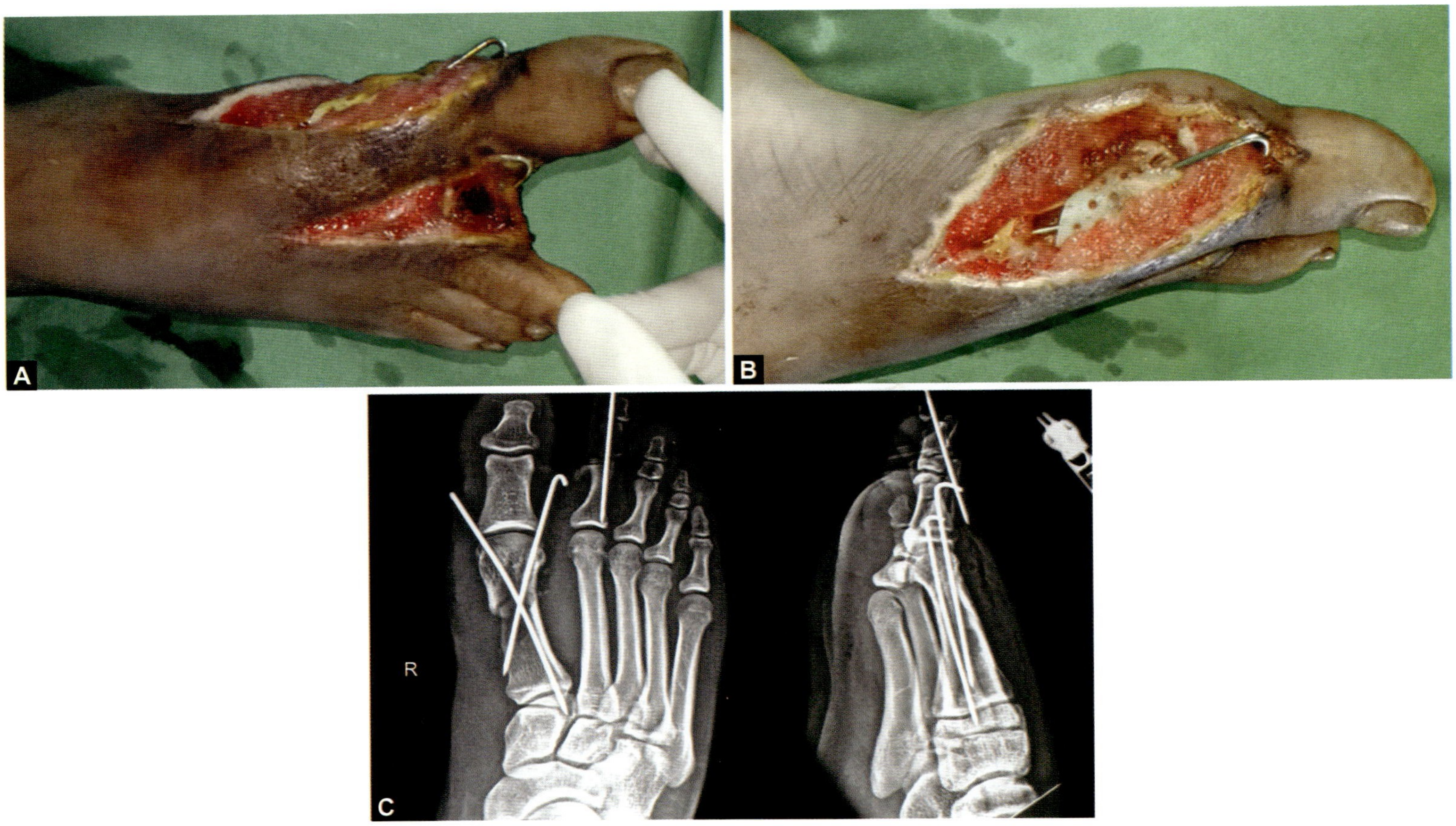

Figs. 11A to C: A right foot crush injury with fractures involving great toe and second toe, with exposed necrotic first metatarsal with K-wire in situ, with second raw area in the first web space with loss of second toe due to gangrene.

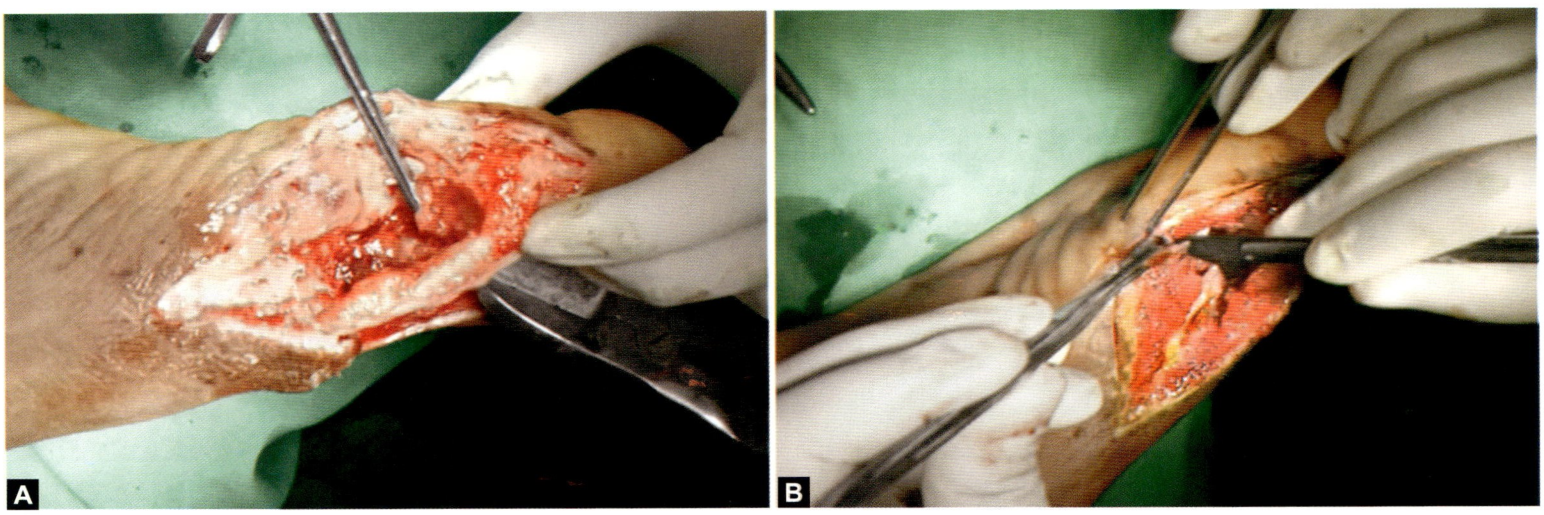

Figs. 12A and B: Surgical debridement of the wound with excision of all the dead and devitalized tissues along with dead bone and K-wires.

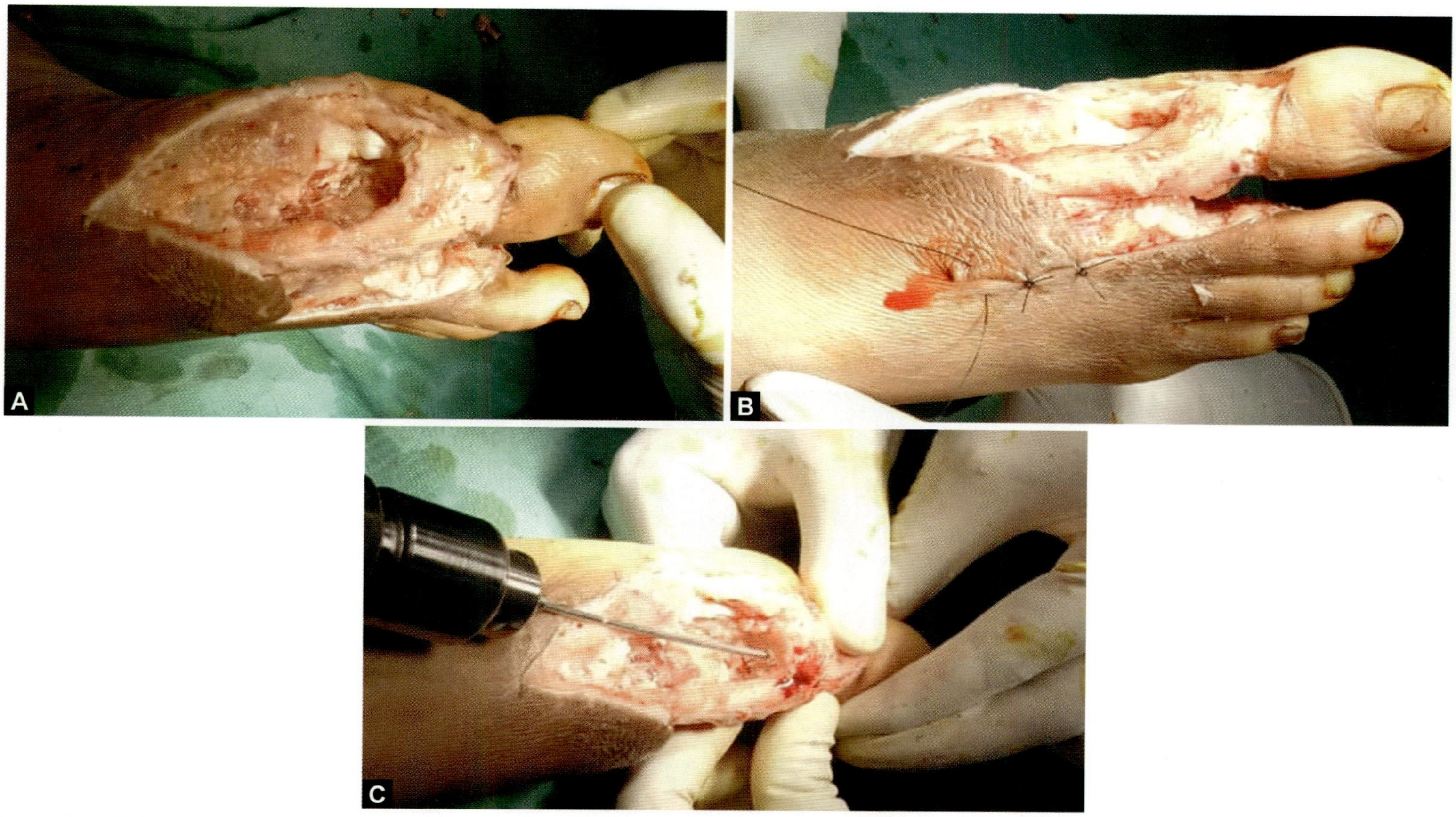

Figs. 13A to C: Completed debridement with a segmental loss of first metatarsal of 4.5 cm. The intervening skin bridge was disconnected and transferred laterally, creating a single defect. The bone gap was bridged with a straight K-wire taking care to maintain the gap and anatomical relations.

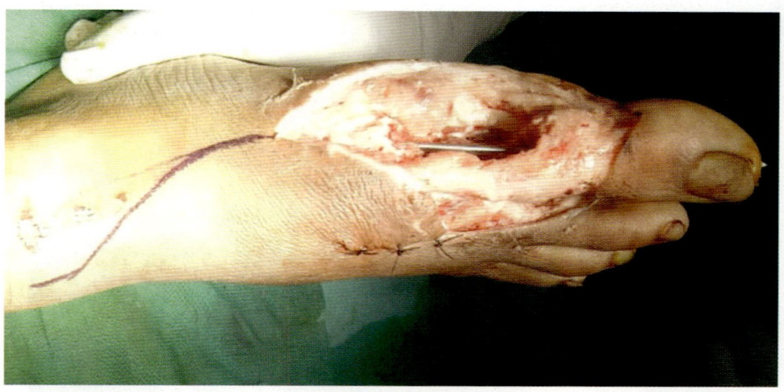

Fig. 14: K-wire in situ across the bone gap, just prior to insertion of the bone cement spacer to maintain the gap and cavity for future bone grafting procedure. The incision is marked to explore the dorsalis pedis vessels as recipient vessels for anastomosis.

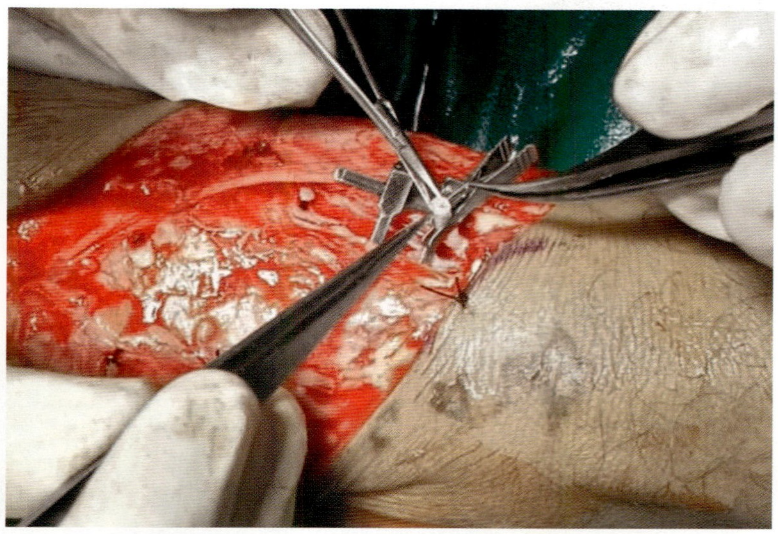

Fig. 15: The vessels are dissected, prepared and the flow is checked to confirm the pulsatile, triphasic flow so as to get a judgment of the pedicle length required and also to shorten the ischemia time.

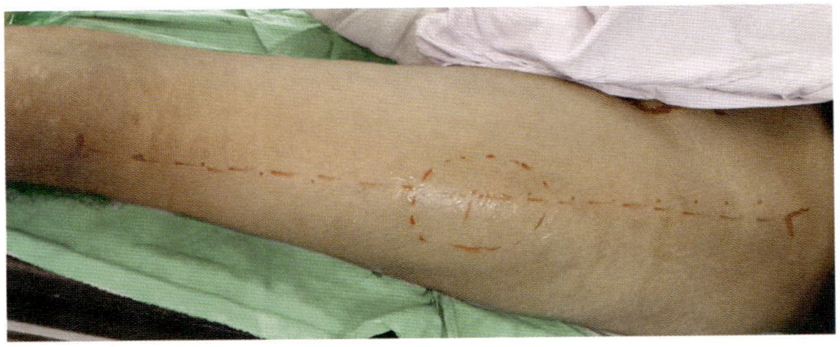

Fig. 16: The axis of the anterolateral thigh flap drawn between anterior superior iliac spine (ASIS) and the superolateral border of patella. A 6 cm diameter circle represents the area of finding perforators from the descending branch of lateral circumflex femoral artery, which is the pedicle of the flap.

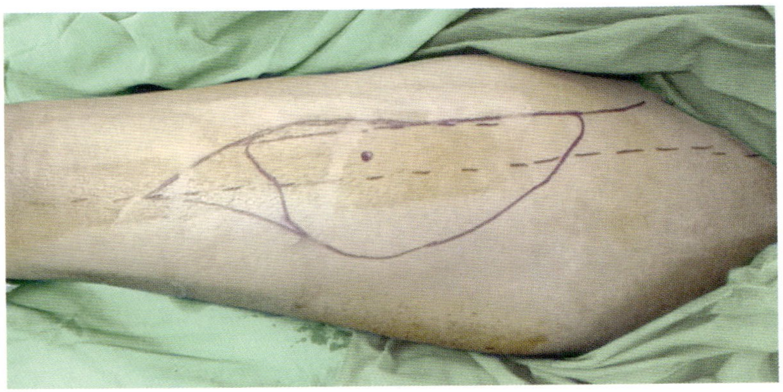

Fig. 17: An exact pattern of the defect is cut and marked on the donor site centered on the vascular axis with proper proximodistal orientation. The ends of the marking are tapered for primary closure. Dot represents the perforator marked with a hand-held Doppler probe.

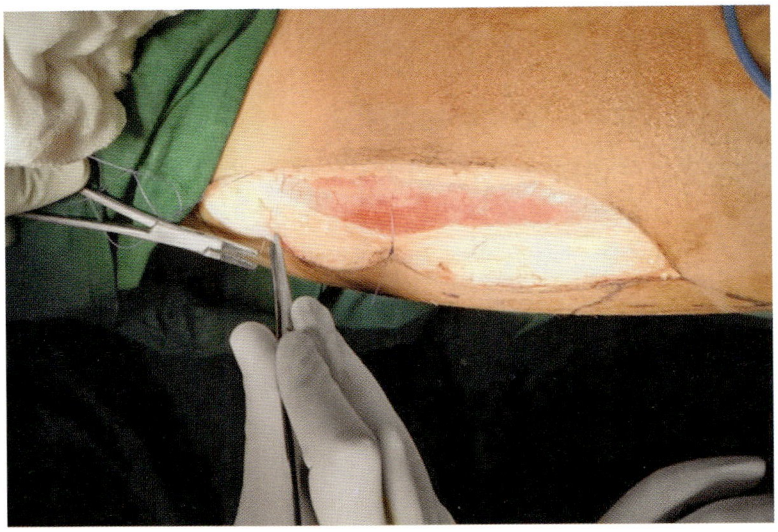

Fig. 18: Anterior approach is most commonly used and the plane of elevation is subfascial, with perforators seen in the septum between rectus femoris and vastus lateralis. Care is taken not to shear the skin and subcutaneous tissue from the fascia.

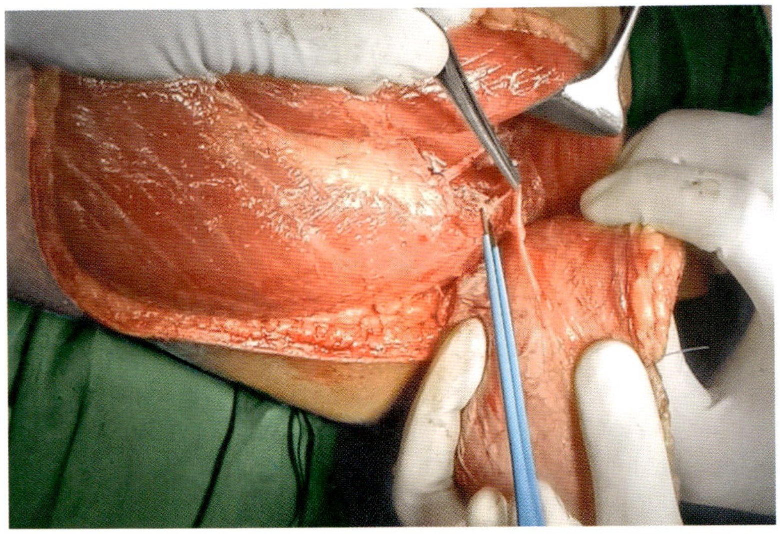

Fig. 19: Perforator dissection toward the main pedicle that is the descending branch of the lateral circumflex femoral vessels. Care is taken to preserve the motor nerves to vastus lateralis and island the entire flap only on the perforator.

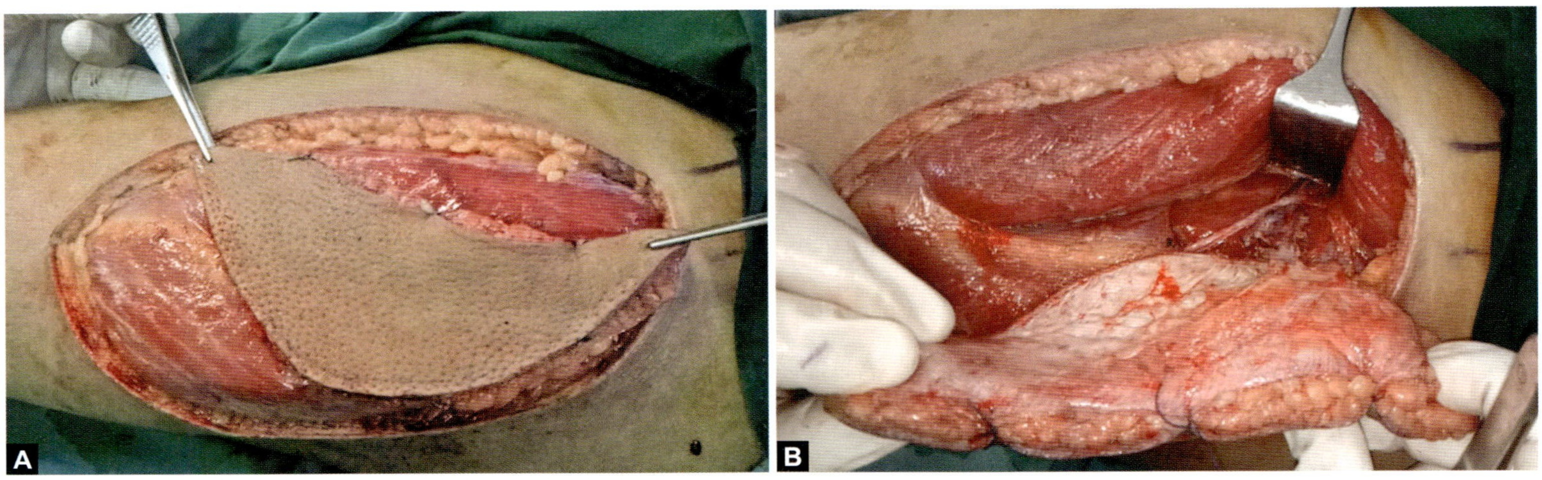

Figs. 20A and B: Completed harvest of the flap with the second image showing the undersurface of the flap and the pedicle going towards the profunda femoris vessels. One can also appreciate the preserved nerve, medial to the pedicle.

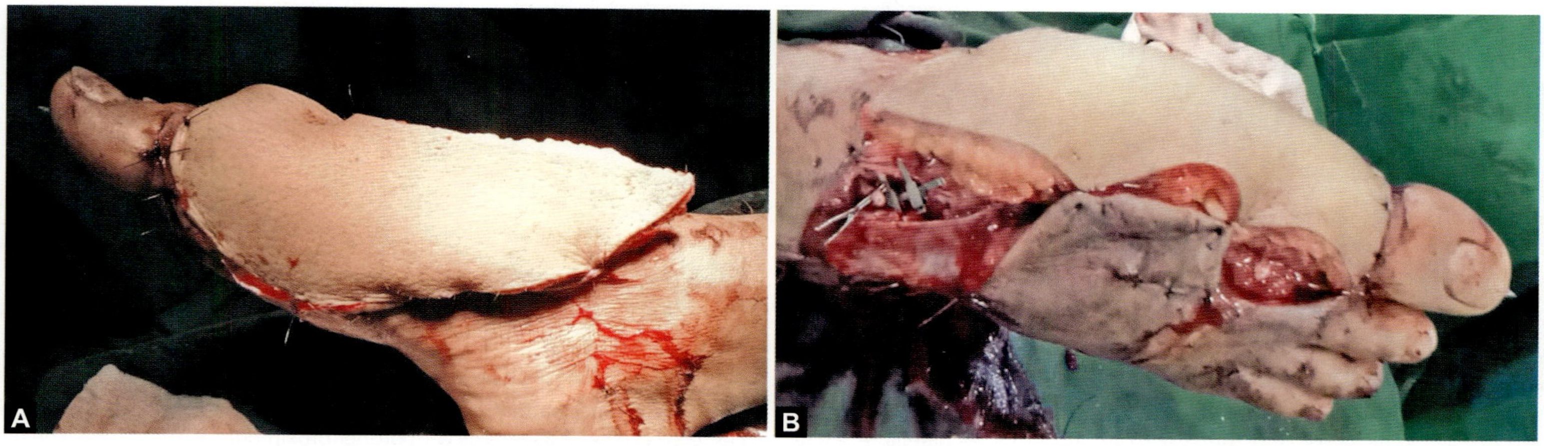

Figs. 21A and B: Flap detached from the donor site, placed in the defect and secured with tagging sutures. The lie of the vessels and the reach is confirmed before starting the microvascular anastomosis.

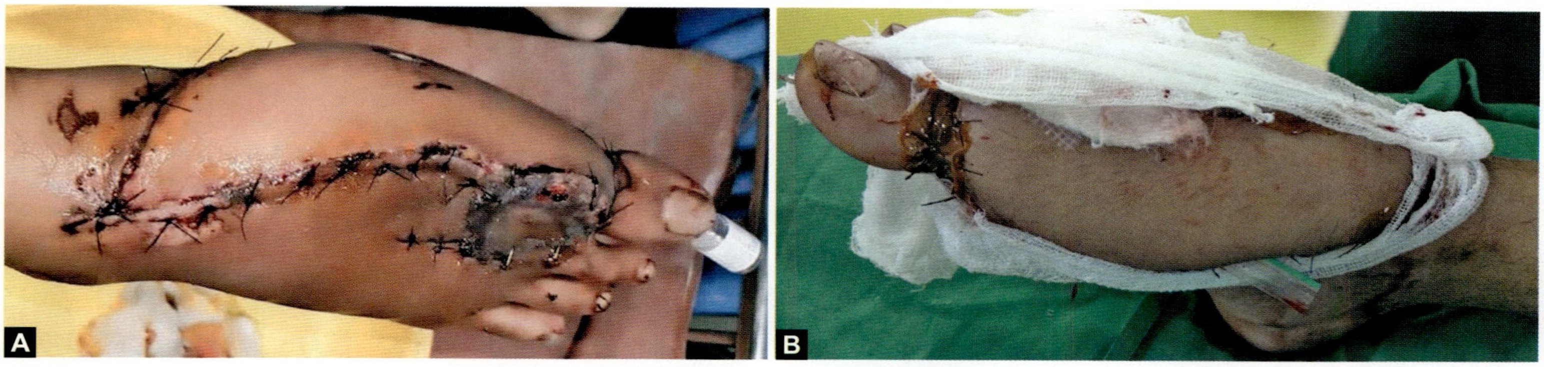

Figs. 22A and B: After completion of the anastomosis and the final inset with a corrugated drain in situ to drain any collection.

plane with the epimysium, taking care not to damage the paratenon in posterior calf to ensure graft take. The cut margins of the skin, subcutaneous tissue and the deep fascia should be at the same level.

As the flap is raised distal to proximal, the location and the axis of the perforators can be carefully noted by the tenting or holes in the deep fascia, or direct visualization in the septum. After the flap has been raised, the ends are grasped and placed into the defect taking care to avoid too much tension, shearing, or separation of the fascia from the overlying subcutaneous tissue. The donor defect after flap transfer is usually covered with a split skin graft.

Common Mistakes

1. Making a surgical plan without assessing of local tissue affected by trauma or infection.
2. General debility, metabolic diseases, malnutrition, anemia, history of smoking, and drug addiction.
3. Poor flap planning and locating the pedicle away from the vascular axis.
4. Improper plane of harvest and not incorporating deep fascia in the flap.
5. Twist and kink at the pedicle, suturing under tension, excessive undermining at the base.
6. Pressure dressing.
7. Inadequate hemostasis, failure to put a drain underneath.

MICROVASCULAR FREE TISSUE TRANSFER

With the advent of microvascular surgery and free tissue transfer with vascular anastomosis, the choices and options for wound coverage have grown manifold. The plastic surgeon who is familiar with the procedure may choose to cover a complex defect post-trauma in difficult anatomical regions like lower one-third and near ankle joint and foot region with a free flap. Some advantages of free flaps are distant donor site outside the zone of trauma with minimum donor site morbidity, single stage complete coverage of the defect with possibility of internal fixation of the underlying fractures or any definitive orthopaedic procedures as we can achieve a durable, well vascularized cover in the same stage and minimum scarring or need of skin grafts thereby reducing chances of postoperative lymphedema and other related complications. However, a free tissue transfer is a demanding surgical procedure with a specific skill set, long-learning curve as well as operative time, higher chances of flap related complications and immediate postoperative concerns that require vigilant monitoring.

We describe here a representative case record of a post-traumatic defect at the medial aspect of forefoot and midfoot region with first metatarsal segmental loss, operated with debridement and bone cement spacer and soft tissue cover with a free anterolateral thigh flap with anastomosis to dorsalis pedis artery and venae comitantes and great saphenous vein.

OPERATIVE STEPS

Debridement

A thorough surgical debridement with excision of all the dead and devitalized tissues and bone under tourniquet and magnification is done first. If any bony intervention or fixation is needed, either in the form of internal or external fixation or spacer, is done. The final defect is determined and a pattern is made for the exact skin and soft-tissue requirement.

Recipient Vessel Preparation

Most commonly used vessels for anastomosis for free flaps in distal leg or foot are the posterior tibial vessels either as end-to-end or end-to-side depending on the foot vascularity on Doppler. But the vessels are to be selected based on the orientation and the location of the defect and zone of trauma; and also ease of reach and lie of the pedicle. The vessel dissection, preparation, and checking the blood flow are preferably done before committing the flap. This confirms the triphasic pulsatile flow, which can sustain the composite tissues of the free flap as well as reduce the ischemia time after the flap is detached.

Marking the Flap

The anterolateral thigh flap is one of the work horse soft-tissue free flaps because of constant reliable anatomy and minimum donor morbidity. This flap is based on the septocutaneous and musculocutaneous perforators from descending branch of lateral circumflex femoral vessels, which are located in the septum between rectus femoris and vastus lateralis muscles. The vascular axis is marked as a line joining the anterior superior iliac spine (ASIS) and the superolateral border of patella, and the perforators are marked using a hand-held Doppler ultrasound, which are usually located within a 6 cm diameter circle centered on the midpoint of this axis. The pattern of the defect is used to mark the skin paddle centered on this axis, with ends tapered for primary closure of the donor defect whenever feasible. Usually, about 8–10 cm of width can be closed primarily, though in some tension.

Anterior Approach of Harvest

Anterior incision should be 1.5–2 cm medial to the vascular axis line, and that is taken first. The rectus femoris muscle is identified after incising the fascia by its bipennate nature, and dissection is continued to identify the perforators entering the deep fascia of the flap located in the septum overlying the vastus lateralis muscle.

Perforator Dissection

After identification of good sizeable perforator, that is dissected from the surrounding tissues toward the main pedicle going deep to the rectus femoris muscle. Care is taken to ensure minimum handling of the perforators as well as preservation of the nerves running along with the pedicle.

Completion of the Harvest

Skin incisions are completed and the flap is skeletonized completely on the perforator by doing dissection in a relatively avascular subfascial plane. Now the bleed in the flap is confirmed to ensure the adequacy of the perforator chosen as well as to rule out any damage to or spasm of the perforators or vessels during dissection.

Inset of the Flap

The flap is then detached from the donor site after clipping the vessels separately, and transferred to the defect.

The flap is secured into the defect with tagging sutures initially so as to adjust the lie and reach of the pedicle to the dissected recipient vessels.

Microvascular Anastomosis

Then, the anastomosis is completed either in loupes or microscope with nonabsorbable suture 8-0/9-0 depending on the size of the vessels. Usually, we prefer to do one artery and one vein, but two veins can also be anastomosed, if easily available and feasible. The bleeding from the flap and the dermal circulation is confirmed (bright red, nonbrisk) and patency of the anastomosis and any leak is also checked.

Closure

Final inset of the flap is completed with loose tagging sutures (simple interrupted or buried mattress) with nonabsorbable suture 3-0. Due care is taken to prevent any undue tension on the sutures and hemostasis in reconfirmed prior to closure. It is advisable to place and secure a corrugated drain at the dependent site to drain out any collections in the immediate postoperative period. Splintage is given to immobilize the ankle joint but taking care not to dorsiflex the foot too much which might result in a kink at the anastomotic site.

POSTOPERATIVE MONITORING

Free flaps need to be monitored every 2 hours in the first 48 hours postoperative period, to ensure the flap perfusion and the patency of the anastomoses. Anything that might suggest either a venous compromise (congestion, brisk dark red bleeding) or an arterial issue (delayed or no bleeding, with pale cold flap) warrants an emergency re-exploration with redoing the anastomoses, if required. Thus, a vigilant monitoring with an early detection of a vascular complication is the only means to salvage a failing free flap.

KEY POINTS

- It is essential to assess the patient as a whole and not just the lower limb trauma or the leg defect.
- Lower limb trauma mandates a multimodality and multidisciplinary care, with early involvement of a reconstructive surgeon.
- Meticulous and adequate debridement is the first stepping stone to a successful and early reconstruction.
- Planning and execution of skeletal fixation and reconstruction are complementary and go hand in hand.
- Early reconstruction and flap cover give the best results and outcomes.

- From a multitude of reconstructive options and flaps available, the choice of procedure depends on variety of factors and tailored according to needs of every patient.

ACKNOWLEDGMENT

"Short Notes in Plastic Surgery" compiled by Dr RL Thatte, Chapter 15A, 15B, http://shortnotesinplasticsurgery.wordpress.com. Department of Plastic and Reconstructive surgery, BJGMC and Sassoon General Hospital, for operative photographs.

SUGGESTED READING

1. Bhattacharya V, Watts R. Ipsilateral fasciocutaneous flaps for leg and foot defects. Indian J Plast Surg. 2003;36(1):30-5.
2. Colohan S, Saint-Cyr M. Chapter 2: Management of lower extremity trauma. In: Neligan PC (Ed). Neligan's Textbook of Plastic Surgery, Volume 4. London: Elsevier; 2018.

Index

Page numbers followed by *b* refer to box, *f* refer to figure, *fc* refer to flow chart, and *t* refer to table.

C

F

G

H

I

P

R

T

U

V

W

X

Z